ENCYCLOPEDIA OF TOXICOLOGY

THIRD EDITION

VOLUME 1

A–DEL

ENCYCLOPEDIA OF TOXICOLOGY

THIRD EDITION

EDITOR-IN-CHIEF

PHILIP WEXLER
US National Library of Medicine, Bethesda, MD, USA

ASSOCIATE EDITORS

MOHAMMAD ABDOLLAHI
Tehran University of Medical Sciences (TUMS), Tehran, Iran

ANN DE PEYSTER
San Diego State University, San Diego, CA, USA

SHAYNE C. GAD
Gad Consulting Services, Cary, NC, USA

HELMUT GREIM
Technical University of Munich, Freising-Weihenstephan, Germany

STACEY HARPER
Oregon State University, Corvallis, OR, USA

VIRGINIA C. MOSER
US Environmental Protection Agency, Research Triangle Park, NC, USA

SIDHARTHA RAY
Manchester University College of Pharmacy, Fort Wayne, IN, USA

JOSE TARAZONA
European Chemicals Agency (ECHA), Helsinki, Finland

TIMOTHY J. WIEGAND
University of Rochester Medical Center and Strong Memorial Hospital, Rochester, NY, USA

VOLUME 1

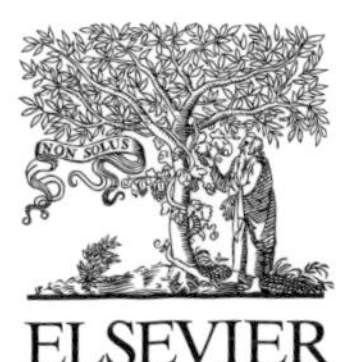

ELSEVIER

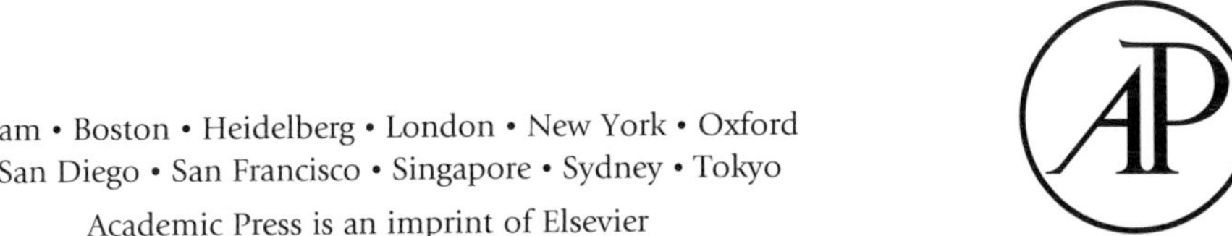

Amsterdam • Boston • Heidelberg • London • New York • Oxford
Paris • San Diego • San Francisco • Singapore • Sydney • Tokyo
Academic Press is an imprint of Elsevier

Academic Press is an imprint of Elsevier
32 Jamestown Road, London NW1 7BY, UK
30 Corporate Drive, Suite 400, Burlington MA 01803, USA
525 B Street, Suite 1800, San Diego, CA 92101-4495, USA

First edition 1998

Second edition 2005

Third edition 2014

The Editor-in-Chief's work on the third edition of the *Encyclopedia of Toxicology* was undertaken as a private citizen, not as a government employee. No official support or endorsement by the US National Library of Medicine or any other agency of the US Federal Government was provided or should be inferred. The views expressed are strictly his own and in no way represent those of the government.

Website links cited in the Encyclopedia were accepted as accurate when first submitted to the publisher, however, the Publisher is unable to ensure that they will continue to remain so.

Notice

No responsibility is assumed by the publisher for any injury and/or damage to persons or property as a matter of products liability, negligence or otherwise, or from any use or operation of any methods, products, instructions or ideas contained in the material herein.

British Library Cataloguing in Publication Data
A catalogue record for this book is available from the British Library

Library of Congress Cataloging-in-Publication Data
A catalog record for this book is available from the Library of Congress

ISBN: 978-0-12-386454-3

For information on all Elsevier publications
visit our website at store.elsevier.com

Printed and bound in the United States of America
14 15 16 17 18 10 9 8 7 6 5 4 3

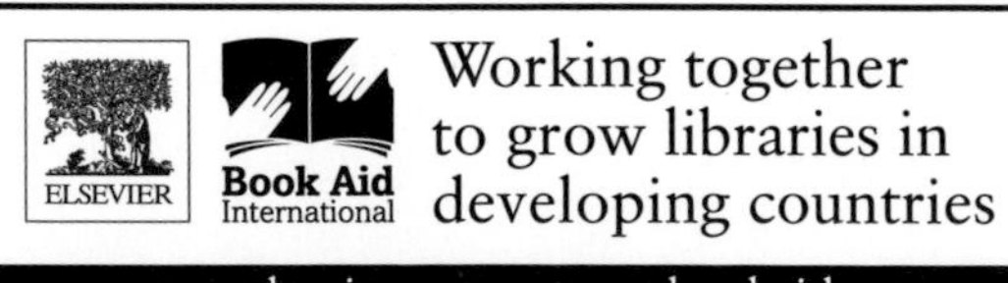

Editorial: Vicky Dyer, Erin Hill-Parks
Production: Justin Taylor

CONTENTS

VOLUME 2

L

N

S

V

FOREWORD

Early humans must have developed, consciously or unconsciously, methods to recognize and avoid toxic plants and poisonous animals, thus inadvertently establishing toxicology as among the earliest applied scientific disciplines with a focus on the health and welfare of the human species. While toxicology's additional emphasis on the environment is more recent and related to population growth and industry, it is no less important. Whatever the validity of this claim to origins in antiquity, toxicology's rapid growth and diversification in recent decades, particularly since the publication of the second edition of this *Encyclopedia of Toxicology*, is undisputed.

Although the US Environmental Protection Agency and the National Institute for Environmental Health Sciences had already initiated studies of new paradigms in risk assessment at the time, it was the 2007 publication of "*Toxicity Testing in the 21st Century: a Vision and a Strategy*" by the National Research Council which gave rise to a huge interest and effort in molecular and cellular approaches to toxicology and their linkages to risk assessment. Studying genome wide effects via microarray techniques and high throughput sequencing are but two fairly recent outgrowths of this emphasis. Research into epigenetics is in its infancy as far as toxicology is concerned but will doubtlessly grow rapidly in importance and application. An equivalent increase in attention is being paid to nanotoxicology, and its practical consequences are now becoming evident. These are but a few of the dramatic developments reflected in this new edition of the *Encyclopedia of Toxicology*, edited so ably by Phil Wexler. We owe him a debt of gratitude for all of his efforts.

Despite many changes in the science of toxicology, what remains unchanged is the need for the toxicological literature to serve many masters. The span from highly specialized researchers and academics in higher education to those who use toxicology in its applied aspects such as clinical and forensic toxicology, agromedicine, risk assessment, consulting and media outreach, is both wide and deep. Clearly, the *Encyclopedia of Toxicology* is a necessary resource for all of these professional groups. It functions as an important locus between the short definitions of dictionaries and the highly detailed narratives of monographs devoted to a single aspect of research. It is an essential work for all toxicologists interested not only in their own area of expertise but also in toxicology as a broader interdisciplinary science and profession. I recommend it without reservation to libraries, not only at institutions of higher learning but also at those of federal, state and private research institutes, as well as to the chemical and related industries. Needless to say, it will be a valued and much used addition to many personal bookshelves.

Ernest Hodgson
Distinguished Professor Emeritus
North Carolina Agromedicine Institute and Toxicology Program
Department of Applied Ecology
North Carolina State University

PREFACE

It has been nearly a decade since the publication of this Encyclopedia's second edition, and in that time toxicology has continued to advance its scientific foundations. The "omics" revolution, along with advances in systems biology, epigenetics, bioinformatics, and computational toxicology are driving toxicology from a discipline dependent upon whole animal testing to one increasingly comfortable with *in vitro* and *in silico* methodologies. This change is taking place both as a humane alternative and as a more practical and cost effective way to deal with the vast number of chemicals for which toxicity data is nonexistent. Adverse outcome pathways are being explored as a means to determine how a direct initiating event at the molecular level can result in an adverse outcome in the biological organism. The 2007 National Research Council publication of *Toxicity Testing in the 21st Century: A Vision and a Strategy* was a seminal event that outlined new technologies in molecular biology and toxicology, and called for a "paradigm shift" to stimulate innovative approaches to testing. The Committee (on Toxicity Testing and Assessment of Environmental Agents) responsible for the report envisioned "a new toxicity-testing system that evaluates biologically significant perturbations in key toxicity pathways by using new methods in computational biology and a comprehensive array of *in vitro* tests based on human biology." On July 11, 2013, the European Union's cosmetic regulation, prohibiting animal testing in the cosmetics industry, came into effect.

Nanotoxicology is another research area which, though certainly not brand new, has come to the fore. Given the quantum size effects and large surface area to volume ratio, materials at this scale may have properties very different from their larger scale counterparts. There remains considerable controversy about the toxic potential of various nanoparticles and debate about how they should be regulated, particularly in products such as cosmetics. Nanotoxicology will continue to be an active area of investigation in the foreseeable future.

Epigenetics, or the study of changes in gene expression over and above those resulting from alterations to DNA proper, has made huge strides in the last several years. Thus, toxicants, behavior, stress and diet have all been shown to play a role in regulating the epigenome. Epigenetic markers have, for example, been shown to influence expression of genes associated with obesity. Epigenetic mechanisms are also being investigated as a possible causative factor in asthma.

In clinical/medical toxicology, the human factor comes directly into play, as do veterinary concerns. This is the branch of toxicology concerned with poisonings. Drugs usually containing a cathinone, marketed as "bath salts," started to be reported to US poison centers in large numbers in 2010. A wide range of effects were noted, ranging from headaches and nausea to hallucinations and paranoia. In 2012, US President Obama signed a bill to ban several types of synthetic drugs including bath salts. Whether this will actually curtail access and use remains to be seen but, regardless, new designer drugs are always just around the corner. The research and clinical communities are, happily, joining forces to probe what has come to be known as "translational toxicology," in which investigating mechanism of action will lead to a better understanding of treatment for people intentionally or accidentally exposed to drugs and other chemicals, and biological agents.

Large scale accidents, regrettably, will continue to plague us. The explosion of the Deepwater Horizon drilling rig in 2010 in the Gulf Coast resulted in the largest offshore oil spill in US history. The long-term effects on the environment and human health, not only of the oil itself, but of the dispersants applied to clean up the oil are still being investigated. After decades of factory pollution and neglect, Lake Tai in China was overtaken by a vast algae bloom and major pollution with cyanobacteria in 2007. Despite a cleanup campaign the situation has barely improved. Generating power from nuclear energy is another sensitive issue that divides even environmental advocates, with some touting and others damning it. The 2011 nuclear accident in Fukushima, Japan, triggered by a major earthquake and massive tsunami, caused over 150,000 residents to evacuate their homes for fear of nuclear contamination – its consequences are still being felt. Toxicologists are increasingly being called upon to assess effects on humans, wild and domestic animals, and the environment, and to offer solutions when such incidents arise. We will always have to contend with emergencies and disasters and must be prepared.

Climate change is another aspect of environmental toxicology which has seen its share of debate in the last decade. Naysayers who deny its existence or reject the human factor, despite the science, may be lesser in number and less vocal but are still being heard. Nonetheless, the Intergovernmental Panel on Climate Change found, in its Fourth Assessment Report, in 2007, that "warming of the climate system is unequivocal", and "most of the observed increase in global average temperatures since the mid-20th century is very likely due to the observed increase in anthropogenic greenhouse gas concentrations." The Fifth Assessment Report should be finalized in 2014. Meanwhile, the Doha Amendment to the Kyoto Protocol was adopted in 2012. Countries which are Parties to the Protocol continue to commit to reducing their greenhouse gas emissions.

Energy production, be it via nuclear, coal, or gas, or even the supposedly more benign solar and wind can result in consequences, expected and unexpected, which have to be dealt with. The continual search for new energy sources and for devising means of extracting energy from existing sources has accelerated as the US and other countries seek energy independence, and has resulted in environmental health dilemmas. Fracking, or hydraulic fracturing, using sand and chemicals to create fractures in rock, has proven an economically viable way to extract oil and gas from previously inaccessible locations. We still fall far short of consensus, though, on fracking's environmental risks. No doubt one of the next great debates on the energy front will be the potential health and, particularly, environmental effects, including global warming, of commercial methane hydrate extraction, once is becomes feasible in the near future.

Accidental and malicious tainting of food, and contamination of consumer products, are of ongoing concern. In 2007, incidents of renal failure in dogs and cats were traced to contaminated pet food from China. Recalls were widespread. The chemical culprit turned out to be melamine, which was added to the wheat gluten to make the food appear higher in protein than it really was. Exported toys from China were found to have high levels of lead in their paint in the same year. Mattel, for example, had to recall 800,000 Barbie doll accessories. And, again in 2007, the head of China's food and drug administration, Zheng Xiaoyu, who, among other things took bribes from the manufacturers of substandard medicines, became the symbol of poor quality control, and paid with his life, as he was executed by lethal injection.

Global security, which includes attentiveness to and curtailment of non-traditional weapons such as are employed in chemical and biological warfare, is another issue which cannot be neglected in the 21st century. Stockpiles of chemicals still exist in many countries. As recently as 2013, there have been allegations of chemical weapons use in Syria. Looking toward the positive, in 2013, Somalia became the 189th State Party to the Chemical Weapons Convention, overseen by the Organisation for the Prohibition of Chemical Weapons (OPCW).

Beyond seeking to reduce and eliminate chemical weapons, managing chemicals on the global level remains a challenge, but slow and steady progress continues to be made. In 2009, nine new chemicals were added to the Stockholm Convention on Persistent Organic Pollutants. Synergies are developing among the Basel, Rotterdam, and Stockholm Conventions, evidenced by a joint meeting of the conferences of the parties in 2013. The Geneva Statement on the Sound Management of Chemicals and Waste, an outcome of this meeting, reaffirmed the three Conventions' commitment to achieving the Millennium Development Goals by 2015 and the sound management of chemicals and hazardous wastes by 2020. 2013 also saw the passage of another global, legally binding treaty, The Minimata Convention on Mercury, which provides controls and reductions across a range of products, processes, and industries where mercury is used, released, or emitted. The European Union's regional legislation, which entered into force in 2007, has worldwide implications for the control of chemicals.

Controversies, public concern (warranted and otherwise) and media shouting over whatever may be the new "chemical of the day," are still with us as, no doubt, they will always be. Whether we talk about phthalates, bisphenol A, or halogenated flame retardants, the press will have a field day. Arsenic, mercury, and lead are sure to fill cocktail party conversation when it goes slack. And the old standbys of tobacco, alcohol, and caffeine are always great silence breakers.

Most of the above topics have been covered, to a greater or lesser extent, in this third edition of the *Encyclopedia of Toxicology*. Since its first edition, the objective was to put toxicology in a larger societal and cultural context. Thus, while the focus here has always been on the science, we have included, in keeping with its encyclopedic nature, important organizations, laws, and history, narratives of accidents and intrigue, and more. In addition, the broad scope of toxicology has been taken into account, and hazards related not only to chemicals, but also to biological agents and radiation, have been considered. The Encyclopedia represents an amalgam of established principles and cutting edge investigations. With toxicology so much a moving target, and the process of paper publication still a lengthy process, it is not possible to create a book which is absolutely exhaustive or up-to-the-second in currency. Nonetheless, we hope it is comprehensive in a practical sense and as timely as possible, and that the gaps are few and far between. The online version, on the other hand, will be the best place to look, between editions, for late breaking developments. We hope you will find this third edition useful.

Philip Wexler

PREFACE TO THE SECOND EDITION

Time passes, but the need for toxicological understanding persists. As much as we might wish for the end of poverty, ignorance, hunger, and exposure to hazardous chemicals, and as much as we work toward these goals, the challenges are formidable, and the end is not in sight. Chemicals and finished products made from chemicals continue to play an ever-present part in our lives. Although it is not evident that the benefits of chemicals always outweigh their risks, there is little doubt that a wide spectrum of chemicals and drugs has enhanced both the duration and quality of our lives. That said, certain of them, in certain situations, are clearly harmful to certain people. Among the fruits of toxicologists' labors is information on how best to eliminate, reduce, or prevent such harm.

The discipline of toxicology has made considerable strides in the 7 years since the first edition of this encyclopedia was published. The understanding of molecular toxicology continues to advance rapidly. Indeed, it is often much easier to generate the data than to find the time to adequately evaluate it. Genomic, proteomic, and other 'omic' technologies are helping us unravel the complex connection between exposure to environmental chemicals and susceptibility to disease. The US National Center for Toxicogenomics, dedicated to research on informatics and computational toxicology, was established in 2000. As a result of this and other research, much more sophisticated approaches are now available for ascertaining chemical safety, and investigating structure–activity relationships. In addition, analytical instrumentation has become more highly refined and sensitive, making it easier to detect and quantitate even smaller amounts of contaminants in biological systems and the environment.

With greater consumer (especially Western) acceptance of complementary and alternative medicine, more people than ever before are being exposed to a vast array of herbal and other plant-based medicinal products. Although toxicologists have always recognized that 'natural' does not necessarily equate with 'safe', not much has been done to assess the hazards of herbal supplements and their interactions with other chemicals. This is beginning to change.

Chemical, biological, and nuclear warfare have always been subjects of interest, sometimes as practical matters, and more often as academic ones. In the light of the events of September 11, 2001, there has been an increased urgency in learning more about nonconventional warfare and its agents, how they operate, and how to protect ourselves from their effects. Toxicology has found itself broadening its scope to deal with this resurgent type of weaponry.

The scope of what constitutes hazards waste, an ever-present downside of the benefits we derive from the manufacture, processing, and use of chemicals and their products, continues to expand as technology moves forward. In the US two million tons of electronic products, including 50 million computers and 130 million cellphones, are disposed of every year. According to the International Association of Electronic Recylers, this number will more than triple by 2010. With such quantities in landfills and rivers, there are bound to be consequences for our air and water. Potential toxicants include lead, cadmium, and beryllium.

Alternatives to animal studies no longer represent a toxicological sideline. While whole animal testing is unlikely to disappear soon, if ever, other methods of determining hazard and safety are increasingly being embraced by the toxicology community and becoming part of mainstream chemical evaluations. *In vitro* approaches (e.g., using cell culture or skin irritation potential) and *in silico* approaches (i.e., using computer programs to estimate toxic properties based on existing data for similar chemicals with or without supplemental chemical and physical property data) are both generating increasing amounts of toxicity information.

The marketplace is seeing an increase in products utilizing nanotechnologies, and nanotechnology research and development is on the upswing. The United States has had an official National Nanotechnology Initiative since 2001. A start has also been made by federal agencies and universities in assessing the environmental and health effects of nanomaterials.

Greater insight into chemical exposures, both actual and anticipated, is helping to develop a more focused picture of the risks these exposures present to humans and the environment. Growing cooperation between toxicologists and exposure assessors is proving vital to strengthening the scientific basis of risk assessment, thus giving risk assessors and managers more credible tools to address the control of chemical hazards.

At the global level, there have been important strides in the control and management of chemicals. The 10-year follow-up to the Rio Earth Summit, the World Summit on Sustainable Development, was held in 2002 in Johannesburg, South Africa. Among the targets it set was to use and produce chemicals by 2020 in ways that do not lead to significant adverse effects on human health and the environment.

The Stockholm Convention to protect human health and the environment from persistent organic pollutants (POPs) became binding on May 17, 2004. POPs tend to be toxic, persistent, accumulative, and capable of traveling long distances in the environment. This Convention seeks to eliminate or restrict the production and use of such chemicals. The Kyoto Protocol, designed to decrease greenhouse gas emissions, has now become an international law, despite the resistance of several countries.

The United States hosts a vibrant and growing community of toxicology professionals who perform innovative toxicological research, and scientists in other countries are making their presence felt equally. Global information sharing and collaborations among these investigators are growing, facilitated by the increased accessibility of the Internet and its enhanced technologies. Significant work is proceeding under the auspices of multinational bodies such as Organisation for Economic Co-operation and Development, the European Commission, and the International Program on Chemical Safety.

Efforts to harmonize and link data and information on toxic chemicals throughout the world have been multiplying. The Globally Harmonized System (GHS) of classification and labeling of chemicals has been adopted and is ready for implementation. This will provide a consistent and coherent approach to identifying hazardous chemicals, as well as provide information on such hazards and protective measures to exposed populations. Meanwhile in the European Union, a regulatory framework known as REACH (Registration, Evaluation and Authorization of Chemicals) has been proposed for the registration of chemical substances manufactured or imported in quantities greater than one ton per year.

Last, but not least, the role that poisons played in personal and political intrigues and vendettas, although it may have peaked with Borgias, by no means ended there. A case in point was the 2004 presidential elections in Ukraine. After a bitterly contested battle for the presidency of Ukraine, Viktor Yushchenko emerged victorious and was inaugurated in January 2005, a happy day for democracy, but with a toxic twist. Yushchenko, according to physicians, suffered severe facial disfigurement (chloracne) and other ailments by being poisoned with large dose of dioxins, allegedly mixed in some soup he consumed. Fortunately he is recovering gradually. Although the full story has not yet emerged, political motivations are suspected.

This second edition has grown from 749 entries submitted by 200 authors to 1057 entries contributed by 392 authors. Virtually all the entries from the first edition have been updated and in some cases entirely new versions of these entries have been written. Among the 308 topics appearing for the first time in this edition are avian ecotoxicology, benchmark dose, biocides, computational toxicology, cancer potency factors, metabonomics, chemical accidents, Monte Carlo analysis, nonlethal chemical weapons, invertebrate ecotoxicology, drugs of abuse, cancer chemotherapeutic agents, and consumer products. Many entries devoted to specific chemicals are also brand new to this edition and the international scope of organizations included has been broadened. Entries describing a number of well-known toxin-related incidents, e.g., Love Canal, Times Beach, Chernobyl, and Three-Mile Island, have been added. In addition to the scientific-based entries, others focus on the societal implications of toxicological knowledge. Among them are Toxicology in Culture, Environmental Crimes, Notorious Poisoners and Poisoning Cases Chemical and Biological Warfare in Ancient Times, and a History of the US Environmental Movement. Thus, this new edition has been expanded in length, breadth, and depth and provides an extensive overview of the many facets of toxicology.

Philip Wexler

PREFACE TO THE FIRST EDITION

There are many fine general and specialized monographs on toxicology, most of which are addressed to toxicologists and students in the field and a few to laypeople. This encyclopedia of toxicology does not presume to replace any of them but rather is intended to fulfill the toxicology information needs of new audiences by taking a different organizational approach and assuming a middle ground in the level of presentation by borrowing elements of both primer and treatise.

The encyclopedia is broad-ranging in scope, although it does not aspire to be exhaustive. The idea was to look at basic, critical, and controversial elements in toxicology, which are those elements that are essential to an understanding of the subject's scientific underpinnings and societal ramifications. As such, the encyclopedia had to cover not only key concepts, such as dose response, mechanism of action, testing procedures, endpoint responses, and target sites, but also individual chemicals and classes of chemicals. Despite the strong chemical emphasis of the book, we had to look at concepts such as radiation and noise, and beyond the emphasis on the science of toxicology, we had to look at history, laws, regulation, education, organizations, and databases. The encyclopedia also needed to consider environmental and ecological toxicology to somewhat counterbalance the acknowledged emphasis on laboratory animals and humans because, in the end, all our connections run deep.

In terms of the chemicals, we the editors of this book made a personal selection based on our own knowledge of those with relatively high toxicity, exposure, production, controversy, newsworthiness, or other interest. The chemicals do not represent a merger of regulatory lists or databases of chemicals; they are what we consider to be, for one reason or another, chemicals of concern to toxicology. The book was not intended as a large-scale compendium of toxic chemicals, several of which already exist.

In the tradition of many standard encyclopedias, scientific and otherwise, the encyclopedia is organized entirely alphabetically. Other than in a few useful but smaller scale dictionaries, this style of arrangement has not been done before for toxicology. This organization, along with a detailed index and extensive cross-references, should help the reader quickly arrive at the needed information.

Next, although this book should be of use to the practicing toxicologist, it is geared more to others who, in the course of their work, study, or for general interest, need to know about toxicology. This would include the scientific community in general, physicians, legal and regulatory professionals, and laypeople with some scientific background. Toxicologists needing to brush up on or get a quick review of a subject other than their own specialty would also benefit from it, but toxicologists seeking an in-depth treatment should instead consult a specialized monograph or journal literature.

The encyclopedia is meant to give relatively succinct overviews of sometimes very complex subjects. Formal references and footnotes were dispensed with because these seemed less relevant to the encyclopedia's goals than a simple list of recommended readings designed to lead the reader to more detailed information on a particular subject entry. The entry on Information Resources leads readers to print and electronic sources of information in toxicology.

First and foremost, thanks go to the Associate Editors and contributors, whose efforts are here in print. Yale Altman and Linda Marshall, earlier Acquisitions Editors for the books, were of great assistance in getting the project off the ground. Tari Paschall, the current Acquisitions Editor, and Monique Larson, Senior Production Editor, both of Academic Press, have with great expertise and efficiency brought it to fruition. Organization and formatting of the original entry manuscripts were handled with skill, patience, and poise by Mary Hall with the help of Christen Bosh and Jennifer Brewster.

My work on the *Encyclopedia of Toxicology* was undertaken as a private citizen, not as a government employee. The views expressed are strictly my own. No official support or endorsement by the US National Library of Medicine or any other agency of the US Federal Government was provided or should be inferred.

Philip Wexler

EDITOR-IN-CHIEF

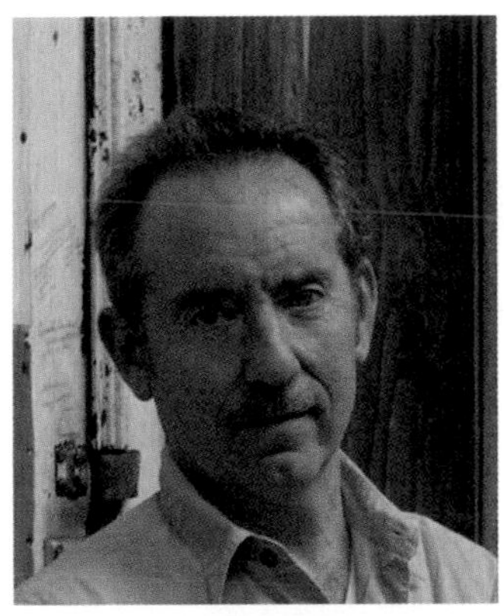

Philip Wexler has been published, taught, and otherwise lectured extensively in the U.S. and abroad on toxicology and toxicoinformatics. He is the Editor-in-Chief of three editions of the *Encyclopedia of Toxicology* (Elsevier. 3rd ed. 2014) and four editions of *Information Resources in Toxicology* (Elsevier. 4th ed. 2009), as well as *Chemicals, Environment, Health: A Global Management Perspective* (CRC Press/Taylor and Francis. 2011). He has served as Associate Editor for Toxicology Information and Resources for Elsevier's journal, *Toxicology* and, in that capacity, edited special issues on Digital Information and Tools. In 2010, he was named the recipient of the US Society of Toxicology's Public Communications Award. He is also overseeing a monographic series on Toxicology History. The first volume, *Toxicology in Antiquity*, is scheduled for publication by Elsevier in 2014.

Mr. Wexler is a Technical Information Specialist at the National Library of Medicine's (NLM) Toxicology and Environmental Health Information Program, within the Specialized Information Services Division (SIS). His career at NLM began as a Fellow of the NLM Associate Program and included a stint with the Reference Services Section. A recipient of the NLM Regents Award for Scholarly or Technical Achievement and the Distinguished Technical Communication Award of the Washington chapter of the Society for Technical Communication, he is team leader for the development of the ToxLearn online multi-module tutorials, a joint activity with the SOT. Mr. Wexler is also project officer for the LactMed file on drugs and lactation, and the IRIS (Integrated Risk Information System) and ITER (International Toxicity Estimates for Risk) risk assessment databases.

Additionally, Mr. Wexler was the guiding force behind, and current federal liaison to, the World Library of Toxicology, Chemical Safety, and Environmental Health (WLT), a free global Web portal that provides the scientific community and public with links to major government agencies, non-governmental organizations, universities, professional societies, and other groups addressing issues related to toxicology, public health, and environmental health. This multilingual resource, fed by information from a roster of international Country Correspondents, has been widely praised for its success in overcoming barriers to the sharing of information between countries, enhancing collaboration, and minimizing duplication.

He is federal liaison to the Toxicology Education Foundation (TEF), past Chair of SOT's World Wide Web Advisory Team, and past President of its Ethical, Legal, and Social Issues Specialty Section. Mr. Wexler led the World Library of Toxicology project prior to its migration to the INND/Toxipedia group, and remains a federal liaison to the project. He was a member of the Education and Communications Work Group of the CDC/ATSDR's National Conversation on Public Health and Chemical Exposure. A co-developer of the Toxicology History Room, he is co-founder and federal liaison to the Toxicology History Association.

ASSOCIATE EDITORS

Mohammad Abdollahi

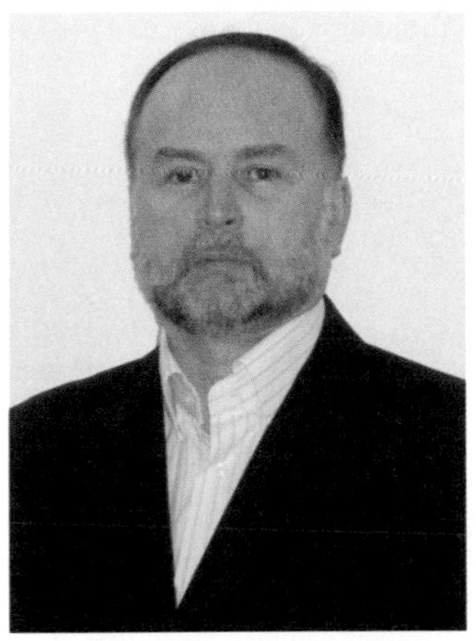

Mohammad Abdollahi acquired a PharmD in 1988 from the Tehran University of Medical Sciences (TUMS) and then completed a PhD in Pharmacology/Toxicology in 1994 from the same university; he completed postdoc training at the University of Toronto in 2001. Since 1988, Mohammad has worked as an academic at TUMS and has studied in the fields of Pharmacology, Toxicology, and Medical Sciences. Since 2003 he has acquired full professor honorship of TUMS. So far, he has contributed to more than 500 papers and 20 books. He is the Editor-in-Chief for two prestigious TUMS journals in the field of Medicine and Pharmacy published by Elsevier and BMC. At international level, he cooperates with the OPCW (Organisation for Prohibition of Chemical Weapons) as a Scientific Advisory Board Member in the Netherlands, the COPE (Committee on Publication Ethics) as a Council Trustee Member in UK, the WHO (World Health Organization) as a Member of the Guideline Developing Group for Prevention of Lead Poisoning in Switzerland, the IAS (Islamic-World Academy of Sciences) as a Fellow, WLT (World Library of Toxicology) as a country correspondent, and some others. At national level, MA has been President of Iranian Society of Toxicology (IranTox) for seven years and was involved in establishing the Drug and Poison Information Centers. He has been the Director of the National Toxicology Examination Board for nine years. Since 2007, MA has been the Dean of Department of Toxicology and Pharmacology in TUMS. Current main research interests of MA are Mechanistic Toxicology, Environmental Toxicology, and Evidence-Based Medicine. He studies to uncover the critical connections between the toxicity of chemicals and the etiology of human diseases.

Ann de Peyster

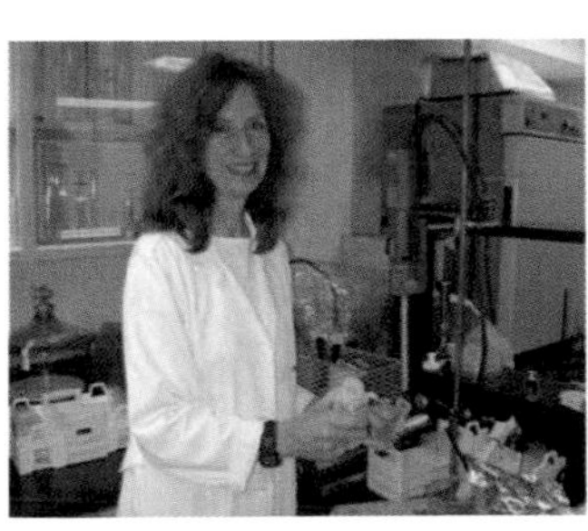

Ann de Peyster joined the faculty of the Graduate School of Public Health at San Diego State University in 1983 to found and direct the Toxicology graduate program after completing her doctorate at U.C. Berkeley. Until 2011 she oversaw development of all aspects of the curriculum and research laboratories; established partnerships with industry and government toxicologists willing to participate in the program; and mentored of dozens of graduate students. Initially holding a joint appointment in SDSU's Department of Biology and the Graduate School of Public Health, she developed and taught a wide variety of laboratory and lecture courses in biology, public health, toxicology and risk assessment, and developed an introductory course in public health research that is now required for public health undergraduates before leaving full-time teaching in 2012. Her main research interests and majority of publications focus on mechanisms of action of chemicals affecting the reproductive system and implications for risk assessment.

In addition to graduate student recruitment and mentoring, she has also served in major administrative roles for the Graduate School of Public Health, including Interim Director (a.k.a. Dean) of the School from 2004–2007. Also active professionally for many years in SETAC, Sigma Xi, and Delta Omega (public health honor society), she has contributed most of her non-academic professional time to the Society of Toxicology. She has devoted special attention to SOT's educational efforts, from K-12 through graduate education, and to the Society's public communications mission. She received the SOT Public Communications Award in 1999 and also served as an SOT Councilor. She is a Fellow of the Academy of Toxicological Sciences and a trustee of the Toxicology Education Foundation.

She continues to pursue other personal and professional interests since resigning her full-time tenured professorship at San Diego State University.

Shayne C. Gad

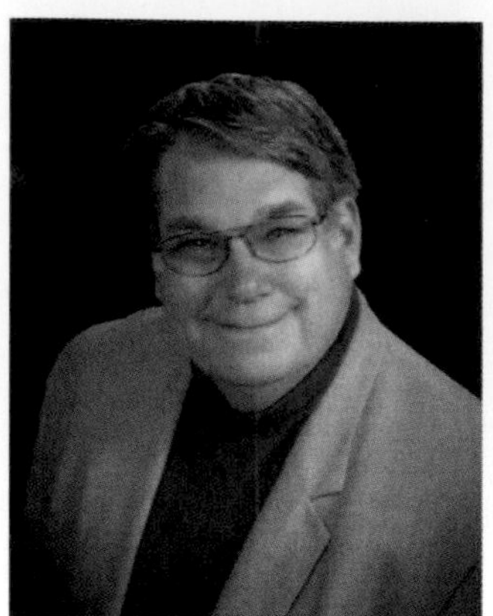

Shayne C. Gad, B.S. (Whittier College, Chemistry and Biology, 1970) and Ph.D. in Pharmacology/Toxicology (Texas, 1977) DABT, ATS, is the principal of Gad Consulting Services, a twenty year old consulting firm with six employees and more than 500 clients (including 300 pharmaceutical companies in the US and 20 overseas). Prior to this, he served in director-level and above positions at Searle, Synergen and Becton Dickinson. He has authored or edited more than 44 published books and more than 350 chapters, articles, and abstracts in the fields of toxicology, statistics, pharmacology, drug development, and safety assessment. He has more than 35 years of broad-based experience in toxicology, drug and device development, statistics, and risk assessment. He has specific expertise in neurotoxicology, *in vitro* methods, cardiovascular toxicology, inhalation toxicology, immunotoxicology, and genotoxicology. Past President of the American College of Toxicology, the Roundtable of Toxicology Consultants and three of SOT's specialty sections, and recipient of the American College of Toxicology Lifetime Contribution Award. He has direct involvement in the preparation of INDs (96 successfully to date), NDA, PLA, ANDA, 510(k), IDE, CTD, clinical data bases for phase 1 and 2 studies, and PMAs. He has consulted for FDA, EPA, and NIH, and has trained reviewers and been an expert witness for FDA, and served as the COO of two pharmaceutical companies while a consultant. He has also conducted the triennial toxicology salary survey as a service to the profession for the last 22 years.

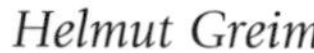

Helmut Greim

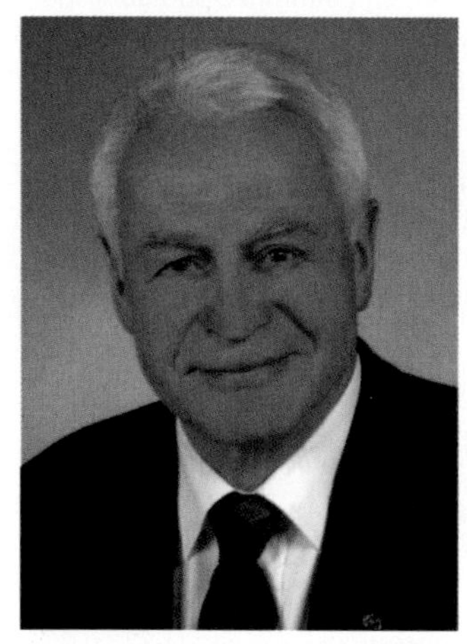

Helmut Greim has studied medicine at the Universities of Freiburg and Berlin, Germany. Thereafter he had research positions in the institutes of Biochemistry and Pharmacology of the Free University of Berlin and of the Institute of Toxicology, University of Tübingen. Between 1970 and 1973 he served as Visiting Research Associate Professor of Pathology, Mount Sinai School of Medicine, City University of New York, and as Visiting Fellow of Pharmacology, Yale University, New Haven, CT. After two years back in Tübingen he was appointed as Director of the Institute of Toxicology of the GSF, a federal Research Institute in Munich. In 1982 he became Professor and Director of the Institute of Toxicology and Environmental Hygiene, Technical University Munich. He retired from these positions in 2003.

His research experience is drug metabolism, toxicokinetics, mechanisms of carcinogenic agents, *in vitro* test systems. Dr. Greim has published over 500 papers in toxicology and risk assessment and has lectured on these subjects in Europe and abroad. Besides many contributions to textbooks he has edited and published two text-books in Toxicology, one in German, the other by Wiley, London (H. Greim and R. Snyder: *Toxicology and Risk Assessment. A comprehensive Introduction*). In June 2012 the book *The cellular response to the genotoxic insult: the question of threshold for genotoxic carcinogens* (H. Greim and R. Albertini) was published by the Royal Society of Chemistry, London.

Dr. Greim has been a member or chair of numerous national and international scientific committees. Since 1983 he was vice Chairman, and in 1998, Chairman of the German Advisory Committee on Existing Chemicals of Environmental Relevance (BUA) of the German Chemical Society until 2007. Since 1982 he has been a member of the Commission for the Investigation of Health Hazards of Chemical Compounds in the Work Areas (MAK-Committee) of the German Research Foundation and has chaired the committee between 1992 and 2007. Between 1996 and 2011 he was a member of the Research Expert Panel of the Research Institute for Fragrance Materials, Hackensack, New Jersey, USA and chairman from 2000 to 2008. Between 1998 and 2008 he was member of the Board of Trustees of the Health and Environmental Safety Institute (HESI) of the International Life Science Institute (ILSI) in Washington and has chaired the Board in 2001 and 2002. Until 2012 he chaired the Scientific Committee on Health and Environmental Risks of the Directorate General (DG) SANCO, Brussels; he is a member of the Scientific Committee on Occupational Exposure Limits of DG EMPLOYMENT, Luxembourg, and since 2008 until the end of 2013 is a member of the Risk Assessment Committee of the European Chemicals Agency in Helsinki.

Dr. Greim was chairman of the Toxicology Section of the German Society of Pharmacology and Toxicology (1982 to 1985), and served as President of the German Society of Pharmacology and Toxicology between 1991 and 1993. In 1998 he organized the International Congress of Pharmacology in Munich.

In 1996 he received the Arnold Lehman Award of the Society of Toxicology, and in 2001 the Herbert Stockinger Award of the American Conference of Governmental Industrial Hygienists.

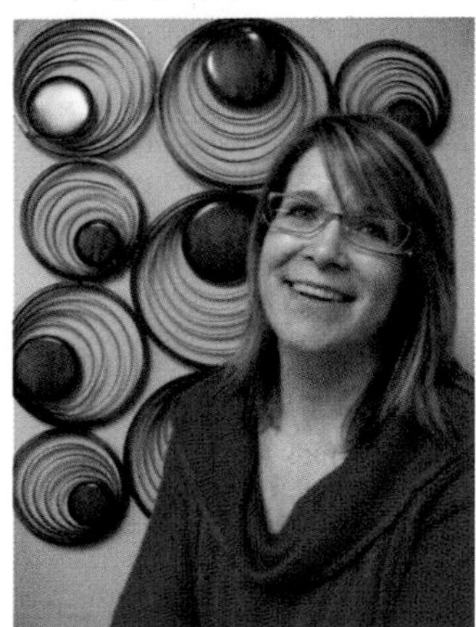

Stacey Harper

Dr. Stacey Harper is an Assistant Professor of Nanotoxicology in a joint position between the Department of Environmental & Molecular Toxicology and the School of Chemical, Biological & Environmental Engineering at Oregon State University (OSU), where she employs *in vivo* approaches to evaluate the biological activity and toxic potential of novel nanomaterials, and has established a collaborative, multidisciplinary research program to develop a knowledgebase of Nanomaterial-Biological Interactions (nbi.oregonstate.edu). She received her doctorate in Biological Sciences from the University of Nevada, Las Vegas in 2003 and was a postdoctoral fellow at the Environmental Protection Agency from 2003–2005, and an NIEHS postdoctoral scholar at Oregon State University from 2005–2009. Dr. Harper currently serves as the co-chair of ASTM International E56 Committee on Nanotechnologies. She was recently awarded an Outstanding New Environmental Scientist award from the National Institute of Environmental Health Sciences and the L.L. Stewart Faculty Scholars award from OSU. From 2011–2012, Dr. Harper served as the president of the Pacific Northwest Association of Toxicologists, a regional chapter of the Society of Toxicology.

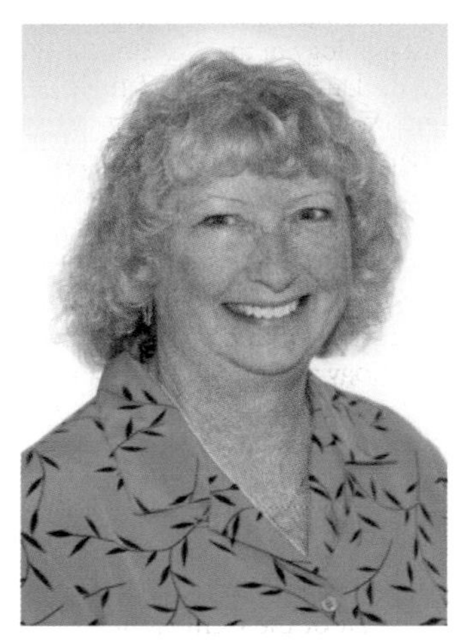

Virginia C. Moser

Dr. Virginia (Ginger) Moser has been at the US Environmental Protection Agency since receiving her PhD in Pharmacology and Toxicology from the Medical College of Virginia in 1983. She has led an active research program there since joining the Laboratory as a National Research Council postdoctoral fellow, and is now a senior toxicologist in the Toxicity Assessment Division of the National Health and Environmental Effects Research Laboratory. She holds adjunct faculty positions at the Integrated Toxicology Program at Duke University, and the Department of Pharmacology and Toxicology, Medical College of Virginia, Virginia Commonwealth University.

Over the years Dr. Moser has focused on using neurobehavioral test methods for both toxicity screening and mechanistic research of a wide variety of environmental chemicals (including pesticides, persistent organic pollutants, and drinking water contaminants) following acute, repeated, and developmental exposures in both rats and mice. Her current research includes evaluating unique susceptibilities of developing and young organisms to neurotoxicants. Dr. Moser was instrumental in validating and promoting the use of neurobehavioral test methods, specifically the functional observational battery (FOB), for toxicity screening. She helped shape the test guidelines for neurobehavioral toxicity testing promulgated by the US EPA, OECD, and FDA, and served as Study Director for an IPCS/WHO international multi-laboratory Collaborative Study on Neurobehavioral Test Methods. She has also been involved with training personnel in contract, chemical, and pharmaceutical testing laboratories in the conduct of these methods, as well as training risk assessors in the interpretation of those data.

Dr. Moser is a Diplomate of the American Board of Toxicology and served on the Executive Board of Directors and as Treasurer of that organization. She is also recognized as a Fellow of the Academy of Toxicological Sciences. She has received many honors from the US EPA, including the Scientific Achievement Award for Human Health Research and the Gold Medal for Exceptional Service. As an active member of numerous scientific societies, she has held elected officer positions, served on planning committees, and organized meetings, symposia, and workshops. She is currently Secretary of the Neurobehavioral Teratology Society, and has served as President and Secretary-Treasurer of the North Carolina Regional Chapter of SOT, Councilor of the International Neurotoxicology Association, and President and Treasurer of the Behavioral Toxicology Society. Currently she serves as associate editor for the *Encyclopedia of Toxicology* (3rd edition), *Neurotoxicology and Teratology*, and *Drug and Chemical Toxicology*, and is on editorial boards for *Toxicological Sciences, Toxicology and Applied Pharmacology*, and *Neurotoxicology*. In addition she has served on NIH, NIEHS, VA, Fogarty, and other grant Study Sections. Over the years she has played integral roles in ILSI/HESI, VCCEP, and OECD expert panels. Within the EPA, she has been involved in numerous pesticide risk assessment workgroups, a member of the IACUC, and many other internal activities. She has over 130 peer-reviewed manuscripts and book chapters published or in press.

José V. Tarazona

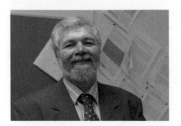

Dr José V. Tarazona is a doctor in veterinary medicine, DVM, and obtained a PhD in toxicology from the University Complutense of Madrid. He started his scientific career on mammalian toxicology as an assistant professor of toxicology at the Veterinary Faculty of Madrid and moved to ecotoxicology and environmental risk assessment as a staff researcher of the Spanish National Institute for Agriculture and Food Research and Technology (INIA). He is currently serving at an EU Agency.

Former Head of the Division of Environmental Toxicology and Director of the Department of the Environment at INIA, he has participated in 33 research projects at the national and European levels mostly as project coordinator or team leader. Coauthor of over 250 scientific papers including 18 books/monographs, covering the development of new (eco)toxicity tests for aquatic and terrestrial organisms; use and validation of biomarkers, bioassays, and other biological alternatives for field monitoring; combination of toxicity thresholds and exposure levels using mathematical models, and the scientific basis of hazard identification and risk assessment of industrial chemicals, pesticides, pharmaceuticals, and complex mixtures.

Involved in the scientific advisory board of the European Union since 1992 as a member of CSTE, CSTEE, SCHER, and ECHA-RAC and also provided scientific advice at the OECD and UN levels; chairing the OECD Expert Group on Chronic Aquatic Hazards and the OECD and UN Expert Groups on Terrestrial Hazards within the GHS strategy, and as a member of the UNEP POPs Review Committee under the Stockholm Convention.

Full member of the Spanish Royal Academy of Veterinary Sciences, former council member of the Society of Environmental Toxicology and Chemistry (SETAC), past president of the Ibero-American Society of Environmental Contamination and Toxicology, and vice president of the Spanish Association of Environmentalist Veterinarian Experts, is also a member of several international scientific societies, and an associate editor of several scientific journals.

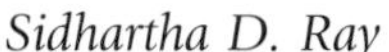

Sidhartha D. Ray

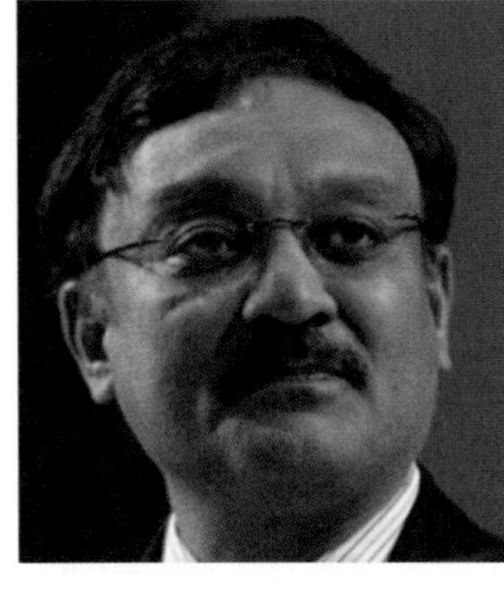

Dr Sidhartha D. Ray is a professor and chair of the Department of Pharmaceutical Sciences of the Manchester College (Est.) School of Pharmacy. He serves on the editorial boards of several high impact-factor international journals: Archives of Toxicology, Oxidative Medicine and Cellular Longevity, and Experimental and Clinical Sciences. His primary research interests are (i) mechanistic toxicology, (ii) drug and chemically induced apoptotic/necrotic cell deaths, and (iii) anti-toxic/anticancer properties of phytochemicals. He has won the two highest academic honors bestowed by an academic institution: Excellence in Teaching and Lifetime Achievement in Scholarship awards. He also received the '2013 Undergraduate Educator of the Year' national award from the Society of Toxicology. He earned his MS and PhD in life sciences from the University of Indore (DAVV), India, and received formal postdoctoral training at Rutgers – The State University of New Jersey, University of California at Santa Cruz, and Medical College of Virginia at Richmond. He is well known: (i) for his groundbreaking discoveries on acetaminophen-induced programmed and unprogrammed cell death in *in vivo* models, (ii) for unraveling anticancer and antitoxic properties of grape seed proanthocyanidin extract against a wide variety of drugs, chemicals and carcinogens, and (iii) for considerably expanding on the knowledge on the safety sciences of drugs, chemicals, and a variety of natural phytochemicals. Dr. Ray is both a dedicated teacher and a formidable scientist who passionately teaches his students how to be "Lifelong Learners"!

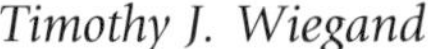

Timothy J. Wiegand

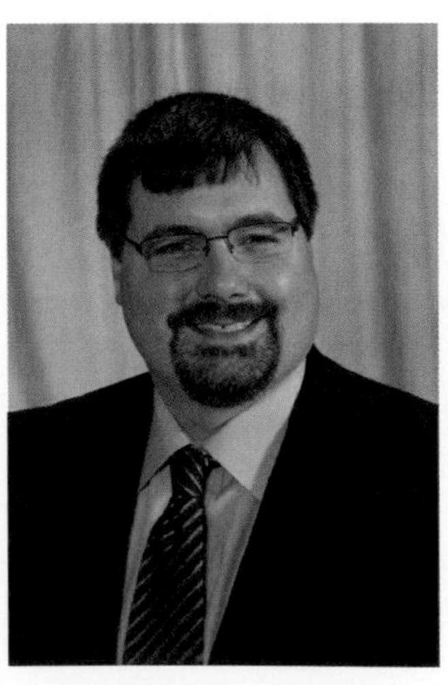

Timothy J. Wiegand, MD, FACMT holds a board certification in internal medicine and medical toxicology. He completed toxicology and clinical pharmacology fellowship training at the University of California, San Francisco in 2006 and is currently the director of toxicology at the University of Rochester Medical Center in Rochester, New York and an associate clinical professor of emergency medicine in the Department of Emergency Medicine at Strong Memorial Hospital and Highland Hospital in Rochester. He is also medical director of Huther-Doyle Chemical Dependency program in Rochester and a consultant toxicologist for the SUNY Upstate Poison Center in Syracuse, New York. He currently serves as the director of the Toxicology Consult Service at Strong Memorial Hospital. The service is responsible for the bedside care of poisoned patients and it is the crux of a toxicology rotation run by him for fellows, residents, and students in both medical and pharmacy training at Strong Memorial Hospital. He has authored numerous chapters in text books and papers in peer-reviewed journals and is an associate editor of the *Encyclopedia of Toxicology*, 3rd edition. His particular areas of interest are in the bedside care of poisoned patients, in the treatment of alcohol, opioid, and other drug withdrawal and dependence syndromes in the interpretation of impairment and intoxication during performance and driving, and in toxicology and pharmacology education and suicide and drug and alcohol abuse prevention.

LIST OF CONTRIBUTORS

A. Abdolahi
Tehran, Iran

A.H. Abdolghaffari
International Campus, Tehran University of Medical Sciences, Tehran, Iran; and Institute of Medicinal Plants, ACECR, Tehran, Iran

M. Abdollahi
Tehran University of Medical Sciences, Tehran, Iran

W.E. Achanzar
Bristol-Myers Squibb Co., Drug Safety Evaluation, New Brunswick, NJ, USA

N.M. Acquisto
University of Rochester Medical Center, Rochester, NY, USA

F.K. Adatsi
Office of Forensic Toxicology Services, Washington, DC, USA

F.A. Adekola
University of Ilorin, Ilorin, Nigeria

D. Agarwal
SB Physiotherapy and Rehabilitation Center, Mawana, India

H. Aizawa
Environment, Health and Safety Division, Organisation for Economic Cooperation and Development, Paris, France

A. Akbar Malekirad
Pharmaceutical Sciences Research Center, Tehran University of Medical Sciences, Tehran, Iran

J.A. Allen
Northwestern University, Chicago, IL, USA

B. Allison
Plankton Ecology and Limnology Laboratory, University of Oklahoma Biological Station, University of Oklahoma, Kingston, OK, USA

N. Alonso Blazquez
National Institute for Agriculture and Food Research and Technology (INIA), Madrid, Spain

R. Altkorn
Oak Brook, IL, USA

M. Amanlou
Tehran University of Medical Sciences, Tehran, Iran

M. Amini
Tehran University of Medical Sciences, Tehran, Iran

S.S. Anand
DuPont Haskell Global Centers for Health and Environmental Sciences, Newark, DE, USA

S.A. Andres
University of Louisville School of Medicine, Louisville, KY, USA

D.J. Angelini
Edgewood Chemical Biological Center, Aberdeen, MD, USA

G. Angelo
Oregon State University, Corvallis, OR, USA

A.M. Api
Research Institute for Fragrance Materials, Inc. (RIFM), Woodcliff Lake, NJ, USA

U. Apte
University of Kansas Medical Center, Kansas City, KS, USA

C.R. Armendáriz
Universidad de La Laguna, Santa Cruz de Tenerife, Spain

S. Asha
Manchester University College of Pharmacy, Fort Wayne, IN, USA

P. Atlason
European Chemicals Agency, Helsinki, Finland

M.S. Attene-Ramos
NIH Chemical Genomics Center, National Center for Advancing Translational Sciences, National Institutes of Health, Bethesda, MD, USA

C.P. Austin
NIH Chemical Genomics Center, National Center for Advancing Translational Sciences, National Institutes of Health, Bethesda, MD, USA

M.A. Babich
U.S. Consumer Product Safety Commission, Rockville, MD, USA

M. Badanthadka
Torrent Research Centre, Gandhinagar, India

M. Baeeri
Pharmaceutical Sciences Research Center, Tehran University of Medical Sciences, Tehran, Iran

K.N. Baer
College of Pharmacy, The University of Louisiana at Monroe, Monroe, LA, USA

A. Baghaei
Faculty of Pharmacy and Pharmaceutical Sciences, Tehran University of Medical Sciences, Tehran, Iran

H. Bahadar
Tehran University of Medical Sciences, Tehran, Iran

B. Balali-Mood
Imperial College London, London, UK

M. Balali-Mood
Newcastle University, Newcastle Upon Tyne, UK; and Medical Toxicology Research Centre, Imam Reza Hospital, Faculty of Medicine, Mashhad University of Medical Sciences, Mashhad, Iran

A.S. Bale
United States Environmental Protection Agency, Washington, DC, USA

B. Ballantyne
Consultant, Charleston, WV, USA

M. Banasik
Instytut Zdrowia Publicznego i Ochrony Środowiska, Warsaw, Poland

C.N. Banks
School of Veterinary Medicine, University of California, Davis, CA, USA

M. Banton
LyondellBasell Corporate HSE/Product Safety, Houston, TX, USA

K.P. Baran
TOX-TK Associates, Inc., Apex, NC, USA

C. Barata
IDAEA—CSIC, Barcelona, Spain

A.C. Barefoot
DuPont Crop Protection, Newark, DE, USA

S.M. Barlow
Brighton, UK

D.B. Barr
Exposure Science and Environmental Health, Rollins School of Public Health, Emory University, Atlanta, GA, USA

F. Barrueto
University of Maryland School of Medicine, Baltimore, MD, USA

C. Barton
Oak Ridge Institute for Science and Education, Oak Ridge, TN, USA

N. Barton
Farmington, NY, USA

M. Battalora
DuPont Crop Protection, Stine-Haskell Research Center, Newark, DE, USA

Z. Bayrami
Tehran University of Medical Sciences, Tehran, Iran

R. Bazl
Tehran University of Medical Sciences, Tehran, Iran

R.D. Beckett
Manchester University College of Pharmacy, Fort Wayne, IN, USA

V. Bečková
National Radiation Protection Institute (SÚRO, v.v.i.), Praha, Czech Republic

S. Beedanagari
Bristol Myers Squibb, New Brunswick, NJ, USA

A.F. Behboudi
Toronto, ON, Canada

L.D. Beilke
Aragon Pharmaceuticals, San Diego, CA, USA

E.M. Beltrán
Laboratory for Ecotoxicology, Spanish National Institute for Agriculture and Food Research and Technology, Madrid, Spain

A. Benson
US Environmental Protection Agency, Washington, DC, USA

L. Bergamo
Università degli Studi di Padova, Padova, Italy

J. Bergueiro
Universidad de Santiago de Compostela, Santiago de Compostela, A Coruña, Spain

F.W. Berman
Toxicology Information Center, Center for Research on Occupational and Environmental Toxicology (CROET), Oregon Health and Science University, Portland, OR, USA

S. Betharia
Manchester University College of Pharmacy, Fort Wayne, IN, USA

S. Bhattacharya
Chittaranjan National Cancer Institute, Kolkata, India

M. Biglar
Tehran University of Medical Sciences, Tehran, Iran

S. Biswas
Birla Institute of Technology and Sciences-Pilani, Hyderabad, India

A.T. Black
Grocery Manufacturers Association, Washington, DC, USA

A.B. Bloomhuff
ACGIH®, Cincinnati, OH, USA

J.R. Bloomquist
Emerging Pathogens Institute, University of Florida, Gainesville, FL, USA

D.L. Bolduc
Armed Forces Radiobiology Research Institute, Bethesda, MD, USA

P.M. Bolger
Annapolis, MD, USA

H.M. Bolt
Leibniz Research Centre for Working Environment and Human Factors (IfADo), Dortmund, Germany

J.A. Bonventre
Oregon State University, Corvallis, OR, USA

H.A. Borek
University of Virginia School of Medicine, Charlottesville, VA, USA

S.J. Borghoff
ToxStrategies Inc., Cary, NC, USA

J.F. Borzelleca
Richmond, VA, USA

M.C. Botelho
National Institute of Health, Porto, Portugal

A.B.A. Boxall
University of York, York, UK

H. Bradford
Tufts University School of Medicine, Boston, MA, USA

P.M. Brady
BNSF Railway, Fort Worth, TX, USA

M. Broderick
California Poison Control System, San Diego, CA, USA

D.A. Brown
Manchester University College of Pharmacy, Fort Wayne, IN, USA

J. Brown
US Environmental Protection Agency, Research Triangle Park, NC, USA

R.D. Bruce

D. Brugge
Tufts University, Boston, MA, USA

K.E. Brugger
DuPont Crop Protection, Newark, DE, USA

M.A. Bryant
Manchester University, North Manchester, IN, USA

M.H. Bucklin
University of Tennessee Medical Center, Knoxville, TN, USA

L.A. Burns-Naas
Drug Safety Evaluation Gilead Sciences, Inc., Foster City, CA, USA

S.A. Burr
Plymouth University Peninsula Schools of Medicine and Dentistry, Plymouth, UK

J.M. Caballero
University of La Laguna, La Laguna, Tenerife, Spain

Z. Cai
University of Louisiana at Monroe, Monroe, LA, USA

E.J. Calabrese
University of Massachusetts, Amherst, MA, USA

M. Calvo
University of Zaragoza, Zaragoza, Spain

J. Cammack
MedImmune, LLC, Gaithersburg, MD, USA

A. Campbell
Western University of Health Sciences, Pharmaceutical Sciences, College of Pharmacy, Pomona, CA, USA

T. Canedy
Orono, ME, USA

F.L. Cantrell
California Poison Control System, San Diego, CA, USA

T. Caquet
INRA, UMR0985 Écologie et Santé des Écosystèmes, Équipe Écotoxicologie et Qualité des Milieux Aquatiques, Agrocampus Ouest, Rennes, France

G. Carbonell
Spanish National Institute for Agriculture and Food Research and Technology, Madrid, Spain

H. Carlson-Lynch
Scarborough, ME, USA

N. Carmichael
European Centre for Ecotoxicology and Toxicology of Chemicals AISBL (ECETOC), Brussels, Belgium

H. Carmo
REQUIMTE/Laboratory of Toxicology, Faculty of Pharmacy, University of Porto, Porto, Portugal

D. Carr
American Association of Poison Control Centers, Alexandria, VA, USA

C.D. Carrington
College Park, MD, USA

F. Carvalho
REQUIMTE/Laboratory of Toxicology, Faculty of Pharmacy, University of Porto, Porto, Portugal

M. Carvalho
REQUIMTE/Laboratory of Toxicology, Faculty of Pharmacy, University of Porto and University Fernando Pessoa, Porto, Portugal

I. de la Casa-Resino
University of Extremadura, Cáceres, Spain

L.J. Cash
Los Alamos National Laboratory, Los Alamos, NM, USA

V. Castranova
National Institute for Occupational Safety and Health, Morgantown, WV, USA

R. Cesnaitis
European Chemicals Agency, Helsinki, Finland

K.D. Chadwick
Bristol-Myers Squibb, Drug Safety Evaluation, New Brunswick, NJ, USA

P. Chakraborty
Chittaranjan National Cancer Institute, Kolkata, India

P.P.K. Chan
PCTS Specialty Chemicals Pte Ltd, Singapore

S. Chang
Wexner Medical Center, Ohio State University College of Medicine, Columbus, OH, USA

R.E. Chapin
Pfizer Global Research and Development, Groton, CT, USA

S. Chateauvieux
Laboratoire de Biologie Moleculaire et Cellulaire du Cancer (LBMCC), Luxembourg

A. Chattopadhyay
Visva-Bharati University, Santiniketan, India

A. Chaumot
IRSTEA Lyon, UR MALY, Ecotoxicologie, Lyon, France

G. Chen
Oklahoma State University, Stillwater, OK, USA

X. Chen
Oak Brook, IL, USA

R.K. Chesser
Texas Tech University, Lubbock, TX, USA

J. Chilakapati
Alcon Laboratories, Fort Worth, TX, USA

K. Chojnacka
Wrocław University of Technology, Wrocław, Poland

K. Chou
Michigan State University, East Lansing, MI, USA

J. Christoforidis
Ohio State University College of Medicine, Columbus, OH, USA

A.K. Clark
California Poison Control System, San Diego, CA, USA

H.J. Clewell
Center for Human Health Assessment, The Hamner Institutes for Health Sciences, Research Triangle Park, NC, USA

S.R. Clough
Haley & Aldrich, Inc., Bedford, NH, USA

P.C.S. Coelho
National Institute of Health, Porto, Portugal

C.R.E. Coggins
Carson Watts Consulting, King, NC, USA

S.M. Cohen
University of Nebraska Medical Center, Omaha, NE, USA

S.D. Cole
Edgewood Chemical Biological Center, Aberdeen, MD, USA

G.B. Corcoran
Wayne State University, Detroit, MI, USA

C. Cornu
European Chemicals Agency, Helsinki, Finland

E. Corsini
DiSFeB, Università degli Studi di Milano, Balzaretti, Milan, Italy

D.A. Cory-Slechta
University of Rochester School of Medicine, Rochester, NY, USA

C. Costa
Portuguese National Institute of Health, Porto, Portugal

L.G. Costa
University of Washington, Seattle, WA, USA

S. Costa
Portuguese National Institute of Health, Porto, Portugal

A. Covaci
University of Antwerp, Antwerp, Belgium

J. Cowden
National Center for Environmental Assessment, US Environmental Protection Agency, Research Triangle Park, NC, USA

K.L. Cumpston
Virginia Commonwealth University Medical Center, Richmond, VA, USA

E. Curfman
Indiana University School of Medicine-Fort Wayne, Fort Wayne, IN, USA

S. Czerczak
Nofer Institute of Occupational Medicine, Łódź, Poland

M.A. Daam
Technical University of Lisbon, Lisbon, Portugal

D.L. Dahlstrom
New Era Sciences, Issaquah, WA, USA

M.A. Darracq
University of California, San Francisco (UCSF), Fresno, CA, USA

A.S. Darwich
School of Pharmacy and Pharmaceutical Sciences, University of Manchester, Manchester, UK

S.R. Das
Oregon State University, Corvallis, OR, USA

J.A. Davis
National Center for Environmental Assessment, US Environmental Protection Agency, Research Triangle Park, NC, USA

I. de la Casa Resino
University of Extremadura, Cáceres, Spain

A.H. de la Torre
Universidad de La Laguna, Santa Cruz de Tenerife, Spain

M. de Lourdes Bastos
REQUIMTE/Laboratory of Toxicology, Faculty of Pharmacy, University of Porto, Porto, Portugal

E. del Río
Universidad Miguel Hernández de Elche, Elche, Spain

S. de Marcellus
Organisation for Economic Co-operation and Development, Paris, France

P.A. Demers
Occupational Cancer Research Centre, Cancer Care Ontario, Toronto, ON, Canada

A. de Peyster
San Diego State University, San Diego, CA, USA

M. Derakhshani
Capilano University, North Vancouver, BC, Canada

S.N. Desai
NINDS-NIH, Bethesda, MD, USA

M.I. de San Andrés Larrea
Universidad Complutense, Madrid, Spain

J. Descotes
Poison Center, Lyon, France

S.S. Devi
Lake Erie College of Osteopathic Medicine, Erie, PA, USA

J.J. Devlin
Centers for Disease Control and Prevention (CDC), Chamblee, GA, USA; and Emory University School of Medicine, Atlanta, GA, USA

P. de Voogt
Institute for Biodiversity and Ecosystem Dynamics, University of Amsterdam, Amsterdam, The Netherlands; and KWR Watercycle Research Institute, Nieuwegein, The Netherlands

L. Devriese
Institute for Agricultural and Fisheries Research, Oostende, Belgium

R.S. DeWoskin
US Environmental Protection Agency, Research Triangle Park, NC, USA

D. de Zwart
National Institute for Public Health and the Environment (RIVM), BA Bilthoven, The Netherlands

M. Diederich
Laboratoire de Biologie Moleculaire et Cellulaire du Cancer (LBMCC), Luxembourg

H.H. Dieter
Federal Environment Agency (UBA, Umweltbundesamt) of Germany, Dessau-Roßlau, Germany

A. Di Guardo
University of Insubria, COMO, Italy

D. Đikić
Faculty of Science, University of Zagreb, Zagreb, Croatia

I. Dincer
University of Ontario Institute of Technology, Oshawa, ON, Canada

V. Dissanayake
Illinois Poison Center, Chicago, IL, USA; and University of Illinois at Chicago, Chicago, IL, USA

S.M. DiZio
California Environmental Protection Agency, Sacramento, CA, USA

T. Dodd-Butera
CSU San Bernardino, San Bernardino, CA, USA

D. Doke
University of Alabama at Birmingham, Birmingham, AL, USA

R.M. Dorsey
Edgewood Chemical Biological Center, Aberdeen, MD, USA

M.M. Dougherty
Upstate Medical University, Syracuse, NY, USA

M.L. Dourson
Toxicology Excellence for Risk Assessment (TERA), Cincinnati, OH, USA

V.J. Drake
Oregon State University, Corvallis, OR, USA

J.H. Duffus
The Edinburgh Centre for Toxicology, Edinburgh, UK

G.G. Dumancas
Oklahoma Medical Research Foundation, Oklahoma City, OK, USA

J.P. Dumbacher
California Academy of Sciences, San Francisco, CA, USA

S.B. DuTeaux
California Air Resources Board, Sacramento, CA, USA

S.T. Dydek
Dydek Toxicology Consulting, Austin, TX, USA

J.A. Dykens
EyeCyte Therapeutics, San Diego, CA, USA

S.R. Eagle
Gad Consulting Services, Cary, NC, USA

D.A. Eastmond
University of California, Riverside, CA, USA

J.D. Easton
Plankton Ecology and Limnology Laboratory, University of Oklahoma Biological Station, University of Oklahoma, Kingston, OK, USA

B.J. Eidemiller
Society of Toxicology, Reston, VA, USA

E.A. Eisen
School of Public Health, University of California, Berkeley, CA, USA

A. Emami
Food and Drug Administration (FDA), Center for Drug Evaluation and Research, Silver Spring, MD, USA

S. Emami
Mazandaran University of Medical Sciences, Sari, Iran

M.R. Embry
ILSI Health and Environmental Sciences Institute, Washington, DC, USA

M.P. Emswiler
Virginia Commonwealth University, Richmond, VA, USA

N.K. Erraguntla
Texas Commission on Environmental Quality, Austin, TX, USA

M. Escribano
Universidad Complutense, Madrid, Spain

S. Espín
University of Murcia, Murcia, Spain

C. Estevan
Universidad Miguel Hernández de Elche, Elche, Spain

J. Estévez
Universidad Miguel Hernández de Elche, Elche, Spain

L. Etemad
Pharmaceutical Research Center, Mashhad University of Medical Sciences, Mashhad, Iran

G.W. Everson
Children's Hospital of Central California, Madera, CA, USA

L.M. Ewers
EWC, Incorporated, Covington, KY, USA

J.H. Fain
Gad Consulting Services, Cary, NC, USA

A.M. Fan
California Environmental Protection Agency, Oakland, CA, USA

F.F. Farris
Manchester University, Fort Wayne, IN, USA

A. Farshchi
Tehran University of Medical Sciences; and food and Drug Laboratory Research Center, Tehran, Iran

O.S. Fatoki
Cape Peninsula University of Technology, Cape Town, South Africa

D. Feakes
OPCW, The Hague, The Netherlands

M. Feasel
Edgewood Chemical Biological Center, Aberdeen, MD, USA

M.J. Fedoruk
University of California, Irvine, CA, USA

I.L. Feitshans
University of Lausanne, Epalinges, Switzerland

G.M. Fent
Oklahoma State University-CVHS, Physiological Sciences, Stillwater, OK, USA

J. Fernández-Tajes
University of A Coruña, A Coruña, Spain

Á.J.G. Fernández
Universidad de La Laguna, Santa Cruz de Tenerife, Spain

C. Fernández
Laboratory for Ecotoxicology, Spanish National Institute for Agriculture and Food Research and Technology, Madrid, Spain

M.D. Fernández Rodríguez
National Institute for Agriculture and Food Research and Technology (INIA), Madrid, Spain

B. Ferrari
IRSTEA Lyon, UR MALY, Ecotoxicologie, Lyon, France

J. Fidalgo
IES Rosalía de Castro Rúa de San Clemente, Santiago de Compostela, A Coruña, Spain

A. Fields
University of Rochester Strong Memorial Hospital, Rochester, NY, USA

G.L. Finch
Drug Safety Research and Development, Worldwide Research and Development, Pfizer Inc., Groton, CT, USA

A. Finizio
University of Milano Bicocca, Milan, Italy

G. Finnveden
KTH Royal Institute of Technology, Stockholm, Sweden

L. Fitzgerald
ToxStrategies, Austin, TX, USA

A. Foroumadi
Tehran University of Medical Sciences, Tehran, Iran

D. Fuentes
Manchester University College of Pharmacy, Fort Wayne, IN, USA

K. Gad
Gad Consulting Services, Cary, NC, USA

S.C. Gad
Gad Consulting Services, Cary, NC, USA

S.E. Gad
Gad Consulting Services, Cary, NC, USA

B. Gadagbui
Toxicology Excellence for Risk Assessment (TERA), Cincinnati, OH, USA

D.W. Gammon
FMC Corporation, Agricultural Chemicals Group, Ewing, NJ, USA

A.J. García-Fernández
University of Murcia, Murcia, Spain

M.C. García Gómez
National Institute for Agriculture and Food Research and Technology (INIA), Madrid, Spain

D.E. Gardner
Inhalation Toxicology Associates, Savannah, GA, USA

A. Garrard
Upstate New York Poison Center, Syracuse, NY, USA

J. Garric
IRSTEA Lyon, UR MALY, Ecotoxicologie, Lyon, France

G. Gautam
West Virginia University School of Medicine, Morgantown, WV, USA

O. Geffard
IRSTEA Lyon, UR MALY, Ecotoxicologie, Lyon, France

M.B. Genter
University of Cincinnati, Cincinnati, OH, USA

A. Gevaart-Durkin
Graduate School of Public Health, San Diego State University, San Diego, CA, USA

N. Ghafouri
California Poison Control System, San Diego Division, San Diego, CA, USA

A.R. Ghazali
Universiti Kebangsaan Malaysia, Kuala Lumpur, Malaysia

K. Ghoreishi
Celgene Corporation, San Diego, CA, USA

B. Ghosh
Harvard University, Boston, MA, USA

S.G. Gilbert
INND (Institute of Neurotoxicology & Neurological Disorders), Seattle, WA, USA

G. Giordano
University of Washington, Seattle, WA, USA

O. Giouleme
Aristotle University of Thessaloniki, Thessaloniki, Greece

M.C.L.R. Gironés
Universidad de La Laguna, Santa Cruz de Tenerife, Spain

F. Gobba
University of Modena and Reggio Emilia, Modena, Italy

S. Goel
Supernus Pharmaceuticals, Rockville, MD, USA

A.R. Gohari
Tehran University of Medical Sciences, Tehran, Iran

J.M. Gohlke
University of Alabama at Birmingham, Birmingham, AL, USA

S. Golbabaei
Amirkabir University of Technology, Tehran, Iran

S.C. Gold
Rutgers School of Law-Newark, Newark, NJ, USA

V.M. Gómez-López
CEBAS-CSIC, Espinardo, Spain

P. Gómez-Ramírez
University of Murcia, Murcia, Spain

A. González-Canga
Agencia Española de Medicamentos y Productos Sanitarios, Madrid, Spain

G.L. González
Universidad de La Laguna, Santa Cruz de Tenerife, Spain

J.E. Goodman
Gradient, Cambridge, MA, USA

E. Gordon
Elliot Gordon Consulting, LLC, Princeton Junction, NJ, USA

T. Gordon
University Medical Center, Tuxedo, NY, USA

R. Gorodetsky
Rochester, NY, USA

J.P. Gray
US Coast Guard Academy, New London, CT, USA

M.D. Green
Wake Forest University School of Law, Winston–Salem, NC, USA

H. Greim
Karlsruher Institut für Technologie (KIT), Karlsruhe, Germany

J.C. Griffiths
Rockville, MD, USA

C.M. Groth
University of Rochester Medical Center, Rochester, NY, USA

P. Guedes de Pinho
REQUIMTE/Laboratory of Toxicology, Faculty of Pharmacy, University of Porto, Porto, Portugal

N. Gupta
Phoenix VA Health Care System, Phoenix, AZ, USA

R.C. Gupta
Murray State University, Hopkinsville, KY, USA

A.J. Gutiérrez
University of La Laguna, La Laguna, Tenerife, Spain

R.C. Guy
Robin Guy Consulting, LLC, Lake Forest, IL, USA

L.T. Haber
Toxicology Excellence for Risk Assessment (TERA), Cincinnati, OH, USA

K. Hacatoglu
University of Ontario Institute of Technology, Oshawa, ON, Canada

K. Hahn
Missouri Poison Center, St. Louis, MO, USA

J.A. Haines
Divonne les Bains, France

P.J. Hakkinen
Institute for Health and Consumer Protection, Ispra, Italy

E.J. Hall
Coastal Valley Veterinary Services, LLC, Old Lyme, CT, USA

G.J. Hall
United States Coast Guard Academy, New London, CT, USA

V.R. Hall
University of Virginia School of Medicine, Charlottesville, VA, USA

K.D. Hambright
Plankton Ecology and Limnology Laboratory, University of Oklahoma Biological Station, and Program in Ecology and Evolutionary Biology, University of Oklahoma, Norman, OK, USA

J.A. Handler
JAH Associates LLC, Wayne, PA, USA

D.K. Hansen
US Food and Drug Administration/National Center for Toxicological Research, Jefferson, AR, USA

K.M. Hanson
Manchester University College of Pharmacy, Fort Wayne, IN, USA

M. Hanson
Faculty of Environment, Earth, and Resources, University of Manitoba, Winnipeg, MB, Canada

L.S. Hardison
University of Virginia Health Systems, Charlottesville, VA, USA

A. Hardisson
University of La Laguna, La Laguna, Tenerife, Spain

S.L. Harper
Oregon State University, Corvallis, OR, USA

A.C. Hartmann
Manchester University, North Manchester, IN, USA

T. Hartung
Center for Alternatives to Animal Testing (CAAT), Johns Hopkins University, Baltimore, MD, USA

A. Hartwig
Karlsruher Institut für Technologie (KIT), Karlsruhe, Germany

S. Hassani
Pharmaceutical Sciences Research Center, Tehran University of Medical Sciences, Tehran, Iran

K.M. Hatlelid
US Consumer Product Safety Commission, Rockville, MD, USA

A.W. Hayes
Spherix, Bethesda, MD, USA; and Harvard School of Public Health, Boston, MA, USA

A.N. Hayes
Pfizer R&D Drug Safety Research & Development, Andover, MA, USA

M.R. Heidari
Kerman University of Medical Sciences, Kerman, Iran

J. Henderson
Michigan State University, East Lansing, MI, USA

B. Henriksen
Creighton University, Omaha, NE, USA

D. Hernández-Moreno
University of Extremadura, Cáceres, Spain

R.C. Hertzberg
US Environmental Protection Agency, Atlanta, GA, USA

T. Hesterberg
Center for Toxicology and Environmental Health, LLC, North Little Rock, AR, USA

M. Heyndrickx
Institute for Agricultural and Fisheries Research, Melle, Belgium

D. Hicks
American Industrial Hygiene Association, Falls Church, VA, USA

R.S. Hikkaduwa Koralege
Oklahoma State University, Stillwater, OK, USA

M.E. Hilburn
Oklahoma State University, Stillwater, OK, USA

P. Hinderliter
Syngenta, Greensboro, NC, USA

E.P. Hines
U.S. Environmental Protection Agency, Research Triangle Park, NC, USA.

B. Hirakawa
Claremont, CA, USA

C.M. Hirata
DuPont Crop Protection, Stine-Haskell Research Center, Newark, DE, USA

S. Ho
School of Pharmacy and Pharmaceutical Sciences, University of Manchester, Manchester, UK

D.W. Hobson
LoneStar PharmTox, LLC, Bergheim, TX, USA

S. Hoffmann
seh consulting + services, Cologne, Germany

A.C. Holloway
McMaster University, Hamilton, ON, Canada

C.P. Holstege
University of Virginia School of Medicine, Charlottesville, VA, USA

E. Holstege
Calvin College, Grand Rapids, MI, USA

S.L. Hon
Grady Health System, Atlanta, GA, USA

M. Honeycutt
Toxicology Division, Texas Commission on Environmental Quality (TCEQ), Austin, TX, USA

S. Hong
Exponent Health Sciences, Irvine, CA, USA

M.D. Hoover
National Institute for Occupational Safety and Health, Morgantown, WV, USA

N.B. Hopf
Institut universitaire romand de Santé au Travail, Institut für Arbeit und Gesundheit, Institute for Work and Health (IST), Lausanne, Switzerland

A.G. Hopp
Edwards Wildman Palmer LLP, Chicago, IL, USA

H. Horiguchi
Akita University, Graduate School of Medicine, Akita, Japan

A. Hosseini-Tabatabaei
University of British Columbia, Vancouver, BC, Canada

A. Hosseini
Iran University of Medical Sciences, Tehran, Iran

M.A. Hostetler
Phoenix Children's Hospital, Phoenix, AZ, USA

C.H. Hsu
Shanghai InnoStar Biotech Co., Ltd., Shanghai, China

F.X. Huang
DuPont Crop Protection, Newark, DE, USA

J.E. Hulla
US Army Corps of Engineers, Sacramento, CA, USA

P. Hultén
Swedish Poisons Information Centre, Stockholm, Sweden

M.L. Hultin
Lansing, MI, USA

H.E. Hurst
University of Louisville, School of Medicine, Louisville, KY, USA

A. Iannucci
Occupational Safety and Health Administration, Washington, DC, USA

S.H. Inayat-Hussain
Universiti Kebangsaan Malaysia, Kuala Lumpur, Malaysia

A.L. Inselman
US Food and Drug Administration/National Center for Toxicological Research, Jefferson, AR, USA

J. Iskander
Centers for Disease Control and Prevention, Atlanta, GA, USA

R.E. Jabbour
Edgewood Chemical Biological Center, MD, USA

M. Jaberidoost
Tehran University of Medical Sciences, Tehran, Iran

M. Jacobs
University of Rochester Medical Center, Rochester, NY, USA

M. Jamei
Simcyp Ltd (a Certara Company), Blades Enterprise Centre, Sheffield, UK

K.P. Jamison
Appalachian College of Pharmacy, Oakwood, VA, USA

M. Janes
La Jolla, CA, USA

D.M. Janz
Toxicology Centre, University of Saskatchewan, Saskatoon, SK, Canada

S.B. Jazayeri
Tehran University of Medical Sciences, Tehran, Iran

A. Jenkins
Texas Commission on Environmental Quality, Austin, TX, USA

M. Jiang
Indiana University School of Medicine—Fort Wayne, Fort Wayne, IN, USA

N. Jin
Cellular and Molecular Biology, Baylor College of Medicine, Houston, TX, USA

K. John
Center for Molecular Toxicology and Carcinogenesis, The Huck Institute of the Life Sciences, Pennsylvania State University, University Park, PA, USA

L. Jones
Toxicology Division, Texas Commission on Environmental Quality (TCEQ), Austin, TX, USA

P.D. Jones
University of Saskatchewan, Saskatoon, SK, Canada

S.A. Jordan
Marketed Health Products Directorate, Health Canada, Ottawa, ON, Canada

A.S. Jurado
CNC – Center for Neuroscience and Cell Biology, University of Coimbra, Coimbra, Portugal

M.P. Kalapos
Theoretical Biology Research Group, Budapest, Hungary

M.A. Kamrin
Williamston, MI, USA

R.W. Kapp
BioTox, Monroe Township, NJ, USA

S. Karami-Mohajeri
Tehran University of Medical Sciences, Tehran, Iran

S. Karanth
Charles River Laboratories, Reno, NV, USA

G. Karimi
Mashhad University of Medical Sciences, Mashhad, Iran

S.A. Katz
Rutgers University, Camden, NJ, USA

W.R. Kem
University of Florida College of Medicine, Gainesville, FL, USA

P. Kempegowda
Ealing Hospital NHS Trust, London, UK

G.L. Kennedy
DuPont Company, Wilmington, DE, USA

J.E. Kester
NewFields, Wentzville, MO, USA

M.R. Khaksar
Pharmaceutical Sciences Research Center, Tehran University of Medical Sciences, Tehran, Iran

S. Kharabaf
Pharmaceutical Sciences Research Center, Tehran University of Medical Sciences, Tehran, Iran

M. Khoobi
Tehran University of Medical Sciences, Tehran, Iran

M.E. Kiersma
Manchester University College of Pharmacy, Fort Wayne, IN, USA

J.M. Kilpinen
European Chemicals Agency, Helsinki, Finland

D.H. Kim
Greenville, NC, USA

S.T. Kim
Life Technologies, Foster City, CA, USA

R.D. Kimbrough
Washington, DC, USA

S.J. Klein
Manchester College, North Manchester, IN, USA

P.L. Knechtges
East Carolina University, Greenville, NC, USA

T.L. Knuckles
West Virginia University School of Medicine, Morgantown, WV, USA

T.B. Knudsen
US Environmental Protection Agency, Research Triangle Park, NC, USA

M.C. Korrapati
Medical University of South Carolina, Charleston, SC, USA

S.E. Koshlukova
California Environmental Protection Agency, Sacramento, CA, USA

P. Kovacic
San Diego State University, San Diego, CA, USA

A. Kraft
National Center for Environmental Assessment, US Environmental Protection Agency, Washington, DC, USA

K. Krafts
University of Minnesota, Minneapolis, MN, USA

P. Krishnan
Pennsylvania State University, University Park, PA, USA

C.L. Kruger
Spherix Consulting, Bethesda, MD, USA

A. Kubic
Illinois Poison Center, Chicago, IL, USA

S. Kulkarni
Novartis Pharmaceuticals, USA

E.S.C. Kwok
California Environmental Protection Agency, Sacramento, CA, USA

B. Laffon
University of A Coruña, A Coruña, Spain

L. Lagadic
INRA, UMR0985 Écologie et Santé des Écosystèmes, Équipe Écotoxicologie et Qualité des Milieux Aquatiques, Agrocampus Ouest, Rennes, France

C.E. Lambert
McDaniel Lambert Inc., Venice, CA, USA

J.R. Landolph
Cancer Research Laboratory, USC/Norris Comprehensive Cancer Center, Keck School of Medicine, Health Sciences Campus, University of Southern California, Los Angeles, CA, USA

R.W. Lange
Bristol-Myers Squibb, Mt. Vernon, IN, USA

P. Lank
Illinois Poison Center, Chicago, IL, USA

P. Lari
Mashhad University of Medical Sciences, Mashhad, Iran

W. Lasley
Center for Health and the Environment, School of Veterinary Medicine, University of California, Davis, CA, USA

V. Lawana
Iowa State University, Ames, IA, USA

C.R. Lazo
Emory University, Atlanta, GA, USA

M.-L. Ledrich
Luxcontrol SA, Esch/Alzette, Luxembourg

F. Le Goff
European Chemicals Agency, Helsinki, Finland

P.J. Lein
School of Veterinary Medicine, University of California, Davis, CA, USA

H.-W. Leung
General Electric Company, Water & Process Technologies, Trevose, PA, USA

Y.L. Leung
Musgrove Park Hospital, Taunton, UK

T.A. Lewandowski
Gradient, Seattle, WA, USA

X. Li
School of Public Health, University of California, Berkeley, CA, USA

J. Liesivuori
University of Turku, Turku, Finland

L. Lim
California Environmental Protection Agency, Sacramento, CA, USA

P. Limaye
Xenometrics LLC, Stilwell, KS, USA

H.H. Lin
University of Rochester Medical Center, Rochester, NY, USA

S.C. Lin
University of California, Riverside, CA, USA

T. Litovitz
Washington, DC, USA

F. Liu
Division of Neurotoxicology, National Center for Toxicological Research/US Food and Drug Administration, Jefferson, AR, USA

J. Liu
Oklahoma State University, Stillwater, OK, USA

M. Lloyd-Smith
National Toxics Network Inc., Bangalow, NSW, Australia

J.C.Y. Lo
San Diego, CA, USA

A.E. Loccisano
Reynolds American Inc., Winston-Salem, NC, USA

P. Logan
3M Company, St. Paul, MN, USA

S. López
Universidad de Santiago de Compostela, Santiago de Compostela, A Coruña, Spain

J. Lord-Garcia
Vallejo, CA, USA

M. Lotti
Università degli Studi di Padova, Padova, Italy

E. Luschützky
European Chemicals Agency, Helsinki, Finland

P. Mahdaviani
Tehran University of Medical Sciences, Tehran, Iran

A. Maier
University of Cincinnati, Cincinnati, OH, USA

G.F. Makhaeva
Institute of Physiologically Active Compounds, Russian Academy of Sciences, Chernogolovka, Russia

I. Malátová
National Radiation Protection Institute (SÚRO, v.v.i.), Praha, Czech Republic

A.A. Malekirad
Payame Noor University, Tehran, Iran

A. Manayi
Tehran University of Medical Sciences, Tehran, Iran

I. Mangas
Universidad Miguel Hernández de Elche, Elche, Spain

M. Mangino
US Environmental Protection Agency, Chicago, IL, USA

R.S. Mangipudy
Bristol-Myers Squibb Co., Drug Safety Evaluation, New Brunswick, NJ, USA

R.D. Maples
Eastern Oklahoma State College, Wilburton, OK, USA

B.J. Marcel
College of Pharmacy, The University of Louisiana at Monroe, Monroe, LA, USA

I. Marigómez
University of the Basque Country (UPV/EHU), Basque, Spain

J.M. Marraffa
Upstate Medical University, Syracuse, NY, USA

E. Martínez-López
University of Murcia, Murcia, Spain

S.M. Mathews
University of Georgia, Atlanta, GA, USA

L.D. Maxim
Everest Consulting Associates, Cranbury, NJ, USA

P.G. Maxwell-Stuart
University of St Andrews, St Andrews, UK

A. Mayor
Stanford University, Palo Alto, CA, USA

B.A. McClane
University of Pittsburgh School of Medicine, Pittsburgh, PA, USA

M.D. McCoole
DuPont Crop Protection, Stine-Haskell Research Center, Newark, DE, USA

D.B. McCormick
Emory University, Atlanta, GA, USA

D. McGregor
Toxicity Evaluation Consultants, Fife, UK

J.M. McKee
Arcadis-US, Brighton, MI, USA

K. McMartin
LSU Health Sciences Center – Shreveport, Shreveport, LA, USA

B. Meek
University of Ottawa, Ottawa, ON, Canada

M. Megharaj
University of South Australia, Mawson Lakes, SA, Australia

H.M. Mehendale
University of Louisiana at Monroe, Monroe, LA, USA

O. Mehrpour
Faculty of Medicine and Medical Toxicology and Drug Abuse Research Center, Birjand University of Medical Sciences, Birjand, Iran

A. Mendes
Portuguese National Institute of Health, Porto, Portugal

J. Méndez
University of A Coruña, A Coruña, Spain

F.-M. Menn
UT–ORNL Joint Institute for Biological Sciences, Center for Environmental Biotechnology, University of Tennessee, Knoxville, TN, USA

S.A. Meyer
College of Pharmacy, University of Louisiana – Monroe, Monroe, LA, USA

I. Michalak
Wrocław University of Technology, Wrocław, Poland

M.P. Míguez-Santiyán
Avda. de la Universidad s/n, Cáceres, Spain

M. Mikulewicz
Medical University of Wroclaw, Krakowska, Wroclaw, Poland

S. Milanez
Oak Ridge National Laboratory, Oak Ridge, TN, USA

B.E. Mileson
Technology Sciences Group Inc., Washington, DC, USA

G.W. Miller
Emory University, Atlanta, GA, USA

S.J. Miller
Grady Health System, Atlanta, GA, USA

S.M. Miller
Virginia Commonwealth University, Richmond, VA, USA

G.C. Millner
Center for Toxicology and Environmental Health LLC, Little Rock, AR, USA

V.C. Minarchick
West Virginia University School of Medicine, Morgantown, WV, USA

A.L. Miracle
Pacific Northwest National Laboratory, Richland, WA, USA

N.S. Mirajkar
Texas Tech University Health Sciences Center, School of Pharmacy, Amarillo, TX, USA

P.E. Mirkes
Washington State University Vancouver, Vancouver, WA, USA

M.S. Mitra
Bristol-Myers Squibb Company, Mount Vernon, IN, USA

V. Mody
South University, Savannah, GA, USA

S. Mogl
Federal Office for Civil Protection FOCP, Spiez Laboratory, Spiez, Switzerland

A. Mohammadirad
Pharmaceutical Sciences Research Center, Tehran University of Medical Sciences, Tehran, Iran

E.-R.E. Mojica
Pace University, New York, NY, USA

L. Molander
Stockholm University, Stockholm, Sweden

A.M. Molina López
Campus Universitario de Rabanales, University of Córdoba, Córdoba, Spain

F. Momen-Heravi
Harvard Medical School, Boston, MA, USA

P. Montague
New Brunswick, NJ, USA

J.P. Monteiro
CNC – Center for Neuroscience and Cell Biology, University of Coimbra, Coimbra, Portugal

F. Monticelli
Paris Lodron University Salzburg, Salzburg, Austria

F. Morceau
Laboratoire de Biologie Moleculaire et Cellulaire du Cancer (LBMCC), Luxembourg

M. Moreno
University of Rochester Medical Center, Rochester, NY, USA

B.W. Morgan
Emory University School of Medicine, Atlanta, GA, USA

S.R. Mortensen
BASF Corporation, Research Triangle Park, NC, USA

V.C. Moser
US Environmental Protection Agency, Research Triangle Park, NC, USA

M. Moshiri
School of Pharmacy, Mashhad University of Medical Sciences, Mashhad, Iran

S. Mostafalou
Tehran University of Medical Sciences, Tehran, Iran

R.A. Moyer
Defense Threat Reduction Agency, Fort Belvoir, VA, USA

K.L. Mumy
Liberty Twp., OH, USA

R. Munday
AgResearch, Hamilton, New Zealand

B.S. Murdianti
Arkansas Tech University, Russellville, AR, USA

A. Murray
Manchester University College of Pharmacy, Fort Wayne, IN, USA

T.M. Murray
Office of Pollution Prevention and Toxic Substances, Washington, DC, USA

T.L. Murta
CSX Transportation, Jacksonville, FL, USA

H. Nadri
Tehran University of Medical Sciences, Tehran, Iran

R. Naidu
University of South Australia, Mawson Lakes, SA, Australia

J.E. Naile
United States Environmental Protection Agency, Athens, GA, USA

D.M. Naistat
College of Science and Engineering, University of Minnesota, Twin Cities, Minneapolis, MN, USA

T. Nakajima
Chubu University, Kasugai, Japan

R.E. Nalliah
Huntington University, Huntington, IN, USA

P. Nance
Toxicology Excellence for Risk Assessment (TERA), Cincinnati, OH, USA

S. Nathan
University of Chicago Medicine, Chicago, IL, USA

L. Navarro
Syngenta Crop Protection, Basel, Switzerland

I.M. Navas
University of Murcia, Murcia, Spain

L.S. Nelson
New York University School of Medicine, NY, USA; and New York City Poison Control Center, NY, USA

C. Nerin
University of Zaragoza, Zaragoza, Spain

J. Newsted
Cardno ENTRIX, East Lansing, MI, USA

S. Nikfar
Faculty of Pharmacy, Tehran University of Medical Sciences, Iran; and Food and Drug Laboratory Research Center, Ministry of Health and Medical Education, Tehran, Iran

A. Nili-Ahmadabadi
Faculty of Pharmacy and Pharmaceutical Sciences Research Center, Tehran University of Medical Sciences, Tehran, Iran

F. Nobay
University of Rochester, Rochester, NY, USA

P. Nony
Center for Toxicology and Environmental Health, LLC, North Little Rock, AR, USA

T.R. Nurkiewicz
West Virginia University School of Medicine, Morgantown, WV, USA

M. Oi
(former OECD Secretariat) Global Environment Bureau, Japanese Ministry of the Environment, Tokyo, Japan

H.K. Okoro
Cape Peninsula University of Technology, Cape Town, South Africa

P.A. Oliveira
University of Trás-os-Montes e Alto Douro, Vila Real, Portugal

L.R. Olsen
University of Copenhagen, Copenhagen, Denmark

A.L. Oropesa Jiménez
University of Extremadura, Cáceres, Spain

S. Othumpangat
National Institute for Occupational Safety and Health, Morgantown, WV, USA

M.V. Pablos
Laboratory for Ecotoxicology, INIA, Madrid, Spain

D. Pakulska
Nofer Institute of Occupational Medicine, Łódź, Poland

M. Pakzad
Faculty of Pharmacy and Pharmaceutical Sciences Research Center, Tehran University of Medical Sciences, Tehran, Iran

E.M. Pallasch
Illinois Poison Center, Chicago, IL, USA

D. Pamies
Universidad Miguel Hernández de Elche, Elche, Spain

H.S. Parihar
Philadelphia College of Osteopathic Medicine, Suwanee, GA, USA

M.S. Parmar
Duquesne University, Pittsburgh, PA, USA

R.J. Parod
BASF Corporation, Wyandotte, MI, USA

P. Paschos
Aristotle University of Thessaloniki, Thessaloniki, Greece

J. Patterson
Toxicology Excellence for Risk Assessment (TERA), Cincinnati, OH, USA

T.J. Patterson
Chevron Energy Technology Company, San Ramon, CA, USA

T.A. Patterson
Regulatory Compliance & Risk Management, National Center for Toxicological Research/US Food and Drug Administration, Jefferson, AR, USA

J. Paulo Teixeira
Portuguese National Institute of Health, Porto, Portugal

A. Pawlaczyk
Lodz University of Technology, Lodz, Poland

M.A. Pearson
Emory University, Atlanta, GA, USA

M.B. Pellerano
New Brunswick, NJ, USA

F. Pellizzato
European Chemicals Agency, Helsinki, Finland

C.M. Perales
Uría Menéndez, Madrid, Spain

T. Peredy
Northern New England Poison Center, Portland, ME, USA

J. Pereira
University of Rochester Medical Center, Rochester, NY, USA

M. Pérez-López
University of Extremadura, Cáceres, Spain

R. Peri
Bristol-Myers Squibb, New Brunswick, NJ, USA

A.S. Persad
US Environmental Protection Agency, Research Triangle Park, NC, USA

H. Persson
Swedish Poisons Information Centre, Stockholm, Sweden

S. Perwaiz
Marketed Health Products Directorate, Health Canada, Ottawa, ON, Canada

M.K. Peterson
Gradient, Seattle, WA, USA

P.J. Pham
Mississippi State University, Mississippi State, MS, USA

T. Pham
Charlotte, NC, USA

B.K. Philip
Bristol-Myers Squibb Company, Mount Vernon, IN, USA

C. Pichery
EHESP (French School of Public Health), Rennes, France

A.J. Pickett
Phoenix Children's Hospital, Phoenix, AZ, USA

B. Piña
IDAEA–CSIC, Barcelona, Spain

K.E. Pinkerton
Center for Health and the Environment, University of California, Davis, CA, USA

R.C. Pleus
Intertox Inc., Seattle, WA, USA

S. Podder
North Eastern Hill University, Shillong, India

M.C. Poirier
National Cancer Institute, National Institutes of Health, Bethesda, MD, USA

A.C. Pomerleau
Emory University School of Medicine, Atlanta, GA, USA

C. Pope
Oklahoma State University, Stillwater, OK, USA

L. Posthuma
National Institute for Public Health and the Environment (RIVM), BA Bilthoven, The Netherlands

J. Potting
Wageningen University, Wageningen, The Netherlands; and KTH Royal Institute of Technology, Stockholm, Sweden

S. Pournourmohammadi
University of Geneva Medical Center, Geneva, Switzerland

S.D. Pravasi
Bristol Myers Squibb (PPD), Hopewell, NJ, USA

R.J. Preston
National Health and Environmental Effects Research Laboratory, US, Environmental Protection Agency, NC, USA

P.A. Prusakov
Mount Sinai Hospital, Chicago, IL, USA

M. Punja
Centers for Disease Control and Prevention, Chamblee, GA, USA

A.C. Puran
University of Rochester Medical Center, Rochester, NY, USA

M.M. Purcell
Upstate Medical University, Syracuse, NY, USA

L. Qian
California Poison Control System – San Diego Division, San Diego, CA, USA

M. Qozi
California Poison Control System San Diego, CA, USA

P.J.E. Quintana
San Diego State University, San Diego, CA, USA

M. Rabiei
Food and Drug Laboratories Research Center, Food and Drug Organization, Tehran, Iran

L.L. Radulovic
Drug Development Preclinical Services, LLC, Ann Arbor, MI, USA

N. Rahmani
Tehran Parks and Green Space Organization, Tehran, Iran

M. Rajabi
Oak Ridge Institute for Science and Education, Oak Ridge, TN, USA

P. Raman
Northeast Ohio Medical University, Rootstown, OH, USA

S. Ramasahayam
Oklahoma State University, Stillwater, OK, USA

M.J. Ramos-Peralonso
Green Planet Environmental Consulting, Madrid, Spain

G.O. Rankin
Physiology and Toxicology, Joan C. Edwards School of Medicine, Marshall University, Huntington, WV, USA

C.V. Rao
NMAM Institute of Technology, Nitte, India

P.S. Rao
Sanofi, Bridgewater, NJ, USA

M. Rashedinia
Mashhad University of Medical Sciences, Mashhad, Iran

A.D. Rath
SCHC, Annandale, VA, USA

D.E. Ray
School of Biomedical Sciences, Medical School, Queen's Medical Centre, University of Nottingham, Nottingham, UK

S.D. Ray
Manchester University, Fort Wayne, IN, USA

N.R. Reed
California Environmental Protection Agency, Sacramento, CA, USA

F. Remião
REQUIMTE/Laboratory of Toxicology, Faculty of Pharmacy, University of Porto, Porto, Portugal

R. Rezaee
Mashhad University of Medical Sciences, Mashhad, Iran

M.A. Rezvanfar
Tehran University of Medical Sciences, Tehran, Iran

N. Rezvani
Graduate School of Nursing, USUHS, Bethesda, MD, USA

L.R. Rhomberg
Gradient, Cambridge, MA, USA

N.K. Riar
University of California, Riverside, Riverside, CA, USA

G. Rice
US Environmental Protection Agency, Cincinnati, OH, USA

J.R. Richardson
Robert Wood Johnson Medical School, Piscataway, NJ, USA; and Environmental and Occupational Health Sciences Institute, Piscataway, NJ, USA

R.J. Richardson
University of Michigan, Ann Arbor, MI, USA

P. Richter
US Food and Drug Administration, Rockville, MD, USA

G. Rider
Oak Brook, IL, USA

H.L. Rivera
University of Maryland School of Medicine, Baltimore, MD, USA

J. Robbens
Institute for Agricultural and Fisheries Research, Oostende, Belgium

D.J. Roberts
Bristol-Myers Squibb, New Brunswick, NJ, USA; and Environmental and Occupational Health Sciences Institute (EOHSI), Piscataway, NJ, USA

L.G. Roberts
Chevron Energy Technology Company, San Ramon, CA, USA

P.J. Robinson
Henry M. Jackson Foundation, 711 HPW/RHDJ Applied Biotechnology Branch, OH, USA

H. Robles
Irvine, CA, USA

B.E. Rodgers
Texas Tech University, Lubbock, TX, USA

K. Rodgers
School of Pharmacy, University of Southern California, Los Angeles, CA, USA

Y.R. Rodriguez
Arizona Department of Environmental Quality, Phoenix, AZ, USA

C. Rodriguez Fernández
Universidad Complutense de Madrid, Ciudad Universitaria, Madrid, Spain

J.R. Roede
Emory University, Atlanta, GA, USA

M.A. Rogawski
School of Medicine, University of California, Davis, CA, USA

L. Rojo
Universidad Miguel Hernández de Elche, Elche, Spain

J.A. Romano
Science Applications International Corporation (SAIC), Frederick, MD, USA; and Tunnell Consulting, Bethesda, MD, USA

S.R. Rose
Virginia Commonwealth University, Richmond, VA, USA

M.A. Rosen
University of Ontario Institute of Technology, Oshawa, ON, Canada

M. Rossol
NY, USA

A. Rostami–Hodjegan
School of Pharmacy and Pharmaceutical Sciences, University of Manchester, Manchester, UK; and Simcyp Ltd (a Certara Company), Blades Enterprise Centre, Sheffield, UK

J.L. Rourke
Dalhousie University, Halifax, NS, Canada

R. Roy
3M Company, St. Paul, MN, USA

S.S. Roy
Chittaranjan National Cancer Institute, Kolkata, India

K.K. Rozman
University of Kansas Medical Center, Kansas City, KS, USA

A.L. Rubin
California Environmental Protection Agency, Sacramento, CA, USA

C. Rubio
University of La Laguna, La Laguna, Tenerife, Spain

R.J. Ruch
College of Medicine and Life Sciences, University of Toledo, Toledo, OH, USA

W.K. Rumbeiha
Iowa State University, Ames, IA, USA

W. Rushton
University of Virginia School of Medicine, Charlottesville, VA, USA

O. Sabzevari
Tehran University of Medical Sciences, Tehran, Iran

M. Saeedi
Tehran University of Medical Sciences, Tehran, Iran

A. Saeid
Wroclaw University of Technology, Wroclaw, Poland

S. Saeidnia
Tehran University of Medical Sciences, Tehran, Iran

S.A. Saghir
Intrinsik Environmental Sciences Inc., Mississauga, ON, Canada; and Aga Khan University, Karachi, Pakistan

K.S. Saili
Oregon State University, Corvallis, OR, USA

H. Salem
Edgewood Chemical Biological Center, MD, USA

M.R. Moyano Salvago
Campus Universitario de Rabanales, University of Córdoba, Córdoba, Spain

J.R. Salvatore
VA Medical Center, Phoenix, AZ, USA

M.D. San Andrés Larrea
Universidad Complutense de Madrid, Ciudad Universitaria, Madrid, Spain

M.I. San Andrés Larrea
Universidad Complutense de Madrid, Ciudad Universitaria, Madrid, Spain

R.D. Sarazan
Data Sciences International (DSI), St. Paul, MN, USA

S. Sardari
Drug Design and Bioinformatics Unit, Biotechnology Research Center, Tehran, Iran

T. Sasaki
Research Laboratories, Maruho Co., Ltd, Kyoto R&D Center, Chudoji, Shimogyo-ku, Kyoto, Japan

S.P. Sawant
Kimberly-Clark Worldwide, Inc., Roswell, GA, USA

V. Schaeffer
Occupational Safety and Health Administration, Washington, DC, USA

L.J. Schep
University of Otago, Dunedin, New Zealand

R.B. Schlesinger
Pace University, New York, NY, USA

S.M. Schneider
Rochester, NY, USA

S.M. Schreffler
Upstate Medical University, Syracuse, NY, USA

M.M. Schultz
The College of Wooster, Wooster, OH, USA

M. Schwartz
Centers for Disease Control and Prevention (CDC), Chamblee, GA, USA

D. Schwela
Stockholm Environment Institute, University of York, York, UK

A.L. Scott
Biogen Idec, Cambridge, MA, USA

B.R. Scott
Lovelace Respiratory Research Institute, Albuquerque, NM, USA

K. Scribner
Center for Toxicology and Environmental Health, LLC, North Little Rock, AR, USA

R.W. Seabury
Upstate Medical University, Syracuse, NY, USA

B. Seco
University of Zaragoza, Zaragoza, Spain

M. Seeley
Gradient, Cambridge, MA, USA

J. Seifert
University of Hawaii, Honolulu, HI, USA

R. Sellamuthu
Indiana University, Indianapolis, IN, USA

T.L. Serex
DuPont Crop Protection, Newark, DE, USA

K. Sexton
University of Texas School of Public Health, Brownsville, TX, USA

S. Shadnia
Shahid Beheshti University of Medical Sciences, Tehran, Iran

A. Shafiee
Tehran University of Medical Sciences, Tehran, Iran

I. Shah
US Environmental Protection Agency, Research Triangle Park, NC, USA

K. Shankar
University of Arkansas for Medical Sciences, Little Rock, AR, USA

L.P. Sheets
Human Safety Regulatory Toxicology, Bayer CropScience, LP, Research Triangle Park, NC, USA

L. Sheppard
Manchester University College of Pharmacy, Fort Wayne, IN, USA

R.N. Shiotsuka
Bayer MaterialScience LLC, Pittsburgh, PA, USA

S. Shirley
Austin, TX, USA

H.A. Shojaei Saadi
Laval University, Québec City, QC, Canada

K.N. Sibbald
University of Virginia School of Medicine, Charlottesville, VA, USA

F.R. Sidell
US Army, Medical Institute of Chemical Defense, Aberdeen Proving Ground, MD, USA

M. Siegrist
Huther Doyle, Rochester, NY, USA

J.E. Simmons
US Environmental Protection Agency, NC, USA

C.J. Sinal
Dalhousie University, Halifax, NS, Canada

P. Singh
Syngenta Crop Protection, LLC, Greensboro, NC, USA

R. Skoglund
3M Company, St. Paul, MN, USA

C. Skonberg
Novo Nordisk A/S, Novo Nordisk Park, Måløv, Denmark

R.J. Slaughter
University of Otago, Dunedin, New Zealand

C.L. Sledge
Emory University Department of Emergency Medicine, Atlanta, GA, USA

J.D. Slothower
Rochester, NY, USA

M. Smith
University of Rochester, Rochester, NY, USA

M.T. Smith
University of California, Berkeley, CA, USA

D.B. Snider
Veterinary Diagnostic Laboratory, College of Veterinary Medicine, Ames, IA, USA

R.G. Snyman
Cape Peninsula University of Technology, Cape Town, South Africa

M. Sobanska
European Chemicals Agency, Helsinki, Finland

M.Á. Sogorb
Universidad Miguel Hernández de Elche, Elche, Spain

F. Soler-Rodríguez
University of Extremadura, Cáceres, Spain

R. Solgi
Pharmaceutical Sciences Research Center, Tehran University of Medical Sciences, Tehran, Iran

K.R. Solomon
Centre for Toxicology, School of Environmental Sciences, University of Guelph, Guelph, ON, Canada

R. Somanathan
Instituto Tecnológico de Tijuana, Tijuana, Mexico

B.R. Sonawane
National Center for Environmental Assessment, Office of Research and Development, US Environmental Protection Agency, Washington, DC, USA

X. Song
Merck & Co., Inc., West Point, PA, USA

M.G. Soni
Soni and Associates Inc, Vero Beach, FL, USA

J. Sorensen
Oak Ridge National Laboratory, Oak Ridge, TN, USA

N.V. Soucy
3M Center, St Paul, MN, USA

R.J. Southard
University of California, Davis, CA, USA

C.B. Spainhour
Spainhour Consulting Services, South Abington Township, PA, USA

P.S. Spencer
Global Health Center and Center for Research on Occupational and Environmental Toxicology, Oregon Health and Science University, Portland, OR, USA

H.A. Spiller
Central Ohio Poison Center, Columbus, OH, USA

B. Spoelhof
Manchester University College of Pharmacy, Fort Wayne, IN, USA

B. Stanard
Frederick, MD, USA

L.W. Stanek
US Environmental Protection Agency, Office of Research and Development/National Center for Environmental Assessment, Research Triangle Park, NC, USA

P.A. Stapleton
West Virginia University School of Medicine, Morgantown, WV, USA

T. Stedeford
US Environmental Protection Agency, Northwest, Washington, DC, USA

J Steidl-Nichols
Drug Safety Research and Development, Pfizer, Groton, CT, USA

M. Stephens
Center for Alternatives to Animal Testing (CAAT), Johns Hopkins University, Baltimore, MD, USA

N.P. Steyn
Human Sciences Research Council, Cape Town, South Africa

J. Stickney
Scarborough, ME, USA

S.J. Stohs
Creighton University Medical Center, Omaha, NE, USA; and Kitsto Consulting LLC, Frisco, TX, USA

D. Stone
Oregon State University, Corvallis, OR, USA

D. Stool
Oak Brook, IL, USA

C.M. Stork
Upstate New York Poison Center, Upstate Medical University, Syracuse, NY, USA

B. Strohm
Delphi, Global EH&S Technical Services, Troy, MI, USA

P.E. Stromberg
Virginia Commonwealth University Medical Center, Richmond, VA, USA

D.W. Sullivan
Gad Consulting Services, Cary, NC, USA

M.R. Sullivan
SCHC, Annandale, VA, USA

L.G. Sultatos
New Jersey Medical School, University of Medicine and Dentistry of New Jersey, Newark, NJ, USA

A. Suryanarayanan
Manchester University College of Pharmacy, Fort Wayne, IN, USA

I. Syed
Harvard Medical School, Boston, MA, USA

D.T. Szabo
US Food and Drug Administration, Rockville, MD, USA

M.I. Szynkowska
Lodz University of Technology, Lodz, Poland

Z. Takacs
ToxinTech, Inc., New York, NY, USA

G. Talaska
University of Cincinnati College of Medicine, Cincinnati, OH, USA

P. Talbot
University of California, Riverside, CA, USA

R.L. Tanguay
Oregon State University, Corvallis, OR, USA

J.V. Tarazona
Spanish Royal Academy of Veterinary Sciences, Madrid, Spain; and Spanish National Institute for Agriculture and Food Research and Technology, Madrid, Spain

J.P. Teixeira
Portuguese National Institute of Health, Porto, Portugal

N.J. Temple
Athabasca University, Athabasca, AB, Canada

W.A. Temple
University of Otago, Dunedin, New Zealand

A. Tena
University of Zaragoza, Zaragoza, Spain

L.K. Teuschler
US Environmental Protection Agency, Cincinnati, OH, USA

EA Thackaberry
Safety Assessment, Genentech, Inc., South San Francisco, CA, USA

K.N. Thakore
California Department of Public Health, Richmond, CA, USA

C. Theodorakis
Texas Tech University, Lubbock, TX, USA

R.E. Thompson
Johns Hopkins Bloomberg School of Public Health, Baltimore, MD, USA

S.L. Thornton
University of Kansas Hospital Poison Control Center, Leawood, KS, USA

D. Ting
California Environmental Protection Agency, Oakland, CA, USA

M.A. Tirmenstein
Bristol-Myers Squibb Co., Drug Safety Evaluation, New Brunswick, NJ, USA

A. Touwaide
Institute for the Preservation of Medical Traditions, Washington, DC, USA

T.G. Towne
Manchester University College of Pharmacy, Fort Wayne, IN, USA

S.A. Traven
University of Virginia School of Medicine, Charlottesville, VA, USA

A. Tritscher
WHO, Geneva, Switzerland

M. Troendle
Richmond, VA, USA

J.E. Trosko
Center for Integrative Toxicology, College of Human Medicine, Michigan State University, MI, USA

W.-T. Tsai
National Pingtung University of Science and Technology, Pingtung, Taiwan

M. Tsai-Turton
Food and Drug Administration, Silver Spring, MD, USA

A. Tsatsakis
University of Crete, Heraklion, Greece

C. Tsitsimpikou
Directorate of Environment, Athens, Greece

A. Tsubura
Department of Pathology II, Kansai Medical University, Moriguchi, Osaka, Japan

T. Tsuda
Okayama University Graduate School of Environmental and Life Science, Okayama, Japan

R.W. Tyl
RTI International, NC, USA

E.M. Udarbe Zamora
A.E.Z.R. Pet Hospital, Petaluma, CA, USA; and Santa Rosa Junior College, Santa Rosa, CA, USA

M.J. Utell
University of Rochester Medical Center, Rochester, NY, USA

M. Vahabzadeh
Medical Toxicology Research Center and Pharmacy School, Mashhad University of Medical Sciences, Iran

V.S. Vaidya
Harvard Medical School, Boston, MA, USA; and Harvard Institutes of Medicine, Boston, MA, USA

V. Valdiglesias
Toxicology Unit, University of A Coruña, A Coruña, Spain

M.A. Valentovic
Physiology and Toxicology, Joan C. Edwards School of Medicine, Marshall University, Huntington, WV, USA

L.G. Valerio
Science and Research Staff, Office of Pharmaceutical Science/Immediate Office, Center for Drug Evaluation and Research, US Food and Drug Administration, Silver Spring, MD, USA

T. Vales
Gad Consulting Services, Cary, NC, USA

L.N. Vandenberg
Tufts University, Medford, MA, USA

P.J. van den Brink
Alterra and Wageningen University and Research Centre, Wageningen, The Netherlands

J. van der Kolk
Eco Conseil, Voorburg, The Netherlands

T.R. Van Vleet
Bristol-Myers Squibb, Mt. Vernon, IN, USA

E. van Vliet
Fetal and Perinatal Medicine Research Group, IDIBAPS, Hospital Clinic, Universitat de Barcelona, Barcelona, Spain

J. Varga
Northwestern University, Chicago, IL, USA

K. Venkateswarlu
Vikrama Simhapuri University, Nellore, India

T. Verslycke
Gradient, Cambridge, MA, USA

B. Versonnen
European Chemicals Agency, Helsinki, Finland

K. Verstraete
Institute for Agricultural and Fisheries Research, Melle, Belgium

M. Vighi
University of Milano Bicocca, Milan, Italy

E. Vilanova
Universidad Miguel Hernández de Elche, Elche, Spain

L. Vincent
The Toxicology Forum, Washington, DC, USA

M. Vincent
Toxicology Excellence for Risk Assessment (TERA), Cincinnati, OH, USA

R. Visser
Organisation for Economic Co-operation and Development, Paris, France

B. Volger
Ceres International, LLC, West Chester, PA, USA

K. von Stackelberg
Harvard School of Public Health, Boston, MA, USA; and NEK Associates LTD, Allston, MA, USA

S.V. Vulimiri
National Center for Environmental Assessment, Office of Research and Development, US Environmental Protection Agency, Washington, DC, USA

M. Wahl
Illinois Poison Center, Chicago, IL, USA; and Northshore University Healthsystems, Evanston, IL, USA

N.J. Walker
National Institute of Environmental Health Sciences, Research Triangle Park, NC, USA

T.D. Walker
US Environmental Protection Agency, Washington DC, USA

D.R. Wallace
Center for Health Sciences, Oklahoma State University, Tulsa, OK, USA

C. Wang
Division of Neurotoxicology, National Center for Toxicological Research/U.S. Food and Drug Administration, Jefferson, AR, USA

G.S. Wang
University of Colorado, Aurora, CO, USA

S.C. Wanna-Nakamura
US Consumer Product Safety Commission, Rockville, MD, USA

R.E. Watson
SNBL USA, Everett, WA, USA

E.V. Wattenberg
Division of Environmental Health Sciences, University of Minnesota, Minneapolis, MN, USA

P.M. Wax
UT Southwestern School of Medicine, Dallas, TX, USA; and American College of Medical Toxicology, Phoenix, AZ, USA

J.A. Weaver
United States Environmental Protection Agency, Washington, DC, USA

N.R. Webber
Westerville, OH, USA

J.A. Weber
Missouri Poison Center, St. Louis, MO, USA

L.P Weber
Veterinary Biomedical Sciences, Saskatoon, SK, Canada

A.J. Weinrich
National Center for Environmental Assessment, Office of Research and Development, US Environmental Protection Agency, Cincinnati, OH, USA

B. Weiss
University of Rochester School of Medicine and Dentistry, Rochester, NY, USA

A. Wennberg
Nutrition and Consumer Protection Division, Food and Agriculture Organization of the United Nations, Viale delle Terme di Caracalla, Rome, Italy

M.J. Wernke
NewFields Companies, LLC, Tallahassee, FL, USA

A. Weston
National Institute for Occupational Safety and Health, Centers for Disease Control and Prevention, Morgantown, WV, USA

P. Wexler
National Library of Medicine, National Institutes of Health, Bethesda, MD, USA

L.D. White
National Institute of Environmental Health Sciences, Research Triangle Park, NC, USA

M.H. Whittaker
ToxServices LLC, Washington, DC, USA

H. Wiedenfeld
Pharmaceutical Institute, University of Bonn, Germany

T.J. Wiegand
Strong Memorial Hospital, University of Rochester Medical Center (URMC), Rochester, NY, USA

D.S. Wikoff
ToxStrategies, Austin, TX, USA

C.P. Wild
IARC, Lyon, France

Y. Will
Pfizer Global R&D, Compound Safety Prediction, World Wide Medicinal Chemistry, Groton, CT, USA

C. Willett
The Humane Society of the United States, Gaithersburg, MD, USA

C.C. Willhite
Risk Sciences International, Ottawa, Ontario, Canada

A. Willis
Toxicology Excellence for Risk Assessment (TERA), Cincinnati, OH, USA

K. Willis
Defense Threat Reduction Agency, Fort Belvoir, VA, USA

B.K. Wills
Virginia Commonwealth University, Richmond, VA, USA

B.W. Wilson
University of California, Davis, CA, USA

J.L. Wittliff
University of Louisville School of Medicine, Louisville, KY, USA

Z.W. Wojcinski
Drug Development Preclinical Services, LLC, Ann Arbor, MI, USA

M.S. Wolfe
National Institute of Environmental Health Sciences, Research Triangle Park, NC, USA

C.S. Wood
Environmental Sciences Division, Oak Ridge National Laboratory, Oak Ridge, TN, USA

G.M. Woodall
US Environmental Protection Agency, National Center for Environmental Assessment, Research Triangle Park, NC, USA

A. Woolley
ForthTox Ltd, Linlithgow, West Lothian, UK

M. Xia
NIH Chemical Genomics Center, National Center for Advancing Translational Sciences, National Institutes of Health, Bethesda, MD, USA

B.J. Ximba
Cape Peninsula University of Technology, Cape Town, South Africa

B. Yan
University of Rhode Island, Kingston, RI, USA

Y. Yanagiba
National Institute of Occupational Safety and Health, Kawasaki, Japan

D. Yang
School of Veterinary Medicine, University of California, Davis, CA, USA

N. Yang
Manchester University College of Pharmacy, Fort Wayne, IN, USA

M. Yoon
Center for Human Health Assessment, The Hamner Institutes for Health Sciences, Research Triangle Park, NC, USA

T. Yorifuji
Okayama University Graduate School of Environmental and Life Science, Okayama, Japan

K. Yoshizawa
Department of Pathology II, Kansai Medical University, Moriguchi, Osaka, Japan

R.A. Young
Knoxville, TN, USA

R.M. Zamor
Plankton Ecology and Limnology Laboratory, University of Oklahoma Biological Station, and Program in Ecology and Evolutionary Biology, University of Oklahoma, Norman, OK, USA

Q.J. Zhao
US Environmental Protection Agency, Cincinnati, OH, USA

HOW TO USE THE ENCYCLOPEDIA

The chemical substances covered in the Encyclopedia represent a highly selective and personal list of those which the editors felt were most noteworthy. Clearly, with around 1000 chemical entries, there was no attempt to approach the 70 million or so unique organic and inorganic chemicals, or even the more than 80,000 chemicals in commerce (the vast majority of which, incidentally, are absolutely barren of toxicity data).

A Note about the format of Entries

Except for chemical substances, the format of entries tends to be free form narrative. Chemical substance entries, on the other hand, follow a loose template including headers such as molecular formula, uses, environmental fate and behavior, toxicokinetics, chronic toxicity, etc. Depending upon the type of chemical, e.g. industrial, pharmaceutical, etc. not every header is relevant. Primary consideration, thus, has been given to organizing the entry in a way that makes sense for the agent in question and the available information on it, rather than adhering tightly to an arbitrary format.

The *Encyclopedia of Toxicology* is a comprehensive and authoritative study encompassing 1160 articles on various aspects of this subject, contained in four volumes. Each article provides a focused description of the given topic, intended to inform a broad range of readers, ranging from students, to research professionals, and interested others.

All articles in the encyclopedia are arranged alphabetically as a series of entries.

1. Contents

Your first point of reference will likely be the contents. The complete contents list appears at the front of each volume providing volume and page numbers of the entry. We also display the article title in the running headers on each page so you are able to identify your location and browse the work in this manner.

You will find "dummy entries" where obvious synonyms exist for entries or for where we have grouped together similar topics. Dummy entries appear in the contents and in the body of the encyclopedia. For example:

Acrylates *see* Acrylic Acid, Ethyl Acrylate; Methyl Acrylate

2. Cross-references

The majority of articles within the encyclopedia have an extensive list of cross-references which appear at the end of each article, for example:

DECANE

See also: Heptane; Hexane; Octane; Pentane; Petroleum Distillates; Propane.

3. Index

The index provides the volume and page number for where the material is located, and the index entries differentiate between material that is a whole article; is part of an article, part of a table, or in a figure.

4. Contributors

A full list of contributors appears at the beginning of each volume.

5. Glossary and Appendix

The *Encyclopedia of Toxicology* contains an extensive list of terms (glossary) used in toxicology, drawn from works produced by the International Union of Pure and Applied Chemistry. The appendix provides information about a selection of online chemical compendia.

ACKNOWLEDGMENTS

First and foremost I want to express my appreciation to the Board of Editors and the 1400 authors whose expertise and dedication have converted the Encyclopedia from a vision to a reality. Elsevier's staff, most particularly its Development Editor, Justin Taylor, have proved invaluable in getting the project off the ground and into their hands and electronic devices.

DEDICATION

For my parents, Yetty and Will, my son, Jake, my wife, Nancy, and our dog, Lola, with love and appreciation to all.

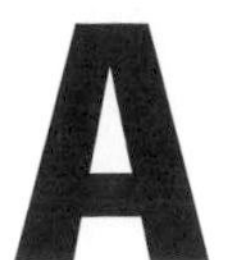

Aberrations of Chromosomes *see* Chromosome Aberrations

Absorption

SA Saghir, Intrinsik Environmental Sciences Inc., Mississauga, ON, Canada; Aga Khan University, Karachi, Pakistan

This article is a revision of the previous edition article by Jules Brodeur and Robert Tardif, volume 1, pp 1–6, © 2005, Elsevier Inc.

Introduction

Absorption is the process by which chemicals (nutrients, essential elements, drugs, and toxicants) enter into the bloodstream after crossing various membranes of the body. The main sites of entry of chemicals are the gastrointestinal (GI) tract, the lungs, and the skin. In drug therapy, other convenient, but less commonly used, portals of entry are the intravenous, subcutaneous, and intramuscular routes. Rates of absorption may vary from one route of administration to the other. In case of intravenous injection, chemicals are directly introduced into the bloodstream and they do not need to cross any membrane; therefore, no absorption phase exists.

Absorption of a chemical from the site of exposure is regulated by biological membranes lining tissues. Membranes are composed of 7–9 nm thick phospholipid bilayers. The hydrophilic ends of the phospholipids project into the aqueous media on each side of the membrane, and the hydrophobic fatty acid tails form a barrier to water in the inner space of the membrane. Proteins are embedded throughout the lipid bilayer for various functions. One of these is to act as active transporters for certain chemicals across the membrane. Proteins can also form small pores through the membrane, serving as aqueous channels allowing passage of water across them.

Before discussing absorption in more detail, it is important to consider mechanisms by which chemicals cross membranes. These mechanisms are of interest for absorption as well as for distribution, metabolism, and excretion – processes of disposition of chemicals.

Chemicals can cross membranes by passive transport, active transport, filtration, and/or endocytosis.

Passive Transport

Passive transport moves chemicals along a concentration gradient by passive and/or facilitated diffusion moving molecules from an area of high concentration to an area of low concentration without any expenditure of cellular energy (**Figure 1**).

Passive Diffusion

This is the mechanism by which lipophilic chemicals move across the membrane by solubilizing within the lipids of the membrane. The driving force for this process is the concentration gradient between the two sides of the membrane, allowing chemicals to move from the side of higher concentration to the side of lower concentration without the expenditure of cellular energy. Passive diffusion continues until concentration gradient of the chemical across membrane exists and is not subject to competition.

Factors that Govern Passive Diffusion

1. *The lipid solubility of a chemical*: This is a characteristic expressed in terms of the ability of a chemical to partition between oil and water phases. The more a chemical dissolves in oil, or its substitute octanol, the more lipid soluble it is and more easily crosses membranes.
2. *The degree of ionization (electrical charge) of a chemical*: As a rule, electrically neutral chemicals permeate more easily through the lipid phase of a membrane due to their higher degree of lipid solubility.
3. *The molecular size of a chemical*: Passive diffusion is normally limited to chemicals with molecular weight $\leq$500 Da. A small molecule will cross membranes more rapidly than a larger one of equal lipophilicity.

Facilitated Diffusion

Facilitated diffusion is similar to passive diffusion with the exception that carrier proteins embedded in the membrane bilayer facilitate the transfer of chemicals across the membrane. Similar to passive diffusion, movement of chemicals across membranes is from the side of high concentration

 http://dx.doi.org/10.1016/B978-0-12-386454-3.00361-4

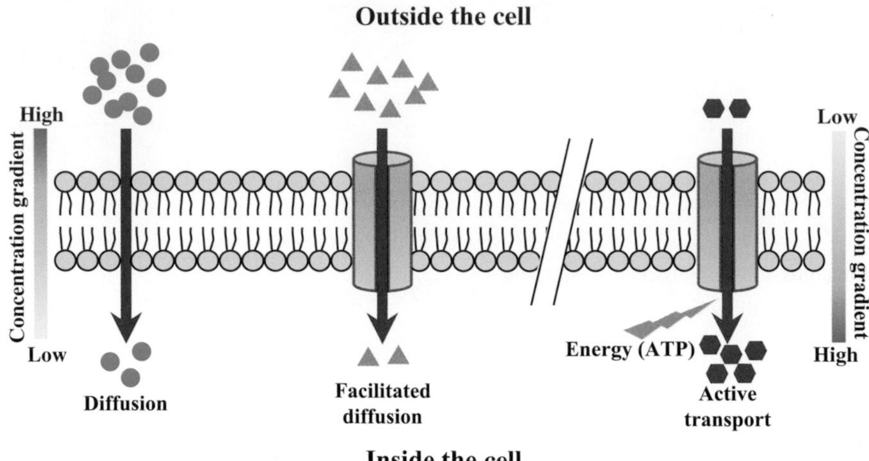

Figure 1 Depiction of simple and facilitated diffusion and active transport of chemicals into the cell through the phospholipid bilayer membrane.

to the side of low concentration without the expenditure of cellular energy. Facilitated diffusion is somewhat specific to chemicals that are able to bind to a carrier protein. Absorption of nutrients such as glucose and amino acids across the epithelial membrane of the GI tract occurs by facilitated diffusion. Since a finite number of carrier proteins are available for transport, the process is saturable at high concentrations of chemicals and competition for transport may occur between molecules of similar structure.

Active Transport

Active transport requires specialized carrier proteins and the expenditure of cellular energy. Carrier proteins allow chemicals to cross the membrane against a concentration gradient or when the phospholipid bilayer of the membrane is impermeable to a chemical (**Figure 1**). The carrier proteins are selective for certain structural features (e.g., ionization state) of chemicals and therefore, saturable. Additionally, chemicals with similar structural features may compete for transport by a given carrier. Active transport is of limited importance for absorption of chemicals; however, it plays an important role in the elimination of chemicals by the liver and the kidneys. A number of tissues (e.g., GI tract, liver, lungs, kidneys, brain, and testes) contain special proteins called efflux transporters (e.g., *P*-glycoprotein, organic anion transporters, organic cation transporters, multidrug and toxic compound extrusion protein, etc.), which actively remove certain absorbed chemicals from the cells. Some efflux transporters are chemical specific and others may accommodate multiple chemicals.

Filtration

Small water-soluble and small charged molecules may cross the GI epithelial membrane through minute pores or water channels (<4 nm) in the membrane. Filtration is an important function for urinary excretion; renal glomeruli possess rather large pores (~70 nm) that allow passage of various solutes (e.g., glucose, small cations and anions) contained in blood into the urine and prevent the loss of larger molecules such as proteins and blood cells.

Endocytosis

Endocytosis is a specialized form of transport by which very large molecules and insoluble materials are engulfed by invagination of the cell membrane, forming intracellular vesicles. For example, absorption of certain dyes by mucosal cells of the duodenum (pinocytosis) is through endocytosis. In the lung, alveolar macrophages scavenge insoluble particles such as asbestos fibers (phagocytosis). These macrophages then seek to eliminate the phagocytized particles through either the mucociliary mechanism or through lymphatic vessels that drain the lungs.

Absorption by the GI Tract

The major role of the GI tract (consisting of mouth, pharynx, esophagus, stomach, small intestine (duodenum, jejunum, ileum), and large intestine) is to provide efficient absorption of essential nutrients contained in ingested foods and liquids. It is also an important route for the absorption of drugs and toxicants. The barrier between the contents of the GI tract (especially in small intestine, where most of the absorption occurs) and the blood vessels consists of epithelium essentially only one cell thick and is easily crossed. The anatomy of the GI tract is illustrated in **Figure 2**.

Absorption occurs mostly by passive diffusion of lipid-soluble nonionized molecules. The degree of ionization is directly dependent on the pH of the GI content influencing absorption of chemicals, with most of the absorption occurring at sites where the chemicals are present in nonionized form. At the low acidic pH of the stomach (1–3), most weak organic acids such as acetylsalicylic acid (aspirin) remain nonionized and diffuse passively across the gastric

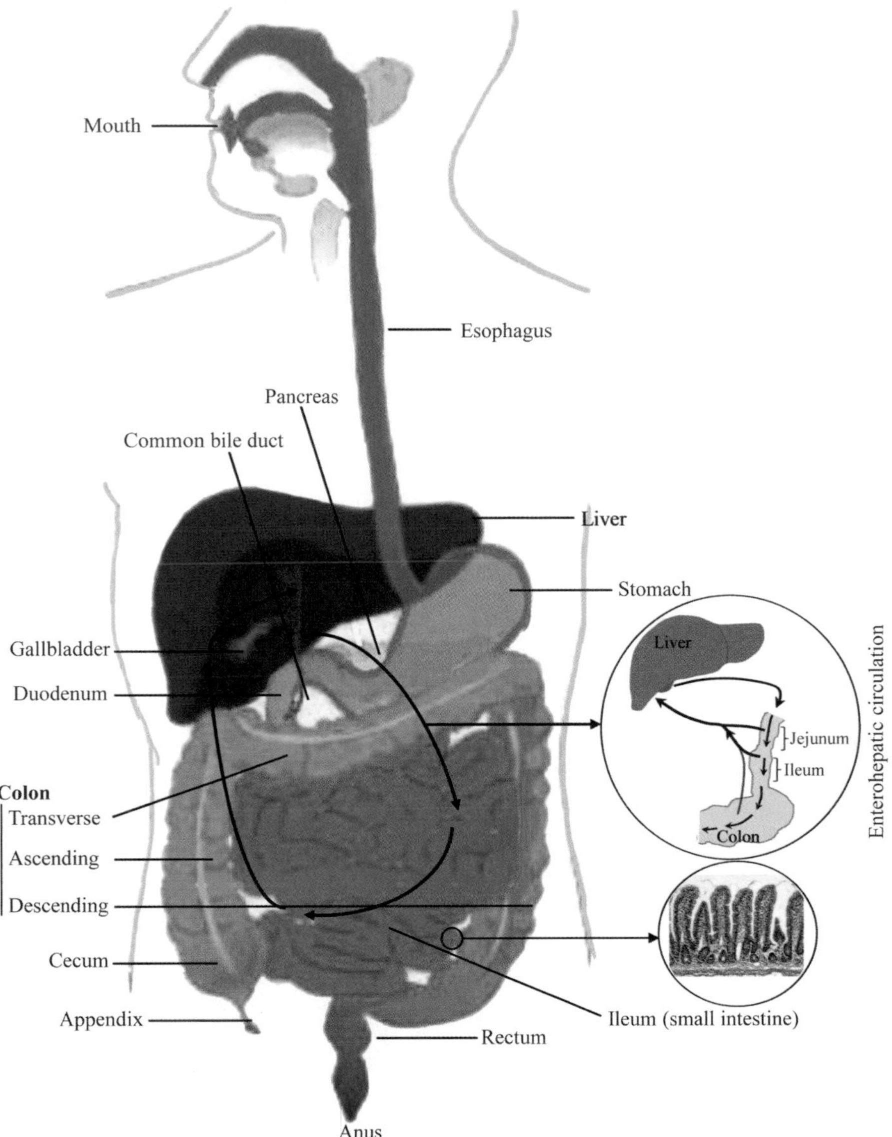

Figure 2 The anatomy of the gastrointestinal tract. Image is a modification of Mariana Ruiz Villarreal, 2006 work, which has been released into the public domain by the author.

mucosa at a rate proportional to the concentration gradient of the nonionized form. On the other hand, weak organic bases will diffuse more easily through the mucosa of the small intestine in which pH is higher (5–8). However, the bulk of absorption does not necessarily occur at the site where pH is optimal for nonionization of chemicals. The very large surface area of the small intestine favors the diffusion of substances even at pH that is not optimal for the degree of nonionization.

The oral cavity, although, has thin epithelium and is rich in blood vessels, favoring absorption; the residence time is usually too brief for any substantial absorption. Absorption of chemicals from stomach is also limited due to its thick mucosal layer and relatively short residence time. Most of the absorption, therefore, occurs in the small intestine, which has a tremendously large surface area due to the presence of villi and microvilli, has more permeable membranes than those in the stomach, and has long residence time.

A small number of chemicals may be absorbed by facilitated diffusion (e.g., antimetabolic nucleotides), active transport (e.g., lead and 5-fluorouracil), or pinocytosis (e.g., dyes and bacterial endotoxins). Chemicals that reach the bloodstream by absorption through the GI tract are transported directly to the liver via the portal circulation, where they normally undergo metabolic biotransformation, mostly to less active (toxic) and in some cases to more active chemical forms, even before gaining access to other tissues of the body; this phenomenon is known as the first-pass effect.

Presence of food in the GI tract is one of the most important factors that modify GI absorption of ingested chemicals. Presence of food in the stomach delays/reduces the absorption of weak organic acids from the stomach. Presence of lipid-rich food delays emptying of the gastric content into the small intestine, delaying the absorption of chemicals.

Chemical interactions in the GI tract between nutrients and drugs may considerably reduce the absorption of some drugs; for example, calcium ions from dairy products form insoluble and nonabsorbable complexes with tetracycline and therefore, the antibiotic works best when taken on an empty stomach. On the other hand, certain drugs are irritants to the GI tract (e.g., nonsteroidal anti-inflammatory drugs and potassium chloride tablets) and must be ingested with food.

Enterohepatic circulation provides an example of a special case of intestinal absorption. Certain chemicals, like methylmercury, after undergoing biotransformation in the liver, are excreted into the intestine via the bile. They then are reabsorbed in the intestine, sometimes after enzymatic modification by intestinal bacteria. This process can markedly prolong the stay of chemicals in the body. It can be interrupted by antibiotics that destroy the intestinal bacterial flora.

Absorption through the Skin

Normal skin represents an effective, but not perfect, barrier against the entry of chemicals. There are two major structural components to the skin – the epidermis (0.05–0.1 mm) and the dermis (1–4 mm) (**Figure 3**). The epidermis is formed of several layers of cells, with the outermost layers, ~10 μm thick, consisting of dried dead cells forming the stratum corneum. The stratum corneum is rich in a filament-shaped protein called keratin, which represents the major structural component of the barrier to passage of chemicals through the skin. Chemicals may move through the various layers of the epidermis by passive diffusion, more slowly through the stratum corneum, but more rapidly through the inner layers of live epidermal cells (stratum lucidum, stratum granulosum, stratum spinosum, and stratum basale).

The stratum corneum is much thicker in areas where considerable pressure and repeated friction occur, like palms and soles; absorption is therefore much slower in these areas.

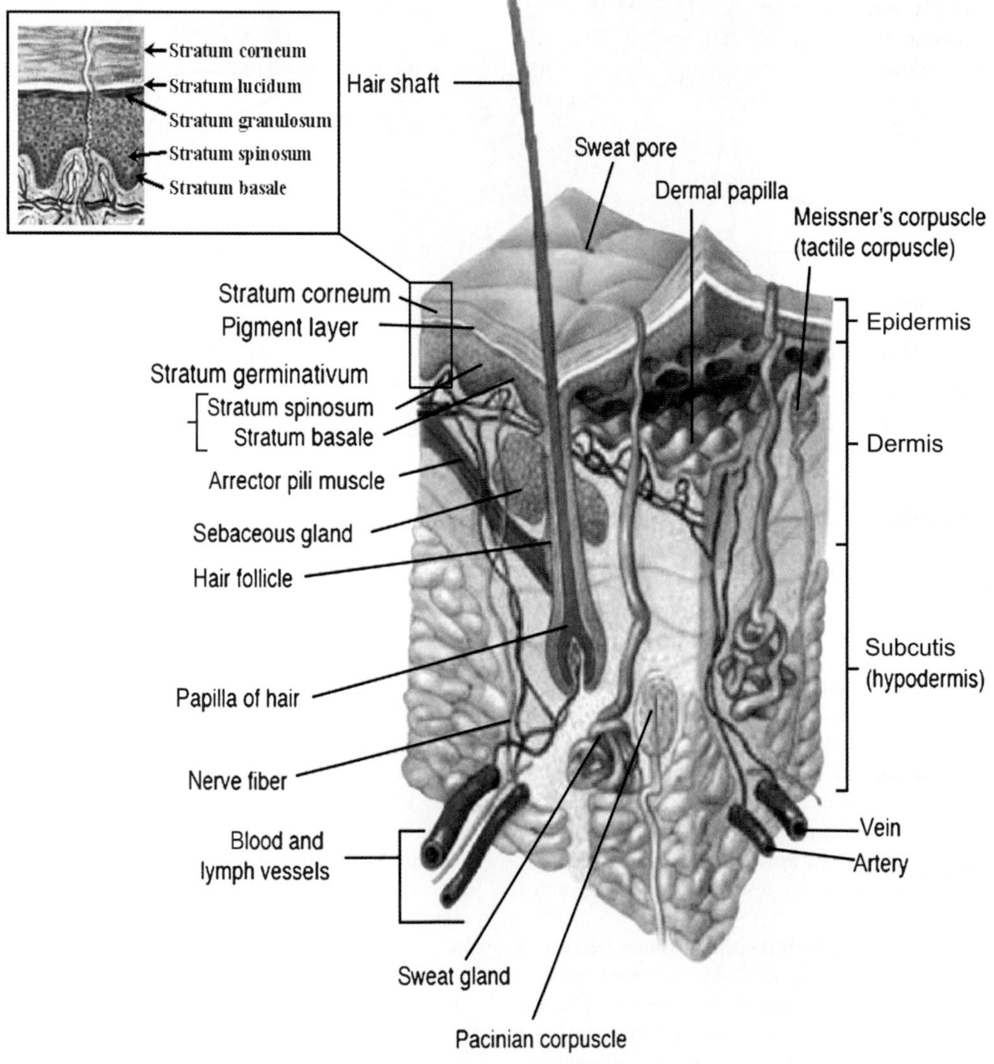

Figure 3 The organization of the skin as a biologic barrier. Image is a modification of the original released into the public domain by the US government.

On the other hand, absorption is much faster from the skin of the scrotum and scalp, for example, due to thin stratum corneum. In general, skin surfaces of the ventral side of the body represent barriers that are easier to cross than those of the dorsal side. Mechanical damage to the stratum corneum by cuts or abrasions of the skin or chemical injury by local irritation with acids or alkalis, for example, is likely to facilitate the entry of chemicals through the skin. This may also be the case in people suffering from certain skin diseases. Similarly, lipid-soluble chemicals are relatively well absorbed through the skin.

The second and the middle layer of the skin is dermis, which consists of connective and fatty tissues and is tightly connected to the epidermis through a basement membrane. The major structural components of dermis are proteins called collagen and elastin, which provide the skin with tensile strength and elasticity. The dermis also contains small blood vessels (capillaries), nerve endings, sebaceous glands, sweat glands, and hair follicles. Small pores in the epidermis allow passage for sweat and oily substances (sebum); these along with hair shafts are not important routes of entry for chemicals. Once a chemical has crossed the epidermis by passive diffusion and gained access to the dermis, diffusion into the bloodstream occurs rapidly. Percutaneous absorption is facilitated by increased peripheral dermal blood flow, which might occur when the ambient temperature is elevated. The presence of elevated sweating increases hydration of the skin and enhances the permeability of the stratum corneum to chemicals, which is of special interest to workers in occupational settings.

Absorption by the Lung

The physiologic role of the lung is to allow gas exchange, extracting oxygen from the ambient air and eliminating carbon dioxide as a catabolic waste. When performing this function, the adult human lung is exposed each day to ~10 000 L of air. The lung becomes an important portal of entry as ambient air contains many airborne chemicals.

Extraneous substances are presented to the lung as gases and vapors, liquid, or solid particles. Following inhalation, they may reach various regions of the respiratory tract, where some fraction will undergo absorption into the bloodstream while the remaining will be either deposited locally or eliminated by exhalation before being absorbed.

In terms of its anatomy and function, the respiratory tract can be divided into three regions: the nasopharyngeal, the tracheobronchial, and the alveolar regions (**Figure 4**). The major absorption takes place in the alveolar region, principally due to its large surface area (80 m^2 in an adult human) and the extreme thinness of the cellular barrier (<1 μm) between the air side of the alveolar sac (lined with epithelial cells) and the lumen of the lung capillaries (lined with endothelial cells).

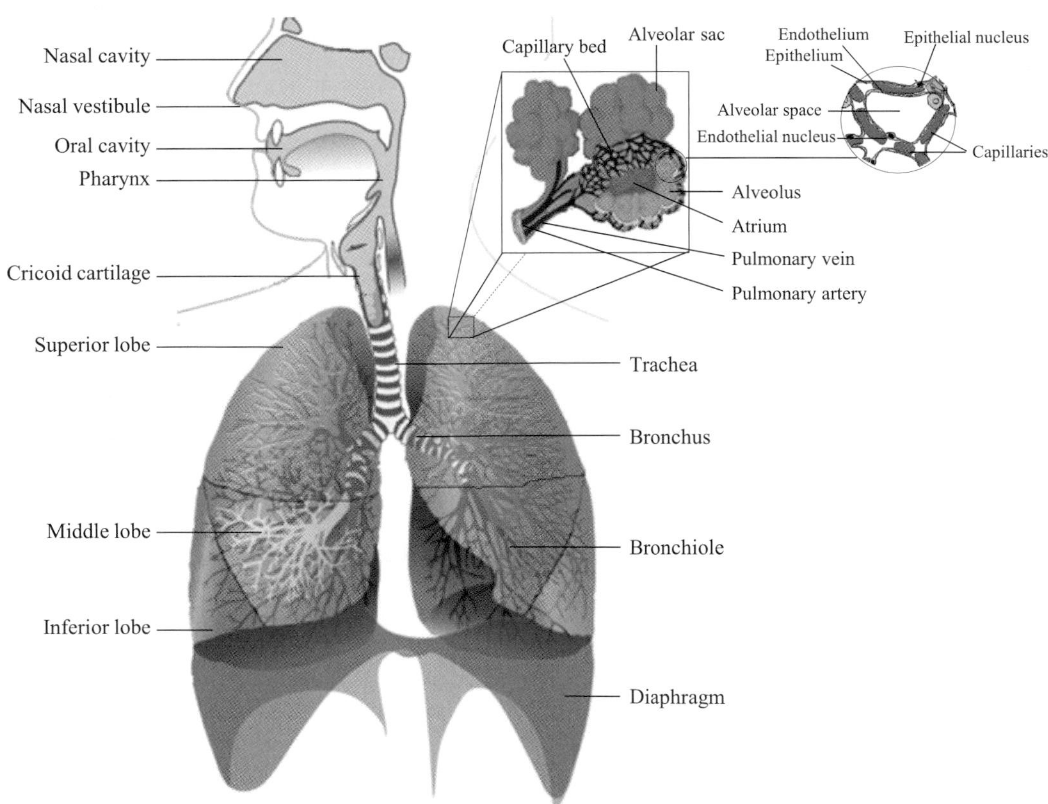

Figure 4 The anatomy of the respiratory tract from trachea to alveolus. Image is a modification of Mariana Ruiz Villarreal, 2007 work, which has been released into the public domain by the author.

When discussing absorption of chemicals through the respiratory tract, it is practical to consider gases and vapors separately from particles.

Gases and Vapors

How much and at what location a gas or vapor will be absorbed in the respiratory tract is determined primarily by the solubility of the agent. The more water-soluble agents (e.g., sulfur dioxide and ketonic solvents) may dissolve in the aqueous fluid lining the cells of the more proximal region of the respiratory tree before reaching the alveolar region. They may then absorb by passive diffusion or pass through membrane pores. When water-soluble gas or vapor is reactive, like formaldehyde, it may form stable molecular complexes with cell components as proximally as in the nasopharyngeal region. By virtue of these mechanisms, the alveolar region of the lung is partially protected against potential injury by certain gases and vapors.

Lipid-soluble gases or vapors diffuse passively through the thin alveolar–vascular cell barrier of the alveolar sac and then dissolve into the blood according to their ability to partition between alveolar air and circulating blood. Substances with high air:blood partitioning are rapidly transported into the bloodstream. For these substances, like styrene and xylene, the amount absorbed is greatly enhanced by increasing the rate and the depth of respiration, as is likely to happen during strenuous physical work. On the other hand, substances with low air:blood partitioning have limited capacity for absorption due to their rapid saturation in blood. For these substances, like the solvents cyclohexane and methyl chloroform, the amount absorbed may be increased only by increasing the blood perfusion (replacement of circulating blood) rate in the lung. This can be achieved during work requiring heavy muscular activity.

Particles

Liquid (e.g., sulfuric acid and cutting fluids) and solid (e.g., silica dusts, asbestos fibers, and microorganisms) particles may become airborne and form respirable aerosols. Depending on their size and diameter, inhaled particles are deposited in different regions of the respiratory system. Once deposited, particles are dissolved locally or moved to other regions of the respiratory tree.

The surface of the cells lining the tracheobronchial tree and the surface of most of the cells lining the nasopharyngeal region are covered with a layer of relatively thick mucus, and cells in the alveolar region are lined with a thin film of fluid. The aqueous environment provided by these surface liquids favors at least partial dissolution and eventually absorption of water-soluble particles, especially those present as liquid droplets. Various defense mechanisms may help remove less soluble particles from their site of deposition.

Particles larger than 5 μm in diameter are usually deposited by inertial impaction on the surface of the nasopharyngeal airways. They may be removed by coughing, sneezing, or nose wiping.

Particles with diameters between 1 and 5 μm are deposited in the tracheobronchial region as a result of either inertial impaction at airway bifurcations or gravitational sedimentation onto other airway surfaces. Undissolved particles may then be removed by the action of the mucociliary defense system working as an escalator. Particles trapped in the mucus are propelled toward the pharynx by the action of thin cilia located on the surface membrane of specialized cells. Once in the pharynx, the particles may be swallowed. The efficiency of the escalator defense system may be greatly impaired by various chemicals, like sulfur dioxide, ozone, and cigarette smoke. They are known to paralyze the activity of the ciliated cells and consequently the upward movement of the mucus.

Particles ranging between 0.1 and 1.0 μm in diameter reach the alveolar region, where they finally hit cellular walls as a result of their random movement within minute air sacs. Removal of particles in this region of the lung is much less efficient. Some of the particles may eventually reach the tracheobronchial escalator system, either as engulfed material within alveolar macrophages or as naked particles transported by the slow movement of the fluid lining the alveoli. Other possible mechanisms involve transport of the particles into the lymphatic system, either within macrophages or by direct diffusion through the intercellular space of the alveolar wall.

Particles smaller than 0.1 μm are not usually deposited in the lung, entering and exiting the airways together with inhaled and exhaled air.

Often, particulate matter acts as a carrier for gases, vapors, and fumes adsorbed onto their surface (solid particles) or dissolved within them (liquid particles); this increases the residence time of such pollutants in specific areas of the lung and imposes an additional task on the pulmonary defense mechanisms.

The most striking example of this synergistic effect is the one observed between sulfur dioxide, a respiratory tract irritant, and suspended particles, both being typical components of urban air pollution. This explains why current guideline values for exposure to sulfur dioxide in the presence of particulate matter are lower than those for exposure to sulfur dioxide alone. Similar concerns can be expressed for combinations comprising exhaust particles from diesel engines and certain carcinogens like polycyclic aromatic hydrocarbons, as well as cigarette smoke and certain other carcinogens like aromatic amines.

Chemicals absorbed by the lung reach the systemic circulation directly and are therefore immediately available for distribution to various tissues of the body.

See also: Biotransformation; Gastrointestinal System; Distribution; Excretion; Pharmacokinetics; Respiratory Tract Toxicology; Occupational Exposure Limits; Skin; Modifying Factors of Toxicity; Toxicity Testing, Dermal; Toxicity Testing, Inhalation.

Further Reading

Inchiosa, M.A., 2006. Toxicokinetics: deposition, absorption, distribution and excretion. In: Salem, S., Katz, S.A. (Eds.), Inhalation Toxicology, second ed. CRC Press, Boca Raton, pp. 405–438.

Lehman-McKeeman, L.D., 2008. Absorption, distribution, and excretion of toxicants. In: Klaassen, C.D. (Ed.), Casarett and Doull's Toxicology: The Basic Science of Poisons, seventh ed. McGraw-Hill, New York, pp. 131–159.

Lu, F.C., Kacew, S., 2009. Absorption, distribution, and excretion of toxicants. Lu's, Basic Toxicology: Fundamentals, Target Organs, and Risk Assessment, fifth ed. Informa Healthcare, New York, pp. 15–30.

Monteiro-Riviere, N.A., 2006. Structure and function of skin. In: Riviere, J.E. (Ed.), Dermal Absorption Models in Toxicology and Pharmacology. CRC Press, Boca Raton, pp. 1–20.

Academy of Toxicological Sciences*

SS Devi, Lake Erie College of Osteopathic Medicine, Erie, PA, USA
HM Mehendale, University of Louisiana at Monroe, Monroe, LA, USA

The Academy of Toxicological Sciences was established in 1981 for the purpose of recognizing and certifying toxicologists. As a nonprofit organization, the mission of the Academy of Toxicological Sciences is to establish a means by which practicing toxicologists are certified based on education (PhD or equivalent doctoral degree and postdoctoral training), professional experience (career advancement), demonstrated achievement (scholarly publications, editorial boards, and awarded grants), proven ability (international honors and awards), and scientific expertise (international scientific boards, committees, and workgroups). The competence and experience of these professional practitioners affect public welfare. Recognition and certification are accomplished by a peer-review process, which is a time-honored mechanism for scientists to evaluate one another based on formal training, proven ability, and experience. Demonstrated achievement, rather than the potential for achievement, is the key to the Academy's evaluation process. Thus, an individual certified as a qualified fellow in toxicology by the Academy of Toxicological Sciences is one who actively practices toxicology and who has been evaluated by the peer-review process according to the Academy's bylaws. As of 2012, there are approximately 250 Academy of Toxicological Sciences certified toxicologists.

Candidates for certification must have a broad knowledge of toxicology and must demonstrate substantive involvement in toxicological activities. To apply, an applicant shall submit an application form and any necessary supporting documentation to the Executive Director of the Academy. The Board of Directors will meet at least three times a year to review both the applications and credentials of the candidates. The criteria for certification in toxicology by the Academy includes education and training, professional experience, and demonstration of scientific recognition.

Successful candidates are certified as Fellows of the Academy of Toxicological Sciences for a period of five years, and may be recertified by submitting an application for review by the Board of Directors.

Contact Details

Academy of Toxicological Sciences Headquarters, 1821 Michael Faraday Drive, Suite 300, Reston, VA 20190, USA. Tel.: +1 703 438 3103.

See also: American Board of Toxicology; American College of Toxicology; The Hamner Institutes for Health Sciences; EUROTOX; The International Society for the Study of Xenobiotics; Society of Environmental Toxicology and Chemistry; International Union of Toxicology; Society of Toxicology.

Relevant Website

www.acadtoxsci.org – Academy of Toxicological Sciences.

* Adapted from information supplied by the Academy of Toxicological Sciences.

 http://dx.doi.org/10.1016/B978-0-12-386454-3.00212-8

Acceptable Daily Intake (ADI)

J Chilakapati, Alcon Laboratories, Fort Worth, TX, USA
HM Mehendale, University of Louisiana at Monroe, Monroe, LA, USA

The acceptable daily intake (ADI) is commonly defined as the amount of a chemical to which a person can be exposed, on a daily basis over an extended period of time, usually without suffering a deleterious effect. It represents a daily intake level of a chemical in humans that is associated with minimal or no risk of adverse effects. It is a numerical estimate of daily oral exposure to the human population, including sensitive subgroups such as children, that is not likely to cause harmful effects during a lifetime. The ADI is expressed in milligrams of the chemical, as it appears in the food, per kilogram of body weight per day (mg kg^{-1} day^{-1}). The US Environmental Protection Agency (EPA) refers to such an exposure level as the risk reference dose (RfD) in order to avoid any implication that any exposure to a toxic material is 'acceptable.' RfDs are generally used for health effects that are thought to have a threshold or low dose limit for producing effects. The ADI concept has often been used as a tool in reaching risk management decisions such as establishing allowable levels of contaminants in foodstuffs and water.

ADI is derived from an experimentally determined no observed adverse effect level (NOAEL). An NOAEL is an experimentally determined dose at which there is no statistically or biologically significant indication of the toxic effect of concern. In an experiment with several NOAELs, the regulatory focus is normally on the highest one, leading to the common usage of the term NOAEL as the highest experimentally determined dose without a statistically or biologically significant adverse effect. In cases in which an NOAEL has not been demonstrated experimentally, the term lowest observed adverse effect level (LOAEL) is used.

ADI values are typically calculated from NOAEL values by dividing by uncertainty (UF) and/or modifying factors (MFs) :

$$\text{ADI (human dose)} = \text{NOAEL (experimental dose)}/\text{UF} \times (\text{MF})$$

In principle, these safety factors (SFs) allow for intraspecies and interspecies (animal to human) variations with default values of 10. An additional uncertainty factor can be used to account for experimental inadequacies, for example, to extrapolate from short-exposure-duration studies to a situation more relevant for chronic study or to account for inadequate numbers of animals or other experimental limitations. Traditionally, an SF of 100 would be used for RfD calculations to extrapolate from a well-conducted animal bioassay (10-fold factor for animal to human) and to account for human variability in response (10-fold factor human-to-human variability).

Modifying factors can be used to adjust the UFs if data on mechanisms, pharmacokinetics, and the relevance of the animal response to human risk justify such modifications. For example, if there is kinetic suggesting that rat and human metabolisms are very similar for a particular compound, producing the same active target metabolite, then, rather than using a 10-fold uncertainty factor to divide the NOAEL from the animal toxicity study to obtain a human relevant RfD, a factor of 3 for that uncertainty factor might be used. Of particular interest is the new extra 10-fold Food Quality and Protection Act factor, added to ensure protection of infants and children.

For other chemicals, with databases that are less complete (e.g., those for which only the results of subchronic studies are available), an additional factor of 10 might be judged to be more appropriate, leading to an SF of 1000. Based on well-characterized responses in sensitive humans, an SF as small as 1 might be selected for certain chemicals, as in the case of the effect of fluoride on human teeth.

Some scientists interpret the absence of widespread effects in the exposed human populations as evidence of the adequacy of the SFs traditionally employed. The RfD approach represents a generally accepted (Food and Drug Administration, National Academy of Sciences, and EPA) method for setting lifetime exposure limits for humans, and the use of 10-fold uncertainty factors (UFs) has some experimental support.

Limitations of RfD

However, there are several limitations in the RfD approach, the net result of which is that exposures resulting in the same RfD do not imply the same level of risk for all chemicals. In addition, the RfD approach does not make use of dose–response information. There are also difficulties in the implications of specific UFs. The default value of 10 for the interspecies UF is a reasonable assumption in some cases, but in other cases may not be appropriate. Such data could be important in estimating levels of concern for public safety. Guidelines have not been developed to take into account the fact that some studies have used larger (smaller) numbers of animals and, hence, are generally more (less) reliable than other studies.

The ADI is generally viewed by risk assessors as a 'soft' estimate, whose bounds of uncertainty can span an order of magnitude. While exposures somewhat higher than the ADI (within reasonable limits) are associated with increased probability of adverse effects, that probability is not a certainty. Similarly, while the ADI is seen as a level at which the probability of adverse effects is low, the absence of all risk to all people cannot be assured at this level.

 http://dx.doi.org/10.1016/B978-0-12-386454-3.00213-X

To reduce uncertainty in calculating RfDs and ADIs, there has been a transition from the use of traditional 10-fold UFs to the use of data-derived and chemical-specific adjustment factors. Current WHO guidance suggests a 4.0- and 2.5-fold factor for the toxicokinetic (TK) and toxicodynamic (TD) interspecies components, respectively, and interindividual TK and TD factors of 3.16.

See also: Benchmark Dose.

Further Reading

Carrington, C.D., Bolger, P.M., 2010. The limits of regulatory toxicology. Toxicol. Appl. Pharmacol. 243 (2), 191–197.

Faustman, E.M., Omenn, G.S., 2001. Risk assessment. In: Klaassen, C.D. (Ed.), Casarett & Doull's Toxicology: The Basic Science of Poisons, sixth ed. McGraw-Hill, New York, pp. 92–94.

Galli, C.L., Marinovich, M., Lotti, M., 2008. Is the acceptable daily intake as presently used an axiom or a dogma? Toxicol. Lett. 180 (2), 93–99.

US Environmental Protection Agency, 1991. Guidelines for developmental toxicity risk assessment. Fed. Reg. 56, 63798–63826.

US Environmental Protection Agency, 1996. Food Quality Protection Act (FQPA). Office of Pesticide Programs, Washington, DC.

Accutane

SC Gad and JH Fain, Gad Consulting Services, Cary, NC, USA

This article is a revision of the previous edition article by Russell Barbare, volume 1, pp 7–9, © 2005, Elsevier Inc.

- Name: Accutane
- Chemical Abstracts Service Registry Number: 4759-48-2
- Chemical/Pharmaceutical/Other Class: Retinoid, 9-*cis* isomer of retinoic acid
- Synonyms: Isotretinoin, 13-*cis*-Retinoic acid, Accutane, Roaccutane, Claravis, Amnesteem, Teriosal
- Molecular Formula: $C_{20}H_{28}O_2$
- Chemical Structure:

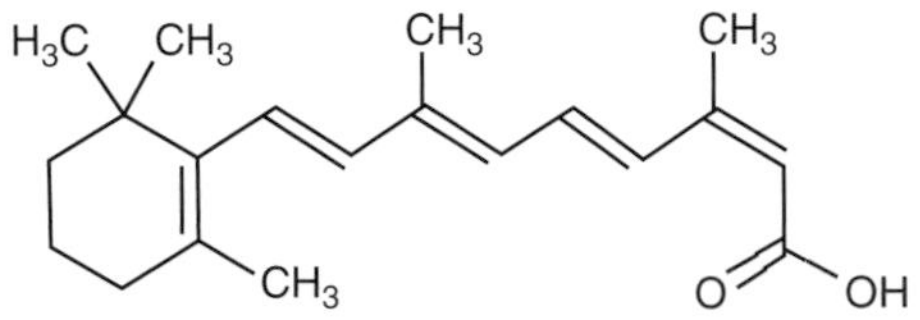

H_3C CH_3 CH_3 CH_3 CH_3 O OH

Background Information

The original patent for Accutane expired in 2002. Held by Hoffmann-LaRoche until that time, it is perhaps now better known by its common name, isotretinoin, although over 100 trade names for the compound now exist. Isotretinoin was originally developed to treat cystic acne, and today this is still its primary use despite several more modern applications of the drug, including a treatment for pancreatic and brain cancers.

Isotretinoin is the 9-*cis* isomer of retinoic acid, a close relative of retinol, or vitamin A. First shown to be an effective treatment for acne in 1982, its development stemmed from advances in knowledge of the effects of vitamin A to reduce or eliminate sebum production. Since that time, however, several instances of deleterious effects became well known, most notably birth defects arising from the use of isotretinoin.

Accutane was removed from distribution by Roche in 2009 after several lawsuits had been filed alleging damages due to side effects, especially in young adult males due to inflammatory bowel disease (IBD).

Uses

The primary use of Accutane (isotretinoin) was the treatment of acne. Its use as an acne treatment is generally limited to severe cases where lesions are at least 5 mm in diameter and appear suppurative or hemorrhagic, or for inflammatory acne and acne conglobata. Less severe acne may be treated with isotretinoin if the patient has a history of dyspigmentation or scarring due to acne. Isotretinoin is generally a last course of treatment in these cases after all other routes have been explored.

Additional uses for Accutane (isotretinoin) include treatments for keratinization such as lamellar ichthyosis, and keratosis follicularis (Darier's disease) in addition to palmoplantar keratoderma and pityriasis rubra pilaris. It is also an effective treatment for severe rosacea and gram-negative folliculitis, and to treat hidradenitis suppurative.

Interestingly, isotretinoin has been shown to significantly reduce inflammation associated with adjuvant arthritis in rats, although this has not been verified to be the case in humans.

Environmental Fate and Behavior

Direct studies focused on the environmental fate of Accutane (isotretinoin) are rare in the literature. The pure compound is insoluble in water, and highly lipophilic. Powders do not aerosolize readily, and volatilization is extremely low. Isotretinoin released into the environment would not be expected to have high mobility in water or soil, and will most likely become deposited in organic materials. Bioaccumulation is possible, but isotretinoin is readily oxidized to form other retinoids or metabolites that are expected to be mitigated via natural biological pathways.

Exposure and Exposure Monitoring

Exposure to Accutane (isotretinoin) occurs primarily from ingestion. Reports of occupational exposure are few, and most occurrences of toxicity from unwanted exposure are due to accidental ingestion of Accutane (or other isotretinoin) tablets. Clearance of the compound is rapid, however, and symptoms are often brief. Symptomatic treatment is recommended, and monitoring is generally qualitative.

Pregnant individuals should be extra cautious to avoid contact with Accutane (isotretinoin), even acute exposure.

Toxicokinetics

Much like its mechanism of toxicity, toxicokinetic profiles for Accutane (isotretinoin) are difficult to determine. Accounts in the literature have focused primarily on the metabolism of the compound.

Accutane (isotretinoin) is rapidly absorbed from the gastrointestinal tract owing to its lipophilicity. When taken with food, this absorption is accelerated. Peak plasma concentrations following an oral dose of isotretinoin occur in the first 30 min; elimination half-life estimates have ranged from 17 to 50 h. Traces of the compound are largely undetectable in most tissues after 24 h, although metabolites may persist in the liver, ureter, ovary, and adrenal and lachrymal glands for at least 7 days.

Accutane (isotretinoin) is distributed systemically almost immediately upon consumption, and is readily isomerized into the all-trans isomer of the compound. Retinoids like Accutane have been shown to regulate gene expression in

 http://dx.doi.org/10.1016/B978-0-12-386454-3.00808-3

a number of systems, and have some influence on the production of steroids. The pharmacological effects of the drug are nonselective once in circulation, and most arise from repeated use of the drug rather than from a single application.

Mechanism of Toxicity

In primates (including humans), isotretinoin (Accutane) is metabolized to a more active form, 13-*cis*-4-oxo-retinoic acid, which is able to move through the placental membrane. On its own, however, Accutane (isotretinoin) is not particularly motile across the placental barrier, and perhaps most interestingly tends not to bind to cellular retinoid-binding proteins or nuclear receptors. The rapid isomerization to the all-trans isomer, the oxidation of Accutane (isotretinoin) to 13-*cis*-4-oxo-retinoic acid, and the relatively high circulation times of these compounds may be important in explaining the teratogenic toxicity of Accutane (isotretinoin).

Some studies have more fully explored the metabolic products of isotretinoin. For example, isotretinoin can be metabolized in the liver by the cytochrome P450 microsomal enzyme system – more specifically the CYP2C8, CYP2C, CYP3A4, and CYP2B6 isoenzymes. The metabolites produced are numerous, including retinoic acid (tretinoin), 4-oxo-isotretinoin, and 4-oxo-retinoic acid (4-oxo-tretinoin). This relatively large array of retinoid metabolites may produce a variety of effects, most notably due to their higher potency as retinoids compared to the parent compound (isotretinoin).

It is possible that these additional metabolites are capable of binding to a variety of retinoid receptors in order to alter gene expression and further transcription or transrepression in protein synthesis, which may be responsible for the toxic effects of isotretinoin.

Acute and Short-Term Toxicity (or Exposure)

Animals

Although exposure to Accutane (isotretinoin) in animals has focused primarily on chronic exposure to elucidate the mechanisms of some of the more pronounced toxic effects of the drug, several studies have examined acute effects as well. These studies focus primarily on the teratogenic effects of Accutane, and most have shown positive, if dose-dependent, relationships with regard to the birth defects associated with exposure.

Lethal dose parameters in several species are available. For rats, mice, and rabbits, oral LD_{50} values of 4, 4, and 2 g kg^{-1}, respectively, have been determined. In Swiss mice, an intraperitoneal injection LD_{50} of 140 mg kg^{-1} day^{-1} has been determined, as well as a gavage dose of 26 g kg^{-1} day^{-1} for 21 days.

Human

In humans, acute effects of Accutane (isotretinoin) have varied greatly. Among the most severe are depression, psychosis, and in rare cases suicidal thoughts and/or attempts. Aggression or violent behavior has also been reported, as well as feelings of sadness, irritability, trouble concentrating, loss of appetite, and unusual tiredness.

It is unclear how this emotional instability arises. These effects appear to be strongly correlated to use of Accutane, since the effects subsided following discontinuing use of the drug, but reappeared when use was reinstated. Some cases of these acute effects were seen to persist after terminating therapy with Accutane (isotretinoin).

Physical symptoms can also occur. For example, pseudotumor cerebri (benign intracranial hypertension) has been observed following treatment with isotretinoin, which may be further complicated with concomitant use of tetracyclines. Early signs can include headache, nausea, vomiting, visual disturbances, and papilledema.

By far the most common acute (as well as chronic) effect of isotretinoin is inflammation of the lips (cheilitis), which occurs in more than 90% of patients using the drug to treat acne. Isotretinoin has also been associated with increases in erythrocyte sedimentation rates, with nearly 40% of patients experiencing this effect. Decreased hemoglobin concentrations decreased hematocrit, decreases in leukocyte and erythrocyte counts, and increased platelet counts have also been observed.

Gastrointestinal effects following the use of isotretinoin (Accutane) have also been reported, including anorexia, increased appetite, and thirst. Inflammatory bowel syndrome has also been associated with the use of Accutane in patients with no prior history of intestinal disorder. Mild gastrointestinal bleeding and weight loss may also occur, though more rarely.

Problems with the eyes, especially vision, may occur with the use of isotretinoin. Conjunctivitis (including blepharoconjunctivitis) and irritation are commonly reported problems associated with its use, while corneal opacity – particularly in patients receiving isotretinoin to treat nodular acne – has also been reported, mostly in patients receiving high doses of the drug. Cataracts and lasting impairments to vision have also been reported.

Chronic Toxicity (or Exposure)

Animal

In animals, chronic toxicity due to isotretinoin has been varied. For example, bone fracture has been observed in mice following 21 consecutive days of oral or intraperitoneal exposure to the drug. Both routes of delivery produced the same effects. Decreases in red blood cell counts were also observed in the study. Further studies have explored the effects of isotretinoin on rats given from one to five times the recommended clinical dose (after normalizing for total body surface area), and found increases in incidences of focal calcification, fibrosis, and inflammation of the myocardium; calcification of pulmonary, coronary, and mesenteric arteries; and metastatic calcification of the gastric mucosa.

Human

In humans, the effects of chronic exposure to isotretinoin (Accutane) are largely extensions of the acute effects of the drug. For example, intracranial hypertension has been reported in patients undergoing therapy with Accutane, as have musculoskeletal effects such as bone or joint pain, muscle aches, arthralgia, and loss of bone density. Osteoporosis, osteopenia, and delayed bone healing have also been reported. Interestingly, nearly 30% of pediatric patients treated with isotretinoin developed back pain ranging from severe to mild, as well as arthralgias. Rarely, chest pain has been observed.

Also associated with the use of isotretinoin has been the appearance of IBD, particularly in those patients with no prior history of gastrointestinal disorders. In some cases, the symptoms of IBD persist after treatment with isotretinoin has been discontinued.

Immunotoxicity

Reports of immunotoxicity associated with the use of Accutane (isotretinoin) have primarily concerned hypersensitivity to other materials. Anaphylactic and other allergic reactions have been reported, including severe allergic vasculitis and cutaneous allergic reactions; extracutaneous involvement and purpura (red patches or bruises) have been observed as well.

Reproductive Toxicity

Accutane (isotretinoin) is a known teratogen and is contraindicated in cases of pregnancy. Fetal abnormalities have been reported in humans and animals. These effects have included central nervous system abnormalities such as hydrocephalus, microcephaly, and cranial nerve deficit. Eye abnormalities such as microphthalmia have been reported, as have heart defects. Parathyroid deficiency and thymus gland abnormalities are also possible effects of exposure to isotretinoin during pregnancy.

Skeletal and tissue abnormalities are commonly associated with the use of Accutane (isotretinoin). These include syndactyly, multiple synostoses, meningomyelocele, malformations of the skull and cervical vertebra, absence of terminal phalanges, and malformations of extremities including the forearm, hip, and ankle. Cleft or high palate, facial dysmorphia, low-set ears, small/absent external auditory canals, and micropinna are other possibilities.

Genotoxicity

Reports of genotoxicity concerning Accutane (isotretinoin) in the literature are few, although some have found evidence of extensive chromosomal modifications (specifically of the skin). It is also possible that Accutane (isotretinoin) may lead to DNA methylation, although there is currently insufficient evidence for this.

Carcinogenicity

Studies have explored the effects of isotretinoin on rats, and found increases in incidences of focal calcification, fibrosis, and inflammation of the myocardium; calcification of pulmonary, coronary, and mesenteric arteries; and metastatic calcification of the gastric mucosa. Few other carcinogenic effects of Accutane (isotretinoin) could be found in the current literature.

Clinical Management

Effects due to the use of Accutane (isotretinoin) should be treated symptomatically. Nausea and vomiting should be treated with metoclopramide. Activated charcoal may be administered; induce vomiting if charcoal is unavailable.

Ecotoxicology

Ecotoxicological information for Accutane (isotretinoin) is relatively rare. This is perhaps due to the ubiquity of retinoids, including isotretinoin, in many biological systems.

One study investigated the effects of isotretinoin and other retinoids on frogs exposed to lake water contaminated with the compounds. Treating the frog embryos at specific developmental stages produced limb abnormalities similar to those suddenly observed in several suspected retinoid contamination sites in the wild.

A 48 h EC_{50} 0.1–0.3 $mg\,l^{-1}$ for *Daphnia magna* has been reported.

Exposure Standards and Guidelines

The Approved Drug Products with Therapeutic Equivalence Evaluations List identifies currently marketed prescription drug products, including isotretinoin, approved on the basis of safety and effectiveness by US Food and Drug Administration under sections 505 of the Federal Food, Drug, and Cosmetic Act.

No further exposure guidelines have been established for Accutane (isotretinoin).

See also: Vitamin A; Vitamin C (Ascorbic Acid); Vitamin D; Vitamin E.

Further Reading

Bigby, M., Stern, R.S., 1988. Adverse reactions to isotretinoin: a report from the Adverse Drug Reaction Reporting System. J. Am. Acad. Dermatol. 18 (3), 543–552.

Charakida, A., et al., 2004. Safety and side effects of the acne drug, oral isotretinoin. Expert Opin. Drug Saf. 3 (2), 119–129.

Csoka, A.B., Szyf, M., 2009. Epigenetic side-effects of common pharmaceuticals: a potential new field in medicine and pharmacology. Med. Hypotheses 73 (5), 770–780.

Fraunfelder, F.W., et al., 2004. Isotretinoin-associated intracranial hypertension. Ophthalmology 111 (6), 1248–1250.

Gardiner, D., Ndayibagira, A., Grün, F., Blumberg, B., 2003. Deformed frogs and environmental retinoids. Pure Appl. Chem. 75 (11–12), 2263–2273.

Nelson, A.M., Zhao, W., Gilliland, K.L., Zaenglein, A.L., Liu, W., Thiboutot, D.M., 2009. Temporal changes in gene expression in the skin of patients treated with isotretinoin provide insight into its mechanism of action. Dermatoendocrinol. 1 (3), 177–187.

Rosa, F.W., et al., June 1986. Teratogen update: vitamin A congeners. Teratology 33, 355–364.

Relevant Websites

http://pubchem.ncbi.nlm.nih.gov/ – Search for 'isotretinoin.'

http://toxnet.nlm.nih.gov – Search for 'isotretinoin' under all databases.

http://www.fda.gov – US Food and Drug Administration (FDA), Center for Drug Evaluation and Research (CDER). Accutane information.

Angiotensin Converting Enzyme (ACE) Inhibitors

HA Spiller, Central Ohio Poison Center, Columbus, OH, USA

- Name: Angiotensin converting enzyme (ACE) inhibitors
- Synonyms: Benazepril, Lotensin® (CAS 86541-75-5); Captopril, Capoten® (CAS 62571-86-2); Enalapril, Vasotec® (CAS 75847-73-3); Enalaprilat, Vasotec IV® (CAS 84680-54-6); Fosinopril, Monopril® (CAS 888 89-14-9); Lisinopril, Prinivil®, Zestril® (CAS 76547-98-3); Quinapril, Accupril® (CAS 85441-61-8); Ramipril, Altace® (CAS 87333-19-5)
- Pharmaceutical Class: Angiotensin converting enzyme (ACE) inhibitors
- Molecular Formula: Benazepril $C_{24}H_{28}N_2O_5$; Captopril $C_9H_{15}NO_3S$; Enalapril $C_{20}H_{28}N_2O_5$; Enalaprilat $C_{18}H_{24}N_2O_5 \cdot 2H_2O$; Fosinopril $C_{30}H_{46}NO_7P$; Lisinopril $C_{21}H_{31}N_3O_5 \cdot 2H_2O$; Quinapril $C_{25}H_{30}N_2O_5$; Ramipril $C_{23}H_{32}N_2O_5$
- Chemical Structures: Lisinopril as example 1 and Captopril (the first synthetic ACE inhibitor) as example 2

Example 1

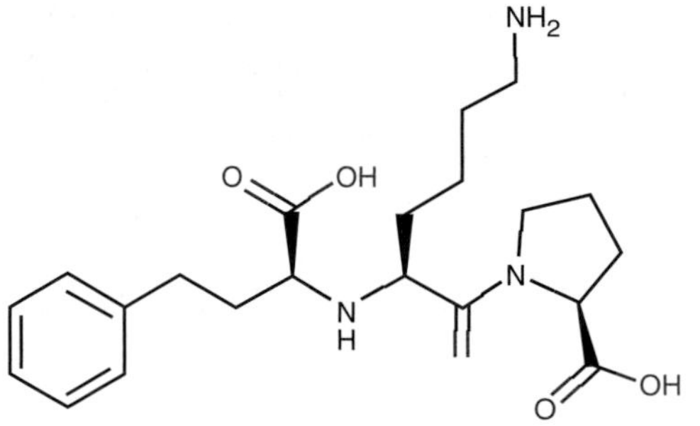

Example 2

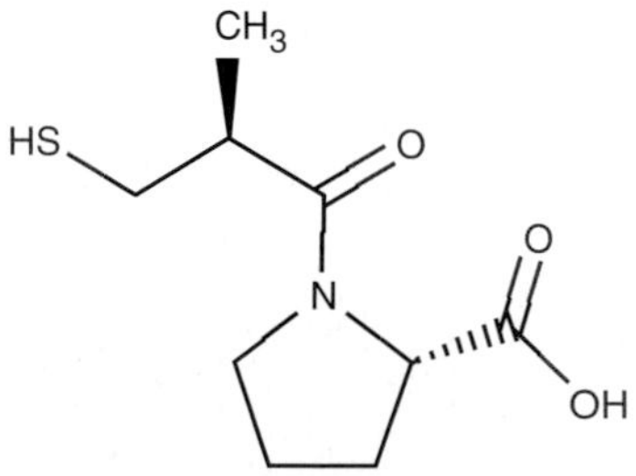

Background (Significance/History)

ACE was discovered in plasma in the 1950s, followed by discovery of bradykinin potentiating factor in the venom of *Bothrops jararaca*, a South American pit viper, in 1965. The first orally active ACE inhibitor, captopril, was developed in 1975 and approved for use by the US Food and Drug Administration in 1981. Captopril was a thiol-containing compound. Enalapril followed captopril and was a compound that lacked the thiol group and potentially side effects associated with this sulfur moiety. There are essentially three groups of ACE inhibitors: (1) those that contain the thiol moiety include captopril, zofenopril, and omapatrilat; (2) those that contain a dicarboxyl group including enalapril, perindopril, lisinopril, ramipril, trandolapril, quinapril, benazepril, and cilazapril; and (3) the phosphorous-containing ACE inhibitors such as fosinopril.

Uses

ACE inhibitors are used in the management of hypertension and congestive heart failure.

Environmental Fate and Behavior Routes

Ingestion is the most common route for both accidental and intentional exposures. Enalaprilat is available for parenteral administration and toxicity could occur via this route as well.

Physicochemical Properties

1. Captopril *as example*
   Molecular weight: 217.29
   Melting point: 104–108 °C
   Solubility: Soluble in water at 0.1 g ml^{-1}, which results in a slightly hazy or colorless solution
   Stability: Stable, although incompatible with strong oxidizing agents
   Refractive index: −127.5° (C 1.7, EtOH)
   p*Ka*: 9.8

Most of the ACE inhibitors contain both proton acceptor and proton donor groups, which may be ionized or protonated, respectively. The dicarboxyl-containing ACE inhibitors behave as strong acids at physiologic (7.4) pH. The thiol-containing captopril is a weak acid with a calculated p*Ka* of 9.55 (experimental 9.8). ACE inhibitors and their metabolites exhibit low lipophilicity.

Calculated Partition Coefficients and Solubility of Certain ACE Inhibitors

Captopril: log P 1.02 and solubility (S g^{-1} dm^{-3}) 4.62
Enalapril: log P 0.09 and solubility (S g^{-1} dm^{-3}) 0.21
Enalaprilat: log P −0.03 and solubility (S g^{-1} dm^{-3}) 0.88
Lisinopril: log P −1.20 and solubility (S g^{-1} dm^{-3}) 0.22
Fosinopril: log P 4.75 and solubility (S g^{-1} dm^{-3}) 1.02

 http://dx.doi.org/10.1016/B978-0-12-386454-3.00686-2

Environmental Fate

No information is currently available on breakdown in soil, groundwater, or surface water. ACE inhibitors are excreted in breast milk in trace amounts. Captopril is distributed into milk in concentrations about 1% of those in maternal blood.

Toxicokinetics

The extent of oral absorption varies from 25% (lisinopril) to 75% (captopril). The rate of absorption also varies from 0.5 h (captopril and enalapril) to 7 h (lisinopril). Reported volumes of distribution range from 0.7 l kg^{-1} (captopril) to 1.8 l kg^{-1} (lisinopril). All of the ACE inhibitors, except for captopril and lisinopril, are metabolized in the liver to active metabolites. Excretion is via both the urine and the feces. The half-life ranges from 1.3 h (enalapril) to 17 h (ramipril).

Mechanism of Toxicity

The ACE inhibitors affect the rennin-angiotensin system. This system has effects on blood pressure as well as fluids and electrolyte balance. Renin modulates the formation of angiotensin I from angiotensinogen. Angiotensin I is then converted via ACE to angiotensin II, primarily in the pulmonary circulation. Angiotensin II is a potent vasoconstrictor that also causes increased aldosterone secretion. Aldosterone is responsible for sodium and water retention. The ACE inhibitors interfere with the conversion of angiotensin I to angiotensin II and, therefore, cause vasodilation as well as sodium and water loss. Angiotensin II is also thought to be inhibited by endogenous beta-endorphin. *In vitro* studies have demonstrated that captopril can inhibit enkephalinase, the enzyme that degrades endorphins. Interference with endorphin metabolism should result in prolonged effects from these opiate-like neurotransmitters. Also, the opiate antagonist naloxone is thought to interfere with beta-endorphins inhibition of angiotensin II. An interaction between angiotensin and bradykinin may also exist. ACE is identical to kinase II, which is responsible for inactivation of bradykinins. Accumulation of bradykinins may cause a decrease in blood pressure by a direct vasodilatory mechanism or through stimulation of prostaglandin release or synthesis. Accumulation of bradykinins may be responsible for the dry cough and angioedema associated with ACE inhibitors.

Acute Toxicity

Human Toxicity

The clinical effects observed following ACE inhibitor poisoning or overdose are a direct extension of their therapeutic effects and would be expected to manifest in 1–2 h postingestion. Maximum hypotensive effect after overdose was noted at 4 h postingestion. Ingestions involving small amounts of ACE inhibitors may result in limited or no toxic effects. Ingestion of more than 20 times the recommended daily dose has resulted in moderate hypotension without sequelae. Clinical effects that may occur include hypotension, usually without a reflex tachycardia and changes in the level of consciousness that are directly related to vascular changes. Only a few cases of profound hypotension have been reported. In each of these cases, blood pressure returned to normal within 24 h of ingestion. There has been a single case of death attributed to an ACE inhibitor alone. A 75-year-old male committed suicide by taking an overdose of ninety 12.5-mg captopril tabs. Postmortem concentrations of captopril were 60.4 mg l^{-1} in this case. Other reported deaths have included coingestants of calcium channel blockers (diltiazem and amlodipine), and toxicity from the calcium channel blocker was believed to be the primary cause of death.

Animal Toxicity

There are limited data, but accidental ingestion of a small amount of ACE inhibitors by companion animals would not expected to be a problem.

Chronic Toxicity

Human

Adverse effects observed at therapeutic doses include cough, dermal reactions, blood dyscrasias, bronchospasm, and hypogeusia. Life-threatening angioedema has been reported, but does not appear to be an IgG-related immune response. Reversible renal failure has been reported with chronic therapy. Clinical effects that may occur include hypotension without a reflex tachycardia, changes in the level of consciousness that are directly related to vascular changes, and hyperkalemia. Hyperkalemia can occur as a response to sodium loss or as a complication of renal failure. Delayed hypotension, at 19 and 25 h, has been observed following ingestion of captopril. Chronic use of a nonsteroidal anti-inflammatory drug with an ACE inhibitor may result in loss of ACE inhibition and reduced efficacy of the antihypertensive effects. There is also increased risk of affecting renal function with this combination.

Reproductive Toxicity

ACE inhibitors are not recommended in pregnancy. Use in the first trimester does not appear to present a significant risk to the fetus, but after this time they have been associated with teratogenicity and severe toxicity. Use of ACE inhibitors has been associated with a decrease in placental blood flow and oxygen delivery to the fetus.

Use of drugs that act on the renin-angiotensin system during the second and third trimesters of pregnancy will decrease renal function and potentially lead to oligohydramnios. This can be associated with fetal lung hypoplasia and skeletal deformations. Use in the first trimester has not been shown to cause fetal abnormalities with increased frequency from other medications with antihypertensive effect.

ACE inhibitors are listed as having potential for toxicity under inclusion of the California Prop 65 Developmental Toxin list. No specific toxicity is documented, however.

Genotoxicity/Mutagenicity

Lisinopril, captopril, quinapril, and benazepril have been studied for mutagenicity using a variety of methods and none have documented evidence of mutagenicity.

Carcinogenicity

Not listed as having carcinogenicity under US Environmental Protection Agency carcinogens, California Prop 65 known carcinogens, International Agency for Research on Cancer carcinogens, US National Toxicology Program carcinogens, or Toxics Release Inventory carcinogen.

Clinical Management

Supportive care, including airway management as well as cardiac and blood pressure monitoring, should be provided to unstable patients. Ingestion of small amounts of an ACE inhibitor in children can be managed with observation at home. Following ingestion of a toxic amount of these agents or recent ingestions involving toxic coingestants, activated charcoal can be used to decontaminate the stomach. Hypotension following ACE inhibitor ingestion has been managed with fluids alone or in combination with vasopressors such as dopamine or norepinephrine. The need for vasopressors after overdose has been infrequent. If profound hypotension resistant to dopamine were to occur, other vasopressors, such as epinephrine and norepinephrine, can be used. Laboratory analysis should be used to monitor electrolytes, especially sodium and potassium. ACE inhibitor serum concentrations are not readily available and have little, if any, clinical utility. Because ACE inhibitors may potentiate the effects of the opiate-like beta-endorphins, some authors have suggested the use of naloxone to reverse their toxicities. Successes and failures with naloxone have been described in case reports. Because naloxone has limited adverse effects, its use could be considered in the management of serious ACE inhibitor toxicity. One case report describes the use of the experimental exogenous angiotensin II to counter severe ACE inhibitor toxicity. The pharmacokinetic characteristics of the ACE inhibitors, limited protein binding, and small volume of distribution make them amenable to hemodialysis. Because major morbidity is rare with these agents, the need for dialysis is questionable.

Angioedema with potential for airway obstruction may not respond to epinephrine and antihistamines. Rapid intubation to protect the airway may be necessary in patients with angioedema.

See also: Beta-Blockers; Calcium Channel Blockers; Cardiovascular System; Gastrointestinal System.

Further Reading

Augenstein, W.L., Kulig, K.W., Rumack, B.H., 1988. Captopril overdose resulting in hypotension. JAMA J. Am. Med. Assoc. 259, 3302–3305.

Christie, G.A., Lucas, C., Bateman, D.N., Waring, W.S., 2006. Redefining the ACE-inhibitor dose response relationship: substantial blood pressure lowering after massive doses. Eur. J. Clin. Pharmacol. 62, 989–993.

Gang, C., Lindsell, C.J., Moellman, J., Sublett, W., Hart, K., Collins, S., Bernstein, J.A., 2013. Factors associated with hospitalization of patients with angiotensin-converting enzyme inhibitor-induced angioedema. Allergy Asthma Proc. 34 (3), 267–273.

Lucas, C., Christie, G.A., Waring, W.S., 2006. Rapid onset of hemodynamic effects after angiotensin converting enzyme-inhibitor overdose: implications for initial patient triage. Emerg. Med. J. 23, 854–857.

Park, H., Purnell, G.V., Mirchandani, H.G., 1998. Suicide by captopril overdose. J. Toxicol. Clin. Toxicol. 28 (3), 379–382.

Remko, M., 2006. Acidity, lipophilicity, solubility, absorption, and polar surface area of some ACE inhibitors. Chem. Pap. 61 (2), 133–141.

Valekar, M., Craig, T.J., 2012. ACE inhibitor-induced angioedema. Curr. Allergy Asthma Rep. 12 (1), 72–78.

Acenaphthene

SJ Klein, Manchester College, North Manchester, IN, USA

This article is a revision of the previous edition article by Sanjay Chanda & Harihara M. Mehendale, volume 1, pp 11–13, © 2005, Elsevier Inc.

- Name: Acenaphthene
- Chemical Abstracts Service Registry Number: CAS 83-32-9
- Synonyms: 1,2-Dihydroacenaphthylene; 1,8-Dihydroacenaphthalene; 1,8-Ethylenenaphthalene; Acenaphthylene; Naphthyleneethylene; Periethylenenaphthalene; Ethylenenaphthylene
- Chemical/Pharmaceutical/Other Class: Arene belonging to the class of polycyclic aromatic hydrocarbons (PAH)
- Molecular Formula: $C_{12}H_{10}$
- Chemical Structure:

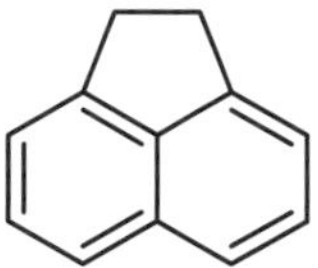

Uses

Acenaphthene is a chemical intermediate used to produce naphthalimide dyes, which are used as fluorescent whitening agents, and used in manufacturing plastics, resins, insecticides, and fungicides.

Background Information

Acenaphthene is a component of crude oil and a product of incomplete combustion of wood, diesel fuel, and garbage, which may be produced and released to the environment during natural fires. Emissions from cigarette smoke, petroleum refining, coal tar distillation, coal combustion, and diesel fueled engines are the major contributors of acenaphthene to the environment. Acenaphthene is used as a chemical intermediate and may be released to the environment via manufacturing effluents and the disposal of manufacturing waste by-products. Because of the widespread use of acenaphthene in a variety of products, acenaphthene may also be released to the environment through landfills, municipal wastewater treatment facilities, and waste incinerators. Acenaphthene should biodegrade rapidly in the environment. The reported biodegradation half-lives for acenaphthene in aerobic soil and surface waters range from 10 to 60 and from 1 to 25 days, respectively. However, acenaphthene may persist under anaerobic conditions or at high concentration due to toxicity to microorganisms. Acenaphthene is not expected to hydrolyze or bioconcentrate in the environment; yet, it should undergo direct photolysis in sunlight environmental media. Acenaphthene is expected to exist entirely in the vapor phase in ambient air.

Environment Fate and Behavior

Routes and Pathways

A Henry's law constant of 1.55×10^{-4} atm m^3 mol^{-1} at 251°C suggests volatilization of acenaphthene from environmental waters may be important. Solubility in water is 100 mg l^{-1}, while solubility in organic solvents such as toluene and ethanol is substantially greater.

Partition Behavior in Water, Sediment, and Soil

A calculated K_{oc} range of 2065–3230 indicates acenaphthene will be slightly mobile in soil. In aquatic systems, acenaphthene can partition from the water column to organic matter contained in sediments and suspended solids.

Environmental Persistency

The reported biodegradation half-lives for acenaphthene in aerobic soil and surface waters range from 10 to 60 and from 1 to 25 days, respectively. However, acenaphthene may persist under anaerobic conditions or at high concentrations due to toxicity to microorganisms.

Bioaccumulation

Acenaphthene is not expected to hydrolyze or bioconcentrate in the environment; yet, it should undergo direct photolysis in sunlit environmental media. The volatilization half-lives from a model river and a model pond, the latter considers the effect of adsorption, have been estimated to be 11 h and 39 days, respectively. The fungus *Cunninghamella elegans* metabolized within 72 h of incubation 64% of acenaphthene present. Acenaphthene is expected to exist entirely in the vapor phase in ambient air. In the atmosphere, the photochemical reactions with hydroxyl radicals, nitrate radical and ozone are likely to be important fate processes.

Exposure and Exposure Monitoring

Routes and Pathways

Skin contact is the most common accidental exposure pathway. Acenaphthene may irritate or burn skin. Exposure can also be through ingestion or inhalation. Its vapor can be poisonous if inhaled. Laboratory animals have developed tumors when exposed to acenaphthene in their food.

Human Exposure

The most probable human exposure would be occupational exposure, which may occur through dermal contact or inhalation at places where acenaphthene is produced or used.

Environmental Exposure

Atmospheric workplace exposures have been documented. Nonoccupational exposures would most likely occur via cigarette smoke, urban atmospheres, contaminated drinking water supplies, and recreational contaminated waterways.

Toxicokinetics

The half-life of acenaphthene in the bluegill fish is less than 1 day. A *Beijerinckia* species and a mutant strain, *Beijerinckia* species strain B8/36, were shown to oxidize acenaphthene. Both organisms oxidize acenaphthene to the same spectrum of metabolites, which included 1-acenaphthenol, 1-acenaphtheneone, 1,2-acenaphthenediol, acenaphthenequinone, and a compound that was tentatively identified as 1,2-dihydroxyacenaphthylene.

Mechanism of Toxicity

5-Nitroacenaphthene causes toxicity by the reduction of the nitro function to the corresponding hydroxylamine. These arylhydroxylamines may be either direct-acting mutagens or may become so following nonenzymic conversion to aryl nitronium ions or they may be esterified to the corresponding electrophilic hydroxamic acid esters. Acenaphthene can bind to hemoglobin to cause methemoglobinemia.

Acute and Short-Term Toxicity (or Exposure)

Animal

Acenaphthene can cause hepatotoxicity in rats and mice. Little information is available regarding acute exposure to acenaphthene. It is biotransformed in the liver. On the basis of a mouse oral subchronic study in which hepatotoxicity was seen as the major effect, the no-observed-adverse-effect level and the lowest-observed-adverse-effect level were 175 and 350 mg kg^{-1} day^{-1}, respectively.

Human

Acenaphthene can be irritating to eyes, skin, and mucous membrane. Acenaphthene may be poisonous if inhaled or absorbed through skin. The vapor may cause dizziness or suffocation. Acenaphthene may cause vomiting if swallowed in large quantity. It can cause methemoglobinemia. There is evidence that acenaphthene is photomutagenic, therefore skin exposure to acenaphthene at the same time as exposure to sunlight is ill-advised.

Chronic Toxicity (or Exposure)

Animal

Rats exposed to acenaphthene at a level of 1271.5 mg m^{-3} for 4 h a day, 6 days per week for 5 months showed toxic effects on the blood, lung, and glandular constituents. The bronchial epithelium showed hyperplasia and metaplasia, which may have been symptoms of the pneumonia that killed a large number of rats during the study. No signs of malignancy appeared during the 8-month postexposure observation period.

Human

Chronic human exposure data are not available. Currently, acenaphthene is under review by US Environmental Protection Agency for evidence of human carcinogenic potential. This does not imply that this agent is necessarily a carcinogen. Experimental evidence up to this point is not conclusive. The nitroderivative of acenaphthene (5-nitroacenaphthene) is a possible carcinogen to humans.

Genotoxicity

Experiments on several strains of bacteria, including *Salmonella Typhimurium* and *Micrococcus pyogenes* var, *aerius* strain FDA209 showed no evidence of mutagenicity.

Carcinogenicity

No evidence of carcinogenicity is available. Some studies have been conducted on a mixture of polyaromatic hydrocarbons that include acenaphthene as one of several components. Individual data on acenaphthene is not available.

Clinical Management

The victim should be moved to fresh air and emergency medical care should be provided. If the victim is not breathing, artificial respiration should be provided; if breathing is difficult, oxygen should be administered. In case of contact with the eyes, the eyes should be flushed immediately with running water for at least 15 min. Affected skin should be washed with soap and water. Contaminated clothing and shoes should be removed and isolated at the site. If methemoglobinemia occurs and is severe, treatment with methylene blue and oxygen is recommended.

Ecotoxicology

Freshwater/Sediment Organisms Toxicity

Treatment of cherry-mazzard hybrid seeds with acenaphthene powder for 10 h inhibited the seed germination and seedling growth. Treatment of *Allium cepa* root meristem cells with acenaphthene vapor for 12–96 h caused anomalies leading to random development of cells.

Marine Organisms Toxicity

Acute toxicity value for bluegill fish was 1700 μg l^{-1} in freshwater and the toxicity to sheepshead minnow was 2230 μg l^{-1} in saltwater. Toxicity to algae occurs at levels as low as 500 μg l^{-1}.

Terrestrial Organisms Toxicity

The oral LD_{50} for rats is reported as 10 mg kg^{-1} and for mice the LD_{50} is 2.1 mg kg^{-1}.

Exposure Standards and Guidelines

CERCLA reportable quantities: Persons in charge of vessels or facilities are required to notify the National Response Center (NRC) immediately, when there is a release of this designated hazardous substance, in an amount equal to or greater than its reportable quantity of 100 lb or 45.4 kg. State drinking water guidelines: Minnesota 400 mg l^{-1} and Florida 20 mg l^{-1}.

See also: Polycyclic Aromatic Hydrocarbons (PAHs); Naphthalene.

Further Reading

Byrne, M., et al., 1985. Exposure and risk assessment for benzo(a)pyrene and other polycyclic aromatic hydrocarbons. GRA&I vol. 3 (21).

Cavallari, J.M., Zwack, L.M., Lange, C.R., Herrick, R.F., McClean, M.D., 2012. Temperature-dependent emission concentrations of polycyclic aromatic hydrocarbons in paving and built-up roofing asphalts. Ann. Occup. Hyg. 56 (2), 148–160.

Harris, J., Perwak, J., Coons, S., 1985. Exposure and risk assessment for benzo(a) pyrene and other polycyclic aromatic hydrocarbons. GRA&I vol. 1 (21).

Jennings, A.A., 2012. Worldwide regulatory guidance values for surface soil exposure to noncarcinogenic polycyclic aromatic hydrocarbons. J. Environ. Manage. 101, 173–190.

Jensen, J., Sverdrup, L.E., 2003. Polycyclic aromatic hydrocarbon ecotoxicity data for developing soil quality criteria. Rev. Environ. Contam. Toxicol. 179, 73–97.

Pothuluri, J.A., et al., 1992. Fungal metabolism of acenaphthene by *Cunninghamella elegans*. Appl. Environ. Microbiol. 58, 3654–3659.

Reisen, F., Arey, J., 2002. Reactions of hydroxyl radical and ozone with acenaphthene and acenaphthylene. Environ. Sci. Technol. 36, 4302–4311.

Staples, C.A., Werner, A.F., 1985. Priority pollutant assessment in the USA: scientific and regulatory implications. Toxic Subst. 6 (4), 186–200.

US Department of Health & Human Services/Agency for Toxic Substances Disease Registry, (1995). Toxicological Profile for Polycyclic Aromatic Hydrocarbons (Update), NTIS# PB/95/264370.

USEPA, 1979. Health Assessment Document: Polycyclic Organic Matter, EPA-600/ 9-79-008.

USEPA, 1980a. Ambient Water Quality Criteria Doc: Acenaphthene (Draft).

USEPA, 1980b. Ambient Water Quality Criteria Doc: Polynuclear Aromatic Hydrocarbons (Draft).

Wilkins, E.S., Wilkins, M.G., 1985. Review of toxicity of gases emitted from combustion pyrolysis of municipal and industrial wastes. J. Environ. Sci. Health A 20 (2).

Yan, J., et al., 2004. Photomutagenicity of 16 polycyclic aromatic hydrocarbons from US EPA priority pollutant list. Mutat. Res. 557 (1), 99–108.

Relevant Websites

http://www.atsdr.cdc.gov – Agency for Toxic Substances and Disease Registry. Toxicological Profile for Acenaphthene.

http://www.inchem.org/documents/ehc/ehc/ehc202.htm – Selected Non-heterocyclic Polycyclic Aromatic Hydrocarbons

Acephate

S Karanth, Charles River Laboratories, Preclinical Services-Nevada, Reno, NV, USA

- Chemical Structure:

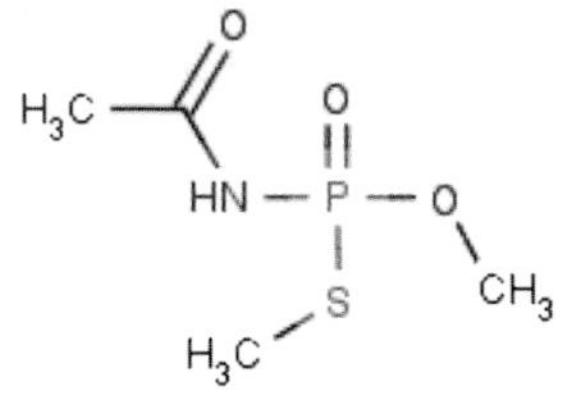

Background

Acephate was first registered in the United States in 1973 as an insecticide on ornamentals. The first food uses (agricultural crops) for acephate were registered in 1974. Acephate is sold as a soluble powder or emulsifiable concentrates or pressurized aerosol; the trade names for products containing acephate include Orthene, Asataf, Pillarthene, Kitron, Aimthane, Ortran, Ortho 12420, and Ortril.

Uses

Acephate is registered for use on a variety of food crops and citrus trees. It is also used commonly in food handling establishments, in horticulture on ornamental plants (cut flowers), and on home lawns and commercial buildings and as seed treatment on cotton and peanuts (seed for planting), on nonbearing crops such as citrus, and on tobacco. It is effective against a wide range of biting and sucking insects, especially aphids.

Environmental Fate

Acephate dissipates rapidly in soil (half-lives of <3 and 6 days). Methamidophos and CO_2 are reported to be the major metabolites in the soil. Acephate is readily degraded in soil by microorganisms and in water it undergoes rapid hydrolysis.

Exposure and Exposure Monitoring

Common routes of acephate exposure include ingestion and inhalation.

Acephate and its metabolite are not persistent under aerobic conditions and are not expected to leach to groundwater. Its rapid degradation makes it nonthreatening to groundwater or surface water.

Toxicokinetics

Acephate is converted to another organophosphate compound, methamidophos, in the body. Studies with ^{14}C-acephate in mammals have shown 75% of the parent compound eliminated in the urine. Other major metabolites include *O,S*-dimethyl phosphorothioate (DMPT, 5%) and S-methyl acetyl phosphoramidothioate (5%).

Mechanism of Toxicity

Acephate exerts its toxicity by inhibiting the enzyme acetylcholinesterase in the synapse and neuromuscular junctions, which leads to accumulation of the neurotransmitter acetylcholine and overstimulation of postsynaptic receptors.

Acute and Short-Term Toxicity

Animal

Acephate is moderately toxic to mammals with an acute oral LD_{50} of 850–950 mg kg^{-1} in rats, whereas its metabolite methamidophos is highly toxic to mammals. The common symptoms of acephate poisoning include salivation, nasal discharge, vomiting, diarrhea, nausea, blurred vision, difficulty in breathing, headache, and muscle weakness. Convulsions, coma, and death may occur in cases of severe acute poisoning.

Human

Acephate exposure can result in cholinesterase inhibition, which causes over excitation of the central and peripheral nervous system. Acephate is nonirritating to skin and slightly irritating to the eyes but is not reported to be a skin sensitizer.

Chronic Toxicity

Animal

Chronic studies in rats and dogs have shown cholinesterase inhibition. Following exposure to acephate in diet (up to 300 mg kg^{-1}), no effects on body weight gain or histopathological changes were observed in rats. Additional chronic dietary exposure studies in rats at concentrations of 0, 2, 5, 10, and 150 ppm for 13 weeks have indicated cholinesterase inhibition in the brain and red blood cells at all doses.

Human

Individuals exposed to acephate for up to 15 months in pilot plant and formulation processes did not show any adverse effects.

Immunotoxicity

Dermal studies in guinea pigs did not show any skin sensitization reaction. Acute acephate exposure in control or

 http://dx.doi.org/10.1016/B978-0-12-386454-3.00090-7

IL-1-challenged rats indicated suppressed blood CD4, CD8, B cells and monocytes, and increased blood neutrophil counts. Subacute acephate exposure at low concentrations has been reported to affect immune responses in avian species.

Reproductive Toxicity

A two-generation reproductive toxicity study in rats indicated various reproductive effects including fetal losses, decreased litter weights at 50 ppm (2.5 mg kg^{-1} day^{-1}) dose level.

Genotoxicity

While *in vivo* studies in mice indicated no mutagenic potential, *in vitro* bacterial and mammalian tests have shown that acephate is weakly mutagenic/genotoxic.

Carcinogenicity

While no human carcinogenicity data are available, acephate is classified as a possible human carcinogen (category C) based on increased incidence of hepatocellular carcinomas and adenomas in female mice.

Clinical Management

In case of dermal exposure, the contaminated area should be washed with plenty of water or showered using soap and shampoo. Eyes should be flushed with water repeatedly for several minutes. Contaminated clothing should be removed and the airway cleared. In case of ingestion, vomiting should be induced. Atropine treatment should be initiated immediately to counteract muscarinic effects. Atropine (adults and children >12 years: 2–4 mg; children <12 years: 0.05–0.1 mg) treatment should be repeated every 15 min until oral and bronchial secretions are controlled and atropinization is achieved. The duration and dosage of atropine treatment should be slowly reduced as the condition of the patient improves. Pralidoxime should be administered slowly at the recommended dosage (adults and children >12 years: 1–2 g; children <12 years: 20–50 mg by IV infusion in 100 ml saline at approximately 0.2 g min). This dosage can be repeated at every 1–2 h intervals initially and at 10–12 h intervals later depending on the condition of the patient. Periodic medical examination and care is required depending on the degree of exposure.

Ecotoxicology

Acephate is considered relatively nontoxic to fish. In field studies, aerial spraying of acephate did not result in significant brain AChE inhibition in trout and salmon in streams near the target area, but a significant AChE inhibition was reported in suckers.

Acephate is considered moderately toxic to upland game birds. The LD_{50} for acephate in mallard ducks is 350 mg kg^{-1}; 140 mg kg^{-1} in pheasants; >5000 ppm for the mallard and 1280 ppm for the bobwhite quail.

Acephate is considered toxic to bees with an LC_{50} of 1.2 μg per bee. In studies of insecticides commonly used in cotton, acephate was shown to be very toxic to adult *Microplitis croceipes* parasitoids, and caused 100% mortality at the lowest recommended field rates.

Exposure Standards and Guidelines

Acceptable daily intake (ADI) = 0–0.01 mg kg^{-1} body weight.

Reference dose (RfD) = 0.004 mg kg^{-1} day^{-1}.

See also: Acetylcholine; Cholinesterase Inhibition; Methamidophos; Neurotoxicity; Organophosphorus Compounds; Pesticides.

Further Reading

Singh, A.K., Jiang, Y., 2002. Immunotoxicity of acute acephate exposure in control or IL-1-challenged rats: correlation between the immune cell composition and corticosteroid concentration in blood. J. Appl. Toxicol. 22, 279.

Tripathia, S.M., Thakera, A.M., Joshib, C.G., Sankhalaa, L.N., 2012. Acephate immunotoxicity in white leghorn cockerel chicks upon experimental exposure. Environ. Toxicol. Pharmacol. 34, 192.

Relevant Websites

http://www.cdpr.ca.gov/docs/risk/toxsums/pdfs/1685.pdf – California Environmental Protection Agency.

http://extoxnet.orst.edu/pips/acephate.htm – EXTOXNET (Extension Toxicology Network), Oregon State University.

http://www.inchem.org/documents/jmpr/jmpmono/v076pr02.htm – International Programme on Chemical Safety.

ftp://ftp.fao.org/docrep/fao/006/y5221E/y5221E00.pdf – Pesticide residues in food (2003).

http://www.epa.gov/opp00001/reregistration/REDs/acephate_red.pdf – US Environmental Protection Agency.

http://www.epa.gov/oppsrrd1/reregistration/acephate/ – US Environmental Protection Agency.

Acetaldehyde

TR Van Vleet and BK Philip, Bristol-Myers Squibb, Mt. Vernon, IN, USA

This article is a revision of the previous edition article by John Sanseverino, volume 1, pp 15–17, © 2005, Elsevier Inc.

- Name: Acetaldehyde
- Chemical Abstracts Service Registry Number: 75-07-0
- Synonyms: Acetic aldehyde, Acetic ethanol, Acetylaldehyde; Ethylaldehyde, Ethanal
- Chemical/Pharmaceutical/Other Class: Aldehydes
- Molecular Formula: C_2H_4O
- Chemical Structure:

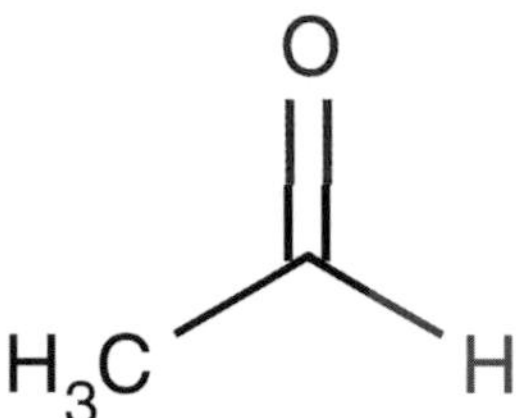

Uses

Acetaldehyde is used in the manufacturing of various chemicals such as acetic acid, pyridine, peracetic acid, pentaerythritol, 1,3-butylene glycol, vinyl acetate resins, synthetic pyridine derivatives, perfumes, flavors, and chloral. Synthetic pyridine derivatives, in particular, account for 40% of acetaldehyde demand. It is also used in the silvering of mirrors, leather tanning, and in fuel compositions, preservatives, paper processing, glues, cosmetics, dyes, plastics, rubber, and as a flavoring agent. Natural sources of acetaldehyde include metabolic intermediate in higher plants, alcohol fermentation, natural combustion, oxidation of hydrocarbons commonly found in the atmosphere, and sugar decomposition in the body. Acetaldehyde is also found in small amounts in alcoholic beverages, plant juices, roasted coffee, and tobacco smoke. Anthropogenic sources include vehicle exhaust, fuel oil, coal, and organic chemical manufacturing.

Environmental Fate and Behavior

Industrial exposures to acetaldehyde are most likely to occur by inhalation with potential for skin and eye contact. Accidental ingestion is also possible. The main source of exposure to acetaldehyde in humans is alcohol consumption and to a lesser extent from air, vehicle exhaust, and from various industrial wastes. Degradation of hydrocarbons, sewage, and solid biological wastes produces acetaldehyde, as well as the open burning and incineration of gas, fuel oil, and coal.

Toxicokinetics

Following inhalation exposure, acetaldehyde is deposited in the nasal cavity and upper respiratory tract, and eventually some traces can be absorbed into the blood and be distributed throughout the body. The uptake of acetaldehyde in the nasal cavity is influenced by its solubility and inspiratory flow rate. Perhaps acetaldehyde uptake in the nasal tissue is dependent on its reaction with tissue substrates that become depleted at high exposure concentrations. Acetaldehyde vapor can be metabolized in the nasal cavity by the mixed-function oxidase and carboxyl esterase systems. The first metabolite of ethanol metabolism is acetaldehyde. Metabolism takes place in the liver to a number of metabolites and some unchanged acetaldehyde gets excreted in the urine and primarily via exhaled breath.

Mechanism of Toxicity

Acetaldehyde is soluble in the mucous membranes of the upper respiratory tract causing irritation of the mucous membranes' sensory nerve endings. It has a general narcotic action and there is also depression of the mucociliary defense system. The direct action of acetaldehyde in the skin and eyes is the result of irritation to these tissues. Large doses may cause death from respiratory paralysis. Acetaldehyde forms stable and unstable adducts with proteins impairing protein function, histone–DNA binding, and inhibition of polymerization of tubulin. Acetaldehyde can react with various macromolecules in the body leading to marked alterations in the biological function of these molecules.

There have been several reports linking metabolism of ethanol to acetaldehyde with the additive potential associated with alcohol consumption. Although these reports are still somewhat controversial, it is possible that acetaldehyde, as a metabolite of ethanol or as a constituent of other products (such as tobacco smoke), may play a contributory role in addictions to these substances. Acetaldehyde exposure produces self-administrative behaviors in animal models.

Acute and Short-Term Toxicity (or Exposure)

Animal

Acute exposure in several species resulted in irritation of respiratory tract, skin, and hypotension. The oral LD_{50} for acetaldehyde in rats has been reported to be 1930 mg kg^{-1} and the 4 h LC_{50} is approximately 13 300 ppm. Acetaldehyde is a severe eye irritant to rabbits at 40 mg and mildly irritating to rabbit skin at 500 mg. Rats exposed to acetaldehyde concentrations ranging from 400 to 5000 ppm via inhalation route (4 week at 6 h day^{-1}, 5 days $week^{-1}$) exhibited slight degeneration of the olfactory epithelium at $\geq$400 ppm and growth retardation and polyuria at 1000 and 2200 ppm.

 http://dx.doi.org/10.1016/B978-0-12-386454-3.00994-5

Human

Acetaldehyde is a metabolic intermediate in humans. It has been identified in food, beverages, and cigarette smoke. Acetaldehyde is metabolized primarily in the liver to a lesser extent in renal tubules by acetaldehyde dehydrogenase. Ethanol-induced liver damage, facial flushing, and developmental effects have been attributed to acetaldehyde. Inhalation exposures to acetaldehyde can result in irritation of eyes and upper respiratory tract. The potent irritant effect of acetaldehyde inhalation (coughing, and burning in the eyes, nose, and throat) typically prevents exposures sufficient to result in depression of the central nervous system. Inhalation at concentrations ranging from 100 to 200 ppm can cause irritation to the mucous membranes. Skin and eye contact with liquid acetaldehyde can produce a burning sensation, lacrimation, and blurred vision.

Chronic Toxicity (or Exposure)

Animal

A 52 week chronic inhalation study in hamsters exposed to 1500 ppm acetaldehyde produced growth retardation, slight anemia, increased enzyme and protein content in the urine, and increased kidney weight. There were distinct histopathological changes in the nasal mucosa and trachea, including hyperplasia, squamous cell metaplasia, and inflammation. Inhalation exposure to acetaldehyde has produced nasal tumors in rats and laryngeal tumors in hamsters. Male and female rats were exposed to acetaldehyde 6 h day^{-1}, 5 days $week^{-1}$ for 28 months at concentrations of 0, 750, 1500, or 3000 ppm. Inhalation exposure to acetaldehyde resulted in dose-related incidence of nasal adenocarcinomas and squamous cell carcinomas of the respiratory epithelium in rats and nasal and laryngeal carcinomas in hamsters. Acetaldehyde is teratogenic in rats and mice. Fetuses from dams injected intraperitoneally with acetaldehyde concentrations ranging from 50 to 100 mg kg^{-1} on day 10, 11, or 12 of gestation produced a significant increase in fetal resorptions, growth retardation, and an increase in malformations, including digital anomalies, cranial and facial malformations, and delayed skeletogenesis. It was concluded that acetaldehyde interfered with placental function via the maternal–placental nutrient exchange, resulting in retarded growth. Overall, there is sufficient evidence in experimental animals for the carcinogenicity and teratogenicity of acetaldehyde. Based on increased incidence of nasal tumors in male and female rats and laryngeal tumors in male and female hamsters after inhalation exposure, IARC classified acetaldehyde as a Group 2B carcinogen (Probable Human Carcinogen).

Human

Acetaldehyde, produced from the metabolism of ethanol, may also be responsible for localized cancers, brain damage in prenatal infants, and growth suppression (in chicken embryos). Acetaldehyde, as a direct result of ethanol metabolism in the body, has been implicated in alcoholic cardiomyopathy and cancer of the digestive tract. Acetaldehyde DNA adducts have been observed in the lymphocytes of human alcohol abusers. Esophageal tumors have been reportedly associated with genetic polymorphisms that result in high acetaldehyde levels after ethanol consumption, but there is inadequate evidence to associate carcinogenicity in humans with acetaldehyde exposure. The levels of acetaldehyde in blood are directly correlated with ethanol consumption.

Genotoxicity

Acetaldehyde has been shown to induce mutagenic changes in many assays. In mammalian *in vitro* assays, acetaldehyde produced sister chromatid exchanges and chromosomal breaks and aberrations in human lymphocytes and in cultured Chinese hamster ovary cells in a dose-related manner. Acetaldehyde at concentrations as low as 3–10 μM inhibited DNA methyltransferase activity *in vitro*. Acetaldehyde caused mutations in *Escherichia coli* systems and *Drosophila melanogaster*. A suppressive effect on rat testicular steroidogenesis was reported at concentration as low as 50 μM (2.2 μg ml^{-1}). Incubation of acetaldehyde (100 mg%) with isolated hepatocytes for 60 min significantly increased lipid peroxide formation.

Clinical Management

The primary risk for exposures of medical importance is via inhalation. Exposures by inhalation should be monitored for respiratory tract irritation, bronchitis, or pneumonitis. Humidified supplemental 100% oxygen should be administered. Gastric lavage may be indicated soon after ingestion of acetaldehyde followed by administration of activated charcoal slurry mixed with a saline cathartic or sorbitol. Exposed eyes should be irrigated with copious amounts of tepid water for at least 15 min. If eye irritation, pain, swelling, lacrimation, or photophobia persists, the patient should be seen in a health care facility.

Exposure Standards and Guidelines

A short-term exposure limit ceiling of 25 ppm for acetaldehyde was recommended to prevent excessive eye irritation, lacrimation, and potential injury to the respiratory tract. The FAO/WHO acceptable daily intake is 0.0–2.5 mg kg^{-1} body weight. The level of use as a food additive (flavorings) is 1–300 ppm.

Further Reading

Eriksson, C., 2001. The role of acetaldehyde in the actions of alcohol. Alcohol. Clin. Exp. Res. 25 (5 Suppl.), 15S–32S.

Peana, A., Muggironi, B., Diana, M., 2010. Acetaldehyde-reinforcing effects: a study on oral self-administration behavior. Front. Psychiatry 1 (23).

Verschueren, K., 2000. Handbook of Environmental Data on Organic Chemicals, third ed. Wiley, New York.

World Health Organization, 1999. Acetaldehyde. World Health Organization, Lyon.

Relevant Websites

http://www.cdc.gov/niosh/npg/npgd0001.html – Centers for Disease Control and Prevention: NIOSH Pocket Guide to Chemical Hazards - Acetaldehyde.

http://www.pesticideinfo.org/Detail_Chemical.jsp?Rec_Id=PC35597 – PAN Pesticides Database - Chemicals: Acetaldehyde.

Acetamide

GL Kennedy, DuPont Company-Consultant, Health and Environmental Sciences, Wilmington, DE, USA

- Chemical Abstracts Service Registry Number: CAS 60-35-5
- Synonyms: Acetic acid amide; Ethanamide; Methanecarboxamide
- Molecular Formula: C_2–H_5–N–O
- Structure:

O
H_3C NH_2

Uses

As a dipolar solvent, acetamide finds many uses as a solvent for both inorganic and organic compounds. The solvency has led to widespread uses in industry including applications in cryoscopy, soldering, and the textile industry. The neutral and amphoteric characteristics allow its use as an antacid in the lacquer, explosives, and cosmetics industries. Its hygroscopic properties make it useful as a plasticizer in coatings, fixtures, cloth, and leather, and as a humectant for paper. It is also a raw material in organic synthesis of methylamine and thioacetamide and as an intermediate in preparation of medicines, insecticides, and plastics.

Environmental Behavior, Fate, Routes, and Pathways

Acetamide will exist as a vapor in the ambient atmosphere. Atmospheric degradation occurs by reaction with photochemically produced hydroxyl radicals. The half-life for this reaction in air is estimated to be 7.6 days. If released to soil, acetamide is expected to have very high mobility and is not expected to adsorb to suspended solids and sediment. Experiments suggest that this chemical may break down in the environment through biodegradation and not through hydrolysis. Volatilization from water surfaces is not expected to be an important fate process based on this compound's estimated Henry's law constant.

Exposure and Exposure Monitoring

Acetamide may be inhaled, swallowed, or absorbed through the skin. In its usual application, inhalation is the most common route of exposure, although dermal contact is always possible.

Toxicokinetics

Oral administration of acetamide in the rat is followed by absorption and 62% is excreted into the urine unchanged in 24 h. Likewise, a large proportion of an oral dose is excreted in the urine unchanged by the dog and the cat. In sheep, absorption of an oral dose is followed by metabolism to CO_2 within 7–12 h. Sequential demethylation of methylacetamide results in acetamide production by rat liver but it is not clear whether this occurs in man. Acetamide is a metabolite of the antiprotozoal drugs metronidazole and ornidazole.

Mechanism of Toxicity

The mechanism of toxicity of acetamide is not known; the response profile is quite different from the better studied dimethyl derivative. Acetamide appears to be in a class of chemicals which, although producing liver cancer in rodents, is less sensitive to inactive in genetic tests looking at formation of micronuclei. The carcinogenic response in rodents appears related to the formation of hydroxylamine from the primary metabolite acetohydroxamic acid.

Acute and Short-Term Toxicity

The oral lethal dose 50 percent (LD_{50}) in rodents ranges from 1 to 7 g kg^{-1} and intravenous LD_{50} in mice and rats is 10 g kg^{-1}. No acute lethality information is available following either dermal or inhalation exposures.

The chemical is considered to be mildly irritating to the skin and eyes. Mild to no irritation to skin or mucous membranes seen in exposed individuals suggests that hydrolysis to lower molecular weight acids, which could cause damage, is not occurring. No other reports could be found in the literature concerning acute toxicity of acetamide in humans.

Chronic Toxicity

The liver appears to be the target of acetamide toxicity although the animal experiments have been limited in the range of endpoints studied. No reports could be found in the literature concerning the potential human health effects of chronic acetamide exposure.

Immunotoxicity

No studies could be found which examine the potential effects of acetamide on the immune system.

Reproductive and Developmental Toxicity

Acetamide is not a developmental toxicant. Although functional reproduction studies have not been completed, no evidence of altered spermatogenesis, hormone changes, or damage to accessory organs was seen in repeat dose studies in rodents.

 http://dx.doi.org/10.1016/B978-0-12-386454-3.00001-4

Genotoxicity

Acetamide was generally inactive in genetic tests *in vitro* including those using *Saccharomyces*, *Salmonella*, and *Aspergillus nidulans*. In a micronucleus test using hamster embryos *in vitro*, the chemical gave weakly positive genotoxic results but these were not confirmed by *in vivo* testing in mouse bone marrow cells. Microtubule assembly involving chromosome segregation can be affected by nonspecific solvent effects from lipophilic agents such as acetamide.

Carcinogenicity

Liver cancers were produced in rats following oral administration of relatively large amounts of acetamide.

Clinical Management

Exposed persons should be removed to fresh air, and medical attention sought as needed for any breathing difficulty. If swallowed, several glasses of water should be given to dilute the chemical; medical attention is needed if large amounts are ingested. For skin contact, the exposed area should be washed with soap and water; medical attention should be sought if irritation develops. For eye contact, water should be used to flush for at least 15 min while lifting the lower and upper eyelids occasionally; immediate medical attention should be sought.

Ecotoxicology

Because of the low bioconcentration potential, no serious effects in the aquatic environment are expected. Acetamide moves through the environment with water and is easily biodegraded as shown in a screening test with sewage inoculum.

Exposure Standards and Guidelines

US Environmental Protection Agency: Listed as a hazardous air pollutant under the Clean Air Act of 1990.

Occupational Safety and Health Administration: No permissible exposure limit (as of October 2003).

US Environmental Protection Agency: Carcinogenic Classification in Group C (possible human carcinogen).

International Agency for Research on Cancer: Classified as a 2B carcinogen (probable human carcinogen with sufficient evidence in laboratory animals).

See also: Clean Air Act (CAA), US; Methylamine; Metronidazole; Thioacetamide.

Further Reading

Kennedy Jr., G.L., 1986. Biological effects of acetamide, formamide, and their monomethyl and dimethyl derivatives. Crit. Rev. Toxicol. 17, 129–182.

Kennedy Jr., G.L., 2001. Biological effects of acetamide, formamide, and their monomethyl and dimethyl derivatives: An update. Crit. Rev. Toxicol. 31, 139–222.

Relevant Website

http://toxnet.nlm.nih.gov – TOXNET, Specialized Information Services, National Library of Medicine. Search for Acetamide.

Acetaminophen

K Shankar, University of Arkansas for Medical Sciences, Little Rock, AR, USA
HM Mehendale, University of Louisiana at Monroe, Monroe, LA, USA

- Name: Acetaminophen
- Chemical Abstracts Service Registry Number: 103-90-2
- Synonyms: APAP, 4′-Hydroxyacetanilide, *P*-hydroxyacetanilide, Acetamide *N*-(4-hydroxyphenyl), *N*-acetyl-*p*-aminophenol, *N*-acetyl-*p*-aminophenol, *P*-acetamidophenol; 4-Acetamidophenol, 4-Acetaminophenol, Paracetamol, Tylenol
- Pharmaceutical Class: Acetaminophen is a synthetic nonopioid congener of acetanilide in the paraaminophenol class
- Molecular Formula: $C_8H_9NO_2$
- Chemical Structure:

HO—C_6H_4—NH—C(=O)—CH_3

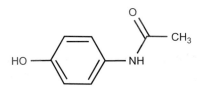

Uses

Acetaminophen is a nonnarcotic analgesic and antipyretic drug. It is used to relieve pain of moderate intensity, such as usually occurs in headache and in many muscle, joint, and peripheral nerve disorders. Headaches are one of the most common indications for the use of acetaminophen. Acetaminophen is used to treat acute tension headaches and mild to moderate migraine, especially in combination with caffeine and aspirin. Acetaminophen is indicated in chronic pain associated with rheumatoid arthritis, back or hip pain, osteoarthritis, dental pain, or acute pain due to soft-tissue injury. Acetaminophen is a suitable substitute for aspirin for its analgesic or antipyretic uses in cases where aspirin is contraindicated (gastric bleeding) or when the prolongation of bleeding time caused by aspirin would be a disadvantage. Acetaminophen has been used in studies of pain relief following obstetric and gynecological procedures, including Caesarean section, hysterectomy, tubal ligation, primary dysmenorrhea, and termination of pregnancy. Acetaminophen is also used to manage chronic pain of cancer, postpartum pain, and postoperative pain after minor surgery. In a double-blind crossover study, the analgesic oral butorphanol, and acetaminophen in combination, showed additive analgesic effects against moderate to severe pain due to metastatic carcinoma over that of the individual drug. Acetaminophen is also widely used as an antipyretic drug to reduce fever.

Background Information

Acetaminophen can be found as the active ingredient in more than 100 over-the-counter products and a number of prescription drugs, alone or in combination with other drugs. The pharmacology and toxicology of this drug have been extensively studied and reviewed. The first clinical use of acetaminophen dates back to 1893 by von Mering (and subsequently by Hinsberg and Treupel, 1894) as an effective antipyretic with comparable pharmacological effects to antipyrine and phenacetin. However, after a hiatus of almost half a century, acetaminophen was rediscovered as the major metabolite of phenacetin and acetanilide in man and was marketed in the United States as a combination with aspirin and caffeine in 1950. In the 1960s and 1970s, concerns about gastrointestinal adverse effects of aspirin and methemoglobinemia of acetanilide only led to increased popularity of acetaminophen as a generally safe antipyretic analgesic. Hepatotoxicity of acetaminophen began to be reported in the late 1960s and has been a topic of intense scientific evaluation to this day. The impact of acetaminophen-induced liver toxicity, accidental or otherwise, will be taken up in later sections.

Routes of Exposure

Acetaminophen is available in several dosage forms, including tablets, capsules, syrups, elixirs, and suppositories. Oral ingestion is the most common route for both accidental and intentional exposure to acetaminophen.

Toxicokinetics

Absorption of acetaminophen occurs in the gastrointestinal tract primarily by passive nonionic diffusion and is highly dependent on several factors, including dose, presence of food and other chemicals, mucosal blood flow, age, body weight, time of day, and coexisting disease condition. At pharmacological doses, acetaminophen is absorbed rapidly, with about 75–95% of the therapeutic oral dose being recovered in the urine by 12–24 h as unchanged acetaminophen or metabolite. A large number of studies have evaluated the pharmacokinetic parameters of acetaminophen in man after oral or intravenous dosing. Most studies consistently report volume of distribution to be between 0.8 and $1\,l\,kg^{-1}$. Total clearance and plasma half-life with therapeutic doses in healthy subjects were usually 3–$5\,ml\,min\,kg^{-1}$ and 1–3 h, respectively. After suprapharmacological or toxic doses, absorption may be delayed after producing peak blood concentrations at approximately 4 h postingestion. In humans, the majority of acetaminophen is metabolized in the liver to glucuronide and sulfate conjugates that are eliminated in the urine. Estimates in humans from urinary metabolites report 50–60% as glucuronide conjugate, 25–35% as sulfate conjugate, and between 2 and 5% of cysteine and mercapturate conjugates each. In young children, the sulfate conjugate predominates. The water-soluble glucuronide and sulfate conjugates are eliminated via the

 http://dx.doi.org/10.1016/B978-0-12-386454-3.00215-3

kidneys. Approximately 2–5% is eliminated in the urine as unchanged acetaminophen. The half-life of therapeutic dose is 1–3 h. In overdose patients, this may be increased to more than 4 h and may even exceed 12 h in patients with severe acetaminophen-induced liver toxicity.

Mechanism of Toxicity

Although a major part of the ingested dose of acetaminophen is detoxified, a very small proportion is metabolized via the cytochrome P450-mixed function oxidase pathway to a highly reactive *n*-acetyl-*p*-benzoquinoneimine (NAPQI). The toxic intermediate NAPQI is normally detoxified by endogenous glutathione to cysteine and mercapturic acid conjugates and excreted in the urine. Recent studies have shown that hepatic P450s, CYP2E1, and to a lesser extent CYP1A2 are responsible for conversion of acetaminophen to NAPQI. In acetaminophen overdose, the amount of NAPQI increases and depletes endogenous glutathione stores. Time course studies have shown that covalent binding of reactive NAPQI and subsequent toxicity occur only after cellular glutathione stores are reduced by 70% or more of normal. Mitochondrial dysfunction and damage can be seen as early as 15 min after a toxic dose in mice, suggesting that this may be a critical to cellular necrosis. The NAPQI is then thought to covalently bind to critical cellular macromolecules in hepatocytes and cause cell death. Recent proteomic studies have identified at least 20 known proteins that are covalently modified by the reactive acetaminophen metabolite. The resulting acetaminophen-cysteine (APAP-CYS) protein adducts can be quantified via a high-pressure liquid chromatography coupled with electrochemical detection (HPLC-EC). Hepatic necrosis and inflammation develop as a consequence of hepatocellular death, which results in development of clinical and laboratory findings consistent with liver failure. A similar mechanism is postulated for the renal damage that occurs in some patients following acetaminophen toxicity.

In the past two decades, several studies have indicated that acetaminophen is a powerful inducer of programmed cell death or apoptosis in addition to necrosis. Acetaminophen-induced apoptosis involves a complex interplay of cell signaling pathways involving the organelles mitochondria, nucleus, and cytoplasm. Key players that propel toxic events leading to various forms of cell deaths are oxidative stress (mediated by BRIs and ROS), intracellular perturbation of Ca^{2+}, and a complex interplay of proteolytic caspases.

Acute Toxicity

Animal

A large body of evidence is available examining the acute toxicity of acetaminophen in animal models. Mice and rats have been widely used to study the toxic effects of acetaminophen. Since the rat is relatively resistant, the mouse has been the most widely used species to study the mechanisms of acetaminophen toxicity and to examine chemicals that potentiate or protect from the toxicity. Hepatotoxicity and nephrotoxicity are the two main effects associated with acute overdose of acetaminophen. Of these, death in most species is due to acute hepatic failure. LD_{50} values range from 350 mg kg^{-1} to 4500 mg kg^{-1} depending on the species and the route of acetaminophen administration, mice (LD_{50} 350–600 mg kg^{-1}) being more far more sensitive than rats, guinea pigs, and rabbits ($LD_{50} > 3$ g kg^{-1}). Death occurs by 12 h after acetaminophen exposure. In mice after a toxic dose, general findings in addition to the severe hepatic necrosis include necrotic changes in the kidney, bronchiolar epithelium, testes, lymphoid follicles of the spleen, and small intestine. Cats are particularly susceptible to acetaminophen intoxication because of their impaired glucuronic acid conjugation mechanism and saturation of their sulfate conjugation pathway. The clinical signs associated with experimental acetaminophen administration to cats included cyanosis followed by anemia, hemoglobinuria, icterus, and facial edema. Laboratory findings in acetaminophen-poisoned cats include methemoglobinemia and an elevated serum alanine aminotransferase activity.

Human

Hepatotoxicity is the primary toxic insult from acute acetaminophen overdose. Acetaminophen overdose accounts for more than 56 000 emergency room visits and is implicated in nearly 50% of all acute liver failure in the United States (U.S. Acute Liver Failure Study Group). Exposure to toxic doses of acetaminophen may be due to intentional (suicidal) or unintentional (accidental). Recent data from Parkland Hospital suggest that greater percentages of unintentional overdose victims suffer from fatal consequences compared to persons attempting suicide (with acetaminophen) primarily due to their characteristic late presentation. Data from the U.S. ALF Study Group show that unintentional overdoses (which are more frequent in liver failure cases) were also larger (median dose of 34 g) compared to suicidal doses, being consumed over several preceding days. There is no clear agreement on a maximum tolerated dose of acetaminophen. Most people tolerate 4–8 g day^{-1} of acetaminophen without any hepatotoxic incidence. However, the risk of severe liver injury may be quite high above the 4 g day^{-1} dose, especially in a group of individuals due to indeterminate idiosyncratic reasons.

The typical clinical manifestations are secondary to hepatic damage. Plasma concentrations should be obtained to determine the probability of acetaminophen-induced hepatotoxicity. The Rumack-Matthews nomogram is used to assess the risk of hepatotoxicity. Levels in excess of 200 μg ml^{-1} of acetaminophen at 4 h postingestion are associated with a high probability of development of hepatotoxicity. A second treatment line 25% lower than the original 200 line was added at the request of the FDA in 1976. While not yet clinically available, newer methods of detecting APAP-toxicity include detection of APAP-cysteine adducts via HPLC-EC and via metabolomic analysis of urine samples (early-intervention pharmacometabolomics). The clinical presentation follows four distinct phases. Gastrointestinal irritation, nausea, and vomiting are present in the first 24 h postingestion. The second stage (24–48 h postingestion) is characterized by the resolution of the initial symptoms, accompanied by elevations of hepatic transaminases. Cases that progress to stage three develop hypoglycemia, coagulopathies, jaundice, and symptoms consistent with hepatic failure. Surviving patients go through a fourth stage of recovery. As toxicity develops, half-life becomes prolonged and transaminases rise and fall. In instances where reliable history of time of ingestion is not available, calculations of body burden may be useful in deciding treatment.

Chronic Toxicity

Animal

In a 2-year feed study, there was no evidence of carcinogenic activity of acetaminophen in male F344/N rats that received 600, 3000, or 6000 ppm acetaminophen for 104 weeks. There was equivocal evidence of carcinogenic activity in female F344/N rats based on increased incidences of mononuclear cell leukemia. Overall, there is inadequate evidence in experimental animals for the carcinogenicity of acetaminophen and is not classifiable as to its carcinogenicity. Acetaminophen was non-mutagenic in the *Salmonella*/mammalian microsome assay at concentrations ranging from 0.1 to 50 mg per plate. In a study to examine the effect of acetaminophen on reproduction and fertility, no changes in the number of pups/litter, viability, or adjusted pup weight were found. Acetaminophen in the diet of Swiss mice reduced weight gain during nursing. Fertility endpoints (ability to bear normal numbers of normal-weight young) were generally not affected.

Human

There is inadequate evidence in humans for the carcinogenicity of acetaminophen and it is not classifiable as to its carcinogenicity. The chronic ingestion of excessive amounts of acetaminophen may produce similar toxicity as a large acute dose but in a more insidious fashion. Age, chronic alcohol abuse, and preexisting disease may be contributing factors. The American Academy of Pediatrics considers use of acetaminophen safe during breast-feeding, and acetaminophen is classified as a category B chemical by the FDA (studies in laboratory animals have not demonstrated a fetal risk, but there are no controlled studies in pregnant women). Acetaminophen should be given with care to patients with impaired kidney or liver function. Acetaminophen should be given with care to patients taking other drugs that affect the liver.

In Vitro Toxicity

Acetaminophen causes cytotoxicity in several cell types; however, the most widely studied cytotoxicity of acetaminophen is in primary hepatocytes or hepatocyte cell lines.

Cytotoxicity in Hepatic Cells

Primary hepatocytes from rats, mice, hamsters, rabbits, dogs, pigs, monkeys, and humans have been shown to be susceptible to acetaminophen *in vitro*. The cytotoxicity of acetaminophen varies considerably depending on species, presumably due to differences in bioactivation and glutathione status. The most obvious morphological effect of acetaminophen in isolated primary hepatocytes is blebbing of the cell membrane. However, electron microscopy has shown that toxicity is associated with progressive loss of microvilli, mitochondrial abnormalities, and appearance of myeloid bodies. Exposure of primary mouse hepatocytes to concentrations of acetaminophen above 1 mM led to significant lactate dehydrogenase leakage in as soon as 3 h. Cytotoxicity of acetaminophen has also been examined using standard liver cell lines, including, PC12 cells, HepG2 cells, and H4IIEC3G^{-} cells, among other cell lines. Immortalized hepatocyte cultures, in many cases, lose their ability to bioactivate acetaminophen and hence are resistant to toxicity. Transient or consistent overexpression of drug-metabolizing enzymes (CYP4502E1 and/or CYP4501A2) leads to increased cytotoxicity of acetaminophen. Acetaminophen is also cytotoxic in cultures of rat liver sinusoidal endothelial cells, Kupffer cells, and mouse fibroblasts.

Cytotoxicity in Other Cells

The cytotoxicity of acetaminophen has been demonstrated in cultures of HeLa cells, L929 and 3T3 murine fibroblasts, chick embryo neurons, rat embryonic and skeletal muscle, peripheral blood lymphocytes, and lung and dermal cells. In addition, cytotoxicity of acetaminophen has been evaluated in the BF-2 fish cell line (see Ecotoxicology).

Clinical Management

Activated charcoal or other gastrointestinal decontamination procedures can be utilized as deemed necessary. Induction of emesis is not recommended as prolonged emesis may interfere with *N*-acetylcysteine (NAC) therapy. The Rumack-Matthew nomogram is utilized to identify proper course of treatment. Blood acetaminophen concentrations of 200 mg l^{-1} (or higher) at 4 h postingestion indicate severe risk of hepatic failure and are treated with a standard NAC treatment regimen. NAC is a glutathione substitute and prevents hepatic damage by quenching the reactive NAPQI. An oral loading dose of 140 mg kg^{-1} (as a 5% solution in soft drink or juice) is followed by 70 mg kg^{-1} given orally as a 5% solution in soft drink or juice every 4 h for an additional 17 doses. An alternative intravenous dosing protocol (20 h regimen) for NAC (Acetadote®; Cumberland Pharmaceuticals) can also be used in patients where oral NAC administration is not possible. A loading dose of 150 mg kg^{-1} NAC (in 200 ml of 5% dextrose in water) is administered over 15 min, followed by 50 mg kg^{-1} NAC in 500 ml of 5% dextrose over the next 4 h. A final dose of 100 mg kg^{-1} NAC is administered in 1000 ml of 5% dextrose over a 16 h period. A longer 72 h treatment regimen with intravenous NAC is recommended in the United States. An injectable form and an extended-release form of NAC are available (Acetadote) for treating patients who developed acetaminophen-induced liver injury. Basic and advanced life-support measures should be utilized as required by the condition of the patient. Studies have also suggested that an increase in alphafetoprotein, a surrogate for hepatic regeneration following injury, is strongly associated with a favorable outcome in patients with acetaminophen-induced liver injury and hence may be used as a supplement to existing prognostic criteria.

Environmental Fate

Acetaminophen was found to be inherently biodegradable and has no bioaccumulation potential. No other information about the environmental fate of acetaminophen is currently available.

Ecotoxicology

The acute toxicity of acetaminophen has been examined in several aquatic species. The LC_{50} value in brine shrimp (*Artemia salina*) examining mortality was reported to be 3820 $\mu mol\,l^{-1}$. The EC_{50} for immobility over a 24 h experiment using water flea (*Daphnia magna*) was 367 $\mu mol\,l^{-1}$. Acetaminophen is classified as not toxic or only slightly to moderately toxic in all fish (fathead minnow, *Pimephales promelas*) and zooplankton species tested. The crustacean fairy shrimp (*Streptocephalus proboscideus*) appears to be highly sensitive to acetaminophen (average LC_{50} of 196 $\mu g\,l^{-1}$).

Other Hazards

Acetaminophen is stable under ordinary conditions of use and storage. In the presence of heat and water, acetaminophen will hydrolyze into acetic acid and p-aminophenol. Incineration can produce carbon monoxide, carbon dioxide, and nitrogen oxides.

Flammability: As with most organic solids, fire is possible at elevated temperatures or by contact with an ignition source.

Explosivity: Fine dust dispersed in air in sufficient concentrations, and in the presence of an ignition source, is a potential dust explosion hazard. The minimum concentration for explosion is 0.25 oz. per cubic feet. The recommended fire-extinguishing media are water spray, dry chemical, alcohol foam, or carbon dioxide. Acetaminophen is capable of generating a static electrical charge. Processes involving dumping of acetaminophen into flammable liquid, inert atmosphere in the vessels or temperatures of flammable liquid should be maintained below its flashpoint.

Exposure Limits

Therapeutic exposure: The total daily dose of acetaminophen should not exceed 4 g. Dosages of acetaminophen over 4–8 g day^{-1} over long periods of time may be associated with higher risk of liver toxicity. Acetaminophen should not be administered for more than 10 days or to young children except upon advice of physician.

Occupational exposure: Mallinckrodt recommends an airborne exposure limit of 5 mg m^{-3}.

Miscellaneous

A special mention of the interaction of acetaminophen and alcohol consumption is warranted. Large numbers of reports in the scientific literature and public media suggest that a potentially high risk of liver toxicity due to acetaminophen exists when consumed following alcohol intake. In a recent review, however, Dr Barry Rumack suggests that only chronic heavy drinkers may be at greater risk following an overdose of acetaminophen and that no potentiation of toxicity occurs at therapeutic doses. However, acetaminophen use during acute or chronic alcohol exposure remains a controversial topic.

See also: Mechanisms of Toxicity; Oxidative Stress.

Further Reading

Bateman, D.N., 2012. Poisoning and self-harm. Clin. Med. 12 (3), 280–282.

Bulku, E., Stohs, S.J., Cicero, L., et al., 2012. Curcumin exposure modulates multiple pro-apoptotic and anti-apoptotic signaling pathways to antagonize acetaminophen-induced toxicity. Curr. Neurovasc. Res. 9 (1), 58–71.

Chun, L.J., Tong, M.J., Busuttil, R.W., Hiatt, J.R., 2009. Acetaminophen hepatotoxicity and acute liver failure. J. Clin. Gastroenterol. 43 (4), 342–349.

DHHS/National Toxicology Program, 1993. Toxicology and Carcinogenesis Studies of Acetaminophen in F344/N Rats and B6C3F1 Mice (Feed Studies). Technical Report Series No. 394, NIH Publication No. 93–2849.

Feucht, C.L., Patel, D.R., 2010. Analgesics and anti-inflammatory medications in sports: use and abuse. Pediatr. Clin. North Am. 57 (3), 751–774.

Gunawan, B.K., Kaplowitz, N., 2007. Mechanisms of drug-induced liver disease. Clin. Liver Dis. 11 (3), 459–475.

Guggenheimer, J., Moore, P.A., 2011. The therapeutic applications of and risks associated with acetaminophen use: a review and update. J. Am. Dent Assoc. 142 (1), 38–44.

Hinson, J.A., Roberts, D.W., James, L.P., 2010. Mechanisms of acetaminophen-induced liver necrosis. Handbook Exp. Pharmacol. 196, 369–405.

James, L.P., Letzig, L., Simpson, P.M., Capparelli, E., Roberts, D.W., Hinson, J.A., Davern, T.J., Lee, W.M., 2009. Pharmacokinetics of acetaminophen-protein adducts in adults with acetaminophen overdose and acute liver failure. Drug Metab. Dispos. 37, 1779–1784.

Jefferies, S., Saxena, M., Young, P., 2012. Paracetamol in critical illness: a review. Crit. Care Resusc. 14 (1), 74–80.

Klein-Schwartz, W., Doyon, S., 2011. Intravenous acetylcysteine for the treatment of acetaminophen overdose. Expert Opin. Pharmacother. 12 (1), 119–130.

Kienhuis, A.S., Bessems, J.G., Pennings, J.L., et al., 2011. Application of toxicogenomics in hepatic systems toxicology for risk assessment: acetaminophen as a case study. Toxicol. Appl. Pharmacol. 250 (2), 96–107.

Malhi, H., Gores, G.J., Lemasters, J.J., 2006. Apoptosis and necrosis in the liver: a tale of two deaths? Hepatology 43 (2 Suppl. 1), S31–S44.

Mazer, M., Perrone, J., 2008. Acetaminophen-induced nephrotoxicity: pathophysiology, clinical manifestations, and management. J. Med. Toxicol. 4 (1), 2–6.

Mehendale, H.M., 2012. Once initiated, how does toxic tissue injury expand? Trends Pharmacol. Sci. 33 (4), 200–206.

Ozkaya, O., Genc, G., Bek, K., Sullu, Y., 2010. A case of acetaminophen (paracetamol) causing renal failure without liver damage in a child and review of literature. Ren. Fail. 32 (9), 1125–1127.

Ruepp, S.U., Tonge, R.P., Shaw, J., Wallis, N., Pognan, F., 2002. Genomics and proteomics analysis of acetaminophen toxicity in mouse liver. Toxicol. Sci. 65, 135–150.

Rumack, B.H., Bateman, D.N., 2012. Acetaminophen and acetylcysteine dose and duration: past, present and future. Clin. Toxicol. (Phila) 50 (2), 91–98.

Starkey Lewis, P.J., Merz, M., Couttet, P., et al., 2012. Serum microRNA biomarkers for drug-induced liver injury. Clin. Pharmacol. Ther. 92 (3), 291–293. http://dx.doi.org/10.1038/clpt.2012.101.

Tujios, S., Fontana, R.J., 2011. Mechanisms of drug-induced liver injury: from bedside to bench. Nat. Rev. Gastroenterol. Hepatol. 8 (4), 202–211.

http://www.fda.gov/NewsEvents/Newsroom/PressAnnouncements/ucm239894.htm – USFDA.

Winnike, J.H., Li, Z., Wright, F.A., et al., 2010. Use of pharmaco-metabonomics for early prediction of acetaminophen-induced hepatotoxicity in humans. Clin. Pharmacol. Ther. 88, 45–51.

Zhao, L., Pickering, G., 2011. Paracetamol metabolism and related genetic differences. Drug Metab. Rev. 43 (1), 41–52.

Acetamiprid

DR Wallace, Center for Health Sciences, Oklahoma State University, Tulsa, OK, USA

- Name of Chemical: Acetamiprid
- CAS RN: 135410-20-7
- Synonyms: Mospilan, Assail, Tristar
- Chemical/Pharmaceutical/Other Class: Neonicotinoid (Pyridylmethylamine) Insecticide
- Molecular Formula: $C_{10}H_{11}ClN_4$
- Chemical Structure: Name: (E)-*N*-[(6-chloro-3-pyridyl) methyl]-*N'*-cyano-*N*-methyl-acetamidine

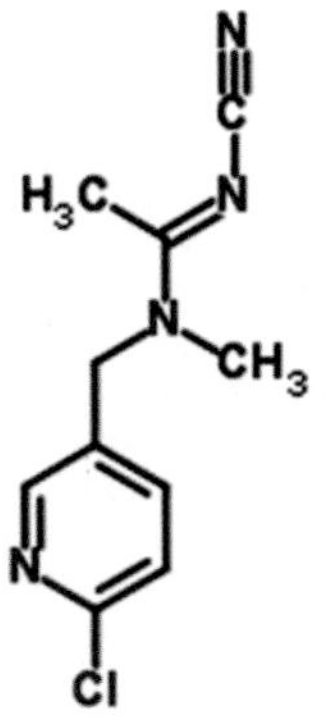

Background

Acetamiprid belongs to the neonicotinoid class of insecticides that were developed in the late 1980s. The precise structure of acetamiprid is that of a chloronicotinyl compound and it has been shown to be a potent agonist at the postsynaptic nicotinic acetylcholine receptors in insects. Numerous studies have shown that acetamiprid exhibits a higher affinity for insect nicotinic receptors compared to its affinity at vertebrate receptors. The primary use for acetamiprid is to control sucking insects such as aphids, which have been known to attack and damage leafy plants. Acetamiprid is available as a ready-to-use (RTU) formulation in addition to wettable powders (WP) and water-dispersible granules. Formulations for dispersal include 99.5% technical, 70% wettable powder end use, 70% water-soluble packet end use, and 0.006% ready-to-use end use product. Acetamiprid can be applied by ground and/or aerial means with sprayers. The application rate should not exceed 0.55 pounds of active ingredient per acre per season. This concentration will be sufficient to control insect populations. Although acetamiprid has shown to have higher affinity for nicotinic receptors in insects compared to mammals, there have been some reports of imidacloprid (another neonicotinoid) undergoing biotransformation in rodents resulting in a compound that has higher affinity for the nicotinic receptor compared to (−)-nicotine. This could potentially lead to toxicity in mammals. There have been no reports of chronic toxicity or of bioactivation of acetamiprid so far in mammals. There has been at least one report where individuals attempted suicide by ingesting a commercial mixture of acetamiprid. There have been no studies which have examined symptomology in humans following acetamiprid exposure, but based on the recorded symptoms in suicide-attempt patients and in other vertebrate species, it appears that primary symptoms include spasms, respiratory distress, and possibly convulsions. A receptor report has shown that acetamiprid can undergo transepithelial absorption across intestinal cells, possibly resulting in toxicity if acetamiprid accumulates within the body. In general, acetamiprid is a relatively safe insecticide with few reported side effects in vertebrates. The persistence of acetamiprid in the environment is low, with quick degradation by soil microbes, or degradation by exposure to ultraviolet (UV) light in soil or in ground water.

Uses

Acetamiprid is used as an insecticide to control sucking-type insects on leafy vegetables and fruits. In many instances, these insects may be resistant to the effects of organophosphorus and other conventional insecticides.

Environmental Fate and Behavior

The primary route of exposure is via diet (food and water). Occupational exposure for individuals who work with this insecticide can occur via dermal contact or inhalation. Acetamiprid exhibits a very short half-life in soil. It is rapidly degraded by aerobic metabolism. Acetamiprid is stable to hydrolysis at environmental temperatures and it photodegrades slowly in water. It is transformed moderately rapidly in aerobic aquatic environments, but only slowly in anaerobic aquatic systems. There appears to be minimal effects on drinking water and due to the rapid breakdown, has not demonstrated the ability to bioaccumulate in wildlife. Due to the rapid breakdown of acetamiprid, it is not expected to be persistent in the environment. Metabolites of acetamiprid will pose a greater risk to the environment, but additional work is needed to determine the fate and toxicity of acetamiprid metabolites.

Exposure and Exposure Monitoring

There are three major routes of acetamiprid exposure: dietary, drinking water, and occupational. By comparing values for drinking water level of comparison vs. drinking water estimated concentration, a potential toxin can be identified in susceptible populations. The Environmental Protection Agency (EPA) has chosen children 1–6 years of age as a primary risk group. Comparing the values for DWLOC and DWEC for acute, short/intermediate, and chronic dietary exposure, the DWLOC/DWEC values are 600/17 ppb, 400/4 ppb, and 80/4 ppb, respectively. Since the DWLOC values are all significantly

 http://dx.doi.org/10.1016/B978-0-12-386454-3.00091-9

higher than the DWEC values, toxicity is not expected to occur. Occupational exposure can occur with individuals who manufacture or handle acetamiprid. A margin of exposure of less than 100 would be considered an occupational risk hazard, and for acetamiprid, the values are greater than 100 except for long-term postapplication exposure which is 90. The value will return to 100 one day following application. Detection of acetamiprid residues on food products, as well as from biological samples, has been accomplished by high-performance liquid chromatography and gas chromatography with mass spectrometry. Recently, immunoassays and the use of liquid chromatography with tandem mass spectrometry have been reported.

Toxicokinetics

Acetamiprid is rapidly and extensively metabolized. Metabolites in urine account for 79–86% of the administered dose. Only 3–7% of acetamiprid is collected unchanged in the urine and feces. Demethylation by Phase I biotransformation is the major pathway, with 6-chloronicotinic acid being the major metabolite. Compounds can then undergo Phase II transformation with glycine conjugation representing the major pathway.

Mechanism of Toxicity

The primary mechanism of acetamiprid toxicity against insects is due to its action at nicotinic cholinergic receptors. The unique nature of the neonicotinoids as insecticides is that the negatively charged cyano (or nitro) group will specifically interact with a cationic binding region that is unique to insects. This action will convey selectivity of action against insects and leave mammalian nicotinic receptors relatively unaffected.

Acute and Short-Term Toxicity

There is little evidence for acetamiprid toxicity in vertebrates. The EPA classifies acetamiprid as both a class II and class III agent. Acetamiprid rating of II was in acute oral studies with rats, II in acute dermal and inhalation studies with rats, and category IV in primary eye and skin irritation studies with rabbits. There is some evidence for contact exposure, dermal irritation, and stomach poisoning following oral ingestion.

Animal

Acute studies in laboratory animals, mainly rats, have demonstrated relatively low toxicity potential for acetamiprid. Oral ingestion appears to elicit the most severe toxicological responses. At dosages in excess of 140 mg kg^{-1}, acetamiprid elicited neurotoxic signs, with animals exhibiting disorders of movement and posture. Surviving animals were free of signs on the following day. The LD_{50} in rats has been reported to be 450 mg kg^{-1} for acetamiprid. Although requiring a large dose for lethality, acetamiprid is still one of the most toxic of the neonicotinoids. The LD_{50} for other compounds such as clothianidin, imidacloprid, and thiamethoxam are 10-fold higher in the rat. Acetamiprid was only slightly toxic following inhalation ($LC_{50} > 1.15$ mg l^{-1}) and weakly toxic following dermal administration ($LD_{50} > 2000$ mg kg^{-1} in rabbit). There was minimal or no irritation of eyes or skin. Some metabolites of acetamiprid exhibited greater toxicity than the parent compound. In other species such as birds and fish, acetamiprid is relatively nontoxic with acute LD_{50} values in birds in excess of 2000 mg kg^{-1} and in excess of 100 ppm in fish. Acetamiprid has been reported by multiple investigators to be moderately toxic in bee populations in that if acetamiprid is applied directly over bees.

Human

No evidence is available for assessing human outcomes following acute exposure to acetamiprid. Signs associated with acute exposure and limits of exposure have been established using data from animal studies. The symptoms associated with rodent toxicity may be applicable to human symptoms and these include lethargy, respiratory distress, reduced movement, and loss of balance with staggering followed by spasms. There have been some reports of acute acetamiprid toxicity in humans following suicide attempts and the symptoms presented by these individuals were similar to what has been reported in other vertebrate toxicity studies. The ingested acetamiprid solutions were 2–18% solutions, but contained many other components that may have contributed to the symptoms observed. Due to the selectivity of acetamiprid for insect nicotinic cholinergic receptors, little human toxicity is expected following normal use.

Chronic Toxicity

Examination of chronic exposure to acetamiprid has utilized animals and little data on chronic human exposure are available. The selectivity of acetamiprid for insect nicotinic receptors would suggest minimal toxicity following chronic exposure.

Animal

Chronic dietary administration of acetamiprid resulted in reduced body and organ weight. Higher doses resulted in neurological dysfunction.

Human

No evidence is available for assessing human outcomes following chronic exposure to acetamiprid. Symptoms associated with chronic exposure and limits of exposure have been established using data from animal studies. Due to the selectivity of acetamiprid for insect nicotinic cholinergic receptors, little human toxicity is expected however.

Immunotoxicity

There have been no reports of immunotoxicity of acetamiprid in humans/vertebrates or other species.

Reproductive Toxicity

There have been no reports of reproductive toxicity of acetamiprid in humans/vertebrates or other species.

Genotoxicity

There have been no reports of genotoxicity of acetamiprid in humans/vertebrates or other species. There has been a report (2007) that indicated that acetamiprid did induce sister chromatid exchange and chromosomal aberrations in human blood lymphocytes (**Kocaman and Topaktas, 2007**).

Carcinogenicity

There was evidence for teratogenic potential in animal studies. There were no positive results in genotoxicity studies using bacterial or mammalian cell assays.

Clinical Management

There are no guidelines for acetamiprid toxicity outside of symptomatic control. Clinical management consists of managing any physical symptoms that are presented after removing the individual from the source of acetamiprid contamination: remove any contaminated clothing and rinse skin or eyes thoroughly with water for 15–20 min. If acetamiprid is inhaled, move the individual to fresh air and monitor breathing, and aid if necessary.

Ecotoxicity

Due to the rapid breakdown of acetamiprid, there is minimal risk to fish or wildlife. Proper labeling could alleviate any additional risk. Specificity for insects significantly reduces any additional toxicity to nontarget organisms. Acetamiprid is only moderately toxic to bees and would pose little threat to endangered species and to nontargeted plants. Acetamiprid does not pose a significant concern for persistence in soil and ground water. Under controlled laboratory conditions, acetamiprid had moderate persistence in soil. But the presence of various microorganisms will reduce the persistence of acetamiprid. A recent report indicated that nearly 95% of acetamiprid is degraded within 15 days of application under normal conditions. Not only has it been reported that soil bacteria can degrade acetamiprid but also the effect of sunlight (UV light) has been shown to degrade acetamiprid. Photolysis of acetamiprid also occurs in solution and contributes to the reduced half-life of acetamiprid in water. Due to rapid degradation and the relatively low potency in vertebrate species, acetamiprid is a relatively safe insecticide.

Exposure Standards and Guidelines

The EPA has established guidelines for toxicological dose and end points for acetamiprid. Using the No Observable Adverse Effect Limit (NOAEL) and uncertainty factor, the reference dose (RfD) can be calculated.

- For acute dietary ingestion for infants and children, NOAEL $= 10\ \text{mg kg}^{-1}$; RfD $= 0.10\ \text{mg kg}^{-1}\ \text{day}^{-1}$.
- Chronic dietary exposure for all populations, NOAEL $= 7.1\ \text{mg kg}^{-1}$; RfD $= 0.07\ \text{mg kg}^{-1}\ \text{day}^{-1}$.
- Short- and intermediate-term incidental exposure to infants and children, NOAEL $= 15\ \text{mg kg}^{-1}\ \text{day}^{-1}$ and for adults NOAEL $= 17.9\ \text{mg kg}^{-1}\ \text{day}^{-1}$.
- Long-term dermal exposure, NOAEL $= 7.1\ \text{mg kg}^{-1}\ \text{day}^{-1}$ with dermal absorption of 30%.
- Short- and intermediate-term inhalation exposure, NOAEL $= 17.9\ \text{mg kg}^{-1}\ \text{day}^{-1}$ and for long-term inhalation exposure, NOAEL $= 7.1\ \text{mg kg}^{-1}\ \text{day}^{-1}$.

See also: Carbamate Pesticides; Imidacloprid; Neonicotinoids; Pyrethrins/Pyrethroids.

Further Reading

Bruneet, J.L., Maresca, M., Fantini, J., Belzunces, L.P., 2008. Intestinal absorption of the acetamiprid neonicotinoid by Caco-2 cells: transepithelial transport, cellular uptake and efflux. J. Environ. Sci. Health B 43, 261–270.
Guohong, X., Guoguang, L., Dezhi, S., Liquing, Z., 2009. Kinetics of acetamiprid photolysis in solution. Bull. Environ. Contam. Toxicol. 82, 129–132.
Gupta, S., Gajbhiye, V.T., 2007. Persistence of acetamiprid in soil. Bull. Environ. Contam. Toxicol. 78, 349–352.
Gupta, S., Gajbhiye, V.T., Gupta, R.K., 2008. Effect of light on the degradation of two neonicotinoids viz acetamiprid and thiacloprid in soil. Bull. Environ. Contam. Toxicol. 81, 185–189.
Health Canada; Pest Management Regulatory Agency; Regulatory Note #REG2002-05.
Hernandez, F., Sancho, J.V., Pozo, O.J., 2005. Critical review of the application of liquid chromatography/mass spectrometry to the determination of pesticide residues in biological samples. Anal. Bioanal. Chem. 382, 934–946.
Imamura, T., Yanagawa, Y., Nishikawa, K., Matsumoto, N., Sakamoto, T., 2010. Two cases of acute poisoning with acetamiprid in humans. Clin. Toxicol. 48, 851–853.
Kocaman, A.Y., Topaktas, M., 2007. *In vitro* evaluation of the genotoxicity of acetamiprid in human peripheral blood lymphocytes. Environ. Mol. Mutagen. 48, 483–490.
Liu, Z., Dai, Y., Huang, G., Gu, Y., Ni, J., Wei, H., Yaun, S., 2011. Soil microbial degradation o neonicotinoid insecticides imidacloprid, acetamiprid, thiacloprid and imidaclothiz and its effect on the persistence of bioefficacy against horsebean aphid Aphis craccivora Koch after soil application. Pest Manag. Sci. 67, 1245–1252.
Mo, J., Pan, C., Zhang, S., Chen, C., He, H., Cheng, J., 2005. Toxicity of acetamiprid to workers of Reticulitermes flaviceps (Isoptera: Rhinotermitidae), Coptotermes formosanus (Isoptera: Rhinotermitidae) and Odontotermes formosanus (Isoptera: Termitidae). J. Pest. Sci. 30, 187–191.
Shi, X.B., Jiang, L.L., Wang, H.Y., Qiao, K., Wang, D., Wang, K.Y., 2011. Toxicities and sublethal effects of seven neonicotinoid insecticides on survival, growth and production of imidacloprid-resistant cotton aphid, Aphis gossypii. Pest Manag. Sci. 67, 1528–1533.
Tomizawa, M., Casida, J.E., 1999. Minor structural changes in nicotinoid insecticides confer differential subtype selectivity for mammalian nicotinic acetylcholine receptors. Br. J. Pharmacol. 127, 115–122.
Tomizawa, M., Casida, J.E., 2003. Selective toxicity of neonicotinoids attributable to specificity of insect and mammalian nicotinic receptors. Ann. Rev. Entomology 48, 339–364.
Tomizawa, M., Casida, J.E., 2005. Neonicotinoid insecticide toxicology: mechanisms of selective action. Ann. Rev. Pharmacol. Toxicol. 45, 247–268.
United States Environmental Protection Agency Federal Register of Environmental Documents.
United States Environmental Protection Agency: Pesticide Fact Sheet.
Watanabe, E., Miyake, S., Baba, K., Eun, H., Endo, S., 2006. Immunoassay for acetamiprid detection: application to residue analysis and comparison with liquid chromatography. Anal. Bioanal. Chem. 386, 1441–1448.

Relevant Websites

http://edis.ifas.ufl.edu/pdffiles/PI/PI11700.pdf.
http://www.epa.gov/fedrgstr/EPA-PEST/2002/March/Day-27/p7098.htm.
www.epa.gov/opprd001/factsheets/acetamiprid.pdf.
http://www.epa.gov/oppsrrd1/REDs/factsheets/mcpa_red_fs.pdf.
http://www.hc-sc.gc.ca/pmra-arla/english/pdf/reg/reg2002-05-e.pdf.

Acetic Acid

SD Pravasi, Bristol Myers Squibb (PPD), Hopewell, NJ, USA

- Name: Acetic acid
- Chemical Abstracts Service Registry Number: 64-19-7
- Synonyms: Glacial acetic acid, Ethylic acid, Pyroligneous acid, Vinegar acid, Methanecarboxylic acid
- Molecular Formula: $C_2H_4O_2$
- Structure:

$$H_3C-C(=O)-OH$$

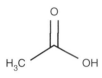

Background (Significance/History)

Acetic acid is present throughout nature as a normal metabolite of both plants and animals. Acetic acid may also be released to the environment in a variety of waste effuents, in emissions from combustion processes, and in exhaust from gasoline and diesel engines. Acetic acid is produced by the decomposition of solid biological wastes and is readily metabolized by living organisms. Using bacteria (*Acetobacter* species), large quantities of vinegar are manufactured by fermenting alcohol employing the following reaction:

$$C_2H_5OH + O_2 \rightarrow CH_3COOH + H_2O$$

Uses

Large quantities of acetic acid are used to make products such as photographic chemicals, pesticides, pharmaceuticals, food preservatives, rubber, and plastics. Acetic acid is also present as the main component of vinegar, albeit at very low concentrations that are harmless to humans. Acetic acid is used in the manufacture of various acetates, acetyl compounds, cellulose acetate, acetate rayon, plastics, and rubber. It is also used in tanning, as laundry sour, in printing calico, and in dyeing silk. It is a solvent for gums, resins, volatile oils, and many other substances. Acetic acid is widely used in commercial organic synthesis.

Environmental Fate and Behavior

Acetic acid is present throughout nature as a normal metabolite of both plants and animals. Acetic acid may also be released to the environment in a variety of waste effuents, in emissions from combustion processes, and in exhaust from gasoline and diesel engines. If released to air, a vapor pressure of 15.7 mmHg at 25 °C indicates acetic acid should exist solely as a vapor in the ambient atmosphere. Vapor-phase acetic acid will be degraded in the atmosphere by reaction with photochemically produced hydroxyl radicals; the half-life for this reaction in air is estimated to be 22 days. Physical removal of vapor-phase acetic acid from the atmosphere occurs via wet deposition processes based on the miscibility of this compound in water. In acetate form, acetic acid has also been detected in atmospheric particulate material. If released to soil, acetic acid is expected to have very high to moderate mobility based upon measured K_{oc} values, using near-shore marine sediments, ranging from 6.5 to 228. No detectable sorption was measured for acetic acid using two different soil samples and one lake sediment. Volatilization from moist soil surfaces is not expected to be an important fate process based upon a measured Henry's law constant of 1×10^{-9} atm m^3 mol^{-1}. Volatilization from dry soil surfaces may occur based upon the vapor pressure of this compound. Biodegradation in both soil and water is expected to be rapid; a large number of biological screening studies has determined that acetic acid biodegrades readily under both aerobic and anaerobic conditions. Volatilization from water surfaces is not expected to be an important fate process based on its measured Henry's law constant. An estimated bacterial colony foraging (BCF) of <1 suggests that the potential for bioconcentration in aquatic organisms is low.

Exposure and Exposure Monitoring

Since acetic acid exists ubiquitously in the environment, the general public is continuously exposed to the compound. Primary routes of exposure to acetic acid are through oral consumption of foods and inhalation of air. Occupational exposure occurs through inhalation and dermal contact.

Toxicokinetics

Acetic acid is absorbed from the gastrointestinal (GI) tract and through the lung. Acetic acid is readily metabolized by most tissues and may give rise to the production of ketone bodies as intermediates. *In vitro* experiments have demonstrated that acetate is incorporated into phospholipids, neutral lipids, sterols, and saturated and unsaturated fatty acids in a variety of human and animal tissue preparations. In catabolism or anabolic synthesis, acetate ion (the anion of acetic acid) is a normally occurring metabolite, for example, in the formation of glycogen, cholesterol synthesis, fatty acid degradation, and acetylation of amines. It is estimated that the plasma level of the acetate ion in humans is about 50–60 μmol l^{-1} (3.0–3.6 mg l^{-1}) and 116 μmol l^{-1} (7 mg l^{-1}) in cerebrospinal fluid. An estimated daily turnover of the acetate ion in humans is about 45 g day^{-1}.

Mechanism of Toxicity

Acetic acid causes toxicity by coagulative necrosis; that is, the acid denatures all tissue proteins to form an acid proteinate. As

 http://dx.doi.org/10.1016/B978-0-12-386454-3.00216-5

a result, both structural and enzymatic proteins are denatured and cell lysis is blocked. Therefore, cell morphology is not greatly interrupted. In addition, an ester is formed which delays further corrosive damage and helps reduce systemic absorption. Thus, damage, especially with small quantities of acid, is frequently limited to local sites of injury to the skin or the GI tract rather than the systemic response.

Acute and Short-Term Toxicity

Animal

Acetic acid is corrosive to skin and gastric mucosa. Repetitive exposure to acetic acid may cause erosion of dental enamel, bronchitis, and eye irritation. Bronchopneumonia and pulmonary edema may develop following acute overexposure. LC_{50} in guinea pig and mouse by inhalation is 5000 ppm h^{-1}, LD_{50} in rat by oral route is 3.53 g kg^{-1}, LD_{50} in mouse is 525 mg kg^{-1}, LD_{50} rabbit oral 1200 mg kg^{-1}. Large oral doses are known to cause narcotic central nervous system depression and death in rats and mice.

Human

Acetic acid is corrosive to skin and gastric mucosa. Liquid or spray mist may produce tissue damage, particularly on mucous membranes of eyes, mouth, and respiratory tract. Spray mist inhalation may produce severe irritation of respiratory tract, coughing, choking, or shortness of breath. It is also known to cause inflammation of the eye and skin. Repetitive exposure to acetic acid may cause erosion of dental enamel, bronchitis, and eye irritation. Bronchopneumonia and pulmonary edema may develop following acute overexposure.

Chronic Toxicity

Animal

In rats, prolonged administration of acetic acid produces hyperplasia in the esophagus and forestomach.

Human

Chronic exposure may result in pharyngitis and catarrhal bronchitis. Ingestion, though not likely to occur in industry, may result in penetration of the esophagus, bloody vomiting, diarrhea, shock, hemolysis, and hemoglobinuria followed by anuria. Pulmonary edema, bronchopneumonia, or chemical pneumonitis may be caused by repeated inhalation. Other toxic effects like dermatitis, erosion of teeth, conjunctivitis, and cumulative systemic injury may also be caused due to prolonged or repeated exposure.

Immunotoxicity

Dibromoacetic acid (DBA) is commonly found in the drinking water as a result of chlorination/ozonation process. Exposure of DBA in mice resulted in no immunotoxic effects at concentrations much larger than those considered acceptable in human drinking water with exception to changes in thymus weight.

Clinical Management

Exposure should be terminated as soon as possible by removal of the patient to fresh air. The skin, eyes, and mouth should be washed with copious water. A 15–20 min wash may be necessary to neutralize and remove all residual traces of the contaminant. Contaminated clothing and jewelry should be removed and isolated. Contact lenses should be removed from the eyes to avoid prolonged contact of the acid with the area. A mild soap solution may be used for washing the skin and as an aid to neutralize the acid but should not be placed into the eye. No cream, ointment, or dressing should be applied to the affected area. Emesis should be avoided in case of ingestion. If a large quantity has been swallowed, gastric lavage should be considered. Dilution with water may be the solution if small quantity of acetic acid is swallowed. Under no circumstances should carbonated beverages ever be used because of large quantities of carbon dioxide gas released that distend the stomach.

Ecotoxicology

Acetic acid is harmful to aquatic life. High concentrations will produce pH levels that are toxic to oxidizing bacteria, thereby inhibiting oxygen demand.

Exposure Standards and Guidelines

Permissible exposure limit – 8-h time-weighted average (TWA): 10 ppm (25 mg m^{-3}).

Threshold limit values – 8-h TWA: 10 ppm. Fifteen-minute short-term exposure limits (STEL): 15 ppm.

National Institute for Occupational Safety and Health recommendations – recommended exposure limit: 10-h TWA: 10 ppm (25 mg m^{-3}).

Recommended exposure limit: 15-min STEL: 15 ppm (37 mg m^{-3}).

Immediately dangerous to life or health: 50 ppm.

Food and Drug Administration Requirements: Acetic acid used as a general purpose food additive in animal drugs, feeds, and related products is generally recognized as safe when used in accordance with good manufacturing or feeding practice.

See also: Vinyl Acetate; 2,4-D (2,4-Dichlorophenoxy Acetic Acid); Chloroacetic Acid.

Further Reading

Deshpande, S.S., 2002. Handbook of Food Toxicology. Marcel Dekker, Inc., 88.4: pp. 262–263.

Schonwald, S., 2004. Medical Toxicology, vol. 147. Lippincott Williams and Wilkins, pp. 918–919.

Relevant Website

http://www.cdc.gov/niosh/idlh/64197.html – Centers for Disease Control and Prevention: NIOSH Publications and Products - Acetic Acid.

http://www.osha.gov – Occupational Safety and Health Administration.

http://www.sci.seastarchemicals.com – Seastar Chemicals Inc.

http://toxnet.nlm.nih.gov – Toxnet (Toxicology Data Network): search under Propargite.

Acetone

MP Kalapos, Theoretical Biology Research Group, Budapest, Hungary

This article is a revision of the previous edition article by Lee R. Shugart, volume 1, pp 27–28, © 2005, Elsevier Inc.

- Chemical Name: Acetone
- Chemical Abstracts Service Registry Number: CAS 67-64-1
- Synonyms: Dimethyl ketone; 2-Propanone; Dimethylketal; Dimethylformaldehyde
- Molecular Formula: $(CH_3)_2CO$
- Chemical Structure:

O
‖
H_3C — C — CH_3

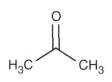

Background

The appearance of acetone in scientific thinking may be traced back to 1798, when John Rollo, an English physician, described a material in human breath of an odor of decaying apples. Later this material was identified as acetone, and it was regarded as a characteristic feature of diabetic coma. By the turn of nineteenth and twentieth centuries, it became widely held that acetone was poorly, if at all, metabolized. This picture started to change from the end of 1940s since experimental data became available showing the incorporation of ^{14}C-carbons of labeled acetone into cholesterol, fatty acids, urea, and glycogen. And the oxidation of acetone to carbon dioxide exhaled in respiratory air was also recognized. The possibility of *in vivo* formation of glucose from acetone in experimental animals was also reported. In 1980, the participation of cytochrome P450 type enzymes in acetone breakdown was discovered. In 1984, the pathways of acetone metabolism in rats were described.

Acetone occurs naturally in plants, trees, volcanic gases, and forest fires, and it is found in vehicle exhaust, tobacco smoke, and landfill sites also. In the metabolic machinery of bacteria and animals, acetone is also present. Industrial processes contribute tonnages of acetone to the environment more than natural processes.

As seen, a long-lasting standard dogma was that acetone was an end product of metabolism in animals and humans. Nonetheless, the pathways described in this article demonstrate the potential for animals and humans to metabolize acetone.

Uses

Acetone has a characteristic odor of decaying apple and a sweetish taste. It is obtained by fermentation (retains a lesser proportion of the acetone market) or chemical synthesis (either as a main product or as a by-product) mainly via the cumene process to produce phenol. The uses of acetone in industry are many and based on its miscibility with water, alcohol, chloroform, ether, and most of the oils. Hence, its largest use is as a solvent in paint, varnishes, lacquers, plastics, and fibers, and a great variety of miscellaneous solvent uses (fats, oils). It is also used to make plastic, fibers, drugs, and other chemicals. In the laboratory, it is used to extract various substances from animal and plant tissues, and as a dehydrating agent. In housekeeping, it is found as a component of detergents and cosmetic products.

Environmental Fate and Behavior

Acetone evaporates rapidly, even from water and soil. Once entered the atmosphere, it is degraded by photolysis, a reaction in which free radicals are involved or removed by wet deposits. It is a significant groundwater contaminant because of its miscibility in water.

Exposure and Exposure Monitoring

Exposure to acetone results mostly from breathing air, drinking water, or coming in contact with products or soil that contains acetone. Significant numbers of workers are potentially exposed to acetone. The general population may be exposed through the use of products such as paints, adhesives, cosmetics, and rubber cement.

There are two main sources of acetone production in animals: the decarboxylation of acetoacetate and the dehydrogenation of isopropanol.

Acetoacetate arises from either lipolysis or amino acid breakdown and its decarboxylation may happen in either an enzyme-catalyzed way or non-enzymatically. The existence of an enzymatic activity has been documented in different rat tissues, and the enzyme, mainly from plasma, has been characterized over the years as to its low substrate affinity and optimal activity at pH 4.5, the loss of activity in the presence of iodoacetate, urea, and $HgCl_2$. Acetone has been found as a competitive inhibitor for the activity. Nevertheless, despite the enhancement of decarboxylation by this 'enzyme,' doubts emerge in regard to its existence as the protein responsible for the enzymatic activity had never been purified to homogeneity. And neither sequencing of the enzyme nor the identification of its coding gene have been done yet, raising the question of what kind of protein this activity in animals can be attributed to. In bacteria, the enzyme, designated acetoacetate decarboxylase (acetoacetate carboxy lyase) and first identified in *Clostridium acetobutylicum*, has been, however, demonstrated in several strains. And also, an enzyme catalyzing the reverse reaction through carbon dioxide fixation has been identified in prokaryotes and named acetone carboxylase. To present knowledge, this enzyme is lacking in animals. The non-enzymatic decarboxylation to acetone of acetoacetate being enhanced by amines was noted as early as 1929.

The reduction of acetone to isopropanol is dominantly catalyzed by alcohol dehydrogenase—type enzymes, and the catalase plays only a subordinate role. The conversion of acetone into isopropanol is a simple oxido-reduction using $NADH + H^+/NAD^+$ as cofactor, and this reaction prefers acetone formation to the reverse reaction.

 http://dx.doi.org/10.1016/B978-0-12-386454-3.00995-7

Two main streams of reactions are known for the degradation of acetone, and the first step in both pathways is the conversion of acetone into acetol by a cytochrome P450 isozyme, designated CYPIIE1 (cytochrome P450 IIE1). This isoenzyme is inducible by the treatment of animals with acetone (believed to be the physiological inducer) and a diverse range of exogenous compounds, as well as by fasting and chemically induced diabetes mellitus. These isozymes are expressed in a wide variety of tissues, among others; in the liver they show a centrilobular distribution.

During acetone degradation, both three-carbon (C_3) and two-carbon (C_2) fragments are produced (**Figure 1**). Indeed, two C_3 pathways have been identified as having pyruvate as a common end product. It is believed that the degradation via methylglyoxal is entirely intrahepatic, while via propanediol extrahepatic step(s) is (are) also suggested to be involved. The only C_2 pathway diverts intermediates of the propanediol route at the level of L-1,2-propanediol. At higher plasma acetone levels (above 4 mM), the C_2 pathway seems to be preferred.

Race differences in acetone metabolism are suggested on the basis of expired air analysis studies.

Toxicokinetics

Acetone entering the blood is carried to all organs in the body. It freely crosses the blood–brain barrier and placenta, and therefore its concentrations in blood and cerebrospinal fluid, and in the body of mother and fetus, are similar in rats. Studies with intravenously administered trace amounts of $[^{11}C]$-acetone to baboons showed a rapid uptake into and a relatively slow clearance from the brain. Patients on ketogenic diet have been reported to exhibit elevated levels of acetone in their plasma and brains.

The elimination half-life for acetone in humans is about 24 h (17–27 h).

The higher the concentration of plasma acetone, the higher the rate of elimination by breath, and the linear relationship between plasma acetone and breath acetone is seen both in starvation and in diabetes up to 4 and 10 mM, respectively. This makes breath acetone a sensitive indicator in controlling diabetes and ketogenic diet. About 7% of endogenous acetone is, however, eliminated in urine, and glucose production starting from acetone may represent about 11% in 21-day starved men. Glucose production from acetone is governed by the liver.

Mechanism of Toxicity

Acetone acts mainly as an irritant affecting the eyes, nose, throat, and respiratory tract. When inhaled or ingested, it is narcotic. It is strongly suggested that acetone leads to narcosis through the potentiation of hyperpolarization of γ-aminobutyric acid receptors, a mechanism that resembles the mode of action of sedatives and ethanol.

Acute and Short-Term Toxicity

Animals

The single oral LD_{50} value for rats is 10.7 ml kg^{-1}, the single skin penetration LD_{50} value for rabbits is >20 ml kg^{-1}, and 30 min is the interval the rats survive when exposed to concentrated vapor inhalation. No irritation is seen in the case of uncovered application of 0.01 ml undiluted sample of acetone on the clipped skin of rabbits, but 0.005 ml of undiluted acetone results in severe burn on rabbit cornea.

When inhaled (12 600–50 600 ppm, 1 ppm equals to 0.0001%) it is narcotic to rodents. The narcotic effect of acetone

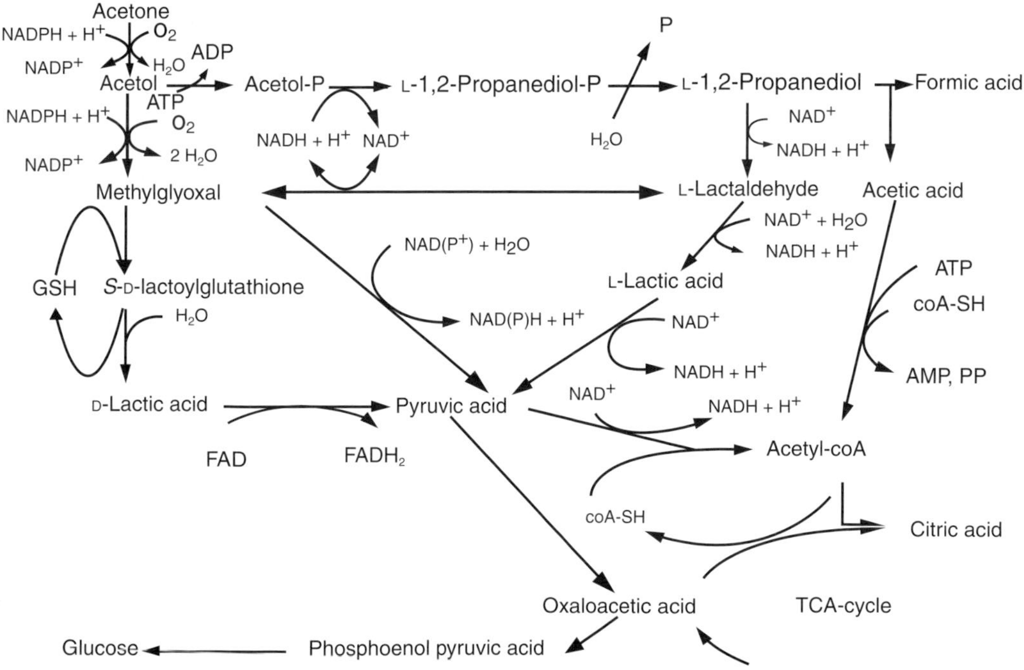

Figure 1 Pathways for acetone metabolism.

is delayed and of considerably longer duration compared to toluene or ethanol. It is fairly distributed in the organs. After inhaling 5% (50 000 ppm) of acetone by guinea-pigs for 5–8 h, congestion of spleen, kidneys, and lungs was observed, and even pulmonary edema occurred.

Application of 1% v/v acetone in drinking water to male mice for a week did not have any influence on body weight, liver weight, blood glucose concentration, and serum glutamate oxaloacetate transaminase activity, but it did decrease hepatic-reduced glutathione levels, and increase CYPIIE1 isozyme activities. Microscopic examinations did not reveal any morphological change in the liver.

The action of externally added acetone on blood glucose concentrations of animals is contradictory. Some investigations reported a rise of blood glucose level after acetone addition, while others failed to corroborate this finding.

Human

Exposure to acetone vapor at a concentration of 1000 ppm for 4 or 8 h does not lead to considerable appearance of tension, tiredness, or any other complaints, but some mild decrements on behavioral performance tests are seen even at 250 ppm acetone concentration. Breathing moderate levels of acetone for short periods of time can, however, cause headache, lightheadedness, confusion, and an elevation in pulse rate. Occupational exposure to acetone results in its detection in urine samples of exposed workers, and there is a linear correlation between exposure and urinary excretion.

Injection of acetone intravenously to humans provoked a drop of blood pressure and drowsiness.

Symptoms following acute acetone ingestion include nausea, vomiting that may progress to hematemesis and gastric hemorrhage, sedation, respiratory depression, ataxia, and paresthesia. Depression resembles alcoholic stupor. Coughing and bronchial irritation may be the only clues to ingestion of quantities that are too small to produce sedation. Swallowing very high levels of acetone can result in unconsciousness and damage to the skin in the mouth. Unconsciousness and even coma accompany high levels of exposure, usually in the case of suicidal or accidental ingestions. Among laboratory data, high levels of acetone are accompanied with a transient elevation of blood glucose and lactate levels, and increased osmolarity and leukocytosis may be seen without any rise of serum levels of hepatic enzymes. Urine test for acetone is strongly positive. Organ damage including liver injury is not evident, suggesting that acetone itself does not exert an immediate toxicity to organs in these suicidal cases, if survived. Since the function of central nervous system is immediately affected by acetone exposure, it is likely that this is the life-threatening factor in acute intoxication and not the metabolic effects of acetone.

Chronic Toxicity

Animals

The application of acetone to rodents (rats and mice, male and female) for 13 weeks resulted in depressed body weight gain (at 50 000 and 100 000 ppm), bone marrow hypoplasia (at 100 000 ppm). Nephropathy at 20 000 and 50 000 ppm as well as hypogonadism at 50 000 ppm developed only in male rats. Acetone treatment during 13 weeks was associated with relative increases in kidney and liver weights above 20 000 ppm. In the case of repeated, daily 4 h inhalation of acetone vapor at concentrations of 12 000 and 16 000 ppm for 10 days to female rats led to a specific alteration of avoidance behavior. In addition, even after a single dose of acetone at the above concentrations, ataxia was produced and a tolerance rapidly developed.

Although acetone inhalation causes bronchial and corneal irritations, indeed the majority of its actions are depressive symptoms, including stupor, dyspnea, fall of body temperature and heart rate, and poor pulse. Its effects are proportional to acetone concentration in the vapor. A decrease of hepatic-reduced glutathione levels and an increased capacity of CYPIIE1 isozymes were noted only when animals were on 1% v/v acetone in drinking water for a week.

No studies are available that would have been undertaken for longer than a 2 week period of time on the toxicity and carcinogenicity of acetone to laboratory animals.

No susceptibility of different age groups of laboratory rats to acetone can be stated.

Human

The relevance to humans of the just-described effects observed in animal studies is questionable, and therefore it is yet unknown if humans would experience such toxicological effects or not. Noteworthy is that under occupational environment exposure to acetone, which frequently happens for longer than a few weeks, these findings show exposed workers do not exhibit more serious long-lasting complaints and only drowsiness, eye and throat irritations, dizziness, headache, or problems with performance are noted. If experienced, the symptoms are transient. However, prolonged or repeated skin contact with acetone may produce severe dermatitis. All in all, acetone is currently not regarded as a genotoxic or mutagenic chemical in humans, and has not been classified as a carcinogen agent either. There is also not any concern for its chronic neurotoxicity.

From a methodological point of view, important shortcomings limiting the use of data for assessing health effects of acetone in humans are that chronic studies were usually undertaken in an occupational environment where the coincidental exposure to other chemicals could not be fully excluded and the proper control groups were sometimes lacking. More important is, however, the note that acetone potentiates the toxicity of consumed ethanol, several medicines, and chemicals, thus enhancing the ignition of the formation of such hazardous materials like methylglyoxal or free radicals.

To sum, only limited information is available, which does not demonstrate conclusive effects either in humans or in experimental animals arising from chronic exposure to acetone. This particularly applies to reproductive toxicity.

Genotoxicity

Acetone of reagent grade was evaluated by the standard plate incorporation method in the Ames *Salmonella* reverse mutation assay with strains TA98, TA100, TA1535, TA1537, and TA1538. Results were negative in these strains. Negative *in vitro* results were also gained in sister chromatid exchange assay, SHE cell transformation assay, and DNA repair-deficient bacterial tests.

Clinical Management

If inhaled intentionally with the purpose of recreational intoxication (usually in combination with other solvents as ingredient of commercial products) or accidentally and if breathing is difficult, the person is moved to fresh air and administered oxygen. For skin contact, the contaminated area is washed with water. For eye contact, water is used for flushing. In case of ingestion, mainly with suicidal intent, intubation, breath assistance, gastric lavages, and hemofiltration may be performed in parallel with forced diuresis.

Acetone provides an antiseizure effect in animal models for epilepsy when administered in millimolar concentrations. No toxicity was noted in these cases. It is suggested that acetone is a factor contributing to the beneficial effects of high-fat, low-carbohydrate ketogenic diets used in clinical practice, particularly to control intractable epilepsies in children.

In experimental animals, no gender differences have been recognized, but it is unknown whether this rule applies to humans too. Nonetheless, sensitive populations have to be considered, especially those suffering diseases in which elevated acetone levels in the plasma may occur (i.e., starvation, diabetes mellitus, alcoholism, inherited disorders of metabolism, etc.).

Ecotoxicology

The LD_{50} of acetone for fish is 8.3 g l^{-1} of water over 96 h. It may also be biodegraded when released into the soil, since it is consumed by microorganisms, but its bioaccumulation and toxicity to aquatic life are not expected.

Other Hazards

Acetone is a volatile, highly flammable liquid, and its vapor may cause flash fire resulting in burns. It has to be kept away from plastic medical products since it violently reacts with those. It potentiates the toxicity of other volatile organic solvents and methylglyoxal, and amplifies the narcotic effects of volatile organic solvents.

Exposure Standards and Guideline

The US National Research Council's Committee on Toxicology recommends 1000 and 200 ppm 24 h emergency exposure limit and 90 day continuous exposure limit for acetone, respectively. The US Department of Labor, Occupational Safety and Health Administration recommends the exposure limit of 1000 ppm for acetone (time-weighted average). The references may differ in various countries.

See also: Acetic Acid; Alcoholic Beverages and Health Effects; Biotransformation; Cumene; Dietary Restriction; Ethanol; Excretion; Formic Acid; Isopropanol; Psychological indices in toxicology; Sedatives.

Further Reading

Arts, J.H., et al., 2002. An analysis of human response to the irritancy of acetone vapors. Crit. Rev. Toxicol. 32, 43–66.

Kalapos, M.P., 2003. On mammalian acetone metabolism: from chemistry to clinical implications. Biochim. Biophys. Acta 1621, 122–139.

Kalapos, M.P., 2006. Acetone metabolism in the liver: two approaches to the same phenomenon. In: Ali, S., Friedman, S.L., Mann, D.A. (Eds.), Liver Diseases: Biochemical Mechanisms and New Therapeutic Insights, first ed. Enfield (NH)-Jersey-Plymouth: Science Publishers, pp. 79–91.

Landau, B.R., Brunengraber, H., 1987. The role of acetone in the conversion of fat to carbohydrate. Trends Biochem. Sci. 12, 113–114.

Relevant Websites

http://www.inchem.org – Acetone: Environmental Health Criteria from the International Program on Chemical Safety.

http://www.atsdr.cdc.gov – Agency for Toxic Substances and Disease Registry. Toxicological Profile for Acetone.

http://www.nap.edu – The National Academies Press. Emergency and Continuous Exposure Limits for Selected Airborne Contaminants. Volume 1.

Acetonitrile

H Robles, Irvine, CA, USA

- Chemical Abstracts Service Registry Number: 75-05-8
- Synonyms: Cyanomethane, Ethane nitrile, Ethanenitrile, Ethyl nitrile, Methanecarbonitrile, Methyl cyanide
- Molecular Formula: C_2H_3N
- Chemical Structure:

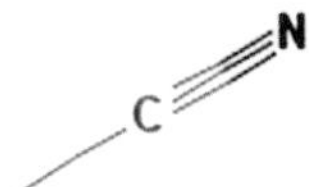

Background

Acetonitrile is a liquid with an etherlike odor. It is a highly polar, volatile solvent used in many different industrial applications. It is widely used in the pharmaceutical, photographic, chemical, and analytical industries. It is useful as an industrial solvent for the separation of olefins, polymers, spinning fibers, and plastics. Other uses include the extraction and refining of copper and by-product ammonium sulfate; used for dyeing textiles and in coating compositions; used as a stabilizer for chlorinated solvents; manufacture of perfumes and cosmetics; and as a general reagent in a wide variety of chemical processes.

Uses

Acetonitrile is used in the chemical industry as an intermediary in the synthesis of several chemicals and products such as acetophene, thiamine, acetamidine, alpha-naphthaleneacetic acid, nitrogen-containing compounds, acrylic fibers, nitrile rubber, pesticides, pharmaceuticals, perfumes, and lithium batteries. It is also used as a polar solvent for both organic and inorganic compounds and in nonaqueous titrations.

Environmental Fate and Behavior

If released to ambient air, acetonitrile will remain in the vapor phase where it will be degraded through reaction with photochemically produced hydroxyl radicals. The half-life of acetonitrile in ambient air has been estimated to be about 620 days. If released to soil, acetonitrile is expected to volatilize rapidly. Biodegradation in soil is not expected to be a major degradation pathway. If released to water, acetonitrile is not likely to adsorb to soil and sediment particles. Acetonitrile is expected to be removed from water bodies through volatilization, as the chemical hydrolysis and bioaccumulation potential for this chemical are low.

Exposure and Exposure Monitoring

Exposure to acetonitrile can occur through the oral, dermal, and inhalation routes. Symptoms of poisoning have been observed in persons exposed through these three routes.

Employees exposed to acetonitrile at potentially hazardous levels should be enrolled in a medical monitoring program. Initially, the employee should undergo a medical examination to establish his/her baseline health conditions. The initial evaluation should include a complete history and physical examination. Persons with history of fainting or convulsive disorders may be at special risk. Examination of the skin (particularly hands and face), eyes, liver, and kidneys should be included. Following initial examination, the employee should be scheduled to undergo annual medical examinations and the above-mentioned tests and examinations should be included.

Blood cyanide concentrations exceeding $0.1\ \mathrm{mg\,l^{-1}}$ of plasma or urine thiocyanate exceeding $20\ \mathrm{mg\,l^{-1}}$ in workers exposed to acetonitrile are indicative of excessive exposure.

Toxicokinetics

Acetonitrile can be acutely lethal when absorbed in high doses. Acetonitrile is metabolized to a hydroxyl metabolite by cytochrome P450 in the liver. Subsequent metabolism through catalase enzymes produces hydrogen cyanide. Once metabolized, the mechanism of action is the same as expected for cyanide poisoning. Onset of cyanide poisoning may be delayed by 3–8 h or more, as metabolism is required to produce the cyanide metabolite. Toxicity may be prolonged for up to 3 days in some cases.

Mechanism of Toxicity

Acetonitrile is slowly metabolized by cytochrome P450 in the liver to produce hydrogen cyanide. Toxicity is produced by the combined effect of circulating acetonitrile and cyanide. Cyanide exerts its toxicological effects by disrupting oxygen utilization at the cellular level. The disruption results in decreased oxygen utilization by body tissues and lactic acidosis.

Acute and Short-Term Toxicity

Animal susceptibility to acetonitrile varies by animal species and route of administration. Overall, animal susceptibility is mediated by the animal's ability to absorb and metabolize acetonitrile into its toxic metabolite, hydrogen cyanide.

Atmospheres containing up to 32 000 ppm acetonitrile are lethal to dogs. In rats, the oral LD_{50} value has been measured to range from $200\ \mathrm{mg\,kg^{-1}}$ (in young rats) to $3800\ \mathrm{mg\,kg^{-1}}$ (age unspecified), whereas the inhalation LC_{50} value has been determined to be 7500 ppm following an 8-h exposure. The acute dermal lethal dose has been investigated in rabbits. The LD_{50} value for the dermal route of exposure has been

 http://dx.doi.org/10.1016/B978-0-12-386454-3.00465-6

determined to be 980 mg kg^{-1}. Subchronic exposures to low concentrations of acetonitrile in the air (665 ppm or less) produced pulmonary inflammation and minor changes in body weights, hematocrit, hemoglobin, and liver and kidney function.

Toxicological effects of acetonitrile are usually delayed, as the chemical has to be metabolized to hydrogen cyanide. However, exposure to high doses may result in rapidly developing loss of consciousness and respiratory failure.

Signs and symptoms of exposure will be determined by the dose of acetonitrile. Onset of symptoms can be expected to be delayed from 2 to 12 h as acetonitrile is slowly metabolized to its toxic metabolite, cyanide. Exposure to low doses will produce nausea, salivation, vomiting, headache, and lethargy. Exposure to higher doses may produce cyanide intoxication characterized by extreme weakness, lethargy, respiratory depression, metabolic acidosis, tachycardia, shock, coma, seizures, and possibly death.

Chronic Toxicity

The toxicological effects of acetonitrile have been attributed to the direct effects of the intact molecule combined with the effects of metabolically generated cyanide ions.

Rats exposed to acetonitrile in air at concentrations ranging from 166 to 665 ppm for 7 h per day for up to 90 days showed no observable effects at dose below 330 ppm. At the maximum dose tested (665 ppm), pulmonary inflammation as well as minor kidney and liver changes were noted in some animals.

Dogs and monkeys exposed to acetonitrile in air for 91 days showed minor variations in body weight, hematocrit, and hemoglobin. The animals were dosed acetonitrile at concentrations averaging 350 ppm for 7 h per day, 3 days per week. Autopsy of the animals revealed some cerebral hemorrhaging as well as pigment-bearing macrophages in some animals.

No reports were found on the chronic toxicological effects of acetonitrile in humans.

Reproductive Toxicity

As in the case of the acute and chronic toxicological effects, the maternal production of cyanide may contribute to the reproductive and developmental toxicities of acetonitrile. Reproductive studies in laboratory animals show fetotoxicity at high acetonitrile doses. However, no teratogenic effects were observed at any dosage level.

Genotoxicity

In vitro studies using rat liver microsomes have demonstrated that the conversion of acetonitrile to cyanide is mediated by cytochrome P450 (P450IIE1).

Acetonitrile was tested for mutagenicity in the *Salmonella*/microsome preincubation assay. The tests were conducted using up to five *Salmonella* strains and in the presence and absence of rat or hamster liver S-9. All tests were negative for mutagenicity including those run at the maximum dose tested (10 mg $plate^{-1}$).

Carcinogenicity

Male and female rats were exposed to acetonitrile by inhalation at doses ranging from 0 up to 400 ppm for 6 h per day, 5 days per week for 2 years. Results of the study were inconclusive regarding the carcinogenic activity of acetonitrile as there was only a marginal increased incidence of hepatocellular adenomas and carcinomas in male rats. Furthermore, there was no evidence of carcinogenic activity in the female rats even at exposures as high as 400 ppm. In a similar study using male and female mice exposed to acetonitrile at doses ranging from 0 up to 200 ppm by inhalation for 6 h per day, 5 days per week for 2 years, no carcinogenic activity was noted in the animals and doses tested. In addition, no epidemiological studies were found that link cancer incidence to acetonitrile exposure.

Clinical Management

The major goal of treatment is to maintain respiration, blood circulation, and vital signs and to prevent further absorption of acetonitrile into the systemic circulation. If ingested, absorption can be prevented or minimized by instituting gastric lavage or by giving activated charcoal and a cathartic. Gastric lavage is effective only if performed soon after ingestion.

Treatment of acetonitrile poisoning is similar to that of cyanide poisoning (*see* Cyanide). This includes immediate therapy with 100% oxygen and assisted ventilation, if necessary. Seizures can be controlled by giving diazepam, phenobarbital, or phenytoin intravenously at appropriate doses. Therapy should also include correction of the metabolic acidosis and to combat cyanide poisoning. Cyanide poisoning is treated by the intravenous administration of sodium nitrite and sodium thiosulfate. Care should be taken to maintain treatment for as long as acetonitrile is being metabolized to cyanide.

Other Hazards

Acetonitrile is highly flammable and will ignite in the presence of flames, sparks, or sufficient heat. Acetonitrile vapors may combine with air to form explosive mixtures. Poisonous gases including hydrogen cyanide and nitrogen oxides are produced in fire.

Ecotoxicology

Toxicity thresholds for protozoa, bacteria, and green algae have been measured to range from 520 mg l^{-1} for *Microcystis aeruginosa* (algae) to 7300 mg l^{-1} for *Scenedesmus quadricauda* (green algae).

The LC_{50} value for acetonitrile in fathead minnow (*Pimephales promelas*) has been measured to be about 1640 $mg\,l^{-1}$ per 96 h in a flow-through bioassay.

The European Union Risk Assessment Report (EURAR, 2002) on acetonitrile summarizes the results of various fish toxicity assays and reports that the 24- to 48-h LC_{50} values were generally higher than 1 $g\,l^{-1}$ for *Oryzias latipes*. The EURAR also states that the lowest reported 48-h LC_{50} values were 730 and 880 $mg\,l^{-1}$ on *Cyprinus carpio* and *Ctenopharyngodon idellus*, respectively.

Exposure Standards and Guidelines

OSHA Permissible Exposure Limit = 40 ppm (70 $mg\,m^{-3}$)
American Conference of Governmental Industrial Hygienists (ACGIH) 8-h Time-Weighted Average = 20 ppm
ACGIH Short-Term Exposure Limit = 60 ppm
National Institute of Occupational Safety and Health Immediately Dangerous to Life or Health = 500 ppm

The United States Environmental Protection Agency Integrated Risk Information System has published a reference concentration for acetonitrile of 0.06 $mg\,m^{-3}$.

Florida State Drinking Water Standard = 42 $\mu g\,l^{-1}$.

See also: Cyanide.

Further Reading

Ellenhorn, M.J., Barceloux, D.G. (Eds.), 1988. Medical Toxicology, Diagnosis and Treatment of Human Poisoning. Elsevier Science Publishing Company, Inc., New York, NY.

European Union Risk Assessment Report. Acetonitrile. CAS No: 75-05-8. EINECS No: 200-835-2, European Commission, Joint Research Centre, EUR.

Hazardous Substances Database (HSDB) (2011) National Library of Medicine (NLM), Specialized Information Service. Online Database. http://toxnet.nlm.nih.gov/cgi-bin/sis/search

Relevant Websites

http://www.epa.gov/ttn/atw/hlthef/acetonit.html. U.S. Environmental Protection Agency's Technology Transfer Network Air Toxics Web Site.

European Chemicals Agency (ECHA). Registered substances: http://apps.echa.europa.eu/registered/registered-sub.aspx

Acetophenone

NV Soucy, 3M Center, St Paul, MN, USA

- Chemical Profile
- Name: Acetophenone
- Chemical Abstracts Service Registry Number: 98-86-2
- Synonyms: Acetylbenzene, Phenyl methyl ketone, 1-Phenylethanone, Benzoyl methide, Hypnone
- Molecular Formula: C_8H_8O
- Chemical Structure:

O
CH3

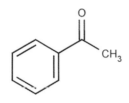

Background

Acetophenone is an aromatic ketone found naturally in fruits, berries, nuts, and meat. Charles Friedel is credited with the first synthetic preparation of acetophenone by the distillation of a mixture of calcium benzoate and calcium acetate in 1857. Acetophenone was described in medical literature as a therapy for the treatment of insomnia under the name of hypnone as early as 1886. In pure form, acetophenone is a colorless, flammable liquid with a sweet odor that has been described as similar to orange blossom or jasmine.

Uses

Acetophenone is used to impart the fragrance of orange blossoms in perfumes, soaps, detergents, and lotions. Concentrations of acetophenone in these products can range as high as 2000 ppm in perfumes and as low as 20–50 ppm in detergents and lotions. Additionally, acetophenone is approved by the U.S. Food and Drug Application as a direct food additive, where its use is primarily as a flavoring agent. The Flavor and Extract Manufacturers Association concluded that acetophenone is generally recognized as safe (GRAS) in 1978 and this status was recently reaffirmed. Acetophenone is used in chewing gum and is added to some tobacco products.

Industrial uses of acetophenone include use as a specialty solvent for plastics and resins, as a catalyst for polymerization of olefins, and as a photosensitizer in organic synthesis. Historically, acetophenone was used as an anesthetic agent, to induce analgesia and also as a hypnotic agent. On the basis of early descriptions of its use, it appears to have been most successful as a therapy for insomnia. Large doses were required to induce sleep and its use as an anesthetic was most successful when used in conjunction with chloroform. The earliest reports of acetophenone in the medical literature date back to 1886 and the primary adverse reaction reported was severe local irritation when injected in patients subcutaneously.

Environmental Fate and Behavior

The production and use of acetophenone as a specialty solvent and fragrance and flavor additive may result in environmental releases to the air, water, and soil. Acetophenone is slightly soluble in water and freely soluble in alcohol, chloroform, fatty oils, and glycerol. The vapor pressure at 25 °C is 0.4 mm Hg, the Henry's law constant is estimated to be 1.04×10^{-5} atm m^3 mol^{-1}, and the octanol/water partition coefficient (log K_{ow}) is 1.58.

If released to the soil, acetophenone is expected to have high mobility, with volatilization from moist soils. If released to the water, volatilization is anticipated from the surface and acetophenone is not anticipated to adsorb to sediment. The potential for bioconcentration in aquatic organisms is predicted to be low. If released to the atmosphere, the half-life is anticipated to be 6 days, with degradation occurring by reaction with photochemically produced hydroxyl radicals.

Exposure and Exposure Monitoring

Ingestion of very low levels of acetophenone is anticipated for the general population through the consumption of natural food products, including fruits, berries, nuts, and meats. Additional ingestion may result from the consumption of processed food products. Dermal exposures may result from the use of soaps, detergents, perfumes, and other cosmetic products. Inhalation and dermal exposures are possible in industrial settings and measurement of hippouric acid in the urine may provide an indication of exposure to acetophenone. The low vapor pressure and good warning properties of acetophenone should reduce the likelihood of overexposure in industrial settings.

Toxicokinetics

Aromatic ketones are rapidly absorbed from the gastrointestinal tract and are primarily metabolized in the liver with urinary excretion. Percutaneous absorption is also a relevant route of exposure. As a simple aromatic ketone, acetophenone administered orally undergoes essentially complete first pass hepatic metabolism and is excreted within 24 h of dosing. Acetophenone is reduced to alpha-methylbenzyl alcohol, which is excreted in the urine as a conjugate of glucuronic acid and this is the major metabolic pathway in animals. Interconversion of aromatic ketones and their corresponding alcohols *in vivo* is common and is observed with acetophenone; the primary metabolite, alpha-methylbenzyl alcohol, is also used as a fragrance and flavoring additive and is oxidized to acetophenone *in vivo*. Alpha-oxidation of acetophenone is an additional metabolic pathway; benzoic acid is an intermediary metabolite in this pathway with further metabolism to hippuric acid which is ultimately excreted in the urine where it can

 http://dx.doi.org/10.1016/B978-0-12-386454-3.01157-X

be used as a biomarker of acetophenone exposure. Acetophenone has been reported to be excreted in human milk.

Mechanism of Toxicity

It is unclear what mechanism is responsible for the central nervous system depression observed following high doses of acetophenone. *In vitro* evaluations have demonstrated that acetophenone suppresses voltage-gated ion channels in olfactory receptor cells and retinal neurons; however, it is unclear if this is related to any of the observed toxicity in animal studies.

Acute Toxicity

The acute oral toxicity of aromatic ketones in general is reported to be low. The oral LD_{50} for acetophenone in the rat ranges from 900 to 3200 mg kg^{-1} indicating a low to moderate potential for acute oral toxicity and signs of toxicity include central nervous system depression. Inhalation acute toxicity studies in animals have produced mixed results. Rats exposed to a saturated atmosphere of acetophenone (~430 ppm) for 8 h did not experience mortality. A 4-h LC_{50} in mice is reported to be ~244 ppm. Acetophenone has a low vapor pressure; therefore, under normal conditions, it is not likely to present as an inhalation hazard. An acute dermal LD_{50} of >20 ml kg^{-1} was reported in guinea pigs indicating a low potential for dermal toxicity. However, dermal absorption is a relevant route of exposure.

Acetophenone is reported to be slightly irritating in rabbit dermal irritation studies following 24-h exposure under occlusive conditions. Irritation was completely reversed after 48 h. In a human patch test conducted in 25 volunteers, 2% acetophenone did not result in skin irritation. In an early study, acetophenone was reported to produce corneal necrosis following instillation of 0.005 ml of a 15% solution of acetophenone; however, in more recent experiments with study designs similar to OECD Test Guideline 405, acetophenone was found to be nonirritating in the rabbit eye. Dermal sensitization has not been reported in humans and acetophenone was not found to have sensitizing potential when evaluated in a guinea pig maximization test or a modified Draize sensitization test.

Respiratory depression was observed in one study in mice, with an airborne concentration of 102 ppm resulting in a 50% reduction in the respiratory rate (RD_{50}) in the exposed animals. Subsequent evaluations in mice of concentrations up to three times this value for 14 days did not result in pathological changes to the nasal passages, trachea, or lungs of the exposed animals. The odor threshold for acetophenone is reported to be between 0.004 and 4.1 ppm, indicating this compound has good warning properties.

Subcutaneous and intravenous administration of acetophenone results in central nervous system depression in multiple animal species. Sleep, analgesia, and anesthesia were the desired effects following administration of acetophenone (hypnone) in humans in the late nineteenth and early twentieth centuries and these effects have been confirmed following intravenous administration in dogs in more modern experiments. Additional effects in dogs included decreased respiration, cardiac modification, low blood pressure, and weak pulse.

Subchronic Toxicity

As with acute toxicity, the primary adverse effects observed following subchronic exposure to acetophenone are neurological in nature. In a combined repeat dose toxicity study and reproductive/developmental screening study, male and female Sprague–Dawley rats were administered 0, 75, 225, or 750 mg kg^{-1} bw day^{-1} of acetophenone by oral gavage for 28 days. Body weight and food consumption were both reduced for males and females in the high dose group; however, hematology and clinical chemistry values were similar between test and control groups. No mortality was observed. At the 750 mg kg^{-1} dose level, male rats had reduced motor activity and reduced forelimb grip strength; these animals also exhibited pre- and post-dose salivation. Male rats from the 225 mg kg^{-1} bw dose group also exhibited pre- and post-dose salivation. The no observed adverse effect level concentration (NOAEL) for neurological effects was 225 mg kg^{-1} bw day^{-1}. The study authors report a systemic NOAEL of 75 mg kg^{-1} bw day^{-1}; however, it is unclear on what basis this NOAEL was determined.

Male and female Osborne–Mendel rats were fed a diet containing 0, 1000, 2500, or 10 000 ppm acetophenone per kg feed for 17 weeks. Dietary concentrations were calculated to be 0, 100, 250, or 1000 mg kg^{-1} bw day^{-1} on the basis of food intake. No effects on body weight, food consumption, or mortality were reported for any of the test groups, and no effects were observed following gross necropsy or microscopic evaluation of liver, kidney, spleen, heart, or testes. There was a loss of acetophenone from the feed formulation in this study. On the basis of data provided by the investigators, the U.S. Environmental Protection Agency (EPA) estimated that the NOAEL (10 000 ppm) corresponded to a daily dose of 423 mg kg^{-1} day^{-1} on the basis of a 15.5% acetophenone loss and estimates of food consumption in rats and an oral reference dose (RfD) was calculated on the basis of these data.

Reproductive Toxicity

Evidence for reproductive and developmental toxicity of acetophenone is limited. In a combined repeat dose toxicity study and reproductive/developmental screening study, male and female Sprague–Dawley rats were administered 0, 75, 225, or 750 mg kg^{-1} bw day^{-1} of acetophenone by oral gavage for 28 days prior to mating. For the reproductive/developmental toxicity portion of the study, doses were continued in pregnant females for a minimum of 14 days through lactation day 3. The number of stillborn pups was significantly increased in the 750 mg kg^{-1} dose group, including one stillborn pup with cleft palate. Scabbing, desquamation, and dermal hypoplasia were observed in the pups from this group that were found dead. Scabbing and desquamation were observed at scheduled necropsy in pups from the 225 and 750 mg kg^{-1} dose groups. Live birth and lactation day 4 viability indices were significantly reduced at the 750 mg kg^{-1} dose. On the basis of these effects, the NOAEL for developmental effects was determined by the study authors to be 75 mg kg^{-1} and the NOAEL for reproductive toxicity was determined to be 750 mg kg^{-1} day^{-1}.

Acetophenone was also administered at 480 mg kg^{-1} bw to the skin of pregnant rats on gestation days 10–15, which includes a portion of the period of organogenesis in the rat. This exposure did not result in any adverse fetal effects.

Genotoxicity

The weight of evidence suggests that acetophenone, like most aromatic ketones, is not genotoxic. Negative results have consistently been obtained in multiple strains of bacteria, with and without metabolic activation, in the Ames assay. Chromosomal aberrations were observed in Chinese hamster ovary cells with metabolic activation, but these effects were not observed when metabolic activation was not present.

Carcinogenicity

No epidemiological studies evaluating the carcinogenic potential of acetophenone exist. In addition, acetophenone has not been evaluated for carcinogenicity in animal studies. The US EPA has classified acetophenone as Group D, not classifiable as to human carcinogenicity.

Clinical Management

Central nervous system depression is the primary effect following large acute doses; therefore, removal to fresh air and respiratory support are suggested; however, human exposures requiring clinical management are not anticipated for acetophenone.

Ecotoxicology

Acute toxicity has been evaluated in the fathead minnow in both static and flow-through assays. The 1- and 24-h LC_{50} are reported to be >200 mg l^{-1}; the 48-h LC_{50} 103 mg l^{-1}, the 72-h LC_{50} 158 mg l^{-1}, and the 96-h LC_{50} are reported to range from 155 to 162 mg l^{-1}.

Exposure Standards and Guidelines

The American Conference of Governmental Industrial Hygienists Threshold Limit Value – Time-Weighted Average is 10 ppm (50 mg m^{-3}).

An oral RfD of 0.4 mg kg^{-1} day^{-1} has been established by the US EPA.

Miscellaneous: Not applicable.

See also: Food Additives; Generally Recognized as Safe (GRAS).

Further Reading

Adams, T.B., McGowen, M.M., Williams, M.C., et al., 2007. The FEMA GRAS assessment of aromatic substituted secondary alcohols, ketones, and related esters used as flavor ingredients. Food Chem. Toxicol. 45, 171–201.

American Conference of Governmental Industrial Hygienists, 2009. TLV Documentation for Acetophenone, Cincinnati, OH.

Beaumetz, D., 1886. Lecture on hypnone. Boston Med. Surg. J. 114 (5), 97–100.

Relevant Website

http://www.epa.gov/iris/index.html – Environmental Protection Agency.

Acetylaminofluorene

I Syed, Harvard Medical School, Boston, MA, USA

This article is a revision of the previous edition article by Sanjay Chanda, Harihara M. Mehendale, volume 1, pp 31–32, © 2005, Elsevier Inc.

- Name: Acetylaminofluorene
- Chemical Abstracts Service Registry Number: 53-96-3
- Synonyms: *N*-fluorene-2-yl-acetamide, *N*-2-fluorenylacetamide, *N*-fluoren-2-yl-acetamide, 2-Acetylaminofluorene, 2-Acetylaminofluorene, *N*-9*H*-fluoren-2-yl-acetamide
- Chemical/Pharmaceutical/Other Class: Aromatic amine
- Molecular Formula: $C_{15}N_{13}NO$
- Molecular Weight: 223.29
- Chemical Structure:

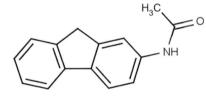

Background Information

2-Acetylaminofluorene (2-AAF) was originally synthesized to be used as a pesticide but due to its profound carcinogenicity it is now purely used in research laboratories for research purposes only. The occupations at greatest risk to acetylaminofluorene exposure are organic chemists, chemical stockroom workers, and biomedical researchers. 2-AAF is a tan-colored compound insoluble in water (melting point. 194 °C). It is soluble in glycols, alcohols, ether, and acetic acid. 2-AAF is no longer produced in commercial quantities anywhere in the world. In 2009, 2-AAF was distributed in small quantities by 17 specialty chemical companies, including 11 in the United States. As per the US Environmental Protection Agency (EPA), environmental release of 2-AAF rose from ~10 000 to ~81 000 lb from 1998 to 2001, and then was contained below 1000 lb in 2003. Although neither the National Institute of Occupational Safety and Health (NIOSH) nor the Occupational Safety and Health Administration (OSHA) has estimated the number of US workers exposed to acetylaminofluorene, perhaps fewer than 1000 workers in 200 laboratories may have come in contact with this compound.

In order to debate 'threshold level,' dose–response relationships, and carcinogenic potential of 2-AAF, a few studies employed very large numbers of female BALB/c StCrlfC3Hf/Nctr mice, and exposed them to low doses of 2-AAF for up to 33 months. Study findings showed two different types of dose–response relationships for urinary bladder neoplasms and liver neoplasms; bladder neoplasms exhibited a minimum effect level (or a nonlinear response) for specific conditions. In contrast, the late-appearing liver neoplasms displayed a nearly linear response that extrapolated directly to zero dose. Time of exposure (18, 24, and 33 months) was shown to be an important factor for incremental positive response. Induction of bladder neoplasms was shown to occur early in the study, but was dependent on the continuous presence of 2-AAF, whereas the liver neoplasms appeared very late in the study but were shown to be induced at a very early point in the exposures and did not require the continuous presence of the carcinogen in order to develop. Results of this type of studies were consistent with 'no threshold concept.' Overall, most studies advocate the importance of the time factor in safety evaluation or risk assessment in carcinogenesis because carcinogen dose, length of exposure, and gender all may play roles in cancer/tumor development.

Uses

Acetylaminofluorene is found as a contaminant in coal gasification processes. It was intended to be used as a pesticide but was never marketed due to its carcinogenicity. It has no known use.

Environmental Fate

According to the US EPA's Toxics Release Inventory, environmental releases of 2-AAF considerably increased from 1998 to 2001, declined to as low as 255 lb in 2003, and have remained below 1000 lb since 2003. However, most of the releases were to hazardous-waste landfills. In 2007, one facility released about 500 lb of 2-AAF to a hazardous-waste landfill and about 250 lb to air. Release of 2-AAF to the environment from artificial sources is probably not significant since less than 20 lb year of this compound are consumed in the United States. If released to soil, 2-AAF is expected to have low mobility. Chemical hydrolysis, oxidation, and volatilization are not expected to be significant. If released to water, 2-AAF may undergo direct photolysis and is expected to strongly adsorb to suspended solids and sediments. Chemical hydrolysis, oxidation, volatilization, and bioaccumulation are not expected to be significant. If released to the atmosphere, 2-AAF may undergo vapor phase adsorption to airborne particulate matter, it may react with photochemically generated hydroxyl radicals (estimated vapor phase half-life$^{1}/_{4}$ 5.92 h) or it may undergo direct photolysis.

Exposure and Exposure Monitoring

Dermal contact is the potential route of exposure in humans apart from inhalation and ingestion. Acetylaminofluorene emits toxic fumes of nitrous oxides when heated to decompose and can be toxic when inhaled.

 http://dx.doi.org/10.1016/B978-0-12-386454-3.00217-7

Toxicokinetics

Acetylaminofluorene is biotransformed in the liver. 2-AAF can stimulate cytochrome P450 1A1 isozyme (CYP1A1) activity, inducing both CYP1A1 and CYP1A2 proteins, whereas 4-acetylaminofluorene modestly increases CYP1A2 but does not influence CYP1A1.

Mechanism of Toxicity

4-Acetylaminofluorene is not carcinogenic; 2-AAF is carcinogenic. 2-AAF can be metabolized to form *N*-hydroxyacetylaminofluorene and 2-aminofluorene, which may covalently bind to the DNA and macromolecules. Ring and *N*-hydroxylation of 2-AAF leads to the formation of water-soluble conjugates like sulfates and glucuronides. The major fraction of urinary metabolites, around 60–80%, consists of sulfate conjugates, and 10–15% of metabolites in urine consist of glucuronides. 2-AAF has been frequently used to demonstrate stages of multistage carcinogenesis following initiation, driven primarily by carcinogen-induced epigenetic alterations (cytosine DNA methylation, histone methylation, and micro-RNA expression).

Acute and Short-Term Toxicity

Animal

A single dose of acetylaminofluorene at 0.1 mg kg^{-1} when injected into mice (DD strain) on gestation days 8–15 produced mainly skeletal defects, cleft lips, cleft palates, and cerebral hernias. The LD_{50} of 4-acetylaminofluorene in mice is 364 mg kg^{-1} by the intraperitoneal route. A single subcutaneous injection of 2-AAF caused liver tumors (hepatocellular tumors) in newborn male mice (**Table 1**).

Human

2-AAF is thought to be carcinogenic to humans. However, no epidemiological study has ever acknowledged evaluating the relationship between human cancer and exposure specifically to 2-AAF.

Chronic and Long-Term Toxicity

Animal

Different species respond differently to chronic administration of 2-fluoroacetylamine. In female mice, dietary administration of 2-AAF caused mammary gland and urinary bladder cancer. In rats, dietary administration of 2-AAF caused liver cancer in both sexes, adenocarcinoma in females and mesothelioma in males. Liver tumors were also observed following dietary administration of 2-AAF to male dogs. In hamsters of both sexes, intratracheal instillation of 2-AAF caused urinary bladder cancer. Intraperitoneal injection of 2-AAF in newborn hamsters until weaning followed by dietary administration, caused urinary bladder and liver cancer, and benign stomach tumors. Fisher 344 rats were fed 0.06% acetylaminofluorene in diet for 4 weeks and then a control diet for 1 week. This schedule was carried out for three cycles (12 weeks). A smaller group was also treated for only one cycle. Rats treated for three cycles showed high incidence of liver, testis, and Zymbal gland tumors. No tumors observed in rats treated for one cycle. When fed to male rats (0.05% of diet) for 3 or 4 weeks, 4-acetylaminofluorene caused proliferation of agranular endoplasmic reticulum and glycogen depletion in hepatocytes. The same treatment when continued for 10 months produced conspicuous morphological alterations in pancreatic granular endoplasmic reticulum together with mitochondrial damage and focal cytoplasmic degradation. No carcinomas were found in any rats administered with 0.000 5% 2-AAF in the diet, for a period of 40 weeks.

Human

Human exposure data are not available. 2-AAF is thought to be 'reasonably anticipated to be a human carcinogen.'

In Vitro Toxicity Data

The mutagenicity of *N*-2-fluorenylacetamide (NFA) was evaluated in *Salmonella* tester strains TA98, TA100, TA1535, TA1537, and TA1538 (Ames test), both in the presence and absence of added metabolic activation by Aroclor-induced rat

Table 1 Some toxic effects of 2-acetylaminofluorene

Organism	*Test type*	*Route*	*Reported dose (normalized dose)*	*Effect*	*Source*
Mouse	LD_{50}	Intraperitoneal	470 mg kg^{-1} (470 mg kg^{-1})		1989. Mutation Research 223, 361.
Mouse	LD_{50}	Oral	810 mg kg^{-1} (810 mg kg^{-1})	Peripheral nerve and sensation: spastic paralysis with or without sensory change Behavioral: altered sleep time (including change in righting reflex) Kidney, ureter, and bladder: other changes in urine composition	1973. Proceedings of the Society for Experimental Biology and Medicine 143, 1117.
Rat	LD_{Lo}	Intraperitoneal	>200 mg kg^{-1} (200 mg kg^{-1})		1985. Archives of Toxicology 56, 151.

Source: http://chem.sis.nlm.nih.gov/chemidplus/jsp/common/Toxicity.jsp – NLM-ChemIDPlus Advanced.

liver S9 fraction. Based on the results of preliminary bacterial toxicity determinations, NFA, diluted with dimethyl sulfoxide (DMSO), was tested for mutagenicity at concentrations up to 1 mg per plate using the plate incorporation assay. NFA caused a positive response in strains TA1535, TA100, and TA98 following metabolic activation.

Genotoxicity

2-AAF is undoubtedly a genotoxic carcinogen. 2-AAF, in addition to exerting its genotoxic effects, often causes a variety of nongenotoxic alterations *in vivo* and *in vitro*.

Carcinogenicity

Administration of 2-AAF caused tumors at several different tissue sites in mice and rats. Dietary administration of 2-AAF caused cancer of the liver (hepatocellular carcinoma) and urinary bladder (transitional-cell carcinoma) in female mice and in rats of both sexes. 2-AAF is carcinogenic to experimental animals, but it is 'reasonably anticipated to be a human carcinogen.'

Clinical Management

In case of contact with material, the eyes should be flushed immediately with running water for at least 15 min, and affected skin should be washed with soap and water. If inhaled, the victim should be moved to fresh air and emergency medical care should be provided. In case of difficulty in breathing, artificial respiration should be provided. Contaminated clothing and shoes should be removed and isolated from the site.

Exposure Standards and Guidelines

As per OSHA, workers' exposure to 2-AAF can be confined by use of engineering controls, work practices, and personal protective equipment, including respirators. NIOSH considers 2-AAF to be a potential occupational carcinogen. NIOSH usually recommends that occupational exposures to carcinogens be limited to the lowest feasible concentration.

Other Hazards

Acetylaminofluorene can be easily ignited by heat, sparks, or flames. Vapors may form explosive mixtures with air. Vapors may travel to the source of ignition and flash back. Most vapors are heavier than air. They can spread along ground and collect in low or confined areas (sewers, basements, tanks). Vapor explosion hazard exists indoors, outdoors, or in sewers.

See also: Carcinogenesis; Cytochrome P450.

Further Reading

Bagnyukova, T.V., Tryndyak, V.P., Montgomery, B., et al., 2008. Genetic and epigenetic changes in rat preneoplastic liver tissue induced by 2-acetylaminofluorene. Carcinogenesis 29 (3), 638–646.

Frith, C.H., Kodell, R.L., Farmer, J.H., 1986. The effects of continued versus discontinued administration of 2-acetylaminofluorene on the morphology and behavior of hepatocellular and urinary bladder tumors in mice. J. Environ. Pathol. Toxicol. Oncol. 7 (1–2), 17–23.

Heflich, R.H., Neft, R.E., 1994. Genetic toxicity of 2-acetylaminofluorene, 2-aminofluorene and some of their metabolites and model metabolites. Mutat. Res. 318 (2), 73–114.

Jain, V., Hilton, B., Patnaik, S., et al., 2012. Conformational and thermodynamic properties modulate the nucleotide excision repair of 2-aminofluorene and 2-acetylaminofluorene dG adducts in the NarI sequence. Nucleic Acids Res. 40 (9), 3939–3951.

Littlefield, N.A., Farmer, J.H., Gaylor, D.W., Sheldon, W.G., 1980. Effects of dose and time in a long-term, low-dose carcinogenic study. J. Environ. Pathol. Toxicol. 3 (3 Spec No), 17–34.

Mu, H., Kropachev, K., Wang, L., et al., 2012. Nucleotide excision repair of 2-acetylaminofluorene and 2-aminofluorene-(C8)-guanine adducts: molecular dynamics simulations elucidate how lesion structure and base sequence context impact repair efficiencies. Nucleic Acids Res. 40 (19), 9675–9690.

Pogribny, I.P., Muskhelishvili, L., Tryndyak, V., et al., 2009. The tumor-promoting activity of 2-acetylaminofluorene is associated with disruption of the p53 signaling pathway and the balance between apoptosis and cell proliferation. Toxicol. Appl. Pharmacol. 235 (3), 305–311.

Pogribny, I.P., Muskhelishvili, L., Tryndyak, V.P., Beland, F.A., 2011. The role of epigenetic events in genotoxic hepatocarcinogenesis induced by 2-acetylaminofluorene. Mutat. Res. 722 (2), 106–113.

Rohrbeck, A., Salinas, G., Maaser, K., et al., 2010. Toxicogenomics applied to in vitro carcinogenicity testing with Balb/c 3T3 cells revealed a gene signature predictive of chemical carcinogens. Toxicol. Sci. 118 (1), 31–41.

Shimada, T., Murayama, N., Yamazaki, H., et al., March 13, 2013. Metabolic activation of polycyclic aromatic hydrocarbons and aryl and heterocyclic amines by human cytochromes P450 2A13 and 2A6. Chem. Res. Toxicol. (Epub ahead of print).

Shpyleva, S.I., Muskhelishvili, L., Tryndyak, V.P., et al., 2011. Chronic administration of 2-acetylaminofluorene alters the cellular iron metabolism in rat liver. Toxicol. Sci. 123 (2), 433–440.

Sigala, F., Kostopanagiotou, G., Andreadou, I., et al., 2004. Histological and lipid peroxidation changes after administration of 2-acetylaminofluorene in a rat liver injury model following selective periportal and pericentral damage. Toxicology 196, 155–163.

Williams, G.M., Iatropoulos, M.J., Jeffrey, A.M., 2004. Thresholds for the effects of 2-Acetylaminofluorene in rat liver. Toxicol. Pathol. 32 (S2), 85–91.

Relevant Websites

http://www.cdc.gov/niosh/docs/81-123/pdfs/0007.pdf – Center for Disease Control and Prevention.

http://www.epa.gov/ttnatw01/hlthef/acetylam.html – Environmental Protection Agency. GOV.

http://ntp.niehs.nih.gov/ntp/roc/twelfth/profiles/Acetylaminofluorene.pdf – National Toxicology Program, 2011. Report on Carcinogens.

http://nj.gov/health/eoh/rtkweb/documents/fs/0010.pdf – New Jersey Department of Health.

https://www.osha.gov/dts/chemicalsampling/data/CH_216800.html – Occupational Safety and Health Administration. GOV.

http://chem.sis.nlm.nih.gov/chemidplus – US National Library of Medicine: ChemIDplus Advanced: Search for Acetylaminofluorene.

Acetylcholine

A Suryanarayanan, Manchester College School of Pharmacy, Fort Wayne, IN, USA

This article is a revision of the previous edition article by Sanjay Chanda and Harihara M. Mehendale, volume 1, pp 33–34, © 2005, Elsevier Inc.

- Name: Acetylcholine
- Chemical Abstracts Service Registry Number: 51-84-3
- Synonyms: Acecoline; Choline acetate; Arterocholine; 2-(Acetoxy)-*N,N,N*-trimethylethanaminium; Ethanaminium; 2-(Acetyloxy)-*N,N,N*-trimethyl
- Chemical Structure:

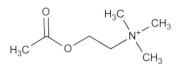

- Molecular Weight = 146.20744

Background Information

Acetylcholine is the endogenous neurotransmitter at cholinergic synapses and neuromuscular junctions in the central and peripheral nervous systems. Acetylcholine is involved in control of behavioral state, posture, cognition and memory, and the autonomous parasympathetic (and preganglionic sympathetic) nervous system. The actions of acetylcholine are mediated through nicotinic and muscarinic cholinergic receptors, which transduce signals via ion channel coupled and G-protein coupled receptor pathways, respectively.

Uses

Acetylcholine is an endogenous neurotransmitter. It was the first neurotransmitter to be discovered. There are commercially available drugs that either block or mimic actions of acetylcholine. Commercial drugs used as cholinergic agonists mimic the action of acetylcholine (e.g. bethanechol, carbachol, and pilocarpine). Cholinesterase inhibitors cause accumulation of acetylcholine and stimulation of the central nervous system, glands, and muscles. Some nerve agents such as the gas Sarin and organophosphate pesticides are examples. Clinically, acetylcholinesterase inhibitors are employed to treat myasthenia gravis and Alzheimer's disease. Acetylcholine receptor antagonists are antimuscarinic agents (atropine, scopolamine), ganglionic blockers (hexamethonium, mecamylamine), and neuromuscular blockers (tubocurarine, pancuronium, succinylcholine).

Exposure Routes and Pathways

Acetylcholine is present in the body as a neurotransmitter. Acetylcholinesterase is the enzyme responsible for breakdown of acetylcholine in the synapse. Any drug classified as cholinergic agonist (which mimics the action of acetylcholine) or anticholinesterase agent (e.g., organophosphorus pesticides, which block the action of acetylcholinesterase and hence stop the breakdown of acetylcholine in the synapse) can increase the level of acetylcholine in the body. Organophosphate poisoning, which is one of the most common cause of poisoning worldwide, causes large amounts of acetylcholine to accumulate in various nerves and receptors. This accumulation leads to muscle weakness, cramps, tachycardia, anxiety, headache, respiratory depression, and death. The most common exposure pathways for the cholinergic agonists are ingestion or eye contact. Acetylcholine chloride is available as an intraocular solution, methacholine chloride is available as a powder, bethanechol chloride is available as tablets, and carbachol is available as an ophthalmic solution. Common exposure pathways to anticholinesterase agents are ingestion, dermal or ocular contact, or inhalation.

Toxicokinetics

Acetylcholine is broken down by the acetylcholinesterase enzyme to choline and acetate. The time required for hydrolysis of acetylcholine is less than a millisecond. If the enzyme is depleted or inhibited, then excessive acetylcholine accumulation in the body can cause toxicity. Symptoms are salivation, lacrimation, urination, diarrhea, muscle tremor, and fasciculation.

Mechanism of Toxicity

Cholinergic agents can increase the acetylcholine level at the synaptic junction and cause rapid firing of the postsynaptic membrane. Antiacetylcholinesterase agents block the acetylcholinesterase enzyme and thus increase the acetylcholine level in the synapse causing rapid firing of the postsynaptic membrane.

Acute and Short-Term Toxicity (or Exposure)

Animal

The clinical signs of excess acetylcholine at nerve endings mimic hyperactivity of the parasympathetic nervous system. Signs relative to the alimentary tract include excess salivation, abdominal pain, vomiting, intestinal hypermotility, and diarrhea. The muscarinic effects of acetylcholine cause bronchoconstriction and an increase in bronchial secretions. The nicotinic effects of acetylcholine consist of involuntary irregular, violent muscle contractions and weakness of voluntary muscles. Death occurs as a result of respiratory failure. Toxicology data for acetylcholine chloride: oral LD_{50} in rat, acute is

 http://dx.doi.org/10.1016/B978-0-12-386454-3.00218-9

2500 mg kg^{-1}, intravenous LD_{50} in mouse is 170 mg kg^{-1}, and LD_{50} in guinea pig is 7.7 mg kg^{-1}.

Human

Acetylcholine agents are contraindicated in persons with asthma, hyperthyroidism, coronary insufficiency, and peptic ulcer. The bronchoconstrictor effect can precipitate asthma, hyperthyroid patients can develop atrial fibrillation, hypotension induced by these agents can reduce coronary blood flow, and gastric acid secretion caused by these agents can aggravate the symptoms of peptic ulcer. Excessive acetylcholine can also cause flushing, sweating, bradycardia, hypotension, abdominal cramps, belching, diarrhea, sensation of tightness in the urinary bladder, involuntary defecation and urination, penile erection, difficulty in visual accommodation, headache, salivation, and lacrimation. It can also cause paralysis of the respiratory muscles. Central nervous system effects include ataxia, confusion, slurred speech, loss of reflexes, Cheyne–Stokes respiration, and finally coma. The time of death after a single acute exposure ranges from 5 min to 24 h depending on the route, dose, and agent of exposure (among other factors).

Chronic Toxicity (or Exposure)

Animal

Animals can lose weight because of the inability to feed and drink because of muscular weakness. Clinical signs in birds include goosestepping, ataxia, wing spasms, wing droop, dyspnea (difficulty in breathing), tenesmus (spasm of anal sphincter), diarrhea, salivation, lacrimation, ptosis (drooping) of the eyelids, and wing-beat convulsions. Susceptibility to organophosphate toxicity varies greatly among individuals of any species and can be increased by frequent repeated mild exposure, which results in greater susceptibility due to exhaustion of the body's store of cholinesterase. No definite postmortem changes are seen and when present are usually secondary to the symptoms; these changes include pulmonary edema, asphyxia, gastroenteritis, and rarely kidney and liver degeneration.

Human

Chronic toxicity can cause polyneuritis, which starts with mild sensory disturbances, ataxia, weakness, and ready fatigability of legs, accompanied by fasciculation, muscle twitching, and tenderness to palpitation. In severe cases, the weakness may progress eventually to complete flaccid paralysis that, over the course of weeks or months, is often succeeded by a spastic paralysis with a concomitant exaggeration of reflexes. During these phases, muscles show marked wasting.

Clinical Management

Exposure should be terminated as soon as possible either by removing the patient or by fitting the patient with a gas mask if the atmosphere remains contaminated. Contaminated clothing should be removed immediately; the skin and mouth should be washed with copious amounts of water. Gastric lavage should be conducted if necessary. Artificial respiration should be administered if required, and administration of oxygen may be necessary. If the convulsion persists, diazepam (5–10 mg intravenously) or sodium thiopental (2.5% intravenously) should be administered, and the patient should be treated for shock. Atropine should be administered in sufficiently large doses, but atropine has no effect on peripheral neuromuscular activation and subsequent paralysis. Pralidoxime (1 or 2 g infused intravenously) should be administered for all peripheral effects. Pralidoxime is an oxime that binds to organophosphate-inactivated acetylcholinesterase to regenerate the enzyme. It is used as an antidote for poisoning by organophosphates or acetylcholinesterase inhibitors (nerve agents), in combination with atropine and diazepam.

See also: Cholinesterase Inhibition; Common Mechanism of Toxicity in Pesticides; Organophosphorus Compounds.

Further Reading

Abdollahi, M., Karami-Mohajeri, S., 2012. A comprehensive review on experimental and clinical findings in intermediate syndrome caused by organophosphate poisoning. Toxicol. Appl. Pharmacol. 258 (3), 309–314.

Brown, M., 2009. Military chemical warfare agent human subjects testing: part 2–long-term health effects among participants of U.S. military chemical warfare agent testing. Mil. Med. 174 (10), 1049–1054.

Brown, J.H., Taylor, P., 1996. Muscarinic receptor agonists and antagonists. In: Hardman, J.G., Limbird, L.E. (Eds.), Goodman and Gillman's Pharmacological Basis of Therapeutics, twelfth ed. McGraw-Hill, New York, pp. 169–276.

Acetylcholinsterase *see* Cholinesterase Inhibition

Acetylene

S Mostafalou and H Bahadar, Tehran University of Medical Sciences, Tehran, Iran

This article is a revision of the previous edition article by Ralph J. Parod, volume 1, pp 34–36, © 2005, Elsevier Inc.

- Name: Acetylene
- Chemical Abstracts Service Registry Number: CAS 74-86-2
- Synonyms: Acetylene, Ethyne, Welding gas, Ethine
- Chemical Class: Aliphatic hydrocarbon C_nH_{2n-2}
- Molecular Formula: C_2H_2
- Chemical Structure:

$$HC \equiv CH$$

Background and Significant History

Acetylene was discovered in 1836 and named by Berthelot in 1860, who studied the properties of this gas. It was used for the first time for lighting in 1892 after the work by Moissan. The oxyacetylene blow pipe was invented in 1901 by Charles, leading to the extensive industrial use of oxyacetylene flame in steel welding, scarfing, surface cementation, oxygen cutting, and hard surfacing.

Uses of Acetylene

About 80% of acetylene production is used as a closed-system manufacturing intermediate for the production of other chemicals. The other chemicals synthesized from acetylene include vinyl chloride monomer, *N*-vinylcarbazole, 1,4-butanediol, vinyl ethers, *N*-vinyl-2-pyrrolidone, vinyl fluoride, *N*-vinylcaprolactam, and vinyl esters. The other use of acetylene as oxyacetylene torches for metal cutting and welding is about 20%.

Environmental Fate and Behavior

Acetylene is released to the environment through various industrial waste streams of industries. Because of the vapor pressure of acetylene (4.04×10^4 mm Hg at 25 °C), it exists in the environment exclusively in the form of gas. The gaseous phase of acetylene is degraded in the environment with photochemically induced hydroxyl radicals; the half-life for this photochemical degradation is approximately 20 days. The estimated K_{oc} of acetylene is 38, and based upon this K_{oc} value, acetylene is expected to possess high mobility if released to soil. Based on the Henry's law constant of 0.022 atm-m^{3}mol^{-1}, derived from vapor pressure 4.04×10^4 mm Hg and water solubility 1200 mg l^{-1}, volatilization from moist soil is the major fate process for acetylene. In soil, biodegradation is not expected to be an important fate process for acetylene, as suggested by 0% biochemical oxygen demand (BOD) in 28 days. Acetylene is not anticipated to be adsorbed by suspended solids and sediments if released to water because of its K_{oc} value. Removal of acetylene from water is expected to be through the volatilization process. The estimated bioconcentration factor (BCF) of 3 for acetylene suggests that the potential for bioaccumulation of acetylene in aquatic organism is low.

Exposure and Exposure Monitoring

Routes and Pathways

Minimal consumer exposure is expected when acetylene is used as a closed-system industrial chemical. However, during welding and scarfing, the major route of exposure is through inhalation of oxyacetylene.

Human Exposure

Human exposure is most likely to occur in workplaces where acetylene is used, and from the atmosphere when released from the other sources. The potential source of exposure for humans is oxyacetylene during welding.

Toxicokinetics

After inhalation, acetylene is rapidly absorbed and eliminated from the body in unchanged form. At normal hematocrit and body temperature, the blood–gas partition coefficient of acetylene is 0.833, which indicates that acetylene has a greater tendency to be eliminated from blood.

Mechanism of Toxicity

Acetylene inactivates the cytochrome p450 enzyme by alkylating the prosthetic heme. Exposure to acetylene causes asphyxiation and depletes atmospheric oxygen.

Acute and Short-Term Toxicity

Animal

- Exposing rats to a concentration of 78% of acetylene (780 000 ppm) for 15 min and inhalation of 90% of acetylene for 2 h caused anesthesia and respiratory failure, respectively.
- Loss of heme and a marked accumulation of porphyrins were observed after exposing the male Wistar rats to 5% acetylene for 18 h.
- Decreased carbon dioxide tension was seen after exposing the rabbits to an acetylene/oxygen mixture containing up to 700 000 ppm of acetylene.

Human

Acetylene at concentrations below a lower explosive limit of 2.5% (25 000 ppm) is not toxic to humans. Varying degrees of temporary and reversible central nervous system depression have been seen after exposure to oxygen containing 10% acetylene. Unconsciousness has been observed in humans after inhaling 33 or 35% acetylene within 7 and 5 min, respectively, and exposure to 80% acetylene has caused complete anesthesia, forced respiration, and hypertension.

Chronic Toxicity

Animals

Significant plasma elevation of aspartate and alanine transaminases has been observed in white rabbits after inhaling crude acetylene at concentration of 58 000 ppm for 10 min at 12-h intervals for a period of 3 weeks. In addition, the catalase activity was depressed in the heart, kidney, and liver tissues. A rise in superoxide dismutase was also observed in the heart tissues.

Human

It is suggested that crude acetylene may have deleterious effects on the blood constituents and vital organs of human in chronic exposures.

Genotoxicity

Sufficient evidence provided by Ames test employing three strains of *Salmonella typhimurium* (TA97, TA98, and TA100) show that acetylene is not genotoxic.

Clinical Management

Ocular Exposure

Remove the patient from the exposure area; irrigate the affected eyes thoroughly with water or 0.9% saline.

Inhalation

After inhaling acetylene gas, the patient needs to be removed from exposure area quickly.

The patient needs to be provided adequate ventilation and oxygen if required. Monitor and manage the patient according to the signs and symptoms.

Ecotoxicology

Aquatic Ecotoxicity

Due to its gaseous nature, acetylene rapidly evaporates from aquatic system to air, and limited data are available about the toxic effects of acetylene on fish.

Other Hazards

Acetylene is a reactive gas and poses a high risk for fire and explosion. Acetylene reacts with active metals such as copper, silver, and mercury to form explosive acetylide compounds. Impurities such as phosphine may be present in acetylene obtained from calcium carbide, which can have deleterious effects on human health.

Exposure Standards and Guidelines

Exposure limits recommended by National Institute of Occupational Safety and Health for acetylene is 2500 ppm as a ceiling.

Miscellaneous

Melting point: −8.07°C.
Boiling point: −8.47°C.
Log p (octanol–water): 0.37.
Vapor pressure: 5240 mm Hg.
Henry's law constant: 0.022 atm-m^3 mol^{-1}.
Water solubility: 1200 mg l^{-1}.

See also: National Institute for Occupational Safety and Health; Pollution, Air in Encyclopedia of Toxicology; Aquatic Ecotoxicology.

Further Reading

American Chemistry Council Acetylene Panel, 2006. Test Plan for Acetylene CAS No.74-86-2, pp. 1–19. www.epa.gov/hpv/pubs/summaries/acetylen/c15005rt2.pdf.

Okolie, N.P., Ozolua, R.I., Osagie, D.E., 2005. Some biochemical and haematological effects associated with chronic inhalation of crude acetylene in rabbits. J. Med. Sci. 5, 21–25.

Screening-Level Hazard Characterization of High Production Volume Chemicals; Acetylene (CAS No. 74-86-2), 2008. Environmental Protection Agency, 1200 Pennsylvania Avenue, NW, Washington, DC 20460-0001. http://www.epa.gov/hpvis/hazchar/74862_Acetylene_HC_INTERIM_June%202008.pdf.

Williams, N.R., Whittington, R.M., 2001. Death due to inhalation of industrial acetylene. J. Toxicol. Clin. Toxicol. 39, 69–71.

Relevant Websites

http://www.hpa.org.uk/webc/HPAwebFile/HPAweb_C/1246260034508 – Health Protection Agency.

http://www.inchem.org – International Programme on Chemical Safety: INCHEM: Acetylene.

http://toxnet.nlm.nih.gov – Toxnet (Toxicology Data Network): search under Toxline for Urea.

http://chem.sis.nlm.nih.gov/chemidplus – US National Library of Medicine: ChemIDplus Advanced: Search for: Acetylene.

Acetylsalicylic Acid

R Gorodetsky, D'Youville College School of Pharmacy, Buffalo, NY, USA

- Name: Acetylsalicylic acid
- Chemical Abstracts Service Registry Number: CAS 50-78-2
- Synonyms: Aspirin, ASA, 2-(Acetyloxy)benzoic acid, 2-Carboxyphenyl acetate
- Molecular Formula: $C_9H_8O_4$
- Chemical Structure:

O
OH
O
O
CH_3

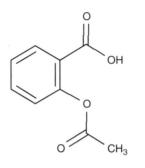

Background

The use of aspirin to treat fever dates back to antiquity with the use of willow bark and leaves. Ever since the active component of willow bark was isolated and marketed in 1899, it has remained one of the most popular medications for the treatment of fever, pain, and inflammation. Aspirin is consistently listed among the agents most often involved in human exposures, and is considered the causative agent in scores of deaths each year.

Uses

Aspirin is used as an analgesic, antipyretic, and anti-inflammatory agent.

Environmental Fate and Behavior

As in humans, the environmental fate of acetylsalicylic acid is pH dependent. Above pH 5.5, acetylsalicylic acid will be the predominant form seen. Anions generally do not volatilize or undergo adsorption to the extent of their neutral counterparts. Although information is limited, aspirin is considered readily biodegradable and is ultimately mineralized to carbon dioxide and water.

Exposure and Exposure Monitoring

Routes and Pathways

Ingestion is the most common route of both accidental and intentional exposures, though rectal exposures have been reported. Toxicity from dermal exposure has not been reported. Intravenous aspirin is available in some countries, though toxicity resulting from this route has not been reported.

Human Exposure

Human exposures to aspirin in the United States are monitored through the National Poison Data System, which draws its information from the poison center system. In 2010, there were nearly 30 000 single-substance exposures to aspirin-containing products reported to US poison centers, and aspirin was involved in 62 fatalities.

Toxicokinetics

Aspirin is rapidly hydrolyzed into salicylate, an active metabolite, in both the gastrointestinal tract and the bloodstream. Both aspirin and salicylate are readily absorbed by passive diffusion across the gastric membrane, with absorption influenced by gastric pH. After a therapeutic dose, peak serum concentrations are typically achieved within 1 h, or within 4–6 h for enteric-coated preparations. Aspirin has a volume of distribution of approximately 0.2 l kg^{-1} and is 90% protein bound. The serum half-life of acetylsalicylic acid is only 15 min, while the half-life of salicylate is approximately 6 h. In overdose, peak serum concentration may be delayed due to pylorospasm, concretions or bezoars, gastric outlet obstruction, or coingestants that slow gastric motility. Peak serum concentrations occurring beyond 24 h postingestion have been reported. The volume of distribution increases to greater than 0.3 l kg^{-1}, and protein binding decreases to less than 75% in overdose, while the kinetics change from first-order elimination to zero-order, with half-lives of 20 h or more. Aspirin metabolites are renally eliminated with 10% as salicylic acid, 75% salicyluric acid, 10% phenolic glucuronide, and 5% acyl glucuronide.

Mechanism of Toxicity

The toxicity of aspirin is multifactorial. Gastrointestinal symptoms such as nausea, vomiting, and abdominal pain occur as a result of both local gastric irritation and stimulation of the medullary chemoreceptor trigger zone. Salicylates directly stimulate the respiratory drive in the brain stem, leading to hyperventilation and respiratory alkalosis. Anion gap metabolic acidosis occurs from a buildup of organic acids as well as the uncoupling of oxidative phosphorylation, which results in an imbalance in ATP consumption and production, resulting in a net buildup of hydrogen ions. Therefore, aspirin often causes a mixed acid–base status. Furthermore, the uncoupling of oxidative phosphorylation results in failure to produce ATP despite increased oxygen utilization, which leads to heat production and hyperthermia. Aspirin interferes with

 http://dx.doi.org/10.1016/B978-0-12-386454-3.00687-4

glucose metabolism and gluconeogenesis, and can cause profound decreases in cerebrospinal fluid glucose concentrations despite normal blood glucose concentrations.

Acute and Short-Term Toxicity

Animal

Animals manifest toxicity to aspirin with similar signs and symptoms to those seen in humans. These may include vomiting and gastric hemorrhage, hyperpnea, respiratory alkalosis, metabolic acidosis, hyperthermia, and seizures. Methemoglobinemia has also been seen in animals following salicylate toxicity.

Human

Acute ingestions of greater than150 mg kg^{-1} may result in toxic effects. Early manifestations of toxicity include nausea, vomiting, and tinnitus, followed by hyperventilation with respiratory alkalosis and concomitant metabolic acidosis. Overall serum pH typically demonstrates alkalosis early in the course of toxicity in adult patients, which may convert to predominant acidosis as the patient's condition deteriorates. Early hyperglycemia may be followed by hypoglycemia or neuroglycopenia. More ominous signs and symptoms associated with severe toxicity include hyperthermia, altered mental status, coma, seizures, cerebral edema, and death. Other symptoms that may be observed include acute lung injury and pulmonary edema, acute renal failure, acute liver injury, and coagulopathies. Signs and symptoms of aspirin toxicity may begin to occur at serum concentrations greater than 30 mg dl^{-1}.

Chronic Toxicity

Animal

Daily doses of acetylsalicylic acid in cats produced toxic hepatitis, vomiting, weight loss, and poor appetite in the low-dose group (33–63 mg kg^{-1} day^{-1}) and anemia, gastric lesions, and death in the high-dose group (81–130 mg kg^{-1} day^{-1}). High doses of aspirin given to mice on day 6 of gestation produced large incidence of lethal deformities.

Human

Chronic salicylism presents similarly to acute toxicity, although more severe symptoms may be present at lower serum concentrations. Chronic salicylism patients will have more profound clinical effects at lower serum salicylate levels compared to patients with acute overdoses. Chronic salicylism is often associated with a delay in diagnosis and higher morbidity and mortality.

Reproductive Toxicity

Aspirin readily crosses the placenta, and if given near term, higher concentrations may be found in the neonate than the mother. Low-dose aspirin given chronically to pregnant patients may be beneficial in certain circumstances (pregnancies complicated by gestational hypertension or systemic lupus erythematosus) and has not been demonstrated to be harmful to the fetus or neonate. However, full-dose aspirin given in the third trimester has been associated with prolonged gestation and labor, premature closure of the ductus arteriosis, and bleeding complications in the neonate. Aspirin used around the time of conception has been associated with an increased risk of spontaneous abortion, and animal models indicate that aspirin may inhibit conception by blocking blastocyst implantation. Currently, there is no enough information to determine if aspirin is a human teratogen. Maternal aspirin overdose in pregnancy poses a serious threat to the fetus.

Carcinogenicity

The Carcinogenic Potency Project at the University of California, Berkeley has had no positive (carcinogenic) experiments with acetylsalicylic acid. Aspirin is not a known human carcinogen.

Clinical Management

Basic and advanced life-support measures should be utilized as necessary. Gastrointestinal decontamination with activated charcoal should be considered for appropriate patients. Patients with altered mental status or recurrent vomiting should not be given activated charcoal unless the airway is protected. Delayed absorption of aspirin is common in overdose, and therefore activated charcoal may be administered late, up to 8 h post-ingestion, and multiple doses may be beneficial. Correction of fluid and electrolyte disturbances is important. Intravenous sodium bicarbonate should be administered to patients manifesting signs and symptoms of salicylate toxicity with a goal of alkalinizing the urine to a pH of 7.5–8. This increases the urinary excretion of salicylate through ion trapping. Hemodialysis should be considered for patients manifesting severe toxicity such as hyperthermia, mental status changes, intractable acidosis, pulmonary edema, or renal failure, and for patients with serum salicylate levels greater than 100 mg dl^{-1} in acute overdose or greater than 60 mg dl^{-1} in chronic overdose.

See also: Charcoal; Salicylates; Pharmacokinetics.

Further Reading

Chyka, P.A., Erdman, A.R., Christianson, G., et al., 2007. Salicylate poisoning: an evidence-based consensus guideline for out-of-hospital management. Clin. Toxicol. 45, 95–131.

Done, A.K., 1960. Salicylate intoxication: significance of measurements of salicylates in blood in cases of acute ingestion. Pediatrics 26, 800–807.

O'Malley, G.F., 2007. Emergency department management of the salicylate-poisoned patient. Emerg. Med. Clin. North Am. 25, 333–346.

Relevant Website

http://health.shorehealth.org/ency/article/002542.htm – Aspirin overdose – Overview.

Acids

A Saeid and K Chojnacka, Institute of Inorganic Technology and Mineral Fertilizers, Wroclaw University of Technology, Wroclaw, Poland

Use

Depending on the type, acids have a wide range of uses. Common examples include acetic acid (in vinegar), sulfuric acid (used in car batteries), and tartaric acid (used in baking). Acids can be liquids (sulfuric acid), solids (anhydrous H_2SO_4, citric acid), or gases (anhydrous HCl, HBr). Strong acids and some concentrated weak acids are corrosive, but there are exceptions, such as carbonic and boric acid, which can be in powder form.

In humans and other mammals, hydrochloric acid is found in the gastric acid (pH usually 1.5–3.5) secreted within the stomach to help hydrolyze proteins and polysaccharides, as well as converting the inactive proenzyme pepsinogen into the enzyme pepsin.

The acidulants malic acid, fumaric acid, and citric acid occur naturally in all living organisms. They all play an integral part in the respiratory processes in living cells. These compounds are formed during cellular metabolism of all living biosystems. The acids provide the cell with energy and the carbon skeletons for the formation of amino acids. The following acids are present in human body and play crucial roles in metabolism: fatty acids, amino acids, nucleic acids, ascorbic acid, and pantothenic acid, also called pantothenate or vitamin B_5. The examples of different acids and their most important toxicological properties are presented in **Table 1**.

Exposure Routes and Pathways

Exposure assessment is a major component of risk assessment. Dermal contact, inhalation, and ingestion are the most common exposure pathways.

Toxicokinetics

Acids can be divided into two groups: organic and inorganic (mineral). Toxicokinetics depends on the type of acid.

Mechanism of Toxicity

The mechanism of toxicity by different acids differs greatly: some are corrosive, other are poisonous, and some are explosive.

Corrosives cause tissue injury by a chemical reaction. Acids cause coagulative necrosis. The acid denatures all tissue protein to form acid proteinates. As a result, both structural and enzymatic proteins are denatured. The vast majority of caustic chemicals are acidic substances that damage tissues by donating a proton in an aqueous solution. The pH of acids is a measure of how easily the chemical donates a proton. This relates to the strength of the acidic substance, and provides some, but not precise correlation with the likelihood of injury. Substances with a pH less than 2 are considered to be strong acids. The severity of tissue injury from acidic substances is determined by the duration of contact: the amount and state (liquid, solid) of the substance involved and the physical properties of the substance, such as pH, concentration, and ability to penetrate tissues. The last reflects the amount of tissue required to neutralize a given amount of the involved substance and is particularly useful for measuring the degree of damage that can be caused by caustics such as phenol, which is a weak acid (nearly neutral pH).

Other acids are dangerous because of toxic rather than acidic qualities. Hydrocyanic acid is a poisonous gas that is difficult to detect. Sulfuric acid is a dangerous dehydrating agent; it can be very dangerous upon contact with eyes, skin, mouth, or other acids. Hydrogen sulfide is highly toxic and forms a complex bond with iron in the mitochondrial cytochrome enzymes, thus preventing cellular respiration. Hydrochloric acid readily releases toxic fumes and can corrode many metals. Picric acid is extremely explosive. Strong acids produce superficial injuries to the esophagus and deep injuries to various parts of the stomach. The mechanism of toxicity depends on the specific type of acid.

Hydrofluoric acid is an interesting case; it is a weak acid (it does not ionize) and as a result can be absorbed by the skin very quickly. Hydrofluoric acid injuries have a potential for both systemic as well as severe local tissue destruction. Once absorbed, it damages tissue, causing severe pain, chemical imbalances, and almost certain death if more than 50 ml are in contact with skin. It interferes with nerve function, meaning that burns may not initially be painful. Accidental exposures can go unnoticed, delaying treatment and increasing the extent and seriousness of the injury (*See* Hydrofluoric Acid).

Among the common laboratory acids, the most dangerous to work with is usually concentrated nitric acid because it reacts strongly with many chemicals, releasing poisonous gases (NO_x). Its fumes can cause explosions, and instantly oxidize flesh, causing severe burns.

Toxicity

Short-term and chronic toxicity (or exposure) both for animal and human cause corrosion of skin and mucosal surface. Repetitive ingestion of acids may induce mucosala forestomach hyperplasia.

Clinical Management

In cases of exposure, therapy should be accurate and immediate. Exposure should be terminated as soon as possible by transfer of the patient to fresh air. A mild soap solution may be used for washing the skin as an aid to neutralize the acid. In the case of ingestion, water and/or milk should be provided (dilution, neutralization). Stimulation to cause vomiting is not advised as this may cause further oral, esophageal, or

 http://dx.doi.org/10.1016/B978-0-12-386454-3.00219-0

Table 1 Examples of acids and their toxicological properties

Name/Formula	*Uses*	*Ecotoxicity fish and invertebrate*	*Mammalian and avian toxicity*	*Teratogenicity and reproductive effects*	*Metabolism and toxicokinetics*	*Legislation*
Sulfuric acid H_2SO_4	• Manufacture of: ○ fertilizers ○ paper ○ glue ○ dyes ○ detergents • Petroleum purification • Metal pickling	• LC_{50} (48 h) flounder: 100–330 mg l^{-1} • LC_{50} (48 h) brown shrimp 60–70 mg l^{-1}	• LD_{50} oral rat 2.14 g kg^{-1} • LC_{50} (2 h) inhalation mouse 320 mg m^{-3} • LC_{50} (2 h) inhalation rat 510 mg m^{-3}	• No effects were observed (dose $\leq$20 mg m^{-3}) for mice • Not confirmed possibility of a carcinogenetic effects in human	• Sulfuric acid is unlikely to accumulate in the body – excreted in the urine	• EC Directive on Drinking Water Quality 80/778/EEC • SO_4^{2-} maximum admissible concentration 250 mg l^{-1} • Recommended level 25 mg l^{-1}
Phosphoric acid H_3PO_4	• Manufacture of: ○ fertilizers ○ phosphate salts ○ polyphosphate ○ detergents ○ catalyst in ethylene • Hydrogen peroxide purification • Flavor acidulant • Synergistic antioxidant and sequestrant in food • Pharmaceutic acid • Dental cements	• LC_{50} (96 h) 'aquatic life' 100–1000 mg l^{-1}	• LC_{50} oral rat 1530 mg kg^{-1} • LC_{50} inhalation mouse 25.5 mg m^{-3} • LC_{50} dermal rabbit 2740 mg kg^{-1}	• No adverse reproductive effects are seen in rats	• After oral absorption eliminated in urine	• Maximum tolerable daily intake (human) is 70 mg kg^{-1}
Acetic acid CH_3CO_2H	• Manufacture of: ○ plastics ○ rubber ○ tanning ○ printing ○ dyeing silks • Acidulant and preservative in foods and solvents for gums, resins, volatile oils	• LC_{50} (96 h) bluegill sunfish 75 mg l^{-1} • LC_{50} (96 h) fathead minnow 88 mg l^{-1} • LC_{50} (24 h) goldfish 423 mg l^{-1} • EC_{50} (24–48 h) *Daphnia magna*, brine shrimp 47–32 mg l^{-1}	• LD_{50} oral rat 3310 mg kg^{-1} • LC_{50} (1 h) inhalation guinea pigs 5000 mg l^{-1} • LD_{50} dermal rabbit 1060 mg kg^{-1}	• Not documented	• Acetic acid shows potential for biological accumulation or food chain contamination	• ACGIH ○ TLV: 25 mg m^{-3} ○ TWA: 15 mg m^{-3} ○ STEL: 37 mg m^{-3} • NIOSH ○ REL: 10 mg m^{-3} ○ TWA: 25 mg m^{-3}, 15 ppm ○ STEL: 37 mg m^{-3}
Benzoic acid $C_7H_6O_2$	• Foodstuff preservative in fast foods and fruit juices • Manufactures of dyestuffs • Antifungal agent	• LC_{50} (96 h) mosquito fish 180 mg l^{-1} • Cell multiplication inhibition test ○ *Pseudomonas sputida* 480 mg l^{-1} ○ *Microcystis aeruginosa* 55 mg l^{-1} ○ *Scenedesmus quadricauda* 1630 mg l^{-1} ○ *Entosiphon sulcatum* 218 mg l^{-1} ○ *Uronema parducci* 31 mg l^{-1}	• LD_{50} oral rat 1700 mg kg^{-1} • LD_{Lo} subcutaneous rabbit 2000 mg kg^{-1} • LD_{Lo} oral human 500 mg kg^{-1}	• Not documented	• Bioconcentration factor in golden ide and *Chlorella fusca* <10 • Human V clearance time 9–15 h • Administered orally, is absorbed from the gastrointestinal tract, conjugated with glycine in the liver to form hippuric (or as benzoylglucuronic acid when taken in high doses) acid, which is rapidly excreted in the urine within 12 h (up to 97% within the first 4 h)	• Commission Regulation (EC) No 877/2003 of 21 May 2003 provisionally authorizing the use of the acidity regulator 'Benzoic acid' in feeding stuffs

pulmonary damage. Clinical treatment in the case of exposure is related with the kind of contact and the type of acid (*See* Hydrofluoric Acid, Phosphoric Acid, Hydrochloric Acid). In the case of sulfuric acid, dilution is inappropriate because of extraordinary thermal effects (*See* Sulfuric Acid). In the case of eye injury, contact lenses should be removed after brief irrigation and then thorough wash should be applied, with 1% calcium gluconate eye drops every 3 h. Immediate ophthalmologic consultation is mandatory.

Ecotoxicology

Ecotoxicological aspects depend on the type of acid. Some acids are introduced into the environment in the form of pesticides and fertilizers. When used in inappropriate ways, they can cause acidification of soil and eutrophication of groundwater.

Another way to introduce acid to the environment is by gaseous oxide acidity: SO_2 from sulfuric acid, NO_2 from nitric acid, and HCl from hydrochloric acid. This is the mechanism of acid rain formation in the atmosphere.

Other Hazards

Other hazards vary depending on the type of acid.

Exposure Standard and Guidelines

Exposure standards and guidelines vary depending on the type of acid (*See* Okadaic Acid, Sulfuric Acid, Nitric acid).

See also: Valproic Acid; Methyl Parathion; Hydrobromic Acid; Hydroiodic Acid; Perfluorooctanoic Acid; Tannic Acid; Butyric Acid; *trans*-Fatty Acids; 5-Nitro-2-Furoic Acid; Phosphoric Acid; Hydrofluoric Acid; Perchloric Acid; Periodic Acid; Picric Acid; Propionic Acid; Peracetic Acid; Acetic Acid; Acrylic Acid; Sulfuric Acid; 2,4-D (2,4-Dichlorophenoxy Acetic Acid); EDTA (Ethylenediaminetetraacetic Acid); Formic Acid; Okadaic Acid; Acetylsalicylic Acid; Boric Acid; Folic Acid; Hydrochloric Acid; Dicarboxylic Acid; Mushrooms, Ibotenic Acid; Chloroacetic Acid.

Further Reading

Crowl, D.A., Louvar, J.F., 2011. Chemical Process Safety: Fundamentals with Applications, third ed. Pearson Education, USA.

Gangolli, S., 2005. Dictionary of Substances and Their Effects, third ed. Royal Society of Chemistry, Cambridge.

Harchelroad Jr., F.P., Rottinghaus, D.M., 2004. Chemical burns. In: Tintinalli, J.E., Kelen, G.D., Stapczynski, J.S., Ma, O.J., Cline, D.M. (Eds.), Emergency Medicine: A Comprehensive Study Guide, sixth ed. McGraw-Hill, New York.

Lewis Sr., R.J., 2007. Hawley's Condensed Chemical Dictionary, fifteenth ed. John Wiley & Sons, New York.

Pohanish, R.P., 2008. Sittig's Handbook of Toxic and Hazardous Chemicals and Carcinogens, fifth ed. William Andrew Publishing, USA.

Pohanish, R.P., Greene, S.A., 2009. Wiley Guide to Chemical Incompatibilities, third ed. John Wiley & Sons, New Jersey.

Smith, J., Hong-Shum, L., 2003. Food Additives Data Book. Blackwell Publishing, UK.

Timbrell, J., 2002. Introduction to Toxicology, third ed. Taylor & Francis, London.

Wentz, D., Wentz, M., Wallace, D.K., 2011. The Healthy Home: Simple Truths to Protect Your Family from Hidden Household Dangers. Vanguard Press, New York.

Relevant Websites

http://www.pesticideinfo.org/Search_Chemicals.jsp – PAN Pesticides Database - Chemicals: Search for Acids.

http://www.hpa.org.uk/webc/HPAwebFile/HPAweb_C/1194947358719 – Health Protection Agency.

http://www.inchem.org/documents/sids/sids/7664939.pdf – OECD Sigs: Sulfuric Acid.

Acifluorfen, Sodium Salt

YR Rodriguez, Arizona Department of Environmental Quality, Phoenix, AZ, USA

- Name: Acifluorfen, Sodium salt
- Chemical Abstracts Service Registry Number: 62476-59-9 (Sodium acifluorfen) 50594-66-6 (Acifluorfen)
- Synonyms: Acifluorfene, Blazer®, Tackle®, Carbofuorfen, 2-Nitro-5-(2-chloro-4-(trifluoromethyl)phenoxy)benzoic acid, 5-(2-Chloro-alpha,alpha,alpha-trifluoro-*p*-tolyloxy)-2-nitrobenzoic acid (IUPAC)
- Molecular Formula: $C_{14}H_7ClF_3NO_5$
- Chemical Structure:

Cl O F F F O N+ O- HO O

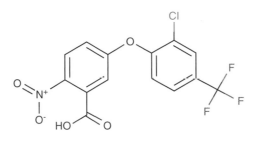

Background

Sodium acifluorfen was first registered in the United States in 1980 as the herbicide Blazer®, by the Rohm and Haas Company. In 1987, the BASF Corporation purchased the registration and supporting data. In 2003, the US Environmental Protection Agency (EPA) conducted an assessment to determine if pesticide products containing the active ingredient sodium acifluorfen were eligible for pesticide reregistration. Results of the US EPA assessment were explained in the Reregistration Eligibility Decision (RED) of sodium acifluorfen. The RED document determined pesticides with the active ingredient of sodium acifluorfen were eligible for reregistration provided certain stipulations listed in the RED document were met, which included additional label requirements to limit the potential for drift. Under the Federal Insecticide, Fungicide, and Rodenticide Act (FIFRA) Section 3, all new pesticides used in the United States must be registered by the Administrator of the US EPA. There are 12 registrations for sodium acifluorfen.

Uses

Sodium acifluorfen is a member of a diphenyl ether group of light-dependent peroxidizing herbicides. Sodium acifluorfen is also a member of the nitrophenyl ether class of herbicides. This class of herbicides can cause rapid disruption of cell membranes in plants. Acifluorfen penetrates into the cytoplasm and causes the formation of peroxides and free electrons (requires light), ultimately destroying the cell membrane. Destruction of the cell membrane prevents translocation to other regions of the plant. In the environment, sodium acifluorfen degrades to acifluorfen (or acifluorfen acid). Additionally, acifluorfen acid is a degradation product of lactofen, another herbicide used on agricultural crops and in forestry. Sodium acifluorfen can be used alone or formulated with similar herbicides. Various formulation types include liquid, ready-to-use, and soluble concentrates. Agricultural crop applications are conducted by aircraft and by broadcast and band treatment using ground equipment. A trigger spray bottle for spot treatment is used by both agricultural and residential applicators. Sodium acifluorfen is primarily used on agricultural crops as a nonselective herbicide for pre- and postemergent control of annual broadleaf weeds and grasses. From 2001 to 2007, the annual US agricultural consumption of sodium acifluorfen was estimated at 300 000 pounds. An estimated 200 000 pounds of the agricultural consumption was applied to soybean crops. Sodium acifluorfen is also used on the agricultural crops peanuts, rice, peas, and strawberries. Sodium acifluorfen is registered for residential use; however, it is limited to spot treatment with ready-to-use formulations. Residential application of sodium acifluorfen is minor compared to agricultural, since it is a nonselective herbicide that kills both weeds and grasses.

Environmental Fate and Behavior

Sodium acifluorfen is directly released into the environment as a pre/postemergent herbicide. In the environment, sodium acifluorfen dissociates to acifluorfen. Sodium acifluorfen has an estimated Henry's law constant of 6.03×10^{-11} atm-m^3 mol^{-1} derived from a vapor pressure of 1.33×10^{-5} mm Hg. Sodium acifluorfen has a water solubility of 62.07 g 100 ml^{-1} (at 20 °C) and an octanol/water partition coefficient of 1.55. Additionally, sodium acifluorfen has a pK_a of 3.86, indicating it will exist in the anion form at pH values from 5 to 9. Acifluorfen has an estimated vapor pressure of 1.5×10^{-8} mm Hg, K_{oc} values from 44 to 684, and an estimated pK_a of 2.07.

The pK_a of sodium acifluorfen indicates the compound will exist in an anion form in the environment. Compared to their neutral counterparts, anion forms do not strongly adsorb to soils containing organic carbon and clay. Anions do not volatilize, therefore it is highly unlikely that acifluorfen will volatilize from dry or moist soil conditions. Additionally, volatilization of sodium acifluorfen from water surfaces is also highly unlikely. The estimated vapor pressure of acifluorfen indicates that it will exist in both the vapor and particulate phases in the ambient air. Based on the K_{oc} value range of 44–684, acifluorfen has a very high to low mobility in soil. Adsorption and desorption are strongly correlated to site-specific soil parameters such as pH and mineral content.

In the environment, sodium acifluorfen dissociates to acifluorfen and sodium. Additionally, acifluorfen acid is a

 http://dx.doi.org/10.1016/B978-0-12-386454-3.01158-1

degradation product of lactofen, another herbicide used on agricultural crops and in forestry. In aerobic soil conditions, acifluorfen has a half-life ranging from 108 to 200 days, and in aerobic aquatic conditions the estimated half-life is 117 days. In anaerobic conditions, acifluorfen has an estimated half-life of 2.75 days. Persistence of the active ingredient in soil will vary based on conditions (i.e., soil pH, soil organic carbon content, and soil iron content). Acifluorfen will undergo photodecomposition in water with a half-life ranging from 21.7 to 352 h depending on water condition (i.e., sediment free, pH, water depth, etc.).

Sodium acifluorfen is expected to be transported by application drift and leaching. A potential method of transport for sodium acifluorfen into surface water is by runoff and erosion from treated soil.

Based on the low octanol/water partition coefficient, neither sodium acifluorfen ($K_{ow} = 3.70$) nor acifluorfen ($K_{ow} = 1.55$) is expected to bioaccumulate in aquatic organisms.

Exposure and Exposure Monitoring

As mentioned in the section Environmental Fate and Behavior, sodium acifluorfen is a nonselective herbicide and is directly released into the environment. The production process of sodium acifluorfen can result in a release to the environment through various waste streams. If acifluorfen reaches groundwater, the compound will persist because of its stability to abiotic hydrolysis. An alternative route to surface water for acifluorfen may come from discharge of acifluorfen-contaminated groundwater into surface water. There is a potential for acifluorfen to persist in surface water if photodegradation does not occur. Its ability to persist in surface waters indicates that runoff is a potential transport mechanism to aquatic and terrestrial organisms.

Occupational exposure to sodium acifluorfen can occur by inhalation and dermal contact at workplaces that produce the compound or during the application process. The label of sodium acifluorfen requires personal protective equipment in the form of a long sleeved shirt, long pants, and chemical resistant gloves. A respirator is not necessary. An occupational handler exposure study indicated there was no risk of concern for occupational handlers.

The general public's exposure can occur through dermal contact with products that contain the active ingredient. Residential use of sodium acifluorfen is as a spot treatment herbicide. Residential applicators are likely to be exposed when using sodium acifluorfen as a spot treatment to driveways, sidewalks, and patios. Health risk is considered to be little or none for residential postapplication exposure because application practices are limited.

Sodium acifluorfen and lactofen are both registered herbicides directly introduced into the environment that degrade to acifluorfen. Monitoring data are available in soil, surface water, and ground water for acifluorfen. Residues of sodium acifluorfen have been detected in 56 of 283 soil samples (up to 0.6 m depth). Residues were detected in samples up to 10 months postapplication. These results indicate that there is a potential for residues to reach groundwater via typical environmental transport. In 1992, acifluorfen residues were reported in the Pesticide in Ground Water Data Base (PGWDB), a summary of groundwater monitoring studies. The PGWDB reported 4 of 1185 sampled wells had concentrations of acifluorfen ranging from 0.003 to 0.025 $\mu g\,l^{-1}$.

The US Geological Survey (USGS) National Water Quality Assessment program conducted a water quality study throughout the United States from 1993 to 2007. Results showed quantifiable residues (estimated and measured) in 173 of 13 524 samples collected. In groundwater, 10 samples displayed residue levels with a maximum measured residue of 0.33 $\mu g\,l^{-1}$. The remaining 163 samples were collected from surface waters with a maximum estimated residue of 2.2 $\mu g\,l^{-1}$ and maximum measured residue of 1.1 $\mu g\,l^{-1}$. Both the surface and groundwater maximum residue results (measured and estimated) were collected from agricultural lands.

Toxicokinetics

Minimal published information can be found about toxicokinetic properties of acifluorfen. Because liver and kidney are known target organs based on animal studies, clearly acifluorfen distributes to those organs. Being just slightly more lipid soluble than water soluble (octanol/water partition coefficient at pH 7 is 1.55), some absorption into the body across lipid membranes can occur following exposure through skin, lungs, or GI tract. Although no detailed information was found about the rate of metabolism or excretion or identities of metabolites, the K_{ow} predicts a fairly short biological half-life in the body and excretion in urine. This would be consistent with the fact that acifluorfen does not bioaccumulate, and also with its relatively low oral, dermal, and inhalation toxicity.

Mechanism of Toxicity

Acifluorfen inhibits the enzyme protoporphyrinogen oxidase, which catalyzes the dehydrogenation of protoporphyrinogen IX to protoporphyrin IX. In the presence of light, accumulated protoporphyrin can generate highly reactive oxygen species and induce membrane lipid peroxidation. The peroxidation of the lipid can result in a chain reaction and cause fragmentation and destruction of the lipid. The consequence of lipid peroxidation for a cell is loss of the membrane function. The primary target organs for sodium acifluorfen are the liver and kidneys. However, there are limited data that suggest cells can synthesize cytochrome P450 for detoxification of sodium acifluorfen. Further study is needed to confirm this.

Acute and Short-Term Toxicity

Sodium acifluorfen has displayed low acute oral, dermal, and inhalation toxicity. Sodium acifluorfen can cause irreversible eye damage. It is not a skin sensitizer, but prolonged or frequent exposure to the skin can cause an allergic reaction. Acute exposure in rabbits indicates sodium acifluorfen is a severe eye irritant and a moderate skin irritant. The US EPA Toxicity Category system, ranging from I (most toxic) to IV (least toxic), classifies sodium acifluorfen for acute eye irritation as a Category I. Based on the US EPA scale, acute skin irritation is a Category II, acute oral and dermal toxicity is a Category III, and acute inhalation toxicity is a Category IV.

Chronic Toxicity

Sodium acifluorfen is a member of the diphenyl ether chemical family. The most common toxicity endpoint with this class of chemicals is liver effects. In subchronic and chronic studies for sodium acifluorfen, the primary target organs were the liver and kidney in mice, rats, and dogs. Subchronic feeding studies in rats and mice displayed a decrease in animal body weight and signs of liver toxicity, which included an increase in liver weight and an increased incidence of cellular hypertrophy. Chronic feeding studies in mice, rats, and dogs displayed reversible liver toxicity, which included acidophilic cells in the liver and an increased liver weight. Chronic feeding studies in mice, rats, and dogs also displayed kidney toxicity, including nephritis/pyelonephritis and increased kidney weight.

Immunotoxicity

Data are limited concerning immunotoxicity. Prolonged or frequent repeated skin exposure to sodium acifluorfen in some individuals can cause an allergic reaction. This endpoint indicates a potential immune system response but further study is needed to define a clear dose–response.

Reproductive Toxicity

Rats exposed to sodium acifluorfen have displayed a decrease in fetal body weight and an increase in anatomical variations. A two-generation reproduction study in rats reported an increase in pup mortality and kidney lesions; however, there were no changes in reproductive parameters. Rats exposed to sodium acifluorfen displayed minimal maternal toxicity, including excess salivation, chromorhinorrhea, piloerection, and urine-stained abdominal fur.

Genotoxicity

Acifluorfen has displayed negative results in genotoxicity studies. Sodium acifluorfen has displayed some weak mutagenic results in an Ames assay with metabolic activation and tumors in rodent studies but not enough evidence to confirm genotoxicity. Studies testing various purity forms of acifluorfen have indicated there is no evidence of induced mutations with or without metabolic activation. Testing has been conducted with purity concentrations of the active ingredient up to 42.8%.

Carcinogenicity

The International Agency for Research on Cancer (IARC) has not classified this herbicide. However, the US EPA Office of Pesticide Programs (OPP) previously classified sodium acifluorfen as a B2 chemical carcinogen (probable human carcinogen). Based on additional studies and reviews, the OPP changed the classification of sodium acifluorfen as "likely to be carcinogenic to humans at high enough doses to cause biochemical and histopathological changes in livers of rodents but unlikely to be carcinogenic at doses below those causing these changes." A study in 60 male and 60 female B6C3F$_1$ mice at doses of 0, 626, 1250, and 2500 ppm for 18 months resulted in decreased body weights in both sexes and an increase in liver tumors in the male mice. At the highest dose level tested (2500 ppm), the liver tumors in the male mice significantly increased above the controls tested and a significant reduction in body weight was recorded. In the female mice, only weight reduction was observed in the highest dose level tested (2500 ppm). Residential uses of sodium acifluorfen are limited to spot treatments only, so therefore carcinogenic effects are not expected to result from residential uses. Chronic occupational exposures are not expected. Typically, sodium acifluorfen is only applied one or two times a year, and therefore, cancer effects in applicators are not expected during the application process.

Clinical Management

Limited data are available on human exposure. However, fatalities have been observed following ingestion of 80 mg kg^{-1}, and health effects are noticeable at 50 mg kg^{-1}. As stated in the section Exposure and Exposure Monitoring section, the primary route of human exposure is by dermal contact or inhalation. If skin contact occurs, remove contaminated clothing, wash the area thoroughly, and repeat washing if necessary. If inhalation exposure occurs, immediately move the individual to fresh air, administer oxygen, and assist ventilation as required. It is highly unlikely to experience toxicity from residual exposure on treated crop products. In the event that an individual has consumed contaminated products over the amount of 40 mg kg^{-1}, perform gastric decontamination by administering activated charcoal slurry.

Ecotoxicology

Sodium acifluorfen is classified as slightly toxic, on an acute basis, to freshwater fish and invertebrates. In an acute study using technical grade sodium acifluorfen, rainbow trout (*Oncorhynchus mykiss*) had an LC$_{50}$ of 17 mg l^{-1}. A chronic study determined the NOAEC to be less than 3.4 mg l^{-1}using fathead minnow (*Pimephales promelas*). The most sensitive acute study using technical grade sodium acifluorfen for freshwater invertebrates was the water flea (*Daphnia magna*), with an LC$_{50}$ of 28.1 mg l^{-1}. There are no available data for chronic freshwater invertebrates.

In terms of acute toxicity, sodium acifluorfen is classified as slightly toxic to saltwater fish. In an acute study using technical grade sodium acifluorfen, sheepshead minnow (*Cyprinodon variegatus*) had an LC$_{50}$ of 39 mg l^{-1}. There are no available data for chronic estuarine/marine fish studies. In acute estuarine/marine invertebrates, sodium acifluorfen is moderately toxic. The most sensitive acute study using technical grade sodium acifluorfen on estuarine/marine invertebrates was the mysid shrimp (*Americamysis bahia*), with an LC_{50} of 3.8 mg l^{-1}. There are no available data for chronic estuarine/marine invertebrates.

Sodium acifluorfen is practically nontoxic to plants with no vascular tissue or vascular system. In a Tier I level study, the concentration of sodium acifluorfen that is equivalent to the maximum label rate (355 μg l^{-1}) caused no growth reduction in algae after 5 days of exposure. In a Tier II level study, the most sensitive nonvascular aquatic plant is *Selenastrum capricornutum*, with an NOAEC greater than 265 ppm. In a Tier II level study, the most sensitive aquatic vascular plant is duckweed, with an EC_{50} of 378 ppb. There is a potential risk to offsite nontarget plants; however, the magnitude is uncertain.

Acute oral toxicity tests indicate that sodium acifluorfen is moderately toxic to birds (quail $LD_{50} = 325$ mg kg^{-1}) and slightly toxic to mammals (rats $LD_{50} = 1540$ mg kg^{-1}). In subacute and chronic studies, sodium acifluorfen is practically nontoxic to birds (quail and mallard $LC_{50} > 10\,000$ ppm).

Other Hazards

Sodium acifluorfen is a strong oxidizer and steps should be taken to avoid contact with all sources of ignition.

Exposure Standards and Guidelines

There are established US tolerances for residues of sodium acifluorfen on peanuts (0.1 ppm), rice – grain (0.1 ppm), rice – straw (0.2 ppm), soybean – seed (0.1 ppm), and strawberries (0.05 ppm). These tolerances are listed in 40 CFR §180.208. There is no Codex maximum residue limit (MRL) for acifluorfen. However, there is one established MRL in Canada, set at 0.02 ppm, for the use of acifluorfen postemergence on soybeans as a control for weeds. Additionally, Brazil has one established MRL on soybeans (dry) at 0.02 ppm.

No Total Maximum Daily Loads have been developed for sodium acifluorfen. Additionally, there is no maximum contaminant level for acifluorfen. The Health Advisories for a 10-kg child is 2 mg l^{-1} (1-day and 10-day), with a Reference Dose of 0.01 mg kg^{-1} day^{-1} and a Drinking Water Equivalent Level of 0.4 mg l^{-1}.

See also: Pesticides; Environmental Risk Assessment, Pesticides and Biocides.

Further Reading

Registration Review – Preliminary Problem Formulation for the Environmental Fate and Ecological Risk, Drinking Water, and Endangered Species Assessments for Sodium Acifluorfen, Docket Number: EPA-HQ-OPP-2010-0931-003, March 24, 2010.

Sodium Acifluorfen, Hazardous Substance Data Bank: http://toxnet.nlm.nih.gov (accessed 7.04.12).

Sodium Acifluorfen: Human Health Assessments Scoping Document in Support of Registration Review, Docket Number: EPA-HQ-OPP-2010-0135-0004, March 23, 2010.

U.S. EPA RED Facts, Sodium Acifluorfen, Docket Number: EPA-738-F-04–001, September 2003.

U.S. EPA Reregistration Eligibility Decision for Sodium Acifluorfen: Case No. 2605 Docket Number: EPA-HQ-OPP-2005-0459, March 2003.

Relevant Website

http://www.epa.gov – U.S. Environmental Protection Agency.

Acrolein

D Pamies and E Vilanova, Universidad Miguel Hernández de Elche, Elche, Spain

This article is a revision of the previous edition article by James M. Garrison, volume 1, pp 40–42, © 2005, Elsevier Inc.

- Name: Acrolein
- Chemical Abstracts Service Registry Number: 107-02-8
- Common Synonyms: 2-Propenal, Acquinite, Acraldehyde, Acraldehydeacroleina
- Molecular Formula: C_3H_4O
- Chemical Structure:

H_2C O H

Background

The first time that acrolein was produced as a commercial product was in the 1930s through the vapor-phase condensation of acetaldehyde and formaldehyde. Another method was developed in the 1940s, which involved the vapor-phase oxidation of propylene. In the 1960s, some advances were found in propylene oxidation process by the introduction of bismuth molybdate-based catalysis, and that became the primary method used for the commercial production of acrolein. Some bioproducts formed for this reaction are acrylic acid, carbon oxides, acetaldehyde, acetic acid, formaldehyde, and polyacrolein. In World War I, it was used as a chemical weapon (pulmonary irritant and lachrymatory agent). Commercial acrolein contains 95.5% or more of the compound, the main impurities being water (<3.0% by weight) and other carbonyl compounds (<1.5% by weight), mainly propanol and acetone. Hydroquinone is added as an inhibitor of polymerization (0.1–0.25% by weight). This product has been classified for its hazard according to the Global Harmonized System (GHS) as described in **Table 1**.

Uses

The main use of acrolein is as an intermediate in the manufacture and synthesis of many organic chemicals like glycerol, polyurethane, polyester resins, methionine, acrylic acid and its esters, and pharmaceuticals. The main additional uses are as a biocide in the control of algae, weeds, and mollusks in recirculating water systems, as a slimicide in the paper industry, and as a biocide in oil wells and liquid petrochemical fuels; it is also used in the cross-linking of protein collagen in leather tanning, as a tissue fixative in histological samples, in the manufacture of colloidal forms of metals, in the production of perfumes, and as a warning agent in methyl chloride refrigerant.

Environmental Fate and Behavior

Exposure Routes and Pathways

The main acrolein route of exposure is through smoke. Acrolein is produced as a by-product of combustion of organic compounds, being present in a large spectrum of different smoke produced by, for example, cigarettes, petrochemical fuels (like gasoline or oil), synthetic polymers, paraffin wax, trees, plants, food, animals, vegetables fats, and building fires. Additional exposure can be linked to traffic accidents or to water treated with biocides that contain acrolein. Improperly handled hazardous waste sites can release acrolein into the nearby environment (air, water, or soil).

Physicochemical Properties

Acrolein is a clear, colorless, or yellow liquid. It is highly flammable at ordinary temperature and very volatile and quickly combusted in air. Its odor is shooting, choking, and strong and can be detected by humans at concentrations in air around 0.25 ppm. It is soluble in water and in organic solvents. It is a very reactive compound in the absence of an inhibitor a highly exothermic polymerization at room temperature (catalyzed by light and air) may occur.

Table 2 shows general relevant physical–chemical properties of acrolein.

Table 1 Classification of acrolein on the basis of the Global Harmony System (GSH)[a]

Hazard class and category code(s)	*Hazard statement code(s)*	*Pictogram, signal word code(s)*
Flam. liq. 2	H225 highly flammable liquid and vapor	GHS02
Acute tox. 2[a]	H330 fatal if inhaled	GHS06
Acute tox. 3[a]	H311 toxic in contact with skin	GHS05
Acute tox. 3[a]	H301 toxic if swallowed	GHS09
Skin corr. 1B	H314 causes severe skin burns and eye damage	Dgr
Aquatic acute 1	H400 very toxic to aquatic life	

[a]Source: From the Annex 6 Table 3.1 in "Regulation (EC) No 1272/2008 of the European Parliament and of the Council of 16 December 2008 on classification, labelling and packaging of substances and mixtures, amending and repealing Directives 67/548/EEC and 1999/45/EC, and amending Regulation (EC) No 1907/2006 (Text with EEA relevance)", Official Journal of the European Union, L 353/, 31.12.2008. Available in Internet (15 November 2013).

Table 2 General physical properties

Physical property	*Value*
Melting point	−87.7 (°C)
Boiling point	52.6 (°C)
Log *P* (octanol–water)	−0.01
Water solubility	2.12E + 05 mg l^{-1} (at 25 °C)
Vapor pressure	274 mm Hg (at 25 °C)
Henry's law constant	1.22E − 04 atm-m^3 $mole^{-1}$ (at 25 °C)
Atmospheric OH rate constant	1.99E − 11 cm^3 molecule-s^{-1} (at 25 °C)

Source: ChemIDplus Advanced data base available in ChemIDplus Advanced data base available in http://chem.sis.nlm.nih.gov/chemidplus/rn/107-02-8 (accessed 15 November 2013). The information is offered by National Library of Medicine (NLM) /NIH (National Institutes of Health). This data base is also available through TOXNET (Toxicology data Network) also offered by NLM: http://toxnet.nlm.nih.gov/cgi-bin/sis/search.

Table 3 Half-life of acrolein in the different environment compartments

Medium	*Reactive*	*Half-life*
Atmosphere	Hydroxyl radical	0.81 days (5 × 10^5 cm^{-3})
	Ozone	41 days (1 × 10^{11} cm^{-3})
	Nitrate radicals	28 days (at 2.4 × 10^8 cm^{-3})
	Nitrogen oxides	3.5 days
Air		10 h
Water		30–100 h
	3-Hydroxypropan-1-al in nonsterile irrigation water	
	pH	Half-life
	6–8	1.7–2.3 days
	5	3.5 days
	7	1.5 days
	10	4 h
	Singlet oxygen	8 years
	Alkyl peroxyl radicals	23 years
	Hexane solvent	UV light > 290 nm
Surface water (river and lakes)		7.6 h–4.6 days
Groundwater	Aerobic and anaerobic degradation	11–56 days
Irrigation canals (herbicide)		7.3–10.2 h
Dry soil		7.5–10.2 h

Source: HSDB (Hazardous Substances Data Bank). The data base is offered by NLM/NIH available in http://toxnet.nlm.nih.gov/.

Partition Behavior in Water, Sediment, and Soil

Modeling studies have been used to characterize the pathways of acrolein and its environment behavior. A steady state, nonequilibrium model (Level III fugacity model) according to Mackay (1991) and Mackay and Paterson (1991) indicates that acrolein has a different behavior depending on the compartment in which it is released. If it is continuously discharged into a specific compartment, most of it can be expected to remain in that compartment.

Environmental Persistence (Degradation/Speciation)

In water-sediment systems, acrolein is degraded by hydrolysis, self-oxidation, and biodegradation. Due to the high volatility and reactivity with soil materials, its accumulation in the environment is not expected. In addition, biotic and abiotic degradation would eliminate this compound rapidly from the soil. The presence in water is mostly related to the use of acrolein as biocide. Acrolein is removed from surface water primarily by reversible hydration, biodegradation by acclimatized microorganisms, and volatilization. In groundwater, acrolein is removed by anaerobic biodegradation and hydrolysis. Therefore, low persistence in water is expected. In the atmosphere, acrolein has a short estimated half-life, and consequently the potential for atmospheric long-range transport is low.

Bioaccumulation and Biomagnification

As expected from its low K_{ow} and high water solubility, acrolein has a low potential for bioaccumulation.

Exposure and Exposure Monitoring

Routes and Pathways

Significant exposures to acrolein are most likely to occur by inhalation, with potential for skin and eye contact, in general through exposure to smoke produced by organic compound combustion. The predominant route of environmental exposure would be inhalation of smoke or automotive exhaust. Some alcoholic drinks such as wine contain a low concentration of acrolein produced by heating of foodstuffs. Ingestion or contact exposure is possible only in accidents or workers who use acrolein as a biocide. However, it can appear in the environment through different waste streams produced, such as aquatic herbicide, warning agent in gases, or fumigant for ground.

Human Exposure

Acrolein can be present in air due to combustion processes (cigarettes, fuels, and other organic combustion). Exposure can be particularly high at smoking places and urban areas with higher automobile traffic. Presence in rural sites is unlikely, and generally the concentration does not exceed 0.1 $\mu g\ m^{-3}$. Humans can be exposed by contact with water treated with slimicides or herbicides. High exposure may be produced by transport accidents of acrolein for commercial uses. Some foods like fried food and roasted coffee can produce small amounts of this product. Acrolein is also found naturally in the body in very small amounts due to the natural formation of the compound by normal lipid oxidation and metabolism of α-hydroxyamino acids.

Environmental Exposure

Levels in outdoor air are usually low (0.2 ppb in urban air and 0.12 ppb in rural air). Even though, one to two orders of magnitude higher levels have been found in several cities and near industrial sources. Acrolein levels in rainwater are also very low. The indoor levels of acrolein in residential houses range from <0.02 to 12 ppb, and are related to tobacco consumption. The acrolein emission generated by a cigarette ranges between 0.06 and 0.22 mg. Presence of acrolein in food is limited.

Toxicokinetics

Acrolein is extensively adsorbed by the inhalation and oral routes. Limited information is available regarding dermal absorption of acrolein. Inhalation is the most frequent route of exposure. Most of the absorption is retained in respiratory tissue, but sometimes part can be absorbed into the blood and distributed throughout the body. Glutathione conjugation is the dominant detoxification pathway. Liver is responsible to transform this metabolism in glyceraldehyde and a number of metabolites (glutathione, cysteine, and *N*-acetylcysteine) that can be excreted in the urine as well as some unchanged acrolein. The majority of free acrolein is excreted by respiratory system in the exhaled breath.

Mechanism of Toxicity

Acrolein reacts directly with protein and nonprotein sulfhydryl groups and with primary and secondary amines. Mercapturic acids, acrylic acid, or glyceraldehyde can also be produced. The last three metabolites have been detected only in *in vitro* experiments. Acrolein affects primarily the respiratory tract, producing irritation in the mucous membranes of the sensory nerve endings. Also, a depression of the mucociliary defense system may appear, depending on the dose. Inhalation may cause hypertension and tachycardia. Concentrated solutions, above 10%, can produce eye irritation, lacrimation, and sometimes ulceration or necrosis. Neurotoxicological effects can also be produced and should be taken in account. Some studies have shown that acrolein can be a possible mediator of oxidative damage in cells and tissues in a wide variety of disease states. The mechanism is not understood.

Acute and Short-Term Toxicity

Animals

Dermal Effects

Like in humans, the eye seems to be the most sensitive target for dermal exposure (0.3 ppm in air). Dogs and monkeys show lacrimation and blinking eyes during intermediate exposure to 3.7 $mg\ kg^{-1}$ while guinea pigs and rodents did not. The levels of acrolein for structural damages in eyes are not known.

Respiratory Effects

Different effects have been reported in animals after exposure to 0.25 ppm acrolein, including reduction in respiratory rate, histological changes in nasal epithelium, reduction in bactericidal activity, high fever, dyspnea, coughing, foamy expectoration, cyanosis, tracheal and alveolar epithelial destruction, pulmonary edema, lung hemorrhage, basal cell metaplasia, and possible death. After vapor acrolein exposure, changes in body and organ weights, hematology, and serum biochemistry have been observed in animals. There is limited evidence that acrolein can depress pulmonary host defenses in mice and rats. Acute inhalation toxicity studies are summarized in **Table 4**.

Oral Effects

Clinical signs in different animals after oral intake are similar and dose related across species. Effects include gastrointestinal

Table 4 Inhalation acute toxicology

Species	*LC_{50} (mg m^{-3})*	*Source*
F-344 rats (male)	6.0 ppm (13.7 mg m^{-3})	Babiuk et al. (1985)
Wistar rats (male)	4.6 ppm (10.5 mg m^{-3})	Bergers et al. (1996)
Wistar rats (male)	9.2 ppm (21.7 mg m^{-3})	Cassee et al. (1996b)
Swiss Webster mice (male)	1.7 ppm (3.9 mg m^{-3})	Kane and Alarie (1977)
Ssc:CF-1 mice (male)	2.9 ppm (6.6 mg m^{-3})	Nielsen et al. (1984)
B6C3F1 mice (male)	1.41 ppm (3.2 mg m^{-3})	Steinhagen and Barrow (1984)
Swiss Webster mice (male)	1.03 ppm (2.4 mg m^{-3})	Davis et al. (1967)

Source: HSDB (Hazardous Substances Data Bank). The data base is offered by NLM/NIH available in http://toxnet.nlm.nih.gov/.

discomfort, vomiting, and stomach ulceration or hemorrhage and edema of the stomach mucosa. The stomach epithelium appears to be the most sensitive target after oral exposure (0.75 mg kg^{-1}). The irritation of the stomach can increase at higher doses (2 mg kg^{-1} and higher). Data are not available to determine if an adaptive effect for chronic oral exposures would be observed at higher dose levels. As in respiratory intake, ingestion of large amounts of acrolein during pregnancy caused similar effects. Nevertheless, there is no evidence of an effect on development of offspring without producing great injury (normally death) in the mother.

Human

Dermal and Ocular Effects

Acrolein causes ocular irritation after contact in the vapor or liquid state. At concentrations of 0.81 ppm in vapors, this compound can cause irritation and produce lacrimation in 20 s and at 1.22 ppm in 5 s. Studies in humans in different vapor-exposure scenarios have shown eye irritation in concentrations of 0.09 ppm. Concentrations of acrolein between 0.5 and 5 ppm caused lacrimation and various degrees of eye irritation in exposure periods of 10 min or less.

Exposure to the skin may produce irritation with erythema, edema, and necrosis, and sensitization can occur from prolonged or repeated contact with acrolein. Volunteers receiving topical applications of a 10% solution of acrolein in ethanol exhibited irritation, papillary edema, polymorphonuclear infiltrates, and epidermal necrosis 48 h after exposure.

Respiratory Effects

Nasal irritation in humans has been observed at levels similar to those seen in animals. Observed effects after exposures as low as 0.25 ppm within 5 min include nasal irritation, discomfort, and reduction in respiratory rate in humans. Human respiratory tracts suffer irritation in the mucous membranes at concentrations higher than 0.3 ppm. Nasal tissue is the most sensitive target, but higher concentrations (2–5 ppm) can extend the effect through the respiratory tract, reaching the alveolar spaces. A reduction in breathing rate was reported by volunteers acutely exposed to levels of 0.3 ppm.

Oral Effects

Human data for oral exposures are not available.

Chronic Toxicity

Animals

There is limited evidence of chronic effects of acrolein in animals. Only two studies have been done. A summary of inhalation acute toxicity effects is shown in **Table 5**.

Human

There is no clear evidence of chronic exposure effects in humans.

Immunotoxicity

Studies in rats and mice with inhalation exposure have shown adverse effects of acrolein in the immune system (including host resistance, pulmonary bacterial clearance, antibody responsiveness, lymphocyte blastogenesis, and respiratory damage).

Reproductive Toxicity

Studies *in vivo* in rats, mice, and rabbits have shown no clear evidence that acrolein can produce effects on the developmental/reproductive toxicity. There are not conclusive evidences of feto/ebriotoxic and teratogen effects. Problems in development have been reported, such as skeletal malformation and reduced weight of offspring, but always related with exposure levels resulting in maternal mortality.

Genotoxicity

There is some evidence that acrolein is able to transcriptionally activate genes responsible for phase II enzymes producing resistance against cell death. This capacity of acrolein can be involved in carcinogenesis in lungs caused by cigarette smoke In the absence of cytotoxicity, acrolein induces gene mutations in bacteria and mammalian cells in culture. The observations of positive mutagenic results in bacterial systems occurred at high concentrations near the lethal dose. Structural chromosomal aberrations have appeared as well in Chinese hamster ovary cells. Acrolein can form adducts with DNA and induce sister chromatid exchange, DNA cross-linking, and mutations under certain conditions. Other *in vitro* evidence has shown how acrolein interferes with DNA repair mechanism somehow. Studies in animals with

Table 5 Inhalation chronic toxicology

Animal	*Exposure*	*Route*	*Time*	*Effect*
Sprague–Dawley rats	8 ppm	Inhalation	1 h day^{-1} for 18 months	Alveoli emphysema
Syrian golden hamsters	0 or 4.0 ppm	Inhalation	7 h $days^{-1}$, 5 days $week^{-1}$, for 52 weeks followed by a 29-week recovery period	Reductions in body weight, increase in relative lung weights and a reduction in relative liver weights in females, as well as slight to moderate histopathological effects in the anterior portion of the nasal passages

Source: Table based in HSBD acrolein monographic information.

exposure to acrolein via drinking water have shown only a single case of a significant tumor. Despite the uncertainties, it may be possible that acrolein could have a weak mutagenicity potential.

Carcinogenicity

There are no adequate human studies on the carcinogenic potential of acrolein. It has been suggested that acrolein is a major etiologic agent for tobacco smoking-related lung cancer. Despite the evidence of the DNA damage produced by acrolein exposure, genotoxicity in mammalian cells has been not proved. There is limited evidence of acrolein carcinogenicity in animal studies, but glyceraldehyde, a potential metabolite of acrolein, is considered to be carcinogenic.

Clinical Management

After inhalation exposure, the respiratory tract should be monitored. Irritation, bronchitis, or pneumonitis can be the first symptoms. Humidified supplemental 100% oxygen should be administered. In case of bronchospasm, treat patients with an aerosolized bronchodilator. Do not induce vomit and keep airway open. For eye contamination, irrigate each eye continuously with 0.9% saline water or tepid water for at least 15 min. If eye irritation, pain, swelling, lacrimation, or photophobia persists after washing with water, the patient should be seen in a health care facility. In some cases, after acrolein ingestion, gastric lavage may be indicated soon after ingestion. If the patient is asymptomatic, administer activated charcoal slurry mixed with saline cathartic or sorbitol 1 g kg^{-1}. If is not possible to apply any of these treatments, administer 5 ml kg^{-1} up to 200 ml of water if the patient can swallow, or milk, but no more than 100 ml for children and 220 ml for adults. For dermal contamination, remove contaminated clothes and wash exposed areas with soap and water. Treat dermal irritation and burns with standard topical therapy.

Ecotoxicology

Aquatic Organism Toxicity

Acrolein is highly toxic to aquatic organisms. There are some studies of the toxicity effect in aquatic environment due to the use of acrolein as herbicide in irrigation canals (**Table 6**). Most algae and weeds have shown high sensitivity to acrolein.

Terrestrial Organisms Toxicity

Most terrestrial crop plants can tolerate irrigation water containing 25 mg acrolein per liter without damage. There are not many data on toxicity relevant to terrestrial wildlife. Data indicate that terrestrial organisms are less sensitive than aquatic organisms to single exposures to acrolein (**Table 7**).

Table 6 Acute toxicity of acrolein to aquatic organisms

Species	*Scientific name*	*% a.i.*	*96 h LC_{50} (ppb)*	*EPA toxicity category*
Bluegill sunfish	*Lepomis macrochirus*	96.4	22	Very highly toxic
Rainbow trout	*Oncorhynchus mykiss*	96.4	<31	Very highly toxic
Water flea	*Daphnia magna*	96.4	<31	Very highly toxic
Sheepshead minnow	*Cyprinodon variegatus*	85.2	430	Highly toxic
Longnose killifish	*Fundulus similis*	100	55	Very highly toxic
Eastern oyster	*Crassostrea virginica*	100	55	Very highly toxic
Eastern oyster	*Crassostrea virginica*	94.7	106	Highly toxic
Brown shrimp	*Penaeus aztecus*	100	100	Highly toxic
Mysid shrimp	*Americamysis bahia*	94.7	500	Highly toxic
Snail	*Australorbis glabratus*	98	10	Very highly toxic
Snail	*Aplexa hypnorum*	50	151	Highly toxic
Snail	*Tanytarsus dissimilis*	50	151	Highly toxic
Mussels	*Mytilus edulis*	100	600 (29 h)	
Carp and threadfin shad			>5	Very highly toxic

Source: Table based in HSBD acrolein monographic information.

Table 7 Acute toxicity of acrolein in terrestrial organisms

Species	*Scientific name*	*Concentration*	*Exposure*	*Effects*
Chicken	*Gallus* sp.	113–454 mg m^{-3}	>27 days	Tracheal damage
Mallards	*Anas platyrhynchos*	9.1 mg kg^{-1}		Intoxication, ataxia, regurgitation, imbalance, and withdrawal
Fruitfly	*Drosophila melanogaster*	4606 mg l^{-1}	4 h	LC_{50}
Crop plants	7 Species	233–4700 μg m^{-3}	Different times	Smog-like leaf damage

Source: Table based in HSBD acrolein monographic information.

Other Hazards

Acrolein is a highly reactive compound and can be polymerized into dimethylaniline in a violent reaction (possible explosively properties) in the presence of strong acids or bases. Care should be taken to prevent mixing with amines, sulfur dioxide, metal salts, and oxidants. Acrolein is sensitive to heat, light, and air.

Exposure Standards and Guidelines

The National Institute for Occupational Safety and Health (NIOSH) recommended exposure limit for an 8- or 10-h time-weighted average (TWA) exposure and/or ceiling. TWA: 0.1 ppm (0.25 mg m^{-3}).

NIOSH short-term exposure limit (STEL): recommended exposure limit for a 15-min period. STEL: 0.3 ppm (0.8 mg m^{-3}).

The Occupational Safety and Health Administration's permissible exposure limit expressed as a TWA; the concentration of a substance to which most workers can be exposed without adverse effect averaged over a normal 8-h workday or a 40-h workweek. TWA: 0.1 ppm (0.25 mg m^{-3})

Miscellaneous

Acrolein is a yellowish liquid with an unpleasant piercing and acrid odor that most people may begin to smell at air concentrations around 0.25 ppm.

See also: Acrylic Acid; Formaldehyde; The Globally Harmonized System for Classification and Labeling of the GHS; Glycerol; Nonlethal Weapons; Clean Water Act (CWA), US; Acetaldehyde.

Further Reading

Abraham, K., Andres, S., Palavinskas, R., Berg, K., Appel, K.E., Lampen, A., September 2011. Toxicology and risk assessment of acrolein in food. Mol. Nutr. Food Res. 55 (9), 1277–1290. http://dx.doi.org/10.1002/mnfr.201100481.

Acrolein. Concise International Chemical Assessment Document 43. World Health Organization. http://www.who.int/ipcs/publications.

Acrolein Data. Chemical Carcinogenesis Research Information System (CCRIS). CCRIS Record Number: 3278.

Bein, K., Leikauf, G.D., 2S. Acrolein – a pul/monary hazard. Mol. Nutr. Food Res. 55 (9), 1342–1360. http://dx.doi.org/10.1002/mnfr.201100279.

Shi, R., Rickett, T., Sun, W., September 2011. Acrolein-mediated injury in nervous system trauma and diseases. Mol. Nutr. Food Res. 55 (9), 1320–1331. http://dx.doi.org/10.1002/mnfr.201100217 (Epub 8 August 2011).

Relevant Website

http://www.atsdr.cdc.gov – Agency for Toxic Substances and Disease Registry. Toxicological Profile for Acrolein.

Acrylamide

G Karimi and M Rashedinia, Mashhad University of Medical Sciences, Mashhad, Iran

This article is a revision of the previous edition article by Ralph J. Parod, volume 1, pp 42–44, © 2005, Elsevier Inc.

- Name: Acrylamide
- Chemical Abstracts Service Registry Number: 79-06-1
- Synonyms: Acrylic acid amide, Ethylenecarboxamide, 2-Propenamide, Propenoic acid amide, Vinyl amide
- Molecular Formula: C_3H_5NO
- Chemical Structure:

$H_2C{=}CH{-}C({=}O){-}NH_2$

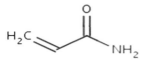

Background

Acrylamide is an odorless, white crystalline solid that initially was produced for commercial purposes by reaction of acrylonitrile with hydrated sulfuric acid.

Acrylamide exists in two forms: a monomer and a polymer. Monomer acrylamide readily participates in radical-initiated polymerization reactions, whose products form the basis of most of its industrial applications. The single unit form of acrylamide is toxic to the nervous system, a carcinogen in laboratory animals and a suspected carcinogen in humans. The multiple unit or polymeric form is not known to be toxic.

In 2002, researchers at the University of Stockholm reported that high levels of acrylamide are formed during the fried or baked high-carbohydrate foods such as potato chips and French fries that are prepared at high temperatures. Because these foods are widely consumed in significant amounts, much interest and concern was generated from the report. Acrylamide has been found in certain foods that have been cooked or processed at high temperatures, above 120 °C.

Acrylamide is formed as a by-product of the Maillard reaction. The Maillard reaction is best known as a reaction that produces pleasant flavor, taste, and golden color in fried and baked foods; the reaction occurs between amines and carbonyl compounds, particularly reducing sugars and the amino acid asparagine. In the first step of the reaction, asparagine reacts with a reducing sugar, forming a Schiff's base. From this compound, acrylamide is formed following a complex reaction pathway that includes decarboxylation and a multistage elimination reaction. Acrylamide formation in bakery products, investigated in a model system, showed that free asparagine was a limiting factor. Treatment of flours with asparaginase practically prevented acrylamide formation. Coffee drinking and smoking are other major sources apart from the human diet.

Uses

Acrylamide is mainly used in the production of polymers and copolymers for various purposes. The monomeric form of acrylamide is primarily used as a chemical intermediate in the production of polyacrylamides, in the synthesis of dyes, in copolymers for contact lenses, and in the construction of dam foundations, tunnels, and sewers. It is also used in research laboratories for gel preparation. The acrylamide gel is used for electrophoresis, a technique for molecular biology and genetic engineering.

Acrylamide polymers are used as additives for water treatment, flocculants, paper making aids, thickeners, soil conditioning agents, sewage and waste treatment, textiles (permanent-press fabrics), production of organic chemicals, and crude oil processing.

Environmental Behavior, Fate

All acrylamide in the environment is synthetic, the main source being the release of the monomer residues from polyacrylamide used in water treatment or in industry. Products and compounds containing polyacrylamide can serve as sources of exposure to residues of acrylamide.

If released to air, the vapor pressure of 0.007 mm Hg at 25 °C indicates that acrylamide will exist solely as a vapor in the ambient atmosphere. Vapor-phase acrylamide will be degraded in the atmosphere by reaction with photochemically produced hydroxyl radicals, and the half-life for this reaction in air is estimated to be 1.4 days. The half-life for the reaction of vapor-phase acrylamide with ozone is estimated to be 6.5 days. Acrylamide is not expected to be susceptible to direct photolysis in sunlight because it does not absorb light with wavelengths >290 nm.

If released to soil, acrylamide is expected to have very high mobility based upon an estimated K_{oc} of 10. Studies suggested that acrylamide is hydrolyzed in soil under aerobic conditions to produce ammonium ion, which is then oxidized to nitrite ion and nitrate ion. Volatilization of acrylamide from dry or moist soil surfaces is not expected to be an important fate process.

If released to water, acrylamide is not expected to adsorb to suspended solids or sediment, based on the K_{oc}. The hydrolysis half-life of acrylamide has been reported as >38 years. The potential for bioconcentration in aquatic organisms is low, and microbial degradation of acrylamide can occur under light or dark, aerobic or anaerobic conditions.

Exposure and Exposure Monitoring

Until the early 2000s, the primary concern about human exposure to acrylamide was in the occupational setting, and guidelines had been established for occupational exposure and levels in drinking water and in foodstuff packaging polymers. The report that acrylamide is formed during high temperature cooking of common human foods has generated interest in the possible carcinogenicity of dietary exposure to acrylamide.

The FDA has estimated overall daily intake levels of acrylamide from exposures in the US diet to be about 0.4 $\mu g\ kg^{-1}\ day^{-1}$ in 2003 and 2004. Estimated daily intake in populations around the world are reasonably similar to the FDA's estimate, with the variability assumed to result from cultural differences in food preferences, processing methods, and consumption levels. Alternate methods for estimating exposure to the general population are based on internal levels of biomarkers of exposure, including levels of hemoglobin (Hb) adducts or urinary metabolites.

The World Health Organization estimates a daily intake of dietary acrylamide in the range of 0.3–2.0 $\mu g\ kg^{-1}$ per body weight for the general population. For high-percentile consumers (90th to 97.5th), daily intakes of dietary acrylamide vary in the range of 0.6–3.5 $\mu g\ kg^{-1}$ per body weight, and as high as 5.1 $\mu g\ kg^{-1}$ per body weight for the 99th percentile consumers.

The daily intakes of dietary acrylamide in children are estimated to be 2–3 times those of adults based on average body weight ratios. The daily intakes of dietary acrylamide for the general population and high consumers (including children) are estimated to be on average 1 and 4 $\mu g\ kg^{-1}$ per body weight, respectively. The main sources of dietary acrylamide are potato chips (16–30%), potato crisps (6–46%), coffee (13–39%), pastry and sweet biscuits (10–20%), and bread and rolls/toast (10–30%). Other food products can account for 10% of the total intake of dietary acrylamide.

In addition, tobacco smoke is a substantial nonfood source of human inhalation exposure to acrylamide for people without occupational exposure. Acrylamide content in mainstream cigarette smoke has been estimated at 1.1–2.34 μg per cigarette.

Toxicokinetics

Studies in animal indicate that acrylamide is readily absorbed by ingestion, by inhalation, and through the skin. No human data on the distribution of acrylamide were identified. Results from several animal studies indicate that, following absorption, radioactivity from radiolabeled acrylamide is distributed among tissues, with no specific accumulation in any tissues other than red blood cells.

About 40% of acrylamide is metabolized by CYP2E1 to the reactive epoxide glycidamide in rats (60% conversion in mice). Glycidamide can be metabolized by epoxide hydrolase or can undergo conjugation with glutathione (GSH). The major pathway of metabolism for acrylamide is its conjugation with reduced GSH by glutathione s-transferase. Elimination occurs mainly in the urine as mercapturic acid conjugates. More than 90% of absorbed acrylamide is excreted in the urine as metabolites. Less than 2% is excreted as unchanged acrylamide. Smaller amounts are excreted in the bile and feces. Approximately 60% of an administered dose appears in the urine within 24 h.

Acrylamide forms different protein adducts, the most important of which are Hb adducts extensively formed at –SH groups and on the amino groups of the N-terminal valines in erythrocytes. The measurement of Hb adducts can give an integrated estimate of the exposure in the previous 3–4 months, because the life span of erythrocytes is about 4 months.

Mechanisms of Action

Acrylamide, the parent compound, is an α,β-unsaturated amide, soft electrophilic toxicant, reacting on thiol groups of proteins (cysteine, homocysteine) and GSH as well as protein-bound –SH groups (kinesin, dynein), whereas the metabolite glycidamide is a harder electrophilic compound, reacting with nucleophilic centers of adenine and guanine in the DNA. It has been shown that acrylamide inhibits the action of brain glutathione s-transferase and reduces the levels of brain GSH. It has also been suggested that acrylamide neurotoxicity is caused by its effects on heavy- and medium-weight neurofilaments, the change it causes on neurotransmitter receptor expression, and through inhibition of neurotransmission. Electrophilic neurotoxins, including acrylamide, can cause protein structure and function changes by oxidation and this can lead to pathway failure and finally nerve cell damage. Therefore, such chemicals at low doses and long-term exposure might be a cause of neurodegenerative diseases such as Alzheimer's disease.

Acute and Short-Term Toxicity

Animal

Determination of the LD_{50} values of acrylamide on laboratory animals indicated that oral LD_{50} value in rat ranging from 124 to 565 $mg\ kg^{-1}$, a dermal LD_{50} value of 400 $mg\ kg^{-1}$ in rat, an intraperitoneal LD_{50} value of 90 $mg\ kg^{-1}$ in rat, an oral LD_{50} value of 107 $mg\ kg^{-1}$ in mouse, an intraperitoneal LD_{50} value of 170 $mg\ kg^{-1}$ in mouse, and an oral LD_{50} value of 150 $mg\ kg^{-1}$ and a dermal LD_{50} value of 1680 $ul\ kg^{-1}$ in rabbit. Acute exposure in 12 h after administration of 50–200 $mg\ kg^{-1}$, poisoned animals displayed impaired hind limb functioning, convulsions, and diffused damage to different sections of the nervous system.

Human

Toxic effects depend on the duration, total dose, and rate of exposure. The effects of acute high-dose exposure can be delayed in onset for several hours. Neurological effects include hallucinations, confusion, tremors, myoclonus, opisthotonos, seizures, memory loss, euphoria, peripheral neuropathy, autonomic nervous system effects, and ataxia. Peripheral neuropathy may appear several weeks following significant acute exposure or following significant chronic exposures.

In severe poisonings, hypotension, peripheral cyanosis, and metabolic acidosis may occur.

Anorexia and gastrointestinal disturbances can be seen in patients with subacute exposure. Pancreatitis, renal toxicity, and oliguria following ingestion have been reported.

Dermal contact is a common route of exposure and may result in skin irritation with numbness, tingling, blistering, and peeling with direct contact of high concentrations. Visual impairment and eye irritation also occur with significant exposure. Inhalation can produce a cough and sore throat.

Chronic Toxicity

Animal

Evidence of neurological effects has been observed following single oral doses of 126 mg kg^{-1} in rats and rabbits and 100 mg kg^{-1} in dogs. Using chronic dosing schedules, it has been observed that cumulative oral doses of 500–600 mg kg^{-1} using daily doses of 25–50 mg kg^{-1} per day are required to produce ataxia in rats, dogs, and baboons. Smaller daily doses do not produce a clinical effect until a larger, cumulative dose is attained. It has been found that the administration of acrylamide at daily doses of 6–9 mg kg^{-1} does not produce evidence of neurotoxicity in rats until a cumulative dose of 1200–1800 mg kg^{-1} is attained, and doses of up to 3 mg kg^{-1} per day for 90 days administered rats do not result in adverse effects. It was reported that rhesus monkeys fed up to 2 mg kg^{-1} per day did not show any adverse clinical effects at 325 days. In the other study, subchronic or prechronic exposure groups of male and female Fischer 344 (F344) rats administered 20 mg kg^{-1} day^{-1} acrylamide in drinking water for 90 days showed dragged rear limbs, decrease in body weight, serum cholinesterase activity, packed cell volume, red blood cells, and hemoglobin values. Slight spinal cord degeneration, atrophy of skeletal muscle, testicular atrophy, and distended urinary bladder were observed.

Human

Long-term acrylamide exposure effects are predominantly sensorimotor and proprioceptive neuropathy with loss of deep tendon reflexes, muscle weakness and wasting, distal extremity numbness, and paresthesias. Excessive sweating and an exfoliative rash are also common with chronic exposure. Also, slight liver function abnormalities have been reported.

Reproductive and Developmental Toxicity

Studies revealed that acrylamide and glycidamide crossed the placenta from maternal to fetal circulation, suggesting fetal exposure if the mother is exposed.

Reproductive toxicity of acrylamide has been observed in male rats; the doses of acrylamide to induce reproductive toxicity were a multiple of those doses to induce neurotoxicity in rodents. The NOAEL for neurotoxicity was 10-fold lower than that for reproductive effects. For morphological changes in nerves of rats, an NOAEL of 0.2 mg kg^{-1} body weight was reported, whereas the NOAEL for reproductive toxicity was indicated with 2 mg kg^{-1} body weight.

In reproductive studies, male rodents showed reduced fertility, dominant lethal effects, and adverse effects on sperm count and morphology at oral doses of acrylamide 47 mg kg^{-1} body weight per day.

Results of repeated dermal exposure studies indicated that 25 mg kg^{-1} day^{-1} or more acrylamide for 5 days on male mice resulted in dominant lethal effects in the progeny, and the reduced number of pregnant females is suggestive of reduced male fertility.

Oral administration of acrylamide, between 7 and 16 days of gestation in rats, decreased the binding of dopamine receptors in the striatal membranes in 2-week-old pups, a fact that may be explained by postnatal exposure through lactation as well as prenatal effects. Degeneration of seminiferous tubules and chromosome aberrations in spermatocytes has been seen in acrylamide-treated male mice. Depressed plasma levels of testosterone and prolactin have also been observed. A statistically significant increase in the incidence of mesothelioma of the scrotal cavity was observed in rats after long-term (2-year) administration of acrylamide in drinking water.

There seems to be a relationship between the neurotoxicity and reproductive toxicity of acrylamide. One theory is that neurotoxicity influences mating behavior. Another theory is that both types of toxicity are mediated through effects on the kinesin motor proteins. These kinesin proteins are found in the flagella of sperm as well as the nervous system and other tissues. Interference with these proteins could reduce sperm motility and fertilization events.

Other mechanisms of acrylamide effects on reproduction in rodents could be from the alkylation of sulfhydryl groups on unique proteins such as protamine in the sperm head and tail. This could affect sperm penetration and induce the preimplantation losses seen in some dominant lethal studies.

Developmental effects associated with oral exposure to acrylamide are restricted to body weight decreases in rats and mice and neurobehavioral changes in the offspring of female Sprague-Dawley rats exposed on gestational day 6–10 to 15 mg kg^{-1} day^{-1}, but not to 10 mg kg^{-1} day^{-1} and in adolescent F344 rats exposed during gestation and lactation and extending through 12 weeks of age at an average dose of 6 mg kg^{-1} day^{-1}, but not at 1.3 mg kg^{-1} day^{-1}. No exposure-related fetal malformations or variations (gross, visceral, or skeletal) were found in Sprague-Dawley rats exposed to doses up to 15 mg kg^{-1} day^{-1} on gestational day 6–20 or in CD-1 mice exposed to doses up to 45 mg kg^{-1} day^{-1} on gestational day 6–17. These doses decreased the maternal weight gain. No signs of hind limb foot splay or other gross signs of peripheral or central neuropathy were noted.

Reproductive toxicity has not yet been observed in humans based on the reported doses.

Immunotoxicity

Studies have demonstrated that acrylamide-induced immunotoxicity produces a significant decrease in the weight of spleen, thymus, and mesenteric lymph nodes in rats. The investigators have also recorded a decrease in cellularity of spleen, thymus, bone marrow, and circulating blood lymphocyte population. Orally administrated acrylamide toxicity appears to decrease ANAE (+) peripheral blood lymphocyte counts and cause histopathological lesions in a dose-dependent manner in ileal Peyer's patches.

ANAE-positive peripheral blood lymphocyte counts significantly decreased, and this decrease can be explained by the effect of acrylamide on the mitotic division of bone marrow cells.

Genotoxicity

The genotoxic, mutagenic, and carcinogenic potentials of acrylamide have been studied extensively. Acrylamide itself reacts rapidly with thiol (–SH) and amino groups; this explains why its primary targets are proteins. Acrylamide has been shown to bind DNA by a Michael-type process *in vitro* with low activity. Nevertheless, there is sufficient evidence in the literature that both acrylamide and its metabolite glycidamide are mutagenic and clastogenic in mammalian cells. Data suggest that mice are more vulnerable to acrylamide tumorigenicity. The metabolic activation of acrylamide is more efficient and the detoxification process is poorer in mice than rats, since mice have higher levels of glycidamide and lower levels of GSH–glycidamide conjugates. Mouse and human cell lines treated with acrylamide or glycidamide showed increased mutation rates, particularly A to G and G to C transitions and G to T transversions. Acrylamide causes induction of the following genotoxic effects:

(1) Gene mutations and chromosomal aberrations in germ cells of mice *in vivo*
(2) Chromosomal aberrations in germ cells of rats *in vivo*
(3) Chromosomal aberrations in somatic cells of rodents *in vivo*
(4) Gene mutations and chromosomal aberrations in cultured cells *in vitro*
(5) Cell transformation in mouse cell lines
(6) Somatic mutation in the spot test *in vivo*
(7) Heritable translocation and specific locus mutations in mice and dominant lethal mutations in both mice and rats
(8) Unscheduled DNA synthesis in rat spermatocytes *in vivo*; but not in rat hepatocytes. However, glycidamide induces unscheduled DNA synthesis in rat hepatocytes

Carcinogenicity

Acrylamide is classified by the International Agency for Research on Cancer as a probable human carcinogen (Group 2A) based on both animal cancer data and *in vitro* and *in vivo* genotoxicity studies. In two 2-year carcinogenicity studies in F344 rats, acrylamide induced neoplasms at multiple organ sites, including thyroid follicular cell tumors (males and females), peritesticular mesotheliomas (males), and mammary tumors (females). In addition, tumors of the brain, oral cavity, uterus, and clitoral gland in female F344 rats were reported in the earlier study in which metabolite covalently binds to DNA, inducing mutations and cell transformation, which eventually leads to the tumors observed in multiple organs.

Studies of human exposure to acrylamide have generally found no association between exposure and cancer risk. Nine studies have examined the association between dietary acrylamide intake and risk of cancers at various sites: colorectal, kidney, bladder, breast, oral, esophageal, larynx, ovarian, endometrial, and prostate.

The only report of a significant association between higher acrylamide intake and cancer risk was for ovarian and endometrial cancer in a cohort of Dutch women.

The absence of positive results in these observational studies, however, cannot be interpreted as proof of no carcinogenicity of acrylamide to humans. Obviously, the conducted studies have potential limitations, including inadequate statistical power due to the small size of study populations and the narrow range of exposure between cases and controls.

Clinical Management

Range of Toxicity

Single or cumulative doses of as little as 50–100 mg kg^{-1} can cause neurologic deficits. Doses of greater than 300 mg kg^{-1} can cause severe CNS and cardiovascular effects acutely.

Antidote and Emergency Treatment

Basic Treatment

Establish a patent airway. Suction if necessary. Watch for signs of respiratory insufficiency and assist ventilations if needed.

Administer oxygen by nonrebreather mask at 10 to 15 l min^{-1}. Monitor for pulmonary edema and treat if necessary. Monitor for shock and treat if necessary. Anticipate seizures and treat if necessary.

Do not use emetics. For ingestion, rinse mouth and administer 5 ml kg^{-1} up to 200 ml of water for dilution if the patient can swallow, has a strong gag reflex, and does not drool. Cover skin burns with dry sterile dressings after decontamination.

Advanced Treatment

Consider orotracheal or nasotracheal intubation for airway control in the patient who is unconscious, has severe pulmonary edema, or is in respiratory arrest. Positive pressure ventilation techniques with a bag valve mask device might be beneficial. Monitor cardiac rhythm and treat arrhythmias as necessary.

Use lactated Ringer's if signs of hypovolemia are present. Watch for signs of fluid overload. Consider drug therapy for pulmonary edema. For hypotension with signs of hypovolemia, administer fluid cautiously. Watch for signs of fluid. Treat seizures with diazepam.

Treatment Overview

Oral Exposure

Ipecac-induced emesis is not recommended because of the potential for CNS depression and seizures. Administer charcoal as slurry (240 ml water/30 g charcoal). Usual doses are 25–100 g in adults/adolescents, 25–50 g in children (1–12 years), and 1 g kg^{-1} in infants less than 1 year old. Gastric lavage should be considered after ingestion of a potentially life-threatening amount of poison if it can be performed soon after ingestion (generally within 1 h). Protect the airway by placing the head down in a left lateral decubitus position or by endotracheal intubation. Control any seizures first.

Contraindications: Loss of airway protective reflexes or decreased level of consciousness in unintubated patients; following ingestion of corrosives; hydrocarbons (high aspiration potential); patients at risk of hemorrhage or gastrointestinal perforation; and trivial or nontoxic ingestion. Pyridoxine use in humans has been reported in a case of acrylamide ingestion, but with unproven effect. In cases of high-dose exposure or in symptomatic patients, pyridoxine use should be strongly considered.

Seizures: Administer a benzodiazepine IV; diazepam (adult: 5–10 mg repeats every 10–15 min as needed; child: 0.2–0.5 mg kg^{-1}, repeat every 5 min as needed) or lorazepam (adult: 2–4 mg; child: 0.05–0.1 mg kg^{-1}).

Hypotension: Infuse 10–20 ml kg^{-1} isotonic fluid. If hypotension persists, administer dopamine (5–20 mcg kg^{-1} min^{-1}) or norepinephrine (adult: begin infusion at 0.5 to 1 mcg min^{-1}; child: begin infusion at 0.1 mcg kg^{-1} min^{-1}); titrate to desired response.

Inhalation Exposure

Move patient to fresh air. Monitor for respiratory distress. If cough or difficulty breathing develops, evaluate for respiratory tract irritation, bronchitis, or pneumonitis. Administer oxygen and assist ventilation as required. Treat bronchospasm with inhaled β_2 agonist and oral or parenteral corticosteroids.

Eye Exposure

Decontamination: Irrigate exposed eyes with copious amounts of room temperature water for at least 15 min. If irritation, pain, swelling, lacrimation, or photophobia persists, the patient should be seen in a health care facility.

Dermal Exposure

Remove contaminated clothing and wash exposed area thoroughly with soap and water. A physician may need to examine the area if irritation or pain persists. Exfoliative rashes can be treated symptomatically.

Ecotoxicology

Acrylamide is moderately toxic to aquatic organisms. In a series of studies, acrylamide exhibited a 96-h LC_{50} value in four freshwater fish of 100–180 mg l^{-1}, a 48-h LC_{50} (immobilization) value of 98 mg l^{-1} in an aquatic invertebrate (*Daphnia magna*), and a 72-h EC_{50} (growth inhibition) value of 33.8 mg l^{-1} in freshwater algae (*Selenastrum capricornutum*). The examination of environmental risk indicates that the risk level for aquatic organisms and wastewater treatment plant microorganisms is less than 1 and therefore negligible. Therefore, the expected low levels of acrylamide released are not expected to result in adverse effects on aquatic organisms.

Exposure Standards and Guidelines

In order to protect workers from adverse health effects due to acrylamide exposure, the American Conference of Governmental Industrial Hygienists (ACGIH) set its threshold limit value, time-weighted average (TLV-TWA) at 30 μg m^{-3} in workplaces.

The US Occupational Safety and Health Administration (OSHA) has set the permissible exposure limit at 300 μg m^{-3}.

Comparing the average daily intake of 1 μg kg^{-1} per body weight of dietary acrylamide by the general population and a dose of 0.30 mg kg^{-1} body weight per day for induction of mammary tumors in rats, according to 2011 Evaluations of the Joint FAO/WHO Expert Committee on Food Additives (JECFA), for the general population and consumers with high exposure, the margin of exposure values are 200 and 50, respectively.

Nevertheless, the significant presence of a known rodent carcinogen in commonly consumed human foods is a legitimate health concern. It is recommended that appropriate efforts be continued to minimize human exposure to acrylamide, especially by reducing acrylamide concentrations in frequently consumed food products. For example, efficient reduction in acrylamide formation has been achieved by using the enzyme asparaginase to selectively remove asparagine prior to heating of cereal and potato products. However, this approach is only applicable to certain foods prepared from liquidized or slurried materials.

See also: Endocrine System; Neurotoxicity; Pollution, Water; Polymers.

Further Reading

Erkekoğlu, P., Baydar, T., 2010. Toxicity of acrylamide and evaluation of its exposure in baby foods. Nutr. Res. Rev. 23, 323–333.

Gargas, M., Kirman, C., Sweeney, L., Tardiff, R., 2009. Acrylamide: consideration of species differences and nonlinear processes in estimating risk and safety for human ingestion. Food Chem. Toxicol. 47, 760–768.

Mei, N., McDaniel, L.P., Dobrovolsky, V.N., Guo, X., Shaddock, J.G., Mittelstaedt, R.A., et al., 2010. The genotoxicity of acrylamide and glycidamide in Big Blue rats. Toxicol. Sci. 115, 412–421.

Praegitzer, S.M., 2011. Acrylamide Formation and Mitigation in Processed Potato Products. Kansas State University.

Toxicological Review of Acrylamide. EPA/635/R-07/009F. www.epa.gov/iris.

WHO, 2011. Evaluation of certain contaminants in food. Seventy-second report of the Joint FAO/WHO Expert Committee on Food Additives. No. 959.

Relevant Websites

http://toxnet.nlm.nih.gov – Toxnet (Toxicology Data Network): search for Acrylamide.

htp://chem.sis.nlm.nih.gov/chemiplus – US National Library of Medicine: ChemIDplus Advanced: Search for Acrylamide.

Acrylates *see* Acrylic Acid; Ethyl Acrylate; Methyl Acrylate

Acrylic Acid

D Brown, Manchester University College of Pharmacy, Fort Wayne, IN, USA

This article is a revision of the previous edition article by Sanjay Chanda & Harihara M. Mehendale, volume 1, pp 45–46, © 2005, Elsevier Inc.

- Name: Acrylic acid
- Chemical Abstracts Service Registry Number: 79-10-7
- Synonyms: Acroleic acid; Aqueous acrylic acid; Ethylene carboxylic acid; Glacial acrylic acid (98% in aqueous solution); 2-Propenoic acid
- Molecular Formula: $C_3H_4O_2$
- Chemical Structure:

H_2C = CH–C(=O)OH

Background

Acrylic acid, also known as prop-2-enoic acid, is an organic molecule with the formula $C_3H_4O_2$, and is the simplest of the unsaturated carboxylic acids. At room temperature, acrylic acid is a colorless liquid with a tart or acrid smell. Industrially, acrylic acid is produced from the oxidation of propene with molecular oxygen. Acrylic acid is highly susceptible to Michael-type reactions, and most of the uses of this chemical involve polymerization reactions. Acrylic acid is used to produce large quantities of acrylic esters.

Uses

Acrylic acid is used as a building block in the production of many types of homopolymeric and copolymeric materials, including various plastics, coatings, adhesives, elastomers, paints, and polishes. Additionally, acrylic acid is used in the production of hygienic medical products, detergents, and wastewater treatment chemicals.

Environmental Fate, Behavior, Routes, and Pathways

Acrylic acid's large-scale use and production results in its release into the environment. The most likely route of exposure is inhalation because acrylic acid has a low vapor pressure. The miscibility of acrylic acid in water combined with its low vapor pressure prevent it from accumulating in the soil. Acrylic acid that is emitted into the atmosphere is degraded photochemically by reaction with hydroxyl radicals. There is no potential for long-range atmospheric transport of acrylic acid because it has an atmospheric lifetime of 1 month.

Acrylic acid rapidly oxidizes when added to water, so the potential to deplete oxygen exists if a large quantity of acrylic acid were released. It has been shown to be oxidized by both aerobic and anaerobic pathways.

Exposure and Exposure Monitoring

Human exposure to acrylic acid is mainly to its vapors, and exposure is primarily confined to production processes as acrylic acid is used in the manufacturing of numerous acrylates. Levels of acrylic acid are monitored in samples by quantification using HPLC.

Toxicokinetics

The excretion half-life of acrylic acid has been found to be 40 min. Both *in vitro* and *in vivo* studies of acrylic acid metabolism have shown that it is extensively metabolized to 3-hydroxyproionic acid, carbon dioxide, and mercapturic acid, all of which are eliminated in expired air and urine. Because of its rapid metabolism, acrylic acid has no potential for bioaccumulation.

Mechanism of Toxicity

Acrylic acid is corrosive, and its toxicity occurs at the site of contact.

Acute and Short-Term Toxicity

Animal

Although a wide range of LD_{50} values has been reported for acrylic acid, it is generally believed to possess low to moderate acute toxicity in the oral route, and moderate acute toxicity in the inhalation and dermal routes. Many of the symptoms of acute toxicity parallel those found in humans.

Human

Acrylic acid is corrosive and irritating to the skin. Exposure to vapor can cause moderate to severe skin and eye irritation. Acrylic acid can also cause forestomach edema. Acute exposure is corrosive to the eyes, nose, throat, and mucous membranes of the upper respiratory and gastrointestinal tracts. Inhalation of vapors produces a burning sensation, cough, nasal discharge, sore throat, labored breathing, headache, nausea, vomiting, confusion, dizziness, and unconsciousness.

 http://dx.doi.org/10.1016/B978-0-12-386454-3.00220-7

Chronic Toxicity

Animal

Animals exposed to acrylic acid via chronic inhalation developed lethargy, weight loss, kidney abnormalities, and inflammation of the upper respiratory tract. Drinking water studies in rats showed a NOAEL of 140 mg kg^{-1} bw per day in decreased weight gain in a 12-month study and a NOAEL of 240 mg kg^{-1} bw per day for histopathological changes in the stomach. Inhalation studies demonstrated a LOAEL of 5 ppm in mice exposed to acrylic acid during 90 days, based on nasal lesions. Analogous studies in rats showed a LOAEL of 75 ppm.

Human

No reports of acrylic acid poisoning of the general public were found.

Reproductive Toxicity

Rats injected with acrylic acid showed signs of teratogenic effects and embryotoxicity.

Genotoxicity

Both positive and negative results have been found in *in vitro* genotoxicity tests. An *in vivo* bone marrow chromosome aberration assay was negative.

Carcinogenicity

The data available do not suggest that acrylic acid is carcinogenic; however, the existing data may be inadequate to conclude that it is not carcinogenic.

Clinical Management

Exposure should be terminated as soon as possible by moving the victim to fresh air. The skin, eyes, and mouth should be washed with copious amounts of water. Contaminated clothing should be removed and isolated. The victim should be kept calm and normal body temperature should be maintained. Artificial respiration should be provided if breathing has stopped. Treatment is usually symptomatic.

Ecotoxicology

Acrylic acid is not thought to pose a threat to ecosystems because of its rapid oxidation to benign chemical species. Bioaccumulation of acrylic acid is low due to its low partition coefficient and rapid oxidation. No evidence of biomagnification of acrylic acid in the food chain was found.

Algae have been found to be the most sensitive to acrylic acid of the aquatic organisms studied, with a no-observed-effect-concentration of 0.008 mg l^{-1}. No studies were found regarding the toxicity of acrylic acid to terrestrial organisms.

Exposure Standards and Guidelines

OSHA has currently set exposure limits for acrylic acid of 10 ppm for an 8-h TWA. However, these are not currently enforced by the agency. The National Institute for Occupational Safety and Health has recommended an exposure limit of 2 ppm for a 10-h TWA.

See also: Acrolein; Acrylamide; Acrylonitrile.

Further Reading

Hellwig, J., Deckardt, K., Freisberg, K.O., 1993. Subchronic and chronic studies of the effects of oral administration of acrylic acid to rats. Food Chem. Toxicol. 3, 1–18.

Klimisch, H.J., Hellwig, J., 1991. The prenatal inhalation toxicity of acrylic acid in rats. Fundam. Appl. Toxicol. 16, 656–666.

Vodicka, P., Gut, I., Frantik, E., 1990. Effects of inhaled acrylic acid derivatives in rats. Toxicology 65, 209–221.

Relevant Websites

http://www.osha.gov/dts/sltc/methods/organic/org028/org028.html
http://www.epa.gov/ttn/atw/hlthef/acrylica.html
http://www.inchem.org/documents/ehc/ehc/ehc191.htm

Acrylonitrile

WE Achanzar and RS Mangipudy, Bristol-Myers Squibb Co., Drug Safety Evaluation, New Brunswick, NJ, USA

This article is a revision of the previous edition article by Raja S. Mangipudy and Harihara M. Mehendale, volume 1, pp. 46–48, © 2005, Elsevier Inc.

- Chemical Abstracts Service Registry Number: CAS 107-13-1
- Synonyms: Acritet; Acrylon, Carbacryl; Cyanoethylene, Propenenitrile; 2-Propenenitrile, Ventox; Vinyl cyanide; TL 314
- Chemical/Pharmaceutical/Other Class: Industrial chemical; Solvent
- Chemical Structure:

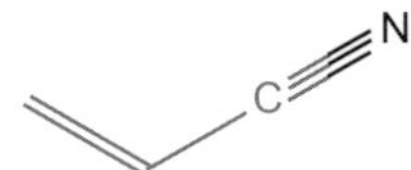

Background

Acrylonitrile is used in the manufacture of acrylic fibers, plastic surface coatings, adhesives, and synthetic rubbers. It was formerly used as a pesticide fumigant for stored grains. It is a chemical intermediate in the synthesis of antioxidants, pharmaceutical dyes, surface-active agents, and in reactions requiring the cyanoethyl group.

Environmental Fate and Behavior

Acrylonitrile is both readily volatile in air and highly soluble in water. These characteristics determine the behavior of acrylonitrile in the environment. The principal pathway leading to the degradation of acrylonitrile in air is photooxidation, mainly by reaction with hydroxyl radicals (OH). Acrylonitrile may also be oxidized by other atmospheric components such as ozone and oxygen. Very little is known about the nonbiologically mediated transformation of acrylonitrile in water. It is oxidized by strong oxidants such as chlorine used to disinfect water. Acrylonitrile is readily degraded by aerobic microorganisms in water.

Exposure and Exposure Monitoring

Occupational exposure to acrylonitrile may occur through inhalation and dermal contact, while the general population may be exposed to acrylonitrile via inhalation of ambient air and dermal contact with products containing acrylonitrile. Measurement of urinary acrylonitrile or the hemoglobin adduct *N*-(2-cyanoethyl)valine are sensitive markers of acrylonitrile exposure.

Toxicokinetics

Acrylonitrile is absorbed by way of inhalation, ingestion, and percutaneously. Rats treated with [^{14}C] acrylonitrile via oral or intravenous route produced radioactivity in the blood, liver, kidneys, lungs, adrenal cortex, and stomach mucosa. Significant amounts are retained in the plasma. Acrylonitrile is metabolized to a lesser extent in humans than in rodents. Acrylonitrile metabolism in humans follows first-order kinetics and acrylonitrile has a half-life of ~8 h. The elimination of acrylonitrile from the plasma of rats is biphasic, with a half-life of 3.5–5.8 and 50–77 h in the a and b phases, respectively. There are four major pathways of metabolism for acrylonitrile: formation of glucuronides, direct reaction with glutathione to form cyanoethyl mercapturic acid, direct reaction with the thiol groups of proteins, and epoxidation to 2-cyanoethylene oxide. *N*-Acetyl-*S*-(2-cyanoethyl)-L-cysteine is a major urinary metabolite in human volunteers exposed to 5–10 mg.

Mechanism of Toxicity

Acrylonitrile owes some of its toxicity to cyanide generation, which inhibits cellular respiration. Preinduction of microsomal mixed function oxidase (MFO) with Aroclor 1254 greatly enhanced the toxicity of acrylonitrile and caused a threefold increase in cyanide levels in rats. Therefore, metabolic activation appears to be necessary in the toxicity of acrylonitrile. The direct reaction of acrylonitrile with the SH groups of proteins and its epoxide metabolite are also expected to be responsible for its effects. Acrylonitrile has also been associated with oxidative stress.

Acute and Short-Term Toxicity

Animal

Acute animal tests in rats, mice, rabbits, and guinea pigs have demonstrated acrylonitrile to have high acute toxicity from inhalation and high to extreme acute toxicity from oral or dermal exposure. Target organs of toxicity include brain, liver, lung, kidney, and gastrointestinal tract.

Human

Workers exposed via inhalation to high levels of acrylonitrile for less than an hour experienced mucous membrane irritation, headaches, nausea, feelings of apprehension, and nervous irritability. Low-grade anemia, leukocytosis, kidney irritation, and mild jaundice were also observed in the workers, with these effects subsiding with the ending of exposure. Symptoms associated with acrylonitrile poisoning include limb weakness, labored and irregular breathing, dizziness and impaired judgment, cyanosis, nausea, collapse, and convulsions. A child died after being exposed to acrylonitrile by inhalation, suffering from respiratory malfunction, lip cyanosis, and tachycardia before death. Several adults exposed to the same concentration of acrylonitrile exhibited eye irritation, but no toxic effects. Acute dermal exposure may cause severe burns to the skin in humans. Deaths have occurred when this compound was used as a room fumigant and pediculicide. Autopsy results suggested cyanide poisoning.

Chronic Toxicity

Animal

In rats chronically exposed by inhalation, degenerative and inflammatory changes in the respiratory epithelium of the nasal turbinates and effects on brain cells have been observed. The reference concentration (RfC) for acrylonitrile is 0.002 $mg\,m^{-3}$ based on degeneration and inflammation of nasal respiratory epithelium in rats. The Environmental Protection Agency (EPA) has calculated a provisional reference dose (RfD) of 0.001 mg per kg of body weight per day for acrylonitrile based on decreased sperm counts in mice.

Human

Headaches, fatigue, nausea, and weakness have been frequently reported in chronically (long-term) exposed workers. Acrylonitrile is a skin sensitizer and repeated dermal exposure to low concentrations may result in allergic dermatitis.

Immunotoxicity

The effects of acrylonitrile on the immune system have not been extensively studied.

Reproductive Toxicity

Fetal malformations (including short tail, missing vertebrae, short trunk, omphalocele, and hemivertebra) have been reported in rats exposed to acrylonitrile by inhalation. In mice orally exposed to acrylonitrile, degenerative changes in testicular tubules and decreased sperm count were observed. No information is available on the reproductive or developmental effects of acrylonitrile in humans.

Genotoxicity

Acrylonitrile is genotoxic in *in vitro* bacterial and mammalian models, although metabolic activation was required. Most *in vivo* cytogenetic studies on intact experimental animals yielded negative results.

Carcinogenicity

Based on experimental animal data, EPA has classified acrylonitrile as a Group B1, probable human carcinogen (cancer-causing agent), while the National Toxicology Program (NTP) has classified acrylonitrile as *reasonably anticipated to be a human carcinogen*. In several studies, an increased incidence of tumors has been observed in rodents exposed by inhalation, drinking water, and gavage. In rats, astrocytomas in the brain and spinal cord and tumors of the Zymbal gland (in the ear canal) have been most frequently reported, as well as tumors of the stomach, tongue, small intestine in both sexes, and mammary gland and blood vessels in females. In mice, tumors were observed in the forestomach and Harderian gland in both sexes and in the ovary and lung in females. In humans, there is insufficient evidence to determine the relationship between acrylonitrile exposure and cancer. A statistically significant increase in the incidence of lung cancer has been reported in several studies of chronically exposed workers. However, data from the US textile worker cohort followed for five decades found no association between acrylonitrile exposure and cancer in any tissue.

Clinical Management

In oral exposure, gastric lavage may be performed soon after ingestion or in patients who are comatose or at risk of convulsing. The volume of lavage return should approximate the volume given. Charcoal slurry, aqueous or mixed with saline cathartic or sorbitol, may be administered. The usual charcoal dose is 30–100 g in adults and 15–30 g in children (1 or 2 $g\,kg^{-1}$ in infants). In case of inhalation exposure, the patient must be moved to fresh air for respiratory distress. If cough or difficulty in breathing develops, evaluation for respiratory tract irritation, bronchitis, or pneumonitis must be performed. For eye exposure, eyes must be washed with copious amounts of tepid water for at least 15 min. If irritation, pain, lacrimation, or photophobia persists, the patient should be removed to a health care facility. For dermal exposure, the exposed area must be washed thoroughly with soap and water.

Ecotoxicology

Acrylonitrile has moderate toxicity to aquatic life. By itself it is not likely to cause environmental harm at levels normally found in the environment. Acrylonitrile can contribute to the formation of photochemical smog when it reacts with other volatile substances in air.

Other Hazards

Acrylonitrile is a reactive chemical that polymerizes spontaneously, when heated, or in the presence of a strong alkali unless it is inhibited, usually with ethylhydroquinone. It can explode when exposed to flame. It attacks copper. It is incompatible and reactive with strong oxidizers, acids and alkalis; bromine; and amines.

Exposure Standards and Guidelines

- Immediately dangerous to life or health Ca (85 ppm)
- Threshold limit value time-weighted average (TLV TWA): 2 ppm confirmed animal carcinogen (skin)
- Emergency Response Planning Guideline (ERPG)-1: 25 ppm
- ERPG-2: 35 ppm
- ERPG-3: 75 ppm

- National Institute for Occupational Safety and Health recommended exposure limit Ca TWA 1 ppm C 10 ppm (15 min) (skin)

See also: Carcinogenesis; Cyanide; Respiratory Tract Toxicology; Occupational Toxicology.

Further Reading

American Conference of Governmental Industrial Hygienists (ACGIH), 1999. TLVs and BEIs: Threshold Limit Values for Chemical Substances and Physical Agents, Biological Exposure Indices. ACGIH, Cincinnati, OH.

Hobbs, C.A., Chhabra, R.S., Recio, L., Streicker, M., Witt, K.L., 2012. Genotoxicity of styrene-acrylonitrile trimer in brain, liver, and blood cells of weanling F344 rats. Environ. Mol. Mutagen. 53 (3), 227–238. http://dx.doi.org/10.1002/em.21680.

National Toxicology Program, 2012. Toxicology and carcinogenesis study of styrene-acrylonitrile trimer in F344/N rats (perinatal and postnatal feed studies). Natl. Toxicol. Program Tech. Rep. Ser. 573, 1–156.

Neal, B.H., Collins, J.J., Strother, D.E., Lamb, J.C., 2009. Weight-of-the-evidence review of acrylonitrile reproductive and developmental toxicity studies. Crit. Rev. Toxicol. 39 (7), 589–612.

Starr, T.B., Gause, C., Youk, A.O., Stone, R., Marsh, G.M., Collins, J.J., 2004. A risk assessment for occupational acrylonitrile exposure using epidemiology data. Risk Anal. 24 (3), 587–601.

Swaen, G.M., Bloemen, L.J., Twisk, J., et al., 2004. Mortality update of workers exposed to acrylonitrile in The Netherlands. J. Occup. Environ. Med. 46 (7), 691–698.

Symons, J.M., Kreckmann, K.H., Sakr, C.J., Kaplan, A.M., Leonard, R.C., 2008. Mortality among workers exposed to acrylonitrile in fiber production: an update. J. Occup. Environ. Med. 50 (5), 550–560.

Thier, R., Lewalter, J., Bolt, H.M., 2000. Species differences in acrylonitrile metabolism and toxicity between experimental animals and humans based on observations in human accidental poisonings. Arch. Toxicol. 74 (4/5), 184–189.

Relevant Websites

http://www.atsdr.cdc.gov – Agency for Toxic Substances and Disease Registry. Toxicological Profile for Acrylonitrile

http://toxnet.nlm.nih.gov – TOXNET, Specialized Information Services, National Library of Medicine. Search for Acrylonitrile.

http://ntp.niehs.nih.gov/ntp/roc/twelfth/profiles/Acrylonitrile.pdf

IPCS, Inchem: 586. Acrylonitrile (WHO Food Additives Series 19); http://www.inchem.org/documents/jecfa/jecmono/v19je13.htm

Acute Health Exposure Guidelines

SB DuTeaux, California Air Resources Board, Sacramento, CA, USA

Introduction

Chemical releases can be sudden and unexpected and, depending on the proximity of population centers, have drastic and even lethal effects. Accidental releases can be the result of natural disasters such as floods or earthquakes. They may involve process failures at industrial facilities, such as valve or line ruptures or failures in chemical containment. Chemicals can also be released through fires and explosions or illegal or uncontrolled dumping. Following the terrorist attacks of 11 September 2001, national security and emergency response experts have also focused on deliberate actions that may result in the release of highly toxic chemicals in areas where people gather, along transportation routes, or into water or food supplies.

Why Focus on Acute Effects?

Planning for and responding to environmental releases of hazardous materials requires a unique set of values designed specifically for either a single acute or short-term exposure. Acute health exposure guidelines differ from those designed to protect from cancer or other chronic effects resulting from long-term chemical exposures.

With unexpected chemical releases, the toxic effects are dependent on three broad factors. First, for toxicity to occur there must be an exposure. If protection measures are such that the population was moved or successfully sheltered-in-place or if the release was remote, the expectation is that very few individuals would be exposed. However, if a population center is located downwind or downstream from the release, a higher number of exposed persons would be expected. Second, effects are dependent on the type of chemical or mixture, the concentration, and the duration of the exposure. Third, with single exposures of relatively high concentrations, the effects are often immediate. Acute effects may occur at the site of contact with the chemical, such as the respiratory tract, eyes, or skin. The effects may also be systemic, affecting a specific organ system such as the cardiovascular or central nervous system.

Besides concern for immediate effects, some chemicals may cause delayed effects. These effects do not have to be observed immediately to be associated with an acute exposure. For example, pulmonary edema caused by inhalation of aluminum phosphide (CASRN: 20859-73-8) may not develop until two or three days after exposure. Delayed effects may also occur following dermal exposure to hydrofluoric acid (CASRN: 7664-39-3) or dimethyl mercury (CASRN: 593-74-8), whose painful and even lethal effects will not be completely evident for days or months after the exposure. Some toxic effects may not completely resolve, leading to long-term or chronic symptomology from a single exposure.

Regulations vs Guidelines

Regulations are considered law. Although differing from country to county and state to state, laws consist of constitutions, legislation, statutes, and codes covering various subject areas. Regulations are generally the official compilation and publication of the adopted rules and can be enforced.

Alternatively, guidelines are statements that determine or suggest a course of action. Guidelines aim to streamline particular processes according to given protocols and are often based on best practice. In government, guidelines are generally used to provide an additional level of safety or protection above that which has the force of law in regulation. By definition, however, following a guideline is never mandatory and is not enforced.

With the exception of occupational standards enforced by Occupational Safety and Health Administration (OSHA), all the other standards described in this article are guidelines.

Acute Health Exposure Guidelines

Most acute health exposure guidelines are designed to protect individuals from increasingly severe adverse effects as a result of a single or short-term exposure. These levels are considered 'guidance' in that there is no federal statute to require protection from these concentrations the way that there are laws for occupational exposure limits. Even so, these values are helpful for community emergency planning, off-site consequence analysis, and knowing what concentration to remediate the impacted area following a hazardous material spill.

Acute exposure guidelines are generally based on a review of available toxicology and epidemiology studies and use a risk assessment methodology that selects a critical endpoint associated with a specific exposure or dose of the chemical. Safety factors may be applied to result in a more conservative value to account for such things as extrapolation of results from animals to humans or intraspecies sensitivity. Exposure durations are generally 8 h or less, with most guidance levels based on an exposure for 1 h. The shortest exposure is 10 min and the longest can extend to 24 h or longer.

Values are generally presented as a matrix of chemical concentrations associated with specific levels of expected injury over a range of defined exposure durations.

Acute Reference Exposure Levels

The Office of Environmental Health Hazard Assessment (OEHHA) within the California Environmental Protection Agency has developed a series of 1-h acute exposure guidelines to address routine release from industrial facilities as well as process upsets or leaks. These acute reference exposure levels, or RELs, provide clear assistance to local officials regarding acute effects of industrial airborne emissions.

 http://dx.doi.org/10.1016/B978-0-12-386454-3.00802-2

Not to be confused with recommended exposure limits developed by the National Institute for Occupational Safety and Health (NIOSH) and also initialized as REL, the OEHHA acute RELs are defined as airborne concentrations of a chemical at which no adverse noncancerous health effects are anticipated including in sensitive subgroups (e.g., infants and children). Acute RELs are designed to protect against exposures lasting no more than 1 h and repeating no more than once every 2 weeks.

OEHHA used the most sensitive relevant health effect reported in the medical or toxicological literature. Data from short-term exposures were used if available. When animal results were based on a different exposure length than the preferred 1-h interval, OEHHA used a modified Haber's law (a mathematical statement relating the concentration of a poisonous gas and how long a gas must be breathed to produce death or other toxic effect) to adjust to the desired exposure duration.

At this writing, acute RELs have been established for over 95 chemicals. A link to OEHHA's REL database is available at the end of the article.

Acute Exposure Guideline Levels

Acute exposure guideline levels (AEGLs) are threshold exposure limits intended to protect the general public including susceptible or sensitive individuals. The values represent airborne concentrations of a chemical substance at or above which individuals may experience an increasing degree or severity of toxic effects, including:

- Notable discomfort (AEGL-1)
- Irreversible or serious long-lasting effects or an impaired ability to escape (AEGL-2)
- Life-threatening effects or death (AEGL-3).

Chemical-specific concentrations are associated with each of five exposure durations (10 and 30 min, 1, 4 and 8 h), and are presented as a matrix of increasing concentration, increasing exposure, and increasing severity of effect.

The development of AEGLs started in 1986 when the US Environmental Protection Agency (EPA) identified approximately 400 extremely hazardous substances based on acute lethality data from rodent studies. This was done in hopes of developing exposure guidelines under the Superfund Amendments and Reauthorization Act of 1986. EPA later requested that the National Research Council (NRC) develop guidelines for establishing AEGLs. The resulting Guidelines for Developing Community Emergency Exposure Levels for Hazardous Substances were published in 1993.

Using the 1993 NRC guidelines report, the National Advisory Committee on AEGLs for Hazardous Substances was convened and included representatives from EPA, Department of Defense, Department of Energy (DOE), Department of Transportation, several state governments, academia, and the chemical industry. From 1996 to October 2011, AEGL values were established for over 300 priority chemicals.

The process for developing AEGLs included a comprehensive search of published scientific literature and unpublished industry and proprietary data and determining the concentrations and exposure durations associated with relevant health effects. From this, a technical support document containing draft AEGL values was developed and sent for review to the AEGL Committee. Following review, a public comment period, and revisions based on scientific merit, the AEGL values would progress from draft, to proposed, to interim, and to final. Final AEGL values may be used on a permanent basis by all federal, state, and local agencies and private organizations.

Since November 2011, a new process has been adopted to finalize the remaining five chemicals on the AEGL priority list. This change is largely due to budgetary constraints, which redirects the remaining work to be done through a subcommittee of the National Academy of Sciences (NAS). Currently, the AEGL program receives technical support from a contractor that is responsible for developing the technical support documents, revising the documents based on federal stakeholder and NAS comment, and posting the final AEGL values.

The AEGL setting process includes transparency of the risk assessment methodology, public participation, and peer-review. The result is federally endorsed guidance criteria for assessing and managing single-exposure emergency events. A link to the searchable AEGL database of over 300 chemicals is available at the end of the article.

Emergency Response Planning Guidelines

Emergency Response Planning Guidelines (ERPGs) are acute exposure guidance values developed by the American Industrial Hygiene Association (AIHA). ERPGs represent maximum chemical concentrations for the general public below which adverse effects are not expected following an exposure for 1 h. Three levels are set for each chemical based on the severity of effect (ERPG-1 for the mildest reversible effects and ERPG-2 and -3 for increasingly severe and irreversible outcomes).

AIHA's ERPG committee gathers information on the chemical properties, experimental animal data, and any available human data. Data are collected from open literature as well as from proprietary and industry sources available only to members. The selection of values is based on review of relevant toxicity data using a risk assessment rationale available in the AIHA ERPG documentation.

The ERPG values have been criticized by some federal and state agency risk assessors as not maintaining transparency in the development of the values and not adhering to a consistent process of derivation. However, many emergency response organizations routinely use these guidelines.

ERPGs have been defined for approximately 145 chemicals at this writing. A link to the current list of AIHA ERPGs is available at the end of the article.

Protective Action Criteria/Temporary Emergency Exposure Limits

The Protective Action Criteria/Temporary Emergency Exposure Limits (PAC/TEELs) are developed by the DOE Subcommittee on Consequence and Protective Actions. DOE requires the use of AEGLs and ERPGs (in order of preference) as emergency exposure limits. Because thousands more chemicals are used and stored across the DOE complex than there are available AEGL or ERPG values, DOE commissioned the development of TEELs so that DOE facilities can conduct required emergency planning for all inventoried chemicals. The combined AEGLs, ERPGs, and TEELs are referred to as PACs.

TEELs are calculated using a mathematical formula to associate chemical concentrations with increasing adverse effects over specified exposure durations. In contrast to the acute exposure guidance levels mentioned earlier, TEEL development uses any available published exposure guidance including occupational exposure limits. This process is generally less rigorous than that used to develop AEGLs or ERPGs. TEELs describe the range of effects following exposure to specific chemical concentrations as such:

- TEEL-1 is an airborne concentration above which it is predicted that the general population, including susceptible individuals, could experience transient and reversible discomfort or irritation or certain asymptomatic, nonsensory effects.
- TEEL-2 is an airborne concentration above which it is predicted that the general population, including susceptible individuals, could experience irreversible or other serious, long-lasting, adverse health effects or an impaired ability to escape.
- TEEL-3 is an airborne concentration above which it is predicted that the general population, including susceptible individuals, could experience life-threatening adverse health effects or death.

TEEL values are subject to change and will be replaced by AEGLs or ERPGs when new values are published. Many TEELs are also updated annually when revised occupational exposure limits are published. PAC/TEELs are currently used across the DOE complex for preplanning, preparedness, and emergency response efforts. Other state, local, and federal agencies also use PAC/TEELs since they provide guidance for thousands of more chemicals than are available from other sources.

A link to the searchable PAC/TEEL database is available in references provided at the end of this article.

Acute Minimal Risk Levels

These values are derived by the Agency for Toxic Substances and Disease Registry and are based on threshold effects derived from animal data or human data when available. The list of compounds for which acute Minimal Risk Levels (MRLs) have been developed is very similar to the priority chemical list for Superfund sites that EPA used when developing the AEGLs. MRLs are available for both inhalation and oral exposure and are based on the most sensitive noncancer effect, including reproductive and developmental endpoints.

The acute MRLs are derived for exposure durations of 1–14 days and are consistent with the EPA reference dose risk assessment methodology. Guidance for developing the acute inhalation MRLs requires that exposures lasting less than 24 h be adjusted to reflect an exposure for 1 day. Although originally developed with the idea of protecting the public from inadvertent releases during Superfund site remediation, the acute MRLs are valuable in any release scenario as guidance values to consider for public exposures ranging from less than an hour to a few hours.

Acute MRLs are available through a link provided at the end of this article.

Provisional Advisory Levels

The Provisional Advisory Levels (PALs) developed by EPA are specifically designed to help inform site-specific decisions following a chemical release, such as to what level the chemical should be cleaned up, when to allow reentry, and when to start reusing a drinking water source. PALs are being developed for both drinking water and inhalation exposures. When completed, the process should result in short-term and subchronic guidance values for 100 high-priority hazardous chemicals and chemical warfare agents.

PALs are a tiered set of threshold inhalation and oral exposure levels for the general public. Three exposure levels are distinguished by severity of toxic effects over a 24-h, 30-day, 90-day, or 2-year exposure durations. The EPA PAL scientific workgroup has devised a risk assessment protocol similar to the AEGL process that considers three health effect levels for defined exposure durations:

- PAL 1 (mild, transient, reversible effect);
- PAL 2 (serious, possibly irreversible effect); and
- PAL 3 (severe effect or lethality).

The development process consists of the following summarized steps: (1) conducting a comprehensive literature search of published and unpublished toxicity data and assessing the toxicokinetic and toxicodynamic data as well as environmental fate and persistence; (2) identifying the critical effect from key studies; (3) calculating air and water concentrations that correspond to adult and child target effect levels; and (4) identifying key uncertainties associated with toxicity information in order to apply appropriate uncertainty factors.

PALs are evaluated by both the EPA PAL scientific workgroup and an external multidisciplinary panel to ensure scientific credibility and wide acceptance. PALs have been developed for over 35 chemicals at this writing. The values are only available by special request. Additional information can be found at http://www.epa.gov/nhsrc/news/news121208.html.

Short-Term Public Emergency Guidance Levels

Short-term public emergency guidance levels (SPEGLs) were developed by the NRC and published in 1986 as one of the first attempts to create public action levels for emergency use. SPEGLs were derived from occupational emergency exposure levels developed by the NRC for military personnel and represent concentrations at or below which no serious impairment is expected including in sensitive groups. Additional safety factors were added to the military levels to protect children and the elderly (SF = 2x) and fetuses and newborns (SF = 10x). Since 1986, there have been tremendous strides in the risk assessment methodologies for developing acute exposures guidelines. As such, SPEGLs are no longer widely used among emergency response agencies for public health protective actions.

Other Values of Interest

Several values that are commonly used to protect workers have been used as a basis of decision making for public health exposures, especially when no other value was readily available. The values are generally designed to protect against repeated exposures over a typical work shift and throughout a working lifetime. Therefore, these values may be more conservative than necessary to protect the general public from one-time exposure and caution is urged when using occupational values to make risk-based decisions to protect the general public. Occupational values of interest include:

- Permissible exposure limits – legal limit values promulgated by OSHA.
- Recommended exposure limits (RELs) – recommended workplace exposure guidelines developed by NIOSH.
- Short-term exposure limits – recommended 15-min exposure limits developed by NIOSH.
- Emergency exposure guidance levels – exposure guidance levels developed by the NRC specifically for military personnel.
- Threshold limit value and time-weighted average (TWA) – developed by American Conference of Governmental Industrial Hygienists (ACGIH) for TWA exposures during a normal 8-h workday (40-h workweek). Short-term and ceiling limit values are also available from ACGIH.

An important set of values to note is the immediately dangerous to life or health (IDLH) concentrations developed by NIOSH. IDLH values are the maximum concentration of a chemical to which a worker without personal protective equipment could be exposed for 30 min or less without escape-impairing symptoms or irreversible health effects. IDLH values are based on the lowest exposure causing death or irreversible health effects in any species. Whenever possible, IDLH values are based on human health effects from short-duration studies. When only lethal dose data from animal studies are available, IDLH values are estimated on the basis of an equivalent exposure to a 70-kg worker breathing at a rate of 50 l per minute for 30 min (equivalent to a dose of 1.5 m^3 of air).

IDLH values remain valuable in the selection of respirators and protection of emergency response entry teams. They were never intended for protecting the general public. However, the widespread use of IDLH values in emergency response requires knowledge of the values and their appropriate application. In 2010, NIOSH proposed updating the IDLH risk assessment methodology to be more consistent with the AEGL process. In this way, NIOSH hopes to ensure a more transparent process and valid scientific rationale for value setting.

A link to over 380 IDLH concentrations is available at the end of the article.

International Acute Exposure Guidelines

Because of the scope of research and resources invested by US federal and state governmental agencies in establishing guidelines for acute exposures, many countries have adopted these values or refer directly to them in their recommendations. However, several countries have developed specific acute exposure guidelines that may be more specific to industries in those countries or population sensitivities. Some examples are explained below.

Canada-Wide Standards

Canada-wide Standards (CWSs) are developed under the authority of the Canada Environmental Standards Sub-Agreement of the Canada Accord on Environmental Harmonization. The Standards Sub-Agreement is a framework for federal, provincial, and territorial environment ministers to work together to address key environmental protection and health risk-reduction issues that require common environmental standards across the country. Governments jointly agree on priorities, develop standards, and prepare complementary work plans to achieve those standards based on the unique responsibilities and legislation of each government. Short-term 1-h and 8-h CWSs are available for benzene, dioxins, furans, mercury, particulate matter, and petroleum hydrocarbons. For example, 1-h and 8-h CWSs for formaldehyde are 123 $\mu g\ m^{-3}$ or 100 ppb and 50 $\mu g\ m^{-3}$ or 40 ppb, respectively.

European Chemicals Agency

The new Classification, Labeling and Packaging (CLP) Regulation entered into force in January 2009 in the European Union and provide a method of classifying and labeling chemicals based on the United Nations' Globally Harmonized System. Part of the CLP Regulation is to ensure that the hazards posed by chemicals are clearly communicated to workers and consumers in the European Union through classification and labeling of chemicals. Under the new standards, industry must establish the potential risks to human health or the environment and classify chemicals in line with the identified hazards prior to placing the chemicals on the market. The hazards are communicated through standard statements and pictograms on labels and safety data sheets. For example, if a substance is characterized as 'acute toxicity category 1 (oral),' the labeling will include the hazard statement 'fatal if swallowed' and the word 'Danger' with a pictogram of skull and crossbones. The CLP regulation does not require independent assessment of acute toxicity if reasonable assessments are available from other governmental institutions.

Public Health England

The Centre for Radiation, Chemical and Environmental Hazards within Public Health England has produced a series of compendia of chemical hazards that provide information to those who may be involved in advising and responding to chemical incidents. For example, the compendium for chlorine provides transportation codes, health effects, and steps for decontamination, plus a summary of acute toxic effects associated with exposures of 1–2900 ppm. The acute effects summary is based on information from Public Health England's National Poisons Information Service. However, the threshold toxicity values provided in the compendium for acute exposures are the aforementioned AEGLs and ERPGs.

Applying the Emergency Exposure Levels to Protect Public Health

It is important to have access to reliable information to quickly protect the public during imminent or threatened chemical releases. There are a myriad of guidelines to use. As such, many response organizations use a hierarchy of available acute exposure guideline. Many federal and state agencies use a hierarchy of exposure guidelines, usually with AEGLs and ERPGs as the first choice depending on their availability for the chemical of concern. In most cases, multiple factors should be considered prior to deciding which guidance level to use, including:

- Potential duration of exposure,
- Extend and spread of spill/release/plume,
- Toxicity of the chemical,
- Chemical and physical characteristics of the chemical,
- Ability to control the release and other site factors,
- Potential for other hazardous conditions (explosions, fire),
- Feasibility of sheltering-in-place,
- Potential evacuation,
- Risk perception and risk communication issues, and
- Special populations at risk.

Acute health exposure guidelines provide a powerful framework for public health or emergency risk management decision making. The use of any one of these guidelines requires professional judgment and situational awareness of the specific chemical release scenario.

See also: Toxicity, Acute; Emergency Response and Preparedness; Occupational Exposure Limits; Clean Air Act (CAA), US; CERCLA; Revised as the Superfund Amendments Reauthorization Act (SARA); Chemical Warfare; The International Conference on Harmonisation.

Further Reading

Adeshina, F., Sonich-Mullin, C., Ross, R.H., Wood, C.S., Dec 2009. Health-based provisional advisory levels (PALs) for homeland security. Inhal. Toxicol. 21 (Suppl. 3), 12–16.

Agency for Toxic Substances and Disease Registry (ATSDR), 1991. Guidance for the Preparation of a Toxicological Profile.

Craig, D.K., et al., 1995. Alternative guideline limits for chemicals without environmental response planning guidelines. AIHA J. 56, 919–925.

National Research Council, 1986. Criteria and Method for Preparing Emergency Exposure Guidance Level (EEGL), Short-term Public Emergency Guidance Level (SPEGL), and Continuous Exposure Guidance Level (CEGL) Documents. Prepared by the Committee on Toxicology. National Academy Press, Washington, DC.

National Research Council, 2001. Standing Operating Procedures for Developing Acute Exposure Guideline Levels for Hazardous Chemicals. Subcommittee on Acute Exposure Guideline Levels, National Research Council, National Academy Press, Washington, DC.

Office of Environmental Health Hazard Assessment, June 2008. Air Toxics Hot Spots Risk Assessment Guidelines: Technical Support Document for the Derivation of Noncancer Reference Exposure Levels. Environmental Protection Agency, Office of Environmental Health Hazard Assessment (OEHHA), California.

US Environmental Protection Agency, 1988. Chemicals in Your Community: A Guide to the Emergency Planning and Community Right to Know Act. Available at: The National Service Center for Environmental Publications (NSCEP) http://www.epa.gov/nscep/index.html.

Relevant Websites

http://www.phmsa.dot.gov/hazmat/library/erg – 2012 Emergency Response Guidebook (ERG) from the US Department of Transportation Pipeline and Hazardous Materials Safety Administration (PHMSA).

http://www.epa.gov/oppt/aegl – Acute Exposure Guideline Levels (AEGL) database.

http://www.atsdr.cdc.gov/toxpro2.html – Acute Minimal Risk Levels (acute MRLs) developed by the Agency for Toxic Substances and Disease Registry (ATSDR).

http://www.oehha.ca.gov/air/allrels.html – Acute Reference Exposure Limits (acute RELs) Database from the California Environmental Protection Agency's Office of Environmental Health Hazard Assessment.

http://www.cameochemicals.noaa.gov/ – CAMEO (Computer-Aided Management of Emergency Operations) Chemicals database from the US Coast Guard, US EPA, and NOAA.

http://www.aiha.org/get-involved/AIHAGuidelineFoundation/EmergencyResponsePlanningGuidelines/Pages/default.aspx – AIHA: Emergency Response Plannign Guidelinest™.

http://www.cdc.gov/niosh/idlh/intridl4.html – Immediately Dangerous to Life or Health (IDLH) values.

http://www.inchem.org – INCHEM, International Programme on Chemical Safety (IPCS) offers access to thousands of searchable full-text documents on chemical risks Poisons Information Monographs, treatment guides, Environmental Health Criteria Monographs, and WHO/FAO Pesticide Data Sheets.

http://www.cdc.gov/niosh/npg – NIOSH Pocket Guide to Chemical Hazards.

http://www.atlintl.com/DOE/teels/teel/search.html – Protective Action Criteria/Temporary Emergency Exposure Limits (PAC/TEELs) database.

http://www.epa.gov/nhsrc/news/news121208.html – Provisional Advisory Limit for Hazardous Agents.

http://toxnet.nlm.nih.gov – TOXNET integrated database of hazardous chemicals, toxic releases and environmental health data from the National Library of Medicine.

http://webwiser.nlm.nih.gov – Wireless Information System for Emergency Responders (WebWISER) from the National Library of Medicine.

Acute Toxicity *see* Toxicity, Acute

Adiponitrile

GL Kennedy, DuPont Company, Wilmington, DE, USA

This article is a revision of the previous edition article by Shashi Ramaiah and Harihara M. Mehendale, volume 1, pp 49–50, © 2005, Elsevier Inc.

- Name: Adiponitrile
- Chemical Abstracts Service Registry Number: 111-69-3
- Synonyms: Hexanedinitrile; Adipic acid dinitrile; Adipic acid nitrile; Adipodinitrile; Adipyldinitrile; 1,4-Dicyanobutane; Hexanedioic acid dinitrile; Tetramethylene cyanide
- Molecular Formula: $C_6H_8N_2$
- Chemical Structure:

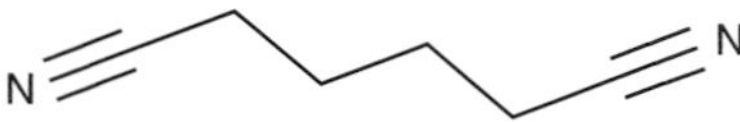

Background

Adiponitrile is an odorless, colorless liquid that decomposes on heating to react violently with strong oxidants. Upon burning, the highly toxic hydrogen cyanide is produced.

Uses

The major use of adiponitrile is as an intermediate in the production of nylon. Lesser uses include that in organic synthesis and in the preparation of adipoguanamine, which is used as an extractant for aromatic hydrocarbons.

Environmental Fate and Behavior

Adiponitrile will exist solely as a vapor in the ambient atmosphere. The chemical can be degraded in air by photochemically produced hydroxyl radicals with a half-life of 23 days. Adiponitrile is expected to have very high mobility in soil, with volatilization from soil or water surfaces not expected to be an important fate process. The chemical is expected to biodegrade in aquatic and soil systems. The potential for bioconcentration in aquatic organisms is low.

Exposure Routes and Exposure Monitoring

In occupational setting, adiponitrile exposure may occur through both inhalation and dermal contact. In the environment, the volatility of adiponitrile is such that it will exist almost exclusively in the vapor state. Ingestion is generally not an important route of exposure.

Toxicokinetics

Following subcutaneous injection to guinea pigs, 79% of the dose was eliminated in the urine as thiocyanate. Dermal application to the guinea pig resulted in the excretion of thiocyanate, with absorption increased by both removal of hair and mild abrasion of the skin. Of the cyanide antidotes, thiosulfate was the most effective. Following absorption, the ratio between the administered adiponitrile and cyanide showed the greater part of the dose existed as cyanide.

Mechanism of Toxicity

The mechanism of adiponitrile's toxicity relates to its ability to release cyanide both *in vitro* and *in vivo*. Cyanide then forms a stable complex with ferric iron in the cytochrome oxidase enzyme. Since this enzyme occupies a central role in the utilization of oxygen in practically all cells, inhibition produces an inhibition of cellular respiration.

Acute and Short-Term Toxicity

Animal

Adiponitrile is highly toxic acutely, with oral LD_{50} values ranging from 22 mg kg^{-1} in the rabbit to 172 mg kg^{-1} in the mouse. The acute dermal toxicity is quite low, being greater than 2000 mg kg^{-1} in the rabbit and when injected subcutaneously to the guinea pig an LD_{50} of 50 mg kg^{-1} was obtained. The LD_{50} in the mouse following intraperitoneal injection was 40 mg kg^{-1}. In male rats, the inhalation LC_{50} for single 4 h periods was 1.71 mg l^{-1}. The material is neither a strong irritant nor a sensitizer in the guinea pig.

Human

In a case history where an individual reported drinking a few milliliters of adiponitrile, the subject felt tightness in the chest, headache, vertigo, and weakness, with difficulty standing. He became cyanotic, respirations were rapid, and he had low blood pressure and tachycardia. The papillary response was barely active and he displayed mental confusion and

 http://dx.doi.org/10.1016/B978-0-12-386454-3.00222-0

tonic-clonic contractures of limbic and facial muscles. In other situations, exposure to skin resulted in irritation and inflammation, with a case reporting massive destruction of the skin of an exposed foot. Vapors are very irritating to the eyes and upper respiratory tract tissues at higher concentrations. The chemical can be fatal when large amounts are absorbed through the skin, swallowed, or inhaled.

Chronic Toxicity

Animal

Repeated inhalation doses of 0.3 mg l^{-1} in rats showed hematologic and kidney changes along with a depressed rate of body weight gain. Slight kidney damage was seen at 0.1 mg l^{-1} and no effects were seen at 0.1 mg l^{-1}. In a 2 year feeding study in rats, degeneration of the adrenal glands in females, but not in males, was the only adverse effect reported. Repeated dermal applications produced histopathologic changes in the liver, kidney, and spleen of guinea pigs.

No effects on reproduction or fertility were seen in rats exposed by inhalation to up to 0.1 mg l^{-1} for 13 weeks. Reduced body weight gain, mortality, and anemia were seen at that concentration. The hematologic changes were reversible. No evidence of fetal abnormalities was seen in rats given oral doses of adiponitrile during gestation although both reduced maternal and fetal weights were seen at the higher doses.

No increase in tumor incidence was reported in a 2 year drinking water study in rats exposed to 50 ppm or in a 3 year feeding study in dogs exposed to 500 ppm.

Human

The effects of longer-term exposure have not been reported. In the workplace, threshold concentrations of up to 2 ppm are considered to be appropriate for those exposed to adiponitrile and such conditions would not be expected to produce any adverse effects, including point of contact irritation. Repeated exposures to higher concentrations would be expected to produce irritation to the eyes, nose, and throat and could potentially aggravate existing respiratory disease. The workplace control limit includes a skin notation that indicates the potential for a significant contribution to the overall exposure by the cutaneous route.

Reproductive Toxicity

No effects on reproduction or fertility were seen in rats exposed by inhalation to up to 0.1 mg l^{-1} for 13 weeks. Reduced body weight gain, mortality, and anemia were seen at that concentration. The hematologic changes were reversible. No evidence of fetal abnormalities was seen in rats given oral doses of adiponitrile during gestation although both reduced maternal and fetal weights were seen at the higher doses.

Genotoxicity

Adiponitrile was not mutagenic to four strains of *Salmonella* both in the presence and in the absence of a metabolic activation system.

Carcinogenicity

No increase in tumor incidence was reported in a 2 year drinking water study in rats exposed to 50 ppm or in a 3 year feeding study in dogs exposed to 500 ppm.

In Vitro Toxicity

Adiponitrile was not mutagenic to four strains of *Salmonella* both in the presence and in the absence of a metabolic activation system.

Clinical Management

In poisoning with most nitrile compounds, the onset of symptoms is generally delayed for up to several hours, thus making a prolonged period of observation in a controlled setting necessary. The initial response may be flushing, tachycardia, tachypnea, headache, and dizziness, which may progress to agitation, stupor, coma, apnea, generalized convulsions, pulmonary edema, bradycardia, hypotension, and death. Severe hypoxic sighs in the absence of cyanosis suggest cyanide poisoning, as cyanosis is generally a late finding and does not occur until the stage of circulatory collapse and apnea.

Oral exposures should consider gastric lavage if symptoms are not present. Do not use emetics and rinse mouth and administer up to 200 ml water for dilution if the patient can swallow, has a strong gag reflex, and does not drool. If symptoms are present, proceed directly to major emergency measures, including use of cyanide antidote kit and other life support systems. Following inhalation exposure, move the patient to fresh air and monitor for respiratory distress. Administer oxygen and assist ventilation as required. All patients should be carefully observed for signs of systemic cyanide poisoning and treat with antidote kit in symptomatic individuals. With dermal contact, remove contaminated clothing and wash the exposed area thoroughly with soap and water. Again, if signs of cyanide poisoning become apparent, treat with antidote. Treat dermal irritation or burns with standard topical therapy.

Ecotoxicity

Lethality in minnows, guppies, and sunfish is seen at concentrations ranging from 775 to 1250 ppm following exposures from 24 to 96 h, indicating relatively low acute toxicity to aquatic species.

Other Hazards

Although among the least toxic of the nitrites, adiponitrile can release cyanide both *in vitro* and *in vivo*; thus it is important to be aware of signs of cyanide poisoning.

Miscellaneous

Adiponitrile should be stored in tightly closed containers in a cool, well-ventilated area. Adiponitrile must be stored to avoid contact with oxidizing agents such as perchlorates, peroxides, permanganates, and fluorine, since violent reactions can occur. Adiponitrile is not compatible with strong acids or reducing agents.

Exposure Standards and Guidelines

Occupational exposure standards and guidelines for adiponitrile include the following:

United States: American Conference of Governmental Industrial Hygienists threshold limit value of 2 ppm (8.8 mg m^{-3}) based on respiratory tract irritation and includes a skin notation. The US National Institute for Occupational Safety and Health recommended exposure limit is 4 ppm (18 mg m^{-3}) as a 10 h time-weighted average.

See also: Cyanide; Nitriles; Volatile Organic Compounds.

Further Reading

Smith, L.W., Kennedy Jr, G.L., 1982. Inhalation toxicity of adiponitrile in rats. Toxicol. Appl. Pharmacol. 65, 257–263.

Relevant Websites

http://nj.gov/health/eoh/rtkweb/documents/fs/0027.pdf – Jersey Hazardous Substances Fact Sheet.

http://toxnet.nlm.nih.gov/cgi-bin/sis/search/f?./temp/~mXaoxz:1 – NLM-HSDB database.

http://www.epa.gov/iris/subst/0515.htm – US Environmental Protection Agency.

Advances in Physiologically Based Modeling Coupled with *In Vitro–In Vivo* Extrapolation of ADMET: Assessing the Impact of Genetic Variability in Hepatic Transporters

S Ho and AS Darwich, School of Pharmacy and Pharmaceutical Sciences, University of Manchester, Manchester, UK
M Jamei, Simcyp Ltd (a Certara Company), Blades Enterprise Centre, Sheffield, UK
A Rostami-Hodjegan, School of Pharmacy and Pharmaceutical Sciences, University of Manchester, Manchester, UK; and Simcyp Ltd (a Certara Company), Blades Enterprise Centre, Sheffield, UK

Background

Research carried out over the last two decades examining the role of transporters on exposure of xenobiotics has revealed the importance of transporter activity and substrate affinity to transporters and metabolizing enzymes for the regulation of substrate disposition in man. Modulation of transporter activity via genetic or epigenetic regulation may provide potential explanation for some of the observed interindividual variability relating to the toxicological effect of xenobiotics, including pesticides, toxins, and medicinal or recreational drugs.

At present, xenobiotics are mainly labeled as being toxic on the basis of outcomes from high dose exposure in animal testing, which does not necessarily translate to adverse toxicological outcomes in man at lower dose levels. Due to a large number of chemicals being subject to sparse toxicological testing in the past and the shift to an earlier testing of drug properties relating to pharmacokinetics (PKs) and toxicity, the use of high-throughput screening has increased in order to cope with increased requirements, where the pharmaceutical industry brings valuable knowledge due to more experience in the area. Automated *in vitro* assays and *in silico* computational methods such as quantitative structure–activity relationship and physiologically based pharmacokinetic (PBPK) modeling play important roles in this process and further bring valuable insight into the assessment of dose-dependent toxicity through *in vitro–in vivo* extrapolation (IVIVE), potentially saving time, cost, and minimizing animal research.

Statins lend themselves well in exemplifying the importance of hepatic transporters on the interindividual variability and dose dependency in relation to toxicological effects of xenobiotics. Being one of the most commonly prescribed drug classes in the world, statins are generally considered well tolerated although they can cause muscle toxicity, myopathy, as an adverse effect where incidents have been observed to increase with the increase in dose. The severity of myopathy ranges from mild myalgia (muscle ache or weakness without creatine kinase (CK) elevation), myositis (muscle symptoms with increased CK levels) to rhabdomyolysis (muscle symptoms with marked CK elevation), a rare but potentially fatal toxicological effect.

Although the PK characteristics of statins vary in large, where, for example, atorvastatin, lovastatin, and simvastatin are mainly metabolized by CYP3A4, whereas pravastatin and rosuvastatin are mainly excreted unchanged, they are all substrates to the organic anion transporter polypeptide (OATP) 1B1, responsible for the active uptake of drug into the liver. The variability in hepatic transporter uptake activity caused by genetic polymorphism is of importance in elucidating the varied extent of toxicological response observed in different populations treated with statins. It has been proposed that a reduction in OATP1B1 transporter activity as a consequence of polymorphism may lead to a reduced hepatic uptake resulting in a reduced drug clearance and an increase in muscle concentrations of some statins potentially leading to the toxicological effect. This is however further complicated by the fact that a number of other transporters exhibit similar functionality to OATP1B1 in the liver whereas several uptake and efflux transporters exist in the muscle tissue.

In this article, the impact of hepatic transporters on systemic and organ exposure and the toxicological impact governed by the PK properties through absorption, distribution, metabolism, excretion, and toxicology (ADMET) processes were described. Further how these PK and toxicokinetic (TK) properties can be investigated through *in vitro* methodology and extrapolated to *in vivo* systems will be explained, allowing PBPK modeling and simulation of the TK impact of altered hepatic active uptake.

Systemic Exposure and Toxicity: 'ADMET'

The exposure of an individual to a certain xenobiotic or drug can be described by the area under the concentration time curve (AUC). The AUC after an orally administered dose (D) is dependent on the proportion of the dose that is absorbed and available in systemic circulation after passage from the gut through the liver (the bioavailability of the drug – F), the clearance (CL), and the dose of the drug, eqn [1]).

$$\mathrm{AUC} = \frac{F \times D}{\mathrm{CL}} \qquad [1]$$

The total CL is defined as the volume of blood which is completely cleared of the xenobiotic per unit time and encompasses clearance by the liver, kidneys, and biliary excretion. In the absence of variation in toxicological effect or pharmacological response (e.g., genetic differences in receptors, underlying effect of disease itself, effects of concomitant drugs), maximum exposure, as measured by maximum concentration of a xenobiotic in blood circulation (C_{max}), and total exposure, as measured by AUC, are often closely linked to the pharmacological as well as concentration-related toxicity or adverse effects. Thus, early determination of the PK characteristics of a drug as in the process of drug development and defining the influence of individual covariates are desirable. A brief description of ADME processes that determine the overall PKs is provided below. This will enable recognition of the separation of elements which are related to human biology and physiology (i.e., system parameters) from those of the drug that, in combination, lead to observed ADMET behavior.

 http://dx.doi.org/10.1016/B978-0-12-386454-3.01058-7

Absorption

Bioavailability (F) is a term often used to describe the absorption of a drug. It is defined as the proportion of an oral dose of a drug which reaches the systemic circulation. It is dependent on a number of factors which are described in eqn [2]:

$$F = f_a \times F_G \times F_H \qquad [2]$$

where f_a is the fraction of the dose entering the gut wall, F_G is the fraction of drug which escapes metabolism in the gut wall and enters the portal vein, and F_H is the fraction of the drug that enters the liver and escapes metabolism, entering systemic circulation. Transporters can potentially affect the absorption of drug from the gastrointestinal tract.

Distribution

Distribution refers to the reversible transfer of drug from one location within the body to another. Distribution of drugs to and from blood and other tissues occurs at various rates and to various extents. Several factors are responsible for the distribution pattern of a drug within the body over time. Some of these are related to the nature of the drug (such as the ability of the drug to cross membranes, plasma protein binding, partitioning into the red blood cells, tissues, and fat) and some others relate to characteristics of the individual (such as the perfusion rate of different tissues by blood, concentration of plasma proteins, hematocrit, body composition). Since the exposure of a given xenobiotic will depend on the amount reaching the site of action and the rate at which it is removed, the above factors are important determinants of dosage regimens.

Metabolism

For the majority of new (and mostly lipophilic) drug compounds, metabolism is a major route of elimination from the body. During preclinical drug development, the quantitative prediction of *in vivo* metabolic clearance from *in vitro* data is arguably one of the most important objectives of *in vitro* metabolism studies.

Excretion

All drugs are ultimately removed from the body, either in the form of their metabolites or in their unchanged form, by excretory organs, mainly the kidneys, and excreted in the urine (although in some instances, excretion may be via the biliary route). Compromised renal function may affect the PKs of the drugs if urinary excretion is a substantial part of the overall elimination.

Organ Exposure and Transporters

Organ- or tissue-specific exposure following an administered drug can be described using the AUC in the studied organ or tissue (AUC_{organ}). Depending on the nature of the organ, being either eliminatory (i.e., liver or kidney) or noneliminatory (i.e., muscle, adipose, or bone), the exposure of the drug to the tissue will be governed by different processes. The net clearance in (CL_{in}) and out (CL_{out}) of a noneliminatory organ is conventionally governed by the substrates' affinity to the specific tissues or organs, or tissue-to-plasma water partition coefficient, and can be considered a passive process as such, thus influencing the overall distribution of the compound in the body (eqn [3]).

$$AUC_{Organ} = \frac{AUC_{System} \times CL_{in}}{CL_{out}} \qquad [3]$$

Due to the practical difficulty in measuring the concentration of xenobiotics in tissue, particularly in humans, mechanism-based approaches to estimate the affinity of various compounds to each tissue have been developed by Poulin and Theil and frequently implemented on physiologically based models. Improved equations by Rodgers and Rowland have allowed for better predictability of ionized molecules based on the assumption of all molecules being dissolved in the intra- and extracellular tissue water and partition into neutral lipids and phospholipids in the tissue cells.

Considering an eliminatory organ CL_{out} can additionally be a component of the systemic elimination of the compound in question from the body. There are numerous drug transporters on the membranes of various tissues. These transporters can influence drug distribution into the tissues particularly for compounds exhibiting permeability limitations to specific tissues where the permeability will act as the rate-limiting step in the distribution to the organ; these compounds will therefore be more dependent on active transport uptake or efflux acting on CL_{in} and CL_{out}, respectively. This will impact the AUC_{organ} but also has the potential of influencing the systemic AUC and subsequently the exposure in other organs. This can be of particular significance in eliminatory organs as transporters can act to increase systemic exposure through transporting altering CL_{in} or CL_{out} of the organ and further affect the amount of the compound in question available for metabolizing enzymes or systemic elimination through the eliminatory organ.

Various Families of Transporters

Transporters are integral proteins which are expressed in the cell membranes. They mediate translocation of endogenous substances and exogenous chemicals in and out of cells using active and passive mechanisms. Transporters are specific in their action, where for example they may facilitate the uptake or excretion of substrates in the intestine or liver. Generally, they can be classified as either influx (uptake into the cell) or efflux (transport out of the cell) transporters.

The disposition of xenobiotics and endogenous substances (e.g., bile acid and cholesterol) is most often associated with two superfamilies of transporters: the solute carrier (SLC) and ATP-binding cassette (ABC) families. They use secondary and tertiary active transport to move chemicals across biological membranes. The OATPs (SLCO), OATs (SLC22A), and organic cation transporters (OCTs, SLC22A) are among the SLC subfamilies. OATPs are found in various tissues, including the liver, intestine, kidney, and brain. They are responsible for the transport of a wide range of endogenous substrates including bile acids, thyroid hormones, steroid conjugates, anionic oligopeptides, eicosanoids, various drugs, and xenobiotic compounds across membranes. Six human OATP families containing eleven human OATP subfamilies have been identified. Among them, OATP1B1 and OATP1B3 are distributed in the liver tissue while OATP1A2 and OATP2B1 are distributed in both liver and intestinal tissues. They participate in the active uptake of compounds from the portal vein into the liver.

Members of the *ABC* family are exclusively considered to be efflux transporters, removing substrate from the cell using primary active transport. They are of importance as they can limit the entry of drugs or facilitate drug removal from the cell in various tissues. The main efflux transporters currently identified include multidrug resistance transporter 1 (MDR1), the canalicular bile salt export pump (BSEP), the multidrug resistance-associated protein (MRP) family, and breast cancer resistance protein (BCRP). MDR1, also refered to as permeability-limiting glycoprotein (P-gp) is encoded by the gene. It is an important efflux transporter involved in oral drug absorption, distribution to tissues, and biliary or urinary excretion of many drugs. P gp was the first drug transporter described, and is known, together with MRPs and some monocarboxylate transporters (MCTs), for giving an MDR characteristic to cancer cells (**Figures 1 and 2**).

Transporter Polymorphism and Impact on 'ADMET'

PKs can be a major source of variability in dose and response relationship. It manifests itself in interindividual differences in the plasma concentration–time profile of a drug. Factors that lead to variability in the ADME parameters are therefore of importance in understanding overall variability in PKs and TKs.

Variability in Absorption

As described previously, absorption is affected by three parameters, f_a, F_G, and F_H. Each of these parameters is sensitive to differences in physiological characteristics between individuals. An important factor affecting f_a is variation in gastrointestinal motility, in particular for drugs with low permeability. F_G is sensitive to the genetics of individual in relation to drug-metabolizing enzymes, diet, and active secretion of the drug back into the gut by the multidrug efflux pumps like P-gp, BCRP or MRP2 that are susceptible to interindividual fluctuations in both abundance and activity. Variability in the first-pass metabolism of the drug by the liver (F_H) is a result of genetic differences in drug metabolism and differences in the physiology of the individual affecting liver blood flow and the size of the liver.

Hepatic transporters mediate transport of substrates in and out of liver, where genetic variation in transporter activity may affect the translocation of substrates. OATP1B1 is involved in the hepatocellular uptake of a variety of endogenous and foreign chemicals. A diverse set of molecules are substrate to OATP1B1, including statins.

OATP1B1 is encoded by the gene *SLCO1B1*. Its protein consists of 670 amino acids with 12 putative membrane-spanning domains, and a large fifth extracellular loop. The OATP1B1 gene is located in chromosome 12 (gene locus 12p12). Numerous sequence variations, such as single nucleotide polymorphisms, have been identified in the *SLCO* gene. These polymorphisms may have significant consequences on PKs, for example, by reducing transporter uptake activity giving rise to interindividual variability in PKs of substrate compounds. OATP1B1 represents the most studied OATP to date.

Studies have shown that the SLCO1B1 c.521T>C variant (*5 or *15 haplotype) may be associated with impaired hepatic uptake and potentially increase the plasma concentration of *OATP1B1* substrates, whereas the *SLCO1B1*1B* haplotype may be associated with an enhanced hepatic uptake and reduced plasma concentrations of some OATP1B1 substrates in Caucasians. Note that genetic differences are found among different racial and ethnic backgrounds. The low-activity haplotypes *5 and *15 have a combined allele frequency of

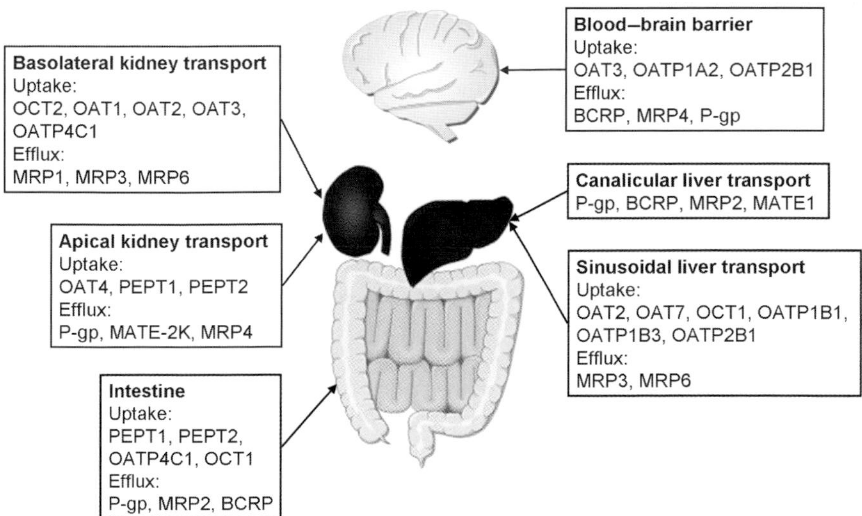

Figure 1 Organ distribution of identified transporters and their functionality in man. Adapted from Zhang, L., Strong, J.M., Qui, W., Lesko, L.J., and Huang, S.M., 2006. Scientific perspectives on drug transporters and their role in drug interactions. Mol. Pharm. 3, 62-69.

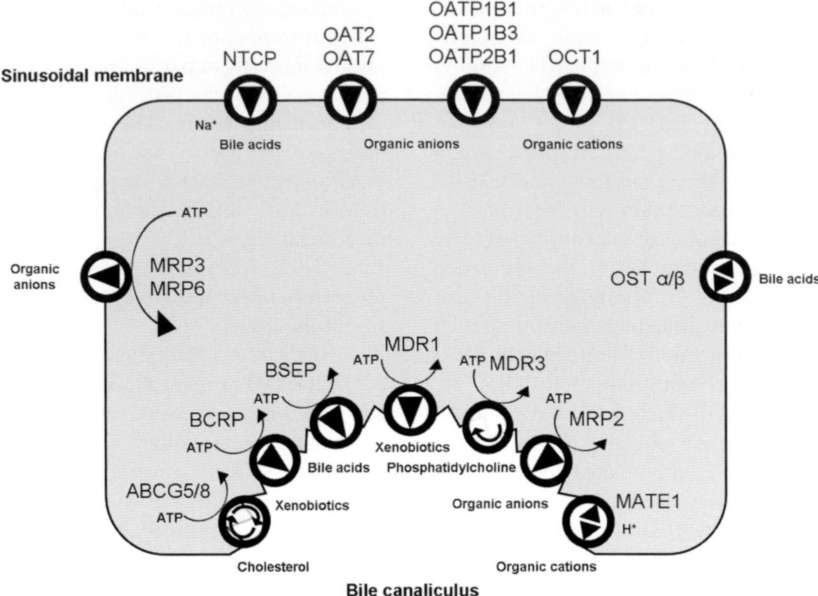

Figure 2 Efflux and uptake transporters located on the sinusoidal (NTCP, OAT2, OAT7, OATP1B1, OATP1B3, OATP2B1 and OCT1) and canalicular membranes (ABCG5/8, BCRP, BSEP, MDR1, MDR3, MRP2 and MATE1) in liver. Direction is indicated by arrows. ABCG5/8 transport cholesterol in and out within the bilayer, whereas MDR3 transport is from the inner to the outer bilayer.

approximately 15-20% in Europeans, 10-15% in Asians, and 2% in sub-Saharan Africans, whereas, the enhanced uptake haplotype *1B has an allele frequency of approximately 26% in Europeans, 39% in South/Central Asians, 63% in East Asians, and as high as 77% in sub-Saharan Africans. As transporters can influence the deposition of drugs and genetic variation in transporters do exist among populations, these give rise to intervariation in response of the same drug.

In Vitro Assessment of Transporter Activity

Tissue volumes and tissue blood flows are essential components of a PBPK model. Correlations between tissue volumes and tissue blood flows should be considered when modeling interindividual variability in drug distribution using PBPK models. There are drug-related characteristics (such as ability to cross membranes, bind to plasma proteins, partition into red blood cells, tissues, or fat, and its specific affinity to influx or efflux transporter proteins) which can influence the dynamics of distribution to various tissues and concentration–time profile of drugs. Many of these can be measured *in vitro* and used for IVIVE purposes. Current IVIVE approaches for assessing the distribution of the drugs to various tissues involve estimation of tissue-to-plasma partition coefficient ($K_{p:t}$) based on affinity to lipids and binding to common proteins present in the tissue interstitial space combined with *in vitro* measurements of blood and plasma protein binding.

Separation of the passive permeability and transporter-mediated flux is an essential element of *in vitro* cell-based studies as these can be used to predict the behavior of the drug *in vivo* (using IVIVE). The active transport kinetics is often described by Michaelis–Menten kinetics (K_m, V_{max}, or CL_{int}, T). The effects of unbound fraction at the binding site cannot be directly measured in most cases; however, delineation via application of models is becoming more popular. These systems together with appropriate modeling are now routinely used to elucidate passive and active transporter processes acting to influence drug permeability. Caco-2 cells grown to confluent monolayers in bicameral filter systems endogenously express the majority of the relevant transporters also expressed in the human intestine *in vivo*. Alternatively, cell line includes Madine Darby Canine Kidney (MDCK II) and Lilly Laboratories Cells – Porcine Kidney Nr. 1 ($LLC\text{-}PK_1$), selected due to their low endogenous transporter expression of mdr1, bcrp, and mrp2. Inhibition of active processes can be an issue knowing the lack of specificity of transporter inhibitors for certain isoforms.

Recently, research has focused on using mathematical models to describe drug concentration time courses at transporter binding sites in order to accurately determine the intrinsic kinetics of active processes. Using a global kinetic approach to simulate the time course of drug concentrations in multiple compartments of the experimental system has been reported in the literature. The models in the last few years have become increasingly more mechanistic (and hence more complex) involving up to five compartments within *in vitro* system to describe the characteristics assumed to be important to the mechanics of drug transport within a two-chamber filter system like the Snap- or Transwell systems. A modeling approach for assessing *in vitro* data can help with recognizing processes that have not been identified to facilitate further work on these as yet unidentified mechanisms acting on the drug. They can help to identify the outliers and supply further guidance toward issues which require extra attention. Examples are provided below to show practical applications.

'PBPK' Modeling of Hepatic Transport

PKs deals with quantitative assessment of the fate of drugs in the body. Mathematical models are necessary to describe and predict concentration–time profiles from data obtained by measuring the drug level in biological fluids such as blood, plasma, and urine. The models can range from simple compartmental analysis to sophisticated PBPK incorporating population-based interindividual variability in physiological parameters.

In PBPK modeling describing liver uptake, the diffusion of the compound into the liver will be limited by the blood flow into the organ as the compound is assumed to not exhibit any permeability limitations into the tissue, and this is referred to as a perfusion-limited organ model. If a compound displays a permeability limitation into the organ, blood flow will no longer be rate-limiting step and the concentration in the organ will rather be dependent on its ability to permeate the tissue, and as described earlier this can be a net effect of diffusion into the tissue, active transporter uptake or efflux.

In order to describe and model the latter scenario, a permeability-limited liver model is required. The permeability-limited liver model divides the liver into three compartments: extracellular water (EW), intracellular water (IW) and capillary blood, where the distribution between the compartments is dynamic as described in **Figure** 3. Sinusoidal transporters will alter the rate at which the drug is transferred between EW and IW, $kt_{\text{EW-in}}$ and $kt_{\text{IW-out}}$.

Transporter kinetics are generally described as an intrinsic clearance equal to the maximal rate ($V_{\max}$) divided by the Michaelis constant (K_{m}) under linear conditions. K_{m} is the substrate concentration at which the rate reaches half of its maximum value ($V_{\max}$).

Transport-mediated uptake or efflux is generally described as an intrinsic clearance (CL_{int}) equal to the maximal rate ($V_{\max}$) divided by the Michaelis constant (K_{m}) under linear conditions using Michaelis–Menten type equations ($V_{\max}$ = maximum flux; K_{m} = substrate concentration giving half $V_{\max}$). A reduction in $V_{\max}$ corresponds to a reduced capacity of active transport.

The CL_{int} is a concentration- and time-dependent variable (eqn [4]), where CL_{int} is in μl min^{-1}, $V_{\max}$ is in per million hepatocytes (pmol) min^{-1}, and K_{m} in μM, respectively:

$$\text{CL}_{\text{int}} = \frac{V_{\max}}{K_{\text{m}} + C_{\text{u}}} \qquad [4]$$

where C_{u} is the unbound concentration at the transporter site. Hence for uptake transporters, it is the unbound concentration in the EW and for efflux transporters it is the unbound concentration in the IW. Usually measuring the unbound concentrations is a challenging task, hence *in silico* methods are developed to estimate these values. In order to predict tissue distribution, recently mechanistic equations have been developed that incorporate compound lipophilicity, binding of compound to plasma and tissue macromolecules, and levels of phospholipids and neutral lipids in plasma and tissues. These models have been further developed accounting for protein binding in the EW and incorporating acidic phospholipids binding for strong bases ($\text{p}K_a > 7.0$).

These equations are developed assuming steady-state condition and instantaneous equilibrium. However, attempts are made to adapt these equations to nonequilibrium conditions and develop models describing transporters functionality in different organs such as liver, brain, and heart. Using a similar approach and without assuming the equilibrium condition, permeability-limited models and equations are developed and implemented within the Simcyp Simulator

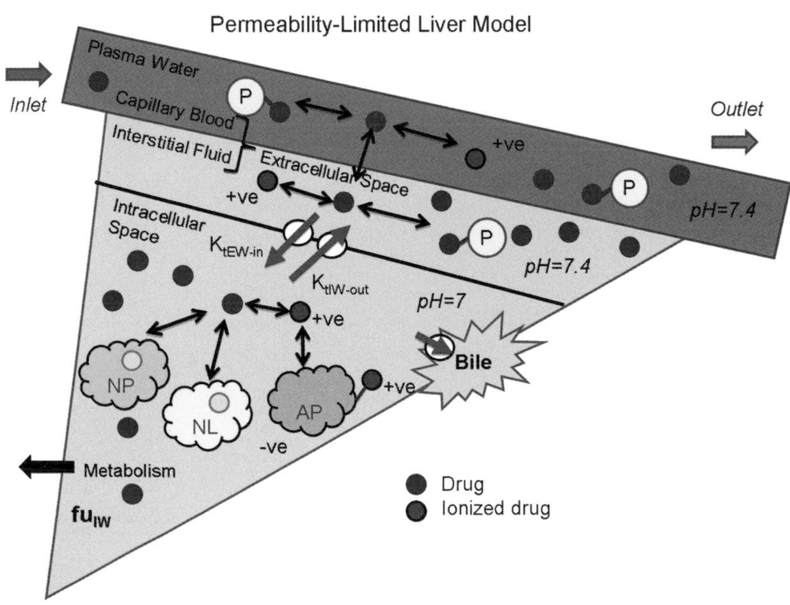

Figure 3 The permeability limited liver model. See text for detailed description.

(since V10). These models are used to estimate the drug unbound fractions in intercellular and EW and predict transporters functionality in different organs including liver, brain, and kidney assuming:

- The tissue is divided into three compartments, namely vascular space and EW and IW spaces.
- The vascular and extracellular compartments are in instantaneous equilibrium though the total concentration in these can be different.
- Only unionized and unbound species can permeate (either passively or actively) through the plasma membrane.
- The movement of the unbound unionized species from the capillary bed (vascular space) to the EW is not a rate-limiting process and the perfusion-limited transition only happens between the EW and IW spaces.
- Passive permeability at the canalicular side of the liver plays a negligible role in biliary secretion.
- Since there are no reports suggesting the presence of drug uptake transporters at the canalicular membrane these are not considered.

The developed models have been used successfully to predict the PK profiles and transporter-mediated interaction of repaglinide, cyclosporine A, clarithromycin, and trimethoprim. These models are also used to simulate the cases described in the following section.

Modeling the transporter activity as a consequence of genetic polymorphism can therefore be done through altering the maximum flux of the transporter and simulating the impact on organ and tissue concentrations as a result of these.

Simulating the Effect of OATP1B1 Polymorphism on the Exposure of Statins

In the following case, how the impact of genetic polymorphism of *SLCO1B1* and OATP1B1 activity and subsequently the TKs of statins can be investigated through a PBPK simulation approach and further give important theoretical insights into the PK parameters governing the systemic and organ exposure of hepatic transporter substrates through sensitivity analysis of OATP1B1 affinity and transport rate is described.

Utilizing a full PBPK distribution model, based on Rodgers and Rowland, coupled with a permeability-limited liver model allowing the implementation of transporter liver uptake, incorporated into the population-based PBPK simulator Simcyp v11 (Simcyp Ltd, Sheffield), concentration time profiles in liver plasma and muscle tissue of atorvastatin, pravastatin, and simvastatin immediate release were simulated at a low, medium, and high therapeutic doses.

A range of affinities and rate of transport values of OATP1B1 substrates were collated from the literature. **Figures 4** and **5** display the distribution of K_m and V_{max}, respectively, for reported substrates. The ranges of V_{max} and K_m values served as a basis for designing the sensitivity analysis simulation study, providing naturally occurring ranges. The genotypic

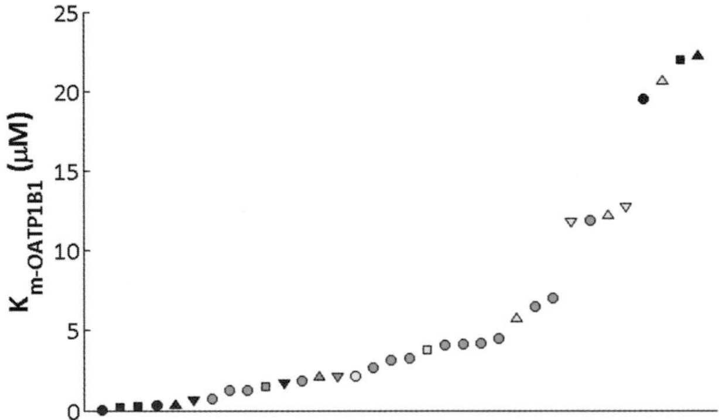

Figure 4 Scatter plot of apparent K_m (μM) values of endogenous and exogenous OATP1B1 substrates where symbol and color coding differentiate substrates.

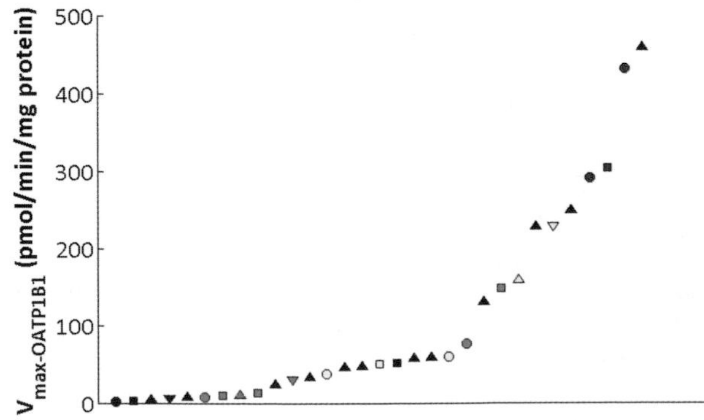

Figure 5 Scatter plot of V_{max} (pmol min^{-1} mg protein^{-1}) values of endogenous and exogenous OATP1B1 substrates where symbol and color coding differentiate substrates.

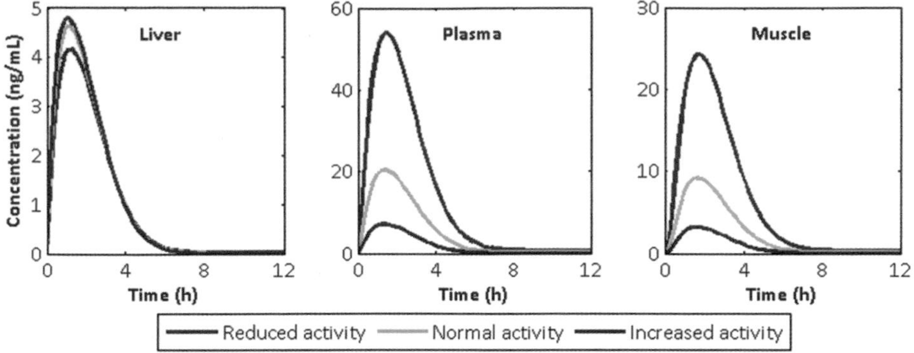

Figure 6 Simulated atorvastatin acid immediate release 40 mg concentration (ng ml^{-1}) time profiles in liver (unbound intracellular concentration), plasma, and muscle tissue at a K_m of 0.4 μM and a V_{max} of 400 pmol min^{-1} million $cells^{-1}$.

polymorphism was implemented through altering V_{max} assigning it a value of one-third of the original value or three times larger to emulate the impact of genetic polymorphism.

Keeping K_m constant and reducing the transporter activity (V_{max}) led to a reduction in the amount of substrate drugs being transported into the hepatocytes. Increased transporter activity led to an increase in drug concentration in the liver, whereas a less active transporter resulted in a higher proportion of drug circulating in plasma. Thus, when a higher amount of drug was taken up into the liver, less would remain in circulation; subsequently, less would be distributed to the muscle tissue. At a high K_m, the substrate affinity to the transporter is high. The available OATP1B1 transporters will be highly occupied by the substrate drug potentially causing saturation. In this scenario, the rate of transport will only have a minor impact on the overall transport.

Atorvastatin Acid

Atorvastatin acid is mainly metabolized in liver by CYP3A4 displays a relatively low passive diffusion clearance (PS_{dif}) into the hepatocytes of 0.017 ml min^{-1} per million cells (CLpd). Due to the low PS_{dif}, the plasma concentration was highly governed by the OATP1B1 transporter activity.

Drug concentration in muscle was highly affected by altering the transporter activity. At a K_m of 0.4 μM and a V_{max} of 400 pmol min^{-1} per million hepatocytes $cells^{-1}$, there was an eightfold difference in the muscle concentration when altering the transporter activity related to the OATP1B1 polymorphism (**Figure 6**). The difference in liver concentration of drug caused by altered transporter activity was less significant when compared with muscle tissue concentration. As atorvastatin acid is metabolized by CYP3A4, an increase in active hepatic drug uptake will be counteracted in the liver by an increase in metabolic clearance, maintaining similar exposure in the liver (**Figure 6**).

Pravastatin

Pravastatin displays a PS_{dif} of 0.397 ml min^{-1} per million cells. The simulated exposure of pravastatin in muscle and liver was higher as compared to plasma. Simulations utilizing parameters reported in literature showed that genotype variation had a reduced impact on the exposure in plasma, liver, and muscle as compared to atorvastatin acid. These findings were similar to the results presented by Kusuhara and Sugiyama, simulating an increase in plasma concentration with a reduced transporter activity whereas drug concentration in plasma was increased and the changes in liver were less significant (**Figure 7**).

Simvastatin

Simvastatin displays a high passive diffusion rate of approximately 74 ml min^{-1} per million hepatocytes cells and the distribution of simvastatin to the liver can therefore be considered perfusion limited. For this reason, the exposure of simvastatin was not affected by altered OATP1B1 transporter activity. Although being highly distributed to the muscle, muscular toxicity is more likely to occur (**Figure 8**).

Conclusion

Using the transporter OATP1B1 and statins as examples, it has been shown how genotypic transporter polymorphism can alter the drug concentration in plasma, liver and muscle to varying extents depending on the PK properties of the substrate. Therefore, there is no simple algorithm for estimating the effect of transporter polymorphism on toxicokinetics, thus forming/providing a compelling argument for the use of PBPK modelling to assess toxicity as a result of transporter polymorphism and simulation in toxicokinetics of polymorphic transporter activity. In conclusion, it was demonstrated that membrane transporter polymorphism can contribute to variability in toxicological effects.

In vitro assays and IVIVE coupled with PBPK modeling and simulation can provide high-throughput, cost-efficient methods for predicting toxicokinetics of xenobiotics in man and have the potential of replacing many animal toxicity studies. *In silico* methods may further be in a better position in predicting active transport effects on the disposition of xenobiotics and their toxicity as compared to current animal models due to observed interspecies variability in abundance and activity of transporters, where accurately predicting the local tissue concentrations may be key to understanding transporter driven toxicity.

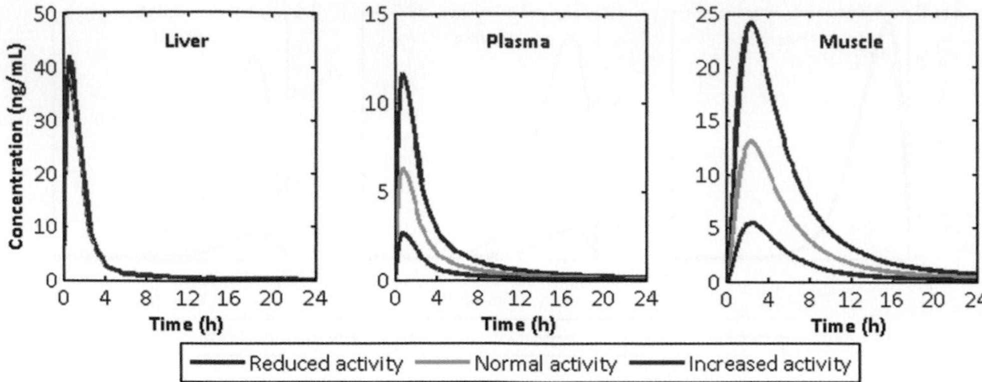

Figure 7 Simulated pravastatin immediate release 20 mg concentration (ng ml^{-1}) time profiles in liver (unbound intracellular concentration), plasma, and muscle tissue at a of K_m 0.4 μM and a V_{max} of 400 pmol min^{-1} million cells^{-1}.

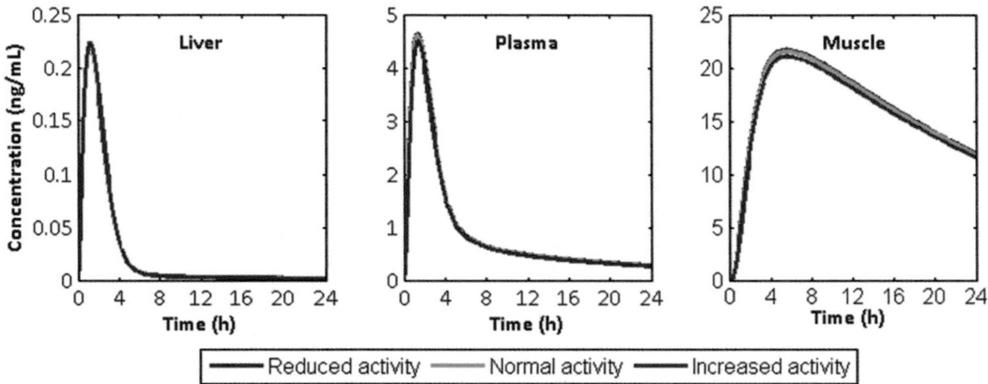

Figure 8 Simulated simvastatin immediate release 40 mg concentration (ng ml^{-1}) time profiles in liver (unbound intracellular concentration), plasma, and muscle tissue at a K_m of 0.4 μM and a V_{max} of 400 pmol min^{-1} million cells^{-1}.

Acknowledgments

The authors wish to thank Dr Sibylle Neuhoff, Simcyp Ltd., Sheffield, for critical review of this article, and Mr James Kay, Simcyp Ltd., Sheffield for his assistance in preparation of the article.

Further Reading

Andersen, M.E., Clewell, H.J., Carmichael, P.L., Boekelheide, K., 2011. Can case study approaches speed implementation of the NRC report: 'toxicity testing in the 21st century: a vision and a strategy?'. ALTEX 28, 175–182.

Dickinson, G.L., Rostami-Hodjegan, A., 2008. Building virtual human populations: assessing the propagation of genetic variability in drug metabolism to pharmacokinetics and pharmacodynamics. In: Bertau, M., Mosekilde, E., Westerhoff, H.V. (Eds.), Biosimulation in Drug Development, first ed. Wiley, Weinheim, Germany, pp. 425–446.

Giacomini, K.M., Sugiyama, Y., 2005. Membrane transporters and drug response. In: Brunton, L.L., Lazo, J.S., Parker, K.L. (Eds.), Goodman & Gillman's: The Pharmacological Basis of Therapeutics, eleventh ed. McGraw-Hill, Columbus, OH, pp. 41–70.

Gui, C., Hagenbuch, B., 2009. Role of transmembrane domain 10 for the function of organic anion transporting polypeptide 1B1. Prot. Sci. 18, 2298–2306.

Jamei, M., Dickinson, G.L., Rostami-Hodjegan, A., 2009. A framework for assessing inter-individual variability in pharmacokinetics using virtual human populations and integrating general knowledge of physical chemistry, biology, anatomy, physiology and genetics: a tale of 'bottom-up' vs 'top-down' recognition of covariates. Drug Metab. Pharmacokinet. 24, 53–75.

Kusuhara, H., Sugiyama, Y., 2009. In vitro-in vivo extrapolation of transporter-mediated clearance in the liver and kidney. Drug Metab. Pharmacokinet. 24, 37–52.

Niemi, M., 2007. Role of OATP transporters in the disposition of drugs. Pharmacogenomics 8, 787–802.

Niemi, M., 2009. Transporter pharmacogenetics and statin toxicity. Clin. Pharmacol. Ther. 87, 130–133.

Pasanen, M.K., Neuvonen, P.J., Niemi, M., 2008. Global analysis of genetic variation in SLCO1B1. Pharmacogenomics 9, 19–33.

Poulin, P., Theil, F.P., 2002a. Prediction of pharmacokinetics prior to in vivo studies. 1. Mechanism-based prediction of volume of distribution. J. Pharm. Sci. 91, 129–156.

Poulin, P., Theil, F.P., 2002b. Prediction of pharmacokinetics prior to in vivo studies. II. Generic physiologically based pharmacokinetic models of drug disposition. J. Pharm. Sci. 91, 1358–1370.

Rodgers, T., Rowland, M., 2007. Mechanistic approaches to volume of distribution predictions: understanding the processes. Pharm. Res. 24, 918–933.

Rostami-Hodjegan, A., 2012. Physiologically based pharmacokinetics joined with in vitro-in vivo extrapolation of ADME: a marriage under the arch of systems pharmacology. Clin. Pharmacol. Ther 92 (1), 50–61.

Shiran, M.R., Proctor, N.J., Howgate, E.M., et al., 2006. Prediction of metabolic drug clearance in humans: in vitro-in vivo extrapolation vs allometric scaling. Xenobiotica 36, 567–580.

van de Waterbeemd, H., Gifford, E., 2003. ADMET in silico modelling: towards prediction paradise? Nat. Rev. Drug Discov. 2, 192–204.

Watanabe, T., Kusuhara, H., Maeda, K., Shitara, Y., Sugiyama, Y., 2009. Physiologically based pharmacokinetic modeling to predict transporter-mediated clearance and distribution of pravastatin in humans. J. Pharmacol. Exp. Ther. 328, 652–662.

Adverse Outcome Pathways: Development and Use in Toxicology

C Willett, The Humane Society of the United States, Gaithersburg, MD, USA

Introduction

Several decades' worth of experience in characterizing chemical toxicity has led to the realization that a new approach is warranted. Such factors as the large number of relatively uncharacterized chemicals that are already in the environment, the need to generate information for extensive regulatory programs such as the European Union's Registration, Evaluation, Authorization and Restriction of Chemical substances (REACH) program, the high cost and slow pace of animal experimentation, and the need to improve the certainty of safety decisions have made it necessary to rethink the traditional approach to hazard and risk assessment, which has generally relied on an extensive array of empirical animal test data. At the same time, advances in biological understanding as well as experimental technologies (e.g., 'omics' tools, stem cell culturing, reconstructed tissues) have allowed the contemplation of dramatically different approaches to understanding disease and toxicology than those traditionally practiced. One such approach couples existing knowledge of normal biology with new chemical and biological information about the consequences of disturbing that biology, leading to a structured, transparent, and hypothesis-based approach to predicting adverse outcomes resulting from those perturbations. This general approach has been variously termed mode-of-action (MoA), toxicity pathway, and adverse outcome pathway (AOP) approaches.

The idea of incorporating mechanistic biochemical information into toxicological assessment is not new; it began with dose–response modeling efforts and MoA frameworks, such as those developed by the International Program on Chemical Safety (IPCS) to determine the human relevance of modes of action of pesticides and industrial chemicals leading to carcinogenicity (and later non-carcinogenic toxicity), and the creation of MoA pathways commonly used in drug development and applied to human disease. The notion of toxicity pathways as articulated by the National Research Council in 2007 in its report, "Toxicity Testing for the 21st Century: a vision and a Strategy", takes this concept a bit further by envisioning a system-wide network of pathways that leads to a predictive, hypothesis-driven assessment paradigm for toxicity in general. The goals of this new approach are to improve efficiency and decrease uncertainty in risk and hazard evaluations. Recently, this concept has been further formalized for toxicological assessment for both human health and ecological endpoints as the AOP and has been taken up by the Test Guidelines Program at the Organization for Economic Cooperation and Development (OECD) as an organizing principle for all test guidelines.

The AOP approach is based on the concept that toxicity results from the chemical exposure and molecular interaction with a biomolecule (e.g., a protein, receptor) – the molecular initiating event (MIE) – followed by a sequential progression of intermediate events through to the eventual toxicological effect or 'adverse outcome' (AO), which is at the individual level for most human health endpoints or at the population level for environmental endpoints (**Figure 1**). The AOP framework codifies this process and allows for the integration of all types of information at different levels of biological organization, from molecular to population level, to provide a rational, biologically based argument (or series of hypotheses) to predict the outcome of an initiating event.

The usefulness of the AOP concept in building a predictive toxicological framework manifests in several ways. In the near term, AOPs can inform chemical grouping or categories and structure–activity relationships, they can aid in increasing certainty of interpretation of both existing and new information, and they can be used to structure integrated testing strategies that maximize useful information gained from

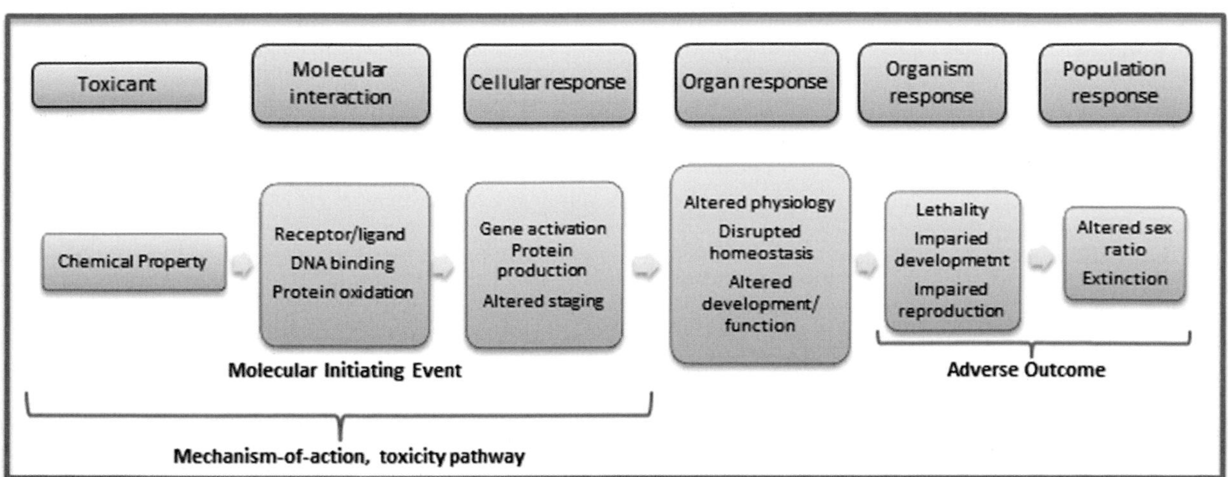

Figure 1 An adverse outcome pathway is a biological map from the molecular initiating event (MIE) through the resulting adverse outcome (AO) that describes both mechanism- and mode-of-action.

 http://dx.doi.org/10.1016/B978-0-12-386454-3.01244-6

minimal testing. In the longer term, AOPs can be used to identify key events for which nonanimal tests can be developed, thereby facilitating transparent, mechanism-based, predictive toxicological assessments with low uncertainty and high human relevance, ultimately without the involvement of animal testing.

Development of an Adverse Outcome Pathway: Where to Begin?

According to the OECD Guidance, an AOP consists of three main elements: one molecular initiating event, one adverse outcome, and any number of intermediate events. While in reality biological processes are actually an interrelated network of multiple processes and an MIE can be associated with a number of AOs (similarly an adverse effect can result from a number of different MIEs), to streamline the development and use of AOPs, OECD has defined an AOP as being a linear pathway from one MIE to one AO. Description of an AOP can begin from any location along the pathway: where you start will depend on the initiator's perspective or expertise. For example, a chemist will likely begin with the MIE and focus on the early part of the pathway, with the likely goal of improving chemical categorization; a bioinformaticist would likely begin in the middle, with a series of gene or protein expression associations or 'fingerprints,' and link outward to either the associated MIE or AO; and a pathologist would begin with an AO and work 'upstream' to link to the causes.

Regardless of how or where the pathway description is initiated, there are a series of questions that should be answered during the pathway characterization, including: How dependable is the information that was used to deduce each step? How well supported are each of the associations between events along the pathway? How complete is the pathway? How many other MIEs or AOs are alternative possibilities surrounding this particular pathway? A full description of an MIE should also include cellular/tissue location – as immediately elicited intermediate events may be similar in two different AOPs but differ in cell type or tissue location (e.g., metabolic transformation of a chemical to an electrophilic species may elicit an MIE for both skin sensitization and liver fibrosis – only in keratinocytes for the former and hepatocytes for the latter). The OECD guidance provides a template and describes the process for evaluating weight-of-evidence for each step in development of an AOP. Similar to the IPCS MoA frameworks, the OECD Guidance suggests evaluating the strength of qualitative and quantitative understanding of each step in the pathway using the using the Bradford-Hill criteria, which assess the strength of association, consistency of the evidence, specificity of the relationship, consistency of temporal relationships and dose–response relationships, biological plausibility, coherence of the evidence, and consideration of alternative explanations.

The European Commission Joint Research Council SEURAT (Safety Evaluation Ultimately Replacing Animal Testing) project has initiated a project to develop two liver toxicity AOPs following the OECD guidance, one for protein alkylation-induced fibrosis and another for liver X receptor activation-induced steatosis.

Two Case Examples of AOPs in Development and Use

Skin Sensitization

Skin sensitization is a relatively simple biological process, yet it involves several cell types and tissues and is a good demonstration of AOP development and use in constructing an integrated testing strategy (**Figure 2**). Sensitization occurs in two phases: the first, the induction phase, is a result of initial contact with an allergen and primes the system; the second, the elicitation phase, is in response to a subsequent exposure and results in an allergic response. As with the local lymph node assay, the sensitization AOP focuses on the induction phase.

The induction phase involves initial contact and penetration of the outer dermis of the skin by a potential sensitizer. Metabolism in the skin can either activate or deactivate the chemical (or have no effect); chemicals that are electrophilic after penetrating the skin are more potent sensitizers than non-electrophiles. The electrophile then interacts irreversibly with nucleophilic sites in proteins (e.g., cysteine and lysine residues) to form a hapten–protein complex in the epidermis – this is the sensitization MIE. In both dendritic cells (antigen-processing cells in the skin) and keratinocytes (the predominant epidermal skin cells), the presence of a hapten–protein complex elicits the production of cytokines that in turn stimulate dendritic cells to migrate to regional lymph nodes and activate T cells there. In the lymph node, hapten–protein fragments are presented in complex with major histocompatibility complex (MHC) molecules by dendritic cells to immature T cells, causing the maturation of memory T cells and the acquisition of sensitivity – this is the key physiologic response of the initiation phase.

The sensitization AOP can be used to design (or organize) an integrated assessment strategy that includes non-test (e.g., quantitative structure activity relationships (QSARs)), in *in vitro* and *in vivo* test results. Such assessment strategies are being developed by a number of research groups.

Estrogen Receptor–Mediated Reproductive Toxicity

Chemicals that bind the estrogen receptor (ER) can either mimic or block estrogenic activity (act as agonists, or antagonists, respectively) by changing expression levels of ER-responsive genes. Subsequent changes in ER-responsive protein levels result in changes at the tissue level (e.g., reproductive organs) and eventually can affect reproductive behavior and capacity (**Figure 3**). In this AOP description (based on measurements in rainbow trout with elements that are generalizable to all vertebrates), the MIE is chemical binding to the estrogen receptor, the first key event is change in gene expression and protein production (measured via ER-responsive reporters *in vitro* or endogenous genes *ex vivo*), a subsequent key event is histopathological changes (e.g., reduced testicular growth, appearance of ova in testes of fish) followed by observation of altered reproductive behavior and sex reversal at the individual level, and finally skewed sex ratios and decreased numbers at the population level.

This AOP provides a biological hypothesis framework for an integrated testing strategy that involves QSAR prediction and measurement of ER binding, measurement of ER transcriptional activity in cells and excised (liver) tissue, histology of

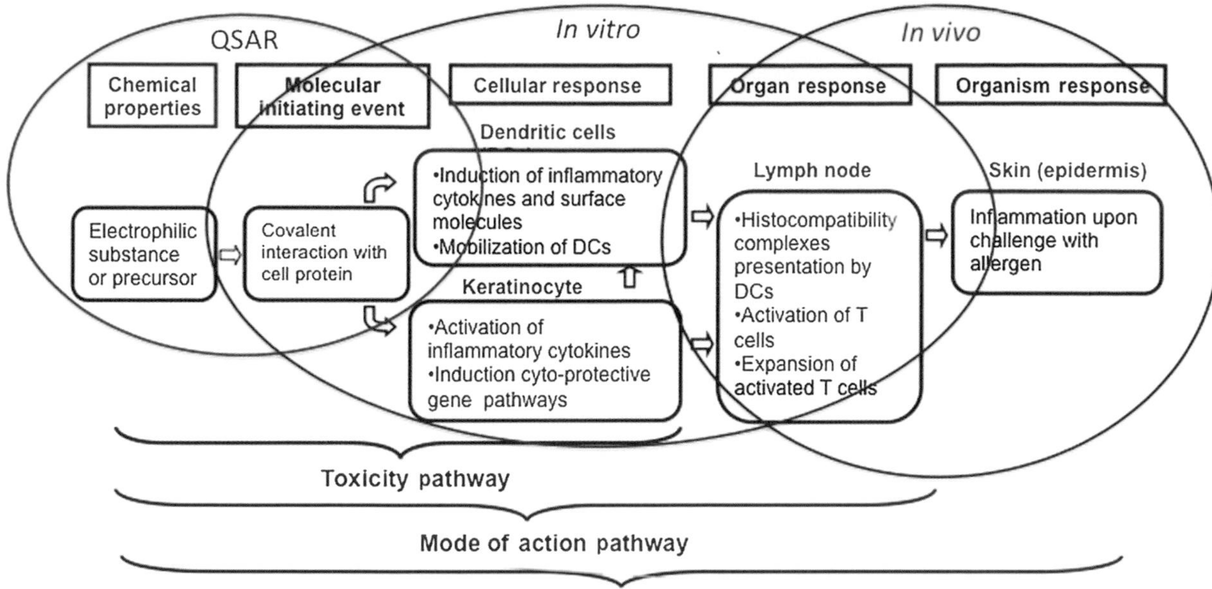

Figure 2 AOP for skin sensitization. Delineated below the diagram are the pathway subtypes: Toxicity pathway as defined by the 2007 National Research Council report, mode-of-action pathway as discussed in the World Health Organization/IPCS guidance, and adverse outcome pathway as defined by Ankley et al., 2010. The types of tests that can currently be used to assess different steps in the pathway are indicated by colored circles. After: Organization for Economic Cooperation and Development (OECD), 2012. The Adverse Outcome Pathway for Skin Sensitization Initiated by Covalent Binding to Proteins, Part 1: Scientific Evidence. Series on Testing and Assessment, No.168.

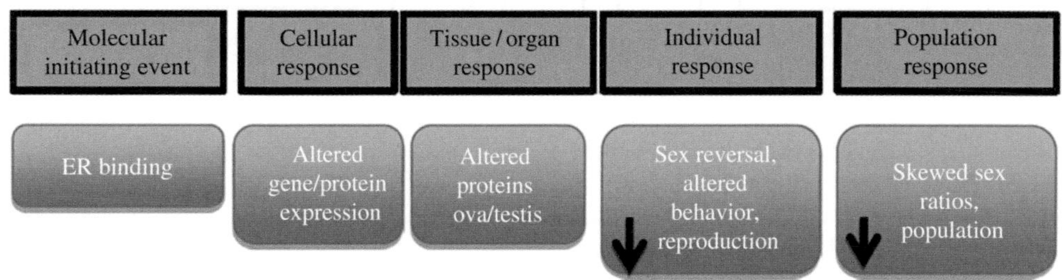

Figure 3 Outline of AOP for estrogen receptor–mediated reproductive toxicity. After: Organization for Economic Cooperation and Development (OECD), 2011. Report of the Workshop on Using Mechanistic Information on Forming Chemical Categories ENV/JM/MONO(2011)8. May 18, 2011. 176 pp.

sexual organs, and measurement of sexual behavior and fecundity.

Using AOPs: How Certain Do You Need to Be?

AOPs have a number of potential uses, including – in the near term – informing chemical categories and structure activity relationships, increasing certainty of interpretation of both existing and new information, and designing integrated testing strategies. The AOPs currently under development differ in detail and complexity and are yet incomplete; nevertheless, they all have utility to improve the hazard and risk assessment process. The level of certainty and completion necessary depends on the intended use of the AOP (**Figure 4**). For example, to use an AOP for building QSARs of MIEs, there must be some solid evidence that the MIE is linked to the AO of interest, but the main focus of certainty would be the chemical and molecular characterization of the MIE itself. To use an AOP for hazard identification or prioritization of chemicals for further testing, strong evidence of the MIE–AO linkage is required, along with substantiation of one or more intermediate events.

Once a number of pathways have been described in sufficient detail, it will also be possible to use them to identifying key events for which tests can be developed; the tests would necessarily address a number of critical steps, thereby ensuring that all possible outcomes are adequately covered. As quantitative information is added to relationships between intermediate events, early events in an AOP can be used directly for risk assessment, without the need to assess the later steps pathway. At this stage, chemical assessment will be streamlined and toxicology transformed from a purely empirical to a predictive science.

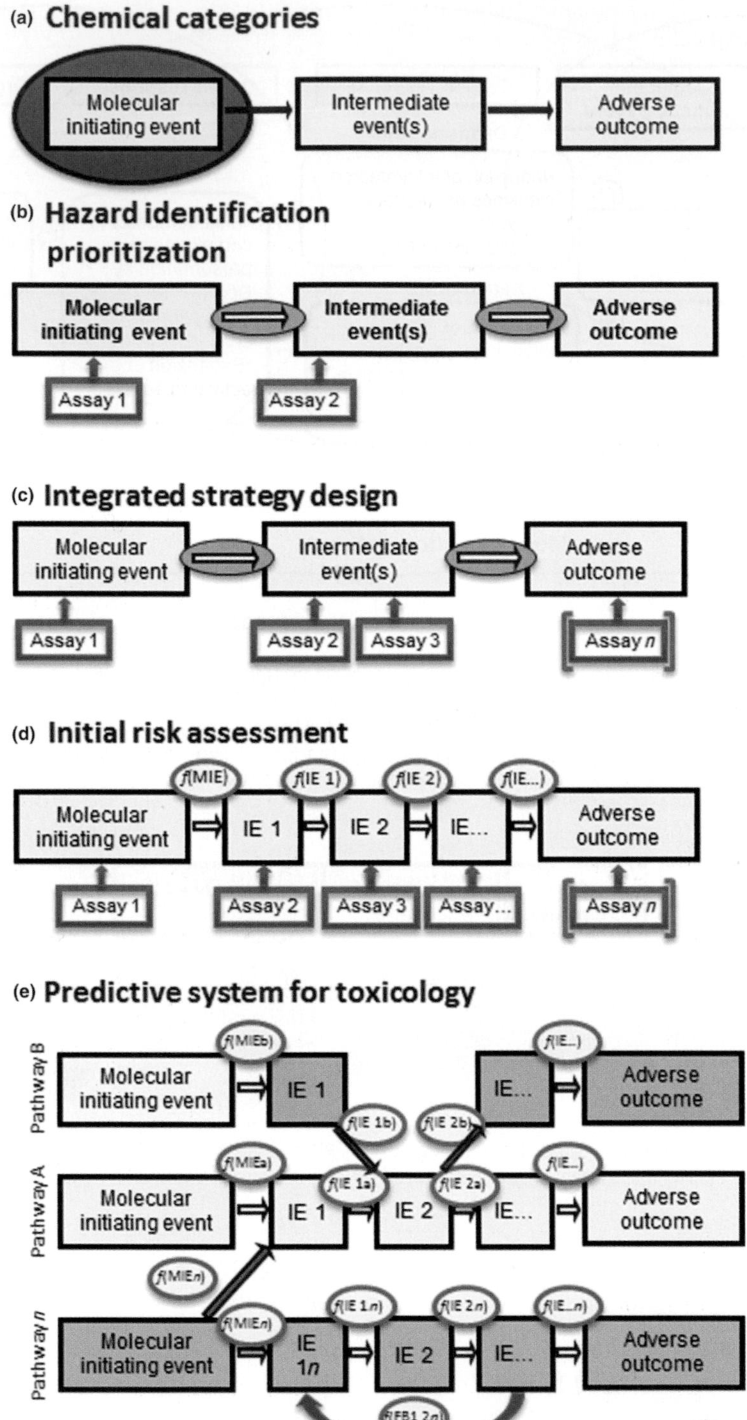

Figure 4 Different uses require different information and levels of certainty. Blue ovals indicate areas of focus; white ovals indicate quantitative relationships.

The Future of AOP Development and Use

A concerted and coordinated effort is required to develop consistent approaches to the development and use of AOPs, along with the necessary databases to support this development. In order to evaluate the relevance, reliability, and robustness of an AOP, it is especially critical to evaluate the empirical and logical premises for the AOP in a transparent way. Toward these goals, the OECD has recently agreed to integrate the AOP approach into the test guidelines program and is currently developing guidance for the development and use of AOPs. This initial guidance to ensure that each AOP is assessed with respect to (1) the qualitative understanding of the AOP, including the concordance of dose–response and temporal relationships among key events; (2) the quality and strength of experimental evidence supporting the AOP, including biological plausibility, coherence, and consistency of the evidence; and finally (3) the quantitative understanding of linkages within the AOP. It is important also to consider the uncertainties, inconsistencies and data gaps in the supporting evidence. The goals of OECD's guidance are to provide consistency in structure and facilitate harmonized use of AOPs.

It is also critical to create a unified knowledge base for AOPs and their supporting evidence, integrating information from all scientific sectors, including toxicology, drug development, disease, medicine, and research. Currently, the Joint Research Council, World Health Organization, and the US Environmental Protection Agency are collaborating to create a series of three databases: an MoA knowledge base to house textual pathway descriptions, a database to house graphical representations, and a database to house *in vitro* results that inform intermediate effects which would serve as building blocks for pathway development.

A publically accessible, harmonized knowledge base that describes AOPs based on integrated toxicological and disease pathway information will allow greatly improved assessment strategy design. Assessment strategies based on transparent, hypothesis-driven evaluation of key steps along an AOP will provide improved predictively (for both human and environmental health) and with greater confidence than current approaches based largely on empirical data from a standard array of animal tests.

See also: High Throughput Screening; *In Vitro–In Vivo* Extrapolation; The Hamner Institutes for Health Sciences; Mechanisms of Toxicity; Biomarkers, Human Health; Mode of Action; Organization for Economic Cooperation and Development; Toxicity Testing, 'Read Across Analysis'; Toxicity Testing in the 21st Century: Approaches to Implementation; Toxicity Testing, Alternatives; QSAR; Environmental Biomarkers; Systems Biology Application in Toxicology; Virtual Models (vM); Evidence-Based Toxicology.

Further Reading

Ankley, G.T., Bennett, R.S., Erickson, R.J., et al., 2010. Adverse outcome pathways: a conceptual framework to support ecotoxicology research and risk assessment. Environ. Toxicol. Chem. 29 (3), 730–741.

Boobis, A.R., Doe, J.E., Heinrich-Hirsch, B., et al., 2008. IPCS framework for analyzing the relevance of a noncancer mode of action for humans. Crit. Rev. Toxicol. 38 (2), 87–96.

Bradbury, S.P., Feijtel, T.C., Van Leeuwen, C.J., 2004. Meeting the scientific needs of ecological risk assessment in a regulatory context. Environ. Sci. Technol. 38, 463A–470A.

Landesman, B., Goumenou, M., Munn, S., et al., 2012. Description of Prototype Modes-of-Action Related to Repeated Dose Toxicity. European Commission, Joint Research Council, Institute for Health and Consumer Protection, Ispra, Italy.

National Research Council, 2007. Toxicity Testing in the 21st Century: A Vision and a Strategy. National Academy of Sciences, Washington, DC.

Organization for Economic Cooperation and Development (OECD), 2011. Report of the Workshop on Using Mechanistic Information on Forming Chemical Categories ENV/JM/MONO(2011)8. May 18, 2011. 176 pp.

Organization of Economic Cooperation and Development (OECD), 2012. The Adverse Outcome Pathway for Skin Sensitization Initiated by Covalent Binding to Proteins, Part 1: Scientific Evidence. Series on Testing and Assessment, No.168.

Organization for Economic Cooperation and Development (OECD), 2013. Guidance Document on Developing and Assessing Adverse Outcome Pathways. Series on Testing and Assessment No. 184.

Schultz, T.W., Diderich, B., Enoch, S., 2011. The OECD Adverse Outcome Pathway Approach. AXLR8–2 Workshop and Progress Report: Alternative Testing Strategies. DG Research and Innovation and AXLR8 Administration, Free University of Berlin, Berlin.

US Environmental Protection Agency, 2006. Presentation to the 39th Joint Meeting of the Chemicals Committee and the Working Party on Chemicals: Experiences Using Integrated Approaches to Fulfil Information Requirements for Testing and Assessment. http://www.oecd.org/env/chemicalsafetyandbiosafety/36286164.pdf (accessed 30.08.12.).

Relevant Websites

http://alttox.org – AltTox, A Comprehensive Resource for Technical and Policy Information on the Development and Use of Alternative Methods.

http://www.seurat-1.eu – European Commission Joint Research Council's SEURAT project.

http://www.thehamner.org/institutes-centers/institute-for-chemical-safety-sciences/toxicity-testing-in-the-21st-century – Hamner Institutes, Institute for Chemical Safety Sciences Toxicity Testing for the 21st Century project.

www.HumanToxicologyProject.org – Human Toxicology Project Consortium.

http://caat.jhsph.edu – Johns Hopkins School for Public Health Center for Alternatives to Animal Testing.

http://search.oecd.org/officialdocuments/displaydocumentpdf/?cote=env/jm/mono(2013)6&doclanguage=en – OECD Guidance on Document on Developing and Assessing Adverse Outcome Pathways.

http://epa.gov/ncct/Tox21 – US EPA Tox21 program.

http://www.epa.gov/ncct/toxcast – US EPA ToxCast program.

Aerosols

WE Achanzar and RS Mangipudy, Bristol-Myers Squibb Co., Drug Safety Evaluation, New Brunswick, NJ, USA

This article is a revision of the previous edition article by Raja S. Mangipudy, volume 1, p 51, © 2005, Elsevier Inc.

- Chemical Abstracts Service Registry Number: N/A
- Synonyms: N/A
- Chemical/Pharmaceutical/Other Class: Aerosols are systems ranging from those of colloidal nature to systems consisting of 'therapeutic packages.' Aerosols are classified as follows:
  - Liquified-gas systems
    - Two-phase: space-spray; surface-coating; dispersion or suspension
    - Three-phase: two-layer; foam; stabilized; quick-breaking
  - Compressed-gas systems
    - Solid-stream dispensing
    - Foam dispensing
    - Spray dispensing
  - Separation of propellant from concentrate systems
    - Piston type
    - Flexible type
    - Atomizer type
    - Mechanical systems
    - Latex diaphragm
- Chemical Structure: N/A

Background

An aerosol is an assembly of particles suspended in the air for a period of time sufficient to allow inhalation or measurement. A large number of agents such as therapeutic compounds, personal hygiene products, pesticides, cleaning agents, lubricants, adhesives, and chemical and biological weapons are intentionally formulated as aerosols to which human exposure can occur either intentionally or accidentally. In addition, many chemicals can be unintentionally dispersed as aerosols under certain conditions such as industrial accidents.

Environmental Fate and Behavior

The environmental fate will be dependent on the specific components of an aerosol.

Exposure and Exposure Monitoring

Human exposure to aerosols primarily occurs via contact with the skin, eyes, or respiratory tract. General exposure monitoring for aerosols entails air sampling to determine the concentration of aerosol components. Depending on the specific compounds involved, biologic monitoring in blood or urine to assess human or animal exposure can be performed.

Numerous common medications with toxic potential are routinely delivered as aerosols. A few of them are listed below:

1. Short-acting bronchodilators (albuterol, pirbuterol, ipratropium)
2. Long-acting bronchodilators (salmeterol, formoterol, tiotropium)
3. Corticosteroids (beclomethasone, triamcinolone, fluticasone, mometasone)
4. Miscellaneous other compounds (cromolyn, acetylcysteine, tobramycin)

Toxicokinetics

Aerosol components can be absorbed primarily via the inhalation or dermal routes, although ingestion can occur if the aerosol contaminates foods or drinks. Inhalation exposure can be affected by factors such as respiratory tract geometry and aerosol properties. Dermal exposure will be affected by skin permeability of the substances. The specific toxicokinetic properties (absorption, excretion, metabolism, half-life) will be dependent on the nature of the aerosol components.

Mechanism of Toxicity

The specific mechanism of toxicity will depend on the nature of the aerosol and the route of exposure. Examples include lung surfactant destruction following inhalation of nonstick cooking spray and bronchoconstriction following trichlorofluoromethane exposure. In some cases, pulmonary toxicity may not result from a specific chemical mechanism but rather from physical perturbation of the lung and a subsequent immunologic response. Dermal toxicity often results from physical damage to the skin or eyes due to the corrosive nature of the aerosol or by eliciting an immune response due to irritation.

Acute and Short-Term Toxicity

Animal

Acute toxicity of a large number of aerosolized compounds has been demonstrated in animals. Effects observed with various compounds include respiratory distress, adverse clinical symptoms, and death. The specific effects are dependent on the aerosol components evaluated.

Human

The following pertains to the general evaluation and treatment of individuals exposed to potentially toxic chemicals via aerosols.

- Exposed individuals should have a careful, thorough medical history and physical examination performed,

 http://dx.doi.org/10.1016/B978-0-12-386454-3.00223-2

looking for any abnormalities. Exposure to chemicals with a strong odor often results in such nonspecific symptoms as headache, dizziness, weakness, and nausea.
- Many chemicals cause irritation of the eyes, skin, and respiratory tract. In severe cases respiratory tract irritation can progress to acute respiratory distress syndrome/acute lung injury, the onset of which can be delayed for up to 24–72 h in some cases.
- Irritation or burns of the esophagus or gastrointestinal tract are also possible if caustic or irritant chemicals are ingested.

The specific components of an aerosol will determine the toxic effects.

Chronic Toxicity

Animal

The chronic effects of aerosol exposure in animals vary greatly depending on the specific aerosol being evaluated. Toxicities observed with various aerosolized compounds include clinical effects, respiratory perturbations, and tumor development.

Human

Chronic effects of aerosol exposure will be determined by the specific components of the aerosol. As an example, there is a well-established relationship between exposure to aerosols and chronic lung diseases such as emphysema, asthma, and lung cancer.

Immunotoxicity

A number of chemical agents produce an allergic hypersensitivity dermatitis or asthma with bronchospasm and wheezing with chronic exposure. The potential for immunotoxicity will depend on the specific aerosol components.

Reproductive Toxicity

The potential for reproductive toxicity will depend on the specific aerosol components.

Genotoxicity

A number of chemicals that humans can be exposed to via aerosols are genotoxic, such as components of fly ash and cigarette smoke. The potential for genotoxicity will depend on the specific aerosol components.

Carcinogenicity

A number of chemicals that humans can be exposed to via aerosols are carcinogenic, such as components of fly ash and cigarette smoke. The potential for carcinogenicity will depend on the specific aerosol components.

Clinical Management

1. Supportive care must be instituted for patients accidentally exposed to aerosol contents via topical, inhalation, or oral routes. A number of chemicals produce abnormalities of the hematopoietic system, liver, and kidneys. Monitoring complete blood count, urinalysis, and liver and kidney function tests is suggested for patients with significant exposure.
2. If respiratory tract irritation or respiratory depression is evident, monitor arterial blood gases, chest X-ray, and pulmonary function tests.
3. Additional measures may need to be taken to address the toxic effects of specific aerosol components.

Ecotoxicology

A number of aerosolized compounds and components such as pesticides and chlorofluorocarbon propellants are known to be harmful to ecologic systems. The potential for ecologic toxicity will depend on the specific aerosol components.

Other Hazards

Aside from potential toxic effects, many aerosols are flammable and/or explosive. Aerosols for consumer use also have inhalant abuse potential (known as 'sniffing' or 'huffing').

Exposure Standards and Guidelines

Exposure standards vary based on the specific aerosol components.

See also: Coal Tar; Occupational Toxicology; Anthrax; Occupational Safety and Health Administration; Respiratory Tract Toxicology; Pollution, Air in Encyclopedia of Toxicology; Recommended Exposure Limits; Carcinogenesis; Sulfur Mustard; Nonlethal Weapons; Skin; V-Series Nerve Agents: Other than VX; VX; Chemical Warfare; Asbestos; Pesticides.

Further Reading

Belej, M.A., Aviado, D.M., 1975. Cardiopulmonary toxicity of propellants for aerosols. J. Clin. Pharmacol. 15, 105–115.
Dolovich, M.B., Dhand, R., 2011. Aerosol drug delivery: developments in device design and clinical use. Lancet 377 (9770), 1032–1045.
National Research Council (U.S.), 2007. Acute Exposure Guideline Levels for Selected Airborne Chemicals, vol. 5. The National Academies Press, Washington, DC.
Sosnowski, T.R., 2011. Importance of airway geometry and respiratory parameters variability for particle deposition in the human respiratory tract. J. Thorac. Dis. 3, 153–155.

Relevant Websites

http://www.epa.gov/ebtpages/airairpollutantsaerosols.html
http://www.aphis.usda.gov; search for "Aerosol" or specific components
http://www.osha.gov/; search for "Aerosol" or specific components
http://www.cdc.gov/niosh/topics/aerosols/pdfs/aerosol_101.pdf
http://www.cdc.gov/niosh/topics/aerosols/pdfs/ACGreport.pdf NIOSH Aerosol Program Assessment Committee Report
http://www.aarc.org/education/aerosol_devices/aerosol_delivery_guide.pdf
http://www.yourlunghealth.org/healthy_living/aerosol/Patient_aerosol_guide.pdf

A-esterase

LG Sultatos, New Jersey Medical School, University of Medicine and Dentistry of New Jersey, Newark, NJ, USA

The phosphorothioate insecticides are a subclass of the organophosphorus insecticides that have been and continue to be used worldwide. Organophosphorus insecticides exert their primary acute toxicity by inhibition of the important enzyme acetylcholinesterase. Interestingly, the phosphorothioates have little capacity to inhibit acetylcholinesterase, but are converted primarily by the liver to potent acetylcholinesterase inhibitors called oxygen analogs or oxons, such as paraoxon (CAS#311-45-5) (**Figure 1**), which are responsible for the cholinergic crisis observed following exposure to phosphorothioate insecticides. Once the oxons have been produced from the parent insecticides, one of the ways in which these highly toxic compounds can be detoxified is through metabolism by enzymes termed A-esterase(s) (**Figure 1**). The term A-esterase originated from researchers over 50 years ago, and was used to refer to enzymes in serum that metabolized carboxylic esters but were insensitive to inhibition by oxons (in contrast to B-esterases are inhibited by oxons). Later this enzyme was shown to detoxify paraoxon in several different species (**Figure 1**), leading to the use of the term A-esterase to refer to enzymes that hydrolyze oxons of phosphorothioate insecticides. Oxons reported to be broken down by A-esterases include paraoxon, methyl paraoxon (CAS#950-35-6), chlorpyrifos oxon (CAS#5598-15-2), methyl chlorpyrifos oxon (CAS#950-35-6), pirimophos methyl oxon (CAS#64709-45-1), and diazoxon (CAS#962-58-3), as well as the organophosphate insecticide dichlorvos (CAS#62-73-7) and the nerve gases sarin (CAS#107-44-8) and soman (CAS#96-64-0). Additionally, the former drug diisopropylflurophosphate (CAS#55-91-4) has been reported to be broken down by A-esterase.

Since the original discovery of A-esterases, many different names have been used for this family of enzymes, including paraoxonase, aryl-ester hydrolase, arylesterase, organophosphate hydrolase, organophosphorus compound hydrolase, and organophosphorus acid anhydrolase. Currently, the most common name for these enzymes is 'paraoxonases,' which has largely replaced the term 'A-esterases.' The name paraoxonase originally described the calcium-dependent hydrolysis of

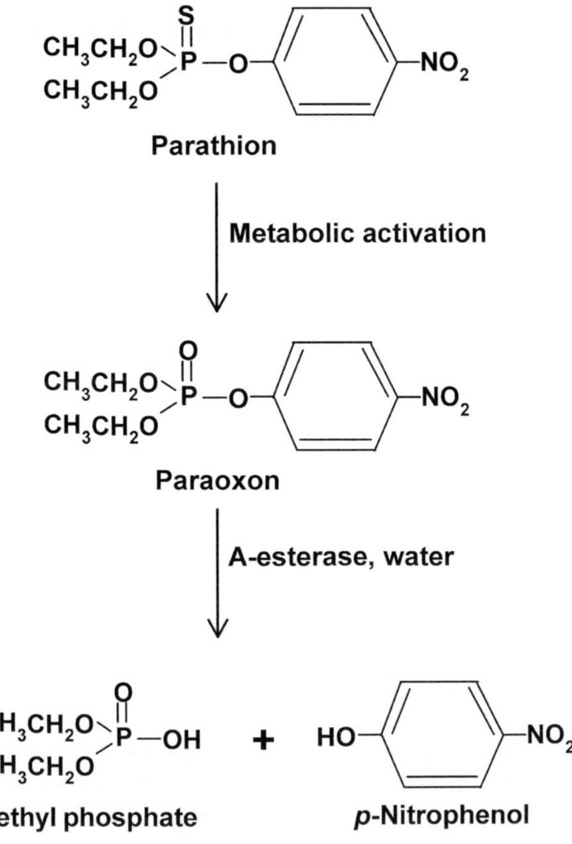

Figure 1 The production of paraoxon (CAS#311-45-5) from parathion (CAS#56-38-2), followed by the detoxification of paraoxon by paraoxonase (A-esterase). It should be noted that parathion is no longer used as an insecticide. The four insecticides that produce oxons that are broken down by paraoxonase (methyl parathion (CAS#298-00-0), chlorpyrifos (CAS#2921-88-2), pirimiphos methyl (CAS#29232-93-7), and diazinon (CAS#333-41-5)) undergo reactions similar to that depicted in this figure.

 http://dx.doi.org/10.1016/B978-0-12-386454-3.00092-0

paraoxon (**Figure 1**) by these enzymes, and paraoxon has been probably the most commonly used substrate to assess activity. More recently, researchers have reported that paraoxon is not a very good substrate, while a variety of lactones are robustly metabolized, prompting the suggestion that paraoxonases should be viewed as lactonases.

In humans, there are three paraoxonases, termed PON1, PON2, and PON3 (all of which have lactonase activity). PON1 has been studied the most, and it is the form that breaks down oxons. While PON1 is synthesized primarily by the liver and is released into the blood where it is associated with high-density lipoproteins, PON1 is widely distributed in many tissues, as evidenced by immunohistochemical studies. Conversely, PON1 mRNA appears to be found only in liver, kidney, and colon, thereby warranting the suggestion that PON1 is delivered to various tissues by high-density lipoproteins.

PON1 activity in human plasma and serum changes as a function of age. Interestingly, studies have shown that preterm babies have lower PON1 activity than term babies, while infants have considerable less activity than adults. In young children, activity seems to increase steadily until at least 7 years of age. Activity of PON1 is generally unchanged over time in adults, except in the elderly where it decreases over time.

PON1 is known to display a single nucleotide polymorphism at position 192, where the presence of a glutamine residue gives rise to a low-activity form toward paraoxon, while the presence of an arginine residue at the same location gives rise to a high-activity form toward paraoxon. Thus, activity of PON1 in an individual is a function of how much enzyme is present, as well as the particular form of the enzyme present. Measurement of PON1-mediated metabolism of paraoxon by serum samples from several hundred subjects reveals a multimodel distribution of activity, reflecting the genetic polymorphism. However, the significance of this polymorphism with regard to other PON1 substrates is unclear, since metabolism of some other substrates, such as chlorpyrifos oxon, displays an unimodal distribution of activity when evaluated in human serum samples from a population of subjects.

Results of studies directed toward understanding the role of PON1 in mediating the toxicity of phosphorothioate insecticides have been mixed. Some researchers have suggested that PON1 activity can influence an individual's susceptibility to phosphorothioate toxicity. Conversely, since the metabolic activity of PON1 toward oxons tends to be low, some researchers have suggested that other detoxifying pathways are more significant at low insecticide exposures, and that PON1 is likely only significant at very high exposures. Moreover, of the approximately 40 organophosphorus insecticides registered with the Environmental Protection Agency, only four produce oxons that have been reported to be substrates for PON1 (chlorpyrifos (CAS#2921-88-2), methyl parathion (CAS#298-00-0), pirimipos methyl (CAS#29232-93-7), and diazinon (CAS#333-41-5)), while one insecticide (dichlorvos) has been reported to be broken down directly by PON1.

In recent years, much effort has been devoted to the discovery of a physiological role for the paraoxonases. A physiological substrate(s) has not yet been identified with certainty, but suggestions include oxidized metabolites of polyunsaturated fatty acids that are similar in structure to lactones, homocysteine thiolactone, and quorum-sensing signaling molecules of *Pseudomonas aeruginosa*. All three forms (PON1, PON2, and PON3) seem to have some role in the prevention of oxidative stress and inflammation, and have been implicated in the modulation of a wide variety of diseases, including atherosclerosis, diabetes, Parkinson's disease, and inflammatory bowel disease. Much more research is required before the implications for human health of PON1, PON2, and PON3 can be fully understood.

See also: Biotransformation; Chlorpyrifos; Diazinon; Methyl Parathion; Pirimiphos Methyl; Dichlorvos; Organophosphate Poisoning; Parathion; Pesticides; Sarin (GB); Soman.

Further Reading

Mackness, B., Mackness, M., Aviram, M., Paragh, G. (Eds.), 2008. The Paraoxonases: Their Role in Disease Development and Xenobiotic Metabolism. Springer, The Netherlands.

Précourt, L.-P., Amre, D., Denis, M.C., et al., 2011. The three-gene paraoxonase family: physiologic roles, actions, and regulation. Atherosclerosis 214, 20–36.

Aflatoxin

MA Tirmenstein and R Mangipudy, Bristol-Myers Squibb Co., Drug Safety Evaluation, New Brunswick, NJ, USA

This article is a revision of the previous edition article by Raja S. Mangipudy and Harihara M. Mehendale, volume 1, pp 54–55, © 2005, Elsevier Inc.

- Chemical Abstracts Service Registry Number: 1402-68-2
- Synonyms: Aflatoxins B1; B2; B3; B4; G1; G2; M1; M2
- Chemical/Pharmaceutical/Other Class: Mycotoxins
- Chemical Structure (Aflatoxin B1):

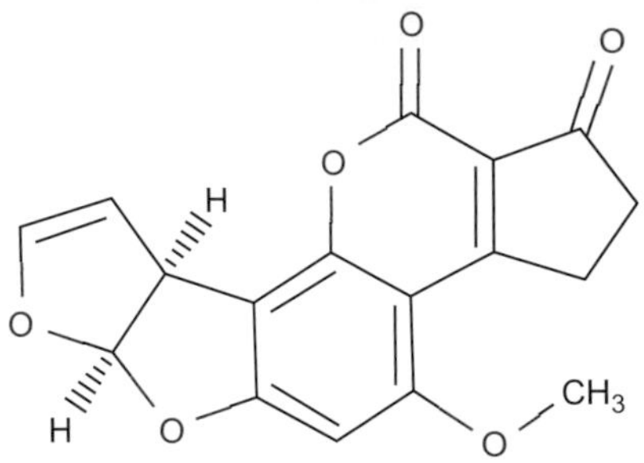

Background

Aflatoxins are naturally occurring bisfuranocoumarin compounds produced from the molds *Aspergillus flavus* and *Aspergillus parasiticus*. The aflatoxins are highly fluorescent. The B refers to blue and the G signifies green fluorescence. M aflatoxins are fungal metabolites present in milk. Aflatoxin B1 is the most common and potent of the aflatoxins. Crops that are affected by aflatoxin contamination include cereals (maize, sorghum, rice, wheat), oilseeds (peanut, sunflower, soybean, cotton), spices (chili peppers, black pepper, coriander, turmeric, ginger), and tree nuts (almond, coconuts, brazil nuts, walnuts, pistachio). Aflatoxin can also be found in the milk, eggs, and meat from animals fed contaminated feed.

Environmental Fate and Behavior

Aflatoxin will exist solely in the particulate phase if released into the ambient atmosphere based on estimated vapor pressure values (1.6×10^{-10} to 7.7×10^{-11} mm Hg) at 25 °C. Particulate-phase aflatoxins would be expected to be removed from the atmosphere by wet and dry deposition. Direct photolysis is also possible since aflatoxins absorb light in the environmental UV spectrum. If released to soil, the aflatoxins are expected to have high to slight mobility based upon K_{oc} values of 3974, 263, and 116. Aflatoxins are not expected to volatilize from dry soil surfaces based upon their vapor pressures. If released into water, the aflatoxins may adsorb to suspended solids and sediment based upon the available K_{oc} values. Estimated BCF values of 2–3 suggest the potential for bioconcentration in aquatic organisms is low. Aflatoxin may also be degraded by photolysis at soil and water surfaces.

Exposure and Exposure Monitoring

Ingestion and dermal contact are possible routes of exposure. Occupational exposure can occur through the handling and processing of aflatoxin-contaminated crops with low-level respiratory exposures to aflatoxin-contaminated dust particles possible. Dust levels of aflatoxin collected at different animal feed production sites ranged from not detectable to 8 μg kg^{-1} dust. Population exposures that have been estimated based on the analysis of aflatoxins in food were calculated for several different countries and ranged up to 2027 ng aflatoxin B1 consumed kg of body weight per day (Southern Guangxi in China sampling 1978–84; source, market samples).

Toxicokinetics

Aflatoxins are well absorbed orally. Exposure to human skin results in slow absorption. Aflatoxins are rapidly cleared from blood. Sixty-five percent of an initial dose of aflatoxin B1 is removed from the blood within 90 min and excreted primarily in the bile. The plasma half-life of aflatoxin is short, and it is excreted slowly as multiple moieties as a result of extensive metabolism. When estimated in human liver homogenates, the parent compound had an estimated half-life of 13 min. *In vitro* liver metabolism studies have shown five different types of metabolic pathways for aflatoxin B1: reduction, hydroxylation, hydration, O-demethylation, and epoxidation. All of these products contain hydroxide groups that allow them to be conjugated with glucuronic acid and sulfate.

Mechanism of Toxicity

Aflatoxin B1 is metabolized to a reactive epoxide (aflatoxin 8,9-epoxide) primarily by the P450 monooxygenase system. In humans, the epoxidation reaction is catalyzed by CYP1A2 and CYP3A4. Once formed, the epoxide can react further to form DNA adducts (aflatoxin-N^7-guanine) and induce mutations and cancer. Alternatively, the epoxide can be detoxified by conjugation with glutathione through the actions of certain glutathione *S*-tranferases. Rats are more susceptible than mice to aflatoxin hepatocarcinogenesis even though both species form the reactive 8,9-epoxide at similar rates. Differences in species susceptibility are hypothesized to relate to increased rates of glutathione conjugation to the aflatoxin 8,9-epoxide in mice compared to rats.

Acute and Short-Term Toxicity

Animal

The oral LD_{50} in monkeys for aflatoxin is 1750 μg kg^{-1} and the LD_{50} in monkeys following intramuscular injection is 2020 mg kg^{-1}.

 http://dx.doi.org/10.1016/B978-0-12-386454-3.00224-4

Human

Acute exposures to aflatoxins resulting in toxicity have been reported in several counties across the globe. In Uganda, fatal hepatic necrosis was reported in a 15-year-old boy who had eaten food contaminated with high concentrations of aflatoxin. In Western India, more than 200 villages experienced an outbreak of a disease affecting humans that was characterized by jaundice, rapidly developing ascites, portal hypertension, and a high mortality rate, with death usually resulting from massive gastrointestinal tract bleeding. The disease was associated with the consumption of badly molded corn containing between 6.25 and 15.6 ppm aflatoxin (average daily intake per victim of 2–6 mg of aflatoxin).

Chronic Toxicity

Animal

Edema and necrosis of hepatic and renal tissues are characteristic of chronic aflatoxin toxicity in experimental animals. Hemorrhagic enteritis and neurological symptoms have also been observed in animals administered aflatoxin. In carcinogenicity studies, aflatoxin produces liver tumors in mice, rats, fish, ducks, marmosets, tree shrews, and monkeys after administration by several routes. In rats, cancers of the colon and kidney were also noted.

Human

Aflatoxin poisoning is difficult to diagnose early in humans. The first clinical symptoms are anorexia and weight loss. Aflatoxins are associated with hepatocellular damage and necrosis, cholestasis, hepatomas, acute hepatitis, periportal fibrosis, hemorrhage, jaundice, fatty liver changes, cirrhosis in malnourished children, and Kwashiorkor. There is evidence of transplacental transport of aflatoxin by the fetoplacental unit. Aflatoxins are proven human carcinogens.

Immunotoxicity

Many animal studies have shown that aflatoxins are immunomodulatory and more specifically that aflatoxin B1 suppresses immune function by affecting T-cell-dependent immunity in several animal species including cattle, poultry, pigs, mouse, rat, and rabbits.

Reproductive Toxicity

The *in vitro* exposure of rat embryos to aflatoxin B1 induced neural tube defects. Aflatoxins have also been shown to be teratogenic in hamsters and mice, causing neural tube closure defects, microcephaly, umbilical hernia, and cleft palate. Although negative teratogenicity studies exist for rats, mice, and commercial livestock, the negative studies involve long-term feeding exposures, while the positive studies involve acute exposure, suggesting that high doses and maternal toxicity may play a role in adverse effects on the offspring. Aflatoxin may be a transplacental carcinogen in the rat. Analysis of aflatoxins in maternal and cord blood samples has also demonstrated the transplacental transport of aflatoxins in humans. Although suspected of playing a role in the early onset of liver cancer in some populations, prenatal exposure has not been demonstrated to be a significant route of exposure to the aflatoxins. Aflatoxins and active carcinogenic metabolites are excreted in breast milk. An estimate of the percentage of the oral dose excreted in milk ranged from 0.09% to 0.43%. A small number of studies have reported that male rats fed aflatoxins developed testicular degeneration and impaired spermatogenesis, although no clear association with aflatoxins and clinical infertility was uncovered in these studies.

Genotoxicity

Aflatoxins are mutagenic in the Ames assay in the presence of metabolic activation (hepatic S9).

Carcinogenicity

Aflatoxins are classified as human carcinogens. There is sufficient evidence in humans for the carcinogenicity of aflatoxin B1 and aflatoxin mixtures. There is also sufficient evidence in animals for the carcinogenicity of aflatoxin mixtures and for aflatoxins B1, G1, and M1.

Clinical Management

Acute aflatoxin toxicity should be treated with decontamination procedures and good supportive care. With chronic ingestion, the primary treatment remains supportive in nature. Elevation of serum alkaline phosphatase is a good indicator of aflatoxin toxicity.

Ecotoxicology

Aflatoxins are highly toxic to many species of animals, including fish and birds.

Other Hazards

Epidemiological and experimental data suggest a synergistic effect of aflatoxin and hepatitis B virus on hepatocellular carcinoma formation.

Exposure Standards and Guidelines

FDA's action levels for aflatoxins in human and animal foods

Product or animal	*Total aflatoxin action level* ($\mu g\,kg^{-1}$)
Human food	20
Milk	0.5
Beef cattle	300
Swine greater than 100 lb	200
Breeding beef cattle, swine, or mature poultry	100
Immature animals	20
Dairy animals	20

See also: Carcinogenesis; Food Safety and Toxicology; Mycotoxins.

Further Reading

Kensler, T.W., Roebuck, B.D., Wogan, G.N., Groopman, J.D., 2011. Aflatoxin: a 50-year odyssey of mechanistic and translational toxicology. Toxicol. Sci. 120 (Suppl. 1), S28–S48.

Mishra, H.N., Das, C.A., 2003. A review on biological control and metabolism of aflatoxin. Crit. Rev. Food Sci. Nutr. 43, 245–264.

Shuaib, F.M., Ehiri, J., Abdullahi, A., Williams, J.H., Jolly, P.E., 2010. Reproductive health effects of aflatoxins: a review of the literature. Reprod. Toxicol. 29, 262–270.

Wild, C.P., Turner, P.C., 2002. The toxicology of aflatoxins as a basis for public health decisions. Mutagenesis 17, 471–481.

Williams, J.H., Phillips, T.D., Jolly, P.E., Stiles, J.K., Jolly, C.M., Aggarwal, D., 2004. Human aflatoxicosis in developing countries: a review of toxicology, exposure, potential health consequences, and interventions. Am. J. Clin. Nutr. 80, 1106–1122.

Relevant Websites

US National Library of Medicine (2007) Hazardous Substances Databank–aflatoxins. http://toxnet.nlm.nih.gov/cgi-bin/sis/htmlgen?HSDB

IARC Monographs–aflatoxins http://monographs.iarc.fr/ENG/Monographs/PDFs/index.php

Air Pollution *see* Pollution, Air in Encyclopedia of Toxicology

Alachlor

MA Tirmenstein and R Mangipudy, Bristol-Myers Squibb Co., Drug Safety Evaluation, New Brunswick, NJ, USA

This article is a revision of the previous edition article by Raja S. Mangipudy and Harihara M. Mehendale, volume 1, pp 58–60, © 2005, Elsevier Inc.

- Chemical Abstracts Service Registry Number: 15972-60-8
- Synonyms: Alachlor; Alanex; Alanox; Alatox 480; Lasagrin; Lasso; Lazo; Metachlor; Methachlor; Pillarzo
- Chemical/Pharmaceutical/Other Class: Herbicide
- Chemical Structure:

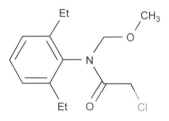

Background

Alachlor is a preemergence herbicide registered by Monsanto in 1969. Alachlor was banned as an herbicide in the European Union in 2006.

Uses

Alachlor is one of the most widely used herbicides in the United States and is used as an herbicide for grasses, broadleaf seeds, corn, sorghum, soybeans, peanuts, cotton, vegetables, and forage crops.

Environmental Fate and Behavior

Alachlor has a low persistence in soil, with a half-life of ≈ 8 days. The main means of degradation is by soil microbes. It has moderate mobility in sandy and silty soils, and thus can migrate to groundwater. The largest groundwater-testing program for a pesticide, the National Alachlor Well Water Survey, was conducted throughout the last half of the 1980s. More than six million private and domestic wells were tested for the presence of alachlor. Less than 1% of all of the wells had detectable levels of alachlor. In the wells in which the compound was detected, concentrations ranged from 0.1 to 1.0 $mg\,l^{-1}$, with the majority having concentrations $\approx 0.2\ mg\,l^{-1}$. Alachlor is relatively stable to hydrolysis and photolysis in water, and degradation in water is not considered as an important environmental fate process. Alachlor appears to be persistent under aquifer biological and geochemical conditions. This means that alachlor can appear in groundwater years after use and can migrate with groundwater away from use areas. Alachlor contamination has resulted in loss of untreated groundwater as a source of drinking water in Florida and other states. The bioaccumulation factor in the channel catfish is 5.8 times the ambient water concentration, indicating that alachlor is not expected to accumulate appreciably in aquatic organisms.

Exposure and Exposure Monitoring

Occupational exposure would be expected to occur through inhalation or dermal contact, although exposure via oral/parenteral route and ocular contact are also possible. Monitoring data indicate that the general population may be exposed to alachlor via inhalation of ambient air and ingestion of food and drinking water contaminated with alachlor.

Toxicokinetics

Alachlor is well absorbed orally. Studies in monkeys have shown dermal penetration of alachlor to be relatively low. Dermal absorption may be linear over time for the duration of exposure. Excretion via kidneys is the major route of elimination in monkeys, but both biliary and urinary excretion occurs at approximately equal extent in rats.

Mechanism of Toxicity

This agent is corrosive and causes skin and eye irritation. Allergic reactions can occur in some individuals with repeated or prolonged skin exposures. In mammals, alachlor appears to form conjugates with glucuronic acid, sulfate, and glutathione (mercapturic acid). It has been postulated that metabolism of alachlor to form the putative carcinogenic metabolite (diethylquinoneimine) is responsible for the production of nasal tumors in rats. Differences in metabolic capacities result in much high levels of diethylquinoneimine in the nasal mucosa of rats compared with other species.

Acute and Short-Term Toxicity

Animal

Alachlor is a slightly toxic herbicide. The LD_{50} of alachlor in rats is between 790 and 1350 $mg\,kg^{-1}$. In the mouse, the LD_{50} is

462 mg kg^{-1}. The dermal LD_{50} in rats is 13 300 mg kg^{-1}, but some of the formulated materials can be more toxic, with dermal LD_{50} values ranging from 7800 to 16 000 mg kg^{-1}. The dermal LD_{50} in rabbits is 3500 mg kg^{-1}. Skin irritation for alachlor is classified as slight to moderate. The inhalation LC_{50} in rats is reportedly greater than 5.1 mg l^{-1} for 4 h of exposure.

Human

Prolonged convulsions were reported following acute oral exposure of a 57-year-old man to alachlor.

Chronic Toxicity

Animal

In a 27-week study, beagle dogs were administered 5–100 mg kg^{-1} day^{-1} for 27 weeks. The 100 mg kg^{-1} day^{-1} dose was reduced to 75 mg kg^{-1} day^{-1} after 3 weeks due to the signs of severe toxicity. In a 6-month dog study, dogs were administered alachlor at 5–75 mg kg^{-1} day^{-1}. Dogs showed liver toxicity at all doses $\geq$5 mg kg^{-1} day^{-1} and indications of anemia were also noted in dogs given doses of $\geq$25 mg kg^{-1} day^{-1}. Mean liver weights of male dogs given 5 mg kg^{-1} day^{-1} alachlor increased 18% above the control value. In 2-year rat studies, alachlor was administered to Long-Evans rats at doses of 14, 42, and 126 mg kg^{-1} day^{-1}. Hepatotoxicity was noted at all dose levels. Doses of 42 and 126 mg kg^{-1} day^{-1} produced irreversible ocular lesions characterized as progressive uveal degeneration syndrome. Ocular lesions have not been observed in other species or in other strains of rats and were considered unique to the Long-Evans rat.

Human

No specific information on the chronic toxicity of alachlor in humans is available. Epidemiology studies in workers manufacturing alachlor indicate no increased mortality rates from cancer or other causes with up to 25 years of follow-up.

Immunotoxicity

Alachlor had no effects on immune function as determined from *in vitro* studies conducted with alachlor incubated with human mononuclear cells isolated from peripheral blood. Alachlor had minimal immunological effects on male rats when it was administered by intraperitoneal injection at doses $\leq$3.75 mg kg^{-1} day^{-1} for 2 weeks.

Reproductive Toxicity

High oral doses (150 or 400 mg kg^{-1} day^{-1}) fed to rats during gestation resulted in maternal and fetal toxicity, but there was no indication that reproduction was affected. Alachlor does not appear to cause reproductive effects. Doses of up to 150 mg kg^{-1} day^{-1} fed to rabbits on days 7 through 19 of pregnancy did not result in any birth defects. Similar studies in rats at doses up to 400 mg kg^{-1} day^{-1} did not result in birth defects, but toxic effects in the mothers and offspring were seen at the highest dose. These data indicate that alachlor is not likely to cause birth defects.

Genotoxicity

Alachlor does not appear to be mutagenic. Mutagenicity assays with a variety of microbial strains at numerous concentrations of alachlor were for the most part negative. In an *in vivo* cytogenetics assay, alachlor was not clastogenic to rat bone marrow cells when administered orally at doses up to 1000 mg kg^{-1}. Alachlor was negative in rat (600 mg kg^{-1}) and mouse (1000 mg kg^{-1}) micronucleus assays. The weight of evidence indicates that alachlor is negative for genotoxicity in mammals.

Carcinogenicity

Rats given high doses of alachlor developed stomach, thyroid, and nasal turbinate tumors. An 18-month mouse study with doses from 26 to 260 mg kg^{-1} day^{-1} had increased benign lung (bronchoalveolar) tumors at the highest dose of alachlor for females but not males. Alachlor is classified by the Environmental Protection Agency (EPA) as unlikely to be carcinogenic to humans at low doses, but likely to be carcinogenic to humans at high doses. Alachlor is a confirmed animal carcinogen with unknown relevance to humans.

Clinical Management

Treatment is symptomatic and supportive. There are no specific antidotes. Ingestion of alachlor is likely to be followed by vomiting and diarrhea due to its irritant properties. In cases of oral exposure, measures to decrease absorption may be useful. Emesis may be induced after careful consideration. For dermal exposure, decontamination by washing the exposed area thoroughly with soap and water is recommended. In cases of inhalation exposure, the victim must be moved to fresh air and monitored for respiratory distress. In cases of eye exposure, the eyes should be irrigated with copious amounts of tepid water for at least 15 min. If irritation, pain, swelling, lacrimation, or photophobia persists, the person should be seen in a health care facility.

Ecotoxicology

- Slightly toxic to mammals, based on a rat study (LD_{50} of 930 mg kg^{-1}).
- Alachlor is slightly to practically nontoxic to wildfowl. Alachlor has a 5-day dietary LC_{50} >5000 ppm in young mallard ducks and bobwhite quail.
- Slightly toxic to honey bees (LD_{50} > 36 μg per bee).
- Slightly to moderately toxic on an acute basis to freshwater aquatic animals (LC_{50}/EC_{50} 1–33 ppm).

- Highly to moderately toxic to freshwater aquatic animals on a chronic basis (NOEC $\geq$0.1 ppm, LOEC $\geq$0.2 ppm).
- Moderately toxic to saltwater fish (LC_{50} 3.9 ppm), moderately toxic to saltwater mycid (LC_{50} 2.4 ppm), and moderately toxic to shellfish (EC_{50} 1.6 ppm).
- Highly toxic to aquatic plants (based on a single species tested: NOEL = 0.35 ppb, LOEL = 0.69 ppb, EC_{50} = 1.64 ppb).

Exposure Standards and Guidelines

- Acceptable daily intake is 0.0025 mg kg^{-1} day^{-1}
- 8-h time weighted average is 1 mg m^{-3}
- Maximum contaminant level is 0.002 mg l^{-1}
- Reference dose is 0.01 mg kg^{-1} day^{-1}

Miscellaneous

The Material Safety Data Sheet should always be referred to for detailed information on handling and disposal.

See also: Common Mechanism of Toxicity in Pesticides; Pesticides.

Further Reading

Gadagbui, B., Maier, A., Dourson, M., Parker, A., et al., 2010. Derived reference doses (RfDs) for the environmental degradates of the herbicides alachlor and acetochlor: results of an independent expert panel deliberation. Regul. Toxicol. Pharmacol. 57 (2–3), 220–234.

Heydens, W.F., Lamb, I.C., Wilson, A.G.E., 2010. Chloroacetanilides. In: Krieger, R. (Ed.), Hayes' Handbook of Pesticide Toxicology, third ed., vol. 1. Elsevier Inc, London, UK, pp. 1753–1769.

Hudson, R.H., Tucker, R.K., Haegele, M.A., 1984. Handbook of Toxicity of Pesticides to Wildlife. Resource Publication 153. US Department of the Interior, Fish and Wildlife Service, Washington, DC.

Johnson, W.O., Kollman, G.E., Swithenbank, C., Yih, R.Y., 1978. RH 6201 (blazer): a new broad spectrum herbicide for postemergence use in soybeans. J. Agric. Food Chem. 26, 285–286.

Kale, V.M., Miranda, S.R., Wilbanks, M.S., Meyer, S.A., 2008. Comparative cytotoxicity of alachlor, acetochlor, and metolachlor herbicides in isolated rat and cryopreserved human hepatocytes. J. Biochem. Mol. Toxicol. 22 (1), 41–50.

Kidd, H., James, D.R. (Eds.), 1991. The Agrochemicals Handbook, third ed. Royal Society of Chemistry Information Services, Cambridge, UK.

Kim, H., Min, J., Park, J., Lee, S., Lee, J., 2011. Erythema multiforme major due to occupational exposure to the herbicides alachlor and butachlor. Emerg. Med. Australas. 23 (1), 103–105.

Lo, Y.C., Yang, C.C., Deng, J.F., 2008. Acute alachlor and butachlor herbicide poisoning. Clin. Toxicol. (Phila) 46 (8), 716–721.

Lu, F.C., 1995. A review of the acceptable daily intakes of pesticides assessed by the World Health Organization. Regul. Toxicol. Pharmacol. 21, 351–364.

Weichenthal, S., Moase, C., Chan, P., 2010. A review of pesticide exposure and cancer incidence in the agricultural health study cohort. Environ. Health Perspect. 118 (8), 1117–1125.

Relevant Websites

Environmental Protection Agency Reregistration Eligibility Decision–alachlor (1998):http://www.epa.gov/oppsrrd1/REDs/0063.pdf

US National Library of Medicine (2009) Chemical Carcinogenesis Research Information System–alachlor http://toxnet.nlm.nih.gov/cgi-bin/sis/htmlgen?CCRIS

US National Library of Medicine (2007) Hazardous Substances Databank–alachlor. http://toxnet.nlm.nih.gov/cgi-bin/sis/htmlgen?HSDB

US National Library of Medicine (2004) Integrated Risk Information System Database–alachlor. http://toxnet.nlm.nih.gov/cgi-bin/sis/htmlgen?IRIS

Chemical Safety Information from Intergovernmental Organizations. http://www.inchem.org/documents/pds/pds/pest86_e.htm

Alar

KD Chadwick and RS Mangipudy, Bristol-Myers Squibb, Drug Safety Evaluation, New Brunswick, NJ, USA

This article is a revision of the previous edition article by Raja S. Mangipudy, volume 1, p 60, © 2005, Elsevier Inc.

- Name: Alar
- Chemical Abstracts Service Registry Number: 1596-84-5
- Synonyms: Aminozide; Daminozide; DMSA; B-995; Kylar; Aminocide
- Molecular Formula: $C_6H_{12}N_2O_3$
- Chemical Structure:

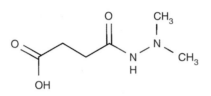

Background and Uses

Alar is a systemic growth regulator approved in the United States for use on ornamental plants such as chrysanthemums, poinsettias, and bedding plants located in enclosed structures such as greenhouses. Alar reduces internode elongation; induces heat, drought, and frost resistance; and produces darker foliage and stronger stems as well as earlier and multiple flowers and fruits. A spray is often applied at the rate of 1500–10 000 ppm. It is a systemic agent (i.e., taken up by the fruit) and cannot be removed by washing or peeling. In 1984, the US Environmental Protection Agency (EPA) initiated a special review of products containing alar based on concerns that alar and its degradant, Unsymmetrical dimethylhydrazine (UDMH), caused tumors. In 1989, the Natural Resources Defense Council released a report entitled "Intolerable Risk: Pesticides in Our Children's Food," which suggested that alar was a 'potent carcinogen' and a threat to children's health due to their proportionally higher consumption of apples and apple products relative to adults. The associated media attention produced the so-called apple scare when products were pulled from shelves. As a result of the negative attention, the sole registrant, Uniroyal Chemical Company, voluntarily canceled all food use registrations for alar in 1989. EPA determined that the remaining nonfood uses of alar did not pose an unreasonable risk to humans.

Environmental Fate and Behavior

Alar does not degrade following contact with water but degrades rapidly in soil resulting in volatile compounds (including formaldehyde) and bound residues; therefore mobility is not considered a concern. In greenhouse studies, alar persistence ranged from 3 to 4 days in different soils. Since alar is registered for greenhouse use only, agricultural runoff into groundwater is not expected to be a concern.

Exposure

Exposure should be limited to dermal and inhalation based on approved usage.

Toxicokinetics

A breakdown product of alar is an asymmetrical 1,1-dimethylhydrazine that is excreted renally.

Acute and Short-Term Toxicity

Alar is of very low acute and subacute toxicity based on oral or inhalation routes of exposure. There is a slightly greater degree of acute toxicity with dermal exposure. EPA considers that alar will not pose unreasonable risks or adverse effects to humans or the environment.

The primary toxic effect seen in animals includes ptosis, central nervous system (CNS) depression, gastrointestinal irritation, and possibly liver function abnormalities.

Reproductive Toxicity

Alar has been shown to produce some maternal toxicity at high doses but did not produce developmental or reproductive toxicity.

Genotoxicity

Neither alar nor UDMH has been shown to be mutagenic.

Carcinogenicity

Concerns about carcinogenicity with UDMH and therefore alar led to the withdrawal of alar for food use in 1989 and the revoking of food tolerances (maximum residue limits) by the EPA in 1990. Two-year bioassays suggested that alar was carcinogenic in female rats (adenocarcinomas of the endometrium of the uterus) and that it increased vascular tumors in the livers of male mice. UDMH caused a slight increase in liver tumors in rats and liver vascular tumors in mice. Since the

 http://dx.doi.org/10.1016/B978-0-12-386454-3.00226-8

presence of UDMH is dependent on alar, and it is classified by the EPA as a 'possible human carcinogen.'

Clinical Management

No human cases have been reported, so treatment recommendations are speculative. Dermal contamination probably requires no treatment other than decontamination. Dietary exposure is not anticipated since alar is no longer approved for food use; however, if ingested, treatment by emesis, gastric lavage, or activated charcoal may be indicated. Patients should be monitored for CNS depression, ptosis (eyelid drooping), and liver function abnormalities if significant amounts (>8 g) have been consumed.

Ecotoxicology

Alar is considered to have very low acute toxicity to mammals, birds, and freshwater fish. It is slightly toxic to aquatic invertebrates.

Exposure Standards and Guidelines

Worker protection standards should be followed including appropriate personal protective equipment and restricted entry intervals.

See also: Pesticides.

Further Reading

Edgerton, L.J., Rockey, M.L., Helen, A., et al., 1967. Colorimetric determination of alar residues in apples. J. Agric. Food Chem. 15 (5), 812–813. http://dx.doi.org/10.1021/jf60153a021.

Fan, A.M., Jackson, R.J., 1989. Pesticides and food safety. Regul. Toxicol. Pharmacol. 9 (2), 158–174.

Finkel, A.M., 1992. Alar: the aftermath. Science 255 (5045), 664–665.

IPCS: INCHEM: http://www.inchem.org/documents/jmpr/jmpmono/v89pr05.htm.

Kimm, V.J., 1991. Alar's risks. Science 254 (5036), 1276.

Kirkland, D., Fowler, P., 2010. Further analysis of Ames-negative rodent carcinogens that are only genotoxic in mammalian cells in vitro at concentrations exceeding 1 mM, including retesting of compounds of concern. Mutagenesis 25 (6), 539–553.

Marshall, E., 1991. A is for apple, alar, and alarmist? Science 254 (5028), 20–22.

Relevant Websites

http://toxnet.nlm.nih.gov - TOXNET, Specialized Information Services, National Library of Medicine. Search for alar.

http://www.epa.gov/pesticides - US EPA website. Search for daminozide.

http://www.cdpr.ca.gov/docs/risk/toxsums/toxsumlist.htm – California EPA Department of Pesticides Regulation. Search for daminozide under Toxicology Data Review Summaries.

INCHEM: http://www.inchem.org/documents/jmpr/jmpmono/v89pr05.htm

Albuterol

SE Gad, Gad Consulting Services, Cary, NC, USA

- Name: Albuterol
- Chemical Abstracts Service Registry Number: 18559-94-9
- Synonyms: Salbutamol, Ventolin, Proventil, Apo-Salvent, Novo-Salmol, Albuterol sulfate; Volmax
- Molecular Formula: $C_{13}H_{21}NO_3$
- Structure:

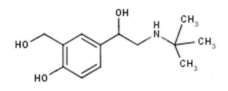

Background

Albuterol is a short-acting β2-adrenergic agonist that is primarily used as a bronchodilator for the treatment of asthma or other pulmonary diseases. It is prepared as a racemic mixture of $R(-)$ and $S(+)$ stereoisomers. The stereospecific preparation of $R(-)$ isomer of albuterol is referred to as levalbuterol. Albuterol may be used for the treatment of hyperkalemia and is found in metered dose inhalers, unit doses for nebulizers, and as an oral syrup and tablets.

Albuterol is a selective β2-adrenergic agonist that primarily causes smooth muscle relaxation. With therapeutic use, adverse effects with albuterol therapy include tachycardia, tremor, hyperactivity, nausea, and vomiting.

Toxicity may result from overstimulation of β-adrenergic activity. In addition, β-adrenergic selectivity is lost, so β-1 effects can be seen. With mild-to-moderate toxicity poisoning/exposure, tachycardia, hypertension, tachypnea, tremor, agitation, nausea, vomiting, hypokalemia, and hyperglycemia may occur. Severe effects include hypotension, dysrhythmias, seizures, and acidosis and are likely to occur only after ingestion.

Uses

Albuterol is used as a bronchodilator in the treatment of asthma or other pulmonary diseases. Off-label uses include treatment of hyperkalemia and in the prevention of premature labor.

The oral adult dose is 2–4 mg three to four times a day. Oral doses for children are 0.1–0.2 $mg\,kg^{-1}$. The inhalational dose is typically 0.1–0.15 $mg\,kg^{-1}$ per dose or 0.5 $mg\,kg^{-1}\,h^{-1}$ for continuous administration.

β-Adrenergic receptors mediate the effects of the sympathetic nervous system throughout the body. β2 Receptors are found on vascular, bronchial, gastrointestinal, and uterine smooth muscle as well as skeletal muscle, hepatocytes, and also the myocardium. Albuterol stimulates adenyl cyclase which catalyzes cyclic adenosine monophosphate (AMP) from adenosine triphosphate (ATP). This mediates bronchodilation and smooth muscle relaxation through activation of protein kinases, leading to phosphorylation of proteins, which in turn increases bound intracellular calcium. The reduced availability of intracellular ionized calcium inhibits actin–myosin linkage, leading to the relaxation of smooth muscle. β2-Adrenergic receptors in the lung also inhibit secretions and decrease histamine release. Stimulation of β2-adrenergic receptors found on the uterine smooth muscle inhibits the onset of labor.

There are no well-controlled studies showing evidence that oral albuterol will stop preterm labor or prevent labor at term and albuterol has not been approved for the management of preterm labor. Serious adverse reactions, including pulmonary edema, have been reported following administration of albuterol to women in labor.

Environmental Fate and Behavior

Albuterol's production and use as a bronchodilator may result in its release to the environment through various waste streams.

Routes and Pathways and Relevant Physicochemical Properties

Melting point: 151 °C (Lunts) and 157–158 °C (Collins),

Octanol/water partition coefficient: log $K_{ow} = 0.64$ (estimated),

Water solubility: $1.43 \times 10^4\ mg\,l^{-1}$,

Henry's law constant = 6.4×10^{-16} atm-$m^3\,mol^{-1}$ at 25 °C,

Soil sediment sorption (log K_{oc}): −1.6 to −1.15, measured.

Partition Behavior in Water, Sediment, and Soil

Solubility

This material contains an active ingredient that for environmental fate predictions has solubility in water.

Volatility

This material contains an active ingredient that will not readily enter into the air from hard surfaces or from a container of the pure substance. This material contains an active ingredient that will not readily enter into air from water.

Adsorption

This material contains an active ingredient that is not likely to adsorb to soil or sediment if released directly to the environment.

Partitioning

This material contains an active pharmaceutical ingredient with octanol/water partition coefficient data that suggest that for

 http://dx.doi.org/10.1016/B978-0-12-386454-3.00809-5

environmental fate predictions, the active pharmaceutical ingredient will not have the tendency to distribute into fats.

Atmospheric Fate

According to a model of gas/particle partitioning of semi-volatile organic compounds in the atmosphere, albuterol, which has an estimated vapor pressure of 8.9×10^{-9} mm Hg at 25 °C, is expected to exist solely in the particulate phase in the ambient atmosphere. Particulate-phase albuterol may be removed from the air by wet and dry deposition.

Terrestrial Fate

Based on a classification scheme, an estimated K_{oc} value of 23 indicates that albuterol is expected to have very high mobility in soil. The pK_{a1} and pK_{a2} of albuterol are 9.2 and 10.7, respectively, indicating that this compound will partially exist protonated in the environment and cations generally adsorb more strongly to suspended solids and sediment than their neutral counterparts. Volatilization of albuterol from moist soil surfaces is not expected to be an important fate process.

Aquatic Fate

Albuterol is not expected to adsorb to suspended solids and sediment. Volatilization from water surfaces is not expected. An estimated bioconcentration factor of 3 suggests that the potential for bioconcentration in aquatic organisms is low.

Environmental Persistency (Degradation/Speciation)

Hydrolysis

This material contains an active pharmaceutical ingredient that has been shown to be chemically stable in water. Hydrolysis is unlikely to be a significant depletion mechanism.

Half-life, neutral: >1 years, measured.

Photolysis

This material contains an active pharmaceutical ingredient that is unlikely to undergo photodegradation.

Ultraviolet/visible spectrum: 225 nm.

Biodegradation

This material contains an active ingredient that is not readily biodegradable (as defined by 1993 Organisation for Economic Cooperation and Development Testing Guidelines).

Aerobic–ready percent degradation: 1%, 28 days, modified Sturm test.

Aerobic–soil percent degradation: 1.3–38.7%, 64 days.

Long-Range Transport

Not known to be transported long-range.

Exposure and Exposure Monitoring

Routes and Pathways

Oral, inhaled, and dermal.

Human Exposure

Occupational exposure to albuterol may occur through dermal contact with this compound at workplaces where albuterol is produced or used. National Institute for Occupational Safety and Health (National Occupational Exposure Survey, 1981–83) has statistically estimated that 744 workers (603 of these are female) are potentially exposed to albuterol in the United States.

Environmental Exposure

Monitoring data indicate that the general population may be exposed to albuterol via ingestion of drinking water and through the use of pharmaceutical products containing albuterol.

Toxicokinetics

Nebulized albuterol has been found more effective than systemic administration. Oral albuterol is readily absorbed from the gut. Sulfate conjugation is the primary metabolic pathway; it is transformed in the liver. There appears to be no direct biotransformation of albuterol in the lungs. Most of an inhaled dose is deposited on the pharynx after inhalation and then swallowed. Albuterol, as both the sulfate and sulfate conjugates (metabolite and unchanged drug), is eliminated via the kidneys. Albuterol follows first-order kinetics. The half-life is 3–5 h with oral dosing, 2–7 h with inhalation, and 5.5–6.9 h with intravenous dosing. Maximum brochodilation occurs within 0.5–2 h, for oral forms in 2–3 h, and sustained-release forms in 6 h.

Absorption may be delayed in large overdoses, especially with sustained-release formulations.

Mechanism of Toxicity

Tachycardia occurs as a reflex to the drop in mean arterial pressure (MAP) or as a result of β-1 stimulus. β-Adrenergic receptors in the locus coeruleus also regulate norepinephrine-induced inhibitory effects, resulting in agitation, restlessness, and hand tremor. Stimulation of nonpulmonary β2 receptors may lead to an increase in heart rate, QT_c interval prolongation, nonspecific T-wave changes, skeletal muscle tremor, and slight increases in blood glucose and nonesterified fatty acids. Hypokalemia is more pronounced in patients receiving intravenous albuterol. Hypotension is also known to occur mostly in overdose. The buildup of cyclic AMP in the liver stimulates glycogenolysis and an increase in serum glucose.

In skeletal muscle, this process results in increased lactate production. Direct stimulus of sodium/potassium ATPase in skeletal muscle produces a shift of potassium from the extracellular space to the intracellular space. Relaxation of smooth muscle produces a dilation of the vasculature supplying skeletal muscle, which results in a drop in diastolic and MAP.

Myocardial ischemia and infarction have been associated with excessive tachycardia in elderly patients. The skin may be warm and pink with evidence of diaphoresis.

Acute and Short-Term Toxicity (Animal/Human)

Signs and symptoms of overdose include exaggeration of common adverse reactions, particularly angina, hypertension, hypokalemia, and seizures. Cardiac arrest may occur.

Animal

Albuterol appears to be relatively benign in animals, similar to human. Agitation, vomiting, and lethargy may be seen. In rats, the oral LD_{50} was more than 2000 mg kg^{-1}, and inhalation LC_{50} could not be determined.

Rodent LD_{50}, intraperitoneal	167–295 mg kg^{-1}
Rodent LD_{50}, intravenous	48.7–57.1 mg kg^{-1}
Rodent LD_{50}, oral	660–2707 mg kg^{-1}
Rodent LD_{50}, subcutaneous	737–2500 mg kg^{-1}

Human

A review of albuterol overdoses revealed that up to 20 times, the oral daily dose produced no deaths. The effects of albuterol overdose are usually mild and benign, although they can be prolonged. Cardiovascular effects are usually limited to a sinus tachycardia and widened pulse pressure. Although there may be a drop in diastolic pressure, the systolic pressure is maintained by increased cardiac output from the trachycardia. Transient hypokalemia can result, caused by a shift of extracellular potassium to the intracellular space with total body stores of potassium generally remaining normal. A transient metabolic acidosis can be seen due to increased lactate production. Restlessness, agitation, tremors apprehension, dizziness, nausea, vomiting, and dilated pupils are common in albuterol overdose.

Diabetes mellitus has been reported in less than 3% of patients receiving albuterol sulfate inhalation aerosol in clinical trials.

Child	TDLo	Oral	0.6–1.85 mg kg^{-1}
Human	TDLo	Intravenous	0.006 mg kg^{-1}
Man	TCLo	Inhalation	0.036 mg kg^{-1} per 6 h
Human	TDLo	Oral	1.6–5.714 mg kg^{-1}

Chronic Toxicity (Animal/Human)

Human

Continued dependence of salbutamol tablets taken in high doses (30–40 tablets daily and 48–64 mg day^{-1}) has led to symptoms of toxic psychosis in one elderly woman and paranoid psychosis in a 52-year-old man. For up to 90 years, 100-mg inhalations of salbutamol daily has been used by asthmatics, who increased doses because they 'needed it' and wanted to 'feel good.' Long-term tolerance develops to bronchodilator action, tremor, tachycardia, prolongation of QT_c interval, hyperglycemia, hypokalemia, and the vasodilator response.

Reproductive Toxicity

Animal

A study in Stride Dutch rabbits at oral doses of 50 mg kg^{-1} (approximately 25 times the maximum recommended daily oral dose for adults on a milligram per square meter basis) found cranioschisis in 7 of 19 (37%) fetuses.

Human

During worldwide marketing experience, various congenital anomalies, including cleft palate and limb defects, have been reported in the offspring of patients being treated with albuterol. Some of the mothers were taking multiple medications during their pregnancies. No consistent pattern of defects can be discerned, and a relationship between albuterol use and congenital anomalies has not been established. Albuterol and albuterol sulfate/ipratropium bromide are classified as Food and Drug Administration Pregnancy Category C by the manufacturer.

Genotoxicity

No evidence of mutagenicity.

Carcinogenicity

Chronic exposure or carcinogenicity studies on Sprague–Dawley rats for 2 years at dietary doses of 2, 10, and 50 mg kg^{-1} of body weight (corresponding to 1/2, 3, and 15 times, respectively, the maximum recommended daily oral dose for adults on a milligram per square meter of body surface area basis of 2/5, 2, and 10 times, respectively, the maximum recommended daily oral dose for children on a milligram per square meter basis) found significant dose-related increases in the incidence of benign leiomyomas for the mesovarium.

Clinical Management

The threshold dose for the development of three or more signs of toxicity is 1 mg kg^{-1} or 3–10 times the recommended daily dose. Toxicity is short lived and does not require specific therapy or hospital admission in most cases.

Children have survived overdoses as large as 100 mg and adults have survived doses up to 240 mg without serious complications. Activated charcoal effectively adsorbs albuterol. The hypokalemia produced reflects a transient shift in potassium location rather than a true deficit of potassium; external replacement therapy is rarely necessary, but can be added to intravenous fluids to support the heart if electrocardiographic changes are noted. A conservative approach to tachycardia is recommended since arrhythmias beyond an increase in rate have not occurred with overdose. Support of blood pressure and control of tachycardia are major therapeutic interventions.

The presence of other dysrhythmias or hypotension indicates a more severe poisoning.

If hypotension is present, intravenous fluid should be used initially. If the hypotension does not respond, a β-adrenergic blocking agent can be used. First-line choices include esmolol or propranolol since the hypotension is often primarily due to the tachycardia. Alternatively, a vasopressor with pure alpha activity such as phenylephrine can be used. Tachycardia can also be treated if necessary with a beta blocker, but this is rarely warranted. Premature ventricular contractions rarely require treatment.

Methylxanthine and other sympathomimetic overdoses can present in a similar manner.

Symptoms may occur after inhalation, but seem to be less common and less serious than when significant amounts have been ingested. Some decontamination may be accomplished by mouth rinsing for materials left on the oral surfaces after use of an inhaler. Material absorbed via inhalation should be treated as with an oral exposure.

If ocular exposure occurs, irrigate exposed eyes with copious amounts of room temperature water for at least 15 min. If irritation, pain, swelling, lacrimation, or photophobia persist, the patient should be seen in a health care facility.

For dermal exposure, remove contaminated clothing and wash exposed area thoroughly with soap and water. A physician may need to examine the area if irritation or pain persists.

Ecotoxicology

Aquatic

Activated sludge respiration.

This material contains an active ingredient that is not toxic to activated sludge microorganisms.

IC_{50}: >830 mg l^{-1}, 3 h.

Daphnid

This material contains an active pharmaceutical ingredient that is not toxic to daphnids.

EC_{50}: 243 mg l^{-1}, 48 h, *Daphnia magna*, static test.

No observed effect concentration: 83.2 mg l^{-1}, 48 h, *Daphnia magna*, static test.

Other Hazards

Interactions

Following single-dose intravenous or oral administration of albuterol to healthy individuals who had received digoxin for 10 days, a 16–22% decrease in serum digoxin concentration was observed. Epinephrine and other orally inhaled sympathomimetic amines may increase sympathomimetic effects and risk of toxicity. MAO inhibitors and tricyclic antidepressants may cause serious cardiovascular effects and risk of toxicity. Propranolol and other beta blockers may antagonize effects of albuterol.

Exposure Standards and Guidelines

None set by regulatory authorities.

See also: Kidney.

Further Reading

Libretto, S.E., 1994. A review of the toxicology of salbutamol (albuterol). Arch. Toxicol. 68 (4), 213–216.

Spangler, D.L., 1989. Review of side effects associated with beta antagonists. Ann. Allergy 62, 59–62.

Alchemy

PG Maxwell-Stuart, University of St Andrews, St Andrews, UK

Alchemy is a science with two faces. One looks outward to the world of matter and seeks either to manipulate aspects of it in such a way as to effect fundamental alterations in its composition, the best-known example of this being the attempt, allegedly successful in several instances, to change lead into gold, or to manufacture an elixir or pill which will preserve or provide good health and prolong a person's life. The other face looks inward and treats the physical processes of the laboratory either as metaphors for spiritual change in the alchemist him or herself or as vehicles with whose help that spiritual change can be made to happen. The origin of alchemy is somewhat obscure. There is a Chinese tradition, whose practice goes back many centuries, an Indian tradition not quite as long but equally distinguished, and a third from Hellenistic Egypt whose Greek word *khémeia* ('a pouring together'), via its Arabic version, supposedly forms the basis of our word 'alchemy' and suggests a derivation from the process of smelting and refining metal ore. Alchemy is sometimes regarded as a proto-chemistry on the grounds that its experiments uncovered white arsenic, silver nitrate, alcohol, ammonium carbonate, potassium sulfate, bismuth, hydrochloric acid, zinc sulfate, ferric chloride, and a host of other substances. It is also often dismissed as though it were chemistry which had taken a wrong turning, but in fact, as its history shows, it was a good deal more complex than that.

Chinese alchemy was encouraged by imperial authority to manufacture gold since gold, which neither rusts nor tarnishes, was clearly not only symbolical of health and long life but also might well, when worn, pass on those desirable properties to the wearer. Metallurgical theory in China, as in the west, said that metals and minerals grow in the earth, slowly over centuries turning from one substance into another, eventually ending as gold. Hence, what the alchemist was trying to do, in theory, was to hasten that natural process and achieve in very short span what 'nature' took time to do. Alongside this, the Chinese alchemist experimented with both inorganic and organic substances to produce elixirs guaranteeing not only long life but also immortality, and one finds some of the great Chinese alchemists – Wei Po-Yang in the second century AD, for example, and Ge Hong and Ko Hung from the third and fourth – writing about their practical craft in combination with appeals to philosophy, astrology, magic, and pharmacology as they sought to elevate alchemy from being merely technical experiments in a laboratory into a more potent, life-changing, life-enhancing total experience. These early days of enthusiasm lasted, on and off, until the fourteenth century, assisted by intermittent imperial patronage, but thereafter interest waned under the increasing weight of public disparagement and, to some extent, Western intellectual influences and so, while alchemy continued to be practiced in China even as late as the twentieth century, public and official support was largely gone.

From China, alchemy seems to have spread to Japan, Tibet, and Burma and it may be that frequent trading contact between China and India opened the way for exchange of ideas on the subject. India certainly had an alchemical tradition of her own, because Indian alchemical works were often translated into Chinese, one of which at least can be dated to the early fifth century AD, and although the high period of Indian alchemy comes much later, in the tenth century, it is clear from their treatises that Indian alchemists were pursuing the same broad aims as their Chinese counterparts: transmutation of less-developed metals into gold and transformation of human bodies into a form which would prolong good health and attain immortality. One of the principal conduits of ideas between China and India, however, was 'Tantrism,' an amalgam of philosophical and religious ideas which suggested that the world of matter was real, not illusory, and that there was, therefore, no barrier between the spiritual and material worlds which could not be broken down by ritual practices designed to channel divine energy into a transformation of the material world. From the fourth or fifth century, then, this Tantrism, which seemed to meld with the philosophical requirements of alchemy, gave Indian a particular coloring and perhaps encouraged the development of elixirs at the expense of transmutation of metals. Tantrism, however, either brought or animated ideas and practices based on hatha yoga on the one hand and magic on the other, and so the Indian alchemist's laboratory might well be a space in which pharmacology met religious worship, distillation shook hands with sexual metaphors, and potentially poisonous substances conjoined with spiritual transcendence. But, as in China, enthusiasm for alchemy, whether gold making or elixir producing, waned somewhat after its early energetic period and although, again as in China, alchemy continues to be practiced in India nowadays, after the thirteenth or fourteenth century, interest and experiment were never quite as intense as they had been.

The history of alchemy further west, however, is rather different. There, Egypt was regarded as the cradle of the science, although attempts to derive 'alchemy' from Arabic *al-* ('the') and Greek *khem* ('black land,' i.e., Egypt) are somewhat dubious. Apart from one source (Pliny the Elder, first century AD) telling us that the Emperor Caligula extracted gold from orpiment, and a highly uncertain tradition that the Emperor Diocletian burned Egyptian alchemists' books in 290, evidence for the practice of alchemy in Egypt is actually rather thin, and it is not until about the second or third century AD that one finds both alchemical texts and references to earlier alchemical practitioners. Pseudo-Demokritos, possibly following Bolos of Mendes from the second century BC, provided practical recipes and mystical observations in his *Physika et Mystika*, as did 'Maria the Prophetess,' a shadowy figure often referred to by later authors as the inventor of certain pieces of alchemical apparatus. Two papyri collections from the third and fourth centuries AD (*Stockholm* and *Leiden X*) contain a mixture of recipes for coloring gemstones, manufacturing dyes, and making alloys which look like gold and silver. Then in the early fourth century came the much-quoted Zosimos, an Egyptian alchemist and mystic, who offered a pseudo-origin for alchemy

 http://dx.doi.org/10.1016/B978-0-12-386454-3.01226-4

in the teaching of angels, and whose references to and descriptions of practical alchemy were made to serve as allegories of a spiritual rather than a laboratorical transformation.

In spite of this, however, it was the practical side of alchemy which received detailed attention in Egypt, as in the later Byzantine Empire and Arabic revival and development of the science, and a tenth-century Byzantine encyclopedist's definition of alchemy as 'the fabrication of silver and gold' underlines the point. Alchemy seems to have come to the Arabs partly at least via Persia (Iran) where Christian communities had preserved both writings and knowledge of the science, and between the eighth and eleventh centuries it enjoyed a golden period, largely under the influence of three great names: Jābir ibn Hayyan (Geber), Abū Bakr Muhammad ibn Zakariya al-Rāzī (Rhazes), and Abū 'Aliāl-Husain ibn Sīnā (Avicenna). The first two of these were practitioners, the third was not, although his negative attitude to alchemy stimulated others to come to its defense, and while Arabic-language alchemical texts depended first on their earlier Greek counterparts, they quickly took over original research. Jābir proposed that metals happen as a result of a combination of 'mercury' and 'sulfur' in certain proportions and under specific celestial influences and that one of the principal aims of the alchemist is to discover the essential characteristics of each metal and bring these into a new balance, thereby altering the composition of the metal in question. Numerological computation was an essential skill in discovering these various balances, and so the alchemist had to be at least a competent mathematician, too. Al-Rāzī, for his part, was particularly interested in pharmacological therapy, and this led him to concentrate on the manufacture of drugs and elixirs, alchemical and non-alchemical, in his laboratory.

Each of these three had treatises attributed to him, so it is sometimes difficult to gauge exactly what opinions he actually had and which were fathered upon him. But it is via the corpus of works bearing their names that alchemy can be said to have passed to the West which then translated them into Latin. These translations began to appear in Spain during the twelfth century, but it was the thirteenth and fourteenth which saw Western fascination with alchemy really burgeon, encouraged by rulers' perpetual need for more money, and one finds that major scholars of the period – Albertus Magnus, St Thomas Aquinas, Roger Bacon, Arnald of Villanova, Ramon Lull – not only expressed interest in alchemy but also had alchemical works foisted upon them, too. Others, such as 'Ortulanus,' author of *True Alchemical Practice* (1386) and the Catalan Franciscan, John of Rupescissa (died 1362), provided practical observations on laboratory processes, although these were often couched in allegorical and metaphorical terms or, as in John's case, mixed with instructions on how to achieve transmutation of metals rendered less obscure because the coming birth of Antichrist and the subsequent arrival of the apocalypse demanded an honesty hitherto veiled in a language of secrets. Once the printing press arrived, knowledge of alchemy spread even more quickly and a readership – interested amateurs and eager professionals – for works of both practice and theory grew in proportion.

Geoffrey Chaucer, author of the *Canterbury Tales* (late 1380s), poked astringent fun at some of the pretensions and obscurities of many alchemical writers, pretensions which lent themselves to parody and satire. His alchemist was poor, dirty, slovenly, and stank of sulfur. He was always borrowing money – hence in part people's suspicions that alchemists merely took one's cash and fobbed one off with metallurgical tricks and nonsense – because alchemy was an expensive occupation. Breakages were frequent and the special equipment was not easy to replace. A fifteenth-century book attributed to Jābir describes various kinds of furnace, for example, which were to be used at different stages of the alchemical process: one for calcinations, another for sublimation, a third for 'descension' (separation of the desired liquefied material from extraneous matter), a fourth for smelting, a fifth for 'solution' (conversion of dry matter into liquid), and a sixth, known as the *athenor*, for 'fixation' (a process to make sure that any desired alteration in the alchemist's material would be stable). Then there were stills, condensers, crucibles, retorts, 'alembics' (a form of still), and evaporating dishes, all of which could be made of pottery or glass, and many of which had very particular shapes and therefore needed to be made or blown to order. The crowded clutter of an alchemist's laboratory can be seen in sixteenth-century woodcuts and seventeenth-century paintings, and the remains of a sixteenth-century alchemical laboratory have been unearthed in Austria, showing that the woodcuts and paintings were accurate in every detail. Over 300 clay crucibles, especially made to resist heat and chemical assault, and shallow ceramic plates called 'scorifiers' have been rescued, restored, and analyzed. What neither pictures nor archaeological relics can do, of course, is convey the stench, the heat, and the noise of these places which were kept going day and night for days and weeks at a time.

Satire and evidence of widespread distrust of alchemists, however, should not mislead one into thinking that alchemy was necessarily spurned or distrusted by everyone. Pope John XXII may have issued a decree against it, but Pope Leo X tolerated it, and monarchs and nobles were keen to support it in the hope of benefiting from the gold and silver they hoped it would produce; indeed, over the centuries there were sufficient apparently successful demonstrations of its abilities to ensure that alchemy would continue to enjoy a large measure of such support. English rulers issued licenses to individual practitioners and encouraged their researches, and the sixteenth and early seventeenth centuries saw at least one King of Denmark, two Electors, one King of Spain, one Queen of Sweden, and two Holy Roman Emperors witnessing public transmutations of base metal into gold before large and potentially skeptical audiences. The curious affair of so-called Rosicrucian pamphlets between 1604 and 1616, which suggested that a secret alchemical brotherhood was poised to reform Europe and introduce a period of peace and prosperity, was also taken seriously and made the science even more alluring. Failure, however, or discovery in the perpetration of fraud resulted in swift punishment. One such alchemist in Germany was tortured with red-hot pincers, then drawn and quartered, and his remains were hung from a public gibbet. Another was hanged on a gold-plated gallows, evidence of his ruler's sardonic sense of humor.

The Philosopher's Stone, as the final transformative substance was usually called, and whose reaction with baser metals caused the desired transmutation, was commonly described as a reddish powder. Producing it involved a lengthy process working with apparently toxic materials and a *prima materia* whose exact identification alchemists kept to themselves or concealed under a variety of extraordinary names. One says 'apparently toxic' because the alchemists' habit of using imagery and metaphorical language and of changing the terms they applied to their working substances means that we now find it difficult to be sure that, for example, when they spoke of 'vitriol,' they meant what we mean by it now. Martin Ruland's *Lexicon of Alchemy* (1612) provides several entries for it, some modified by reference to color. Thus, 'metallic vitriols are the salts of metals'; 'red vitriol is the perfect sulfur of the philosophers at the red stage'; 'white vitriol is white galitzen stone'; 'Roman vitriol is green atrament'; and for 'atrament,' he gives 32 separate definitions including ink (made from soot) and various forms of iron and copper sulfate. To add to the confusion, modern commentators regard 'oil of vitriol' as referring to sulfuric acid, which would make working with it highly dangerous.

Mercury, one of the three substances most commonly referred to by alchemists along with sulfur and salt, was certainly known as the material recognized by that name nowadays. It was used as a life-prolonging elixir, an ingredient in cosmetics, and was employed by at least some alchemists who sought to 'purify' it by cleansing it with distilled sal ammoniac or copperas or vinegar. On the other hand, developing alchemical theory proposed that just as humans are composed of spirit, soul, and body, so metals consist of mercury, sulfur, and salt. "Mercury is the spirit, sulphur is the soul, and salt is the body," wrote the Swiss physician and alchemist Paracelsus in 1537. So when alchemical texts mention mercury, do they mean the chemical element or the metallic principle? "You must always be careful to distinguish what is generally and particularly stated concerning mercury," warned Ruland, "as to whether it be about ordinary mercury or about our [*i.e. alchemical*] mercury. Do not make a mistake, otherwise the information will be useless." Likewise, sulfur presents two general possibilities. Ruland again: "Ordinary sulphur, by whatever name we call it, remains an enemy of all metals. It consumes, blackens, and destroys. But philosophical [*i.e. alchemical*] sulphur is life-giving, matures and blackens, but does not destroy." Hence it follows that 'salt' had more than one meaning and, indeed, was applied as a general term to various substances including borax (*sal albus*), sal ammoniac, niter, saltpeter, alum, mercury, urine, calcinated tartar, and common rock salt. Trying to identify the components of alchemical experiments at any given time is thus fraught with difficulty, and it is quite possible that some commentators have been overconfident in their assertions that *X* alchemical substance is what we know as *Y*.

Paracelsus (1493–1541) illustrates this well. He recognized a wide variety of substances under a single alchemical principle: for example, his 'salt' seems to have included potassium nitrate, the vitriols of copper, iron, and magnesium, and the salts generated by mercury, arsenic, antimony, and lead. To him, alchemy was most important as an adjunct of medicine, and he was convinced that the human body acted as a kind of alchemical laboratory, separating pure substances from impure. "Everything," he wrote in his *Volumen Medicinae Paramirum* (*c.*1520), "is perfect in itself, but both a poison and a benefit to something else," and elsewhere, "Arsenic is the most poisonous of substances and a drachm of it will kill a horse. But fire it with salt of nitre and it is no longer a poison." Hence if a toxic substance is introduced into the body, (while taking nourishment, for instance), its effects can be combated by the administration of another poison whose therapeutic action purifies the affected organ or organs and therefore cures the illness or at least offers some kind of palliation. In order for the curative or palliative poison to work beneficially, of course, its dosage should be very small. This was crucial. "Only the dose allows something to avoid being poisonous," he wrote, and clearly this must have been true of his use of *arcanum vitrioli* ('the secret thing enclosed in vitriol') mixed in wine to treat epilepsy, His 'oil of vitriol,' on the other hand, which he employed for skin complaints of various kinds, seems to have been corrosive and therefore very painful. Once again, however, it may be difficult to elicit from his descriptions exactly what it was he would use in his recipes. "There are many kinds of vitriol," he says, noting that "[it] offers a complete cure of jaundice, sands and stones, fevers, worms and falling-sickness ... [as well as] for surgical diseases such as hereditary scabies, leprosy, ringworm, etc. .... These are vigorously attacked by vitriol, which cures them from the root" (*Diseases Which Deprive People of Their Reason*, written *c.*1528). Not surprisingly, therefore, Paracelsus appears to have had a reputation among his contemporaries for poisoning his patients, and has been given another by moderns, 'the Father of Toxicology.'

Alchemists, then, dealt with substances which were often highly toxic but, like Paracelsus, were concerned more with the ultimate uses to which their derivatives could be put rather than the poisonous properties those substances contained. So in view of the dubious nature of many of those substances, it is not surprising to find that alchemists were convinced they had to reduce their basic ingredients by fire, liquefy them, and distil them over and over again, many hundreds of times. This rendered them 'safe.' Then practitioners carefully watched for distinctive changes, usually signified in rapid changes of color known as the 'Peacock's Tail' before the material finally settled into the desired red. These procedures fell into three principal stages: (1) the black stage during which the basic material was broken down ('died') and reconstituted as something different; (2) the multiple color stage; and (3) the red stage out of which the Stone emerged, and it was during the course of these procedures that medicinal elixirs and tinctures were usually obtained. 'Rectified aqueous alcohol,' for example, was to be dripped slowly over the residue left after producing the Stone, and this would result in a golden-reddish clear liquid which, taken in wine, was said to cure any ailment. Metaphorical language – that of death, marriage, birth, and regeneration – was used to describe these various stages, as was that of sacramental theology, and so alchemical writings frequently offer a combination of chemistry and Christian mysticism. It is this which seems to account for the deep interest and unwearied experimental efforts of such people as Andreas Libavius, George Starkey ('Eugenius Philalethes'), Robert Boyle, and Isaac Newton, and even Emmanuel Swedenborg who was hostile to alchemy pursued his chemical experiments in the light of his deeply particular and personal religious convictions. Newton, on the other hand, was deeply devoted to alchemy and doggedly pursued it for mainly religious reasons, on the grounds that if alchemy could show that there was some kind of universal spirit responsible for both creation and the workings of creation, it would provide important evidence for God's active presence in the universe.

But the eighteenth century did alchemy few favors. Charlatans continued to flourish, as did secret and not so secret societies offering pseudo-mystical experiences to their members. Worried that these might tarnish the respectability of the growing number of scientific bodies both within and outwith academic circles, experimenters began to withdraw from the wider rough and tumble and concentrate on more limited, more specialized, less controversial fields of inquiry. Even so, alchemy was still being practiced at Harvard in the early years of the century, although by the middle of the nineteenth chemists had carefully and successfully distinguished themselves from alchemists, and interested observers such as Ethan Hitchcock, an adviser to Abraham Lincoln, preferred to regard alchemy as a spiritual discipline rather than a laboratory activity. Many in the nineteenth and the twentieth centuries agreed with him, and yet that did not stop dedicated individuals from persisting with practical alchemical work. Theodore Tiffereau, for example, conducted experiments between 1854 and 1855 to transmute Mexican silver into gold using, among other materials, nitric acid, hyponitrous acid, nitrogen peroxide, and concentrated sulfuric acid, with trace amounts of gold to act as reagents. He was followed in the 1890s by Stephen Emmens who attempted much the same kind of process and persuaded the United States Mint to buy a large quantity of the gold thus produced.

Between 1908 and 1920 when he published the results of his work, François Jollivet-Castelot also transmuted silver into gold by using orpiment, antimony sulfide, tellurium, nitric acid, and a little pure silica, along with gold reagents, these experiments being replicated by others, apparently with some degree of success. But while the early twentieth century saw continued efforts to produce alchemical gold, the attention of alchemists was beginning to turn toward spagyric medicine and the manufacture of health-giving elixirs. Husband and wife Richard and Isabella Ingalese, for example, while claiming to have made the Philosopher's Stone between 1917 and 1920, made the more astonishing report that in 1917 they had succeeded in producing the white stone of the philosophers – an alchemical product preliminary to the final red Stone – and had used this to resuscitate a dead woman who then lived for a further 7 years. In England, Archibald Cockren worked on various transmuting tinctures during the 1930s, producing among others one which he called 'philosophic gold,' until at last he was successful in manufacturing the red Stone itself. Armand Barbault in France during the 1960s and 1970s worked with dew, earth, and plants as his basic materials, adding powdered gold at one stage in the process with a view to producing a series of transformative elixirs, and likewise Albert Riedel (better known as 'Frater Albertus'), basing his alchemy on Paracelsus's proposition that matter consists of three principles – spirit/mercury, sulfur/soul, and body/salt – worked mainly with plants to produce therapeutic elixirs.

The twentieth century also saw a growing interest in promoting alchemy as a system of spiritual exploration and regeneration, sometimes, however, working alongside laboratory experiments. This, for Frater Albertus, was one crucial difference between alchemy and chemistry. Another was that 'any poison can be removed alchemically from any herb or metal and its healing and curing properties set free.' These principles, too, were important for Jean Dubuis, nuclear physicist and alchemist, who founded *Les Philosophes de Nature* in 1979, and for various online alchemical organizations such as the Paracelsus College and the Spagyricus Institute. But has alchemy ever genuinely succeeded in the transmutation of baser metal into gold? By way of answer, history points to three medallions in the Kunsthistorisches Museum in Vienna, one silver and two gold, which claim to be the results of transmutations successfully performed before witnesses in 1675, 1677, and 1716, and another example in the British Museum in London, dated 1814.

See also: Chemical Interactions; The History of Toxicology; Antimony; Bismuth; Copper; Gold; Lead; Mercury; Metals; Silver; Sulfuric Acid.

Further Reading

Alchemy website. www.levity.com/alchemy/.
Ball, P., 2006. The Devil's Doctor: Paracelsus and the World of Renaissance Magic and Science. William Heinemann, London.
Burland, C.A., 1967. The Arts of the Alchemist. Weidenfeld & Nicolson, London.
Crisciani, C., 2002. Il papa e l'alchimia. Viella, Roma, Italy.
Dobbs, B.J.T., 1975. The Foundations of Newton's Alchemy. Cambridge University Press, Cambridge.
Greiner, F., 1998. Aspects de la tradition alchimique au xviie siècle. SEHA-ARCHE, Paris–Milan.
Maxwell-Stuart, P.G., 2008. The Chemical Choir: A History of Alchemy. Continuum, London.
Moran, B.T., 2005. Distilling Knowledge: Alchemy, Chemistry, and the Scientific Revolution. Harvard University Press, Cambridge, MA.
Newman, W.R., 2006. Atoms and Alchemy. University of Chicago Press, Chicago and London.
Newman, W.R., Principe, L.M., 2002. Alchemy Tried in the Fire. University of Chicago Press, Chicago and London.
Nummendal, T., 2007. Alchemy and Authority in the Holy Roman Empire. University of Chicago Press, Chicago and London.
Patai, R., 1994. The Jewish Alchemists. Princeton University Press, Princeton, NJ.
Principe, L.M., 1998. The Aspiring Adept: Robert Boyle and His Alchemical Quest. Princeton University Press, Princeton, NJ.
Roberts, G., 1994. The Mirror of Alchemy. The British Library, London.
Szydlo, Z., 1994. Water Which Does Not Wet Hands. Polish Academy of Sciences, Warsaw, Portland.

Alcoholic Beverages and Health Effects

K Shankar, University of Arkansas for Medical Sciences, Little Rock, AR, USA
HM Mehendale, University of Louisiana at Monroe, Monroe, LA, USA

Human consumption of alcoholic beverages dates back to the earliest periods of recorded history. Beer was a widely popular beverage in ancient Egypt in the 2nd millennium BC, as was wine in the Greek and Roman civilizations. Distillation of alcohol, originally developed by the Arabs, was quickly adapted among all regions of the world, including Europe, Asia, and the Far East, as early as the thirteenth and fourteenth centuries. A variety of alcoholic beverages are legally consumed in most countries, and more than 100 countries have implemented laws regulating their production, sale, and consumption; however, most countries have set the minimum age at which a person may legally buy or drink alcohol containing products. This minimum allowable drinking age varies in countries, averaging to 18 years in most areas. Today, approximately 60% of the adult US population consumes alcohol, having had at least 12 drinks in the past year. Although most people who drink do it safely, approximately 18.2 million Americans or 7.6% of the population meet the diagnostic criteria for alcohol use disorder. Alcohol abuse may be the number one health issue in the United States with annual cost estimates of more than US $185 billion a year (NIAAA estimate of 1998). More than one-half of American adults have a close family member who has or has had alcoholism. Almost 2.7 million violent crimes (or one in every three violent crimes) and 16 000 traffic accidents can be directly linked to alcohol. Alcohol consumption has consequences for the health and well-being of those who drink and, by extension, the lives of those around them. Because alcoholism affects many aspects of our society, clearly alcoholism has enormous social implications including burden on social and health services. Epidemiological studies with twins, families, and adoptive families clearly indicate an important role for an individual's genetics in determining the likelihood for developing alcoholism. The Centers for Disease Control and Prevention (CDC) has developed an online resource called the Alcohol-related Disease Impact software to estimate the impact of alcohol-related deaths and years of potential life lost.

In the United States, a 'drink' is considered to be 0.5 ounces (oz) or 15 g of alcohol, which is equivalent to 12 oz of beer, 8 oz of malt liquor, 5 oz of wine, or 1.5 oz of 80 proof distilled spirits (gin, rum, vodka, and whiskey). According to the Dietary Guidelines for Americans, jointly issued by the US Department of Agriculture and the US Department of Health and Human Services, moderate drinking is no more than two standard drinks per day for men and no more than one per day for women. Moderate drinking may be defined as drinking that does not generally cause problems, either for the drinker or for society. The term is often confused with 'social drinking,' which refers to drinking patterns that are accepted by the society in which they occur. However, social drinking is not necessarily free of problems. The National Institute on Alcohol Abuse and Alcoholism further recommends that people aged 65 and older limit their consumption of alcohol to one drink per day. Alcoholism, also known as 'alcohol dependence,' is a disease that includes four symptoms: (1) **Craving:** A strong need, or compulsion, to drink. (2) **Loss of control:** The inability to limit one's drinking on any given occasion. (3) **Physical dependence:** Withdrawal symptoms, such as nausea, sweating, shakiness, and anxiety, that occur when alcohol use is stopped after a period of heavy drinking. (4) **Tolerance:** The need to drink greater amounts of alcohol in order to 'get high.'

Health Effects of Alcohol Abuse

Effects of Alcohol on the Liver

Alcohol abuse significantly contributes to liver-related morbidity and mortality worldwide. Long-term alcohol use is the leading cause of illness and death from liver disease. There are three phases of alcohol-induced liver damage: alcoholic fatty liver, which is usually reversible with abstinence; alcoholic hepatitis or inflammation; and alcoholic cirrhosis or scarring of the liver. Patients with both alcoholic cirrhosis and hepatitis have a death rate of more than 60% over a 4-year period. The prognosis is bleaker than the outlook for many types of cancers. As many as 900 000 people in the United States suffer from cirrhosis and some 26 000 of these die each year. The risk for liver disease is related to how much a person drinks: the risk is low at levels of alcohol consumption but steeply increases with higher levels of consumption. Because effects of alcohol are dose-related and because of the steepness at which the adverse effects are observed, **moderation** is emphasized in social or occasional drinking. Gender also plays a role in the development of alcohol-induced liver damage. Some evidence indicates that women are more susceptible to the cumulative effects of alcohol on the liver.

Alcohol Consumption and Obesity

Obesity has reached epidemic proportions in many Western countries and its incidence continues to grow the world over. The etiology of obesity is complex and both diet and genetics play important roles. Since a gram of alcohol provides 7.1 kcal of energy and comes just after fat as a potential source of energy, it is possible that calories from alcohol contribute to body-weight gain. Furthermore, alcohol cannot be stored and hence is oxidized right after consumption, sparing fat and carbohydrates. In consumers, alcohol calories can vary from 0 to 25% of total daily calories and are frequently added over calories from food and other beverages. Currently it is unclear, however, whether alcohol consumption is a risk factor for weight gain because studies performed to date show positive, negative, and no association. Overall the evidence that alcohol may increase weight gain is evident only in studies with high levels of drinking. Moreover, light to moderate drinking especially of red wine may protect from weight gain.

 http://dx.doi.org/10.1016/B978-0-12-386454-3.00227-X

Cancer and Alcohol Abuse

Alcohol has been linked to a number of cancers, including cancers of the head and neck, digestive tract, and breast. Alcohol is clearly established as a cause of cancer of various tissues in the airway and digestive tract, including the mouth, pharynx, larynx, and esophagus. There is convincing evidence that alcohol consumption increases the risk of breast cancer. Research suggests that the risk of cancers is associated with both the concentration of alcohol and the number of drinks consumed. Alcohol acts synergistically with tobacco to dramatically increase the risk of cancers above that of alcohol or tobacco alone. An increased risk of stomach cancer among alcohol drinkers has been identified in several but not the majority of studies. The link between alcohol use and chronic gastritis is clear, although the progression from chronic gastritis to neoplasia is less well understood and involves factors in addition to alcohol. Only weak positive association between alcohol use and cancers of the colon, rectum, and breast exists.

Cardiovascular Health and Alcohol Use

Cardiovascular diseases account for more deaths among Americans than any other group of diseases. Of all causes of death, coronary heart disease (CHD) is the leading cause of death among Americans. Several large prospective studies throughout the world suggest a reduced risk of CHD with alcohol use over a wide range of consumption levels. However, in these studies the apparent protective effects of alcohol against CHD were realized at low to moderate levels of alcohol (ranging from one to two drinks per week to one to two drinks per day). However, the risk increased at drinking levels above five drinks a day for men and two drinks a day for women. Both the type of alcoholic beverage consumed and the pattern of drinking (small amounts every day versus large amounts on only one or two days a week) influence protection against CHD. Long-term alcohol consumption is known to induce megamitochondria formation in heart tissue, thus compromising optimal functioning of cardiac myocytes. The relationship between alcohol consumption and stroke risk suggests that heavy drinking increases the risk of stroke, especially in women. However, evidence suggesting that moderate level of alcohol consumption protects from stroke is at best equivocal. In addition, it appears that a high level of alcohol consumption increases blood pressure, a critical risk factor for stroke. Hypertension could be another consequence.

Alcohol and the Skeleton

An association between alcohol intake and accidental injury is well established. The risk of falling is tripled in those having a blood alcohol concentration (BAC) of 0.1–0.15% and 60 times higher in those with a BAC of 0.16% or higher, compared with those whose BAC is 0.1% or lower. Beyond the risks of falling, however, emerging evidence suggests alcoholics may also suffer from a generalized skeletal fragility, leading to alcohol-induced osteopenia. Although the degree to which alcohol contributes to the osteopenia in the general population is not clear, but data from experimental animal studies suggest that alcohol can disrupt the tightly coupled processes of bone formation and resorption.

Fetal Alcohol Syndrome

Fetal alcohol syndrome (FAS) is a set of birth defects caused by maternal consumption of alcohol during pregnancy. FAS is considered the most common preventable cause of mental retardation. The annual cost of FAS according to the 10th Special Report to the US Congress on Alcohol and Health estimated the annual cost of FAS in 1998 to be $2.8 billion.

Miscellaneous Impacts of Alcohol Consumption

Alcohol is converted by alcohol dehydrogenase (ADH) to acetaldehyde, which is converted by aldehyde dehydrogenase to acetic acid, then to CO_2 and water in the Krebs cycle. The rate of metabolism is zero order – i.e., it is not concentration dependent (about $7\ g\ h^{-1}$) at BACs $> 0.02\ g\ l^{-1}$. Cytochrome P450 ethanol oxidation by CYP2E1, CYP3A4, and CYP2E1 is inducible and greater in chronic heavy drinkers, accounting for an increased rate of metabolism at high BACs. Ethanol metabolism produces reduced NAD (NADH), and in turn NADH reduces ability of liver to produce UDP-glucuronic acid, necessary for glucuronidation of morphine and other drugs. Individuals on morphine-containing medications are faced with such situations. In contrast, acute ethanol can inhibit CYP3A4, thus increasing morphine effects. Chronic ethanol induces CYP3A4, increasing morphine metabolism and thus reducing its effects. Likewise, chronic ethanol induces a number of cytochrome P450 isozymes (2E1, 3A4, and 1A2), and CYP3A4 and CYP1A2 can contribute to an increased rate of methadone metabolism in alcoholics, leading to reduced methadone efficacy. Alcoholics can also develop severe liver disease leading to an alteration in methadone disposition (Kreek, 1988). A majority of the literature supports the notion that alcohol-containing beverages can considerably influence metabolism of drugs and chemicals in the body (Ray and Mehendale, 1990).

It is important to recognize that a number of alcoholic beverages may naturally contain small amounts of *n*-butanol, a four-carbon alcohol, due to fermentation. Detectable amounts are found in beer, grape brandies, wine, whisky, and a variety of food products. It is also formed during deep frying of corn oil, cottonseed oil, trilinolein, and triolein, and is often used as an ingredient in processed and artificial flavorings. Improperly processed country liquors are the main source of contamination.

See also: Ethanol; Fetal Alcohol Spectrum Disorders; Immune System; Liver.

Further Reading

Agrawal, A., Freedman, N.D., Cheng, Y.C., et al., 2012. Measuring alcohol consumption for genomic meta-analyses of alcohol intake: opportunities and challenges. GENEVA Consortium. Am. J. Clin. Nutr. 95 (3), 539–547.

Centers for Disease Control and Prevention (CDC). Alcohol-Related Disease Impact (ARDI). Atlanta, GA: CDC. Available at: http://www.cdc.gov/alcohol/ardi.htm.

de Leiris, J., Besse, S., Boucher, F., 2010. Diet and heart health: moderate wine drinking strengthens the cardioprotective effects of fish consumption. Curr. Pharm. Biotechnol. 11 (8), 911–921.

Giacosa, A., Adam-Blondon, A.F., Baer-Sinnott, S., et al., 2012. Alcohol and wine in relation to cancer and other diseases. Eur. J. Cancer Prev. 21 (1), 103–108.

Hughes, K., Quigg, Z., Eckley, L., et al., 2011. Environmental factors in drinking venues and alcohol-related harm: the evidence base for European intervention. Addiction 106 (Suppl 1), 37–46. http://dx.doi.org/10.1111/j.1360-0443.2010.03316.x.

NIAAA Resources on Alcohol Consumption and Alcohol-Related Problems. http://www.niaaa.nih.gov/publications.

Ray, S.D., Mehendale, H.M., 1990. Potentiation of CCl_4 and $CHCl_3$ hepatotoxicity and lethality by various alcohols. Fund. Appl. Toxicol. 15 (3), 429–440.

Salaspuro, M., 2011. Acetaldehyde and gastric cancer. J. Dig. Dis. 12 (2), 51–59. http://dx.doi.org/10.1111/j.1751-2980.2011.00480.x.

Sayon-Orea, C., Martinez-Gonzalez, M.A., Bes-Rastrollo, M., 2011. Alcohol consumption and body weight: a systematic review. Nutr. Rev. 69 (8), 419–431. http://dx.doi.org/10.1111/j.1753-4887.2011.00403.x.

Singer, M.V., Feick, P., Gerloff, A., 2011. Alcohol and smoking. Dig. Dis. 29 (2), 177–183.

Smoliga, J.M., Baur, J.A., Hausenblas, H.A., 2011. Resveratrol and health – a comprehensive review of human clinical trials. Mol. Nutr. Food Res. 55 (8), 1129–1141. http://dx.doi.org/10.1002/mnfr.201100143.

Tariba, B., 2011. Metals in wine–impact on wine quality and health outcomes. Biol. Trace Elem. Res. 144 (1–3), 143–156.

U.S. Substance Abuse and Mental Health Services Administration. http://www.samhsa.gov/.

10th Special Report to the U.S. Congress on Alcohol and Health. U.S. Department of Health and Human Services. http://pubs.niaaa.nih.gov/publications/10report/intro.pdf.

Alcoholism *see* Alcoholic Beverages and Health Effects

Alcohols *see* Alcoholic Beverages and Health Effects; Allyl Alcohol; Benzyl Alcohol; Ethanol

Aldicarb

VC Moser, Toxicity Assessment Division, NHEERL/ORD, US Environmental Protection Agency, NC, USA

This article is a revision of the previous edition article by Paul R. Harp, volume 2, pp 64–66, © 2005, Elsevier Inc.

The views expressed in this paper are those of the author and do not necessarily reflect the views or policies of the US Environmental Protection Agency.

- IUPAC Name: [(E)-(2-methyl-2-methylsulfanylpropylidene) amino] *N*-methyl carbamate
- Synonyms: Aldicarbe; Temik®; ENT 27093; UC21149; RCRA waste number P070; AI3-27093; OMS 771; NCI C08640; SHA 098301
- Chemical Structure:

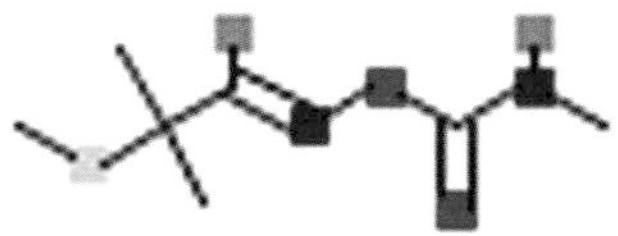

Background

Aldicarb was introduced in 1970, and within a decade its use was restricted due to high levels of water contamination and food residues. In 1981, aldicarb was classified as a restricted use pesticide (used only by certified applicators), and in 1984 was placed under US EPA Special Review. Aldicarb is one of the most potent *N*-methyl carbamate insecticides, and has undergone extensive field, laboratory, and human studies.

Uses

Aldicarb is a systemic insecticide and nematicide used on a variety of agricultural crops, including cotton, potatoes, and citrus. It is commercially sold only as a granular formulation (primarily containing 15% active ingredient), which is to be incorporated into the soil to provide maximum efficacy and to minimize hazard to birds and other wildlife. Dietary risk and ground water contamination have been the primary concerns for the use of aldicarb. Following recent assessments based on additional toxicity data, the US EPA determined that residues found in citrus and potatoes may pose unacceptable dietary risks to infants and children. Subsequently, discussions with the current registrant resulted in additional risk mitigation measures and lowered application rates for remaining uses, leading to a voluntary phase-out of all uses in the United States by 2018.

Environmental Fate and Behavior

Aldicarb rapidly degrades to the sulfoxide and sulfone forms, which are moderately persistent. These chemicals are highly soluble in water and mobile in soil. They have been detected at high levels in ground water and have contaminated wells and drinking water supplies. Breakdown and persistence in soil and water depends on bacteria, sunlight, moisture, and a number of other factors, leading to wide variations in estimates of environmental exposures. Being a systemic insecticide, residues have also been detected in food products.

Exposure and Exposure Monitoring

Environmental measures of aldicarb exposure should include parent, sulfoxide, and sulfone; indeed, maximum residue levels are expressed as the sum of these. Water contamination is monitored through the US National Primary Drinking Water Regulations.

Toxicokinetics

Toxicokinetic parameters are similar across species. Aldicarb is rapidly and well-absorbed through the oral, dermal, and inhalation routes of exposure. Upon uptake, it is quickly metabolized and excreted. Oxidation reactions rapidly convert aldicarb to aldicarb sulfoxide, which is as toxic as the parent, with slower and lesser formation of the less-toxic sulfone. Hydrolysis pathways yield inactive oximes and nitriles. Limited studies suggest that aldicarb is detoxified to some extent by carboxylesterases. Animal studies have indicated aldicarb and its metabolites are widely distributed to tissues, including fetal tissue. Tissue accumulation has not been reported. The major route of excretion is urinary, with at least 80% of the dose eliminated within 24 h. A minor route of biliary elimination undergoes enterohepatic recirculation, and small amounts are excreted in feces and milk.

 http://dx.doi.org/10.1016/B978-0-12-386454-3.00093-2

Mechanisms of Toxicity

Aldicarb (and its sulfoxide metabolite) binds and inhibits acetylcholinesterase, the enzyme responsible for metabolizing the neurotransmitter acetylcholine at cholinergic nerve terminals. The resultant accumulation of synaptic acetylcholine causes overstimulation of the cholinergic pathways and produces central and peripheral toxicities. This action leads to signs of cholinergic crisis, including sweating, nausea, dizziness, miosis, blurred vision, abdominal pain, vomiting, and diarrhea, progressing to tremors, convulsions, and death. The acetylcholinesterase inhibition is readily reversible with rapid reactivation occurring through spontaneous decarbamylation, and recovery of function is evident within minutes to hours. Recent *in vitro* and *in vivo* studies have suggested that aldicarb could damage tissue *via* oxidative stress, which may play an additional role in its toxicity.

Acute and Short Term Toxicity

Animal

Signs of acute exposure in animals are due to acetylcholinesterase inhibition and mirror effects of other *N*-methyl carbamates. Aldicarb is very potent, with lethality associated with cholinesterase inhibition occurring at doses less than 1 mg kg^{-1} in most species. There is evidence from comparative studies in rats that the young may be more sensitive than adults to these acute effects. Aldicarb is not a skin irritant and does not cause dermal sensitization.

The signs of acute exposure to aldicarb in animals are consistent with dose-dependent cholinergic stimulation. High-dose exposures produce frank toxicity and cholinergic signs, whereas lower exposures result in more subtle physiological (e.g., heart rate), neuromuscular (e.g., motor function), and behavioral (e.g., cognition) changes. In laboratory studies, these changes may be detected with a variety of behavioral assessments.

Human

Humans exposed to aldicarb show the same toxic signs and symptoms as seen with experimental animals, with rapid onset and recovery. Mild cases of exposure, sufficient to produce sweating, headache, and nausea, may be confused with the flu. The ingestion of contaminated foods and accidental exposures to workers have resulted in a number of human poisoning incidents, some quite severe. Several outbreaks of food poisoning, involving up to hundreds of affected individuals, have implicated improperly treated crops, e.g., cucumbers, watermelons, and bananas.

Chronic Toxicity

Animal

With repeated exposures, acetylcholinesterase inhibition remains the predominant form of toxicity, and there is little evidence of progressive or chronic effects. Aldicarb does not inhibit neurotoxic esterase (NTE) and does not produce delayed neuropathy. When administered in water or diet, higher doses may be tolerated compared to acute (bolus) administration.

Human

Data on chronic toxicity are not available. The few epidemiological studies in the literature do not show causal relationships between aldicarb exposure and long-term adverse outcomes.

Immunotoxicity

Several immunotoxicity studies report contradictory results using a measure of antibody production (humoral immunity), and other studies suggest alterations in macrophage function. Thus, immunological findings are inconclusive.

Reproductive Toxicity

Several developmental studies, including multigenerational, in laboratory animals showed no evidence of embryotoxicity, fetotoxicity, or teratogenicity at doses that are not overtly maternally toxic.

Genotoxicity

Although a few mutagenicity assays were positive with aldicarb, the weight of evidence from a range of *in vitro* and *in vivo* studies support conclusions that aldicarb is not a mutagen.

Carcinogenicity

Studies show that aldicarb is not carcinogenic.

Clinical Management

Persons providing medical assistance should avoid contact with contaminated clothing, which should be removed and discarded. Exposed dermal areas should be cleaned thoroughly with soap and water, and eyes should be flushed with generous amounts of clean water for at least 15 min. If the patient is not in a life-threatening condition, and is treated soon after exposure, activated charcoal may be used to reduce absorption from the gastrointestinal tract. Gastric lavage should be considered if more toxic quantities have been ingested, if possible within 1 h of exposure.

Emergency management should not be delayed. Support for the airway, breathing, and circulation of the patient is most important. Patients may have excessive secretions, bronchorrhea, bronchospasm, and weakness of respiratory muscles; intubation and mechanical ventilation may be necessary. Muscarinic effects (e.g., salivation, lacrimation) may be reduced by administration of atropine, with repeated high doses until pulmonary secretions dissipate. Benzodiazepines may be used to control seizure. The use of pralidoxime is controversial, but may be useful if poisoning includes organophosphorus compounds. Some clinical reports suggest it is contraindicated for carbamate-only poisoning, whereas others have reported that it is effective in reducing morbidity and mortality in severe poisonings. Furosemide may be useful for pulmonary edema that continues after atropinization.

Plasma or RBC cholinesterase measurements may be used to indicate the type of agent involved, but due to the rapid reversibility of the inhibition produced by carbamates, such laboratory assays may not be accurate and in fact could be misleading. Metabolite analysis of a urine sample may allow confirmation of the pesticide.

Ecotoxicity

Aldicarb is extremely toxic to birds, and moderately toxic to fish, bees, and wildlife. Exposures of nontarget species occur from contaminated water or consumption of applied granules. Bioaccumulation in the environmental and bioconcentration in tissues are low.

Exposure Standards and Guidelines

The US EPA acute reference dose for aldicarb is 0.001 $mg\,kg^{-1}$, based on RBC cholinesterase inhibition studies in humans. With incorporation of an additional factor to assure safety to infants and children, the US EPA population adjusted dose becomes 0.00027 $mg\,kg^{-1}$. The Joint FAO/WHO Meeting on Pesticide Residues established an acceptable daily intake value of 0.003 $mg\,kg^{-1}$, but this has not been reevaluated in 10 years. The proposed US EPA maximum contaminant level (MCL) for aldicarb and its sulfoxide in drinking water is 0.003 $mg\,l^{-1}$, and for aldicarb sulfone is 0.004 $mg\,l^{-1}$; for each chemical the MCL goal is 0.001 $mg\,l^{-1}$.

See also: Carbamate Pesticides; Cholinesterase Inhibition; Common Mechanism of Toxicity in Pesticides; Neurotoxicity.

Further Reading

Baron, R.L., 1994. A carbamate insecticide: A case study of aldicarb. Environ. Health Perspect. 102 (Suppl. 11), 23–27.

Goldman, L.R., Beller, M., Jackson, R.J., 1990. Aldicarb food poisonings in California, 1985–1988: Toxicity estimates for humans. Arch. Environ. Health 45, 141–147.

Gupta, R.C., 2006. Toxicology of Organophosphate and Carbamate Compounds. Elsevier, New York.

Moore, D.R., Teed, R.S., Rodney, S.I., Thompson, R.P., Fischer, D.L., 2010. Refined avian risk assessment for aldicarb in the United States. Integr. Environ. Assess. Manag. 6, 83–101.

Moore, D.R., Thompson, R.P., Rodney, S.I., Fischer, D., Ramanarayanan, T., Hall, T., 2010. Refined aquatic risk assessment for aldicarb in the United States. Integr. Environ. Assess. Manag. 6, 102–118.

Pelekis, M., Emond, C., 2009. Physiological modeling and derivation of the rat to human toxicokinetic uncertainty factor for the carbamate pesticide aldicarb. Environ. Toxicol. Pharmacol. 28, 179–191.

Risher, J.F., Mink, F.L., Stara, J.F., 1987. The toxicologic effects of the carbamate insecticide aldicarb in mammals: A review. Environ. Health Perspect. 72, 267–281.

Ritter, W.F., 1990. Pesticide contamination of ground water in the United States: A review. J. Environ. Sci. Health Part B 25, 1–29.

Wolfe, M.F., Seiber, J.N., 1993. Environmental activation of pesticides. Occup. Med. 8, 561–573.

Relevant Websites

http://www.epa.gov/oppsrrd1/REDs/factsheets/aldicarb_fs.html – background and recent regulatory actions in US.

http://www.inchem.org/documents/jmpr/jmpmono/v92pr03.htm – information from the International Programme on Chemical Safety.

http://www.epa.gov/pesticides/safety/healthcare/handbook/Chap05.pdf – recognition and treatment of carbamate poisoning.

Aldosterone *see* Corticosteroids

Aldrin

M Honeycutt and S Shirley, Austin, TX, USA

This article is a revision of the previous edition article by Benny L. Blaylock, volume 1, pp 66–68, © 2005, Elsevier Inc.

Background

- Chemical Abstracts Service Registry Number: CAS 309-00-2
- RTECS: IO2000000
- Chemical Name: 1,2,3,4,10,10-Hexachloro-1,4,4α,5,8,8α-hexahydro-1,4-*endo,exo*-5,8-dimethanonaphthalene, abbreviated HHDN
- Molecular Formula: $C_{12}H_8Cl_6$
- Relative Molecular Mass: 364.91
- Chemical Structure:

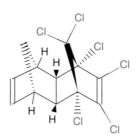

- Trade Names: Aldocit, Aldrex, Aldrosol, Compound 118, Drinox, ENT 15,949, Hexachlorohexahydro-endo, exo-dimethanonaphthalene, HHDN, Kortofin, Octalene, OMS 194, Seedrin

Uses

Aldrin (CAS 309-00-2) is a synthetic organochlorine pesticide, and was used as a broad-spectrum soil insecticide for protection of food crops, and as seed dressing for the control of pests such as ants and termites. In 1972, the US Environmental Protection Agency (USEPA) canceled all but three specific uses: subsurface termite control, dipping of nonfood plant roots and tops, and completely contained moth-proofing in the manufacturing processes. In 1987, all uses were voluntarily canceled by the manufacturer. Aldrin has not been produced domestically since 1974, or imported after 1985.

Environmental Fate and Behavior

Relevant Physicochemical Properties

Aldrin is a crystalline solid with a melting point of 104–105.5 °C. It has a vapor pressure of 1.2×10^{-4} mm Hg at 25 °C, a log organic carbon partition coefficient of 7.67, and is practically insoluble in water (0.027 mg l^{-1} at 27 °C, also reported as 0.2 mg l^{-1} at 25 °C). Aldrin has a log octanol–water partition coefficient of 6.50 and a density of 1.6–1.7 g cc^{-1}, at 20 °C.

Partition Behavior in Water, Sediment, and Soil

Consistent with its intended use on insects in soil, aldrin is not very water soluble. It binds to sediment, but rarely leaches into deeper soil layers and groundwater. Aldrin is volatile and readily degrades to dieldrin in the environment. When aldrin is applied to silty loam soil, the amount detectable in 1.7 years will have declined by 25% of the amount applied. Aldrin is estimated to have a half-life in soil of 1.5–5.2 years, depending on the composition of the soil.

Environmental Persistence

Persistence is defined in terms of the half-life of a substance in the soil. For aldrin, this has been determined to be 2–15 years. Aldrin is largely converted via biological or abiotic mechanisms to dieldrin, which is significantly more persistent. Both aldrin and dieldrin are absorbed into the food chain. Residues may remain in the soil for a long period, if contaminated plant and animal materials are added to the topsoil. Aldrin and dieldrin are retained in the fatty materials of sewage sludge, and in fish emulsions used as fertilizers. Topical soil application of these materials makes these compounds available to grazing animals, which ingest some soil when they crop grass. Aldrin may be volatilized from sediment, and redistributed by air currents, contaminating distant areas. Nationally, levels of aldrin have declined since agricultural uses were discontinued.

Long-Range Transport

The atmospheric photooxidation half-life of aldrin is estimated to be between 55 min and 9.1 h. Aldrin may be volatilized from sediment and redistributed by air currents, contaminating distant areas. Aldrin has been detected in organisms in the Arctic waters and in sediments in the Great Lakes basin, suggesting long-range transport from southern agricultural regions.

Bioaccumulation and Biomagnifications

Aldrin is reported by Environment Canada to have a Bioconcentration Factors of 350–44 600. However, aldrin is

 http://dx.doi.org/10.1016/B978-0-12-386454-3.00094-4

rapidly converted to dieldrin, which is significantly more persistent. Dieldrin readily bioaccumulates in terrestrial and aquatic organisms. Biomagnification factors ranging from 2.2 (in rainbow trout) to 16 (in herring gulls) have been reported for dieldrin. Bioconcentration factors for dieldrin in various aquatic organisms range from 400 to 68 000, indicating that dieldrin shows moderate to significant bioaccumulation in various aquatic species.

Exposure and Exposure Monitoring

Routes and Pathways

As aldrin has not been used in the United States since 1987, new releases should not occur, and only rarely might be observed at hazardous waste treatment facilities. Potential exposures via drinking water and diet are likely higher than exposures from air or soil. The primary route of exposure to aldrin by the general public is dietary intake. Since aldrin is no longer used throughout most, if not all, of the world, inhalation exposure during application is not a significant source of exposure for the general public. Drinking water exposure is also not a significant source of exposure for the general public.

Human Exposure

General population exposure to aldrin may occur through the diet, but detection of aldrin residue in foods has decreased over time. Inhalation exposure may occur among people living in residences where aldrin was applied historically as a pesticide. Aldrin is absorbed following ingestion, inhalation, and dermal application. After absorption, aldrin is metabolized to dieldrin so rapidly that aldrin is rarely detected.

In the Centers for Disease Control and Prevention's Fourth National Report on Human Exposure to Environmental Chemicals, aldrin was not detected in blood samples for years 2001–02 (limit of detection 5.94 $ng\,g^{-1}$) for the 2278 individuals sampled. For 2003–04, aldrin was not detected (limit of detection 7.8 $ng\,g^{-1}$) for the 1946 individuals tested.

Environmental Exposure

Aldrin binds strongly to soil particles and is very resistant to leaching into groundwater. Volatilization is an important mechanism of loss from the soil. Due to its persistent nature and hydrophobicity, aldrin is known to bioconcentrate, but mainly as its conversion product, dieldrin. Aldrin is readily metabolized to dieldrin in both animals and plants, and therefore aldrin residues are rarely present in animals, and then only in very small amounts.

Toxicokinetics

Because of its relatively rapid metabolic conversion to dieldrin, aldrin is infrequently observed in human tissue, and there is little information on its distribution. The initial and principal biotransformation of aldrin following oral exposure is the relatively rapid, mixed function oxidase-mediated epoxidation to dieldrin.

In some extrahepatic tissues (e.g., lung) that contain relatively little cytochrome P-450 activity, *in vitro* studies suggest that aldrin may be epoxidized to dieldrin via an alternate, prostaglandin endoperoxide synthase pathway, one which is dependent on arachidonic acid rather than on nicotine adenine dinucleotide phosphate (NADPH).

Although data from humans are extremely sparse, one excretion study conducted on workers occupationally exposed to aldrin identified 9-hydroxy dieldrin, as a fecal metabolite. Animal studies have collectively demonstrated the following metabolites of dieldrin to be among the most significant: pentachloroketone, 6,7-trans-dihydroxydihydroaldrin and its glucuronide conjugate, 9-hydroxy dieldrin and its glucuronide conjugate, and aldrin dicarboxylic acid. The appearance and proportions of these metabolites can vary by species, strain, and sex, as can the overall rates of aldrin biotransformation.

Mechanism of Toxicity

Human health effects from aldrin at low environmental doses, or at biomonitored levels from low environmental exposures, are unknown. At high doses, aldrin blocks inhibitory neurotransmitters in the central nervous system (CNS). This action can cause hyperexcitation, leading to symptoms such as muscle twitching and seizures. Both *in vitro* experiments using rat brain membranes and intravenous or intraperitoneal administration of aldrin to rats have shown that aldrin can inhibit the activity of gamma aminobutyric acid (GABA) receptors by blocking influx of chloride through the $GABA_A$ receptor–ionophore complex.

Acute and Short-Term Toxicity

The toxicity of aldrin is essentially identical to dieldrin and similar to other cyclodiene insecticides. The doses at which aldrin is acutely lethal in experimental animals are quite similar to lethal dieldrin doses. Oral LD_{50} values for single doses of aldrin in rats ranged from 39 to 64 $mg\,kg^{-1}$. The CNS is the primary target with convulsions being the primary symptom. Patients may also experience headache, irritability, dizziness, nausea, vomiting, hyperexcitability, and coma. Onset of symptoms may occur within minutes to hours of ingestion.

Chronic Toxicity

When humans have been exposed for longer periods to lower doses of these compounds, neurotoxic symptoms have included headache, dizziness, general malaise, nausea, vomiting, and muscle twitching or myoclonic jerking. The available literature does not include other significant adverse health effects in humans resulting from longer-term or chronic exposure to aldrin.

Immunotoxicity

Very little, if any, data exist regarding aldrin immunotoxicity in humans or in animals. More data, though still limited, has been collected on the immunotoxicity of dieldrin.

Reproductive Toxicity

Reproductive effects of aldrin in humans have not been examined, though one study reported aldrin levels in blood and placental tissues of women who had premature labor or spontaneous abortions were significantly higher than in women with normal deliveries. However, this study had severe limitations and should be interpreted with caution. Decreased fertility was observed in some animal studies at doses as low as 0.63 mg aldrin per kg per day administered orally. Reproductive effects observed in other studies included decreased sperm count, degeneration of germ cells, decreased weights of seminal vesicles and prostate and coagulating glands, decreased seminiferous tubule diameter, decreased plasma and testicular testosterone, decreased prostatic fructose content and acid phosphatase activity, and decreased plasma luteinizing hormone and follicular stimulating hormone.

Developmental effects of aldrin have not been studied in humans, though effects (external malformations, skeletal anomalies, cleft palate, webbed foot, and open eye) in mice and hamsters occurred after exposure to $>25\,mg\,kg^{-1}$. However, some developmental studies have failed to find these effects. Decreased postnatal survival has also been observed in offspring in a three-generation study in rats at doses as low as 0.125 mg aldrin per kg per day. Maternal mortality was not seen in this study at this level. A similar decrease in postnatal survival has also been seen in mice and dogs.

Genotoxicity

Aldrin is not mutagenic in the Ames Assay, nor does it induce plasmid DNA breakage in *Escherichia coli* (although it was tested only in the absence of S9 metabolic activation). Gene conversion in *Saccharomyces cerevisiae* was not noted in the presence or absence of exogenous metabolic activation, though it has been reported to induce reverse mutation in this organism. The mouse dominant lethal assay, *in vivo* induction of mice micronuclei, and *Drosophila melanogaster* sex-linked recessive lethal mutation results were either not significant or negative. *In vivo* clastogenic responses seen in mouse bone marrow cells occurred at levels that were also cytotoxic.

Carcinogenicity

The International Agency for Research on Cancer (IARC) categorizes aldrin as a Group 3 chemical – unclassifiable as to human carcinogenic potential. The USEPA classifies aldrin as a probable human carcinogen (B2), because of its carcinogenicity in mice. However, the human relevance of the murine data is questionable. The available data indicate that dieldrin does not act directly on DNA, but induces a carcinogenic response through nongenotoxic mechanisms.

Cancer bioassays in several strains of mice and rats have shown an increase in the incidence of hepatocellular hyperplasia, hepatocellular carcinomas, and/or hepatomas with chronic exposure. A number of cancer bioassays in rats have produced mostly negative results, though some of these studies had severe limitations. Dieldrin appears to act as a liver tumor promoter in mice, increasing DNA synthesis and causing oxidative damage.

Clinical Management

Medical treatment in the case of exposure is symptomatic and supportive. Convulsions and hypoxia are the symptoms most likely to be observed. If aldrin is ingested, careful gastric lavage is recommended, being careful to avoid aspiration into the lungs. If not in a hospital setting, vomiting should be immediately induced, followed by administration of activated charcoal and magnesium or sodium sulfate. Milk is contraindicated.

Ecotoxicology

Freshwater–Sediment Organism Toxicity

Aldrin exhibits a wide range of toxicity in freshwater aquatic organisms, with invertebrates being the most sensitive group. Values for 96-h LC_{50}s range from 1 to 200 $\mu g\,l^{-1}$ for aquatic insects and from 2.2 to 53 $\mu g\,l^{-1}$ for fish. Generally, LC_{50} values for aldrin are very similar to those for dieldrin where the same species were tested. Aldrin and dieldrin are often considered together since aldrin is rapidly converted in tissues and in environmental media to dieldrin. Most long-term and bioaccumulation studies have been conducted with dieldrin.

Marine Organism Toxicity

Saltwater fish species are acutely sensitive to aldrin, with 48-h or 96-h LC_{50} values ranging from 2 to 7 $\mu g\,l^{-1}$ for six species. Generally, LC_{50} values for aldrin are very similar to those for dieldrin where the same species were tested. Estuarine invertebrates are acutely sensitive to aldrin, with LC_{50} or EC_{50} values ranging from 0.4 to 33 $\mu g\,l^{-1}$. Aldrin and dieldrin are often considered together, since aldrin is rapidly converted in tissues, and in environmental media to dieldrin. Most long-term and bioaccumulation studies have been conducted with dieldrin.

Terrestrial Organism Toxicity

Aldrin LC_{50}s of 2.6 ppm (24 h) and 2.4 ppm (48 h) were reported in Rana hexadactyla from waterborne exposures. LC_{50} values in avian species range from 6.6 ppm (female Bobwhite Quail) to 520 ppm (female Mallard duck). Aldrin and dieldrin are often considered together, since aldrin is rapidly converted in tissues, and in environmental media to dieldrin. Most long-term and bioaccumulation studies have been conducted with dieldrin.

Other Hazards

Aldrin is not explosive and does not have a flash point.

Exposure Standards and Guidelines

The USEPA developed an oral reference dose of 0.00003 mg kg^{-1} day^{-1} for aldrin, which was last revised in 1988. The USEPA also developed an oral slope factor of 17 mg kg^{-1} day^{-1} and a drinking water unit risk factor of 0.00049 μg l^{-1} day^{-1}, which was last revised in 1993. The USEPA has not developed a drinking water Maximum Contaminant Level and Maximum Contaminant Level Goal for aldrin. However, USEPA has a 10-day drinking water health advisory level of 0.3 μg l^{-1} and a lifetime drinking water health advisory level of 0.002 μg l^{-1} for aldrin. The Agency for Toxic Substances and Disease Registry (ATSDR) developed an acute oral minimal risk level (MRL) of 0.002 mg kg^{-1} day^{-1} and a chronic oral MRL of 0.00003 mg kg^{-1} day^{-1} for aldrin in 2002. The American Conference of Governmental Industrial Hygienists (ACGIH) has a threshold limit value as an 8 h time-weighted average of 0.25 mg m^{-3} in 1996 and gave it a 'skin' notation, meaning dieldrin can be absorbed in toxicologically relevant amounts through the skin. ACGIH gave aldrin an A3 carcinogenicity classification, which confirmed Aldrin as an animal carcinogen with unknown relevance to humans. The Occupational Safety and Health Administration also has 8 h time-weighted permissible exposure limit of 0.25 mg m^{-3} and a 'skin' notation, last reviewed in 2002. The National Institute for Occupational Safety and Health has a recommended exposure limit of 0.25 mg m^{-3} as a 10 h time-weighted average and a 'skin' notation and an Immediately Dangerous to Life or Health level of 25 mg m^{-3}, both of which were last reviewed in 2010.

Miscellaneous

Aldrin is corrosive to metals, owing to the slow formation of hydrogen chloride during storage. It is also noncombustible as the substance itself does not burn, but may decompose upon heating to produce corrosive and/or toxic fumes.

Aldrin and dieldrin are cyclodienes, and are made by a chemical process known as the Diels–Alder reaction, hence their names.

See also: Neurotoxicity; Organochlorine Insecticides; Resistance to Toxicants.

Further Reading

Agency for Toxic Substances and Disease Registry (ATSDR), Toxicological Profile for Aldrin. US Department of Health and Human Services, Public Health Service, Atlanta, GA.

International Programme on Chemical Safety (IPCS), 1989. Environmental Health Criteria for Aldrin and Dieldrin Geneva. World Health Organization, Geneva, Switzerland.

Swaen, G.M., de Jong, G., Slagen, J.J., van Amelsvoort, L.G., 2002. Cancer mortality in works exposed to dieldrin and aldrin: and update. Toxicol. Ind. Health 18 (2), 63–80.

United States Environmental Protection Agency (USEPA), 2003. Procedures for the Derivation of Equilibrium Partitioning Sediment Benchmarks (ESBs) for the Protection of Benthic Organisms: Dieldrin EPA/600/R-02/010. Office of Research and Development, Washington, DC.

Relevant Websites

http://www.atsdr.cdc.gov/.
http://www.epa.gov/IRIS/.
http://www.osha-slc.gov.
http://toxnet.nlm.nih.gov/.

Algae

KD Hambright and RM Zamor, Plankton Ecology and Limnology Laboratory, University of Oklahoma Biological Station, and Program in Ecology and Evolutionary Biology, University of Oklahoma, Norman, OK, USA
JD Easton and B Allison, Plankton Ecology and Limnology Laboratory, University of Oklahoma Biological Station, University of Oklahoma, Kingston, OK, USA

This article is a revision of the previous edition article by Keiko Okamoto and Lora E. Fleming, volume 1, pp 68–76, © 2005, Elsevier Inc.

Toxins discussed in this article are produced by microscopic, aquatic organisms commonly known as harmful algae, including unicellular, coenobial, and colonial species of Bacteria (Cyanobacteria) and Eukarya. Algae are generally autotrophic and rely on photosynthesis for their energy, but many species can also obtain energy heterotrophically from external dissolved and particulate organic sources via osmotrophy (direct absorption and uptake of organic molecules from the surrounding water), phagotrophy (ingestion of prey or other food particles), dasmotrophy (cell membranes of prey are perforated by extracellular toxins, inducing osmosis and leakage of organic compounds available for uptake or incorporation), and a variety of other heterotrophic strategies. Algae that are capable of both auto- and heterotrophy are known as mixotrophs. Included in algae are organisms also commonly referred to as phytoplankton, dinoflagellates, red and brown tides, diatoms, cyanobacteria, blue-green algae, and golden algae, of which some produce very potent toxins. This article focuses on the following algal toxins that are fairly well characterized in terms of adverse effects known to occur in humans and laboratory animals: azaspiracids, brevetoxins, ciguatoxins, maitotoxins, domoic acid (DA), okadaic (or okadeic) acid, saxitoxins, aplysiatoxins, anatoxins, microcystins, nodularins, and cylindrospermopsins. Azaspiracids, brevetoxins, ciguatoxins, maitotoxins, and okadaic acid are all classified chemically as polyether toxins. Domoic acid is a cyclic amino acid and saxitoxin is a purine alkaloid. A secondary focus is provided at the end of this article in which other less-studied, primarily ichthyotoxic, algal and cyanobacterial toxins with suspected human health concerns are mentioned briefly.

Commonly used synonyms for these sources and types of toxicity include azaspiracid shellfish poisoning (AZP) caused by at least 12 azaspiracid analogs; neurotoxic shellfish poisoning (NSP) caused by at least 10 known brevetoxins; ciguatera fish poisoning (CFP or Ciguatera) caused by more than 20 ciguatoxin congeners, gambiertoxins, and maitotoxins; amnesic shellfish poisoning (ASP) caused by one or more of three DA derivatives; paralytic shellfish poisoning (PSP) caused by at least 24 derivatives of saxitoxins; diarrhetic shellfish poisoning (DSP) caused by okadaic acid and dinophysistoxins; plus many other less-characterized toxins too numerous for detail in this brief overview (e.g., cyclic imines, golden algal toxins, karlotoxins, *Pfiesteria* toxins, pectenotoxins, and yessotoxins); and finally, red tides; harmful algal blooms (HAB), dinoflagellate blooms, cyanotoxins, and phycotoxins.

Exposure Routes and Pathways

A major route of human exposure to algal toxins is through the consumption of contaminated seafood products. The consumption of contaminated clams, mussels, scallops, oysters, and other shellfish causes shellfish-associated diseases (ASP, AZP, DSP, NSP, and PSP). Consuming contaminated large reef fish, like barracuda and grouper, causes ciguatera. Consumption of puffer fish with saxitoxin through shellfish feeding has resulted in cases of PSP.

Inhalation exposure of airborne toxins is also known to occur. For example, *Karenia brevis* which produces brevetoxin is relatively fragile and easily broken apart, particularly in wave action along beaches, thus releasing the toxin. During an active near-shore bloom (a.k.a., red tide), the water and aerosols of salt spray can contain toxins and cellular fragments, both in the droplets and attached to salt particles. These airborne particulates can cause respiratory irritation in humans on or near beach areas and can be carried inland under certain wind and other environmental conditions. The use of particle filter masks or retreat from the beach to indoors may provide protection from such airborne toxins. Similar airborne exposure in scientific laboratories that study toxigenic algae has been implicated in human toxicity.

Ciguatera, caused by ingested ciguatoxins and maitotoxins, can reportedly be sexually transmitted. There are also reports of acute health effects of ciguatera toxin in the fetus and newborn child exposed through placental and breast milk transmission from the mother. Domoic acid (ASP) has been shown to enter the placenta, accumulate in the amniotic fluid, enter the brain tissue of prenates, and can be transferred to milk in mammals.

Humans can also be exposed to cyanobacteria and their toxins through direct skin contact or by drinking contaminated water. Other possible routes of exposure include inhalation of contaminated aerosols, consumption of contaminated food, and even through dialysis. Therefore, occupational exposures for fisherman, watermen, and scientists, as well as recreational exposures for the general public, are all possible.

Toxicokinetics

The fate and metabolism of algal toxins is unclear and understudied; however, it is known that the absorption of both lipophilic and hydrophilic algal toxins occurs rapidly from the gastrointestinal and respiratory tracts. For example, to evaluate brevetoxin toxicokinetics from acute inhalation exposure up to

 http://dx.doi.org/10.1016/B978-0-12-386454-3.00983-0

7 days, 12-week-old male F344/Crl BR rats were exposed to a single dose of 6.6 mg kg^{-1} of the brevetoxin PbTx-3 through intratracheal instillation. More than 80% of the PbTx-3 was rapidly cleared from the lung and distributed by the blood throughout the body, particularly the skeletal muscle, intestines, and liver with low but constant amounts present in blood, brain, and fat. Approximately 20% of the toxin was retained in the lung, liver, and kidneys for up to 7 days.

Domoic acid can be absorbed orally at 5–10% of the administered dose. Domoic acid is distributed to the blood, but penetration of the blood–brain barrier is poor. Domoic acid is excreted unchanged in the urine with no evidence of metabolization. Impaired renal function can result in increased blood serum concentrations, residence time, and risk. Elimination half-life ranges from 20 min in rodents to 114 min in monkeys.

Postmortem examinations of patients that have died from PSP via saxitoxin found toxins in blood, urine, bile, cerebrospinal fluid, liver, lung, kidney, stomach, spleen, heart, brain, adrenal glands, pancreas, and thyroid glands with evidence of conversion of saxitoxin to neosaxitoxin and of gonyautoxin 2–3 to gonyautoxin 1–4. There is some evidence for human metabolism of saxitoxin through glucuronidation, a detoxification pathway in humans for metabolically converting xenobiotics to water-soluble metabolites, with excretion occurring in urine and feces.

Absorption of many of the cyanobacterial toxins occurs rapidly from the gastrointestinal tract. Microcystins are selectively transported from the gut and blood into the liver, where they can become concentrated. Microcystins in the liver can persist for up to 6 days; others found in the kidney can remain detectable for up to 24 h.

Acute and Chronic Toxicity and Mechanisms of Action: Algal Toxins

In general terms, people suffering from signs and symptoms of illnesses associated with eating seafood (invertebrates and fish) contaminated with algal toxins typically present the acute onset of gastrointestinal symptoms within minutes to 24 h. Victims may also exhibit a wide range of signs and symptoms involving many organ systems, including respiratory (difficulty breathing), peripheral nervous system (numbness and tingling), central nervous system (hallucinations and memory loss), and cardiovascular system (fluctuating blood pressure and cardiac arrhythmia). These signs and symptoms, depending on the particular disease, may last from hours to months. There are no records of human illnesses from consumption of invertebrates or fish contaminated with freshwater algal or bacterial toxins, although there is evidence of bioaccumulation of bacterial toxins in fish.

In addition to consumption of contaminated seafood, humans can be exposed to both marine and freshwater algal and bacterial toxins through airborne aerosols and with direct contact with water containing toxins and toxin-producing algae and bacteria, including drinking contaminated water.

Chronic algal toxin exposure remains mostly unstudied, although some limited information about specific toxins is included in the descriptions that follow. On the other hand, exactly how some of these toxins affect cells and tissues (mechanism of action) have received considerable attention from researchers.

Azaspiracids

Azaspiracid 1 (AZA1, Chemical Abstracts Service (CAS) Registry Number 214899-21-5, $C_{47}H_{71}NO_{12}$) and its 11 analogues, AZA2–AZA12, are polyether, lipophilic toxins produced by the dinoflagellate *Azadinium spinosum*. AZA1–AZA3 tend to be the dominant compounds found in shellfish, followed by AZA4 and AZA5. AZA6–AZA11 are typically minor components and believed to be bioconversion products of the main AZA analogues. Chromatographic studies suggest as many as 32 different analogues, but these are yet to be properly characterized. AZA, first detected in 1995 when consumers of blue mussels (*Mytilus edulis*) imported to the Netherlands from Ireland became ill, accumulates in various bivalve shellfish species, including clams, cockles, scallops, and oysters, and also in crabs. Cases of AZP have since been reported from numerous European countries, including Norway, Sweden, Ireland, England, France, Spain, and Portugal, and Morocco and eastern Canada.

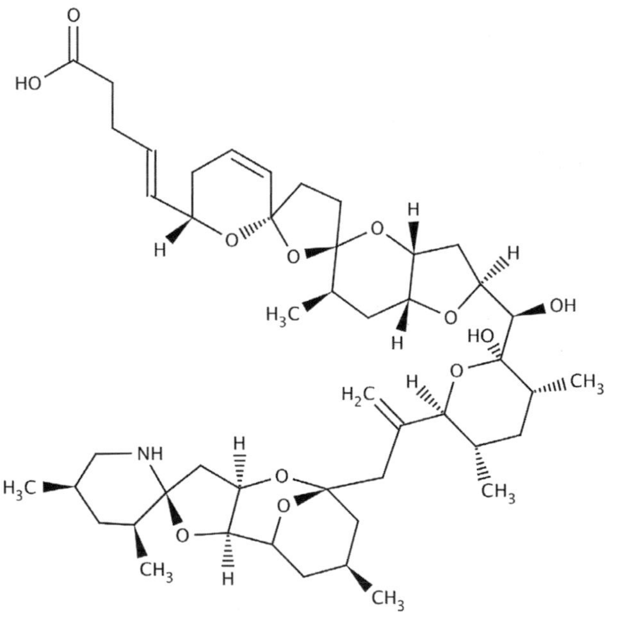

Azaspiracid

In general, AZA poisoning is rare. Symptom manifestation of acute AZP occurs within hours of ingestion of contaminated shellfish and includes nausea, vomiting, severe diarrhea, and stomach cramps, which are similar to the symptoms associated with DSP. Illness may persist for several days, and full recovery was established for the 1997 Arranmore Island incident. No long-term effects or illnesses have been reported.

Intraperitoneal (IP) minimum lethal dose of partially purified AZA in mice was 150 μg kg^{-1} and of purified AZA1, AZA2, and AZA3, the minimum lethal doses were 200, 110, and 140 μg kg^{-1}, respectively. The oral minimum lethal dose of

AZA varies between 250 and 450 μg kg^{-1}, depending on mouse age. Toxicological studies conducted using mice revealed that AZA targets the liver, lung, pancreas, thymus, spleen (T and B lymphocytes) and digestive tract. AZA1 has been shown to be cytotoxic to a range of cell types, particularly neurons, and a potent teratogen to finfish. AZA4 inhibits plasma membrane Ca^{2+} channels. Chronic effects observed in mice after oral administration of AZA were interstitial pneumonia, shortened villi in the stomach and small intestine, fatty changes in the liver, and necrosis of lymphocytes in the thymus and spleen.

Brevetoxins

Brevetoxin A (PbTx-1, CAS 98225-48-0, $C_{49}H_{70}O_{13}$) and its analogues, PbTx-2, PbTx-3, PbTx-4, PbTx-5, PbTx-6, PbTx-7, PbTx-8, and PbTx-9, are cyclic polyether, lipophilic toxins produced by *K. brevis*, formerly known as *Gymnodinium breve*, and *Ptychodiscus brevis*. PbTx-1 and PbTx-1 are believed to be the parent algal toxins from which PbTx-3 through PbTx-9 are derived. PbTx-2 is the most common form, while PbTx-1 is the most potent of the brevetoxins. Brevetoxins are known to accumulate in various shellfish species, such as oysters, clams, and mussels. They are not toxic to shellfish but are toxic to fish, marine mammals, birds, and humans, in which consumption of brevetoxin-contaminated shellfish causes NSP. Most cases of NSP have occurred in the coastal waters of New Zealand and in the Gulf of Mexico during 'red tide' events, but NSP intoxication has been identified worldwide.

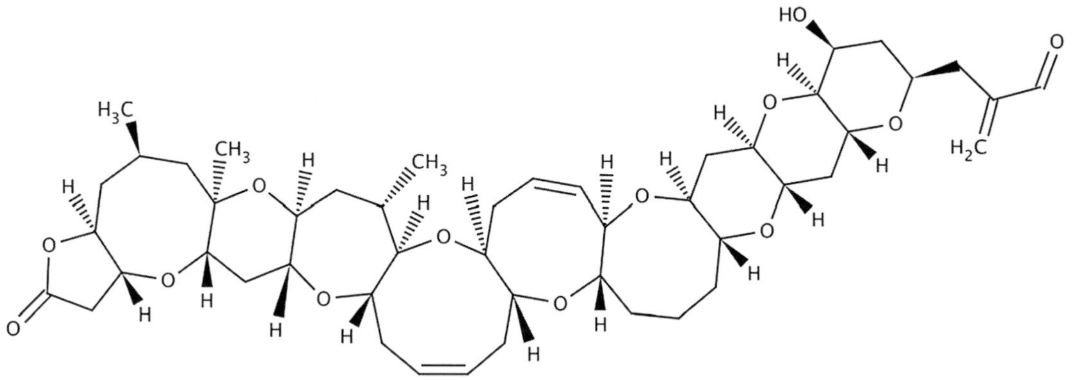

neurologic symptoms following ingestion of contaminated shellfish (a.k.a., NSP) and (2) an apparently reversible upper respiratory syndrome (conjunctival irritation, copious catarrhal exudates, rhinorrhea, nonproductive cough, and bronchoconstriction) following inhalation of contaminated aerosols. Recovery is reportedly complete in a few days, although persons with chronic pulmonary disease such as asthma may experience more severe and prolonged respiratory effects. In addition, skin and eye irritation by environmental exposures among people living or visiting Florida during *K. brevis* bloom has been reported. NSP and the respiratory irritation associated with aerosolized brevetoxins have both been reported along the Gulf of Mexico as well as far north as North Carolina; similar brevetoxin-associated syndromes have been reported in New Zealand.

After oral ingestion, brevetoxin poisoning (or NSP) is characterized by a combination of gastrointestinal and neurologic signs and symptoms. The incubation period ranges from 15 min to 18 h. Gastrointestinal symptoms include abdominal pain, vomiting, and diarrhea. Neurological symptoms include paresthesias, reversal of hot and cold temperature sensation, vertigo, and ataxia. Inhalational exposure to brevetoxin results in cough, dyspnea, and bronchospasm. Persons exposed to aerosolized brevetoxins may suffer shortness of breath, sneezing, and other allergy and asthma-like symptoms. Those with preexisting airway disease appear most likely to be affected. During swimming, direct contact with the toxic blooms may take place and eye and

Brevetoxin A

Brevetoxins are neurotoxins which activate voltage-sensitive sodium channels causing sodium influx and nerve membrane depolarization. Brevetoxins cause biphasic cardiovascular response with hypotension and bradycardia followed by hypertension and tachycardia. The respiratory arrest induced by a lethal dose results mainly from depression of the central respiratory center. Although evidence suggests that brevetoxins affect mammalian cortical synaptosomes and neuromuscular preparations, the majority of toxic effects associated with brevetoxins predominantly appear to result from the substantial and persistent depolarization of nerve membranes. In the lung, brevetoxin appears to be a potent respiratory toxin involving both cholinergic and histamine-related mechanisms.

The two forms of brevetoxin-associated clinical effects first characterized in Florida are (1) an acute gastroenteritis with

nasal membrane irritation can occur. No fatalities have been reported but there are a number of cases, which led to hospitalization.

Fish, birds, and mammals are all susceptible to brevetoxins. In Japanese medaka fish (*Oryzias latipes*), brevetoxins induce embryonic toxicity and developmental abnormalities. The fish are killed apparently through lack of muscle coordination and paralysis, convulsions, and death by respiratory failure. In the mosquito fish (*Gambusia affinis*) bioassay, the lethal dose (LD_{50}) is reported at 0.011 mg l^{-1}. Exposed birds die acutely with neurologic and hematologic effects. Brevetoxins were implicated in the deaths of manatees in Florida during a widespread bloom of *G. breve*. At necropsy, the animals did not appear to be unhealthy, and they had recently fed. High levels of brevetoxin were found by histochemical stain in cells throughout the body, particularly macrophages.

The mouse LD_{50} of brevetoxins ranges 170–400 μg kg^{-1} body weight (bw) IP, 94 μg kg^{-1} bw intravenously, and 520–6600 μg kg^{-1} bw orally.

Ciguatoxins

Ciguatoxin 1 (CTX-1, CAS 11050-21-8, $C_{60}H_{86}O_{19}$) and its analogues (more than 20 identified to date) are lipid-soluble polyether compounds produced by members of the dinoflagellate genus *Gambierdiscus*, not only including *Gambierdiscus toxicus* but also many other 'cryptic' *Gambierdiscus* species. Unlike open-water red tides, *Gambierdiscus* spp. tend to be benthic or epiphytic, often associated with the quiet waters of mangrove systems, leeward sides of coral reefs, and even man-made structures including petroleum platforms and artificial reefs that serve as benthic habitat within the euphotic (lighted) zone and fish aggregation areas. The most commonly reported marine toxin disease in the world is CFP or ciguatera. CFP outbreaks typically occur in a circumglobal belt extending approximately from latitude 35 N to 34 S, which includes Hawaii, the South Pacific including Australia, the Caribbean, and the Indo-Pacific, although the transport of contaminated fish and tourism have led to cases of CFP in both North America and Northern Europe. Ciguatoxins accumulate in benthic-feeding organisms and pass up the food chain, bioconcentrating in top-predator (apex, piscivorous) reef fishes, especially in fatty tissues, liver, viscera, and eggs. Ciguatoxins are relatively heat stable, remaining toxic after cooking and following exposure to mild acids and bases. Ciguatoxins arise from biotransformation in the fish of precursor gambiertoxins and less polar ciguatoxin. The primary Pacific ciguatoxin is Pacific ciguatoxin 1 (P-CTX-1) and the primary Caribbean form is C-CTX-1.

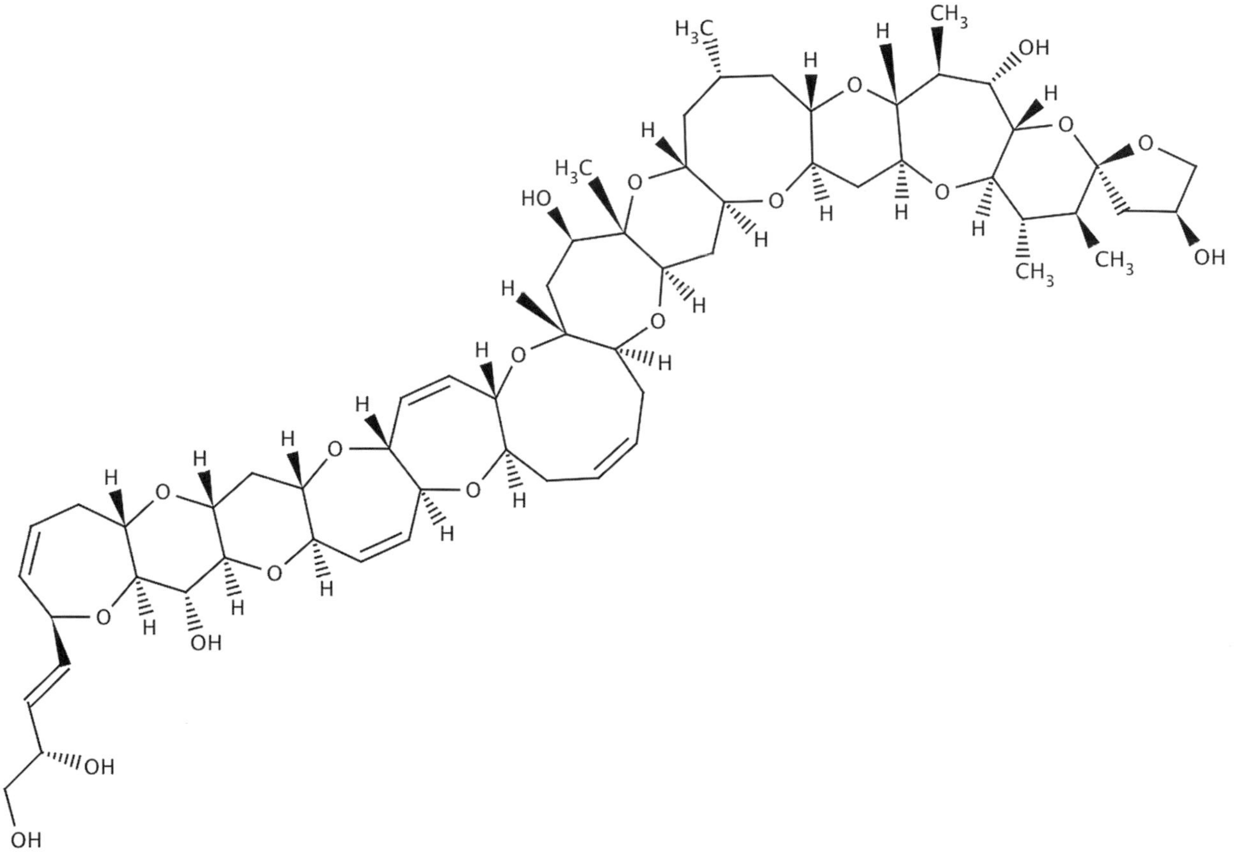

Ciguatoxin-1

Ciguatera presents primarily as an acute neurologic disease manifested by multiple gastrointestinal (diarrhea, abdominal cramps, and vomiting) and cardiovascular (arrhythmias and heart block) signs and symptoms within a few hours of contaminated fish ingestion, followed by neurologic manifestations (paresthesias, pain in the teeth, pain on urination, blurred vision, and temperature reversal) within hours to days. Neurologic symptoms may precede the gastrointestinal symptoms in Pacific CFP. Acute fatality usually due to respiratory failure, circulatory collapse, or arrhythmias is reported. Lethality is usually seen with ingestion of the most toxic parts of fish (liver, viscera, roe). The minimal lethal dose for a person weighing 165 lbs is less than 1 μg kg^{-1}. Those surviving ciguatera intoxication, especially in the Caribbean, suffer for weeks to months with debilitating neurologic symptoms, including profound weakness, temperature sensation changes, pain, and numbness in the extremities. Affected mothers have been reported to transmit ciguatoxins through breast milk, and some evidence suggests that the disease may also be transmitted through semen.

Chronic ciguatera can present as a psychiatric disorder of general malaise, depression, headaches, muscular aches, and peculiar feelings in extremities for several weeks to months. This may be due to prolonged debilitating paresthesias ranging from extreme fatigue to pain in the joints and changes in temperature sensation that can last from weeks to months and possibly to years. It is reported anecdotally that those with chronic symptoms seem to have recurrences of their symptoms with the ingestion of fish (regardless of type), ethanol, caffeine, and nuts up to 3–6 months from initial ingestion of ciguatera. Ciguatoxins are reported to induce developmental toxicity in Japanese medaka fish (*O. latipes*).

Lipid-soluble ciguatoxins and brevetoxins have immunologic cross-reactivity and thus have similar epitopic sites and mechanisms of action, as described in the previous section. Ciguatoxins activate voltage-sensitive sodium ion channels in nerve and muscle tissues, leading to cell membrane instability. P-CTX-1 is the most polar and toxic form of ciguatoxins, causing CFP in humans ingesting fish with levels at or above 0.1 $\mu g\,kg^{-1}$ fish flesh. The LD_{50} in mice for ciguatoxin P-CTX-1, P-CTX-2, and P-CTX-3 is 0.25, 2.3, and 0.9 $\mu g\,kg^{-1}$ bw when injected IP. The minimal lethal dose for a person weighing 165 lbs is less than 1 $\mu g\,kg^{-1}$. C-CTX-1 is less polar and 10 times less toxic than P-CTX-1.

Maitotoxins

Maitotoxin (MTX-1, CAS 59392-53-9, $C_{164}H_{256}O_{68}S_2Na_2$) and its analogues (MTX-2 and MTX-3) are water-soluble polyether compounds produced by the dinoflagellate *G. toxicus.* Maitotoxin precursors are also produced by *Prorocentrum* spp., *Ostereopsis* spp., *Coolia monotis, Thecadinium* spp., and *Amphidinium carterae.* Maitotoxins, named from the ciguateric fish *Ctenochaetus striatus* called 'Maito' in Tahiti from which maitotoxin was first isolated, are biotransformed to ciguatoxins by herbivorous fishes and invertebrates that graze on *G. toxicus.* Like ciguatoxins, maitotoxins bioaccumulate as they move up the food chain into higher trophic levels.

Maitotoxin is yet another toxin which is believed to cause ciguatera but with different symptoms than those caused by ciguatoxins. In smooth muscle and skeletal muscle exposed *in vitro,* maitotoxins cause calcium ion-dependent contraction. Maitotoxins increase the calcium ion influx through excitable membranes, causing cell depolarization, hormone and neurotransmitter secretion, and breakdown of phosphoinositides (important in regulating the function of integral cell membrane proteins). The calcium-dependent action of maitotoxins occurs in the absence of sodium ions and in the presence of tetrodotoxin, precluding the participation of sodium channels.

MTX is considered one of the most potent toxins (by weight) known with a mouse LD_{50} of 0.13 $\mu g\,kg^{-1}$ IP.

Domoic Acid

Domoic acid (DA, CAS 14277-97-5, $C_{15}H_{21}NO_6$), identified as the causative agent of ASP, is primarily produced by diatoms of the genus *Pseudo-nitzschia* but is also produced by members within the diatom genera *Amphora* and *Nitzschia* and some members within the red algae genera *Alsidium, Amansia, Chondria, Digenea,* and *Vidalia.* It was first isolated from the red alga *Chondria armata,* commonly known as 'Domoi', in 1959 and was used as an effective anthelmintic. Domoic acid consists of a proline ring, three carboxyl groups, and an imino group that can appear in five charged states depending on pH. It is

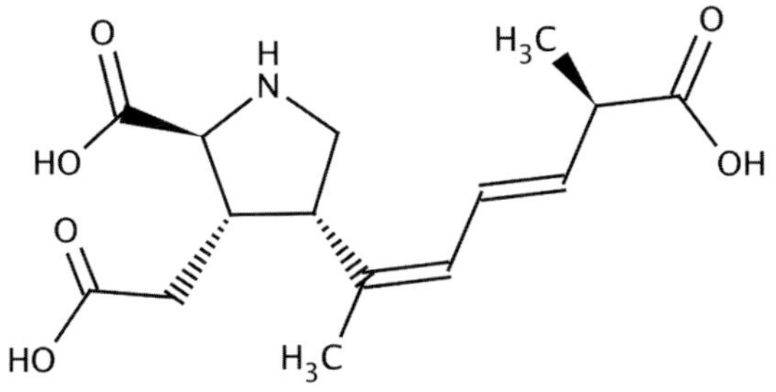

Domoic acid

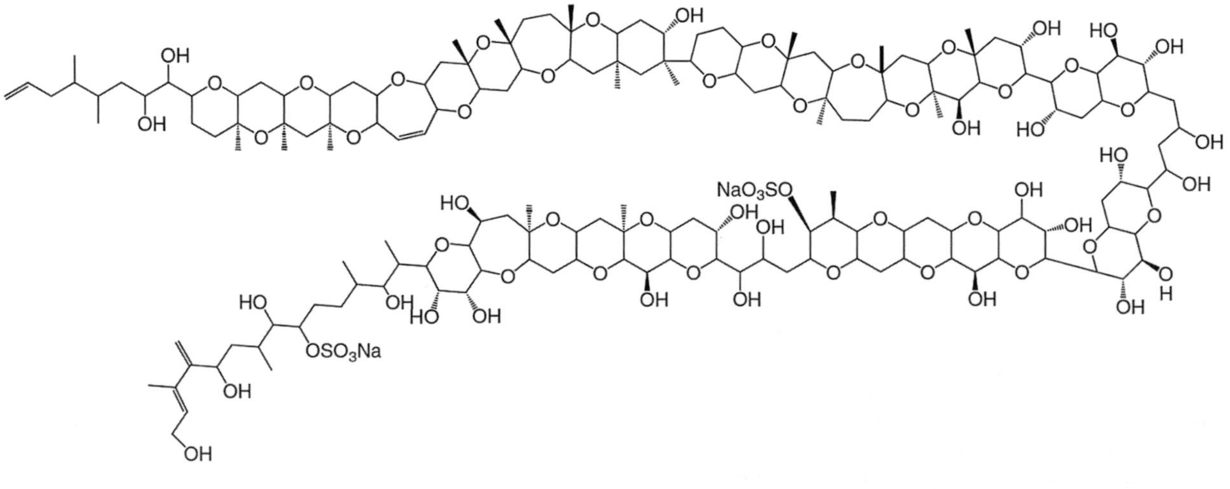

Maitotoxin

a water-soluble amino acid (nonprotein) and is structurally similar to kainic acid, glutamic acid, and aspartic acid.

The toxin accumulates in the hepatopancreas of mussels, scallops, and other filter-feeding shellfish. Heat-stable neurotoxic DA is similar in structure to the excitatory dicarboxylic amino acid, kainic acid, and has an antagonistic effect at the glutamate receptor. Domoic acid interacts with glutamate receptors on nerve cell terminals, causing excitotoxicity that can lead to neuronal cell damage or death from an excessive influx of Ca^{2+}. This is caused by coactivation of the -amino-3-hydroxy-5-methyl-4-isoxazolepropionic acid (AMPA), *N*-methyl-D-aspartate (NMDA), and especially kainate receptors for which DA has a high affinity. For the kainate receptors, the efficacy with which DA binds is thought to be the result of a nondesensitization of the channel.

In 1998, DA toxicity was reported in California sea lions. Predominantly neurological signs were observed, which included severe seizures that resulted in opisthotonus (spasm in which the head, neck, and back are arched backward), then death. Domoic acid has also been implicated in the deaths of marine mammals and birds in the Pacific Northwest of the US coast.

short-term memory. In some cases, confusion, memory loss, disorientation, and even coma are reported. In addition, seizures and myoclonus are observed acutely. Permanent neurologic sequelae, especially cognitive dysfunction, were reportedly most likely in persons who developed neurologic illness within 48 h, males, in older patients (>60 years) and in younger persons with preexisting illnesses such as diabetes, chronic renal disease, and hypertension with a history of transient ischemic attacks.

The mouse LD_{50} of DA is 3.6 mg kg^{-1} when injected IP.

Okadaic Acid

Okadaic acid (okadeic acid, ocadaic acid, OA, CAS 78111-17-18, $C_{44}H_{68}O_{13}$) and its analogues dinophysistoxin-1 (DTX-1, CAS 81720-10-7, $C_{45}H_{70}O_{13}$) and dinophysistoxin-2 (DTX-2, CAS 139933-46-3 $C_{44}H_{68}O_{13}$) are lipophilic, polyether toxins produced by various dinoflagellates in the genera *Prorocentrum* (e.g., *P. lima*, *P. arenarium*, *P. hoffmannianum*, *P. maculosum*, *P. faustiae*, *P. levis*, and *P. belizeanum*) and *Dinophysis* (e.g., *D. acuta*, *D. acuminata*, *D. caudata*, *D. fortii*, *D. miles*, *D. norvegica*, *D. rapa*, and *D. sacculus*).

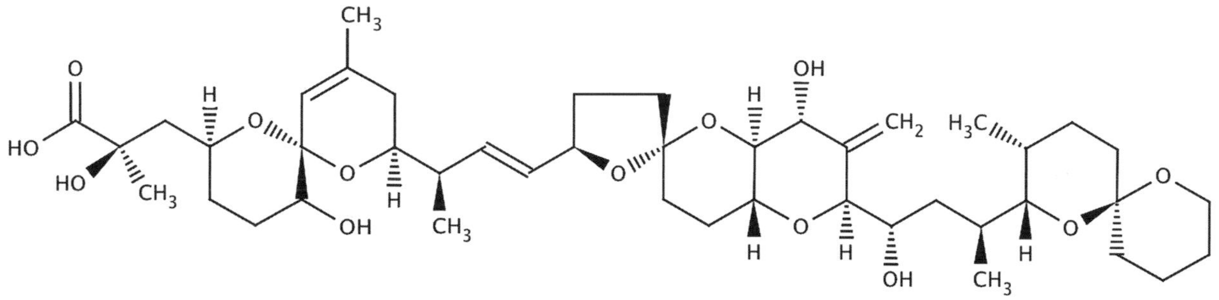

Okadaic acid

DA exposure studies have been conducted on monkeys, mice, rats, birds, and fish including IP injections, direct brain injections, and intravenous, intraarterial, intrauterine, and oral dosing. Symptoms include vomiting, seizures, and memory loss in humans, vomiting in monkeys, scratching and seizures in mice, tremors in birds, and spiral swimming in fish.

Human toxicity results primarily from consuming contaminated shellfish and one of the most prominent features of human toxicity is memory loss, hence the name 'amnesic shellfish poisoning.' ASP was first described from an outbreak in Canada in 1987 during which 143 people became affected and 4 died from eating contaminated shellfish cultivated from Prince Edward Island. Since that time, DA contamination of shellfish stocks and the associated ASP has become a global problem coming to the attention of numerous monitoring programs and food safety regulatory agencies (including the World Health Organization) in affected coastal regions of Europe, Australia, and New Zealand, the east coast of Asia and Japan, and the west coast of North America.

The acute symptoms of ASP caused by DA include vomiting, abdominal cramps, diarrhea, severe headache, and loss of

Toxins within the OA group are responsible for provoking DSP in humans after the consumption of shellfish that have accumulated these toxins in their digestive gland. OA was originally isolated from marine sponges of the genus *Halichondria* and DTX-1 and -2 were first isolated from mussels. OA and DTXs are polyketide compounds containing furane- and pyrane-type ether rings and an alpha-hydroxycarboxyl function differing only in the number or position of the methyl groups. Many derivatives of these parent toxins have been described after being found in shellfish and algae, including OA esters, okadaates, OA-diol-esters (e.g., acylated derivatives with fatty acids in the DTX-3 group, primarily with hexadecanoic acid, diol-esters formed in the unsaturated diols, and esterfication of the diol-esters with sulfated chains with or without and amide function in the DTX-4 and DTX-5a-c groups) and other compounds that comprise changes to the OA backbone (e.g., norokadanone, 19-epi-OA, and belizeanic acid). Prorocentrin is another compound that shows similarity with OA that is produced by *P. lima*. Of particular interest is the fact that significant portions of the toxins found in bivalves are the acylated derivatives. These derivatives may be a product of animal metabolism not produced directly by the algae and they show increased liposolubility when compared to their parent toxins.

DSP was first identified in 1978 after a series of food poisonings resulting from eating contaminated mussels and scallops in the Tohoku district of Japan affected 164 individuals. DSP outbreaks have been predominantly reported in Japan, Europe, and Australia, but cultures of *P. lima* isolated from the gulf of California and Mexico are capable of producing toxin. Thus the problem is generally considered to be a worldwide phenomenon. Toxins within the OA group can withstand mildly acidic to strongly basic pH but degrade rapidly in strong mineral acids. However, without acid, OA group compounds are largely stable to heat and are not degraded with normal cooking procedures and contaminated foods may serve to buffer against degradation of the toxins by the gastric juices. Compounds within the OA group produce toxic effects on hydrolysis within the human digestive tract. They are inhibitors of the serine/threonine protein phosphatases 1 (PP1) and 2A (PP2A), enzymes responsible for dephosphorylation of proteins, which are essential to metabolic processes in eukaryotic cells. Symptoms of DSP poisoning are nausea, diarrhea, vomiting, and abdominal pain starting within 3–12 h of initial consumption. Although originally the cause of the symptoms of diarrhea were thought to be caused by sodium secretion of intestinal cells, an increase in the paracellular permeability of intestinal cells by the toxins is now thought to be the likely cause of diarrhea. The Report of the Joint Food and Agriculture Organization of the United Nations, Intergovernmental Oceanographic Commission of United Nations Educational, Scientific, and Cultural Organization (UNESCO), and World Health Organization ad hoc Expert Consultation on Biotoxins in Bivalve Molluscs established a lowest observed adverse effect level (LOAEL) of 1 μg OA kg^{-1} bw. They established a provisional acute reference dose of 0.33 μg OA kg^{-1} bw. Most individuals recover within 3 days, and there have been no reported long-term effects or deaths reported due to acute DSP poisoning. However, these toxins have been shown to be tumor promoters and ancillary evidence has associated these toxins with digestive cancer. Additionally, there is evidence for cytotoxicity and potentially genotoxicity including formation of unspecific DNA adducts.

The LD_{50} for mouse injected IP for OA is 0.2–0.225 mg kg^{-1} bw, for DTX-1 is 0.16 mg kg^{-1} bw, for DTX-2 is 0.35 mg kg^{-1} bw, and for DTX-3 is 0.2–0.5 mg kg^{-1} bw. However, IP doses have been shown to have little effect on the digestive tract, primarily affecting the liver. Lethal oral doses have been reported for mouse from 2 to 10 times higher than the IP dose.

Saxitoxins

Saxitoxins (STXs, PSTs, CAS 35523-89-8, $C_{10}H_{17}N_7O_4$) are group of neurotoxic purine alkaloids that are responsible for causing PSP in humans after consumption of contaminated shellfish or other seafood, particularly lobster and puffer fish (not to be confused with poisonings caused by tetrodotoxin). STXs responsible for most reports of PSP are primarily produced by dinoflagellates of the genera *Alexandrium* (*A. fundyense*, *A. catenella*, *A. tamarense*, *A. hiranoi*, *A. monilatum*, *A. minutum*, *A. lusitanicum*, *A. tamiyavanichii*, *A. taylori*, and *A. peruvianum*), *Gymnodinium* (*G. catenatum*), and *Pyrodinium* (*P. bahamense*) but can also be produced by some species of cyanobacteria (see below) in the genera *Anabaena* (*A. circinalis* and *A. lemmermannii*), *Aphanizomenon* (*A. gracile* and *A. issatschenkoi*), *Cylindrospermopsis* (*C. raciborskii*), *Lyngbya* (*L. wollei*), *Planktothrix*, and *Rivularia*. There are suggestions that saxitoxins may actually have a bacterial origin, but the evidence is inconclusive at this point.

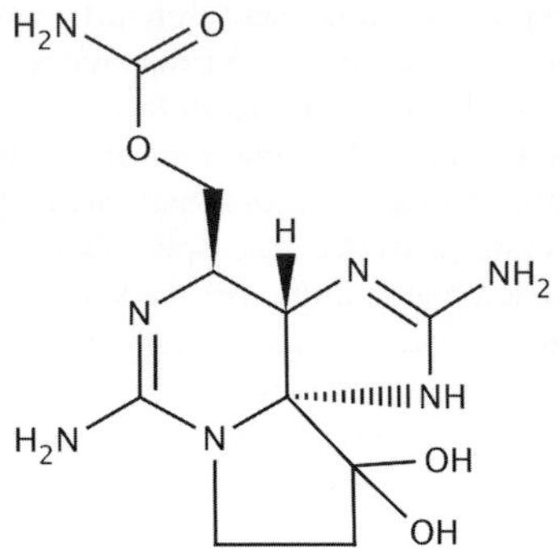

H_2N O O H N NH_2 N NH H_2N N OH OH

Saxitoxin

Substitutions with different hydroxyl, carbamyl, and sulfate functional groups at four sites along the backbone structure have resulted in the identification of at least 24 saxitoxin-like compounds that can vary by more than three orders of magnitude in toxicity. The most toxic of these are the carbamate toxins (saxitoxin (STX), neosaxitoxin (NEO), and gonyautoxins 1–4 (GTX)) followed by the decarbamoyl toxins (dcSTX, dcNEO, dcGTX 1–4, not common) and the *N*-sulfocarbamoyl toxins (B1 [GTX5], B2 [GTX6], and C1–C4), respectively. A fourth group of toxins, the hydroxybenzoate toxins, are produced by *G. catenatum* (GC 1–3), but more research needs to be conducted to determine the extent of their toxicity. Saxitoxin is the most well-studied member of this group.

The first PSP event on record occurred in 1927 in San Francisco, USA, coinciding with a bloom of the *A. catenella*, affecting 102 people and causing 6 deaths. However, saxitoxin was first isolated from butter clams, *Saxidomus giganteus*. The problem is now known to be a worldwide, having been reported in 27 locations by 1990. STXs are heat and acid stable, thus cooking the seafood does not denature the toxins. Saxitoxin acts by specifically and selectively binding to voltage-gated sodium channels on excitable cells functionally blocking sodium conductance and preventing impulse generation in peripheral nerves and skeletal muscles. STX exposure studies have been conducted on cats, chickens, dogs, guinea pigs, monkeys, mice, rats, birds, and rabbits including IP injections, intravenous injections, inhalation, and oral dosing. Saxitoxin can also block action potentials directly in skeletal muscles. Symptoms of poisoning generally occur within 30 min of consuming contaminated seafood including tingling sensations of the lips, mouth, and tongue, numbness of extremities, paresthesias, weakness, ataxia, floating/dissociative feelings, nausea, shortness of breath, dizziness, vomiting, headache, dysphagia, dysarthria, diastolic and systolic hypertension, and death. Death is caused by asphyxiation. Onset of symptoms has been reported as starting within a few minutes of seafood consumption, and death has been reported within 3–4 h of consumption. Medical treatment consists of providing respiratory support and fluid therapy. Humans typically start to recover within 12–24 h with no long-lasting effects; however, little if anything is known about the chronic effects of these toxins. Currently, STX is strictly regulated by the Organization for the Prohibition of Chemical Weapons listed as a schedule 1 chemical intoxicant.

The Report of the Joint Food and Agriculture Organization of the United Nations, Intergovernmental Oceanographic Commission of UNESCO, and World Health Organization ad hoc Expert Consultation on Biotoxins in Bivalve Molluscs established an LOAEL of 2 μg STX kg^{-1} bw and a provisional acute reference dose of 0.7 μg STX kg^{-1} bw. Generally, the action limit for STX for most seafood and shellfish is 0.8 mg STX equivalents per kilogram of tissue that has been accepted by many regulatory agencies worldwide. This standard has been in place for approximately 50–60 years. Recently, the European Food Safety Authority suggested a level of 75 μg STX equivalents per kilogram of tissue. The mouse bioassay is the primary determinant of PSP toxins in shellfish for most regulatory agencies. The LD_{50} for mice injected peritoneally for STX is 0.008 mg kg^{-1} bw, injected intravenously is 8.5 mg kg^{-1} bw, and administered orally is 263 mg kg^{-1} bw.

Acute and Chronic Toxicity and Mechanisms of Action: Cyanobacterial Toxins

There are at least 13 different genera of cyanobacteria that have been shown to produce toxins, often several different toxins per species. The main toxin-producing genera include *Anabaena, Aphanizomenon, Cylindrospermopsis, Gloeotrichia, Hapalosiphon, Lyngbya, Microcystis, Nodularia, Nostoc, Oscillatoria, Schizothrix, Spirulina,* and *Synechocystis*. Toxic blooms of cyanobacteria with associated animal poisonings have been reported in all continents except Antarctica. There have been frequent reports of thirsty domestic animals and wildlife consuming fresh water contaminated with toxic cyanobacterial algal blooms and dying within minutes to days from acute neurotoxicity and/or hepatotoxicity. Mammals and birds appear to be more susceptible to cyanobacterial algal toxins than aquatic invertebrates and fish, with some species variability. Prolonged morbidity and mortality have been reported in animals exposed to cyanobacterial algae in the wild.

There are individual case reports of persons exposed through swimming to cyanobacterial algal blooms with skin irritation and allergic reactions (both dermatologic and respiratory) with continued positive reaction on skin testing. In particular, urticaria (hives), blistering, and even deep desquamation of skin in sensitive areas like the lips and under swimsuits have been reported, especially with *Lyngbya majuscula* in tropical areas. Consumption of or swimming in cyanobacterial toxin-contaminated waters has also yielded increased case reports of gastrointestinal symptoms, especially diarrhea. One severe outbreak in Brazil was associated with lethality from hepatotoxicity in dialysis patients exposed to water contaminated with microcystins; another outbreak in Australia was also associated with lethality from hepatorenal syndrome in children and adults exposed to contaminated drinking water. In addition to gastrointestinal and dermatologic symptoms, eye irritation, asthma, and 'hay fever symptoms' have been reported repeatedly with exposure to contaminated recreational water exposure in the United States, Canada, the United Kingdom, and Australia. The chronic effects of exposure to small quantities of cyanobacterial algal toxins are still under study. In the mid-1980s, studies were done in China, where people were drinking untreated water contaminated with cyanobacterial algal toxins. It was found that drinking contaminated pond and ditch water was associated with high rates of liver cancer. When the quality of drinking water sources was improved in these areas, the rate of liver cancer decreased. The incidence of liver cancer attributable to cyanobacterial algal toxins in the United States is unknown.

Aplysiatoxins

Aplysiatoxins (CAS 52659-57-1, $C_{32}H_{47}BrO_{10}$) and debromoaplysiatoxins are alkyl phenols produced by *Lyngbya gracilis, L. majuscula, Calothrix crustacean, Nostoc muscorum, Schizothrix calcicola,* and *S. muscurom*.

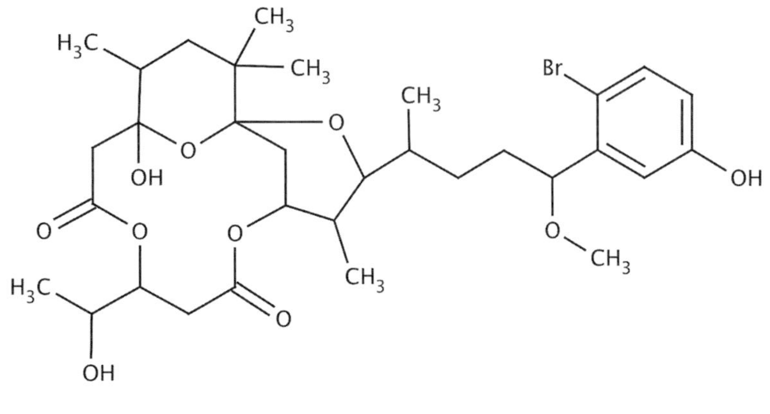

Aplysiatoxin

Aplysiatoxins can cause severe skin dermatitis and are potent tumor promoters and protein kinase C activators. Aplysiatoxins and debromoaplysiatoxins from blue-green algae attached to seaweed (*Gracilaria coronopifolia*) are suspected of causing gastrointestinal symptoms, including diarrhea, nausea, and vomiting in a poisoning case in Hawaii in 1994. Mouse studies have shown small intestinal bleeding and large intestinal edema following toxic injections of aplysiatoxin.

The mouse LC_{50} of aplysiatoxin is 118 $\mu g\,kg^{-1}$, IP.

Anatoxins

Anatoxins, are alkaloid neurotoxins, represented here by anatoxin-A (CAS 64285-06-9, $C_{10}H_{15}NO$) and anatoxin-A (S) (CAS 103170-78-1, $C_7H_{17}N_4O_4P$), produced by species of the genera *Anabaena, Planktothrix, Cylindrospermum, Aphanizomenon,* and *Phormidium.*

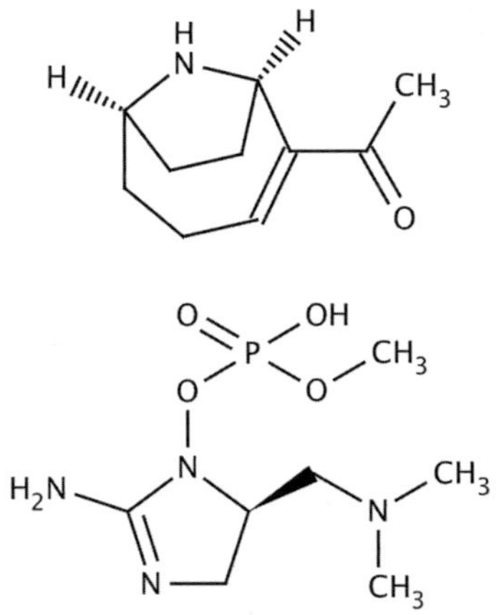

Anatoxin-A and Anatoxin-A (S)

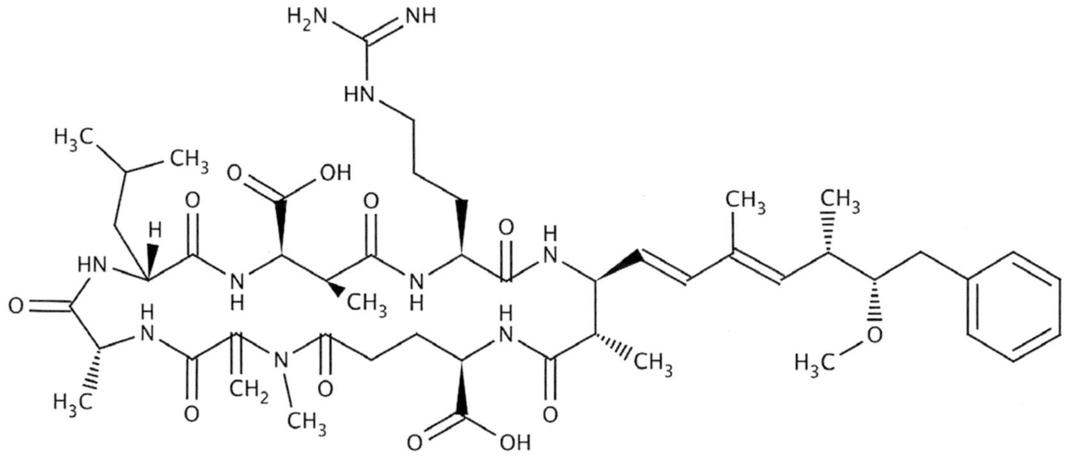

Microcystin-LR

To date, only cattle, dog, and bird poisonings have been documented. Anatoxin-A acts like the neurotransmitter acetylcholine, except that it cannot be degraded by acetylcholinesterase. Anatoxin-A (S) is a natural organophosphate that binds to acetylcholinesterase enzymes, resulting in uncontrolled muscle hyperstimulation. Hypersalivation, lacrimation, and urinary incontinence, signs of parasympathetic stimulation, characterize anatoxin-A (S) poisoning.

Anatoxin-A and Anatoxin-A (S) have mouse LC_{50} of 250 and 40 $\mu g\,kg^{-1}$, IP.

Saxitoxins

Saxitoxin and neosaxitoxin are both neurotoxins that may also be classified as cyanobacterial toxins. See above for details.

Microcystins

Microcystins, of which there are at least 80 variants, are based on a cyclic heptapeptide structure. Toxic variants contain the unique hydrophobic amino acid, 3-amino-9-methoxy-10-phenyl-2,6,8-trimethyl-deca-4(*E*),6(*E*)-dienoic acid (ADDA), and are represented by the prototype compound microcystin-LR or cyanoginosin LR; CAS 101043-37-2, $C_{49}H_{74}N_{10}O_{12}$. Microcystins are produced by a wide variety of planktonic cyanobacteria, including *Microcystis aeruginosa, M. virdis, M. ichthyoblabe, M. botrys, Planktothrix agardhii, P. rubescens, P. mougeotii, Anabaena flos-aquae, A. cirinalis, A. lemmermannii, Nostoc* spp., and *Snowella lacustris,* as well as the benthic cyanobacteria *Hapalosiphon hibernicus* and *Oscillatoria limosa.*

Experimentally, acute high-dose administration of microcystin can lead to death from hepatoencephalopathy within hours. Chronic administration of sublethal amounts of *Microcystis* (a cyanobacterial algae which produces microcystin) extracts in drinking water to mice resulted in increased mortality with chronic active liver disease, even at fairly low doses and in relatively short time periods in the laboratory. Studies in mice have also shown that some cyanobacterial algal toxins cause precancerous damage to both the liver and the bowel. In the laboratory experimental animals, teratogenic activity has been demonstrated with oral administration of *Microcystis* extracts; ~10% of otherwise normal neonatal mice had small brains with extensive hippocampal neuronal damage.

Poisoning by microcystins can lead to visual disturbances, nausea, and vomiting. Acute exposure can lead to liver failure and death within hours to days. Microcystins inhibit protein phosphatases, particularly PP1 and PP2A, resulting in hyperphosphorylation of many cellular proteins, including the hepatocellular cytoskeleton, causing loss of cell-to-cell contact and intrahepatic hemorrhaging. Other effects include altered mitochondrial membrane permeability, generation of reactive oxygen species, and initiation of programmed cell death (apoptosis). Microcystins are also believed to cause damage to cell DNA by the activation of endonucleases and have been linked to human liver and colon cancer. Microcystin-LR has an LC_{50} of 60 $\mu g\,kg^{-1}$ IP in mice.

Nodularins

Nodularin (CAS 118399-22-7, $C_{41}H_{60}N_8O_{10}$), a cyclic pentapeptide toxin similar to microcystin, was first isolated from *Nodularia spumigena*. Because this species tends to inhabit brackish waters, humans generally are at low risk to exposure through drinking waters.

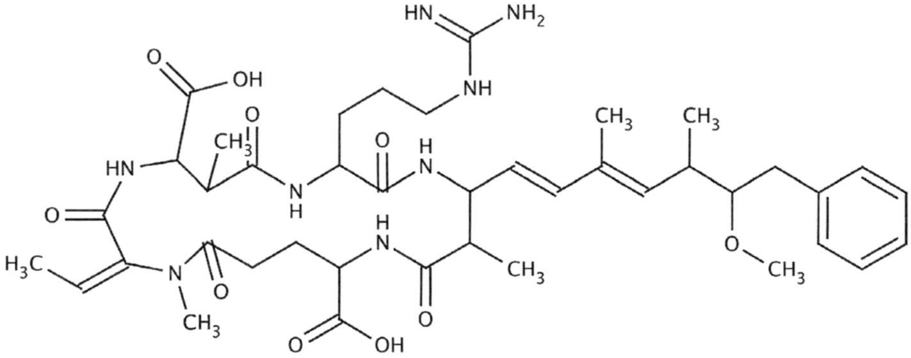

Nodularin

ADDA is present in nodularins, as in microcystins, but other amino acids are different. For example, dehydroalanine is replaced by *N*-methyl-dehydrobutyrine. The presence of ADDA results in similar phosphatase inhibition and the many subsequent effects as seen in microcystins. The smaller size of nodularins prevents the molecule from binding covalently to active sites (as seen in microcystins), allowing nodularins to affect other sites in cells, and possibly explaining observed carcinogenic effects. Nodularin has a mouse LC_{50} of 60 $\mu g\,kg^{-1}$, IP.

Cylindrospermopsin

Cylindrospermopsin (CAS 143545-90-8, $C_{15}H_{21}N_5O_7S$), a cyclic guanidine alkaloid, with at least three variants, is produced by *Cylindrospermopsis raciborskii, Aphanizomenon ovalisporum, Anabaena bergii, Umezakia natans, Raphidiopsis curvata*, and other unidentified species.

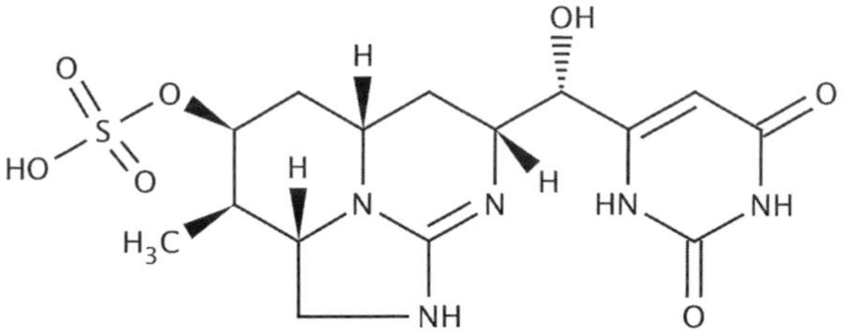

Cylindrospermopsin

Cylindrospermopsins are included in the cyanobacterial hepatoxin group which blocks protein synthesis. Acute exposure to cylindrospermopsin results in lipid accumulation in the liver followed by hepatocellular necrosis. Other organs are also affected with widespread necrosis of the tissues of the kidneys, bladder, ureter, and spleen. Cylindrospermopsin has a delayed toxicity, with an LC_{50} of 2100 $\mu g\,kg^{-1}$ IP in mice at 24 h, but 200 $\mu g\,kg^{-1}$ after 5 days.

Other Cyanobacterial Toxins

A large variety of other toxins are produced by cyanobacteria but are not as well documented. These include lyngbyatoxin (dermatotoxic), endotoxins, and other substances as yet undescribed, including additional tumor promoters.

Acute and Chronic Toxicity and Mechanisms of Action: Other Toxins

Numerous other algal toxins have been described. Many are believed to play important roles in prey capture and predator avoidance. These compounds tend to be ichthyotoxic, but their toxicity to humans is less certain than the toxins described above.

Cyclic Imines

Cyclic imines, including gymnodimine (GYM), spirolides (SPX), pinnatoxins (PnTx), prorocentrolide, and spirocentrimine, are fast-acting toxins. The presence of this group of compounds in shellfish was discovered because of their very high acute toxicity in mice upon IP injections of lipophilic extracts. All the cyclic imines for which data are available are toxic to mice after IP administration. Mouse LC_{50} values for GYMs range 6.5–100 μg kg^{-1}, for SPX, 6.5–8 μg kg^{-1}, and for PnTx, 16–45 μg kg^{-1}. There is no evidence that any of the cyclic imines have been responsible for toxic effects in humans.

Dinophysistoxin

See OA.

Golden Algal Toxins

Blooms of algal genera within the Prymnesiophyceae, notably species of *Prymnesium, Chrysochromulina,* and *Phaeocystis,* and the Raphidophyceae, primarily species of *Chattonella, Heterosigma,* and *Fibrocapsa,* are well known for massive fish kills that have led to great economic losses, but no cases of human toxicity have been reported. Four species of *Prymnesium* are reported to be toxic to vertebrates or invertebrates and toxicity in two other species is suspected. Several hemolytic compounds termed 'prymnesins' have been described in *P. parvum,* but have yet to be fully characterized. These include several galactolipids and two polyoxy-polyene-polyethers (prymnesin-1 and -2). Mouse LC_{99} values for prymnesins-1 and prymnesins-2 were 50 and 80 μg kg^{-1}; LC_{50} values for the fish *Tanichthys albonubes* were 8 and 9 nM.

A different assemblage of ichthyotoxic polyunsaturated fatty acids and their conjugated galactoglycerolipid progenitors, consisting primarily of stearidonic acid (LC_{50} = 21.9 μM, 10- to 14-day-old fry of the fish *Pimephales promelas*), and including docosahexanoeic acid (LC_{50} = 4.7 μM), arachinodonic acid (LC_{50} = 9.2 μM), pinolenic acid (LC_{50} = 18.2 μM), and eicosapentaenoic acid (LC_{50} = 23.6 μM), was identified in laboratory cultures of *P. parvum.* Some of these toxins were present in bloom and fish kill sites, but below toxic concentrations. Instead a different, yet-characterized, ichthyotoxic fatty acid was detected. Cytotoxicity to a human (MDA-MB-435) cancer cell line was observed for one of the fatty acids isolated from *P. parvum* in cultures (GAT 512A, IC_{50} = 24.2 μM).

Chrysochromulina polylepis produces two compounds, one hemolytic and one ichthyotoxic. The hemolytic compound was characterized as a galactolipid, 1-acyl-3-digalacto-glycerol. Small amounts of a polyunsaturated fatty acid, octadecapentaenoic acid, were also detected.

Karlotoxins

Karlotoxins are water-soluble hemolytic, cytotoxic, and ichthyotoxic compounds produced by the dinoflagellate *Karlodinium veneficum.*

Pfiesteria Toxins

The dinoflagellate *Pfiesteria* spp. is believed to produce and release into the environment potent extracellular toxins, or exotoxins, referred to generally as *Pfiesteria* toxins (PfTx) that have been linked to mass fish mortalities and human disease in mid-Atlantic estuaries. Learning impairments have been seen as long as 10 weeks after a single acute exposure to *Pfiesteria* in Sprague–Dawley rats. A hydrophilic toxin (PfTx) isolated from *P. piscicida* cultures when applied locally to the ventral hippocampus on repeated acquisition of rats in the radial-arm maze impaired choice accuracy and early learning which was persistent across 6 weeks of testing after a single administration of the toxin.

Adverse health effects, including cognitive disturbance, were found in humans following accidental exposure to *P. piscicida* in laboratory facilities. Cognitive deficits have also been described in people believed to be exposed to *Pfiesteria* through sea spray in coastal Maryland during a *Pfiesteria* bloom. These adverse health effects have been termed Possible Estuary-Associated Syndrome by the Centers for Disease Control and Prevention, symptoms of which include cognitive and visual contrast sensitivity deficits, pulmonary impairment, gastrointestinal disruptions, and immunologic dysfunction.

Pectenotoxins

Pectenotoxins (PTXs) are a group of polyether macrolides produced by the dinoflagellates of the genus *Dinophysis* (*D. fortii, D. acuminata, D. acuta, D. caudate, D. rotunda, D. norvegica*). PTXs have also been detected in *Protoperidinium divergens, P. depressum,* and *P. crassipes.* PTXs are suspected to be DSP toxins because they are detected with the same extraction methods and bioassays used for OA and were first isolated from the scallop, *Patinopecten yessoensis.* There is no evidence of adverse acute or chronic health effects of pectenotoxins in humans. IP injection of PTXs in mice leads to liver necrosis. The mouse LC_{50} values (IP) for PTXs range between 250 and 770 μg kg^{-1} for PTX1, 2, 3, 4, 6, and 11 and greater than 5000 μg kg^{-1} for PTX7, 8, 9, and 2-SA. Toxicity in other PTX analogues has not been demonstrated.

Yessotoxins

Yessotoxins (YTXs) are disulfated polycyclic polyethers that resemble brevetoxins, produced by the dinoflagellate *Lingulodinium polyedrum.* Like PTX, YTX was first isolated from the digestive glands of the scallop *P. yessoensis* and are suspected to be DSP toxins because they are detected with the same extraction methods and bioassays used for OA. There have been no reports of ill effects in humans attributable to YTX. IP injection of YTXs in mice leads to cardiac muscle damage. Mouse LC_{50} values (IP) range between 80 and 750 μg kg^{-1} for YTX and its analogues.

Clinical Management

Very little clinical research has been conducted to determine effective treatments. Medical care is primarily supportive.

Medical treatment of CFP has been to a large extent symptomatic; a variety of agents, including vitamins, antihistamines, anticholinesterases, steroids, and tricyclic antidepressants, have been tried with limited results. If given within 3 days of exposure, intravenously, mannitol (1 mg kg^{-1} given rapidly over 1 h) has been demonstrated in a single-blinded control trial to resolve acute symptoms and prevent chronic symptoms, although repeated administrations may be necessary if symptoms return; a more recent clinical trial did not find an effect;

Table 1 US FDA action levels in seafood for natural toxins associated with shellfish and fish poisoning

Poisoning	*US FDA action level*
PSP	0.8 ppm (80 μg per 100 g) saxitoxin equivalents
NSP	0.8 ppm (20 mouse units per 100 g) brevetoxin-2 equivalents
DSP	0.16 ppm total OA equivalents (i.e., combined free OA, dinophysistoxins, acyl-esters of OA, and dinophysistoxins)
ASP	20 ppm domoic acid, except in the viscera of Dungeness crab, where the action level is 30 ppm
CFP	0.01 ppb P-CTX-1 equivalents for Pacific ciguatoxin and 0.1 ppb C-CTX-1 equivalent for Caribbean ciguatoxin
AZP	0.16 ppm azaspiracid equivalents

Source: US FDA. (April 2011). Fish and Fishery Products Hazards and Controls Guidance, fourth ed. Department of Health and Human Services, Public Health Service Food and Drug Administration, Center for Food Safety and Applied Nutrition, Office of Food Safety.

however, this trial included subjects treated long after the initial 3-day window. Gut emptying and decontamination with charcoal have been recommended, although often the severe ongoing vomiting and diarrhea prevent this. Atropine is indicated for bradycardia and dopamine or calcium gluconate for shock. It is recommended that opiates and barbiturates be avoided since they may cause hypotension, and opiates may interact with maitotoxins. Amitriptyline (25–75 mg b.i.d.) and similar medications do seem to have some success in relieving the symptoms of chronic ciguatera such as fatigue and paresthesias. It is possible that nifedipine may be appropriate as a calcium channel blocker to counteract the effects of maitotoxins. Anecdotal food avoidance as mentioned above is also recommended. In addition, there is no immunity to these illnesses, and recurrences of actual ciguatera in the same individual appear to be worse than the initial illnesses. A rapid, accurate diagnosis and treatment of CFP within the first 72 h after exposure may be critical in preventing some of the neurologic symptoms that might otherwise become chronic and debilitating. The treatment of DSP caused by OA is symptomatic and supportive. In general, hospitalization is not necessary; fluid and electrolytes can usually be replaced orally.

Supportive measures are the basis of treatment for PSP that is caused by saxitoxins, especially ventilatory support in severe cases. In animals, artificial respiration is the most effective treatment. Up to 75% of severely affected persons die within 12 h without supportive treatment. When the ingestion of contaminated food is recent, gut decontamination by the gastric lavage and administration of activated charcoal or dilute bicarbonate solution is recommended. Care must be taken concerning aspiration with the neurologically compromised patient. In general, the only treatment available for exposure to cyanobacterial algal toxins is supportive medical treatment after complete removal from exposure. If the exposure was oral, administration of activated carbon to decrease gut absorption may be efficacious if given within hours of exposure. Based on past outbreaks, monitoring of volume, electrolytes, liver, and kidney function should all be considered in the case of acute gastroenteritis associated with some of the cyanobacterial algal toxins.

Exposure Standards and Guidelines

Global seafood safety standards have not been established. In the United States, US Food and Drug Administration (FDA) enacted the Hazard Analysis and Critical Control Points (HACCP) program of 1997. The FDA has established action levels in suspected seafood for the toxins causing some of the shellfish poisonings (see **Table 1**). When an action level is reached, the HACCP plan must be followed to prevent unsafe products from reaching the consumer.

See also: Ciguatoxin; Okadaic Acid; Saxitoxin.

Further Reading

Dominguez, H.J., Paz, B., Daranas, A.H., Norte, M., Franco, J.M., Fernández, J.J., 2010. Dinoflagellate polyether within the yessotoxin, pectenotoxin, and okadaic acid toxin groups: characterization, analysis and human health implications. Toxicon 56, 191–217.

Etheridge, S.M., 2010. Paralytic shellfish poisoning: seafood safety and human health perspectives. Toxicon 56, 108–122.

FAO/IOC/WHO 2005. Report of the Joint FAO/IOC/WHO ad hoc Expert Consultation on Biotoxins in Bivalve Molluscs. Food and Agriculture Organization of the United Nations, Intergovernmental Oceanographic Commission of UNESCO, World Health Organization, Oslo, Norway, September 26–30, 2004.

Granéli, E., Turner, J.T. (Eds.), 2006. Ecology of Harmful Algae. Springer, Berlin, Germany.

Hallegraeff, G.M., Anderson, D.M., Cembella, A.D. (Eds.), 2003. UNESCO Manual on Harmful Marine Algae. UNESCO/WHO, Geneva, Switzerland.

Hudnell, H.K. (Ed.), 2008. Cyanobacterial Harmful Algal Blooms: State of the Science and Research Needs. Springer, New York.

Hui, Y.H., Kits, D., Stanfield, P.S. (Eds.), 2001. Seafood and Environmental Toxins. Dekker, New York.

Kirkpatrick, B., Fleming, L.E., Squicciarini, D., et al., 2004. Literature review of Florida Red Tide: implications for human health. Harmful Algae 3 (2), 99–111.

Lefebvre, K.A., Robertson, A., 2010. Domoic acid and human exposure risks: a review. Toxicon 56, 218–230.

Lehane, L., Lewis, R.J., 2000. Ciguatera: recent advances but the risk remains. Int. J. Food Microbiol. 61, 91–125.

Plakas, SM., Dickey, R.W., 2010. Advances in monitoring and toxicity assessment of brevetoxins in molluscan shellfish. Toxicon 56, 137–149.

Relevant Websites

http://oceanservice.noaa.gov/hazards/hab/ – Harmful Algal Blooms: Simple Plants with Toxic Implications. National Oceanic and Atmospheric Administration, National Ocean Service,

http://yyy.rsmas.miami.edu/groups/ohh/ – University of Miami. Oceans and Human Health Center.

http://www.whoi.edu/science/B/redtide/species/speciestable.html – US Fish, Shellfish and Wildlife Affected by Toxic or Harmful Microalgal Species. Woods Hole Oceanographic Institution, The Harmful Algae Page.

http://www-cyanosite.bio.purdue.edu – A Webserver for Cyanobacterial Research. Purdue University, Department of Biological Sciences.

http://www.issha.org – The International Society for the Study of Harmful Algae (ISSHA).

Alkalies

V Lawana, Iowa State University, Ames, IA, USA

This article is a revision of the previous edition article by Sanjay Chanda and Harihara M. Mehendale, volume 1, pp 76–77, © 2005, Elsevier Inc.

- Name: Alkalies
- Chemical Abstracts Service Registry Number: N/A (ID: D000468000)
- Synonyms: Base, Basic solutions, Alkaline solutions/mixtures
- Molecular Formula: N/A
- Chemical Structure: N/A

Background

Alkalies are amongst the oldest forms of chemical reagents that are being used in countless number of experimental and therapeutic settings. Their application varies from preparation of surgical equipment to manufacturing of disinfectants. Alkalies are usually an inorganic class of chemicals. Physiologically, alkalies also play a crucial role in maintaining proper pH in body compartments (e.g., kidney-urine); however, such mechanisms are usually controlled and regulated within the body. A number of compounds with alkaline properties have tremendous therapeutic value (**Table 1**).

With reference to alkalies, a syndrome called milk-alkali syndrome develops from drinking too much milk (which is high in calcium) and taking certain antacids, especially calcium carbonate or sodium bicarbonate (baking soda), over a long period of time. Calcium deposits in the kidneys and in other tissues can occur in milk-alkali syndrome, and high levels of vitamin D can worsen this condition. Although extremely rare today, milk-alkali syndrome often used to be a side effect of peptic ulcer disease treatment with antacids containing calcium. Sophisticated medications that do not contain calcium are used today for treating ulcers. Individuals on calcium carbonate in an attempt to prevent osteoporosis sometimes face this condition (even in those taking as little as 2 g of calcium per day). The best way to reduce calcium overload is to eliminate milk and other forms of calcium such as in antacids. Damage may be permanent in kidney failure patients.

Uses

Alkalies are widely used compounds. They are used in antacid preparation to treat gastric as well as systemic acidosis. Depending on specific alkali, they are also used in bleaches, cleaning agents, detergents, unslaked lime, etc.

Environmental Fate

In cases of a solid alkali spill on soil, groundwater pollution occurs. Precipitation will dissolve some of the solid and create an aqueous solution of that alkali, which then would be able to infiltrate the soil. However, prediction of the concentration and properties of the solution produced would be difficult.

Exposure Routes and Pathways

Usual exposure routes include dermal exposure, oral ingestion (usually accidental), and nasal inhalation.

Toxicokinetics

Toxicokinetics varies depending on the type of alkali. These are in general small molecular weight molecules and undergo weak dissociation in gastric acid pH. In general, they are readily converted into salt depending on the microenvironment.

Mechanism of Toxicity

Alkalies usually act by altering pH of the extracellular fluid. They exhibit their toxic effects by liquefaction necrosis, meaning that they damage the cell membrane, and thus cell integrity is ruptured. This causes cell lysis. (This is why they are used in lysis buffer preparations for various biochemical

Table 1 Useful therapeutic properties of some well-known alkaline compounds

Name of compound	*Disease treatment*
Alkalies	Hypercalcemia, leishmaniasis
Alkalies	Renal insufficiency
Aluminum hydroxide	Status epilepticus
Aluminum hydroxide	Acute kidney injury
Aluminum hydroxide	Seizures
Lithium carbonate	Seizures
Magnesium hydroxide	
Nickel hydroxide	Reperfusion injury; wounds and injuries; Crohn's disease
Potassium hydroxide	Dermatitis, irritant

Source: http://ctdbase.org – Comparative Toxicogenomics database; Mount Desert Island Biological Lab.

 http://dx.doi.org/10.1016/B978-0-12-386454-3.00228-1

assays.) Intracellular alkalinization is more serious; such conditions alter intracellular redox balance and alter metabolic pathways, ultimately breaking down cellular homeostasis.

Acute and Short-Term Toxicity

Animals

The toxicity of alkalies in animals is the same as that of humans.

Human

Alkalies can cause skin irritation and skin burns. Also, they cause damage to mucosal membrane and eyes almost immediately on contact. However, the absence of burns, irritation, erythema, or other such signs in the oral or circumoral area does not necessarily indicate that esophageal injury does not exist. Inhalation of the fumes may cause pulmonary edema or pneumonitis.

Chronic Toxicity

Animals

Toxic manifestations of alkalies in animals are the same as that of humans.

Human

Chronic exposure to any alkali is generally not beneficial and causes severe toxicity. Burns that appear to be mild at the time of injury can sometimes go on to cause opacification, vascularization, ulceration, or perforation. Direct exposure is always injurious, and prolonged alkalinization of any biological material can induce irreversible changes.

Carcinogenicity

There is no evidence of as alkali-mediated tumorogenetic effects.

Clinical Management

Exposure should be terminated as soon as possible by removing the victim to fresh air. The skin, eyes, and mouth should be washed with copious amounts of water. A 20–30 min wash may be necessary to neutralize and remove all residual traces of the contamination. Contaminated clothing and jewelry should be removed and isolated. Treatment may require instillation of a local anesthetic to treat the blepharospasm (spasmodic winking from involuntary contraction of the orbicular muscle of the eyelids). Oral ingestion requires immediate dilution therapy with water or milk. Antidotes such as vinegar or lemon juice are absolutely contraindicated. Emesis should be avoided in case of ingestion.

Ecotoxicology

These chemicals are easily degradable in environment and form salts readily. They are not known to have any profound ecotoxic impact except in exceptional circumstances such as accidental spills.

Exposure Standards and Guidelines

The guidelines given here are for sodium hydroxide (common alkali).

US Occupational Safety and Health Administration standards: permissible exposure limit: 8 h time-weighted average is 2 mg m^{-3}.

Threshold limit values: ceiling limit is 2 mg m^{-3}.

US National Institute for Occupational Safety and Health recommendations: recommended exposure limit is 2 mg m^{-3}.

See also: Potassium; Sodium.

Further Reading

Klassen, C.D., Casarett, L.J., Doull, J., 2013. Casarett and Doull's Toxicology: The Basic Science of Poisons, eighth ed. McGraw-Hill, New York.

Marcus, W.L., 1994. Lithium: a review of its pharmacokinetics, health effects, and toxicology. J. Environ. Pathol. Toxicol. Oncol. 13 (2), 73–79.

Mohammadi, Z., Dummer, P.M., 2011. Properties and applications of calcium hydroxide in endodontics and dental traumatology. Int. Endod. J. 44 (8), 697–730.

NIOSH, 1975. Criteria Document: Sodium Hydroxide. DHEW, NIOSH, pp. 76–105.

Olmedo, H., Herrera, M., Rojas, L., et al., Comparison of the adjuvant activity of aluminum hydroxide and calcium phosphate on the antibody response towards Bothrops asper snake venom.

Ortiz-Santaliestra, M.E., Fernández-Benéitez, M.J., Marco, A., 2012. Density effects on ammonium nitrate toxicity on amphibians. Survival, growth and cannibalism. Aquat. Toxicol. 110–111, 170–176.

Picolos, M.K., Orlander, P.R., 2005. Calcium carbonate toxicity: the updated milk-alkali syndrome; report of 3 cases and review of the literature. Endocr. Pract. 11 (4), 272–280.

Sato, Y., Taki, K., Honda, Y., Takahashi, S., Yoshimura, A., 2013. Lithium toxicity precipitated by thyrotoxicosis due to silent thyroiditis: cardiac arrest, quadriplegia, and coma. Thyroid 23 (6), 766–770.

Relevant Website

http://ctdbase.org/detail.go?type=chem&acc=D000468&view=disease – Comparative Toxicogenomics database.

Alkyl Halides

S Kulkarni, Novartis Pharmaceuticals, USA

This article is a revision of the previous edition article by Swarupa G. Kulkarni and Harihara M. Mehendale, volume 1, pp 77–79, © 2005, Elsevier Inc.

- Name: Alkyl Halides
- Chemical Abstracts Service Registry Number: None as a group
- Synonyms: Methyl bromide, Methyl chloride, Methyl iodide, Dichloromethane, Tetrachloroethane, Carbon tetrachloride, Trichloroethene, Trichloroethylene, A number of fluorinated hydrocarbons (e.g., Freons), Halogenated hydrocarbons, Haloalkanes
- Molecular Formula: $R(X)_n$, where R is a hydrocarbon alkyl group and X is a halogen. One or more halogens may be present in one compound

Uses

Many halogenated hydrocarbons have important commercial applications. Alkyl halides are important intermediates in synthesis, as solvents in the laboratory and industry, and as dry cleaning fluids. They also find use as anesthetics and refrigerants. For example, trichloroethene is a common dry cleaning solvent. The fluorinated hydrocarbons (Freons) are used as refrigerants, industrial solvents, fire extinguishers, local anesthetics, and glass chillers, but mainly as propellants in aerosol products. Methyl bromide, methyl chloride, and methyl iodide are used as refrigerants in chemical synthesis and as fumigants. Methyl bromide is used with carbon tetrachloride in fire extinguishers. Methyl chloroform is used as a solvent for cleaning and degreasing, and in paint removers. Dichloromethane is used in paint removers and as an industrial solvent. Tetrachloroethane is used as a solvent in industry and occurs as a contaminant in other chlorinated hydrocarbons. It is occasionally present in household cleaners. Carbon tetrachloride is used as a solvent and intermediate in many industrial processes.

Exposure Routes and Pathways

Inhalation, dermal, and ocular contact are common routes of exposure.

Toxicokinetics

Fluorocarbon compounds are lipid soluble and, thus, generally well absorbed through the lung. Absorption after ingestion is much lower than after inhalation. Most of the fluorinated hydrocarbons are immediately absorbed via inhalation.

There is a significant accumulation of fluorocarbons in the brain, liver, and lungs compared to blood levels, signifying a tissue distribution of fluorocarbons similar to that of chloroform. Fluorocarbons are concentrated in body fat where they are slowly released into blood at a concentration that should not cause any risk of cardiac sensitization. Fluorocarbons are excreted primarily by the lungs.

Acute and Short-Term Toxicity (or Exposure)

Animal

Deliberate ocular exposure in rabbits to liquid Freon 12 produced effects related to the duration of exposure. Severe corneal damage with opacity occurred following exposure for 30 s. In dogs, inhalation of fluorinated hydrocarbon vapors causes bradycardia followed by deterioration to ventricular fibrillation in some animals.

Human

Freons are very toxic when inhaled in high concentrations or for extended periods. Inhalation of fluorinated hydrocarbons such as those caused by leaking air conditioners or refrigerators usually results in transient eye, nose, and throat irritation. Palpitations and lightheadedness are also seen. Headache was a common complaint, reported in 71% of 31 workers exposed to bromotrifluoromethane in one incident. Inhalation of halides at sufficient concentrations associated with deliberate abuse, or spills or industrial use occurring in poorly ventilated areas, has been associated with ventricular arrhythmias, pulmonary edema, and sudden death. Fluorinated hydrocarbons are believed to cause arrhythmias by sensitizing the myocardium to endogenous catecholamines. Freon solvents are used as degreasers. Dermal contact with fluorinated hydrocarbons may result in defatting, irritation, contact dermatitis, or skin injury. Severe frostbite was reported as a rare effect of severe Freon exposure. Mucosal necrosis and perforation of the stomach developed in one patient after ingesting a small amount of trichlorofluoromethane. Fluorocarbons containing bromine are more toxic than the corresponding chlorine compounds. There is a significant interpatient variation following exposure to fluorocarbons and it is difficult to predict symptoms following exposure. Compounds like dibromochloropropane, in which occupational exposure has affected male fertility, have now been removed from the market. Following acute exposure to methyl bromide, chloride, or iodide, nausea and vomiting, blurred vision, vertigo, weakness or paralysis, oliguria or anuria, drowsiness, confusion, hyperactivity, coma, convulsions, and pulmonary edema are noted. Pulmonary edema and bronchial pneumonia are most often the cause of death. Skin contact causes irritation and vesiculation.

Methyl chloroform and dichloromethane are central nervous system (CNS) depressants. Methyl chloroform sensitizes the myocardium to catecholamine-induced arrhythmias. Following exposure to tetrachloroethane, irritation of the eyes

 http://dx.doi.org/10.1016/B978-0-12-386454-3.00229-3

and nose, followed by headache and nausea, is observed. Cyanosis and CNS depression progressing to coma may appear after 1–4 h.

Chronic Toxicity (or Exposure)

Animal

Some of the chlorinated hydrocarbon solvents such as methylene chloride and chloroform have caused cancer in several species of experimental animals and are suspect human carcinogens.

Human

A syndrome of impaired psychomotor speed, impaired memory, and impaired learning has been described in workers with chronic occupational exposure to fluorinated hydrocarbons. Skin irritation and defatting dermatitis upon prolonged or repeated contact with the skin to trichloromonofluoromethane have been reported. An excess of CNS symptoms was seen in a group of workers chronically exposed to trichloromonofluoromethane. Repeated exposure to methyl bromide, methyl chloride, and methyl iodide will cause blurring of vision, numbness of the extremities, confusion, hallucinations, somnolence, fainting attacks, and bronchospasm. Chronic toxicity has not been reported with dichloromethane. Headache, tremor, dizziness, peripheral paresthesia, and anesthesia have been reported after chronic inhalation or skin exposure to tetrachloroethane. The US National Institute of Occupational Safety and Health recommends that methyl chloride, methyl bromide, and methyl iodide be considered as potential occupational carcinogens and that methyl chloride be considered a potential occupational teratogen.

Clinical Management

This management is intended for use in the absence of a specific treatment protocol for a product or a chemical. Symptomatic and supportive care is the primary therapy. The general approach to a poisoned patient is to first assess the vital signs of the patient followed by assessing the route of administration for potential toxicity. Measures to prevent further absorption of the compound may be useful. Victims of inhalation exposure should be moved from the toxic environment and administered 100% humidified supplemental oxygen with assisted ventilation as required. Exposed individuals should have a careful and thorough medical examination performed to look for abnormalities. Patients with fluorohydrocarbon poisoning should not be given epinephrine or similar drugs because of the tendency of fluorohydrocarbon to induce cardiac arrhythmia, including ventricular fibrillation. Monitoring including complete blood count, urine analysis, and liver and kidney function tests is suggested for patients with significant exposure. Activated charcoal or gastric lavage may be indicated to prevent further absorption. Exposed eyes should be irrigated with copious amounts of tepid water for at least 15 min. If irritation, pain, swelling, lacrimation, or photophobia persists after 15 min of irrigation, an ophthalmologic examination should be performed.

Environmental Fate

Highly chlorinated/fluorinated compounds are not expected to biodegrade rapidly.

Miscellaneous

Alkyl halides are practically insoluble in water. They are miscible in all proportions with liquid hydrocarbons and are, in general, good solvents for many organic substances. Most of the common organic halides are liquids. Like alkanes, halogen compounds are insoluble in and inert to cold concentrated sulfuric acid. In a series of alkyl halides, the boiling point rises with an increase in molecular weight due to the presence of either a heavier halogen atom or a larger alkyl group. Bromides boil at temperatures distinctly higher than the corresponding chlorides, and iodides are higher boiling than the bromides. Increase in the halogen content decreases their flammability. In contact with an open flame or very hot surface, fluorocarbons may decompose into highly irritant and toxic gases such as chlorine, hydrogen fluoride, or chloride, and even phosgene. Alkyl halides can be prepared by addition of the halogen or hydrogen halides to alkenes as well as by substitution of a halogen for hydrogen in an alkane. The most important method of preparing alkyl halides is by reaction between an alcohol and a hydrogen halide.

See also: Carbon Tetrachloride; Catecholamines; Chloroform; Freons; Methyl Bromide.

Further Reading

Kharasch, E.D., 2008. Adverse drug reactions with halogenated anesthetics. Clin. Pharmacol. Ther. 84, 158–162.

Relevant Websites

http://toxnet.nlm.nih.gov – TOXNET, Specialized Information Services, National Library of Medicine.

http://www2.chemistry.msu.edu/faculty/reusch/virttxtjml/alhalrx1.htm – Occurrence of Alkyl Halides..

Allergenicity Testing *see* Toxicity Testing, Sensitization

Allyl Alcohol

SP Sawant, Kimberly-Clark Worldwide, Inc., Roswell, GA, USA
HS Parihar, PCOM School of Pharmacy, Suwanee, GA, USA
HM Mehendale, University of Louisiana at Monroe, Monroe, LA, USA

This article is a revision of the previous edition article by Sharmilee P. Sawant & Harihara M. Mehendale, volume 1, pp. 80–81, © 2005, Elsevier Inc.

- Name: Allyl alcohol
- Chemical Abstracts Service Registry Number: 107-18-6
- Synonyms: 1-Propen-3-ol, 2-Propenol, 2-Propen-1-ol, Vinyl carbinol
- Molecular Formula: C_3H_6O
- Chemical Structure:

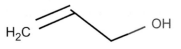

Background

Allyl alcohol (CAS # 107-18-6) is a colorless liquid with a pungent, mustard-like odor, soluble in water, and with a chemical structure of $CH_2{=}CHCH_2OH$. It is synthesized by the hydrolysis of allyl chloride or isomerization of propylene oxide. It is used as a raw material in manufacturing of various polymers, pharmaceuticals, pesticides, and other allyl compounds.

Uses

Industrial solvent, herbicide, and fungicide.

Environmental Fate and Behavior

Allyl alcohol is a colorless water soluble liquid. The melting point, boiling point, vapor pressure, and the octanol–water partition coefficient ($\log K_{ow}$) are $-129\,°C$, $97\,°C$, 26.1 mm Hg at $25\,°C$, and 0.17, respectively. The Henry's law constant is 4.99×10^{-6} atm-m^3 mol^{-1}. Allyl alcohol's production, its use as an industrial solvent and as a raw material/intermediate in the preparation of pharmaceuticals, polymers, organic chemicals, in the manufacture of glycerol and acrolein, and in the production of insecticides and herbicides, may result in its release to the environment. The vapor pressure of allyl alcohol, 26.1 mm Hg at $25\,°C$, indicates that if released in the air, it will exist mainly as a vapor in the ambient atmosphere. If released to soil, allyl alcohol is expected to have very high mobility based upon an estimated K_{oc} of 1.3 and will be distributed mainly in the water and soil. If released into water, allyl alcohol will stay in the water and is not expected to adsorb to suspended solids and sediments. Allyl alcohol is stable in water since it lacks functional groups that hydrolyze under environmental conditions and hence hydrolysis is not expected to be an important environmental fate process. In an aerobic biodegradation study, allyl alcohol was found to readily degradable (82–86%) in 14 days. The estimated bioconcentration factor of 3.2 based on the low $\log K_{ow}$ indicates that the potential to bioaccumulate in aquatic organisms is expected to be low.

Exposure and Exposure Monitoring

Occupational exposure to allyl alcohol may occur through inhalation and dermal contact where allyl alcohol is produced or used. Monitoring data indicate that the general population may be exposed to allyl alcohol via inhalation of ambient air or ingestion of food.

Toxicokinetics

Allyl alcohol is metabolized via two alternative oxidative pathways leading to the formation of acrolein or the epoxide glycidol. The epoxide may then be converted to glycerol by epoxide hydrolase. The conversion of allyl alcohol to acrolein is mediated by alcohol dehydrogenase (ADH) and then may be further oxidized to acrylic acid by Nicotinamide adenine dinucleotide- or Nicotinamide adenine dinucleotide phosphate-dependent enzymes in the liver cytosol or microsomes or to glycidaldehyde by a microsomal enzyme with subsequent conversion to glyceraldehyde by epoxide hydrolase. Alternatively, acrolein may react directly both enzymatic and nonenzymatic reactions to form stable adducts with glutathione (GSH) or other low molecular weight thiol compounds prior to excretion in the urine as mercapturate. Both glycidol and glycidaldehyde are substrates for lung and liver cytosolic GSH-S-transferases.

Mechanism of Toxicity

Allyl alcohol is inactive per se and its toxic effect is mediated by its ADH oxidation to form acrolein, which is responsible for the hepatotoxic action. The toxicity of the alcohol (or its metabolite acrolein) is dependent on the concentration of GSH. After

 http://dx.doi.org/10.1016/B978-0-12-386454-3.00230-X

severe depletion of GSH, the reactive metabolite of allyl alcohol can bind to essential sulfhydryl groups in the cellular macromolecules, leading to structural and functional changes that may lead to cell death. In this case, the appearance of lipid peroxidation could be merely the consequence of cell death. In the liver, Kupffer cell activation has been implicated in playing a prominent role during progression of toxicity.

Acute and Short-Term Toxicity

The oral LD_{50} values reported in rat and mice are 64, 70, and 99–105 mg kg^{-1} and 85 and 96 mg kg^{-1}, respectively. The dermal LD_{50} (rabbit) is 89 mg kg^{-1}. The inhalation of LC_{50} in rat and mouse are 76 ppm per 8 h and 500 mg m^{-3} per 2 h, respectively. The LD_{50} values reported in rats and mice following intraperitoneal administration are 37 and 60 mg kg^{-1}, respectively. Studies have shown that allyl alcohol is slightly irritating to skin and irritating to the eyes in rabbits. Allyl alcohol is not a skin sensitizer in guinea pigs. Acute exposure to allyl alcohol causes liver and kidney damage in animals. Allyl alcohol is classified as a periportal hepatotoxicant since it selectively damages the periportal region of the liver. Studies have shown that in adult rats, allyl alcohol produces a moderate to marked periportal necrosis with attendant inflammation and hemorrhage, and also decreases hepatic cytochrome P450, benzphetamine *N*-demethylation, and ethoxyresorufin *O*-deethylation activities by about 30%. In immature rats, it lowered both cytochrome P450 activity (30%) and ethoxyresorufin *O*-deethylation (75%). Benzphetamine *N*-demethylation was not significantly affected in immature rats. Intraperitoneal administration of 1.5 mmol kg^{-1} allyl alcohol to starved Swiss albino mice causes the development of hemolysis in nearly 50% of the animals. Other toxic effects include renal necrosis, pulmonary edema, and central nervous system effects at higher dose levels.

The most important adverse effects of occupational exposures to allyl alcohol are upper respiratory tract irritation and burning of the eyes. The substance may cause effects on the muscles, resulting in local spasms and aching. The appearance of these effects may be delayed after exposure.

Chronic Toxicity

Chronic exposure to allyl alcohol can cause liver and kidney damage.

Reproductive Toxicity

A reproductive/developmental toxicity study was conducted using both sexes of Sprague–Dawley rats. The rats were dosed 2, 8, or 40 mg per kg bodyweight per day via oral gavage. The male rats were dosed from 14 days before mating for a total of 42 days and the female rats were dosed 14 days before mating and throughout mating and a pregnancy period to day 3 of lactation. Clinical findings reported in parental animals at 40 mg per kg bodyweight per day were salivation, lacrimation, irregular breathing, decrease in locomotor activity in both sexes, and loose stools in males. Histopathological examination at 40 mg per kg bodyweight per day revealed atrophy of the thymus and hyperplasia of luteal cells in the ovary in females. In the livers, necrosis, fibrosis, and proliferation of bile ducts, hypertrophy, brown pigmentation in perilobular hepatocytes, and diffuse clear cell changes were observed in male and female rats at 40 mg per kg bodyweight per day. Reproductive effects such as extension of estrous cycle length and increases in estrous cycle were reported in females at 40 mg per kg per bodyweight per day. In offspring, a decrease in viability index on day 4 and total litter loss (from one dam) was reported at 40 mg per kg bodyweight per day. The lowest observed adverse effect level was reported as 40 mg per kg bodyweight per day based on parental and reproductive/developmental toxicity and a no observed adverse effect level is reported as 8 mg per kg bodyweight per day.

Genotoxicity

Several *in vivo* and *in vitro* genotoxicity studies have been conducted. Three out of seven *in vitro* genotoxicity assays including bacterial and mammalian cells gave positive results for these assays. Three *in vivo* genotoxicity assays, *in vivo* tests for chromosomal mutations (rat bone marrow and mouse erythrocyte micronuclei tests), and *in vivo* dominant lethal tests, produced negative results. Thus, based on the *in vitro* assays and *in vivo* tests, there is equivocal evidence that allyl alcohol is genotoxic.

Carcinogenicity

Allyl alcohol is classified as A4 (not classifiable as human carcinogen) by the American Conference of Governmental Industrial Hygienists.

Clinical Management

Exposure should be terminated as soon as possible by removal of the patient to fresh air. Skin, eyes, and mouth should be washed with copious amounts of water. Contaminated clothing should be removed. A mild soap solution may be used for washing the skin, but should not be used in the eye. Dilution with water may be effective if small amounts are swallowed until additional medical attention is available.

Ecotoxicology

The toxicity of allyl alcohol has been investigated in aquatic animals and plants. Several studies have shown that allyl alcohol causes acute toxicity in fish (medaka and fathead minnow), daphnia magna, polychaete, and green algae, and chronic toxicity in daphnia magna. Based on these studies, allyl alcohol is toxic to aquatic organisms and plants.

Exposure Standards and Guidelines

The Occupational Safety and Health Administration general industry permissible exposure limit: 2 ppm, 5 mg m^{-3} 8-h time-weighted average (TWA) (skin).

The National Institute for Occupational Safety and Health recommended exposure limit: 2 ppm 10-h TWA, 4 ppm 15-min short-term exposure limit (skin).

American Conference of Governmental Industrial Hygienists threshold limit value is 8-h TWA: 0.5 ppm, skin.

See also: Liver.

Further Reading

Atzori, L., Dore, M., Congiu, L., 1989. Aspects of allyl alcohol toxicity. Drug Metabol. Drug Interact. 7, 295–319.

Auerbach, S.S., Mahler, J., Travlos, G.S., Irwin, R.D., 2008. A comparative 90-day toxicity study of allyl acetate, allyl alcohol and acrolein. Toxicology 253 (1–3), 79–88.

Irwin, R.D., Jul 2006. NTP technical report on the comparative toxicity studies of allyl acetate (CAS No. 591-87-7), allyl alcohol (CAS No. 107-18-6) and acrolein (CAS No. 107-02-8) administered by gavage to F344/N rats and B6C3F_1 mice. Toxic. Rep. Ser. 48, 1–73. A1–H10.

Li, A.A., Fowles, J., Banton, M.I., Picut, C., Kirkpatrick, D.T., 2012. Acute inhalation study of allyl alcohol for derivation of acute exposure guideline levels. Inhal. Toxicol. 24 (4), 213–226.

Tukov, F.F., Maddox, J.F., Amacher, D.E., Bobrowski, W.F., Roth, R.A., Ganey, P.E., 2006. Modeling inflammation-drug interactions in vitro: a rat Kupffer cell-hepatocyte coculture system. Toxicol. In Vitro 20 (8), 1488–1499.

Relevant Websites

http://toxnet.nlm.nih.gov/cgi-bin/sis/search/r?dbs+hsdb:@term+@rn+@rel+107-18-6 – Hazardous Substances Data Bank for Allyl Alcohol.

http://chem.sis.nlm.nih.gov/chemidplus/ProxyServlet?objectHandle=Search&actionHandle=getAll3DMViewFiles&nextPage=jsp%2Fcommon%2FChemFull.jsp%3FcalledFrom%3D&chemid=0000107186&formatType=_3D – Organisation for Economic Co-operation and Development- Screening Information Datasheet for Allyl Alcohol (2-PROPEN-1-OL CAS N: 107-18-6) ChemIDplus advanced for allyl alcohol.

http://www.epa.gov/chemrtk/hpvis/rbp/Allyl%20Alcohol_Web_SuppDocs_August%202008.pdf – United States Environmental Protection Agency Supporting Document for Risk Based Prioritization.

Allylamine

NV Soucy, 3M Center, St Paul, MN, USA

Chemical Profile

- Name: Allylamine
- Chemical Abstracts Service Registry Number: 107-11-9
- Synonyms: 2-Propen-1-amine, 2-Propenylamine, 3-Amino-1-propene, 3-Aminopropene, Monoallylamine
- Molecular Formula: C_3H_7N
- Chemical Structure:

H_2N–CH_2–CH=CH_2

Background

Allylamine is a primary unsaturated alkylamine and in this review refers to monoallylamine. Allylamine can also be used generically to describe the secondary (diallyl-) and tertiary (triallyl-) amine derivatives of monoallylamine, as well as other more complex alkylamines. Allylamine is a colorless, flammable liquid and is volatile and reactive with oxidizing materials. Allylamine has a strong ammonia odor, is acutely toxic by all routes of exposure, and produces cardiotoxicity in a manner that has been well characterized by *in vivo* and *in vitro* methods. In addition to its use as an industrial chemical, allylamine is utilized as a model compound for basic research investigations into mechanisms of cardiovascular disease based on the nature of the cardiac and vascular lesions observed following allylamine exposure.

Uses

Allylamine is used as an industrial solvent and in organic synthesis, including rubber vulcanization, synthesis of ion-exchange resins, and as an intermediate in pharmaceutical synthesis. Derivatives of allylamine are utilized as both veterinary and human pharmaceuticals, including the antifungal agent terbinafine. Allylamine has been used since the 1940s as a research tool for investigations of cardiovascular disease, with the earliest studies using allylamine to induce initial vascular injury in animal models of atherogenesis. Additionally, allylamine has been used to model myocardial infarction and vascular injury in animal models of human cardiovascular disease.

Environmental Fate and Behavior

The production and use of allylamine as an industrial solvent may result in environmental releases to the air, water, and soil. Allylamine is freely soluble in water, alcohol, chloroform, and most solvents. The vapor pressure at 20 °C is 198 mm Hg, the Henry's law constant is estimated to be 9.95×10^{-6} atm m^3 mol^{-1}, and the octanol/water partition coefficient (log K_{ow}) is estimated to be 0.21.

If released to the soil, allylamine is expected to have very high mobility, with volatilization from dry soils. If released to the water, volatilization is anticipated from the surface and allylamine is not anticipated to adsorb to sediment. The potential for bioconcentration in aquatic organisms is predicted to be low. If released to the atmosphere the half-life is anticipated to be 6.9 h, with degradation occurring by reaction with photochemically produced hydroxyl radicals.

Exposure and Exposure Monitoring

Occupational exposures to allylamine are possible via inhalation, dermal, and ingestion. Environmental releases from industrial sources could also result in human exposures. Allylamine has been associated with tobacco; it is unclear if it is a natural component of tobacco, a pyrolysis product in tobacco smoke or an additive in the production of tobacco products.

Toxicokinetics

Allylamine is rapidly absorbed across the gastrointestinal tract when ingested; it primarily distributes to the aorta and coronary arteries with lesser distribution to the liver and kidney and is excreted in the urine, with up to 60% of a single oral dose excreted within 24 h. Allylamine is metabolized to acrolein and hydrogen peroxide by a semicarbazide-sensitive amine oxidase (SSAO) that catalyzes essentially the same reaction catalyzed by monoamine oxidase and is highly active in vascular tissue. Acrolein is further metabolized to 3-hydroxypropylmercapturic acid through glutathione conjugation, and this is the primary urinary metabolite.

Mechanism of Toxicity

Allylamine exposure results in myocardial damage and intimal proliferation of vascular smooth muscle cells in multiple animal species. The mechanism for these distinctive cardiovascular lesions is believed to be related to its bioactivation to acrolein and possibly hydrogen peroxide. Several lines of evidence support this hypothesis; SSAO is highly active in vascular tissue where allylamine predominantly distributes, incubation of homogenates of vascular tissue with allylamine results in the generation of acrolein and hydrogen peroxide,

 http://dx.doi.org/10.1016/B978-0-12-386454-3.01160-X

and pretreatment with a semicarbazide inhibitor of SSAO reduces or eliminates the hypercontraction and vasospasm associated with allylamine exposure *in vitro*. Researchers have taken advantage of the distinctive lesions that result from various exposures to allylamine and have used it as chemical tool to induce animal models of cardiovascular dysfunction that resemble human disease.

Acute and Short-Term Toxicity

Animal

Allylamine is acutely toxic in multiple animal species regardless of the route of administration. The oral LD_{50} in the rat is reported to be 106 mg kg^{-1}, the 4-h inhalation LC_{50} in the rat is reported to be 286 ppm, and the dermal LD_{50} in rabbits is reported to be 35 mg kg^{-1}. Unlike other aliphatic amines, where acute toxicity increases with the addition of side chains, the acute toxicity of allylamine decreases as side chains are added, with a 10-fold decrease in acute oral toxicity for triallylamine. Signs of toxicity following these acute exposures include eye, skin, and respiratory irritation, pulmonary edema, and myocardial lesions. Allylamine is a severe eye and skin irritant, with some studies indicating the potential for corrosive effects. There are no data to suggest that allylamine is a dermal sensitizing agent.

Respiratory depression was observed in mice, with an airborne concentration of 9 ppm resulting in a 50% reduction in the respiratory rate (RD_{50}) in the exposed animals. Subsequent evaluations in mice of concentrations up to 27 ppm for 14 days did not result in pathological changes to the nasal passages, trachea, or lungs of the exposed animals.

Human

The odor threshold for allylamine is reported to be 2.5 ppm in human volunteers, with dose-related increases in the incidence of eye irritation, nose irritation, and pulmonary discomfort. Central nervous system effects included headache and nausea and were observed at all dose levels with no apparent dose-related effect. At 14 ppm, the irritant effects to the eyes, nose, and respiratory system became intolerable to the test subjects. Case reports indicate that chest pain and respiratory irritation have been reported following occupational accidents and exposures.

Chronic Toxicity

Animal

When administered by parenteral routes of exposure, the pathological lesions induced by allylamine primarily are associated with the heart, aorta, and coronary arteries. However, when administered intravenously, allylamine has also been associated with hepatic cellular vacuolization, thickening of the pulmonary artery, and vascular sclerosis of the kidney. These extracardiac lesions all seem to have a vascular component which is further data to support a common mechanism of toxicity.

Human

At least one study has investigated cardiovascular effects in workers exposed to allylamine; however, no associations were observed.

Reproductive Toxicity

No data are available for this end point. The National Toxicology Program testing status for allylamine indicates that a conventional teratology study has been completed in rats; however, the results are not discussed and test data and report are not yet available.

Genotoxicity

Genotoxicity studies have been conducted in multiple bacterial strains with and without metabolic activation and all of the results have been negative.

Carcinogenicity

No epidemiological studies evaluating the carcinogenic potential of allylamine exist. In addition, allylamine has not been evaluated for carcinogenicity in animal studies. Acrolein, the active metabolite, has been evaluated for carcinogenicity by the Environmental Protection Agency but the data were judged to be inadequate for classification.

Clinical Management

On the basis of animal data, allylamine is anticipated to be acutely toxic by all routes of exposure. Occupational accidents are the most likely source of life-threatening exposures. Removal from exposure and supportive clinical care are recommended in the case of overexposure.

Exposure Standards and Guidelines

Occupational exposure guidelines are not established for allylamine. The National Research Council has established acute exposure guideline levels (AEGLs) for the general public which are applicable to emergency exposures ranging from 10 min to 8 h. The AEGL-1, the threshold for irritation and other sensory effects which would be transient and reversible upon cessation of exposure, is set at 0.42 ppm for exposures ranging from 10 min to 8 h. The AEGL-2, the threshold above which the general population could experience irreversible effects, including impairment of the ability to escape, is set at 3.3 ppm for 10 min to as low as 1.2 ppm for 8 h. The AEGL-3, the threshold above which the general population could experience life-threatening health effects and death, is set at 150 ppm for 10 min to as low as 2.3 ppm for 8 h.

See also: Acrolein; Allyl Alcohol; Cardiovascular System.

Further Reading

Boor, P.J., Hysmith, R.M., 1987. Allylamine cardiovascular toxicity. Toxicology 44, 129–145.

National Research Council, 2007. Acute Exposure Guideline Levels for Selected Airborne Chemicals, vol. 6. National Academies Press, Washington, DC.

Relevant Websites

http://www.epa.gov/iris/index.html – US Environmental Protection Agency.

http://ntp.niehs.nih.gov – National Toxicology Program: Search for Allylamine.

Allyl Formate

SP Sawant, Kimberly-Clark Worldwide, Inc., Roswell, GA, USA
HM Mehendale, University of Louisiana at Monroe, Monroe, LA, USA

- Name: Allyl formate
- Chemical Abstracts Service Registry Number: 1838-59-1
- Synonyms: Allyl alcohol, Formate, Formic acid, Allyl ester, 2-Propenyl ester
- Molecular Formula: $C_4H_6O_2$
- Chemical Structure:

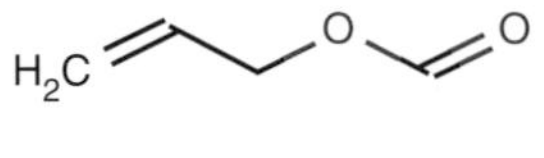

Background

Allyl formate (CAS # 1838-59-1) is a clear, colorless liquid. It is slightly soluble in water. It is reported to cause liver and kidney injury in animals. The most common effect in humans following occupational exposure to allyl formate exposure is upper respiratory tract irritation.

Uses

It is used as a solvent in spray lacquers, enamels, varnishes, and latex paints and as an ingredient in paint thinners and strippers, varnish removers, and herbicides. It is also used in liquid soaps, cosmetics, industrial and household cleaners, and dry-cleaning compounds.

Exposure and Exposure Monitoring

The substance can be absorbed into the body by inhalation and dermal contact, and by ingestion.

Toxicokinetics

Allyl formate is rapidly cleaved *in vivo* by nonspecific esterases to allyl alcohol. Allyl alcohol is metabolized via two alternative oxidative pathways leading to the formation of acrolein or the epoxide, glycidol. The epoxide may then be converted to glycerol by epoxide hydrolase. The conversion of allyl alcohol to acrolein is mediated by alcohol dehydrogenase, which may then be further oxidized to acrylic acid by nicotinamide adenine dinucleotide- or nicotinamide adenine dinucleotide phosphate-dependent enzymes in the liver cytosol or microsomes or to glycidaldehyde by a microsomal enzyme with subsequent conversion to glyceraldehyde by epoxide hydrolase. Alternatively, acrolein may react directly both enzymatically and nonenzymatically to form stable adducts with glutathione (GSH) or other low molecular weight thiol compounds prior to excretion in the urine as mercapturate.

Mechanism of Toxicity

Allyl formate is cleaved by nonspecific esterases to allyl alcohol, which is then oxidized by alcohol dehydrogenases to the reactive acrolein, which is responsible for the hepatotoxic action. The toxicity of allyl alcohol via its metabolite acrolein is dependent on the concentration of GSH. After depletion of GSH, the reactive metabolite of allyl alcohol can bind to essential sulfhydryl groups in the cellular macromolecules, leading to structural and functional modifications, which can be responsible for hepatic injury. Appearance of lipid peroxidation signals events that follow toxication mechanisms initiated by acrolein, and subsequent and continued lipid peroxidation could be merely the consequence of the cell death.

Acute and Short-Term Toxicity

Animal

The LD_{50} reported following oral administration in rats and mice is 125 and 96 mg kg^{-1}, respectively. The LC_{50} reported following inhalation exposure in rats and mice is 980 and 610 mg m^{-3}, respectively. Acute exposure to allyl formate causes liver and kidney damage. Allyl formate is classified as a periportal hepatotoxicant since its metabolite, acrolein, selectively damages the periportal region of the liver in rodents.

Human

The most important adverse effect of occupational exposures to allyl formate is upper respiratory tract irritation.

Chronic Toxicity

Animal

Chronic exposure to allyl formate can cause liver and kidney damage.

Human

Long-term exposure may lead to liver or kidney damage.

Clinical Management

Exposure should be terminated as soon as possible by removal of the patient to fresh air. Skin, eyes, and mouth should be washed with copious amounts of water. Contaminated clothing should be removed. A mild soap solution may

 http://dx.doi.org/10.1016/B978-0-12-386454-3.00231-1

be used for washing the skin, but should not be placed in the eye. Dilution with water may be effective if small amounts are swallowed before medical attention is sought.

Ecotoxicology

The substance is reported to be very toxic to aquatic organisms.

See also: Acrolein; Allyl Alcohol.

Further Reading

Athersuch, T.J., Keun, H., Tang, H., Nicholson, J.K., 2006. Quantitative urinalysis of the mercapturic acid conjugates of allyl formate using high-resolution NMR spectroscopy. J. Pharm. Biomed. Anal. 40 (2), 410–416.

Droy, B.F., Davis, M.E., Hinton, D.E., 1989. Mechanism of allyl formate-induced hepatotoxicity in rainbow trout. Toxicol. Appl. Pharmacol. 98, 313–324.

Rees, K.R., Tarlow, M.J., 1967. The hepatotoxic action of allyl formate. Biochem. J. 104, 757–761.

Yap, I.K., Clayton, T.A., Tang, H., et al., 2006. An integrated metabonomic approach to describe temporal metabolic disregulation induced in the rat by the model hepatotoxin allyl formate. J. Proteome Res. 5 (10), 2675–2684.

Alpha Blockers

SM Miller and KL Cumpston, Virginia Commonwealth University, Richmond, VA, USA

- Name: Alpha blockers
- Chemical Abstracts Service Registry Numbers: 19216-56-9, 63590-64-7, 74191-85-8, 106133-20-4
- Synonyms: Cardura, Carduran, Hytrin, Minipress, Flomax
- Chemical/Pharmaceutical/Other Class: Selective alpha-1 adrenergic antagonists
- Molecular Formulae: $C_{19}H_{21}N_5O_4$, $C_{19}H_{25}N_5O_4$, $C_{23}H_{25}N_5O_5$, $C_{20}H_{28}N_2O_5S$
- Chemical Structures:

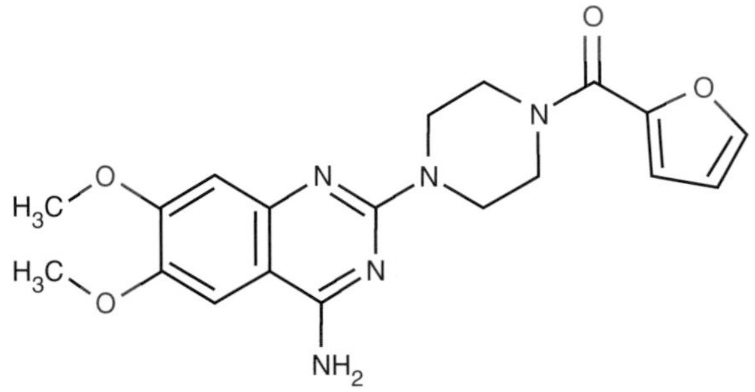

Prazosin

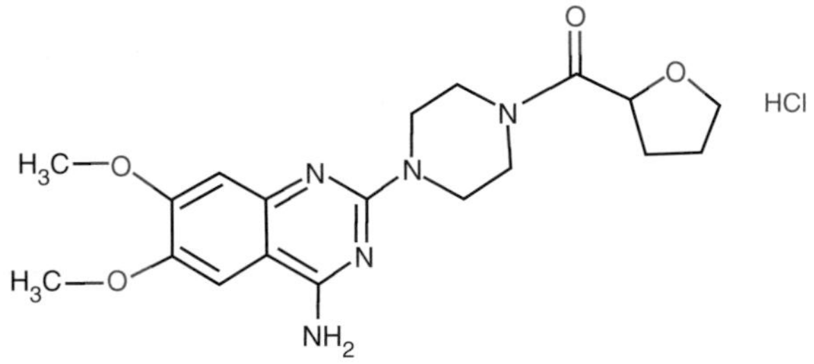

Terazosin

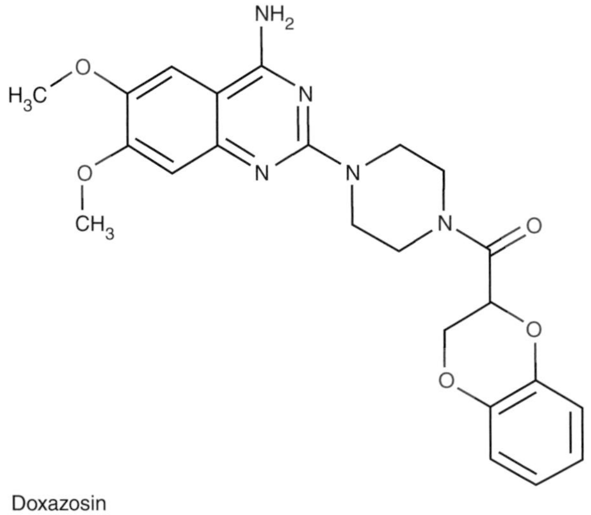

Doxazosin

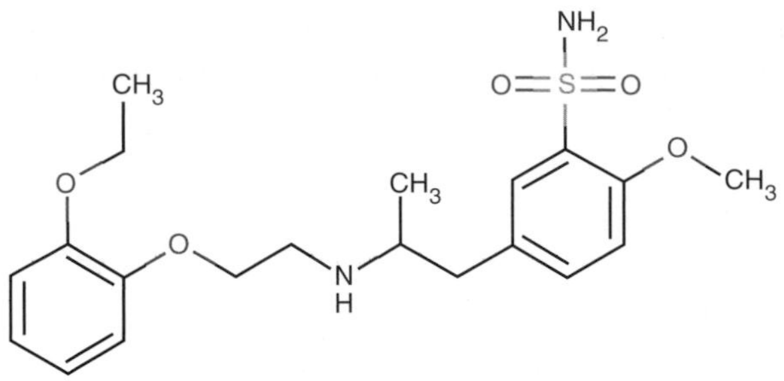

Tamsulosin

Uses

Alpha receptor antagonists can be selective or nonselective for alpha-1 and 2 receptors in peripheral smooth muscle. Selective alpha-1 antagonists such as prazosin, terazosin, and doxazosin will be the focus of this article and are used for several different modalities including treatment for urinary dysfunction secondary to benign prostatic hyperplasia (BPH) and primary hypertension. Prazosin has also been studied in the treatment of alcohol dependence. A large trial, 'Clinical Trial of the Adrenergic Alpha-1 Antagonist Prazosin for Alcohol Dependence,' will be completed in 2013. Tamsulosin and alfuzosin are used primarily for the treatment of BPH.

Background

Prazosin, terazosin, and doxazosin are alpha antagonists used for the control of blood pressure and for constriction of the prostate in the treatment of prostatic hypertrophy. Prazosin is also used as a sympatholytic and is under study for use in certain disease states including for the treatment of alcohol dependence, posttraumatic stress disorder, and severe nightmares and sleep disturbances.

Exposure Routes and Pathways

Ingestion and injection are more common routes of accidental and intentional toxicity.

Toxicokinetics

Prazosin has a bioavailability of around 60% hepatic metabolism, 97% protein binding, volume of distribution of 0.5 l kg^{-1}, and a half-life of around 2–3 h. Terazosin is approximately 90% protein bound, extensively metabolized by the liver and achieves peak concentration around 1 h after oral

 http://dx.doi.org/10.1016/B978-0-12-386454-3.00714-4

ingestion. The volume of distribution for prazosin is 25–30 l, and it has a half-life of 9–12 h. Doxazosin has a bioavailability of 65%, with 98% protein binding, and it achieves a peak concentration 2–3 h after immediate-release forms are taken orally. There is an extensive hepatic metabolism, and it has a half-life of approximately 22 h. Tamsulosin has more than 90% bioavailability, achieves peak concentrations in 4–8 h, undergoes extensive hepatic metabolism, 76% renal excretion, and has a half-life of 9–13 h.

Mechanism of Toxicity

The alpha antagonists produce arterial smooth muscle relaxation, vasodilation, and a reduction of the blood pressure. Excessive vasodilation causes hypotension and can lead to reflex tachycardia and sometimes somnolence when affecting the central nervous system (CNS).

Acute and Short-Term Toxicity (or Exposure)

Human

Alpha-1 blockers can produce significant symptoms of postural hypotension, including light-headedness, syncope, or palpitations, particularly after the first dose or if the dosing is rapidly increased. Hypotension and CNS depression ranging from lethargy to coma have been reported in overdose. Tachycardia is most often seen, but cases of bradycardia have been reported and are thought to be associated with a sympatholytic effect seen with the alpha antagonists in some patients. Priapism can occur as a side effect.

Reproductive Toxicity

Doxazosin, prazosin, and terazosin are classified as Food and Drug Administration pregnancy category C.

Clinical Management

Patients who are awake after a significant ingestion can be treated with activated charcoal. Basic and advanced life-support measures should be implemented. Airway management is not generally required but patients should be monitored for decrease in mental status. For hypotension, patients should receive intravenous fluid boluses. A vasopressor with alpha-1 agonism properties like norepinephrine or phenylephrine may counteract the alpha-1 antagonism, leading to vasoconstriction and increase in blood pressure.

See also: Mechanisms of Toxicity; Pharmacokinetics; Isopropanol; Poisoning Emergencies in Humans; Cardiovascular System.

Further Reading

Cubeddu, L.X., 1988. New alpha 1-adrenergic receptor antagonists for the treatment of hypertension: role of vascular alpha receptors in the control of peripheral resistance. Am. Heart J. 116, 133–162.

Froehlich, J.C., Hausauer, B.J., Federoff, D.L., Fischer, S.M., Rasmussen, D.D., 2013. Prazosin reduces alcohol drinking throughout prolonged treatment and blocks the initiation of drinking in rats selectively bred for high alcohol intake. Alcohol. Clin. Exp. Res. 37 (9), 1552–1560.

Kim, A.K., Souza-Formigoni, M.L., 2013. Alpha 1-adrenergic drugs affect the development and expression of ethanol-induced behavioral sensitization. Behav. Brain Res. 256C, 646–654 (Epub ahead of print).

Lenz, K., Druml, W., Kleinberger, G., 1985. Acute intoxication with prazosin: case report. Hum. Toxicol. 4, 53–56.

Lip, G.Y.H., Ferner, R.E., 1995. Poisoning with anti-hypertensive drugs: alpha adrenoreceptor antagonists. J. Hum. Hypertens. 9, 523–526.

Robbins, D.N., Crawford, E.D., Lackner, L.H., 1983. Priapism secondary to prazosin overdose. J. Urol. 130, 975.

Satar, S., Sebe, A., Avci, A., et al., 2005. Acute intoxication with doxazosin. Hum. Exp. Toxicol. 24 (6), 337–339.

Seak, C.J., Lin, C.C., 2008. Acute intoxication with terazosin. Am. J. Emerg. Med. 26 (1), 117–126.

Relevant Website

http://clinicaltrials.gov/ct2/show/NCT00167687 – Prazosin Alcohol Dependence IVR Study at ClinicalTrials.gov.

Aluminosilicate Fibers

LD Maxim, Everest Consulting Associates, Cranbury, NJ, USA
MJ Utell, University of Rochester Medical Center, Rochester, NY, USA

- Name: Aluminosilicate fiber
- Chemical Abstracts Service Registry Number: 142844-00-6
- Synonyms: Refractory ceramic fiber (RCF), aluminosilicate wool (ASW).
- Molecular Formula: No specific ChemID formula: This fiber is produced by melting a mixture of alumina (Al_2O_3) and silica (SiO_2) in approximately equal proportions. Other inorganic oxides, such as ZrO_2, Cr_2O_3, B_2O_3, and TiO_2, are sometimes added to alter the properties (e.g., the maximum end-use temperature) of the resulting product. International Agency for Research on Cancer (IARC) and NIOSH provide illustrative composition ranges for aluminosilicate fibers. Compositions vary by manufacturer and intended end use; detailed data can be found in manufacturer's technical and safety data sheets. Standard fibers range in reported composition (percentage by weight) from 40 to 55% alumina and 45 to 65% silica (exclusive of minor ingredients). Higher-temperature (sometimes termed zirconia aluminosilicate) fiber compositions range in composition from 28 to 40% alumina, 43 to 56% silica, and 14 to 18% zirconia.
- Structure: No specific ChemID structure: Amorphous fibers of variable dimensions.

Background

Aluminosilicate fibers (commonly called refractory ceramic fibers (RCFs) in the United States) are amorphous fibers belonging to a class of materials termed synthetic vitreous fibers (SVFs), also termed man-made mineral fibers or man-made vitreous fibers. This class of materials also includes glass wool, rock (stone) wool, slag wool, mineral wool, and special-purpose glass fibers. Fibers can be classified in various ways, such as natural versus synthetic, organic versus inorganic, and crystalline versus amorphous. Several fiber taxonomies have been proposed; **Figure 1** shows the taxonomy of SVFs.

Aluminosilicate wools (ASWs) were first invented in the early 1940s and commercialized in the 1950s in the United States and somewhat later in other countries. Substantial energy price increases beginning in the 1970s increased the economic benefits of energy conservation and the market for these fibers.

ASWs are SVFs produced by melting (at $\sim 1925\,^{\circ}C$) alumina, silica, and other inorganic oxides, and then blowing or spinning these melts into fibers. These fibers can also be produced by melting blends of calcined kaolin, alumina, and silica. The bulk fibers produced by this process can be used directly for some applications, but are more commonly converted into other physical forms, including blanket, modules (folded blanket capable of being installed rapidly in industrial furnaces), paper, felt, board, vacuum formed parts, textiles, and putties or pastes. Conversion to various physical forms takes place at locations where aluminosilicate fibers are produced, facilities operated by converters (producers of intermediate goods) or end users. Primary manufacturing facilities for aluminosilicate fibers are located in North and South America, Europe, and Asia. Conversion facilities and end users are distributed throughout the industrialized world.

Uses

ASWs have several desirable properties for use as high-temperature insulating materials, including low thermal conductivity, low heat storage (low volumetric heat capacity), thermal shock resistance, lightweight, good corrosion resistance, and ease of installation. Depending upon the fiber composition, the maximum end-use temperature for ASWs can be as high as $1430\,^{\circ}C$ ($2600\,^{\circ}F$). Because of this capability, these fibers are also included in the class of high-temperature insulating wools (HTIWs). Benefits of the use of ASW insulation include reduced energy costs and reduced greenhouse gas emissions. The energy savings can be substantial when compared to conventional high-temperature insulation such as insulating firebrick.

Applications and markets for ASWs are principally industrial and vary by product form and country including furnace linings and components in the cement, ceramic, chemical, fertilizer, forging, foundry, glass, heat treating, nonferrous metals, petrochemical, power generation (cogeneration), and steel industries. ASWs are used for passive fire protection applications where thin, lightweight materials are needed to prevent flame penetration. ASWs are also used to a minor degree in emission control applications such as heat shield insulation, catalytic converter support mat, and filtration media for air bag inflators. Though sometimes referred to in the literature as a substitute for asbestos, aluminosilicate fibers are not typically used in asbestos applications. Aluminosilicate fibers are priced substantially higher than various types of asbestos and have maximum end-use temperatures substantially greater than those for asbestos (which vary depending upon the product but are typically $\leq 850\,^{\circ}C$).

Environmental Fate and Behavior

Aluminosilicate fibers are white fibrous solids, soluble to a degree in human lung fluid (see below). The usual physicochemical parameters relevant to fate and transport (e.g., solubility, vapor pressure, octanol–water partition coefficient, and Henry's law constant) are not applicable or relevant; vapor pressure, octanol–water partition coefficient, and Henry's law constant are exceedingly low and not measurable. Fibers are capable of being transported in the air and are removed by gravitational settling. The Member State Support Document

 http://dx.doi.org/10.1016/B978-0-12-386454-3.01161-1

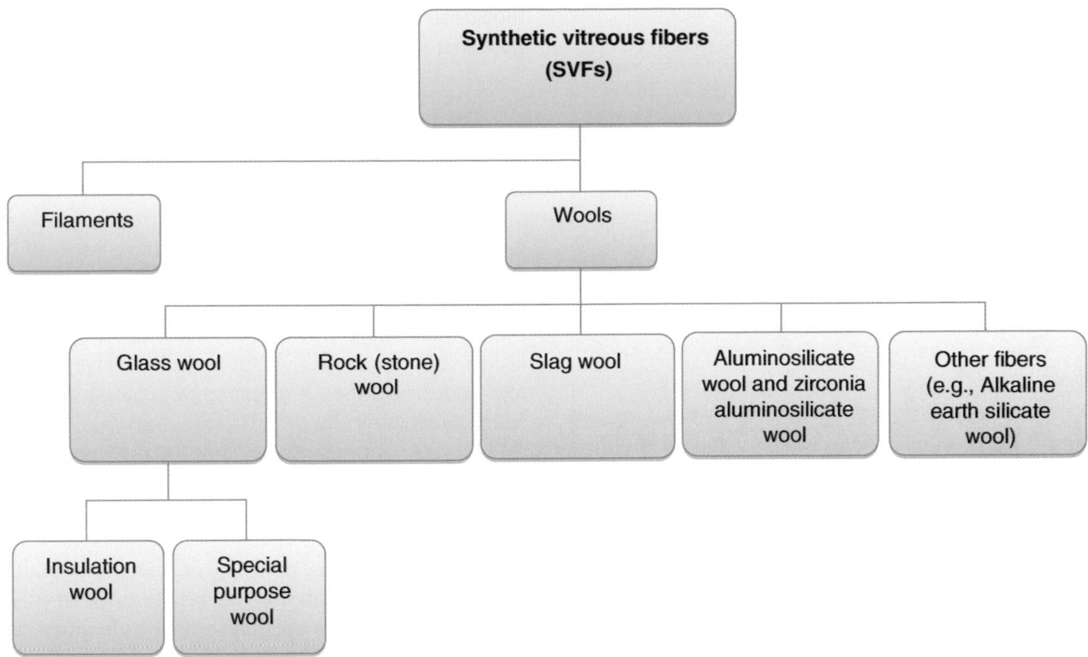

Figure 1 Taxonomy of synthetic vitreous fibers (SVFs). Reproduced from International Agency for Research on Cancer (IARC)., 2002. IARC Monographs on the Evaluation of Carcinogenic Risks to Humans, vol. 81, Man-made Vitreous Fibres, IARC, Lyon, France.

submitted to the European Chemicals Agency in favor of listing aluminosilicate fibers as a substance of very high concern (SVHC) notes that environmental fate and hazard data were not relevant.

Exposure and Exposure Monitoring

Possible pathways for human exposure include ingestion, inhalation, and dermal contact. There are only limited data on ASW concentrations in the environment, typically in the vicinity (fence line) of manufacturing facilities and at one landfill. Arithmetic mean fence line boundary concentrations range from beneath the detection limit to .02 fibers per milliliter ($f\,ml^{-1}$). The greatest exposure to aluminosilicate (and other) SVFs occurs from inhalation by workers who manufacture, convert, use, or remove these fibers. It is estimated that approximately 30 000 workers in the United States are occupationally exposed to ASWs and a similar number in Europe. As of this writing, no estimates are available for the size of the exposed population in Asia.

The ASW industry has developed a comprehensive (now nearly worldwide) product stewardship program (PSP) to identify and manage risks associated with production or use of these fibers. In the United States, this voluntary program is overseen by the Occupational Safety and Health Administration. Two components of the PSP are directed to measuring and controlling occupational exposures to aluminosilicate and related HTIWs. These efforts are well documented. As part of the PSP, industrial hygienists from ASW producers monitor exposures (including 8-h time-weighted average (TWA) respirable fiber concentrations) at plants operated by producers and also at customer facilities. Data collected by this program include TWA fiber concentrations, jobs (partitioned into eight functional job categories (FJCs)), tasks within jobs, exposure controls, and use of personal protective equipment (PPE). Key results of the exposure monitoring program include the following: (1) exposures vary by FJC and task within FJC; exposures are the highest for removal of after-service insulation, (2) for comparable jobs exposures are slightly lower at plants operated by producers, but the gap has narrowed over the years, and (3) weighted (by number of workers in each FJC) fiber concentrations have decreased over the years and now average between .2 and .3 $f\,ml^{-1}$, absent any correction for protection associated with the use of PPE. However, there is substantial variability in TWA fiber concentrations – even within a specific FJC and plant the coefficient of variation σ/μ is typically >1.0.

Figure 2 shows weighted arithmetic mean time trends in TWA fiber concentrations in the United States.

Toxicokinetics

The deposition and clearance of ASW and other fibers have been extensively studied, which has resulted in the development of a generally accepted paradigm of fiber toxicology often described as 'the 3 Ds' for dose, dimension, and durability. The inhaled dose depends upon the concentration of respirable fibers (fibers capable of reaching the alveolar region, typically those with diameters less than approximately 3.0 μm for humans) and the exposure duration. Fiber dimensions are important in several respects: (1) fiber dimensions (chiefly diameter) determine whether a fiber is respirable, (2) fiber dimensions determine the fraction of fibers deposited in the alveolar region via diffusion, sedimentation, and impaction, (3) fiber dimensions (diameter and length) affect the rate of

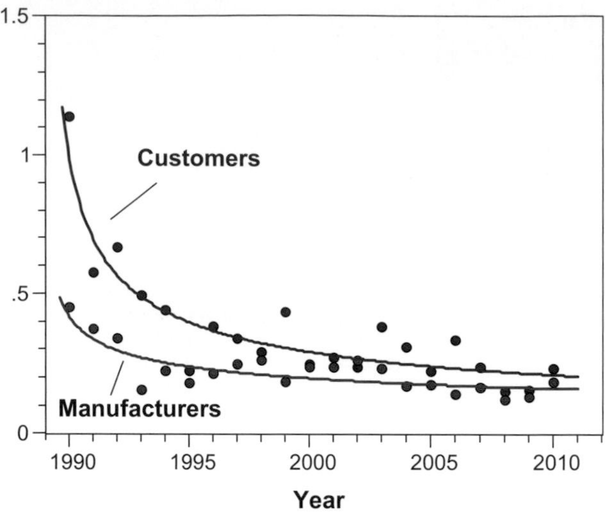

Figure 2 Time trends in weighted average TWA fiber concentrations at manufacturer and customer facilities.

clearance of fibers from the lung, and (4) fiber length affects the apparent toxicity of the fiber (other things being equal). Finally, the toxicokinetics of a fiber depends upon its rate of clearance from the lung. Clearance from the alveolar region takes place by three mechanisms including (1) removal of short (say <20 μm or approximately the diameter of an alveolar macrophage (AM) in humans) fibers by phagocytosis of AMs, (2) dissolution of both short and long fibers in lung fluids, and (3) breakage of long fibers, which in the case of aluminosilicate and other SVFs is chiefly transverse breakage, creating shorter fibers capable of being removed by AMs. The temporal pattern of lung burden of long fibers (e.g., those >20 μm long although this threshold is not a 'bright line') is believed to be a key determinant of the biological effects of exposure to SVFs. Clearance rates of fibers are estimated *in vitro* by measured dissolution rates (and derivatively a dissolution rate constant K_{dis}) in simulated lung fluid or *in vivo* from short-term animal inhalation studies. Data on fiber clearance from laboratory animals after cessation of exposure often indicate that a 'two-pool' model fits best. The weighted halftime for clearance of long fibers ($WT_{0.5}$) – a key measure of biopersistence – is found to correlate well with the results of animal cancer bioassays. Fibers with greater biopersistence are more likely to result in tumors in animal bioassay studies.

One study presents a mathematical model to calculate the deposition fractions of ASWs (using fiber dimensions similar to those measured in occupational exposure studies) in humans as approximately .08 and .16, respectively, for nose and mouth breathing. Dissolution rates (typically measured in nanograms per square centimeter per hour) from *in vitro* studies have been measured for many SVFs, including aluminosilicate fibers, and correlate well with weighted halftimes derived from *in vivo* studies. The biopersistence of aluminosilicate fibers, as measured by the weighted halftime of fibers >20 μm long from inhalation studies, is approximately 53 days, which shows that ASW is more biopersistent than many SVFs, but comparable to those for other SVFs including one type of rock wool, E-glass, and 475 glass. The biopersistence of aluminosilicate fibers is substantially lower than that for crocidolite asbestos (~800 days), which suggests that the toxic effects of aluminosilicate fibers are likely to be markedly less than those for this form of asbestos.

Mechanism of Toxicity

Numerous *in vitro* and *in vivo* studies have been conducted on both natural and synthetic fibers to try to understand and measure cytotoxicity, mutagenicity, and genotoxicity. Many of these studies have proven inconclusive, so mechanism(s) of action are still unclear. Other studies have indicated that aluminosilicate fibers are less active biologically than various forms of asbestos.

Acute and Short-term Toxicity (Animal/Human)

Aluminosilicate fibers have a recognized potential to cause mild mechanical irritation to the respiratory tract (nose, throat, and lungs), eyes, and skin of exposed individuals, a property typically listed on safety data sheets.

Chronic Toxicity (Animal/Human)

Aluminosilicate fibers have been evaluated in several chronic animal studies with various routes of exposure (inhalation, intratracheal instillation, intrapleural injection, and intraperitoneal injection). Of greatest potential relevance are the results of chronic inhalation studies, which indicated that rats and hamsters exposed to aluminosilicate fibers developed fibrosis and tumors. Interpretation of the results is made more difficult by the fact that the experiments employed an aluminosilicate fiber with a high and nonrepresentative content of particulate material, believed to be an artifact of the test sample preparation method, resulting in lung overload. Acknowledging this complication, IARC nonetheless concluded that there was sufficient evidence for carcinogenicity of aluminosilicate fibers in experimental animals, resulting in a cancer classification of Group 2B. Other regulatory or advisory agencies have reached similar conclusions. As noted above, ASW has been classified as an SVHC in Europe.

The aluminosilicate fiber industry has sponsored several epidemiological studies on workers exposed to these fibers. The studies evaluated/measured symptoms, X-rays, pulmonary function, and mortality. Collectively, these studies indicated that exposed workers (1) exhibited symptoms (e.g., dyspnea) similar to those reported in other dust-exposed populations, (2) developed statistically significant, but not clinically significant, deficits in certain measures of pulmonary function in a cross-sectional study, but no excessive decline in a later longitudinal study, and (3) a dose-related increase in pleural plaques, but no interstitial fibrosis. The mortality study indicated that there was no incremental lung cancer and no cases of mesothelioma. (The mortality study indicated that there was a statistically significant association with cancers of the urinary organs, an unexpected finding, which may be due to chance.) The mortality study is ongoing.

Immunotoxicity

There are limited reports indicating that aluminosilicate fibers are immunotoxic. Additionally, depending upon the end-use temperature and duration, the hot face of aluminosilicate fiber insulation that has reached the end of its service life may form crystalline quartz, cristobalite, or tridymite. Respirable crystalline silica (RCS) is known to be immunotoxic.

Reproductive and Developmental Toxicity

Reproductive toxicity screening was conducted as part of Regulation, Evaluation, Authorisation and Restriction of Chemicals (REACH) submittal for these fibers. Results were negative: at what was regarded as the maximum usable dose there were no adverse reproductive effects seen with RCF administered by gavage. Exposure to reproductive organs is extremely unlikely.

Genotoxicity

For the purposes of compiling a complete REACH registration dossier for RCF/ASW, Covance (an independent quality-assured toxicology testing facility) conducted studies to determine the genotoxic potential of ASW. The studies concluded that in standard regulatory mutagenicity tests using five different histidine-requiring strains of *Salmonella typhimurium* (TA98, TA100, TA1535, TA1537, and TA102), ASW at concentrations up to 5000 μg per plate did not induce gene mutations. And, in a standard regulatory *in vitro* cytogenicity assay using duplicate cultures of Chinese hamster ovary cells, ASW up to and including a maximum practicable concentration of 1000 $\mu g\,ml^{-1}$ did not induce micronuclei in either pulse or continuous exposure regimes. Study authors concluded that ASW has no mutagenic activity in standard test systems for this endpoint. (Note: In the absence of positive *in vitro* mutagenicity results, *in vivo* genotoxicity testing is not normally required and was not conducted.)

The genotoxicity of aluminosilicate fibers has been evaluated by two agencies (Health Council of the Netherlands and SCOEL) that identified and reviewed the available literature. These agencies concluded that results of the applicable studies and the information that inflammation is the underlying mechanism of fiber carcinogenicity strongly indicate that the genotoxic effects observed in some (but not other) studies of aluminosilicate were secondary. One consequence of this conclusion is the possibility of a dose threshold for observed carcinogenic effects (see below).

Carcinogenicity

Exposure to aluminosilicate fibers has been shown to cause interstitial fibrosis, lung cancer, and mesothelioma in laboratory animals (hamsters and rats) exposed by various routes, including nose-only inhalation. As noted above, the ongoing epidemiology studies of occupationally exposed cohorts have not resulted in any interstitial fibrosis, incremental lung cancer, or mesothelioma.

Aluminosilicate fibers have been classified variously as (1) possibly carcinogenic to humans (Group 2B) by IARC, (2) reasonably anticipated to be a human carcinogen by the National Toxicology Program, (3) according to Regulation (EC) No 1272/2008 under the CLP Regulation (classification, labeling, and packaging of substances and mixtures) ASW has been classified as a 1B carcinogen ('presumed to have carcinogenic potential for humans, classification is largely based on animal evidence'), and (4) classification according to directive 67/548/EEC aluminosilicate fibers have been classified as a Category 2 carcinogen ('substances which should be regarded as if they are carcinogenic to man').

Ecotoxicity

The ecotoxicity of aluminosilicate fibers has not been studied. However, these fibers are inorganic, inert, stable, and not soluble in water (solubility $<1\ mg\,l^{-1}$) and as such are unlikely to have a detrimental effect on the environment.

Other Hazards

As noted above, ASWs are made using silica as an ingredient. However, crystalline silica is not present in any ASW product as sold or installed. When amorphous ASWs are used in high-temperature applications, depending upon the end-use temperature and duration, ASW can devitrify and form crystalline quartz, cristobalite, and tridymite, some of which may be respirable. Thus, the possible hazard is associated only with handling after-service insulation. Exposure to RCS has been linked to adverse respiratory effects, including silicosis and lung cancer. RCS is classified as a known human carcinogen by IARC.

Typically, formation of RCS from ASW is limited to the surface of the hot face of the after-service insulation. The ASW industry monitors RCS exposures for removal of after-service insulation as part of its stewardship program. In most cases, exposure monitoring indicates that RCS concentrations are beneath the analytical limits of detection. Statistical analyses suggest that average levels of RCS are beneath occupational exposure limits (OELs) in force in the United States as of December 2012.

Exposure Standards and Guidelines

Numerous countries and organizations have recommended or mandated OELs for ASW. **Table 1** provides a sample of applicable values as of December 2012.

The industry's recommended exposure limit (where more stringent OELs are not in force) for ASW is $.5\,f\,ml^{-1}$ based on feasibility and prudence, not demonstrated risk. The National Institute for Occupational Safety and Health has reviewed several risk analyses on occupational exposure to ASW and reported that incremental working lifetime risk estimates range from .073 to 1.2/1000 at an OEL of $0.5\,f\,ml^{-1}$. Calculated risks depend upon the models and assumptions.

Table 1 Specific OELs for aluminosilicate fiber

Country	*Occupational exposure limit (OEL) (f ml^{-1})*
Austria	.5
Belgium	.5
Canada	.2–1[a]
Czech Republic	1
Denmark	1
Finland	.2
France	.1
Italy	.2
The Netherlands	.5
Norway	.1
Poland	1
Slovakia	2
Spain	.5
Sweden	.2
Switzerland	.25
UK	1
USA	.5
Japan	1
SCOEL[b]	.3

[a]OELs vary by territory for Canada.
[b]Scientific Committee on Occupational Exposure Limits.
Sources: Diverse, including the ECFIA website (www.ecfia.eu/has_elv.htm).

See also: Occupational Toxicology; Aerosols; Respiratory Tract Toxicology; Pollution, Air in Encyclopedia of Toxicology; Toxicity Testing, Inhalation; Silica, Crystalline

Further Reading

Agency for Toxic Substances and Disease Registry (ATSDR), September, 2004. Toxicological Profile for Synthetic Vitreous Fibers. US Department of Health and Human Services. Available online at: Public Health Service, Agency for Toxic Substances and Disease Registry, Washington, DC. http://www.atsdr.cdc.gov/toxprofiles/tp.asp?id=908&tid=185.

Bernstein, D.M., 2007. Synthetic vitreous fibers: a review toxicology, epidemiology and regulations. Crit. Rev. Toxicol. 37 (10), 839–886.

Health Council of the Netherlands, Dutch Expert Committee on Occupational Standards (DECOS), 2011. Refractory Ceramic Fibres: Evaluation of the Carcinogenicity and Genotoxicity. Subcommittee on the Classification of Carcinogenic Substances of the Dutch Expert Committee on Occupational Safety (DECOS), a Committee of the Health Council of the Netherlands, No. 2011/29, The Hague, November 15, 2011. 45 pp.

International Agency for Research on Cancer (IARC), 2002. IARC Monographs on the Evaluation of Carcinogenic Risks to Humans. In: Man-made Vitreous Fibres, vol. 81. IARC, Lyon, France.

LeMasters, G.K., Lockey, J.E., Yiin, J.H., Hilbert, T.J., Levin, L.S., Rice, C.H., 2003. Mortality of workers occupationally exposed to refractory ceramic fibers. J. Occup. Environ. Med. 45, 440–450.

Lockey, J., LeMasters, G., Rice, C., Hansen, K., Levin, L., Shipley, R., Spitz, H., Wiot, J., 1996. Refractory ceramic fiber exposure and pleural plaques. Am. J. Respir. Crit. Care. Med. 154, 1405–1410.

Mast, R.W., Maxim, L.D., Utell, M.J., Walker, A.M., 2000. Refractory ceramic fiber: toxicology, epidemiology, and risk analyses – a review. Inhal. Toxicol. 12, 359–399.

Maxim, L.D., Allshouse, J., Fairfax, R.F., Lentz, T.J., Venturin, D., Walters, T.E., 2008. Workplace monitoring of occupational exposure to refractory ceramic fiber – a 17-year retrospective. Inhal. Toxicol. 20, 289–309.

Maxim, L.D., Hadley, J.G., Potter, R.M., Niebo, R., 2006. The role of fiber durability/biopersistence of silica-based synthetic vitreous fibers and their influence on toxicology. Regul. Toxicol. Pharmacol. 56, 42–62.

Maxim, L.D., Venturin, D., Allshouse, J.N., 1999. Respirable crystalline silica exposure associated with the installation and removal of RCF and conventional silica-containing refractories in industrial furnaces. Regul. Toxicol. Pharmacol. 29, 44–63.

McKay, R.T., LeMasters, G.K., Hilbert, T.J., Levin, L.S., Tice, C.H., Borton, E.K., Lockey, J.E., 2011. A long term study of pulmonary function among U.S. refractory ceramic fiber workers. Occup. Environ. Med. 68 (2), 89–95.

National Institute for Occupational Safety and Health (NIOSH), 2006. Criteria for a Recommended Standard, Occupational Exposure to Refractory Ceramic Fibers. Department of Health and Human Services, Centers for Disease Control Prevention, National Institute for Occupational Safety and Health, Atlanta, GA, 203 pp.

National Research Council (NRC), 2000. Review of the U.S. Navy's Exposure Standard for Manufactured Vitreous Fibers, Subcommittee on Manufactured Vitreous Fibers, Committee on Toxicology, Board on Environmental Studies and Toxicology, Commission on Life Sciences, National Research Council. National Academy Press, Washington, DC, 47 pp.

Scientific Committee on Occupational Exposure Limits (SCOEL). 2011. Recommendation from the Scientific Committee on Occupational Exposure Limits for refractory Ceramic fibers. European Commissions, Employment, Social Affairs, and Inclusion, SCOEL/SUM/165, September, 2011.

Utell, M.J., Maxim, L.D., 2010. Refractory ceramic fiber (RCF) toxicity and epidemiology: a review. Inhal. Toxicol. 22 (6), 500–521.

Yu, C.P., Zhang, L., Oberdörster, G., Mast, R.W., Maxim, D., Utell, M.J., 1995. Deposition of refractory ceramic fibers (RCF) in the human respiratory tract and comparison with rodent studies. Aerosol. Sci. Technol. 23, 291–300.

Relevant Websites

http://www.osha.gov/SLTC/syntheticmineralfibers/index.html – Safety and Health Topics: Synthetic Mineral Fibers. U.S. Occupational Safety and Health Administration, Washington, DC.

http://www.atsdr.cdc.gov/toxprofiles/tp.asp?id=908&tid=185 – Toxicological Profile For Synthetic Vitreous Fibers. US Department of Health and Human Services, Public Health Service, Agency for Toxic Substances and Disease Registry, Washington D.C.

http://www.ecfia.eu/ – A European focused association of manufacturers and users addressing health, safety and environmental aspects of the manufacture, use and disposal of High Temperature Insulation Wools (HTIW).

http://www.htiwcoalition.org/ – The HTIW Coalition represents the North American High Temperature Insulation Wool (HTIW) industry in matters relating to health and safety.

http://www.epa.gov/iris/subst/0647.htm – The US Environmental Protection Agency Integrated Risk Information System website for Refractory Ceramic Fibers.

http://ntp.niehs.nih.gov/ntp/roc/twelfth/profiles/CeramicFibers.pdf – National Toxicology Program, Department of Health and Human Services, *Report on Carcinogens, Twelfth Edition* (2011), Ceramic Fibers (Respirable Size).

Aluminum

SC Gad, Gad Consulting Services, Cary, NC, USA

- Chemical Abstracts Service Registry Number: 7429-90-5
- Synonyms: Aluminum, Molten, Metana, Aluminum powder, Pyrophoric
- Molecular Formula: Al
- Valence States: +1, +2, +3

Background

Although aluminum was one of the last metals to be commercialized, it has been recognized for centuries. Aluminum was first recognized by the Romans as an astringent substance, and they called it 'alum.' By the middle ages it was manufactured as 'alum stone,' a subsulfate of alumina and potash. In 1825, Hans C. Øersted was able to isolate a few drops of the raw material, and by 1886 it had patents from both Charles Martin Hall of the United States and Paul-Louis-Toussaint Heroult of France. Aluminum was commercialized in industry by the end of the nineteenth century.

Uses

Aluminum can be used in several different ways, either alone or compounded, and in a variety of forms, including powder. Aluminum is frequently used in food packaging, and also in utensils and electrical conductors. Aluminum compounds are widely used in industry, in the form of alums in water treatment and alumina in abrasives and furnace linings. However, aluminum is used alone very rarely since it is such a soft metal. It is often combined with other metals to create a stronger, more durable metal. These combinations are called aluminum alloys. Aluminum alloys are used extensively in aircraft. Aluminum and aluminum salts can also be found in many consumer products such as antiperspirants, food additives, antacids, astringents, and buffered aspirins. Powdered aluminum is used to make explosives and fireworks.

There has been concern about the exposures resulting from leaching of aluminum from cookware and beverage cans; however, aluminum beverage cans are usually coated with a polymer to minimize such leaching. Leaching from aluminum cookware becomes potentially significant only when cooking highly basic or acidic foods, for example, in one study, tomato sauce cooked in aluminum pans was found to accumulate 3–6 mg aluminum per 100 g serving.

Aluminum is absorbed from the soil by many plants that humans consume. The amount that a person would inhale depends on where they reside, and aluminum levels are much higher in industrial and urban areas. Another route of exposure is through skin contact with soil, water, and with aluminum metal.

Aluminum is a good conductor of both heat and electricity. These properties make it suitable for industrial purposes. Aluminum is used in alloys with copper, zinc, manganese, and magnesium.

Environmental Fate and Behavior

- Routes and pathways relevant physicochemical properties
  Melting point = 660 °C.
  Boiling point = 2450 °C.
  Specific gravity = 2.708 g cm^{-1}.
  Solubility: insoluble in H_2O, HNO_3. Soluble in HCl, H_2SO_4.
- Partition behavior in water, sediment, and soil
  The contribution of aluminum from drinking water is about 100 μg day^{-1}.
  Air aluminum concentrations vary between 20 and 500 ng m^{-3} in rural settings and 1000 and 6000 ng m^{-3} in urban areas. Humans exposed to ambient aluminum concentrations of 2000 ng m^{-3} and particle size <5 μm and who have a normal ventilator volume of 20 m^3 day^{-1} would inhale 40 μg aluminum day^{-1}.
- Environmental persistence
  Aluminum cannot be degraded in the environment in its elemental state, but can undergo various precipitation or ligand exchange reactions. The solubility of aluminum in the environment depends on the ligands present and the pH.
- Long-range transport
  The major feature cycle of aluminum include leaching of aluminum from geochemical formations and soil particulates to aqueous environments, adsorption onto soil or sediment particulates, and wet and dry deposition from the air to land and surface water.
- Bioaccumulation and biomagnification
  Aluminum does not bioaccumulate to a significant extent. Thus, certain plants can accumulate high concentrations of aluminum. Plant matter like tea leaves may contain >5000 mg kg^{-1} of aluminum. Lycopodium, some fern species, and members of genera *Symplocos* or *Orites* may contain high levels of aluminum. It does not appear to accumulate to any significant degree in cow's milk or beef tissue, and it is therefore not expected to undergo biomagnification in terrestrial food chains.

Exposure and Exposure Monitoring

Aluminum is the most abundant metal, and the third most abundant element in the Earth's crust. Human exposure to this metal is common and unavoidable. However, intake is relatively low because aluminum is highly insoluble in many of its naturally occurring forms. Humans are always exposed to some form of aluminum by eating food, drinking water, ingesting aluminum-containing medicinal products, or just breathing air. The average human intake is estimated to be 30–50 mg day^{-1}. This intake comes primarily from foods, drinking water, and pharmaceuticals. Food additives can contain aluminum; due to certain additives, processed cheese and cornbread are two major contributors to high aluminum exposures in the American diet. Some common over-the-counter medications such as antacids

 http://dx.doi.org/10.1016/B978-0-12-386454-3.00810-1

and buffered aspirin contain aluminum, and can increase intake significantly.

Toxicokinetics

Less than 1% of that taken into the body orally is absorbed from the gastrointestinal tract. Aluminum can increase the absorption of other chemicals such as fluoride, calcium, iron, and phosphates. Most of the aluminum absorbed into the body will eventually end up in the bones or lungs. Aluminum that is not absorbed by the bones or lungs is excreted by the kidneys.

Mechanism of Toxicity

Aluminum binds diatomic phosphates and possibly depletes phosphate, which can lead to osteomalacia. High aluminum serum values and high aluminum concentration in the bone interfere with the function of vitamin D. The incorporation of aluminum in the bone may interfere with deposition of calcium; the subsequent increase of calcium in the blood may inhibit release of parathyroid hormones by the parathyroid gland. The mechanism by which aluminum concentrates in the brain is not known; it may interfere with the blood brain barrier.

Acute and Short-Term Toxicity (or Exposure)

Animal

Acutely, aluminum itself has minimal systemic toxicity. Overall, animals become weaker and less active due to exposure.

Human

Aluminum has not been shown to alter the immune system in humans exposed by the oral or inhalation routes. Skin sensitization may occur.

Chronic Toxicity (or Exposure)

Animal

Cats and rabbits are aluminum sensitive, and have showed neurotoxic effects from aluminum. There is no evidence that aluminum exposure will affect reproduction. Toxicity of aluminum in animals differs from humans because animals are much more sensitive to high exposures. Monkeys on a low calcium, high aluminum diet showed neurological disease similar to those of amyotrophic lateral sclerosis and Parkinsonism. Rats and hamsters showed signs of lung damage after breathing large amounts of aluminum dust. Death often occurred after the inhalation of air highly concentrated with the chemical.

Human

Fibrosis of the lung may occur through inhalation of aluminum dust particles. Aluminum has been associated with encephalopathy, bone disease, and anemia related to dialysis. It has also been thought that aluminum may be a cofactor in the etiopathogenesis of some neurodegenerative diseases, including Alzheimer's disease. Direct evidence, however, cannot link the two together. Aluminum toxicity has been well recognized in patients with renal failure. Also, an increased concentration of aluminum in infant formulas and in solutions for home parenteral nutrition has been associated with neurological consequences and metabolic bone loss.

Immunotoxicity

There are insufficient data on the immunotoxicity effects of aluminum.

Reproductive Toxicity

When $AlCl_3$ was orally administered in various species such as rat, guinea pigs, and rabbits, maximum doses of 27 mg Al kg^{-1} for 20–30 days resulted in 'slight' gonadal toxicity. Oral doses of 100–200 mg Al kg^{-1} given for 6 months resulted in decreased numbers and motility of spermatozoa and proliferation of testicular interstitial cells at highest doses. The highest doses (100 and 200 mg Al kg^{-1} for $>$ 4 weeks) via intraperitoneal injection of soluble aluminum nitrate nonahydrate in male rats before mating decreased pregnancy rates and weight loss in males. A dose of 200 mg kg^{-1} significantly decreased epididymal spermatocytes and testicular spermatid, and decreased organ weight as well. Considering the use, the forms of aluminum, and the amount encountered in daily life, the capacity should appear to be considerable in the safe margins between unacceptable reproductive events and daily conditions of usage or ingested aluminum.

Genotoxicity

Several studies indicate that various species of aluminum compounds or complexes are capable of interaction with DNA contained in chromosomes, which might lead to abnormalities in their configuration and replication. *In vitro* experiments indicate that aluminum-induced DNA binding and cross-linking resulted in clastogenic effects, led to configuration changes, and altered sister chromatid exchange, ineffective or reduced DNA replication, and circular dichroism of DNA. It is also suggested that accumulation of aluminum in cell nuclei potentially alters protein–DNA interactions and calmodulin biosynthesis. Theoretically, the altered configuration of calmodulin can affect calcium modulation of the second messenger system that is activated by neurotransmitters. Other *in vitro* effects suggest aluminum-induced chromatid alteration. The alternation and generalization of transformed cells to normal, untreated cells are unknown.

Carcinogenicity

Aluminum is not classifiable as a human carcinogen; the American Conference of Governmental Industrial Hygienists

(ACGIH) classifies it as group A4. Most animal studies have failed to demonstrate carcinogenicity attributable to aluminum powder or several aluminum compounds. In 1987, the International Agency for Research on Cancer (IARC) concluded that there is sufficient evidence that certain exposures occurring during aluminum production cause cancer of the lung and bladder.

Clinical Management

Aluminum overload has very few treatment options. Besides symptomatic treatment, deferoxamine is used as a chelating agent.

Ecotoxicology

Aluminum occurs naturally in soil, water, and air. It is redistributed or moved by natural and human activities. High levels in the environment can be caused by the mining and processing of its ores and by the production of aluminum metal, alloys, and compounds. Small amounts of aluminum are released into the environment from coal-fired power plants and incinerators. Virtually all food, water, and air contain some aluminum, which nature is well adapted to handle.

Exposure Standards and Guidelines

The ACGIH and the Occupational Safety and Health Administration (OSHA) in the United States have the following airborne exposure limit:

- *ACGIH threshold limit value*: Aluminum oxide: 10 mg m^{-3} (time-weighted average (TWA)) inhalable (total) particulate matter containing no asbestos and <1% crystalline silica, A4. Soluble salts as Al: 2 mg m^{-3} (TWA).
- OSHA permissible exposure limit: Alpha alumina (aluminum oxide): 15 mg m^{-3} total dust, 5 mg m^{-3} respirable fraction. Aluminum as metal: 15 mg m^{-3} total dust, 5 mg m^{-3} respirable fraction.

See also: Metals.

Further Reading

Ae, N., Arihara, J., Okada, K., Srinivasan, A. (Eds.), 2011. Plant Nutrient Acquisition: New Perspectives: The Role of the Root Cell Wall in Aluminum Toxicity. Springer Verlag, Tokyo Japan, pp. 201–226.

Becaria, A., Campbell, A., Bondy, S.C., 2002. Aluminum as a toxicant. Toxicol. Ind. Health 18 (7), 309–320.

Bingham, E., Cohrssen, B. (Eds.), 2012. Patty's Toxicology, sixth ed., vol. 2. Wiley, New York, pp. 354–406.

Mailloux, R.J., Lemire, J., Appanna, V.D., 2011. Hepatic response to aluminum toxicity: dyslipidemia and liver diseases. October. Exp. Cell. Res. 317 (6), 2231–2239.

Nordberg, G.F., Fowler, B.A., Nordberg, M., Friberg, L.T., 2007. Handbook on the Toxicology of Metals, third ed. Associated Press, London.

Wier, H.A., 2012. Aluminum toxicity in neonatal parenteral nutrition: what can we do?. January. Ann. Pharmacother. 46 (1), 137–140.

Relevant Websites

http://www.inchem.org – Aluminum (Environmental Health Criteria).

http://www.aluminum.org – The (US) Aluminum Association Website.

http://www.atsdr.cdc.gov – Agency for Toxic Substances and Disease Registry. Toxicological Profile for Aluminum.

Aluminum Phosphide

M Abdollahi, Faculty of Pharmacy and Pharmaceutical Sciences Research Center, Tehran University of Medical Sciences, Tehran, Iran
O Mehrpour, Faculty of Medicine and Medical Toxicology and Drug Abuse Research Center, Birjand University of Medical Sciences, Birjand, Iran

This article is a revision of the previous edition article by Christopher H. Day, volume 1, pp 84–86, © 2005, Elsevier Inc.

- Name: Aluminum phosphide
- Chemical Abstracts Service Registry Number: 20859-73-8
- Synonyms (Various Brand Names): Celphos, Alphos, Quickphos, Phosfume, Phostoxin, Talunex, Degesch, Synfume, Chemfume, Phostek, Delicia
- Molecular Formula: AlP
- Chemical Structure:

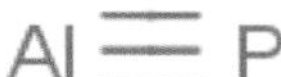

Uses

The primary use for AlP is as a fumigant to control insects and rodents in both food and nonfood crops in indoor environments. It is also used in the control of rodents outdoors via application to their burrows or in grain storage areas. Due to the extremely common use of this compound for protecting rice, it is also called rice tablet in some countries. AlP is formulated in solid form and is available for use as a tablet, pellet, or dust. It is marketed as dark gray 3-g tablets consisting of AlP (56%) and carbamate (44%), under brand names such as Celphos, Alphos, Quickphos, Phosfume, Phostoxin, Talunex, Degesch, Synfume, Chemfume, Phostek, and Delicia in porous hags or blister packs.

Exposure Routes and Pathways

AlP is usually formulated as dark gray or dark yellow crystals that have an odor similar to decaying fish or garlic. Most lethal exposures to AlP occur via the oral route with suicidal intent. Because it is a solid material, dermal absorption of AlP is unlikely. AlP is highly reactive with water, such that any contact with moisture results in decomposition to phosphine gas. Phosphine gas is colorless, flammable, and explosive at room temperature. Therefore, the primary exposure route is via inhalation and absorption by the lungs. Exposure is also possible through ingestion of commodities, such as grains and nutmeats, treated with AlP; these foods may contain residues of phosphine gas. Residues of phosphine gas in treated commodities are expected to be <0.004 ppm (limit of detection in several studies) following aeration.

Toxicokinetics

Phosphine gas is rapidly absorbed through the lungs following inhalation. Following ingestion of AlP, phosphine is released as soon as AlP or other phosphide salts come into contact with hydrochloric acid in the stomach. Phosphine is quickly absorbed and readily transferred to the bloodstream. Many large organs are affected following exposure, suggesting that phosphine is effectively distributed throughout the body. *In vitro* studies suggest that phosphides are absorbed as microscopic particles of unhydrolyzed salt that permanently interact with free hemoglobin and hemoglobin in intact erythrocytes (rat and human) to produce a hemichrome (a methemoglobin derivative resulting from distorted protein conformation). In addition, Heinz bodies (denatured hemoglobin aggregates) are formed when phosphide concentration *in vitro* exceeds 1.25 $\mu g\ ml^{-1}$. Reports of *in vivo* phosphide poisoning showed intravascular complications such as hemolysis and methemoglobinemia, which support the involvement of erythrocytes in the biotransformation of phosphine in humans. Phosphine is excreted in the urine as hypophosphite and is also exhaled in the unchanged form. There is evidence that unexpired phosphine may be metabolized to phosphates, hypophosphite, and phosphite.

Mechanism of Toxicity

Phosphine is known to bind to and inhibit cytochrome oxidase and changes the valence of the hem component of hemoglobin. Oxidative stress is one of the main mechanisms of action of AlP toxicity, which boosts extramitochondrial release of free oxygen radicals resulting in lipid peroxidation and protein denaturation of the cell membrane in various organs. Furthermore, AlP reduces glutathione, which is one of the main antioxidant defenses. AlP causes toxic stress, accompanied by changes in glucose metabolism. It also disrupts protein synthesis and enzymatic activity, particularly in the lung and heart cell mitochondria, which leads to blockage of the mitochondrial electron transport chain. Phosphine may cause denaturing of various enzymes; it is involved in cellular respiration and metabolism, and may be responsible for denaturation of the oxyhemoglobin molecule.

Acute and Short-Term Toxicity

Animal

Acute exposure to elevated levels of phosphine gas by animals (horses and rats) can result in lethargy, shallow breathing, immobility, agitation, ataxia, convulsions, seizures, profuse sweating, tachycardia, tachypnea, pyrexia, ataxia, widespread muscle tremors, hepatic encephalopathy, and death. Clinically relevant laboratory findings include hypoglycemia, high plasma concentrations of lactate and ammonia, and increased

 http://dx.doi.org/10.1016/B978-0-12-386454-3.00467-X

activity of gamma-glutamyl transpeptidase, aspartate aminotransferase, and alkaline phosphatase. The lethal concentration 50% (LC_{50}) after inhalation for 4-h inhalation for phosphine gas in rats has been found to be $15\,mg\,m^{-3}$ (11 ppm), although a more recent study showed no mortality in male and female rats exposed to a single 6-h exposure to $15\,mg\,m^{-3}$ suggesting that the 4-h inhalation LC_{50} for rodents may exceed $15\,mg\,m^{-3}$.

Human

Acute oral exposure in humans has resulted in severe metabolic acidosis, pulmonary edema, various cardiovascular abnormalities such as dysrhythmia, transient atrial fibrillation, ST-T wave changes and conduction defects, left ventricular heart failure, sinus tachycardia, severe and refractory hypotension, and refractory cardiogenic shock. These may result in cerebral anoxia, which usually presents as drowsiness, delirium, and coma following inadvertent or voluntary ingestion. These effects are likely caused by the formation and subsequent toxicity of phosphine gas liberated in the stomach following contact with water. Other adverse effects that have been noted in humans following accidental or suicide-related intake of aluminum phosphide include gastrointestinal effects such as abdominal pain and vomiting, severe thirst, hepatic effects such as hyperemia and hepatic dysfunction, renal effects such as profound proteinuria, anuria, and renal failure, and neurological effects such as restlessness and loss of consciousness. Also some electrolyte and metabolic abnormalities may occur, such as changes in blood levels of sodium, potassium, and glucose as well as severe acidosis. Hepatitis, pancreatitis, acute adrenocortical insufficiency, acute tubular necrosis, and disseminated intravascular coagulation are less common findings. The mortality rate in adults who have ingested 500 mg of AlP or more is between 30% and 100%. The higher the blood phosphine level, the higher the mortality. Patients with blood phosphine levels equal to or less than 1.067 ± 0.16 mg survived, and this dose seems to be the lethal threshold of phosphine toxicity. Poor prognosis is indicated by hyperglycemia, high simplified acute physiology score (SAPS II), hypotension, acidosis, leukocytosis, hyperuricemia, electrocardiographic (ECG) abnormalities, high acute physiology and chronic health evaluation score (APACHE II), low Glasgow coma scale score, acute renal failure, low prothrombin rate, hyperleukocytosis, methemoglobinemia, use of vasoactive drugs, lack of vomiting after ingestion, and use of mechanical ventilation.

Chronic Toxicity

Animal

In chronic studies with rats, exposure to AlP-fumigated chow ($4.5\,mg\,m^{-3}$ phosphine) resulted in a decrease in food intake, body weight, hemoglobin level, red blood cells, hematocrit, and an increases in platelet counts. Following a 4-week recovery period, symptoms were absent in many of the exposed rats, suggesting apparent reversibility. Neither AlP nor phosphine gas exhibits carcinogenic, reproductive, or developmental effects in animals.

Human

There is evidence that long-term phosphine exposure by individuals involved in the application of pesticides resulted in chromosome damage. Chronic exposure to very low levels of phosphine may result in altered motor, visual, and speech skills. Neither AlP nor phosphine gas exhibits carcinogenicity in humans, or results in reproductive or developmental effects. Although definitive evidence is lacking, it is assumed that phosphine is an inhibitor of oxidative phosphorylation *in vivo*.

In Vitro Toxicity Data

Phosphine has been reported as negative for induction of reverse gene mutations up to cytotoxic doses in the Ames assay (*Salmonella typhimurium*). Increased chromosomal aberrations were reported in Chinese hamster ovary (CHO) cells exposed to doses of about 2500 or 5000 ppm of phosphine without activation with the S9 fraction. Chromosomal aberrations in CHOs were also reported in cells tested with S9 activation at 2500 ppm, but not at 5000 ppm.

Clinical Management

An antidote proper for phosphine poisoning is still unavailable. If the victim has ingested AlP, emesis should not be induced. Phosphine gas will be produced in the stomach when AlP contacts the resident gastric fluids. A slurry of activated charcoal may be administered at $1\,g\,kg^{-1}$ body weight although no study has proved its efficacy in humans. Any victim who has ingested AlP should be immediately transported to a medical facility for treatment and monitoring. Gastric lavage with potassium permanganate, activated charcoal + sorbitol solution, and coconut oil can be performed as the first emergency step. Potassium permanganate (1:10 000 solution) oxidizes phosphine gas in the stomach to phosphate, and reduces the amount of lethal phosphine gas. Cardiac monitoring should include blood pressure and ECG to prevent dysrhythmia and maintain tissue perfusion and oxygenation. Another necessary step in the management of AlP poisoning is early treatment of shock with fluid and vasoactive agents (norepinephrine or phenylephrine, dopamine, and dobutamine) to control central venous pressure (CVP) or pulmonary artery wedge pressure (PAWP).

Anti-arrhythmic agents, direct current (DC) cardioversion, and a temporary pacemaker should be used to control dysrhythmia. Some reports suggest the efficacy of trimetazidine and digoxin in the management of AlP cardiotoxicity. Trimetazidine has recently proven to be effective in stopping ventricular ectopic beats and preserving oxidative metabolism. In addition, digoxin can be used to stabilize left ventricular heart failure. For metabolic acidosis, intravenous sodium bicarbonate should be considered, whereas severe acidosis, volume overload, or renal failure may require hemodialysis. However, hemodialysis is probably not very effective in removing phosphine. Rescuers need to be aware of any solid phosphide contamination on the victim's clothing, skin, or hair, which will produce phosphine following contact with water, as well as any vomitus which could give off phosphine gas. Preventive measures might help control the risk of poisoning in humans, such as limited access to phosphide compounds, regulations to ban its use as a pesticide, and keeping health professionals abreast of the latest knowledge about early management of phosphide poisoning.

Environmental Fate

Once exposed to water or in the presence of high ambient humidity, AlP generates phosphine gas. Therefore, atmospheric dissipation is expected to be the primary fate process for phosphine. In addition to phosphine being generated from the reaction of AlP with water, the other reaction product is aluminum hydroxide, a common constituent of clay. If the liberated phosphine (PH_3) burns, it will produce phosphorus pentoxide (P_2O_5), which forms orthophosphoric acid (H_3PO_4) when exposed to water.

Ecotoxicology

Very limited ecotoxicological data are available on the effects of phosphine; very few data were found for the effects of AlP on wildlife. One study reported that turkeys and chickens exposed to phosphine gas at concentrations of 211 and 224 mg m^{-3} for 74 and 59 min, respectively, exhibited dyspnea, organ swelling, convulsions, and death. These types of effects are unlikely in the unconfined atmospheric conditions to which most birds and wildlife are exposed in nature. However, if misapplied or disposed of incorrectly, phosphine gas liberated from the decomposition of AlP could represent a significant hazard to nontarget wildlife exposed to the gas in burrows or other confined spaces. Under most circumstances, exposure to aquatic organisms would be unlikely due to the limited use of AlP in terrestrial environments. Two studies of aquatic toxicity are available in the literature. Both studies were acute tests on fish (snakehead catfish and rainbow trout). The reported lethal concentration (LC_W) values were 0.10 and 0.004 mg l^{-1} for the snakehead catfish and rainbow trout, respectively. These results indicate that phosphine is highly toxic to these fish species. Although there are very few data for other bird or fish species, it is possible that other members of these taxa may be similarly sensitive to the effects of phosphine due to an anticipated similar mode of action.

No chronic ecotoxicity data exist for AlP or phosphine in the available literature.

Other Hazards

Any individual previously exposed to AlP should check with their doctor before taking vitamins that contain phosphorus supplements.

Exposure Standards and Guidelines

Several agencies have established exposure standards or guidelines for AlP as phosphine (summarized in **Table 1**). Generally, a standard or guideline represents the concentration that if met will prevent an adverse effect from occurring at low exposure doses, and will therefore necessarily prevent the occurrence of the more serious effects that are known to occur at higher doses. The chronic reference concentration (RfC) of 0.0002 ppm (0.0003 mg m^{-3}) for phosphine was set to prevent decreases in body weight in the general population over a lifetime of exposure. The American Conference of Governmental Industrial Hygienists threshold limit value of 0.3 ppm was set to prevent irritation and adverse effects to the central nervous system and gastrointestinal tract in workers exposed for 8 h day^{-1} throughout their working life.

Table 1 Summary of exposure standards and guidelines for phosphine

Agency	*Standards and guidelines (ppm)*	*Averaging time*
US EPA	RfC (0.000 2)	24 h a day for a lifetime
OSHA	PEL (0.3)	8 h a day over working lifetime
ACGIH	TLV–TWA (0.3)	8 h a day over working lifetime
ACGIH	ERPG-2 (0.5)	1 h
NIOSH	IDLH (50)	NA

US EPA, United States Environmental Protection Agency; OSHA, Occupational Safety and Health Administration; NIOSH, National Institute for Occupational Safety and Health; ACGIH, American Conference of Governmental Industrial Hygienists; RfC, reference concentration; PEL, permissible exposure limit; TLV, threshold limit value; TWA, time-weighed average; ERPG-2, Emergency Response Planning Guideline; IDLH, immediately dangerous to life or health; NA, not applicable.

See also: Phosphine; Phosphorus.

Further Reading

Gurjar, M., Baronia, A.K., Azim, A., Sharma, K., 2011. Managing aluminum phosphide poisonings. J. Emerg. Trauma Shock 4, 378–384.

Mehrpour, O., Alfred, S., Shadnia, S., et al., 2008. Hyperglycemia in acute aluminum phosphide poisoning as a potential prognostic factor. Hum. Exp. Toxicol. 27, 591–595.

Mehrpour, O., Singh, S., 2010. Rice tablet poisoning: a major concern in Iranian population. Hum. Exp. Toxicol. 29, 701–702.

Mehrpour, O., Farzaneh, E., Abdollahi, M., 2011. Successful treatment of aluminum phosphide poisoning with digoxin: a case report and review of literature. Int. J. Pharmacol. 7, 761–764.

Mehrpour, O., Jafarzadeh, M., Abdollahi, M., 2012. A systematic review of aluminium phosphide poisoning. Arh. Hig. Rada. Toksikol. 63, 61–73.

Proudfoot, A.T., 2009. Aluminium and zinc phosphide poisoning. Clin. Toxicol. (Phila) 47, 89–100.

Shadnia, S., Rahimi, M., Pajoumand, A., Rasouli, M.H., Abdollahi, M., 2005. Successful treatment of acute aluminium phosphide poisoning: possible benefit of coconut oil. Hum. Exp. Toxicol. 24, 215–218.

Shadnia, S., Mehrpour, O., Abdollahi, M., 2008. Unintentional poisoning by phosphine released from aluminum phosphide. Hum. Exp. Toxicol. 27, 87–89.

Shadnia, S., Sasanian, G., Allami, P., Hosseini, A., Ranjbar, A., Amini-Shirazi, N., Abdollahi, M., 2009. A retrospective 7-years study of aluminum phosphide poisoning in Tehran: opportunities for prevention. Hum. Exp. Toxicol. 28, 209–213.

Shadnia, S., Mehrpour, O., Soltaninejad, K., 2010. A simplified acute physiology score in the prediction of acute aluminum phosphide poisoning outcome. Indian J. Med. Sci. 64, 532–539.

Shadnia, S., Soltaninejad, K., Hassanian-Moghadam, H., Sadeghi, A., Rahimzadeh, H., Zamani, N., Ghasemi-Toussi, A., Abdollahi, M., 2011. Methemoglobinemia in aluminum phosphide poisoning. Hum. Exp. Toxicol. 30, 250–253.

Relevant Websites

http://curriculum.toxicology.wikispaces.net/2.2.10.30+Phosphorus+and+phosphides
http://www.inchem.org/documents/pims/chemical/pim865.htm
http://toxnet.nlm.nih.gov/cgi-bin/sis/search

Amantin, α- *see* Mushrooms, Cyclopeptide

Amdro

JR Bloomquist, Emerging Pathogens Institute, University of Florida, Gainesville, FL, USA

This article is a revision of the previous edition article by Jamaluddin Shaikh, volume 1, pp 87–88, © 2005, Elsevier Inc.

- CAS RN: CAS 67485-29-4
- Synonyms: Tetrahydro-5,5-dimethyl-2(1H)-pyrimidinone [3-[4-(trifluoromethyl)phenyl]-1-[2-[4-(trifluoromethyl) phenyl]ethenyl]-2-propenylidene]hydrazone; AC 217,300; Andropro; Combat; Hydramethylnon
- Molecular Formula: $C_{25}H_{24}F_6N_4$ (494.5 g mol^{-1})
- Chemical Structure:

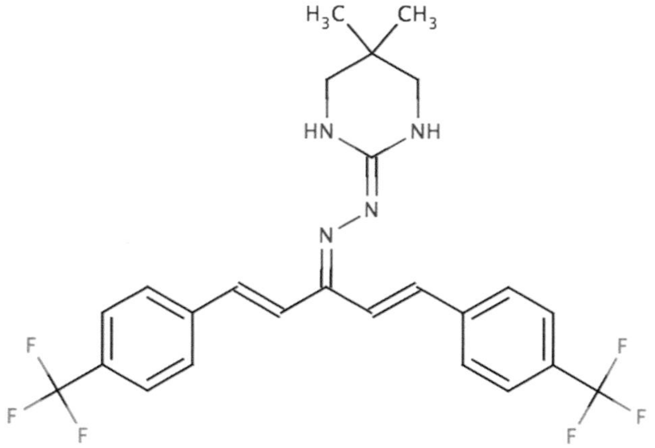

H3C CH3 HN NH N N F F F F F F

Background

Amidinohydrazones were synthesized as experimental insecticides by American Cyanamid Co. in the late 1970s, and Amdro was selected for commercial development. Amdro is typically formulated as tan to yellow granules having an odor of vegetable oil. Amdro is a slowly acting stomach poison. It is selective for insects with chewing or sponging mouthparts, and has low activity when applied topically or as a surface contact insecticide. Insects exposed *via* ingestion show no signs of intoxication for the first 24 h, but subsequently stop feeding and become lethargic. Insects become moribund after 3–4 days of exposure, but death can be further delayed for several more days. Injected doses, however, are toxic to both sensitive and insensitive insect species, indicating that pharmacokinetic differences are responsible for selectivity. The unusual penetration/disposition of Amdro is therefore a critical determinant in its biological activity and has limited its commercial uses as an insecticide. However, the slow action of Amdro is essential to its effectiveness against ants and cockroaches. For ants, an effective chemical needs to be distributed throughout the colony by foraging workers prior to overt toxicity. In cockroaches, significant mortality of first instar nymphs resulted from ingesting the feces of exposed adults, where the slow action of Amdro allows the adults to return to harborages before they die. The nymphal ingestion of Amdro *via* coprophagy is a unique property of the chemical that enhances its ability to reduce cockroach populations.

Uses

Amdro is used as an insecticide, and is typically formulated as a bait. A granule bait formulation is applied to lawns to control fire ants. It usually works in 7–14 days when applied as a mound treatment, and 2–3 weeks when broadcast. A 0.1% Amdro bait is typically applied at 1–2 pounds acre^{-1} when used on larger fields. If applied to pastureland, a 7-day waiting period should be observed before cutting or baling hay. Outdoor plastic ant stakes or indoor plastic bait stations are also used with Amdro as general ant killers. For cockroach control in homes, warehouses, restaurants, etc., Amdro is applied within a plastic bait station or with a gel applicator syringe. The bait is dispensed in areas where cockroaches congregate, such as kitchens, under appliances, etc. The use of plastic bait stations reduces chemical exposure of children and pets.

Environmental Behavior, Fate, Routes, and Pathways

Amdro has the following physico-chemical properties. Its water solubility is 6 ppb, but it is freely soluble in acetone and somewhat soluble in ethanol and methanol. It has a P_{OW} value of 204 at pH 7 and 20 °C. Amdro binds to soil organic matter and photolysis on the soil surface is biphasic, with half-lives of 4 days and about 30 days. It has half-lives for aerobic soil metabolism of 385 days, and for anaerobic aquatic metabolism of 445–552 days. Thus, Amdro on soil surfaces appears to be nonpersistent and immobile, while subsurface residues are more persistent, but still immobile, so its expected environmental transport is limited. Amdro has little potential to leach into groundwater, due to its low water solubility, propensity to bind to soil organic matter,

 http://dx.doi.org/10.1016/B978-0-12-386454-3.00095-6

and the fact that it photodegrades in water with a half-life of under 1 h.

Amdro displays a tendency to accumulate in fish tissues, with reported bioconcentration factors of 1300× in whole fish, 780× in fillet, and 1900× in viscera. Tissue clearance of Amdro residues was slow, with 48–63% eliminated after a 14-day period, but considering its current limited outdoor use, low aqueous solubility, photodegradation in water, and high soil sorption affinity, the compound is expected to display little bioaccumulation in the environment.

Exposure and Exposure Monitoring

Ingestion is the primary route of exposure for deployed uses, while occupational exposure may occur *via* inhalation and dermal routes. Dermal absorption in rats was about 1% of the applied dose in 10 h. Nontarget exposures to humans and pets *via* Amdro baits are low. Exposures *via* food and drinking water contamination are negligible.

Toxicokinetics

Consistent with studies in cockroaches, Amdro is not well absorbed *via* the oral route in rats and is also poorly metabolized. Rats eliminated over 90% of the dose in the feces, and over 70–85% as parent compound, within 36 h. Urinary metabolites were 1–4% of the total administered compound, composed primarily of a cinnamic acid and a substituted *p*-toluic acid as the two main polar metabolites. Unmetabolized parent compound was also the most abundant chemical species found in sampled tissues, including the liver.

Mechanism of Action

Amdro's slow action would suggest a nonneuronal site of action. It inhibits mitochondrial respiration at micromolar concentrations in intact Chinese hamster ovary cells, as well as isolated mitochondrial preparations, *in vitro*. Sequential isolation of coupling sites with specific substrates showed that it was the most potent and effective inhibitor when succinate was used as the electron donor. Thus, coupling site III (cytochrome b to c_1 complex) is the primary target site. A number of environmental and metabolic degradation products were also examined and shown to be inactive, confirming that Amdro itself is the toxophore.

Acute and Short-Term Toxicity

Amdro belongs to EPA toxicity class III. The oral lethal dose 50 percent (LD_{50}) in male and female rats was 817–1502 mg kg^{-1} (1146 mg kg^{-1} combined). Signs of intoxication were ataxia, diuresis, anorexia, nasal bleeding, bloody tears, and salivation. The acute dermal LD_{50} in rabbits was >2000 mg kg^{-1}. The acute (4 h) inhalation lethal concentration 50 percent (LC_{50}) in rats was 2.9 mg l^{-1}, with overall similar clinical signs, but also with rales, labored breathing, and yellow material on the fur. Amdro is not a dermal irritant or a skin sensitizer, but is a mild eye irritant.

Chronic Toxicity

A 6-month feeding study in dogs reported increased incidence of soft stools, mucoid stools, and diarrhea at the highest level of exposure (3.0 mg kg^{-1} day^{-1}), when given for 26 weeks. However, food consumption and weight gain were normal, and although there was increased liver size, histopathological examination found no abnormalities. Dietary exposures of up to 200 ppm in rats found a reduction in body weight and food consumption with no effect on survival, even at the highest dosage. Dose-dependent amyloidosis of the kidney occurred in females at 50 and 100 ppm. Amdro is not a neurodevelopmental toxicant and is not teratogenic in either rats or rabbits. Little is known regarding chronic effects of Amdro in humans.

Reproductive and Developmental Toxicity

No reports of reproductive effects in humans have appeared. Overall, negative effects of Amdro on development of offspring in animal studies only occurred at doses producing maternal toxicity. Effects on males were more potent. In rat feeding studies, the reproductive toxicity, no observable adverse effect level (NOAEL) was 25 ppm (1.66 mg^{-1} kg^{-1} day^{-1} for males), based on the histological findings in the testes, which included degeneration of the germinal epithelium and aspermia, as well as increased cellular debris in the epididymides. At 75 ppm (5.05 mg^{-1} kg^{-1} day^{-1} in males), male reproductive performance was reduced, as evidenced by lower pregnancy rates and smaller litters. The NOAEL for offspring toxicity was taken as 75 ppm, the highest dose tested.

Genotoxicity

Amdro was negative in *Salmonella typhimurium*/*Escherichia coli* reverse gene mutation assays, *Schizosaccharomyces pombe* P1 forward gene mutation assay, Chinese hamster ovary chromosome aberration, and *Saccharomyces cerevisiae* D4 mitotic gene conversion assay.

Carcinogenicity

Based on an increase in lung adenomas and lung adenomas/carcinomas in female mice from 25 to 100 ppm exposures in the diet, Amdro has been classified as a Group C possible human carcinogen by the US Environmental Protection Agency.

Clinical Management

When dermally exposed to Amdro, remove contaminated clothing and wash the exposed area with soap and water. Any persistent irritation of the skin should be examined by a physician. For eye exposures, irrigate exposed eyes with plenty of water (room temperature) for at least 15 min. If there is persistent irritation, pain, swelling, lacrimation, or photophobia, seek medical attention. In case of oral exposure to Amdro, drink 1–2 glasses of water and induce vomiting, and/or administer activated charcoal as a slurry (240 ml water/30 g charcoal). If seizures are present, seek medical attention, where standard doses of benzodiazepines, such as diazepam or lorazepam, are administered, as needed, for suppression of symptoms. If seizures recur, phenobarbital or propofol may be used. Patients should be monitored for hypotension, dysrhythmias, respiratory depression, and the need for endotracheal intubation, as well as hypoglycemia, electrolyte disturbances, and hypoxia.

Ecotoxicology

Amdro is practically nontoxic to birds, with oral LD_{50} values in mallard duck and bobwhite quail of 2510 and 1825 mg kg^{-1}, respectively. Amdro is moderately to highly toxic to fish. The LC_{50} (4 days) values for Amdro in fathead minnow (*Pimephales promelas*), rainbow trout (*Onchorhyncus mykiss*), and channel catfish (*Ictalurus punctatus*) are ca. 75, 160, and 100 ppb, respectively. For the water flea (*Daphnia magna*) and third instar larval midge (*Chironomus plumosus*) the LC_{50} (2 days) values are 1140 and 140 ppb, respectively. A more recently reported value for *D. magna* LC_{50} is 130 ppb, more in line with the *Chironomus* result. Amdro is of low toxicity to honey bees in a standard acute contact assay, consistent with its known action as a stomach poison. Its toxicity to aquatic algae (4-day LC_{50}) is 5 ppb to *Chlorella* spp. and 18 ppb to *Dunaliella tertiolecta*. The LC_{50} to the marine haptophyte (*Isochrysis galbana*) occurs at 2.9 and 0.24 ppb in the marine diatom *Skeletonema costatum* (4-day values in each case).

Exposure Standards and Guidelines

Although chronic human exposures were judged to be unlikely, a NOAEL of 1 mg kg^{-1} day^{-1} was established. This NOAEL was used to derive a reference dose for Amdro, which is 0.01 mg kg^{-1} day^{-1}, where lifetime exposures at this level are not expected to cause a risk to human health. A factor in this calculation is that dietary residues for Amdro are negligible, and accordingly, no residues were found in goat milk or tissues after 8 days in the diet at 0.2 mg kg^{-1}, or in cow milk or tissues at 0.05 mg kg^{-1} for 21 consecutive days. Although agricultural uses for Amdro are limited to ant control, residue tolerances have been set for forage grasses, hay, and pineapple at 0.05 ppm, meaning that Amdro residues up to this level are still considered acceptable for animal and human consumption.

See also: Pesticides.

Further Reading

Hollingshaus, J.G., 1987. Inhibition of mitochondrial electron transport by hydramethylnon: A new amidinohydrazone insecticide. Pesticide Biochemistry and Physiology 27, 61–70.

Silverman, J., Vitale, G.I., Shapas, T.J., 1991. Hydramethylnon uptake by Blattella germanica (Orthoptera: Blattellidae) by coprophagy. J. Econ. Entomol. 84 (1), 176–180.

Relevant Websites

http://pmep.cce.cornell.edu – Cornell University.

www.epa.gov/oppsrrd1/REDs/2585red.pdf – EPA Hydramethylnon Eligibility Decision (RED) Fact Sheet.

http://extoxnet.orst.edu – Extension Toxicology Network, Oregon State University.

http://www.fluoridealert.org – Fluoride Action Network Pesticide Project.

http://npic.orst.edu/ – National Pesticide Information Center, Oregon State University and USEPA.

http://toxnet.nlm.nih.gov/ – TOXNET Toxicology Data Network, National Library of Medicine.

American Academy of Clinical Toxicology

LD Beilke, Aragon Pharmaceuticals, San Diego, CA, USA

This article is a revision of the previous edition article by Christopher P. Holstege, volume 4, pp 485–486, © 2005, Elsevier Inc.

Overview

The American Academy of Clinical Toxicology (AACT) was established in 1968 by a group of physicians and scientists with the goal of advancing the diagnosis and treatment of poisonings. In 1974, the AACT established the American Board of Medical Toxicology to certify physicians in the specialty of clinical toxicology, which was recognized as a subspecialty in 1992 by the American Board of Medical Specialties. In 1985, a second certifying board, the American Board of Applied Toxicology (ABAT) was established for nonphysician peer recognition.

Today, the AACT is an international organization whose membership comprises clinical and research toxicologists, physicians, veterinarians, nurses, pharmacists, analytical chemists, industrial hygienists, poison information center specialists, and allied professionals.

Mission Statement

The AACT is a multidisciplinary professional organization uniting scientists and clinicians in the advancement of research, education, prevention, and treatment of diseases caused by chemicals, drugs, and toxins.

The founders of the AACT established the Academy to:

- Promote the study of health effects of poisons on humans and animals.
- Unite into one group scientists and clinicians whose research, clinical, and academic experience focus on clinical toxicology.
- Foster a better understanding of the principles and practice of clinical toxicology.
- Encourage development of new therapies and treatment in clinical toxicology.
- Facilitate information exchange among individual members and organizations interested in clinical toxicology.
- Define the position of clinical toxicologists on toxicology-related issues.

American Board of Applied Toxicology

The ABAT was established by the AACT to provide special recognition to professionals (other than practicing physicians) who demonstrate exceptional knowledge, experience, and competence in applied clinical toxicology. An examination is administered periodically and is open to AACT members who meet the qualifications. Candidates who pass the examination are awarded the status of Diplomate of the American Board of Applied Toxicology.

Resources/Publications

As a result of an earlier collaboration regarding gastrointestinal decontamination, the Academy now collaborates with the European Association of Poisons Centres and Clinical Toxicologists (EAPCCT) to develop position statements on various clinical toxicology-related topics, such as snake envenomation and ipecac syrup. These position statements were systematically developed (and are routinely updated) as clinical guidelines intended for the in-hospital treatment of the poisoned patient. As the need arises, an ad hoc committee is appointed to develop an Academy position paper. These position statements/papers are published in Clinical Toxicology. Clinical Toxicology is the official journal of the AACT, the EAPCCT, and the American Association of Poison Control Centers.

The Academy also regularly publishes a newsletter, AACTion Newsletter, which can be accessed on the Academy website.

Special Interest Groups

Special interest sections of the AACT provide individuals with the opportunity to interact with professionals who have similar interests and to participate in specific educational and research forums. The AACT maintains six Specialty Sections: Acute & Intensive Care Toxicology, Pediatric Toxicology, Occupational & Environmental Toxicology, Medical Legal, Envenomations, and Herbs & Dietary Supplements. A full description of each interest group can be found on the AACT website.

Annual Scientific Meetings

The AACT coordinates the North American Congress of Clinical Toxicology, a forum for presentations on clinical and applied research. Special symposia and technical training courses also are conducted.

Research Awards

AACT Research Award Grant – The goal of this grant program is to provide competitive funding for clinical research that encourages the development of new therapies and treatment and adds to the understanding of the principles and practice of clinical toxicology.

Lampe–Kunkel Memorial Award for Research on Natural Products of Toxicology – The goal of this grant program is to provide competitive funding for original research to investigate some aspect of toxicity due to naturally occurring phenomenon (i.e., plants, mushrooms, algae, insects, snakes).

AACT Junior Investigator Research Grant Program – This is a research grant program that supports clinical toxicology research and the development of new investigators' research skills, with an emphasis on the mentoring of new researchers.

 http://dx.doi.org/10.1016/B978-0-12-386454-3.00688-6

Contact AACT

National Office, 6728 Old McLean Village Drive, McLean, VA 22101, 703-556-9222 (voice); 703-556-8729 (fax). E-mail: admin@clintox.org, URL: http://www.clintox.org/index.cfm.

See also: American Board of Toxicology; American College of Toxicology; Society of Toxicology; American Association of Poison Control Centers; American College of Medical Toxicology; Poisoning Emergencies in Humans; Drug and Poison Information Centers; The European Association of Poisons Centres and Clinical Toxicologists (EAPCCT).

Relevant Websites

http://www.clintox.org/index.cfm – AACT.
http://www.clintox.org/ABAT_Main.cfm – ABAT.
http://www.aapcc.org/ – American Association of Poison Control Centers.
http://www.calpoison.org/ – California Poison Control System.

American Association of Poison Control Centers

D Carr, American Association of Poison Control Centers, Alexandria, VA, USA

This article is a revision of the previous edition article by Christopher P. Holstege, volume 4, p 487, © 2005, Elsevier Inc.

Overview

The American Association of Poison Control Centers (AAPCC) represents and supports the network of 57 poison centers in the United States in the interests of poison prevention and in the treatment of poison exposures. The AAPC maintains the National Poison Data System, the largest poison information and surveillance database in the United States, which collects and monitors adverse incidents across the nation every 19 min and alerts federal, state, and local agencies of noteworthy events. The AAPCC conducts national outreach and education in partnership with the individual poison centers. The AAPCC sets accreditation standards for poison center operations and certifies poison specialists who respond to inquiries from the public, health-care providers, and emergency response personnel. In 2010, the 57 poison centers across the United States received approximately 4 million calls; 2.4 million of these calls were related to exposures and the rest were requests for information. The AAPCC has established the following national toll-free number for poisoning emergencies: 800-222-1222. (For a complete listing of poison centers, refer to www.aapcc.org.)

Mission

The AAPCC advances poison centers in their public health mission through information, advocacy, education, and research. Poison centers reduce the morbidity and mortality from unintentional poisonings by responding to calls for assistance related to foodborne toxins, medications, animal and environmental toxic events, and hazards.

Membership Criteria

Membership categories of the AAPCC include US Poison Center Member, Poison Prevention Education Center, Associate Institutional Member, Canadian Associate Institutional Member, Animal Poison Center, Industry Product Surveillance Service of Industry Poison Center, Individual Member, Honorary Member, and Sustaining Member.

Key Activities

The activities of the AAPCC include the following:

- Accreditation of regional poison centers and certification of poison center personnel.
- Interaction with private and governmental agencies whose activities influence poisoning and poison centers.
- Development of public and professional education programs and materials.
- Collection and analysis of national poisoning data.
- Promotion and support of legislation to improve poison prevention practices and programs.
- Participation on and partnerships with national coalitions and committees to advance public safety and poison prevention.

Publications

The AAPCC publishes the following:

- Annual Report of the American Association of Poison Control Centers' National Poison Data System published every December in *Clinical Toxicology* and available on the Association's website.
- The Association's newsletter, *The Poison Line*, published six times a year.
- An online discussion forum called 'Patient Management Guidelines for Poisonings.'
- Clinical Toxicology is the official journal of the American Association of Poison Control Centers (and the American Academy of Clinical Toxicology and the European Association of Poisons Centres and Clinical Toxicologists).

Meetings

Each year, the Association holds a national conference of poison center leaders that addresses scientific issues related to poisoning and poison prevention. AAPCC also conducts business meetings and holds committee meetings at this conference.

Awards and Grants

The AAPCC offers research awards to educators and specialists in poison information. Awards for best original scientific poster and best original scientific platform are presented annually at the North American Congress of Clinical Toxicology.

 http://dx.doi.org/10.1016/B978-0-12-386454-3.00689-8

American Board of Toxicology

SS Devi, LECOM School of Pharmacy, Bradenton, FL, USA
HM Mehendale, University of Louisiana at Monroe, Monroe, LA, USA

The American Board of Toxicology, Inc. (ABT) certifies individuals in general toxicology through a process that evaluates expert knowledge as demonstrated by education, experience, and passage of a comprehensive written examination. Certified individuals are initially recognized by being designated as Diplomates of the ABT for a period of 5 years.

ABT objectives are to encourage the study of the science of toxicology and to stimulate its advancement by promulgation of standards for professional practice. It is ABT's policy that Diplomates demonstrate a continual commitment to excellence in the science of toxicology. Successful achievement of these goals as outlined by the Board will result in an individual maintaining recognition as a Diplomate by the ABT.

The ABT has identified three performance criteria by which a Diplomate will be evaluated pursuant to recertification. These criteria are (1) Active Practice of Toxicology, (2) Continuing Education, and (3) Maintaining Expert Knowledge in General Toxicology. Each Diplomate, at the beginning of the fourth year of their current certification, will be required to apply for recertification. ABT will review activities in each of the three performance areas and notify the Diplomate of acceptable progress or deficiencies that need to be addressed. If, in the opinion of the Board, a Diplomate is not compliant with each of the three criteria at the end of the fifth certification year, that Diplomate may be required to successfully pass the formal certification examination. Diplomates who are compliant with each of the three performance criteria will be certified for an additional 5 years.

Active Practice of Toxicology: Active practice is defined as performing, directing, or managing toxicology activities such as research, testing, teaching, clinical practice, or regulation.

Continuing Education: A successful program of continuing education may encompass myriad diverse activities. The study of published texts, periodicals, or scientific journals germane to toxicology is a means by which Diplomates routinely maintain or expand their knowledge of toxicology. Other evidence of a commitment to continued education is attendance at specific programs where toxicology themes are presented in a comprehensive or in-depth manner. Such programs are often held during general or annual meetings of the Society of Toxicology, American College of Toxicology, Federation of American Societies for Experimental Biology, Environmental Mutagen Society, Teratology Society, American Association for Cancer Research, or Chapter Meetings of the Society of Toxicology. Attendance Forum or Target Organ Conferences also provide opportunities to maintain or expand a Diplomate's knowledge of toxicology.

Maintaining Expert Knowledge of General Toxicology: It is held that an objective mechanism is required for the Diplomate and ABT to gauge the success of their efforts to maintain expert knowledge in general toxicology. A recertification examination prepared by the ABT is to serve in this evaluation process during the first two recertification cycles. Diplomates will have the opportunity to privately complete the recertification examination during the fourth year of their certification period using their own reference material as needed. The completed examination will be graded by ABT. The Diplomate must answer 80% of the questions on each of the three parts correctly in order to pass. Subsequent recertification cycles will require the submission of examination questions for the test bank.

Summary of Recertification Process: Each Diplomate maintains a personal file of activities germane to the Active Practice and Continuing Education criteria for certification, that is, name of meeting attended, number of hours, title, topics, faculty, etc. Each Diplomate is required to be recertified every 5 years in order to maintain the Diplomate status.

Contact Details

American Board of Toxicology, P.O. Box 30054, Raleigh, NC 27622, USA. Tel.: +1 919 841 5022. URL: http://www.abtox.org/HomePage.aspx.

See also: American Board of Toxicology; American College of Toxicology; The Hamner Institutes for Health Sciences; EUROTOX; The International Society for the Study of Xenobiotics; Society of Environmental Toxicology and Chemistry; International Union of Toxicology; Society of Toxicology.

Relevant Website

http://www.abtox.org – American Board of Toxicology - home page.

 http://dx.doi.org/10.1016/B978-0-12-386454-3.00232-3

American College of Medical Toxicology

PM Wax, UT Southwestern School of Medicine, Dallas, TX, USA and American College of Medical Toxicology, Phoenix, AZ, USA
TJ Wiegand, University of Rochester Medical Center, Rochester, NY, USA

Published by Elsevier Inc.
This article is a revision of the previous edition article by Christopher P. Holstege, volume 4, p 489, © 2005, Elsevier Inc.

Overview

The American College of Medical Toxicology (ACMT) is a 501(c)6 nonprofit organization that was established in 1993 as the primary organization to serve physicians who are medical toxicologists. As of 2013, ACMT is the largest organizations of Board-certified medical toxicologists in the world. The organization's goal is to support quality medical care for persons exposed to potentially harmful pharmaceuticals and chemicals and to support training of the physicians who provide this care.

Mission Statement

The mission of ACMT is to "advance quality care of poisoned patients and public health through physicians who specialize in consultative, emergency, environmental, forensic, and occupational toxicology."

Governance

ACMT is governed by a 13-member Board of Directors. The ACMT national headquarters is located in Phoenix, Arizona, and is supported by a five-member staff.

Membership

Full membership in ACMT is restricted to those physicians who are Board-certified in medical toxicology. Membership is also available to fellows-in-training, residents and medical students, international members, and affiliate members. As of 2013, ACMT had grown to more than 650 members.

Resources/Publications

The *Journal of Medical Toxicology* (JMT) is the official journal of ACMT and is published quarterly by Springer. This international, peer-reviewed journal is dedicated to advancing the science and practice of medical toxicology. JMT is indexed by the library of medicine and is available online through many libraries around the world.

ACMT Newsletter is a bimonthly newsletter for ACMT members appearing six times a year. The newsletter features member news, current news and popular culture in toxicology, president's report, current information on billing and reimbursement in toxicology, and information about conferences and events in toxicology.

Committees/Sections

Operationally, ACMT is organized into committees and sections. ACMT committees include people whose primary focus is on education, practice, guideline development, research, media, fellowship program support, membership, nominations, and awards. ACMT also supports sections on addiction medicine, government, industry, legal and consultative, medication management, military, and a recent graduate section.

Scientific Meetings

ACMT hosts its Annual Scientific Meeting each spring. Highlights of this meeting include original research presentations, a fellow research forum, an open mike forum, cutting edge plenary lectures, and practice and career development sessions. Abstracts presented at the Annual Scientific Meeting are published in JMT. ACMT also organizes periodic courses on forensic toxicology, chemical terrorism, and emerging drug epidemics, and is a contributing society to the North American Congress of Clinical Toxicology each fall.

The Toxicology Investigators Consortium Case Registry

Established in 2010, ACMT developed and hosts the Toxicology Investigators Consortium (ToxIC) Case Registry. This registry is the largest database of toxicology patients treated by medical toxicologists in the world. More than 35 sites from the United States and other parts of the world contribute cases to this registry. As of September 2013, almost 24 000 cases have been entered into this registry. JMT publishes the annual reports from the ToxIC Case Registry.

Awards

ACMT in conjunction with the Medical Toxicology Foundation supports awards in research innovation, education innovation, and young physician development in medical toxicology.

See also: American Board of Toxicology; American College of Toxicology; American Academy of Clinical Toxicology; Poisoning Emergencies in Humans; Drug and Poison Information Centers; The European Association of Poisons Centres and Clinical Toxicologists (EAPCCT).

 http://dx.doi.org/10.1016/B978-0-12-386454-3.00690-4

Further Reading

Wax, P.M., Kleinschmidt, K.C., Brent, J., ACMT ToxIC Case Registry Investigators, Dec 2011. The toxicology investigators consortium (ToxIC) registry. J. Med. Toxicol. 7 (4), 259–265.

Wiegand, T.J., Wax, P.M., Schwartz, T., Finkelstein, Y., Gorodetsky, R., Brent, J., Toxicology Investigators Consortium Case Registry Investigators, Dec 2012. The toxicology investigators consortium case registry – the 2011 experience. J. Med. Toxicol. 8 (4), 360–377.

Relevant Website

http://www.acmt.net/ – American College of Medical Toxicology (ACMT) website.

American College of Toxicology

RC Guy, Robin Guy Consulting, LLC, Lake Forest, IL, USA

This article is a revision of the previous edition article by Harihara M. Mehendale, volume 4, pp 489–490, © 2005, Elsevier Inc.

Overview

The American College of Toxicology (ACT) is a worldwide professional organization comprising toxicologists and those in toxicology-related fields. It was founded in 1977 and incorporated in 1979 (in Illinois). The office is located in Bethesda, Maryland. The ACT is incorporated as a not for profit organization. Members must adhere to the ACT Bylaws and the Code of Ethics. The ACT has its own professional journal: The *International Journal of Toxicology*, published by Sage Publications.

Mission

The mission of the ACT is to educate, lead, and serve professionals in toxicology and related disciplines by promoting the exchange of information and perspectives on applied toxicology and safety assessment.

Strategic Objectives

The strategic objectives of ACT are

- Focus on interdisciplinary exchange of scientific information, especially because scientific information is used in regulations;
- Sponsor scientific and educational programs in toxicology;
- Present the ideals and opinions of its membership;
- Disseminate information of the results of toxicological research, standards, and practices through the College journal and newsletter;
- Serve in other capacities in which the College can function more efficiently as a group than as individuals.

Leadership and Membership

The ACT's Executive Council is composed of the President, President-Elect, Vice President, Past President, Secretary, and Treasurer. In addition, there are nine Council members. The Executive Director manages the overall operation of the organization.

Officials and Committee members are voted into their respective offices by other Full members. The Presidential track is filled by succession of 1-year term. Members vote on a Vice President, who after the term moves into the President-Elect position, which, in turn, leads to the President, followed by the Past-President. The Secretary and the Treasurer each serve a 2-year term. The councilors serve a 3-year term.

The ACT has seven types of membership: Full, Associate, Distinguished Fellow, Student, Emeritus, Honorary, and Corporate. The three major types of individual memberships are as follows.

Full

Any person who is qualified, by virtue of training and experience, and is actively involved in toxicology through administration, teaching, research, or safety assessment, and who is functioning as a scientist or professional in toxicology is eligible for Full membership. Full members must have 5 years of experience directly related to toxicology and fulfill one or more of the following requirements: formal advanced training in toxicology or related field, at least one peer-reviewed publication on a topic relevant to toxicology, or board certification in a subject relevant to toxicology. *Full membership must be sponsored by two Full members of the College.* One of the sponsors for the Full member can be associated with the same institution/organization of the candidate. The second sponsor must be from outside the candidate's organization. The membership application to support candidacy as a Full member must be completed in its entirety.

Associate

Any person who is qualified, by virtue of training and experience, and is actively involved in toxicology through administration, teaching, research, or safety assessment functioning as a scientist or professional and who has, at a minimum, an earned baccalaureate degree from a recognized college or university, or who has training and experience in toxicology, shall be eligible for election as an Associate member. Associate members must have 2 years of experience directly related to toxicology. Time spent pursuing an advanced degree in toxicology will count toward total experience. Associate membership must be sponsored by one Full member of the College who can represent the same institution/organization as the candidate. The membership application to support candidacy as an Associate member must be completed in its entirety. Associate members can upgrade their membership status to Full membership upon completing a membership application for Full status and submitting it through the Executive Director for approval by the Membership Committee. Associate members are eligible to serve on committees.

Student

Any student engaged in studies leading to a degree in the field of toxicology or a field impinging upon toxicology shall be eligible for Student membership upon recommendation of their academic advisor. Student members shall pay no membership fees or other assessments (excluding the annual meeting registration fee) but cannot vote or hold elective office. Student members shall not receive the College's Journal, unless purchased annually.

 http://dx.doi.org/10.1016/B978-0-12-386454-3.00233-5

Annual Meeting

Annual meetings locations usually alternate between the eastern and the western parts of the United States, to decrease the amount of time regulators need to travel at least every other year. Symposia are diverse and tailored to the needs of the toxicologic community, although most symposia are focused on the practical and regulatory aspects of toxicology, as opposed to pure research.

The ACT makes numerous awards at the annual meeting, usually held in November. These include

ACT Distinguished Scientist Award – An individual (not necessarily a member of ACT) who has made outstanding contributions to toxicology and its relationship to the regulation of chemicals, and the improvement of public health. The DSA winner becomes the Luncheon Speaker at the November 2012 annual meeting in Orland, Florida.

ACT Service Award – Recognizes an individual for their long-term dedication to the ACT including but not limited to service to the College (e.g., councilor, officer, and committee member), frequent participation and contribution to the annual meeting (speaker, chairperson, and organizing committee), and long-standing support of the College's activities. The recipient of the ACT Service Award must be a member of ACT.

ACT Young Professional Award – Recognizes an ACT member in good standing with no more than 10 years of full-time employment experience since completing their highest degree (time spent in postdoctoral training is not considered toward the 10 years of experience). Nominee must have demonstrated outstanding service to the College, including serving as an officer, councilor, committee member, and/or frequent participation and contribution at the annual meeting or any other College activity (i.e., speaker, chairperson, organizing committee, etc.).

ACT President's Award for Best Paper Published in the *International Journal of Toxicology* – Each year, the *International Journal of Toxicology* recognizes the authors of the best paper published in the journal. The award consists of a check for $1000 and a citation certificate. The award is announced and presented at the Annual Conference of the ACT during the Monday Luncheon Award Ceremonies.

Marshall Steinberg Memorial Award – This prize is given at the discretion of the International Pharmaceutical Excipients Council of the Americas (IPEC) Foundation Board of Directors to reward those individuals who have made outstanding contributions in the area of safety and toxicology for excipients. This prize recognizes achievements in the field of pharmaceutical excipients that includes but is not limited to (1) research that contributes to the safety of excipients; (2) investigations that establish test methods and standards that enhance the safety of excipients; (3) studies that support the development of new excipients or novel uses for existing excipients that provide or ensure greater safety in their use in pharmaceuticals; and (4) toxicology research that improves the overall safety of excipients or finished pharmaceuticals.

Furst Award – This award, through a generous contribution from the late Dr Arthur Furst, is given to the Best Student Paper presented at the annual meeting. It consists of a Travel Award and plaque.

Student Travel Awards are also awarded to deserving students to assist in travel to the annual meeting.

The ACT also presents webinars and courses throughout the year. Two of the courses, Toxicology for Industrial and Regulatory Scientists and Pathology for Non-Pathologists, are highly successful courses.

Toxicology for Industrial and Regulatory Scientists is taught by distinguished experts, and is designed to provide a basic training in toxicology. Participants obtain an overall understanding of the principles of nonclinical safety evaluation with emphasis on the practical application of these principles and interpretation of nonclinical safety data.

Pathology for Non-Pathologists is also cosponsored by The Society of Toxicologic Pathology. Topics change yearly and primarily focus on at least one organ system.

See also: Food Safety and Toxicology; The International Conference on Harmonisation; Micronucleus Assay; Mouse Lymphoma Assay; Safety Pharmacology; Toxicity, Acute; Toxicity Testing, Carcinogenesis; Toxicity, Subchronic and Chronic; Toxicity Testing, Developmental; Toxicity Testing, Mutagenicity; Toxicity Testing, Reproductive; Toxicity Testing, Sensitization; Toxicity Testing, Validation.

Relevant Websites

www.actox.org – American College of Toxicology.

http://www.actox.org/Journal/IntlJournalofToxicology/tabid/5180/Default.aspx – International Journal of Toxicology.

ACGIH® (American Conference of Governmental Industrial Hygienists)

DL Dahlstrom, New Era Sciences, LLC, Issaquah, WA, USA
AB Bloomhuff, ACGIH®, Cincinnati, OH, USA

This article is a revision of the previous edition article by Andrew Maier, volume 4, pp 491, © 2005, Elsevier Inc.

History

The independent National Conference of Governmental Industrial Hygienists (NCGIH) convened on 27 June 1938, in Washington, DC. Representatives to the conference included 76 members, representing 24 states, three cities, one university, the US Public Health Service, the US Bureau of Mines, and the Tennessee Valley Authority. This meeting was the culmination of concerted efforts by John J. Bloomfield and Royd S. Sayers.

NCGIH originally limited its full membership to two representatives from each governmental industrial hygiene agency. In 1946, the organization changed its name to the American Conference of Governmental Industrial Hygienists (ACGIH®) and offered full membership to all industrial hygiene personnel within the agencies as well as to governmental industrial hygiene professionals in other countries.

At its first meeting, NCGIH created nine standing committees. The committees were charged to address the important industrial hygiene issues of the pre-war era: appraisal methods; relationships with industry, labor, the medical profession, and other agencies; technical standards; education; uniform reporting of occupational diseases and other illnesses among workers; administrative development of state activities; industrial health code; legislation; and personnel. Over the next five decades, some of these committees evolved and expanded, assuming different titles; some became the purview of other organizations or agencies; and some achieved their goals and ended their active roles.

Undoubtedly the best known of ACGIH®'s activities, the Threshold Limit Values for Chemical Substances (TLV®-CS) Committee was established in 1941. This group was charged with investigating, recommending, and annually reviewing exposure limits for chemical substances. It became a standing committee in 1944. Two years later, the organization adopted its first list of 148 exposure limits, then referred to as Maximum Allowable Concentrations. The term Threshold Limit Values (TLVs®) was introduced in 1956. The first *Documentation of the Threshold Limit Values* was published in 1962 and is now in its seventh edition. Today's list of TLVs® includes 642 chemical substances and physical agents, as well as 47 biological exposure indices (BEIs®) for selected chemicals.

In 1961, ACGIH® began co-sponsoring an annual conference, the American Industrial Hygiene Conference and Exposition (AIHce), with the American Industrial Hygiene Association (AIHA).

ACGIH® Today

What began as a limited membership base has grown to the all-encompassing categories of today. Membership is open to all practitioners in industrial hygiene, occupational health, environmental health, and safety domestically and abroad. In September 2000, ACGIH® bylaws were amended, allowing members who are not government or academic employees greater voting rights as well as the opportunity to serve on the ACGIH® Board. During this time, ACGIH® has grown and expanded without losing sight of its original goal, "to encourage the interchange of experience among industrial hygiene workers and to collect and make accessible such information and data as might be of aid to them in the proper fulfillment of their duties."

Today, nine ACGIH® committees focus their energies on a range of topics: agricultural safety and health, air sampling instruments, bioaerosols, biological exposure indices, industrial ventilation, international, small business, threshold limit values for chemical substances (TLV®-CS), and threshold limit values for physical agents (TLV®-PA).

The tradition of reliable working committees has served ACGIH® exceptionally well. Through the efforts of its committees, ACGIH® has been able to provide critical information and has recommended practices to industrial hygienists worldwide. This history of sharing knowledge, based on careful study and independent judgment, has garnered international respect and accolades for ACGIH®.

Mission

Since its founding in 1938, ACGIH® has gone through many changes. Its membership has grown and diversified; its interests and projects have multiplied; names and faces in the organization have changed. Despite these changes, ACGIH® has not lost sight of its original objectives, which are reflected in today's organizational mission: *ACGIH® is a member-based organization that advances occupational and environmental health.*

Membership Criteria

There are ~3000 members worldwide. The main membership categories are regular and associate. Regular members are occupational hygiene, occupational health, environmental health, or safety professionals whose primary employment is with a government agency or an educational institution. Associate members are people who are engaged in the occupational hygiene, environmental health, occupational health or safety professions, but are not eligible for regular membership. Other membership categories include student, retired, honorary, and organizational.

Key Activities, Publications, Databases, and Services

ACGIH® supports its mission by developing scientific guidelines for the use of occupational and environmental health and

 http://dx.doi.org/10.1016/B978-0-12-386454-3.00584-4

safety professionals and developing and sponsoring numerous educational activities that facilitate the exchange of ideas, information, and techniques. These courses, symposia, webinars, and workshops are all vehicles for achieving the ultimate goal of worker health and safety.

The best known of the ACGIH's committee activities is the *Threshold Limit Values for Chemical Substances and Physical Agents and Biological Exposure Indices* book (better known as the *TLVs®* and *BEIs®*). These occupational exposure criteria are widely used around the world as the basis for occupational health protection. Today's list of TLVs® includes 658 chemical substances and 17 physical agents, as well as 47 biological exposure indices (BEIs®) for selected chemicals.

Two other ACGIH® committees have created publications that are recognized as the preeminent professional references in their respective fields: *Industrial Ventilation: A Manual of Recommended Practice*, first published in 1951, and *Air Sampling Instruments for Evaluation of Atmospheric Contaminants*, which debuted in 1960. The Ventilation Manual, now known as *Industrial Ventilation: A Manual of Recommended Practice for Design* (the Design Manual), is now in its 27th edition and has a companion, *Industrial Ventilation: A Manual of Recommended Practice for Operation and Maintenance* (the O&M Manual). The ASI Manual is in its 9th edition. Twenty-two monographs that will be included in a future ACGIH® *Signature Publication*, entitled *Air Sampling Technologies: Principles and Applications*, are available as downloadable documents. These represent the latest air sampling principles and practices.

The other ACGIH® committees have also published valuable professional reference texts. Some of these include: *Bioaerosols: Assessment and Control* (1999); *A Guide for Control of Laser Hazards, 4th Edition* (1990); and *Particle Size-Selective Sampling for Particulate Air Contaminants* (1999).

ACGIH® offers approximately 400 publication titles, including their well-known *Signature Publications*. Topics include industrial hygiene, environmental health, safety and health science, medical/toxicology, hazardous materials/waste, workplace controls, indoor air quality, physical agents, ergonomics, distance learning, computer resources, downloadable TLV® and BEI® *Documentation* and other downloadable products, and professional development. All of ACGIH®'s publications can be ordered online at www.acgih.org/store.

In addition to its publications, ACGIH® has supported numerous educational activities that facilitate the exchange of ideas, information, and techniques. These courses, symposia, webinars, and workshops are all vehicles for achieving the ultimate goal of worker health and safety.

ACGIH® also supports its mission through the sponsorship of conferences and seminars. Today, the American Industrial Hygiene Conference and Exposition (AIHce) is one of the world's premier conferences for occupational and environmental safety and health professionals. It attracts an international attendance of almost 8000 each year. ACGIH® committees and individual members contribute their expertise in professional development courses, technical sessions, and poster sessions.

ACGIH®'s dedication to information dissemination is also evident through its commitment to the *Journal of Occupational and Environmental Hygiene*, which it publishes jointly with the American Industrial Hygiene Association (AIHA).

In 1998, ACGIH® formed the Foundation for Occupational Health & Safety (FOHS). FOHS was established to complement the work of the American Industrial Hygiene Foundation (AIHF). The FOHS mission includes:

- Sponsoring research, education, and the publication of scientific information.
- Providing a vehicle for financial support of the improvement and enhancement of occupational and environmental health and safety and the general public health.
- Disseminating the results of valuable research findings and assuring a heightened quality of continuing education in occupational safety and health.

More information about FOHS can be found at www.fohs.org.

Related Organizations

- American Industrial Hygiene Association (AIHA)
- International Occupational Hygiene Association (IOHA)
- (US) National Institute for Occupational Safety and Health (NIOSH)
- (US) Occupational Safety and Health Administration (OSHA).

See also: National Institute for Occupational Safety and Health; Occupational Safety and Health Administration; American Industrial Hygiene Association; Industrial Hygiene.

American Industrial Hygiene Association

D Hicks, American Industrial Hygiene Association, Falls Church, VA, USA

About American Industrial Hygiene Association

The American Industrial Hygiene Association (AIHA®) is one of the largest international associations serving the needs of occupational and environmental health and safety professionals practicing industrial hygiene in industry, government, labor, academic institutions, and independent organizations. AIHA was founded in 1939.

What We Do

AIHA is devoted to achieving and maintaining the highest professional standards for our members. Working with the American Board of Industrial Hygiene, we promote certification of industrial hygienists. Our education programs are second to none, and offer opportunities to occupational and environmental health and safety professionals to maintain credentials in their respective fields. AIHA operates several highly recognized laboratory accreditation programs, based on the highest international standards, ensuring the quality of the data used in making critical worker protection decisions.

Mission

Creating knowledge to protect worker's health.

Vision 2020

Elimination of workplace illnesses.

Core Values

We prevent illnesses and injuries: AIHA members strive to prevent occupational illness and injury as a fundamental principle of the industrial hygiene and related occupational and environmental health and safety professions.

We advocate and develop science-based policy and practice: AIHA members advocate for the profession and develop sound science-based public policy and practice through collaboration across scientific and technical communities to ensure that safe and healthy environments are provided for all workers and communities.

We respect workers and communities: AIHA members respect the rights of workers and communities to have healthy and safe environments.

We support employers and employees: AIHA members recognize and support that operational excellence is complementary to both business and industrial hygiene and related occupational and environmental health and safety goals and priorities.

We respect our members: AIHA's Board of Directors, volunteers, members, and staff conduct the business of the Association with respect for diversity of opinion, transparent, and open communication, and with due consideration of each member's limited volunteer time.

Industrial Hygienists

The goal of the industrial hygienist is to keep workers, their families, and the community healthy and safe. They play a vital part in ensuring that international, federal, state, and local laws and regulations are followed in the work environment.

Typical roles of the industrial hygienist include the following:

- Investigating and examining the workplace for hazards and potential dangers.
- Making recommendations on improving the safety of workers and the surrounding community.
- Conducting scientific research to provide data on possible harmful conditions in the workplace.
- Developing techniques to anticipate and control potentially dangerous situations in the workplace and the community.
- Training and educating the community about job-related risks.
- Advising government officials and participating in the development of regulations to ensure the health and safety of workers and their families.
- Ensuring that workers are properly following health and safety procedures.

Journal

The *Journal of Occupational and Environmental Hygiene* (JOEH) is published to enhance the knowledge and practice of occupational and environmental hygiene and safety. Available primarily online, JOEH is a joint, peer-reviewed publication of AIHA® and American Conference of Governmental Industrial Hygienists (ACGIH®).

Conference

The American Industrial Hygiene Conference and Expo (AIHce) is the 'must attend' event for thousands of industrial hygiene and occupational and environmental health and safety professionals each spring. AIHce is the source for professional development and networking for over 75 years. Engaging general sessions, innovative technical sessions, comprehensive professional development courses, and a bustling Expo Hall

 http://dx.doi.org/10.1016/B978-0-12-386454-3.00585-6

provide the opportunity to refresh skills and earn certification maintenance points.

Related Organizations

- ACGIH
- International Occupational Hygiene Association
- National Institute for Occupational Safety and Health (US)
- Occupational Safety and Health Administration (US)

Contact Details

American Industrial Hygiene Association (AIHA)
3141 Fairview Park Drive, Suite 777
Falls Church, VA 22042, USA
Tel.: +1 703 849 8888
URL: http//www.aiha.org

See also: National Institute for Occupational Safety and Health; Occupational Safety and Health Administration; Occupational Safety and Health Act, US; ACGIH® (American Conference of Governmental Industrial Hygienists).

Further Reading

Castleman, B.I., 1999. Castleman global corporate policies and international "double standards" in occupational environment health. Int. J. Occup. Environ. Health 5, 61–64.
Kromhout, H., 2002. An international perspective on occupational health and hygiene. Int. J. Occup. Environ. Health 8, 111–112.
Kyle, A.D., 2011. Environmental health tracking. Encyclopedia of Environ. Health, Amserdam, The Netherlands: Elsevier B.V. pp. 424–432.
LaDou, J., 2003. International occupational health. Int. J. Hyg. Environ. Health 206 (4–5), 303–313.

Americium

I Malátová and V Bečková, National Radiation Protection Institute (SÚRO, v.v.i.), Praha, Czech Republic

Background

Americium is a transuranic radioactive chemical element located in the periodic table below the lanthanide element europium, and thus by analogy named after another continent, America. Americium was discovered in 1944 by the group of Glenn T. Seaborg. They produced americium by bombarding plutonium 239 with high energy neutrons. This formed ^{240}Pu, which was itself bombarded with neutrons and changed into ^{241}Pu, which then decayed into ^{241}Am through beta decay. This work was carried out at the University of Chicago's Metallurgical Laboratory, now known as Argonne National Laboratory. The discovery of americium was announced only in 1945 because during the Manhattan project all discoveries were classified.

At present altogether 18 isotopes of americium are known; however, only three of them with a sufficiently long half-life are significant from the point of view of their radiotoxicity. **Table 1** shows the half-lives and energies and how these three long-lived americium radioisotopes are formed.

Americium (Am) is the seventh member of the actinoid series, with electron configurations in its ground and ionized states analogous to those of its lanthanide homolog, europium (Eu). The solution chemistries of these two elements, however, show substantial differences, with the major ones being the difficulties in preparing Am(II) and the absence of Eu(IV), Eu(V), and Eu(VI).

Metallic americium is silvery-white. It slowly tarnishes in dry air and dissolves in acids, but it is resistant to alkalis. Americium dioxide, the most used form in production of americium sources, is a black crystalline compound, insoluble in water, soluble in acids.

Commercial nuclear power reactors produce kilogram quantities of both ^{241}Am and ^{243}Am with an isotopic composition dependent on reactor burn-up. Because of the complex composition of fission products in burnt-up fuel, ^{241}Am is produced from old plutonium, from which the ^{241}Am ingrown from ^{241}Pu is separated by means of solvent extraction and ion exchange.

Americium can be detected by gamma spectrometry through its gamma energy line 59.5 keV. The most common and sensitive measuring technique is alpha spectrometry with silicon detectors or pulse ionization chamber.

Uses

Only ^{241}Am and ^{243}Am have practical use. In some of americium isotopes, spontaneous fission occurs and some of them have large cross section for absorption of thermal neutrons resulting thus in a small critical mass for a sustained nuclear reaction. This is favorable for portable nuclear weapons and also for a small nuclear reactor. However, scarcity and high price hinder wider application of americium as a nuclear fuel. Americium-243 is used as a tracer in radiochemical applications and analysis. Americium-241 has wider use as a source in ionization chambers in smoke detectors, discharge arresters, and industrial gauges. It is also used as a source of alpha particles for production of neutrons in AmBe neutron sources. Americium-241 is also used as standard source for gamma and alpha spectrometry and for X-ray fluorescent spectroscopy when its gamma energy line 59.5 keV excites K X-rays of the lighter elements.

Environmental Behavior, Sources, Routes and Pathways

Environmental Presence

Americium-241 is the most important radioisotope of americium from the point of view of the occurrence in environment. The other long-lived isotope ^{243}Am is produced in nuclear reactors in smaller activity compared to ^{241}Am. The activity of ^{242m}Am (half-life 160 years) that originated in

Table 1 Physical properties of long-lived americium isotopes

Radioisotope	*Half-life (y)*	*Decay mode*	*Energy/Intensity*	*Specific activity (Bq/g)*	*Production*
^{241}Am	432.2	α	5486 keV/0.845	1.27E+11	^{241}Pu $\beta-$decay
		α	5443 keV/0.130		
		γ	59.5 keV/0.359		
		SF	4.10E-12		
^{242m}Am	141	α	5142 keV/0.00027	3.88E+11	^{241}Am(n.γ)
		α	5207 keV/0.004		
		IT	0.9954		
^{243}Am	7370	α	5275 keV/0.874	7.38E+09	^{238}U multiple neutron capture
		α	5233 keV/0.11		
		γ	74.66 keV/0.68		^{239}Pu multiple neutron capture
		SF	3.70E-09		

SF – spontaneous fission.
IT – internal transition.

 http://dx.doi.org/10.1016/B978-0-12-386454-3.01162-3

nuclear weapons tests was nearly six orders of magnitude lower in comparison with ^{241}Pu activity from which ^{241}Am in-grows. Americium-241 is produced in nuclear power plants during activation of ^{239}Pu and ^{240}Pu by neutrons, which is followed by beta decay of ^{241}Pu ($T_{1/2} = 14.35$ years). This means that also in burned-up fuel ^{241}Am is produced by decay of ^{241}Pu a long time after the fuel is removed from a nuclear reactor. Maximum of in-grown activity of ^{241}Am from ^{241}Pu arises after 70 years. Americium-243 is produced from short-lived ^{243}Pu arising from bombardment of ^{239}Pu and ^{238}U by neutrons, so it is not produced after shutdown of a nuclear reactor.

Americium-241 is detectable in very small activities over the whole Northern Hemisphere as the result of nuclear weapons tests in the atmosphere in the 1950s and beginning of the 1960s. Very sensitive methods, including radiochemical separation from large samples, are necessary for detection of ^{241}Am in soil, which may be present in concentrations of 20–40 Bq m^{-2}. Airborne releases and effluents to the hydrosphere from nuclear power plants also contain very small activities of transuranic elements, including americium-241, but even very sensitive detection methods can detect it directly in releases only (at tenths of kBq to a few kBq per year), not in the environment. Existing americium contamination is concentrated in the areas used for the atmospheric nuclear weapons tests conducted between 1945 and 1980, as well as at the sites of nuclear incidents, such as the Chernobyl disaster in 1986. For example, the analysis of the debris at the testing site of the first US hydrogen bomb in Enewetak Atoll revealed high concentrations of various actinoids including americium. The glassy residue left on the desert floor where atomic bombs were tested in Alamogordo, New Mexico, Kazakhstan, and the Maralinga desert in Australia contain traces of ^{241}Am. Elevated levels of americium were also detected at the crash site of a US B-52 bomber, which carried four hydrogen bombs, in 1968 in Thule, Greenland and at the location of a similar incident in Palomares, Spain. Other potential sources of ^{241}Am are two sunken nuclear submarines in the Barents Sea: 'Komsomolets' with a reactor and two nuclear torpedoes and 'Kursk' with a reactor and probably with nuclear weapons as well. Also 17 reactors dumped in the Kara Sea are potential sources of transuranic elements, including ^{241}Am. Places in which nuclear weapon industries were located both in the United States and in Russia have increased content of ^{241}Am in soil and, therefore, also in airborne aerosols from resuspension. Examples of such locations are Hanford and Rocky Flats in the United States, and Chelyabinsk and Kyshtym in Russia.

During monitoring of the environment around Chernobyl after the 1986 nuclear reactor failure, the most attention was paid to ^{239}Pu. As the total activity of ^{239}Pu and ^{241}Pu released from the Chernobyl power plant are known, and the fate of both plutonium isotopes in the environment is the same, it can be assumed that the ratio of their respective activities at the time of deposition was the same as in total release. In-growth of ^{241}Am from ^{241}Pu can be calculated from the activity of ^{241}Pu. In the 30-km diameter zone around Chernobyl for which an estimated deposition of ^{239,240}Pu was higher than 3.7 kBq m^{-2}, the in-growth of ^{241}Am 30 years after the accident is about 40 kBq m^{-2}.

Partition Behavior in Water, Sediment, and Soil

Americium's behavior in the environment cannot be isolated from that of plutonium as a precursor of ^{241}Am. Behavior of Am and Pu in marine environments has been thoroughly studied in the Irish Sea, where low-level radioactive wastes from the Sellafield site, once a plutonium production plant and now a nuclear reprocessing station, have been discharged since the early 1950s. ^{241}Am discharges peaked there in the early 1970s. Those studies show that americium sorbs on particulates and adsorbs to sediments, thus being quickly removed from water column.

In sorption and desorption in an environmental system, presence of organic matter in water and sediment plays an important role complexing americium and enhancing its transportability. Bicarbonate and/or carbonate complexes are dominant in sea water or underground water with low organic carbon content, whereas in fresh waters of low calcium concentration complexation reactions with humic and fulvic material are dominant. Investigation of plutonium and americium subsurface transport in the vicinity of locations contaminated with radioactive waste showed that traces of the actinoides were detected in groundwater 3.4 km from the point of discharge at Los Alamos National Laboratory, United States or 4 km from the Mayak Production Association, Russia. Here, the mechanism of transport is explained not only by natural conditions, but also by man-induced presence of organic substances in the wastes. The role of colloid formation and complexation in transport of americium in water has still been a subject of investigation and discussion.

Fate of americium in soil is closely related to its behavior in water. In soil, americium forms strong complexes with soil organic matter. In soils poor in organic matter americium resides in upper layers. On the other hand, if soluble complexes with organic matter are formed, mobility of americium and its bioavailability are enhanced. As ^{241}Pu is a precursor of ^{241}Am, plutonium retention in soil must also be taken into consideration. In most soils, americium is more mobile (less adsorbed to soil) than plutonium. Bioavailability is characterized by concentration ratios (CR) defined as Bq kg^{-1} in organisms per Bq kg^{-1} in soil or Bq kg^{-1} in organisms per Bq l^{-1} in water. Concentration ratios for root uptake of americium from soil are in the order of 10^{-6}–10^{-2}. Roots and leaves accumulate considerably more americium than fruit and grain. The uptake is higher from acidic and organic rich soils.

Accumulation of Am from water into fish flesh is low – CR in the order 10^{-3}–10^{-1}, depending on organic matter content in water, though Am is concentrated in seaweed (CR $\sim 1.10^2$) and in shellfish, particularly in shells.

Environmental Persistence (Degradation, Speciation) and Long-Range Transport

Activity of ^{241}Am in the environment is decreasing with its physical half-life only. When in-growth from ^{241}Pu takes place, its activity is increasing up to 50 years and afterward decreasing with ^{241}Am half-life. Long-range transport of ^{241}Am in the air depends on its origin and size of aerosol. Aerosol size is characterized by its Activity Median Aerodynamic Diameter (AMAD). Long-range transport of aerosol particles is described by many models of atmospheric dispersion which use particles of defined size – usually AMAD 1 μm is used. The dependence of long-range transport on size of particles was seen very well in the Chernobyl accident: Particles connected with dispersed fuel which had bigger AMAD (^{239}Pu, ^{241}Pu, ^{90}Sr) were deposited near the place of origin, whereas small particles with AMAD 1 μm and less were transported over very long distances. ^{241}Am was also deposited in the vicinity of the Chernobyl power plant, and its activity is increasing by decay of ^{241}Pu.

Human Exposure and Exposure Monitoring

Knowledge of human exposure with ^{241}Am is derived from descriptions of real cases of occupational internal contamination, which occurred at many places. The most serious case occurred during separation of ^{241}Am from irradiated fuel in 1976, when a worker was exposed to few hundreds GBq through the skin and inhalation. Another thoroughly studied case was inhalation with a lower intake probably from the year 1965. Both these workers from the United States, were followed during their life by *in vivo* measurement and excreta bioassay, and donated their bodies to the US Transuranium and Uranium Registry. Radiochemical analysis of different organs and tissues of these two donors and many other volunteers who were internally contaminated during their life contributed to the knowledge of behavior of americium in human body. *In vivo* studies and excretion bioassay of many internally contaminated workers followed for longer time also make a significant contribution to the knowledge of kinetics of americium in the human body long time after the intake.

Monitoring of Human Exposure

Intake of americium-241 by humans can be detected directly by *in vivo* measurements of the body by whole body counters equipped with detectors sensitive to low energy gamma radiation. Suitable devices are semiconductor high purity germanium detectors with special thin windows or scintillation phoswich (sandwich from NaI(Tl) and CsI(Tl)) detectors. Usually, special configuration is used for detection of ^{241}Am in individual organ or tissues, for example, lungs, liver, or skeleton through measurements of skull or knee. Doses to tissues and organs are then derived with the use of biokinetic models, enabling estimation of intake of ^{241}Am and afterward, through tabulated values for doses per unit intake in sievert per becquerels. Detection of internal contamination by direct *in vivo* measurement is much less sensitive than bioassay of excreta. Urine and feces are commonly analyzed, but blood and tissues are also assayed, though more rarely. Post mortem analyses can be performed on bones and inner organs.

Toxicokinetics

Behavior of americium in human body depends on the path of intake which could be by inhalation, ingestion or directly to the blood stream by injection, or by a wound. When Am is inhaled as aerosol, its behavior in the respiratory tract depends on the size of aerosol and inhaled compound. As a rule, aerosol with AMAD larger than 10 μm is eliminated by extrathoracic pathways and goes to the alimentary tract. Entry and deposition in the individual parts of respiratory tract are governed only by the size distribution of the aerosol particles. Absorption into blood depends on the physicochemical form of the radionuclide deposited in the respiratory system. Most Am compounds are described as the class M of solubility in lungs – it means that 10% of materials from lungs is absorbed to blood with half-life of 10 min and 90% with half-life of 140 days. About 70% of the deposit in the alveolar–interstitial region reaches body fluids. Americium is deposited from blood mainly in liver and bones, a part is excreted through feces and urine. Fecal excretion is important in a relatively short time after the entry of americium into the respiratory system when americium is still in lungs; later on, urinary excretion is about three times as high as the fecal one.

After an ingestion intake, nearly 90% is excreted via feces during the first 3 days because the absorption to blood from small intestines is very low. Only after about 50 days urinary excretion prevails. When the entry of americium to the organism occurs through a wound or by injection, about 30% goes to the skeleton and less than 10% is excreted. Americium belongs to so-called bone-seeking elements and among them, to bone surface seekers. It was found that after the entry to the organism, Am is deposited mainly on the bone surfaces; however, later on is covered by new bone. According to experiments with Beagle dogs the distribution among different bones varies with injection levels, some of which were high enough to induce radiation effects. Excretion of americium from humans is very slow, with the exception of an early phase. Content of americium in a skeleton over time increases up to about 3–5 years after intake. Three years after an injection, about 50% of injected activity is in the skeleton. After inhalation, about 4% of inhaled activity is in the skeleton. Afterward, activity in the skeleton and also excreted activity decreases, with the half-life of about 70 years.

Mechanism of Toxicity

The mechanism of action of radioactive elements is usually described by their radiotoxicity rather than their chemical toxicity. Exposure of internal human tissues to americium-241 occurs only after ^{241}Am enters human body, as the range of effects of alpha radiation in tissue is only about a few tens of micrometers. In such cases, cells could be damaged by absorption of energy of alpha particles. When the dose is great enough, cells are damaged to such extent that they cannot repair themselves. When too great a cell population is affected, then adverse effects occur in that tissue. ^{241}Am stays in human and other mammalian organisms for a very long time, so occurrence of stochastic (late) effects is much more probable.

Acute and Short-Term Toxicity (Animal/Human)

Acute effects of intake of americium were studied in Beagle dogs; however, most attention was devoted in these experiments to their morbidity and life span. When higher activities of ^{241}Am were injected to Beagle dogs, sharp decreases in retention in liver occurred after 100 days after the injection and deposition in skeleton increased. It is assumed that this phenomenon is due to radiation damage of liver that then releases americium to accumulate in other parts of the body. Some studies were also conducted on smaller laboratory animals (mice and rats), but it was felt that it is very difficult to extend such data to humans.

In a case of human contamination that followed an explosion of about 100 GBq ^{241}Am, immediate treatment reduced contamination to approximately 200 MBq, and, after one day, to about 40 MBq. Persistent adverse effects in blood – specifically clinical lymphopenia and thrombocytopenia – were observed. Survival of the individual was probably due to intense and long-term chelation therapy with diethylenetriaminepentaacetic acid (DTPA) and through medical care. In dogs exposed to about 60 Bq kg^{-1}, leukopenia and elevated hematopoietic activity were reported.

Chronic Toxicity (Animal/Human)

When chronic exposure to low doses of ionizing radiation occurs, late (stochastic) effects occur. Bone surfaces, red bone marrow, lymph nodes, and liver obtain the largest doses from americium intakes. When chronic inhalation exposure takes place, doses to parts of the respiratory tract also contribute significantly to committed effective dose.

Carcinogenicity

Beagle dogs were internally contaminated either by injection or by inhalation and their health status was followed over their life span. Health effects of transuranic elements, including americium, were compared with the health effects caused by intakes of ^{226}Ra and ^{224}Ra for extrapolation purposes; that is, for these two radionuclides some relevant data on occurrence of malignancies in humans already existed. Osteosarcomas and other malignancies were found in the exposed animals. In people with internal contamination with ^{241}Am of different activity levels, no malignancy was found that could be connected to exposure; however, the number of human exposures is very small.

Clinical Management

Decrease of body burden of americium (^{241}Am) in people with internal contamination is possible with the intravenous administration of chelating agents. Commonly used calcium and/or zinc salts of DTPA are especially useful when the entry of americium into the body is through a wound. When inhalation intake is concerned, significant decrease of americium in liver is possible provided that repeated intravenous injection or infusion with DTPA takes place. The content of americium in skeleton or in lungs is affected only marginally. DTPA increases excretion through urine about 50 times, but only for a short time (about one day); therefore, protracted application has to be used. Decrease in occurrence of osteosarcoma was observed in Beagle dogs treated with DTPA in comparison with controls injected with ^{241}Am only; however, no significant decrease in bone retention was observed.

Exposure Standards and Guidelines

Limits of exposure of workers from intake of ^{241}Am are the same as for all other radionuclides. For workers, they are 20 mSv per year averaged over 5 consecutive years or 50 mSv in any single year provided that the dose over five consecutive years does not exceed 100 mSv. For the general population, the limit is 1 mSv in a year or, in special circumstances, an effective dose of up to 5 mSv in a single year provided that the average dose over 5 consecutive years does not exceed 1 mSv per year. The limits for internal contamination are valid for committed effective dose; that is, 50 years integral effective dose rate for workers and 70 years integral for the general population. Annual intake of ^{241}Am can be calculated from tabulated dose coefficients which give dose per unit intake in sieverts per becquerel (Sv/Bq). For ingestion intake, the limit is about 2×10^{-7} (Sv/Bq) and for inhalation about 2×10^{-5} (Sv/Bq); it means that for exposure 1 mSv per year, ingestion intake could not exceed 5000 Bq per year or inhalation intake 50 Bq per year.

Ecotoxicology

Experiments with transfer of americium from fresh and marine water to fish were performed with the aim to investigate impacts on the human food chain. Effects of americium on the environment are not known, because in the polluted areas americium always occurs together with other radionuclides. Generally, adverse effects of artificial radionuclides present in the environment on biota were not observed.

Funding

Project of the Ministry of the Interior of the Czech Republic, "Research of advanced methods for detection, assessment and consequential management of radioactive contamination," identification code VF20102015014.

See also: Plutonium; Radiation Toxicology, Ionizing and Nonionizing.

Further Reading

Choppin, G.R., 2006. Actinide speciation in aquatic systems. Mar. Chem. 99 (1–4), 83–92.

Environmental Protection: Transfer Parameters for Reference Animals and Plants. In: ICRP Publication 114, Ann, vol. 39, 2009. ICRP (6).

Hengé-Napoli, M.H., Stradling, G.N., Taylor, D.M. (Eds.), 2000, Decorporation of radionuclides from human body. Rad. Prot. Dosimetry, vol. 87, p. 1. Special Issue.

International Basic Safety Standards for Protection against Ionizing Radiation and for the Safety of Radiation Sources. IAEA Safety Series No. 115, 1996. International Atomic Energy Agency, Vienna. ISBN:92-0-104295-7.

Runde, W.H., Schulz, W.W., 2006. Americium. In: Morss, L.R., Edelstein, N.M., Fuger, J., Katz, J.J. (Eds.), The Chemistry of the Actinide and Transactinide Elements, third ed. Springer, pp. 1265–1395.

Sokolik, G.A., Ovsiannikova, S.V., Ivanova, T.G., Leinova, S.L., 2004. Soil-plant transfer of plutonium and americium in contaminated regions of Belarus after the Chernobyl catastrophe. Environ. Int. 30 (7), 939–947.

Tolmachev, S.Y., Ketterer, M.E., Hare, D., Doble, P., James, A.C., 2011. The US transuranium and uranium registries: forty years' experience and new directions in the analysis of actinides in human tissues. Proc. Radiochim. Acta 1, 173–181.

Relevant Websites

http://www.atsdr.cdc.gov/ToxProfiles/tp156.pdf – Agency for Toxic Substances and Disease Registry. Toxicological Profile for Americium.

http://www.epa.gov/radiation/radionuclides/americium.html – US Environmental Protection Agency Protection/ Radiation.

http://janus.northwestern.edu/dog_tissues/reports/red_book.pdf – US Food and Drug Administration:Aristolochic Acid: Letter to Industry.

Ames Test

RC Guy, Robin Guy Consulting, LLC, Lake Forest, IL, USA

The Ames bacterial reverse mutation test uses strains of *Salmonella typhimurium* and *Escherichia coli* that require amino acids (histidine or tryptophan, respectively) to detect point mutations and frameshift mutations. The reverse mutation allows the *S. typhimurium* or *E. coli* strains to restore the functional capability of the bacteria to synthesize the specific amino acid on their own, independent of amino acid content in the medium. The test is the most commonly used reverse mutation test. The Ames test was developed by and named for Bruce Ames of the University of California at Berkeley.

Point mutations are base-pair substitutions; that is, a base change in DNA of at least one DNA base pair. In a reverse mutation test, this change may occur at the site of the original mutation or at a second site in the bacterial genome. Frameshift mutations are the addition or deletion of one or more base pairs in the DNA, thereby changing the reading frame in the RNA.

Mutations in oncogenes and tumor suppressor genes of somatic cells can be involved in tumor formation. The Ames test is rapid, sensitive, inexpensive, and relatively easy for a microbiology laboratory to perform. This test can be used on a wide variety of materials, including volatile compounds.

Many compounds that are positive in the Ames test are mammalian carcinogens and a huge database exists; however, there is not an exact correlation between the Ames test and carcinogenicity. Even with the addition of a metabolic activation system, this prokaryotic system cannot precisely replicate a mammalian cell *in vivo*. Correlation may be dependent on chemical class. Care should be taken to avoid conditions that would lead to results not reflecting authentic mutagenicity. As in mammalian *in vitro* systems, positive results that do not reflect authentic mutagenicity may arise from a variety of possible changes, including pH, osmolality (very high concentrations of test article), or high levels of cytotoxicity (Scott, et al., 1991).

The Ames test is recommended by International Conference on Harmonisation (ICH) and International Organization for Standardization (ISO) guidelines as part of standard genetic toxicology batteries. The other assays include the mouse lymphoma and *in vivo* micronucleus tests. This bacterial reverse mutation test may not be appropriate for the evaluation of certain classes of chemicals, for example, highly bactericidal compounds (e.g., certain antibiotics), any of which may interfere with cell division or replication, and possibly some peptides. In such cases, mammalian mutation tests may be more appropriate.

The most commonly used tester strains are *S. typhimurium* TA1535, TA1537, TA98, and TA100 and *E. coli* WP_2 *uvrA*. Other strains may be used as long as there are historical data that support the findings. The *S. typhimurium* strains have a mutation on their histidine operon as follows:

TA1535 (hisG46)
TA1537 (hisC3076)
TA98 (hisD3052)
TA100 (hisG46)

The histidine mutation prevents the *S. typhimurium* strains from synthesizing histidine, and, therefore, prevents the growth of the cell. All the *S. typhimurium* strains have additional mutations of the *rfa* and *uvrB* genes. The *rfa* gene has a loss of one of the enzymes responsible for the synthesis of part of the lipopolysaccharide layer of the cell wall, which increases the cell's permeability to certain chemical classes. The *uvrB* gene contains a deletion that causes a deficit in the DNA excision-repair system, which causes increased sensitivity to certain chemicals. Strains TA98 and TA100 also have an R-factor, in this case the pKM101 plasmid, which further causes increased sensitivity to certain chemicals. TA1537 and TA98 are reverted back to their original histidine-independent state by frameshift mutations. TA1535 is reverted back by base-pair mutations and TA100 is reverted back by both frameshift and base-pair mutations.

The tryptophan mutation prevents the *E. coli* WP_2 *uvrA* strain from synthesizing tryptophan. A revertant can occur by a base change.

Cultures of established cell lines or cell strains should be used. These should be karyotyped.

Tests conducted *in vitro* generally require the use of an exogenous source of metabolic activation. S9 is the most commonly used exogenous source of metabolic activation. S9 is a rat liver homogenate prepared from the livers of rodents treated with enzyme-inducing agents such as Aroclor 1254. This metabolic activation system simulates the metabolic characteristics of a mammal under *in vivo* conditions. Therefore, a typical assay should determine the mutagenic potential of a chemical in the absence and presence of a metabolic activation system (S9). For both metabolic situations, a negative (solvent) and the appropriate positive control should be tested concurrently.

The Ames test consists of a preliminary phase to find the dose range and the final mutagenicity phase. For the preliminary phase, more details of the procedure are described below, but each strain, with and without S9, is plated onto a single plate with 9–10 concentrations. The maximum dose level recommended is 5000 μg per plate (or 5 μl per plate for a liquid test substance) when not limited by solubility or cytotoxicity. The vehicle used may include sterile water, dimethylsulfoxide (DMSO), or ethanol. Cytotoxicity is usually determined after 24–48 h of incubation.

For the main mutagenicity assay, suspensions of bacterial cells are exposed to approximately five concentrations of the test material in the presence and in the absence of an exogenous metabolic activation system. If no toxicity was observed in the preliminary study to find the dose range, concentrations of up to 50 μl or 5000 μg per plate should be used. Triplicate plates per concentration per strain with and without metabolic activation are standard. Negative and positive controls are used as appropriate.

The two most popular methods are the plate incorporation method and the preincubation method. In the plate

 http://dx.doi.org/10.1016/B978-0-12-386454-3.00811-3

incorporation method, these suspensions are mixed with an overlay (top) agar and plated immediately onto minimal medium (bottom agar). In the preincubation method, the suspension mixture is incubated and then mixed with a top agar before plating onto minimal medium. For both techniques, after 2 or 3 days of incubation, normal-sized, revertant colonies are counted and compared with the number of spontaneous revertant colonies on solvent control plates. Independent repeats are recommended by the ICH guidelines. Certain modifications of the methods need to be incorporated for specific types of test articles. The ICH guidance S2(r1) recommends, based on experience with testing pharmaceuticals, that a single Ames test is considered sufficient when it is clearly negative or positive, and carried out with a fully adequate protocol including all strains with and without metabolic activation, a suitable dose range that fulfills criteria for top dose selection, and appropriate positive and negative controls.

Negative (solvent) and positive controls must be utilized for a valid study. A historical database must be maintained for these results. The positive control concentration must be documented, as different solvents and concentrations are required for different strains and metabolic activation conditions. Examples of positive control substances include:

Absence of exogenous metabolic activation

- Sodium azide [CAS no. 26628-22-8] for TAl535 and TAl00
- 2-Nitrofluorene [CAS no. 607-57-8] TA98, TA1538
- 9-Aminoacridine [CAS no. 134-50-9] TAl537, TA97 and TA97a
- 4-Nitroquinoline [CAS no. 56-57-5] WP2 uvrA

Presence of exogenous metabolic activation

- 2-Anthramine for all strains

To ensure that the results of an assay are valid, specific criteria have been determined. Both positive and negative (solvent) control values should reasonably be within the normal historical data for the laboratory. Tester strains must be identified and have a characteristic number of spontaneous revertants per plate for the vehicle controls. A minimum of three nontoxic concentrations must be evaluated.

Once the data are available for analyses, evaluation of the results follows. There are several criteria for determining a positive result, such as a concentration-related increase over the range tested and/or a reproducible increase at one or more concentrations in the number of revertant colonies per plate in at least one strain with or without a metabolic activation system. The concentration-related increase would be three times the mean vehicle control value for strains TA1535, TA1537, and TA1538 and two times the mean vehicle control value for TA98, TA100, and WP_2 *uvrA*. The biological relevance of the results should be considered first.

A negative test is when the results do not meet the above criteria and the test material is thereby considered to be not mutagenic.

The Ames test is a sensitive predictor of mutagenicity in mammals, but it should not be used in a vacuum. The Ames test should be used in a battery of *in vitro* and *in vivo* tests for predicting the genetic toxicity potential of test materials. The ICH developed a revised guidance, S2(R1), to assist in the preparation of a genetic toxicology battery and the conduct of studies. This guidance merges the old ICH S2A and S2B. The purpose of the revision was to optimize the standard genetic toxicology battery for prediction of potential human risks, and to provide guidance on interpretation of results.

The US Food and Drug Administration (FDA) has posted a template for the *In Vitro* Bacterial Reverse Mutation (Ames) Test (FDA, 2004).

See also: The International Conference on Harmonisation; Micronucleus Assay; Mouse Lymphoma Assay; Toxicity Testing, Mutagenicity.

Further Reading

Ames, B.N., McCann, J., Yamasaki, E., 1975. Methods for detecting carcinogens and mutagens with the *Salmonella*/mammalian-microsome mutagenicity test. Mutat. Res. 11, 347–364.

FDA, 2004. Template for the In Vitro Bacterial Reverse Mutation (Ames) Test http://www.fda.gov/Food/GuidanceComplianceRegulatoryInformation/GuidanceDocuments/FoodIngredientsandPackaging/ucm094212.htm (accessed 22.01.12.).

Federal Insecticide, Fungicide and Rodenticide Act. http://www.epa.gov/oecaagct/lfra.html (accessed 27.06.12.).

Gatehouse, D., Haworth, S., Cebula, T., Gocke, E., Kier, L., Matsushima, T., Melcion, C., Nohmi, T., Yenitt, S., Zeiger, E., 1994. Recommendations for the performance of bacterial mutation assays. Mutat. Res. 312, 217–233.

ICH, 2011. ICH Harmonised Tripartite Guideline; Guidance on Genotoxicity Testing and Data Interpretation for Pharmaceuticals Intended for Human Use S2(R1) http://www.ich.org/fileadmin/Public_Web_Site/ICH_Products/Guidelines/Safety/S2_R1/Step4/S2R1_Step4.pdf Current Step 4 version dated 9 November 2011 (accessed 22.01.12.).

Kier, L.D., Brusick, D.J., Auletta, A.E., Yon Halle, E.S., Brown, M.M., Simmon, V.F., Dunkel, V., McCann, J., Mortelmans, K., Prival, M., Rao, T.K., Ray, V., 1986. The *Salmonella typhimurium*/mammalian microsomal assay: a report of the U.S. Environmental Protection Agency Gene-tox program. Mutat. Res. 168, 69–240.

Maron, D.M., Ames, B.N., 1983. Revised methods for the *Salmonella* mutagenicity test. Mutat. Res. 113, 173–215.

Scott, D., Galloway, S.M., Marshall, R.R., Ishidate, M., Brusick, D., Ashby, J., Myhr, B.C., 1991. Genotoxicity under extreme culture conditions. A report from ICPEMC task group 9. Mutat. Res. 221, 147–204.

Relevant Websites

http://www.epa.gov/oecaagct/lfra.html – Federal Insecticide, Fungicide and Rodenticide Act (Environmental Protection Agency; www.epa.gov)

www.fda.gov – Food and Drug Administration.

www.ich.org – Good Laboratory Practices International Conference on Harmonization.

Aminobiphenyl, 4-

H Robles, Irvin, CA, USA

- Chemical Abstracts Service Registry Number: 92-67-1
- Synonyms: 4-ADP, 4-Biphenylamine, *p*-Phenylaniline, *p*-Xenylamine, Xenylamine
- Chemical Formula: $C_{12}H_{11}N$
- Chemical Structure:

H_2N—(biphenyl structure)

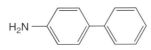

Background

4-Aminobiphenyl was formerly used as a rubber antioxidant and in the manufacture of azo dyes. Due to its carcinogenicity 4-aminobiphenyl is no longer produced commercially. It is found in tobacco smoke.

Uses

4-Aminobiphenyl is not produced commercially. However, it is used in research as a cancer-causing agent.

Environmental Fate and Behavior

4-Aminobiphenyl may have been released into the environment during its production and use as a rubber antioxidant and dye intermediate; however, sources suggest that it was no longer in significant production by the early 1970s. 4-Aminobiphenyl is easily oxidizable and probably undergoes photolysis but there is little actual data on these processes. If released on land it is expected to adsorb moderately to soil, probably binding to humic materials, and undergo redox reactions. If released to surface water, it is expected to adsorb to sediment, and probably undergo photolysis and oxidation. It may be degraded by oxidation by alkoxy radicals, which are photochemically produced in eutrophic waters, with an estimated half-life of 14 days. 4-Aminobiphenyl is biodegradable and biodegradation may well occur in both soil and water but there are no rates available for soil or surface waters. It has a low potential for bioconcentration. In the atmosphere, degradation should occur due to direct photolysis, oxidation by ambient oxygen, and photochemically produced hydroxyl radicals (estimated half-life 6–7 h in the vapor phase).

Exposure and Exposure Monitoring

Because 4-aminobiphenyl is found in tobacco smoke, one of the major routes of exposure for the general population is the passive and active inhalation of tobacco smoke. Laboratory personnel working with 4-aminobiphenyl without adequate personal protection may also be exposed occupationally by the dermal and inhalation routes.

Toxicokinetics

4-Aminobiphenyl is converted to its active metabolite, *N*-hydroxy-4-aminobiphenyl, in the liver and the bladder. In the liver, 4-aminobiphenyl is subjected to *N*-hydroxylation and *N*-glucuronidation to produce *N*-glucuronide-4-aminobiphenyl. This metabolite accumulates in the urine of the bladder where, under acidic pH conditions, it is hydrolyzed to its active metabolite. 4-Aminobiphenyl can also be activated directly in the bladder mucosa. The active metabolite is believed to produce cancer through its reaction with cellular DNA. In animal studies, the observed incidence of 4-aminobiphenyl adducts with bladder epithelium DNA correlated well with the observed bladder tumor incidence.

Mechanism of Toxicity

4-Aminobiphenyl is one of a number of chemicals that cause methemoglobinemia, or conversion of hemoglobin to methemoglobin, which reduces the ability of the blood to carry oxygen to the tissues. In addition, the active metabolite (see above) is believed to produce cancer through its reaction with cellular DNA. In animal studies, the observed incidence of 4-aminobiphenyl adducts with bladder epithelium DNA correlated well with the observed bladder tumor incidence.

Acute and Short-Term Toxicity

Acute overexposure is known to produce methemoglobinemia and urinary tract damage. Signs and symptoms of overexposure include headache, lethargy, cyanosis, hematuria (bloody urine), a bluish tint of the skin and mucus membranes as well as a burning sensation in the urinary tract. The oral LD_{50} has been reported to be 500 mg kg^{-1} in rats and 25 mg kg^{-1} in dogs.

Chronic Toxicity

The target organ of toxicity is the bladder. Chronic overexposure is known to produce bladder damage and cancer. Signs and symptoms of bladder damage may include painful urination and the presence of blood and pus in the urine.

There is sufficient epidemiological and animal toxicological data to classify 4-aminobiphenyl as a carcinogen. In humans, occupational exposure has been shown to produce bladder tumors. In animals, chronic administration has produced tumors in the bladder, mammary gland, gastrointestinal tract, and liver of exposed animals.

 http://dx.doi.org/10.1016/B978-0-12-386454-3.00002-6

Reproductive Toxicity

There is no published information on the reproductive toxicity of 4-aminobiphenyl. However, it has been shown to cross the placenta in humans and has been detected in fetal blood. Thus, 4-aminobiphenyl has the potential to cause methemoglobinemia in both the mother and the fetus. Acute and/or chronic methemoglobinemia may compromise the health and survival of the fetus.

Genotoxicity

4-Aminobiphenyl can form chemical addition products (adducts) with DNA and hemoglobin. Formed adducts can lead to cancer development. For example, levels of 4-aminobiphenyl–hemoglobin adducts found in tobacco smokers are reported to be proportional to bladder cancer risk. Reports also show 4-aminobiphenyl can induce unscheduled DNA synthesis and mutations in cultured mammalian cells and microorganisms. 4-Aminobiphenyl is also reported to promote chromosome aberrations and sister chromatid exchanges in laboratory mice.

Carcinogenicity

Epidemiological studies have found 4-aminobiphenyl to be a human carcinogen. The incidence of bladder tumors in workers occupationally exposed to 4-aminobiphenyl was reported to range from 11% to 17% of the exposed population. Because epidemiological studies provide sufficient evidence of the direct relationship between 4-aminobiphenyl exposures and cancer incidence, the International Agency for Research on Cancer has classified 4-aminobiphenyl as a Group 1 carcinogen.

Oral administration of 4-aminobiphenyl to dogs, mice, and rabbits has been shown to produce bladder and liver cancer. Oral administration has also produced mammary tumors in rats.

Clinical Management

4-Aminobiphenyl is not produced commercially and is not a major ingredient in consumer products. Therefore, it is highly unlikely a person would accidentally ingest or be exposed to sufficiently high doses to prompt a medical emergency. Treatment options consist of patient decontamination; collection of blood and urine chemistry; treatment of methemoglobinemia (if present); and life support, as needed. Because the clinical management for overexposure varies depending on the dose absorbed, route of administration, the patient's age and health status, time elapsed since exposure, etc., medical practitioners treating a patient suspected of 4-aminobiphenyl overexposure should consult clinical specialists or other published literature for treatment options.

Ecotoxicology

Currently, no significant risks to the ecosystem should be expected with this compound. It has not been in production for several decades and, as discussed in more detail in the section on environmental fate, 4-aminobiphenyl biodegrades if released into the environment.

Other Hazards

Flammability is low to moderate when exposed to heat, flames (sparks), or powerful oxidizers. 4-Aminobiphenyl autoignites at temperatures of 450 °C. When strongly heated, 4-aminobiphenyl emits toxic fumes.

Exposure Standards and Guidelines

The National Institute for Occupational Safety and Health (NIOSH) considers 4-aminobiphenyl to be a potential occupational carcinogen.

The American Conference of Governmental Industrial Hygienists (ACGIH) has classified 4-aminobiphenyl as a confirmed human carcinogen.

Special precautions must be taken when working with 4-aminobiphenyl. Personnel handling 4-aminobiphenyl must obey and follow industrial hygiene and health protection requirements for handling potentially carcinogenic substances. At a minimum, 4-aminobiphenyl exposures should be limited to the lowest feasible concentration through the use of engineering controls, work practices, and personal protective equipment, including impervious and disposable gowns and gloves as well as eye and respiratory protection. In addition, working area and working instruments must be especially designed for handling potentially harmful substances.

See also: Carcinogenesis; Carcinogen–DNA Adduct Formation and DNA Repair; Toxicity Testing, Carcinogenesis.

Further Reading

Klaassen, C.D., 2008. Casarett & Doull's Toxicology, The Basic Science of Poisons, seventh ed. McGraw-Hill, New York.
National Toxicology Program, 2011. Twelfth Report on Carcinogens: 4-Aminobiphenyl (92-67-1). http://ntp.niehs.nih.gov/ntp/roc/twelfth/profiles/Aminobiphenyl.pdf.
Sax, N.I., Lewis, R.J., 1989. Dangerous Properties of Industrial Materials, seventh ed. Van Nostrand Reinhold, New York.

Relevant Websites

http://www.epa.gov/ttnatw01/hlthef/aminobip.html – US EPA 4-aminobiphenyl.
http://toxnet.nlm.nih.gov/cgi – National Library of Medicine TOXNET - search for aminobiphenyl.

Aminoglycosides

TG Towne, Manchester University College of Pharmacy, Fort Wayne, IN, USA

This article is a revision of the previous edition article by Abraham Dalu, volume 1, pp 93–96, © 2005, Elsevier Inc.

- Representative Compounds: Amikacin; Gentamicin; Kanamycin; Neomycin; Netilmicin; Paromomycin; Streptomycin; Tobramycin
- Chemical Abstracts Service Registry Number: 57-92-1 (streptomycin)
- Synonyms: (For streptomycin – Agrept, Agrimycin, Gerox, NSC-14083, Streptcen)
- Molecular Formula: $C_{21}H_{39}N_7O_{12}$
- Structure: Aminoglycoside antimicrobials have many dissimilar structures; therefore, it is impossible to represent the entire class with a single structure. The structure shown here is streptomycin, the first aminoglycoside antimicrobial:

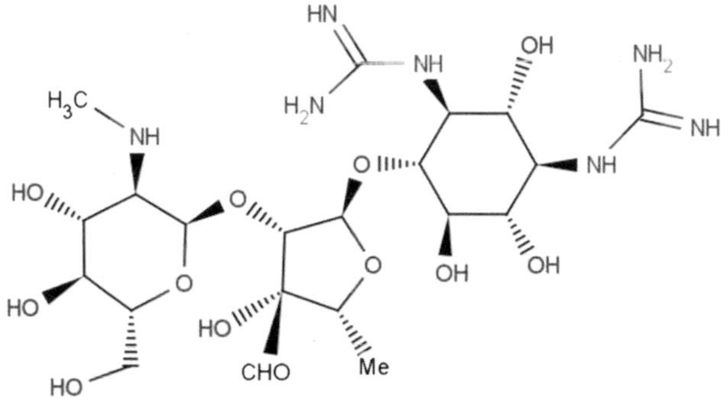

Background (Significance/History)

Aminoglycosides are hydrophilic sugars that possess amino and hydroxyl functionalities. They are polycationic species at physiological pH, meaning they bind to negatively charged molecules such as DNA and RNA. Since their introduction into clinical use and despite the advent of newer agents (carbapenems, monobactams, fluoroquinolones), aminoglycoside antibiotics continue to play an important role in the treatment of severe infections, particularly those due to aerobic, Gram-negative bacilli. Several factors account for their durability and continued clinical usefulness: therapeutic efficacy, synergy with β-lactam antibiotics, low rates of development of true antibiotic resistance, and low drug cost. Their main drawback has been the occurrence of (reversible) nephrotoxicity and ototoxicity in a significant number of patients (5–25%).

The first aminoglycoside, streptomycin was isolated from *Streptomyces griseus* in 1943; neomycin was isolated from *Streptomyces fradiae*. This antibiotic was very effective against tuberculosis. However, one of the main drawbacks to streptomycin is its toxicity, especially to cells in the inner and middle ear and the kidney. Furthermore, some strains of tuberculosis are resistant to treatment with streptomycin. Therefore, medical researchers have put considerable effort into identifying other antibiotics with streptomycin's efficacy, but without its toxicity. Gentamicin, isolated from *Micromonospora* in 1963, was a breakthrough in the treatment of Gram-negative bacillary infections, including those caused by *Pseudomonas aeruginosa*. Other aminoglycosides were subsequently developed, including amikacin (Amikin), netilmicin (Netromycin), and tobramycin (Nebcin), which are all currently available for systemic use in the United States.

Uses

Aminoglycosides are a group of potent antibiotics primarily used to treat certain infections caused by aerobic, Gram-negative bacteria. They are used in the treatment of severe infections of the abdomen, urinary tract, skin and soft tissue, bone, cervix, blood, eye ear, lungs, and heart. In general, gentamicin, tobramycin, and amikacin are used in similar circumstances, often interchangeably. Of these, gentamicin is the aminoglycoside used most often because of its low cost and reliable activity against Gram-negative aerobes. Tobramycin may be the aminoglycoside of choice for use against *P. aeruginosa* because of its greater *in vitro* activity. Amikacin is used against bacteria that are resistant to other aminoglycosides, since its chemical structure makes it less susceptible to inactivating enzymes. Aminoglycosides are also effective against mycobacterial species.

In certain cases, such as with infective endocarditis, aminoglycosides are used synergistically with β-lactam antibiotics to enhance the bactericidal action of the agents against Gram-positive bacteria. In addition, some of the aminoglycosides have been widely used for preparation of the bowel for surgery and as an adjunct to the therapy of advanced stages of hepatic encephalopathy. A more recent utilization of these agents has been aerosolization via nebulizer for direct delivery to lung tissue. This has been shown to be an effective means of antibiotic delivery for patients with cystic fibrosis and those with other difficult to treat Gram-negative bacteria in their lungs.

Aminoglycosides are ineffective against anaerobic bacteria (bacteria that cannot grow in the presence of oxygen), viruses, or fungi. Only one aminoglycoside, paromomycin, is used against parasitic infection.

Environmental Fate and Behavior

Aminoglycosides are water-soluble compounds that are naturally occurring products of bacteria found in the soil. They are highly polar compounds and under acidic conditions may become positively charged by protonation. This positive charge may lead to adsorption to clay and soil materials, which under normal parameters are negatively charged. They are readily degraded in the environment and relatively minor persistence and accumulation.

Exposure and Exposure Monitoring

Exposure to aminoglycosides is primarily encountered via the intravenous or inhaled route for the treatment of infection.

Unlike many other antibiotics, monitoring of drug concentration in the serum is critical for these agents both to improve efficacy and minimize toxicity. Environmental exposure occurs in very low concentrations as a natural product of bacterial species primarily found in the soil.

Toxicokinetics

Aminoglycosides are poorly absorbed from the gastrointestinal or respiratory tract. The extent of absorption varies with a specific agent, ranging from as low as 0.2% to as high as 9%. Protein binding of aminoglycoside is from as low as 0–3% to as high as 11% depending on the agents. The volume of distribution for aminoglycosides ranges from 0.16 to 0.34 l kg^{-1}. Greater than 90% of aminoglycosides are excreted unchanged through the kidney. After parenteral administration, aminoglycosides are primarily distributed within the extracellular fluid. Thus, the presence of disease states or iatrogenic situations that alter fluid balance may necessitate dosage modifications. When used parenterally, adequate drug concentrations are typically found in bone, synovial fluid, and peritoneal fluid. Penetration of biological membranes is poor because of the drug's polar structure. Intracellular concentrations are also usually low, with the exception of the proximal renal tubule. Endotracheal administration results in higher bronchial levels compared with systemic administration, but differences in clinical outcome have not been consistent.

Following parenteral administration of an aminoglycoside, subtherapeutic concentrations are usually found in the cerebrospinal fluid, vitreous fluid, prostate, and brain. Aminoglycosides are rapidly excreted by glomerular filtration, resulting in a plasma half-life of therapeutic doses ranging from 1.5 to 3.2 h in a patient with 'normal' renal function and 30–60 h in patients with impaired kidney function. The half-life of aminoglycosides in the renal cortex is ~100 h, so repetitive dosing may result in renal accumulation and toxicity.

Mechanism of Toxicity

The mechanism of toxicity for aminoglycosides has not been fully explained and is therefore unclear. It is known that the drug attaches to a bacterial cell wall and is drawn into the cell via channels made up of a protein, porin. Once inside the cell, aminoglycoside attaches to the 30S bacterial ribosomes. Ribosomes are the intracellular structures responsible for manufacturing proteins. This attachment either inhibits protein biosynthesis or causes the cell to produce abnormal, ineffective proteins. The bacterial cell cannot survive with this impediment. This explanation, however, does not account for the potent bactericidal properties of these agents, since other antibiotics that inhibit the synthesis of proteins (such as tetracycline) are not bactericidal. Recent experimental studies show that the initial site of action is the outer bacterial membrane. The cationic antibiotic molecules create fissures in the outer cell membrane, resulting in leakage of intracellular contents and enhanced antibiotic uptake. This rapid action at the outer membrane probably accounts for most of the bactericidal activity.

Energy is needed for aminoglycoside uptake into the bacterial cell. Anaerobes have less energy available for this uptake, so aminoglycosides are less active against anaerobic bacteria (bacteria that cannot grow in the presence of oxygen), viruses, and fungi. And only one aminoglycoside, paromomycin, is used against parasitic infection. Like all other antibiotics, aminoglycosides are not effective against influenza, the common cold, or other viral infections.

Acute and Short-Term Toxicity (To Include Irritation and Corrosivity)

Animal

Several investigators have assessed the toxic effects of high doses of aminoglycosides in animals. Studies with dogs, rabbits, rats, and guinea pigs treated with doses ranging from 7.5 to 120 mg kg^{-2} day^{-1} in single or divided doses for 10–29 days suggest that less frequent aminoglycoside administration is associated with less nephrotoxicity as assessed by serum creatinine levels, the glomerular filtration rate, and histopathology. A single study in rats assessing ototoxicity based on cochlear histology reported a lack of toxicity regardless of administration frequency.

Human

Because the body does not metabolize aminoglycosides, aminoglycoside activity is unchanged by induction or inhibition of metabolic enzymes, such as those in the cytochrome p450 system. Certain medications may increase the risk of renal toxicity with aminoglycoside use (e.g., diuretics, radiographic contrast exposure, ACE inhibitors, nonsteroidal anti-inflammatory drugs, other nephrotoxic medications, concomitant use of amphotericin and cisplatin).

All aminoglycosides have a downside: They can cause ototoxicity. In the case of systemic gentamicin, ototoxicity appears to be primarily related to the duration of treatment, the course exceeds 10–14 days. It is also important to realize that gentamicin-induced ototoxicity tends to be primarily vestibular, although cochleotoxicity is seen as well. Overdoses may result in renal damage or ototoxicity (deafness and vertigo), and rarely neuromuscular blockade and hypersensitivity reactions depending on the dose and duration. Nephrotoxicity receives the most attention, perhaps because of easier documentation of reduced renal function, but it is usually reversible. Nephrotoxicity results from renal cortical accumulation resulting in tubular cell degeneration and sloughing. Examination of urine sediment may reveal a dark-brown, fine, or granulated casts consistent with acute tubular necrosis but not specific for aminoglycoside renal toxicity. Although serum creatinine levels are frequently monitored during aminoglycoside use, an elevation in serum creatinine is more likely to reflect glomerular damage rather than tubular damage. In most clinical trials of aminoglycosides, however, nephrotoxicity has been defined by an elevation of serum creatinine. Periodic monitoring of serum creatinine concentrations may alert the clinician to renal toxicity. Retinopathy, visual loss, and conjunctival necrosis have also been associated with this class of antibacterial agent. Irreversible damage of the auditory and vestibular functions of the eighth cranial nerve can occur, but this is thought to be related to dose and duration of treatment.

Chronic Toxicity

Human

Chronic topical application of 1% neomycin to a large wound precipitated severe hearing loss in an adult within 3 weeks of the application. Serious toxicity is a major limitation to the usefulness of the aminoglycosides, and all drugs in this class share the same spectrum of toxicity.

Immunotoxicity

Hypersensitivity reactions have been noted in patients receiving therapy with aminoglycoside antibiotics by a variety of routes (inhaled, intravenous, oral). These reactions have included rash, urticaria, stomatitis, pruritus, generalized burning, fever, eosinophilia, lacrimation, itching and edema of the eyelid, conjunctival erythema anaphylaxis, exfoliative dermatitis, toxic epidermal necrosis, erythema multiforme, and Stevens–Johnson syndrome. Cross-allergenicity has been reported with these agents. In addition, a common additive to intravenous formulations of aminoglycosides, sodium metabisulfite, can cause an allergic-type response. Though not exclusively limited to persons with asthma, they are particularly susceptible to this allergy. If allergic, these patients may experience coughing/wheezing, shortness of breath, bronchoconstriction, rapid swelling of the skin, flushing, tingling sensations, and even shock.

Granulocytopenia has been noted in some patients following the administration of aminoglycosides; however, a causal relationship has not been fully established.

Reproductive Toxicity

Aminoglycosides readily cross the placental barrier, leading to detectable serum levels in a developing fetus. In several case reports, the agent streptomycin has been implicated in total and irreversible bilateral deafness in children born to mothers who received the agent during pregnancy. While other aminoglycosides have not been reported as having these effects, as a class the agents are FDA pregnancy category D, meaning there is evidence for human fetal risk, but potential benefits may warrant the use during pregnancy despite the risks.

Genotoxicity

The mutagenicity of aminoglycoside antibiotics has been evaluated in both *Salmonella typhimurium* and *Saccharomyces cerevisiae*. None of the aminoglycosides demonstrated mitotic crossing-over, point mutations, or mitotic gene conversion. Additionally, tests to induce forward point mutations in Chinese hamster ovary cells at concentrations ranging from 128 to 5000 $\mu g\ ml^{-1}$ did not report any mutagenic activity. All studies performed to assess the genotoxicity of the aminoglycoside, streptomycin, against human lymphocytes have determined there is either no evidence of the toxicity or the results were inconclusive.

Carcinogenicity

None of the aminoglycosides are listed by International Agency for Research on Cancer, National Toxicology Program, or Occupational Safety and Health Administration as known carcinogens.

Clinical Management

Management of toxic doses or an overdose of an aminoglycoside should begin with prompt assessment respiratory and cardiovascular function and support when necessary. This may be critical if the patient experiences neuromuscular blockade leading to respiratory paralysis. For patients who have received an intravenous injection of these agents, managing renal function is also important. Proper hydration with a urine output of 3–5 $ml\ kg^{-1}\ h^{-1}$ should help to reduce the potential for nephrotoxicity in patients with normal hydration status and kidney function. Routine analysis of fluid balance, serum creatine, and serum trough values should be performed. In patients with serum trough levels that are prolonged, hemodialysis may be considered. If patients experience ototoxicity, discontinuation of the aminoglycoside is the only way to reduce the potential for irreversible damage. Risks and benefits must be weighed carefully with this approach. Systemic toxicity with inhaled aminoglycosides is rare; however, large doses, when inhaled, may cause severe bronchospasm in patients. These patients should be managed with inhaled β-2 adrenergic agonists, such as albuterol, and other respiratory supportive care.

Ecotoxicity

As products that are or were originally derived from bacteria found commonly in the soil, their potential for ecotoxicity exists only if major releases of large quantities occurred. Little to no data exist describing this type of toxicity for aminoglycoside antibiotics.

See also: Ciprofloxacin; Kidney; Chloramphenicol; Erythromycin; Metronidazole; The Penicillins; Rifampin; Cephalosporins.

Further Reading

Avent, M.L., Rogers, B.A., Cheng, A.C., Paterson, D.L., 2011. Current use of aminoglycosides: indications, pharmacokinetics and monitoring for toxicity. Intern. Med. J. 41 (6), 441–449.

Gilbert, D.N., Leggett, J.E., 2010. Aminoglycosides. In: Mandell, G.L., Bennett, J.E., Dolin, R. (Eds.), Mandell, Douglas and Bennett's Principles and Practices of Infectious Diseases. Churchill Livingston Elsevier, Philadelphia, pp. 359–384.

Aminopyridine, 4- (4-AP)

RC Gupta, Murray State University, Hopkinsville, KY, USA

This article is a revision of the previous edition article by David Roane, volume 1, pp 96–97, © 2005, Elsevier Inc.

- Name: Aminopyridine, 4- (4-AP)
- Chemical Abstracts Service Registry Number: CAS 504-24-5
- Synonyms: Avitrol; 4-AP; 4-Pyridinamine; 4-Pyridamine; Pyridine-4-amine; Fampridine™
- Chemical/Pharmaceutical/Other Class: Avicides; Aminopyridine pesticides; K^+ channel blocker; Apoptosis inducer
- Molecular Formula: $C_5H_6N_2$
- Chemical Structure:

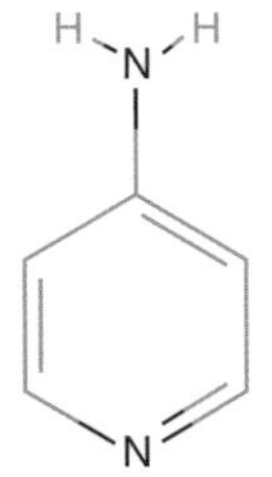

Background

In the 1960s, avicides were developed to kill or repel the birds that destroy crops and grain, ruin the look of beautiful buildings and monuments, and are hazardous to airplane flights. 4-Aminopyridine (4-AP) was developed by the Phillips Petroleum Company and marketed in 1963 as an avicide under the name Avitrol. Avitrol has also been used as a bird repellent. Currently, it is a product of the Avitrol Corporation (Tulsa, Oklahoma, USA). Avitrol is the most popular avicide that is registered at the US Environmental Protection Agency for the control of certain pest birds that feed on cattle feedlots, field corn, wheat, sorghum, sunflowers, peanuts, pecans, grain, feed processing plants, etc. In recent years, the use of Avitrol has been banned in many cities of the United States, including New York, San Francisco, and Boulder, because of its toxicity to nontarget species. Many incidents of Avitrol poisonings have been reported in birds, and domestic, wild, and zoo animals. Secondary poisoning is very common in nontarget birds and dogs. Avitrol has been involved in many suicidal cases. Currently, 4-AP is a compound of significant interest, because it is therapeutically indicated in neurological diseases such as multiple sclerosis. As an experimental compound, 4-AP is used as a K^+ channel blocker, Ca^{2+} activator, and apoptosis inducer (**Figure 1**).

Uses

4-AP is commonly marketed as Avitrol to control the overpopulation of certain birds, including pigeons, red-winged blackbirds, blackbirds, cowbirds, grackles, sparrows, starlings, gulls, and crows. However, its use for controlling birds has been criticized by the Humane Society of the United States. 4-AP has received much attention because of its application as a pharmacological drug in neurological diseases, and as an experimental K^+ channel blocker, Ca^{2+} channel activator, and apoptosis inducer.

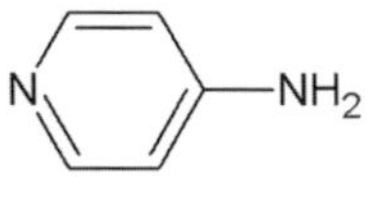

Figure 1 Chemical structure of 4-AP.

Environmental Fate and Behavior

4-AP is adsorbed to soil particles and is moderately persistent in the environment. It has been reported to be slowly metabolized by soil microorganisms. The rate of disappearance varies with the organic content of soils, and the disappearance half-time has been reported to range from 3 to 32 months. Movement from upper soil layers is thought to be minimal due to strong soil adsorption, and the compound is not expected to represent a significant threat to groundwater.

Exposure Routes and Pathways

As an avicide, 4-AP is mixed into grain and set out as bait. It elicits toxicity to all grain-consuming birds. Oral exposure can occur with the misuse of impregnated grain. Any grain-consuming organisms, including livestock, are at risk of accidental ingestion. Human exposure is also possible in industrial and manufacturing settings and in circumstances where individuals (e.g., applicators) may be exposed during avicide use. Upon contact, 4-AP is also absorbed through the skin. In clinical settings, patients are deliberately exposed to 4-AP for its therapeutic effects. Because chronic dietary intake of 4-AP is expected to be negligible, prolonged human exposure is unlikely.

Toxicokinetics

4-AP, like other aminopyridines, is rapidly absorbed from the gastrointestinal tract into circulation. 4-AP can also be absorbed following dermal exposure. The compound is readily metabolized in the liver, and approximately 90% of the administered dose (oral or intravenous) is excreted unchanged in the urine. 4-AP is not known to accumulate in the body.

Mechanism of Toxicity

4-AP produces toxicity through multiple mechanisms. At toxic doses, 4-AP blocks voltage-sensitive K^+ ion channels and increases acetylcholine levels at the synapses and neuromuscular junctions. This results in hyperactivity, convulsions, and seizures. 4-AP also causes excess methemoglobin formation,

 http://dx.doi.org/10.1016/B978-0-12-386454-3.00096-8

and methemoglobin is unable to carry oxygen to the tissues, thereby causing respiratory distress. Death occurs due to cardiac and respiratory arrest. Because 4-AP blocks voltage-sensitive K^+ channels in neurons, it has the capacity to enhance action potential conduction in demyelinated tissue with therapeutically beneficial results. For example, a compound, Fampridine®/Fampyra®, is indicated as a therapeutic agent in the treatment of multiple sclerosis. 4-AP is also being investigated for its ability to improve neuronal signaling in patients with partial spinal cord injuries.

Acute Toxicity

4-AP is toxic to man, animals, birds, fish, and wildlife.

Animals

The oral LD_{50} in rats is ~20 mg kg^{-1}. The LD_{50} for dermal exposure in rabbits is 326 mg kg^{-1}. The commercially available, technical grade 4-AP contained in the avicide product, Avitrol, has a reported oral LD_{50} of 28.7 mg kg^{-1} in rats and 3 mg kg^{-1} in dogs. 4-AP is also an eye irritant.

In mammals, 4-AP produces symptoms similar to those of epileptic seizures. Doses near the LD_{50} exert a usual sequence of symptoms, including hyperexcitability, salivation, tremors, muscle incoordination, and convulsions. Death results from cardiac and respiratory failure. Most of these symptoms are associated with hypercholinergic activity. In general, onset of signs occurs within 10–15 min and death occurs within 15 min to 4 h.

Humans

Reported toxicities are of an acute nature. Signs and symptoms in humans include paresthesia, sweating, dizziness, nausea, ataxia, tremors, dyspnea, tachycardia, weakness, diaphoresis, altered mental status, hypertension, thirst, tonic–clonic convulsions, and seizures. Avitrol produces toxic effects similar to those described for 4-AP. Avitrol also causes metabolic acidosis, leukocytosis, and elevation of serum enzymes (glutamic oxaloacetic transaminase, lactate dehydrogenase, and alkaline phosphatase). Death occurs due to cardiac and respiratory failure. Because 4-AP is a nervous system stimulant, it has been suggested that individuals with a history of convulsive disorders may be at increased risk. Convulsions are reported to be responsive to benzodiazepines. 4-AP has been reported to cause severe poisoning in adult humans at doses less than 60 mg. The dosages used for therapeutic purposes in human trials are 20–30 mg day^{-1} in divided doses over extended periods. In one reported study, six patients were given 24 mg intravenously without experiencing serious side effects.

Chronic Toxicity

Animals

Long-term exposure may affect liver and nervous system functions. Long-term dietary exposures increase brain weights.

Humans

There are several cases of acute toxicity of 4-AP due to accidental or intentional exposure. There are, however, no data available to report long-term effects of low-dose exposure to 4-AP.

Reproductive Toxicity

No adverse reproductive outcomes were noted in a study in quail, but otherwise there are no data available.

Genotoxicity

4-AP was negative in several mutagenicity assays.

Clinical Management

Pancuronium is a pharmacologic antidote and is recommended in severely poisoned human patients. Propranolol appears to block some of the cardiac toxicity of 4-AP. Seizures can be treated with diazepam. In severe cases, phenobarbital or phenytoin can be given if there is no response to diazepam. General symptomatic and supportive treatment is rewarding. Bicarbonate should be added to the fluid therapy to treat acidosis.

Ecotoxicology

Birds

Avitrol produces toxicity in birds in a dose-dependent manner; that is, birds exposed to a low dose exhibit utter distress calls, whereas with higher doses, they become incapacitated and die. Birds exposed to Avitrol usually show an onset of signs within 5–15 min and signs of severe intoxication for a period of 30–60 min. Intoxicated birds rarely recover, and when they do it is observed within 15 h. The oral acute LD_{50} values (expressed as milligram per kilogram body weight) for Avitrol are reported to be 10–12 for chickens, 8 for gulls, 3 for crows, 5.6 for pheasants, 15 for bobwhite quail, 8 for mourning doves, 3.8–4 for sparrows, 5–6 for starlings, 4–7 for pigeons, 9 for blackbirds, and 3.2 for boat-tailed grackle. LC_{50} values of 4-AP for *Coturnix* quails, mourning doves, and mallard ducks are 447, 316, and 722 ppm, respectively.

Fish

4-AP is moderately toxic to fish. The LC_{50} in bluegill is reported to be 3.2–3.4 mg l^{-1}.

Exposure Standards and Guidelines

No observed effect level of 4-AP is reported to be 200 ppm in dogs and 3 ppm in rats. Acceptable daily intake is reported to be 0.0015 mg kg^{-1} day^{-1}.

See also: Pesticides.

Further Reading

Gupta, R.C., 2012. Avitrol. In: Gupta, R.C. (Ed.), Veterinary Toxicology: Basic and Clinical Principles. Academic Press/Elsevier, Amsterdam, pp. 712–715.

Johnson, N.C., Morgan, M.W., 2006. An unusual case of 4-aminopyridine toxicity. J. Emerg. Med. 30, 175–177.

King, A.M., Menke, N.B., Katz, K.D., Pizon, A.F., 2012. 4-Aminopyridine toxicity: a case report and review of the literature. J. Med. Toxicol. 8, 314–321.

Pickett, T.A., Enns, R., 1996. Atypical presentation of 4-aminopyridine overdose. Ann. Emerg. Med. 3, 382–385.

US Environmental Protection Agency, 1980. Pesticide Registration Standard: 4-Aminopyridine: Avitrol. Office of Pesticides and Toxic Substances, Washington, DC.

Wu, Z.Z., Li, D.P., Chen, S.R., Pan, H.L., 2009. Aminopyridines potentiate synaptic and neuromuscular transmission by targeting the voltage-activated calcium channel β subunit. J. Biol. Chem. 284, 36453–36461.

Relevant Websites

http://pmep.cce.cornell.edu – Pesticide Management Education Program.

http://www.avitrol.com – Avitrol - Bringing balance to an unbalanced environment.

Amiodarone

JM Marraffa, Upstate Medical University, Syracuse, NY, USA

This article is a revision of the previous edition article by Elizabeth J. Scharman, volume 1, pp 98–99, © 2005, Elsevier Inc.

- Name: Amiodarone
- Chemical Abstracts Service Registry Numbers: 1951-25-3; 19774-82-4 (hydrochloride)
- Synonyms: Amiodarone hydrochloride; Cordarone®; Nexterone®; (2-(4-[2-Butyl-1-benzofuran-3-yl)carbonyl]-2,6-diiodopheoxy)ethyl)diethylamine
- Chemical/Pharmaceutical/Other Class: Class III antiarrhythmic agent, an iodinated benzofuran derivative antiarrhythmic
- Molecular Formula: $C_{25}H_{29}I_2NO_3$
- Chemical Structure:

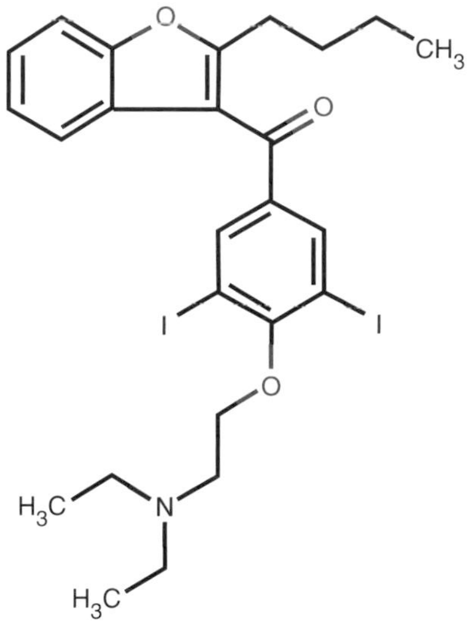

Background

Amiodarone was synthesized by chemists working with the plant extract of Khella (*Ammi visnaga*), which is a common plant in North Africa. Scientists had noted that extracts of this plant called khellin were effective in attenuating angina in individuals taking it for other reasons and attempted to extract an active component from the plant. Amiodarone was ultimately synthesized in 1961 by Belgian chemists working on preparations derived from khellin. Amiodarone gained widespread use in Europe by 1980 and was approved in the United States by the Food and Drug Administration in 1985 for the treatment of arrhythmias.

Uses

Amiodarone has a major place in the management of both acute and chronic ventricular and supraventricular arrhythmias. It is one of the most commonly used and prescribed antiarrhythmic drugs. Amiodarone is indicated in life-threatening, recurrent, ventricular tachycardia or fibrillation when other interventions, such as epinephrine, have failed. It is also used in the management of supraventricular tachyarrhythmias, including atrial fibrillation, atrial flutter, and paroxysmal reentrant supraventricular tachycardia. Amiodarone serves a prominent place in advanced cardiac life support algorithms for numerous unstable rhythms. For unstable rhythms, amiodarone is used in the parenteral (intravenous) form. Oral amiodarone is used for chronic therapy once a patient is stabilized.

Environmental Fate and Behavior

Exposure Routes and Pathways

Accidental and intentional overdoses of amiodarone are not prevalent, and only a few cases are reported in the literature. If overdose does occur, however, ingestion is the most common route of exposure. Amiodarone is available in oral form as well as for parenteral administration, and toxicity can occur by either route.

Physicochemical Properties

Appearance of amiodarone is as a crystalline powder or in solution; it is a clear to pale-yellow micellar solution. Its pH is 3–4 for a 5% aqueous solution.

Its molar mass is 645.311 6 g.

Human Exposure

Amiodarone and its metabolites are distributed into milk in concentrations much higher than maternal plasma concentrations. Data indicate that amiodarone and the major metabolite *N*-desethylamiodarone milk-to-plasma ratios range from 2.3 to 9.1 and from 0.8 to 3.8, respectively.

Toxicokinetics

Following oral administration, amiodarone is slowly and variably absorbed from the gastrointestinal tract. The oral bioavailability varies greatly, with a range of 22–86% (average of 50%). The reason for the variable bioavailability is not known but postulated to be due to metabolism of drug in the gut lumen, first-pass metabolism in the liver, and poor dissolution characteristics of the drug. If amiodarone is ingested with foods, in particular those high in fat content, the rate and extent of absorption are increased.

The peak plasma concentration of amiodarone occurs within 3–7 h (range: 2–12 h) after oral administration. The

 http://dx.doi.org/10.1016/B978-0-12-386454-3.00691-6

onset of action, however, is delayed for 2–3 days and up to 1–3 weeks post drug initiation. Although not clearly established, the maximal antiarrhythmic effect occurs within 1–5 months after initiation of oral therapy. The antiarrhythmic effect generally persists for 10–150 days after withdrawal of therapy.

Amiodarone is extensively metabolized to an active metabolite, *N*-desethylamiodarone. The apparent volume of distribution is 65.8l kg^{-1} (range: 18.3–147.7 l kg^{-1}). After chronic administration, amiodarone and its metabolite are extensively distributed to adipose tissue and many other organs, including the liver, lung, spleen, and skeletal muscle. Amiodarone is extensively bound to plasma proteins, mainly albumin. The drug and its metabolite cross the placenta and are distributed into breast milk.

The metabolism of amiodarone is not fully elucidated but appears to be at least biphasic. After a single i.v. dose of amiodarone, the terminal elimination half-life is on average, 25 days (range: 9–47 days). The elimination half-life of *N*-desethylamiodarone is equal to or longer than the parent drug. The half-life appears to be much more prolonged following multiple doses rather single doses. After chronic oral administration, the drug appears to be eliminated in a biphasic manner with an initial elimination half-life of about 2.5–10 days, which is followed by a terminal elimination half-life averaging 53 days (range: 26–107 days).

The exact metabolism of amiodarone has not been fully described, but the drug appears to be extensively metabolized in the liver by *N*-deethylation to *N*-desethylamiodarone. The excretion of amiodarone and its metabolite is not fully described, though it appears that it is nearly completely excreted in the feces as unchanged drug and *N*-desethylamiodarone presumably via biliary elimination.

Amiodarone and its major metabolite are not amenable to hemodialysis for drug removal.

Mechanism of Action

Amiodarone displays electrophysiologic characteristics of all four classes within the Vaughan-Williams classification scheme. It is a sodium channel blocker with relatively fast on–off kinetics; it has nonselective beta-adrenergic antagonist activity, blocks potassium channels, and has a small degree of calcium channel antagonist activity. Its most prominent activity is potassium channel blockade and, therefore, is classified as a Class III antiarrhythmic agent. It delays repolarization via prolongation of the action potential duration and effective refractory period; decreases AV conduction; depresses sinus node and junctional automaticity; acts as a noncompetitive alpha- and beta-receptor inhibitor; and slows automaticity of Purkinje fibers. Despite its popularity and frequency of use, amiodarone is a complex drug and displays unusual pharmacologic effects and pharmacokinetics. Even more peculiar is the multisystem organ adverse events attributed to amiodarone. The exact mechanisms of these adverse events remain unclear. Fatal complications of amiodarone include acute respiratory distress syndrome (ARDS), pulmonary fibrosis, cirrhosis, and bradycardia leading to cardiac arrest. Amiodarone pulmonary toxicity is probably related to a combination of different mechanisms, including a cytotoxic effect on pneumocytes; an immune mediated mechanism in genetically predisposed patients; and possibly an effect on the angiotensin enzyme system. This results in a disruption of lysosomal membranes by amiodarone and a release of toxic oxygen radicals leading to apoptosis of lung epithelial cells.

Acute and Short-Term Toxicity

Animal

The oral LD_{50} dose of amiodarone hydrochloride is >3000 mg kg^{-1} in rats and dogs. The intravenous LD_{50} dose of amiodarone hydrochloride is 170 mg kg^{-1} in rats and 5000 mg kg^{-1} in dogs.

Human

There is no published/established oral toxic dose of amiodarone. The determination of toxicity is based on observation and clinical effects. Symptoms include nausea; vomiting; bradycardia; hypotension; heart block; QT prolongation with torsade de Pointes being a rare effect; and tremor and ataxia.

Chronic Toxicity (or Exposure)

Animal

Chronic studies in rats demonstrate an increase in carcinogenicity risk for thyroid tumors. The effects are dose related and have been described at doses as low as 5 mg kg^{-1}. Daily doses of 90 mg kg^{-1} in pregnant rats showed reduced fertility. Daily doses in rabbits of 25 mg kg^{-1} showed no change in fertility or effects on the fetus. However, higher daily doses of 75 mg kg^{-1} resulted in an increased rate of spontaneous abortion in these rabbits.

Human

Acute administration of amiodarone is generally well-tolerated by patients; however, chronic administration can result in severe and devastating adverse effects. The exact mechanisms of these adverse effects remain postulated and not clearly elucidated. Severe bradycardia has been reported to occur. Hypo- and hyperthyroid have been reported with an unclear mechanism of toxicity.

Pulmonary toxicity has been reported to occur in up to 5% of treated patients. The development of lung toxicity appears to be associated with older age, duration of treatment, cumulative dose, high levels of the metabolite, history of cardiothoracic surgery, use of iodinated contract media, and probably preexisting lung disease. The devastating pulmonary toxicity may develop as early as the first few days of treatment to several years later. The onset of this toxicity can be either insidious or rapidly progressive. Pulmonary fibrosis has resulted in death.

Other side effects include elevated liver function tests; uncommonly fulminant hepatitis; fatigue; tremor; dizziness; ataxia; corneal micro deposits (which usually do not affect vision); optic neuropathy/neuritis, which can lead to blindness; blue-gray skin discoloration, especially in areas exposed to the sun; and skin necrosis, which rarely has occurred.

Immunotoxicity

Reproductive Toxicity

Amiodarone hydrochloride had reproductive effects in rats when given at a dosage of 90 mg kg^{-1} day^{-1} to male and female rats at 9 weeks prior to mating. In rabbits, at doses of 5, 10, and 25 mg kg^{-1} day^{-1} maternal deaths occurred in all groups. Embryotoxicity occurred at doses of 10 mg kg^{-1} and above. No teratogenicity occurred at any doses. In rats, amiodarone has been found to be teratogenic at doses of 100 mg kg^{-1} day^{-1} given intravenously.

Amiodarone is pregnancy category D. Amiodarone and its major metabolite desethylamiodarone are distributed into maternal plasma, cord plasma, infant plasma, placental tissue, and breast milk. There have been case reports of neonatal hypothyroidism in infants whose mothers were taking amiodarone during pregnancy.

Genotoxicity

Amiodarone HCl has not been shown to be mutagenic in Ames, micronucleus, and lysogenic induction tests.

Carcinogenicity

Thyroid tumors have occurred after oral administration in rats, including follicular adenoma and carcinoma. The incidence of thyroid tumors in rats was higher than the incidence in controls with doses as low as 5 mg kg^{-1} day^{-1}.

Clinical Management

In patients with intentional overdose of amiodarone, treatment is mainly supportive. Amiodarone is adsorbed to activated charcoal and it should be considered in patients with large, intentional ingestions. There is little experience in managing patients with intentional overdoses of amiodarone because this is not commonly reported. In such cases, treatment is largely based on symptoms. Vasopressors should be considered for blood pressure support. Atropine should be considered if symptomatic bradycardia occurs. Hemodialysis to remove amiodarone has little benefit.

Patients with toxicity secondary to therapeutic, chronic use of amiodarone should be managed supportively as well. Patients on chronic amiodarone therapy should be routinely followed and have continued monitoring, including liver function tests, thyroid function tests, eye exams, chest radiographs, and pulmonary function tests. In patients demonstrating adverse effects, a risk versus benefit assessment should be performed to determine whether amiodarone therapy should be continued. In patients that develop pulmonary toxicity, discontinuation of therapy should be strongly considered. In patients with severe pulmonary toxicity and ARDS, discontinuation of therapy is necessary and consideration of corticosteroids should be employed.

Exposure Standards and Guidelines

The exposure limits for amiodarone hydrochloride include an 8 h time-weighted average of 70 μg m^{-3} (Hospira EEL).

See also: Iodine.

Further Reading

Bogazzi, F., Tomisti, L., Bartalena, L., Aghini-Lombardi, F., Martino, E., 2012. Amiodarone and the thyroid: a 2012 update. J. Endocrinol. Invest. 35 (3), 340–348.

Erdogan, H.I., Gul, E.E., Gok, H., Nikus, K.C., 2012. Therapy-resistant ventricular tachycardia caused by amiodarone-induced thyrotoxicosis: a case report of electrical storm. Am. J. Emerg. Med. 30 (9), 2092.e5–2092.e7.

Martin, C.M., 2012. Thyroid dysfunction and the elderly patient: a primer for pharmacists. Consult. Pharm. 27 (10), 682–688.

Papiris, S.A., Triantafillidou, C., Kolilekas, L., Markoulaki, D., Manali, E.D., 2010. Amiodarone: review of pulmonary effects and toxicity. Drug Saf. 33 (7), 539–568.

Van Cott, T.E., Yehle, K.S., Decrane, S.K., Thorlton, J.R., 2013. Amiodarone-induced pulmonary toxicity: case study with syndrome analysis. Heart Lung 42 (4), 262–266.

Relevant Websites

http://www.aafp.org/afp/2003/1201/p2189.html – Amiodarone: Guidelines for Use and Monitoring.

http://heartdisease.about.com/od/drugsforheartdisease/a/amiodarone_lung.htm – Amiodarone Lung Toxicity.

http://heartdisease.about.com/library/weekly/mcurrent.htm – Detailed History of Amiodarone in Particular the Development and FDA Approval in 1985.

http://emedicine.medscape.com/article/129033-overview – Thyroid Dysfunction Induced by Amiodarone Therapy an *eMedicine* (Medscape) Reference Article.

http://www.uptodate.com/contents/amiodarone-pulmonary-toxicity – UpToDate Article on Amiodarone Pulmonary Toxicity.

Amitraz

VC Moser, Toxicity Assessment Division, NHEERL/ORD, US Environmental Protection Agency, Research Triangle Park, NC, USA

This article is a revision of the previous edition article by Jamaluddin Shaikh, volume 2, pp 99–100, © 2005, Elsevier Inc.

The views expressed in this paper are those of the author and do not necessarily reflect the views or policies of the US Environmental Protection Agency.

- IUPAC Name: *N,N′*-[(methylimino)dimethylidyne]di-2,4-xylidine
- Synonyms: BTS 27419, BAAM®, Taktic®, Mitac®, Preventic®, Ovasyn®
- Molecular Formula: $C_{19}H_{23}N_3$
- Chemical Structure:

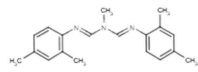

Background

Amitraz has been used as an insecticide and acaricide on crops, livestock, and pets since the mid-1970s. While there are a number of synthesized formamidine chemicals, only a few are marketed as pesticides. These chemicals stimulate the light organ of the firefly, causing it to glow, confirming their actions as octopamine receptor agonists in insects.

Uses

Amitraz is a contact insecticide and acaricide used to control psylla, whiteflies, and mites on cotton and pear crops; and mites, lice, and ticks on livestock, wildlife, and pets. It is applied via spray-dip machines, low-pressure ground sprayers, dip or hand spray, or in impregnated dog collars. The registrant has canceled the use of amitraz on cotton and pear in the United States.

Environmental Fate and Behavior

Amitraz is rapidly degraded (aerobic soil $t_{1/2}$ of about 1 day) to several transformation products, and contamination of ground or surface waters is not a concern. On the other hand, the degradates are moderately persistent in aquatic and terrestrial environments, and are relatively immobile in soil.

Exposure and Exposure Monitoring

Humans may be exposed to amitraz residues in foods or occupationally; however, the highest potential for residential exposures involves its use as a tick dip and in pet collars resulting in dermal or incidental oral ingestion.

Toxicokinetics

Amitraz is rapidly and well-absorbed via oral exposure. After a single dose, onset of effects is rapid (within hours of dosing). A major metabolite, *N′*-(2,4-dimethylphenyl)-*N*-methylformamidine (BTS-27271), has been shown to have the same biological activity of amitraz in mammalian systems. Several subsequent metabolites include hydrolysis and conjugated products that are excreted primarily in urine, and to lesser extent in feces. Metabolism is similar across species, including humans.

Kinetic studies of single, low doses indicate that amitraz is eliminated within hours after a single dose, but behavioral and pharmacological studies suggest dose dependency. Following a low dose (5 mg kg^{-1}), greater than half of a dose is gone within 24 h, whereas higher doses (50–75 mg kg^{-1}) require several days. Similarly, behavioral studies show that effects of lower doses are reversible within hours to days, whereas higher doses produced effects that were still evident after 8 days.

Mechanisms of Toxicity

Formamidines produce behavioral changes in target pests, including altered feeding and mating behaviors, representing a novel mode of pesticidal and pestistatic actions. Similarity between the target insect octopamine receptors and mammalian α_2-adrenoreceptors gives support for the mechanism of toxicity produced by amitraz, which is mediated through the noradrenergic nervous system. Specifically, amitraz-induced bradycardia, mydriasis, sedation, intestinal stasis, hyperglycemia, and even lethality were blocked using pharmacological antagonists of the α_2-adrenoreceptors (e.g., yohimbine, piperoxan, atipamezole), but not by blockers of the α_1-adrenoreceptors, or of other neurotransmitter receptors. This relative selectivity has been confirmed both *in vivo* and *in vitro* using receptor binding assays. Monoamine oxidase inhibition, a known action of other formamidine chemicals, was only measured at highly toxic doses of amitraz. In addition to these neurological actions, amitraz and other formamidines are anti-inflammatory and antipyretic by means of blocking prostaglandin E2 synthesis.

Acute and Short-Term Toxicity

Animal

Amitraz is moderately toxic by dermal exposure and slightly toxic by oral exposure or inhalation. It is nonirritating and does not cause skin sensitization. Dogs and baboons are the most sensitive with oral LD_{50} values around 100–250 mg kg^{-1},

 http://dx.doi.org/10.1016/B978-0-12-386454-3.00097-X

rats are somewhat less sensitive with LD_{50} values around 500–800 mg kg^{-1}, and mice are least sensitive with LD_{50} values >1600 mg kg^{-1}.

Acute neurotoxic signs include hypothermia, periods of excitability and aggression, ataxia, and decreased spontaneous activity. High doses produce tremors, convulsions, and signs of hypothalamic depression. Other pharmacological actions include slowed gastrointestinal transit, which can exacerbate colic in horses. In addition to laboratory animal studies, there are a number of reports on adverse effects following amitraz use in dogs and horses, which appear to be very sensitive.

Human

Studies in human volunteers reported nervous system effects, including excitation followed by sedation, disorientation, hypothermia, and decreased heart rate and blood pressure: these signs mirror those observed in laboratory animal studies. Humans appear to be the most sensitive species.

Chronic Toxicity

Animal

Neurotoxic effects (central nervous system (CNS) depression, hyperexcitable and aggressive behaviors, and hypothermia) were evident in subchronic and chronic studies in rodents and nonrodents; indeed, these signs are similar across species, sexes, and routes of administration. The effects at low doses do not appear to accumulate with repeated exposure, but repeated higher doses intensify the hyperreactivity syndrome. Higher doses in several species also produce decreased weight gain, hyperglycemia, and liver and kidney toxicity. Dosing for just a few days induced hepatic microsomal enzyme levels and activities. Altered hormone levels (e.g., 17β-estradiol, testosterone) may result from altered metabolism; decreased hormone release and weak antiestrogenic activity have also been reported *in vitro*.

Human

Little is known regarding the chronic effects of amitraz in humans.

Immunotoxicity

Dosing for 1 month increased adrenal weight, decreased splenic plaque-forming cells, and attenuated delayed-type hypersensitization reaction in rats.

Reproductive Toxicity

In rat and rabbit developmental studies, embryotoxicity (increased fetal death, decreased size), and teratogenicity (fetal visceral and skeletal abnormalities) were observed at doses lower than or equal to those producing maternal toxicity (clinical signs, decreased weight gain). A rat multigenerational study showed reduced litter size and pup survival in all three generations. Special reproductive studies indicated prolonged estrus cycling in rats but not in mice, although changes in hormone levels and relative lengths of proestrus to diestrus were noted in the latter species. Decreased male fertility, increased resorptions, and changes in reproductive organ weights were indicative of adverse effects on fertility and reproductive systems in mice.

Prenatal exposure of rats resulted in altered ages of physical developmental landmarks (vaginal opening, fur development, incisor eruption, righting reflex) and changes in open-field behavior in the offspring for up to 1 month of age. Pre- and postnatal exposures also resulted in long-term changes in noradrenergic, serotonin, and dopamine neurochemistry.

Genotoxicity

The results of several studies indicate that amitraz is not mutagenic and does not cause DNA damage.

Carcinogenicity

Mouse studies have reported lymphoreticular, lung, or liver tumors at the highest dose tested, which produced considerable toxicity, in females only. No findings of carcinogenicity have been reported in rats. The data are generally noncompelling, and the US Environmental Protection Agency (US EPA) has classified it as 'suggestive evidence of carcinogenicity.'

Clinical Management

With dermal exposure, areas exposed to amitraz should be washed with soap and water. Eyes should be washed with copious amounts of clean water. Symptoms include skin rashes, eye and oral irritation, coughing, nausea, headache, sore throat, and sweating. These minor effects are rapidly reversible. Accidental ingestion of sufficient amounts leads to depressed respiration, hypotension, bradycardia, miosis, gastric stasis, hyperglycemia, and coma. These signs and symptoms are somewhat similar to cholinesterase inhibitor poisoning and have sometimes been misdiagnosed as such. Gastric lavage or activated charcoal is indicated immediately. Symptomatic treatments and supportive care (intubation and assisted ventilation) are usually effective. Although α_2-antagonists (e.g., yohimbine) have been shown to block amitraz effects in animal studies, this treatment has not been explored in clinical cases.

Ecotoxicity

The parent amitraz is only slightly toxic to several avian species (8-day LD_{50} values >1000 ppm in diet), but causes reproductive toxicity (eggshell cracking, decreased viability of embryos and chicks). On the other hand, amitraz is highly toxic to fish (96-h LC_{50} values 1–10 ppm) and aquatic invertebrates. The degradates of amitraz, which are more environmentally stable, tend to have the reverse toxicity pattern. Amitraz is practically nontoxic to bees.

Exposure Standards and Guidelines

The US EPA dietary reference dose (RfD) for amitraz is $0.0125 \text{ mg kg}^{-1} \text{ day}^{-1}$, based on an acute no-effect level (NOEL) of 0.125 mg kg^{-1} in a human neurotoxicity study; with the inclusion of an additional factor to assure safety to infants and children, the US EPA population adjusted dose becomes $0.00125 \text{ mg kg}^{-1} \text{ day}^{-1}$. Due to the reversibility of acute doses, the US EPA determined that this endpoint is appropriate for exposures of all durations. The Joint FAO/WHO Meeting on Pesticide Residues established an acute RfD value of 0.01 mg kg^{-1}, based on the same human study, as well as an acceptable daily intake (ADI) value of $0.01 \text{ mg kg}^{-1} \text{ day}^{-1}$, based on the NOEL of $1.3 \text{ mg kg}^{-1} \text{ day}^{-1}$ for developmental effects in rats.

See also: Behavioral Toxicology; Developmental Toxicology; Neurotoxicity; Pesticides.

Further Reading

Avsarogullari, L., Ikizceli, I., Sungur, M., Sözüer, E., Akdur, O., Yücei, M., 2006. Acute amitraz poisoning in adults: Clinical features, laboratory findings, and management. Clin. Toxicol. (Philadelphia) 44, 19–23.

Costa, L.G., Olibet, G., Murphy, S.D., 1988. Alpha 2-adrenoceptors as a target for formamidine pesticides: *In vitro* and *in vivo* studies in mice. Toxicol. Appl. Pharmacol. 93, 319–328.

Costa, L.G., Olibet, G., Wu, D., Murphy, S.D., 1989. Acute and chronic effects of the pesticide amitraz on α_2-adrenoceptors in the mouse brain. Toxicol. Lett. 47, 135–143.

Evans, P.D., Gee, J.D., 1980. Action of formamidine pesticides on octopamine receptors. Nature 287, 60–62.

Hollingworth, R.M., 1976. Chemistry, biological activity, and uses of formamidine pesticides. Environ. Health Perspect. 14, 57–69.

Hollingworth, R.M., Murdock, L.L., 1980. Formamidine pesticides: Octopamine-like actions in a firefly. Science 208, 74–76.

Institoris, L., Banfi, H., Lengyel, Z., Papp, A., Nagymajtenyi, L., 2007. A study on immunotoxicological effects of subacute amitraz exposure in rats. Hum. Exp. Toxicol. 26, 441–445.

Kim, J.C., Shin, J.Y., Yang, Y.S., Shin, D.H., Moon, C.J., Kim, S.H., Park, S.C., Kim, Y.B., Kim, H.C., Chung, M.K., 2007. Evaluation of developmental toxicity of amitraz in Sprague-Dawley rats. Arch. Environ. Contam. Toxicol. 52, 137–144.

Knowles, C.O., Benezet, H.J., 1981. Excretion balance, metabolic fate and tissue residues following treatment of rats with amitraz and *N′*-(2,4-dimethylphenyl)-*N*-methylformamidine. J. Environ. Sci. Health, Part B. Pesticides, Food Contam. Agric. Wastes B16, 547–555.

Moser, V.C., 1991. Investigations of amitraz neurotoxicity in rats: IV. Assessment of toxicity syndrome using a functional observational battery. Fundam. Appl. Toxicol. 17, 7–16.

Palermo-Neto, J., Sákaté, M., Flório, J.C., 1997. Developmental and behavioral effects of postnatal amitraz exposure in rats. Braz. J. Med. Biol. Res. 30, 989–997.

Smith, B.E., Hsu, W.H., Yang, P.C., 1990. Amitraz-induced glucose intolerance in rats: Antagonism by yohimbine but not by prazosin. Arch. Toxicol. 64, 680–683.

Relevant Websites

http://www.epa.gov/pesticides/reregistration/amitraz/ – background and recent regulatory actions in US.

http://www.inchem.org/documents/jmpr/jmpmono/v098pr02.htm – information from the International Programme on Chemical Safety.

http://www.cdpr.ca.gov/docs/risk/rcd/amitraz.pdf – risk characterization document from California Environmental Protection Agency.

Amitrole

R Sellamuthu, Indiana University, Indianapolis, IN, USA

- Name: Amitrole
- Chemical Abstracts Service Registry Number*: 61-82-5
- Synonyms*: 1H-1,2,4-Triazol-3-amine; 1H-1,2,4-Triazol-3-ylamine; 2-Amino-1,3,4-triazole; 2-Aminotriazole; 3-AT
- Molecular Formula*: $C_2H_4N_4$
- Chemical Structure*:

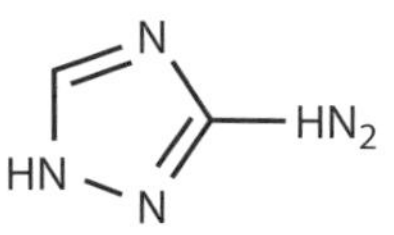

*All from ChemIDplus.

Background

Amitrole is not a naturally occurring chemical. It is a white to yellowish crystalline powder first synthesized in 1898 by allowing aminoguanidine to react with formic acid. It was manufactured for commercial use in the United States in the late 1940s. Amitrole was introduced as an herbicide in the United States in 1948 and was restricted to postharvest applications in food crops. However, misuse of amitrole and detection of residues were reported in cranberry crops in the late1950s. This incident is also known as the Cranberry Crisis of 1959. These incidents led to enforcement of the Delaney Clause law, which prohibited the addition of any potentially carcinogenic chemicals to food. In 1996, new regulations implemented in the Food Quality Protection Act changed how pesticides in foods were regulated; however, meanwhile, the US Environmental Protection Agency canceled the registration of amitrole use on food crops and restricted use to nonfood crops.

Uses

Amitrole is a triazole compound used as nonselective herbicide. It has broad spectrum of activity and is primarily used on outdoor areas, specifically nonagricultural areas, on orchids and roadsides to control annual grasses, deep-rooting weeds (annual and perennial broad leaf), grasses, aquatic weeds in drainages and marsh land, and poison ivy. It is combined with other herbicides and applied as a total herbicide in postharvest applications and before annual sowing of certain crops. In addition, amitrole is used on soils of non-crop land and interrow weed control in vineyards, excluding animal grazing land and water sources. Amitrole is also reported to be used as a reagent in photography and a plant growth regulator. Commercial amitrole is available in various forms. Water-soluble granules containing 86% amitrole are most commonly used throughout the world.

Environmental Fate and Behavior

Amitrole is a nonvolatile, crystalline powder, readily soluble in water (280 g l^{-1} at 25 °C), and is also soluble in polar solvents such as ethanol, methanol, and chloroform. Amitrole is stable in water. Amitrole levels have been estimated in various environmental compartments. However, water and soil are the only compartments that contribute to the environmental fate of amitrole. Amitrole does not enter into the atmosphere because of its low vapor pressure. Excessive application of amitrole above the recommended level on soil leads to contamination of soil and leaching, depending on the soil type. The leached-out amitrole contaminates the surface as well as groundwater. Leaching behavior is affected by the presence of dissolved organic matter despite the high water solubility.

Amitrole is persistent in pond water and moist soil. Most of the amitrole present in soil is readily degraded by microbes (mineralization) under aerobic conditions, which is the major degradation pathway. Other routes such as abiotic mechanisms contribute less to the degradation process. Laboratory studies indicated that amitrole is moderately persistent with an aerobic half-life of 26 days in soil and 57 days in water. However, amitrole is more persistent in water under anaerobic conditions with more than a 1 year half-life. Studies also demonstrated that photodegradation of amitrole is slow in soil but stable in water. There will be no bioaccumulation or biomagnification of amitrole expected because of high water solubility, a very low log K_{ow}, and nonpersistence in animals.

Exposure and Exposure Monitoring

When used according to recommended guidelines, amitrole is not released into the environment from manufacturing units. Processing mechanisms such as dry crushing and bagging in manufacturing plants release appreciable quantities of amitrole into the surroundings, with the concentrations as high as 100 μg m^{-3} causing risk of potential exposure to workers by inhalation exposure. In addition, inhalation exposure is likely to occur in living areas due to herbicide spraying in the vicinity. There is no known dietary exposure reported due to the restricted use on nonfood crops.

The potential exposure to amitrole is minimal in humans because of restricted use on nonfood crops. However, workers especially in manufacturing units (mixers and loaders) and workers applying the herbicide in the agricultural fields have been exposed to amitrole. The potential routes of occupational exposure to amitrole occur through inhalation, accidental ingestion, and dermal and eye contact. Human exposure data were limited; only a few occupational exposure surveys from the United States, Sweden, and Finland reported that workers were exposed to amitrole during handling processes. Thyroid

 http://dx.doi.org/10.1016/B978-0-12-386454-3.01163-5

function tests are employed routinely to monitor the workers for exposure to amitrole.

Toxicokinetics

In general, amitrole is rapidly and almost completely absorbed from gastrointestinal tracts and lungs, and excreted in urine without any change within 24 h. Metabolic transformation in mammals is minimal. One study reported the ingestion of amitrole (20 mg kg^{-1}) by a woman followed by complete excretion of unchanged compound in urine (1 g l^{-1}). Amitrole level in blood was elevated (13 mg l^{-1}) 12 h after ingestion of a herbicide containing a mixture of amitrole and ammonium thiocyanate, and finally resulted in death of the victim.

Amitrole is readily absorbed from the gastrointestinal tract immediately after ingestion in mice, rats, and dogs. Amitrole was absorbed by the dermal route as high as 30%. All absorbed compounds were accumulated in liver of mice and rats. Distribution studies in mice demonstrated that administered amitrole (given by gavage and intravenous route) is distributed in bone marrow, spleen, thymus, and liver. Amitrole is metabolized in the liver, and 50% is metabolized within 3 h in a dose-dependent manner. In rodents, the unchanged form of amitrole is eliminated in urine, and blood levels are drastically reduced within 24 h. Metabolic studies in rats detected three metabolites in urine. Concentrations of eliminated metabolites were higher after 24 h post-dosing with low levels of amitrole.

Mechanism of Toxicity

The thyroid gland is the main target organ in rats, mice, and dogs. Amitrole inhibits thyroid peroxidase enzyme, which is involved in thyroxine hormone (T_4) synthesis. *In vitro* studies demonstrated that thyroid peroxidase and prostaglandin-H-synthase produced the reactive metabolites from amitrole, which irreversibly bind with and inactivate thyroid peroxidases. As a result, T_4 formation is reduced in blood. Reduced level of T_4 acts on the pituitary gland via negative feedback mechanism and increases thyrotropin (TSH) secretion from the pituitary gland. TSH stimulates the thyroid gland, and absence of negative feedback inhibition of TSH by T_4 contributes to the thyroid gland growth. This mechanism is responsible for thyroid tumors, specifically follicular cell adenoma and carcinoma, in rats exposed to amitrole.

Acute and Short-Term Toxicity

Amitrole is classified as slightly toxic based on laboratory animal studies. Amitrole caused a mixed response from symptoms of no poisoning to death after ingestion by humans, depending on the dose and chemical present in the herbicide mixture. However, dry, nonproductive cough and development of diffuse, severe alveolar damage in lungs (following exposure to 19% amitrole), and inhibition of iodide uptake in thyroid gland (following exposure to 10–100 mg) were reported after acute short-term exposure. Associated symptoms of acute toxicity in humans include skin rash, vomiting, diarrhea, and nosebleeds. Amitrole is a nonirritant if exposure is less than 8 h and slightly irritating after 24 h exposure among volunteers. Some workers have developed mild dermatitis.

Table 1 LD_{50}/LC_{50} values of amitrole and its relative toxicity in laboratory animals

Species	*Dose LD_{50}/LC_{50}*	*Relative toxicity*
Rat	LD_{50} oral: >4000–25 000 mg kg^{-1}	Slightly toxic
Rat	4 h Inhalation LC_{50} oral: >439 mg m^{-3}	Slightly toxic
Rat	LD_{50} dermal: 2500 mg kg^{-1}	Slightly toxic
Mice	LD_{50} oral: 11 000–14 700 mg kg^{-1}	Slightly toxic
Rabbit	LD_{50} dermal: >10 000 mg kg^{-1}	Slightly toxic

The LD_{50}/LC_{50} values of amitrole and relative toxicities for laboratory animals are listed in **Table 1**.

Signs of acute toxicity induced by high doses of amitrole were depression, dyspnea, diarrhea, ataxia, convulsions, coma, and death. Amitrole poisoning in most of the species caused symptoms of diarrhea, edema of lung, and hemorrhages of various organs. Studies of amitrole in rabbits led to the designation of slightly toxic and practically nontoxic for eye irritation and dermal toxicity, respectively. Dermal application of amitrole in rabbits and rats produced mild erythema. Eye irritation was reported in rabbit (conjunctival sac route) but not in rats (inhalation exposure).

Chronic Toxicity

Long-term exposure studies indicated that amitrole is nonhazardous to workers who have adequate protection in the workplace. Chronic exposure to amitrole induced goiter and tumors of thyroid, pituitary, and liver in humans. There have been no reported signs of amitrole toxicity in humans, but symptoms reported in laboratory animal studies include dyspnea, muscle spasm, ataxia, anorexia, salivation, skin dryness, and reduction in thyroid functions.

Dogs fed with high concentrations (13 and 32 mg kg^{-1} body weight per day) for more than a year developed hypertrophy of pituitary gland, enlarged thyroid gland, follicular hyperplasia, reduced T_3 and T_4 levels, and mild anemia. Continuous feeding of 100 mg kg^{-1} amitrole produced goiter in both sexes of rats (within 3 months) and in mice (18 months) but not in golden hamsters. In general, amitrole did not induce toxicity in hamsters and rabbits. These results demonstrated the difference in sensitivity to amitrole. In addition, tumors developed in rats and mice, which are discussed below.

Immunotoxicity

A single case report described allergic contact dermatitis in a human after exposure to amitrole for 6 months and positive patch test. Dermal application of amitrole in guinea pigs produced a sensitizing effect.

Reproductive Toxicity

Amitrole is classified as Pregnancy Category C chemical. Reproductive and developmental effects of amitrole in humans are not available. Low levels of dietary amitrole (1.25 mg or 5 mg kg^{-1} day^{-1}) given to rats did not induce adverse effects in reproduction. Feeding of high doses of amitrole (36 or 75 mg kg^{-1} day^{-1}) to rats caused delayed growth and hyperplasia of thyroid gland in parents as well as pups; atrophy of spleen and thymus in pups; and increased mortality of pups after weaning without affecting fertility of parents. Teratogenic effect also was reported in pups of rats exposed to high doses of amitrole during pregnancy.

Genotoxicity

Human data on genotoxic effects are lacking. Most of the *in vitro* genotoxicity studies of amitrole were negative. Amitrole does not cause chromosomal aberrations in Chinese hamster lung cells or human lymphocytes. Induction of sister chromatid exchange in Chinese hamster cells was observed without a dose–response relationship. Similarly, there are no positive test reports for genotoxic effects of amitrole from *in vivo* studies.

Carcinogenicity

One cohort study reported that Swedish railroad workers who were exposed to amitrole and other herbicide for 45 days developed cancer later in their life. However, workers exposed to amitrole alone did not get cancer, which led to the conclusion that amitrole did not induce cancer in that other study involving humans with concurrent exposure to other agents. Several studies demonstrated the carcinogenic potential of amitrole in rodents and classified it as a probable human carcinogen, Group B2. As discussed in mechanisms of toxicity section, amitrole inhibits thyroxine synthesis by non-genotoxic mechanism and stimulates TSH secretion continuously to cause hyperplasia of follicular epithelial and induce follicular cell adenoma and follicular cell carcinoma in rats. These tumors were reported in chronic exposure to amitrole (>2.5 mg kg^{-1} day^{-1}) by inhalation and dermal routes. Amitrole also induced liver tumors and pituitary tumors in mice, and pituitary tumors in rats, by non-genotoxic mechanisms.

Clinical Management

General emergency managements for dermal, inhalation, and oral exposure are recommended by the US National Institute for Occupational Safety and Health (NIOSH).

Table 2 LD_{50}/LC_{50} values of amitrole and its relative toxicity in other species

Species	*Dose LD_{50}/LC_{50}*	*Relative toxicity*
Mallard duck	LD_{50} 2000 mg kg^{-1}	Slightly toxic
Quail	LD_{50} >2150 mg kg^{-1}	Practically nontoxic
Honeybee	LD_{50} >10 μg bee	Practically nontoxic
Trout (96 h)	LC_{50} Oral: >1000 mg l^{-1}	Practically nontoxic
Soil microflora	At 10x normal application rate	No adverse effect

Ecotoxicology

Amitrole present in water sources can be toxic to birds, fishes, and other aquatic species. LD_{50} values of amitrole for some nonmammalian species are listed in **Table 2**.

Exposure Standards and Guidelines

Several countries have established occupational exposure limits, time weighted average (TWA) 0.2 mg m^{-3}, and other guidelines for amitrole. The following agencies in the USA set exposure limits for amitrole in occupational settings.

1. Occupational Safety and Health Administration (OSHA) permissible exposure limit 8 h TWA: 0.2 mg m^{-3}
2. NIOSH recommended exposure limit 8 h TWA: 0.2 mg m^{-3}
3. American Conference of Governmental and Industrial Hygienists (ACGIH) assigned threshold limit value: 0.2 mg m^{-3} as a TWA for a normal 8 h workday and a 40 h work week

OSHA and NIOSH limits are based on the risk of cancer associated with exposure to amitrole, and the ACGIH limits are based on the risk of systemic and reproductive effects associated with exposure to amitrole.

See also: Atrazine; Common Mechanism of Toxicity in Pesticides; Triazines.

Further Reading

IARC, 2001. Amitrole. In: Some Thyrotropic Agents. IARC Monographs on the Evaluation of Carcinogenic Risk of Chemicals to Humans, vol. 79. International Agency for Research on Cancer, Lyon, France, pp. 381–410.

Amitroptyline *see* Tricyclic Antidepressants

Ammonia

RJ Parod, BASF Corporation, Wyandotte, MI, USA

- Chemical Abstracts Service Registry Number: 7664-41-7
- Synonyms: Anhydrous ammonia; Liquid ammonia; Spirit of hartshorn
- Molecular Formula: N–H_3
- Chemical Structure: NH_3

Background

Ammonia is a naturally occurring compound which is a key component of the global nitrogen cycle and all living organisms. It is generated in nature primarily by the decay of plant and animal matter and is used as an essential nutrient by all mammals to synthesize nucleic acids and proteins and to maintain acid–base balance. Nitrogen fixation by current industrial processes approximates that produced naturally by biological processes and lightening strikes.

Uses

Commercial production of ammonia is primarily via a modified Haber–Bosch process in which atmospheric nitrogen is combined with hydrogen obtained from natural gas under high temperature and pressure conditions, a process termed nitrogen fixation. About 80% of the commercially produced ammonia is used in fertilizers with the remainder used in a variety of applications such as plastics, synthetic fibers and resins, pharmaceuticals, explosives, refrigeration, and household cleaners.

Environmental Fate and Behavior

With a vapor pressure of 8611 hPa at 20 °C, ammonia is a gas under normal environmental conditions. In the atmosphere, ammonia is estimated to have a half-life of several days. The primary fate process is the reaction of ammonia with acid air pollutants and removal of the resulting ammonium (NH_4^+) compounds by dry or wet deposition. Rain washout and reaction with photochemically produced hydroxyl radicals also contribute to the atmospheric fate of vapor–phase ammonia. In water, ammonia acting as a weak base ($pK_a = 9.25$) will exist in equilibrium with the ammonium ion. Ammonia will volatilize to the atmosphere due to its high vapor pressure in water (2878 hPa at 25 °C) while the ammonium ion will be removed via uptake by aquatic plants, adsorption to sediments, and microbial transformation to nitrites (NO_2^-) and nitrates (NO_3^-). In soil, the same general processes will occur. As a result, ammonia does not readily leach through soil. However, nitrate can leach through soil due to its high water solubility and if present at a high enough concentration may cause methemoglobinemia in infants. Due to the multiple physical and biological transformation processes that exist in nature, ammonia is not expected to accumulate in the environment or living organisms.

Exposure and Exposure Monitoring

Ammonia is a gas under normal environmental conditions; thus, human exposures typically occur via inhalation. Dermal and oral exposures are also possible as ammonia has high water solubility. Background concentrations of ammonia in air (1 ppb), water (30 ppb), and soil (3 ppm) are low but can increase by orders of magnitude in areas of fertilizer production and application, sewage treatment, and livestock confinement.

Toxicokinetics

Unionized ammonia freely diffuses through tissue cells and forms ammonium hydroxide (NH_4OH) upon contact with tissue water; in the blood, ammonium ion (99%) and ammonia (1%) exist in a dynamic equilibrium as predicted by pH partitioning for a weak base ($pK_a = 9.25$). During short-term ($\leq$2 min) human exposures to $\leq$500 ppm ammonia, most ($\geq$83%) of the inspired ammonia is retained within the upper airways. This absorption process may be adaptive or saturable because most of the ammonia inspired during longer exposures (10–27 min) is exhaled with only 4–30% being retained within the upper airways and available for systemic absorption. This scrubbing of the inspired air by the upper respiratory tract protects the deeper lung from damage by ammonia. Ammonia or ammonium ion is well-absorbed by the gastrointestinal tract, and almost 100% of the ammonia produced endogenously in the human digestive tract (60 mg kg^{-1} day^{-1}) is absorbed and metabolized in the liver to urea and glutamine. The brain can also convert ammonia to glutamine. Due to first-pass metabolism in the liver, little ammonia from the gut reaches the systemic circulation, and toxicologically significant amounts of ammonia in blood (>1 μg ml^{-1}) probably occur only in severe disease states where the metabolism of ammonia by the liver and the excretion of metabolites by the kidney are compromised. It is unlikely that a significant amount of the ammonia contacting the skin is absorbed. Ammonia that reaches the circulation is

 http://dx.doi.org/10.1016/B978-0-12-386454-3.00468-1

distributed throughout the body where it can be used in protein synthesis or as a buffer. Most of the absorbed ammonia is excreted in the urine as urea, with minimal amounts excreted in the feces or expired air.

Mechanism of Toxicity

The primary immediate effect of ammonia exposure is burns to the skin, eyes, and respiratory tract. Ammonia dissolves in tissue water and forms ammonium hydroxide that breaks down cellular proteins, saponifies cell membrane lipids resulting in cell disruption and death, and initiates an inflammatory response that further damages surrounding tissues. Under pathological conditions (e.g., cirrhosis) that impair the metabolic capability of the liver, ammonia can enter the brain, overwhelm the limited capacity of astrocytes to metabolize ammonia, and result in a potentially fatal disorder called hepatic encephalopathy.

Acute and Short-Term Toxicity

Animal

The 1 h inhalation lethal concentration 50 percent (LC_{50}) values in mice and rats receiving whole-body exposures were ~4200 and 14 000 ppm, respectively. The rat oral lethal dose 50 percent (LD_{50}) of aqueous ammonia is 350 mg kg^{-1}, while that to ammonium salts is ≥2000 mg kg^{-1}. A 20% solution of aqueous ammonia was corrosive to rabbit skin, while a 10% solution was not.

Human

Ammonia has an odor threshold ranging from 1 to 5 ppm. Acute changes in respiratory function are not seen in workers exposed to 9 ppm ammonia for 8 h. Exposures between 20 and 25 ppm can cause complaints and discomfort in some workers unaccustomed to ammonia exposure but have little effect on pulmonary function or odor sensitivity. Concentrations of 100 ppm caused definite irritation of the respiratory tract and eyes, and exposures at 250 ppm ammonia are bearable for 30–60 min. Severe irritation of the respiratory tract, skin, and eyes has been observed following ammonia exposures ranging from 400 to 700 ppm. Exposure to 2500–4500 ppm ammonia can be fatal within 30 min. Immediate fatalities appear to be the result of airway obstruction, particularly laryngeal edema, and glottic spasm, while infections and other secondary complications appear to be the cause of fatality among those who survive for several days to weeks.

Chronic Toxicity

Animal

Ammonia is considered as an irritant gas that generally causes severe local effects in the absence of systemic toxicity. While there are no guideline studies on ammonia, some information can be obtained from non-guideline studies on surrogate ammonium salts since once absorbed the ammonium ion and ammonia exist in equilibrium. When male and female rats were exposed to ammonium sulfate in the diet (≤1975 mg kg^{-1} day^{-1}) for 13 weeks, neither body weight, food consumption, or hematological and clinical parameters were affected. Although kidney and liver weight changes were noted, these effects occurred only at the highest dose and in the absence of histopathological changes. Diarrhea was seen in males at the highest dose while females were unaffected. The no observable adverse effect levels (NOAELs) were 866 mg kg^{-1} day^{-1} (m) and 1975 mg kg^{-1} day^{-1} (f). In a combined repeated-dose/reproduction/developmental study similar to an Organization for Economic Cooperation and Development (OECD) 422 protocol, rats were exposed by gavage to ammonium phosphate at doses up to 1500 mg kg^{-1} day^{-1}. At the two highest doses, alkaline phosphatase was increased and total blood protein was decreased resulting in a NOAEL of 250 mg kg^{-1} day^{-1}.

Human

No health effects were observed in volunteers exposed to ammonia (25–100 ppm) for 6 h day^{-1} over a period of 6 weeks; after 2–3 weeks of exposure, volunteers were inured to the eye, nose, and throat irritation noted at these concentrations. There were no differences in pulmonary function or respiratory and cutaneous symptoms between soda ash workers exposed for an average of 12 years to a mean time-weighted average (TWA) of 9.2 ppm ammonia and those exposed to a mean of 0.3 ppm ammonia. The NOAEL obtained in this worker population was used by the US Environmental Protection Agency under its Integrated Risk Information System program to establish a reference concentration of 0.07 ppm for the general population chronically exposed to ammonia.

Immunotoxicity

While studies in animals have shown that exposures to ammonia (25–100 ppm) can decrease resistance to bacterial infection, there is no evidence that the secondary infections accompanying the dermal and respiratory lesions seen after human exposures to ammonia are due to an effect on immune function.

Reproductive Toxicity

There are no data on the effect of ammonia in animals or humans. However, data on related ammonium compounds in animals suggest that ammonia does not affect either reproduction or development. For example, histological lesions were not seen in the reproductive organs of rats exposed to ammonium sulfate (≤1975 mg kg^{-1} day^{-1}) via the diet for 13 weeks. Similarly, reproductive and developmental parameters in a screening study similar to an OECD 422 protocol were not affected when male and female rats were exposed to diammonium phosphate (≤1500 mg kg^{-1} day^{-1}) via gavage.

Genotoxicity

Data from *in vitro* and *in vivo* mutagenicity and clastogenicity tests of ammonia, aqueous ammonia (NH_4OH), and ammonium salts following guideline protocols are negative. Positive and negative results have been reported in nonguideline studies, the former sometimes occurring only at cytotoxic doses.

Carcinogenicity

There are no data in animals or humans on the carcinogenic potential of ammonia following either inhalation or dermal exposures. In a 2-year drinking water study in mice given 193 mg ammonia kg^{-1} day^{-1} as NH_4OH, carcinogenic effects were not observed in mice and the spontaneous development of breast cancer commonly seen in C4H mice was not affected. In a study of the role of ammonia generated by *Helicobacter pylori* on the development of gastric lesions, 0.01% ammonia in drinking water ($\sim$42 mg ammonia kg^{-1} day^{-1}) increased the incidence and severity of gastric tumors induced in rats that had been pretreated with *N*-methyl-*N′*-nitro-*N*-nitrosoguanidine, a known stomach carcinogen in experimental animals. This dose is more than 100-fold greater than the daily dose of ammonia ingested by humans in food and water. There are no data in humans on the carcinogenic effects of ammonia or ammonium compounds following oral exposure.

Clinical Management

Exposures by inhalation should be monitored for respiratory tract irritation, upper airway obstruction, bronchitis, or pneumonitis. Humidified supplemental 100% oxygen should be administered to help soothe bronchial irritation. Oxygen, in combination with intubation and mechanical ventilation, may be required in severe cases. Exposed eyes and skin should be irrigated immediately with copious amounts of water; eyes should be washed for at least 30 min or until the eye reached neutral pH as tested in the conjunctival sac. If eye irritation, pain, swelling, lacrimation, or photophobia persist, the patient should be seen in a health care facility.

Ecotoxicology

The toxicity of ammonia is commonly evaluated using ammonium salts that dissociate in water to ammonia and ammonium cation. Unionized ammonia is considered the more toxic of the two moieties. As predicted by pH partitioning, the toxicity of ammonium salts increases with increasing pH due to the higher fraction of unionized ammonia. Unionized ammonia levels are lower at high ionic strengths which can impact the toxicity of ammonia in estuarine and marine environments. The toxicity of unionized ammonia also increases with decreasing temperature. The 96-h LC_{50} values for ammonium compounds in a variety of fish species range between 6.9 and 175 mg total ammonia per liter depending on pH and temperature; the unionized ammonia levels under these conditions typically range between 0.16 and 3.4 mg l^{-1}. The 48-h effective concentration 50% (EC_{50}) values for a variety of aquatic invertebrates exhibit similar ranges. While data on the toxicity of ammonia to aquatic plants are limited, available data indicate they are more tolerant to ammonia than fish or invertebrates.

Other Hazards

Ammonia has lower and upper explosive limits of 15 and 28% by volume in air, respectively.

Exposure Standards and Guidelines

International occupational exposure limits (OELs) generally range between 20 and 25 ppm as an 8-h TWA. The American Conference of Governmental Industrial Hygienists has established an 8-h TWA OEL for ammonia of 25 ppm with a 15-min excursion limit of 35 ppm. National Institute of Occupational Safety and Health recommends a 10-h TWA OEL of 25 ppm with a 15-min excursion limit of 35 ppm and indicates that 300 ppm ammonia is immediately dangerous to life or health. OSHA has a permissible exposure limit of 50 ppm for an 8-h TWA.

See also: ACGIH® (American Conference of Governmental Industrial Hygienists); Ames Test; Chromosome Aberrations; Developmental Toxicology; Dose–Response Relationship; Aquatic Ecotoxicology; Ecotoxicology, Aquatic Invertebrates; Environmental Exposure Assessment; Environmental Protection Agency, US; Gastrointestinal System; Genetic Toxicology; LD_{50}/LC_{50} (Lethal Dosage 50/Lethal Concentration 50); Mechanisms of Toxicity; Mode of Action; National Institute for Occupational Safety and Health; Occupational Exposure Limits; Occupational Safety and Health Administration; Organization for Economic Cooperation and Development; Oral/Dermal Reference Dose (RfD)/Inhalation Reference Concentration (RfC); Respiratory Tract Toxicology; Risk Assessment, Human Health; Toxicity Testing, Aquatic; Toxicity Testing, Carcinogenesis; Toxicity Testing, Developmental; Toxicity Testing, Mutagenicity; Toxicity Testing, Reproductive; Toxicity, Acute; Toxicity, Subchronic and Chronic; Pharmacokinetics.

Further Reading

ATSDR, 2004. Toxicological Profile for Ammonia. Available at http://www.atsdr.cdc.gov/toxprofiles/tp126.pdf

US EPA, 2009. Draft 2009 Update, Aquatic Life Ambient Water Quality Criteria for Ammonia – Freshwater. EPA-822-D-09-001.

WHO, 1986. Environmental Health Criteria No. 54: Ammonia. Available at http://www.inchem.org/documents/ehc/ehc/ehc54.htm

Relevant Websites

Agency for Toxic Substances and Disease Registry. http://www.atsdr.cdc.gov –

European Chemicals Agency. Registered substances: Ammonia,Anhydrous http://apps.echa.europa.eu/registered/registered-sub.aspx - Information on

National Institute for Occupational Safety and Health (NIOSH) http://www.cdc.gov/niosh/topics/ammonia/

Organization for Economic Cooperation and Development OECD) Existing Chemicals Database. SIDS Initial Assessment Report on Ammmonia http://webnet.oecd.org/Hpv/UI/SIDS_Details.aspx? –

Ammonium Nitrate

PS Rao, Sanofi, Bridgewater, NJ, USA

- Name: Ammonium nitrate
- Chemical Abstracts Service Registry Number*: 6484-52-2; 893438-76-1; 95255-40-6
- Synonyms*: Ammonium nitrate; Ammonium nitricum; Ammonium saltpeter; Ammonium(I) nitrate (1:1); Caswell No. 045; EINECS 229-347-8; EPA Pesticide Chemical Code 076101; German saltpeter; HSDB 475; Herco prills; Merco prills; Nitram; Nitrate d'ammonium; Nitrate d'ammonium (French); Nitrate of ammonia; Nitrato amonico; Nitrato amonico (Spanish); Nitric acid, ammonium salt; Norway saltpeter; UNII-T8YA51M7Y6; Varioform I
- Molecular Formula: $H_4N_2O_3$
- Chemical Structure:

$$HO-N^{+}(=O)-O^{-} \quad NH_4^{+}$$

Introduction

Ammonium nitrate is found as colorless or white to gray crystals or odorless beads with a molecular weight of 80.06 and a specific gravity of 1.725 g cm^{-1}. It has a melting point of 169.51 °C and boils at 2101 °C with evolution of nitrous oxide. Heating may cause violent combustion or explosion. The substance decomposes on heating or producing toxic fumes (nitrogen oxides). The substance is a strong oxidant and reacts with combustible and reducing materials. It forms chloramines on chlorination and is incompatible with acetic acid; acetic anhydride, hexamethylene tetramine acetate, and nitric acid mixture; ammonia; aluminum, calcium nitrate, and formamide mixture; metals; alkali metals; and combustible agents.

Texas City Disaster

One of the worst industrial disasters in the US history occurred on 16 April 1947, when a ship, named *SS Grandcamp*, exploded at the docks in Texas City near Galveston. A French-owned vessel, carrying explosive ammonium nitrate produced during wartime for explosives and later recycled as fertilizer, detonated 2300 tons of $H_4N_2O_3$, caught on fire, and eventually exploded when attempts were made to extinguish the fire. During this tragedy, not only the entire dock area but also the nearby Monsanto Chemical Company, other smaller companies, grain warehouses, and numerous oil and chemical storage tanks all got destroyed. Smaller explosions and fires were ignited by flying debris along the industrial area and throughout the city. The concussion of the explosion was felt as far away as Port Arthur, and thousands of residences and buildings throughout Texas City were destroyed. Burning wreckage ignited everything within miles, including dozens of oil storage tanks and chemical tanks. The nearby city of Galveston was covered with an oily fog that left deposits over every exposed outdoor surface.

During this ongoing tragedy, another nearby docked ship called *SS High Flyer*, carrying ammonium nitrate, was also ignited by the first explosion and exploded about 16 h later. The entire disaster took approximately 576 lives, 398 of whom were identified and 178 listed as missing. Almost all persons in the dock area – firemen, ships' crews, and spectators – were killed, and most of the bodies were never recovered; 63 bodies were buried unidentified. The number of injured ranged in the thousands, and loss of property totaled about $67 million (over $1 billion today). Litigation over the Texas City disaster was finally settled in 1962, when the US Supreme Court refused to review an appeals court ruling that the Republic of France, owner of the Grandcamp, could not be held accountable for any claims resulting from the explosion. The disaster brought changes in chemical manufacturing and new regulations for the bagging, handling, and shipping of chemicals. A positive result of the Texas City disaster was widespread disaster response planning to help organize plant, local, and regional emergency response teams.

Uses

Ammonium nitrate is used commonly in fertilizers; in pyrotechniques, herbicides, and insecticides; and in the manufacture of nitrous oxide. It is used as an absorbent for nitrogen oxides, an ingredient of freezing mixtures, an oxidizer in rocket propellants, and a nutrient for yeast and antibiotics. It is also used in explosives (especially as an oil mixture) for blasting rocks and in mining. Nitrates and nitrites are used to cure meats and to develop the characteristic flavor and pink color, to prevent rancidity, and to prevent growth of *Clostridium botulinum* spores in or on meats.

Mechanisms of Action

Nitrate and nitrites can combine with secondary amines to form dimethylnitrosamines, which are acutely toxic and cause centrilobular necrosis, fibrous occlusion of central veins, and pleural and peritoneal hemorrhages in animals. In the body nitrates are converted to nitrites, which can oxidize hemoglobin to methemoglobin and lead to cyanosis.

Ammonia and alkali metal are formed when ammonium nitrate reacts with metal hydroxides, releasing:

i) $NH_4NO_3 + NaOH \rightarrow NH_3 + H_2O + NaNO_3$

ii) $NH_4NO_3 + KOH \rightarrow NH_3 + H_2O + KNO_3$

Hydrochloric acid can react with ammonium nitrate to give rise to ammonium chloride and nitric acid: $NH_4NO_3 + HCl \rightarrow NH_4Cl + HNO_3$

 http://dx.doi.org/10.1016/B978-0-12-386454-3.00235-9

No residue is found when ammonium nitrate is heated:

$$NH_4NO_3 \Delta\rightarrow N_2O + 2H_2O$$

Ammonium nitrate is also formed in the atmosphere from emissions of NO, SO_2, and NH_3 and is a secondary component of particulate matter.

Acute and Short-Term Toxicity

Animal

LD_{50} Rat oral: 2085 mg kg^{-1}

LD_{50} Rat dermal: >5000 mg kg^{-1}

LD_{50} Rat inhalation: >88.8 mg l^{-1}

Methemoglobinemia, which can lead to anoxia and death in extreme cases, is the primary acute toxic effect of oral exposure to inorganic nitrates in all the animals tested. Ruminant animals are the most susceptible species. Toxicity depends on a number of factors, including the conversion of nitrates to nitrites; the ability of the various animals to enzymatically reduce methemoglobin; the amount of vitamins A, C, D, and E in the diet; and the nutritional state of the animal. Acute nitrate toxicity in cattle has been reported following the ingestion of water containing ≥500 ppm nitrate or feed containing ≥5000 ppm nitrates. Nitrate is rapidly converted to nitrite in the rumen and is immediately absorbed in large amounts into the bloodstream. Animals can die within a few hours of initial ingestion of a high nitrate feed. If cattle are fed once a day, maximum· met-hemoglobin level occurs ~8 h after feeding. When cattle are fed twice daily, maximum levels occur 4–5 h after feeding. With once-a-day feeding, a larger quantity of feed is consumed at once and a greater amount of nitrate is released from the feed in a short period of time. Therefore, the once-a-day feeding program results in higher total methemoglobin levels than twice-a-day feeding.

Signs of acute poisoning in cattle are increased heart rate, muscle tremors, vomiting, weakness, blue-gray mucous membranes, excess saliva and tear production, depression, labored or violent breathing, staggering gait, frequent urination, low body temperature, disorientation, and an inability to get up. Animals are often found in a lying position after a short struggle. In most cases of acute poisoning, animals are found dead before any signs of toxicity are observed.

Human

Ammonium nitrate is irritating to the eyes, nose, throat, and mucous membranes. Inhalation of this compound can cause severe lung congestion, coughing, difficulty in breathing, and increased acid urine. Exposure to large amounts can cause systemic acidosis and abnormal hemoglobin. It is considered to have low toxicity since it causes reversible tissue changes that disappear when exposure stops.

In the body, nitrates are converted to nitrites, which can oxidize hemoglobin to methemoglobin and lead to cyanosis. Nitrates also cause unconsciousness, dizziness, fatigue, shortness of breath, nausea, and vomiting. The skin is warm and sweaty and later becomes cold due to vasodilation. It causes coronary blood vessel contraction, bradycardia, atrial fibrillation, cardiac ischemia, headache, convulsions, and diarrhea. Nitrate transferred through breast milk causes methemoglobinemia in infant. Infants are more predisposed to nitrate-related toxicity than adults due to decreased ability to secrete gastric acid, higher levels of fetal hemoglobin, and diminished enzymatic capability to reduce methemoglobin to hemoglobin.

No data are available on the teratogenicity or mutagenicity of ammonium nitrate.

Chronic Toxicity (or Exposure)

Animal

Chronic nitrate toxicity is a form of nitrate poisoning where the clinical signs of the disease are not observed. It is more common to see a reduction in weight gain, lower milk production, depressed appetite, and a greater susceptibility to infections. These production-related problems or losses are not often recognized and will occur when nitrate levels are at 0.5–1.0% of the daily feed consumption. Chronic nitrate poisoning can cause abortions within the first 100 days of pregnancy because nitrates interfere with the implantation of the egg in the uterus. When implantation fail, the fetus dies and is resorbed. During the first trimester of pregnancy, no obvious signs of an abortion are seen. Reproductive problems may also occur due to a nitrate- or nitrite-induced hormone imbalance, but most are usually not recognized as feed related.

Calves affected by nitrate poisoning during the last three months of gestation are usually born one to four weeks premature, and most appear normal but die within 18–24 h of birth. Surviving newborn calves that are affected by nitrate poisoning may have convulsions and seizures.

Human

Chronic ingestion of 5 mg kg^{-1} day^{-1} is considered unacceptable. Common findings associated with nitrate poisoning include unconsciousness, dizziness and fatigue, shortness of breath, nausea, vomiting, coma, cyanosis, dyspnea, and pallor.

Clinical Management

Absorption should be prevented by dilution with 4–8 ounces of milk or water or by gastric lavage in patients who are comatose or at a risk of convulsing. Charcoal or saline cathartic may also be given. Emesis may be induced if initiated within 30 min of ingestion. Methylene blue is used to treat methemoglobinemia. Diazepam is administered (maximum rate 5 mg min^{-1}) to control seizures. Recurrent seizures are controlled by phenytoin or phenobarbital. An EKG should be monitored while administering phenytoin. Dopamine or norepinephrine is administered to control hypotension.

In cases of mild nitrate toxicity (blood methemoglobin levels <20%), asymptomatic patients do not require treatment other than avoiding ingestion or inhalation of substances that cause methemoglobinemia. In symptomatic patients with moderate or severe toxicity and hypoxia or dyspnea, 100% oxygen should be administered immediately to saturate fully all remaining normal hemoglobin. Specific therapy for methemoglobinemia consists of intravenous administration of methylene blue at a dose of 1–2 mg kg^{-1} body weight (0.1–0.2 ml kg^{-1} body weight of a 1% solution in saline) over a 5- to 10-min period. Within 15 min of methylene blue administration, cyanosis will usually begin obviously to improve. If no response to the initial injection occurs within 15 min in seriously ill patients, or within 30–60 min in moderately ill patients, a second methylene blue dose of 0.1 ml kg^{-1} body weight can be given. Caution is advised because methylene blue can slightly worsen methemoglobinemia when given in excessive amounts. In general, the total dose administered during the first 2–3 h should not be >0.5–0.7 ml kg^{-1} of body weight. Methylene blue should not be administered to a patient with known glucose-6-phosphate dehydrogenase (G-6-PD) deficiency because severe hemolytic anemia can develop. For severe, life-threatening methemoglobinemia, especially when the patient responds poorly to methylene blue therapy or when the patient has G-6-PD deficiency, treatment options include exchange transfusion and hyperbaric oxygen therapy. During treatment in the hyperbaric chamber, sufficient oxygen can be dissolved directly in the blood to support life; reversible binding to hemoglobin is not required. Blood transfusion might be required if massive hemolysis develops. In persons with severe hemolysis, maintaining a brisk urine flow and alkalinizing the urine by administration of sodium bicarbonate might help protect against renal injury from erythrocyte breakdown products. Patients with severe poisoning who are experiencing seizures or cardiac arrhythmias might require anticonvulsant or antiarrhythmic therapy.

Ecotoxicology

Invertebrate EC_{50}: *Daphnia magna*, 48 h period – 555 mg l^{-1};

Algae EC_{50}: *Scenedesmus quadricauda*, 72 h period – 83 mg l^{-1}; fish (LC_{50}): Chinacook salmon, rainbow trout, bluegill, 96 h period – 420–1360 mg NO_3 l^{-1}.

Ammonia is a toxic hazard to fish and maybe harmful to animals on direct ingestion. Ammonium nitrate is nonpersistent and noncumulative when applied using normal agriculture practices. Ammonium nitrate is very soluble in water. Upon decomposition, ammonium nitrate will release ammonium and nitrate ions. The NO_3^- ion is mobile. The NH_4^+ ion is adsorbed by soil. It is not listed as a marine pollutant.

Exposure Standards and Guidelines

The nitrate limit in drinking water was established as a safeguard against infantile acquired methemoglobinemia. The US Environmental Protection Agency's maximum contaminant level (MCL) for nitrates is 10 ppm. The MCL for nitrites is 1 ppm.

See also: Nitrous Oxide.

Further Reading

Boukerche, S., Aouacheri, W., Saka, S., 2007. Toxicological effects of nitrate: biological study in human and animal. Ann. Biol. Clin. (Paris) 65 (4), 385–391.

Camargo, J.A., Alonso, A., Salamanca, A., 2005. Nitrate toxicity to aquatic animals: a review with new data for freshwater invertebrates. Chemosphere 58 (9), 1255–1267.

Heindel, J.J., Chapin, R.E., Gulati, D.K., et al., 1994. Assessment of the reproductive and developmental toxicity of pesticide/fertilizer mixtures based on confirmed pesticide contamination in California and Iowa groundwater. Fundam. Appl. Toxicol. 22, 605–621.

National Academy of Sciences, 1981. The Health Effects of Nitrite, Nitrate and N-nitroso Compounds. National Academy Press, Washington.

US Environmental Protection Agency, 1987. Nitrate/Nitrite Health Advisory. US Environmental Protection Agency, Office of Drinking Water, Washington.

US Environmental Protection Agency, 1990. National Pesticide Survey: Summary Results of Pesticides in Drinking Water Wells. US Environmental Protection Agency, Office of Pesticides and Toxic Substances, Washington.

Yang, R., 1993. NTP technical report on the toxicity studies of pesticide/fertilizer mixtures administered in drinking water to F344/N rats and B6C3F1 mice. Toxic. Rep. Ser. 36, 1–G3.

Relevant Websites

http://www.1.agric.gov.ab.ca – Alberta Agriculture and Rural Development.

http://www.dhs.gov/ammonium-nitrate-security-program – US Dept. of Homeland Security - Ammonium Nitrate Security Program.

http://www.neochim.bg/files/SDS_NPK_en.pdf – Neochim Plc - Safety Data Sheet NPK AN based, compound fertilizer.

http://www.toxnet.nlm.nih.gov – Toxnet (Toxicology Data Network): search for Ammonium Nitrate.

Amobarbital *see* Barbiturates

Amphetamines

EM Pallasch, Illinois Poison Center, Chicago, IL, USA
M Wahl, Illinois Poison Center, Chicago, IL, USA and Northshore University Healthsystems, Evanston, IL, USA

This article is a revision of the previous edition article by Michael Wahl, volume 1, pp 108–109, © 2005, Elsevier Inc.

- Name: Amphetamines
- Chemical Abstracts Service Registry Number: 300-62-9
- Synonyms: Phenethylamine; racemic β-phenylisopropylamine (**Figure 1**). Phenethylamines are a large group of structurally similar agents that includes the amphetamines, hallucinogenic tryptamines, and the cathinones. Amphetamines and cathinones have similar activities, but are technically subsets of phenethylamines. Slang terms for this group of stimulants include uppers, meth, speed, ice, dexies, and crank.
- Chemical/Pharmaceutical/Other Class: Central nervous system stimulant
- Molecular Formula: $C_9H_{13}N$
- Chemical Structure:

CH_3
|
—CH_2CHNH_2

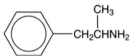

History

The first amphetamine was originally developed in 1887 by Edeleano, a Romanian chemist working in Germany. It became available in the form of an inhaler for use as a nasal decongestant under the name Benzedrine in the 1930s. It was marketed for the treatment of narcolepsy and appetite suppression and was also used off-label for schizophrenia, morphine addiction, alcoholism, and behavioral issues in children. In the 1940s, methamphetamine and amphetamine were used by soldiers during World War II to fight combat fatigue and amphetamine is currently permitted for use to promote wakefulness in battle. Amphetamines were readily available over the counter and by prescription until the dangers of use, abuse, and addiction such as palpitations, convulsions, and psychosis were recognized. The drug was classified as a schedule II substance under the federal Controlled Substances Act in 1970. Amphetamines

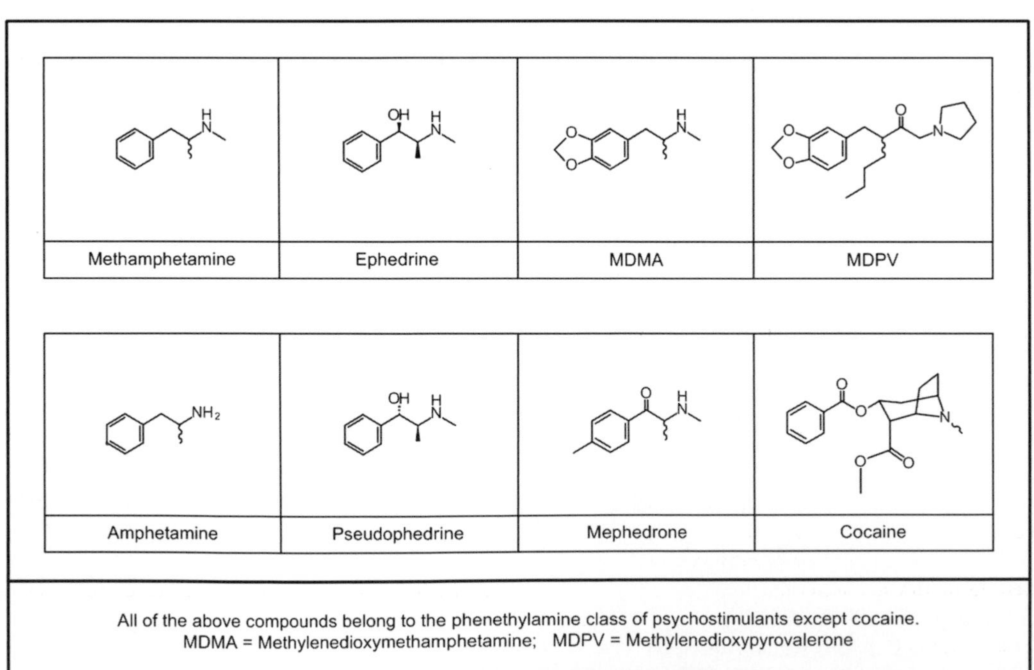
Methamphetamine
Ephedrine
MDMA
MDPV
Amphetamine
Pseudophedrine
Mephedrone
Cocaine
All of the above compounds belong to the phenethylamine class of psychostimulants except cocaine.
MDMA = Methylenedioxymethamphetamine; MDPV = Methylenedioxypyrovalerone

Figure 1 Structures of methamphetamine and selected other psychostimulants. Source: Vearrier, D., Greenberg, M.I., Ney Miller, S., Okaneku, J.T., Haggerty, D.A. 2012. Methamphetamine: history, pathophysiology, adverse health effects, current trends, and hazards associated with the clandestine manufacture of methamphetamine. Disease-a-Month 58 (2), 33–92.

 http://dx.doi.org/10.1016/B978-0-12-386454-3.00692-8

remained a popular drug of abuse leading to illegal production and criminal activity. Motorcycle gangs would conceal methamphetamine in the crankcases of their bikes, leading to the popular slang term 'crank.' Methamphetamine abuse resurged in the 1980s and 1990s along with 'designer drugs' such as methylenedioxymethamphetamine (MDMA). These drugs were popularized in clubs and 'rave' parties, prompting the Methamphetamine Control Act of 1996. In 2005 a federal law was enacted to regulate the sale of the precursors of methamphetamine (pseudoephedrine, ephedrine). The law limits the purchaser to a maximum of 3.6 g of pseudoephedrine per day and requires identification and the signature of the purchaser at the pharmacy counter. Newer designer drugs known as 'bath salts' comprised of amphetamine-like chemicals, cathinone derivatives (e.g., methylenedioxypyrovalerone and mephedrone) are emerging drugs of abuse prompting lawmakers to create and amend regulations prohibiting the manufacture and sale of these amphetamine-like compounds.

Uses

Amphetamines are advocated for use in a wide variety of conditions but are medically approved for the treatment of attention-deficit hyperactivity disorder, narcolepsy, and weight loss. Amphetamines are also popular drugs of abuse available in several forms for different routes of abuse.

Environmental Fate and Behavior

Physicochemical Properties

Amphetamine is a clear to colorless liquid in freebase or white crystalline substance as a salt. As a liquid it slowly volatilizes and has a characteristic amine odor. Amphetamine base is slightly soluble in water, soluble in alcohol and ether. The melting point of amphetamine is 300 °C with some decomposition occurring.

Exposure Routes and Pathways

Amphetamines are most commonly administered orally when prescribed. Certain amphetamines of abuse (i.e., methamphetamine) are injected, smoked, or snorted (insufflations) as well. Exposure to methamphetamine can occur through environmental contamination as well and children and other individuals on-site at a methamphetamine production center (including a 'mom-and-pop' lab in a house) can be exposed through the environment at a clandestine lab. In fact 15% of children simply around individuals who use methamphetamine will test positive for the drug and nearly 100% of children in a clandestine lab environment will have methamphetamine detectable in their system.

Therapeutic dosing for amphetamine ranges from 5 to 60 mg per day in adults and 5–40 mg per day in children of 6 years of age and older. Peak plasma concentrations are dependent on the route of exposure. Absorption from the gastrointestinal tract is rapid producing peak concentrations in approximately 2–3 h vs 30 min when used intravenously or intramuscularly. Delayed release preparations will take longer time to reach peak concentrations. Absorption into the lungs via smoking reaches the brain within 7 s. More than 50% of a dose undergoes hepatic metabolism, and about 30% is excreted unchanged in urine. The amount of nonmetabolized drug recovered in urine is greater with acidic urine. The half-life ranges from 8 to 30 h.

Toxicokinetics

Amphetamines are generally well absorbed from the gastrointestinal tract in therapeutic doses. Several commercially available amphetamines are formulated as sustained or delayed release products. Peak steadystate serum levels are expected within 30 min after intravenous injection and within 2–3 h after ingestion of immediate release products. In overdose and with exposure to sustained release products, delays in absorption are expected. Amphetamines have a volume of distribution of approximately 3–5 $l\ kg^{-1}$ with low protein binding. These agents are extensively metabolized through hepatic and renal pathways via cytochrome P450 enzymes. Cytochrome CYP2D6 may be responsible for some amphetamine-related drug toxicity. Substrate competition or inhibition at this metabolic site may increase the half-life of amphetamines. Many metabolites have amphetamine activity. Elimination can vary greatly. Some amphetamines have primary renal elimination with the rate of elimination depending upon the urine pH (e.g., amphetamine). With others, less than 1% of the parent compound is renally excreted (e.g., methylphenidate). Half-lives vary as well with intravenous methylphenidate at 1–2 h and chlorphentermine at 5 days.

Mechanism of Toxicity

Amphetamines are indirect acting sympathomimetics, producing their effects by inhibiting the transporters of dopamine, norepinephrine, and serotonin at the presynaptic nerve terminal (**Figure 2**). This increases the release of norepinephrine, dopamine, and serotonin and increased norepinephrine levels at central synapses, which further stimulates alpha and beta receptors. Some amphetamines also inhibit monoamine oxidase, preventing the breakdown of catecholamines. These mechanisms combine to produce the sympathomimetic and central nervous system (CNS) effects seen with amphetamine abuse.

Acute and Short-Term Toxicity (or Exposure)

Animal

Amphetamine toxicity in animals manifests itself in a similar way as humans. Expected signs and symptoms include hypertension, tachycardia, seizures, coma, and hyperthermia. Rhabdomyolysis may also result and leads to renal failure if not treated aggressively.

Human

Toxicity in humans will follow the expected sympathomimetic toxidrome. CNS effects include hypervigilance, agitation,

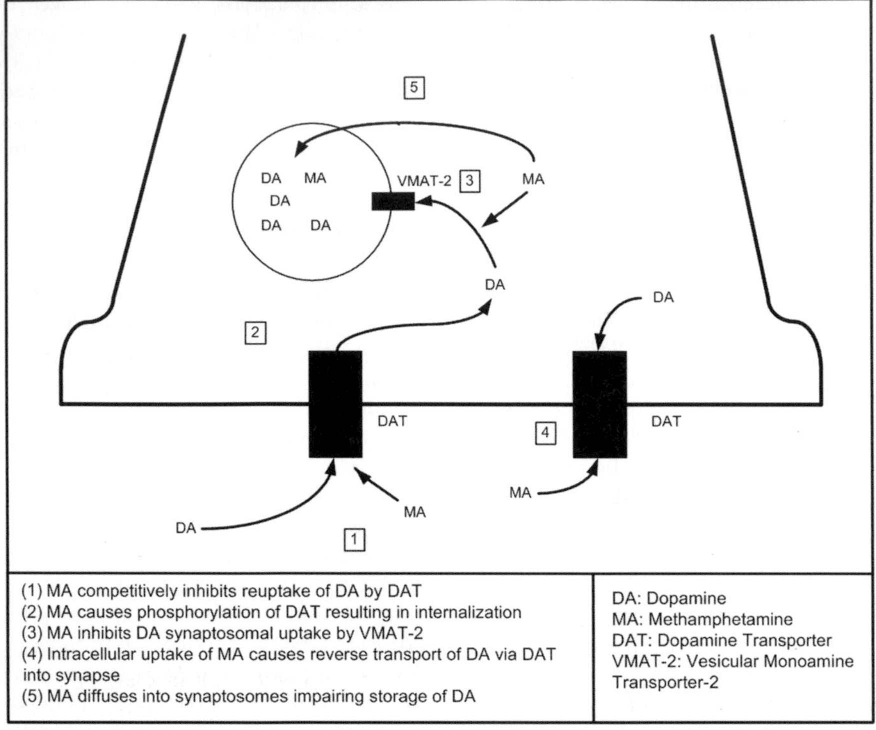

Figure 2 Mechanism of action of methamphetamine on dopamine neurotransmission. MA, methamphetamine; DA, dopamine; DAT, dopamine transporter; VMAT, vesicular monoamine transporter-2. Source: Vearrier, D., Greenberg, M.I., Ney Miller, S., Okaneku, J.T., Haggerty, D.A. 2012. Methamphetamine: history, pathophysiology, adverse health effects, current trends, and hazards associated with the clandestine manufacture of methamphetamine. Disease-a-Month 58 (2), 33–92.

restlessness, decreased appetite, irritability, stereotyped repetitive behavior, and insomnia with low doses. Patients may develop psychosis due to dopaminergic effects. With larger exposures, confusion, panic reactions, aggressive behavior, hallucinations, seizures, delirium, coma, and death can occur. Intracranial bleeding can result from untreated hypertension. Trauma is common secondary to behavior changes and impaired judgment. Frequent use results in fatigue, paranoia, and depression. Cardiovascular effects include tachycardia, hypertension, chest pain, myocardial ischemia or infarction, dysrhythmias, cardiovascular collapse, and death. Other effects include rhabdomyolysis, increased respiratory rate, flushing, diaphoresis, and dilated pupils. Hyperthermia may lead to multisystem organ failure. Serotonin syndrome is also possible in overdose of certain amphetamines alone or in combination with other serotonergic agents. Symptoms include altered mental status, hyperthermia, rigidity, and autonomic instability.

Chronic Toxicity (or Exposure)

Animal

Animal models describe changes in behavior with toxicity and withdrawal. Chronic dosing of animals leads to stereotypic, compulsive behaviors of searching and examining in higher animals, sniffing and biting movements in lower animals. There has been no increased carcinogenic activity in rats and mice fed varying doses of amphetamine over studies as long as 2 years.

Human

Chronic use may result in paranoia, psychosis, bruxism, compulsive behavior, and cardiomyopathy. Acute withdrawal may lead to headache, anxiety, and depression.

In Vitro Toxicity Data

Several amphetamines have been shown to have monaminergic neurotoxic properties. Recent studies of PC12 dopaminergic cells have shown increased activity of capsase-3 and mitochondrial cytochrome c release. These findings suggest that amphetamines (particularly substituted amphetamines) may induce apoptosis, possibly via a mitochondrial pathway.

Reproductive Toxicity

Amphetamines do not appear to cause congenital abnormalities when taken during pregnancy; however, intrauterine growth retardation, premature delivery, and maternal and fetal morbidity is significantly increased when abuse of amphetamines occurs during pregnancy. A mild withdrawal syndrome has also been reported after delivery with amphetamine use during pregnancy. Most studies of long-term follow-up of children exposed to amphetamines during pregnancy have found no significant chronic behavioral changes. Adverse effects *in utero* to the vasoconstrictive effects of amphetamines have been reported including cerebral injury. Poor outcomes occurring during amphetamine exposure during pregnancy may also be due to factors other than the drug itself including multiple drug use, poor maternal health, socioeconomic factors, and other lifestyle variables.

Genotoxicity

Amphetamines are not thought to be mutagenic.

Carcinogenicity

Amphetamines are not carcinogenic in humans. Some amphetamines have been shown to have beneficial effects in the treatment of certain cancers, in particular hematologic malignancies.

Clinical Management

After assessment of airway, breathing, and circulation with necessary supportive care, decontamination of the gastrointestinal tract should be undertaken for substantial recent ingestions. If patients present within an hour of ingestion or have taken a modified release product, consider activated charcoal; a 10:1 ratio of activated charcoal per gram of ingested substance may be administered to patients who are awake and alert and can protect their airway. Gastric lavage may be recommended in potentially life-threatening ingestions that present within 60 min of ingestion. Determination of specific toxic doses is difficult in chronic users of amphetamines due to the development of tolerance. Oxygen and benzodiazepines should be administered as needed for agitation, shortness of breath, or chest pain. Increased blood pressure can be managed with benzodiazepines. Although vasodilators such as nitroprusside have been recommended, reflex tachycardia is a common result. Beta blockers are not recommended for use in overdose due to possible unopposed alpha adrenergic effects, which may lead to exacerbation of symptoms, i.e., worsening hypertension. Benzodiazepines may be necessary for agitated or combative patients. Benzodiazepines, cooling, and rehydration are standard treatments for patients with increased temperature and rhabdomyolysis. Hyperthermia is a poor prognostic sign and should be aggressively treated.

Clinical Management and Suggested Diagnostic Tests

Electrolytes, urinalysis, complete blood count, urine toxicology screen, creatine kinase, and cardiac enzymes are helpful laboratory tests for evaluation. In patients with severe toxicity monitor arterial blood gas (ABG), liver function tests, coagulation studies and disseminated intravascular coagulation panel.

Exposure Standards and Guidelines

Amphetamine is a Comprehensive Environmental Response, Compensation and Liability Act (CERCLA) hazardous substance and subjects to the release reporting requirement of CERCLA section 103, 40 CFR parts 302 and 355. It is an extremely hazardous substance and subjects to reporting requirements when stored in amounts of 1000 lbs or greater (the threshold planning quantity).

Miscellaneous

Drug Screening

Qualitative tests such as immunoassays may have false positive results for products containing ephedrine and pseudoephedrine. Other substances, such as labetalol and ranitidine, may cross-react with antiamphetamine antibodies, giving a false positive test result as well. Selegiline, a selective monoamine oxidase inhibitor type B, is partially metabolized to amphetamine and thus will give a positive result by most analytical methods. Additionally some newer designer drugs such as MDMA may not react with antiamphetamine antibodies and will result in a negative test. Limitations such as these may make clinical interpretations more difficult and imprecise. A confirmatory test, such as gas chromatography–mass spectrometry, offers greater specificity and sensitivity and may be the best choice in avoiding false positives and false negatives.

See also: Drugs of Abuse; Benzodiazepines; Methylenedioxymethamphetamine; Poisoning Emergencies in Humans.

Further Reading

Baselt, R.C., 2002. Disposition of Toxic Drugs and Chemicals in Man, sixth ed. Biomedical Publications, Foster City, CA. 64–66.

Biaggioni, I., Robertson, D., 2009. Adrenoceptor agonists & sympathomimetic drugs (Chapter 9). In: Katzung, B., Masters, S.B., Trevor, A.J. (Eds.), Basic and Clinical Pharmacology, eleventh ed. McGraw-Hill (Access Medicine).

Blanckaert, P., van Amsterdam, J., Brunt, T., van den Berg, J., Van Durme, F., Maudens, K., Van Bussel, J., 2013. 4-methyl-amphetamine: a health threat for recreational amphetamine users. J. Psychopharmacol. 27 (9), 817–822.

Chiang, W., 2010. Amphetamines. In: Flomenbaum, et al. (Eds.), Goldfrank's Toxicologic Emergencies, ninth ed. McGraw-Hill, New York, NY, pp. 1078–1090.

German, C.L., Fleckenstein, A.E., Hanson, G.R., 2013. Bath salts and synthetic cathinones: an emerging designer drug phenomenon. Life Sci.. S0024-3205(13) 00424–4.

Kraemer, T., Maurer, H.H., 2002. Toxicokinetics of amphetamines: metabolism and toxicokinetic data of designer drugs, amphetamine, methamphetamine and their N-alkyl derivatives. Ther. Drug Monit. 24 (2), 277–289.

McCann, U.D., Ricaurte, G.A., 2004. Amphetamine neurotoxicity: accomplishments and remaining challenges. Neurosci. Biobehav. Rev. 27, 821–826.

POISINDEX® System: Amphetamines. Klasco, R.K. (Ed.), POISINDEX® System. Thomson Reuters, Greenwood Village. Colorado Edition Expires (04/2012).

Prosser, J.M., Nelson, L.S., 2012. The toxicology of bath salts: a review of synthetic cathinones. J. Med. Toxicol. 8 (1), 33–42.

Vearrier, D., Greenberg, M.I., Ney Miller, S., Okaneku, J., Haggerty, D.A., 2012. Methamphetamine: history, pathophysiology, adverse health effects, current trends, and hazards associated with the clandestine manufacture of methamphetamine. Dis. Mon. 58 (2), 33–92.

Relevant Websites

http://emedicine.medscape.com/article/812518-overview – Amphetamine toxicity – Medscape reference an online resource on diagnosis, mechanism of toxicity, clinical management and treatment of amphetamine toxicity.

http://health.utah.gov/meth/index.html – Utah Department of Health - Methamphetamine.

http://www.drugabuse.gov/sites/default/files/drugfacts_bath_salts_final_0_1.pdf – National Institute on Drug Abuse (NIDA) information on bath salts (cathinones).

http://www.aiha.org/aihce06/handouts/po118vandyke.pdf – National Jewish Medical Center power point resource on methamphetamine particle size and persistence after methamphetamine cook.

http://www.dtsc.ca.gov/SiteCleanup/ERP/upload/OEHHA_Memo-Nov2007.pdf – Office of Environmental Health Hazard Assessment for children's exposure to methamphetamine surface residue in use and clandestine laboratory environment.

www.erowid.org/ – Online resource for intoxicating plants and drugs – information and resources including journal articles, timelines, media, prohibition sites, harm reduction, subjective user reports and chemical information.

Amyl Nitrite

A Kubic and M Wahl, Illinois Poison Center, Chicago, IL, USA

This article is a revision of the previous edition article by Michael Wahl, volume 1, pp 110–111, © 2005, Elsevier Inc.

- Name: Amyl Nitrite
- Chemical Abstracts Service Registry Number: 110-46-3
- Synonyms: 3-methylbutyl nitrite; 3-methylbutyl ester; Isopentyl alcohol nitrite; Aspiral; Nitramyl; Isoamyl nitrite; 3-methyl-1-nitrosoxybutane; Nitrous acid, Poppers (colloquial, street slang)
- Molecular Formula: $C_5H_{11}NO_2$
- Chemical Structure:

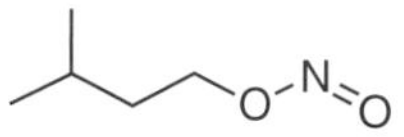

Background/Uses

Amyl nitrite had been used clinically as early as 1867, when the Scottish physician Sir Thomas Brunton used it as a vasodilator as treatment for angina pectoris in his patients. In the late 1880s, a protective effect on cyanide toxicity in canines was noted when amyl nitrite was inhaled postexposure. Amyl nitrite has been used clinically in a multicomponent cyanide antidote kit and is also a recreational drug of abuse ('poppers').

Environmental Fate and Behavior

Routes

A volatile liquid, amyl nitrite is slightly soluble in water and is commonly supplied in ampoules that are broken and administered by inhalation. Inhalation is likely the most common route of exposure, though reports of ingestion of the liquid itself have been seen. Amyl nitrite may also be absorbed through the skin when skin comes in contact with the liquid.

Stability

Amyl nitrite is an unstable compound. It is air and light sensitive and flammable. Amyl nitrite forms explosive mixtures with air or oxygen, and it is incompatible with oxidizing agents and reducing agents.

Physicochemical Properties

Clear to yellowish liquid with a fruity odor.

Molar mass 117.15 g mol^{-1}.

Density 0.872 g cm^{-3} liquid (25 °C).

Boiling point 99 °C, 372 K, 210 °F.

Solubility is slightly soluble to insoluble in water.

Flash point of 50 °F (10 °C).

Refractive index 1.3871.

Partition coefficient (log P (octanol/water)), 2.8.

Amyl nitrite is highly flammable and reactive. It is an explosion and fire hazard.

Disposition in Body

Amyl nitrite is absorbed rapidly from mucous membranes after inhalation but rapidly inactivated by hydrolysis. Amyl nitrite is inactivated after ingestion owing to hydrolysis in the gastrointestinal tract.

Toxicokinetics

Amyl nitrite is rapidly absorbed from the lungs, and hydrolyzed to nitrite ion and its corresponding alcohol. Approximately two-thirds of the ion is metabolized by the body, while the remaining one-third is excreted unchanged in the urine. When amyl nitrite is ingested, it undergoes hydrolysis in the stomach.

Mechanism of Toxicity

The primary mechanism of toxicity develops from the powerful oxidative effects of nitrites on hemoglobin. Methemoglobinemia, which develops when the iron atom in hemoglobin loses one electron to an oxidant, causing a change from the ferrous (2^+) state to the ferric (3^+) state, may cause cellular hypoxia. When methemoglobin levels exceed 10–15%, cyanosis may be evident. Nitrites also cause vasodilation by direct action on smooth muscle. Physical effects include decreases in blood pressure, headache, flushing of the face, increased heart rate, dizziness, and relaxation of involuntary muscles, especially of the blood vessels and the anal sphincter.

Amyl nitrite may be irritating to the lungs and throat when breathed in. With exposure to the skin, amyl nitrite has irritant properties. It can also be readily absorbed, causing systemic effects with skin contact.

Acute and Short-Term Exposure

Human

Breathing amyl nitrite can cause irritation of the lungs and throat, with coughing and shortness of breath developing. Exposure occurs either through breathing in or through contact with the skin. Nausea, vomiting, central nervous system (CNS) depression, and dizziness can occur shortly after exposure. Amyl nitrite may cause symptoms consistent with methemoglobinemia and vasodilation. Previously healthy patients who develop symptoms of methemoglobinemia may present initially with cyanosis, progressing to dizziness, fatigue, nausea, vomiting, and headache. As the methemoglobin level rises, symptoms of dyspnea, severe lethargy, and confusion may develop, culminating in possible coma, seizures, and death as the levels approach or exceed 70%. A hallmark sign of methemoglobinemia is the characteristic chocolate brown color of the blood apparent in a blood sample. Hemolysis and hemolytic anemia may be noted in patients with G6PD deficiency. Vasodilation may cause throbbing headache and hypotension.

Amyl nitrite may increase cerebral and intraocular pressure with acute exposure. It is contraindicated in patients with cerebral hemorrhage and glaucoma.

Animal

Symptoms are usually consistent with methemoglobinemia, including tachypnea, weakness, and cyanotic or chocolate brown mucous membranes in equine or porcine species. Increases in intraocular pressure have been reported in some animals.

Chronic Toxicity

Human

Chronic exposure to amyl nitrite can cause tolerance and reduced effect to the vasodilating properties of this chemical. Decrements in vision in chronic 'poppers' users have been reported with disruption in the outer segments of the fovea reported as the mechanism in these patients. Vision returns with cessation of recreational nitrite use.

Animal

Chronic exposure in equine populations is suggested to cause infertility, abortion, stunted growth, and immunosuppression in animals. Studies in mice have shown that amyl nitrite reacts with amines to form nitrosamines, which are highly carcinogenic.

Immunotoxicity

In vitro tests show volatile nitrites, including isobutyl and amyl nitrite, to have significant immunosuppressive effects to human lymphocytes.

Reproductive Toxicity

Nitrites are excreted in breast milk, and may cause symptoms of methemoglobinemia in infants. Infants may be at greater risk for nitrite toxicity due in part to the lack of complete development of the NADH methemoglobin reductase enzyme system until the age of approximately 6 months.

Use of amyl nitrite in pregnancy can cause significant harm to the fetus because maternal blood flow is significantly reduced through reductions in systemic vascular resistance, which results in less blood flow through the placenta. Amyl nitrite is pregnancy category C.

Carcinogenicity

While not known to be carcinogenic in humans, the metabolized byproducts of many nitrites when metabolized further into *N*-nitroso compounds have been found to be highly carcinogenic in some animal species.

Clinical Management

The most common route of exposure will be via inhalation. Since the onset of effects is within 30 s when inhaled and lasts 3–5 min, effects due to vasodilation and decreases in systemic vascular resistance should be transient and self-limited. In patients with orthostatic hypotension, their head should be of low posture and movement of their extremities and raising of their extremities will hasten recovery. If amyl nitrite is ingested, nausea and vomiting may occur and should be treated with antiemetic agents as needed. Patients with CNS depression should be evaluated for head injury from falling and supported as needed with attention to the airway and breathing. Vomiting after amyl nitrite ingestion may lead to aspiration. A chest X-ray is indicated in these patients. Patients with concern for methemoglobinemia will need further care and monitoring. Arterial blood gas, complete blood count, and methemoglobin levels should be determined in all symptomatic patients along with close monitoring of vital signs and electrocardiogram. Treatment with methylene blue may be considered in patients with severe methemoglobinemia, though its use in patients with known G6PD deficiency is controversial. If seizures develop, initial control should be with a benzodiazepine with addition of phenobarbital if necessary for recurrent or refractory symptoms. Hypotension may be treated initially with intravenous fluid boluses. This effect is usually short-lived and dissipates rather quickly as the half-life of amyl nitrite is only minutes.

Exposure Standards and Guidelines

The US Environmental Protection Agency considers a maximum contaminant level goal of nitrites in drinking water to be less than 1 mg l^{-1}. World Health Organization guidelines for nitrites recommend levels less than 3 mg l^{-1} short term and, provisionally, levels less than 0.2 mg l^{-1} long term.

No occupational exposure limits have been set for amyl nitrite.

Miscellaneous

Amyl nitrite is typically supplied in 0.3 g in 0.3 ml capsules or ampoules. The liquid is covered by a special mesh that allows for crushing between the fingers and subsequent inhalation by patients with angina pectoris. Amyl nitrite is highly flammable as a liquid and should be kept away from flames.

See also: Butyl Nitrite; Cyanide; Poisoning Emergencies in Humans.

Further Reading

Audo, I., El Sanharawi, M., Vignal-Clement, C., Villa, A., Morin, A., Conrath, J., Fompeydie, D., Sahel, J.A., Gocho-Nakashima, K., Goureau, D., Paques, M., 2011. Foveal damage in habitual popper users. Arch. Ophthalmol. 129 (6), 703–708.

Edwards, R.J., Ujma, J., 1995. Extreme methemoglobinemia secondary to recreational use of amyl nitrite. J. Accid. Emerg. Med. 12, 138–142.

Howland, M.A., 2006. Sodium and amyl nitrites. In: Flomenbaum, et al. (Eds.), Goldfrank's Toxicologic Emergencies, eighth ed. McGraw-Hill, New York, NY, pp. 1725–1727.

Klasco, R.K. (Ed.), POISINDEX® System: Amyl Nitrite. POISINDEX® System. Thomson Reuters, Greenwood Village, Colorado (Edition Expires (4/2012)).

Modari, B., Kapadia, Y.K., Kerins, M., Terris, J., 2002. Methylene blue: a treatment for severe methaemoglobinaemia secondary to misuse of amyl nitrite. Emerg. Med. J. 19, 270.

Neuberger, A., Fishman, S., Golik, A., 2002. Hemolytic anemia in a G6PD deficient man after inhalation of amyl nitrite ("poppers"). Isr. Med. Assoc. J. 11, 1085–1086.

Newell, G.R., Adams, S.C., Mansell, P.W., Hersh, E.M., 1984. Toxicity, immunosuppressive effects and carcinogenic potential of volatile nitrites: possible relation to Kaposi's sarcoma. Pharmacotherapy 4 (5), 284–291.

Reggad, A., Ficko, C., Andriamanantena, D., Flateau, C., Rapp, C., 2012. Acute hemolytic anemia in an HIV patient after inhalation of amyl nitrite. Med. Mal. Infect. 42 (12), 619–620.

Relevant Websites

http://emedicine.medscape.com/article/814287-treatment – Medscape *eMedicine* content on cyanide intoxication and treatment including the cyanide antidote kit with amyl nitrite.

www.epa.gov – United States Environmental Protection Agency – For EPA information on amyl nitrite.

http://www.erowid.org/chemicals/inhalants/inhalants_info1.shtml – Vault of Erowid content on inhalants – amyl nitrite.

www.who.int/en/ – World Health Organization.

Anabolic Steroids

SP Sawant, Kimberly-Clark Worldwide, Inc., Roswell, GA, USA
HS Parihar, PCOM School of Pharmacy, Suwanee, GA, USA
HM Mehendale, University of Louisiana at Monroe, Monroe, LA, USA

This article is a revision of the previous edition article by Sharmilee P. Sawant and Harihara M. Mehendale, volume 1, pp 111–113, © 2005, Elsevier Inc.

Introduction

Anabolic steroids, also known as anabolic androgenic steroids (AAS) or performance enhancing drugs, are the endogenously or exogenously synthesized derivatives of the male sex hormones (androgens), particularly testosterone, that enhance the anabolic effects of androgens and decrease or eliminate the androgenic effects. Some of the examples of exogenous anabolic steroids are nandrolone, oxandrolone, and trenbolone and endogenous anabolic steroids are testosterone, androstenediol, androstenedione, and dehydroepiandrosterone. These agents show both beneficial and harmful effects, depending on the exposure levels.

Many organs and systems of the body, including the reproductive system, muscle, bone, hair follicles in the skin, liver, kidneys, the hematopoietic system, and the central nervous system, are affected by the action of androgens. The actions of anabolic steroids can be classified under two categories, namely, androgenic and anabolic. The androgenic effects of these steroids can be generally considered as those associated with masculinization such as growth of the testes, external genitalia and male accessory reproductive glands (prostate, seminal vesicles, and bulbourethral), deepening of the voice due to enlargement of the larynx, hair growth (in the pubic, limb, chest, and facial region), an increase in sebaceous glands activity that may result in acne, and neuropsychiatric or behavioral effects such as increased aggressiveness. The anabolic effects are associated with protein building in skeletal muscle and bone, which may increase physical strength and body mass. In males, androgens are necessary for sustaining reproductive function, development and maintenance of skeletal muscle and bone, and cognitive function.

Testosterone has been modified structurally with an intention to afford synthetic anabolic steroids that enhance the anabolic effects of androgens and decrease or eliminate the androgenic effects. Anabolic steroids were first developed in the late 1930s in an effort to treat hypogonadism and chronic wasting. During World War II, they were given to German soldiers to enhance their aggressiveness. Their use rapidly spread and after World War II athletes were openly using anabolic steroids for performance enhancement. Tightly controlled scientific studies have shown that testosterone and its derivative, nandrolone decanoate, and enanthate increase athletic performance by building muscle mass and strength.

Mechanisms of Action

Anabolic steroids are reported to exert their actions by genomic and nongenomic mechanisms.

1. Anabolic steroids bind to androgen receptors intracellularly to form the steroid–receptor complex, and this complex translocates to the nucleus. In the nucleus, the complex interacts with the steroid response elements, resulting in gene activation, and transcription, resulting in mRNA synthesis, and consequently translation, resulting in protein synthesis. The resultant proteins cause alteration in cell function, growth, or differentiation.
2. Modulation of androgen receptor activation is due to intracellular metabolism of anabolic steroids. Certain anabolic steroids, particularly derivatives of testosterone, are designed to improve their protein anabolic effects and reduce the androgenic effects. For example, nandrolone is reported to be converted by 5α-reductase enzyme to a metabolite that binds with weaker affinity to the androgen receptor in androgenic tissues and thus reducing androgen receptor–mediated response of nandrolone in androgenic tissues. In the skeletal muscle, since the 5α-reductase enzyme activity is negligible, the parent compound, nandrolone, binds with stronger affinity to the androgen receptor, thus mediating the anabolic effects.
3. An anticatabolic effect mediated by interference with glucocorticoid receptor expression.
4. Affecting the genome-dependent and genome-independent pathways in brain such as modulation of the gamma-amino butyric acid (GABA) receptor function in the central nervous system resulting in behavioral effects.

Clinical Applications

Many anabolic steroids are used as therapeutic agents. In general, anabolic steroids have been indicated for treating renal failure, bone marrow failure, anemia, delayed puberty, and children with reduced growth. Testosterone preparations are used in male hypogonadism, in hormone replacement therapy, and as male contraception. Males with decreased circulating testosterone associated with chronic diseases or conditions, for example, those with severe burn injuries or acquired immunodeficiency syndrome (AIDS)-associated wasting, may benefit from the use of anabolic steroids. The anabolic steroid nandrolone decanoate is reported to be effective in treating sarcopenia in patients receiving dialysis. Oxandrolone is indicated to stimulate muscle protein anabolism in older women.

Human Toxicity and Adverse Effects

There are several reversible and irreversible adverse/side effects associated with the use of anabolic steroids. Nonmedical use of anabolic steroids such as increasing physical strength and

 http://dx.doi.org/10.1016/B978-0-12-386454-3.00236-0

improving body composition has been associated with several adverse effects. These adverse effects are function of steroids used, the dose, duration of use, and route of administration. Some of the minor side effects associated with anabolic steroids use include headache, gastrointestinal irritation, stomach pain, and oily skin.

In men, anabolic steroids have been reported to reduce sperm production, cause testicular atrophy (shrinking of testicles), impotence, temporary infertility, and irreversible gynecomastia. Other effects include increased frequency and duration of erection, premature sexual development, development of breast, and difficulty or pain while urinating. In women, anabolic steroids use is reported to cause changes in or cessation of menstrual cycle, increase in body hair, clitoral enlargement, decrease in breast size and body fat, deepening of voice, and decrease in scalp hair (baldness).

The cardiovascular effects of anabolic steroids are dose dependent. Long-term use of anabolic steroids has been reported to cause hypertension, stroke, heart attack, cardiac arrhythmias, and sudden death due to cardiac failure. Anabolic steroid use had also been reported to cause premature and permanent termination of growth among adolescents. Long-term use of anabolic steroids has also been associated with liver injury, hepatitis, development of fatal cysts, hepatocellular carcinoma, and hepatic angiosarcoma. Anabolic steroids cause growth of sebaceous glands and increased secretion of natural oil sebum resulting in oily skin and acne.

Anabolic steroid use is also associated with psychiatric and behavioral effects. They are reported to increase aggressiveness, particularly when high doses are taken. Other effects reported are depression, mood swings, fatigue, restlessness, loss of appetite, and mania.

Lastly, use of anabolic steroids has been indicated to develop dependency due to feeling of well-being associated with its use. Also, abusers taking a dose of anabolic steroids are also at risk to develop dependency due to withdrawal symptoms such as depression and fatigue when they stop taking anabolic steroids.

Control of Anabolic Steroids

Anabolic steroids are controlled substances in several countries, including Australia, Argentina, Brazil, Canada, the United Kingdom, and the United States. The US congress passed the Anabolic Steroid Enforcement Act in 1990, which declared anabolic steroids a controlled substance (Schedule III, Controlled Substance Act). In 2003, the Controlled Substance Act was amended to include prohormones (steroid precursors) since they may potentially act as steroid hormones. The Anabolic Steroid Control Act of 2004 was introduced, which took effect in January 2005, and it reclassified prohormones as controlled substances by amending sections of the Controlled Substance Act and the Anabolic Steroid Enforcement Act of 1990.

The International Olympic Committee (IOC) Medical Commission introduced anabolic steroids as a banned class in 1974 in order to control doping in human sport. In 1999, various governments, intergovernmental organizations, and other public and private bodies fighting against doping in human sport in concert with IOC started the World Anti-Doping Agency (WADA). All the rules and detailed technical documents concerning anabolic steroids (and other drugs) are constantly evolving under WADA and up-to-date information can be found at the WADA web site (http://www.wada-ama.org/en/).

Clinical Management

Current knowledge is based largely on the case studies and reports from physicians who have worked with patients undergoing steroid withdrawal. These reports indicate that supportive therapy is sufficient in some cases. Patients are educated about what they may experience during withdrawal and are evaluated for suicidal thoughts. If symptoms are severe or prolonged, medications, or hospitalization may be needed. Some medications restore the disrupted hormonal system due to steroid abuse. Other medications target specific withdrawal symptoms such as antidepressants to treat depression and analgesics for headaches and muscle and joint pains. Some patients exhibiting psychiatric and behavioral effects require assistance beyond simple treatment of withdrawal symptoms and are treated with behavioral/psychiatric therapies.

See also: Androgens; Behavioral Toxicology; Dietary Supplements.

Further Reading

Amsterdam, J.V., Opperhuizen, A., Hartgens, F., 2010. Adverse health effects of anabolic-androgenic steroids. Regul. Toxicol. Pharmacol. 57, 117–123.

Fitch, K., 2012. Proscribed drugs at the Olympic Games: permitted use and misuse (doping) by athletes. Clin. Med. 12 (3), 257–260.

Fact sheets on anabolic steroids can be ordered free, by calling NIDA (National Institute of Drug Abuse) Infofax at 1-888-NIH-NIDA (1-888-644-6432) or, for those with hearing impairment, 1-888-TTY-NIDA (1-888-889-6432). Information on steroid abuse also can be accessed through the NIDA Steroid Abuse Web Site (http://www.steroidabuse.org/).

Giannoulis, M.G., Martin, F.C., Nair, K.S., Umpleby, A.M., Sonksen, P., 2012. Hormone replacement therapy and physical function in healthy older men. Time to talk hormones? Endocr. Rev. 33 (3), 314–377.

Golestani, R., Slart, R.H., Dullaart, R.P., et al., 2012. Adverse cardiovascular effects of anabolic steroids: pathophysiology imaging. Eur. J. Clin. Invest. 42 (7), 795–803.

Kersey, R.D., Elliot, D.L., Goldberg, L., et al., 2012. National Athletic Trainers' Association position statement: anabolic-androgenic steroids. J. Athl. Train. 47 (5), 567–588.

Kicman, A.T., 2008. Pharmacology of anabolic steroids. Br. J. Pharmacol. 154, 502–521.

Marshall-Gradisnik, S., Green, R., Brenu, E.W., Weatherby, R.P., 2009. Anabolic androgenic steroids effects on the immune system: a review. Cent. Eur. J. Biol. 4 (1), 19–23.

Maung, A.A., Davis, K.A., 2012. Perioperative nutritional support: immunonutrition, probiotics, and anabolic steroids. Surg. Clin. North Am. 92 (2), 273–283.

Nyberg, F., Hallberg, M., 2012. Interactions between opioids and anabolic androgenic steroids: implications for the development of addictive behavior. Int. Rev. Neurobiol. 102, 189–206.

Oberlander, J.G., Henderson, L.P., 2012. The Sturm und Drang of anabolic steroid use: angst, anxiety, and aggression. Trends Neurosci. 35 (6), 382–392.

Pope, H.G., Ionescu-Pioggia, M., Pope, K.W., 2001. Drug use and life style among college undergraduates: a 30-year longitudinal study. Am. J. Psychiatry 158 (9), 1519–1521.

Rane, A., Ekström, L., 2012. Androgens and doping tests: genetic variation and pit-falls. Br. J. Clin. Pharmacol. 74 (1), 3–15.

Salvador, J.A.R., Carvalho, J.F.S., 2013. Anticancer steroids: linking natural and semi-synthetic compounds. Nat. Prod. Rep.. http://dx.doi.org/10.1039/C2NP20082A.

Scarth, J.P., Kay, J., Teale, P., 2012. A review of analytical strategies for the detection of 'endogenous' steroid abuse in food production. Drug Test. Anal. 4 (Suppl. 1), 40–49.

Stohs, S.J., Ray, S.D., 13 Sep 2012. A review and evaluation of the efficacy and safety of *Cissus quadrangularis* extracts. Phytother. Res.. http://dx.doi.org/10.1002/ptr.4846 [Epub ahead of print].

Strano-Rossi, S., Fiore, C., Chiarotti, M., Centini, F., 2011. Analytical techniques in androgen anabolic steroids (AASs) analysis for antidoping and forensic purposes. Mini Rev. Med. Chem. 11 (5), 451–458.

Relevant Websites

http://www.medicinenet.com/anabolic_steroid_abuse/article.htm – MedicineNet.com.

http://www.drugabuse.gov/drugs-abuse/steroids-anabolic – National Institute of Dramatic Art.

http://teens.drugabuse.gov/facts/facts_ster1.php – National Institute of Dramatic Art Teens.

http://www.vanderbilt.edu/AnS/psychology/health_psychology/anabolic_steroids.htm – Vanderbilt University.

Analytical Toxicology

SC Gad, Gad Consulting Services, Cary, NC, USA

Analytical toxicology is the use of qualitative and quantitative chemical, immunological, and physical techniques in sample preparation, separation, assay calibration, detection and identification, and quantification for toxicological research and testing. Examples of the objectives of such analysis include:

- Determining the levels of exposure to potential toxicants via air, water, or food.
- Verifying exposure levels to doses for animals in experimental studies.
- Determining levels of xenobiotics and their metabolites in animal studies.
- Screening blood and urine for the presence of illicit drugs or their metabolites.
- Measuring levels of endogenous compounds and molecules to evaluate organ function and damage (clinical chemistry).
- Identifying metabolites and macromolecular adjuncts to identify mechanisms of action.
- Evaluating and quantitating the formation and distribution of antibodies.

The diagnosis and treatment of health problems induced by chemical substances and the closely allied field of therapeutic drug monitoring rely on analytical toxicology, and advances in the field have added both power and problems to toxicology, dual gifts of increases in sensitivity and specificity. Although the analytes are present in matrices similar to those seen in forensic toxicology, the results must be reported rapidly to be of use to clinicians in treating patients. This requirement of a rapid turnaround time limits the number of chemicals that can be measured because methods, equipment, and personnel must all be available for an instant response to toxicological emergencies. Investigations for an 'unknown' drug or poison are usually carried out on specimens of urine (30 ml for qualitative tests) and blood (10 ml for quantitative tests). No preservatives should be added to urine specimens and blood samples should be heparinized.

Occupational and regulatory toxicology requires strict analytic procedures for implementation or monitoring. In occupational toxicology, the analytical methods used to monitor threshold limit values and other means of estimating the exposure of workers to toxic hazards may utilize simple, nonspecific, but economical screening devices. However, to determine the actual exposure of a worker, it is necessary to analyze blood, urine, breath, or another specimen by employing methods similar to those used in clinical or forensic toxicology. For regulatory purposes, a variety of matrices (e.g., food, water, and air) must be examined for extremely small quantities of analytes. Frequently, this requires the use of sophisticated methodology with extreme sensitivity. Both of these applications of analytical toxicology impinge on forensic toxicology because an injury or occupational disease in a worker can result in a legal proceeding.

Other applications of analytical toxicology occur frequently during the course of experimental studies. Confirmation of the concentration of dosing solutions and monitoring of their stability often can be accomplished with the use of simple analytical techniques. The bioavailability of a dose may vary with the route of administration and the vehicle used. Blood concentrations can be monitored as a means of establishing this important parameter. In addition, an important feature in the study of any toxic substance is the characterization of its metabolites as well as the distribution of the parent drug, together with its metabolites, to various tissues. This requires sensitive, specific, and valid analytical procedures. Similar analytical studies can be conducted within a temporal framework to gain an understanding of the dynamics of the absorption, distribution, metabolism, and excretion of toxic chemicals.

Analysis of Common Toxic Substances

Analytical toxicology is intimately involved in many aspects of experimental and applied toxicology. Because toxic substances include all chemical types and their measurement may require the examination of biological or nonbiological matrices, the scope of analytical toxicology is broad. Nevertheless, a systematic approach and a reliance on the practical experience of generations of forensic toxicologists can be used in conjunction with the sophisticated tools of analytical chemistry to provide the data needed to understand the hazards of toxic substances more completely. As Paracelsus states: "All substances are poisons: There is none which is not a poison." Analytical toxicology potentially encompasses all chemical substances. Forensic toxicologists learned long ago that when the nature of a suspected poison is unknown, a systematic, standardized approach must be used to identify the presence of most common toxic substances. An approach that has stood the test of time was first suggested by Chapuis in 1873 in *Elements de Toxicologie*. It is based on the origin or nature of the toxic agent. Such a categorization can be characterized as follows:

1. gases,
2. volatile substances,
3. corrosives,
4. metals,
5. anions and nonmetals,
6. nonvolatile organic substances, and
7. miscellaneous.

In addition to considering the descriptive classification of the substance, one must determine the method for separating a toxic agent from the matrix in which it is collected and embedded. The matrix is generally a biological specimen such as a body fluid or a solid tissue. The agent of interest may exist in the matrix in a simple solution or may be bound to protein and other cellular constituents. The challenge here is to separate the toxic agent in sufficient purity and quantity to permit it to be characterized and quantified. At times, the parent compound is no longer present in large enough amounts to be separated. In such cases, known metabolites may indirectly provide measure of the parent substance. With other

 http://dx.doi.org/10.1016/B978-0-12-386454-3.00812-5

substances, interaction of the poison with tissue components may require the isolation or characterization of a protein adduct. Methods for separation have long provided a great challenge to analytical toxicologists. Only recently have methods become available which permit direct measurement of some analytes without prior separation from the matrix.

The following sections provide a closer look at analytical toxicological issues related to substance class.

Gases

Gases are most simply measured by means of gas chromatography. Some gases are extremely labile, and the specimen must be collected and preserved at temperatures as low as that of liquid nitrogen. Generally, the gas is carefully liberated by incubating the specimen at a predetermined temperature in a closed container. The gas, freed from the matrix, collects over the specimen's 'headspace,' where it can be sampled and injected into the gas chromatograph. Other gases, such as carbon monoxide, interact with protein, or the adduct can be measured independently, as in the case of carboxyhemoglobin.

Volatile Substances

Volatile substances are generally liquids of a variety of chemical types. Gas–liquid chromatography is the simplest approach for simultaneous separation and quantitation in many cases. The simple alcohols can be measured by injecting a diluted body fluid directly onto the column of the chromatograph. A more common approach is to use the headspace technique, as is done for gases, after incubating the specimen at an elevated temperature.

Corrosives

Corrosives include mineral acids and bases. Many corrosives consist of ions that are normal tissue constituents. Clinical chemical techniques can be applied to detect these ions when they are in great excess over normal concentrations. Because these ions are normal constituents, the corrosive effects at the site of contact of the chemical, together with other changes in blood chemistry values, can confirm the ingestion of a corrosive substance.

Metals

Metals are encountered frequently as occupational and environmental hazards. Elegant analytical methods are available for most metals even when they are present at extremely low concentrations. Classical separation procedures involve destruction of the organic matrix by chemical or thermal oxidation. This leaves the metal to be identified and quantified in the inorganic residue. Unfortunately, this prevents a determination of the metal in the oxidation state or in combination with other elements, as it existed when the metal compound was absorbed. For example, the toxic effects of metallic mercury, mercurous ion, mercuric ion, and dimethyl mercury are all different. Analytical methods must be selected which determine the relative amount of each form present to yield optimal analytical results.

Toxic Anions and Nonmetals

Toxic anions and nonmetals are a difficult group for analysis. Some anions can be trapped in combination with a stable cation, after which the organic matrix can be destroyed, as with metals. Others can be separated from the bulk of the matrix by dialysis, after they are detected by colorimetric or chromatopathic procedures. Still others are detected and measured by ion-specific electrodes. There are no standard approaches for this group, and other than phosphorus, they are rarely encountered in an uncombined form.

Nonvolatile Organic Substances

Nonvolatile organic substances constitute the largest group of substances that must be considered by analytical toxicologists. This group includes drugs, both prescribed and illegal, pesticides, natural products, pollutants, and industrial compounds. These substances are solids of liquids with high boiling points. Thus, separation procedures generally rely on differential extractions, either liquid–liquid or solid–solid in nature. These extractions often are not efficient, and recovery of the toxic substance from the sample matrix may be poor. When the nature of the toxic substance is known, immunoassay procedures are useful because they allow a toxicologist to avoid using separation procedures. Such compounds can be classified as organic strong acids, organic weak acids, organic bases, organic neutral compounds, or organic amphoteric compounds.

Analytical Chemistry in Environmental Toxicology

There are many cases in which toxic agents are either present in an environment (or the life forms in an environment) or that they may be. This may pose special problems to an analytical chemist:

1. Accurately measuring exposure levels above ambient background levels.
2. Detection and accurate measurement of moieties in complex and natural matrices (i.e., seawater, soils, aquatic, and terrestrial organisms).
3. Identification and quantification of complex mixtures of chemical moieties at low levels.

Miscellaneous

Finally, a miscellaneous category must be included to cover the large number of toxic agents that cannot be detected by the routine application of the methods described previously. Venoms and other toxic mixtures of proteins or uncharacterized constituents fall into this class. Frequently, if antibodies can be grown against the active constituent, immunoassay may be the most practical means of detecting and measuring these highly potent and difficult to isolate substances.

Unfortunately, unless highly specific monoclonal antibodies are used, the analytical procedure may not be acceptable for forensic purposes. Frequently, specific analytical procedures must be developed for each analyte of this type. At times, biological endpoints are utilized to semiquantify the concentration of the isolated product.

Analytical Techniques

Due to increased levels of sensitivity of analytical techniques and a range of legal requirements (including Good Laboratory Practices and issues in potential litigation), particular care must be taken in collecting and handling samples to both avoid contamination and maintain a chain of custody of samples and sample records. There are a vast variety of techniques now employed in analysis:

- Chromatography
- Thin layer, gas, high-performance liquid chromatography
- Mass spectrometry
- Photometry/spectroscopy
- Spectrometry (ultraviolet, infrared, and visible light)
- Flame photometry, atomic absorption, nuclear magnetic resonance spectroscopy, electron spin resonance spectrophotometry, Raman spectroscopy
- Immunoassays
- Radioimmunoassay, enzyme immunoassay, fluorescent immunoassay
- Isotopic labeling
- Positron emission tomography
- Magnetic resonance imaging

Newer and more complex material analysis techniques are:

- Accelerator mass spectrophotometry
- Atomic absorption spectroscopy
- Auger electron spectroscopy
- Controlled potential coulometry
- Crystallographic texture measurement
- Electrogravimetry
- Electrometric titration
- Electron probe X-ray microanalysis
- Elemental and functional group analysis
- Extended X-ray absorption fine structure
- Ferromagnetic resonance
- Field ion microscopy
- High temperature combustion
- Image analysis
- Inert gas fusion
- Inductively coupled plasma
- Ion chromatography
- Low energy electron diffraction
- Low energy ion scattering spectroscopy
- Mass spectrometry
- Molecular fluorescence spectrometry
- Mossbauer spectroscopy
- Neutron activation analysis
- Neutron diffraction
- Optical emission spectroscopy
- Optical metallography membrane electrodes
- Particle induced X-ray emission potentiometric
- Radial distribution function analysis
- Radio analysis
- Rutherford backscattering spectroscopy
- Scanning electron microscopy
- Secondary ion mass spectroscopy
- Single crystal X-ray diffraction
- Small angle X-ray and neutron scattering
- Spark source mass spectrometry
- Transmission electron microscopy
- Voltammetry
- Wet analytical chemistry
- X-ray diffraction residual stress techniques
- X-ray photoelectron spectroscopy
- X-ray powder diffraction
- X-ray spectrometry
- X-ray topography

See also: International Society of Exposure Science; Microarray Analysis.

Further Reading

Analytical toxicology for clinical, forensic and pharmaceutical chemists. In: Brandenberger, H., Maes, R.A.A. (Eds.), Clinical Biochemistry, vol. 5. Walter de Gruyter Inc, Berlin.

Baselt, R.C., 2011. The Disposition of Toxic Drugs and Chemicals in Man, ninth ed. Biomedical Publications, Seal Beach, CA, pp. 1900.

Blanke, R.V., Decker, W.J., 1999. Analysis of toxic substances. In: Tietz, N.W. (Ed.), Textbook of Clinical Chemistry, third ed. Saunders, Philadelphia, pp. 1670–1744.

Caldwell, W.S., Byrd, G.D., deEthizy, J.D., Warthen, G.D., 2008. Modern instrumental methods for studying mechanisms of toxicity. In: Hayes, A.W. (Ed.), Principles and Methods of Toxicology, fifth ed. CRC Press, Boca Raton, FL, pp. 2041–2112.

Flanagan, R.J., et al., 2007. Fundamentals of Analytical Toxicology. John Wiley and Sons, Chichester, England.

Maurer, H.H., 2010. Analytical toxicology. EXS 100, 317–337.

Stahr, H.M., 1991. Analytical Methods in Toxicology. Wiley, New York, pp. 328.

Relevant Websites

http://www.jatox.com – Journal of Analytical Toxicology. Preston Publications, Niles, IL.

http://www.who.int/pcs/publications/training_poisons/basic_analytical_tox/en/index.html – WHO basic analytical tox

Ancient Warfare and Toxicology

A Mayor, Stanford University, Palo Alto, CA, USA

Historical Use of Natural Toxins

In antiquity, natural toxins were exploited to make poison weapons for waging the earliest forms of biological and chemical warfares. A wide range of substances, from toxic plants and venomous insects and reptiles to infectious agents and noxious chemicals, were weaponized in ancient Europe, the Mediterranean, North Africa, the Middle East, Central Asia, India, China, and in the Americas. Evidence for the concept and practice of toxic warfare can be traced back thousands of years. For example, cuneiform tablets from about 1200 BC record that the Hittites of Asia Minor deliberately drove plague victims into enemy territory.

Such practices did not require a scientific understanding of toxicology, epidemiology, and chemistry, or depend on advanced technology, but were based on centuries of observation and experimentation with easily available toxic materials. Strategies based on insidiously attacking an opponent's biological vulnerabilities with poisonous agents could be advantageous while the facing troops were superior in number, courage, skill, or technology. Yet the use of toxic weapons also entailed practical and ethical dilemmas in antiquity.

The first poison projectiles were probably devised for hunting and then turned toward war. The bow and arrow was a highly effective delivery system for toxins at an early date, since a mere scratch from a treated point could be fatal.

Toxic Weapons in Mythology

The concept of poisoned projectiles is embedded in the ancient Greek language, since the word for 'poison', toxicon, is derived from toxon, the word for 'arrow'. Greek mythology offers further evidence of the antiquity of the concept. The great hero of myth, Hercules, for example, invented biological weaponry when he dipped his arrows in the venom of the *Hydra* monster, a many-headed serpent. Homer's *Iliad*, an oral epic first written down in the eighth century BC, contains indirect allusions to the use of toxic projectiles in the legendary Trojan War. Homer's descriptions of black (rather than red) blood oozing from wounds, battlefield doctors sucking out poisons, and never-healing wounds are all hallmarks of snake venom poisoning. In the *Odyssey*, Homer describes the Greek hero Odysseus smearing lethal plant juices on arrows intended for enemies. According to myth, Odysseus himself died from a wound inflicted by a spear tipped with the toxic spine of a marbled stingray, a common species in the Mediterranean.

The epic poem recounting the legendary history of Rome, the *Aeneid* by Virgil, also refers to poisoned spears wielded by the early Romans, and poisoned weapons appear in the mythological epic of India, the *Rigveda*. Myth and legend likely reflect the early invention of biological arms in various cultures and they also offered models for the actual practice of biological warfare.

Plant Poisons in Biological Warfare

About 24 toxic Eurasian plant species, often employed as medicines in tiny dosages, were collected to make arrow poisons or other biological weapons used in historical battles. One of the most popular plant drugs was hellebore, identified by the ancients as black hellebore (probably the Christmas rose of the buttercup Ranunculaceae family, *Helleborus niger*) and white hellebore (the lily family, Liliaceae). The unrelated plants are each laden with powerful chemicals that cause severe vomiting and diarrhea, muscle cramps, delirium, convulsions, asphyxia, and heart attack. Hellebore was one of the arrow drugs used by the Gauls, among other groups, and it was also used to poison wells.

Another favorite biowar toxin was aconite or monkshood (also called wolfsbane). Aconitum (buttercup family) contains the alkaloid aconitine, a violent poison, which in high doses causes vomiting and paralyzes the nervous system, resulting in death. Aconite was employed by the archers of ancient Greece and India, and its use in warfare continued into modernity. For example, during the war between the Spanish and the Moors in 1483, Arab archers wrapped aconite-soaked cotton around their arrowheads. Nepalese Gurkhas poisoned wells with aconite in the nineteenth century, and during World War II, Nazi scientists created aconitine-treated bullets.

Henbane (*Hyoscyamus niger*), a sticky, bad-smelling weed containing the powerful narcotics hyoscyamine and scopolamine, was also collected as arrow poison in antiquity. Henbane causes violent seizures, psychosis, and death. Other plant juices used on projectiles included hemlock (*Conium maculatum*), yew (*Taxus baccata*), rhododendron, and several species of deadly nightshade or belladonna, which causes vertigo, extreme agitation, coma, and death. The fact that the Latin word for deadly nightshade was *dorycnion*, 'spear drug', suggests that it was smeared on weapons at a very early date, as noted by Pliny the Elder, a natural historian of the first century AD.

Snake Venom in Biological Warfare

Snake venom was another well-known arrow poison. Since snake venom is digestible, it could be safely used for hunting because the venom did not make game harmful to eat, but the venom in the bloodstream of an enemy brought a painful death or a never-healing wound. Numerous poisonous snakes exist around the Mediterranean and in Africa and Asia.

According to the Greek and Roman writers, archers who steeped their arrows in serpents' venom included the Gauls, the Dacians and Dalmatians (of the Balkans), the Sarmatians of Persia (now Iran), the Getae of Thrace, Slavs, Armenians, Parthians between the Indus and Euphrates, Indians, North Africans, and the Scythian nomads of the Central Asian steppes. According to the ancient Greek geographer Strabo, the arrow

 http://dx.doi.org/10.1016/B978-0-12-386454-3.00996-9

poison concocted by the Soanes of the Caucasus was so noxious that its mere odor was injurious. Strabo also reported that people of what is now Kenya dipped their arrows 'in the gall of serpents', while the Roman historian Silius Italicus described the snake venom arrows used by the archers of Libya, Morocco, Egypt, and Sudan. Ancient Chinese sources show that arrow poisons were also in use in China at early dates. In the Americas, Native Americans used snake, frog, and plant poisons on projectiles for hunting and warfare.

Complex recipes for envenomed arrows are recorded in Greek and Latin texts. One of the most dreaded arrow drugs was concocted by the Scythians, who combined snake venom and bacteriological agents from rotting dung, human blood, and putrefying viper carcasses bloated with feces. Even in the case of a superficial arrow wound, the toxins would begin taking effect within an hour. Envenomation accompanied by shock, necrosis, and suppuration of the wound would be followed by gangrene and tetanus and an agonizing death.

Several snake species contributed the venom used by the Scythians, including the steppe viper *Vipera ursinii renardi*, the Caucasus viper *Vipera kaznakovi*, the European adder *Vipera berus*, and the long-nosed or sand viper *Vipera ammodytes transcaucasiana*. In ancient India, one of the most feared poisons was derived from the rotting flesh and venom of the white-headed Purple Snake, described by the natural historian Aelian (third century AD). His detailed description suggests that the Purple Snake was the rare, white-headed viper discovered by modern herpetologists in the late 1880s, *Azemiops feae*.

Different snake venoms tipped the arrows encountered by the army of Alexander the Great in his conquest of India in 327–325 BC. According to the historians Quintus Curtius, Diodorus of Sicily, and others, the defenders of Harmatelia (Mansura, Pakistan) had smeared their arrows and swords with an unknown snake poison. Most modern historians assume cobra poison, but the ancient historians' detailed description of the gruesome deaths suffered by Alexander's men points to the deadly Russell's viper. Even the slightly wounded went immediately numb and experienced stabbing pain and wracking convulsions. Their skin became cold and livid and they vomited bile. Black froth exuded from the wounds and then purple-green gangrene spread rapidly, followed by death. Death from cobra venom is relatively painless, from respiratory paralysis, but the Russell's viper causes numbness, vomiting, severe pain, black blood, gangrene, and death – as described by Alexander's historians.

Poisoning Water and Food

Tainting water and food was another ancient biological tactic. A legendary Greek account set in about 1000 BC tells how King Cnopus conquered Erythrae (in what is now Turkey) by drugging a bull and tricking the enemy into eating the poisoned meat. The earliest historically documented case of poisoning drinking water occurred in Greece in about 590 BC, during the First Sacred War. Athens and allied city-states made war on the strongly fortified city of Kirrha, which controlled the road to Delphi, the site of the famous Oracle of Apollo. According to several ancient Greek historians, Kirrha had offended the God and was therefore to be totally destroyed. During the siege, the league of allies gathered a great quantity of hellebore and placed it in the water pipes supplying Kirrha. The soldiers guarding Kirrha's walls – and the entire population – fell violently ill and the allies easily overran the city and wiped out combatants and civilians alike. After the war, Athens and her allies had second thoughts and agreed among themselves not to interfere with water supplies should they ever find themselves at war with each other.

Roman commanders also poisoned wells. Manius Aquillius, for example, ended a long-drawn-out war to quell insurrections in the Roman province of Asia Minor in 129 BC, by pouring poison into the springs supplying the rebelling cities. According to the Roman historian Florus, however, his victory was dishonorable because of the resort to underhanded biological tactics.

The Carthaginian generals Himilco and Maharbal overcame enemies in North Africa by tainting wine with mandrake, a heavily narcotic root of the deadly nightshade. In North America, Native Americans poisoned enemy's drinking water with rotting animal skins. In ancient India, numerous recipes for poisoning enemy food and water are given in the *Arthashastra*, a warfare manual dating to the fourth century BC, written by Kautilya, the advisor of King Chandragupta.

In 65 BC, naturally occurring toxic honey was used against the army of the Roman general Pompey during the war against King Mithradates VI of Pontus. In the Black Sea region, Mithradates' allies set out tempting honeycombs along the Romans' route and hid. The honey was made by wild bees that gathered nectar from rhododendron blossoms, which contain devastating neurotoxins. As the legionnaires succumbed to the sweet treat, collapsing with vertigo, vomiting, and diarrhea, the enemy ambushed and slaughtered about 1,000 of Pompey's men.

Stinging Insects and Biting Snakes in Biological Warfare

Stinging insects such as wasps, deadly vipers, and scorpions could also be drafted for war. Perhaps, as early as Neolithic times, hives filled with furious bees were thrown at enemies, who were driven into chaos by the painful stings; and later, catapults were used to hurl beehives. The ancient Maya of Central Mexico created ingenious booby traps to repel besiegers on their fortress walls, consisting of dummy warriors whose gourd heads were filled with hornets.

In the second century BC, the Carthaginian general Hannibal devised a plan of filling clay pots with live vipers during a naval battle against Pergamum, in which he was outnumbered. The enemy sailors were panicked and easily defeated when the catapulted pots smashed on their ships' decks, releasing masses of snakes.

At the fortified city of Hatra (Iraq), in AD 198–199, besieging Roman legions led by Emperor Septimius Severus were forced to retreat after the Hatreni defended their walls with insect bombs. They had packed terracotta pots with scorpions (arthropods), assassin bugs, and other poisonous insects from the surrounding desert. The historian Herodian wrote that as the insects rained down on the Romans scaling the walls, they "fell into the men's eyes and exposed parts of their bodies, digging in, biting, and stinging the soldiers, causing severe injuries." The terror effect would be impressive, no matter how many men were actually stung. Scorpion stings inject a complex combination of toxins, causing intense pain, thirst, great agitation, muscle spasms, convulsions, slow pulse, irregular breathing, and torturous death. Assassin bugs, predatory, bloodsucking insects with sharp beaks, inflict an extremely painful bite and inject a lethal nerve poison that liquefies tissues. It is possible that *Paederus* beetles were also collected by the Hatreni. Pederin, the virulent poison secreted by predatory Staphylinidae (rove) beetles was well-known in ancient India and China. One of the most powerful animal toxins in the world, pederin is a blistering agent on the skin and eyes, and in the bloodstream its toxicity is more potent than cobra venom.

Contagions as Biological Warfare Agents

Many historians have considered the Mongols' ploy of catapulting of bubonic plague victims over the walls at Kaffa on the Black Sea in 1346 to mark the beginning of biological warfare. But an empirical understanding of contagion developed much earlier in history. In Mesopotamia in 1770 BC, for example, cuneiform tablets warned that disease could be spread by fomites, infectious pathogens on clothing, bedding, and other items. Legends about King Solomon suggested that he hid plague in sealed jars in the Temple of Jerusalem to infect Babylonian and Roman invaders. During the Peloponnesian War (fourth century BC), the Athenians suspected that the Spartans had spread plague (apparently smallpox) by poisoning their wells. In ancient India, Kautilya's *Arthashastra* suggested ways of infecting enemies with illnesses such as fevers, wasting lung disease, and rabies.

In Roman times, historians such as Seneca and Dio Cassius deplored "man-made pestilence," the malicious transmission of plagues by saboteurs who pricked victims with infected needles during the reigns of Domitian and Commodus in the first and second centuries AD. The Great Plague of AD 165–180, probably smallpox, was spread from Babylon (modern Iraq) to Syria, Italy, and Germany by Roman soldiers returning from the war to control Mesopotamia. According to historians of the era, the epidemic began when some Roman soldiers looted a treasure chest in an enemy temple in Babylonia. The implication of the historical accounts, that the chest was booby trapped with plague-laden items, is plausible. The local population would have had some immunity to the epidemic, while the invading Roman army would have been vulnerable. At the very least, the reports demonstrate that the notion of deliberately spreading epidemics among the enemy was widely contemplated by that time.

Toxic Aerosols and Incendiaries as Chemical Weapons

Asphyxiating clouds of smoke, dust, and gases were effective chemical weapons in antiquity. One of the earliest documented examples of toxic aerosols occurred during the Peloponnesian War in 429 BC, when Sparta besieged the city of Plataea. As reported by the historian Thucydides, the Spartans created a massive fire next to Plataea's city walls, and fueled the conflagration with liberal quantities of resinous pine tree sap and sulfur. The combination of pitch and sulfur created clouds of toxic sulfur dioxide gas, fumes that can be fatal when inhaled in large amounts. A few years later, in 424 BC, the Spartans' allies the Boiotians invented a 'flamethrowing' machine to propel noxious smoke from charcoal, resin, and sulfur used against the walled city of Delium.

Archaeologists have discovered physical evidence to show that in AD 256, the Sassanians attacking Roman-held Dura-Europos (on the modern border of Iraq and Syria) created a similar incendiary mixture that resulted in a deadly gas enveloping a siege tunnel, killing 19 Romans and 1 Sassanian.

The Greek strategist Aeneas the Tactician, writing in 360 BC, suggested the use of incendiaries made with pitch, hemp, and sulfur. Roman historians tell how burning chicken feathers created irritating, choking fumes propelled by bellows into siege tunnels.

In 80 BC, the Roman general Sertorius deployed choking clouds of dust to defeat the Characitani of Spain, who had taken refuge in inaccessible caves. The fine white soil in the area consisted of limestone and gypsum. Sertorius ordered his soldiers to pile great heaps of the powder in front of the caves. When the wind was right, the Romans stirred up the dust and raised great clouds of caustic lime powder, a severe irritant to the eyes and lungs. The Characitani surrendered.

A similar dust was used in China to quell an armed peasant revolt in AD 178, when 'lime chariots' equipped with bellows blew limestone powder into the crowds. The powdered lime interacts with the moist membranes of the eyes, nose, and throat with corrosive, burning effect, blinding and suffocating the victims.

In the Middle East, where petroleum is abundant, naphtha (the volatile and toxic light fraction of oil) was ignited and poured on attackers. The ancient Indians and Chinese added 'fire chemicals' to their incendiaries, explosive saltpeter or nitrite salts, a key ingredient of gunpowder, and they also mixed a great variety of plant, animal, and mineral poisons, such as arsenic and lead, in smoke and fire bombs. In the New World and in India, the seeds of toxic plants and hot peppers were burned to rout attackers.

Practical and Ethical Issues

The toxicity of plants, venoms, and other poisons used in armaments posed perils to those who wielded them, and the mythology and the history of poison weapons is rife with examples of accidental self-injury and unintended collateral damage. The use of windborne toxins also involved 'blowback' problems, as acknowledged by Kautilya in his *Arthashastra*. He advised that protective salves and other remedies be applied before deploying poisonous smokes. Toxic weapons are notoriously difficult to control and often resulted in the destruction of noncombatants as well as soldiers, especially in siege situations.

The use of poisons in warfare led to a search for antidotes. Ancient sources list hundreds of substances that are believed to counteract specific weaponized poisons, from rust filings to poultices made from medicinal plants. It was also believed that one could become invulnerable to toxins by ingesting minute amounts of various poisons over time. Mithradates VI of Pontus (d. 63 BC) was an early experimenter in creating a 'universal antidote', later known as mithridatium and ingested by Roman emperors such as Nero and Marcus Aurelius, and later by European royalty, to gain immunity to poisoning.

The use of toxic weapons was surrounded by ambivalence in antiquity, though there were few rules of war governing their use. Weapons that delivered hidden poisons to make an enemy defenseless or experience excessive suffering aroused moral criticism in many cultures, even as their use was rationalized in numerous recorded instances. Ancient Greeks considered poisoned projectiles a cowardly weapon, for example, yet their mythic heroes, Hercules and Odysseus, resorted to such arms, and well poisoning and toxic aerosols were used in historical Greek conflicts. Poisoned arrows and tainting water and food supplies were deplored by many Romans, yet their generals occasionally turned to such strategies. The Hindu *Laws of Manu* (dating to 500 BC) recommended spoiling the enemy's food and water but forbade the use of poisoned arrows. In the same era, Kautilya's *Arthashastra* extolled the advantages of poisoning projectiles, food, and water and asphyxiating foes with chemical and disease-laden clouds of smoke. Notably, Kautilya stressed the deterrent effect of publicizing the horrid ingredients of one's toxic arsenal, a strategy also embraced by the Scythians and others in broadcasting their recipes for poison arrows. Sun Tzu's *Art of War* (500 BC) praised deceptive terror strategies based on fire and Chinese treatises give myriad recipes for toxic aerosols and incendiaries. On the other hand, humanitarian codes of war in China (450–200 BC) forbade ruses of war and harming noncombatants.

Self-defense was often a rationale for the use of toxic weapons. Besieged cities and desperate populations overcome by overwhelming invaders turned to biological weapons as a last resort. Some commanders used poisons in frustration to break stalemates or long sieges. Other situations, such as holy wars, quelling rebellions, and fighting people considered 'barbarians', encouraged the indiscriminate use of bioweapons against entire population. The threat of horrifying toxic weapons could discourage would-be attackers or bring quick capitulation. Some commanders had no compunctions about using any weapons at hand, and in some cultures poison arrows were the customary weapons in both hunting and warfare.

The scope of human ingenuity in weaponizing natural forces in antiquity is impressive, and many of the ancient examples anticipated, in substance or principle, almost every basic form of biological and chemical weapon known today, from spreading plague to poisoning water. For example, asphyxiating smokes were precursors of mustard and other toxic gases first used in World War I. Red hot sand catapulted onto Alexander the Great's men in the fourth century BC is analogous to modern thermite bombs of World War II. The burning, adhering effects of ancient petroleum incendiaries were reproduced in the modern invention of napalm so notorious during the Vietnam War. Even the advanced stench and noise weapons, the so-called calmatives in mists or water supplies, and top secret insect and animal-based weapons developed by modern military scientists all have antecedents in the ancient world.

Nor are the dangers of self-injury and disposing of poison weapons anything new. The ancient myth of the *Hydra* with its ever-proliferating heads is a fitting symbol of the dilemmas off creating toxic arms. Faced with the problem of disposing of the immortal central head of the *Hydra*, Hercules buried it deep in the ground and placed a huge boulder as a marker over the spot. A similar geological solution is used today to dispose off toxic and nuclear weapons material, with burial deep underground in the deserts of New Mexico and Nevada, necessitating warnings to future generations about the perils of biochemical agents. A model for avoiding the proliferation of toxic weaponry is also found in Greek myth. The archer who inherited Hercules' *Hydra*-venom arrows had experienced grievous injury from the arrows himself, before he deployed them against the Trojans. After the Trojan War, he dedicated the poisonous arrows to a temple of Apollo, the god of healing, rather than passing them on to the next generation of warriors.

See also: Animals, Poisonous and Venomous; Chemical Warfare Delivery Systems; Chemical Warfare During WW1; Plants, Poisonous; Toxicology in the Arts, Culture, and Imagination.

Further Reading

James, S., 2011. Stratagems, combat, and "chemical warfare" in the siege mines of Dura-Europos. American Journal of Archaeology 115, 69–101.

Jones, D., 2007. Poison Arrows: North American Indian Hunting and Warfare. University of Texas Press, Austin, TX.

Kautilya, 1992. Arthashastra (Trans. L.N. Rangarajan). Penguin Classics, Delhi.

Lockwood, J., 2009. Six-Legged Soldiers: Using Insects as Weapons of War. Oxford University Press, Oxford, UK.

Mayor, A., 2009. Greek Fire, Poison Arrows and Scorpion Bombs: Biological and Chemical Warfare in the Ancient World. Overlook Press, New York, NY.

Sawyer, R., 2007. The Tao of Deception: Unorthodox Warfare in Historic and Modern China. Basic Books, New York, NY.

Androgens

PS Rao, Sanofi, Bridgewater, NJ, USA

This article is a revision of the previous edition article by Prathibha S. Rao and Harihara M. Mehendale, volume 1, pp 121–125, © 2005, Elsevier Inc.

- Name: Androgens
- Chemical Abstracts Service Registry Number: D00072800
- Synonym: Male sex hormones
- Chemical Structure: Testosterone (middle) is a potent androgen; most androgens (middle) and estrogens are produced from biotransformation of cholesterol (left)

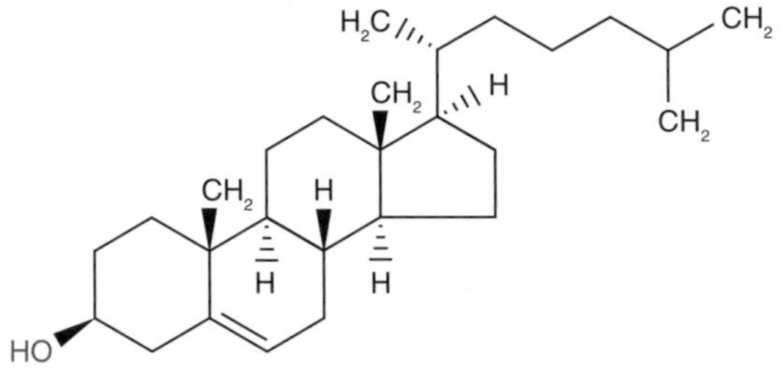

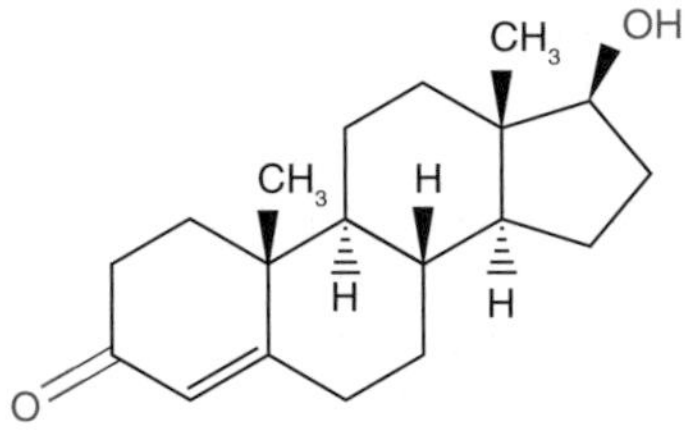

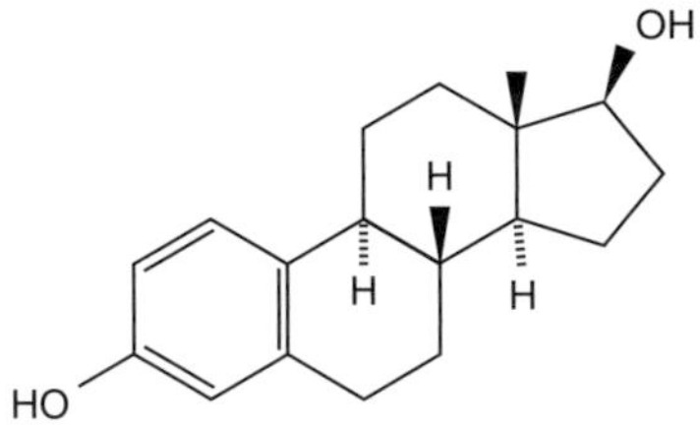

Background

A subset of androgens, adrenal androgens, includes any of the 19-carbon steroids synthesized by the adrenal cortex, the outer portion of the adrenal gland (zonula reticularis – innermost region of the adrenal cortex), that function as weak steroids or steroid precursors, including dehydroepiandrosterone (DHEA), dehydroepiandrosterone sulfate (DHEA-S), and androstenedione.

Besides testosterone, other androgens include the following:

Dehydroepiandrosterone (DHEA): a steroid hormone produced in the adrenal cortex from cholesterol. It is the primary precursor of natural estrogens. DHEA is also called dehydroisoandrosterone or dehydroandrosterone.

Androstenedione (Andro): an androgenic steroid produced by the testes, adrenal cortex, and ovaries. While androstenediones are converted metabolically to testosterone and other androgens, they are also the parent structure of estrone.

Androstenediol: the steroid metabolite that is thought to act as the main regulator of gonadotropin secretion.

Androsterone: a chemical by-product created during the breakdown of androgens, or derived from progesterone, that also exerts minor masculinizing effects, but with one-seventh the intensity of testosterone. It is found in approximately equal amounts in the plasma and urine of both males and females.

Dihydrotestosterone (DHT): a metabolite of testosterone, and a more potent androgen than testosterone in that it binds more strongly to androgen receptors. It is produced in the adrenal cortex.

Uses

Androgens/systemic testosterone are primarily indicated in males as replacement therapy when congenital or acquired endogenous androgen absence or deficiency is associated with primary or secondary hypogonadism. Primary hypogonadism includes conditions such as testicular failure due to cryptorchidism, bilateral torsion, orchitis, or vanishing testis syndrome; orchidectomy; Klinefelter's syndrome; chemotherapy; or toxic damage from alcohol or heavy metals. Hypogonadotropic hypogonadism (secondary hypogonadism) conditions include idiopathic gonadotropin or luteinizing-hormone-releasing hormone deficiency or pituitary-hypothalamic injury as a result of tumors, trauma, or radiation and are the most common forms of hypogonadism seen in older adults.

Acute and Short-Term Toxicity

Animal

Six adult male baboons received weekly intramuscular injections of 200 mg testosterone enanthate (equivalent to 8 mg kg^{-1} body weight) for up to 28 weeks, while two control animals received weekly injections of the vehicle only. Quantitative increases in the weight and volume of both prostatic lobes were seen after 15 weeks of treatment, and by week 28 there was an increase in stromal tissue with papillary ingrowth or invagination of glandular epithelium in the caudal lobe of the prostate. The serum concentrations of testosterone and dihydrotestosterone were significantly elevated, from 10 and 2–3 ng ml^{-1} to 30–40 and 5–6 ng ml^{-1}, respectively. The androstenedione concentrations were increased by three to four times and that of estradiol from 20 to 80–90 pg ml^{-1}. From this study, it was concluded that these steroids play a direct role in inducing early benign prostate hypertrophy in baboons and that their observations were similar to those in human benign prostate hypertrophy.

 http://dx.doi.org/10.1016/B978-0-12-386454-3.00237-2

Human

Androgens may have a virilizing effect in women. The undesirable manifestations include acne, growth of facial hair, and coarsening of the voice. Profound virilization and serious disturbances in the growth and osseous development can occur when androgens are given to children. The capacity of androgens to enhance epiphyseal closure in children may persist for several months after discontinuation of the drug. All androgens should be used with great care in children. Androgens should not be used during pregnancy since they cross the placenta and cause masculinization of the female fetus. Feminizing effects, particularly gynecomastia, can occur in men who receive androgens. The feminizing effects are particularly severe in children and men with liver disease.

Water retention due to sodium chloride (salt) is a common manifestation that leads to weight gain. Edema is also found in patients with cardiac heart failure, renal insufficiency, liver cirrhosis, and hypoproteinemia. When large doses are used to treat neoplastic diseases, compounds with 17-alkyl substitutions can cause cholestatic hepatitis; at high doses, jaundice is the most common clinical feature with accumulation of bile in the bile capillaries. Jaundice usually develops after 2–5 months of therapy. It can be detected by increases in plasma aspartate aminotransferase and alkaline phosphatase.

Obstructive sleep apnea (OSA) causes a mild lowering of blood testosterone concentrations that is rectified by effective continuous positive airway pressure (CPAP) treatment. Although testosterone treatment has precipitated OSA and has potential adverse effects on sleep in older men, the prevalence of OSA precipitated by testosterone treatment remains unclear. It appears to be a rare idiosyncratic reaction among younger hypogonadal men but the risk may be higher among older men as the background prevalence of OSA rises steeply with age. Hence, screening for OSA by asking about daytime sleepiness and partner reports of loud and irregular snoring, especially among overweight men with large collar size, is wise for older men starting testosterone treatment although not routinely required for young men with classical hypogonadism.

Chronic Toxicity (or Exposure)

Animal

The effects of subcutaneously injected or implanted testosterone and its esters have been reviewed extensively. The working group convened by the International Agency for Research on Cancer concluded that "there is sufficient evidence for the carcinogenicity of testosterone in experimental animals. In the absence of adequate data in humans, it is reasonable, for practical purposes, to regard testosterone as if it presented a carcinogenic risk to humans." The relevance of animal models to human prostate disorders has been reviewed. Besides humans, dogs are the only animals that develop prostatic cancer and benign prostatic hyperplasia at a high frequency. In this model, long-term treatment with androgens and estrogens is required to produce hyperplasia, although such synergism is not observed in other species. ACI rats spontaneously develop histologically evident prostatic cancer, which does not progress to clinically relevant disease when pharmacologically relevant amounts of exogenous androgen are administered. Prostate cancer has been induced only in the Noble and Lobund–Wistar strains of rat.

The role of hormones, including androgens, in the development of mammary neoplasia in rodents and their relevance to human risk assessment has been reviewed. Endogenous androgens are necessary for mammary development in rodents, and it was noted that rodent models mimic some but not all the complex external and endogenous factors involved in initiation, promotion, and progression of carcinogenesis. Tumor type and incidence are influenced by the age, reproductive history, and the endocrine milieu of the host at the time of exposure. The spontaneous incidence of tumors differs in different strains of rats and mice. In rats, most spontaneous neoplasias, with the exception of leukemia, occur in endocrine organs or organs under endocrine control. Russo and Russo concluded that mechanism-based toxicology is not yet sufficient for human risk assessment and the approach should be coupled to and validated by conventional long-term bioassays.

Fischer 344 rats were given 3,20-dimethyl-4aminobiphenyl (a prostate carcinogen) at 50 mg kg^{-1} body weight 10 times at 2 week intervals, and then, from week 20, testosterone propionate and/or diethylstilbestrol by subcutaneous silastic implant for 40 weeks, as seven cycles of 30-day treatment and 10-day withdrawal. Intermittent administration of testosterone resulted in suppression of the development of ventral prostate adenocarcinomas and slight (nonsignificant) increases in the incidences of invasive carcinomas of the lateral prostate and seminal vesicles. Diethylstilbestrol completely suppressed tumorigenesis, and the combination with testosterone propionate inhibited prostate tumor development.

Hydroxyprogesterone caproate was given intramuscularly every other week at an average dose of 13 mg to 19 female rabbits, and testosterone ethanate was given intramuscularly every other week at an average dose of 15 mg to 21 animals; both treatments were given for up to 763 days. Rabbits treated with progesterone developed numerous endometrial cysts, sometimes associated with atypical hyperplasia; active mammary secretion was also seen. Treatment with testosterone induced two adenomatous polyps of the endometrium in one animal, but no other noteworthy endometrial changes were found, and one control animal developed similar polyps. Neither significantly altered other tissues such as the ovary, adrenal, thyroid, or pituitary gland. No precancerous endometrial changes or cancers were found.

Human

With prolonged treatment, as in long-term use of androgens in mammary carcinoma, male pattern baldness, excessive body hair, prominent musculature, and hypertrophy of the clitoris may develop and may be irreversible. Patients receiving the 17a-alkyl substituted androgens may develop hepatic adenocarcinoma; the complications may be more common in people with Fanconi's anemia.

Chronic Poisoning

Ingestion: Hepatic damage, manifest as derangement of biochemical tests of liver function and sometimes severe enough to cause jaundice; virilization in women; prostatic hypertrophy, impotence and azoospermia in men; acne, abnormal lipids, premature cardiovascular disease (including stroke and myocardial infarction), abnormal glucose tolerance, and muscular hypertrophy in both sexes; psychiatric disturbances can occur during or after prolonged treatment.

Parenteral exposure: Virilization in women; prostatic hypertrophy, impotence, and azoospermia in men; acne, abnormal lipids, premature cardiovascular disease (including stroke and myocardial infarction), abnormal glucose tolerance, and muscular hypertrophy in both sexes. Psychiatric disturbances can occur during or after prolonged treatment. Hepatic damage is not expected from parenteral preparations.

Course, prognosis, cause of death: Patients with symptoms of acute poisoning are expected to recover rapidly. Patients who persistently abuse high doses of anabolic steroids are at risk of death from premature heart disease or cancer, especially prostatic cancer. Nonfatal but long-lasting effects include voice changes in women and fusion of the epiphyses in children. Other effects are reversible over weeks or months.

Genotoxicity

Testosterone and its esters are not mutagenic in bacteria. This also holds for methylnortestosterone (MENT) (Organon, unpublished data). The anabolics trenbolone, fluoxymesterone, and oxymetholone were found negative in bacterial and mammalian cell systems with equivocal results at highly toxic concentrations for trenbolone in the mouse lymphoma L5178Y TK system.

Carcinogenicity

See Chronic Toxicity (Animal) section above.

Toxicokinetics

Injected as oil, androgens are so quickly absorbed, metabolized, and excreted that the effect is very small. Esters of testosterone are more slowly absorbed and are more effective. The majority of the androgens is inactivated primarily in the liver and involves oxidation of the hydroxy groups and reduction of the steroid ring. Alkylation at the 17-position retards hepatic metabolism and hence is effective orally.

About 90% of the androgens are excreted in the urine; 6% appear in the feces after undergoing enterohepatic circulation. Small amounts are also excreted as soluble glucuronide and sulfate conjugates. Many of the synthetic androgens have a longer half-life. Unaltered compounds are excreted in the urine and feces.

Clinical Management

Edema due to salt retention is generally treated with diuretics targeted at increased sodium excretion.

Environmental Fate

Hormones excreted in animal waste have been measured in surface and groundwater associated with manure that is applied to the land surface. Limited studies have been done on the fate and transport of androgenic hormones in soils. There were weak correlations of sorption with soil particle size, organic matter, and specific surface area. Testosterone was the dominant compound present in the soil column effluents; although it was found that testosterone degraded more readily than 17β-estradiol, it appeared to have a greater potential to migrate in the soil because it was not strongly absorbed.

Ecotoxicology

The Endocrine disruption in the marine environment (EDMAR) program investigated evidence of changes associated with endocrine disruption in marine life and, if so, the possible causes and potential impacts. It followed on from work that demonstrated that flounder in some UK estuaries had changes consistent with endocrine disruption. Male flounder from some industrialized estuaries showed strong vitellogenin induction. Caught sand gobies exhibited no vitellogenin induction or intersex, but feminization of secondary sexual characteristics was observed in male gobies in some estuaries. Viviparous blennies in some estuaries showed induction of vitellogenin, and incidence of intersex. Toxicity identification and evaluation (TIE) procedures deployed on the Tyne and Tees estuaries identified three natural (steroidal) and two industrial (surfactant and phthalate) estrogenic compounds as possible causes of the observed effects. A study utilizing fathead minnows was conducted to study the differences in the reproductive biology between groups of minnows from a stream directly below the effluent outfall from a feedlot, from a stream that receives runoff from an agricultural field with disbursed cattle, and from uncontaminated areas upstream from the two previous sample areas. The size, sex hormone levels, and gonads of the sampled fish were tested for the effects of trenbolone-β, an active synthetic anabolic steroid. The female fish near the contaminated areas were found to have higher levels of androgens in their systems and smaller distances between internal organs than those from upstream. Similarly, male minnows had smaller testicles and closer internal organs than those from uncontaminated waters. No pathology was apparent in the ovaries or testicles of the fish collected in the contaminated water.

Other Hazards

For men and women, the use of male steroids (androgens) – either the hormone testosterone or the synthetic anabolic steroids – may also increase the risk of coronary artery disease. These drugs lower high-density lipoprotein (HDL) (the good) cholesterol levels, increase low-density lipoprotein (LDL) (the bad) cholesterol levels, and cause high blood pressure. All of these effects may contribute to having a heart attack at an early age or to having a stroke. What effects the use of anabolic steroids early in life has later in life are unclear. Although mind-altering drugs typically are those that have potential for abuse, several other drugs that do not alter the mind (or do so only occasionally) are often taken without medical need, even when doing so endangers the quality of life or health and safety of the user. Using a drug this way is considered drug abuse. People who stop abusing any of these drugs do not experience withdrawal symptoms, but they may experience medical problems when the drug is discontinued abruptly (problems that are usually preventable if discontinuation is supervised by a doctor). Anabolic steroids are very similar to the hormone testosterone. They have many physical effects on the body, including muscle growth and increased strength as well as increased energy level. Thus, anabolic steroids are often abused to gain a competitive edge in sports. Users are often athletes, typically football players, wrestlers, or weight lifters, and almost all users are male. Very high doses of anabolic steroids may cause erratic mood swings, irrational behavior, and increased aggressiveness (often called steroid rage). Anabolic steroids can damage the liver and cause jaundice. Regular use of any amount also tends to increase body hair. Acne commonly gets worse with anabolic steroid use and is one of the few side effects for which an adolescent may visit a doctor. Laboratory tests can measure anabolic steroid breakdown products in the urine. Up to 6% of boys in high school, including nonathletes, have used anabolic steroids at least once. A particular problem with anabolic steroid use in adolescents is early closure of the growth plates at the ends of bones, resulting in permanent short stature. Other side effects are common to both adolescents and adults.

See also: Endocrine System; Reproductive System, Female; Radon; Toxicity Testing, Reproductive.

Further Reading

Anderson, P.D., Johnson, A.C., Pfeiffer, D., et al., 2012. Endocrine disruption due to estrogens derived from humans predicted to be low in the majority of U.S. surface waters. Environ. Toxicol. Chem. 31 (6), 1407–1415.

Connell, J.M., Rapeport, W.G., Beastall, G.H., Brodie, M.J., 1984. Changes in circulating androgens during short term carbamazepine therapy. Br. J. Clin. Pharmacol. 17 (3), 347–351.

De Oliveira, D.H., Fighera, T.M., Bianchet, L.C., Kulak, C.A., Kulak, J., 2012. Androgens and bone. Minerva Endocrinol. 37 (4), 305–314.

Dhillon, V.S., Singh, J., Singh, H., Kler, R.S., 1995. In vitro and in vivo genotoxicity of hormonal drugs. VI. Fluoxymesterone. Mutat. Res. 342, 103–111.

Eliassen, A.H., Spiegelman, D., Xu, X., et al., 2012. Urinary estrogens and estrogen metabolites and subsequent risk of breast cancer among premenopausal women. Cancer Res. 72 (3), 696–706.

Fontana, K., Rocha, T., da Cruz-Höfling, M.A., 2012. Regulation of neuronal and endothelial nitric oxide synthase by anabolic–androgenic steroid in skeletal muscles. Histol. Histopathol. 27 (11), 1449–1458.

Hickey, T.E., Robinson, J.L., Carroll, J.S., Tilley, W.D., 2012. The androgen receptor in breast tissues: growth inhibitor, tumor suppressor, oncogene? Mol. Endocrinol. 26 (8), 1252–1267.

Higgins, J.P., Heshmat, A., Higgins, C.L., 2012. Androgen abuse and increased cardiac risk. South. Med. J. 105 (12), 670–674.

Kanayama, G., Kean, J., Hudson, J.I., Pope Jr., H.G., 2012. Cognitive deficits in long-term anabolic–androgenic steroid users. Drug Alcohol Depend. http://dx.doi.org/http://dx.doi.org/10.1016/j.drugalcdep.2012.11.008 pii: S0376-8716(12)00449-8. (Epub ahead of print).

Kayani, M.A., Parry, J.M., 2008. The detection and assessment of the aneugenic potential of selected oestrogens, progestins and androgens using the in vitro cytokinesis blocked micronucleus assay. Mutat. Res. 651 (1–2), 40–45.

Kersey, R.D., Elliot, D.L., Goldberg, L., et al., 2012. National Athletic Trainers' Association position statement: anabolic–androgenic steroids. J. Athl. Train. 47 (5), 567–588.

Lee, H.R., Hyun, S.H., Jeung, E.B., Choi, K.C., 2012. 193 Bisphenol A and phthalate enhanced the growth of prostate cancer cells and altered tgf-β signaling molecules via an estrogen receptor or androgen receptor-dependent pathway in in vitro and in vivo models. Reprod. Fertil. Dev. 25 (1), 245–246.

Meyer, K., Korz, V., 2012. Age dependent differences in the regulation of hippocampal steroid hormones and receptor genes: relations to motivation and cognition in male rats. Horm. Behav. pii: S0018-506X(12)00292-9. http://dx.doi.org/http://dx.doi.org/10.1016/j.yhbeh.2012.12.002.

Oettel, M., 2003. Testosterone metabolism, dose–response relationships and receptor polymorphisms: selected pharmacological/toxicological considerations on benefits versus risks of testosterone therapy in men. Aging Male 6, 230–256.

Schulman, C., Irani, J., Aapro, M., 2012. Improving the management of patients with prostate cancer receiving long-term androgen deprivation therapy. BJU Int. 109 (Suppl. 6), 13–21. http://dx.doi.org/10.1111/j.1464-410X.2012.11216.x.

Secreto, G., Venturelli, E., Meneghini, E., Carcangiu, M.L., 2012. Androgen receptors and serum testosterone levels identify different subsets of postmenopausal breast cancers. BMC Cancer 12 (1), 599.

Secreto, G., Zumoff, B., 2012. Role of androgen excess in the development of estrogen receptor-positive and estrogen receptor-negative breast cancer. Anticancer Res. 32 (8), 3223–3228.

Simon, J.A., 2001. Safety of estrogen/androgen regimens. J. Reprod. Med. 46, 281–290.

Smith, H.S., Elliott, J.A., 2012. Opioid-induced androgen deficiency (OPIAD). Pain Physician 15 (3 Suppl.), ES145–ES156.

Wood, R.I., Armstrong, A., Fridkin, V., Shah, V., Najafi, A., Jakowec, M., 2012. Roid rage in rats? Testosterone effects on aggressive motivation, impulsivity and tyrosine hydroxylase. Physiol. Behav. pii: S0031-9384(12)00411-8. http://dx.doi.org/10.1016/j.physbeh.2012.12.005.

Yesalis, C.E., Kennedy, N.J., Kopstein, A.N., Bahrke, M.S., 1993. Anabolic–androgenic steroid use in the United States. J. Am. Med. Assoc. 270, 1217–1221.

Relevant Websites

http://www.inchem.org – International Programme on Chemical Safety: INCHEM: Search for Androgens.

http://www.merck.com – Merck - company website.

Anesthetics

F Liu and C Wang, Division of Neurotoxicology, National Center for Toxicological Research/U.S. Food and Drug Administration, Jefferson, AR, USA
TA Patterson, Regulatory Compliance & Risk Management, National Center for Toxicological Research/U.S. Food and Drug Administration, Jefferson, AR, USA

This article is a revision of the previous edition article by Jeffrey W. Allen, volume 1, pp 125–134, © 2005, Elsevier Inc.

An anesthetic is a chemical that produces a state of anesthesia. The term 'anesthesia' is Greek in origin, meaning 'without sensation.' It is a medical technique generally used to induce a loss of sensation to stimuli on patients who undergo surgery or other medical procedures to avoid pain or distress they may otherwise experience. Anesthetics can be generally categorized into two classes based on their functions: general anesthetics and local anesthetics.

General Anesthetics

General anesthetics are used to induce general anesthesia, which is a balanced state of unconsciousness, accompanied by the absence of pain sensation and paralysis of skeletal muscle over the entire body. General anesthetics are either gases or volatile liquids that evaporate as they are inhaled through a mask along with oxygen, or anesthetic agents that are administered intravenously. **Table 1** lists commonly used general anesthetics.

The precise mechanism of general anesthesia is not yet fully understood. Most of the currently used general anesthetics may act by enhancing the activity of the inhibitory neurotransmitter γ-aminobutyric acid (GABA) in the central nervous system (CNS), or by antagonizing the effect of the excitatory neurotransmitter, *N*-methyl-D-aspartate (NMDA), on NMDA receptors. Narcotic anesthetics are an important adjunct for general anesthesia. Their analgesic functions are mediated by opioid receptors in the CNS, spinal cord, and periphery. There are three principal classes of opioid receptors: mu, delta, and kappa. Narcotics may be administered intravenously, intrathecally, or into epidural space. There are four categories of narcotics: natural alkaloids of opium, synthetic derivatives of morphine, synthetic agents resembling the morphine structure, and narcotic antagonists used as antidotes in cases of narcotic overdose. Fentanyl (also known as fentanil) is a commonly used synthetic narcotic due to its better lipid solubility, more rapid onset of action, more potent anesthetic effect, absence of histamine release, and independence of renal function for drug clearance. Sufentanil and alfentanil are two examples of newer synthetic narcotics.

Inhalation Anesthetics

Inhalation anesthetics are compounds that enter the body through the lungs and are carried by the blood to tissues. An ideal inhalation anesthetic should have ample potency, low solubility in blood and tissues, resistance to physical and metabolic degradation, and a protective effect and lack of injury to vital tissues. The potency of an inhalation anesthetic is determined by the minimum alveolar concentration (MAC), which is the concentration of an inhaled vapor in the lung, at steady state, at which 50% of subjects do not react to a standard surgical stimulus at 1 atm. A potent volatile anesthetic has a lower MAC value. Some inhalation anesthetics have been reported to cause seizure and agitation and to irritate the airways. Sevoflurane has an intermediate solubility in blood and tissues and does not cause respiratory irritation, circulatory stimulation, or hepatotoxicity. Therefore, sevoflurane is currently the most popular anesthetic agent in North America for anesthesia induction by inhalation. The depth of anesthesia induced by inhalation anesthetics can be adjusted rapidly by altering the anesthetic-to-oxygen ratio inhaled by the patient.

Table 1 Commonly used general anesthetics

Generic name	*CAS Registry number*	*Chemical formula*	*Dosage forms/routes*
Desflurane	57041-67-5	$C_3H_2F_6O$	Volatile liquid/inhalation
Enflurane	13838-16-9	$C_3H_2ClF_5O$	Volatile liquid/inhalation
Etomidate	33125-97-2	$C_{14}H_{16}N_2O_2$	Injectable/injection
Halothane	151-67-7	$C_2HBrClF_3$	Volatile liquid/inhalation
Isoflurane	26675-46-7	$C_3H_2ClF_5O$	Volatile liquid/inhalation
Ketamine hydrochloride	1867-66-9	$C_{13}H_{17}Cl_2NO$	Injectable/injection
Methohexital sodium	22151-68-4	$C_{14}H_{17}N_2NaO_3$	Injectable/injection
Midazolam hydrochloride	59467-96-8	$C_{18}H_{14}Cl_2FN_3$	Injectable/injection; syrup/oral
Nitrous oxide	10024-97-2	N_2O	Gas/inhalation
Propofol	2078-54-8	$C_{12}H_{18}O$	Injectable/injection
Sevoflurane	28523-86-6	$C_4H_3F_7O$	Volatile liquid/inhalation
Thiopental sodium	71-73-8743	$C_{11}H_{17}N_2NaO_2S$	Injectable/injection

 http://dx.doi.org/10.1016/B978-0-12-386454-3.00003-8

Intravenous Anesthetics

Similar to inhalation anesthetics, an ideal intravenous anesthetic agent should have a rapid onset of action; be quickly cleared from the circulation and CNS to facilitate the adjustment of depth of anesthesia; protect vital tissues; and not affect the circulatory system or have other adverse effects. Among these agents, propofol is commonly used for the intravenous induction of general anesthesia. Propofol has a rapid onset of action because it is lipid-soluble and distributes quickly into the CNS and other tissues. It has a greater degree of safety than other intravenous general anesthetics due to its faster clearance. Propofol acts to potentiate the inhibitory effects of GABA receptors in the CNS.

Ketamine is labeled a dissociative anesthetic because the anesthetized patient feels consciously detached from the environment before losing consciousness. The dissociative state is indicated by sedation, amnesia, immobility, and marked analgesia. In adult patients, ketamine produces postoperative effects (such as sensory illusions and vivid dreams); therefore, it is not routinely administered to adults. However, it is useful for anesthetizing children, patients in shock, and trauma casualties in war zones where anesthesia equipment may be difficult to obtain. Ketamine acts as a noncompetitive antagonist of NMDA receptors.

Intravenous anesthesia is suggested for the induction of anesthesia but not for the maintenance of anesthesia. Administration of multiple doses by intravenous injection or a continuous intravenous infusion could result in drug accumulation and delays in recovery from anesthesia.

Uses and Exposure Routes and Pathways

In modern medicine it is very common to use both inhalation and intravenous general anesthetics to achieve balanced anesthesia. The combination of both classes of anesthetics maximizes the benefits of each drug and minimizes the dose of both drugs, thus reducing side effects from the anesthesia. Moreover, the patients can better tolerate a combination of anesthetics compared with an individual anesthetic.

Toxicokinetics

Inhalation anesthetics undergo very little metabolism. They are largely eliminated in the exhaled air by the lungs. Only a small portion of inhalation anesthetics is metabolized in the body. The inhalation anesthetic nitrous oxide is not metabolized in the body. Sevoflurane is an inhalation anesthetic commonly used in clinics, and metabolism studies suggest that approximately 5% of the sevoflurane dose may be metabolized. Cytochrome P450 2E1 is the principal isoform identified for sevoflurane metabolism. Intravenously injected propofol has a high rate of total body clearance; it is rapidly and extensively metabolized in the liver and at extrahepatic sites. Propofol metabolites are inactive glucuronide and sulfate derivatives. Intravenously administered ketamine is metabolized in the liver by the microsomal enzyme system involving hydroxylation and demethylation. The principal metabolite of ketamine is norketamine, which lacks a methyl group compared with ketamine. The concentration of norketamine is about one-third that of ketamine. The cyclohexanone ring of ketamine also undergoes oxidative metabolism to form the second metabolite, dehydronorketamine. The high lipid solubility of ketamine results in a rapid onset of action.

Intravenous fentanyl is extensively used in anesthesia and analgesia. It is metabolized by cytochrome P450 CYP3A4 to norfentanyl, hydroxypropionyl fentanyl, and hydroxypropionyl norfentanyl. None of the metabolites are active. About 75% of administered fentanyl is excreted as metabolites in the urine, and 9% is excreted in the stool.

Acute and Short-Term Toxicity of General Anesthetics

Inhalation anesthetics can be toxic to the liver, kidney, or blood cells. The inhalation anesthetic with the most incidence of liver injury is halothane, followed by isoflurane, then desflurane. Respiratory depression occurs with all inhalation anesthetics. Malignant hyperthermia is a rare condition caused by an allergic response to a general anesthetic. The signs of malignant hyperthermia include rapid irregular heartbeat; breathing problems; high fever; and muscle tightness or spasms. These reactions can occur following the administration of general anesthetics, especially halothane. Reduced blood pressure generally can be observed when halothane is administered; however, other inhalation anesthetics can have the same effects, although to a lesser extent.

Preclinical data since 2002 indicate that general anesthetics can have acute and sometimes long-lasting effects on the developing CNS by increasing neuron apoptosis. Rodent and nonhuman primate models have demonstrated that the neurotoxic effects of anesthetics on developing brains are related to the route of administration and are dose-dependent, exposure duration-dependent, and developmental stage-dependent; the brain growth spurt period is the most vulnerable time. These factors are important because they can help identify thresholds of exposure for producing neurotoxicity in the developing nervous system. These findings have called into question the safety of general anesthetics in the pediatric population. However, existing human data are insufficient to support or refute the possibility that neurotoxic effects observed in animals could occur in children.

Chronic Toxicity (Animal/Human)

A recent study reported that prolonged anesthetic (ketamine) exposure during the brain growth spurt period caused long-lasting cognitive deficits in rhesus monkeys, providing evidence of chronic neurotoxic effects of general anesthetics. Elderly patients are another group who are at higher risk of cognitive deficits after surgery and anesthesia. The International Study of Postoperative Cognitive Dysfunction has established the existence of postoperative cognitive dysfunction (POCD) in the elderly.

Mechanism of Toxicity

The mechanisms by which general anesthetics cause acute and prolonged neurotoxic effects are not clear. One of the hypotheses for the developing brain, regarding the acute neurotoxic effects of anesthetics by antagonizing NMDA receptors, suggests that continually blocking NMDA receptors with NMDA receptor antagonists, such as ketamine, may induce a compensatory upregulation of NMDA receptors on the neurons. The upregulation of NMDA receptors allows for the accumulation of toxic levels of intracellular free calcium. Consequently, neurons are more vulnerable to the excitotoxic effects of endogenous glutamate after NMDA receptor antagonist withdrawal.

The underlying mechanisms for POCD in the elderly remain unknown. *In vitro* studies demonstrated that some inhalation anesthetics (i.e., isoflurane, isoflurane plus nitrous oxide, sevoflurane, etc.) induced apoptosis and increased amyloid-beta (Aβ) formation (Aβ is a protein fragment of an amyloid precursor protein; a healthy brain is able to break down and eliminate it, but in Alzheimer's disease, the fragments accumulate to form hard, insoluble plaques), providing a potential link between anesthesia administration and Alzheimer's disease.

Carcinogenesis, Mutagenesis, and Impairment of Fertility

In general, inhalation anesthetics are freely transferred to fetal tissues. Animal studies on enflurane did not reveal evidence of carcinogenic or mutagenic effects. Reproduction studies conducted in rats and rabbits at doses up to four times the human dose of enflurane did not reveal evidence of impaired fertility or fetal harm. Isoflurane, enflurane, and sevoflurane do not show teratogenic potential.

Chronic occupational exposure to anesthetic gases in operating rooms during pregnancy has raised concern that such exposure may cause birth defects and spontaneous abortions, but there has been no direct evidence of a correlation between occupational exposure and congenital abnormalities. At present, with good scavenging and low-level exposure to waste, anesthetic gases do not appear to be a risk during occupational exposure.

Clinical Management

Although evidence from preclinical studies indicates the neurotoxic effects of general anesthesia on developing animal brains, there is no direct evidence that anesthetics are unsafe for children. Parents of children requiring surgery should consult anesthesiologists or other qualified physicians for advice about an individual child's situation. During general anesthesia, respiratory and cardiovascular functions should always be monitored. Necessary actions should be taken immediately to resolve any depressant effects.

Local Anesthetic Agents

Local anesthetic agents can cause reversible local anesthesia by inducing the absence of pain sensation without affecting consciousness. All local anesthetics consist of three components: an aromatic portion, an intermediate chain, and an amine group. The intermediate chain, which connects the aromatic and amine portions, is composed of either an ester or an amide linkage. Thus, the local anesthetics are further classified into two categories: esters and amides. Anesthetics such as benzocaine, chloroprocaine, cocaine, cyclomethycaine, dimethocaine/larocaine, piperocaine, propoxycaine, procaine/novocaine, proparacaine, and tetracaine are esters. Examples of amides include articaine, bupivacaine, cinchocaine/dibucaine, etidocaine, levobupivacaine, lidocaine/lignocaine, mepivacaine, prilocaine, ropivacaine, and trimecaine. Both classes of local anesthetics act mainly by preventing sodium influx through voltage-gated sodium channels in the neuronal cell membrane into the cytoplasm, thus preventing the local membrane from depolarization. Therefore, an action potential cannot be generated and spread; the signal conduction is inhibited, thereby effecting local anesthesia. In general, all nerve fibers are sensitive to local anesthetics. However, nerve fibers that have a smaller diameter are more readily blocked than those with larger diameter. For instance, the pain sensation, transmitted by small and unmyelinated nerves, can be blocked more rapidly than other sensations. In addition, local anesthetics have a greater binding affinity to sodium channels, which are in an activated state. An active neuron is more sensitive to local anesthetics. This is referred to as state-dependent blockade.

Lipid solubility of anesthetics is the most important factor in determining the intrinsic anesthetic potency, which is influenced by the aromatic portion of the molecule. The duration of anesthesia is determined by the extent of local anesthetics binding to proteins, which are immersed in lipids of the membrane. The greater the binding affinity to nerve proteins the longer the anesthetic activity will persist.

Uses and Exposure Routes and Pathways

Local anesthetic agents are administered to the areas around the nerves to be blocked (skin, subcutaneous tissues, intrathecal, and epidural spaces). Their activities vary considerably. Topical anesthesia is the administration of local anesthetics to the skin or other body surface. Most anesthetics are barely absorbed through intact skin, and the effectiveness of anesthesia is affected. Eutectic mixtures, such as 2.5% lidocaine and 2.5% prilocaine (EMLA), improve the effectiveness of the anesthetic on intact skin by lowering the melting temperature of the mixture compared with that of each individual anesthetic.

Infiltration anesthesia is the injection of local anesthetics into the tissue to be anesthetized. Amide anesthetics with a moderate duration of action are commonly used (i.e., lignocaine, prilocaine, and mepivacaine) to cause infiltration anesthesia for minor surgical procedures.

Epidural anesthesia is the administration of local anesthetics to the epidural space between the dura mater and the periosteum lining the vertebral canal. The conduction is blocked at the intradural spinal roots and the absence of pain sensation can be achieved. Spinal anesthesia is the application of local anesthetics into the cerebrospinal fluid at the site of the lumbar spine.

Intravenous local anesthesia is the injecting of local anesthetics into a vein of a limb (a leg, foot, or lower arm, hand) that has been exsanguinated and blocked by a tourniquet. The anesthesia is limited to the area that is excluded from blood circulation. One restriction that should be kept in mind is that bupivacaine and etidocaine should never be used for intravenous local anesthesia due to the risk of cardiotoxicity.

Toxicokinetics

All local anesthetics are weakly alkaline. They exist in both nonionized and ionized forms. The term pK_a of a weak base is defined as the pH at which both forms exist in equal amounts. At physiological pH (7.4), local anesthetics are more ionized than nonionized (as their pK_a values are >7.4). However, the proportions vary among the anesthetics. Nonionized anesthetics can pass through the lipid cell membrane more rapidly than ionized ones. Therefore, an anesthetic agent that has a higher proportion of nonionized form will reach the target site more quickly and will have a faster onset of blocking.

Ester and amide anesthetics are metabolized through different routes. The metabolism of esters (except cocaine) is through hydrolysis in plasma by the enzyme pseudocholinesterase and they have a short half-life. Cocaine is hydrolyzed in the liver. Ester metabolite excretion is through the kidney. The amides undergo enzymatic degradation by microsomal enzymes located in the liver. This is a slower process, hence the half-life of amides is longer and they can accumulate if given repeatedly.

Acute and Short-Term Toxicity of Local Anesthetics

Allergic reactions to local anesthetics are rare. Esters produce the most anesthetic-induced allergic reactions due to their metabolite, *para*-aminobenzoic acid (PABA), a well-known allergen. Hypersensitivity to amide local anesthetics is seldom observed. Since there is no cross-allergy between esters and amides, amides can be used as alternatives in patients who show hypersensitivity to esters. Therefore, amides are now more commonly used than esters.

Local anesthetics may be toxic if sufficient amounts are absorbed into the systemic circulation or administered improperly. The toxicity can be at local and systemic levels. The local adverse effects of anesthetics may include prolonged anesthesia and paresthesias, which may become irreversible.

Systemic toxicological effects of local anesthetics involve the central nervous, cardiovascular, and immune systems. In general, the CNS is more sensitive to local anesthetics than the cardiovascular and immune systems. Therefore, symptoms and signs of CNS disturbances usually occur earlier, showing excitatory effects in the brain before the depressant effects. Myocardial depression and bradycardia indicate the effects of local anesthetics on the cardiovascular system. On very rare occasions (<1%), immunoglobulin E (IgE)–mediated allergic reactions can occur.

CNS toxicity is usually related to the intrinsic potency of the anesthetics. Procaine is least potent and least toxic following a rapid intravenous injection. Bupivacaine, tetracaine, and etidocaine are the most potent compounds in terms of intrinsic anesthetic and CNS convulsive activity. Lidocaine, mepivacaine, and prilocaine are intermediate in anesthetic potency and convulsive activity.

Chronic Toxicity (Animal/Human)

Local anesthetics can easily cross the placenta by passive diffusion. There is now general agreement that properly conducted epidural anesthesia does not cause neurobehavioral changes in the newborn.

Carcinogenesis

Long-term studies in animals to evaluate carcinogenic potential have not been conducted on most local anesthetics. A minor metabolite of lidocaine, 2,6-xylidine, has been found to be carcinogenic in rats.

Mutagenesis and Impairment of Fertility

Mutagenic potential or the effects on fertility of most local anesthetics has not been reported, although animal experiments have reported decreased pup survival in rats and an embryocidal effect in rabbits when bupivacaine hydrochloride was administered to these species in doses comparable to 9 and 5 times, respectively, the maximum recommended daily human dose. However, there are no adequate and well-controlled studies in pregnant women of the effects of the same agent on the developing fetus.

Clinical Management

Administration of local anesthetic agents should be stopped if a patient shows any signs or symptoms of toxicity during anesthesia. An intravenous lipid emulsion treatment, called lipid rescue, has been shown to be effective in treating cardiotoxicity based on animal evidence and human case reports. The use of lipid rescue has been encouraged in the United Kingdom and officially promoted as a treatment by the Association of Anesthetists of Great Britain and Ireland.

Disclaimer

This document has been reviewed in accordance with U.S. Food and Drug Administration (FDA) policy and approved for publication. Approval does not signify that the contents necessarily reflect the position or opinions of the FDA. The findings and conclusions in this report are those of the authors and do not necessarily represent the views of the FDA.

See also: Neurotoxicity; Benzodiazepines; Cocaine; Opium and the Constituent Opiates; Lidocaine; Nitrous Oxide.

Further Reading

American Society of Health-System Pharmacists, 2010. AHFS Drug Information 2010. ASHP, Bethesda, MD.

Miller, K.W., Roth, S.H. (Eds.), 1986. Molecular and Cellular Mechanisms of Anesthetics. Springer, New York.

Miller, R.D., 2004. Miller's Anesthesia, sixth ed. Churchill Livingstone, Philadelphia, PA.

Wang, C., Slikker Jr., W., 2011. Developmental Neurotoxicology Research: Principles, Models, Techniques, Strategies and Mechanisms. John Wiley, Hoboken, NJ.

Relevant Website

http://www.iars.org – International Anesthesia Research Society

Aneuploidy

DA Eastmond, University of California, Riverside, CA, USA

Aneuploidy is a condition ōin which the chromosome number of a cell or individual differs from a multiple of the haploid complement for that species. In common terms, an aneuploid cell has one or more chromosomes in addition to or less than what is normal for that cell type; for example, a human somatic cell with 45 or 47 chromosomes rather than 46, the normal diploid number. Similarly, an aneuploid human germ cell possesses ≤22 or ≥24 chromosomes rather than the haploid chromosome number of 23. In cytogenetics, aneuploidy is considered one type of numerical chromosome aberration. The other type of aberration is polyploidy, where the chromosome number of a cell is increased by a multiple of the haploid complement for the species (e.g., a human cell with 69 or 92 chromosomes rather than the diploid 46 would be considered polyploid). Aneuploid cells may be further described as hyperploid (having additional chromosomes), hypoploid (possessing fewer chromosomes), or as having trisomy (possessing three copies of one chromosome), or monosomy (with a single copy of a chromosome). In some cases, researchers have expanded the definition of aneuploidy to include partial or segmental aneuploidies, conditions resulting from structural rearrangements in which portions of chromosomes have been added to or lost from a cell. In this article, aneuploidy is used based on its original and more widely accepted definition, which involves the loss or gain of entire chromosomes.

Aneuploidy occurring in germ cells and early embryos is a major cause of morbidity and mortality in humans. It is associated with infertility, pregnancy loss, congenital malformations and mental retardation. Congenital aneuploidy involving autosomal chromosomes affects approximately 0.15% of all live births, and aneuploidy involving the sex chromosomes affects another 0.175%. In addition, the frequency of chromosomal abnormalities is much higher among pregnancies that terminate at birth (~5%) or during gestation (~50% in fetuses dying between weeks eight and eleven of gestation). In most cases, these abnormalities are believed to have contributed to the embryonic and fetal deaths. Overall, chromosome abnormalities are estimated to be responsible for ~30% of lost pregnancies, with aneuploidy accounting for roughly 75% of the total. As a consequence, it has been estimated that approximately 13 000 aneuploid babies are born each year in the United States and that another 150 000 to 200 000 chromosomally abnormal embryos are spontaneously aborted. Among the surviving offspring, the most common type of congenital aneuploidy is Down syndrome, which results from trisomy of chromosome 21 and occurs in approximately 1 in 800 newborns (0.13%). Similarly, Klinefelter syndrome (XXY), YY males (XYY), triple X females (XXX), and Turner syndrome (XO) are congenital aneuploidies of the sex chromosomes that individually affect approximately 0.05–0.005% of live births. Because most of these individuals are infertile and exhibit developmental abnormalities, aneuploidy is responsible for a significant portion of the recognized cases of infertility, congenital malformations, and mental retardation. Indeed, aneuploidy has been reported to be the leading genetic cause of mental retardation in the United States.

Nonrandom patterns of numerical aberrations are frequently observed in cancer cells, implicating aneuploidy in carcinogenesis. Associations between aneuploidy and neoplastic development have also been observed in patients with congenital and familial predispositions for cancer, as well as in patients with cancers resulting from chemical exposures. Similar results have been observed in animals and cellular systems in which the nonrandom gain or loss of specific chromosomes has been associated with tumorigenesis or neoplastic transformation. These patterns have been seen in tumors occurring spontaneously as well as those induced by chemical, radiation, or viral agents.

Although chromosomal changes appear to be a secondary effect related to cell proliferation or genomic instability in some tumors, a growing body of molecular and cytogenetic evidence indicates that the induction of aneuploidy plays an important role in neoplastic transformation. This has perhaps been best characterized in the case of retinoblastoma (RB) where it has been shown that the loss of the allele containing the functional Rb tumor suppressor gene frequently occurred through a mechanism involving nondisjunction of chromosome 13. Similarly, alterations in gene dosage resulting from aneuploidy are believed to contribute to the development of many other cancers. However, recent studies involving both humans and animals have indicated that the relationship between aneuploidy and cancer is complex. Although changes in chromosome number have been clearly associated with increased incidences of some cancers, aneuploidy has also been shown to reduce the incidence of cancer in other tissues. For example, individuals with Down syndrome have an increased risk of myeloid and lymphoid leukemia early in life but exhibit decreased risks of solid tumors as they age. Similar combinations of carcinogenic and anticarcinogenic effects have also been seen in animal studies.

Mechanistically there are many ways by which aneuploidy can occur. Almost any process that interferes with mitosis or meiosis during cell division can affect chromosome segregation and result in aneuploidy. In germ cells, aneuploidy appears to originate in part from aberrant meiotic recombination, premature separation of sister chromatids, and possibly altered DNA methylation. During carcinogenesis, aneuploidy has been reported to result from mechanisms including spontaneous errors of mitosis, chemical interference with the mitotic spindle, viral integration resulting in chromosomal instability, as well as mutations affecting the kinetochore, the centrosome, or other cellular structures and organelles.

 http://dx.doi.org/10.1016/B978-0-12-386454-3.00004-X

The ability of chemicals to interfere with proper chromosome segregation has been an area of considerable concern within genetic toxicology. Many chemical and physical agents including those used as pesticides, pharmaceuticals, consumer products, and industrial chemicals have been shown to induce aneuploidy *in vitro* and/or *in vivo*. Indeed, drugs such as vincristine sulfate and griseofulvin are used specifically because of their ability to induce aneuploidy, which gives them cytostatic or cytotoxic properties. Despite the common use of aneugenic chemicals, the extent to which aneuploidy induced by these agents contributes to cancer and reproductive dysfunction in the general population remains uncertain. However, due to the established involvement of aneuploidy in carcinogenesis and in adverse reproductive outcomes, there continues to be concern about the safety of aneuploidy-inducing agents.

Many different assays have been developed to detect aneuploidy, all of which have significant limitations. The conventional approach has been to count the number of chromosomes in metaphase preparations of dividing cells. Unfortunately, this restricts the detection to actively dividing cells, which may not be present in the tissue of interest. In addition, this technique is laborious and prone to technical artifacts, such as chromosome loss during metaphase preparation. The micronucleus assay, particularly as modified with antibodies or probes to detect centromere-containing micronuclei, has emerged as a simple way to detect aneugenic agents. Although valuable, this assay is only able to detect chromosome loss and breakage, and may not detect agents that specifically induce nondisjunction or chromosome gain. Other techniques involving fluorescence in situ hybridization with DNA probes allow chromosome gains to be detected in many tissues but are relatively insensitive unless multiple probes and other modifications are used. As a result, efforts to develop assays or combinations of assays that will allow the efficient detection of aneugenic agents are continuing.

See also: Ames Test; Analytical Toxicology; Carcinogen–DNA Adduct Formation and DNA Repair; Chromosome Aberrations; Dominant Lethal Assay; Host-Mediated Assay; Molecular Toxicology: Recombinant DNA Technology; Mouse Lymphoma Assay; Sister Chromatid Exchanges; Toxicity Testing, Mutagenicity.

Further Reading

Aardema, M.J., Albertini, S., Arni, P., et al., 1998. Aneuploidy: a report of an ECETOC task force. Mutat. Res. 410, 3–79.

Cavenee, W.K., Koufos, A., Hansen, M.F., 1986. Recessive mutant genes predisposing to human cancer. Mutat. Res. 168, 3–14.

Golbus, M.S., 1981. Chromosome aberrations and mammalian reproduction. In: Mastroianni, L., Biggers, J.D. (Eds.), Fertilization and Embryonic Development In Vitro. Plenum Press, New York, pp. 257–272.

Hasle, H., 2001. Pattern of malignant disorders in individuals with Down's syndrome. Lancet Oncol. 2, 429–436.

Hunt, P.A., Hassold, T.J., 2002. Sex matters in meiosis. Science 296 (5576), 2181–2183.

Hecht, F., Hecht, B.K., 1987. Aneuploidy in humans: Dimensions, demography, and dangers of abnormal numbers of chromosomes. In: Vig, B.K., Sandberg, A.A. (Eds.), Aneuploidy, Part A: Incidence and Etiology. Alan R Liss, New York, pp. 9–49.

Hook, E.B., 1985. The impact of aneuploidy upon public health: Mortality and morbidity associated with human chromosome abnormalities. In: Dellarco, V.L., Voytek, P.E., Hollaender, A. (Eds.), Aneuploidy Etiology and Mechanisms. Plenum Press, Ltd., New York, pp. 7–33.

Mohrenweiser, H.W., 1991. Germinal mutation and human genetic disease. In: Li, A.P., Heflich, R.H. (Eds.), Genetic Toxicology. CRC Press, Boca Raton, FL, pp. 67–92.

Oshimura, M., Barrett, J.C., 1986. Chemically induced aneuploidy in mammalian cells: mechanisms and biological significance in cancer. Environ. Mutagen. 8, 129–159.

Schuler, M., Rupa, D.S., Eastmond, D.A., 1997. A critical evaluation of centromeric labeling to distinguish micronuclei induced by chromosomal loss and breakage *in vitro*. Mutat. Res. 392, 81–95.

Weaver, B.A., Silk, A.D., Montagna, C., Verdier-Pinard, P., Cleveland, D.W., 2007. Aneuploidy acts both oncogenically and as a tumor suppressor. Cancer Cell 11, 25–36.

Angiotensin-Converting Enzyme Inhibitors *see* Angiotensin Converting Enzyme (ACE) Inhibitors

Aniline

SC Gad, Gad Consulting Services, Cary, NC, USA

- Chemical Abstracts Service Registry Number: 62-53-3
- Synonyms: Phenylamine; Aminobenzene; Blue oil
- Molecular Formula: C_6H_7N
- Chemical Structure:

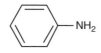

Background

First produced in 1826 by Otto Unverdorben through destructive distillation of indigo, the first industrial use was as a purple dye, Mauveine, formulated by William Henry Perkin accidentally in an attempt to isolate quinone. The name aniline was given in deference to the indigo-yielding plant, Indigofera suffruticosa, commonly named anil.

Uses

Intermediate in dyestuff production and in the manufacture of pharmaceuticals, photographic developers, shoe polish, resins, varnish, perfumes, and organic chemicals.

Environmental Fate and Behavior

Although largely a synthetic chemical, aniline is produced from the burning of vegetation; therefore fires and especially wildfires must be considered a minor source.

Aniline degrades in the atmosphere primarily by reaction with photochemical-produced hydroxyl radicals, with a half-life of 1–2 h. The reaction products include potentially harmful substances such as nitrosamines, nitrobenzene, formic acid, nitrophenols, phenol, nitrosobenzene, and benzidine. At ground level, VOCs react with other air pollutants and contribute to the formation of potentially harmful concentrations of ozone in the lower atmosphere.

Aniline's short half-life in air means that the likelihood of long-range transport is low.

A bioconcentration factor (BCF) for aniline has been calculated at 91, indicating that the compound has the potential to moderately accumulate and magnify in the ecosystem.

Exposure and Exposure Monitoring

Exposure to the eyes or skin likely lead to irritation at the site, and dermal absorption of aniline is high, contributing to systemic toxicity. Aniline is also well absorbed by the inhalation and ingestion routes, either of which can rapidly lead to severe systemic toxicity.

Results of exposure include methemoglobinemia, destruction of red blood cells, as well as various cardiopulmonary effects, such as ischemia and arrhythmias. The overall toxic effects are largely a result of this methemoglobinemia, affecting cardiopulmonary and CNS systems.

Environmental exposure is limited owing to the short half-life of aniline. Aniline's density is greater than that of ambient air, so it can accumulate in low-lying areas, which can increase exposure. In the event that aniline enters water it survives significantly longer.

Toxicokinetics

Aniline is rapidly absorbed by the skin, lungs, and gastrointestinal tract of experimental animals. After intravenous injection of radiolabeled aniline to rats, radioactivity is distributed throughout the body. Highest concentrations were found in the blood, liver, kidney, urinary bladder, and gastrointestinal tract. The major urinary metabolites in various animal species tested are *o*-, *p*-amino-phenol, and their conjugates. *p*-Aminophenyl- and *p*-acetylaminophenylmercapturic acids are also excreted in rats and rabbits. *N*-Hydroxylation of aniline by liver microsomes from several species has been observed *in vitro*. The formation of phenylhydroxylamine from aniline appears to be the reactive metabolite responsible for its toxic activity.

Mechanism of Toxicity

The formation of phenylhydroxylamine from aniline appears to be the reactive metabolite responsible for its toxic activity.

Acute and Short-Term Toxicity (or Exposure)

Animal

Moderate skin and severe eye irritant in rabbits; reproductive toxin in mice. Rat LCLo 250 ppm h^{-1}; dermal LD_{50}

 http://dx.doi.org/10.1016/B978-0-12-386454-3.00813-7

1400 mg kg^{-1}; mouse oral LD_{50} 464 mg kg^{-1}. Aniline is a mutagen and clastogen, being positive in the *in vivo* mouse micronucleus and sister chromatid exchange assays. DNA strand breakage was induced in the livers and kidneys of rats exposed *in vivo*.

Human

Human acute LDLo is 350 mg kg^{-1}. Systemic exposure leads to methemoglobin formation, and metabolic formation of aniline from a number of drugs leads to methemoglobinemia associated with their use. Normal systemic levels should be <1 mg l^{-1}.

Toxic oil syndrome (TOS) is a multisystemic disease that occurred in epidemic proportions in Spain in 1981 caused by the ingestion of rapeseed oil denatured with aniline. It was one of the largest intoxication epidemics ever recorded. This oil had been illegally sold as olive oil, and many aniline-derived oil components have been identified in the oil. The pathological findings in TOS showed primary endothelial injury, with cell proliferation and perivascular inflammatory infiltrates, and an immunological mechanism has been directly implicated in this illness.

Chronic Toxicity (or Exposure)

Animal

Aniline can cause methemoglobin formation, and liver and endocrine effects. It causes kidney, urethra, bladder, and hematological neoplasia. For example, aniline administered to rats for 5, 10, or 20 days resulted in splenic congestion, increased hematopoiesis and hemosiderosis, and bone marrow hyperplasia, and the dietary intake of aniline hydrochloride by rats for 104 weeks at levels of 10, 30, or 100 mg kg^{-1} diet is associated with an increased incidence of primary splenic sarcomas. Several species of animals exposed to 5 ppm of aniline vapor daily for 6 months resulted in no effects other than a slight increase in methemoglobin in the blood of rats. Repeated subcutaneous injections of 1.25 mg aniline in lard produced no tumors in mice that survived 2 years, and no tumors were observed after 15 months in mice given eight subcutaneous injections of aniline (5 mg in olive oil), or after 12 months in mice given 13 subcutaneous injections of aniline hydrochloride.

Human

The World Health Organization, International Agency for Research on Cancer, has evaluated the data for aniline and has placed aniline in its group 3 'classification of carcinogenicity,' that is, aniline is not classifiable as to its carcinogenicity to humans.

Immunotoxicity

There are insufficient data on the immunotoxicity of aniline.

Reproductive Toxicity

Aniline is positive in the *in vitro* sister chromatid exchange and mouse lymphoma assays. Further, results for cytogenetic effects in Chinese hamster ovary cells were positive for both chromosome aberrations and sister chromatid exchanges. Aniline can also cross the placental barrier, inducing methemoglobinemia in the fetus as well as mother, which is less easily reversed in the fetus. Aniline is not currently included on lists of harmful teratogens, although additional data are necessary for conclusive results.

Genotoxicity

Although aniline per se is not mutagenic in the Ames *Salmonella typhimurium* assay system, the urine of rats that received aniline orally was mutagenic for *S. typhimurium* when the assay was performed in the presence of liver microsomes from PCB-induced rats.

Carcinogenicity

The IARC has rated aniline as group 3, or not classifiable as to its carcinogenicity in humans. EPA groups classified aniline as B2, a probable human carcinogen, and the ACGIH has classified it A3, a confirmed animal carcinogen that has unknown relevance in humans.

Clinical Management

Immediate removal from exposure is necessary, followed by cardiopulmonary support as well as oxygen. There is no risk of secondary contamination to rescuers. Methemoglobin levels should be managed and/or reduced with suitable agents such as methylene blue. In cases of ingestion, do not induce emesis; activated charcoal can be administered at 1 g kg^{-1}.

Ecotoxicology

Aniline is very toxic to aquatic organisms; for example, there was an inhibiting effect of 20–40 ppm aniline on the pigmentation of *Xenopus laevis* embryos, and a concentration as low as 1 ppm on the body size of young toads. Investigation of the death of pine trees in the United States found air pollution from aniline as the most likely causal agent for needle necrosis and abscission.

Other Hazards

Exposure Standards and Guidelines

The American Conference of Governmental Industrial Hygienists has established an 8-h time-weighted average of

2 ppm. The US Occupational Safety and Health Administration permissible exposure limit is 5 ppm.

Miscellaneous

Aniline has a characteristic fishy odor that is perceptible at 1 ppm, below the exposure standards.

See also: Carcinogen–Dna Adduct Formation and Dna Repair; Genetic Toxicology.

Further Reading

Bingham, E., Cohrssen, B., Powell, C.H. (Eds.), 2001. Patty's Toxicology, fifth ed. vol. 8. Wiley, New York, pp. 1210–1211.
Centers for Disease Control and Prevention, CDC, 2012 Feb. Severe methemoglobinemia and hemolytic anemia from aniline purchased as 2C-E (4-ethyl-2,5-dimethoxyphenethylamine), a recreational drug, on the Internet – Oregon, 2011. MMWR 61 (5) 85–88.
Dom, N., Knapen, D., Blust, R., 2012 Jan. Assessment of aquatic experimental versus predicted and extrapolated chronic toxicity data of four structural analogues. Chemosphere 86 (1), 56–64.
Oh, M., Kim, S., 2012 Jan. Preparation and electrochemical characterization of polyaniline/activated carbon composites as an electrode material for supercapacitors. J. Nanosci. Nanotechnol. 12 (1), 519–524.
Ruiz-Mendez, M.V., Posada de la Paz, M., Abian, J., et al., 2001. Storage time and deodorization temperature influence the formation of aniline-derived compounds in denatured rapeseed oils. Food Chem. Toxicol. 39, 91–96.

Relevant Websites

http://www.atsdr.cdc.gov – Agency for Toxic Substances and Disease Registry. Toxicological Profile for Aniline.
http://toxnet.nlm.nih.gov – TOXNET, Specialized Information Services, National Library of Medicine. Search for Aniline.
www.ec.europa.eu/food/fs/sct/out186.endpf - Scientific comittee on Toxicity, Ecotoxicity and The Environment (CSTEE) Opinion on the results of the risk assessment of Aniline

Animal Models

SC Gad, Gad Consulting Services, Cary, NC, USA

The use of animals in experimental medicine, pharmacological study, and toxicological assessment is a well-established and essential practice. Whether serving as a source of isolated cells or tissues, a disease model, or as a prediction for drug or other xenobiotic action in humans, experiments in animals have provided the necessary building blocks that permitted the explosive growth of medical and biological knowledge in the latter half of the twentieth century. Animal experiments also have served rather successfully as identifiers of potential hazards to and toxicity in humans for synthetic chemicals with many intended uses.

Animals have been used as models for centuries to predict what chemicals and environmental factors would do to humans. The earliest uses of experimental animals are lost in prehistory, and much of what is recorded in early history about toxicology testing indicates that humans were the test subjects. The earliest clear description of the use of animals in the scientific study of the effects of environmental agents appears to be by Priestley (1792) in his study of gases. The first systematic use of animals for the screening of a wide variety of agents was published by Orfila (1814) and was described by Dubois and Geiling (1959) in their historical review. This work consisted of dosing test animals with known quantities of agents (poisons or drugs) and included the careful recording of the resulting clinical signs and gross necropsy observations. The use of animals as predictors of potential ill effects has grown since that time.

Current Animal Studies

The current regulatory required use of animal models in toxicity or safety testing began by using them as a form of instrument to detect undesired contaminants. For example, canaries were used by miners to detect the presence of carbon monoxide – a case in which an animal model is more sensitive than humans. By 1907, the US Food and Drug Administration started to protect the public by the use of a voluntary testing program for new coal tar colors in foods. This was replaced by a mandatory program of testing in 1938, and such animal testing programs mandated by regulations have continued to expand until recently.

The knowledge gained by experimentation on animals has undoubtedly increased the quality of our lives, an observation that most reasonable people would find difficult to dispute, and has also benefited animals. As is the case with many tools, animals have sometimes been used inappropriately, and modifications in use have evolved slowly. These unfortunate instances have helped fuel an increasingly vituperative animal rights movement. This movement has encouraged a measure of critical self-appraisal on the part of scientists concerning the issues of the care and usage of animals. The Society of Toxicology, for example, has established an Animals in Research Committee, and has published guidelines for the use of animals in research and testing. In general, the purpose of this committee is to foster thinking on the four Rs of animal-based research: reduction, refinement, research into replacements, and responsibility (protecting humans from avoidable harm).

The media commonly carry reports that present that most (if not all) animal testing and research is not predictive of what will happen in humans and, therefore, such testing is unwarranted. Many of the animal rights groups also present this argument at every opportunity and reinforce it with examples that entail seemingly great suffering in animals but that add nothing to the health, safety, and welfare of society. This is held to be especially the case for safety testing and research in toxicology. Animal rights activists try to 'prove' this point by presenting examples of failure; for example, thalidomide may be presented as an example without pointing out that, in the case of thalidomide, there was lack of adequate testing (or of interpretation of existing test results) before marketing. In light of the essential nature of animal research and testing in toxicology, this is equivalent to seeking to functionally disarm us as scientists. Our primary responsibility (the fourth R) is to provide the information to protect people and the environment, and without animal models we cannot discharge this responsibility.

When confronted with this argument, all too many toxicologists cannot respond with examples to the contrary. Indeed, many may not even fully understand the argument at all. Also, very few are familiar enough with some of the history of toxicity testing to be able to counter with examples in which it has not only accurately predicted a potential hazard to humans, but also has directly benefited both humans and animals. There are, however, many such examples. Demonstrating the actual benefit of toxicology testing and research with examples that directly relate to the everyday lives of most people and not esoteric, basic research findings (which are the most exciting and interesting products to most scientists) is not an easy task. Examples that can be seen to affect neighbors, relatives, and selves on a daily basis would be the most effective. The problem is that toxicology is, in a sense, a negative science. The things we find and discover are usually adverse. Also, if the applied end of our science works correctly, then the results are things that do not happen (and therefore are not seen).

If we correctly identify toxic agents (using animals and other predictive model systems) in advance of a product or agent being introduced into the marketplace or environment, then generally it will not be introduced (or will be removed) and society will not see death, rashes, renal and hepatic diseases, cancer, or birth defects, for example. Also, because these things already occur at some level in the population, it seems that seeing less of them would be hard to firmly tie to the results of toxicity testing that rely on animals. In addition, the fact that animals are predictive models for humans is controversial.

 http://dx.doi.org/10.1016/B978-0-12-386454-3.00814-9

Origins of Predictive Animal Testing

The actual record of evidence for the predictive value of animal studies and how they have benefited humans and domestic animals are reviewed in the following. However, the negative image needs to be rebutted. First, it must be remembered that predictive animal testing in toxicology, as we now know it, arose largely out of three historical events.

The "Lash Lure" Case

Early in the 1930s, an untested eyelash dye containing i-pheylenediamine (Lash Lure) was brought onto the market in the United States. This product (as well as a number of similar products) rapidly demonstrated that it could sensitize the external ocular structures, leading to corneal ulceration with multiple cases of loss of vision and at least one fatality.

The Elixir of Sulfanilamide Case

In 1937, an elixir of sulfanilamide dissolved in ethylene glycol was introduced into the marketplace. One hundred and seven people died as a result of ethylene glycol toxicity. The public response to these two tragedies helped prompt the US Congress to pass the Federal Food, Drug, and Cosmetic Act of 1938 (FD&C Act). This law mandated the premarket testing of drugs for safety in experimental animals. It is a fact that since the imposition of animal testing, as a result of these two cases, no similar occurrence has happened, even though society uses many more consumer products and pharmaceuticals today than during the 1930s.

Thalidomide

The use of thalidomide, a sedative-hypnotic agent, led to some 10 000 deformed children being born in Europe. This in turn led directly to the 1962 revision of the FD&C Act, requiring more stringent testing. Current testing procedures (or even those at the time in the United States, where the drug was never approved for human use) would have identified the hazard and prevented this tragedy. In fact, tragedies like this have not occurred in Europe or the United States except when the results of animal tests have been ignored. **Table 1** presents an overview of cases in which animal data predicted adverse effects in humans.

Birth defects, for example, have occurred with isotretinoin (Accutane) where developmental toxicity had been clearly established in animals and presented on labeling, but the drug has continued to be used by potentially pregnant women.

Choosing an Animal Model

Choosing the appropriate animal model for a given problem is sometimes guesswork and often a matter of convenience. One often uses a species with which one is most familiar and for which there is extensive prior experience, with little consideration as to whether the chosen species is actually the most appropriate for the problem at hand. For example, the rat is probably a poor model for studying the chronic toxicity of any new nonsteroidal anti-inflammatory drug (NSAID) because the acute gastrointestinal toxicity will probably mask any other toxic effects. The guinea pig is less sensitive to most NSAIDs than the rat and closer in sensitivity to humans and thus would be a more appropriate species for investigating the chronic (non-gastrointestinal) toxicity of an NSAID. This practice of not rationally choosing an appropriate species for an experiment undoubtedly results in questionable science. This alone should be considered a waste of animals and resources. It results also in additional, and sometimes duplicative, experiments. It is common, for example, to default to using primates for evaluating proteins when they are often not a good model.

Research into replacements for test animals, such as cellular cultures, organs harvested from slaughterhouses, *in silico* (computer) modeling, and physical/chemical systems, has been extensive. Although each of these has their utility and they have reduced animal usage in both certain geographic regions (such as the EU) and product areas (cosmetics and consumer products being notable examples), regrettably, changes in

Table 1 Animal models that predicted adverse effects of xenobiotics in humans

Agent	*Effect*	*Animal species*	*In human*
Thalidomide	Phocomelia	Rat	No/yes
Accutane	Developmental toxicity of CNS (neural tube defects)	Rat, rabbit, dog, primate	Yes
AZT	Bone marrow depression	Rat, dog, monkey	Yes
Valproic acid	Cleft palate	Rat, mouse, rabbit	Yes
Cyclosporine	Nephropathy, reversible immune response suppression (essential aid to organ transplantation)	Rat, monkey	Yes
Benoxaprofen (Oraflex)	Hepatotoxicity	No	Yes
	Photosensitivity	Guinea pig	Yes
Zomepirac (Zomax)	Anaphylactic shock	No	Yes
MPTP	Parkinsonism	Monkey	Yes
Cyclophosphamide	Hemorrhagic cystitis	Rat, dog	Yes
Mercury	Encephalopathy	Rat, monkey	Yes
Diethylene glycol	Nephropathy	Rat, dog	Yes
Razoxin	Myelomonocytic leukemia	Mouse	Yes

testing requirements in other areas (such as medical devices) have simultaneously caused an increase in animal usage.

Alternatives will not fully replace animals for the foreseeable future. Some degree of animal use will continue, while the future is bright for ongoing progress with the three Rs, based on new technology and science, for example, building on the quite recent development of transgenic and knockout models for research on various diseases to go along with xenograft and other types of animal models. New models such as telemeterized larger animal species have also now achieved broad use, and hold the promise of both providing more meaningful data for human identifying and evaluating human risks and of serving to reduce the number of animals required and used. At the same time, most transgenic animal usage has been additional to existing programs, actually serving to increase animal usage owing to these models largely being seen as a means to answer new questions. However, society's increasing aversion to risks is a powerful driver in the other direction.

See also: Analytical Toxicology; *In Vitro* Tests; *In Vivo* Tests; Society of Toxicology; Thalidomide; Toxicity Testing, Alternatives; Toxicity Testing, Aquatic; Toxicity Testing, Behavioral; Toxicity Testing, Carcinogenesis; Toxicity Testing, Dermal; Toxicity Testing, Developmental; Toxicity Testing, Inhalation; Nonmammalian Models in Toxicology Screening.

Further Reading

Boelsterli, U.A., 2003. Animal models of human disease in drug safety assessment. J. Toxicol. Sci. 28, 109–121.

Boverhoff, D.R., et al., 2011. Transgenic animal models in toxicology: historical perspectives and future outlook. Toxicol. Sci. 121 (2), 207–233.

Gad, S.C. (Ed.), 2006. Animal Models in Toxicology, second ed. Dekker, New York.

Relevant Websites

http://www.toxicology.org - Society of Toxicology, Animals in Research.

http://dels.nas.edu - US National Academy of Sciences, Institute of Laboratory Animal Research (ILAR). Animal Models & Strains Search Engine.

Animals, Poisonous and Venomous

T Dodd-Butera, CSU San Bernardino, San Bernardino, CA, USA
M Broderick, California Poison Control System, San Diego, CA, USA

Background

Phylum Arthropoda is the largest phylum in the animal kingdom. Many of the species are nontoxic. However, class Arachnida contains spiders. Spiders have venom, but the black widow, brown recluse, and hobo spiders are responsible for a more significant number of toxicity events in humans.

Black Widow Spider: *Lactrodectus mactans* (see Figure 1)

Introduction

Black widow spiders can be found in dark spaces of trash, closets, woodpiles, and other areas in and around the home. The female spider is dangerous to humans and larger than the male. The spider is noted for a black color that is shiny, with a rounded abdomen and a red hourglass mark on the ventral surface (**Figure 1**).

Toxicity

The black widow spider produces neurotoxic venom, due in part to the alpha latrotoxin in the protein. Exposure is usually through a painful bite, although the bite may occasionally go unnoticed until symptoms develop. The mechanism of action of black widow spider venom involves binding of the gangliosides and glycoproteins of the motor end plate in the neuromuscular junction, which affects the opening of sodium channels and the release of acetylcholine (Ach) and norepinephrine. This results in excessive stimulation and allows for penetration and circulation of the venom into the lymphatic system.

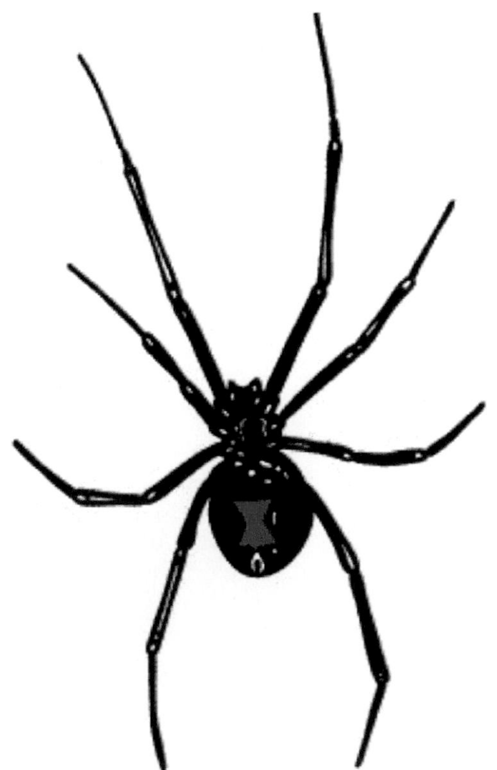

Figure 1 Black widow spider. http://www.calpoison.org/public/spiders.html#1.

A black widow spider bite may appear as a pale target area, surrounded by redness. Extreme muscle cramping and pain may develop in the back, abdomen, shoulders, and thighs, within minutes to hours of the bite. Weakness, headache, anxiety, restlessness, nausea, and vomiting may also occur. Other potential symptoms include itching, difficulty breathing, and increased blood pressure. 'Facies lactrodectismica' is characterized by unique facial sweating and grimacing. Death has occurred, but is rare. Sensitive populations, such as the very young and the elderly, are at the greatest risk for toxicity, in addition to those with blood pressure problems and chronic illnesses. Depending on the severity, symptoms may last for several days.

Treatment

Initial treatment should consist of washing the bite area carefully. Having the telephone number of a regional poison control center by the phone is helpful in order to obtain accurate poison information and to decrease anxiety in an emergency. Medical attention should be sought, especially in members of high-risk groups. Black widow spider antivenin is available, however, is not always necessary. Effective results have been achieved using *Lactrodectus* antivenin; however, in rare cases, anaphylaxis and serum sickness have been reported. Symptomatic and supportive treatment, with observation in a health care facility, may be more appropriate, and can be determined by a health care provider. Hypertension and pain control may require medication. Monitoring the site of the bite for proper healing and follow-up is important, as in tetanus prophylaxis, when indicated. Patients should be educated about possible preventive measures to be taken in order to avoid black widow spider habitats, when possible.

Another example of a spider causing lactrodectism is the redback spider (*Latrodectus hasseltii*), which is the leading spider envenomation requiring antivenom in Australia. The spider is usually 10 mm in length and has a prominent, globular abdomen bearing either a red, orange, or brown stripe. The male redback spider rarely causes envenomation.

Brown Recluse Spiders: *Loxosceles reclusa* (see Figure 2)

Introduction

The violin or fiddleback spider is a small (1/2 inch long), brown spider with a violin-shaped mark on the dorsum surface

 http://dx.doi.org/10.1016/B978-0-12-386454-3.00984-2

of the cephalothorax. It has six (not eight) eyes, and the tail segment has no markings. Any markings on the tail end of a spider, eliminate the potential that it is *L. reclusa*. Sometimes spider bites are erroneously attributed to the brown recluse spider, but there are a number of insects and spider bites, which can cause tissue wounds. Exposure is through a bite with potential envenomation, which may go unnoticed, so sometimes the spider is unseen. This can lead to confusion about the source of toxicity and symptoms. The brown recluse spider may be found in quiet, dark places, such as woodpiles and basements, where it can go undisturbed (**Figure 2**).

Toxicity

Loxosceles venom contains hyaluronidase, alkaline phosphatase, 5-ribonucleotide phosphohydrolase, and sphingomyelinase D. Sphingomyelinase D is a component of the cytotoxic venom, with a molecular weight of 32 000 Da. Sphingomyelinase causes release of choline and *N*-acylsphingosine phosphate from the red blood cell membrane, which stimulates platelet aggregation and dermonecrosis.

Initially, a local lesion may appear, with swelling at the site of the bite. The bite can take on a 'bull's-eye' appearance, with a central blister that breaks open, and can leave a skin ulcer, which develops a scab. Ulceration with delayed healing may occur. The ulcer can worsen with pain and expanding tissue damage. Initially, a red itchy rash presents within 24–48 h after the spider bite. Symptoms can progress systemically to include nausea, vomiting, fever, muscle aches, and potentially, hemolytic anemia, and disseminated intravascular coagulation (DIC).

Treatment

Most of these spider bites do not result in serious toxicity. Initial treatment consists of washing the affected bite area. Having the telephone number of a regional poison control center by the phone is helpful in order to obtain accurate poison information and to decrease anxiety in an emergency. If symptoms of infection develop, or the area develops an ulcer that does not heal, a medical consultation should be sought. There is no antivenin for *L. reclusa*, and treatment is symptomatic and supportive, particularly for signs of infection. If a wound becomes deep and infected, antibiotics and surgical options may be considered, in addition to medical management of complications. There is no proven preventive measure to avoid dermonecrosis, thus observation of affected areas is indicated. Surgery for abscess formation, or corrective measures for tissue damage may be indicated. Victims of envenomation who are susceptible to infection or have conditions, which impair healing are at risk and should be monitored carefully. Prevention is difficult, but shaking out items carefully and avoiding areas where *Loxosceles* reside, if possible, may be helpful to minimize envenomation potential.

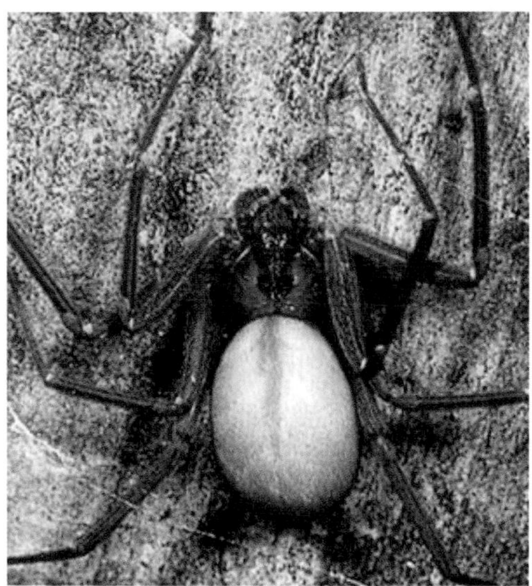

Figure 2 Brown recluse spider. http://www.calpoison.org/public/spiders.html#1.

Hobo Spiders

Introduction

There is a group of spiders, whose bites look similar to a brown recluse spider bite. Some of the spiders in this group include the running spider, jumping spider, wolf spider, tarantula, sac spider, orb weaver spider, and the northwestern brown spider, also known as the hobo spider.

Tegenaria agrestis (hobo spiders) are found in Europe and the Pacific Northwestern United States. *Tegenaria agrestis* spiders are brown with gray markings and approximately 10 mm in length. Hobo spiders are found in woodpiles, basements, and moist areas.

Toxicity

Envenomation from a painless bite by *T. agrestis* may result in necrosis, similar to *L. reclusa*. Unlike the previous spiders discussed, male hobo spiders are more venomous than females. The hobo spider often causes a bite that leaves an open, slow-healing wound. Local symptoms of blistering may occur after envenomation. Scarring and healing may range from 1 month to 3 years, in more severe cases.

Treatment

Treatment is symptomatic and supportive for wound care (similar to *Loxosceles*) and hematological complications. Recommendations for treatment include keeping the affected area clean and observing for signs of infection. Consultation with a health care provider is recommended if the bite becomes infected, systemic symptoms worsen, or if the symptoms do not resolve.

Funnel Web Spiders

Introduction

Funnel web spiders (encompassed within the genera *Atrax* and *Hadronyche*) are found in southeastern Australia, but may be found in other parts of the world, if kept as exotic pets. They are part of a group of spiders known as 'mygalomorphs,' which have fangs that penetrate in a downward fashion. Bites may be deadly, particularly in the male spider of this group. Funnel web spiders may live on the ground, in the trees, rocks, or piles of leaves. They may also wander into areas around swimming pools, so precaution should be taken in these areas, to avoid envenomation. Gardening was found to be an activity highly associated with these types of spider bites.

Toxicity

Funnel spider venom is harmful in humans and other primates, but not necessarily all mammals. The venom is a complex mixture; however, the neurotoxic components that contribute to symptoms are known as the Ç-atracotoxins. These may slow sodium current inactivation, with resultant firing of action potentials. The excessive release and eventual depletion of sympathetic neurotransmitters lead to a biphasic symptomatic response, which may range from mild to severe toxicity. The first phase is characterized by local effects, including a painful bite site, with swelling, redness, and fang marks. General symptoms during this first phase can also include perioral numbness, severe facial and tongue spasms, piloerection, nausea, vomiting, abdominal cramps, salivation, lacrimation, and profuse sweating. Difficulty in breathing may be experienced, along with high blood pressure, an irregular heartbeat, and mental confusion. In the second phase, which may occur several hours after cessation of secretions, victims of envenomation can experience extremely low blood pressure, decreased respirations, noncardiogenic pulmonary edema, and cardiac arrest.

Treatment

Envenomations may result in mild, moderate, or severe symptoms. Medical attention should be sought, in the event of an identified funnel web spider bite. Antivenin may be required in cases of severe envenomation. If needed, this will be administered in a health care setting by a health care provider, with careful patient monitoring. There have been no reports of human fatalities since the use of antivenin, in the 1980s.

Scorpions

Introduction

Globally, approximately 1500 species of scorpions are identified, though not all are considered dangerous to humans. Scorpionism is a public health problem in certain areas of the world. These include Africa (South, north-Saharan, and Sahelian sections), Near and Middle East, South India, Mexico and South Latin America, east of the Andes, which involves an estimated 2 billion people at risk. Poisonous scorpions can also exist in the United States, including the *Centruroides sculpturatus* (*exilicauda*) and *Centruroides gertschii* variety (see **Table 1**). Scorpion stings frequently occur during hot, summer months in various regions.

Table 1 Selected venomous scorpions and areas inhabited

Area	*Selected species*
North Africa	*Androctonus australis*, *Leiurus quinquestriatus* and *Androctonus*, *Mauretanicu*, *Androctonus aeneas*, *B. occitanus* and *Hottentota* (=*Buthotus*) *franzwerneri*
Subsaharan Africa	*Parabuthus granulates*, *A. australis*, *A. aeneas*, *Buthus occitanus* and *H. franzwerneri*
Near and Middle East	*Androctonus* and *Leiurus genera*
India	*Hottentota* (=*Mesobuthus*) *tumulus*
Arizona (USA)	*Centruroides sculpturatus* (=*Centruroides exilicauda*)
Mexico	*Centruroides limpidus*, *C. sufussus*, and *C. limpidus tecomanus*

Toxicity

All scorpions have venomous apparatus in common that consist of a vesicle with a pair of joined glands, included in the bulbous segment of the telson. This is situated in the postabdomen, just anterior to a stinger. The venom vesicle is surrounded by a layer of striated muscle, which regulates ejection; and thus, there is a potential for 'dry' stings without venom. Stings may result accidently, from stepping on the stinger, or through aggressive grabbing of the prey with the scorpion's anterior pincers, and then stabbing the victim.

The venom may contain hyaluronidase, phospholipase, acetylcholinesterase, and other digestive enzymes and neurotoxins, which affect sodium channels and prolong action potentials. Swift reaction of catecholamine release has been attributed to the dramatic cholinergic symptoms. There are also species of scorpions that may cause disruption to bleeding. Envenomations by *Tityus*, *Buthus*, *Androctonus*, and *Leiurus* species have been reported to cause pulmonary edema, cardiovascular collapse, DIC, renal failure, and fatalities. Children under 6 years of age are particularly vulnerable to systemic symptoms.

Treatment

Variable amounts of venom may be ejected from the telson, so dose from injection is uncertain and treatment must be based on evaluation of patient symptoms. In the *Centruroides* species, stings produce severe pain, when the area is 'tapped.' There is a potential for a range of symptoms, as noted above, and is dependent on species of scorpion, age and health of victim. Local wound care is commonly required, but the potential symptoms of restlessness, impaired vision, neurotoxic, cardiovascular, and respiratory symptoms mandate that treatment be supportive and appropriate to the level of severity. In certain species, administration of antivenin is appropriate, when available, and is a decision made by the health care provider. Pain management is also important to alleviate suffering in the victim. Prevention strategies include shaking out shoes, sleeping bags, and tents, and careful attention when in an area of scorpions, particularly at night.

Hymenoptera

Introduction

The order Hymenoptera includes families of venomous insects, known as honeybees, bumblebees, wasps, hornets, yellow jackets, and ants. Female insects have the venom located in their posterior abdomen. Bites and stings from this group may cause allergic reactions, and sometimes rapid death from anaphylactic reactions.

Toxicity

Hymenoptera venom contains combinations of various enzymes, with different methods of stinging the victim (see Table 2). Some insects deposit the stinger in the victim, causing insect death, while others are capable of stinging the victim multiple times. Ants have the potential to inject venom through a stinger, or some may spray venom from the posterior abdomen after biting the victim.

Treatment

Dose of venom varies, as each sting may empty the contents of the venom gland or deliver a fraction of the contents. In addition, some insects may inflict multiple stings, while others die with one. Response to venom is also variable, as noted; hypersensitivity in some individuals may occur, and result in fatalities. Further, a fire ant nest may contain thousands of insects, which deliver a sting rapidly, if disturbed. This increases the dose of venom. Thus, treatment should be based on the victim's symptoms, as it is difficult to estimate dose and exposure. Victims of bites and stings generally present with complaints of pain, with swelling and redness surrounding the site. Multiple stings may produce vomiting, diarrhea, decreased blood pressure, muscle breakdown, and death. Swelling of the upper airway is a hazard, but rarely occurs with one sting, in individuals without hypersensitivity. Allergic reactions are generally rapid, and the victim should be monitored closely in a health care facility and treated for anaphylaxis, if needed. Occasionally, delayed sensitivity may occur, including fever, arthralgias, and potentially severe illness, so further monitoring by a health care provider may be needed. Keeping the area clean and free of pain and infection are important in milder cases. There is no available antivenin, so treatment is symptomatic and supportive. Individuals with known sensitivity may carry an emergency kit containing epinephrine, under the advice of a health care provider.

Snakes

Introduction

There are approximately 3000 types of snakes that exist around the world, with an estimated 600 types that are venomous. Reports from databases of the World Health Organization estimate a range of 20 000–94 000 deaths occurring, annually, from snakebites. Snakes exist on every continent, with the exception of Antarctica.

Toxicity

Snakes are classified in the phylum Chordata, subphylum Vertebrata, class Reptilia, order Squamata, suborder Serpentes. There are 14 families, but Colubridae, Elapidae, Hydrophidae, Viperidae, Crotalinae, and Viperinae are the families and subfamilies of poisonous snakes (see Figure 3).

The dose and exposure to venom vary due to the complexity of multiple components, the amount injected, and the type of snakebite. Approximately 20% of snakebites do not involve injection of venom. These are known as 'dry' bites. With envenomations in humans, effects vary from cytotoxic, neurotoxic, and hemotoxic events, which are dependent on species, seasonal, and geographic factors. Potential symptoms include tissue destruction, paralysis, and extensive bleeding. Victims are often young, and face the potential of lifelong disability, even when the snakebite does not result in fatality.

Treatment

An important aspect of treatment for all snake envenomations is access to health care facilities, with available providers, medical care, and antivenin (as needed). Symptomatic and supportive care can be lifesaving, and must be in consultation with a health care provider, especially familiar with snakebites. Calm, but rapid removal of the victim to a health care facility is an essential component of treatment. Some select specifics are provided below.

Crotalinae: Envenomations leave fang marks similar to puncture wounds, with a potential for progressive edema and ecchymosis. Initially, stinging and burning pain may occur. Victims are generally observed for 8–12 h, however, to ascertain the extent of injury and toxicity. Swelling of the affected area is particularly important to observe for and may be followed by nausea, vomiting, hypotension, and cardiovascular collapse, in extreme cases. Health care providers observe for generalized fasciculations, muscle weakness, and blood clotting disorders, coupled with deteriorating medical conditions in the victim, in order to determine the appropriate use of antivenin.

Table 2 Order hymenoptera stings

Family	*Type of insect*	*Stinger*	*Death of insect (yes or no)*
Apidae	Honeybee	Remains in the victim	Yes
Bombidae	Bumblebees	Remains intact	No, multiple stings possible
Vespidae	Wasps, hornets, yellow jackets	Remains intact	No, multiple stings possible
Formicidae	Ants	Stinger injection or spray	No

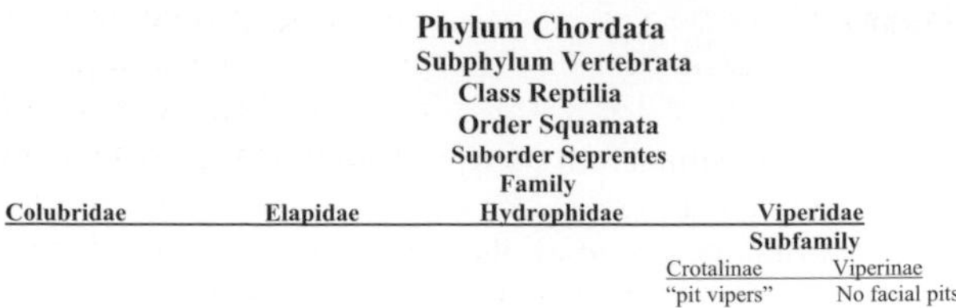

Figure 3 Classification of selected poisonous snakes.

Elapidae: These snakes have small mouths and fixed fangs in the rear of the mouth, which require chewing on the victim, in order to envenomate. Symptoms can occur in a few hours, or may be delayed. These include minimal initial swelling and tingling, which may progress to nausea, vomiting, weakness, and mental confusion. Neurological symptoms can predominate, and respiratory arrest may occur, for which rapid respiratory support is an important treatment. Antivenin may be utilized by a health care provider if bleeding disorders or neurotoxicity occurs.

Treatment of snakebites *does not* include the use of a tourniquet, or making cuts over the site of the bite. Accidental envenomation may occur even when the snake is dead, and can happen when attempting to identify the type of snake involved, so caution should be exercised. In addition, careful attention to surroundings in the outdoors and observing for signs of warning in areas where snakes are present are important prevention measures.

Venomous Lizards

Introduction

The Gila monster (*Heloderma suspectum*), order Squamata, is found in desert areas such as the southwestern United States and Mexico. It is large, orange and black in color, with a length of up to 2 feet, and weight of approximately 5 pounds. They are large, timid, creatures, spending most of their time in underground burrows.

Toxicity

Though bites are rare, Gila monsters are known for their tenacity when they bite. In the event of a bite, they may need to be forcibly disengaged from victims. Unlike snakes, Gilas do not inject venom with fangs, but rather fasten onto victims, releasing neurotoxins through grooves in their teeth. Venom contains enzymes, hyaluronidase, phospholipase A, and serotonin, with a mixture of additional components.

Treatment

Envenomation does not always occur with bites. Symptoms following envenomation include pain, swelling, and possible anaphylactic reactions. Venom is a mild neurotoxin, so symptomatic and supportive care for the victim is indicated for treatment, under the supervision of a health care provider, when necessary.

Poison Dart Frogs

Introduction

Poison dart frogs, family Dendrobatidae, inhabit rainforests and other warm, moist climates. Only poisonous frogs from the genus *Phyllobates*, especially the species *Phyllobates terribilis*, *Phyllobates bicolor*, and *Phyllobates aurotaenia*, secrete batrachotoxin, the toxin used to poison the tips of darts for hunting by South American tribes, such as the Naonama, Choco, and Cuna groups from Columbia. The toxin is taken up through the diet of the frog and is secreted onto the skin.

Toxicity

Batrachotoxin, found in the skin glands of the *Phyllobates* frogs, is a steroidal alkaloid, which protects the frogs by producing toxic effects in the mouths of predators. The toxin acts by preventing voltage-gated sodium channels from closing in nerves. It is very potent and specific with doses of less than 0.1 μg eliciting convulsions, muscle contractions, salivation, and death. Other symptoms include respiratory paralysis and muscular paralysis.

Treatment

While there are currently no effective treatments or antidotes for batrachotoxin poisoning, certain anesthetics and antagonists can be used to reverse membrane depolarization. Tetrodotoxin can also be used to treat batrachotoxin poisoning through antagonistic effects on sodium flux.

Platypus

Introduction

The platypus is a monotreme mammal found in Australia and Tasmania, and is one of the very few venomous mammals. The platypus has webbed feet, a large duck-billed snout, and a beaverlike tail. Platypuses do not have teeth, but the males are venomous, with stingers on their rear feet.

Toxicity

The ankle spurs of male platypuses produce a venom comprised of defensin-like proteins, nerve growth factor, and natriuretic peptides. Three of these proteins are unique to the platypus. Although the defensin-like proteins are not lethal to humans, victims experience such excruciating pain that they may become incapacitated. The pain is associated with mast cell degeneration. The toxin is a C-type natriuretic peptide, and has been associated with calcium-dependent nociceptor action. The envenomation is also associated with an extended hyperalgesia.

Treatment

Treatment is symptomatic and requires medical attention for pain relief; functional impairment of the affected envenomation area can also persist and requires medical monitoring. No antivenom is available.

Pitohuis

Introduction

The pitohuis, genus *Pitohui*, family Pachycephalidae, are brightly colored, poisonous birds of New Guinea and the only birds known to be poisonous to humans, as established by the scientist Jack Dumbacher in 1989. The most toxic species includes the Hooded and Variable *Pitohui*. Similar to the toxin of the poison dart frog, the toxin is found on the skin, and also on the feathers of some birds. It is postulated that the toxin in the Pitohui serves as a defense against parasites and predators. Although poisonous to humans, the birds are still consumed on New Guinea using a specific method of cooking and skinning. Just like the poison dart frogs, the pitohuis get the toxins from their diet, namely the beetle Choresine.

Toxicity

Batrachotoxin is a potent steroid alkaloid associated with both the poison dart frog and the *Pitohui* bird. The mechanism of toxicity is through modulation of voltage-gated sodium channels, and subsequent depolarization of nerves and muscles. In toxic exposures, symptoms may include arrhythmias and eventual cardiac failure.

Pumiliotoxins are also found in the poisonous dart frog, but are less toxic than batrachotoxins. They also involve calcium and sodium dependent mechanisms (which are not yet fully elucidated). Difficulties with locomotion after exposure contribute to myotoxicity, and may include partial paralysis and/or clonic movements.

Treatment

There is no specific antidote for exposure to these toxins. Treatment for human exposures would be symptomatic and supportive, requiring urgent medical attention in the event of cardiotoxicity.

Slow Loris

Introduction

The slow loris, family Lorisidae, genus *Nycticebus*, is a nocturnal arboreal primate found in Vietnam, Indonesia, and the rainforests of Malaysia. They are considered to be an endangered species as of 2012 and are listed on the IUCN Red List. Their diet consists of insects, bird eggs, small vertebrates, and fruit.

Toxicity

The slow loris is the only venomous primate. Slow lorises have a toxic bite due to a toxin that is produced by the licking a gland on their inner elbow, the brachial organ. Saliva from the slow loris is required to activate the secretion from the arm gland. However, very little else is known about the chemical nature of the toxin. The slow loris bite is reported to be painful in humans with symptoms including burning of the tongue and throat, hypotension, muscle convulsions, heart and respiratory problems, unconsciousness, and even death through anaphylaxis shock.

Treatment

Vaccination against tetanus and antibiotics is often given to bite victims. Treatment is symptomatic for bites and anaphylaxis.

See also: Snakes; Plants, Poisonous (Humans); Poisonous (animals); Marine Venoms and Toxins; Spiders; Scorpions.

Further Reading

Bentur, Y., Taitelman, U., Aloufy, A., 2003. Evaluation of scorpion stings: the poison; center perspective. Vet. Hum. Toxicol. 45, 108–111.

Isbister, G.K., Fan, H.W., 2011. Spider bite. Lancet 378 (9808), 2039–2047.

Kasturiratne, A., Wickremasinghe, A.R., de Silva, N., Gunawardena, N.K., Pathmeswaran, A., Premaratna, R., Savioli, L., Lalloo, D.G., de Silva, H.J., 2008. The global burden of snakebite: a literature analysis and modelling based on regional estimates of envenoming and deaths. PLoS Med. 5 (11), e218.

Mebs, D., 2002. Venomous and Poisonous Animals: A Handbook for Biologists, Toxicologists and Toxinologists, Physicians and Pharmacists. CRC Scientific Publishing, Boca Raton, FL.

Olson, K.R. (Ed.), 2007. Poisoning and Drug Overdose, fifth ed. Lange Medical Books/McGraw Hill, New York.

Zhao, M., Gao, X., Wang, J., He, X., Han, B., 2013. A review of the most economically important poisonous plants to the livestock industry on temperate grasslands of China. J. Appl. Toxicol. 33 (1), 9–17. http://dx.doi.org/10.1002/jat.2789.

Relevant Websites

http://www.toxinology.com – Clinical Toxinology Resources (University of Adelaide).

http://www.nlm.nih.gov/medlineplus/ency/ – Medline Plus: Search for Funnel Web Spider.

http://animals.nationalgeographic.com/animals/reptiles/gila-monster/ – National Geographic: Gila Monster.

http://www.ipm.ucdavis.edu/PMG/PESTNOTES/ – University of California Agriculture & Natural Resources Pest Notes Library.

http://toxicology.ucsd.edu/modules.htm – University of California, San Diego: Medical Toxicology.

Animal Testing Alternatives *see* Toxicity Testing, Alternatives

Animal Venoms in Medicine

Z Takacs, ToxinTech, Inc., New York, NY, USA
S Nathan, University of Chicago Medicine, Chicago, IL, USA

Introduction

Venomous animals occur in most animal phyla, including Cnidaria (sea anemones, jellyfishes, corals), Mollusca (marine snails, cephalopods), Annelida (leeches), Arthropoda (arachnids, insects, centipedes), Echinodermata (sea urchins, starfishes), and Chordata (fishes, reptiles, mammals). They are distributed throughout the Earth, inhabit a wide range of ecosystems, and have an evolutionary history dating back hundreds of millions of years. This broad evolutionary and environmental space has resulted in an extraordinarily diverse and powerful arsenal of molecules, yet all aiming toward one common goal: disablement of key physiological processes within seconds (**Figure 1**).

Venom Definition

'Venom' is defined as an animal secretion (by a specialized apparatus that is functionally and morphologically a separate unit within the body) used in feeding and/or defense, evolved to be delivered via physical trauma (by the parenteral route; e.g., by fang, harpoon, chelicerae) to an other animal causing a toxic (regardless of how weak or strong in magnitude but biologically beneficial for the producing organism) effect. (For simplicity, 'toxin' in this article refers to any venom component.)

Biology

Animal venoms evolved to harm, immobilize, or kill a wide spectrum of prey, predator, or adversary (e.g., intraspecific competition) species. In these target organisms, toxins aim at physiologically key and vulnerable body functions: neuromuscular signaling, vascular hemostasis, and the cardiovascular system, among others. Interfering with these functions allows for quick and powerful pharmacological intervention in a phylogenetically broad range of taxa.

Venom is a complex mixture of proteins, peptides, and low-molecular weight organic and inorganic components, all acting synergistically. The peptidic components are enzymatic or nonenzymatic and are typically responsible for most, although not all, of the main pharmacological characteristics of crude venom. Venom from a single species is a mixture of about 50–200 different components (near-extreme examples: 7–8 gene products in Tiger rattlesnake (*Crotalus tigris*), up to 600 peptide masses in Sydney funnel-web spider (*Atrax robustus*)), and composition varies among and within species. Toxin molecules can be monomeric or homo/heteromultimeric

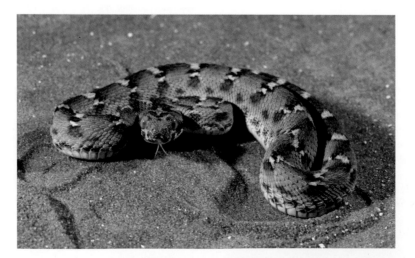

Figure 1 The manufacturer of a life-saving drug in the Arabian desert. The GPIIb/IIIa receptor antagonist toxin echistatin isolated from the Saw-scaled viper (*Echis carinatus*) venom served as a template for tirofiban (AGGRASTAT®) to treat unstable angina and non-Q-wave myocardial infarction (Photo: Dr Zoltan Takacs).

 http://dx.doi.org/10.1016/B978-0-12-386454-3.01241-0

complexes held together by covalent or noncovalent interactions.

History of Venoms in Medicine

Long before the current era of medicine, the life of Mithridates VI of Pontus (in 67 BC) is believed to be saved by Scythian shamans in present-day Turkey using viper (Viperidae) venom. The Ayurvedic texts of Susruta Samhita and Charaka Samhita (dates uncertain: first and second centuries AD) mention animal venoms in the context of medical use. Leech and bee venoms as therapeutic agents dates back thousands of years to a number of ancient cultures from the Far East to the Mediterranean region.

Modern experimental medicine credits two Italians as early pioneers of toxinology: Francesco Redi (1626–97) to show that it is not the snake's spirit that kills but its venom, and Felix Fontana (1730–1805) to show that viper venom affects blood. Around 1905, hirudin extract from the European medicinal leech (*Hirudo medicinalis*) was used as the first parenteral anticoagulant. Trials in 1934 with locally applied Russell's viper (*Daboia russelii*) venom diluted at 1:10 000 showed "success to stop haemorrhage following dental extraction." In 1938, Russell's viper venom was offered as a coagulant under the name Rusven. In 1936, "hämokoagulase" was purified from the Brazilian pit viper Jararaca (*Bothrops jararaca*), and this venom fraction is still in use today for hemorrhage.

In 1963, prolonged clotting defects were reported after Malayan pit viper (*Calloselasma rhodostoma*) bites, an observation that led to the isolation of a toxin called ancrod, and by 1968, turning it into a defibrinogenating therapeutic. Another milestone occurred in 1981 with the US Food and Drug Administration (FDA) approval of the antihypertensive agent captopril, derived from the Jararaca (*B. jararaca*) venom. This was the first example of reduction of a toxin to a small-molecule mimic, and also the pharmaceutical company Squibb's first billion-dollar drug. Venoms have also been instrumental for discoveries in many fields of basic science, for example, nucleic acid, ion channel, and nerve growth factor research, to name only a few.

Toxins as Drug Templates

Evolutionary Aspect

Despite the vast number of toxins in nature's venoms, peptidic toxins fall into a handful of protein scaffolds encoded by gene superfamilies. The length of the peptide, the number and relative position of disulfide bonds, the signal peptide, and other sequence determinants are highly conserved and signatory for a scaffold. Consequently, within a scaffold, the primary, secondary, and tertiary structures are extensively conserved, yet discrete amino acid substitutions along the peptide backbone are present and confer novel biological function.

Toxin genes typically evolve from genes of other body proteins with nontoxic physiological functions expressed in tissues other than the venom gland. For example, three-finger toxin scaffold widespread in elapid snakes (Elapidae: cobras, mambas, sea snakes, etc.) is homologous to the Ly-6 superfamily of proteins, present from Cnidaria to Chordata. Lynx1 peptide, a member of the Ly-6 superfamily, is an endogenous physiological neuromodulator in the mammalian central nervous system, with no toxic function. Subtle amino acid changes on this scaffold theme, however, generated an amazingly different and wide range of molecules (now called toxins) with unique biological activities targeting the muscle-type or neuronal nicotinic acetylcholine receptors (nAChRs), muscarinic acetylcholine (ACh) receptors, voltage-gated Ca^{2+} (Ca_V)-1 channels, acid-sensing ion channel, acetylcholinesterase, platelet integrin GPIIb/IIIa, coagulation factor VIIa, and others.

The actual process of toxin evolution occurs by gene duplication, gene conversion, alternative splicing, and various forms of gene domain multiplication, or loss. The new gene is typically subject to rapid diversification by accelerated evolution and positive selection. Amino acid substitution rate correlates with surface accessibility of residue that is a driver for novel specificity, and toxin genes rank among the most rapidly evolving protein-coding genes in Metazoa. The process is mostly attributed to the predator–prey arms race, and the same protein scaffolds are often convergently recruited into the venom arsenal by different animal taxa. There is also evidence that toxin genes could potentially revert back to nontoxic physiological function.

The end result is an astonishing array of unique toxins – each with a distinct, however subtle or pronounced, pharmacological property – based on a handful of evolution-tested, robust molecular scaffolds.

Chemistry

In medical applications, peptidic toxins could be used either in their native (natural or synthetic) form or as a modified molecule (peptidomimetic – a molecule that mimics the desired action of the native peptide). In the native form, they bear high potency, and the conformationally restrained structure may minimize binding to nontargets, resulting in high selectivity. As venoms are meant to be injected into foreign tissues, intrinsic sequence properties and posttranslational modifications (disulfide bonds, inhibitory cysteine knot, C-terminal amidation, etc.) often confer an inherent stability to toxins against degradation by proteases. Toxins are also soluble, a benefit in peptide therapeutics. Low accumulation in tissues and low toxicity are further advantages of peptidic drugs.

Undesirable aspects of using peptidic drugs are the need for parenteral administration (low oral bioavailability), susceptibility to proteolysis, short half-life, immunogenicity including triggering allergic reactions, and synthetic production issues (e.g., quantity, posttranslational modification). Toxin size and charge may also be limiting factors. At present, protein therapeutics are typically restricted to cell surface and extracellular targets. Furthermore, employing toxins directly purified from crude venom poses a challenge for quality control. To some degree, venom composition, including toxin sequence, varies (e.g., due to geographical origin of the specimen), and venom extraction, toxin purification/purity are also variables that must be controlled.

Reducing native toxins to peptide or nonpeptide (small molecule) peptidomimetic could offer more desirable pharmacokinetic properties such as increased bioavailability, enable membrane transport, and counter enzymatic degradation. However, designing peptidomimetics has many challenges. In successful therapeutic examples when toxins have been reduced to peptidomimetics, the structural elements responsible for activity (pharmacophore) were located in a continuous segment along the peptide backbone. Yet, in other toxins, the pharmacophore domain is contiguous in space rather than along the peptide backbone thus making it more problematic to develop mimics. The approach to develop captopril from the native toxin was one of the early examples of successfully reducing peptides to small molecules based on structure–activity relationship. Biomedical utilization of the nonpeptidic components of animal venoms remains less explored.

Pharmacology

The major advantage of toxins is that evolution perfected them to act on many of the same target molecules whose control is needed for therapeutic medical intervention. Often different scaffolds, from different taxa, are aimed at the same target molecule but with somewhat different binding sites. Toxin sequence diversity enables subtle distinction among target subtypes or the interaction with entirely different classes of targets, and thus induces an extremely wide variety of biological activities.

Enzymes, cell surface receptors of various types, including ion channels, control a wide range of key physiological processes and thus are among the major target classes for drugs. Hydrolases, G-protein-coupled receptors (GPCRs), and Ca^{2+} channels, are examples of the most prominent drug targets. For the very same reason – controlling key physiological processes – the enzymes/enzymatic pathways and cell surface receptors are also the principal target for animal toxins. Toxin targets with medical relevance include, but are not limited to, ligand-gated nAChRs, *N*-methyl-D-aspartate receptors, 5-hydroxytryptamine$_3$ receptors, and Ca_V, voltage-gated Na^+ (Na_V), and voltage-gated K^+ (K_V) channels, an array of GPCRs (e.g., α-adrenergic, muscarinic ACh, neurotensin, endothelin, and vasopressin receptors), and the norepinephrine transporter. A myriad of other regulator molecules of blood coagulation, platelet aggregation, and cardiovascular system are also major toxin targets, such as prothrombin, fibrinogen, integrin, angiotensin-converting enzyme (ACE), complement component C3, to name but a few. Nucleotides and lipids are also targeted by toxins.

Typically, a particular toxin scaffold interacts with a restricted number of target types and/or subtypes, such as a subset of K_V channels. This target-biased nature of toxin scaffolds makes them an ideal starting pool to select drug leads, templates on which further optimization can be performed. The structure of toxin targets is also evolutionarily conserved across species. This means toxins that work in a nonhuman species will likely, but not always, have a similar effect on molecules in humans.

Toxins often tend to have pharmacological properties that are required or beneficial for a lead compound: high affinity, potency, specificity (distinction among receptor types) and selectivity (distinction among receptor subtypes), therapeutic efficacy, and suitable mechanism of action. Other times, one or more of these factors are clearly not met, and further screening or optimization is needed. Safety, pharmacokinetics, and delivery also have to be addressed.

Current Medical Application of Animal Venom Toxins

Diagnostics

Toxins are used in approximately 15 diagnostic assays in clinical hemostasis laboratories and as a test for myasthenia gravis. All toxins are originated from snake venoms (**Table 1**).

The vertebrate hemostatic system, a delicate interaction among thrombocytes (known also as platelets in mammalian vertebrates), endothelial cells, subendothelial structures, and plasma proteins is easily vulnerable to disruptive biochemical or biophysical factors. This very system is a major and multipoint target for toxins that can lead to lethal thromboembolic events or hemorrhage (**Figure 2**). The mechanism of action of toxins is often extremely similar to the corresponding physiological clotting factor, and they can activate or inactivate numerous phases of blood coagulation. Importantly, however, because of acting independently from cofactors, or by being resistant to inhibitors, or to proteolytic degradation, the target organism's own control mechanisms are ineffective against the action of toxins. As a result, toxins with defined mechanisms of action, restricted substrate specificity, and unaffected by the inhibitory pathways are valuable sources of diagnostic tools.

Current diagnostics are mostly enzymatic toxins; nonenzymatic examples are BOTROCETIN® or α-bungarotoxin. They are typically purified directly from the crude venom, thus subject to taxonomic, geographic variability, and possibly misidentification. For example, geographical variability in Russell's viper venom (*D. russelii*) has been attributed to variability in the test results. Additionally, presence of toxin isoforms in a single venom could complicate test reproducibility.

While some tests have limited use, venoms are used, for example, to identify factor V Leiden mutation, one of the most common hereditary procoagulant states. Dilute Russell's viper venom time is widely used to detect lupus anticoagulants, a major risk factor for arterial and venous thrombosis, accounting for ~15% of patients with thromboembolic events. The availability of direct diagnosis (e.g., by sequencing) is expected to overtake the utilization of some toxin-based tests.

Therapeutics

Toxins are used in approximately 15 different medications (**Table 2**). Drugs from toxins include potentially life-saving (e.g., eptifibatide, captopril, enalapril), first-in-class (e.g., ACE inhibitors, incretin peptide mimetics), and some of the top-selling medications in the history of medicine (e.g., captopril/ ACE inhibitors). Toxins as drugs are either used as a natural toxin purified directly from crude venom (e.g., batroxobin), synthetic version of the natural toxin (e.g., exenatide, ziconotide), or as a peptide (e.g., eptifibatide) or nonpeptide (e.g.,

Table 1 Clinical diagnostics derived from animal venom toxins

Test/Reagent name	*Species origin*	*Mechanism of action*	*Test for*
anti-Ca_v2 antibodies assay	Geography cone snail (*Conus geographus*) or Magician's cone snail (*Conus magus*)	radioiodinated (*Cg*) ω-conotoxin GVIA or (*Cm*) ω-conotoxin MVIIC binding to $Ca_v2.2$, 2.1 respectively	Lambert-Eaton myasthenic syndrome
Anti-nAChR antibodies assay	Many-banded krait (*Bungarus multicinctus*) or 'Cobras' (*Naja* spp.)	Radioiodinated (*Bm*) α-bungarotoxin or (*N*) cobratoxin binding to nAChR	Myasthenia gravis
Anti-nAChR antibodies assay	Monocellate cobra (*Naja kaouthia*)	Eu^{3+}-α-cobratoxin binding to nAChR	Myasthenia gravis
BOTROCETIN®	Neuwied's lancehead (*Bothrops neuwiedi*) or Jararaca (*Bothrops jararaca*)	Induces von Willebrand factor (vWF) dependent platelet aggregation	von Willebrand factor (vWF) level
Factor V activator (RVV-V)	Russell's viper (*Daboia russelii*)	Activates factor V	Factor V determination
PEFAKIT® PiCT®	Russell's viper (*Daboia russelii*)	Activates factor V	Anticoagulant activity based on factor Xa and/or factor IIa inhibition
PEFAKIT® APC-R Factor V Leiden	Russell's viper (*Daboia russelii*); and Tiger snake (*Notechis scutatus*)	(*Dr*) activates factor V; and (*Ns*) activates prothrombin	Factor V Leiden mutation (FV:Q506)
PROTAC®	Copperhead (*Agkistrodon contortrix*)	Activates protein C	Protein C and protein S levels
PROC® GLOBAL	Copperhead (*Agkistrodon contortrix*)	Activates protein C	Protein C and protein S pathway abnormalities
CRYOCHECK™ CLOT C™	Copperhead (*Agkistrodon contortrix*); and Russell's viper (*Daboia russelii*)	(*Ac*) activates protein C; and (*Dr*) activates factor X	Protein C activity
CRYOCHECK™ CLOT S™	Copperhead (*Agkistrodon contortrix*); and Russell's viper (*Daboia russelii*)	(*Ac*) activates protein C; and (*Dr*) activates factor X	Protein S activity
REPTILASE® Time	Common lancehead (*Bothrops atrox*) or Brazilian lancehead (*Bothrops moojeni*)	Cleaves Aα-chain of fibrinogen	Fibrinogen level and function; heparin contamination
Textarin time	Eastern brown snake (*Pseudonaja textilis*)	PL dependent prothrombin activator	Activated protein C resistance; lupus anticoagulants
Textarin/ecarin ratio	Eastern brown snake (*Pseudonaja textilis*); and Saw-scaled viper (*Echis carinatus*)	(*Pt*) PL dependent prothrombin activator; and (*Ec*) activates prothrombin to meizothrombin in the absence of PL	Confirmation of lupus anticoagulants
Ecarin clotting time	Saw-scaled viper (*Echis carinatus*)	Activates prothrombin to meizothrombin in the absence of PL	Direct thrombin inhibitors; prothrombin quantification; lupus anticoagulants
Factor X activator (RVV-X)	Russell's viper (*Daboia russelii*)	Activates factor X	Lupus anticoagulants; distinguishing between factor VII and factor X deficiency
SPECTROZYME® FXa	Russell's viper (*Daboia russelii*)	Activates factor X	Factor X activity
STACLOT® APC-R	Western rattlesnake (*Crotalus oreganus*)	Activates factor X	Activated protein C resistance
Stypven time (Russell's viper venom time)	Russell's viper (*Daboia russelii*)	Activates factor X	Factor VII or X deficiency
Dilute Russell's viper venom time (dRVVT)	Russell's viper (*Daboia russelii*)	Activates factor X	Lupus anticoagulants
Dilute Russell's viper venom confirm DVVCONFIRM®	Russell's viper (*Daboia russelii*)	Activates factor X; extra PL corrects dRVVT	Confirmation of lupus anticoagulants
Taipan snake venom time	Taipan (*Oxyuranus scutellatus*)	Prothrombin activator, stimulated by PL	Lupus anticoagulants

Note: Order is based on the molecular weight of the principal (or first) toxin molecule responsible for activity. The extent of utilization, test name, and classification varies. Per classification, some tests may overlap. Test variations exist (e.g., Taipan snake venom time/ecarin time). Only one brand name (in parentheses) is provided as an example. PL, phospholipid.

tirofiban, captopril) peptidomimetic of the natural toxin. In 'hemocoagulases,' a crude venom fraction containing two natural toxins is utilized.

Currently drugs are derived from the venoms of various species of vipers (Viperidae), the European medicinal leech (*H. medicinalis*), Gila monster (*Heloderma suspectum*), and the marine snail Magician's cone (*Conus magus*). Representative indications include unstable angina, type 2 diabetes mellitus, hypertension, congestive cardiac failure, prevention of hemorrhage during surgery, and chronic pain. As an example of the impact venom-based agents have had on medicine, two out of the three available agents in the platelet glycoprotein

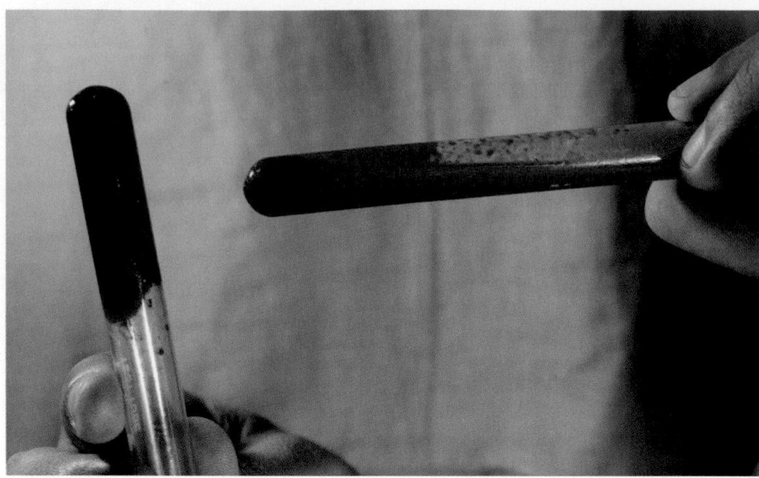

Figure 2 Viper venom targets blood coagulation. 20 min whole blood clotting test. Left: Healthy control. Right: Adult patient in Nepal, bitten by a suspected Mountain pit viper (*Ovophis monticola*) and displays signs of consumption coagulopathy (Photo: Dr Zoltan Takacs).

inhibitor class of drugs are snake venom derived (**Figure 3**). These agents constitute cornerstone therapy for the most lethal types of heart attacks (e.g., ST segment elevation). Only captopril and other ACE inhibitors are taken orally, the rest have to be administered parenterally, and/or, in limited cases, topically. BYDUREON® is formulated in biodegradable polymeric microspheres that encapsulate exenatide and provide extended release.

Globally, tens of millions of patients are treated with drugs derived from toxins, with many lives saved. The annual global sales figures (in 2013) range between US$~27 million for PRIALT® and US$~698 million for BYETTA®/BYDUREON®, while ACE inhibitors as a class was the fourth most widely prescribed medicine in the United States (2009).

Other Biomedical Applications

Animal venoms have a number of other biomedical applications outside the scope of this text. There is one cosmetic derived from a neurotoxin of the Wagler's pit viper (*Tropidolaemus wagleri*) acting on the nAChR. It is marketed to smoothen wrinkle lines when rubbed on the facial skin. Venoms are also the starting materials to manufacture antivenom for the clinical management of animal venom poisoning, responsible for ~20 000–100 000 fatalities a year, globally. Toxins are also used for preparative applications, for example, to produce defibrinogenated plasma or meizothrombin, and for attempts to develop pesticides. In various basic science disciplines, toxins are essential research tools, which, in turn, also fuels the development of toxin-derived medications.

Toxin-Derived Drugs in Advanced Stages of Development

A number of toxins and toxin-derived compounds are in various stages of development ranging from the experimental phase to clinical trials. Examples in clinical trials in 2014 include Eastern green mamba (*Dendroaspis angusticeps*) cenderitide (CD-NP) for congestive cardiac failure, Sun anemone (*Stichodactyla helianthus*) ShK-186 for various autoimmune diseases, and Common vampire bat (*Desmodus rotundus*) desmoteplase to treat acute ischemic stroke. CD-NP elegantly builds on the evolutionary relationship of nontoxin and toxin body proteins. It is a chimeric human-mamba peptide that exhibits more desirable pharmacology than either of the templates, the human C-type natriuretic peptide or *Dendroaspis* natriuretic peptide. ShK-186 is a result of a decade-long work that generated hundreds of analogs of the K^+ channel-blocking toxin ShK to improve target selectivity and stability. Desmoteplase is a recombinant form of *Desmodus* salivary plasminogen activator $\alpha 1$ with high fibrin specificity isolated from the bat saliva.

Efforts in the clinical phase are also under way in China to develop alternatives to the natural toxin ingredients of batroxobin and hemocoagulase, currently purified from snakes living in South America. Strategies include recombinant toxin production and competing products that are based on toxins isolated from the venom of the Chinese moccasin (*Deinagkistrodon acutus*) and other species native to the Far East.

Medical Potential of Animal Venoms

A combination of key parameters make animal toxins an unparalleled arsenal for biomedical applications: immense diversity, inherent biological properties, advances in technology to isolate, screen, engineer, and formulate/deliver peptides and derived peptidomimetic compounds.

The global diversity of venomous animals ranges about 100 000–170 000 species. Collectively, it is estimated that there are more than 20 million unique animal toxins existing in nature. Approximately, the number of crude venoms screened for various biological activities is in the many hundreds, toxins known to science is in the scale of 10 000, while it is likely no more than 1000 toxins have been studied in detail. This effort resulted in about 15 medications. The sheer magnitude of these

Table 2 Drugs derived from animal venom toxins

Drug name	*Species origin*	*Mechanism of action*	*Indication*
Captopril (CAPOTEN®)	Jararaca (*Bothrops jararaca*)	Angiotensin-converting enzyme inhibitor	Hypertension, cardiac failure
Enalapril[a] (VASOTEC®)	Jararaca (*Bothrops jararaca*)	Angiotensin-converting enzyme inhibitor	Hypertension, cardiac failure
Exenatide (BYETTA®)	Gila monster (*Heloderma suspectum*)	Glucagon-like peptide-1 receptor agonist	Type 2 diabetes mellitus
Exenatide (BYDUREON®)	Gila monster (*Heloderma suspectum*)	Glucagon-like peptide-1 receptor agonist (extended release)	Type 2 diabetes mellitus
Ziconotide (PRIALT®)	Magician's cone snail (*Conus magus*)	$Ca_v2.2$ channel antagonist	Management of severe chronic pain
Bivalirudin (ANGIOMAX®)	European medicinal leech (*Hirudo medicinalis*)	Reversible direct thrombin inhibitor	Anticoagulant in percutaneous coronary intervention
Lepirudin (REFLUDAN®)	European medicinal leech (*Hirudo medicinalis*)	Binds irreversibly to thrombin	Anticoagulation in heparin-associated thrombocytopenia; related thromboembolic disease
Desirudin (IPRIVASK®)	European medicinal leech (*Hirudo medicinalis*)	Selective and near-irreversible inhibitor of thrombin	Prevention of venous thrombotic events
Tirofiban (AGGRASTAT®)	Saw-scaled viper (*Echis carinatus*)	Antagonist of fibrinogen binding to GPIIb/IIIa receptor	Acute coronary syndrome
Eptifibatide (INTEGRILIN®)	Pigmy rattlesnake (*Sistrurus miliarius*)	Prevents binding of fibrinogen, von Willebrand factor, and other adhesive ligands to GPIIb/IIIa receptor	Acute coronary syndrome; percutaneous coronary intervention
Batroxobin (DEFIBRASE®)	Common lancehead (*Bothrops atrox*) or Brazilian lancehead (*Bothrops moojeni*)	Cleaves Aα-chain of fibrinogen	Acute cerebral infarction; unspecific angina pectoris; sudden deafness
Platelet gel (PLATELTEX-ACT®)	Common lancehead (*Bothrops atrox*)	Cleaves Aα-chain of fibrinogen	Gelification of blood for topical applications in surgery
Fibrin sealant (VIVOSTAT®)	Brazilian lancehead (*Bothrops moojeni*)	Cleaves Aα-chain of fibrinogen	Autologous fibrin sealant in surgery
Thrombin-like enzyme	Chinese moccasin (*Deinagkistrodon acutus*) or Siberian pit viper (*Gloydius halys*) or Ussuri mamushi (*Gloydius ussuriensis*)	Fibrinogenase	'Antithrombotics'; 'defibrinating agent for the treatment and prevention of thromboembolic diseases'
Hemocoagulase (REPTILASE®)	Common lancehead (*Bothrops atrox*) or Jararaca (*Bothrops jararaca*) or Brazilian lancehead (*Bothrops moojeni*)	Cleaves Aα-chain of fibrinogen; factor X and/or prothrombin activation	Prophylaxis and treatment of hemorrhage in surgery
Medicinal leech therapy	Medicinal leech (*Hirudo verbana*) or other Hirudinida species	Inhibit platelet aggregation and the coagulation cascade	Skin grafts and reattachment surgery

Note: Order is based on the complexity (disulfide bonds, sequence length) of the lead toxin molecule or venom fraction, less complex first. The extent of utilization, drug name, and drug classification varies. Per classification, drugs may overlap. In some cases, species origin is uncertain, and available references are limited. Drug misnaming is known to occur in the industry. Only one brand name (in parentheses) is provided as an example. List does not include terminated and/or data-deficient agents, such as ancrod (ARVIN®), ximelagatran (EXANTA®), and 'hemocoagulase' *Daboia russelii* and *Gloydius ussuriensis.*

[a]Enalapril and other ACE inhibitors are regarded as later-generation derivatives of captopril.

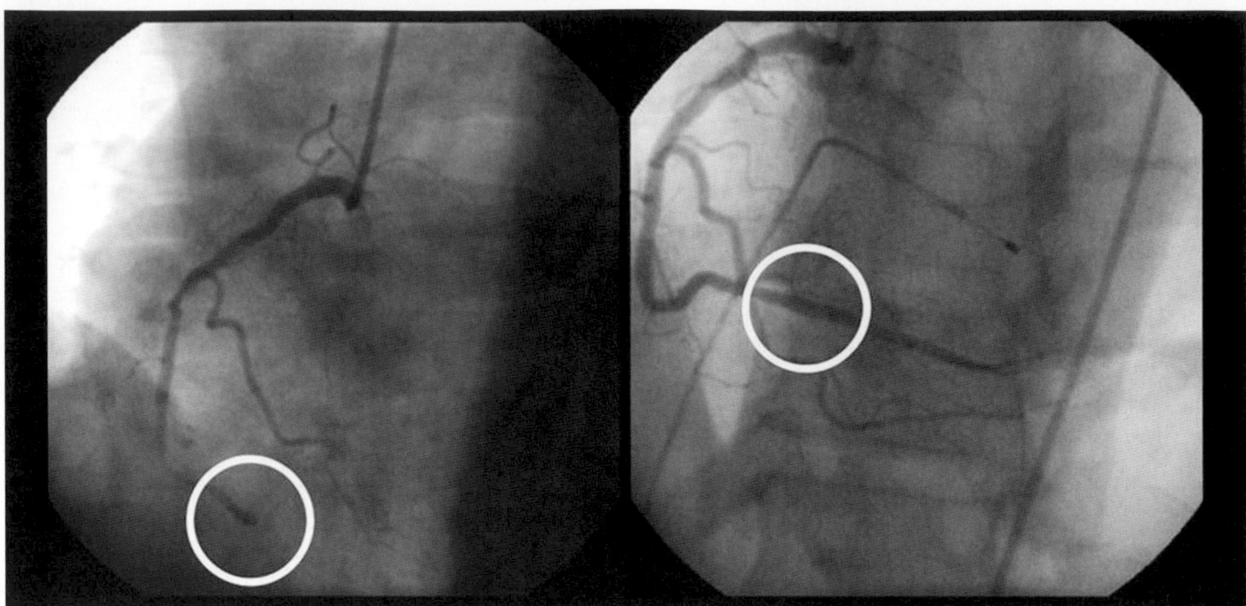

Figure 3 Viper venom–based eptifibatide in a heart attack patient. Left: The presence of occlusive thrombus (blood clot, circled) within a coronary artery and resulting diminishment or cessation of blood flow, is the hallmark finding on angiography in patients afflicted with a heart attack. After direct (intracoronary) and systemic (intravenous) administration of eptifibatide to promote disaggregation of accumulated blood platelets, the occluded segment of clot is first mechanically disrupted using a balloon catheter and then, definitively addressed via placement of a coronary stent (miniature metal scaffold). Right: The final result (previously occluded segment circled) reveals patency of the right coronary artery with restoration of flow into the branch vessels, facilitated by eptifibatide (Angiogram: Dr Sandeep Nathan).

numbers reflects the untapped potential in nature's venoms for medicine.

Pharmaceutical target identification and validation, and establishing novel and robust chemical starting points are among the biggest challenges in drug discovery. Given their evolutionary origin/diversity and pharmacology, animal toxins possess vast potential to address these and related challenges. As examples of potential impact, five of the seven pharmacological sites on the Na_V channels are defined by animal toxins, and 10% of the first 30 toxins isolated from marine snail venoms have reached at least phase I clinical trials.

With advances in genomics, proteomics, and bioinformatics, along with the diverse array of high-throughput screening methods, we are reaching the stage where the large-scale screening of toxins is a reality and the limiting factor is less of a technological challenge but more of actually accessing samples from nature. A major facilitating factor is the requirement for less venom/tissue samples for proteomic and genomic characterization.

Advances in production of target-focused toxin libraries, engineering protein scaffolds, reducing the native toxins to peptidomimetics, formulating/delivering peptidic toxins by nanotechnology or by other means are all opening up new avenues. For example, melittin, a toxin from the European honeybee (*Apis mellifera*), forms pores on lipid membranes, although somewhat indiscriminately. Nanoparticles carrying melittin and polyethylene glycol (PEG; as molecular spacers) on their surface attenuate HIV-1 infectivity. Cells, much bigger in size than HIV-1, are not affected, due to steric restriction to melittin by PEG.

Since toxins affect an extremely diverse set of targets and organs, their potential extend to many different types of conditions, for instance, cardiovascular diseases, cancer, diabetes, autoimmune and nervous system disorders. Relevant global market forecasts, for example, for glucagon-like peptide-1 agonists for diabetes is US$6 billion (by 2015) and for overall autoimmune disease therapeutics is $59 billion (by 2018). Time span between lead toxin identification and FDA approval varies between 7 years (eptifibatide) and 25 years (ziconotide).

Lastly, extracting biological samples necessitate an ethical and legal responsibility. Proper scientific sampling of venoms should not have a detrimental effect on species and habitats. Yet, the results obtained from it should, ideally, be shared with communities, conservation efforts at the site of origin, and possibly beyond. A drug from venom could be seen as an ultimate gift by nature, and should be positioned, locally and globally, for efforts to conserve biological diversity.

See also: Angiotensin Converting Enzyme (ACE) Inhibitors; Botulinum Toxin; Cardiovascular System; Centipedes; Ciguatoxin; Cosmetics and Personal Care Products; Dose–Response Relationship; Drug and Poison Information Centers; Marine Venoms and Toxins; Neurotoxicity; Saxitoxin; Scorpions; Shellfish Poisoning, Paralytic; Snakes; Spiders; Tetrodotoxin; 'Toxic' and 'Nontoxic': Confirming Critical Terminology Concepts and Context for Clear Communication; Toxicology.

Further Reading

Cushman, D.W., Ondetti, M.A., 1999. Design of angiotensin converting enzyme inhibitors. Nat. Med. 5, 1110–1112.

Escoubas, P., King, G.F., 2009. Venomics as a drug discovery platform. Expert Rev. Proteomics 6, 221.

Ferreira, S.H., 2000. Biodiversity, sustainability and drug development. In: Rocha-Miranda, C.E. (Ed.), Transition to Global Sustainability: The Contribution of Brazilian Science. Academia Brasileira de Ciencias, Rio de Janeiro, pp. 171–177 (Chapter 10).

Fox, J.W., Serrano, S.M., 2007. Approaching the golden age of natural product pharmaceuticals from venom libraries: an overview of toxins and toxin-derivatives currently involved in therapeutic or diagnostic applications. Curr. Pharm. Des. 13, 2927–2934.

Han, T.S., Teichert, R.W., Olivera, B.M., Bulaj, G., 2008. *Conus* venoms – a rich source of peptide-based therapeutics. Curr. Pharm. Des. 14, 2462–2479.

King, G.F., 2011. Venoms as a platform for human drugs: translating toxins into therapeutics. Expert Opin. Biol. Ther. 11, 1469–1484.

Kini, R.M., Clemetson, K.J., Markland, F.S., McLane, M.A., Morita, T. (Eds.), 2010. Toxins and Hemostasis: from Bench to Bedside. Springer, Dordrecht.

Lewis, R.J., Garcia, M.L., 2003. Therapeutic potential of venom peptides. Nat. Rev. Drug Discov. 2, 790–802.

Mackessy, S.P. (Ed.), 2009. Handbook of Venoms and Toxins of Reptiles. CRC Press/ Taylor & Francis Group, Boca Raton, FL.

Marsh, N., Williams, V., 2005. Practical applications of snake venom toxins in haemostasis. Toxicon 45, 1171.

Marsh, N.A., 2001. Diagnostic uses of snake venom. Haemostasis 31, 211–217.

Mebs, D., 2002. Venomous and Poisonous Animals: A Handbook for Biologists, Toxicologists and Toxinologists, Physicians and Pharmacists. Medpharm, Stuttgart.

Richard, T., Layer, R.T., McIntosh, J.M., 2006. Conotoxins: therapeutic potential and application. Mar. Drugs 4, 119–142.

Stocker, K.F., 1990. Medical Use of Snake Venom Proteins. CRC Press, Boca Raton, FL.

Stocker, K.F., 1998. Research, diagnostic and medicinal uses of snake venom enzymes. In: Bailey, G.S. (Ed.), Enzymes from Snake Venom. Alaken, Fort Collins, CO, pp. 705–736.

Vetter, I., Davis, J.L., Rash, L.D., Anangi, R., Mobli, M., Alewood, P.F., Lewis, R.J., King, G.F., 2011. Venomics: a new paradigm for natural products-based drug discovery. Amino Acids 40, 15–28.

Antagonism *see* Chemical Interactions

Anthracene

PS Rao, Sanofi, Bridgewater, NJ, USA

- Name: Anthracene
- Chemical Abstracts Service Registry Number: 120-12-7
- Synonyms: AI3-00155, Anthracene, Anthracen, Anthracen (German), Anthracin, Bis-alkylamino anthracene, CCRIS 767, EINECS 204-371-1, Green oil, HSDB 702, NSC 7958, Paranaphthalene, Tetra Olive N2G, UNII-EH46A1TLD7
- Molecular Formula: $C_{14}H_{10}$
- Chemical Structure:

Background

Anthracene is one of a group of chemicals called polycyclic aromatic hydrocarbons (PAHs). PAHs are often found together in groups of two or more. They can exist in more than 100 different combinations, but the most common are treated as a group of 15. PAHs are found naturally in the environment but they can also be made synthetically. Anthracene can vary in appearance from a colorless to pale yellow crystal-like solid. PAHs are created when products like coal, oil, gas, and garbage are burned but the burning process is not complete. Very little information is available on the individual chemicals within the PAH group; the majority of the information is for the entire PAH group. Anthracene is a solid white to yellow crystal, has a weak aromatic odor, and sinks in water. Its characteristics are boiling point, 3421 °C; melting point, 2181 °C; molecular weight, 178.22; density/specific gravity, 1.25 at 27 and 41°C; octanol–water coefficient, 4.45. It is soluble in absolute alcohol and organic solvents. Maximum absorption occurs at 218 nm.

Uses

Most of the PAHs are used to conduct research. Like most PAHs, anthracene is used to make dyes, plastics, and pesticides. It has been used to make smoke screens and scintillation counter crystals. (A scintillation counter is used to detect or count the number of sparks or flashes that occur over a period of time.)

Mechanisms of Action

Acute and Short-Term Toxicity

Animal

LD_{50} Mouse oral: $>17\ g\ kg^{-1}$
LD_{50} Mouse ip: $430\ mg\ kg^{-1}$
LD_{50} Rat oral: $>160\,000\ mg\ kg^{-1}$
LD_{50} Rat dermal: $>1320\ mg\ kg^{-1}$

Human

Anthracene is photosensitizing. It can cause acute dermatitis with symptoms of burning, itching, and edema, which are more pronounced in the exposed bare skin regions. Other symptoms are lacrimation, photophobia, edema of the eyelids, and conjunctival hyperemia. The acute symptoms disappear within several days after cessation of contact. Systemic effects of industrial anthracene manifest themselves by headache, nausea, loss of appetite, slow reactions, and adynamia.

Chronic Toxicity (or Exposure)

Animal

Anthracene showed no mutagenic activity in *Salmonella typhimurium* TA100 and TA98 with and without addition of rat liver microsomes (S9) and no carcinogenic activity in Swiss albino mice. A significant increase in the formation of nonneoplastic melanotic tumors was observed among first- and second-generation progeny of *Drosophila melanogaster* that had been exposed chronically as larvae to low concentrations of anthracene.

Human

Chronic exposure to anthracene may lead to inflammation of the gastrointestinal tract, patchy areas of increased yellow-brown pigment changes, loss of skin pigment, thinning or patchy thickening of skin, skin warts, skin cancer, and pimples. Repeated breathing of fumes, especially from heated anthracene, may cause a chronic bronchitis with cough and phlegm. Repeated exposure of male scrotum can cause skin thinning and increased skin pigmentation. Oral reference dose (RfD) = $1000\ mg\ kg^{-1}\ day^{-1}$ (UF = 3000).

 http://dx.doi.org/10.1016/B978-0-12-386454-3.00238-4

Clinical Management

No specific treatments have been prescribed. The patient should be moved to fresh air in case of respiratory distress.

Ecotoxicology

The substance is very toxic to aquatic organisms. The substance may cause long-term effects in the aquatic environment.

Exposure Standards and Guidelines

No occupational exposure limits have been established for anthracene. However, safe work practices should always be followed.

See also: Coke Oven Emissions; Polycyclic Aromatic Hydrocarbons (PAHs).

Further Reading

Anthracene IARC Summary & Evaluation, 1983. vol. 32.

Bonnet, J.L., Guiraud, P., Dusser, M., 2005. Assessment of anthracene toxicity toward environmental eukaryotic microorganisms: *Tetrahymena pyriformis* and selected micromycetes. Ecotoxicol. Environ. Saf. 60 (1), 87–100.

Bos, R.P., Theuws, J.L.G., Jongeneelen, F.J., Henderson, P.T., 1988. Mutagenicity of bi-, tri- and tetra-cyclic aromatic hydrocarbons in the "taped-plate assay" and in the conventional *Salmonella* mutagenicity assay. Mutat. Res. 204, 203–206.

Choia, J., Oris, J.T., 2003. Assessment of the toxicity of anthracene photo-modification products using the topminnow (*Poeciliopsis lucida*) hepatoma cell line (PLHC-1). Aquat. Toxicol. 65 (3), 243–251.

Huang, X.-D., McConkey, B.J., Sudhakar Babu, T., Greenberg, B.M., 1997. Mechanisms of photoinduced toxicity of photomodified anthracene to plants: inhibition of photosynthesis in the aquatic higher plant *Lemna gibba* (*duckweed*). Environ. Toxicol. Chem. 16 (8), 1707–1715.

McCloskey, J.T., Oris, J.T., 1991. Effect of water temperature and dissolved oxygen concentration on the photo-induced toxicity of anthracene to juvenile bluegill sunfish (*Lepomis macrochirus*). Aquat. Toxicol. 21 (3–4), 145–156.

Relevant Websites

http://www.atsdr.cdc.gov – Agency for Toxic Substances and Disease Registry. Toxicological Profile for Anthracene.

http://www.1.nature.nps.gov – US Dept of the Interior: National Park Service.

http://www.speclab.com – Spectrum Laboratories Inc.

http://www.state.nj.us – State of New Jersey.

http://rais.ornl.gov – The Risk Assessment Information System.

http://toxnet.nlm.nih.gov – Toxnet (Toxicology Data Network): search for Anthracene.

Anthrax

K Shankar, University of Arkansas for Medical Sciences, Little Rock, AR, USA
HM Mehendale, University of Louisiana at Monroe, Monroe, LA, USA.

Epidemiology

Anthrax is a zoonotic disease with worldwide distribution. Anthrax is caused by *Bacillus anthracis*, a Gram-positive, spore-forming, rod-shaped bacterium that primarily infects herbivores such as cattle and deer. The earliest known description of anthrax is found in the Book of Genesis, in which the fifth plague is said to have killed Egyptian cattle. Further, there are numerous descriptions of anthrax in animals and humans in Hindu, Greek, and Roman literature. Between 20 000 and 100 000 cases of anthrax have been estimated to occur worldwide. Human anthrax is most common in enzootic areas in developing countries, among people who work with livestock, eat undercooked meat from infected animals, or work in establishments where wool, goatskins, and pelts are stored and processed. West Africa is the most affected part in the world. Anthrax is also a significant problem in other parts of Africa, Central America, Spain, Greece, Turkey, and the Middle East. In economically advanced countries, where animal anthrax is controlled, incidence in humans is rare. Further infections have been dramatically reduced by the vaccination of high-risk individuals and improvements in industrial hygiene. Incidence in the United States declined to less than one case per year until the recent biological terrorism attacks in the fall of 2001.

Microbiology

Bacillus anthracis is nonmotile, catalase-positive, nonhemolytic on blood agar and frequently occurs in long chains. Virulent forms are surrounded by a capsule. Sporulation occurs in soil and on culture media but not in living tissue. Spores are highly resistant to ultraviolet light, extreme high temperatures, high pH, drying, high salinity, and routine methods of disinfection.

Molecular Mechanism of Toxicity

Anthrax toxin is composed of three proteins: protective antigen (PA; 83 kDa), lethal factor (LF; 90 kDa), and edema factor (EF; kDa). Individually, none of the three proteins are toxic but they interact synergistically with at least one of the others. PA and LF (called lethal toxin, LeTx) can cause lethal shock in experimental animals, and a mixture of PA and EF (edema toxin, EdTx) induces edema at the site of injection. Since two discrete units of the toxin are required for its action, the term binary toxin has been used to label this and other bacterial toxins. Anthrax is unique from other binary toxins in that the binary moieties (EF and LF) interact only after being secreted from the bacteria. Further, EF and LF enter the cell via a single PA protein. Assembly of the three toxin proteins is initiated when PA binds to a proteinaceous cellular receptor and is activated by a member of the furin family of cellular proteases. The exact mechanisms of internalization of the toxin moieties are subjects of scientific inquiry. Inside the cellular cytoplasm, EF (a calcium and calmodulin-dependent adenylate cyclase) causes a dramatic increase in intracellular cAMP concentrations, and LF acts proteolytically to cleave certain MAPK kinases.

Clinical Forms of Anthrax

Anthrax mainly occurs in three forms: cutaneous, inhalation, and gastrointestinal. Exposure to *B. anthracis* most likely in an occupational setting is the cause of cutaneous anthrax. The incubation period varies from 1 to 12 days. In most cases the disease remains localized to the skin lesion. Major diagnostic characteristic is the development of edema around the lesion. The fatality rate is 20% without and less than 1% with antibiotic treatment. Inhalation anthrax is the most lethal form of anthrax resulting from inhalation of pathogenic endospores. The U.S. Department of Defense estimates that the lethal dose in humans is approximately 8000–10 000 spores. The illness is biphasic after exposure to large numbers of spores. The first phase is characterized by a 'flu-like' illness with nonproductive cough. After several days of apparent improvement there is a sudden onset of rapidly progressive respiratory failure, acute dyspnea, circulatory collapse, and pleural effusion. The mortality rate is very high, despite supportive care and antibiotics, generally within 24 h of the onset of the second stage due to toxemia and suffocation. Gastrointestinal anthrax, although rare, occurs after an incubation period of 1–7 days following ingestions of *B. anthracis* via contaminated food or drink. Mortality rates are estimated to be between 25 and 60% unless treatment is begun early enough. Severe abdominal pain, fever, nausea, vomiting, and bloody diarrhea are manifested during the disease. Death occurs due to toxemia and shock.

Clinical Treatment

Prompt clinical diagnosis and treatment with effective antimicrobial drugs are necessary for successful treatment of anthrax. Several historical strains produce an inducible β-lactamase and are resistant to penicillin. Ciprofloxacin (400 mg intravenously twice daily) and possibly other quinolones or doxycycline (200 mg intravenously twice daily) should be used as initial therapy. The duration of treatment for inhalation anthrax should be 60 days. Corticosteroid therapy should be considered for patients with inhalation anthrax associated with meningitis or severe edema. Supportive therapy should be initiated to prevent shock, fluid and electrolyte imbalance, and loss of airway patency. The U.S. Centers for Disease Control and Prevention has approved Ciprofloxacin, doxycycline, and penicillin G procaine for treatment of all age groups. Levofloxacin is FDA approved for treatment of inhalational anthrax (postexposure) in adults 18 years or older.

 http://dx.doi.org/10.1016/B978-0-12-386454-3.00239-6

Treatment with oral Ciprofloxacin or doxycycline for 7–10 days is recommended for localized or uncomplicated cases of naturally acquired cutaneous anthrax, such as that associated with exposure to animals with anthrax or to products such as hides from animals with anthrax. Immunotherapy is not very common.

Potential for Use as a Biological Weapon

Anthrax is classified as a Category A biological weapon (most dangerous) along with smallpox, plague, *Clostridium botulinum* toxins, filoviruses, etc. *Bacillus anthracis* has several biological, technical, and virulence characteristics that make it an attractive weapon for bioterrorism. These include easy procurement from a variety of sources and relative ease to grow, process, and store. The World Health Organization estimates that 50 kg of weapon-grade anthrax spores released by an aircraft over an urban population of 5 million would result in 250 000 cases of mainly inhalation anthrax.

See also: Bio Warfare and Terrorism: Toxins and Other Mid-Spectrum Agents; Botulinum Toxin; Chemical Warfare; Chemical Warfare Delivery Systems; Immune System.

Further Reading

Artenstein, A.W., Opal, S.M., 2012. Novel approaches to the treatment of systemic anthrax. Clin. Infect. Dis. 54 (8), 1148–1161.

Bouzianas, D.G., 2010. Current and future medical approaches to combat the anthrax threat. J. Med. Chem. 53, 4305–4331.

Collier, R.J., Young, J.A., 2003. Anthrax toxin. Annu. Rev. Cell Dev. Biol. 19, 45–70.

Ghosh, N., Tomar, I., Goel, A.K., 2012. A field usable qualitative anti-PA enzyme linked immunosorbent assay for serodiagnosis of human anthrax. Microbiol. Immunol. http://dx.doi.org/10.1111/1348-0421.12014 (Epub ahead of print).

Hicks, C.W., Sweeney, D.A., Cui, X., Li, Y., Eichacker, P.Q., 2012. An overview of anthrax infection including the recently identified form of disease in injection drug users. Intensive Care Med. 38 (7), 1092–1104.

Kaur, M., Bhatnagar, R., 2011. Recent progress in the development of anthrax vaccines. Recent Pat. Biotechnol. 5 (3), 148–159.

Oncu, S., Oncu, S., Sakarya, S., 2003. Anthrax – an overview. Med. Sci. Monit. 9, 276–283.

Putzer, G.J., Koro-Ljungberg, M., Duncan, R.P., Dobalian, A., 2013. Preparedness of rural physicians for bioterrorist events in Florida. South. Med. J. 106 (1), 21–26. http://dx.doi.org/10.1097/SMJ.0b013e31827caed2.

Steelfisher, G.K., Blendon, R.J., Brulé, A.S., et al., 2012. Public response to an anthrax attack: a multiethnic perspective. Biosecur. Bioterror. 10 (4), 401–411.

Wang, D.B., Tian, B., Zhang, Z.P., et al., 2012. Rapid detection of *Bacillus anthracis* spores using a super-paramagnetic lateral-flow immunological detection system. Biosens. Bioelectron.. http://dx.doi.org/10.1016/j.bios.2012.10.088 (pii: S0956-5663(12)00782-8, Epub ahead of print).

Anticholinergics

JP Gray, U.S. Coast Guard Academy, New London, CT, USA
SD Ray, Manchester University, Fort Wayne, IN, USA

This article is a revision of the previous edition article by Swarupa G. Kulkarni, and Harihara M. Mehendale, volume 1, pp 146–148, © 2005, Elsevier Inc.

- Name: Anticholinergics
- Synonyms: Parasympatholytics; Cholinergic blockers; Sympatholytics; Antispasmodics

Background (Significance/History)

Acetylcholine is a neurotransmitter synthesized in neurons and secreted in response to neuronal stimuli; upon release into the synaptic cleft, it activates acetylcholine receptors and is rapidly degraded by acetylcholinesterase enzymes. Acetylcholine is capable of activating two major classes of receptors, muscarinic acetylcholine receptors (MAChRs) and nicotinic acetylcholine receptors (NAChRs), named for their differential selectivity for the xenobiotic compounds muscarine and nicotine, respectively.

Whereas MAChRs are primarily located in the autonomic ganglia, organs innervated by the parasympathetic division of the autonomic nervous system, and the central nervous system (CNS), NAChRs are located at neuromuscular junctions and autonomic ganglia. Although they respond to the same neurotransmitter, MAChRs are G protein-linked receptors and NAChRs are ion channel receptors, providing a structural basis for their differential sensitivities to nicotine and muscarine.

Anticholinergics antagonize the activities of acetylcholine and vary in their selectivity for acetylcholine receptors (AChRs), mechanism of action, distribution, and blood–brain barrier penetration. A wide variety of anticholinergic compounds exists with specific sites of action. Examples of common anticholinergic compounds are as follows: (see **Table 1**; antimuscarinic: atropine, benztropine, biperiden, ipratropium, oxitropium, glycopyrrolate, oxybutynin, chlorphenamine, diphenhydramine, dimenhydrinate, orphenadrine, etc.; antinicotinic agents: bupropion, tubocurarine, dextromethorphan, mecamylamine, doxacurium, etc.). In addition to physostigmine, nicotine also counteracts anticholinergics by activating NAChRs. Anticholinergics drugs are extensively used in a variety of conditions (gastrointestinal disorders, dizziness, sinus bradycardia, insomnia, genitourinary disorders, pulmonary disorders, etc.). Treating asthma, chronic obstructive pulmonary disease (COPD), and pupil diation are few of the commonest. Intentional overdose, inadvertent ingestion, medical noncompliance, or geriatric polypharmacy are the prime causes of anticholinergic syndrome.

Uses

Atropine, the prototypical MAChR inhibitor (anticholinergic), is an alkaloid derived from nightshade that acts as a competitive antagonist of MAChRs. Atropine blocks the MAChR receptor M2 in the heart, which is normally stimulated by the vagus nerve of the parasympathetic nervous system, resulting in an increased heart rate, useful for the treatment of bradycardia. Atropine reverses symptoms of nerve agent exposure, known as SLUDGE syndrome (salivation, lacrimation, urination, defecation, gastrointestinal motility, and emesis). Atropine does not cross the blood–brain barrier. Scopolamine, identical in structure with the exception of an additional oxygen atom, acts like atropine, but also depresses the CNS. Together with opioids, scopolamine can induce 'twilight sleep.'

Three major subtypes of MAChR exist. M1 receptors are found in the CNS and autonomic ganglia. M1 anticholinergics are used to treat gastric secretion abnormalities and airway restriction. M2 receptors occur in the atria and are important for tachycardia. M3 receptors are located on smooth muscle cells of the airway and are important for airway contraction. These receptors differ in sensitivity to various antimuscarinic compounds.

Many other anticholinergic drugs are used to treat a variety of symptoms, depending on their selectivity for MAChRs or NAChRs, and on their distribution-dependent localization to various target organs (**Table 1**). Most drugs target the muscarinic receptors. Uses include as antihistamines (hydroxyzine and diphenhydramine, also known as benadryl), pupil dilation for eye exams (tropicamide and cyclopentolate), chronic obstructive pulmonary disease (ipratropium and tiotropium), gastric acid secretion inhibition (pirenzepine), irritable bowel syndrome (dicyclomine and mebeverine), motion sickness (dimenhydrinate), Parkinsonian symptoms (trihexyphenidyl, benzatropine, and procyclidine), and urinary bladder spasms and urge incompetence (flavoxate, oxybutynin, tolterodine, solifenacin, and darifenacin).

Very few drugs target NAChRs. One example is curare, a paralytic used as a muscle relaxant for surgery. At higher doses, it can inhibit breathing and can cause a temporary paralytic 'locked-in' syndrome.

Anticholinesterase chemicals including the pesticide parathion and nerve agent soman inhibit acetylcholinesterase, an enzyme required for removal of acetylcholine from synaptic junctions. Anticholinergics such as atropine are used to treat anticholinesterase exposure by increasing activity of the AChRs. Oxime drugs such as pralidoxime counteract nerve agents by reactivating cholinesterases; they only function against nerve agents. However, oximes only work against organophosphate inhibitors of acetylcholinesterase.

Environmental Fate and Behavior

Atropine and scopolamine, both natural products, have no significant environmental impact. Other anticholinergics are not recognized environmental pollutants.

 http://dx.doi.org/10.1016/B978-0-12-386454-3.00240-2

Table 1 Common anticholinergic drugs

Drug	*Disease/target*	*Receptor*[a]
Atropine	Nerve agent exposure	NS – not specific
Scopolamine	CNS	NS – not specific
Dicyclomine	Intestinal spasms	NS – not specific
Mebeverine	Intestinal spasms	N.D.
Propantheline	Intestinal spasms	N.D.
Glycopyrrolate	Intestinal spasms	N.D.
Hydroxyzine	Antihistamine	N.D.
Diphenhydramine	Antihistamine	M2
Tropicamide	Mydriasis	N.D.
Cyclopentolate	Mydriasis	N.D.
Ipratropium	COPD/asthma	NS – not specific
Tiotropium	COPD	M3
Pirenzepine	Gastric acid secretion	M1
Telenzepine	Gastric acid secretion	M1
Flavoxate	Urinary symptoms	N.D.
Oxybutynin	Urinary symptoms	M1, M3
Tolterodine	Urinary symptoms	NS – not specific
Trospium	Urinary symptoms	NS – not specific
Darifenacin	Urinary symptoms	M3
Solifenacin	Urinary symptoms	M3
Oxybutynin	Urinary symptoms	M2, M3
Darifenacin	Urinary symptoms	M3
Trihexyphenidyl/ Benzhexol	Parkinsons	M1
Benzatropine	Parkinsons	N.D.
Procyclidine	Parkinsons	N.D.
Gallamine	Muscle relaxant	M2
Methoctramine		M2
AFDX-116		M2
Imipramine	Urinary symptoms	M3
Pilocarpine		M2
Pralidoxime	Cholinesterase regenerator	N/A
Diacetylmonoxime	Cholinesterase regenerator	N/A

[a]Note that specificity for receptor is also affected by ADME.
M1, nerves; M2, heart, nerves, smooth muscle; M3, glands, smooth muscle, endothelium; N.D., not determined.

Toxicokinetics

Atropine is a tertiary anticholinergic, which refers to the nitrogen within the molecule. Tertiary anticholinergics are capable of distributing throughout the CNS, whereas quaternary anticholinergics primarily target peripheral tissues. Overall anticholinergics have a diverse distribution profile due to the diversity of chemical structures making up this class of drug.

Elimination of anticholinergics is also widely variable. Atropine has a half-life of 2 h, with most excreted unchanged in the urine.

Mechanism of Toxicity

Most anticholinergics are competitive inhibitors of acetylcholine for binding to the AChR. Atropine and other tertiary amines can cross the CNS and the placenta (found in breast milk in small quantities). It is oxidized primarily in the liver, and apparently metabolized in the liver to tropic acid, tropine, and possibly esters of tropic acid and glucuronide conjugate. Antimuscarinics, in contrast, are mainly eliminated in urine as unchanged drug and its metabolites. Following oral administration, substantial amounts of antimuscarinics may be eliminated in feces as unabsorbed drug.

Acute and Short-Term Toxicity

Target organ systems of anticholinergics include the CNS, eye, cardiovascular system, respiratory system, gastrointestinal tract, genitourinary tract, and sweat glands. These target organs differ widely depending on the agent's biodistribution and selectivity for MAChRs. Atropine overexposure is particularly dangerous to children who are susceptible to hyperthermia.

Overexposure to anticholinergics can result in elevated body temperature, elevated heart rate, dry mouth, difficulty in urination, constipation, drowsiness, dizziness, and increased pupil size, in the absence of bowel sounds and diaphoresis. A common pneumonic device used is, 'Blind as a bat, mad as a hatter, red as a beet, hot as Hades, dry as a bone, the bowel and bladder lose their tone, and the heart runs alone.'

Chronic Toxicity

Chronic exposure to anticholinergics was shown to adversely affect the progression of Alzheimer disease, and is contraindicated in elderly patients due to the risk for dementia. Chronic exposure of rabbits to intramuscular atropine at 10% of the LD_{50} for 100 days resulted in toxicity in half of the animals exposed. A number of toxicological symptoms were noted including weight loss, edema of organs, hepatitis, and pulmonary thrombosis. Death was caused by convulsions and respiratory failure, and failure to maintain food intake.

Genotoxicity

Atropine and diphenhydramine are not noted genotoxicants. Atropine was not a mutagen in an *Escherichia coli* assay.

Carcinogenicity

Atropine promoted carcinogenesis in rat stomach by *N*-methyl-*N*′-nitro-*N*-nitrosoguanidine.

Clinical Management

Anticholinergics typically act as partial agonists for acetylcholine receptors. Physostigmine, a reversible inhibitor of acetylcholinesterase, can be given (0.5–1 mg) intravenously to block degradation of acetylcholine, which in turn activates NAChR and MAChR by competing for binding to the receptors with the anticholinergic compounds. Due to a very narrow therapeutic index, the drug must be administered carefully to prevent overactivation of AChRs, which would result in symptoms consistent with nerve agent exposure. It must also be delivered frequently due to the short half-life of the compound. Some recommend that instead of using physostigmine, overdose of atropine be treated symptomatically, due to the difficulty in the administration of physostigmine and the toxicity associated with inappropriate administration.

While benzodiazepines were previously used to treat agitation induced by anticholinergic overdose, this treatment is becoming less popular, and it has not been shown to be effective in treatment of anticholinergic-induced delirium. Physostigmine has been shown to also help both agitation and delirium, working within 15–20 min of treatment. Since anticholinergic drugs are prescribed for a wide range of medical conditions, such as acid reflux, Parkinson's disease, high blood pressure, and urinary incontinence, care must be taken while administering these drugs because they may impair cognition.

Physostigmine salicylate is the best antidote for anticholinergic toxicity. Most patients are safely treated without it, but it is recommended when tachydysrhythmia (abnormal heart rhythm with a rate greater than 100 bpm) with subsequent hemodynamic compromise, intractable seizure, severe agitation or psychosis, or some combination thereof is present. Physostigmine is contraindicated in patients with cardiac conduction disturbances on electrocardiogram.

Ecotoxicology

Atropine sulfate is not toxic in three different freshwater invertebrates, with EC_{50} and LC_{50} above 300 mg l^{-1}.

See also: Cholinesterase Inhibition; Gastrointestinal System; Neurotoxicity; G-Series Nerve Agents; Nerve Agents; V-Series Nerve Agents: Other than VX.

Further Reading

Derinoz, O., Emeksiz, H.C., September 2012. Use of physostigmine for cyclopentolate overdose in an infant. Pediatrics 130 (3), e703–e705. http://dx.doi.org/10.1542/peds.2011-3038.

Dhote, F., Carpentier, P., Barbier, L., et al., 2012. Combinations of ketamine and atropine are neuroprotective and reduce neuroinflammation after a toxic status epilepticus in mice. Toxicol. Appl. Pharmacol. 259 (2), 195–209.

Gore, A., Brandeis, R., Egoz, I., et al., 2012. Efficacy assessment of various anticholinergic agents against topical sarin-induced miosis and visual impairment in rats. Toxicol. Sci. 126 (2), 515–524.

Hail, S.L., Obafemi, A., Kleinschmidt, K.C., 2013. Successful management of olanzapine-induced anticholinergic agitation and delirium with a continuous intravenous infusion of physostigmine in a pediatric patient. Clin. Toxicol. (Phila). 51 (3), 162–166.

Karimi, S., Dharia, S.P., Flora, D.S., Slattum, P.W., 2012. Anticholinergic burden: clinical implications for seniors and strategies for clinicians. Consult. Pharm. 27 (8), 564–582.

Leone Roberti Maggiore, U., Salvatore, S., Alessandri, F., et al., 2012. Pharmacokinetics and toxicity of antimuscarinic drugs for overactive bladder treatment in females. Expert Opin. Drug Metab. Toxicol. 8 (11), 1387–1408.

Nebes, R.D., Pollock, B.G., Perera, S., Halligan, E.M., Saxton, J.A., 2012. The greater sensitivity of elderly APOE ε4 carriers to anticholinergic medications is independent of cerebrovascular disease risk. Am. J. Geriatr. Pharmacother. 10 (3), 185–192.

Pieper, M.P., 2012. The non-neuronal cholinergic system as novel drug target in the airways. Life Sci. 91 (21–22), 1113–1118.

Rai, B.P., Cody, J.D., Alhasso, A., Stewart, L., December 2012. Anticholinergic drugs versus non-drug active therapies for non-neurogenic overactive bladder syndrome in adults. Cochrane Database Syst. Rev. 12 (12), CD003193. http://dx.doi.org/10.1002/14651858.CD003193.pub4.

Schultz, M.K., Wright, L.K., Stone, M.F., et al., 2012. The anticholinergic and antiglutamatergic drug caramiphen reduces seizure duration in soman-exposed rats: synergism with the benzodiazepine diazepam. Toxicol. Appl. Pharmacol. 259 (3), 376–386.

Travers, A.H., Milan, S.J., Jones, A.P., Camargo Jr., C.A., Rowe, B.H., December 2012. Addition of intravenous beta(2)-agonists to inhaled beta(2)-agonists for acute asthma. Cochrane Database Syst. Rev. 12 (12), CD010179. http://dx.doi.org/10.1002/14651858.CD010179.

Vande Griend, J.P., Linnebur, S.A., 2012. Inhaled anticholinergic agents and acute urinary retention in men with lower urinary tract symptoms or benign prostatic hyperplasia. Ann. Pharmacother. 46 (9), 1245–1249.

Wilson, M.E., Lee, G.K., Chandra, A., Kane, G.C., 2011. Central anticholinergic syndrome following dobutamine-atropine stress echocardiography. Echocardiography 28 (10), E205–E206.

Zant, J.C., Rozov, S., Wigren, H.K., Panula, P., Porkka-Heiskanen, T., 2012. Histamine release in the basal forebrain mediates cortical activation through cholinergic neurons. J. Neurosci. 32 (38), 13244–13254.

Relevant Websites

http://www.atsdr.cdc.gov/ – Agency for Toxic Substances & Disease Registry: search for Cholinesterase Inhibitors.

http://emedicine.medscape.com/article/812644-overview – Emedicine – Anticholinergic Toxicity.

http://www.ncbi.nlm.nih.gov/pubmed/19046488 – US National Library of Medicine (PubMed): Use of anticholinergic therapy in men.

http://www.ncbi.nlm.nih.gov/pubmed/19552610 – US National Library of Medicine (PubMed): Drugs with anticholinergic properties: a potential risk factor for psychosis onset in Alzheimer's.

http://www.ncbi.nlm.nih.gov/pubmed/21635190 – US National Library of Medicine (PubMed): Drugs with anticholinergic properties: a current perspective on use and safety.

Antidotes

S Shadnia, Shahid Beheshti University of Medical Sciences, Tehran, Iran
LS Nelson, New York University School of Medicine, New York, NY, USA; and New York City Poison Control Center, New York, NY, USA

Background

Poisoning in adults accounts for almost 13.8% of all admissions to the ICU. In addition, two-thirds of the reported poisoning exposures occur in the pediatric age group (<20 years).

Antidotes are compounds that alter the action of a poison in the body to prevent, reverse, or mitigate the toxic effects. Examples of mechanisms by which antidotes work include competition at a receptor site, alteration of a metabolic process, engaging a counter-regulatory physiologic process, or hastening the excretion or detoxification of a toxin. Although antidotes are generally beneficial in intoxicated patients, some of them are themselves toxic and should be used only when indicated.

N-Acetylcysteine

Available forms:

Oral solutions: 10% (100 mg ml^{-1}; 4, 10, 30 ml); 20% (200 mg ml^{-1}; 4, 10, 30 ml).
Injection solution: 20% (200 mg ml^{-1}; 30 ml).

Indications:

Poisoning with:

1. Acetaminophen
   1.1. Patients with a history of a single acute overdose of more than 140 mg kg^{-1} of acetaminophen or a serum level on or above the treatment line on the Rumack-Matthew nomogram (e.g., over 150 mg dl^{-1} at 4 h postingestion).
   1.2. The acetaminophen level must be drawn between 4 and 24 h postingestion.
2. *Amanita phalloides* mushroom.
3. Chlorinated hydrocarbon.
4. Monochloroacetic acid.
5. Cyclophosphamide.
6. Doxorubicin.

Dosage:

1. Oral dosage:
   1.1. The loading dose is 140 mg kg^{-1} orally for both adults and children.
   1.2. Maintenance dose is 70 mg kg^{-1} orally, every 4 h for 17 doses in both adults and children.
   1.3. NAC solutions of 10 or 20% can be diluted in water or soft drinks such as fruit juice or soda to a 5% solution.
   1.4. If the patient vomits within 1 h of any dose, the dose should be repeated.
   1.5. No increase in oral NAC dose is required when it is coadministered with activated charcoal.
2. Intravenous (IV) dosage:
   2.1. Loading dose of 150 mg kg^{-1} diluted in 200 ml DW5% infused over 60 min, followed by 50 mg kg^{-1} in 500 ml D5W infused over 4 h and 100 mg kg^{-1} in 1000 ml D5W infused over 16 h.

Atropine Sulfate

Available forms:

Injection solutions as sulfate: 0.05 mg ml^{-1} (5 ml); 0.1 mg ml^{-1} (5, 10 ml); 0.4 mg per 0.5 ml (0.5 ml); 0.4 mg ml^{-1} (0.5, 1, 20 ml); and 1 mg ml^{-1} (1 ml).
AtroPen (Prefilled autoinjector for intramuscular (IM) injection): 0.5 mg per 0.7 ml (0.7 ml-blue label); 1 mg per 0.7 ml (0.7 ml-dark red label); 2 mg per 0.7 ml (0.7 ml-green label).

Indications:

1. Intoxication with organophosphorus or carbamate cholinesterase inhibitors, including pesticides (e.g., parathion, carbaryl), nerve agents (e.g., sarin), or medicinals (e.g., physostigmine).
2. Cholinomimetic agents, such as pilocarpine.
3. Intoxication with mushrooms containing muscarine (Inocybe or Clitocybe).

Dosage:

1. Loading dose:
   1.1. *Adults*: 1–5 mg IV with a doubling dose every 3–5 min to achieve and maintain full atropinization. Organophosphorus pesticides usually require more than a single dose of atropine.
   1.2. *Children*: 0.02–0.05 mg kg^{-1} IV with a doubling dose for every 3–5 min to achieve and maintain full atropinization.
2. Maintenance dose:
   2.1. *Adults*: IV infusion of 10–20% of the loading dose per hour.
   2.2. *Children*: Infusion rates of 0.02–0.08 mg kg^{-1} h^{-1}.
   2.3. The atropine can be diluted in 0.9% sodium chloride.

Considerations:

1. Full atropinization is indicated by complete clearing of rales and drying of pulmonary secretions. Tachycardia is not a contraindication to continued dosing to meet pulmonary endpoints.
2. Adequate oxygenation is very important in hypoxic patients who may be at risk of ventricular fibrillation if atropine is given.
3. Careful suctioning of oral and tracheal secretions may be necessary until atropinization is achieved.
4. Gradual withdrawal of atropine is done by lengthening intervals between doses while checking lung bases for rales and observing patient for return of cholinergic signs.

 http://dx.doi.org/10.1016/B978-0-12-386454-3.01064-2

Activated Charcoal

Available forms:

Oral suspensions: 12.5 g per 60 ml; 15 g per 72 ml; 25 g per 120 ml; 50 g per 240 ml.

Indications:

Nearly all chemicals are adsorbed to activated charcoal. Activated charcoal is generally administered to most poisoned patients to reduce the amount absorbed into the systemic circulation. Contraindications include concerns for airway protection (e.g., coma) or integrity of the gastrointestinal tract (e.g., caustics).

Dosage:

1. *Adults*: 1 g kg^{-1} body weight, up to 100 g.
2. *Children*: 0.5–1 g kg^{-1}.

Considerations:

Heavy metals, iron, lithium, potassium, alcohols, and fluoride are not adsorbed to activated charcoal limiting its effectiveness.

Calcium Gluconate or Chloride

Available forms:

Injection solution: 10% (100 mg ml^{-1}) (10, 50, 100, and 200 ml).
Tablets: 500, 650, and 975 mg.
Powder: 347 mg per tablespoon.

Indications:

1. Calcium channel blockers intoxication.
2. Hyperkalemia.
3. Beta blockers intoxication.
4. Hydrofluoric acid (HF) and fluoride intoxication.
5. Hypermagnesemia.
6. Black widow spider envenomation.

Dosage:

1. *Adults*: 3 g (30 ml of 10% calcium gluconate), or 1 g (10 ml of 10% calcium chloride) over 5–10 min.
   1.1. Repeat the dose every several minutes as necessary.
   1.2. In the case of cardiac arrest, the dose should be infused over 10–20 s.
2. *Children*: 60 mg kg^{-1} (0.6 ml kg^{-1} of 10% calcium gluconate) or 20 mg kg^{-1} (0.2 ml kg^{-1} of 10% calcium chloride) over 5–10 min.
   2.1. Repeat the dose every several minutes as necessary.
   2.2. In the case of cardiac arrest, the dose should be infused over 10–20 s.
3. In the case of mild to moderate dermal toxicity due to HF/fluoride exposure, the salts of calcium are used.
   3.1. Topical calcium gluconate gel for dermal exposure of HF <20%.
      3.1.1. Apply 2.5% gel (can be made with surgical lubricant and aqueous calcium salt) to the exposed area for 15 min.
      3.1.2. Consider the use of subcutaneous injection of calcium gluconate (10%), if there is a failure to respond to calcium gluconate gel.
   3.2. Subcutaneous calcium gluconate (10%) for dermal exposure of HF >20%.
      3.2.1. Infiltrate each square centimeter of the exposed area with 0.5 ml of 10% calcium gluconate.
4. In the case of significant burn due to HF/fluoride exposure, calcium salts may be administered intravenously (for systemic toxicity) or intraarterially (for hand burns predominantly).
   4.1. Ten milliliters of 10% calcium gluconate plus heparin 5000 units in a total volume of 40 ml is administered intravenously.
   4.2. Ten milliliters of 10% calcium gluconate in 50 ml of 0.9% sodium chloride solution is intraarterially infused over 4 h.

Levocarnitine

Available forms:

Capsule: 250 mg.
Tablets: 330, 500 mg.
Oral solution: 100 mg ml^{-1} (118 ml).
Injection solution: 200 mg ml^{-1} (5, 12.5 ml).

Indications:

1. Valproic acid/sodium valporate-induced hyperammonemia.
2. Valproic acid/sodium valporate-induced elevated aspartate and alanine transaminases.
3. Acute metabolic disorders resulting from L-carnitine deficiency.

Dosage:

1. *Clinically well patients*: 100 mg kg^{-1} day^{-1}per os
   1.1. The maximum dose is up to 3 g day^{-1}.
   1.2. The daily dose is given in every 6 h intervals.
2. *Clinically ill patients*: Loading dose of 100 mg kg^{-1} up to 6 g intravenously infused over 30 min followed by 15 mg kg^{-1} every 4 h through IV infusion over 10–30 min.
3. In acute metabolic disorders resulting from L-carnitine deficiency, the loading dose of 50–500 mg kg^{-1} IV is administered followed by the daily dose divided into every 4 h doses.
   3.1. Maximum daily dose is up to 6 g in addition to the loading dose.

Considerations:

1. For patients with end-stage renal disease, 10–20 mg kg^{-1} by slow IV bolus over 2–3 min after completion of dialysis is indicated.
2. In acute overdose of valproic acid/sodium valporate without hepatic enzyme abnormalities or symptomatic hyperammonemia, prophylactic administration of L-carnitine is not generally performed but can be considered.
   2.1. One hundred milligrams per kilogram per day up to 3 g, given in divided doses every 6 h, are administered intravenously.

Cyanide Antidote Kit

Contents:

Amyl nitrite: 0.3 ml ampule.
Sodium nitrite: 3% ampule (300 mg per 10 ml).
Sodium thiosulfate: 25% vial (12.5 g per 50 ml).

Indications:

Suspected cyanide poisoning.

Dosage:
1. Break ampule of amyl nitrite and allow patient to inhale for 15 s; then, take away for 15 s and repeat this.
   1.1. Use a fresh ampule every 3 min.
2. Injection of sodium nitrite 3%, 300 mg IV infusion over 5 min (children: 0.2 ml kg^{-1} of a 3% concentration up to 300 mg).
3. Sodium thiosulfate: 12.5 g (50 ml of a 25% concentration) infused IV over 10–30 min or as a bolus (children: 0.5 g kg^{-1}, max 12.5 g)

Considerations:
1. Avoid sodium nitrite when carboxyhemoglobin is expected to be elevated (as in fire victim). Administration of thiosulfate alone, in stated doses, is appropriate in this situation.
2. Monitor methemoglobin concentrations in patients receiving nitrites.
3. Hydroxocobalamin preferred, if available.

Deferoxamine

Available forms:

Powder for injection: 2 g and 500 mg.

Indications:

Acute and chronic iron toxicity (due to transfusion-dependant anemias).

Dosage:
1. *Intermittent*: 1 g IM followed by 500 mg at 4 and 8 h post-ingestion and then 4–12 h as necessary (maximum: 6 g day^{-1}).
2. *Infusion*: Initiate at 5 mg kg^{-1} h^{-1}, titrate to 15 ml g^{-1} kg^{-1} h^{-1} IV (max 8 g day^{-1}) mild to moderate: administer for 6–12 h and reassess; Severe toxicity: administer 24 h and reassess.

Digoxin-Specific Antibody Fragments

Available forms:

IV powder for solution; 38 mg.

Indications:

Digoxin and all digitalis-like glycoside poisoning (unproven for most other than digoxin).

Dosage:
1. Acute ingestion: 10–20 vials.
2. Chronic ingestion in adults: 3–6 vials.
3. Chronic ingestion in children: 1–2 vials.

Dimercaprol (British Anti-Lewisite, BAL)

Available forms:

IM oil; 10%

Indications:

Arsenic, gold, lead, and mercury poisoning.

Dosage:

Four milligrams per kilogram every 4 h, deep IM, up to 3 g day^{-1}.

Considerations:
1. Formulated in peanut oil; painful IM injection and caution with allergy.
2. Not used for organic mercury poisoning.
3. Being replaced by succimer for most indications given the latter's oral route; except lead encephalopathy.
4. Start 4 h before $CaNa_2$ EDTA.

Edetate Calcium Disodium (Calcium Disodium EDTA, $CaNa_2$ EDTA)

Available form:

Injection solution: 200 mg ml^{-1}.

Indications:

Lead encephalopathy or other significant clinical effects.

Dosage:

Twenty-five to seventy-five milligrams per kilogram per day IV infusion over 8–12 h for 5 days (up to 2–3 g day^{-1}).

Considerations:
1. Dimercaprol (BAL) should be administered 4 h prior to starting this dose for lead neurotoxicity/ encephalopathy.
2. Caution with preparations: Disodium EDTA (Na_2 EDTA can cause fatal hypocalcemia).
3. Adequate hydration is important prior to therapy.

Ethanol

Available forms:

Oral solution: 20%.
IV Infusion: 10%.

Indication:

Methanol or ethylene glycol poisoning.

Dosage:
1. Loading dose:
   1.1. *Oral*: 0.8 g kg^{-1} ethanol 20%.
   1.2. *IV*: 0.8 g kg^{-1} ethanol 10% over 1 h.
2. Maintenance:
   2.1. *Oral* 20%: 80 mg kg^{-1} h^{-1} if ethanol naive (not ethanol tolerant).
   2.2. *IV* 10%: 80 mg kg^{-1} if ethanol naive (not ethanol tolerant).

Considerations:
1. Monitor serum ethanol concentrations and maintain at approximately 100 mg dl^{-1}.

2. Patients with tolerance to ethanol (e.g., alcoholics) require higher maintenance infusions, generally about double that of naive patients.
3. Ethanol infusions may cause irritation to the vein. Prolonged oral use irritates the gastric mucosa.
4. Fomepizole is preferred, if available.

Flumazenil

Available form:

IV solution: 0.1 mg ml^{-1}.

Indication:

Reversal of benzodiazepine-induced sedation.

Dosage:
1. *Adults*: Initial dose of 0.2 mg IV over 30 s. If there is no response, an additional 0.3 mg is administered. Repeated dosing with 0.5 mg can be used, administered every 1–2 min, up to a total dose of 3 mg.
2. Pediatric dose of 0.01 mg kg^{-1} (0.1 ml kg^{-1}) IV with a maximum dose of 1 mg.

Considerations:
1. It should not be administered in patients with seizure producing agents (e.g., tricyclic antidepressants) or those likely to be dependent on benzodiazepines (i.e., may precipitate withdrawal).
2. It is of limited benefit in patients with benzodiazepine overdose.

Folinic Acid (Leucovorin)

Available form:

Tablets: 5, 10, 15, and 25 mg.
Powder for injection: 50, 100, 200, 350 mg.
Solution for injection: 10 mg ml^{-1}.

Indications:

Methotrexate, methanol, and folic acid antagonist toxicity.

Dosage:
1. For methanol poisoning: 1–2 mg kg^{-1} IV every 4–6 h until methanol is eliminated and acidosis resolves.
2. If methotrexate dose is unknown, 100 mg m^{-2} every 4–6 h until the serum methotrexate level is less than 10^{-8} mol l^{-1}.

Considerations:

'Leucovorin rescue' for methotrexate chemotherapy follows specific guidelines based on the dose of methotrexate.

Fomepizole

Available form:

IV solution: 1 g ml^{-1}.

Indication:

Methanol or ethylene glycol poisoning.

Dosage:

A loading dose of 15 mg kg^{-1} IV followed by 10 mg kg^{-1} every 12 h for four doses and 15 mg kg^{-1} every 12 h until ethylene glycol or methanol concentrations are below 20 mg dl^{-1}.

Glucagon

Available form:

Injection powder for solution: 1 mg.

Indication:

Calcium channel blocker and beta-blocker toxicity.

Dosage:
1. *Loading dose*: 50 μg kg^{-1} (3–5 mg) infused in 1–2 min, titrate up to 10 mg.
2. *Continuous infusion*: 2–5 mg h^{-1} up to10 mg h^{-1}.

Considerations:

Vomiting common, a concern in patients with unprotected airways.

Hydroxocobalamin

Available forms:

IM solution: 1000 μg ml^{-1}.
IV powder for solution: 5 g.

Indication:

Suspected cyanide poisoning.

Dosage:
1. *Adults*: 5 g (2 × 2.5 g vials) over 15 min (approximately 15 ml min^{-1}).

Repeated additional 5 g IV doses over 15 min to 2 h may be administered up to a total dose of 10 g.

2. *Children*: 70 mg kg^{-1} up to 5 g.

Considerations:
1. Sodium thiosulfate 12.5 g is generally administered subsequently, or concomitantly through a different intravenous line.
2. Red discoloration of skin and body fluids occur.
3. Interference with certain laboratory tests, such as cooximetry for carbon monoxide, is expected.

Insulin

Available forms:

Regular insulin; injection solution: Many strengths.

Indications:

Calcium channel blocker and beta-blocker toxicity.

Dosage:
1. *Bolus*: Regular insulin 1 U kg^{-1} IV with 0.5 g kg^{-1} glucose.
2. *Maintanance*: Regular insulin 0.5 U kg^{-1} h^{-1} (up to 2.5 U kg^{-1} h) with 0.5 g kg^{-1} h^{-1} dextrose infusion.

Considerations:

1. Hypoglycemia should be expected and carefully monitored.
2. Onset of cardiovascular effect is approximately 30 min

Intravenous Lipid Emulsion

Available form:

Twenty percent (100, 250, 500, 1000 ml).

Indications:

Calcium channel blocker, tricyclic antidepressant, and local anesthetics toxicity (and others).

Dosage:

1. *Loading dose*: 1.5 ml kg^{-1} IV over 2–3 min, repeat bolus dose every 3–5 min up to 3 ml kg^{-1}.
2. *Maintenance dose*: 0.25–0.5 ml kg^{-1} min for 30–60 min.

Considerations:

Current understanding is that lipid provides a sink to draw lipophilic toxins from their target tissues.

Usually reserved for rescue therapy in critically ill patients not responding to appropriate medical therapy.

D-Penicillamine

Available form:

Oral capsule: 250 mg.

Indications:

Lead, mercury, copper, and arsenic toxicity.

Dosage:

Fifteen to forty milligrams per kilogram orally in four divided doses (up to max 500 mg) 4 times a day for 5 days.

Considerations:

1. Currently of limited use.
2. Caution in patients with penicillin allergy.

Methylene Blue

Available form:

IV solution: 1% (10 mg ml^{-1}).

Indication:

Methemoglobinemia.

Dosage:

One to two milligrams per kilogram (0.1–0.2 ml kg^{-1} of 1% solution) IV very slowly over several minutes. Maximum dose should not exceed 7 mg kg^{-1} (0.7 ml kg^{-1}).

Naloxone

Available forms:

Injection solution: 0.4 and 1 mg ml^{-1}.

Indication:

Confirmed or suspected overdose with opioids.

Dosage:

1. *Apnea*: 2 mg IV stat.
2. *Respiratory depression; non-opioid-dependent patients*: 0.5–2 mg IV, subcutaneous (SQ), IM, IN (intranasally).

Opioid-dependent patients: 0.05–0.1 mg IV, SQ, IM, IN, with slow upward titration while ventilating and oxygenating patient.

Repeat dosing every 2–3 min if the initial response is inadequate. If there is no response after 10 mg, reconsider the diagnosis of opioid toxicity.

Considerations:

Excessive dose may precipitate opioid withdrawal, which may be severe and life threatening.

Octreotide

Available forms:

Injection solution: 50, 100, 200, 500, and 1000 μg ml^{-1}.

Indication:

Sulfonylurea-induced hypoglycemia.

Dosage:

1. *Adults*: 50 μg every 6 h SQ.
2. *Children*: 1.25 μg kg^{-1} every 6 h SQ (up to 50 μg).

Considerations:

Not for insulin-induced hypoglycemia.

Oxygen

Available form:

O_2 100%

Indications:

1. Carbon monoxide toxicity.
2. Pulmonary irritant toxins.

Dosage:

1. Depending on response of patient, 100% oxygen for 1 h and then decrease gradually.
2. For carbon monoxide, administration may be needed for prolonged period, up to 72 h, if hyperbaric oxygen therapy not performed.

Physostigmine

Available forms:

Injection: 1 mg ml^{-1} in 2 ml ampules and 1 ml prefilled syringes.

Indications:

Toxicities associated with anticholinergic syndrome.

Dosage:

1. *Adults*: 1–2 mg over 2–3 min
2. *Children*: 0.02 mg kg^{-1} IV over at least 5 min

Considerations:

1. Administration too rapidly may cause cholinergic crisis or seizures.
2. Dose can be repeated after 5 min for inadequate response and the absence of cholinergic signs.

Pralidoxime Chloride

Available forms:

Powder for injection: 1 g per 20 ml vials.
Auto-injectors: 600 mg ml^{-1}.

Indications:

1. Organophosphate insecticide poisoning.
2. Anticholinesterase overdosage (neostigmine, pyridostigmine).

Dosage:

1. *Initial dose*: 30 mg kg^{-1} IV bolus over 30 min (up to 2 g).
2. *Maintanance dose*: 8 mg kg^{-1} h^{-1} IV infusion.

Protamine Sulfate

Available form:

Injection: 10 mg ml^{-1}.

Indication:

Heparin overdose.

Dosage:

One milligram of protamine will neutralize 100 U (1 mg) of heparin.

Prussian Blue

Available form:

Capsules: 500 mg.

Indication:

Thallium or cesium contamination.

Dosage:

Total daily dose of 9 g in three 3 g divided doses.

Pyridoxine (Vitamin B_6)

Available forms:

Tablet: 20, 25, 50, 100, 250, and 500 mg.
Injection: 100 mg ml^{-1} in 10 and 30 ml vials.

Indications:

1. Isoniazid overdose related toxicity, particularly seizure or coma; and
2. ethylene glycol poisoning.

Dosage:

One gram for each gram of isoniazid ingested up to 70 mg kg^{-1} (max 5 g) IV infusion at 0.5 g min^{-1} until seizure stops, with remainder intravenously infused over 4–6 h.

Sodium Bicarbonate

Available forms:

Tablet: 325 (3.9 meq), 500 (6 meq), 520 (6.2 meq), and 650 (7.7 meq) mg.

Solution for injection:

4.2% (0.5 meq/ml) in 2.5-, 5-, and 10 ml syringes.
5% (0.6 meq ml^{-1}) in 500 ml containers.
7.5% (0.9 meq ml^{-1}) in 50 ml vials.
8.4% (1 meq ml^{-1}) in 10- and 50 ml vials.

Oral powder: 20.9 (na/0.5 tsp) in 120-, 240-, 480-, and 2400 g container.

Indications:

1. Tricyclic antidepressant, type I antidysrhythmic, and quinidine toxicity (to provide a sodium ion bolus and alkalinize the blood).
2. Aspirin or methanol poisoning (to alkalinize the blood and urine).

Tricyclic antidepressant, type I antidysrhythmic, and quinidine toxicity (to provide a sodium ion bolus and alkalinize the blood).

Aspirinor methanol poisoning (to alkalinize the blood and urine).

Dosage:

1. *Initial dose*: 1–2 meq kg^{-1} IV bolus
2. *Maintenance dose*: 150 meq diluted in 850 ml D5W, 1–3 ml kg^{-1} h^{-1} IV infusion and titrate to serum pH up to 7.55.

Succimer (Dimercaptosuccinic Acid, DMSA)

Available forms:

Capsules: 100 mg.

Indications:

Lead, arsenic, and mercury poisoning.

Dosage:

Adults: 10 mg kg^{-1} PO Q8H for 5 days followed by 10 mg kg^{-1} twice a day for 14 days. Can be repeated after 2-week drug holiday.

Considerations:

1. Best studied for lead, and lead dosing used for other metals.
2. Endpoint of therapy not well established but blood metal concentrations in or near the normal range and improvement in clinical toxicity are accepted.

Thiamine

Available forms:

Tablet: 5, 10, 25, 50, 100, 250, and 500 mg.
Elixir: 250 μg 5 ml^{-1}.
Injection: 100 mg ml^{-1} in 1 ml ampules and prefilled syringes and 1-, 2-, 10-, and 30 ml vials.

Indication:

Ethylene glycol poisoning.

Dosage:

One hundred milligram IM or IV. (Oral route should be avoided because of its unpredictable absorption).

Vitamin K_1 (Phytonadione)

Available forms:

Tablet: 5 mg.
Injection: 2, 10 mg ml^{-1}.

Indications:

Warfarin and rodenticide anticoagulants.

Dosage:

1. Twenty-five to fifty milligrams orally 3–4 times a day for 1–2 days
2. In life-threatening bleeding: 10 mg 2–4 times a day

Considerations:

For life-threatening bleeding, vitamin K is generally insufficient and other interventions such as plasma or clotting factors are required.

Antivenom

Antivenom, an antitoxin that counteracts specific venom, is a necessary treatment for most venomous poisonings. For example, snake antivenom immunoglobulins are the only specific treatment for snakebites. Most antivenoms can reverse or prevent morbidity and reduce mortality from venom. Antivenoms are antibodies produced by another animal in response to a venomous insult. The antibodies are typically harvested from the blood of the animal and purified as antivenom for treatment.

See also: Environmental Risk Assessment, Secondary Poisoning; Poisoning Emergencies in Humans; Notorious Poisoners and Poisoning Cases; Plants, Poisonous (Humans); Plants, Poisonous (Animals); American Association of Poison Control Centers.

Further Reading

Bebarta, V.S., Pitotti, R.L., Borys, D.J., Morgan, D.L., February 2011. Seven years of cyanide ingestions in the USA: critically ill patients are common, but antidote use is not. Emerg. Med. J. 28 (2), 155–158. http://dx.doi.org/10.1136/emj.2009.089896.

Ghannoum, M., Gosselin, S., January 2013. Enhanced poison elimination in critical care. Adv. Chronic Kidney Dis. 20 (1), 94–101. http://dx.doi.org/10.1053/j.ackd.2012.09.002.

Nelson, L.S., Lewin, N.A., Howland, M.A., Hoffman, R.S., Goldfrank, L.R., Flomenbaum, N.E., 2010. Goldfrank's Toxicologic Emergencies, ninth ed. McGraw Hill, New York.

Nurulain, S.M., July 2012. Different approaches to acute organophosphorus poison treatment. J. Pak. Med. Assoc. 62 (7), 712–717.

Patel, S.R., October–December 2013. Toxicologic emergencies in the intensive care unit: management using reversal agents and antidotes. Crit. Care Nurs. Q. 36 (4), 335–344. http://dx.doi.org/10.1097/CNQ.0b013e3182a10cbd.

Potempa, J., Travis, J., Golonka, E., Shaw, L., December 31, 2006. Poison-antidote systems in bacteria: the co-evolution of functional counterparts. Cell Mol. Biol. (Noisy-le-grand) 52 (4), 18–22.

Schaper, A., Ceschi, A., Deters, M., Kaiser, G., March 2013. Of pills, plants, and paraquat: the relevance of poison centers in emergency medicine. Eur. J. Intern. Med. 24 (2), 104–109. http://dx.doi.org/10.1016/j.ejim.2012.11.013.

Relevant Websites

http://www.who.int/ipcs/publications/training_poisons/guidelines_poison_control/en/index7.html – World Health Organization Guidelines for Poison Control.

http://www.who.int/gho/phe/chemical_safety/poisons_centres/en/index.html – World Health Organization, World Directory of Poison Centres.

Antimony

SC Gad, Gad Consulting Services, Cary, NC, USA

- Name: Antimony
- Chemical Abstracts Service Registry Number: 7440-36-0
- Synonym: Stibium
- Chemical/Pharmaceutical/Other Class: Metals
- Molecular Formula: Sb
- Valence States: 0, −3, +3, +5

Background Information

Antimony (Sb) has been known since antiquity, and its early use as a cosmetic continues even today. Often mixed with lead or other heavy metals, this mascara-type cosmetic is known as kohl. Believed to possess powers to shield the eye from the sun and disease, it served purposes in both cosmetics and mysticism. Antimony has been found in many artifacts in the Middle East, and seems to have been used in the creation of small personal ornamentation or vessels.

Uses

Antimony is used in white metal, which is any of a group of alloys having relatively low melting points. White metal usually contains tin, lead, or antimony as the chief component (e.g., the alloys Britannia and Babbitt). Antimony is used as a hardening alloy for lead, especially in storage batteries and cables, bearing metal, type metal, solder, collapsible tubes and foil, sheet and pipe, semiconductor technology, and pyrotechnics. It is also used in thermoelectric piles and for blackening iron or coatings. Antimony-containing compounds are used in materials for refrigerators, air conditioners, aerosol sprays, paints, and flameproofing agents. Approximately half of the antimony used in the United States is recovered from lead-based battery scrap. Antimony is also used medicinally, e.g., antimony potassium tartrate (APT) as an emetic and the more soluble pentavalent antimony compounds such as sodium stibogluconate and stibosamine as antiparasitic agents to different leishmaniasis vectors. The pentavalent forms are more physiologically tolerated than the trivalent forms.

Environmental Fate and Behavior

Antimony is found naturally in the Earth's crust and can be released into the environment as windblown dust or sea spray or from volcanic eruptions or forest fires. However, the emission of antimony into the environment is overwhelmingly the result of human activity, with the emission of antimony trioxide, tetroxide, and pentoxide forms being the most significant. Antimony trioxide is emitted as a result of coal burning, or with fly ash when antimony-containing ores are smelted. Humans are exposed to low amounts of antimony from the air, drinking water, and food contaminated with soil. Antimony concentration in the atmosphere is thought to be 1.4–55 ng m^{-3}. The more water soluble forms of antimony are very mobile in aqueous media while the less soluble forms of antimony are found attached to particles of soil, clay, and sediment in rivers and lakes. The concentration of antimony in the Pacific Ocean was found to be 0.2 $\mu g\, l^{-1}$ and in the Rhine river at 0.1 $\mu g\, l^{-1}$. The trivalent state of antimony is the form most often released by anthropogenic activities. In terms of soil concentrations, it was reported by a US Geological Survey to be less than 1–8 ppm in soil, with an average of 0.48 ppm. Studies have estimated an exposure of less than 5 $\mu g\, day^{-1}$ on average from food and water and appears to be significantly higher than exposure by inhalation. Antimony does not bioaccumulate in food sources. The food contamination from soil is thought to be in the low $\mu g\, kg^{-1}$ wet weight range. Drinking water contamination of antimony is thought to be from the metal plumbing and fittings, in which case it is thought to be the less toxic antimony(V) form. The US Environmental Protection Agency standard for antimony in the drinking water is 6 $\mu g\, l^{-1}$. Occupational exposures to antimony as well as therapeutic administration are more likely to be higher and thus may produce toxic effects.

Exposure and Exposure Monitoring

The emission of antimony into the human environment is overwhelmingly the result of human activity, with the emission of antimony trioxide being the most significant source. Antimony trioxide is emitted as a result of coal burning, or with fly ash when antimony-containing ores are smelted. In addition, medicines containing antimony are administered orally. Antimony is present in food and drinking water, mostly in the low $mg\, kg^{-1}$ wet weight range or less, including vegetables grown on Sb-contaminated soils. Daily oral uptake of Sb ranges from 10 to 70 $mg\, day^{-1}$ and appears to be significantly higher than exposure by inhalation. Absorption is poor via the gastrointestinal (GI) route, though onset of symptoms is rapid if sufficient exposure is reached and can result in death. Antimony poisoning symptoms are quite similar to those of arsenic, including vomiting, diarrhea, colic, and metallic taste, but it is far less toxic. Due to the poor absorption of antimony by the GI tract, exposure to antimony is primarily of concern via the inhalation route, particularly in workplaces in which antimony is used. Air concentrations of up to 10 mg m^{-3} have been recorded in workplaces where antimony is used, particularly smelting works and abrasives production. Worldwide, airborne antimony concentrations are approximately 0.001 $\mu g\, m^{-3}$.

Toxicokinetics

Normally, antimony is absorbed slowly when ingested or administered orally. Absorption of all valent states of antimony in the GI tract is low with 5–20% absorption seen in animal studies. Four people with involuntary intoxication of APT

 http://dx.doi.org/10.1016/B978-0-12-386454-3.00815-0

showed an absorption rate of 5%. Antimony is more readily absorbed through the respiratory tract. Antimony can concentrate in lung tissue, the thyroid gland, the adrenal glands, the kidneys, and the liver. The trivalent compounds of antimony concentrate in the red blood cells and liver, and the pentavalent compounds concentrate in the blood plasma. Both forms are excreted in feces and urine, but generally, more trivalent compounds are excreted in urine and more pentavalent compounds in feces. Presumably by reacting with the sulfhydryl groups, antimony can inhibit oxidative and phosphorylating enzymes like monoamine oxidase, succinoxidase, pyruvate brain oxidase, and phosphofructokinase. Inhibition of these enzymes can alter activities such as glucose metabolism and nerve transmission. Ten percent of the trivalent form is excreted by the kidney in 24 h; 50–60% of the pentavalent form is found in the urine within 24 h.

Mechanism of Toxicity

The toxicity of Sb is a function of the water solubility and the oxidation state of the Sb species under consideration. Antimony(III) is generally more toxic than antimony(V) and inorganic forms are thought to be more toxic than organic forms. Stibane gas (SbH_3) when inhaled is the most toxic. Antimony toxicity often parallels that of arsenic, although antimony salts are less readily absorbed than arsenic. It is presumed that antimony, like arsenic, complexes with sulfhydryl groups of essential enzymes and other proteins. By analogy, antimony can uncouple oxidative phosphorylation, which would inhibit the production of energy necessary for cellular functions. Antimony's trivalent compounds are more toxic than its pentavalent compounds.

Acute and Short-Term Toxicity (or Exposure)

Animal

Minimal intraperitoneal lethal dose for rats injected with antimony metal was shown to be 10 mg 100 g^{-1} weight. Animals showed dyspnea, weight loss, hair loss, and myocardial insufficiency. Post mortems showed cardiac lesions with liver and spleen damage. Death was attributed to myocardial edema. The LD_{50} for APT in rabbit and rats is about 115 mg kg^{-1} and about 600 mg kg^{-1} in mice. A study where 400 mg kg^{-1} APT was given to mice and rats for 14 days showed stomach and liver lesions.

Human

Accidental poisonings can result in acute toxicity, which produces vomiting and diarrhea similar to arsenic poisoning. Most information regarding antimony toxicity has been obtained from industrial exposures. Occupational exposures usually occur through inhalation of dusts containing antimony compounds. Six workers exposed to antimony trisulfide (used as a pigment and in match production) at concentrations greater than 3.0 mg m^{-3} in a factory that produces grinding wheels experienced heart complications and died, and the rest of the population working in the environment showed limited cardiovascular changes. Inhalation of antimony hydride (stibine gas) can lead to hemolytic anemia, renal failure, and hematuria. Stibine gas is produced when antimony alloys are treated with acids. Minimal oral lethal doses of APT in children are thought to be 300 mg and adults 1200 mg.

Chronic Toxicity (or Exposure)

Animal

Rats exposed to a dose level of 4.2 mg m^{-3} airborne antimony trioxide dust for 1 year were reported to develop lung tumors; at a dose level of 1.6 mg m^{-3}, lung tumors were not found. Guinea pigs exposed to airborne antimony trioxide developed interstitial pneumonia. Oral feeding of antimony to rats does not induce an excess of tumors or teratogenesis.

Human

Inhalation of antimony compounds produces different effects at different concentrations. Chronic inhalation of low concentrations causes rhinitis and irritation of the trachea. At high concentrations, acute pulmonary edema occurs, and bronchitis may occur (the bronchitis may lead to emphysema). Inhaled antimony concentrates in lung tissue; as a result, pneumoconiosis with obstructive lung disease has been recorded. The available data on antimony as a human carcinogen are inconclusive. In addition, a temporary skin rash, called 'antimony spots,' can occur in persons chronically exposed to antimony in the workplace. Reoccurring oral exposure to therapeutic doses of antimony(III) was associated with optic nerve destruction, uveitis, and retinal bleeding. The symptoms of exposure included headache, coughing, anorexia, troubled sleep, and vertigo.

Immunotoxicity

Transient immunologic reactions, including tachyphylaxis and anaphylactoid reactions, may occur. Increased polymorphonuclear neutrophils and cytokines have been measured in persons exposed to zinc oxide fumes. Very little information is available on the immunotoxicity of antimony.

Reproductive Toxicity

A few studies suggest that antimony can cause reproductive toxicity. A study in rats given antimony trioxide at 209 mg m^{-3} for 63 days inhibited the ability of two-thirds of the rats to conceive. Rabbits given metallic antimony of 5–55 mg every other day for 30, 60, or 90 days showed an increase in abortions. Women working at an antimony metallurgic plant where they were exposed to antimony trioxide, antimony pentasulfide, and metallic antimony showed higher rates of spontaneous abortions and menstruation difficulties.

Genotoxicity

The compounds $SbCl_3$ and $SbCl_5$ were reported to be genotoxic in the rec-assay with *Bacillus subtilis*. Sb(III)acetate enhanced the simian-adenovirus-7-mediated transformation of SHE-cells, and enhanced rates of chromosomal breaks in human leukocytes after treatment with APT. However, another study showed that $SbCl_3$ did not induce DNA/protein-crosslinks in V79-cells and peripheral human lymphocytes. In a study done on workers exposed to antimony trioxide, increased oxidative damage to DNA was seen in the workers compared to controls, though there was not an increase in sister chromatid exchange or micronuclei. Overall, due to the lack of human studies, antimony genotoxicity in humans is inconclusive.

Carcinogenicity

The International Agency for Research on Cancer categorizes antimony as a possible carcinogen (group 2B). While current data on carcinogenicity of antimony in humans have been inconclusive, rat studies done with antimony trioxide and antimony trisulfide have shown lung tumor formation. An increase in the incidence of lung cancer has been reported in workers exposed to APT dust, but not other cancers.

Clinical Management

The oil-soluble BAL (British anti-Lewisite; 2,3-dimercaptopropanol) administered intramuscularly appears to be the antidote of choice for antimony poisoning. The antidotal action of BAL depends on its ability to prevent or break the union between antimony and vital enzymes.

Ecotoxicology

Soil toxicity studies show EC_{20} values for the following invertebrates: *Enchytraeus crypticus* (enchytraeid), 194 mg kg^{-1} dry weight (dw); *Folsomia candida* (springtail), 81 mg kg^{-1} dw; and *Eisenia fetida* (earthworm), 30 mg kg^{-1} dw. These values are well above the background concentrations for antimony in US soils.

Exposure Standards and Guidelines

The American Conference of Governmental Industrial Hygienists (ACGIH) and the Occupational Safety and Health Administration (OSHA) in the United States have the following airborne exposure limits:

OSHA Standard: Permissible exposure limit – 8 h time-weighted average (TWA) = 0.5 mg m^{-3}.

ACGIH threshold limit value: 8 h TWA = 0.5 mg m^{-3} (antimony and compounds, as Sb). ACGIH classifies antimony as a suspected human carcinogen.

In the United States, antimony is listed as a Clean Air Act hazardous air pollutant generally known or suspected to cause serious health problems. Antimony and its compounds are listed as Clean Water Act toxic pollutants, subject to effluent limitations. The Federal Drinking Water Standards is 6 $\mu g\ l^{-1}$.

See also: Antimony Trioxide; Metals.

Further Reading

Fowler, B.A., et al., 2013. Antimony, sixth ed., vol. 1. In: Patty's Toxicology, pp. 491–497.

Lylenda, C.A., Fowler, B.A., 2007. Antimony. In: Nordberg, G.F., Fowler, B.A., Nordberg, M., Friberg, L.T. (Eds.), Handbook on the Toxicology of Metals, third ed. Academic Press, San Diego, pp. 353–366.

Sundar, S., Chakravarty, J., 2010. Antimony toxicity. Int. J. Environ. Res. Publ. Health 7 (12), 4267–4277.

Winship, K.A., 1987. Toxicity of antimony and its compounds. Adverse Drug React. Acute Poisoning Rev. 2, 67–90.

Relevant Websites

http://www.atsdr.cdc.gov – Agency for Toxic Substances and Disease Registry. Toxicological Profile for Antimony.

http://www.echemportal.org/echemportal/index?pageID=0&request_locale=en – eChem Portal Homepage, Search for: 'Antimony.'

http://toxnet.nlm.nih.gov/ – Toxnet Homepage, Search for: 'Antimony.'

Antimony Trioxide

SC Gad, Gad Consulting Services, Cary, NC, USA

- Chemical Abstracts Service Registry Number: 1309-64-6
- Synonyms: Antimony white, Antimony oxide, Antox, Thermogrand B, ATO, Diantimony trioxide, Antimony (3+) oxide
- Chemical/Pharmaceutical/Other Class: Metal oxide
- Molecular Formula: Sb_2O_3
- Chemical Structure:

$$\left[Sb^{3+}\right]_2 \left[O^{2-}\right]_3$$

Background Information

Antimony trioxide (ATO) is a white, odorless, crystalline powder. This amphoteric oxide is not readily soluble in water, but will dissolve in sodium hydroxide solution or in mineral acids. In nature, it is found as the orthorhombic mineral valentinite and the octahedral mineral senarmontite. ATO is an industrial chemical produced worldwide with a 2005 production estimate of 120 000 tons per year. Several processes are used to produce ATO, with the most common being the smelting of stibnite ore at very high temperatures to produce a crude antimony trioxide, which is then further purified by sublimation to separate out other components like arsenic trioxide, a common contaminant in antimony ores.

Uses

Commercially, the most common use for antimony trioxide is to provide flame-retardant properties to textiles, paper, rubber, adhesives, and plastics. Added to ceramics and glass, ATO adds opacity, hardness, and resistance to acids. It is also used as a turbidifier in white enamel, pigments, and munitions and as a catalyst in the production of polyethylene terephthalate (PET plastic).

Environmental Fate and Behavior

Antimony trioxide is a form of antimony that is released into the atmosphere primarily from human activities in high-temperature industrial processes such as coal burning or with fly ash when antimony-containing ores are smelted. Antimony trioxide is the most significant form of antimony present in the atmosphere. The combustion of products coated with ATO for its flame-retardant properties and fossil fuel combustion will also release ATO into the atmosphere. Antimony compounds suspend to air particles and, with a half-life of 30–40 days in the air, are capable of traveling long distances through the atmosphere. Current estimates of atmospheric antimony are around 0.001 $\mu g\ m^{-3}$. ATO is a form of antimony that is relatively insoluble in water. The presence of ATO in bodies of water is due to its absorption onto clays, dirt, and other sediment, especially in areas where sediments accumulate, such where a contaminated river flows into a reservoir, lake, or river bend. Soil persistence of ATO is expected to be higher near production facilities or waste disposal sites.

Exposure and Exposure Monitoring

The most significant source of human exposure occurs occupationally to workers exposed to dust and fumes such as in ATO smelting plants, or in plants making or using antimony trioxide in other ways. Occupational exposure to ATO occurs mainly through inhalation, though mucociliary action may cause gastrointestinal effects. Lung, eye, and dermal irritations have been reported. Occupational exposure can be monitored by urine testing.

Toxicokinetics

Animals fed ATO showed antimony in the thyroid, lungs, adrenal glands, blood, heart, hair, spleen, kidneys, and liver. Clearance from these tissues over time showed tissue-specific differences, with slower clearance from blood, lungs, liver, and spleen. In another study, ATO persisted the longest in the thyroid. The low solubility of antimony trioxide causes antimony trioxide particles to persist longer in lung tissue when inhaled than other soluble forms of antimony. That ATO can be absorbed through the lungs into the body is based on evidence of finding elevated antimony concentrations in the urine and blood of antimony smelting workers. Women working in antimony smelting plants have shown elevated antimony in placenta, cord blood, urine, and breast milk. Evidence also shows a relatively long half-life of antimony trioxide in the lungs of exposed workers. ATO has been detected in the lungs of these workers long after exposure has been terminated. Animal studies have shown that antimony retention in the lungs depends on the size of the particle (with larger particles being cleared more rapidly) as well as the solubility of the antimony compound. While persistence of antimony in lung tissue has been demonstrated in humans, antimony trioxide is thought to be cleared from other affected organs such as liver and kidney more rapidly. Trivalent antimony readily leaves the plasma but remains in the circulation bound to erythrocytes and is excreted in the bile after conjugation with glutathione.

Mechanism of Toxicity

Antimony (Sb) toxicity often parallels that of arsenic, although antimony salts are less readily absorbed than arsenic. It is presumed that antimony, like arsenic, complexes with sulfhydryl groups of essential enzymes and other proteins. By analogy, antimony can uncouple oxidative phosphorylation, which would inhibit the production of energy necessary for cellular functions. Mechanisms of toxicity of the ATO form of antimony are not as readily apparent.

Acute and Short-Term Toxicity (or Exposure)

Animal

Antimony trioxide has an oral LD_{50} in rats of >20 000 mg kg^{-1}. The relatively low toxicity of this compound is due to its extremely low solubility in water. Mouse intraperitoneal $LD_{50} = 172$ mg kg^{-1}. Studies where cats and dogs were exposed orally to ATO at 100 mg kg^{-1} showed no toxic effects; however, animal studies done on acute exposure to ATO by inhalation did show toxicity. For instance, studies on guinea pigs exposed to 45 mg kg^{-1} ATO by inhalation for 33–106 h exhibited interstitial pneumonitis and fatty degeneration of the liver. Inconsistent hematological effects of ATO inhalation on animals were also reported. Antimony trioxide is a mild eye irritant in rabbits.

Human

In humans, the primary sites affected by antimony trioxide acute toxicity are pulmonary and gastrointestinal. Other sites affected are heart, liver, kidney, and mucous membrane. Antimony spots have been reported, which is a rash consisting of pustules and papules near sweat and sebaceous glands on skin. Symptoms related to human exposure to antimony trioxide in the workplace are mainly irritation of mucous membranes in eyes, mouth, nose, throat, and upper respiratory tract. It has been reported that smelter workers exposed to antimony trioxide frequently experienced symptoms of rhinitis, pharyngitis, laryngitis, gastroenteritis, pneumonitis, and bronchitis. Other common symptoms listed were weight loss, nausea, diarrhea, vomiting, and abdominal cramps. A particular incident was reported where numerous people became ill after drinking lemonade that had been left in a white enamel tub overnight. The illness was thought to have been caused by the antimony trioxide that had leached into the acidic lemonade from the tub. The tub contained 2.88% of antimony trioxide while the resulting lemonade had 0.013% antimony. Acute symptoms included nausea, vomiting, burning stomach pain, and colic. Most recovered within 3 h.

Chronic Toxicity (or Exposure)

Animal

Given the prevalence of human occupational exposure to ATO, numerous animal studies have been done to assess chronic ATO inhalation exposure. Animals chronically exposed to antimony trioxide showed myocardial damage and fatty degeneration of the liver as well as incidences of anemia, decreased white cell count, and polymorphonuclear leukocyte reduction. Chronic exposure leads to reproductive and developmental effects.

Human

Antimony pneumoconiosis (or antimoniosis) is a frequent outcome in workers chronically exposed to antimony trioxide through inhalation. This often symptomless condition is characterized by diffuse punctate spots of less than 1 mm seen on lung X-rays. A study done on workers in antimony smelting plants who were exposed to ATO dust at antimony concentrations of 0.08–138 mg m^{-3} for 1–15 years showed no significant problems with pulmonary function. Pneumoconiosis was present in 3/13 of the workers, with five additional workers with suspected pneumoconiosis. Other studies done on people with chronic occupational exposure to ATO showed that the number of spots shown on X-rays correlated with the amount of time the person was exposed and the concentration of ATO retained in the lungs. They found these lung changes could occur only after a few years of exposure to ATO. In another study, 51 workers who worked at a smelting plant for 9–31 years and were exposed to dust particles containing up to 88% antimony trioxide and 8% antimony pentoxide showed pneumoconiotic changes after 10 years of employment there. The most common symptom among workers was chronic coughing and frequent symptoms included conjunctivitis, upper airway inflammation, chronic bronchitis, chronic emphysema, and pleural adhesions. No malignant lesions were found in this study.

Reproductive Toxicity

It was reported that women working in an antimony smelting plant had higher incidences of spontaneous abortions, higher rates of late stage abortions, higher rates of premature births, and more gynecologic problems than a control group of women. Fumes that the women were exposed to were thought to contain mostly antimony trioxide with antimony pentasulfide and metallic dust. Other reproductive effects included lower birth weights of the offspring and at 3 months and 1 year. Increases in antimony content of blood, urine, breast milk, and placenta relative to control, unexposed group were noted.

Genotoxicity

The *in vivo* genotoxicity of antimony trioxide was studied using single- and repeat-dose mouse bone marrow micronucleus tests, and the rat liver unscheduled DNA synthesis assay. All three studies were negative. In contrast, chromosomal damage by antimony trioxide was reported in mouse bone marrow cells after repeat dosing but not after single dosing. Positive results were observed with antimony trioxide in the *in vitro* cytogenetic assay with human lymphocytes and the sister chromatid exchange assay with V79-cells, but not in the L5178Y mutation assay. Thus ATO may be considered clastogenic with *in vitro* studies.

Carcinogenicity

Antimony trioxide has been classified by the American Conference of Governmental Industrial Hygienists (ACGIH) as group A2, a suspected human carcinogen and by the International Agency for Research on Cancer into group B2 (potential carcinogen). In a rat study, doses of antimony trioxide as high as 4.5 mg m^{-3} delivered by inhalation for 12 months did not produce cancer. However, other studies did show increased lung tumors in rats exposed to 4.2 mg m^{-3} antimony trioxide 6 h day^{-1}, 5 days $week^{-1}$ for 1 year. The inconsistencies in the animal studies as well as a lack strong evidence in humans are the reasons behind these classifications. Studies done by Health Canada suggest that ATO could be a 'threshold carcinogen.' It may not cause lung tumors due to DNA effects, but due to impaired lung clearance, particle overload, and subsequent inflammatory response leading to fibrosis and tumor formation.

Clinical Management

The oil-soluble BAL (British anti-Lewisite; 2,3-dimercaptopropanol) administered intramuscularly appears to be the antidote of choice for antimony poisoning. The antidotal action of BAL depends on its ability to prevent or break the union between antimony and vital enzymes.

Ecotoxicology

ATO does exhibit some potential to persist in the environment, especially in soils and aquatic sediments. The levels of ATO are not thought to be high enough to be considered hazardous to aquatic or terrestrial organisms. The potential for bioaccumulation is low.

LD_{50} for *Lepomis macrochirus* (bluegill sunfish) is >530 mg l^{-1} 96 h^{-1} and the LD_{50} for *Pimephales promelas* (fathead minnow) is >833 mg l^{-1} 96 h^{-1}.

Exposure Standards and Guidelines

US Occupational Safety and Health Administration standard for antimony: 0.5 mg m^{-3} 8 h exposure limit for 40 h workweek.

ACGIH threshold limit value: 8 h time-weighted average: 0.5 mg m^{-3} (antimony and compounds, as Sb).

In the United States, antimony is listed as a Clean Air Act hazardous air pollutant generally known or suspected to cause serious health problems. Antimony and its compounds are listed as Clean Water Act toxic pollutants, subject to effluent limitations. The Federal Drinking Water Standard is 6 mg l^{-1}.

See also: Antimony; Metals.

Further Reading

Fowler, B.A., Madden, E.F., Chou, S., 2012. Arsenic, antimony, and bismuth. Patty's Toxicol. 475–510.

Leonard, A., Gerber, G.B., 1996. Mutagenicity, carcinogenicity and teratogenicity of antimony compounds. Mutat. Res. 366 (1), 1–8.

Lylenda, C.A., Fowler, B.A., 2007. Antimony. In: Nordberg, G.F., Fowler, B.A., Nordberg, M., Friberg, L.T. (Eds.), Handbook on The Toxicology of Metals, third ed. Academic Press, San Diego, pp. 353–366.

Pohanish, R.P. (Ed.), 2002. Sittig's Handbook of Toxic and Hazardous Chemicals and Carcinogens. Noyes Publishing, imprint of William Andrew Publishing, Norwich, NY, pp. 719–721.

Relevant Websites

http://www.echemportal.org/echemportal/page.action?pageID=9 – eChem Portal Substance Search page, search for 'antimony trioxide' or CASRN.

www.EPA.gov – Environmental Protection Agency homepage, search for: 'antimony trioxide.'

http://toxnet.nlm.nih.gov/ – Toxnet homepage, search for: 'antimony trioxide' or CASRN.

Anxiolytics

D Fuentes and SD Ray, Manchester University College of Pharmacy, Fort Wayne, IN, USA
CP Holstege, University of Virginia School of Medicine, Charlottesville, VA, USA

- Name: Benzodiazepines
- Chemical Abstracts Service Registry Number: Representative compounds are listed below

Compounds	*CASRN*
Diazepam	439-14-5
Chlordiazepoxide	58-25-3
Flurazepam	17617-23-1
Clonazepam	1622-61-3
Midazolam	59467-70-8
Alprazolam	28981-97-7

- Synonyms: Representative listed below

Diazepam: Anxicalm®; Valium®; Trazepam®; 1-Methyl-5-phenyl-7-chloro-1,3-dihydro-2*H*-1,4-benzodiazepin-2-one; 7-Chloro-1-methyl-5-phenyl-2*H*-1,4-benzodiazepin-2-one
Chlordiazepoxide: Librium®; Angirex®; Elenium®; 3*H*-1,4-Benzodiazepin-2-amine, 7-chloro-*N*-methyl-5-phenyl, 4-oxide; 7-Chlor-2-methylamino-5-phenyl-3*H*-1,4-benzodiazepin-4-oxide
Flurazepam: Flurazepam®; Dalmane-R®; Dalmadorm®; 7-Chloro-1-(2-(diethylamino)ethyl)-5-(2-fluorophenyl)-1,3-dihydro-2*H*-1,4-benzodiazepin-2-one; 7-Chloro-1-(2-(diethylamino)ethyl)-5-(2-fluorophenyl)-1*H*-1,4-benzodiazepin-2(3*H*)-one
Clonazepam: Klonopin®; Clonex®; Solfidin®; 1,3-Dihydro-7-nitro-5-(2-chlorophenyl)-2*H*-1,4-benzodiazepin-2-one; 2*H*-1,4-Bbenzodiazepin-2-one, 5-(2-chlorophenyl)-1,3-dihydro-7-nitro-
Midazolam: Versed®; Midazolamum®; Dormicum®; 8-Chloro-6-(*o*-fluorophenyl)-1-methyl-4*H*-imidazo(1,5-a)(1,4)benzodiazepine; 8-Chlor-6-(2-fluorphenyl)-1-methyl-4*H*-imidazo(1,5-a)(1,4) benzodiazepine
Alprazolam: Xanax®; Alpronax®; V; 8-Chloro-1-methyl-6-phenyl-4*H*-s-triazolo(4,3-a)(1,4)benzodiazepine; 4*H*-(1,2,4) Triazolo(4,3-alpha)(1,4)benzodiazepine, 8-chloro-1-methyl-6-phenyl-

- Molecular Formula:

Diazepam: C_{16}–H_{13}–Cl–N_2–O	(molecular weight 284.75)
Chlordiazepoxide: C_{16}–H_{14}–Cl–N_3–O	(molecular weight 299.76)
Flurazepam: C_{21}–H_{23}–Cl–F–N_3–O	(molecular weight 387.88)
Clonazepam: C_{15}–H_{10}–Cl–N_3–O_3	(molecular weight 315.71)
Midazolam: C_{18}–H_{13}–Cl–F–N_3	(molecular weight 325.77)
Alprazolam: C_{17}–H_{13}–Cl–N_4	(molecular weight 308.77)

- Chemical Structure:

Diazepam (CASRN : 439-14-5)

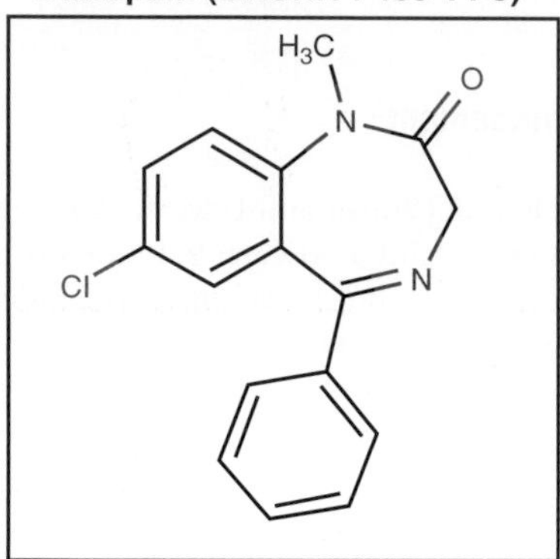

Chlordiazepoxide (CASRN : 58-25-3)

H3C
NH
N
Cl
N
O

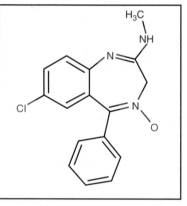

Flurazepam (CASRN : 17617-23-1)

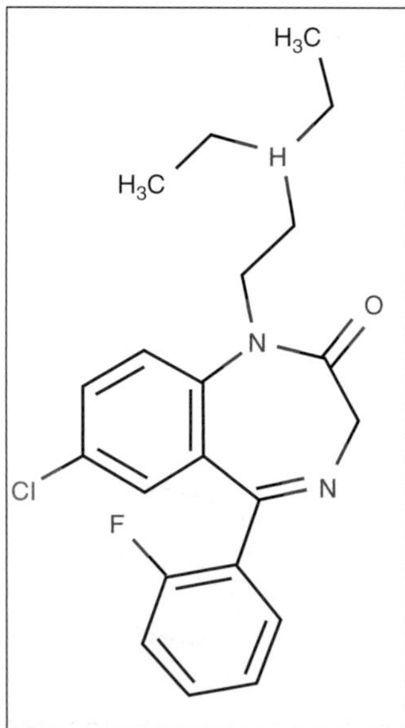

 http://dx.doi.org/10.1016/B978-0-12-386454-3.00241-4

Clonazepam (CASAN : 1622-61-3)

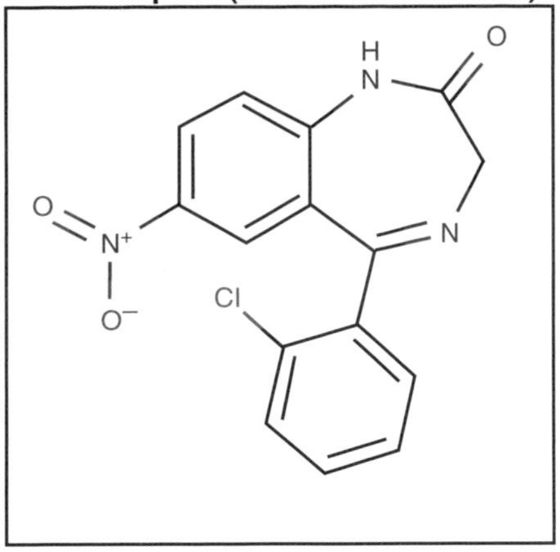

Midazolam (CASRN : 59467-70-8)

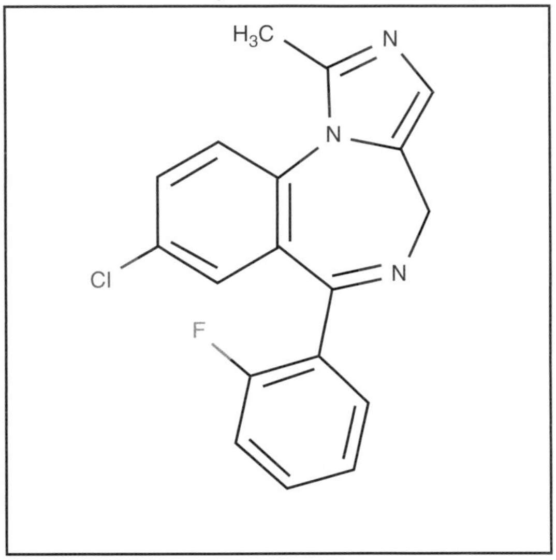

Alprazolam (CASRN : 28981-97-7)

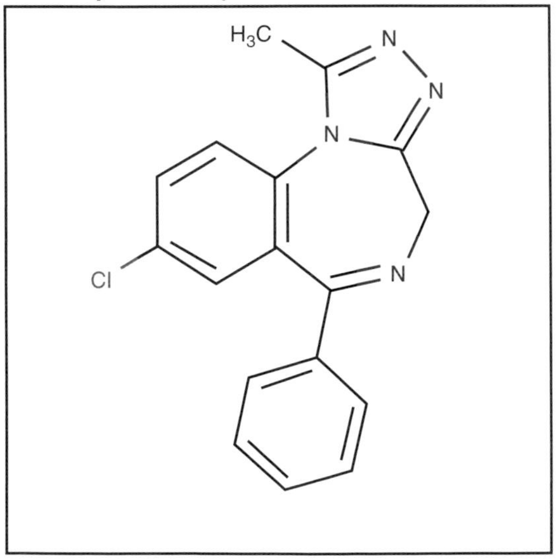

Background

Benzodiazepines (BZD) are a very large family of central nervous system (CNS) medications. This group consists of diazepam, chlordiazepoxide, flurazepam, clonazepam, midazolam, and alprazolam. Some of the brand names in this category, Valium®, Dalmane®, Librium®, Klonopin®, Xanax®, and Versed®, have been around for a long time. All BZDs are classified as schedule IV controlled substances, capable of causing dependence, tolerance, and abuse. Chronic exposure-associated toxic effects are secondary to the presence of the drug and metabolites and include depressed mental status, ataxia, vertigo, dizziness, fatigue, impaired motor coordination, confusion, disorientation, and anterograde amnesia. Paradoxical effects of psychomotor excitation, delirium, and aggressiveness also occur. These chronic effects are more common in the elderly, children, and patients with renal or hepatic disease.

Diazepam (Valium®), a BZD derivative, is a frontrunner in this family; it is very well known for its psycholeptic and anxiolytic actions. It is a crystalline solid, very slightly soluble in water, soluble in alcohol, and freely soluble in chloroform. It is primarily used in treatment of anxiety disorders, seizures, and status epilepticus. Liver cytochrome P450 enzymes metabolize diazepam and very little unchanged drug is eliminated in the urine. Hepatic *n*-demethylation results in the formation of the active metabolite desmethyldiazepam (or nordiazepam). This metabolite is hydroxylated to form oxazepam, which is conjugated to oxazepam glucuronide (minor metabolite is temazepam). The main active substances found in blood are diazepam and desmethyldiazepam. Urinary excretion of diazepam is primarily in the form of sulfate and glucuronide conjugates, and accounts for the majority of the ingested dose. Diazepam is excreted in the breast milk in significant amounts and in sweat in nanogram quantities. Valium is contraindicated in patients with a known hypersensitivity to diazepam, pediatric patients, and patients with myasthenia gravis, severe respiratory insufficiency, severe hepatic insufficiency, pregnancy, and sleep apnea syndrome. Diazepam is not classifiable as to its carcinogenicity in humans (Group 3). The most commonly encountered adverse events are ataxia, euphoria (3%, rectal gel), incoordination (3%, rectal gel), somnolence, rash (3%, rectal gel), and diarrhea (4%, rectal gel).

Chlordiazepoxide (Librium®) is metabolized extensively in the liver and has a very long half-life. Besides its use as an anxiolytic, it is also used in alcohol withdrawal syndromes. The liver injury from BZD is probably due to a rarely produced intermediate metabolite. As with other BZD, chlordiazepoxide therapy is not associated with serum aminotransferase or alkaline phosphatase elevations, and clinically apparent liver injury from this BZD has been reported but is very rare. The typical anxiolytic activity of the BZDs is mediated by their ability to enhance gamma-aminobutyric acid (GABA)-mediated inhibition of synaptic transmission through binding to the $GABA_A$ receptor. Use of chlordiazepoxide in the United States began in 1960s, and it enjoyed popularity for many years. It is not a commonly prescribed BZD anymore, having been replaced by other BZDs with more favorable pharmacokinetics, half-life, and tolerance. The most common side effects of chlordiazepoxide are dose related and include drowsiness, lethargy, ataxia, dysarthria, and dizziness. Tolerance develops to most of these side effects and to the anxiolytic effects as well. A few deaths have been reported at doses greater than 700 mg with chlordiazepoxide.

Flurazepam (Dalmane®), also available in hydrochloride form, is available in multiple generic forms and formerly under the brand name of Dalmane®. Use of flurazepam in the United States began in 1970 for the short-term management of insomnia. Like chlordiazepoxide, flurazepam was an extensively prescribed medication for sleep but no longer has the same popularity. It is an orally administered BZD for treating insomnia. Flurazepam exposure has not been reported to be associated with serum aminotransferase or alkaline phosphatase elevations; clinically apparent liver injury from Flurazepam has been reported but is very rare. Flurazepam is metabolized extensively in the liver to its active metabolite, which is then excreted in the urine. The sedating and soporific activity of this compound follows the BZD rules as described previously. Flurazepam, is contraindicated during pregnancy (US Food and Drug Administration (FDA) category X). Safety and efficacy of flurazepam in children younger than 15 years of age have not been established. The residual effects of a single dose are more prominent after diazepam, lorazepam, and nitrazepam than after flurazepam and triazolam. During repeated administration, the effects of flurazepam may persist for over 10 h.

Clonazepam (Klonopin®) was approved as an antiepileptic agent in the United States in 1997; more than 20 million prescriptions are filled annually. Clonazepam is currently indicated for management of absence seizures and myoclonic seizures in children as well as generalized seizure disorders in both adults and children. Clonazepam is effective in status epilepticus, but diazepam and lorazepam are preferable because of their longer half-lives. Clonazepam is also used for restless leg syndrome, dysarthria, tic disorders, panic disorder, and acute mania. Side effects of clonazepam are dose related and include drowsiness, lethargy, ataxia, dysarthria, and dizziness. Tolerance develops to these side effects, but tolerance may also develop to the antiseizure effects. Clonazepam as with other BZD is rarely associated with serum alanine transaminase (ALT) elevations, and clinically apparent liver injury from clonazepam is extremely rare formation. Overdose of clonazepam may produce many adverse effects, such as, somnolence (~37% of patients), confusion, ataxia, diminished reflexes, or coma. FDA pregnancy risk factor analysis has categorized Klonopin as category D. Klonopin metabolites are excreted by the kidneys; to avoid their excess accumulation, caution should be exercised in the administration of the drug to patients with impaired renal function.

Midazolam (Versed®) acts at the level of the limbic, thalamic, and hypothalamic regions of the CNS through potentiation of GABA (inhibitory neurotransmitter), primarily by decreasing neural cell activity in all regions of CNS. Anxiety is decreased by inhibiting cortical and limbic arousal. Midazolam promotes relaxation through inhibition of spinal motor reflex pathway, and also depresses muscle and motor nerve function directly. It also acts as an anticonvulsant and augments presynaptic inhibitions of neurons, limiting the spread of electrical activity. Midazolam has twice the affinity for benzodiazepine receptors than does diazepam and has more potent amnesic effects. It is short acting and roughly three to four times more potent than diazepam. It may cause fetal toxicity when administered to pregnant women, but potential benefits from use of the drug may be acceptable in certain conditions despite the possible risks to the fetus. Midazolam crosses the placenta and is distributed into amniotic fluid in animals and humans (FDA pregnancy category D). Midazolam has been detected in maternal venous serum, umbilical venous serum, umbilical arterial serum, and amniotic fluid in humans. However, it is not known whether midazolam is distributed into milk. It is primarily metabolized in the liver and gut by human cytochrome P450 IIIA4 (CYP3A4) to its pharmacologic active metabolite, α-hydroxymidazolam, followed by glucuronidation of the α-hydroxyl metabolite that is present in unconjugated and conjugated forms in human plasma. The α-hydroxymidazolam glucuronide is then excreted in urine. No significant amount of parent drug or metabolites is extractable from urine before beta-glucuronidase and sulfatase deconjugation, indicating that the urinary metabolites are excreted mainly as conjugates. Midazolam is also metabolized to two other minor metabolites: 4-hydroxy metabolite (about 3% of the dose) and 1,4-dihydroxy metabolite (about 1% of the dose) are excreted in small amounts in the urine as conjugates. Decreased respiratory rate (23%) and apnea (15%) are the two prime adverse effects.

Alprazolam (Xanax®) is an orally available benzodiazepine used predominantly for therapy of anxiety and panic disorders. Alprazolam came into use in the United States in 1981, and more than 40 million prescriptions are filled every year. Extended-release forms are available for this drug. The most common side effects of alprazolam are dose related and include drowsiness, lethargy, ataxia, dysarthria, and dizziness. Tolerance develops to these side effects, but tolerance may also develop to the anxiolytic effects. Alprazolam like other BZD is rarely associated with serum ALT elevations, and clinically apparent liver injury from alprazolam is extremely rare. Liver injury is usually mild to moderate in severity and self-limited. Alprazolam is metabolized in rat and human liver by P4503A1 and P4503A4, respectively, to 4-hydroxy alprazolam (4-OHALP, pharmacologically less active) and alpha-hydroxy alprazolam (alpha-OHALP, pharmacologically more active), and relative amounts of alpha-OHALP formed in the brain have been found to be higher than in liver.

BZD overdose in adults frequently involves coingestion of other CNS depressants, which act synergistically to increase toxicity. The elderly and very young children are more susceptible to the CNS depressant action. Intravenous administration of even therapeutic doses of BZDs may produce apnea and hypotension. Dependence may develop with regular use of BZDs, even in therapeutic doses for short periods, whereas physical and psychological dependence when administered at high doses for prolonged periods of time. If BZD are discontinued abruptly after regular use, then withdrawal symptoms may develop.

The clinical manifestations of the withdrawal syndrome are similar to those associated with withdrawal of other sedative hypnotic and CNS depressant drugs. The long half-life and presence of active metabolites result in delayed onset of symptoms. The symptoms include anxiety, insomnia, irritability, confusion, anorexia, nausea and vomiting, tremors, hypotension, hyperthermia, and muscular spasm. Severe withdrawal symptoms include seizures and death. The treatment to prevent withdrawal and minimize any symptoms is to slowly reduce the dose of diazepam over 2–4 weeks.

Uses

Anxiolytics are extensively used medications, primarily for preoperative relief of anxiety, for conscious sedation, as hypnotics in the treatment of insomnia, for short-term relief of symptoms of anxiety, or for the management of anxiety disorders. BZDs are also used for the management of agitation associated with alcohol withdrawal, for their anticonvulsant properties, and as skeletal muscle relaxants. BZDs are preferred over barbiturates since these are less likely to produce tolerance and physical dependence and are remarkably safe in large suicidal doses.

Environmental Fate and Behavior

Most BZDs have identical environmental fate and behavior. They are classified as schedule IV substances. Diazepam has been discussed here. Diazepam's release to the environment is via its production and use as a tranquilizer. BZDs such as diazepam may also be of natural origin, with research showing their presence in mammalian brain tissue and in various plant products. If released to air, an estimated vapor pressure of 2.8×10^{-8} mmHg at 25 °C indicates diazepam will exist in both the vapor and particulate phases in the atmosphere. Atmospheric reaction generated by photochemically produced hydroxyl radicals typically degrades vapor-phase diazepam; the half-life for this reaction in air is estimated to be 40 h. Particulate-phase diazepam will be removed from the atmosphere by wet or dry deposition. Diazepam does not contain chromophores that absorb at wavelengths >290 nm, and therefore is not expected to be susceptible to direct photolysis by sunlight. If released to soil, diazepam is expected to have very moderate to low mobility based on K_{oc} values ranging from 192 to 630. Volatilization from dry and moist soil surfaces is not expected to be an important fate process. C^{14}-labeled diazepam exhibited a biodegradation half-life of greater than 365 days when incubated using a water/sediment sample, suggesting that biodegradation is not an important environmental fate process. Volatilization from water surfaces is not expected to be an important fate process based on this compound's estimated Henry's Law constant. This group has moderate potential for bioconcentration in aquatic organisms. Hydrolysis is not expected to be an important environmental fate process since this compound lacks functional groups that hydrolyze under environmental conditions. Occupational exposure to diazepam may occur through inhalation and dermal contact with this compound at workplaces where diazepam is produced or used. Monitoring data indicate that the general population may be exposed to diazepam via dermal contact with contaminated water. Exposure to diazepam among the general population may be also among those administered the drug.

Toxicokinetics

As examples, diazepam and lorazepam are well absorbed from the gut. Lorazepam taken orally reaches peak concentrations in approximately 2 h and has a 90% bioavailability. Some of these agents are also absorbed quickly via intramuscular routes. Diazepam given intramuscularly reaches peak concentrations within approximately 2 h. Plasma concentration of the BZDs and their metabolites exhibits considerable interpatient variation. Onset and duration of action vary depending on the BZD and the route of administration. BZDs are widely distributed in body tissues and cross the blood–brain barrier. Generally, BZDs and their metabolites cross the placenta. The concentration of diazepam in fetal circulation has been reported to be equal to or greater than the maternal plasma concentration. The drugs and their metabolites are distributed into milk. BZDs and their metabolites are highly bound to plasma proteins. Lorazepam possesses a protein binding capacity of 85–91%, while diazepam is bound to proteins at 95–98%. Lorazepam is metabolized via the hepatic system via conjugation and undergoes extensive and rapid metabolism, subject to enterohepatic recirculation. Lorazepam's major metabolite is lorazepam glucuronide as 3-*O*-phenolic glucuronide. Diazepam is metabolized via the hepatic system through P450 enzymes, CYP2C19 and CYP3A4, undergoing extensive oxidation and demethylation, as well as 3-hydroxylation and glucuronidation. Metabolites of diazepam include 3-hydroxydiazepam (temazepam) and 3-hydroxy-*N*-diazepam (oxazepam). A variety of other BZD agents, including chlordiazepoxide, clorazepate, flurazepam, quazepam, clonazepam, midazolam, alprazolam, and triazolam, undergo a variety of metabolic processes and form metabolites.

For example, about 70% of flurazepam is converted to metabolites during its first pass through the intestine and liver. There are at least six nonconjugated metabolites of the drug, of which five are more potent in various activities than is flurazepam. The active metabolites in flurazepam are desalkylflurazepam and *N*-1-hydroxyethylflurazepam; the active substances in the blood include hydroxyethylflurazepam (flurazepam aldehyde) and desalkylflurazepam. Clinically, the desamino (group at position 1 converted to HOC_2H_4–) and desalkyl (group at position 1 removed) metabolites are of major significance. Not only are they an order of magnitude more potent than is flurazepam in animal tests, but also they reach higher concentration in plasma than does flurazepam.

Clonazepam, on the other hand, is rapidly and completely absorbed after oral administration. Absolute bioavailability of clonazepam is ~90%. Plasma concentrations of clonazepam peak within 1–4 h after oral administration. Clonazepam is approximately 85% bound to plasma proteins. Clonazepam is highly metabolized, with less than 2% unchanged. Clonazepam is excreted in the urine. Biotransformation occurs mainly by reduction of the 7-nitro group to the 4-amino derivative. This derivative can be acetylated, hydroxylated, and glucuronidated. Cytochrome P450 isozyme CYP3A is thought to be involved in clonazepam oxidation and reduction. The elimination half-life of clonazepam is typically 30–40 h. Clonazepam kinetics are dose independent throughout the dosing range. There is no evidence that clonazepam induces its own metabolism or that of other drugs in humans.

Mechanism of Toxicity

The advantage of using BZDs is that they have a larger therapeutic index. The exact sites and mode of action of the BZDs have not been elucidated. Pharmacologically, these agents act on the BZD binding site on the chloride channels of GABA, an inhibitory neurotransmitter receptor in the CNS. Action on this receptor increases the frequency of the chloride channel opening, which hyperpolarizes the cells and prevents nerve firing and stimulation. CNS depression results from this effect via depression of the reticular activating system and spinal cord reflexes. Allosteric interaction of central BZD receptors with $GABA_A$ receptors and subsequent opening of chloride channels are involved in eliciting the CNS effects of the drugs. These drugs appear to act at the limbic, thalamic, and hypothalamic levels of the CNS. In usual therapeutic doses, BZDs appear to have very little effect on the autonomic nervous system, respiration, or cardiovascular system. In mild to moderate toxicity, CNS depression may occur, as well as respiratory depression, especially when coingested with other sedative/hypnotic agents. Symptoms of severe toxicity include respiratory depression or arrest, coma, hypotension, and hypothermia, especially with coingestion of other CNS-depressing agents. These do not produce extrapyramidal side effects or interfere with the autonomic nervous system function.

Acute and Short-Term Toxicity (or Exposure)

Animal

The toxic effects of diazepam, chlordiazepoxide, and nitrazepam on the spermatozoa of mice disclosed different types of abnormalities involving both shape and size of the sperm head. The incidences of abnormal sperm heads were significantly high after diazepam treatment. All three drugs produced maximum effects at week 6.

LD_{50} values for some of the well-known BZDs are as follows:

Diazepam
LD_{50} rat oral 352–710 mg kg^{-1}
LD_{50} mouse oral 48–278 mg kg^{-1}
LD_{50} mouse s.c. 300 mg kg^{-1}
LD_{50} mouse i.p. 47–220 mg kg^{-1}
LD_{50} rat i.p. 46 500 μg kg^{-1}
LD_{50} rat s.c. 6350 μg kg^{-1}
LD_{50} mouse skin 800 mg kg^{-1}
LD_{50} mouse i.v. 25 mg kg^{-1}
LD_{50} mouse parenteral 150 mg kg^{-1}
LD_{50} rabbit i.v. 9 mg kg^{-1}

Chlordiazepoxide
LD_{50} rat oral 548 mg kg^{-1}
LD_{50} rat i.p. 143 mg kg^{-1}
LD_{50} rat i.v. 165 mg kg^{-1}
LD_{50} mouse oral 260 mg kg^{-1}
LD_{50} mouse i.p. 207 mg kg^{-1}
LD_{50} mouse s.c. 392 mg kg^{-1}
LD_{50} mouse i.v. 95 mg kg^{-1}

Flurazepam
LD_{50} mouse i.p. 290 mg kg^{-1}
LD_{50} mouse oral 870 mg kg^{-1}
LD_{50} mouse i.v. 84 mg kg^{-1}

Clonazepam
LD_{50} mouse i.p. 13 300 mg kg^{-1}
LD_{50} rat i.p. 14 200 mg kg^{-1}
LD_{50} mouse oral 2 g kg^{-1}
LD_{50} rat oral >15 g kg^{-1}

Midazolam
LD_{50} mouse i.m. 50 mg kg^{-1}
LD_{50} mouse i.v. 50 mg kg^{-1}
LD_{50} rat oral 215 mg kg^{-1}
LD_{50} rat i.v. 75 mg kg^{-1}
LD_{50} rat i.m. 50 mg kg^{-1}

Alprazolam
LD_{50} mouse oral 1020 mg kg^{-1}
LD_{50} rat oral >2000 mg kg^{-1}
LD_{50} mouse i.p. 540 mg kg^{-1}
LD_{50} rat i.p. 610 mg kg^{-1}

i.p.: intraperitoneally; i.v.: intravenous; i.m.: intramuscular; s.c.: subcutaneous.

Human

BZDs primarily target the CNS, causing respiratory depression and consciousness. The BZDs have a low order of toxicity unless ingested with other CNS depressants. Deep coma is rare. The BZDs have been known to cause dose-dependent adverse CNS effects. BZD overdosage may result in sedation, somnolence, impaired coordination, slurred speech, confusion, coma, and diminished reflexes. Diplopia, dysarthria, ataxia, and intellectual impairment are not uncommon. Hypotension, seizures, respiratory depression, and apnea may also occur. Although cardiac arrest has been reported, death from overdose of BZDs in the absence of concurrent ingestion of alcohol and other CNS depressants is rare. Outcomes are usually favorable when used alone. Deep coma and other manifestations of severe CNS depression are rare.

Anxiolytic and possibly paradoxical CNS stimulatory effects of BZDs are postulated to result from release of previously suppressed responses (disinhibition). After usual doses of BZD for several days, the drugs cause a moderate decrease in rapid eye movement (REM) sleep. REM rebound does not occur when the drugs are withdrawn. Stages 3 and 4 sleep is markedly reduced by usual doses of the drugs; the clinical importance of these sleep stage alterations has not been established.

The onset of impairment of consciousness is relatively rapid in BZD poisoning. Onset is more rapid following larger doses and with agents of shorter duration of action. The most common and initial symptom is somnolence. This may progress to coma Grade I or Grade II following very large ingestions.

Classification of coma has been describes as follows:

Coma Grade I: Depressed level of consciousness, response to painful stimuli, deep tendon reflexes and vital signs intact
Coma Grade II: Depressed level of consciousness, no response to painful stimuli, deep tendon reflexes and vital signs intact
Coma Grade III: Depressed level of consciousness, no response to painful stimuli, deep tendon reflexes absent. Vital signs intact
Coma Grade IV: Coma grade III plus respiratory and circulatory collapse

Source: IPCS-InChem.

Severe anaphylactic reactions following intravenous administration of diazepam have been reported. Intravenous formulations of lorazepam and diazepam may contain propylene glycol, which may contribute to these types of reactions. Effects are merely extensions of pharmacological effects. Nausea, vomiting, dizziness, drowsiness, miosis, and gastric distention may be seen. A few deaths have been reported at doses greater than 700 mg with chlordiazepoxide.

There is a broad spectrum of signs and symptoms associated with acute benzodiazepine toxicity. Lethargy, ataxia, nystagmus, diplopia, amnesia, slurred speech, confusion, hypotonia, hypotension, hypothermia, coma, respiratory depression, and death have been reported. Rarely, paradoxical excitation may occur at lower does. Toxic doses for each agent have not been clearly established. When large doses of lorazepam have been infused chronically, there are multiple reports of the development of a syndrome consisting of a hyperosmolar state with metabolic acidosis and cardiovascular compromise. This syndrome has been attributed to propylene glycol, the diluent in lorazepam.

Chronic Toxicity (or Exposure)

Animal

A number of repeated-dose studies have been carried out. In general, toxic effects have not been remarkable. In a 3-month study in rats and a 6-month study in dogs, some increase in liver size was seen, together with an increase in blood cholesterol; in the dogs an elevation of plasma alanine aminotransferase activity was observed. There was no increase in tumor frequency after feeding diazepam to rats and mice for 104 and 80 weeks, respectively.

Human

Tolerance and psychological and physical dependence may occur following prolonged use of BZDs. Such effects may occur following short-term use of BZDs, particularly at high doses. Drowsiness, ataxia, slurred speech, and vertigo may be seen on dependence. Withdrawal symptoms, including anxiety, agitation, tension, dysphoria, anorexia, insomnia, sweating, blurred vision, irritability, tremors, and hallucinations, may be seen. Milder withdrawal symptoms such as insomnia have also been reported. Since some BZDs and their metabolites have long elimination half-lives, withdrawal symptoms may not occur until several days after the drug has been discontinued. With all BZD agents, patients should be warned that development of withdrawal symptoms may occur if using these agents on a chronic basis. Patients may require a carefully designed tapering regimen if they are to abandon BZD after chronic use.

Chronic use of flurazepam is often followed by tolerance and decrease in effectiveness. The most common side effects of flurazepam are dose related and include daytime drowsiness, lethargy, and dizziness. Flurazepam and other BZDs are classified as schedule IV controlled substances, capable of causing dependence, tolerance, and abuse. Only a few case reports of acute liver injury from flurazepam have been published and mostly before 1980. The latency to onset of acute liver injury has varied from 2 to 6 months and the pattern of liver enzyme elevations was cholestatic.

Among all BZDs, alprazolam is the most frequently prescribed medication in several continents. It has also been hypothesized that alprazolam is relatively more toxic than other BZDs. The paradoxical effects associated with alprazolam are aggression, rage, twitches, tremor, mania and agitation, and hyperactivity. The other effects include slurred speech, suicidal ideation, disinhibition, change in libido, skin rash, anterograde amnesia, concentration problems, and urinary retention.

Clinical Management

Basic and advanced life-support measures should be implemented as necessary. Gastrointestinal decontamination procedures should be used as appropriate, based on the patient's level of consciousness and history of ingestion. Activated charcoal can be used to adsorb the benzodiazepines however significant CNS depression or coma are contraindications for the administration of charcoal in a simple benzodiazepine overdose due to the risk of aspiration. The patient's level of consciousness and vital signs should be monitored closely. Obtunded patients with reduced gag reflex should be intubated to prevent pulmonary aspiration. Respiratory support, including oxygen and ventilation, should be provided as needed. If hypotension occurs, it should be treated with standard measures including intravenous fluids, Trendelenburg positioning, and dopamine by intravenous infusion. Forced diuresis, hemoperfusion, and hemodialysis are of no value in benzodiazepine toxicity. If withdrawal signs and symptoms develop, treatment should focus on either benzodiazepine or phenobarbital therapy with a gradual dose reduction.

Flumazenil (Romazicon) is a benzodiazepine antagonist, which can reverse the CNS depressant effects of these agents. It should be used with caution in acute intentional benzodiazepine overdoses. Because acute benzodiazepine overdoses generally result in only mild toxicity, it has limited clinical utility in this setting. Flumazenil's use in the acute benzodiazepine intoxicated patient may lead to an unnecessarily long observation period after fumazenil's infusion. This observation is necessary to be certain that reoccurrence of benzodiazepine toxic effects do not occur after flumazenil is metabolized. Flumazenil must be used with caution in mixed drug overdoses as seizures can develop, particularly if tricyclic antidepressants have been coingested. Also, it can induce potentially serious benzodiazepine withdrawal in dependent patients.

Reproductive Toxicity

BZDs should be avoided during the first trimester and at delivery. Malformation and CNS dysfunction have been described in infants born of mothers using BZDs during pregnancy. Both animal data and human epidemiological studies suggest that BZDs are teratogens.

Mutagenicity

Diazepam has been reported to have mutagenic activity in the *Salmonella typhimurium* tester train TA100 in the Ames test, and to be genotoxic in a mouse bone marrow micronucleus test. Little or no effect was seen in an assay for chromosomal aberrations, performed in Chinese hamster cells in vitro.

Carcinogenicity

There is no evidence of carcinogenicity in humans. In vitro studies suggest that alprazolam, bromazepam, and lorazepam, at concentrations equivalent to oral doses, exhibit statistically significant genotoxicity in human lymphocyte cultures.

Exposure and Exposure Monitoring

Miscellaneous

This class of compounds includes the BZDs like diazepam (Valium) and oxazepam (Serax), chlordiazepoxide (Librium), flurazepam (Dalmane), clonazepam (Klonopin), midazolam (Versed), alprazolam (Xanax), and triazolam (Halcion).

See also: Barbiturates; Neurotoxicity.

Further Reading

Anwar, M.J., Pillai, K.K., Khanam, R., et al., 2012. Effect of alprazolam on anxiety and cardiomyopathy induced by doxorubicin in mice. Fundam. Clin. Pharmacol. 26 (3), 356–362.

Bergmann, R., Kongsbak, K., Sørensen, P.L., Sander, T., Balle, T., 2013. A unified model of the GABA(A) receptor comprising agonist and benzodiazepine binding sites. PLoS One 8 (1), e52323 (Epub 7 January 2013).

Chouinard, G., 2004. Issues in the clinical use of benzodiazepines: potency, withdrawal, and rebound. J. Clin. Psychiatry 5, 7–12.

Debruyne, D., Pailliet-Loilier, M., Lelong-Boulouard, V., et al., 2010. Therapeutic drug monitoring of clonazepam. Therapie 65 (3), 219–224.

Ekonomopoulou, M.T., Akritopoulou, K., Mourelatos, C., Iakovidou-Kritsi, Z., 2011. A comparative study on the cytogenetic activity of three benzodiazepines in vitro. Genet. Test. Mol. Biomarkers 15 (6), 373–378.

Fukasawa, T., Suzuki, A., Otani, K., 2007. Effects of genetic polymorphism of cytochrome P450 enzymes on the pharmacokinetics of benzodiazepines. J. Clin. Pharm. Ther. 32 (4), 333–341.

Gaudreault, P., Guay, J., Thivierge, R.L., Verdy, I., 1991. Benzodiazepine poisoning. Clinical and pharmacological considerations and treatment. Drug Saf. 6 (4), 247–265.

Grimsley, A., Gallagher, R., Hutchison, M., et al., 2013. Drug–drug interactions and metabolism in cytochrome P450 2C knockout mice: application to troleandomycin and midazolam. Biochem. Pharmacol. 86 (4), 529–538.

Howland, R.H., 2010. Potential adverse effects of discontinuing psychotropic drugs. J. Psychosoc. Nurs. Ment. Health Serv. 48 (9), 11–14.

Istaphanous, G.K., Loepke, A.W., 2009. General anesthetics and the developing brain. Curr. Opin. Anaesthesiol. 22 (3), 368–373.

Krüger, S., 2012. Psychopharmacological treatment of mood and anxiety disorders during pregnancy. Handb. Exp. Pharmacol. 214, 279–305, 2012.

Lader, M., 2011. Benzodiazepines revisited – will we ever learn? Addiction 106 (12), 2086–2109.

Levine, M., Ruha, A.M., 2012. Overdose of atypical antipsychotics: clinical presentation, mechanisms of toxicity and management. CNS Drugs 26 (7), 601–611.

Lima, S.A., Tavares, J., Gameiro, P., de Castro, B., Cordeiro-da-Silva, A., 2008. Flurazepam inhibits the P-glycoprotein transport function: an insight to revert multidrug-resistance phenotype. Eur. J. Pharmacol. 581 (1–2), 30–36.

Mandrioli, R., Mercolini, L., Raggi, M.A., 2010. Metabolism of benzodiazepine and non-benzodiazepine anxiolytic–hypnotic drugs: an analytical point of view. Curr. Drug Metab. 11, 815–829.

Moroz, G., 2004. High-potency benzodiazepine: recent clinical results. J. Clin. Psychiatry 65, 13–18.

Mumma, B.E., Shellenbarger, D., Callaway, C.W., et al., 2009. Neurologic recovery following cardiac arrest due to benzodiazepine and opiate toxicity. Resuscitation 80 (12), 1446–1447.

Riddle, M.A., Bernstein, G.A., Cook, E.H., Leonard, H.L., March, J.S., Swanson, J.M., 1999. Anxiolytics, adrenergic agents and naltrexone. J. Am. Acad. Child Adolesc. Psychiatry 38, 546–556.

Riss, J., Cloyd, J., Gates, J., Collins, S., 2008. Benzodiazepines in epilepsy: pharmacology and pharmacokinetics. Acta Neurol. Scand. 118 (2), 69–86.

Skolnick, P., 2012. Anxioselective anxiolytics: on a quest for the Holy Grail. Trends Pharmacol. Sci. 33 (11), 611–620.

Sun, T., Hu, G., Li, M., 2009. Repeated antipsychotic treatment progressively potentiates inhibition on phencyclidine-induced hyperlocomotion, but attenuates inhibition on amphetamine-induced hyperlocomotion: relevance to animal models of antipsychotic drugs. Eur. J. Pharmacol. 602 (2–3), 334–342.

Vrzal, R., Kubesova, K., Pavek, P., Dvorak, Z., 2010. Benzodiazepines medazepam and midazolam are activators of pregnane X receptor and weak inducers of CYP3A4: investigation in primary cultures of human hepatocytes and hepatocarcinoma cell lines. Toxicol. Lett. 193 (2), 183–188.

Yuksel, A., Erdur, B., Kortunay, S., Ergin, A., 2013. Assessment of propofol, midazolam and ziprasidone, or the combinations for the prevention of acute cocaine toxicity in a mouse model. Environ. Toxicol. Pharmacol. 35 (1), 61–66.

Relevant Websites

https://aapcc.s3.amazonaws.com/pdfs/annual_reports/2011_NPDS_Annual_Report.pdf – American Association of Poison Control Centers.

http://bnf.org – British National Formulary.

http://www.inchem.org/documents/pims/pharm/pim181.htm – International programme on Chemical Safety.

http://emedicine.medscape.com/article/813255-overview#a0101 – MedScape.

http://chem.sis.nlm.nih.gov/chemidplus – US National Library of Medicine: ChemIDplus Advanced: Search for: Anxiolytics.

http://toxnet.nlm.nih.gov/cgi-bin/sis/search/r?dbs+hsdb:@term+@rn+@rel+439-14-5 – National Library of Medicine-Hazardous Substances Data Bank.

http://toxnet.nlm.nih.gov/cgi-bin/sis/search/r?dbs+hsdb:@term+@rn+@rel+58-25-3 – National Library of Medicine-Hazardous Substances Data Bank.

http://toxnet.nlm.nih.gov/cgi-bin/sis/search/r?dbs+hsdb:@term+@rn+@rel+17617-23-1 – National Library of Medicine-Hazardous Substances Data Bank.

http://toxnet.nlm.nih.gov/cgi-bin/sis/search/r?dbs+hsdb:@term+@rn+@rel+28981-97-7 – National Library of Medicine-Hazardous Substances Data Bank.

http://livertox.nlm.nih.gov/Chlordiazepoxide.htm – National Library of Medicine-Livtox (Chlordiazepoxide).

http://livertox.nlm.nih.gov/Flurazepam.htm – National Library of Medicine-Livtox (Flurazepam).

http://toxnet.nlm.nih.gov/ – Search for Alprazolam or 2-Chlorodiazepam.

Apoptosis

DA Brown, N Yang and SD Ray, Manchester University College of Pharmacy, Fort Wayne, IN, USA

Definition

Apoptosis (Ap oh' tosis or A 'pop tosis: Greek 'apo,' meaning leaf; 'ptosis,' meaning falling off), a form of cell death, is a genetically regulated self-orchestrated naturally occurring cell death process that is active during the course of development and induced during pathological conditions for the overall benefit of the organism. In contrast, necrosis (necroh' sis), another form of cell death, typically affects groups of contiguous cells, and an inflammatory reaction usually develops in the adjacent viable tissue in response to the released cellular debris.

Introduction

Cell death is a necessary event in the life of a multicellular organism. There are two major forms of cell death, designated apoptosis and necrosis, with the former being the most common cell death pathway. Since apoptosis is a result of tightly regulated, genetically controlled, self-orchestrated processes, it is often referred to as programmed cell death (PCD). In contrast, necrosis is termed unprogrammed cell death since it occurs accidentally in an unplanned manner. It has recently been suggested that a third type of cell death, termed apocrosis or aponecrosis, exists. Cells dying by this mechanism display signs of both apoptosis and necrosis. This is thought to arise from the incomplete execution of biochemical cascades associated with apoptosis.

PCD was first described by C. Vogt in the middle of the nineteenth century through observations on the morphology of dying cells during metamorphosis in amphibians. By 1885, there were numerous publications accounting similar morphological changes in the tissues of metamorphosing insects. Studies performed in the 1960s by Australian pathologist John Kerr on ischemic liver injury reported the existence of two types of cell death: what was then known as classical necrosis, and another form, where scattered cells were converted into small round masses of cytoplasm, often containing specks of condensed nuclear chromatin. Kerr subsequently coined this newly discovered type of cell death apoptosis. Since then, an enormous amount of research has been performed investigating the cellular and molecular mechanisms involved in apoptosis.

Apoptosis exists in a delicate and tightly controlled balance with mitosis. Research done in the field of PCD in the past few decades has produced a wealth of information regarding the precise, highly controlled cellular and molecular events that occur during apoptosis. The following sections aim to highlight these processes and to share recent developments in the field.

What Is Cell Death?

Generally, cell death or loss of cell viability can be regarded as an irreversible failure of vital cellular functions coupled with irreparable structural damage. Therefore, cell death is considered a near equilibrium terminal end stage, and can be induced by a variety of physiological or nonphysiological conditions, such as ischemia, hypoxia, exposure to certain drugs and chemicals, immune reactions, infectious agents, high temperature, radiation, and various disease states. Cellular exposure to these conditions, either *in vivo* or *in vitro*, could be either apoptogenic (apoptosisinducing) or necrogenic (necrosis inducing). The biological and medical implications of cell death are becoming increasingly evident as more information is learned concerning these processes.

Morphology of Apoptosis

The assignment of apoptosis as the mechanism involved in a cell's death can be greatly facilitated by observing morphological changes. These can be observed by light and electron microscopy. A readily apparent morphological change is a decrease in cell size; the cytoplasm becomes denser and the organelles are more tightly packed. Pyknosis, a classis sign of apoptosis, also occurs, resulting from condensation of chromatin. Histological staining usually shows single cells or small clusters or cells. Subcellular changes can be observed with electron microscopy.

A hallmark feature of apoptosis is plasma membrane blebbing. This is followed by separation of cell fragments into apoptotic bodies in a process called budding. The integrity of the organelles is maintained at this point and an intact plasma membrane encloses these apoptotic bodies. These are phagocytosed by macrophages, parenchymal cells, and neoplastic cells and subsequently degraded in phagolysosomes. Apoptosis usually does not yield to inflammation because apoptotic cells or apoptotic bodies do not release cellular contents, are quickly phagocytosed, and the engulfing cells do not produce inflammatory factors mediators in response to phagocytosis.

Apoptosis versus Necrosis

Apoptosis and necrosis occur via distinct mechanisms and give different morphologies. However, it is not always easy to distinguish between the two based on simple histological observations. Necrosis is typically referred to as accidental cell death and is an uncontrolled, passive process. Usually large fields of cells are affected. In contrast, apoptosis is a tightly regulated, energy-dependent process that usually affects individual or clusters of cells.

Morphologically, necrosis is associated with cell swelling, formation of cytosolic vacuoles, distended endoplasmic reticulum, swollen or ruptured mitochondria, cytoplasmic blebs, ruptured lysosomes, and eventual cell membrane disruption. This results in the release of cytoplasmic contents into the surrounding area, triggering inflammatory responses.

Despite these two paths of cell death having distinct mechanisms and morphologies, it is possible for a cell to undergo both processes at once, in a hybrid cell death process. This is referred to as the 'apoptosis–necrosis continuum.' Two features influencing the position of this continuum are the availability of

 http://dx.doi.org/10.1016/B978-0-12-386454-3.00242-6

caspases and intracellular ATP. The path by which a cell dies is controlled in part by the nature of the death signal, type of tissue, and the physiological environment (**Table 1**).

Biochemical Features of Apoptosis

Apoptotic cells display characteristic biochemical changes. Protein cleavage, protein cross-linking, breakdown of DNA, and phagocytic recognition are readily observed. Caspases, which are ubiquitously expressed as inactive proenzymes, are activated. This activation begins a protease cascade, where one caspases activates another, and serves to amplify the apoptotic signaling pathway, leading to rapid cell death.

Since their discovery several years ago, 10 major types of caspases have been reported. These are broadly grouped into initiators (caspases-2, -8, -9, -10), effectors or executioners (caspases-3, -6, -7), and inflammatory caspases (caspases-1, -4, -5). Additionally, several more caspases have been identified, including caspase-11 (involved in cytokine maturation during septic shock), caspase-12 (related to apoptosis caused by β-amyloid), caspase-13 (a bovine gene), and caspase-14 (thought to be important to embryonic development). Caspases have proteolytic activity and can cleave proteins at aspartic acid residues; the specificities of caspases are due to recognition of nearby amino acids. Activation of caspases appears to send the cell on an irreversible path toward cell death.

An additional biochemical feature of apoptosis is the expression of specific cell surface markers that aid in the phagocytic recognition of apoptotic bodies by adjacent cells. One such marker is phosphatidylserine, normally facing inward in the cell's plasma membrane. During apoptosis, phosphatidylserine is oriented to the outside of the cell, where it is a well-known recognition ligand for phagocytes. Proteins also serve as recognition markers, including annexin I and calreticulin.

Apoptotic Mechanisms

Apoptosis is a tightly controlled, energy-driven process involving a carefully orchestrated series of molecular events. The cell death process can be divided into two stages: induction and execution. The induction phase relies on death-inducing signals to stimulate proapoptotic signal transduction cascades. Induction of apoptosis has been shown to proceed by two main apoptotic pathways: the intrinsic, or mitochondrial pathway, and the extrinsic, or death receptor pathway. Recent

Table 1 Sequence of cellular events associated with apoptosis contrasted with those associated with necrosis

Characteristic	*Apoptosis*	*Necrosis*
Distribution	Affects individual cells scattered throughout the tissue	Affects massive and contiguous cells
Adhesion between cells and to basement membrane	Lost early	Lost but late
Cellular morphology	Chromatin condensation (karyorrhexis) followed by margination as large crescents to the periphery of the nuclear membrane; fragmentation in large masses (convolution). See **Figure 2b**	Irregular clumping of chromatin, pyknosis or karyolysis, nucleolysis occasionally precedes collapse of nuclear membrane; cells occasionally maintain their boundaries with some or no organelles. See **Figure 2c**
	Loss of cell volume (cytoplasmic compaction)	Very early swelling of cell, ballooning occurs frequently
Damage to organelles, e.g., mitochondrion	Late (organelles mostly retain integrity), occasionally organellar swelling and bleb formation on cell surface appear very late (organelles found in blebs)	Very early swelling of organelles; cells disintegrate and lyse, appear chaotic, form blebs early (organelles are not found in blebs)
DNA breakdown pattern	Internucleosomal cleavage (ladder-like pattern on agarose gel)	Random or irregular damage (appears as a smear on gel)
Release of lysosomal enzymes	Absent	Present
Duration of biochemical and morphological changes	Minutes to hours	Hours to days
Ultimate outcome	Forms apoptotic bodies, occasionally containing intact organelles	Swelling, disintegration, dissolution
Cell removal	Usually phagocytosis by all types of resident and nonresident cells	Usually cells are not removed
Inflammation	Absent	Present
Energy requirement and overall regulation	Strictly energy dependent, very tightly regulated, signaling dependent, can easily be delayed but can be inhibited with difficulty	Energy and signaling independent, occasionally energy dependent, can be blocked prior to irreversible changes (e.g., plasma membrane leakage)
Genomic control	Strictly dependent	Usually independent
Scar formation	Absent	Present
Cellular osmotic regulation	Intact	Lost leading to cell swelling

evidence suggests that these two are linked. It has been shown that T-cells can initiate apoptosis through either granzyme A or B. The events triggering apoptosis via the intrinsic, extrinsic, and granzyme B pathways are different; however, the execution of apoptosis uses the same biochemical machinery, the caspases. Apoptosis induced by granzyme A utilizes a parallel, caspase-independent pathway. **Figure 1** outlines the major events occurring during these apoptotic pathways.

Extrinsic Pathway

Apoptosis induced by these pathways is initiated by the activation of transmembrane receptors, known as death receptors, by death ligands. This growing group of death receptors (and death ligands) belongs to the tumor necrosis factor (TNF) receptor superfamily and is characterized by the presence of extracellular cysteine-rich domains. The death receptors have an intracellular death domain which couples receptors to the apoptosis-inducing machinery. Notable death ligands/receptors include FasL/FasR, TNF-α/TNFR1, Apo3L/DR3, Apo2L/DR4, Apo2L, DR5, lymphocyte-associated receptor of death, TNF-related apoptosis-inducing ligand (TRAIL-R1), and TRAIL-R2. Activation of death receptors is controlled in many cases by the inducible *de novo* expression of the respective death ligands such as CD95L, TNF, or TRAIL. Besides death domains, there are also death effector domains involved downstream of the process.

A classic example of the sequence of events in an extrinsic pathway can be described by TNF-α and its receptor, TNFR1. Upon binding of TNF-α to trimeric TNFR1, there is a recruitment of cytosolic adapter proteins, including TNF receptor-1-associated death domain protein (TRADD), Fas-associated protein with death domain (FADD), and receptor interacting protein (RIP). TRADD binds to the death domain of TNFR1. After binding, FADD interacts with procaspase-8, inducing autocatalytic activation to form the death-inducing signaling complex containing active caspase-8. Subsequent activation of caspase-3 triggers the execution phase of apoptosis.

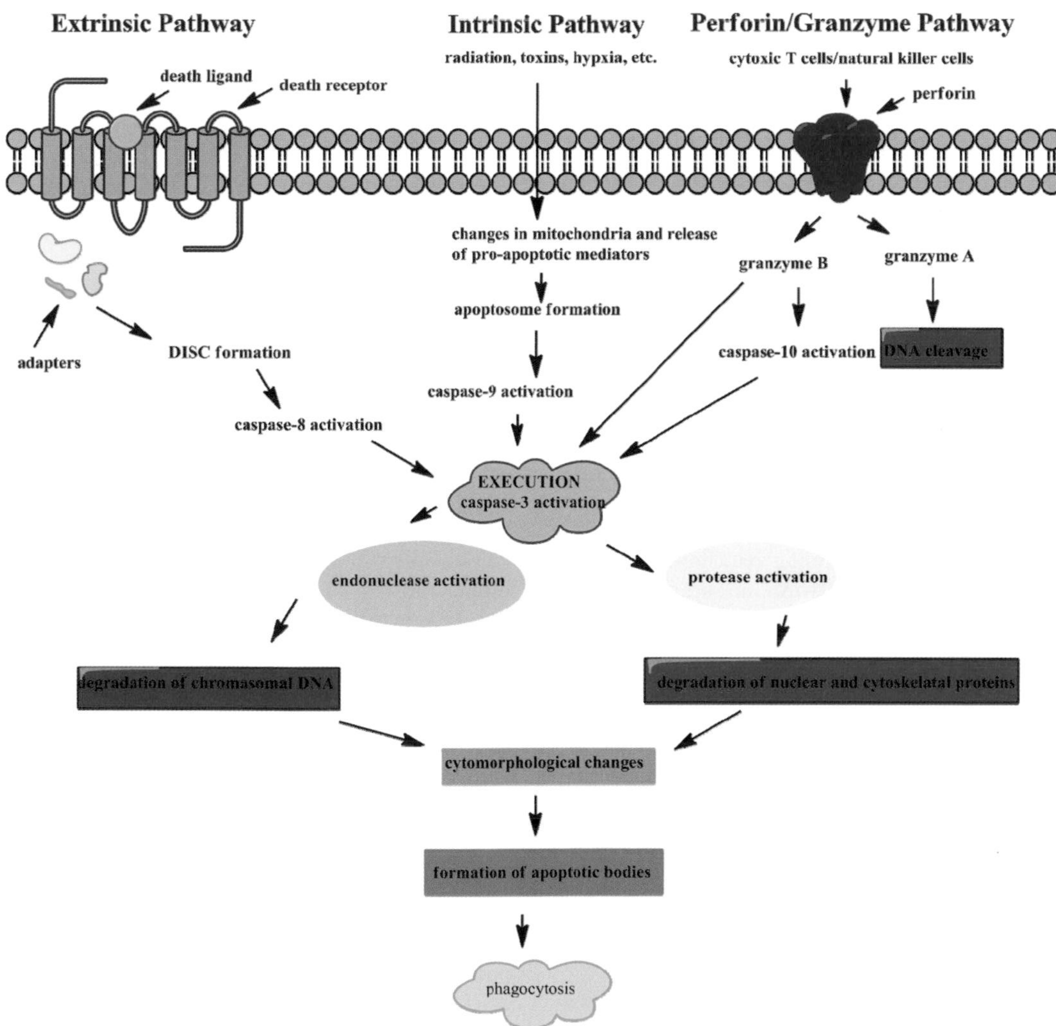

Figure 1 Schematic diagram showing possible apoptotic pathways. Induction of apoptosis can be achieved via the extrinsic, intrinsic, and perforin/granzyme pathways. Each pathway requires different stimuli and caspases to initiate apoptosis. However, these initiation pathways all end with the activation of caspase-3, beginning the execution phase of apoptosis. Activation of endonucleases and proteases result in the degradation of nuclear DNA and nuclear and cytoskeletal proteins. This gives rise to the classic cytomorphological changes seen in apoptotic cells, including cell shrinkage, chromatin condensation, formation of cytoplasmic blebs, and apoptotic bodies. Phagocytosis of the apoptotic bodies is the final step.

Perforin/Granzyme Pathway

A major pathway used to clear virus-infected or transformed cells is the perforin/granzyme pathway. In this pathway, sensitized cytotoxic T-lymphocytes (CTLs) and natural killer cells secrete perforin, a protein that induces the formation of pores in the plasma membrane of target cells. These pores allow cytoplasmic granules containing the serine proteases granzyme A and B (originating from the CTL) to enter the target cell.

Granzyme B cleaves various proteins at an aspartate residue and activates procaspase-10 and cleaves factors such as inhibitor of caspase-activated DNAse (ICAD). Granzyme B can directly activate caspase-3. It has also been shown that granzyme B can use the mitochondrial pathway to amplify the cell death signal, through cleavage of Bid and release of cytochrome *c*.

Granzyme A plays a role in CTL-induced apoptosis through the activation of a caspase-independent pathway. Granzyme A causes DNA nicking by activating DNAse NM23-HI (a tumor suppressor), and causing apoptotic DNA degradation. DNAse NM23-HI plays a vital role in the prevention of cancer by inducing tumor cell apoptosis.

Intrinsic Pathway

There are a variety of nonreceptor-mediated stimuli that can trigger the intrinsic apoptotic pathway. These stimuli produce intracellular signals that originate from the mitochondria and act directly on cellular targets, and can act in either a positive or a negative manner. Negative signals could be hormone or growth factor deprivation, redox imbalance, radiation (ultraviolet light, x-rays), chemotherapeutic drugs, toxins, hypoxia, viral infection, and oxidative stress. These factors cause a loss of apoptotic suppression and an induction of apoptosis.

These stimuli cause changes in the inner membrane of mitochondria. The mitochondrial permeability transition pore opens, and this results in a loss of mitochondrial transmembrane potential, and leakage of proapoptotic proteins. One group of such proteins, including cytochrome *c*, Smac/DIABLO, and the serine protease HtrA/Omi, activate the caspase-dependent mitochondrial pathway. A second group of proteins, which include apoptosis-inducing factor (AIF), endonuclease G, and, caspase-activated DNAse (CAD), are released later during apoptosis, when the cell has committed to die. AIF and endonuclease G behave in a caspase-independent fashion and, upon release from the mitochondria, travel to the nucleus and cleave chromatin and initiate chromatin condensation (stage I). CAD also travels to the nucleus, where is it cleaved by caspase-3 and initiates oligonucleosomal DNA fragmentation and advanced chromatin condensation (stage II condensation).

Execution Pathway

The intrinsic and extrinsic pathways are distinct in terms of how they induce apoptosis, but they both end at the execution phase. This phase of apoptosis is initiated by the activation of the execution caspases. These caspases (caspases-3, -6, -7) activate cytoplasmic endonucleases, which degrade nuclear material, and proteases that break down nuclear and cytoskeletal proteins. The stereotypical, morphological, and biochemical changes observed during apoptosis are caused by degradation of substrates such as cytokeratins, PARP, the nuclear protein NuMA, the plasma membrane cytoskeletal protein alpha fodrin, and others.

Considered the most important executioner caspase, caspase-3 can be activated by any of the initiator caspases, such as caspase-8, -9, and -10. The inhibitor of endonuclease CAD, ICAD, is cleaved by caspase-3. Active CAD then degrades chromosomal DNA in the nucleus and induces chromatin condensation. Caspase-3 also plays a role in the reorganization and breakdown of the cell into apoptotic bodies.

The last stage in apoptosis is phagocytosis. This stage is initiated by changes in membrane symmetry and externalization of recognition molecules, including phosphatidylserine. The emergence of phosphatidylserine on the outside of the cell facilitates noninflammatory phagocytotic recognition, which is efficient and results in no release of cellular material.

Regulation of Apoptosis

These apoptotic mitochondrial events are controlled by a family of proteins known as Bcl-2. In both pathological as well as physiological conditions, Bcl-2 family gene products have emerged as a critical regulator of apoptosis. For instance, expression of the Bcl-2 protein has been shown to directly prevent apoptosis by enhancing cellular antioxidant capacity, possibly through scavenging reactive oxygen radicals, or indirectly by counteracting oxidative stress. The other potential mechanisms of this gene include a role in regulation of intracellular calcium, nuclear transport, and control of signal transduction pathways. Other members of the Bcl-2 family include Bcl-X (Bcl-XL and Bcl-XS), Mcl-1, Bax, A1, Bag, Bak, Bad, Bcl-w, and Ced-9.

Recently, the protein p53, referred to by many as the 'guardian of the genome' has received considerable attention for its role in apoptosis. This is a tumor-suppressor protein that helps organisms cope with DNA damage by either stalling cell division or inducing cell death. The p53 tumor suppressor limits cellular proliferation by inducing cell cycle arrest and apoptosis in response to cellular stresses such as DNA damage, hypoxia, and oncogene activation. Many apoptosis-related genes that are transcriptionally regulated by p53 have been identified. These are candidates for implementing p53 effector functions. In response to oncogene activation, p53 mediates apoptosis through a linear pathway involving Bax transactivation, Bax translocation from the cytosol to membranes, cytochrome *c* release from mitochondria, and caspase-9 activation, followed by the activation of caspases-3, -6, and -7. p53-mediated apoptosis can be blocked at multiple death checkpoints, by inhibiting p53 activity directly, by Bcl-2 family members regulating mitochondrial function, by blocking caspase-9 activation, and by caspase inhibitors. Understanding the mechanisms by which p53 induces apoptosis, and the reasons why cell death is bypassed in transformed cells, is of fundamental importance in cancer research, and has great implications in the design of anticancer therapeutics. **Table 2** highlights important pro- and antiapoptotic genes, and **Figure 2** depicts a schematic representation of apoptotic regulatory pathways.

Table 2 Summary of proapoptotic and antiapoptotic genes

Proapoptotic genes				*Antiapoptotic genes*			
Extrinsic pathways		*Intrinsic pathways*		*Extrinsic pathways*		*Intrinsic pathways*	
Death receptors	*Other factors*	*Bcl-2 family*	*Other factors*	*Death receptors*	*Other factors*	*Bcl-2 family*	*Other factors*
FAS/CD95	TRADD	BAX	Cytochrome *c*	TRAILR3/DcR1	FLIP	BCL-2	c-IAP1
TNFR1	TRAF2	BAK	Smac/Diablo	TRAILR4/DcR2	FAIM	BCL-XL	c-IAP2
TNFR2	DAXX	BCL-XS	AIF	DcR3	c-IAP1	BCL-W	XIAP
Apo3/DR3	FADD	BIK/NBK	Apaf-1		c-IAP2	BAG	NAIP
TRAILR1/DR4	Caspase-8	BIM/BOD	Endo G		XIAP	MCL-1	Survivin
TRAILR2/DR5	Caspase-3	BAD	Caspase-9		NAIP	A1/BFL-1	Livin
DR6	Caspase-6	BID	Caspase-3		Survivin	BOO/DIVA	ILP2
	Caspase-7	BLK	Caspase-6		Livin	NR-13	BRUCE
		BOK/MTD	Caspase-7		ILP2	CED-9	
		EGL-1			BRUCE		
		HRK					
		NOXA					
		PUMA					

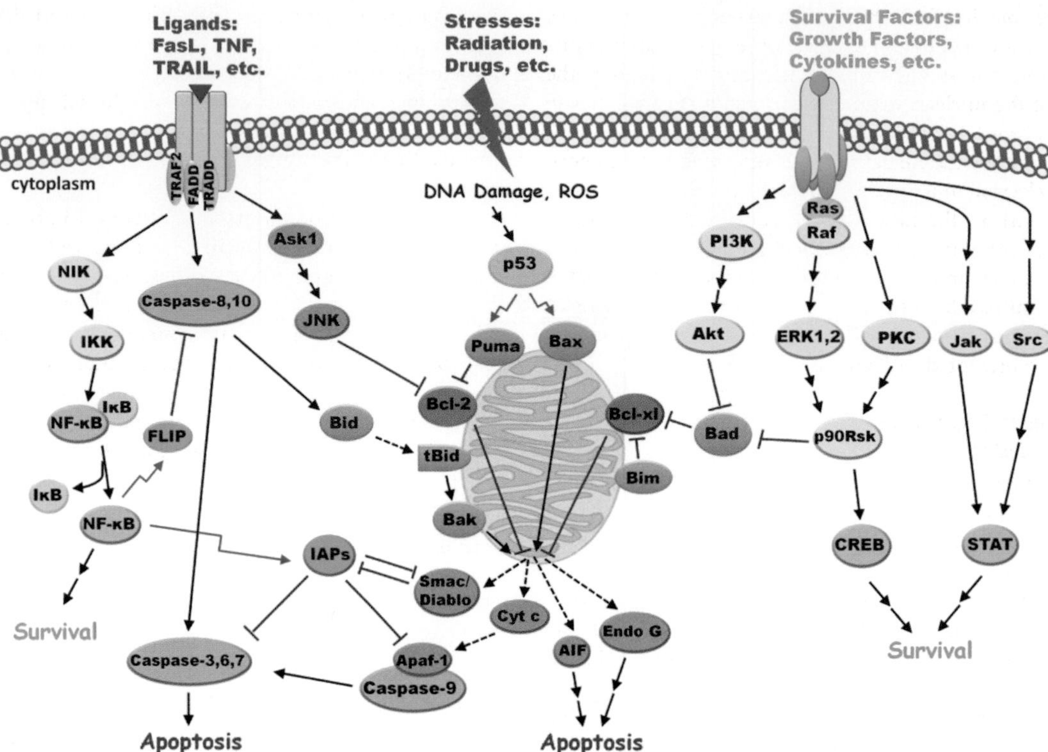

Figure 2 Overview of cellular pathways of apoptosis and survival. Apoptosis is triggered either by the binding of death receptors to their ligands (extrinsic pathways) or by a variety of stresses including radiation and drugs (intrinsic pathways). Apoptosis is inhibited by three types of antiapoptotic proteins (FLIPs, IAPs, and antiapoptotic Bcl-2 family members) and survival signals which are activated by growth factors and cytokines. The functions of proteins in color: transcription factors (blue), caspases (purple), proapoptotic Bcl-2 family members (orange), antiapoptotic Bcl-2 family members (brown), survival-related proteins (olive green), other apoptosis-related protein (rose), and other antiapoptosis-related factors (green). The meanings of symbols are arrow (→), direct activation; consecutive arrows (→ →), multistep activation; zigzag arrow (↯), transcription activation; dashed arrow (···>), translocation; and T-shaped line (⊥), direct inhibition. FLIP, FLICE (Caspase-8) inhibitory protein, and IAP, inhibitor of apoptosis.

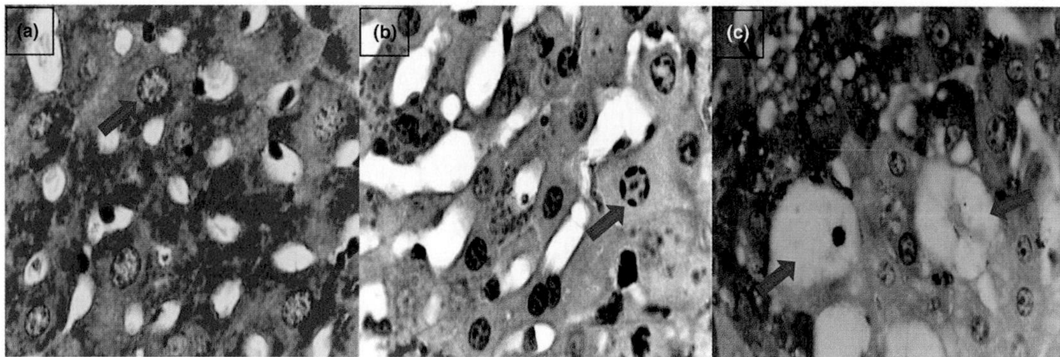

Figure 3 Light photomicrographs (PAS-stained; X1000) of liver sections showing architecture of a normal hepatocyte with a normal nucleus (Panel a: see arrow), apoptotic hepatocyte with an apoptotic nucleus (Panel b: see arrow; in the vicinity of normal, damaged, and glycogen depleted hepatocytes), and necrotic hepatocytes with necrotic changes (see Panel c: a liver cell with a nucleus with disintegrated cytoplasm and another liver cell without a nucleus with disintegrated cytoplasm; arrows indicate both necrotic cells). Liver injury and apoptosis were induced by a single hepatotoxic dose of acetaminophen (500 mg kg^{-1}, intraperitoneal). Source: Ray and Jena, Arch. Toxicol. 73: 594–606, 2000; Ray, Proc. Soc. Free Rad. Res., 2004.

Histological Stages of Apoptosis

Tissues undergoing apoptosis proceed through four steps.

Step I: Cellular Shrinkage

The earliest changes observed include the loss of cell junctions and other specialized plasma membrane structures such as microvilli. In intact organs or tissues, a withdrawal mode from the surrounding sets in. Typically, the cytoplasm begins to shrink following the cleavage of lamins and actin filaments, and in some instances cytoplasm becomes hypertrophied.

Step II: Nuclear or Chromatin Condensation

This is the most noticeable distinguishing feature of apoptosis, which shows stereotypical changes. This stage goes through very complex biochemical and molecular changes. At this stage, chromatin condenses, fragments in an orderly fashion into one or more large (or small) masses, and migrates toward the periphery of the nuclear membrane (in many cases the nuclei of apoptotic cells take on a 'horse-shoe' like appearance). As the process continues, the nucleus breaks into several fragments. Under an electron microscope, these fragments appear very dense and dark in the near total absence or loss of volume regulation of other organelles, such as the mitochondria. The contraction of cytoplasmic volume is apparently associated with loss of intracellular fluid and ions. Photomicrographs of normal (Panel a), apoptotic (Panel b), and necrotic (Panel c) liver cells are presented in **Figure 3**.

Step III: Cellular Fragmentation and Formation of Apoptotic Bodies

Cells committed to apoptosis continue to shrink, packaging themselves into a form that allows for easy engulfment by all types of cells. The cell transiently adopts a deeply convoluted outline and shows extensive surface blebbing. In order to promote their phagocytosis by macrophages, apoptotic cells often elicit biochemical changes on the plasma membrane surface that appeal the macrophage response. One such change is the translocation of phosphatidylserine from the inner leaflet of the cell to the outer surface. Lysophosphatidylcholine generated as a result of caspase-3-mediated activation of the Ca^{2+}-independent phospholipase-A_2 renders cells vulnerable to phagocytosis. Membrane changes can often be observed morphologically through the appearance of membrane blebs or blisters which often appear toward the end of the apoptotic process. Subsequently, the cell breaks up into several membrane bound smooth-surfaced 'apoptotic bodies' that contain a variety of tightly compacted organelles and some nuclear fragments. Under the microscope, appearance of apoptotic bodies is a common feature used by trained pathologists to identify apoptosis in any tissue.

Step IV: Phagocytosis of Apoptotic Cells or Bodies

Apoptotic bodies show a great diversity in size, and shape, and there is no limit to the number of apoptotic bodies formed from one cell. Apoptotic bodies are typically phagocytosed by 'professional phagocytes' (macrophages) or neighboring cells serving as 'semiprofessional' phagocytes (glomerular mesangial cells, Kupffer cells, or liver cells). These phagocytic cells are responsible for removing apoptotic cells from tissues in a clean and tidy fashion that avoids many of the problems associated with necrotic cell death. Although professionally trained engulfing cells are typically members of the reticuloendothelial system (mononuclear phagocytes, such as macrophages, phagocytes etc.), any other normal or abnormal cell capable of phagocytosis may participate in cell clearance process. The endocytosed apoptotic debris is rapidly degraded by a series of enzymes within lysosomes, and the adjacent cells move around or, if necessary, proliferate to replace the gap created by the just deleted apoptotic cell.

Physiological Role of Apoptosis

Cell death by apoptosis has been reported in many organisms, including plants, nematodes, insects, fish, birds, amphibians, and mammals. Apoptosis plays critical role in development. For example, many transitory organs and tissues are removed by apoptosis, including phylogenetic vestiges in higher vertebrates, tails and gills of insects, and the tail fin of tadpoles. Additional biological architectures are shaped by apoptosis and include limbs, the central nervous system, and many internal organs.

The execution of apoptosis is of critical importance in the survival of many organisms, and most cells appear to be capable of undergoing PCD. Apoptosis occurs in most tissues in an organism and on a regular basis. For instance, a cell whose DNA is damaged by ultraviolet radiation from sunlight is either repaired or jettisoned via apoptosis-assisted peeling. Apoptosis is the mechanism by which natural killer cells nonspecifically kill virally infected cells, stimulating the infected cell to undergo PCD. Additionally, without selective destruction of self-recognizing T-cells, animals would lack cellular immunity. These beneficial aspects of apoptosis are responsible for removing an estimated 50–70 billion cells daily from the average human adult. Indeed, the requirement of death to support life is a vital, if not paradoxical, biological theme.

Pathological Role of Apoptosis

Aberrations in normal apoptotic functioning can be detrimental to organisms and have been implicated in a number of diseases. Cancer, for example, is a result of too little apoptosis. Cancer cells typically have mutations in key genes that allow them to ignore normal cellular signals that control growth. The result is uncontrolled proliferation and the formation of tumors.

There are diseases that are the result of too much apoptosis. In neurodegenerative disorders, such as Alzheimer's disease and Parkinson's disease, apoptosis is thought to be responsible for much of the cell death and loss of neurons. Apoptosis also plays a role in many autoimmune diseases. For example, in rheumatoid arthritis, proliferation of synovial cells is thought to result from resistance to apoptotic stimuli.

As apoptosis plays a large role in the development and progression of numerous diseases, exploiting this cell death process has large therapeutic potential. Selectively inducing cancer cells to undergo apoptosis would provide a treatment for cancer. Modulating apoptosis in various parts of the body, such as the joints, muscles, and central nervous system, would be beneficial to the treatment of autoimmune, inflammatory, neurodegenerative disorders, and viral infections.

Toxicology and Apoptosis

The interaction of toxicants and apoptosis is complex and the mechanisms of interaction are likely to differ among different toxicants. The apoptosis-inducing potential of a variety of drugs, chemicals, and carcinogens has been intensively investigated from a mechanistic standpoint. Decades of research have focused on the ability of carcinogens to induce cell transformation; however, although it is not entirely true, many investigators share the notion that carcinogens antagonize (or alter) or mutate the apoptotic pathway and improve the

Table 3 Examples of apoptosis inducers

Drugs/chemicals	*Physical insults*	*Microbes*	*Cytokines*	*Withdrawal from trophic factors*
Acetaminophen, ethanol, chloroform, CCl_4, furosemide, dimethylnitrosamine, doxorubicin, chemotherapeutic agents, glucocorticoids, glutamate, calcium, azide, hydrogen peroxide, propanollol, TCDD, okadaic acid, lead nitrate, vincristin, vinblastin, TPA, PMA, BAP, PAHs, quinones, free radicals (superoxide, hydroxyl)	Neutrons, X-rays, β-rays, γ-rays, ultraviolet-radiation, heat shock	HIV-1, Sindbis Baculo virus, Influenza virus-A, Human Papilloma virus, Reo virus, Epstein–Barr virus, Escherichia spp., Yersinia spp., Salmonella spp., Propionibacterium spp., Fungal toxins (ochratoxin A and fumonisins)	TNF-α, TGF-β, Several interleukins	Glucose, growth factors (interleukin-2, interleukin-3, interleukin-10, interleukin-13, granulocyte-macrophage colony stimulating factor, granulocyte stimulating factor, fibroblast growth factor, transforming growth factor β1, neurotrophic factor), hormones (estrogen, androgen, progesterone, ACTH)

chances of cell survival. On the contrary, many carcinogens are powerful inducers of apoptosis. These issues have been addressed at great length during the recent years. A short list of classic apoptogens is listed in **Table 3**. Treatment of cells with certain pharmacologic agents may not result in either classic apoptosis or classic necrosis. The formation of micronuclei, aberrant mitoses, a mitotic arrest, and other cellular perturbations can result in cell death that may be nonapoptotic/nonnecrotic in nature.

Assays for Apoptosis

Apoptosis proceeds as a result of a tightly controlled signaling cascade that is regulated at numerous points. As such, it is possible to assay the activities of the proteins involved. Since many features of apoptosis and necrosis overlap, it is often crucial to utilize more than one assay to confirm that apoptosis is the cell death mechanism. Typically, assays are chosen that evaluate an early and a late apoptotic event. These experiments evaluate cytomorphological alterations, measure DNA fragmentation, detect caspases, cleaved substrates, regulators, inhibitors, membrane alterations, and employ mitochondrial assays.

Common experimental techniques used in the detection of apoptosis include flow cytometry, fluorescence microscopy, DNA fragmentation assay, agarose gel electrophoresis, bright field and electron microscopy, TUNNEL assay (Tdt-Utp Nick End Labeling), western blot analysis, and DNA microarray.

Summary

Apoptosis is a process of cell death that follows a series of carefully controlled, energy-driven events. Apoptotic cells are recognized by distinct biochemical and morphological features that separate them from necrotic cells. Caspases are thought to be instrumental to induction and execution of apoptosis. A large amount of information is known regarding the key biochemical, molecular, and genetic processes that operate during apoptosis; however, there is much to learn about the regulation and interactions of the many components involved. An understanding of the molecular mechanisms of apoptosis is crucial because this process of PCD plays a vital role in physiology, pathophysiology, organ toxicity, and cancer. This is the only known cell death process that can be turned on or off and/or delayed by maneuvering specific genes. Several clinical trials are in progress to control cancer via regulation of apoptosis.

See also: Cell Cycle.

Further Reading

Amaral, J.D., Xavier, J.M., Steer, C.J., Rodrigues, C.M., 2010. The role of p53 in apoptosis. Discov. Med. 9, 145–152.

Bulku, E., Stohs, S.J., Cicero, L., Brooks, T., Halley, H., Ray, S.D., 2012. Curcumin exposure modulates multiple peo-apoptotic and anti-apoptotic signaling pathways to antagonize acetaminophen-induced toxicity. Curr. Neurovasc. Res. 9, 58–71.

Crawford, E., Wells, J., 2011. Caspase substrates and cellular remodeling. Ann. Rev. Biochem. 80, 1055–1087.

Elmore, S., 2007. Apoptosis: a review of programmed cell death. Toxicol. Pathol. 35, 495–516.

Favaloro, B., Allocati, N., Graziano, V., Dillio, C., De Laurenzi, V., 2012. Role of apoptosis in disease. Aging (Albany NY) 4 (5), 330–349.

Galluzzi, L., Aaronson, S.A., Abrams, J., 2009. Guidelines for the use and interpretation of assays for monitoring cell death in higher eukaryotes. Cell Death Differ. 16, 1093–1107.

Green, D.R., 2011. Means to an End. Cold Spring Harbor Laboratory Press, New York.

Kepp, O., Galluzzi, L., Lipinski, M., Yuan, J., Kroemer, G., 2011. Cell death assays for drug discovery. Nat. Rev. Drug Discov. 10, 221–237.

Orrenius, S., Nicotera, P., Zhivotovsky, B., 2012. Cell death mechanisms and their implications in toxicology. Toxicol. Sci. 119 (1), 3–19.

Kerr, J.F., Wyllie, A.H., Currie, A.R., 1972. Br. J. Cancer 26 (4), 239–257.

Ray, S.D., Corcoran, G.B., 2009. Apoptosis and cell death. In: Ballantyne, B. (Ed.), General and Applied Toxicology, third ed. John Wiley, UK.

Ray, S.D., Mumaw, V.R., Raje, R.R., Fariss, M.W., 1996. Protection of acetaminophen-induced hepatocellular apoptosis and necrosis by cholesteryl hemisuccinate pretreatment. J. Pharmacol. Exp. Ther 279 (3), 1470–1483.

Vandenabeele, P., Galluzzi, L., Vanden Berghe, T., Kroemer, G., 2010. Molecular mechanisms of necroptosis: an ordered cellular explosion. Nat. Rev. Mol. Cell Biol. 11, 700–714.

Zitvogel, L., Kepp, O., Kroemer, G., 2010. Decoding cell death signals in inflammation and immunity. Cell 140, 798–804.

Relevant Websites

http://www.cellsalive.com/ – CELLS alive.

http://bioinf.gen.tcd.ie/cgi-bin/casbah/casbah.pl – The CASBAH.

http://www.celldeath-apoptosis.org/ – The International Cell Death Society.

Aquatic Ecotoxicology *see* Aquatic Ecotoxicology

Aquatic Toxicity Testing *see* Toxicity Testing, Aquatic

Aramite

S Goel, Supernus Pharmaceuticals, Rockville, MD, USA
D Agarwal, S. B. Physiotherapy and Rehabilitation Center, Mawana, India

This article is a revision of the previous edition article by Swarupa G. Kulkarni, Harihara M. Mehendale, volume 1, pp 167–168, © 2005, Elsevier Inc.

- Name: Aramite
- Chemical Abstracts Service Registry Number: 140-57-8
- Synonyms: Aracide; (RS)-2-(4-tert-butylphenoxy)-1-methylethyl 2-chloroethyl sulfite; 2-Chloroethyl 2-[4-(1,1-dimethylethyl)phenoxy]-1-methylethyl sulfite; 2-(*p*-Butyl phenoxy)-1-methylethyl-2-chloroethylsulfite; Sulfurous acid, 2-(*p*-*t*-butylphenoxy)-1-methylethyl-2-chloroethyl ester; Orthomite
- Molecular Formula: $C_{15}H_{23}ClO_4S$
- Chemical Structure:

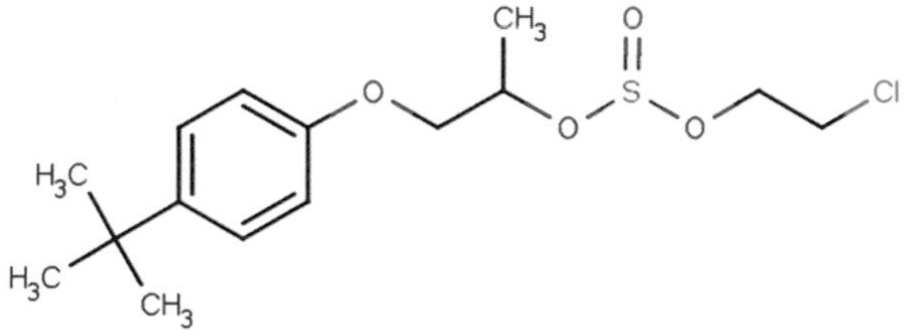

Background

Aramite is a synthetic chlorinated hydrocarbon with molecular weight of 334.87 and density of 1.143 at 20 °C. It is a clear, light-colored oil with melting point of 37.3 °C and boiling point of 175 °C at 0.1 mm Hg. The technical grade aramite is a dark amber liquid. Aramite is soluble at 0.000 1% (practically insoluble) in water but is miscible in many organic solvents. It was sold as mixture in organic solvents at different strengths for further dilution and use. Aramite was used as a pesticide (acaricide) to control mites in plants and animals. Aramite was initially introduced to market around 1950. It was mostly used between 1950 and 1954 in greenhouses in the United States. Its manufacture and use were voluntarily discontinued due to its carcinogenic potential according to a US Environmental Protection Agency (EPA) notice dated 12 April 1977. However, there are reports of bans of aramite use in a few European countries, in 1987 (Lithuania), 1996 (Poland), and 1999 (Estonia). There is no information on the production, import, registration, marketing, stockpiling, and use of aramite in Russia. Occupational exposure through dermal contact and inhalation was possible during its use.

Uses

Aramite was formerly used in control of mites (miticide) in citrus fruits, vegetables, and animals. Active mite stage was most sensitive to aramite toxicity. The death in mites was due to paralysis and disorganized movements of appendages, leading to detachment from the plant. Insects and mites other than *Tetracychidae* are not as sensitive to aramite. Mites exposed in the field to up to 21 applications were not found to develop resistance in mites, unlike other organochlorines where insects develop resistance rapidly. Aramite is rendered inactive when mixed with lime and other alkaline materials. Aramite was used in combination of other pesticides to control a wide range of mite species.

Environmental Fate and Behavior

Aramite can be released directly into the environment through its use as an acaricide (miticide); however, this use has been discontinued. If released to soil, aramite is expected to have no mobility. Volatilization from moist soil surfaces is not expected to be an important fate process based on an estimated Henry's Law constant of 1.9×10^{-7} atm m^3 mol^{-1}. Biodegradation data for aramite are not available, and if released into water, aramite is expected to adsorb to suspended solids and sediments based upon the estimated K_{oc} of $2.0 \times 10^{+4}$. Volatilization from water surfaces is not expected to be an important fate process based on this compound's estimated Henry's Law constant. Aramite's potential for bioconcentration in aquatic organisms is very high. Functional groups of aramite are susceptible to hydrolysis; however, insufficient data are available to predict the relative importance or occurrence of chemical or biological degradation processes in water or soil. Aramite is hydrolyzed by alkalies and may contribute to degradation in soil or water. If released into air, aramite is expected to be physically removed by wet and dry deposition processes.

Exposure and Exposure Monitoring

Although exposure through oral consumption of contaminated vegetables and fruits is possible, it should no longer be occurring since the use of aramite has been discontinued voluntarily on the basis of carcinogenicity according to the US EPA. Occupational exposure through dermal contact and inhalation of aerosols and dusts is possible during application.

Toxicokinetics

The information on the extent and rate of absorption of aramite is not available. However, indirect evidence from toxicity studies suggests that aramite is absorbed in the stomach in rodents and dogs. Limited pharmacokinetic from a single study in rat indicates that aramite is metabolized to at least two compounds and eliminated in urine. One of them was identified as 1-(*p*-tert-butylphenoxy) 2-propanol. The above suggests that one of the sulfite ester bonds in aramite is hydrolyzed during metabolism. No further information on distribution and excretion of aramite is available.

Mechanism of Toxicity

Aramite causes mutation in glutathione-*S*-transferases (GST) gene *GSTM1* that encodes enzyme involved in its detoxification. The mutation can impact the activity of enzyme and lead to toxicity. Aramite causes increase in enzymes in rat plasma indicative of liver and intestinal damages, including glutamic oxaloacetic transaminase (GOT), glutamic pyruvic transaminase (GPT), acid phosphatase (ACP), and alkaline phosphatase (ALP) activities.

Acute and Short-Term Toxicity

Animal

A large oral dose causes central nervous system depression of long duration in laboratory mammals. The principal autopsy finding was hemorrhagic syndrome particularly involving the lungs. Undiluted aramite and its concentrated solution are irritating to the skin and conjunctiva of experimental animals. Aramite has been found to give electroretinographic indications of intoxication of retinal photoreceptors when injected into mice and when applied to the eyeball. The oral LD_{50} is 3.9 g kg^{-1} in rats and guinea pigs, and 2 g kg^{-1} for mouse.

Human

Acute exposure to aramite in an undiluted form may cause skin and eye irritations.

Chronic Toxicity

Animal

Aramite causes increase in enzymes in rat plasma indicative of liver and intestinal damages, including GOT, GPT, ACP, and ALP activities. It causes mutation in GST gene *GSTM1* that encodes enzyme involved in its detoxification. Carcinogenic potential in rats was evaluated at doses 100, 200, 400, 500, 1580, and 5000 ppm (mg kg^{-1} diet) in diet for 2 years in two or more studies. At 5000 ppm, all rats died by 96 weeks of treatment. In mice, carcinogenicity was evaluated at 100, 200, and 400 ppm in diet. Increased incidence of liver tumors and/or neoplastic nodules in three strains of male and female rats and in one strain of a male mouse and extrahepatic biliary system tumors (e.g., bile duct adenomas) were noted in dogs following chronic oral exposure. In mice, hepatomas were reported. Aramite was not found to be carcinogenic upon dermal application in mice at up to 10 mg aramite in acetone. The mean survival time of low dose versus control mice was 452 versus 386 days.

Carcinogenicity of aramite was also evaluated in a 3.5 year study in dogs. The animals in this study were dosed aramite in diet at 0, 500, or 828–1420 ppm. Neoplastic nodules in liver, cancer of biliary system, and adenosarcomas of gall bladder and extrahepatic ducts were reported.

Human

This compound is classified as a probable human carcinogen (classification B2) based on increased tumors in animals and insufficient human data. No data are available on the number of workers who were actually or potentially exposed to aramite during its manufacture and formulation. The lowest published lethal dose/concentration in humans is 429 mg kg^{-1}.

Reproductive Toxicity

Chronic exposure to aramite at 1580–5000 ppm in diet in rats decreased F_0 pups body weights at weaning. The survival during lactation of F_0 and F_1 pups was decreased in rats fed with 5000 ppm and in F_2 rats fed with 500, 1580, and 5000 ppm. The F_0 rats fed with aramite at 5000 ppm failed to develop pregnancies, without affecting the indices of fertility and reproduction in all three F_0, F_1, and F_2 generations.

Genotoxicity and Carcinogenicity

Aramite was negative in a dominant lethal effect assay for genotoxicity following a single intraperitoneal dose of 200–500 mg kg^{-1} in mice. Aramite is classified as a Group B2 carcinogen (probable human carcinogen) by US EPA based on data from animal bioassays. This classification is based on the increased incidence of liver tumors and/or neoplastic nodules in strains of rats and mice, and tumors of extrahepatic biliary system in dogs. No carcinogenic data for aramite are available for humans.

Clinical Management

Common practices used in the event of poisoning include, for example, skin decontamination for dermal exposure with soap and water, irrigation of eyes with copious amount of saline in ocular exposure, and moving the subject to fresh air in the event of exposure via inhalation. In the event of oral poisoning, if detected soon after ingestion, attempts could be made to induce vomiting to expel the stomach content and the aramite, followed by medical attention. If significant time has passed, then immediate medical attention should be sought. Chemical analysis of an appropriate sample will help confirm the aramite poisoning. Gas chromatography and mass spectrophotometry methods are used for analysis.

Exposure Standards and Guidelines

Aramite was voluntarily canceled on the basis of carcinogenicity in a notice dated 12 April 1977, thereby revoking any tolerance established for aramite or its residues. Reference dose for aramite for chronic oral exposure is 0.05 mg kg^{-1} day^{-1} and a reportable quantity for chronic (noncancer) toxicity was set at 1000 ppm.

Ecotoxicology

Aramite inhibits the germination and growth of petunia pollen tubes of terrestrial flora at 1000 ppm.

Aramite concentrations of 0.9 ppm in mites can cause acute toxicity in birds. However, young birds such as bobwhites, *Colinus virginianus*, Japanese quails, *Coturnix c. japonica*, and ring-necked pheasant can consume dietary levels of 5000 ppm for 5 days without mortality.

The 96 h LC_{50} of aramite generally ranged from 43 to 387 μg l^{-1} in fish species such as *Daphnia magna*, *Gammarus fasciatus*, rainbow trout, and bluegill. Shorter 26 h LD_{50} for water flea is 0.069 mg l^{-1}. The 48 h EC_{50} for *D. magna*, *Caldoceran*, and *Serrasalmus serrulatus* is 0.16–0.18 mg l^{-1}. The 96 h LC_{50} for scud, *Gammarus lacustris*, is 0.06 mg l^{-1}.

Miscellaneous

Aramite is a clear, light-colored liquid with a melting point of −31.7 °C and a boiling point of 175 °C at 0.1 mm Hg. It is noncorrosive and has a specific gravity of 1.145 at 20 °C. It is practically insoluble in water and is miscible with many organic solvents. When heated to decomposition, it emits highly toxic fumes of chlorides and oxides of sulfur.

See also: Pesticides.

Further Reading

Al-Badraan, A.I., Al-Sarry, M.H., Al-Karishy, K.J., 2011. Histopathological changes and metabolic gene polymorphism caused by aramite exposure in experimental rats. Afr. J. Biotechnol. 10, 11682–11695.

Aramite-revocation of tolerance; establishment of zero tolerance. Food and Drug Administration. Fed. Regist., 1958, 225.

Carricaburu, P., Lacroix, R., Claude, J.R., Lacroix, J., 1979. Electroretinographic study during acute aramite intoxication of the white mouse. Toxicol. Eur. Res. 2 (4), 195–198.

Claude, J.R., Huyen, V.N., Warnet, J.M., Blanc, F., 1975. [Primary liver carcinogenesis induced by the pesticide 2-(4-tert-butylphenoxy0-1-methylethyl 2-chloroethyl sulphite (Aramite)]. C. R. Acad. Sci. Hebd. Seances Acad. Sci. D 281 (9), 599–604.

Full, C., 2011. Report on "The pesticides selected for immediate priority action: a compilation and evaluation of the information given by the contracting parties with the focus on use and legislation". Helsinki Commission, Baltic Marine Environment Protection Commission.

Health and Environmental Effects Document for Aramite, 1989. Office of Solid Waste and Emergency Response, US Environment Protection Agency. ECAO-CIN-G083, 1989.

Johnson, W.W., 1980. Handbook of Acute Toxicity of Chemicals to Fish and Aquatic Vertebrates, p. 19.

Smith, F.F., 1960. Resistance of green house spider mites to acaricides. Misc. Publ. Entomol. Soc. Am. 2, 5–11.

Relevant Websites

http://www.drugfuture.com/toxic/q129-q58.html – Environmental Protection Agency.

http://toxnet.nlm.nih.gov/cgi-bin/sis/htmlgen?HSDB – National Institutes of Health-National Library of Medicine-Hazardous Substances Data Bank-Aramite.

http://nj.gov/health/eoh/rtkweb/documents/fs/0150.pdf – New Jersey Department of Health.

http://www.pesticideinfo.org/Detail_Chemical.jsp?Rec_Id=PC33708#Toxicity – Pesticide Action Network, USA.

http://toxnet.nlm.nih.gov/ – Toxnet (Toxicology Data Network): Search for Aramite.

http://www.epa.gov/iris/subst/0473.htm – US Environmental Protection Agency.

Aristolochic Acids

SA Jordan and S Perwaiz, Marketed Health Products Directorate, Health Canada, Ottawa, ON, Canada

Chemical Profile

- Name: Aristolochic Acids
- Unless otherwise specified, the term aristolochic acids refer to a mixture of aristolochic acid I and its demethoxylated derivative, aristolochic acid II.
- Aristolochic Acid I
- Chemical Abstract Service Registry Number: 313-67-7
- Chemical Abstract Service Name: 8-Methoxy-6-nitrophenanthro[3,4-d]-1,3-dioxole-5-carboxylic acid
- Synonyms: 3,4-Methylenedioxy-8-methoxy-10-nitro-1-phenanthrenecarboxylic acid; 8-Methoxy-3,4-methylenedioxy-10-nitrophenanthrene-1-carboxylic acid; Aristinic acid; Aristolochic acid A; Aristolochine
- Molecular Formula: $C_{17}H_{11}NO_7$
- Structure:

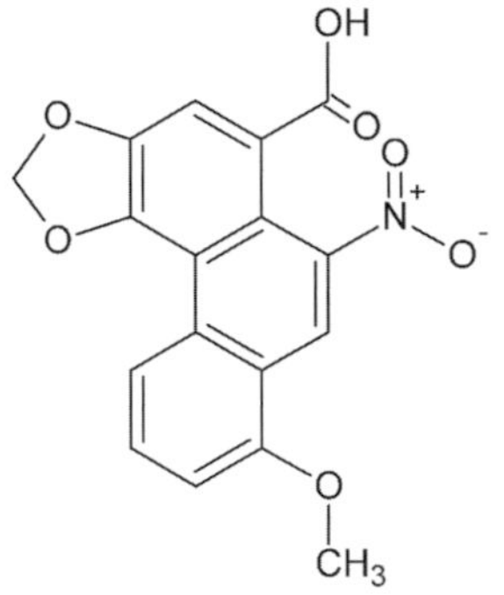

- Aristolochic Acid II
- Chemical Abstract Service Registry Number: 475-80-9
- Chemical Abstract Service Name: 6-Nitrophenanthro[3,4-d]-1,3-dioxole-5-carboxylic acid
- Synonyms: Aristolochic acid B; 3,4-Methylenedioxy-10-nitrophenanthrene-1-carboxylic acid
- Molecular Formula: $C_{16}H_9NO_6$
- Structure:

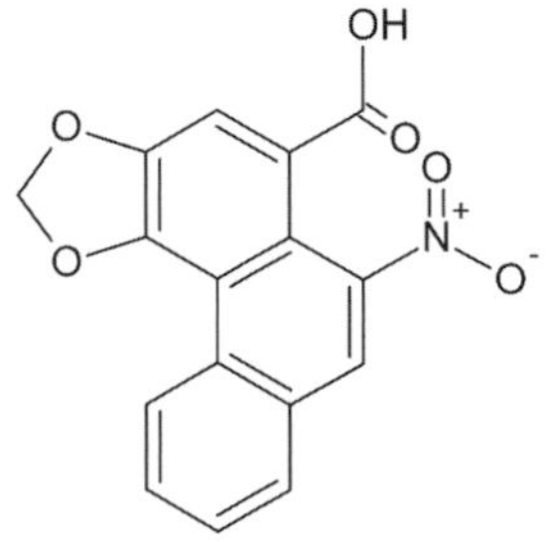

Background

Aristolochic acids (AAs) are a group of nitrophenanthrene carboxylic acids which occur in a variety of plants of the genus *Aristolochia* and *Asarum*. Although a variety of AAs exist (including AA I, Ia, II, III, IIIa, IV, IVa), the main representative members of this group of phytochemicals are AA I and AA II, as they have been the compounds which have been studied the most, and are found in the highest concentrations in the plants where AAs occur.

The toxic nature of these compounds was raised to international attention after cases of toxicity in humans occurred in Belgium in the early 1990s. Severe renal damage was noted in over 100 persons in that country, who used a Chinese medicine for weight loss. The product in question was meant to contain the plant *Stephania tetrandra* (family Menispermaceae), but instead contained *Aristolochia fang ji* (family Aristolochiaceae).

Human cases of renal toxicity similar to those in Belgium, and associated with the use of herbal medicines containing AAs, have been noted elsewhere in Europe, and also in Asia and North America. The toxicity caused by the AAs was originally termed Chinese herb nephropathy (CHN). As a result of the severe toxicity caused by AAs, many countries have either banned the use of plants containing these chemicals or severely restricted their use (e.g., only allowed in extremely dilute homeopathic products). The term CHN has now been replaced with the more general term 'aristolochic acid nephropathy' (AAN).

Interest in AAs has also arisen due to the fact that they have been implicated in Balkan endemic nephropathy (BEN), speculated to be due to the contamination of flour made from wheat contaminated with the seeds of *Aristolochia clematis*.

Uses

AAs have no industrial use. They are constituents of certain plants that have been used medicinally since ancient times. The use of plants of *Aristolochia* and *Asarum* species in traditional medicine is varied and ranges from use in childbirth, fever, snakebites and scorpion stings, infection, inflammation, and diarrhea. AAs themselves have also been reported to have antiviral and antibacterial effects, and also antitumor effects. Human trials were conducted in the 1960s for their potential antitumor effects, but these studies were halted when renal toxicity was observed. Other modern uses of the plant extracts were discontinued once it became clear that the AAs were mutagenic and carcinogenic. Purified AAs are also used for research or reference standard purposes.

Environmental Fate and Behavior

AAs are not volatile and have melting points ranging from 281 to 286 °C. They are slightly soluble in water and soluble in acetic acid, acetone, aniline, alkalis, chloroform, diethyl ether, and ethanol, but insoluble in benzene and carbon disulfide.

 http://dx.doi.org/10.1016/B978-0-12-386454-3.01164-7

AAs are present in many plant species growing in the natural environment throughout the world. The compounds are bound up in the plant tissue, so are not considered to be problematic from the environmental point of view.

On the other hand, commercially available free AAs are considered environmentally stable in nature and, therefore, they may persist in the environment (water/soil) if inadvertently released in sewers or waterways. However, the magnitude of use of free AAs is very limited, and would not be of environmental concern.

Exposure and Exposure Monitoring

Plants containing AAs are mainly used as herbal medicines. AAs may also be found as a contaminant in other herbal products. Exposure to AAs could occur either by the intentional use of AA-containing plants or by the use of medicines in which some ingredients have been substituted by plants containing AAs, or where such plants have been mistakenly added.

The possibility for exposure to AAs in food also exists. It has been suggested that contamination of wheat flour by *Aristolochia* species growing as weeds adjacent to wheat fields might be responsible for BEN. Indeed, seeds of *A. clematitis* have been found commingled with wheat grain during harvest in regions where BEN is endemic. Because *Aristolochia* species are widely distributed and wheat can be traded internationally, there is the theoretical potential for exposure outside of the region of harvest; however, no literature exists on this subject. Furthermore, there is no evidence published in the scientific literature to show that bioaccumulation or biomagnification of AAs within a food chain is of any significance.

Although occupational exposure to AAs has not been documented in the published scientific literature, herbalists or gardeners may be potentially exposed to AAs while using AA-containing plants. Oral exposure from these sources would be negligible; however, dermatitis has been observed from direct contact with the leaves of some AA-containing plants.

Regulatory agencies have not established allowable levels of AAs in food or therapeutic products as these constituents are widely prohibited for human use by international regulators. For instance, the European Agency for the Evaluation of Medicinal Products warned European Union Member States to "take steps to ensure that the public is protected from exposure to AAs arising from the deliberate use of *Aristolochia* species or as a result of confusion with other botanical ingredients." Exposure has been reduced in many (but not all) countries due to strict regulation of AA-containing herbs used in traditional medicine. Such products continue to be used, however, and are available for purchase over the Internet.

Toxicokinetics

No data were found on the absorption of AAs following dermal or inhalation exposure. This is not surprising, since the main route of exposure in humans is by the oral route (i.e., the consumption of herbal medicines). After oral administration, AAs appear to be widely distributed, as evidenced by the finding of AA–DNA adducts in the kidney, ureter, bladder, liver, stomach, small intestine, brain, and lung of patients exposed to these substances. Similarly, in rodent models, DNA adducts have been found in the kidney, bladder, liver, brain, and lung. Adducts were also noted in the forestomach of rodents administered AAs.

Phase I metabolism produces a number of metabolites of AAs in experimental animals. Among the animals studied (rats, mice, guinea pigs, rabbits, and dogs), the dog (beagle) is the closest to the human, in terms of phase I metabolism. Although definitive studies have not been conducted in humans, so far only aristolactam I and II have been detected. The lactams are produced by nitroreduction from AA I and II, respectively, and their formation is catalyzed by both cytosolic and microsomal enzymes. In experimental animals, *O*-demethylation and denitration also occur. Despite interspecies differences in phase I metabolites, all species produce aristolactams I and II, and these are the compounds responsible for the carcinogenicity of the AAs. Phase I metabolites of AAI in rats are excreted within approximately 24 h. Metabolites of AAII remain present in urine after 72 h. The aristolactams are excreted in both urine and feces. Phase II metabolites in animals are primarily the glucuronides of AAIa and aristolactam I.

Mechanism of Toxicity

The aristolactam metabolites of AAI and AAII are further metabolized to cyclic *N*-acylnitrenium ions, which represent the ultimate carcinogens (see Carcinogenicity, below). These ultimate carcinogens are able to bind to DNA bases (specifically purine nucleotides). The principle DNA adduct in humans is 7-(deoxyadenosin-N^6-yl)aristolactam I (dA–AAI), but adducts associated with deoxyguanosine also occur. Although AA–DNA adducts can be found in various organs, the main toxicity in exposed individuals is noted in the urinary tract in both experimental animals and humans. These adducts are associated with the urothelial carcinogenicity of the AAs, but there is also speculation that they are responsible for the renal fibrosis that is seen in AAN.

Postulated mechanisms for the noncarcinogenic renal toxicity include reduced capacity to repair renal tubular cell damage and loss of blood vessels around the renal tubules (resulting in hypoxia and tubular epithelial damage). Some evidence also points to a transformation of renal tubular epithelial cells to myofibroblasts. Evidence suggests that such effects may be similar in both experimental animals and humans exposed to AAs. AAs have been linked to increased intercellular calcium with possible initiation of apoptosis. Mitochondrial perturbation may also occur in renal tubular epithelial cells.

Further information on the genotoxicity and carcinogenicity of the AAs is provided below.

Acute and Short-Term Toxicity

Direct contact with the leaves of *Asarum canadense* (Canadian snakeroot or wild ginger) has been reported to cause dermatitis in humans. It is unclear whether this effect is due to the presence of AAs or other constituents.

Oral LD_{50} values for AAs in rats were found to be 203 and 184 mg kg^{-1} bw in males and females, respectively. By the intravenous route, the corresponding values were 83 and 74 mg kg^{-1} bw in males and females, respectively. Studies in mice have shown lower LD_{50} values, suggesting some variation in acute toxicity between rodent species.

Short-term toxicity in animals is noted in a variety of organs. Oral administration of AAs has been shown to produce hyperkeratosis and hyperplasia of the epithelium in the forestomach of rodents. Gastric mucosal fibrosis was noted in rabbits. Changes in the forestomach of rats can be seen within 24 h of exposure, leading to papillomas in the epithelium after 14 days of exposure.

Hepatotoxicity is not a major effect produced by AAs. In oral exposure, AAs are not themselves necrogenic; however, hepatocellular necrosis occurs after intravenous administration to experimental animals. AAs are also able to act as initiating agents in rat liver.

The main toxicity seen in animals and humans is renal toxicity. The carcinogenic aspect of this organ-specific toxicity is discussed below. In animals, a single or short-term administration of a mixture of AAI and AAII has been shown to cause renal tubular necrosis, independent of the route of administration. Oral, short-term, repeated exposure produces a dose-dependent renal toxicity in animals, with doses ranging from 2.5 mg kg^{-1} bw (9 days) to 50 mg kg^{-1} bw (3 days). Most effects are seen in the range of 20–30 mg kg^{-1} bw. Renal fibrosis has also been observed in some (but not all) studies. Some animal studies have shown long-term reversibility of renal toxicity upon cessation of treatment. There is some evidence in animals that the renal toxicity is due to AAI, but not AAII.

In humans, acute renal failure has resulted from excessive use of some AA-containing herbal remedies, and renal toxicity was noted after short-term administration in early clinical trials of purified AAs as antitumor agents. It is interesting to note that oral doses of AAs causing renal effects in humans (about 1 mg kg^{-1} bw) are lower than that which cause similar effects in animals.

Chronic Toxicity

Long-term toxicity studies have been conducted in a variety of animal species, using mixtures of AAI and AAII, AAI only, or extracts of AA-containing plants. The main findings have been tumor induction in a variety of organs. Tumors have been consistently induced by AA exposure in the forestomach, renal cortex, renal pelvis, and urinary bladder of rats. In the one-rat study which used a simulated weight-loss regimen (mimicking the human exposure to AAs from the Belgian slimming product noted above), only forestomach tumors were observed. The comparison between studies is made difficult due to the variety of test materials and routes of administration, and the sample sizes. A single study in rodents (intraperitoneal route, up to 21 months of exposure) demonstrated renal and gastric fibrosis.

In humans, long-term intake of AAs (e.g., from herbal remedies) results in a characteristic syndrome of toxicity (AAN) characterized by a rapid progressing nephropathy involving extensive cortical interstitial fibrosis with marked loss of renal tubules. Glomerular sclerosis is also a part of the pathological picture of the condition. The severity of the condition has resulted in patients undergoing hemodialysis and renal transplantation. While the disease can progresses rapidly, end-stage renal failure has been shown to occur months to years after cessation of exposure to AA-containing herbal remedies.

See below for a discussion on the renal carcinogenesis associated with the AAs.

Immunotoxicity

The amount of research into the effects of AAs on the immune system is limited. AA (specific type unknown) has been described as being able to stimulate immune reactions by acting as a phagocytosis stimulating agent. Treatment of rats with AA has been shown to significantly upregulate gene expression in the kidney, related to immune response. Such effects did not occur in the liver, which may contribute to the organ-specific nature of the toxicity of the AAs. No research has been conducted to systematically study specific immune effects related to AA exposure in animals.

Reproductive Toxicity

Only a limited amount of information exists on the potential reproductive effects of AAs. Some studies in rats (acute exposure of a single high dose (200 mg kg^{-1} bw) of a mixture of AAI and AAII) have shown a severe reduction in spermatogenesis, regressive changes in the germinal epithelium, and degeneration products in epididymal tubules. Dose-related testicular degeneration has also been noted after 4 weeks of exposure to 5 or 25 mg kg^{-1} bw AA in rats.

Genotoxicity

Both AAI and AAII are direct acting mutagens in *Salmonella* tester strains TA100 and TA1537, but weakly mutagenic in strains lacking nitroreductase activity. This observation matches with the fact that the major metabolic route for the production of aristolactams is nitroreduction. Only the nitro group of the AAs is important for their mutagenicity in *Salmonella*.

The AAs are genotoxic mutagens. The aristolactam metabolites of the AAs are metabolized to a cyclic *N*-acylnitrenium ion that is able to form adducts with the purine nucleotides of DNA. The major, and most stable of these adduct is dA–AAI. AA–DNA adducts are found in many tissues of both animals and humans exposed to AAs. The adduct dA–AAI is extremely persistent, being present in human tissue at least 10 years after exposure to AAs.

In rodents, the major DNA mutation is an A:T to T:A transversion in one codon in the *H-ras* gene, a mutation that is seen in all forestomach tumors in that species. In humans, a similar transversion occurs in the *TP53* tumor suppressor gene in urothelial tissue.

Carcinogenicity

There is clear and unequivocal evidence that AAs are carcinogenic to animals and humans. The International Agency for

Research on Cancer has classified plant species of the genus *Aristolochia* as being carcinogenic to humans (Group 1), and naturally occurring mixtures of AAs to be probably carcinogenic to humans (Group 2A). Urothelial tumors of the renal pelvis, ureters, and urinary bladder are the most prominent tumor type in persons exposed the AAs. Based on the Belgian cohort of AA-exposed individuals, about 50% of those persons affected by AAN developed urothelial tumors in the upper urinary tract, within 6 years of exposure. The carcinogenicity appears to be dose related; patients consuming 200 g of AA-containing herbs had an increased risk of developing cancer. Even so, the risk of cancer was increased in patients who were exposed to AAs, but who lacked the characteristics of AAN. Upper urinary tract cancers appear to be increasing in certain regions of the world such as Taiwan, over the past two decades. This increase has been suspected to be due to an increase in the use of *Aristolochia* species to replace herbs in the traditional Chinese medicine plant groups of Fang chi and Mu tong. These substitutions were banned in China in 2003, and many countries have banned the use of *Aristolochia* species in herbal medicines except, in some cases, in highly dilute homeopathic medicines, where no starting material would remain.

Clinical Management

The cessation of exposure to AA-containing products is unlikely to result in a reversal of the toxic effects, as renal toxicity and cancer have occurred in individuals who stopped using AA-containing products months to years before a diagnosis. Severe toxicity may result in hemodialysis or even renal transplantation. As some patients developed urothelial cancer in the absence of classic AAN symptoms, some authors have recommend the removal of the kidneys and ureters of all patients with AAN, even in the absence of urothelial tumors.

Ecotoxicology

Information is lacking on the ecotoxicology of the AAs. As these compounds occur naturally in the environment, they are not considered an environmental concern.

Exposure Standards and Guidelines

Exposure controls for AA have been set by a variety of authorities. These authorities have set time-weighted average values of between 5 and 15 mg m^{-3} for AAI as inert or nuisance dust (total dust or respirable fractions).

As noted above, international regulatory authorities have set limits to the types of allowable products that can contain AAs or have banned them altogether.

See also: Carcinogenesis; Dietary Supplements; Kidney; Natural Products; Plants, Poisonous (Humans).

Further Reading

Arlt, V.M., Stiborova, M., Schmeiser, H.H., 2002. Aristolochic acid as a probable human cancer hazard in herbal remedies: a review. Mutagenesis 17, 265–277.

Chen, M., Su, M., Zhao, L., Jiang, J., Liu, P., et al., 2006. Metabonomic study of aristolochic acid-induced nephrotoxicity in rats. J. Proteome Res. 5, 995–1002.

Chen, C.H., Dickman, K.G., Moriya, M., Zavadil, J., Sidorenko, V.S., et al., 2012. Aristolochic acid-associated urothelial cancer in Taiwan. Proc. Natl. Acad. Sci. USA 21, 8241–8246. Published ahead of print, 9 April, doi10.1073/pnas.1119920109.

Cosyns, J.P., 2003. Aristolochic acid and 'Chinese herbs nephropathy': a review of the evidence to date. Drug Saf. 26, 33–48.

Cosyns, J.P., Jadoul, M., Squifflet, J.P., De Plaen, J.F., Ferluga, D., et al., 1994. Chinese herbs nephropathy: a clue to Balkan endemic nephropathy? Kidney Int. 45, 1680–1688.

Cosyns, J.P., Dehoux, J.P., Guiot, J., Goebbels, R.M., Robert, A., et al., 2001. Chronic aristolochic acid toxicity in rabbits: a model of Chinese herbs nephropathy? Kidney Int. 59, 2164–2173.

Debelle, F.D., Vanherweghem, J., Nortier, J., 2008. Aristolochic acid nephropathy: a worldwide problem. Kidney Int. 74, 158–169.

De Broe, M.E., 2012. Chinese herbs nephropathy and Balkan endemic nephropathy: toward a single entity, aristolochic acid nephropathy. Kidney Int. 81, 513–515.

Mengs, U., 1987. Acute toxicity of aristolochic acid in rodents. Arch. Toxicol. 59, 328–331.

National Toxicology Program, 2008. Report on Carcinogens Background Document for Aristolochic Acids. National Toxicology Program, Research Triangle Park, NC.

Schmeiser, H.H., Stiborova, M., Arlt, V.M., 2009. Chemical and molecular basis of the carcinogenicity of Aristolochia plants. Curr. Opin. Drug. Discov. Devel. 12, 141–148.

Relevent Websites

http://monographs.iarc.fr/ENG/Monographs/vol100A/mono100A.pdf – International Agency for Research on Cancer (IARC) monograph on plants containing aristolochic acid.

http://ntp.niehs.nih.gov/ntp/roc/twelfth/profiles/AristolochicAcids.pdf – National Toxicology Program Report on Carcinogens, 12th Edition.

http://www.fda.gov/food/recallsoutbreaksemergencies/safetyalertsadvisories/ucm095290.htm – US Food and Drug Administration:Aristolochic Acid: Letter to Industry.

Arsenical Vomiting Agents

R Jabbour and H Salem, Edgewood Chemical Biological Center, MD, USA
B Ballantyne[†]
SA Katz, Rutgers University, Camden, NJ, USA

This article is a revision of the previous edition article by Harry Salem, Bryan Ballantyne, and Sidney A. Katz, volume 1, pp 171–172, © 2005, Elsevier Inc.

- Name: Adamsite (DM)
- Chemical Abstracts Service Registry Number: 578-94-9
- Synonyms: Diphenylaminearsine; Diphenyl-amino-chlorarsine; 10-Chloro-5,10-dihydrophenarsazine; White Cross Gas; Phenarsazine chloride (see **Table 5**)
- Molecular Formula: $C_{12}H_9AsClN$
- Chemical Structure:

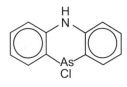

Background (Significance/History)

Adamsite (DM) was first synthesized in 1915 by a German chemist Heinrich Wieland, and again in 1918 by a US chemist Robert Adams who named it adamsite. DM is a yellow-green, odorless crystalline solid at room temperature with low volatility. It is insoluble in water and relatively insoluble in organic solvents.

Uses

DM has been used as a vomiting agent and as a riot-control agent. It is considered insufficiently toxic for use in war, but too potent for control of civilian disturbances. Thus, it was banned in 1930 for use against civilians. Adverse health effects due to exposure are generally self-limiting, resolving within 30 min, and do not require specific therapy. Prolonged exposure or exposure to high concentrations may result in more severe adverse health effects, serious illness, or death. DM has found extensive use as a pesticide for treatment of wood against insects.

Environmental Fate and Behavior

DM has an estimated K_{oc} value of 5750 which indicates a lack of mobility once it is released into sediment. Also, its volatility from moist soil and water is not expected to be significant. Its environmental fate is based upon its estimated Henry's law constant of 3.3×10^{-8} atm-m^3 mol^{-1}. DM was reported to hydrolyze slowly under alkaline conditions to bis(diphenylaminoarsine)oxide in moist alkaline soils. DM is not expected to volatilize from dry soil surfaces based upon its vapor pressure of 2×10^{-13} mmHg at 20 °C. With such low vapor pressure, once released into air it will exist as particulates at ambient pressure and could be removed from air through wet and dry deposition. DM release into water will be expected to adsorb to suspended solids and sediment based upon its estimated K_{oc}. DM's effect on aquatic life could be extrapolated from its estimated bioconcentration factor (BCF) value of 263, which indicates high potential for accumulation in aquatic organisms. There are no available data for arsenical vomiting agents on their biodegradation. The hydrolysis of solid DM is generally considered negligible due to the formation of an oxide coating. However, in the aerosol state it hydrolyzes more rapidly. DM lacks chromospheres capable of light absorption beyond 290 nm, which makes it less susceptible to undergo photolysis when exposed to sunlight.

Exposure and Exposure Monitoring

Arsenical vomiting agents typically are disseminated as aerosols. Normally DM is a solid, but upon heating it vaporizes and then condenses to form an aerosol. It is toxic through inhalation, ingestion, and skin contact. It irritates the eyes and respiratory tract, but not necessarily the skin. The primary route of absorption is through the respiratory system. The effects of the vomiting agents by any route of exposure are slower in onset but have prolonged systemic effects. As a result of this delay, less early warning signs are present and as such exposure to large amount of vomiting agents is possible. Systemic signs and symptoms subsequently follow the initial irritation and could consist of headache, nausea, vomiting, diarrhea, abdominal cramps, and mental status changes. These signs and symptoms often last for several hours after exposure.

Since arsenical vomiting agents are banned from use, human exposure to them is rare and no literature report was found past the 1960s addressing human exposure. However, potential human exposure to arsenical vomiting agents could be possible due to laboratory accidents, terrorist attacks, or military conflicts. Moreover, there are few reported studies dating back to 1922–58 in which human subjects were exposed to dosages ranging from 4.6 to 144 mg min m^{-3}. The majority of exposures occurred by inhalation and typically led to symptoms of ocular, nasal, and respiratory tract irritation. Nonspecific gastrointestinal symptoms (e.g., vomiting or diarrhea) were also observed. In those studies dating from 1922 to 1958, a few human subjects were exposed to DM agents at

[†] Deceased.

 http://dx.doi.org/10.1016/B978-0-12-386454-3.00587-X

different concentrations not exceeding the maximum safe dose of 100 mg min m^{-3}. The human subjects were then examined before, immediately after, and 2–4 days after exposure. It was determined that the concentration necessary to produce irritation in 50% of the subjects (ECt_{50}) at 2 min was 38 mg min m^{-3} for DM. The 3 min ECt_{50} value was 19 mg min m^{-3} for DM. The Ct value for DM agent that is necessary to cause nausea and vomiting was estimated at 370 mg min m^{-3}. The accidental DM agent exposure of 22 sleeping men in barracks had been cited. The estimated reported concentration was 1130–2260 mg min m^{-3}, for exposure duration of 5 min (by a first source) or 30 min (by a second source). For a 5-min exposure, the dosage was estimated to be 5650–11 300 mg min m^{-3} and for a 30-min exposure, it was 33 900–67 800 mg min m^{-3}. This event resulted in one death from the DM inhalation. The postmortem findings were severe airway and lung damage, similar to those observed with death from chloroacetophenone (CN) exposure. Another source reported severe pulmonary injury and death after accidental exposure to high concentrations of DM in confined spaces, but no details were given.

Toxicokinetics

By any route of administration, the effects are slower in onset but with prolonged systemic effects than that of typical riot-control agents such as *o*-chloro-benzylmalononitrile (CS). Vomiting agents are irritants upon initial exposure. The slow onset for DM allows for the absorption of much more DM before a warning is perceived. The estimated threshold concentrations for irritation of the throat, lower respiratory tract, and initiation of the cough reflex are 0.38, 0.50, and 0.75 mg m^{-3}, respectively.

Mechanism of Toxicity

DM's primary action is on the upper respiratory tract, causing irritation of the nasal mucosa and nasal sinuses, burning in the throat, tightness and pain in the chest, and uncontrollable coughing and sneezing. It also causes eye irritation and burning, with tearing, blepharospasm, and injected conjunctiva.

DM is more toxic than other riot-control agents; the LCt_{50} for humans has been estimated to be 11 000 mg min m^{-3}. The amount that is intolerable for humans has been estimated by some to be 22 mg min m^{-3} and by others to be 150 mg min m^{-3}. The threshold for irritation in humans is about 1 mg m^{-3}, but some people have tolerated exposures of 100–150 mg min m^{-3}.

This class of compounds is unique among the riot-control agents because the effects do not appear immediately on exposure or seconds afterward, but rather several minutes later. The other characteristic of these compounds is that there may be more prolonged systemic effects, including headache, mental depression, chills, nausea, abdominal cramps, vomiting, and diarrhea, which last for several hours after exposure. The LCt_{50} necessary to cause nausea and vomiting has not been established, but is estimated to be about 370 mg min m^{-3}.

DM is considered less effective as a riot-control or incapacitating agent than CS and CN, and it has been conjectured that there are greater differences in susceptibility among people to DM than to the other agents. DM, like CS, is considered to be a cholinesterase inhibitor, which may be responsible for its lacrimatory effect. DM also has a direct effect on gastric activity, but the evidence suggests that the lethal effect is respiratory related.

Acute and Short-Term Toxicity

Various animal species including monkeys have been exposed to DM. Following acute exposures, the animals exhibited ocular and nasal irritation, hyperactivity, salvation, labored breathing, ataxia, and convulsions.

Histopathology did not reveal any abnormalities at exposure dosages of below 500 mg min m^{-3}. At higher dosages, animals that died or were killed demonstrated hyperemia of the trachea, pulmonary congestion and edema, and pneumonia. These effects were consistent with exposure to pulmonary irritants. DM toxicity for various animals and its acute exposure guideline levels (AEGL) values are given in Tables 1 and 2.

Monkeys have been exposed to varying concentrations and durations and were examined after 3–30 h after exposure. At Ct dosage of 2565 mg min m^{-3} no death was observed with any monkey during the exposure examination period. The signs and symptoms at this dosage included edema of trachea, bronchial mucosa, and superficial tracheitis.

In monkeys a Ct of 8540 mg min m^{-3} resulted in ocular and nasal conjunctival congestion, facial erythema, and decreased responses, all of which were resolved within 24 h. Exposure to the high dosage of 28 765 mg min m^{-3} resulted in hyperactivity, copious nasal discharge, conjunctival congestion, marked respiratory distress, as well as gasping and gagging in all the exposed monkeys. Eight of these exposed monkeys died within 24 h of exposure. Necropsy of these animals revealed

Table 1 DM toxicity values

Species	*LCt_{50} (mg min m^{-3})*	*Intravenous LD_{50} (mg kg^{-1})*
Mouse	22 400	17.9
Rats	3700	14.1
Guinea pig	7900	2.4

Theoretical dose calculated from respiratory volume, LCt_{50}, and estimated percent retention.

Table 2 Derived AEGL values for DM6

Time	*AEGL 1 (discomfort)*	*AEGL 2 (impaired escape)*	*AEGL 3 (life threatening/death)*
10 min	0.20 mg m^{-3}	9.7 mg m^{-3}	21 mg m^{-3}
30 min	0.041 mg m^{-3}	6.8 mg m^{-3}	17 mg m^{-3}
60 min	0.016 mg m^{-3}	2.6 mg m^{-3}	6.4 mg m^{-3}
4 h	0.0022 mg m^{-3}	0.36 mg m^{-3}	0.91 mg m^{-3}
8 h	0.00083 mg m^{-3}	0.14 mg m^{-3}	0.34 mg m^{-3}

congestion and extremely edematous lungs. Microscopic examination revealed ulceration of the tracheobronchial tree and pulmonary edema.

Studies were also conducted in which monkeys were exposed to low target concentrations of 100 and 300 mg m^{-3} DM for 2–60 min and 2–40 min, respectively. The signs of toxicity increased as the duration increased, characteristic of exposure to irritants. At the maximum dosage of 13 200 mg min m^{-3}, the animals exhibited nausea and vomiting, oral and nasal discharge, and conjunctival congestion. Only blinking was noted below 1296 mg min m^{-3}.

The effects of DM on the gastrointestinal tract were suggested as a possible cause of death. Dogs were dosed both intravenously and orally with lethal doses of DM, while central venous pressure, right ventricular pressure, cortical electric activity, alveolar CO_2, respiratory rate, heart rate electrocardiogram, and gastric activity were monitored. DM caused a marked elevation of both amplitude and rate of gastric activity for 15–20 min, and then returned to normal. Pretreatment with trimethobenzamide, an effective antiemetic for peripheral and centrally acting emetics, did not prevent DM gastric activity. However, pretreatment with chlorpromazine was effective. The authors concluded that DM affects the stomach directly, and that the primary cause of death following exposure to DM is its effects on the lungs.

The effects of DM on the eyes and skin of rabbits were also studied. DM was suspended in corn oil and instilled into the eyes of rabbits in doses of 0.1, 0.2, 0.5, 1.0, and 5.0 mg. No effect was observed at 0.1 mg, but mild conjunctivitis was observed at 0.2 mg. At 0.5 mg, mild blepharitis was also seen. Corneal opacity persisted over the 14-day observation period in rabbit eyes that were dosed with 1.0 and 5.0 mg. Corn oil suspensions of DM (100 mg ml^{-1}) were placed on the clipped backs of rabbits at doses of 1, 10, 50, 75, and 100 mg. Necrosis of the skin was observed at 10 mg and higher. The skin sensitization potential of DM in guinea pigs was negative.

Immunotoxicity

There is no direct study reported in literature that addresses DM immunotoxicity; however, several studies reported showed that arsenic-containing compounds decreased significantly the hemoglobin level, total erythrocyte count, and total leukocyte count in animals.

Reproductive Toxicity

No direct study of DM is available on its effect on the reproductive system. However, study with arsenic compound such as arsine gas, AsH_3, showed no adverse impact on the developmental reproductive system of mice.

Carcinogenicity

No available data showing the classification of DM in terms of its carcinogenicity have been reported. However, other arsenic-containing compounds such as arsine, AsH_3, are classified by the International Agency for Research on Cancer as category-1, which is a carcinogenic classification to human in terms of individual compound or in a mixture.

Clinical Management

Exposure to DM often occurs through inhalation and typically leads to symptoms of ocular, nasal, and respiratory tract

Table 3 Ecotoxicological data of arsenic warfare agents

Parameters	*Data*	*References*
Molecular weight	277.57 g mol^{-1}	
Ecotoxicology		
Fish	Not soluble	SRC, 2002
PNEC	1×10^{-2} mg l^{-1}	Voie et al., 2001
Accumulation		
$BCF_{estimated}$	262	SRC, 2002
Absorption/distribution		
Solubility in water	Not soluble	Blanch et al., 2001
Density	1.65 g cm^{-3}	SRC, 2002
H	3.26×10^{-8} atm-m^3 mol^{-1}	
K_{oc}	5.75×10^{-3}	
Log K_{ow}	4.05	

PNEC, predicted no-effect concentration.

Table 4 Comparative derived AEGL levels for arsenical vomiting agents

	DM (mg m^{-3})	ED (mg m^{-3})	MD (mg m^{-3})	PD (mg m^{-3})	DA (mg m^{-3})
AEGL-1 (nondisabling)					
10 min	0.2	NR	NR	NR	NR
30 min	0.041	NR	NR	NR	NR
1 h	0.016	NR	NR	NR	NR
4 h	0.0022	NR	NR	NR	NR
8 h	0.00083	NR	NR	NR	NR
AEGL-2 (disabling)					
10 min	9.7	0.17	0.63	0.37	1.1
30 min	6.8	0.057	0.14	0.12	0.79
1 h	2.6	0.029	0.053	0.061	0.39
4 h	0.36	NR	0.015	NR	0.098
8 h	0.14	NR	0.0063	NR	0.049
AEGL-3 (lethality)					
10 min	21	0.52	1.9	1.1	3.4
30 min	17	0.17	0.42	0.37	2.4
1 h	6.4	0.086	0.16	0.18	1.2
4 h	0.91	NR	0.044	NR	0.3
8 h	0.34	NR	0.019	NR	0.15

NR, not reported.

Table 5 Nomenclature and molecular structure of arsenical vomiting agents

Common name	*Military designator*	*Chemical name/synonyms*	*CAS*	*Structure*
Adamsite	DM	Diphenylaminechlorarsine Diphenylaminochloroarsine Diphenylaminechlororarsin Diphenylaminearsine 10-Chloro-5, 10-dihydrochlorphenarsazine Phenarsazine chloride 5-Aza-10-arsenaanthracene chloride	578-94-9	H N As Cl
Diphenylchloroarsine	DA	Diphenylchloroarsine Diphenylarsinous chloride Clark I Blue Cross	712-48-1	Cl As
Diphenylcyanoarsine	DC	Diphenylarsinouscyanide Clark II	23525-22-6	N C As
Ethyldichloroarsine	ED	Ethyldichloroarsine	598-94-9	Cl As Cl
Phenyldichloroarsine	PD	Phenyldichloroarsine Dichlorophenylarsine Phenyl-arsenous dichloride	696-28-6	Cl As Cl
Methyldichloroarsine	MD	Methyldichloroarsinc Methyl-arsonous dichloride Dichloromethylarsine Dichloridemethylarsine Methyldichlorarsine	593-89-5	As Cl Cl

irritation. Also, gastrointestinal symptoms such as vomiting are often observed with DM exposure. DM poisoning has a rapid onset but signs and symptoms could take several minutes to develop and could potentially last for hours. Rapid manifestation of cough, nose and throat irritation, vomiting, or dyspnea is a strong indication of DM poisoning. There is no diagnostic laboratory protocol to determine exposure to DM. For further discussion refer to Centers for Disease Control Emergency Preparedness and Response for DM.

Ecotoxicology

An estimated K_{OC} value (distribution coefficient between water and organic carbon) of 5.75×10^3 indicates that DM will adsorb to sediments. DM is practically insoluble in water. The agent hydrolyzes very slowly in water, where the products are hydrochloric acid and bis(diphenylaminoarsine)oxide. The decomposition product, bis(diphenylaminoarsine)oxide has similar toxicity as DM. The relevant ecotoxicological reports in the literature address the European dumpsites after World War II. Large quantities of chemical warfare agents of which one-third included arsenical compounds were dumped in European waters after World War II in an area within the Lithuanian economic zone. A study conducted by the Lithuanian Center of Marine Research showed that DM and other arsenical compounds are preserved in the seabed. The same study suggested that DM would spread very slowly from the chemical munitions source and only contaminated local sediments. Such

Table 6 Chemical, physical, environmental, and biological properties of CS, CN, and DM

Properties	*o-Chlorobenzylidene malononitrile (CS)*	*1-Chloroacetophenone (CN)*	*Diphenylaminearsine (DM)*
Chemical and physical			
Boiling point	310 °C	248 °C	410 °C with decomposition
Vapor pressure	0.00034 mmHg at 20 °C	0.0041 mmHg at approximately 20 °C	4.5×10^{-11} mmHg at 25 °C
Density			
Vapor	–	5.3[a]	–
Liquid	–	1.187 g ml^{-1} at approximately 58 °C	–
Solid	Bulk: 0.24–0.26 g cm^{-3} Crystal: 1.04 g cm^{-3}	1.318 g cm^{-3} at approximately 20 °C	Bulk: <1 g cm^{-3} Crystal: 1.65 g cm^{-3} at 20 °C
Volatility	0.71 mg m^{-3} at 25 °C	34.3 mg m^{-3} at approximately 20 °C	Not of practical significance
Appearance/odor	White crystalline powder with pungent odor (pepper)	Fragrant (like apple blossoms)	Yellow-green, odorless, crystalline substance
Solubility			
In water	Insoluble	Insoluble	0.0064 g/100 g at room temperature
In other solvents	Organic solvents; complete	Organic	Best: acetone, 13.03 g/100 g at 15 °C
Environmental and biological			
Detection	No detector	No detector	No detector
Persistency			
In soil	Varies	Short	Persistent
On materiel	Varies	Short	Persistent
Skin decontamination	Soap and water	Soap and water	Soap and water
Biologically effective amount			
Aerosol (mg min m^{-3})	LCt_{50}: 60 000 ICT_{50}: 3–5	LCt_{50}: 7000–14 000 ICT_{50}: 20–40	LCt_{50}: 11 000–35 000 ICT_{50}: 22–150; nausea, vomiting: approximately 370

LCt_{50}, the concentration.
[a]Compared with the density of air.

observations could be used as indicators of leakage of chemical warfare agents from dumped containers. The concentrations for total arsenic in sediments have been reported from 9 to 480 mg kg^{-1}. The highest concentration was found in the samples from the dumpsite in Skagerrak (Netherlands), in which high concentrations of Clark I, triphenylarsine, and bis(diphenylarsine)oxide were found in the same samples. Also, at the Skagerrak dumpsite, the arsenic concentration level of 18–210 mg kg^{-1} could be found several centimeters below the bottom–water interface. Deeper sediment horizons (10–11 cm) at the Gotland (Liepaja-Latvia) dumpsite had elevated arsenic contents with concentrations up to 100 mg kg^{-1}. Arsenical compound pollution was not observed in the upper layers of sediments and in the bottom water at this site at the Gotland dumpsite. The aquatic life in the dumpsite area did not show drastic changes in the presence of arsenical compounds and data collected were not conclusive to provide definitive correlation between aquatic environment and contamination by arsenical compounds including DM, see **Table 3**.

Other Hazards

Due to the fact that some arsenical vomiting agents have uses in industries for various purposes, there is a concern about their impact on environment and natural resources. Their disposal should follow at all local, state, and federal rules and regulations. This disposal is similar to 'destruction of chemical weapons,' which includes conversion of chemicals in an essentially irreversible way to a form unsuitable and less toxic chemical by-products. For those nonchemical warfare processes that use certain arsenical agents, it is highly recommended to utilize alternative chemical products with less inherent propensity for occupational exposure or environmental contamination. Ultimate disposal of the chemical must consider the material's impact on air quality; potential migration in soil or water; toxicological impacts on human, animal, aquatic, and plant life; and should conform to all environmental and public health rules and regulations.

Exposure Standards and Guidelines

Table 4 represents the derived AEGL data collected from animal exposure experiments.

Miscellaneous

Species Variability for AEGL Values

Although these derived AEGL values are based on results from limited animal species exposed to arsenical vomiting agents, the available data do not indicate variability in the toxicodynamics of those agents across species. However, the reported data from which those AEGL values are derived indicate species variability but it is ambiguous to what degree the variability can be attributed to varying experimental parameters, protocols, and techniques (**Tables 5** and **6**).

See also: Arsenic; Riot Control Agents; Chemical Warfare.

Further Reading

Agency for Toxic Substances and Disease Registry (ATSDR) Agency for Toxic Substances and Disease Registry, 2002. DHHS-PHS, Washington, DC. Toxicological profile for arsenic.

Franke, C., et al., 1994. Chemosphere 29, 1501–1514.

Garnaga, G., Stankevičius, A., 2005. Arsenic and other environmental parameters at the chemical munitions dumpsite in the Lithuanian economic zone of the Baltic sea. Environ. Res. Eng. Manage. 3 (33), 24–31.

Glasby, G.P., 1997. Disposal of chemical weapons in the Baltic Sea. Sci. Total Environ. 206, 267–273.

http://www.bt.cdc.gov/agent/adamsite/casedef.asp.

McNamara, B.P., Owens, E.J., Weimer, J.T., Ballard, T.A., Vocci, F.J., 1969. Toxicology of Riot Control Chemicals – CS, CN, and DM. U.S. Army Medical Research Laboratory, Edgewood Arsenal, MD. Technical Report EATR 4309.

Meylan, W.M., Howard, P.H., 1995. J. Pharm. Sci. 84, 83–92.

Meylan, W.M., et al., 1999. Environ. Toxicol. Chem. 18, 664–672.

Morrissey, R.E., Fowler, B.A., Harris, M.W., Moorman, M.P., Jameson, C.W., Schwetz, B.A., 1990 Aug. Arsine: absence of developmental toxicity in rats and mice. Fundam. Appl. Toxicol. 15 (2), 350–356.

Organization for the Prohibition of Chemical Weapons, 2007. Convention on the Prohibition of the Development, Production, Stockpiling and Use of Chemical Weapons and Their Destruction, p. 87 http://www.opcw.org/chemical-weapons-convention.

Owens, E.J., McNamara, B.P., Weimer, J.T., et al., 1967. Toxicology of DM. Medical Research Laboratories, Edgewood Arsenal, MD. Tech. Report 4108.

Patra, P.H., Bandyopadhyay, S., Bandyopadhyay, M.C., Mandal, T.K., 2013. Immunotoxic and genotoxic potential of arsenic and its chemical species in goats. Toxicol. Int. 20, 6–10.

Salem, H., Olajos, E.J., Katz, S.A., 2001. Riot-control agents. In: Somani, S.M., Romano Jr, J.A. (Eds.), Chemical Warfare Agents: Toxicity at Low Levels. CRC Press, Boca Raton, FL.

Sidell, F.R., 1997. Riot control agents. In: Zajtchuk, R., Bellamy, R.F. (Eds.), Textbook of Military Medicine: Medical Aspects of Chemical and Biological Warfare. Office of the Surgeon General at TMM Publications, Borden Institute, Walter Reed Army Medical Center, Washington, DC, pp. 307–324.

Sidell, F.R., et al. (Eds.), 1997. Medical Aspects of Chemical and Biological Warfare, p. 319.

Striker, G.E., Streett, C.S., Ford, D.F., Herman, L.H., Helland, D.R., 1967. A Clinicopathological Study of the Effects of Riot Control Agents on Monkeys. III. Diphenylaminochloroarsine (DM) Grenade. U.S. Army Medical Research Laboratory, Edgewood Arsenal, MD. Technical Report 4070.

Tørnes, J.A., Voie, Ø.A., Ljønes, M., Opstad, A.M., Bjerkeseth, L.H., Hussain F., 2002. Investigation and Risk Assessment of Ships Loaded with Chemical Ammunition Scuttled in Skagerrak. TA-1907/2002.

USEPA. Acute Exposure Guideline Levels (AEGLs): Adamsite Results. Last Updated on November 27, 2007. Available from, as of March 27, 2008: http://www.epa.gov/oppt/aegl/pubs/rest134.htm.

Walker, A.M., Stevens, J.J., Ndebele, K., Tchounwou, P.B., 2010. Arsenic trioxide modulates DNA synthesis and apoptosis in lung carcinoma cells. Int. J. Environ. Res. Public Health 7, 1996–2007.

Relevant Websites

http://www.atsdr.cdc.gov/ – Agency for Toxic Substances and Disease Registry.

http://toxnet.nlm.nih.gov/cgi-bin/sis/htmlgen?CTD – Elucidates molecular mechanisms by which environmental chemicals affect human disease © 2004–2010 Mount Desert Island Biological Laboratory.

http://www.epa.gov/oppt/aegl/pubs/chemlist.htm – EPA related literature web site that provide information about standard exposure and guidelines for environmental contaminants.

http://www.cdc.gov/nceh/ – National Center for Environmental Health (NCEH), plans, directs, and coordinates a national program to maintain and improve the health of the American people.

http://toxnet.nlm.nih.gov/index.html – National Library of Medicine databases on toxicology, hazardous chemicals, environmental health, and toxic releases.

http://sis.nlm.nih.gov – (US) National Library of Medicine, Specialized Information Services, Chemical Warfare Agents.

http://www.bt.cdc.gov – (US) Centers for Disease Control and Prevention, Agency for Toxic Substances and Disease Registry, Chemical Agents.

Arsenic

RW Kapp, Jr., BioTox, Monroe Township, NJ, USA

- Name: Arsenic
- Chemical Abstracts Service Registry Number: 7440-38-2
- Synonyms: Arsen; Arsenic black; Gray arsenic; Arsenicals
- Molecular Formula: As
- Valence States: 0, 3^+, 5^+
- Chemical Structure: N/A

Background

The word arsenic has several derivations including from the Syriac word (al) *zarniqa* (ܐܠ ܙܐܪܢܝܩܐ), the Persian word zarnikh, (زرنيخ), and the Greek word arsenikon (Αρσενικόν). It is also related to the similar Greek word *arsenikos* (Αρσενικός), meaning 'masculine' or 'potent.' The word was subsequently adopted into Latin as arsenicum and ultimately into French and English as arsenic. Arsenic compounds have been known since the days of Ancient Greece and Rome when arsenic sulfide or orpiment (As_2S_3) was used by physicians to heal and by murderers to poison. Arsenic compounds were mined by the early Chinese, Greek, and Egyptian civilizations who found it could be produced from its ores easily that made it one of the first recognized as an element by early alchemists. Alchemy existed from about 500 BC to about the end of the sixteenth century. Alchemists were on a quest to turn various metals into precious metals such as gold and searching for ways to have eternal life. While most of alchemy was shrouded in mysticism and magic, a number of early techniques were later found to be useful in modern chemistry. The discovery of arsenic is credited to alchemist Albert the Great (Albertus Magnus 1193–1280), a German Dominican friar who achieved fame for his advocacy in the peaceful coexistence of science and religion. He heated As_2S_3 with soap and formed elemental arsenic. The first directions for the preparation of the metalloid arsenic, however, are found in the writings of Paracelsus (1493–1541), the father of modern toxicology.

Uses

Dioscorides, a Greek physician, described arsenic as a poison in the first century. Its ideal properties for sinister uses included its lack of color, odor, or taste when mixed in food or drink and its easy access that made it readily available to all classes of society. The primary current use of arsenic is for strengthening alloys of copper and lead for car batteries. Arsenic is found in semiconductor electronic devices and in the production of chemicals such as chromated copper arsenate, monosodium methyl arsenate (MSMA), and disodium methyl arsenate (DSMA) used for treating wood products, herbicides, and insecticides. 4-Hydroxy-3-nitrobenzenearsonic acid is added to animal food as a method of disease prevention and growth stimulation. Arsenic compounds have been used as medicines, including arsphenamine and neosalvasan that were indicated for syphilis and typanosomiasis but have been superseded by modern antibiotics. Arsenic trioxide has been used in a variety of ways over the past 500 years, but recently in the treatment of acute promyelocytic leukemia. Potassium arsenite was used in Fowler's solution for the treatment of psoriasis, malaria, chorea, and syphilis until the 1950s. Lewisite is an organoarsenic compound once manufactured in the United States and Japan as a chemical weapon that caused severe blistering and lung irritation.

Environmental Behavior, Fate, Routes, and Pathways

Arsenic is an odorless, tasteless semimetallic compound, whose symbol is As; the atomic number is 33; and the density is 5.7 g cm^3 at 14 °C. Arsenic appears in three allotropic forms: yellow, black, and gray; the stable form is a silver-gray, brittle crystalline solid. Atmospheric arsenic is a mixture of the trivalent and pentavalent forms and comes from various sources: volcanoes and microorganisms release volatile methylarsines, and anthropogenic sources including nonferrous metal mining and smelting, pesticide application, coal combustion, wood combustion, and human waste incineration. Arsenic cannot be destroyed in the environment so it remains persistent. It can change form or become attached to or separated from particles. Arsenic in water can undergo a number of transformations, including oxidation–reduction reactions, ligand exchange, precipitation, and biotransformation with many factors influencing the effectiveness of the processes including pH, temperature, salinity, season, distribution, and composition of the biota, and the nature and concentration of natural organic matter.

Soluble forms move with the water and may be carried to long distances. Thus, arsenic can get into lakes, rivers, or underground water by dissolving in rain or snow or through the discharge of industrial wastes. Arsenic may be adsorbed from water onto sediments or soils. However, because many arsenic compounds tend to partition to soil or sediment, they tend to concentrate in upper soil layers indefinitely.

Bioconcentration of arsenic occurs in algae and lower invertebrates. Both bottom-feeding and predatory fish can accumulate contaminants found in water. The major bioaccumulation transfer is between water and algae, at the base of the food chain that has a strong impact on the concentration in fish. Bottom-feeders are readily exposed to the greater quantities of arsenic, which accumulate in sediments. No differences were found for arsenic existing between bottom-feeders and predators in tissue levels of metals and other contaminants. Therefore, biomagnification in aquatic food chains does not appear to be significant.

Exposure and Exposure Monitoring

Arsenic naturally occurs in soil and will be present in the atmosphere as airborne dust. Arsenic released from

 http://dx.doi.org/10.1016/B978-0-12-386454-3.00817-4

combustion processes will occur as highly soluble oxides. Gaseous alkyl arsenic compounds are released from soil that has been treated with inorganic arsenic compounds as a result of biogenic processes. Arsenic occurs in seawater and vegetation and is released into the atmosphere in sea salt spray and forest fires. Atmospheric levels of arsenic in remote locations range from 1 to 3 mg m^{-3} while concentrations in urban areas may range from 20 to 100 ng m^{-3} with higher concentrations (>1000 ng m^{-3}) in the vicinity of industrial sources. Arsenic released to air exists mainly in the form of particulate matter.

Arsenic is widely distributed in the Earth's crust, which contains about 3.4 ppm arsenic. It is found in nature in minerals such as realgar (As_4S_4), orpiment (As_2S_3), and arsenolite (As_2O_3), and rarely in its elemental form. There are over 150 arsenic-bearing minerals. Elemental arsenic is not soluble in water. Arsenic complexes with iron, aluminum, and magnesium oxides are found in soil surfaces. Natural levels of arsenic in soil range from 1 to 40 mg kg^{-1} although higher levels may occur in mining areas, at waste sites, near high geological deposits of arsenic-rich minerals or from pesticide application.

In aquatic systems, inorganic arsenic occurs in trivalent and pentavalent forms. Concentrations of arsenic in open ocean seawater are typically 1–2 μg l^{-1}. Arsenic is widely distributed in surface freshwaters, and concentrations in rivers and lakes are generally ≤10 μg l^{-1}, although individual samples may range up to 5 mg l^{-1} near anthropogenic sources. Arsenic levels in groundwater average about 1–2 μg l^{-1} except in areas with sulfide mineral deposits where arsenic levels range up to 3 mg l^{-1}. Arsenic has also been detected in rainwater at average concentrations of 0.2–0.5 μg l^{-1}.

Arsenic is found in many foods at concentrations ranging from 20 to 140 μg kg^{-1}. Total arsenic concentrations may be higher in certain seafoods. However, about 85–>90% of the arsenic in the edible parts of marine fish and shellfish is organic arsenic (e.g., arsenobetaine, arsenochloline, dimethylarsinic acid - commonly called 'fish arsenic') which is relatively nontoxic to humans.

Mean dietary intakes of total arsenic of 50.6 μg day^{-1} (range of 1.01–1081 μg day^{-1}) and 58.5 μg day^{-1} (range of 0.21–1276 μg day^{-1}) are reported in females and males, while the dietary intake of inorganic arsenic has been estimated to range from 1 to 20 μg day^{-1}. The predominant dietary source of arsenic is seafood.

An example of widespread environmental exposure to toxic levels of arsenic would be drinking water wells in Bangladesh during the 1980s and 1990s. Intentional spousal poisoning is infrequently not detected in time for successful medical intervention.

Toxicokinetics

Kinetics and metabolism of arsenicals in animals and humans are complex as a result of differences in physicochemical properties and bioavailability of the various forms of arsenic. Arsenic metabolism is also characterized by large qualitative and quantitative interspecies differences. Both arsenate and arsenite are generally well absorbed by both the oral and inhalation routes, while organic arsenic in soil is absorbed to a lesser extent than solutions of arsenic salts. The rate of absorption of insoluble arsenic is much lower than that of more soluble forms. Once absorbed, arsenites are oxidized to arsenates and methylated ultimately producing dimethylated arsenic metabolites. The rate and relative proportion of methylation production varies among species. Most arsenic is excreted in the urine as a mixture of monomethylarsonic acid (MMA) and dimethylarsinic acid (DMA). Smaller amounts are excreted in feces.

Mechanism of Toxicity

Trivalent arsenic exerts its toxic effects mainly by disrupting ATP production by inhibiting lipoic acid, which is a cofactor for pyruvate as well by replacing phosphate which uncouples oxidation phosphorylation. This inhibits the electron transport chain in the mitochondria and the ultimate synthesis of ATP. Hydrogen peroxide production is also increased, which, it is speculated, has potential to form reactive oxygen species and oxidative stress. These metabolic interferences lead to death from multisystem cell death and organ failure. The activity of enzymes is due to the functional groups on amino acids such as the sulfhydryl group on cysteine or coenzymes such as lipoic acid, which has vicinal thiol groups. Trivalent inorganic arsenicals readily react with sulfhydryl groups such as cysteine creating a strong complex between arsenic and vicinal sulfhydryl reagents. These actions inhibit not only the formation of Acetyl-CoA but also the enzymes succinic dehydrogenase and pyruvate. Arsenite inhibits the binding of steroids to the glucocorticoid receptor, but not other steroid receptors. The probable mechanism of toxicity of pentavalent inorganic arsenate is its reduction to a trivalent form, arsenite, which is more toxic than the arsenate. Thus, a variety of mechanisms lead arsenic to impair cell respiration and subsequently diminish ATP formation.

Acute and Short-Term Toxicity

Acute data are mixed showing a variety of target organs. Inorganic arsenic is acutely toxic and ingestion of large doses leads to gastrointestinal symptoms, disturbances of cardiovascular, respiratory and central nervous system functions, multiorgan failure, and eventually death. In survivors, bone marrow depression, hemolysis, hepatomegaly, melanosis, polyneuropathy, and encephalopathy may be observed. Nausea, vomiting, and diarrhea are very common symptoms in humans following oral exposure to inorganic arsenicals, both after acute high-dose exposure and after repeated exposure to lower doses; these effects are likely due to a direct irritation of the gastrointestinal mucosa. Acute, high-dose exposure can lead to encephalopathy, with clinical signs such as confusion and hallucinations.

Chronic Toxicity

Chronic exposure of humans to inorganic arsenic in the drinking water is causally related to increased risks of cancer in the skin, lungs, bladder, and kidneys, as well as other skin changes such as hyperkeratosis and pigmentation changes. Six-month dietary dog studies showed a dose-dependent decrease in feed consumption and body weights and increased levels of aspartate aminotransferase suggesting heptatoxicity at 4 and 8 mg kg^{-1} day^{-1} of arsenite; however, no confirmatory histopathology was noted. Histological alterations in kidney and liver were observed in rats exposed to 50 μg sodium arsenate per ml for 320 days in drinking water. There is evidence that chronic arsenic exposure to humans can cause hypertension and cardiovascular disease, diabetes, cerebrovascular disease, and long-term neurological effects.

Immunotoxicity

No direct studies were located regarding immunological and lymphoreticular effects in humans or animals after oral exposure to organic arsenicals; however, there was no evidence of immunosuppression detected in mice chronically exposed to arsenate. Occupational data suggest that workers may be sensitized to arsenic, however, the data are not confirmed. Dermal studies in guinea pigs did not yield evidence of a sensitization reaction to inorganic arsenic.

Reproductive Toxicity

Animal data suggest that arsenic may cause changes to the reproductive organs of both sexes, including decreased organ weight and increased inflammation of reproductive tissues. Animal studies of oral inorganic arsenic exposure have reported developmental effects, but only at maternally toxic concentrations. The most sensitive species was the rabbit, which had increased resorptions and decreased viable fetuses/litter at 1.5 mg As kg^{-1} day^{-1} and a developmental no observable adverse effect level (NOAEL) of 0.4 mg As kg^{-1} day^{-1}.

Exposure to arsenic in drinking water has been associated with adverse reproductive outcomes showing increases in spontaneous abortions in women drinking water at 0.008 mg As kg^{-1} day^{-1} for 5–10 years and water at 0.006 mg As kg^{-1} day^{-1}. Chronic exposure of women to arsenic in the drinking water has been associated with infants with low birth weights. Similar associations have been made between late fetal mortality, neonatal mortality, and postneonatal mortality and exposure to $\leq$0.86 mg l^{-1} of arsenic in drinking water.

Genotoxicity

An increased incidence of chromosomal abnormalities was detected in rats orally administered with 4 mg kg^{-1} day^{-1} of sodium arsenate for 2–3 weeks, but no consistent increase in chromosomal aberrations was detected in bone marrow cells or spermatogonia from mice orally administered with 50 mg kg^{-1} day^{-1} of sodium arsenite for $\leq$8 weeks.

Studies in human fibroblasts, lymphocytes and leukocytes, mouse lymphoma cells, Chinese hamster ovary cells, and Syrian hamster embryo cells demonstrate that *in vitro* arsenic exposure can induce chromosomal aberrations and sister chromatid exchange. *In vitro* studies in humans, mouse, and hamster cells have been positive for DNA damage.

Several tests indicate that DMA and roxarsone may cause chromosome aberrations, mutations, and DNA strand breaks; *in vitro* studies with MMA did not find significant increase in the occurrence of chromosome aberrations, bacterial mutations, or unscheduled DNA synthesis. An increased number of DNA strand breaks were detected in lung and other tissues of mice and rats orally administered with 1500 mg kg^{-1} DMA.

Carcinogenicity

Mice exposed to arsenic in drinking water containing 500 μg pentavalent arsenic l^{-1} for 2 years showed increased incidence in tumors of the lung, liver, gastrointestinal tract, and skin. Rats exposed to high levels of DMA show increased incidence of urinary bladder cancer. Arsenic exposure via drinking water is causally related to cancer in the lungs, kidney, bladder, and skin in humans. Drinking water arsenic concentrations of 50 μg l^{-1} have been associated with increased risks of cancers of the bladder and lung.

Arsenic is a known human carcinogen by both the inhalation and oral exposure routes. Cumulative exposure to 0.75 mg m^{-3} year has been associated with an increased risk of cancer of the lung. Miners exposed to arsenic trioxide have been reported to have higher risk of lung cancer. Increased incidence of lung cancer has also been observed among chemical plant workers who are primarily exposed to arsenate. In humans exposed chronically by the oral route, skin tumors are the most common type of cancer. In addition to skin cancer, there are reports that indicate ingestion of arsenic also increases the risk of bladder and lung tumors and to a lesser extent, liver, kidney, and prostate tumors.

Clinical Management

Arsenite inhibits the binding of steroids to the glucocorticoid receptor, but not other steroid receptors, therefore, binding of arsenite to protein at nonessential enzyme sites is thought to be a detoxication mechanism. Acute arsenic intoxication can be treated with chelating agents such as dimercaprol (British anti-Lewisite or BAL), and D-penicillamine. Although body burden is not reduced, chelators bind free arsenic and serve to reduce the biologically active arsenic. Chelation therapy is most effective when instituted within a few hours after exposure. Vomiting should also be induced with Ipecac in the alert patient. Activated charcoal and gastric lavage are useful followed by electrolyte replacement if indicated.

Treatment of chronic arsenic poisoning is accomplished using BAL prescribed in dosages of 5 mg kg^{-1} up to 300 mg every 4 h for the first day; followed by the same dosage every 6 h for the second day; the following 8 days the dose is administered every 8 h.

Ecotoxicology

Arsenic is moderately to highly toxic in studies conducted on amphibians, fish, and invertebrates and terrestrial biota. Arsenic compounds cause acute and chronic effects that include lethality, inhibition of growth, photosynthesis and reproduction, and behavioral effects. Inorganic arsenicals are more toxic than organic arsenicals and arsenite is more toxic than arsenate. The mode of toxicity and mechanism of uptake of arsenate by organisms differ considerably explaining the interspecies differences in organism responses. The 96 h LC_{50}s for freshwater fish for trivalent arsenic range from 10.8 to 91 mg l^{-1} and from 4.8 to >360 mg l^{-1} for pentavalent arsenic. Biomagnification in aquatic food chains has not been observed. Terrestrial plants may accumulate arsenic by root uptake from the soil or by adsorption of airborne arsenic deposited on the leaves.

Bioconcentration of arsenic compounds in freshwater organisms is lower than for marine organisms. Marine organisms normally contain arsenic residues ranging from <1 to >100 mg kg^{-1}, predominantly as organic arsenic chemicals such as arsenosugars (macroalgae) and arsenobetaine (invertebrates and fish). Bioaccumulation of organic arsenic compounds, after their biogenesis from inorganic forms, occurs in aquatic organisms. Some species accumulate substantial levels, with mean concentrations of ≤3000 mg kg^{-1} at arsenical mine sites. In marine fish, 96 h LC_{50}s range from 12.7 to 28.5 mg trivalent arsenic l^{-1} and from 21.4 to 157 mg pentavalent arsenic l^{-1}. Acute toxicity for the organic arsenical MMA ranges from 1.9 to 1412 mg organoarsenic l^{-1}.

Exposure Standards and Guidelines

Minimal Risk Levels (MRLs)

Inhalation

- No acute-, intermediate-, or chronic-duration inhalation MRLs were derived for inorganic arsenic or organoarsenic compounds.

Oral

- An MRL of 0.005 mg As kg^{-1} day^{-1} has been derived for acute-duration oral exposure (≤14 days) to inorganic arsenic.
- No intermediate-duration oral MRL was derived for inorganic arsenic.
- An MRL of 0.000 3 mg As kg^{-1} day^{-1} has been derived for chronic-duration oral exposure (≥1 year) to inorganic arsenic.
- No acute-duration oral MRL was derived for MMA.
- An MRL of 0.1 mg MMA kg^{-1} day^{-1} has been derived for intermediate-duration oral exposure (15–364 days) to MMA.
- An MRL of 0.01 mg MMA kg^{-1} day^{-1} has been derived for chronic-duration oral exposure (≥1 year) to MMA.
- No acute- or intermediate-duration oral MRLs were derived for DMA.
- An MRL of 0.02 mg DMA kg^{-1} day^{-1} has been derived for chronic-duration oral exposure (≥1 year) to DMA.

Arsenic Regulations

Regulating body	*Standard*	*Classification*
International		
IARC	Carcinogenicity	Group 1
WHO	Air quality	1.5×10^{-3} unit risk
	Drinking water	0.01 mg l
German – MAK	Carcinogenicity	Class 1
United States		
ACGIH	TLV	0.01 mg m^{-3}
	Carcinogenicity	TLV-A1
NIOSH	REL	0.002 mg m^{-3}
	IDLH	5 mg m^{-3}
	Carcinogenicity	Ca
OSHA	PEL organic As	0.5 mg m^{-3}
	PEL inorganic As	10 μg m^{-3}
	PEL organic As – industry + shipyards	0.5 mg m^{-3}
	Carcinogenicity	Ca
EPA	Drinking water equivalent level (DWEL)	0.01 mg l^{-1}
	Drinking water unit risk	5×10^{-5} μg l^{-1}
	Water – maximum contaminant level	0.01 mg l^{-1}
	Residue tolerance – DMA	2.8 ppm
	Residue tolerance – MMA	0.35–0.9 ppm
	Carcinogenicity	Group A
	Inhalation unit risk	4.3×10^{-3} μg m^{-3}
	RfC	No data
	RfD	3×10^{-4} mg kg^{-1} day^{-1}
FDA	Bottled drinking water	0.01 mg l^{-1}
NTP	Carcinogenicity	Known human carcinogen (K)
USDA	Prohibited in organic crop production	Arsenic

Arsenic Compounds

Arsenic metal per se is rarely encountered in nature or in other than in the metals or electronic components industries. Rather, most human and environmental exposure is to a range of inorganic and organic arsenic compounds.

Inorganic arsenic compounds are generally more toxic than organic ones, but less prone to bioaccumulation. They are known to cross the placental barrier, though increased methylation decreases toxicity in pregnant women. Chronic exposure to inorganic moieties also greatly increases risk for cardiovascular disease and mortality.

The most important inorganic compounds are arsenic trioxide (which occurs in minerals and elsewhere in nature), and arsine gas (AsH_3), which occurs primarily in nonferrous metal refineries, but is also used for doping semiconductor chips. Both of these are trivalent valence compounds. Arsine is a colorless, inflammable gas with a garlic odor. It is a powerful hemolytic poison that is readily absorbed upon inhalation.

Arsenic trioxide is readily absorbed from the stomach, and is a common cause of environmental exposure. It is frequently used in the treatment of lumber and can thereby cause widespread exposure. It is also used as a precursor for most organic and inorganic arsenic compounds created for other uses.

Common organic arsenic compounds are arsanilic acid, methylarsonic acid, and arsenobetaine (which is commonly found as it accumulates in seafood).

Testing for arsenic levels in humans involves sampling from hair, nails, and urine. To determine whether there has been inorganic exposure, urine must be tested for monomethylarsonic acid (MMA), and dimethylarsinic acid (DMA).

See also: Arsenical Vomiting Agents; Arsine; Metals; Neurotoxicity; Notorious Poisoners and Poisoning Cases; Pollution, Soil; Pollution, Water.

Further Reading

Abernathy, C.O., Calderon, R.L., Chappell, W.R. (Eds.), 2012. Arsenic: Exposure and Health Effects. Abernathy-Dordrecht, The Netherlands, Springer Science + Business Media Dordrecht.

Arsenic and Arsenic Compounds, Environmental Health Criteria 224, 2001. World Health Organization, Geneva.

Agency for Toxic Substance and Disease Registry (ATSDR), 2007. Toxicological Profile for Arsenic. US Department of Health and Human Services, Public Health Services, GA.

Bolt, H.M., 2012. Arsenic: an ancient toxicant of continuous public health impact, from iceman Ötzi until now. Arch. Toxicol. 86 (6), 825–830.

Caravati, E.M., 2004. Arsenic and arsine gas. In: Dart, R.C. (Ed.), Medical Toxicology, third ed. Lippincott Williams & Wilkins, Philadelphia, pp. 1393–1401.

Huang, C., Ke, Q., Costa, M., Shi, X., 2004. Molecular mechanisms of arsenic carcinogenesis. Mol. Cell. Biochem. 255 (1–2), 57–66.

Hughes, M.F., Beck, B.D., Chen, Y., Lewis, A.S., Thomas, D.J., October 2011. Arsenic exposure and toxicology: a historical perspective. Toxicol. Sci. 123 (2), 305–332.

International Programme on Chemical Safety, 2001. Arsenic and Arsenic Compounds, Environmental Health Criteria 224. WHO, Geneva.

International Water Association, 2012. Arsenic Contamination in the World: An International Sourcebook. International Water Association, London, UK.

Jomova, K., Jenisova, Z., Feszterova, M., Baros, S., Liska, J., Hudecova, D., Rhodes, C.J., Valko, M., March 2011. Arsenic: toxicity, oxidative stress and human disease. J. Appl. Toxicol. 31 (2), 95–107.

Masotti, A., 2013. Arsenic: Sources, Environmental Impact, Toxicity and Human Health – A Medical Geology Perspective. Nova Science Publishing Inc., Hauppauge, NY.

Nordberg, G.F., Fowler, B.A., Nordberg, M., Friberg, L.T., 2007. Handbook on the Toxicology of Metals, third ed. Elsevier, London, UK.

Pimparkar, B.D., Bhave, A., October 2010. Arsenicosis: a review of recent advances. J. Assoc. Physicians India 58, 617–624, 629.

States, J.C., Barchowsky, A., Cartwright, I.L., Reichard, J.F., Futscher, B.W., Lantz, R.C., October 2011. Arsenic toxicology: translating between experimental models and human pathology. Environ. Health Perspect. 199 (10), 1356–1363.

US Department of the Interior, 1998. Guidelines for Interpretation of the Biological Effects of Selected Constituents in Biota, Water, and Sediment: Arsenic.

Yedjou, C., Tchounwou, P., Jenkins, J., McMurray, R., August 2010. Basic mechanisms of arsenic trioxide (ATO)-induced apoptosis in human leukemia. J. Hematol. Oncol. 3, 28.

Relevant Websites

http://www.atsdr.cdc.gov/ – Agency for Toxic Substances and Disease Registry.

http://www.epa.gov/ – Environmental Protection Agency.

http://toxnet.nlm.nih.gov – Toxnet (Toxicology Data Network): search under HSDB for Arsenic.

Arsine

D Pakulska and S Czerczak, Nofer Institute of Occupational Medicine, Łódź, Poland

This article is a revision of the previous edition article by Felix Ayala-Fierro, volume 1, pp 173–176, © 2005, Elsevier Inc.

- Chemical Abstracts Service Registry Number: 7784-42-1
- Synonyms: Agent SA, Arsenic hydride, Arsenic trihydride, Arseniuretted hydrogen, Arsenous hydride, Arsenowodor [Polish], Arsenwasserstoff [German]
- Chemical Formula: AsH_3
- Chemical Structure:

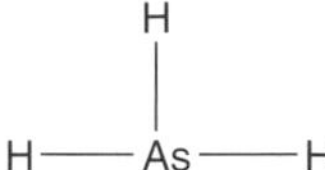

- Conversion Factors: $1\ ppm = 3.24\ mg\ m^{-3}$; $1\ mg\ m^{-3} = 0.31\ ppm$

Background (Significance/History)

Arsine is a highly toxic but nonirritating gas. Its garlic odor occurs only at concentrations that are hazardous to health and life (0.5 ppm; $1.6\ mg\ m^{-3}$) and above. Arsine was first obtained in 1775. The first case of arsine poisoning was reported in 1815, when Scheele, a German chemist exposed to a low concentration of arsine in his laboratory, died 9 days later. During World War II, arsine was investigated as a warfare agent but was never used on the battlefield. The current occupational exposure limit for arsine in most European countries is 0.05 ppm ($0.2\ mg\ m^{-3}$). In 2003, American Conference of Governmental Industrial Hygienists (ACGIH) placed threshold limit values (TLVs) of arsine under revision, because the Occupational Safety and Health Administration in the United States (OSHA), the National Toxicological Program (NTP), and the International Agency for Research on Cancer (IARC) classified its metabolites (arsenic and arsenic compounds) as human carcinogens and proposed a new threshold limit value-time weighted average (TLV-TWA) of 0.003 ppm and designated it as an A1-confirmed human carcinogen. In 2004, ACGIH placed arsine on the "notice of intended changes" list, with a proposed value of 0.005 ppm ($0.016\ mg\ m^{-3}$). This value as well as an A4 designation "not classifiable as a human carcinogen", was accepted in 2007 and is still valid.

Uses

Arsine is mainly used in the semiconductor industry to manufacture microchips. It is applied for epitaxial growth of gallium arsenide and as a dopant to ultrapure crystals to increase electrical conductivity for silicon-based electronic devices. This compound is also used for the production of light-emitting diodes and glass dyes.

The use of arsine is increasing continuously throughout the world.

Environmental Fate and Behavior

Arsine is relatively stable in air and may travel in the atmosphere from a point of emission to remote areas, especially at night before it is converted into nonvolatile oxidized compounds, which may be further removed by particulate matter or deposited back to the soil. Since arsine is decomposed by the action of ultraviolet rays, its stability is reduced during the day. Arsine is moderately soluble in water (20 ml per 100 ml at 20 °C). After entering the water, arsine is likely to be oxidized to other arsenic compounds, of which only a small percentage remain in the water; the rest are deployed along the zone of sediment, where they can undergo biomethylation by microorganisms.

Exposure and Exposure Monitoring

Human Exposure

The major route of human exposure to arsine is inhalation. This gas is heavier than air, so dangerous concentrations can be reached very quickly in enclosed, poorly ventilated, or low-lying areas. Most cases of exposure to arsine occur during the use of acids and crude metals, one or both of which contain arsenic as an impurity. Exposure to arsine occurs mainly in an occupational setting where the gas is accidentally formed during industrial processes involving mining, smelting, refining, soldering, galvanizing, and to a lesser extent during use of the gas itself. Arsine poisoning has been also reported during the use of herbicides containing arsenic compounds, and also in home circumstances where arsine is created by fungal action in paints, wallpaper, and mattresses that contained arsenic compounds. Arsine intoxication is often unexpected, since even very small amounts of arsenic can produce dangerous quantities of arsine. The preferred biomarker of exposure to arsine is urine. It was estimated that total arsenic concentrations in urine in excess of $50\ \mu g\ l^{-1}$ ($0.67\ \mu mol\ l^{-1}$) corresponded with arsine concentrations in the air above $15.6\ \mu g\ m^{-3}$. Other biomarkers, which however are nonspecific for arsine, include arsenic concentration in blood, hair, and nails.

Environmental Exposure (Monitoring Data in Air, Water, Sediment, Soil, and Biota)

Data on the occurrence of arsine per se in any of the environmental compartments is not available.

Toxicokinetics

Following inhalation, arsine is absorbed through the lungs. Since the gas is lipid soluble, it easily crosses the alveolar and

 http://dx.doi.org/10.1016/B978-0-12-386454-3.00005-1

capillary membranes of the lungs. Due to water solubility (20 ml per 100 ml at 20 °C) arsine pulmonary retention time is short compared with insoluble arsenic compounds. Arsine easily passes into the blood circulation where its concentration increases rapidly. Distribution to the liver, kidneys, spleen, and other organs is much slower. After absorption, arsine is oxidized to trivalent arsenic and pentavalent arsenic. Trivalent arsenic is subsequently methylated to monomethylarsonate and dimethylarsinate. Arsine as water-soluble gas is rapidly excreted in the form of metabolites via urine. The highest urinary excretion occurs within the first 24 h (about 60% of absorbed arsenic) following an acute exposure to arsine. Half-life of arsine in humans is 2–4 days.

Mechanism of Toxicity

Arsine acts predominantly as a hemolytic agent. Hemolysis appears to be dependent on membrane disruption as a result of arsine reactions with sulfhydryl groups and from formation of hydrogen peroxide and adducts with oxyhemoglobin. Failure of the kidneys and other organs is probably not only due to the effects of red blood cell debris slugging within the microcirculation but also to a direct toxic effect on the organs.

Acute and Short-Term Toxicity

Animal

The acute lethal effect of arsine is dose- and time-dependent. The longer the exposure time, the lower the lethal concentration 50% (LC_{50}) values. The rat LC_{50} values for exposure for 0.5, 1 and h are 777.6 mg m^{-3} (240 ppm), 576.72 mg m^{-3} (178 ppm), and 145.6 mg m^{-3} (45 ppm), respectively. Among test animals, mice appear to be the most sensitive to arsine. The 10 min LC_{50} values for rats, rabbits, and mice are 390 mg m^{-3} (120 ppm), 650 mg m^{-3} (200 ppm), 250 mg m^{-3} (77 ppm), respectively. Arsine toxicity involves mainly erythrocytes and the hematopoietic system. The main effect of acute toxicity is hemolysis, which was found in *in vivo* and *in vitro* studies. Results of blood tests of female mice conducted 24 h after exposure for 1 h in the range of concentrations: 16.2–84.2 mg m^{-3} (5–26 ppm) revealed a linear decrease in hematocrit with increasing gas concentration, a decrease in the number of erythrocytes, significant increases in circulating reticulocytes, changes in osmotic fragility, and an increase in leukocyte levels. An increase in relative spleen weights was found in mice exposed to 1.6, 8.1, and 16 mg m^{-3} (0.5, 2.5, 5 ppm) for 6 h.

Human

Arsine is a nonirritating gas. In acute exposure, it acts as a strong hemolytic agent, which can lead to death due to damage to the kidneys and other organs. The lethal effect of arsine is dependent on the level and duration of exposure. Exposure to 9.72–32.4 mg m^{-3} (3–10 ppm) may induce symptoms within a few hours; a concentration of 32.4–194.4 mg m^{-3} (10–60 ppm) may exert a hazardous effect within 30–60 min and a concentration of 810 mg m^{-3} (250 ppm) is immediately fatal. Since the odor of arsine is detectable only at a concentration of 1.6 mg m^{-3} (0.5 ppm) and above, and arsine is not irritating, the affected person may not feel discomfort during exposure. The latency period ranges from 0.5 to several hours after exposure. The longer and higher the level of the exposure, the shorter the latency period. First symptoms include headache, weakness, chills, fever, difficulty breathing, tachycardia, chest pain, abdominal pain, muscle pain, pale skin, nausea, and diarrhea. During breathing, the smell of garlic can occur. Within a few hours after exposure, discoloration of urine up to a port wine hue and unusual slate-bronze skin color may be observed. Hematuria is usually found 4–6 h after exposure, followed by oliguria and anuria, and less frequently, proteinuria. Jaundice is usually seen within 24–48 h after exposure. In addition, enlargement and tenderness of the liver and spleen, and costovertebral angle tenderness may occur. Vertical white lines on the nails (Mees' lines) can be observed 2–3 weeks after exposure. The most commonly described clinical symptom of arsine poisoning is hemolytic anemia with intensity depending on the concentration and time of exposure. Blood testing shows increased white blood cell count and free hemoglobin, and variation in the size and shape of red blood cells, Heinz bodies, and ghost cells, which demonstrates the ongoing damage to erythrocytes. Within a few days after exposure, signs of central nervous system disorders may develop, such as anxiety, memory impairment, confusion, and, within 1–2 weeks, signs of peripheral nerve damage. Dermal contact with liquefied compressed gas may result in frostbite injury. There are no data available on the toxic effects of arsine on the skin and eyes.

Chronic Toxicity

Animal

The effects of chronic arsine toxicity in animals are similar to those observed in acute toxicity and relate to erythrocytes and the hematopoietic system, including splenomegaly and hemolytic anemia, indicated by decreases in erythrocyte count, hematocrit, and hemoglobin concentration as well as increase in the leukocyte level, and the appearance of Heinz bodies in erythrocytes.

Other effects include alterations in immune system function that have been noted in animals exposed for prolonged periods of time. Although the reproductive and developmental toxicity has not been completely studied, studies on rats exposed to 8.1 mg m^{-3} (2.5 ppm) arsine for 6 h per day on gestation days 6–15 exhibited increased fetal body weight.

Human

Chronic exposure to very small concentrations of arsine may cause cumulative hemolytic damage leading to anemia. The degree of anemia is proportional to the duration of arsine exposure. Repeated exposure to arsine may also damage the kidney, liver, heart, and nervous system. The symptoms of chronic poisoning are similar to those observed in acute poisoning, except that the latency period from exposure to first symptoms is longer. The symptoms include intense focal headache, nausea, low-grade fever, paresthesia, anemia, hepatic and renal impairment, and characteristic fingernail changes (Mees' lines). A decrease in hemoglobin concentration and the presence of basophilic granulocytes in red blood cells are observed.

Reproductive Toxicity

Limited data are available on the reproductive and developmental effects of arsine in humans. A few occupational studies showed an increase in the rate of miscarriage among women who work in the semiconductor industry, in which arsine is used to produce microchips. However, due to exposure to multiple chemicals, it is not possible to assess clearly the role of arsine in the observed increase in rate of miscarriage.

Genotoxicity

Although there are no data available on the genotoxicity of arsine per se, data concerning other inorganic arsenic compounds indicate its genotoxicity.

Carcinogenicity

There are no human and animal data to assess the carcinogenicity of arsine per se. However, arsine decomposes in the body into compounds some of which are recognized by the International Agency for Research on Cancer as known human carcinogens (IARC Group 1); therefore, presently, an increase in the risk of cancer due to prolonged exposure to arsine cannot be excluded. ACGIH is of the opinion that arsine is unlikely to cause lung cancer due to its short pulmonary retention time compared with insoluble arsenic compounds but may present a systemic risk to other organs.

Clinical Management

In acute exposure, immediate medical assistance may be critical. The victim should be moved immediately to fresh air and away from the source of exposure. All persons suspected to be exposed to arsine should be transported to medical facilities for evaluation. Persons who experience the garlic odor should be transported first. Acute arsine exposure by humans is usually fatal without appropriate therapy. There is no antidote for arsine, but the effects can be treated.

No specific test is available for arsine exposure; however, arsine exposure may lead to detection of increased arsenic levels in urine ($>50\,\mu g\,l^{-1}$ for a spot test or $>50\,\mu g$ for a 24-h urine test) and signs of hemolysis (e.g., hemoglobinuria, anemia, and decreased haptoglobin) may indicate arsine poisoning. Initial therapy should be directed to supporting respiratory, vascular, and renal function. In the case of respiratory distress, the victim should receive oxygen. The use of diuretics to maintain urinary flow is an important consideration and should be performed under medical control. If hemolysis develops, urinary alkalization should be initiated. Hemodialysis should be considered if renal failure is severe. According to the NIOSH guidelines, treatment for severe acute arsine poisoning should include immediate blood exchange transfusion to replace hemolyzed red blood cells and remove arsine and hemoglobin–arsine complexes. Other blood purification methods include plasma exchange, which effectively removes toxins, fragments of red blood cells, and metabolites of arsine that accumulate in the blood and can cause serious damage to the kidneys and other organs. It is recommended to provide red blood cell exchange as soon as possible and, in addition, plasma exchange. Although BAL (British anti-Lewisite, dimercaprol) and other chelating agents are acceptable for arsenic poisoning, they are not effective antidotes for arsine poisoning and are not recommended. Administration of dimercaprol has no effect on arsine hemolysis, but it lowers blood arsenic levels resulting from arsine exposure. The use of chelators must be carefully evaluated due to their potential side effects. In case of contact with liquefied compressed gas, frosted skin should be gently washed with water; clothing should be gently removed from the affected area.

Other Hazards

Arsine and arsine gas/air mixtures are flammable and explosive and may be ignited by heat, sparks, or flames. The explosive limits (% by volume in air) are 4.5% (lower limit) and 78% (upper limit). The gas may travel along the ground and migrate to distant ignition sources and flash back. Arsine as a result of flow and agitation can cause generation of electrostatic charges. Arsine is stable at room temperature and begins to decompose to arsenic and hydrogen at about 230 °C with complete decomposition at about 300 °C. Arsine gives off arsenic oxides (posing a risk to health) in a fire that can accumulate or move with the wind in the form of dust. Arsine is a strong reducing agent and reacts vigorously with oxidizers such as potassium permanganate, sodium hypochlorite, oxygen, ozone, chlorine, fluorine, and nitric oxide. Arsine is not known to polymerize.

Exposure Standards and Guidelines

In many European countries (e.g., Austria, Belgium, France, Spain, Switzerland, United Kingdom) as well as in USA-OSHA, the TWA for an 8-h exposure has been established at the level of 0.05 ppm ($0.2\,mg\,m^{-3}$), taking into account mainly hemolytic properties of arsine (**Table 1**). In 2003, ACGIH placed the TLVs of arsine under revision, because OSHA, NTP, and IARC classified its metabolites (arsenic and arsenic compounds) as human carcinogens. Since 2007, ACGIH accepted 0.005 ppm ($0.016\,mg\,m^{-3}$) as the TLV-TWA (based mainly on the relationship between arsine inhalation in humans and the urinary arsenic concentrations). In support of these values, ACGIH indicated that compliance with this value should reduce the risk of hemolysis and hemolysis-related effects on spleen, liver, and kidney function. Due to lack of sufficient data, the substance was designated as A4-not classifiable as a human carcinogen. In Germany, due to an inadequate database, especially the lack of data on genotoxicity and carcinogenicity, the compound is listed in Section IIb of the list of MAK and BAT values that refer to substances for which no MAK value can be established at present. NIOSH has classified arsine as a potential occupational carcinogen.

Miscellaneous

Since the arsine odor threshold is about 10-fold higher than the TLV, it cannot be regarded as an adequate indicator of the

Table 1 Workplace hygiene standards for arsine

Agency/Country	*TLV-TWA*	*STEL*	*Other*
ACGIH	0.005 ppm (0.016 mg m^{-3})	n.e.	
NIOSH	n.e.	n.e.	IDLH: 3 ppm
NIOSH	n.e.	n.e.	Ceiling: 0.002 mg m^{-3} (15 min sampling period)
OSHA	0.05 ppm (0.2 mg m^{-3})	n.e.	PEL - TWA
European Union	n.e.	n.e.	
Austria	0.05 ppm (0.2 mg m^{-3})	0.25 ppm (1 mg m^{-3})	
Belgium	0.05 ppm (0.16 mg m^{-3})	n.e.	
Denmark	0.01 ppm (0.03 mg m^{-3})	0.02 ppm (0.06 mg m^{-3})	
France	0.05 ppm (0.2 mg m^{-3})	0.2 ppm (0.8 mg m^{-3})	
Germany (AGS)	0.005 ppm (0.016 mg m^{-3})	0.04 ppm (0.128 mg m^{-3})	
Germany (DFG)	substance for which no MAK values can be established at present		
Hungary	0.2 mg m^{-3}	0.8 mg m^{-3}	
Poland	0.02 mg m^{-3}	n.e.	
Spain	0.05 ppm (0.16 mg m^{-3})	n.e.	
Sweden	0.02 ppm (0.05 mg m^{-3})	n.e.	
Switzerland	0.05 ppm (0.16 mg m^{-3})	n.e.	
United Kingdom	0.05 ppm (0.16 mg m^{-3})	n.e.	

Abbreviations: ACGIH, American Conference of Governmental Industrial Hygienists; AGS, Ausschuss für Gefahrstoffe (Committee on Hazardous Substances); DFG, Deutsche Forschungsgemeinschaft (German Research Foundation); IARC, International Agency for Research on Cancer; IDLH, immediately dangerous to life or health; MAK, maximum concentration in workplace; NIOSH, US National Institute of Occupational Safety and Health; NTP, US National Toxicology Program; OSHA, US Occupational Safety and Health Administration; PEL, permissible exposure limit; STEL, short-term exposure; TLV-TWA, threshold limit value–time-weighted average; n.e. - not established.

presence of arsine in the air. Arsine is generally shipped in cylinders as a liquefied compressed gas.

See also: Kidney; Blood; Arsenic.

Further Reading

ACGIH, 2007. Documentation of Threshold Limit Values for Arsine. American Conference of Governmental Industrial Hygienists, Cincinnati (OH).

ACGIH, 2011. TLVs and BEIs. American Conference of Governmental Industrial Hygienists, Cincinnati (OH).

Ayala-Fierro, F., Barber, D.S., Rael, L.T., Carter, D.E., 1999. In vitro tissue specificity for arsine and arsenite toxicity in the rat. Toxicol. Sci. 52, 122–129.

Ayala-Fierro, F., Baldwin, A.L., Wilson, L.M., Valeski, J.E., Carter, D.E., 2000. Structural alterations in the rat kidney after acute arsine exposure. Lab. Investigation 80 (1), 87–97.

Hatlelid, K.M., Brailsford, C., Carter, D.E., 1996. Reactions of arsine and hemoglobin. J. Toxicol. Environ. Health 47 (2), 145–157.

International Agency for Research on Cancer, 1987. Arsine IARC Monographs on the Evaluation of Carcinogenic Risks on Humans, (Suppl. 7), Overall Evaluations of Carcinogenicity: An Updating of IARC Monographs Volumes 1 to 42, p. 100. Lyon, France: IARC.

Klimecki, W.T., Carter, D.E., 1995. Arsine toxicity: Chemical and mechanistic implications. J. Toxicol. Environ. Health 46, 399–409.

Mestrot, A., Merle, J.K., Broglia, A., Feldmann, J., Krupp, E.M., 2011. Atmospheric stability of arsine and methylarsines. Environ. Sci. Technol. 45 (9), 4010–4015.

Mestrot, A., Merle, J.K., Broglia, A., Feldmann, J., Krupp, E.M., 2011. Field fluxes and speciation of arsines emanating from soils. Environ. Sci. Technol. 45 (5), 1798–1804.

Pakulska, D., Czerczak, S., 2006. Hazardous effects of arsine: A short review. Int. J. Occup. Med. Environ. Health 19 (1), 36–44.

Rael, L.T., Ayala-Fierro, F., Carter, D.E., 2000. The effect of thiols and thiol-inhibitors compounds on arsine-induced toxicity in the human erythrocyte membrane. Toxicol. Sci. 55 (2), 468–477.

Song, Y., Wang, D., Li, H., Hao, F., Ma, J., Xia, Y., 2007. Severe acute arsine poisoning treated by plasma exchange. Clin. Toxicol. (Philadelphia) 45 (6), 721–727.

Winski, S.L., Barber, D.S., Rael, L.T., Carter, D.E., 1997. Sequence of toxic events in arsine-induced hemolysis in vitro: Implications for the mechanism of toxicity in human erythrocytes. Fund. Appl. Toxicol. 38, 123–128.

Relevant Websites

http://www.asiaiga.org/docs/AIGA%20050_08%20Code%20of%20Practice_Arsine.pdf – AIGA (Asia Industrial Gases Association) Globally Harmonized Document 050/08 (JIMGA-TS/36/08/E).

http://www.atsdr.cdc.gov/MHMI/mmg169.html – ATSDR Arsine, Agency for Toxic Substances & Disease Registry, Department of Health and Human Services.

http://bioterrorism.slu.edu/blood/quick/arsines.pdf – Chemical Terrorism Fact Sheet Blood Agents – Arsines (Arsenic Hydride, AsH3), A Division of Saint Louis University School of Public Health.

http://www.inchem.org/documents/cicads/cicads/cicad47.htm – CICAD (2002) Concise International Chemical Assessment Document 47, Arsine: Human Health Aspects, World Health Organization, Geneva.

http://www.epa.gov/oppt/aegl/pubs/results2.htm – EPA (Environmental Protection Agency) Arsine Results, Acute Exposure Guideline Levels.

http://bgia-online.hvbg.de/LIMITVALUE/WebForm_ueliste.aspx – GESTIS - International limit values for chemical agents.

http://www.hpa.org.uk/web/HPAwebFile/HPAweb_C/1202487024075 – HPA (Health Protection Agency) Compendium of chemical hazards: Arsine and Stibine.

http://www.inchem.org/documents/icsc/icsc/eics0222.htm – ICSC: 0222, Arsine (ICSC), International Chemical Safety Cards, The International Programme on Chemical Safety.

http://monographs.iarc.fr/ENG/Monographs/vol23/volume23.pdf – IARC Monograph "Arsenic and Arsenic Compounds".

http://emedicine.medscape.com/article/833740-workup – Medscape. Arsine Poisoning Workup.

http://www.cdc.gov/Niosh/npg/npgd0040.html – NIOSH (2011) Pocket Guide to Chemical Hazards, Arsine, The National Institute for Occupational Safety and Health.

Arts, Crafts, Theater, and Entertainment

M Rossol, NY, USA

This article is a revision of the previous edition article by Angelique Dosh, volume 1, pp 176–178, © 2005, Elsevier Inc.

Introduction/background

Arts and crafts work clearly has been a part of human history since before the walls of caves were painted and before stone, wood, and pottery items were handcrafted. This tradition only faltered during the industrial revolution when mass production methods eliminated the need for hand-made household furnishings and when photography made it unnecessary for artists to depict real people and places.

Then a late nineteenth century English poet and artist, William Morris, articulated a philosophy stressing the importance of the dignity and humanity of the work of craftsmen. Widely considered the founder of the Arts and Crafts Movement, his philosophy affected nearly every aspect of household design from architecture to pottery and continues to do so. Today, public and private educational institutions, at nearly all levels, are likely to teach painting, drawing, printmaking, photography (chemical and/or digital), ceramics, and wood working. Schools with strong art programs may have sculpture programs that offer welding, casting bronze and iron, plastic resin work, and stone carving. College craft classes may include jewelry, textile dying and weaving, glass blowing, stained glass, book binding, lead type setting, and more. Graduates from these schools often set up small cottage industries or home studios. A few will become major figures in the art world with scores of employees doing the actual production of their sculptures, glass, prints, or other art works.

In addition, many ethnic groups in underdeveloped countries and indigenous people in industrial countries engage heavily in art and craft production both to raise their economic status and to keep their traditions alive. Ethnic and folk art are widely represented at the highest levels of gallery and auction art sales.

But whether in a developing country or in a prestigious university graduate art program, traditional arts and crafts still involve materials, equipment, and processes that were used hundreds or even thousands of years ago. Some of these processes involve highly toxic substances. For example, all countries exempt art and craft paints from the consumer regulations that restrict the lead content of household paints. It is recognized worldwide that lead and many other toxic metal-containing pigments are required if painted art objects are to remain unfaded over decades or centuries.

A new source of art materials is also being exploited worldwide in arts and crafts. Sometimes lauded as recycling, artists use trash, found objects, and junk yard refuse. For example, galleries exhibit baskets woven from discarded brightly colored, lead-filled, vinyl-coated telephone cable wires. Other examples include jewelry cast from the lead and cadmium solder alloys melted out of old computer parts and sculptures cut from aluminum cans.

Both modern and ancient industrial process are used by artists and craftspeople from universities to cottage industries. They use machines to shape wood, plastics, and stone, they weld and braze, they cast bronze and iron in small foundries, they blacksmith, blow glass, cast plastic resins, and more. (Some new industrial art processes involve relatively hazard-free computer art and digital photography methods. These are not covered in this article.)

The challenge for the toxicologist is to understand that the catalog of art and craft materials is essentially endless. Detailed lists of materials and equipment used should be solicited from patients who are artists or craftspeople. And every nonartist patient should be asked about their hobbies and the art or craft activities of other household members.

Toxicity of Art Materials

Inorganic Pigments and Colorants

About half of the pigments in all adult art materials are inorganic, meaning they are metal compounds or minerals. These commonly contain lead, cadmium, chromium, cobalt, mercury, manganese, antimony, titanium, copper, and zinc. This includes the pigments in oils, acyclics, watercolors, printmaking inks, and even colored pencils.

Ceramic glazes and metal enamel colorants are based on the same metals except that these colorants may also contain a wider variety of metals including nickel, selenium, vanadium (yellow), and rare earth metals (e.g., lanthium, tantalum). Stained glass is colored with the same metals but also may include significant percentages of arsenic (in some opaque whites) and small amounts of uranium (dichroic or carnival glass). Fluxes, which are substances that are used to affect the temperature at which ceramic glazes, metal enamels, and glass fuse or melt, commonly contain lead, barium, lithium, boron, sodium, and potassium.

Organic Pigments and Dyes

There are roughly 2000 commercially available organic pigments and dyes, any of which may be used in art materials and craft textile dyes. Only a relative handful of these organic colorants have ever been studied for toxicity. Many should be assumed to be carcinogens based on their structure. Included are those based on aniline (Chemical Abstracts Service Registry Number (CAS) 62-53-3), benzidine (CAS 92-87-5), 3,3′-dichlorobenzidine (CAS 91-94-1), *o*-toluidine (CAS 95-53-4), and anthraquinone (CAS 84-65-1). Some artists derive their dyes and pigments from natural sources. The toxicity of a colorant is not related to its origins and many toxic colorants (e.g., anthraquinones) are found in nature.

Exposure to Pigments and Dyes

The mere presence of toxic pigments, dyes, metal compounds, or minerals in an art material is not significant unless exposure to them occurs. This is most likely when powdered materials are used, drawings are made with dusty chalk-like pastels, dry paint is sanded or burned, or paints and dyes are air-brushed or sprayed. Exposure to ceramic glaze chemicals during use is almost inevitable because the glazes dry to a powder when applied and dust usually is found throughout glazing areas. Exposure to glass pigments can occur when pieces are shaped by grinding dry (a dust) or wet (creates an airborne mist). Both glass and ceramic glaze metals can become airborne as invisible fumes when heated in kilns or furnaces and can subsequently settle on surfaces in the studio.

However, even without obvious exposure scenarios, the use of toxic art materials in homes or living spaces can be assumed to provide significant exposure over time.

Solvents and Exposure

Exposure to solvents by inhalation is unavoidable during use since they evaporate into the air. Some also absorb through the skin. Many different solvents are used in arts and crafts. Traditional art painting, for example, commonly involves various petroleum distillates or turpentine (CAS 8006-64-2). The toxicity of these materials can vary widely from highly refined aliphatic petroleum distillates with an American Conference of Governmental Industrial Hygienists (ACGIH) threshold limit value (TLV)-time-weighted average (TWA) in the range of 300 ppm to more toxic and sensitizing solvents such as turpentine with a TLV-TWA of 20 ppm.

Hundreds of other solvents are used as diluents, carriers, degreasers, and cleaners. The most common types are ketones, aromatic hydrocarbons, alcohols, amines, and glycol ethers. In addition, some exotic solvents are used such as pine oil (alpha-pinene, CAS 80-56-8) and citrus oil (D-limonene, CAS 5989-27-5, DFG MAK 20 ppm). Toxicologists should note that these natural solvents may have lower TLVs than most synthetic ones.

Oils and Waxes

Many art processes involve oils and waxes such as in oil-based paints, wax resists in ceramics and batik textile dyeing, lost wax casting, and encaustic painting in which wax is the vehicle or binder in which the pigments are suspended. These oils and waxes release toxic decomposition products when heated or burned including aldehydes such as acrolein (CAS 107-02-8), formaldehyde (CAS 50-00-0), and a host of hydrocarbons.

Plastic Resins

Common two-component plastic products used primarily in sculpture or crafts include (1) polyester resins that contain styrene (CAS 100-42-5, TLV-TWA 20 ppm) and are cured with organic peroxides; (2) acrylates; (3) epoxy resins often cured with complex amines and diluted with diglycidyl ethers; and (4) two-component urethane products cured with diisocyanates (TLV-TWA 0.005 ppm). These monomers, curing agents, and diluents are often highly toxic. Sensitization reactions such as allergic dermatitis and asthma are well known to be associated with amine curing agents and isocyanates.

Preformed plastic sheets and foam are also machined and hot-wire cut into shapes. The burning plastics release hundreds of chemicals including the monomers and additives such as phthalates and chlorinated and brominated fire retardants. The very popular vinyl polymer hand-molded clays use to make jewelry and small objects contain between 3 and 25% free phthalates. The users are exposed to phthalates by skin contact during forming and by inhalation when they are driven off into the air when they are heated in kitchen ovens as the product literature directs. (Hidden Hazards: Health Impacts of Toxins in Polymer Clays, commissioned by the Vermont Public Interest Research Group. It can be obtained by visiting the Web site http://www.vpirg.org or writing to VPIRG, 141 Main Street, Suite 6, Montpelier, VT 05602, USA.)

Metals

Common metal products used include lead solders for crafts and stained glass, cadmium-fluxed silver and gold solders, nickel–silver casting alloys, beryllium/copper alloys still found in some sculpture and jewelry alloys, and a host of complex alloys used in bronze, brass, white metals, and more. Artists machining or welding junk metals may inadvertently be exposed to toxic alloys and solders never intended for art or craft processes.

Minerals

Ceramics, stone and lapidary carving, and glass work involve exposure to minerals. Silica is present in most minerals and clays. Asbestos can contaminate some industrial talcs used in ceramics, steatites, and soap stones used in sculpture, one form of jade (nephrite), serpentine, and some vermiculites. Lead is a common contaminant in sculpture stones such as dolomite. Uranium and other radioactive metals are present in some granites. Toxicologists whose patients are exposed to stone dusts need to identify the source since their composition varies significantly from quarry to quarry.

Photochemicals

Traditional black and white photography is still done in many art schools. It involves the use of developers such as hydroquinone, acetic acid to stop the reaction, and chemical washes to clean and harden the print. Most of the liquid chemical baths also contain sulfite preservatives. The resulting airborne darkroom chemicals commonly include sulfur dioxide from the preservatives, acetic acid, and formaldehyde from some hardeners. Some types of photo resists and film cleaners also contain solvents.

Toning is also done in which silver is replaced with other metals. Some toners give off hydrogen sulfide and involve chemicals such as selenium, chromium, palladium, and uranium.

Historic photo processes are also taught in many schools. These may use dichromates, ferri-and ferrocyanides, silver nitrate (CAS 7761-88-8), mercury compounds, and more.

Other Processes and Materials

Art and craft processes also include woodworking, leather working, welding and foundry work, and anodizing and cyanide plating (see sections on wood dust, various metals, cyanide plating chemicals). Toxicologists should consider that the exposures can be exacerbated by the close quarters and poor ventilation often found in the artist's studio, cottage industry, or school art department.

Ceramic kilns, glass and foundry furnaces, welding torches, forges, and other high-heat processes can expose workers to combustion gases and decomposition byproducts, metal fumes, infrared radiation, and heat.

Legislation

In the 1980s, consumer labels in most countries only required warnings on products capable of causing acute effects as determined by lethal dose 50% (LD_{50}) and lethal concentration 50% (LC_{50}) animal tests. For example, these tests were required under the United States Federal Hazardous Substances Act and the Canadian Federal Hazardous Products Act. Since these acute animal tests do not detect chronic effects, products with significant chronic hazards commonly were not labeled with warnings. Even products containing powdered asbestos could be sold without warnings. For example, asbestos-containing products such as instant paper maches and clays, even for children, were routinely labeled as nontoxic in the United States.

The gross inadequacy of the laws in the United States resulted in the passing of the Labeling of Hazardous Art Materials Act (LHAMA) in 1988. LHAMA requires warning labels on products containing known chronically hazardous substances. This law applies to "any raw or processed material, or manufactured product, marketed or represented by the producer or repackager as intended for and suitable for users ..." These users are defined as "artists or crafts people of any age who create, or recreate in a limited number, largely by hand, works which may or may not have a practical use, but in which esthetic considerations are paramount" [16 Code of Federal Regulations 1500.14(b)(8)(i)(B)(1) and (2)]. This broad definition means the law is applied to paints, inks, marking pens, pencils, ceramic clays and glazes, metals and solders intended for jewelry making, face paints for children, and much more.

The LHAMA requires a toxicologist to assess the potential hazards of a list of ingredients provided by the manufacturer and to determine which specific label warnings, if any, are needed to provide sufficient information for consumers to use the product safely. The rules for this process were developed in a standard of the American Society for Testing and materials (ASTM D 4236) which was incorporated into the law. However, the manufacturer pays the toxicologist for certification that the product is properly labeled which creates a conflict of interest. As a result, LHAMA has serious deficiencies:

1. Substances requiring labeling must be known to possess chronic hazards. Yet most organic pigments and dyes used in art materials have never been tested for chronic hazards. In this case, the toxicologist can label these untested products as nontoxic by default, even if the product contains ingredients that are in chemical classes suspected to cause cancer.
2. A powerful impetus to label products as nontoxic exists due to a common public school practice of requiring nontoxic labels as a condition of purchase. A toxicologist who chooses not to allow the nontoxic label on potentially hazardous art material will exclude their client's products from the lucrative school market.
3. Some tests used by certifying toxicologists to determine toxicity are faulty. For example, a test in which materials are placed in acid is sometimes used to determine if the toxic substances in the product will be released in the digestive tract (ASTM D 5517). This test does not consider that, in addition to acid and water, digestive tracts use bases, enzymes, cellular activities, heat, and movement to dissolve materials. Only after there were poisonings and a death from accidental ingestion of lead ceramic glazes labeled as nontoxic were these tests abandoned by certifying toxicologists. Acid tests are still used to evaluate some other types of art products.
4. Faulty methods are used by some toxicologists to estimate exposures during art making. They often do not consider the artist's intimate contact with their materials, crowded classrooms, tiny home studios, poor ventilation, lack of sinks, and other conditions common to home studios and schools.
5. The hazards of materials used in ways other than the label directs are not considered. Artists and teachers traditionally use materials creatively. For example, melting crayons for candle making or batik fabric resists causes these nontoxic products to release highly toxic gases and fumes from decomposition of the wax and from some of the pigments.
6. Consumers and even consulting toxicologists (unless they sign a confidentiality agreement) cannot easily find out what chemicals are in US art materials. Instead, they are told that a toxicologist has evaluated the product and determined that exposure will not be significant if the product is used as directed. The material safety data sheets also usually are not helpful. While they are supposed to list toxic materials in amounts over 1.0% or carcinogens in amounts over 0.1% by weight, they usually refer instead to the toxicologist's certification.

It is clear that in the United States, consumers and consulting toxicologists would be better served by proper material safety data sheets than laws such as LHAMA. And if the United Nations' Globally Harmonized Safety Data Sheet format is adopted worldwide, the disclosure of potentially toxic substances in art materials should be greatly improved.

Theatrical and Entertainment Materials

Many art and craft materials are also used by theater and entertainment workers. Scenic artists paint sets, dye huge back drops, sculpt, and cast plastics. Set construction is done with carpentry and welding. Designers of costumes and sets may use water colors, markers, or oils to depict their concepts. Costume makers and wardrobe attendants work with textiles, fabric dyes and paints, detergents, and flame retardants. Prop makers work with thrift shop and junk materials, and all manner of paints, plastics, wood, textiles, and adhesives. One major difference is that sets and props are not designed to last hundreds of years. This means they can be painted with ordinary consumer paints or theatrical paints that are based on common polymer latex paints, rather than toxic archival art materials.

However, there are some exposure to materials that are completely unique to theater and entertainment workers. Two of these are make up and atmospheric special effects.

Makeup

A number of studies show that beauticians and cosmetologists suffer a higher incidence of health problems (see Cosmetics and Personal Care Products). No similar studies have been made of diseases of theatrical makeup artists, but it is clear that they are exposed to some of the same chemicals. In addition, they are exposed to the solvents, minerals, dyes and pigments, and preservatives.

Inhalation of makeup ingredients

Face powders, makeup, and rouges are likely to contain minerals such as talc, kaolin (and other clays), chalk (CAS 1317-65-3), zinc oxide (CAS 1314-13-2), titanium dioxide (CAS 13463-67-7), mica, and bismuth oxychloride (CAS 7787-59-9). These minerals are usually harmless by skin contact or ingestion. However, air-brushing of cosmetics is commonly done in theater and the inhalation route cannot be discounted by toxicologists.

Airbrush applicators cannot control the fine airbrush mist to specific areas of the face or insure that none of the mist is inhaled by the client and the makeup artist. Dressing rooms in which large numbers of performers or chorus members are being made up can be seen to have a foggy atmosphere from airbrush overspray.

There are standards for exposure by inhalation in most countries limiting worker exposure to talc, kaolin, and titanium dioxide. These minerals are likely to be present in nanoparticle size in cosmetics, which is generally recognized as a more toxic form. For example, the National Institute for Occupational Safety and Health (NIOSH) has set two different recommended exposure limits (RELs) for titanium dioxide: 2.4 $mg\,m^{-3}$ for respirable particles and 0.3 $mg\,m^{-3}$ for nanoparticles. There may be additional hazards from inhaled pigments, dyes, and preservatives in make up that might be considered.

Special effect makeup

Putty, wax, beeswax, and morticians' wax can all be used to build up a part of the face for theatrical purposes. Collodion (CAS 9004-70-0) can be used to fake age or scars. Natural rubber latex can be made to function in many of these ways, and it also acts as a glue or adhesive, as does spirit gum. Spirit is a term applied to alcohol solvents (usually ethyl alcohol) and gum can mean any exudate of a number of plants or trees. Spirit gums today are usually a mixture of natural and synthetic resins.

As the need for extremely complex special effects makeup including whole head masks and prostheses increases, two-component urethane and other resins may be used by make up artists. These are often used in shops and studios that are not sufficiently ventilated to preclude exposure to the monomers and curing agents. Many people are allergic to some components of these products. Others may have reactions to removal of the spirit gums or masks when they are pulled off the skin or by the solvents used to clean the skin afterward.

Atmospheric Special Effects

Atmospheric fog, smoke, and haze (an effect that is only seen when strong lights beam through them) are unique theatrical hazards. No other industry deliberately pollutes the air of its workers or the air breathed by its customers (the audience). And some of the workers are dancers and singers who are actually highly trained athletes whose inhalation risks are increased by their activities. Performers may also be children or the elderly. Audience members can also include people with disabilities and respiratory illnesses.

Most of the chemical mist aerosols used for these effects are in the range of 10 to 1 μm in diameter and highly respirable. There are three primary types used today: the glycols (including glycerin), mineral oils, and cryogenic gases.

Glycols

These are also called dihydric alcohols except for glycerin, which is a trihydric alcohol. Chemicals used in these effects may include

- ethylene glycol (CAS 107-21-1, used primarily in the past)
- diethylene glycol (CAS 111-46-6)
- butylene glycols (1,2-, 1,3-, and 1,4-butanediol, CAS 584-03-2, 107-88-0, 110-63-4)
- triethylene glycol (CAS 112-27-6)
- polyethylene glycol (E 200, made by Dow Chemical, used in the past)
- polypropylene glycols (not commonly used)
- mono-propylene glycol (propylene glycol; 1,2-propandiol, CAS 57-55-6)
- dipropylene glycols (CAS 25265-71-8, 110-98-5, 108-61-2)
- glycerin (glycerol; 1,2,3-propanediol, CAS 56-81-5)

All these glycols and glycerine are hygroscopic and can dry and irritate the skin and cause pain and redness in the eyes. It is presumed this quality is also the reason there is a high incidence of acute laryngitis and tracheitis among performers in a study of Actor's Equity performers. Asthma may also be related to exposure. Two case reports of occupational asthma either caused by or exacerbated by glycol theatrical fog in an opera singer and a stage hand were also reported in 1996 by the New Jersey Department of Health. Another study found reduced levels of lung function (both forced expiratory volume in 1 s (FEV_1) and forced vital capacity (FVC)) associated with working within 10 feet of the fog machine, and both acute and chronic upper airway irritation associated with increased exposure to both glycol and oil mist effects. (The 99-page report to Safety and Health in Arts, Production, and Entertainment (SHAPE, now renamed ActSafe) by the University of British Columbia School of Occupational and Environmental Hygiene provides data on the size of the aerosols, the concentrations workers in different jobs experienced, and health effects. The health effects included reduced levels of lung function (both FEV_1 and FVC) associated with working within 3 m of the fog machine, and both acute and chronic upper airway irritation associated with increased exposure to both the glycol and oil mist fogs. Some effects were observed at concentrations below the ACGIH TLV for oil mist or the standard set for glycols by the American National Standard Institute (ANSI) standards.)

Glycerine mist has an ACGIH TLV-TWA of 10 mg m^{-3} to protect workers from physical irritation of the upper respiratory tract. Propylene glycol has a Workplace Environmental Exposure Limit TWA of 10 mg m^{-3} set by the American Industrial Hygiene Association. There is not enough data on most of the other glycols to set limits.

Petroleum distillates and oils

Many types of oils and petroleum-derived chemicals have been used over the years. Most of the flammable neurotoxic distillates are no longer used. They have been replaced by higher molecular weight oils such as the following:

- Mineral oils of various grades such as white mineral oil, cosmetic, medicinal, and food grades (e.g., baby oil). In the past, industrial grades (e.g., cutting oils) were used.
- Kerosene and various grades of fuel oil (e.g., no. 2 fuel oil used in the 1980s).
- Vegetable oils (are used but are not common).

Some grades of fuel and cutting oils can contain significant amounts of toxic impurities. Even very refined, nontoxic mineral oils (baby oil) can cause effects by inhalation. While refined mineral oil can be safely ingested (used as a laxative) and is soothing to the skin, inhalation of large amounts can cause life-threatening chemical pneumonia. The ACGIH TLV-TWA for respirable highly refined oil mists is 5 mg m^{-3}.

Vegetable oils can cause allergies in some people and they can cause the same irritant effects as petroleum oils.

Cryogenic gases and water

The two most common cryogenic fogs use carbon dioxide (dry ice) and liquid nitrogen. In some cases, other inert gases such as argon are used. They all rely on the extreme coldness of either the ice or gases when first released from compressed gas cylinders to create fog by condensing water vapor from the air. Wherever this water-mist fog is found, high levels of the cryogenic gas are present. Inadequate stage and orchestra pit ventilation used with these effects has caused adverse effects on the breath control of musicians and singers.

Liquid air fog, a combination of liquid nitrogen and liquid oxygen, is being used in some new applications. This product will eliminate the oxygen deprivation problem. However, there is a risk that the nitrogen, which boils at a lower temperature than oxygen, will boil off first leaving the oxygen. High levels of oxygen released from such a machine can create a fire hazard.

Water mists are also used, especially for outdoor venues. The water must not be left standing before use or inhalation of disease-causing microorganisms can occur. Fresh potable water that is high in minerals may also produce an irritating dust as the mist dries in the air.

Real smoke

Even in countries where it is banned, smoking is usually permitted on stage. Some performers smoke herbal cigarettes instead. From a scientific standpoint, all types of cigarettes are health hazards. It is the chemicals released from burning leaves that cause cancer, not nicotine. All burning hydrocarbons release cancer-causing and toxic substances. Substances used to create smoke on stage or on movie locations outdoors include

- frankincense (olibanum gum, bee smokers)
- rosin
- charcoal
- paper
- naphthalene (CAS 91-20-3) and anthracene (CAS 120-12-7) used outdoors for black smoke
- rubber tires (used outdoors)
- lead azide (CAS 13424-46-9) for fake car explosions with a black smoke

Inorganic chloride fumes

Most of these chloride products were developed originally to study airflow patterns in ventilation systems. They were never intended for theatrical purposes. Nevertheless, these products are still being used by some special effects people. The products may include

- ammonium chloride (CAS 12125-02-9)
- titanium tetrachloride (CAS 7550-45-0) outdoor use, highly irritating
- zinc chloride (CAS 7646-85-7)
- calcium chloride (CAS 10043-52-4), tin chloride (CAS 7789-67-5), and other chlorides

Dusts and powders

These are often used to simulate conditions such as after an earthquake, explosion, or dust storm. Currently, the following types of dusts are used in theatrical and film productions. Mineral dusts such as fuller's earth, vermiculite, and talc are used. Some of these products contain respirable silica, which can cause lung damage, asbestos (tremolite), or other fibrous minerals (attapulgite in some fuller's earth) that are associated with asbestos-like diseases. In 1998, a New York union camera operator was overexposed repeatedly for 2 days on a film location to fuller's earth and developed a partially disabling fibrotic lung condition for which workers compensation was obtained.

Organic dusts such as wood dust, wheat and other grain flours, and starch have also been used. The organic dusts are likely to cause irritation and allergies. Wood dust should never be used since it is sensitizing, toxic, and most wood dusts have a TLV-TWA of 1 mg m^{-3}. Baker's asthma is a well-known occupational disease that affects people exposed to flour.

Pyrotechnic smoke

Theatrical pyrotechnics are potentially capable of creating ear-damaging sound, eye-damaging light, and airborne toxic chemicals in their smoke. Hundreds of chemicals can be used in indoor and outdoor pyrotechnics. Each chemical has one or more function in the chemical reactions that occur on combustion. Most common pyrotechnic mixtures consist of an oxidizer, a fuel, a source of carbon, and various additives such as chlorine donors to enhance color and other chemicals to modify appearance or sound.

Compounds such as oxides and chlorides of almost any metal in the periodic table can be present in pyrotechnic emissions. Indoor pyrotechnics should not use the most toxic metals such as arsenic, mercury, and lead, but outdoor effects commonly contain these and other toxic metals.

The metals most often found in dust left from pyrotechnics include compounds of potassium, titanium, sulfur, calcium, iron, and aluminum. These are alkaline in nature and irritate the respiratory system. Silicon oxides are often present as well.

In addition to metal compounds, gases such as sulfur oxides, nitrogen oxides, chlorine, and hydrochloric acid, and many other irritating gases can be present. Carbon monoxide and carbon dioxide are also present.

Legislation and Standards

Almost every country has occupational regulations that apply to worker exposure of one or more of these chemicals. However, enforcement is rarely seen in this industry. However, some theatrical unions ban or restrict the use of certain effects.

Standards have been set for exposure to the glycol and oil mist fogs by the Entertainment Services Technology Association (ESTA). (ESTA has merged with the PLASA, formerly known as the Professional Lighting And Sound Association, and their joint standards can be found at http://www.plasa.org/standards/.) These standards have now been granted approval by the ANSI and assigned the following numbers:

- ANSI E1.23 – 2006: Design and Execution of Theatrical Fog Effects [includes recommendations for use of glycols, glycerin, mineral oils, nitrogen, oxygen and carbon dioxide fog];
- ANSI E1.5 – 2003: Entertainment Technology - Theatrical Fog Made With Aqueous Solutions of Di- And Trihydric Alcohols;
- ANSI E1.29-2009: Product Safety Standard for Theatrical Fog Generators [that use water, glycol, glycerin, or mineral oil].

The standards require monitoring or other precautions to insure that glycol TWAs are below 10 mg m^{-3} and oil TWAs are below 5 mg m^{-3}. ESTA is currently working on a standard for dust effects. It is unlikely that these standards are being followed in most productions.

The National Fire Protection Association (NFPA) has applicable standards for pyrotechnics and flame effects:

- NFPA 1126: Standard for the Use of Pyrotechnics Before a Proximate Audience;
- NFPA 160: Standard for the Use of Flame Effects Before a Proximate Audience.

These standards only address safety hazards. For example, the only mention of smoke in NFPA 1126 is that it should not be do dense that it obscures exit signs.

Other Theatrical Hazards

New technology applied to theatrical production has introduced lasers, holographs, black lights, strobe lights, ear-damaging sound levels and more. Some of these have adverse effects on performers.

See also: Acrolein; Asbestos; Benzidine; Cadmium; Cosmetics and Personal Care Products; Glycol Ethers; Limonene; Metals; Phthalates; Talc; Toluidines; Turpentine; Wood Dusts.

Further Reading

Dement, J.M., Zurnwalde, R.D., Garnbel, J.F., et al., 1980. NIOSH Technical Report: Occupational Exposure to Talc Containing Asbestos (Morbidity, Mortality, and Environmental Studies of Miners and Millers. NIOSH.

Rossol, M., 2001. The Artist's Complete Health and Safety Guide, third ed. Allworth Press, New York (4th edition expected 2012).

Rossol, M., 2011. The Health & Safety Guide for Film, TV & Theater, second ed. Allworth Press, New York.

Arts and Toxicology *see* Toxicology in the Arts, Culture, and Imagination

Asbestos

M Lotti and L Bergamo, Università degli Studi di Padova, Padova, Italy

This article is a revision of the previous edition article by Xuannga Mahini, volume 1, pp 179–182, © 2005, Elsevier Inc.

Name, formula, and Chemical Abstracts Service Registry Number: Asbestos (1332-21-4); Serpentine group: Chrysotile (White Asbestos), $Mg_3(Si_2O_5)(OH)_4$ (12001-29-5); Amphibole group: Amosite (Grunerite or Brown Asbestos), $(MgFe^{2+})_7Si_8O_{22}(OH)_2$ (12172-73-5); Crocidolite (Blue Asbestos), $Na_2Fe^{3+}(MgFe^{2+})_3(Si_8O_{22})(OH)_2$ (12001-28-4); Tremolite, $Ca_2Mg_5Si_8O_{22}(OH)_2$ (14567-73-8); Actinolite, $Ca_2(MgFe^{2+})_5Si_8O_{22}(OH)_2$ (77536-66-4); Anthophyllite, $Mg_7(Si_8O_{22})(OH)_2$ (17068-78-9)

Background

Asbestos refers to a heterogeneous variety of fibrous hydrated silicate minerals subdivided into two groups differing in mineralogic properties and chemical composition: amphiboles and serpentines. The amphibole family (straight fibers) consists of crocidolite (blue asbestos), amosite, anthophyllite, and tremolite (brown asbestos). Crysotile (curved and flexible fibers, white asbestos) is the only serpentine and accounts for over 90% of all commercial asbestos. Mining of asbestos began toward the end of the nineteenth century in Canada, Australia, South Africa, and the United States and peaked in the 1970s of the following century when the greatest consumption occurred in the United States, United Kingdom, France, Australia, and other industrialized countries. Asbestos has been extensively manufactured because of its high tensile strength, flexibility, resistance to chemical and thermal degradation, and high electrical resistance, thus leading to a variety of occupational exposures. These included miners and millers and workers engaged in the production of materials made from asbestos, in construction and insulation industries, in shipyards, and others. Nonoccupational exposures also occurred including environmental and domestic ones. Exposures to asbestos fibers cause fibrotic and malignant diseases of the lung and pleura, including asbestosis, pleural plaques, and both lung and pleural cancers. Lung and pleural fibrosis were first associated with asbestos exposure during the 1930s, lung cancer after World War II, and pleural cancer in the 1960s.

Mining and consumption declined during the last decades of the twentieth century because of the awareness of the dangers of asbestos exposures. At first, there were stringent controls that led to the eventual banning of asbestos in most industrialized countries, although exposures may still occur occasionally, due to the large amount of insulation and construction materials left over from previous times. The disease of asbestosis is found very rarely nowadays in these countries, whereas asbestos-related malignancies are still encountered, due to the long latency from exposure to the onset of disease.

However, asbestos is still being mined in several countries such as Canada, Russia, and China, used locally, and also exported to countries in Asia, Africa, and the former Eastern bloc, where there is little or no regulation. Estimates of the World Health Organization indicate that 125 million people worldwide are currently exposed to asbestos.

Uses

Asbestos minerals have been used in over 3000 commercial applications. Asbestos may be present in insulation materials in factories, buildings such as schools and homes, ships, cement and sheeting, paint, brake linings and friction pads, railroad machinery, roofing materials, water pipes, and various appliances. In the past, asbestos was woven to manufacture fireproofing materials and even used in cigarette filters.

Environmental Behavior, Fate, Routes, and Pathways

Asbestos fibers are chemically inert and do not undergo significant degradation in the environment. Small diameter fibers can remain suspended in the air and water for a long time and can be transported by wind and water. Asbestos fibers are not able to move through the soil and are generally not broken down into other compounds in the environment.

Exposure and Exposure Monitoring

Inhalation is the principal route of exposure to asbestos. Other routes may include ingestion through food and drink or by swallowing inhaled asbestos cleared from the lungs. The sampling of asbestos fibers which are longer than 5 μm can be monitored in the air of the personal breathing zone. The sampling procedure consists in drawing volume of air (between 25 and 2400 l) through a cassette containing a mixed cellulose ester membrane filter. A phase-contrast microscope is used to recognize asbestos fibers and a transmission electron microscope (TEM) is used to distinguish from nonasbestos fibers. Scanning transmission electron microscope is less accurate than TEM for fiber detection. TEM is also used to count the fibers in lung tissue, bronchoalveolar lavage (BAL), and sputum.

Toxicokinetics

The most common route of entry into the body is by inhalation. The larger and curly shaped fibers are removed by the cilia of tracheobronchial tree, whereas fibers less than 10 μm in length can enter the distal respiratory airways. Here, smaller fibers may be engulfed by alveolar macrophages and transported to lymph nodes. Most fibers remain as they are or as asbestos bodies (ratio 5000–10 000:1), the latter resulting from the coating of fibers with hemosiderin and proteinaceous material. Amphibole fibers have a relatively small cross-sectional diameter with a needle-like shape and tend to be readily transported to the periphery of the lung. These characteristics are thought to account for the higher pathogenicity of amphiboles, as compared with that of chrysotile. In addition, the different toxicities of fibers also correlate with their persistence and clearance from the lung. The estimated half-life of crocidolite and amosite fibers in the lung is in the range of several years and that of chrysotile in the range of months.

Fibers are usually found at a higher concentration in the pleura than in the lung parenchyma, although they are not distributed homogeneously. There are also high concentrations of fibers in the anthracotic areas of the parietal pleura.

Fibers may also reach the peritoneum by direct translocation across the gut wall after ingestion or swallowing of the inhaled asbestos cleared from the lungs.

Mechanisms of Action

Certain physical and physicochemical properties of fibers, including shape, surface, structure, and chemical composition, relate to asbestos toxicities. Chemical differences such as the nature of cations present in the particles lead to differences in the overall shape and persistence of asbestos fibers in the lung.

It is not yet clear as to whether asbestos fibers have a direct carcinogenic effect on lung and pleural cells or if they cause cancer indirectly. Asbestos fibers cause inflammation and generate reactive oxygen and nitrogen species leading to fibrosis and DNA damage. Asbestos fibers cause mutations on certain chromosomes and aneuploidia, besides epigenetic effects such as changes in miRNA expression and DNA hypermethylation.

Acute and Short-Term Toxicity

Animal

Animals exposed to asbestos developed pleural mesothelioma. In rats exposed to high concentrations of asbestos for a short period (from 7 h up to 1 day, inhalation) or long period (up to 2 years) of time, similar mesothelioma incidence and latencies were observed. Rats with inhalation exposure to chrysotile for 90 days did not develop lung fibrosis at low asbestos concentrations, but slight lung fibrosis occurred at higher doses. Five-day inhalation studies conducted with tremolite and amosite describe the incidence of lung fibrosis in rats. Single dose intrapleural injection of asbestos in rats is able to produce mesotheliomas.

Human

Very short exposures to asbestos (a few months) may correlate with an increased risk in developing pleural plaques and mesothelioma decades later. Only in exceptional circumstances and after very high exposures, has there been a report of both asbestosis and lung cancer.

Chronic Toxicity

Animal

Lung fibrosis in many animal species (pigs, rats, hamsters, monkey) has been observed after chronic inhalation of both chrysotile and amphiboles. The incidence and the severity of the fibrosis are dose related. The disease is progressive after cessation of exposure. In rat studies, chrysotile asbestos and longer fibers (>5 μm) were more fibrogenic than shorter ones.

Human

Chronic exposures to asbestos fibers cause nonmalignant and malignant diseases of the lung and pleura. Asbestosis is a fibrosis of the lung interstitium that may occur after intense and prolonged exposures to all types of asbestos fibers. The most common respiratory symptom associated with asbestosis is insidious onset dyspnea, typically beginning on exertion. Cough, phlegm, and symptoms of chronic bronchitis are frequent by the time the disease progresses and symptoms are associated with an accelerated decline of ventilatory function. After cessation of exposure the disease may remain static or progress.

Pleural abnormalities associated with asbestos include acute pleural effusion, diffuse and circumscribed pleural thickening (pleural plaques), and rounded atelectasis. Exudative or hemorrhagic acute pleural effusions are rare and they could be asymptomatic or associated with fever and pleuritic pain. Pleuritis might result in diffuse pleural thickening and rounded atelectasis. Pleural plaques are indicators of past exposure to asbestos representing a result of localized inflammation. They are usually bilateral, localized at diaphragmatic pleura, and calcified, appearing with latency of more than 10 years and without relationship with the intensity and duration of exposure. Pleural plaques are asymptomatic and do not evolve into malignancy.

The clinical evaluation of nonmalignant asbestos-related diseases includes history of exposure, physical examination, chest imaging studies, and pulmonary function tests.

Plain chest X-ray could detect advanced asbestosis and pleural thickening. However, conventional computed tomography (CT) and high resolution CT scan are superior to chest films in identifying parenchymal lesions and pleural plaques. Honeycombing and the thickening of septa and interlobular fissures are characteristics of asbestosis and in order to grade both pneumoconiosis severity and pleural changes, films are classified by the International Labour Organization.

Lung function abnormalities in asbestosis are restrictive (reduction of all lung volumes), although signs of airway obstruction are often observed, possibly due to concurrent exposures to smoking and irritants or to asbestos itself. Restrictive abnormalities can also be detected in cases of diffuse pleural thickening, whereas pleural plaques are usually not associated with changes in lung function. Detection of asbestos bodies and fibers in BAL and biopsies indicates exposure and may confirm the diagnosis of asbestosis.

Genotoxicity

In Vitro

Asbestos produces genetic damage and morphologic transformation of hamster cells. Asbestos fibers cause chromosomal aberrations, i.e., aneuploidy (usually polyploidy), fragmentation, breaks, rearrangements, gaps, dicentrics, inversions, and rings. Cell treated with asbestos suspension showed reduced p53 protein expression. Asbestos is not mutagenic in *Escherichia coli* and *Salmonella typhimurium* assays.

In Vivo

In rats treated with crocidolite intraperitoneally, DNA deletions have been observed in peritoneal tumors. In inhalation and intratracheal instillation studies, an increased mutation frequency was described in lung cells.

Studies on asbestos-exposed workers showed that the number of chromosomal aberrations and the rate of sister chromatid exchanges were significantly elevated.

Carcinogenicity

Lung tumor and pleural mesothelioma have been described only in rats. Inhalation studies described a linear relationship between exposure to asbestos and lung cancer incidence. Mesothelioma was also induced in rats after injection or implantation of asbestos into the pleural or peritoneal cavities.

Chronic exposure to asbestos is among the known causes of lung cancer. Cumulative exposures that have been shown to double the risk correspond to 25 fibers $\times$ ml^{-1} years, i.e. concentration of fibers in the air multiplied for the years of exposure. This exposure is similar to that correlating with the development of asbestosis. However, it is still debated as to whether the presence of asbestosis is a requirement or not for lung cancer development. Epidemiological studies show that high exposures to asbestos and tobacco smoking have multiplicative effects. Latency period for lung cancer is 20–30 years. Presenting symptoms may include chronic cough, hemoptysis, chest pain, dyspnea, and weight loss. Diagnostic procedures include detailed occupational history, chest imaging, bronchoscopy with BAL, and histopathology. Both BAL and surgical samples may be useful for the attribution of a lung tumor to asbestos exposure when high concentrations of both asbestos bodies and fibers are found, although reported counts are quite variable. Asbestos fibers have been associated with any type of cancer histotype. Prognosis after surgery and/or chemotherapy does not differ from that of the respective histotype of lung cancer.

Mesothelioma is a malignant disease arising from pleura (60–65%), peritoneum (25%), and other mesothelial membranes. The relationship of asbestos exposure with the development of malignant mesothelioma has been well established, and the disease occurs even after minor degrees of exposure. However, in about 20% of the patients no history of definite exposure to asbestos can be identified. Uncommon causes of mesothelioma include irradiation and perhaps the SV40 virus. The risk of the disease may depend on several factors including the type of fibers, duration and intensity of exposure, timing of exposure in a person's life, and time since first exposure. This latency period is 35–40 years or more. Unlike the instance of lung cancer, smoking does not increase the risk of mesothelioma in asbestos-exposed individuals. The most frequent presenting symptoms of mesothelioma are nonspecific and related to the local effects of the tumor. Common presentation of pleural mesothelioma includes effusion, dyspnea, and chest pain and that of peritoneal mesothelioma includes abdominal distension with ascites. Diagnostic procedures rely on a comprehensive occupational and environmental history, imaging, pleuroscopy, laparoscopy, histopathology, and biomarkers such as blood osteopontin and mesothelin family proteins. Differential diagnosis with epithelial and sarcomatous tumors requires panels of specific immunostaining. Prognosis is poor and death occurs often within a few months of diagnosis, irrespectively from surgical and/or chemotherapy treatment.

Several other malignancies have been recently associated in epidemiological studies with chronic asbestos exposures including laryngeal and ovarian cancers.

Clinical Management

There is no specific treatment for asbestosis and other fibrotic manifestations of asbestos toxicity although symptomatic treatment with steroids and antibiotics may be necessary in advanced cases of asbestosis.. Surgical and chemotherapeutic treatments of asbestos-related malignancies do not differ from the current ones for these tumors.

Exposure Standards and Guidelines

Asbestos is considered a human carcinogen by regulatory agencies worldwide. Existing exposure levels in Western countries are as follows: Occupational Safety & Health Administration: 0.1 fiber cm^{-3}; 8 h time-weighted average (TWA) for respirable fibers with a length-to-diameter ratio of at least 3 to 1, as determined using phase-contrast illumination: 1 fiber cm^{-3} excursion level (30 min). National Institute for Occupational Safety and Health: 0.1 fiber cm^{-3} 10 h TWA. American Conference of Industrial Hygienists: 0.1 fiber cm^{-3} 8 h TWA. European Union: 0.1 fiber cm^{-3} as a TWA.

Specific regulations exist to control the release of asbestos from building demolition/renovation and to manage waste containing asbestos.

See also: Chromosome Aberrations; Occupational Toxicology; Occupational Safety and Health Administration; Carcinogenesis; International Agency for Research on Cancer; Respiratory Tract Toxicology; Erionites; Occupational Exposure Limits.

Further Reading

American Thoracic Society, 2004. Diagnosis and initial management of non-malignant diseases related to asbestos. American Journal of Respiratory and Critical Care Medicine 170, 691–715.

Asbestos, asbestosis and cancer: the Helsinki criteria for diagnosis and attribution. Scandinavian Journal on Work and Environmental Health 23, 1997, 311–316.

Banks, D.E., Shi, R., McLarty, J., et al., 2009. American College of Chest Physician consensus statement on the respiratory health effects of asbestos. Results of the Delphi Study. Chest 135, 1619–1627.

IARC Monographs Vol. 2, 1973. Vol. 14, 1977. Suppl. 7 1987.

Lotti, M., Bergamo, L., Murer, B., 2010. Occupational toxicology of asbestos-related malignancies. Clinical Toxicology 48, 485–496.

Robinson, B.W.S., Chahinian, A.P. (Eds.), 2002. Mesothelioma. Martin Dunitz, London, UK, p. 336.

Roggli, V.L., Oury, T.D., Sporn, T.A. (Eds.), 2004. Pathology of Asbestos-Associated Disease. Springer, New York, NY, p. 421.

Tossavainen, A., 2000. International Expert Meeting on new advances in the radiology and screening of asbestos-related diseases. Scandinavian Journal on Work and Environmental Health 26, 449–454.

Relevant Websites

IARC http://www.iarc.fr
NIOSH http://www.cdc.gov/NIOSH
OSHA http://www.osha.gov
ACGIH http://www.acgih.org

Asia Pacific Association of Medical Toxicology (APAMT)

WA Temple, University of Otago, Dunedin, New Zealand
JA Haines, Chemin de la Creuse, Divonne les Bains, France

Historical Development of the Association

The Asia Pacific Association of Medical Toxicology (APAMT) is an international association that was established by a group of medical toxicologists at the Joint International Programme on Chemical Safety (IPCS)/World Health Organization (WHO)/ World Federation of Associations of Poison Control and Clinical Toxicology Centres Workshop on Prevention and Management of Poisoning by Toxic Substances, held in Kuala Lumpur, Malaysia, 29 November–2 December 1989. Representatives from 27 countries participated at this meeting. Professor Ralph Edwards, the then director of the New Zealand National Poison Information Centre, was elected as the founding president of the association. Other APAMT officers included Dr Julian White (Australia), Dr Madhi Balali-Mood (Iran), Dr Ossy Kasilo (Zimbabwe), and Professor Ravindra Fernando (Sri Lanka) as vice presidents; Professor Tariq Abdul Razak (Malaysia) as secretary general; Dr Wayne Temple (New Zealand) as treasurer; Dr Don Ferry (New Zealand) as coordinating secretary.

The secretariat of the association initially resided in New Zealand with Dr Ferry until the appointment of Dr Kenneth Hartigan-Go (Philippines) as coordinating secretary in November 1991 at an association meeting held during the IPCS working group on Natural Toxins in Singapore. The secretariat remained in the Philippines until 2006, then transferred to Sri Lanka where Professor Andrew Dawson (president 2006–08) was based with the South Asian Clinical Toxicology Research Collaboration.

In late 2011, the secretariat of APAMT moved to Penang, Malaysia, at the National Poison Centre, Universiti Sains Malaysia.

Initially, members kept in contact through a newsletter, prepared by the coordinating secretariat at the Philippine National Poisons Centre in Manila. Originally, foreseen to be a quarterly newsletter, the first two (volume 1, nos. 1 and 2) were issued in mid-1992; then two issues (volume 2, nos. 1 and 2) appeared in the first half of 1993. There was then a gap until the last quarter of 1994 when a single issue (volume 3, no. 1) appeared. Another single issue with the same number appeared in August 1996 containing the constitution.

A constitution for the association was drafted at the INTOX-4 meeting in Adelaide and was circulated during 1992 and examined at an APAMT symposium on Experience of Poison Control Centres in the Asia-Pacific Region, held that year in September in Quebec, Canada, during the 5th annual meeting of the INTOX Project. The approved constitution was published in Volume 3 of the newsletter in 1996. It was subsequently revised after 2004.

The APAMT logo is shown below.

Past and Current Structure

APAMT Past Presidents

Professor Ralph Edwards (first president) 1989–1991
Professor Ravindra Fernando (Sri Lanka) 1991–1994
Professor Madhi Balali-Mood (Iran) 1994–2001
Dr Jou-Fang Deng (Taiwan) 2001–2006
Professor Andrew Dawson (Australia) 2006–2008
Dr Winai Wananukul (Thailand) 2008–2010

APAMT Board Members 2012

Dr Chen-Chang Yang, President (Taiwan)
Dr Andrew Dawson (Australia)
Dr Winai Wananukul (Thailand)
Dr Jou-Fang Deng (Taiwan)
Dr Wayne Temple (New Zealand)
Dr Reza Afshari (Iran)
Dr Michael Eddelston (Scotland)
Dr I. Gawarammana (Sri Lanka)
Dr Surjit Singh (India)
Dr Hossein Hassanian (Iran)

APAMT Objectives

The general objective of the association is the promotion of all aspects of chemical safety, poison control, and treatment, within the Asia Pacific region. In pursuance of this general goal, the association proposed to establish and maintain cooperation with governmental organizations, professional bodies, and other groups or individuals concerned with toxicological

 http://dx.doi.org/10.1016/B978-0-12-386454-3.01101-5

problems, in order to facilitate action designed to reduce or eliminate risks and optimize treatment or management of poisoning; to assemble studies, observations, and data essential to the understanding of poisoning; to promote and conduct scientific research and investigations for the study of poisoning; to supply information and advice in this field through information centers in the Asia Pacific region; to foster professional education in the field of toxicology; and to collaborate with international institutions and particularly the WHO.

APAMT Activities and Achievements

At the early stages of the association, membership was open to professionals working in poison centers and related activities in countries of the Asia Pacific region and in countries outside the region where no association of toxicologists recognized by the then World Federation of Associations of Poison Control and Clinical Toxicology Centres (WFAPCCT) existed (the agreement among the international and national bodies constituting the WFAPCCT subsequently fell into abeyance). Initially, memberships from 16 countries were represented.

The association has been very active in the promotion of poison control and treatment by participating in the INTOX Project of the IPCS/WHO/United Nations Environment Programme (UNEP)/International Labour Organisation (ILO). The efforts of Dr John Haines, formerly with the IPCS, in facilitating INTOX workshops brought together many members of APAMT at these occasions and allowed for meetings of the association to be held prior to the more formalized general assemblies that were subsequently held during the APAMT congresses. APAMT formally recognized Dr Haines for this work by making him the first honorary fellow during the association's ninth congress in Hanoi in 2010.

The association has also supported national and international seminars and workshops on poison control such as the International Seminar and Workshop on Prevention and Management of Poisoning by Toxic Substances which was held on 16 September 1996 in Jakarta, Indonesia.

APAMT is currently participating in the South Asian Clinical Toxicology Research Collaboration (SACTRC). The general objective of the collaboration is to promote clinical research, particular in toxicology and toxinology, within the South Asian region (Sri Lanka, India, Pakistan, Maldives, Bangladesh, and Nepal). These objectives include increasing research capacity through postgraduate training and the establishment of Sri Lanka as an international centre of clinical research excellence. SACTRC was formally established in 2004 following a Wellcome Trust grant awarded to Dr Michael Eddleston, a current APAMT board member. Many of the collaborators were actively involved in research on poisoning and envenoming in South Asia over the preceding decade. Several APAMT board members of APAMT are actively involved in SACTRC research and have presented their findings at APAMT congresses.

Two meetings of experts on poisoning and chemical safety, significant in promoting poison control in the region, were held in Colombo, Sri Lanka, July 1997 and Kathmandu, Nepal, May 1999, respectively of the South Asian Association for Regional Cooperation (SAARC), an organization of South Asian nations, founded in December 1985 and dedicated to economic, technological, social, and cultural development. It was through the influence of the APAMT's second president, Ravindra Fernando, that the issues of poisoning in the region were brought to the SAARC political forum; senior government officials were made more aware of the issues and could better respond to initiatives in their own countries.

Congresses

APAMT made an active contribution to the fifth World Conference of the WFAPCCT, which was held during November 1994 in Taipei, Taiwan.

The first APAMT scientific congress was held together with the fifth Iranian Congress of Toxicology and Poisonings in Teheran, Iran, from 27–30 September 1997. Although this congress was actually the first standalone congress held by the APAMT, there was some confusion that the Taiwanese meeting had also been an APAMT congress. The resultant misunderstanding led to the next congress being billed as the third congress when it was actually the second.

The third congress of the APAMT was held during 11–15 November 2001 in Penang, Malaysia.

The fourth congress of the APAMT took place during 24–26 November 2004 in Manila, Philippines.

The fifth APAMT congress was held during 6–8 August 2006 in Colombo, Sri Lanka.

The sixth APAMT congress took place during 12–14 December 2007 in Bangkok, Thailand.

The seventh APAMT congress was held during 7–10 December 2008 in Chandigarh, India.

The eighth APAMT congress was held during 20–22 October 2009 in Beijing, China.

The ninth APAMT congress took place during 17–19 November 2010 in Hanoi, Vietnam.

The tenth congress of the APAMT was held during 11–14 November 2011 in Penang, Malaysia,

The eleventh APAMT congress is scheduled to take place from 29 November to 1 December 2012, at the Hong Kong Academy of Medicine, Hong Kong.

Cooperative Activities

There has been regular involvement of members of the association representing the medical toxicology professional community in international fora and activities: Intergovernmental Forum on Chemical Safety (IFCS), International Conference on Chemicals Management (ICCM), Strategic Approach to International Chemicals Management (SAICM) regional and intersessional activities, and intergovernmental negotiations on new initiatives (e.g., mercury).

Association members have also contributed to strengthening the capacity for poison control, including training in the region. Dr Wayne Temple is working in conjunction with the WHO on a SAICM Quick Start Fund project to establish desktop poison information centers in the Pacific Islands.

A SACTRC-initiated proposal for a distance learning Masters program in clinical toxicology was agreed to in December 2007 and course delivery began in June 2008 at the Sri Lankan Post Graduate Institute of Medicine (PGIM). APAMT members have contributed significantly to this program. Members have also contributed to e-learning activities including Wikitox.

Future directions of the association will include greater involvement in international and interprofessional issues: strengthening capacity for health and environmental surveillance to toxic exposures under conditions of the region; timely publication of critically reviewed data; encouraging young professionals to participate in national and international meetings to present their work and learn from others; and taking a proactive role as an interlocutor at international level to stakeholder debate of policy issues relating to sound management of chemicals and waste.

See also: World Health Organization/International Programme on Chemical Safety (WHO/IPCS).

Further Reading

Dawson, A.H., Buckley, N.A., 2011 Feb. Toxicologists in public health – following the path of Louis Roche (based on the Louis Roche lecture "An accidental toxicologist in public health", Bordeaux, 2010). Clinical Toxicology (Philadelphia) 49 (2), 94–101.

Relevant Websites

http://www.asiatox.org – Asia Pacific Association of Medical Toxicology (APAMT).

http://www.prn.usm.my/apamten – 10th Scientific Congress of the Asia Pacific Association of Medical Toxicology (APAMT).

www.sactrc.org/ – South Asian Clinical Toxicology Research Collaboration.

Aspartame

RC Guy, Robin Guy Consulting, LLC, Lake Forest, IL, USA

- Name: Aspartame
- Chemical Abstracts Service Registry Number: 22839-47-0
- Synonyms: L-α-aspartyl-L-phenylalanine 1-methyl ester, NutraSweet
- Chemical/Pharmaceutical/Other Class: Dipeptide methyl ester
- Molecular Formula: $C_{14}H_{18}N_2O_5$
- Structure:

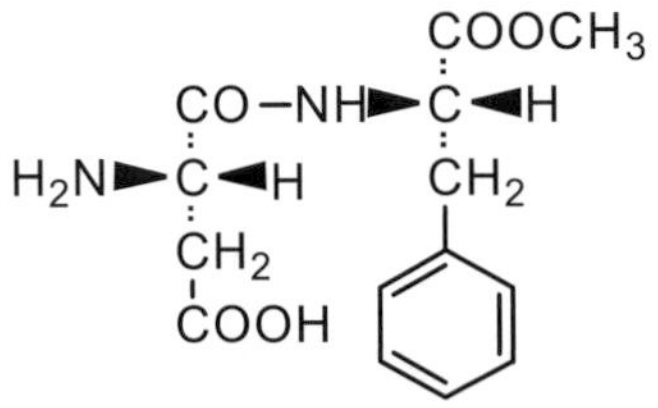

Background Information

Based on the lack of toxicity in animal studies, a no-observed effect level of at least 4000 mg kg^{-1} body weight per day was established by the Joint FAO/WHO Expert Committee on Food Additives (JECFA), the European Food Safety Authority (EFS, formerly the Scientific Committee on Food (SCF)), and the Health Protection Branch of Health and Welfare Canada. As a result, an acceptable daily intake (ADI) of 40 mg kg^{-1} body weight was set by these agencies. The Food and Drug Administration set the ADI at 50 mg kg^{-1} body weight based on both animal and human studies (Butchko et al., 2002; JECFA, 1980; SCF, 2002; Tschanz et al., 1996). Aspartame is a high-intensity sweetener approved for use in over 90 countries and in more than 6000 products (Magnuson et al., 2007). Aspartame is nontoxic at dosages up to 4000 mg kg^{-1} day^{-1} and is not carcinogenic (Magnuson et al., 2007).

Uses

High-intensity sweetener, flavor enhancer.

Exposure Pathways

Oral.

Toxicokinetics

Aspartame is hydrolyzed entirely in the gastrointestinal tract to its constituent amino acids, aspartate and phenylalanine, and methanol. These are then absorbed by the body and utilized via the same metabolic pathways as when these same constituents are derived from common foods; they are found in common foods in much larger quantities than from aspartame in foods or beverages.

Mechanisms of Toxicity

Aspartame is nontoxic. However, individuals with the rare, genetic disease, phenylketonuria (PKU), cannot properly metabolize phenylalanine. Such individuals are detected by testing at birth and placed on special low-phenylalanine diets to control their blood phenylalanine concentrations. Thus, PKU individuals need to be aware that aspartame is a source of phenylalanine.

Animal Toxicity

Aspartame is nontoxic, carcinogenic, mutagenic, or teratogenic and has no effect on reproduction. Carcinogenicity studies with aspartame have failed to reveal any dose–response between aspartame and tumors (Butchko et al., 2002; FDA, 2007; NCI, 2009 SCF, 2002; Stegink and Filer, 1984; Tschanz et al., 1996).

Human Toxicity: Acute

Aspartame is nontoxic when administered as an acute dose in humans. Humans were administered aspartame at dosages up to 200 mg kg^{-1} body weight as a single bolus dose. Blood concentrations of aspartic acid, phenylalanine, and methanol were well below any levels considered potentially harmful. The toxic effects of methanol in humans are due to accumulation of its metabolite, formate. Blood formate concentrations did not increase after this abusive bolus dose of aspartame (equal to the amount in about 28 liters of beverage with aspartame consumed at once or about 65–70 times the amount of aspartame people consume daily at the 90th percentile). Urinary excretion of formate increased significantly in samples collected 0–4 and 4–8 h after aspartame ingestion. Therefore, the rate of formate formation did not exceed the rate of formate excretion, even after this very large bolus dose (Butchko et al., 2002; Stegink and Filer, 1984; Tschanz et al., 1996).

Human Toxicity: Chronic

Aspartame was tested in studies of up to 27 weeks duration in healthy adults, children, and adolescents, obese subjects, individuals with diabetes, and individuals heterozygous for PKU. The results of these studies show that there was no

 http://dx.doi.org/10.1016/B978-0-12-386454-3.00818-6

accumulation of plasma aspartate, phenylalanine, or methanol in humans following long-term exposure (Butchko et al., 2002; Stegink and Filer, 1984; Tschanz et al., 1996).

In a 6-month study in healthy adults, subjects were given 75 mg kg^{-1} body weight per day of aspartame or placebo (provided as three divided doses daily). This daily dose provided approximately the same amount of aspartame as 10 liters of a soft drink sweetened with 100% aspartame. There was no accumulation of blood or plasma aspartate, phenylalanine, methanol, or formate over the course of the study. In addition, urinary formate excretion did not increase, indicating no significant increase of formate formation. There were no adverse experiences and no effects on physical examinations, including vital signs, EKGs, ophthalmologic examinations, or biochemical parameters after aspartame compared to placebo.

See also: Food Additives; Food and Drug Administration, US; Food, Drug, and Cosmetic Act, US; Food Safety and Toxicology; Joint FAO/WHO Expert Meetings (JECFA and JMPR).

References

Butchko, H., et al., 2002. Aspartame: review of safety. Regul. Toxicol. Pharmacol. 35 (2), S3–S92.

FDA, 2007. FDA Statement on European Aspartame Study. http://www.fda.gov/Food/FoodIngredientsPackaging/FoodAdditives/ucm208580.htm 20 April 1997.

Joint FAO/WHO Expert Committee on Food Additives, 1980. Aspartame: Toxicological Evaluation of Certain Food Additives, WHO Food Additive Series No. 15, pp. 18–86. JECFA, Geneva.

Magnuson, B.A., et al., 2007. Aspartame: a safety evaluation based on current use levels, regulations, and toxicological and epidemiological studies. Crit. Rev. Toxicol. 37, 629–727.

National Cancer Institute (NCI), 2009. Artificial Sweeteners and Cancer. http://www.cancer.gov/cancertopics/factsheet/Risk/artificial-sweeteners.

Scientific Committee on Food (SCF), 2002. Opinion of the Scientific Committee on Food. Update on the Safety of Aspartame. European Commission. Health and Consumer Protection Directorate-General. http://ec.europa.eu/food/fs/sc/scf/out155_en.pdf 10 December 2002.

Stegink, L.D., Filer Jr, L.J. (Eds.), 1984. Aspartame: Physiology and Biochemistry. Marcel Dekker, New York.

Tschanz, C., Butchko, H., Stargel, W., Kotsonis, F., 1996. The Clinical Evaluation of a Food Additive: Assessment of Aspartame. CRC Press, Boca Raton, FL.

Further Reading

Australia New Zealand Food Authority (ANZFA), 1997. Information Paper. Aspartame: Information for Consumers. June, 1997.

Department of Health, 1998. 1996 Annual Report of the Committees on Toxicity, Mutagenicity, and Carcinogenicity of Chemicals in Food, Consumer Products and the Environment, United Kingdom. pp. 56–57.

Food and Drug Administration (FDA), 1981. Aspartame: commissioner's final decision. Fed. Regist. 46, 38285–38308.

Food and Drug Administration (FDA), 1983. Food additives permitted for direct addition to food for human consumption; aspartame. Fed. Regist. 48 (132), 31376–31382.

Food and Drug Administration (FDA), 1984. Food additives permitted for direct addition to food for human consumption: aspartame. Fed. Regist. 49, 6672–6677.

Food and Drug Administration (FDA), 1996. FDA Statement on Aspartame. FDA Talk Paper, 18 November, 1996.

French Food Safety Agency (AFSSA), 2002. Assessment Report. Opinion on the Possible Link between the Exposition of Aspartame and the Incidence of Brain Tumours in Humans, Maisons-Alfort. 7 May, 2002. www.afssa.fr/avis/index.asp?id_dossier=1815.

Health and Welfare Canada, 1981. Aspartame. Health Protection Branch, Ottawa. 31 July,1981. Information Letter No. 602.

Health Canada, 2003. Chemical Health Hazard Assessment on the Safety of Aspartame. http://www.hc-sc.gc.ca/food-aliment/cs-ipc/chha-edpcs/e_aspartame01.html (19 February 2003).

Joint FAO/WHO Expert Committee on Food Additives, 1981. International Program on Chemical Safety (IPCS). Toxicological Evaluation of Certain Food Additives. WHO Technical Report Series No. 699. Geneva, pp. 28–32.

Leon, A.S., Hunninghake, D.B., Bell, C., Rassin, D.K., Tephly, T.R., 1989. Safety of long-term large doses of aspartame. Arch. Intern. Med. 149, 2318–2324.

Ministry of Agriculture, Fisheries, and Food (MAFF), 1982. Food Additives and Contaminants Committee Report on the Review of Sweeteners in Food. Committee on Toxicity of Chemicals in Food, Consumer Products and the Environment. FAC/REP/34:HMSO 1982.

Scientific Committee on Food (SCF), 1997. Minutes of the 107th Meeting of the Scientific Committee on Food Held on 12–13 June, 1997. Brussels, pp. 9–10.

Scientific Committee on Food (SCF), 1985. Food Science and Techniques. Reports of the Scientific Committee on Food (Sixteenth Series). Commission of the European Communities, Luxembourg.

Tephly, T.R., 1999. Comments on the purported generation of formaldehyde and adduct formation from the sweetener aspartame. Life Sci. 65, 157–160.

Aspririn *see* **Acetylsalicylic Acid**

Astemizole

A Shafiee and M Khoobi, Tehran University of Medical Sciences, Tehran, Iran

This article is a revision of the previous edition article by Michael D. Reed, volume 1, pp 187–188, © 2005, Elsevier Inc.

- Name: Astemizole
- Chemical Abstracts Service Registry Number*: 68844-77-9
- Synonyms*: Alermizol; Astesen; Esmacen; Laridal; Hismanal; 1-[(4-Fluorophenyl)methyl]-*N*-[1-[2-(4-methoxyphenyl) ethyl]-4-piperidinyl]-1*H*-benzimidazol-2-amine; Paralergin; Retolen; Waruzol
- Molecular Formula*: ($C_{28}H_{31}FN_4O$)
- Chemical Structure*:

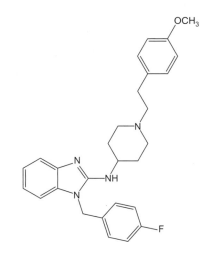

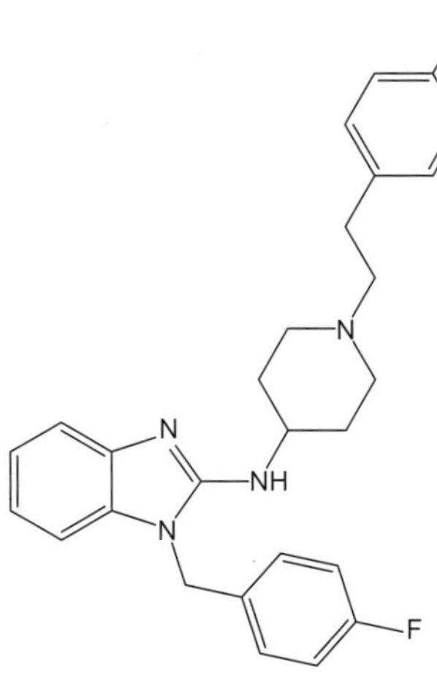

*All from ChemIDplus.

Background

Astemizole as a non-sedating selective histamine H_1-antagonist ($IC_{50} = 4$ nM) has been widely utilized to relieve seasonal or all-year allergic rhinitis, chronic urticaria, conjunctivitis, and other allergic symptoms.

Janssen Pharmaceutica discovered astemizole in 1977, and it was marketed under the brand name Hismanal and approved by the US Food and Drug Administration in 1988. It was first sold in North American markets in the mid-1980s ('Astemizole Hismanal') by Janssen Pharmaceutica (now Johnson and Johnson) and voluntarily withdrawn by this company from global markets in 1999. Astemizole can inhibit nose and bronchial reaction in people exposed to histamine and allergens. Several studies revealed that astemizole has an antimalaria activity and selectivity for 5-HT, dopamine, and muscarinic acetylcholine receptors. Some clinical studies showed that astemizole did not cause drowsiness or sedation in patients. Unlike the most first-generation antihistamines, astemizole as a second-generation antihistamine cannot penetrate into the central nervous system and therefore causes fewer adverse side effects. Binding of astemizole to the H_1-receptor in place of histamine results in fewer allergic symptoms. More detailed studies have shown that astemizole can reduce the release of mediators in allergic reactions like prostaglandins, leukotrienes, and histamine from mast cells.

A study on the effect of astemizole on the Ca^{2+} fluxes in rat basophilic leukemia (RBL-2H3) cells revealed that it can increase the intracellular calcium concentration through releasing intracellular Ca^{2+} stores and also inhibit the Ca^{2+} influx via store-operated Ca^{2+} channels. Astemizole can inhibit human ether-a-go-go-related gene (hERG) potassium ion channel currents in the mid to high nanomolar range. Inhibition was selective for hERG compared to a number of other cloned K^+ channels.

Moreover, astemizole can suppress the expression of cyclins after 6–8 h costimulation with IGF-1. After treatment with astemizole, QT prolongation and increase in the Na^+–K^+ interval of the electrocardiogram-like waves can be observed. Several studies show proarrhythmic effects of desmethylastemizole as a dominant compound in serum, which is the principal cause of long QT syndrome and Torsades de Pointes. These fatal side effects led to its withdrawal from the markets.

However, recent studies show that using astemizole along with radiotherapy could be beneficial to destroy prostate cancer cells through an autophagic-facilitated mechanism. It can be introduced as a novel intervention for the treatment of prostate cancer.

Astemizole is currently used in 30 countries where malaria is endemic, including Vietnam, Thailand, and Cambodia. It was found that astemizole is a potent anti-malarial agent against both chloroquine-sensitive and chloroquine-resistant parasites *in vitro* and *in vivo*. Several studies have been focused on the synthesis of astemizole analogs to improve antimalarial activity and reduce hERG-related and other side effects of the parent drug.

Uses

Astemizole is prescribed usually for the therapy of allergic reactions, including rhinitis, asthma, conjunctivitis, and chronic idiopathic urticaria. It is used as a histamine-1 (H-1) receptor antagonist in medical condition. Astemizole and

 http://dx.doi.org/10.1016/B978-0-12-386454-3.00694-1

desmethylastemizole (its metabolites) are known as a potent hERG potassium ion channels. Astemizole was developed as a radioligand for the hERG K^+ channel-binding assay and PET imaging of T-pathology. Recent studies revealed that astemizole could be used clinically as a radiotracer for neuroimaging in Alzheimer's disease diagnosis, due to its aggregated tau protein binding ability.

In addition, it is a new promising anticancer drug owing to its ability to inhibit potassium channel, which is involved in cancer cell growth. Histamine can either promote or inhibit cell proliferation depending on the cell type; thereby the role of histamine in the cell proliferation is disputable. Astemizole is a new antimalarial agent showing activity against both chloroquine-sensitive and multidrug-resistant parasites. It also has been found to have anti-prion activity.

Environmental Behavior, Fate, Routes, and Pathways

Astemizole is soluble in ethanol and DMSO (25 mg ml^{-1}), chloroform, methanol, and water (partly soluble). It is very toxic to organisms in the aquatic environment due to its long-term adverse effects. It is not recommended to concomitant usage of astemizole-like compounds such as fluconazole, metronidazole, miconazole, and ketoconazole.

Exposure and Exposure Monitoring

Human are typically exposed to astemizole by ingestion. In a cohort study, 114 women exposed to astemizole were matched with 114 women exposed to known nonteratogens such as acetaminophen and dental radiographs. Two major malformations were found in both groups. Daily administration of 10 mg kg^{-1} astemizole to female Wistar rats during the pregnancy caused pinna detachment delay, reduced fertility, and the startle reflex.

Toxicokinetics

After oral administration, astemizole is absorbed quickly, although its onset of action is late. Administration of astemizole with meals can reduce the rate, but not the overall extent of enteric absorption. Astemizole can bind to plasma protein about 97%; therefore, its duration of action is long. It distributes extensively within the body fluids and secretes in the milk. It does not cross the blood–brain barrier in a significant extent.

Astemizole has a cardiotoxic effect, producing a dangerous arrhythmia known as TdP. Astemizole undergoes extensive first-pass hepatic metabolism via cytochrome P450 (CYP450) enzymes (primarily 3A4). Therefore, drugs interacting with CYP3A4 can affect astemizole systemic exposure and toxic potential. Its metabolism gives three primary and active metabolites: desmethylastemizole, norastemizole, and 6-hydroxydesmethylastemizole. A study on the excretion and biotransformation of astemizole shows that its metabolites are slowly excreted in the urine and feces. Desmethylastemizole with a long elimination time (9–13 days) is the dominant metabolite of astemizole, which is generated by oxidative *O*-demethylation of the parent drug. It can potently block the repolarization of K^+ current (IKr). Norastemizole is a second metabolite of astemizole, which is generated by oxidative *N*-dealkylation of the parent drug. Astemizole and its metabolites are reported to be H_1-receptor antagonists. Norastemizole has low concentrations in the serum and exhibits more potent blockade on the H_1-receptor than desmethylastemizole and astemizole. Astemizole and its metabolites can block the hERG channels.

Asymptomatic liver enzyme elevations, edema, epistaxis, myalgia, bronchospasm, depression, palpitation, photosensitivity, pruritus, paresthesia, angioedema, and rashes may occur in treating patients with astemizole. Some other side effects associated with astemizole are stomach upset (nausea, diarrhea, or constipation), allergic reaction, faintness, increased heart rate, uncommonly irregular heart rhythms, lung swelling, incoordination, and disordered sleep and dreaming. Astemizole can also cause adverse cardiac effects at high doses, probably due to an action on H_3-receptors.

Mechanisms of Action

Cardiotoxicity (Torsades de Pointes arrhythmia) is the main and serious toxicity related with astemizole administration. The exact mechanism of the cardiotoxicity is not exactly clear, though it is believed to be similar to terfenadine. Astemizole and its primary metabolite desmethylastemizole may be able to inhibit cardiac delayed potassium rectifier (Ikr) channels likewise terfenadine does. The Ikr channel is the potassium channel involved in repolarization of cardiac cells and therefore its blockade can decrease the outflow of cellular potassium, resulting in dysrhythmia and most notably Torsades de Pointes.

Furthermore, norastemizole and 6-hydroxyastemizole can also inhibit Ikr channels at much lower amounts than the parent drug. Overdose of astemizole in patients with hepatic and renal dysfunction leads to accumulation of astemizole and its metabolites. In this condition, the patients are disposed to astemizole-induced cardiotoxicity.

Acute and Short-Term Toxicity

Human

Unlike first-generation antihistamines, astemizole is a 'non-sedating' agent and does not comprise the anticholinergic properties. Patients with astemizole overdose are usually fully awake or only slightly sedated. Following astemizole ingestion, serious cardiac effects, including prolongation of the QT interval, arrhythmias, arrest, hypotension, palpitations, syncope, dizziness, and death, could be observed in the patients. These cardiotoxic effects are usually associated with doses higher than recommended and/or increased plasma concentrations of the drug and its active metabolites. Although at the recommended dose and two or three times the recommended dose, cardiotoxic effects may occur rarely. Administration of the drug along with the inhibitors of the CYP3A4, including the azole antifungals, macrolide antibiotics, selective serotonin reuptake inhibitors (SSRIs) and antiretroviral drugs, considerably increases the risk of astemizole-induced cardiotoxicity.

Chronic Toxicity

There was limited evidence that indicates repeated or long-term occupational exposure can have an effect on organs or biochemical systems. There has been some concern about carcinogenic and mutagenic effect of astemizole; however, there are not enough data to make an assessment. There is also poor evidence about sensitization reaction by skin contact. Hypersensitivity reactions including bronchospasm, hives (urticaria), deep dermal wheals (angioneurotic edema), running nose (rhinitis), and blurred vision would be observable after exposure to small quantities of the drug. Anaphylactic shock and skin rash (non-thrombocytopenic purpura) would also be expected.

Cross-sensitivity with other chemical agents that have caused prior sensitization could be observed. Astemizole did not show carcinogenic effect using oral doses less than 80 mg kg^{-1} day^{-1} for 24 and 18 months in rats and mice, respectively.

Micronucleus, dominant lethal, sister chromatid exchange, and Ames tests have shown no mutagenicity. Teratogenic effects were not detectable in rats at oral doses up to 130 times the recommended dose. Fertility was not affected in rats at oral doses of up to 40 times the recommended human dose.

Animal

At lower doses (50 times the recommended human dose), no toxicity was observed in the mothers or pups; conversely, toxic effects were noticeable on the unborn rat pups at higher doses of 100 times the recommended human dose, as well as in the mothers.

Immunotoxicity

Growing evidences have focused on the role of astemizole and histamine receptors (HRs) antagonists in immune modulation. However, the roles of HRs agonists are still unclear.

Genotoxicity

Astemizole did not show genotoxic and carcinogenic effects in most of various cytogenetic test systems.

Carcinogenicity

Based on carcinogenicity investigations on Swiss mice and Wistar rats exposed to astemizole, this compound is not capable of promoting tumor growth and it is not tumorigenic.

Clinical Management

Basic and advanced life-support measures should be utilized as necessary. Using activated charcoal may be beneficial following oral ingestion. Since the drug is rapidly absorbed from the intestine, the efficacy of activated charcoal and/or gastric lavage will depend on the time these therapies are used after the ingestion. Further, the effectiveness of multidose activated charcoal would appear limited considering the drug's extensive V_d ($\sim$250 l kg^{-1}) and high protein binding (97%). Close EKG monitoring should be instituted immediately and continued for a minimum of 24 h.

Exposure Standards and Guidelines

Astemizole can considerably improve calcitriol's growth-inhibitory effects (3–11 fold, $p < .01$). Mean IC_{20} values were 1.82 ± 2.41 nM and 1.62 ± 0.75 μM for calcitriol (in estrogen receptor negative cells) and astemizole, respectively.

See also: Chloroquine/Hydroxychloroquine; Methylenedioxymethamphetamine.

Further Reading

Bartra, J., Valero, A.L., Cuvillo, A., Dávila, I., Jáuregui, I., Montoro, J., Mullol, J., Sastre, J., 2006. Interactions of the H[1] antihistamines. J. Investig. Allergol. Clin. Immunol. 16, 29–36.

Borowiec, A.-S., Hague, F., Gouilleux-Gruart, V., Lassoued, K., Ouadid-Ahidouch, H., 2011. Regulation of IGF-1-dependent cyclin D1 and E expression by hEag1 channels in MCF-7 cells: the critical role of hEag1 channels in G1 phase progression. Biochim. Biophys. Acta 1813, 723–730.

Brambilla, G., Mattioli, F., Robbiano, L., Martelli, A., 2011. Genotoxicity and carcinogenicity studies of antihistamines. Arch. Toxicol. 85, 1173–1187.

Briggs, G.G., Freeman, R.K., Yaffe, S.J., 2011. Drugs in Pregnancy and Lactation. Lippincott Williams & Wilkins, p. 102.

Chestnut, D.H., Polley, L.S., Wong, C.A., Tsen, L.C., May 15, 2009. Chestnut's Obstetric Anesthesia: Principles and Practice. Elsevier Health Sciences.

Fischer, M.J.E., Paulussen, J.J.C., de Mol, N.J., Janssen, L.H.M., 1998. Dual effect of the anti-allergic astemizole on Ca^{2+} fluxes in rat basophilic leukemia (RBL-2H3) cells: release of Ca^{2+} from intracellular stores and inhibition of Ca2+ release-activated Ca^{2+} influx. Biochem. Pharmacol. 55, 1255–1262.

Heideman, S.M., Samaik, A.P., 1996. Arrhythmias after astemizole overdose. Pediatr. Emerg. Care 12, 102–104.

Hu, W.-W., Yang, Y., Wang, Z., Shen, Z., Zhang, X.-N., Wang, G.-H., Chen, Z., 2012. H1-antihistamines induce vacuolation in astrocytes through macroautophagy. Toxicol. Appl. Pharmacol. 260, 115–123.

Kasurka, C.B., Sekeroglu, Z.A., Sekeroglu, V., 2011. Evaluation of the genotoxicity and cytotoxicity of fexofenadine in cultured human peripheral blood lymphocytes. Toxicol. *In Vitro* 25, 1480–1484.

Oprea, T.I., Bauman, J.E., Bologa, C.G., Buranda, T., Chigaev, A., Edwards, B.S., Jarvik, J.W., Gresham, H.D., Haynes, M.K., Hjelle, B., Hromas, R., Hudson, L., Mackenzie, D.A., Muller, C.Y., Reed, J.C., Simons, P.C., Smagley, Y., Strouse, J., Surviladze, Z., Thompson, T., Ursu, O., Waller, A., Wandinger-Ness, A., Winter, S.S., Wu, Y., Young, S.M., Larson, R.S., Ch, Willman, Sklar, L.A., 2011. Drug repurposing from an academic perspective. Drug Discov. Today Ther. Strateg. http://dx.doi.org/10.1016/j.ddstr.2011.10.002.

Rampe, D., Brown, A.M., 2013. A history of the role of the hERG channel in cardiac risk assessment. J. Pharmacol. Toxicol. Methods. http://dx.doi.org/10.1016/j.vascn.2013.03.005.

Riss, P.J., Brichard, L., Ferrari, V., Williamson, D.J., Fryer, T.D., Hong, Y.T., Baron, J.-C., Aigbirhio, F.I., 2013. Radiosynthesis and characterization of astemizole derivatives as lead compounds toward PET imaging of T-pathology. Med. Chem. Commun. 4, 852–855.

Rojo, L.E., Alzate-Morales, J., Saavedra, I.N., Davies, P., Maccioni, R.B., 2010. Selective interaction of Lansoprazole and astemizole with tau polymers: potential new clinical use in diagnosis of Alzheimer's disease. J. Alzheimers Dis. 19, 573–589.

Snyder, R.D., 1998. A review and investigation into the mechanistic basis of the, genotoxicity of antihistamines. Mutat. Res. 411, 235–248.
Ten Eick, A.P., Bhmer, J.L., Reed, M.D., 2001. Safety of antihistamines in children. Drug Saf. 24, 119–147.
Vanparys, P., Fabry, L., Leonard, A., Marsbroom, R., 1982. Mutagenicity tests with astemizole *in vitro* and *in vivo*. Arch. Toxicol. 50, 167–173.

Relevant Website

www.drugs.com – Drug information online.

Atrazine

J Liu, Oklahoma State University, Stillwater, OK, USA

Atrazine (1912-24-9) is a commonly used herbicide to control pre- and postemergence grasses and broadleafed weeds.

- Molecular Formula: $C_8H_{14}ClN_5$
- Chemical Structure:

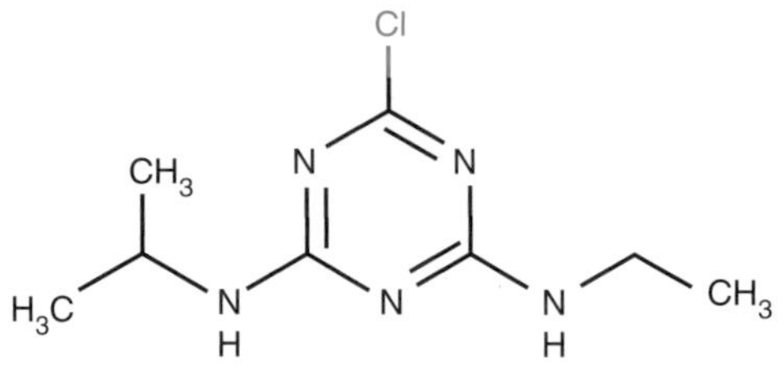

Uses

For decades, atrazine has been one of the most heavily used agricultural herbicides in the United States and is used extensively worldwide to control pre- and postemergence grasses and broadleafed weeds. The annual usage of atrazine in US agriculture has been ranked number two among conventional pesticides (behind glyphosate) based on active ingredients used (70–80 millions of pounds annually) over approximately the last decade. Atrazine is primarily used on various field crops such as corn (approximately 75% of the field corn acreage grown in the United States), sorghum, sugarcane, etc. It is also used in industrial applications.

Environmental Fate and Behavior

Atrazine is highly persistent in the environment due to its resistance to abiotic hydrolysis (stable at pHs 5, 7, and 9) and to direct aqueous photolysis (stable under sunlight at pH 7). Moreover, the compound has a limited volatilization potential and is only moderately susceptible to aerobic biodegradation, which is the main route of dissipation of atrazine. A colder climate makes atrazine even more persistent in the environment. Atrazine does not get adsorbed to soil particles strongly and therefore has a relatively high potential to contaminate ground and surface waters despite its moderate solubility in water.

Exposure and Exposure Monitoring

The ocular and dermal routes are the primary exposure pathways. Ingestion and inhalation are other possible routes of exposure.

Toxicokinetics

Atrazine has the potential to be absorbed through the gastrointestinal tract, through the intact skin, and by inhalation. The percentage absorbed through dermal application is increased with time and decreased with dose. However, the majority (65–95%) of atrazine applied on the skin was recovered in the water used for washing or was found associated with the skin at the site of exposure. Once absorbed, it follows first-order distribution kinetics and undergoes *N*-dealkylation and dechlorination of the triazine ring. The highest level of atrazine is noted in the red blood cell followed by lungs, liver, spleen, and kidneys. The half-life of atrazine in the tissues is <31–39 h. Urinary excretion is the major route of elimination in mammals. A small amount is also excreted in the feces. The major metabolite in both urine and feces is diaminochlorotriazine.

Mechanism of Toxicity

The triazine herbicides are selective inhibitors of the Hill reaction in plant photosynthesis. In mammals, atrazine disrupts luteinizing hormone (LH) and prolactin secretion through direct action on the hypothalamus–pituitary axis.

In vitro, atrazine was found to strongly potentiate arsenic trioxide-induced cytotoxicity and transcriptional activation of stress genes in transformed human hepatocytes, while atrazine itself did not show any significant effects.

Acute and Short-Term Toxicity (or Exposure)

Animal

Atrazine has low acute toxicity in mammals and falls into toxicity category III or IV. The oral LD_{50} in rats is $>2\ g\ kg^{-1}$. The dermal LD_{50} and inhalation LC_{50} (1 h) values in rats are $>3\ g\ kg^{-1}$ and 700 mg m^3, respectively. The oral LD_{50} values in mice and rabbits are 1.8–4.0 g kg^{-1} and 750 mg kg^{-1}, respectively. Atrazine was negative in primary skin irritation and dermal sensitization tests. Rats exposed to high dosages of atrazine showed changes in arousal and motor function, dyspnea, hypothermia, and spasms. With lethal oral dosages, death occurred rapidly (within 12–24 h). A 90-day subchronic oral study in rats and 21-day dermal study in rabbits provided no observed adverse effect levels (NOAELs) of 3.3 and 100 mg kg^{-1} day^{-1}, respectively.

Human

There have been relatively few recorded cases of human poisonings among occupationally exposed workers in the United States. One death was reported following extensive dermal exposure. Dermal exposure to atrazine can cause skin rash, erythema, blisters, and edema. Ocular irritation, chest pains, and a feeling of tightness in the chest, nausea, and dizziness have also been reported after ocular, oral, or inhalation exposures.

 http://dx.doi.org/10.1016/B978-0-12-386454-3.00098-1

Chronic Toxicity (or Exposure)

Animal

About 40% of rats died, with signs of respiratory distress and paralysis of the limbs following oral administration of 20 mg kg^{-1} day^{-1} atrazine for 6 months. Structural and chemical changes were noticed in various organs including heart, liver, ovaries, etc. Dogs treated with 3.65 mg kg^{-1} day^{-1} atrazine in the diet for 52 weeks showed various treatment-related cardiac changes including EKG alterations, moderate to severe atrial dilation, and enlarged hearts. Histopathology revealed cardiac myolysis and focal atrophy. The NOAEL for atrazine in dogs of both sexes was established at about 5 mg kg^{-1} day^{-1}.

Human

The carcinogenic effect of high doses of atrazine noted in female Sprague–Dawley rats is a strain-, sex-, and tissue-specific response that appears to have low biological relevance in humans due to the differences in the endocrine control of reproductive senescence. While considerable debate still exists on the carcinogenic potential of atrazine, the potential impact of chronic exposure on human health appears more likely on reproduction and development via effects on endocrine signaling and not carcinogenicity.

Immunotoxicity

Atrazine has been reported to cause changes in immunological parameters in adult female B6C3F1 mice. Acute atrazine (100–300 mg kg^{-1}, ip) exposure decreased the percentage of $CD4^+$ and $CD8^+$ T cells in the thymus and the nucleated cells in the spleen. Splenic NK cell activity and the IgG1/IgG2α responses to KLH were all decreased by atrazine in a dose-dependent manner. Both acute and chronic (28 days) exposure to atrazine caused changes in white blood cell count and lymphocyte phenotypes in the blood and spleen. NK cell activity was decreased to a greater extent with chronic exposure. Prenatal/lactational exposure has been shown to cause changes in immune function in adult offsprings in a gender- and age-specific manner.

Reproductive Toxicity

Prenatal developmental toxicity study in female Sprague–Dawley rats exposed to atrazine during gestation day 6 through day 15 demonstrated maternal and developmental NOAELs of 25 mg kg^{-1} day^{-1}. Using both Long–Evans and Sprague–Dawley female rats, atrazine was found to disrupt the hypothalamic control of pituitary-ovarian function as indicated by alteration in LH and prolactin serum levels. Females treated with atrazine (75, 150, and 300 mg kg^{-1} day^{-1} for 21 days by gavage) showed irregular cycles and repetitive pseudopregnancies. Maternal exposure to atrazine during lactation may result in prostatitis in adult male offspring due to atrazine's suppressive effect on suckling induced prolactin release.

Genotoxicity

Based on evidence derived from a large array of assays such as bacterial reverse mutation test, mammalian bone marrow chromosome aberration test, dominant lethal assay, and UDS assay, atrazine was concluded to lack mutagenic potential.

Carcinogenicity

When CD-1 mice of both sexes were treated with atrazine in the diet at dose levels of 10–3000 ppm daily for 91 weeks, no treatment-related increase in tumor incidence was noted when compared with controls. Neither male or female Fischer 344 rats nor male Sprague–Dawley rats given atrazine at a maximum tolerated dose in the diet for 24 months exhibited any increase in the incidence of tumors of any type. However, mammary tumors were observed in female Sprague–Dawley rats after 24 months of dietary administration of high levels of atrazine. The mechanism of tumorigenesis in female Sprague–Dawley rats appears to be mediated via suppression of the LH 'surge,' leading to persistent elevation of estrogen and prolactin. The differences in response to the carcinogenic effect of high levels of atrazine observed in mice versus rats and male (and of primary importance, humans) versus female Sprague–Dawley rats appears due to differences in endocrine control mechanisms affecting reproductive senescence and the development of the mammary tumors during aging.

Clinical Management

Treatment is symptomatic.

Ecotoxicology

Atrazine, with acute oral LD_{50} values of 4900 mg kg^{-1}, is practically nontoxic to birds. The compound is slightly toxic to aquatic animals. Rainbow trout and midge, the most sensitive freshwater species tested, have 96 and 48 h LC_{50} values of 5.3 and 0.72 mg l^{-1}, respectively. The most sensitive marine animals tested were the spot fish (*Leiostomus xanthurus*) with a 96 h LC_{50} value of 8.5 mg l^{-1} and the copepod (*Acartia tonsa*) with a 96 h LC_{50} value of 88 mg l^{-1}. Atrazine has low acute toxicity potential in bees (oral $LD_{50} > 100$ μg per bee).

Exposure Standards and Guidelines

The US EPA and the JMP acute reference dose (RfD) is 0.1 mg kg^{-1} day^{-1}, and chronic RfD is 0.018 mg kg^{-1} day^{-1}. The ACGIH TLV-TWA for atrazine is 5 mg m^{-3}.

See also: Pesticides; Pollution, Water.

Further Reading

Cooper, R.L., Stoker, T.E., Tyrey, L., Goldman, J.M., McElroy, W.K., 2000. Atrazine disrupts the hypothalamic control of pituitary-ovarian function. Toxicol. Sci. 53 (2), 297–307.

Grube, A., Donaldson, D., Kiely, T., Wu, L., 2011. Pesticides Industry Sales and Usage: 2006 and 2007 Market Estimates. U.S. Environmental Protection Agency.

Jowa, L., Howd, R., 2011. Should atrazine and related chlorotriazines be considered carcinogenic for human health risk assessment? J. Environ. Sci. Health Part C 29, 91–144.

Pruett, S.B., Fan, R., Zheng, Q., Schwab, C., 2009. Patterns of immunotoxicity associated with chronic as compared with acute exposure to chemical or physical stressors and their relevance with regard to the role of stress and with regard to immunotoxicity testing. Toxicol. Sci. 109 (2), 265–275.

Rowe, A.M., Brundage, K.M., Barnett, J.B., 2007. Developmental immunotoxicity of atrazine in rodents. Basic Clin. Pharmacol. Toxicol. 102, 139–145.

Simpkins, J.W., Swenberg, J.A., Weiss, N., Brusick, D., Eldridge, J.C., Stevens, J.T., Handa, R.J., Hovey, R.C., Plant, T.M., Pastoor, T.P., Breckenridge, C.B., 2011. Atrazine and breast cancer: a framework assessment of the toxicological and epidemiological evidence. Toxicol. Sci. 123, 441–459.

Stevens, J.T., Sumner, D.D., 1991. Herbicides. In: Hayes Jr., W.J., Laws Jr, E.R. (Eds.), Handbook of Pesticide Toxicology. Academic Press, New York, pp. 1381–1383.

Stevens, J.T., Breckenridge, C.B., Wetzel, L., 1999. A risk characterization for atrazine: oncogenicity profile. J. Toxicol. Environ. Health A 56 (2), 69–109.

Stoker, T.E., Robinette, C.L., Cooper, R.L., 1999. Maternal exposure to atrazine during lactation suppresses suckling-induced prolactin release and results in prostatitis in the adult offspring. Toxicol. Sci. 52 (1), 68–79.

Tchounwou, P.B., Wilson, B.A., Ishaque, A.B., Schneider, J., 2001. Atrazine potentiation of arsenic trioxide-induced cytotoxicity and gene expression in human liver carcinoma cells (HepG2). Mol. Cell. Biochem. 222 (1–2), 49–59.

Relevant Websites

http://ace.orst.edu.

http://www.epa.gov/oppsrrd1/reregistration/atrazine/atrazine_update.htm.

http://www.who.int/water_sanitation_health/dwq/chemicals/atrazine/en/.

Atropine

AL Scott, Biogen Idec, Cambridge, MA, USA

- Name: Atropine
- Chemical Abstracts Service Registry Number: 51-55-8
- Synonyms: AtroPen; Atropine sulfate; Benzeneacetic acid, alpha-(hydroxymethyl)-8-methyl-8-azabicyclo(3,2,1)oct-3-yl ester, endo-(+-)-; DL-Hyoscyamine; Tropine tropate
- Chemical/Pharmaceutical/Other Class: Antimuscarinic agent; Anticholinergic agent
- Molecular Formula: $C_{17}H_{23}NO_3$
- Chemical Structure:

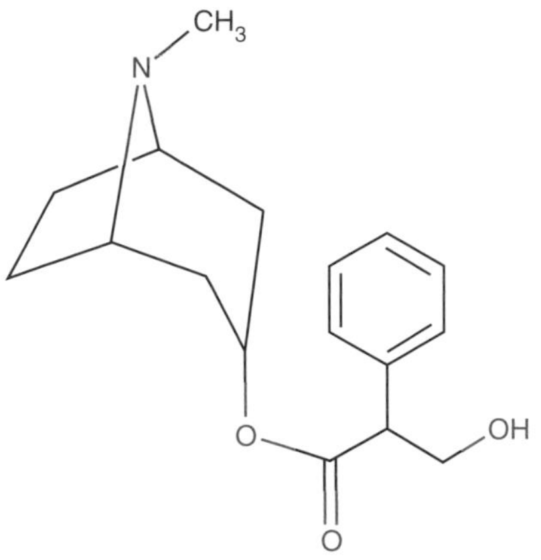

Background

Atropine is the racemic mixture of L- and D-hyoscyamine and possesses 50% of the antimuscarinic potency of L-hyoscyamine. Atropine is derived from the components of the belladonna plant and is also present in other plants from the Solanaceae family. Women in ancient times often dripped the plant's juices into their eyes, causing mydriasis and thereby enhancing their beauty. In Italian, belladonna translates to 'beautiful lady.' In the United States, the atropine autoinjector has been in use since 1973 for the treatment of exposures to chemical warfare nerve agents and insecticides.

Uses

Atropine is used in the management of sinus bradycardia with hemodynamic instability and in the treatment of peptic ulcer disease, irritable bowel syndrome, urinary incontinence, and organophosphate and carbamate poisoning. It is also present in ophthalmic preparations to induce mydriasis and cyclopegia. Atropine is often administered preoperatively to decrease secretions.

Environmental Fate and Behavior

Free atropine is only slightly soluble in cold water. It melts at 115 °C but decomposes upon boiling.

Environmental monitoring of atropine is not routinely performed by regulatory bodies. Hazardous short-term degradation products are not likely to occur. Accidental environmental exposure may occur through unintentional ingestion of toxic plants of the Solanaceae family, such as the deadly nightshade.

Exposure and Exposure Monitoring

Ingestion is the most frequent route of exposure. Exposure can also occur following instillation of eye solutions and via subcutaneous, intramuscular, intravenous, and inhalation routes. Accidental overdosage may occur when atropine is administered for the treatment of organophosphate or carbamate insecticide poisoning.

Monitoring of atropine levels in blood or bodily fluids is not employed in standard exposure management. Environmental monitoring of atropine is not a common practice.

Toxicokinetics

In therapeutic doses, atropine is well absorbed. In toxic doses, absorption may be prolonged secondary to decreased gastric motility. Atropine is 18% bound to plasma protein and its volume of distribution ranges from 2 to 4 l kg^{-1}. Atropine is metabolized in the liver to tropic acid, tropine, esters of tropic acid, and glucuronide conjugates. Elimination follows first-order kinetics. Approximately 30–60% is excreted unchanged in the urine. Drug clearance is dependent on glomerular filtration. The elimination half-life is 2–3 h in adults but may be longer in children.

Mechanism of Toxicity

Atropine competitively antagonizes acetylcholine at the neuroreceptor site. Atropine prevents acetylcholine from exhibiting its usual action but does not decrease acetylcholine production. Cardiac muscle, smooth muscle, and the central nervous system are most affected by the antagonism of acetylcholine.

Acute and Short-Term Toxicity

Animal

Animals are at risk for anticholinergic poisoning from atropine. Toxicity is similar to that in humans. Gastrointestinal decontamination and supportive care should be employed.

There is interspecies variability and variability based on the route of exposure to atropine. The rat LD_{50} oral is 500 mg kg^{-1}; the LD_{50} intraperitoneal is 280 mg kg^{-1}; and the LD_{50} IV is 73 mg kg^{-1}.

 http://dx.doi.org/10.1016/B978-0-12-386454-3.00695-3

Human

Overdosage of atropine results in signs and symptoms consistent with the anticholinergic toxidrome. Signs and symptoms have been reported following the ingestion of as few as four to five drops of 4% ocular atropine solution. Patients exhibit warm, flushed, and dry skin as a result of peripheral vasodilatation. Mydriasis occurs due to antagonism of acetylcholine in the muscles of the iris. Urinary retention, thirst, delirium, hallucinations, and decreased bowel sounds may occur. Tachycardia with ensuing hypertension can appear secondary to vagal blockade. The anticholinergic toxidrome may be delayed and can occur in cycles. Severe intoxications may progress to seizures, coma, and arrhythmias.

Chronic Toxicity

Animal

A juvenile pygmy sperm whale (*Kogia breviceps*) was treated with several doses of atropine to relieve symptoms of pyloric stenosis. The animal developed signs and symptoms of anticholinergic toxicity including hyperexcitability, ascending weakness, vomiting, and aspiration of seawater. Symptoms resolved after administration of physostigmine.

Human

Chronic ingestion of greater than therapeutic amounts of atropine may produce symptoms of the anticholinergic toxidrome.

Immunotoxicity

Atropine is not known to cause specific immunotoxic effects. As with exposure to any agent, humans may be at risk for hypersensitivity reactions to atropine.

Reproductive and Developmental Toxicity

Atropine Carries FDA Pregnancy Category C Rating

Atropine may be used during pregnancy as a preoperative, preanesthetic agent to reduce salivation and bronchial secretions. Atropine rapidly crosses the human placenta. In one study of 44 healthy pregnant women, a maximum umbilical to maternal vein ratio of 1.27 was observed 6 min after administration of 0.01 mg kg^{-1} intravenously. The corresponding umbilical and maternal vein atropine levels were 22 and 17 nmol l^{-1} respectively. Intramuscular injection produced lower concentrations.

Another study administered labeled atropine intravenously prior to delivery to quantify placental transfer and fetal distribution of the drug. The concentrations in the umbilical vein 1 and 5 min after injection were 12 and 93%, respectively, of the corresponding maternal value. Concentrations in the umbilical artery were approximately 50% of those in the umbilical vein during the same period.

Studies have shown that administration of atropine to a pregnant woman during the last trimester can mask the effects of vagal stimulation on the fetal heart, producing tachycardia within 5–30 min after injection. Limited data have shown that atropine can suppress fetal breathing, although fetal hypoxia has not been observed. Atropine could reduce lower esophageal sphincter pressure enough to predispose the newborn to aspiration. Uterine contractility does not appear to be significantly affected by atropine, perhaps due to a decrease in the sensitivity of muscarinic receptors on myometrial tissue during pregnancy.

Multiple prospective cohort studies have monitored tens of thousands of mother–child pairs in which the mother was exposed to atropine during pregnancy. Overall, these data do not support an association between the use of atropine and congenital defects.

Anticholinergic agents can inhibit lactation in animals, via inhibition of growth hormone and oxytocin secretion. These agents can also reduce serum prolactin in nonnursing women, but decreased prolactin levels in an established nursing mother should not affect her ability to breast-feed. In theory, long-term use of atropine may reduce milk production or milk letdown, but a single systemic or ophthalmic dose should not interfere with breast-feeding.

Genotoxicity

Studies of the mutageniticity of atropine in *Escherichia coli* have demonstrated no effects on cell DNA. Atropine is not expected to cause chromosome abnormalities at clinically relevant doses.

Carcinogenicity

No large-scale or long-term studies have been performed examining the carcinogenicity of atropine. In one isolated rat study, 25 μg kg^{-1} administered twice daily for 5 days to virgin female rats demonstrated no carcinogenic effect.

Clinical Management

Basic and advanced life support measures should be utilized as necessary for atropine exposure. Gastric decontamination procedures should be employed based on the patient's history and current symptomatology. Activated charcoal can be given to adsorb atropine. The mainstay of treatment is supportive care. Physostigmine, a cholinesterase inhibitor, can be given to patients to reverse signs and symptoms of the anticholinergic toxidrome. However, the administration of physostigmine may be contraindicated in the patient who has also been exposed to a tricyclic antidepressant, or another agent known to cause QRS interval widening on the EKG. Extracorporeal elimination measures are ineffective in atropine overdose for toxin removal.

Ecotoxicology

Significant intra- and interspecies variations exist among animals surrounding the toxicity of atropine and other belladonna alkaloids. Rabbits, guinea pigs, and birds are resistant to their effects due to internal detoxifying mechanisms. Horses, cattle, and goats are also reportedly resistant to ingested but not injected belladonna. Pigs are susceptible to effects from ingested belladonna compounds.

Signs of acute intoxication are similar in all mammalian species.

Exposure Standards and Guidelines

Published guidelines or occupational standards for atropine exposure are not commonly employed. Exposures are managed with first aid measures and symptomatic and supportive care.

See also: Anticholinergics; Carbamate Pesticides; G-Series Nerve Agents; Organophosphorus Compounds; Poisoning Emergencies in Humans.

Further Reading

Bucaretchi, F., Prado, C.C., Branco, M.M., et al., 2012. Poisoning by illegal rodenticides containing acetylcholinesterase inhibitors (chumbinho): a prospective case series. Clin. Toxicol. 50, 44–51.

Chia, A., Chua, W.H., Cheung, Y.B., et al., 2012. Atropine for the treatment of childhood myopia: safety and efficacy of 0.5%, 0.1%, and 0.01% doses (atropine for the treatment of myopia 2). Ophthalmology 119, 347–354.

Gaire, B.P., Subedi, L., March 2013. A review on the pharmacological and toxicological aspects of *Datura stramonium* L. J. Integr. Med. 11 (2), 73–79.

Hoefnagel, D., 1961. Toxic effects of atropine and homatropine eye drops in children. N. Engl. J. Med. 264, 168–171.

Mercey, G., Verdelet, T., Renou, J., et al., 2012. Reactivators of acetylcholinesterase inhibited by organophosphorus nerve agents. Accounts of Chemical Research 45, 756–766.

Robenshtok, E., Luria, S., Tashma, Z., Hourvitz, A., 2002. Adverse reaction to atropine and the treatment of organophosphate intoxication. Isr. Med. Assoc. J. 4, 535–539.

Avian Ecotoxicology *see* Avian Ecotoxicology

Avermectin

GM Fent, Oklahoma State University-CVHS, Stillwater, OK, USA

This article is a revision of the previous edition article by Katherine K. Williamson, volume 1, pp 192–194, © 2005, Elsevier Inc.

Background

The avermectins are a group of related, 16-member, naturally occurring or semisynthetic macrocyclic lactone endectocides. They are produced from the fermentation products of the soil-dwelling actinomycete, *Streptomyces avermitilis,* and effectively control a wide variety of both endo- and ectoparasites. The avermectins are used extensively around the world in veterinary and human medicine to control parasitic infections and in agriculture/horticulture to control insects on many crops and ornamentals.

The avermectins exert their therapeutic effects through binding to glutamate-gated chloride channels, causing a flaccid paralysis and death of the parasite. The avermectins were initially believed to work by increasing the release of GABA in the parasite. However, the main mechanism of actions for the avermectins is now believed to be selective high-affinity binding to glutamate-gated chloride channels in neural and muscle and cells. There is also evidence that the avermectins interact with GABA receptors but the higher concentrations required for this interaction are higher than those required for the glutamate-mediated effects.

- Name: Avermectin
- Chemical Structure:

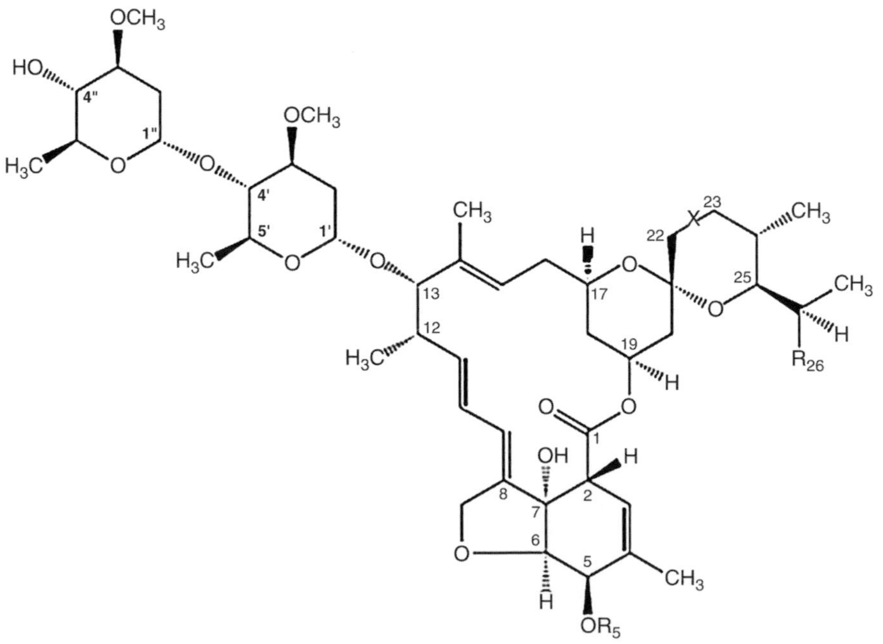

Components A: $R_5 = CH_3$ Components a: $R_{26} = C_2H_5$ Components 1: X = –CH=CH–

Components B: $R_5 = H$ Components b: $R_{26} = CH_3$ Components 2: X = –CH_2–CH(OH)–

 http://dx.doi.org/10.1016/B978-0-12-386454-3.00099-3

Uses

Veterinary Medicine

Avermectins are used extensively in veterinary medicine to control a number of parasitic organisms in both livestock and companion animals. They are approved for use in domestic and wild ruminants, horses, swine, dogs, and cats. The avermectins effectively control gastrointestinal nematodes, ticks, mites, lice, cattle grubs, and lungworms. Ivermectin, the most widely used and studied of the avermectins, has a wide therapeutic index with recommended dosage of 0.2 mg kg^{-1} in cattle and horses, 0.006 mg kg^{-1} in dogs for the prevention of heartworm infection, and 0.2–0.4 mg kg^{-1} to treat intestinal parasites. Several veterinary formulations are available and include abamectin (avermectin b_1), ivermectin (22,23-dihydro-avermectin b_1), eprinomectin (4′-epi-acetylamino-4″-deoxyavermectin b_1), doramectin [25-cyclohexyl-5-*o*-demethyl-25-de(1-methylpropyl) avermectin a_{1a}], and selamectin [25-cyclohexyl-25-de (1-methylpropyl)-5-deoxy-22,23-dihydro-5-(hydroxyimino)-avermectin B_{1a}].

Human Medicine

Ivermectin is used to treat onchocerciasis, lymphatic filariasis, strongyloidiasis, and cutaneous larval migrans and is an effective treatment for scabies in humans.

Environmental Fate and Behavior

Ivermectin is the most widely studied of the avermectins, and this section refers to ivermectin unless otherwise stated. Ivermectin is neutral at all pH values, has an estimated melting point of 349.8 °C, a vapor pressure of $<1.5 \times 10^{-9}$, and a water solubility of approximately 4 mg l^{-1}. Due to its very low water solubility, ivermectin and the other avermectins have little mobility and are unlikely to leach into groundwater. Degradation occurs primarily through photolysis both within the soil and in water; microbial breakdown also contributes to the loss of avermectins from the soil. The half-life is approximately 1 week when it is applied to the soil surface and is approximately 2 weeks to 2 months if dark, aerobic conditions are present. Some recent literature reports regarding the environmental risk assessment of ivermectin indicate a possible need for additional risk assessment evaluations of ivermectin. For additional information on this topic, the reader is directed to the further reading section.

Exposure and Exposure Monitoring

Accidental exposure can occur via the respiratory, dermal, and oral routes or by an injection stab.

Toxicokinetics

The toxicokinetics of ivermectin depend on the route of administration, product formulation, and the species. Following oral administration in humans, ivermectin is highly protein bound, has a large volume of distribution, and has a plasma half-life of 16 h. It is metabolized by hepatic CYP3A4 to multiple metabolites. In cattle, the half-life of a single intravenous dose is 2.8 days and increases to 8 days following subcutaneous injection. In simple-stomached animals, the oral bioavailability is 95% but drops to 25–33% in ruminant animals. Ivermectin is excreted in the milk, and residues may remain in the liver for up to 14 days; therefore, label withdrawal times should be closely followed.

Mechanism of Toxicity

The avermectins exert their therapeutic effects through high-affinity binding to glutamate-gated chloride channels; this binding causes an irreversible increase in chloride conductance, hyperpolarization, and flaccid paralysis of the parasite. These effects do not appear to occur in mammals, giving the avermectins a large margin of safety. However, at higher doses, the avermectins also interact with other chloride channels, including GABA and glycine-dependent channels. These interactions do occur in mammals and are believed to be responsible for the neurotoxicity seen in mammals.

Acute and Short-Term Toxicity

In animals, signs of neurotoxicity may develop in the case of extreme overdose or at lower doses in ivermectin-sensitive breeds of dogs. Clinical signs of toxicity include mydriasis, depression, ataxia, and tremor and in severe cases coma and death. Certain breeds of dogs (collies and others) have an increased sensitivity to these drugs. This increased sensitivity is likely due to the absence or partial absence of a *P*-glycoprotein in the blood–brain barrier that is responsible for drug transport from the brain back into the blood. A 4 base-pair deletion in the MDR1 gene has been shown to be responsible for this deficiency in several breeds of collie dogs and some Australian shepherds.

In humans, toxicity is usually related to a hypersensitivity reaction (Mazzotti reaction) caused by dying microfilaria. Clinical signs include fever, pruritus, arthralgia, myalgia, postural hypotension, edema, lymphadenopathy, headache, sore throat, and stomach upset. Other clinical signs that may also be seen include rash, dizziness, seizure, dyspnea, ataxia, and urticaria.

Chronic Toxicity

In animals, repeated low-dose exposure to avermectins appears to cause greater toxicity compared to a single high dose. Dogs dosed orally with 0.5 and 1 mg kg^{-1} day^{-1} for year showed signs of weight loss, lethargy, recumbency, tremor, and mydriasis. Effects on weight (increased gain or loss) and tremor were also seen following chronic exposure to abamectin in rats and mice.

Little is known about the chronic toxicity of the avermectins in humans.

Reproductive Toxicity

Ivermectin has been used safely in breeding cattle, but abamectin caused reproductive effects in rats given 0.40 mg kg^{-1} day^{-1}.

This suggests that there is a potential for reproductive effects at high enough doses, and the World Health Organization recommends against the use of ivermectin for mass administration in pregnant women and during the first week of lactation.

Genotoxicity

Ivermectin was negative in Ames mutagenesis assays.

Carcinogenicity

Rats and mice fed the maximum tolerated dose of abamectin for 24 months did not have increased tumor incidence, and abamectin is not considered carcinogenic in rats or mice.

Clinical Management

Treatment of intoxication with one of the avermectins should focus on decontamination and supportive care. Following recent oral ingestion emesis, activated charcoal, and a saline cathartic are beneficial at limiting absorption. In severe cases of intoxication in animals, the use of physostigmine has been report to be beneficial in the supportive care of these animals. In humans suffering from a Mazzotti-like reaction due to microfilaria die-off, the use of analgesics and antihistamines is beneficial. In severe cases, glucocorticoids may be required.

Ecotoxicology

The avermectins are relatively nontoxic to birds but are highly toxic to fish, aquatic invertebrates, and honeybees. The LD_{50} and the dietary LC_{50} in bobwhite quail is 2 g kg^{-1} and 3102 ppm, respectively. Mallard ducks fed up to 12 ppm abamectin in their diets for 18 weeks showed no evidence of adverse effects on reproduction. In rainbow trout, bluegill sunfish, sheepshead minnow, catfish, and carp, the 96 h LC_{50} was 3.2, 9.6, 15, 24, and 42 ppb, respectively. In pink shrimp, eastern oysters, and blue crab, the 96 h LC_{50} for abamectin is 0.0016, 430, and 153 mg l^{-1}, respectively. The 48 h LC_{50} in *Daphnia* was 0.34 ppb. In a 28 day bioaccumulation study, abamectin did not bioaccumulate in bluegill sunfish. In bees, the 24 h contact LC_{50} for abamectin is 2 ng per bee, and it has an oral LD_{50} of 9 ng per bee.

Exposure Standards and Guidelines

In the United States, the acceptable daily intake (ADI) and reference dose (RfD) are 0.0001 and 0.0004 mg kg^{-1} day^{-1}, respectively. In the EU, the ADI and RfD are 0.0025 and 0.005 mg kg^{-1} day^{-1}, respectively.

See also: Selamectin; Pesticides.

Further Reading

Lanusse, C.E., Lifschitz, A.L., Imperiale, F.A., 2009. Macrocyclic lactones: endectocide compounds. In: Riviere, J.E., Papich, M.G. (Eds.), Veterinary Pharmacology and Therapeutics, ninth ed., pp. 1119–1144.

Liebig, M., Fernandez, A.A., et al., 2010. Environmental risk assessment of ivermectin: a case study. Integr. Environ. Assess. Manag. 6 (1), 567–587.

Lu, F.C., 1995. A review of the acceptable daily intakes of pesticides assessed by the World Health Organization. Regul. Toxicol. Pharmacol. 21, 351–364, 10-13.

McCarthy, J., Loukas, A., Hotez, P.J., 2011. Chemotherapy of helminth infection. In: Brunton, L., Chabner, B., Knollman, B. (Eds.), Goodman and Gilman's the Pharmacological Basis of Therapeutics, twelfth ed., pp. 1443–1461.

Trailovic, S.M., Nedeljkovic, J.T., 2011. Central and peripheral neurotoxic effects of ivermectin in rats. J. Vet. Med. Sci. 73 (5), 591–599.

U.S. Environmental Protection Agency, 1995. Integrated Risk Information System Database. Washington, DC, pp. 10–14.

Relevant Websites

http://ec.europa.eu/food/plant/protection/evaluation/database_act_subs_en.htm – European Commission: Health and Consumers - EU Pesticides database.

http://ec.europa.eu/food/plant/protection/evaluation/existactive/list-abamectin_en.pdf – Review report for the active substance abamectin Finalised in the Standing Committee on the Food Chain and Animal Health at its meeting on 11 July 2008 in view of the inclusion of abamectin in Annex I of Directive 91/414/EEC.

http://www.epa.gov/iris/subst/0381.htm – US Environmental Protection Agency: Integrated Risk Information System - Avermectin B1.

http://extoxnet.orst.edu/pips/abamecti.htm – Extension Toxicology Network, Oregon State University. Abamectin Pesticide Information Profile.

Azathioprine

S Espín and AJ García-Fernández, University of Murcia, Murcia, Spain

This article is a revision of the previous edition article by Eric M. Silberhorn, volume 1, pp 196–200, © 2005, Elsevier Inc.

- Name: Azathioprine
- Chemical Abstracts Service Registry Number (CAS RN)*: 446-86-6
- Synonyms*: 6-((1-Methyl-4-nitro-1*H*-imidazol-5-yl)thio)-1*H*-purine, Azamune, Azanin, Azasan, Imuran
- Molecular Formula*: $C_9H_7N_7O_2S$
- Chemical Structure*:

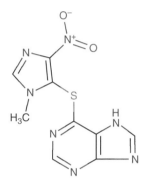

*All from ChemIDplus.

Background

Azathioprine is a thiopurine immunosuppressant drug to prevent rejection of allogeneic organ transplants and to manage many immunological diseases. It is a chemical analog of the physiologic purines and antimetabolite (an inhibitor of purine synthesis), and is a prodrug for 6-mercaptopurine (6-MP). The two drugs were developed originally by George Hitchings and Gertrude Elion as antileukemia agents in 1954. Azathioprine was first used in human transplantation in 1962. Nowadays, thiopurines are used for their anti-inflammatory and immunosuppressant effects.

Uses

Azathioprine is an immunosuppressive agent used to prevent rejection of allogeneic kidney and other organ transplants (i.e., from genetically different donors). This drug is also used to manage severe rheumatoid arthritis in adults and a variety of immunological diseases, such as systemic lupus erythematous, autoimmune hemolytic anemia, chronic active hepatitis, ulcerative colitis, Crohn's disease, dermatomyositis, pemphigus vulgaris, polyarteritis nodosa and idiopathic thrombocytopenia. It has also been found to be an effective steroid sparing agent.

The drug is generally used in combination with other immunosuppressive therapy, including local radiation therapy, corticosteroids, and other cytotoxic agents. It is considered to be a prodrug that converts after absorption into 6-MP, an important component of treatment programs for acute lymphocytic leukemia in children and adults.

Environmental Fate and Behavior

Azathioprine is an odorless powder, has crystal form at room temperature, and has a pale-yellow color. Azathioprine has a molecular weight of 277.3 g mol^{-1}, its melting point ranges from 243 to 244 °C, the vapor pressure is 2.41×10^{-12} mm Hg at 25 °C, and the dissociation constant (pK_a) is 8.2. Its octanol/water partition coefficient (Log K_{ow}) is 0.1. The drug is insoluble in water (water solubility 0.272 g l^{-1} at 25 °C), very slightly soluble in ethanol and chloroform, sparingly soluble in dilute mineral acids, and soluble in dilute alkaline solutions.

Azathioprine is stable in neutral or acid solutions, with maximum stability at pH 5.5–6.5, but is hydrolyzed to 6-MP in alkaline solutions, especially on warming. Hydrolysis to 6-MP also occurs in the presence of sulfhydryl compounds such as cysteine.

Exposure and Exposure Monitoring

Exposure routes to azathioprine during medical treatment are ingestion and intravenous injection. Azathioprine is typically administered in tablet form (25, 50, 75, and 100 mg). Following renal transplantation, azathioprine may initially be given by intravenous route to patients unable to tolerate oral medication. However, oral therapy should replace parenteral therapy as soon as possible. The injectable form is presented as the sodium salt in 100 mg vials. The usual dose for kidney-transplant patients is 3–5 mg kg^{-1} day^{-1}, which may be reduced to 1–3 mg kg^{-1} day^{-1} for maintenance. For rheumatoid arthritis, the initial dose is 1 mg kg^{-1} day^{-1}, and the dose may be increased to 2.5 mg kg^{-1} day^{-1}. For inflammatory bowel disease, the adult dosage ranges from 1.5 to 3.0 mg kg^{-1} day^{-1}.

Occupational exposure to azathioprine may occur via inhalation of dust during production, formulation, and packaging of the drug. A study developed at a pharmaceutical plant in South Africa showed that the highest median concentrations of azathioprine dust measured were 0.26 mg m^{-3} in the breathing zone and 0.07 mg m^{-3} in personal air samples. From 1981 to 1983, the National Institute for Occupational Safety and Health conducted the National Occupational Exposure Survey involving on-site visits to 4490 establishments. The survey estimated that 1849 workers, including 880 women, were potentially exposed to azathioprine.

Toxicokinetics

Azathioprine is readily absorbed from the gastrointestinal tract, with 16–50% absorbed in healthy guts. It is rapidly distributed throughout the body and reaches peak plasma concentrations within 1–2 h after administration. Azathioprine is maximum

30% bound to plasma proteins, and very small amounts enter the brain. It crosses the placenta, and trace amounts of the 6-MP metabolite have been detected in fetal blood.

Azathioprine is rapidly converted to 6-MP. Approximately 88% of azathioprine is metabolized *in vivo* by both nonenzymatic and enzymatic degradation by sulfhydryl compounds such as glutathione to 6-MP, presumably in the liver and erythrocytes. The plasma half-life of azathioprine is approximately 12–15 min, while that of 6-MP is approximately 30 min to 4 h. Bioactivation of 6-MP occurs enzymatically to form the active metabolites 6-thioguanine nucleotides (6-TGN) and 6-methylmercaptopurine. The active metabolites 6-TGN, responsible for the therapeutic action, are formed intracellularly and appear to have long half-lives. Moreover, 6-MP may be oxidized to 6-thiouric acid (6-TU) by xanthine oxidase, or methylated to 6-methylmercaptopurine by thiopurine methyltransferase (TPMT). The level of TPMT activity has been considered responsible for the variation in the therapeutic efficacy and toxicity of azathioprine. Patients with low TPMT enzyme activity should have excessive production of active 6-TGN, leading to toxic accumulation. However, patients with high TPMT activity should present lower 6-TGN levels and lack of response to therapy.

Small amounts of azathioprine and 6-MP are excreted intact. In the 24 h period after administration up to 50% of the dose is excreted in the urine, but only 10% is excreted as the parent drug, and 12% of the dose is excreted unchanged in the feces. Published reports have found minimal 6-MP excretion into breast milk.

Mechanism of Toxicity

The conversion of azathioprine to 6-MP is believed to contribute to many of the pharmacological and toxicological effects of azathioprine. Mainly through its metabolites, azathioprine inhibits purine biosynthesis and DNA, RNA, and proteins synthesis. This drug may also inhibit mitosis and coenzyme formation and functioning, interfering with cellular metabolism. The exact mechanism of azathioprine and 6-MP immunosuppressive action has not been determined and may be multifactorial. A triple mechanism has been proposed: (1) the induction of a very specific apoptotic pathway in lymphocytes, (2) the incorporation of the active metabolites 6-TGN into DNA resulting in DNA damage and the impairment in its repair system that induces the activation of nonspecific apoptotic pathways in proliferating lymphocytes, and (3) the inhibition of *de novo* purine biosynthesis by methylmercaptopurine nucleotides. Besides, an *in vitro* study conducted with rat hepatocytes concluded that azathioprine toxicity involves depletion of reduced glutathione, which leads to mitochondrial injury with profound depletion of ATP and cell death by necrosis. Cell death was prevented by potent antioxidants, glycine, and blocking the mitochondrial permeability transition pore.

Acute and Short-Term Toxicity

According to Regulation (EC) No 1272/2008, azathioprine is placed in Category II regarding skin and eye irritation. Azathioprine is also classified in Category IV in the acute oral toxicity. The lethal dose to 50% of exposed individuals (LD_{50}) after oral dosing is 535 mg kg^{-1} in rats and 1389 mg kg^{-1} in mouse. After intraperitoneal administration, the LD_{50} is 300 mg kg^{-1} in rats and 273 mg kg^{-1} in mouse. The LD_{50} after intraduodenal administration is 630 mg kg^{-1} in rats and 2437 mg kg^{-1} in mouse. Studies with animals have shown that the hematopoietic system is affected by azathioprine with depression of granulopoiesis, megakaryocytes and, as a result, platelet formation. Reversible hepatotoxicity has been observed in dogs at doses of 5 mg kg^{-1} day^{-1}, while a dose of 10 mg kg^{-1} for 10 days produced death from agranulocytosis. The lymphatic system is also affected in monkeys, with atrophy of the lymphoid tissue at doses of 1 mg kg^{-1} day^{-1}.

Since azathioprine is a myelotoxic and hepatotoxic immunosuppressive agent, bone marrow and liver are the main targets, but gastrointestinal tract, kidney, lungs, central nervous system, and skin may also be affected. Signs of acute overdose in humans include bone marrow suppression manifested by leukopenia (in 2–3 days) or, less frequently, macrocytic and megaloblastic anemia, and thrombocytopenia, which may result in prolongation of clotting time and eventual hemorrhage. Severe pancytopenia has been observed in about 1% of patients who receive more than 2.5 mg kg^{-1}. Leukopenia is the main toxic effect that may occur after therapeutic doses and overdoses of azathioprine. Myelosuppression is dose dependent and typically observed after 7–14 days of therapy. Infections are very common in transplant patients receiving azathioprine. The drug may also affect liver (elevation in liver enzymes and cholestasis) and kidney (renal failure, acute tubular necrosis) function, but these organs usually returned to normality after discontinuation of the drug.

Other signs of acute overdose are gastrointestinal tract disturbances such as vomiting or nausea, hypermotility, abdominal pain, and diarrhea, which appear mainly at higher doses. Other symptoms may include fever, weakness, joint pain, lower back or side pain, skin rash or red spots on skin, unusual bleeding or bruising, painful or difficult urination, and blood in urine or stools. In skin and eyes, azathioprine causes irritation, and if inhalation occurs, upper respiratory tract and mucous membrane irritation may happen.

Chronic Toxicity

Chronic azathioprine exposure studies with animals show weight loss, diarrhea, tachypnea, and ear duct squamous-cell carcinomas in rats (150 mg kg^{-1} for 52 weeks); lymphomas in mice (100 mg kg^{-1} for 6, 7, or 10 months depending on the study); leukemia and lung adenomas in mice (40 or 10 mg kg^{-1} daily on days 1–4 after birth); bone marrow depression in dogs and rats (4 and 45 mg kg^{-1} per day, respectively); and lymphomas and uterine hemangioendotheliomas in mice (20 mg kg^{-1} during 94 weeks).

In humans, azathioprine may cause bone marrow depression reflected mainly as leukopenia. Long-term immunosuppression may increase susceptibility to infections such as herpes simplex, herpes zoster, and verrucae. Azathioprine may also increase the development of tumors such as non-Hodgkin's lymphoma, squamous-cell carcinoma, mesenchymal tumors, and hepatobiliary carcinoma. There are also reports of chronic liver disease (hepatitis), portal hypertension, hepatic veno-occlusive disease, and hemangioma of the liver after azathioprine therapy. Acute pancreatitis was also reported following long-term treatment. Acute restrictive lung disease, interstitial nephritis, and a case of progressive leukoencephalopathy after 4 years of azathioprine therapy were reported. Skin rash, alopecia, and urticaria were also documented. Prolonged or repeated exposure in humans may cause allergic reactions (dermatitis or asthma) in sensitive individuals if inhaled, ingested, or in contact with skin.

Immunotoxicity

Azathioprine affects *in vitro* lymphocyte proliferation, macrophage cytotoxicity, and natural killer cell activity in experimental animals. Immunotoxicological effects of azathioprine in rats are reductions in the organ weights such as thymus and spleen, and decreased number of white blood cells. Bone-marrow cell counts were reported to be significantly reduced, attributed to the decrease in the number of lymphocytes and granulocytes. Histopathologically, azathioprine produced a decrease of lymphocytes in the thymus and spleen.

Azathioprine may also inhibit the *in vitro* lymphocyte proliferation and the mixed lymphocyte reaction in humans. The drug impaired T-helper function as well as B cell differentiation of peripheral blood, lymph node, and spleen lymphocytes. Azathioprine produces bone marrow suppression normally manifested by leukopenia in treated patients. The drug may reduce gammaglobulin synthesis, natural killer cell activity, and antibody-dependent cellular cytotoxicity in patients with rheumatic disorders or renal transplant recipients. Maternal use of azathioprine during pregnancy has been reported to suppress immune function in human infants. In this sense, lymphopenia, decreased immunoglobulin G and M levels, cytomegalovirus infection, and a decreased thymic shadow have been reported in one infant whose mother had received 150 mg of azathioprine daily. However, most of these anomalies were reversed before one year of age. Pancytopenia and severe immunodeficiency were also reported in a premature infant whose mother received 125 mg of azathioprine daily.

Reproductive Toxicity

Teratogenic effects, including cleft palates, open-eye, skeletal malformations, and decreased thymus size, have been reported in the offspring of mice injected intraperitoneally during the period of organogenesis with the equivalent of 4–13 times the maximum human therapeutic dose of azathioprine. Increased frequencies of cleft palates, ocular anomalies, and limb malformations also occurred among the offspring of rabbits injected intraperitoneally in doses equivalent to 2–6 times those used in humans. This drug induced embryolethality and growth retardation in the offspring of rats and mice injected intraperitoneally during the period of organogenesis in doses equivalent to up to 4 times the human therapeutic dose, but no malformations were noted in the surviving fetuses. Azathioprine also caused temporary depression in spermatogenesis and reduction in sperm viability and sperm count in mice at doses 10 times the human therapeutic dose.

The US Food and Drug Administration classified azathioprine in category D (positive evidence of human fetal risk). The data currently available in humans are both limited and conflicting. Although there are no well-controlled studies in pregnant women, some studies have reported that azathioprine may cause fetal harm when administered during pregnancy. Effects associated with prenatal exposure to azathioprine, such as spontaneous abortions and low birth weight, appear to be increased in pregnancies of renal transplant recipients treated with the drug, particularly if the woman requires a high dose therapy. Exposure to azathioprine during pregnancy has been associated with a slight increase in the frequency of anomalies in infants, including hydrocephalus, anencephaly, microcephaly, hypospadias, malformed hand and face, polydactyly, cleft palate, pulmonary artery stenosis, and congenital heart disease. The incidence of pregnancy-related complications (spontaneous abortions and congenital abnormalities) has also been shown to increase when fathers used azathioprine or 6-MP within 3 months before conception. In contrast, some studies suggested that treatment with azathioprine/6-MP before or at conception or during pregnancy for other conditions such as inflammatory bowel disease appears to be safe. A recent study in 2012, the largest study so far with over 100 prospectively ascertained pregnancies of spouses of male patients exposed to azathioprine or 6-MP, concluded that no specific adverse effects were observed after paternal treatment with the drug and, although data are still limited, there is no need for termination of pregnancy or invasive diagnostics only because parents were treated with these drugs.

Genotoxicity

Azathioprine was positive in the Ames mutagenicity assay using *Salmonella typhimurium* strain TA100, both with and without metabolic activation. Negative results were found for the TA98 strain under similar test conditions. Both azathioprine and 6-MP have been found to be mutagenic in various mammalian *in vitro* and *in vivo* assays. In animals treated *in vivo*, azathioprine induced dominant lethal mutations in mice and chromosomal aberrations in rabbit lymphocytes and Chinese hamster bone-marrow cells. The drug did not induce sister chromatid exchanges in Chinese hamster bone-marrow cells and in human lymphocytes *in vitro*. In humans, prenatal exposure to azathioprine or 6-MP has been associated with chromosomal aberrations in offspring, such as chromatid breaks and deletions. However, the number of reported children conceived by parents treated with the drug is too small to conclude the possible mutagenic effects of azathioprine.

Carcinogenicity

The International Agency for Research on Cancer (IARC) considered there to be sufficient evidence in experimental animals for the carcinogenicity of azathioprine. Squamous-cell ear duct carcinoma was observed in rats orally exposed to azathioprine (100 mg kg^{-1} for 52 weeks) and malignant thymic lymphomas were found in mice exposed to azathioprine by subcutaneous or intramuscular injection (100 mg kg^{-1} several times per week for 6, 7, or 10 months, depending on the study). Besides, leukemia was observed in mice exposed to azathioprine by intraperitoneal route (40 mg kg^{-1} daily on days 1–4 after birth), and lung adenomas were found in mice intraperitoneally exposed to the drug (10 mg kg^{-1} daily on days 1–4 after birth). Oral exposure in female mice (20 mg kg^{-1} during 94 weeks) produced lymphomas and uterine hemangioendotheliomas.

Azathioprine is 'known to be a human carcinogen' by the National Toxicology Program based on sufficient evidence of carcinogenicity from studies in humans, and is classified in Group 1 as 'carcinogenic to humans' by the IARC.

Two large prospective epidemiological studies reported that kidney-transplant patients treated almost routinely with azathioprine and prednisone presented high incidences of non-Hodgkin's lymphoma, squamous-cell carcinoma, mesenchymal tumors, and hepatobiliary carcinoma. An increased risk of the same cancers, although to a lesser extent than in the transplant patients, has been found in patients treated with this drug for other diseases such as rheumatoid arthritis, systemic lupus and other collagen disorders, inflammatory bowel disease, and certain skin and renal diseases. A recent study of more than 45 000 patients with inflammatory bowel disease published in 2013 has found an increased rate of overall cancer among users of azathioprine compared with controls. This study confirmed an increased risk of lymphoid tissue cancer and additionally found a significantly increased risk of urinary tract cancer associated with azathioprine.

Clinical Management

There is no specific antidote for azathioprine. The azathioprine safety data sheet indicates the general treatment. Do not induce vomiting if swallowed unless directed to do so by medical personnel, remove to fresh air if inhalation occurred, wash with soap and water in case of skin contact, and flush eyes with plenty of water for at least 15 min if eye contact occurred. The recommendations for workers are to use personal protection such as safety glasses, lab coat, dust respirator, and gloves. It is also necessary to use process enclosures and local exhaust ventilation.

In treated patients, leukopenia induced by azathioprine and other side effects are usually reversible with discontinuation of treatment or a dose reduction. Administration of azathioprine with food or in a divided dose may help to reduce the incidence of gastrointestinal upset. Treatment for an overdose is symptomatic and has included gastric lavage.

Azathioprine contraindications are hypersensitivity to the drug, impaired hepatic or bone marrow function, severe infections, pancreatitis, pregnancy, and lactation. Although women taking azathioprine are advised to not breastfeed their infants, more recent data suggest that this may be safe. Other relative contraindications to azathioprine use are renal failure, viral hepatitis, human immunodeficiency virus infection, previous varicella zoster virus exposure, and premalignancy.

Regarding drug interactions, azathioprine dose should be reduced to one-quarter of the original dose when administered with allopurinol, as allopurinol inhibits xanthine oxidase activity, which affects the metabolism of 6-MP. However, it is better not to use these two drugs together. Azathioprine may reduce the anticoagulant effect of warfarin and may alter the effect of certain neuromuscular blocking agents. Administration with medicines that may have a myelosuppressive effect, such as penicillamine, should be avoided. The use of angiotensin-converting enzyme inhibitors to control hypertension has been shown to potentiate the effects of azathioprine. Aminosalicylate derivatives (sulphasalazine, mesalazine, or olsalazine) inhibit the TPMT enzyme and may potentiate azathioprine toxicity.

Exposure Standards and Guidelines

The regulatory authorities of the EU and the American Conference of Industrial Hygienists have not established occupational exposure limits for azathioprine. The healthcare company GlaxoSmithKline established an occupational exposure limit of 3 mg m^{-3} measured as the 8 h time weighted average limit (TWA). The Working Conditions Regulations in the Netherlands established an occupational exposure limit of 0.005 mg m^{-3} measured as 8 h TWA.

See also: Carcinogenesis; Carcinogen Classification Schemes.

Further Reading

Arnott, I.D.R., Watts, D., Satsangi, J., 2003. Azathioprine and anti-TNFα therapies in Crohn's disease: a review of pharmacology, clinical efficacy and safety. Pharmacol. Res. 47, 1–10.

Cara, C.J., Pena, A.S., Sans, M., Rodrigo, L., Guerrero-Esteo, M., Hinojosa, J., García-Paredes, J., Guijarro, L.G., 2004. Reviewing the mechanism of action of thiopurine drugs: towards a new paradigm in clinical practice. Med. Sci. Monit. 10 (11), RA247–254.

Hoeltzenbein, M., Weber-Schoendorfer, C., Borisch, C., Allignol, A., Meister, R., Schaefer, C., 2012. Pregnancy outcome after paternal exposure to azathioprine/6-mercaptopurine. Reprod. Toxicol. 34 (3), 364–369.

International Agency for Research on Cancer (IARC), 2012. Monographs of the Evaluation of Carcinogenic Risks to Humans. In: A Review of Human Carcinogens: Pharmaceuticals, vol. 100A. p. 435. Available at: http://monographs.iarc.fr/.

International Programme on Chemical Safety (IPCS), 1996. Azathioprine. Poison Information Monographs PIM 053. Available at: http://www.inchem.org/.

Matsumoto, K., Sekita, K., Ochiai, T., Takagi, A., Takada, K., Furuya, T., Kurokawa, Y., Saito, Y., Teshima, R., Suzuki, K., et al., 1990. Evaluation of immunotoxicity testings using azathioprine-treated rats: the international collaborative immunotoxicity study (azathioprine). Eisei Shikenjo Hokoku 108, 34–39.

Meggitt, S.J., Anstey, A.V., Mohd Mustapa, M.F., Reynolds, N.J., Wakelin, S., 2011. British Association of Dermatologists' guidelines for the safe and effective prescribing of azathioprine 2011. Br. J. Dermatol. 165, 711–734.

Pasternak, B., Svanström, H., Schmiegelow, K., Jess, T., Hviid, A., 2013. Use of azathioprine and the risk of cancer in inflammatory bowel disease. Am. J. Epidemiol..

Polifka, J., Friedman, J., 2002. Teratogen update: azathioprine and 6-mercaptopurine. Teratology 65, 240–261.

U.S. Department of Health and Human Services, 2011. Report on Carcinogens, twelfth ed. Public Health Service, National Toxicology Program. Available at: http://ntp.niehs.nih.gov/.

Waksman, J.C., Delgado, J.H., 2004. Immunosuppressants. In: Dart, R.C. (Ed.), Medical Toxicology, third ed. Lippincott Williams and Wilkins, Philadelphia, USA. (Chapter 170).

Relevant Website

http://actor.epa.gov/actor/faces/ACToRHome.jsp – ACToR (Aggregated Computational Toxicology Resource) (2012). Chemical Summary: Azathioprine (446-86-6).

Azinphos-Methyl

S Karanth, Charles River Laboratories, Reno, NV, USA

- Name: Azinphos-methyl
- Chemical Structure:

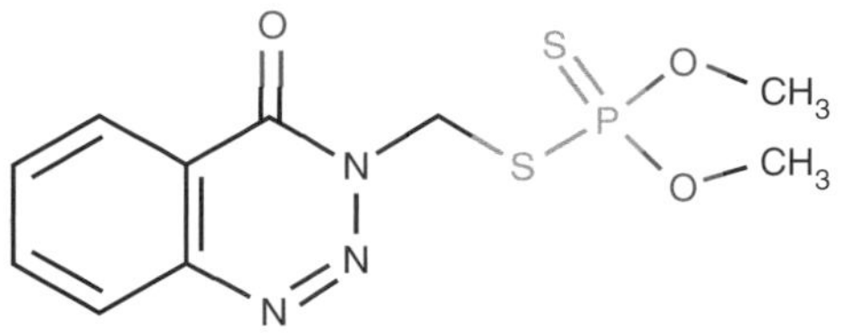

Background

Azinphos-methyl (AZM) was initially registered as an insecticide in the United States in 1959. Because of its health risks to farm workers, pesticide applicators, and aquatic ecosystems, the US Environmental Protection Agency issued a final decision on 16 Nov 2006, to phase out the remaining uses of AZM by 30 Sep 2012. AZM is sold under the trade names Gusathion®, Guthion®, and Methyl-Guthion®.

Uses

AZM is a broad-spectrum, nonsystemic insecticide and acaricide commonly used on a number of fruit, vegetable, and nut crops. It is not used in residential and public health pest control.

Environmental Fate

AZM adsorbs strongly to soil particles, and it has high potential to reach surface water through both spray drift and runoff. In sterile soil, its half-life is almost 1 year. Biodegradation and evaporation are the primary routes of elimination from soil, but it is also degraded by ultraviolet light. Degradation is more rapid at higher temperatures. AZM has a short half-life in surface waters (2 days). Hydrolysis is more prominent under alkaline conditions, but the compound is relatively stable in water below pH 10. The half-life on crops is 3–5 days under normal conditions.

Exposure and Exposure Monitoring

Common routes of AZM exposure include dermal, inhalation, and ingestion. Persistence of AZM is generally low under field conditions. It is fairly immobile in soil, it has low water solubility and low leaching potential, and is unlikely to contaminate groundwater.

Toxicokinetics

AZM is readily absorbed and distributed throughout the body following exposure. Mixed-function oxidase-mediated oxidative desulfuration of the parent compound produces the active metabolite, azinphos methyloxon. Other major metabolites include dimethylphosphorothioic and dimethylphosphoric acids and desmethyl azinphos-methyl.

Mechanism of Toxicity

Like other organophosphate insecticides, AZM exerts toxicity by inhibiting the enzyme acetylcholinesterase (AChE). AZM requires bioactivation for its biological action. The parent compound is activated to the potent 'oxon' by microsomal mixed-function oxidase enzymes, which in turn elicits toxicity by inhibiting AChE in synapse and neuromuscular junctions. AChE inhibition leads to overstimulation of cholinergic receptors on postsynaptic neurons, muscle cells, and/or end organs and consequent signs and symptoms of cholinergic toxicity.

Acute and Short-Term Toxicity

Animal

Acute toxicity studies in laboratory animals have shown that AZM is highly toxic to mammals. Oral and dermal LD_{50} values in laboratory rats are 4–16 and 88–220 mg kg^{-1}, respectively.

Human

Because of its high acute toxicity, low doses (>1.5 mg day^{-1}) of AZM can lead to severe poisoning. Most common signs and symptoms of acute poisoning include salivation, excessive sweating, stomach pain, vomiting, and diarrhea. Inhalation of dust or aerosol containing AZM can lead to wheezing, tearing of the eyes, blurred vision, and tightness in the chest. Eye contact with concentrated solutions of AZM can be life threatening.

Chronic Toxicity

Animal

Laboratory rats can tolerate a dietary dose of 0.5 mg kg^{-1} day^{-1} for 2 months without any adverse effects. Repeated long-term exposure to AZM can lead to memory loss and irritability.

Human

AChE inhibition caused by AZM can persist for a long time (2–6 weeks). Repeated chronic exposure may therefore result in prolonged AChE inhibition that may lead to flu-like illnesses.

Immunotoxicity

A dietary study in rats at doses up to 125 mg kg^{-1} day^{-1} for 3 weeks resulted in general toxicological and immunological

 http://dx.doi.org/10.1016/B978-0-12-386454-3.00101-9

changes at 125 mg kg^{-1} day^{-1} including increased mortality rate, decreased body weight, decreased relative spleen, pituitary, and mesenteric lymph node weights, and unspecified histopathological changes in the thymus, pituitary, adrenal glands, and testes. It is unclear if the immunological changes are due to the direct or indirect effects of AZM.

Reproductive Toxicity

A dietary reproductive toxicity study in rabbits indicated no effects on litter size, number of stillbirths, sex ratios, fetal weight, fetal development, or pup survival up to 30 days.

Genotoxicity

AZM is not mutagenic.

Carcinogenicity

AZM is classified as a 'not likely' human carcinogen.

Clinical Management

General decontamination procedures should be immediately initiated in case of AZM exposure. For skin decontamination, the exposed area should be washed with plenty of water or soap, and shampoo can be used during showering. In case of eye contamination, the eyes should be flushed with water repeatedly for several minutes. The contaminated clothing should be removed and the airway cleared. In case of ingestion, vomiting should be induced. Atropine treatment should be initiated immediately to counteract muscarinic effects. Atropine (adults and children >12 years: 2–4 mg; children <12 years: 0.05–0.1 mg) treatment should be repeated every 15 min until oral and bronchial secretions are controlled and atropinization is achieved. The duration and dosage of atropine treatment should be slowly reduced as the condition of the patient improves. Pralidoxime (2-PAM) should be administered slowly at the recommended dosage (adults and children >12 years: 1–2 g; children <12 years: 20–50 mg by IV infusion in 100 ml saline at ~0.2 g min^{-1}). This dosage can be repeated every 1–2 h intervals initially and at 10–12 h intervals later depending on the condition of the patient.

Ecotoxicology

AZM is highly toxic to fish and other aquatic organisms and moderately toxic to birds. It is also considered to pose minimal acute or chronic risk to wildlife. AZM is acutely toxic to a variety of wildlife species, including amphibians, crustaceans, molluscs, and many beneficial insects such as honey bees.

Exposure Standards and Guidelines

Acceptable daily intake = 0–0.002 5 mg kg^{-1} body weight.
Reference dose = 0.001 49 mg kg^{-1} day.

See also: Acetylcholine; Atropine; Biotransformation; Cholinesterase Inhibition; Food Quality Protection Act; Neurotoxicity; Organophosphorus Compounds; Pesticides.

Further Reading

Carrier, C., Brunet, R.C., 1999. A toxicokinetic model to assess the risk of azinphosmethyl exposure in humans through measures of urinary elimination of alkylphosphates. Toxicol. Sci. 47, 23–32.
Meyers, S.M., Wolff, J.O., 1993. Comparative toxicity of azinphos-methyl to house mice, laboratory mice, deer mice, and gray-tailed voles. Arch. Environ. Contam. Toxicol. 26, 478–482.

Relevant Websites

http://www.atsdr.cdc.gov/substances/index.asp – Agency for Toxic Substances & Disease Registry: search for "Azinphos Methyl".
http://www.cdpr.ca.gov/docs/risk/rcd/azmrcdre_98.pdf – California Department of Pesticide Regulation.
http://www.epa.gov/opp00001/reregistration/REDs/azm_red.pdf – Environmental Protection Agency.
http://www.epa.gov/oppsrrd1/REDs/azinphosmethyl_ired.pdf – Environmental Protection Agency.
http://www.epa.gov/opp00001/reregistration/azm/phaseout_fs.htm – Environmental Protection Agency.
http://pmep.cce.cornell.edu/profiles/extoxnet/24d-captan/azinphos-methyl-ext.html – Extoxnet: Azinphos Methyl.

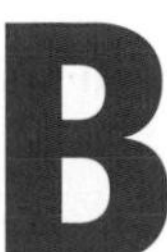

Bacillus cereus

HS Parihar, Philadelphia College of Osteopathic Medicine, Suwanee, GA, USA

This article is a revision of the previous edition article by Lee R. Shugart, volume 1, p 203, © 2005, Elsevier Inc.

Introduction

Bacillus cereus (*B. cereus*) is classified as a gram-positive, aerobic or facultative anaerobic, spore former, motile, pathogenic, and opportunistic bacterium capable of producing resistant endospores in the presence of oxygen. *B. cereus* is widely distributed in the environment, namely soil, where spores persist under adverse conditions. *B. cereus* can grow over a wide temperature range (8–55 °C), but it is not well suited to tolerate low pH values (minimum 5–6) or water content (minimum water activity 0.95).

B. cereus endospores are resistant to heat, radiation, disinfectants, and desiccation, and their adhesive characters facilitate their attachment to processing equipment and resistance to cleaning procedures. These organisms frequently contaminate clinical environments, biotechnological processes, and food production. *B. cereus* is known to be a causative organism for a wide range of opportunistic infections, both in immunocompromised and in immunocompetent patients, causing two distinct foodborne illness syndromes, namely diarrhea and emesis, and a wide range of opportunistic infections such as severe endophthalmitis, bacteremia, septicemia, endocarditis, pneumonia, meningitis, gastritis, and cutaneous infections. *B. cereus* infection can produce enterotoxins in the human small intestine, causing diarrheal food poisoning. *B. cereus* intoxication leads to the production of a toxin, cereulide, causing emesis.

Food Safety and Public Health Implications

B. cereus endospores are present in a wide variety of foods, including rice and pasta, milk and dairy products, infant foods, meat products, spices, fresh vegetables, seafood, ready to eat foods, dried foods such as spices, milk powders, and cereal products. Food products such as meat products, soups, vegetables, sauces, and dairy products are often associated with diarrheal food poisoning. Whereas rice and pasta are associated with the emetic type of syndrome.

Dried foods such as spices, milk powders, and cereal products are often quite heavily contaminated with *B. cereus* spores, and in presence of moisture, these spores may germinate, leading to spoilage or food poisoning. Food spoilage not only manifests as changes in texture or the production of off-flavors, it can also simply be caused by unwanted microbial growth in commercially sterile products. Such problems cause significant financial losses, despite the contributions of modern food technology and preservation techniques. Recent concerns are the tolerance, adaptation, or resistance of spores or vegetative cells of some species to conditions of low temperature or low pH that were previously presumed to stop growth, or to treatments such as ultrahigh heat treatment that were expected to inactivate all living material.

Use of *B. cereus* in probiotics is also an area of concern. This concern in the use of aerobic endospore formers in probiotic preparations, both for humans and for other animals, arises from the potential of these organisms to disseminate any antibiotic resistance genes that they might carry. The European Commission's Scientific Committee on Animal Nutrition has accordingly discouraged the use of strains from the *B. cereus* group, because of their potential to cause illness in humans and animals, and has deemed certain other animal products as unsafe because of the dangers of disseminating resistance to clinically important antibiotics such as erythromycin and lincosamides (e.g., lincomycin and clindamycin).

Mechanism of Toxicity

B. cereus is known to produce a variety of protein toxins of which three have been implicated in diarrheal illness. These enterotoxins are believed to cause diarrhea by damaging the integrity of ileal epithelial cell membranes. Diarrheal illness is characterized by abdominal pain with watery diarrhea 8–16 h after ingestion of the contaminated food, and it is associated with a diversity of foods from meats and vegetable dishes to pastas, desserts, cakes, sauces, and milk. Symptoms usually resolve within 24–48 h. In some cases, bloody diarrhea and necrotic enteritis have also been noted, and some outbreaks have included fatalities, particularly in children, with cases of liver failure, liver failure with brain edema, and brain edema with liver necrosis.

The three enterotoxins implicated in diarrheal illness are chromosomally encoded and classified as:

1. Hemolysin BL (Hbl) is a proteinaceous toxin that causes osmotic lysis by forming a transmembrane pore.

 http://dx.doi.org/10.1016/B978-0-12-386454-3.00997-0

2. Nonhemolytic enterotoxin (Nhe) is a three-part, proteinaceous, pore-forming toxin that is structurally similar to Hbl.
3. Cytotoxin K (CytK) is a single-component, β-barrel, pore-forming toxin.

Nhe is known to be the most dominant toxin in diarrheal illnesses. However, since most strains produce more than one enterotoxin, it is difficult to determine the *in vivo* potency of an individual toxin. Hence, it is most likely that combinations of toxins may act synergistically.

The main factor for the emetic food poisoning syndrome is cereulide. Cereulide is a small ring-formed dodecadepsipeptide comprising a ring of four amino- and/or oxyacids (D-*O*-Leu-D-Ala-L-*O*-Val-L-Val). It is produced in larger amounts at lower incubation temperatures (12–22 °C). Cereulide production by *B. cereus* has not been demonstrated at temperatures below 12 °C. This emetic toxin is very stable molecule and it can withstand high-temperature heat treatment, especially during cooking procedures such as frying, roasting, and microwaving. It shows remarkable stability also when exposure to wide pH conditions (2–11) and protease enzymes such as pepsin and trypsin. Thus accumulation of cereulide in food is a major risk because it cannot be destroyed easily by food processing or digestion.

Various environmental factors such as temperature and atmospheric composition and other factors such as nutrients of food, carbon source, amino acids, pH, cations, and food consistency have significance in *B. cereus* toxicity.

Temperature: Cereulide production occurs in the temperature range of 8–40 °C (optimal temperature between 20 and 30 °C). Hence keeping food at room temperature is considered to be most dangerous.

Atmospheric composition: Oxygen is essential for cereulide production; thus, reduced O_2 levels or replacing head space atmosphere in food packaging with nitrogen gas will aid in prevention of *B. cereus* emetic food poisoning. However, anaerobic conditions result in slower bacterial growth but increased enterotoxin production.

Nutrients and food properties: Non-acidic foods with high water and starch content generally lead to increased production of cereulide.

Carbon source (starch): Emetic *B. cereus* strains produce high amounts of cereulide in many farinaceous foods, such as mashed potatoes, cooked rice, noodles, spaghetti, bread, and pastries. Glucose is required in low to moderate concentration for enterotoxin production.

Amino acids: It has been demonstrated that emetic *B. cereus* strains require the amino acids L-leucine, L-valine, and L-threonine for growth. Since leucine (E641) and valine are also frequently used as flavor enhancers in food items, caution is needed in regard to emetic food poisoning by *B. cereus*.

pH: Cereulide production is inhibited by low pH values. Acidification of food by addition of a dressing like mayonnaise, ketchup, or vinegar decreased the bacterial growth and cereulide concentration in these foods.

Enterotoxins: Nhe is the most common and most important virulence factor of *B. cereus*.

Conclusions

B. cereus is a pathogenic and opportunistic pathogen widely distributed in the environment. Its spores are found in many packaged, processed, and improperly stored cooked food items are responsible for food spoilage and poisoning due to toxin production. These spores can germinate and the vegetative cells multiply under improper storage or packaging conditions. Regulation of toxin production in *B. cereus* is a complex process that is still not completely understood. However, various environmental parameters that affect the toxin expression in *B. cereus* have been identified. Controlled temperature storage, acidification of food products, lowering moisture control, modified atmosphere packaging, etc., are some methods to prevent *B. cereus* outgrowth and toxin production in foods to avoid both emetic and diarrheal food poisoning and maintain food safety standards. As these toxins can be produced by all the other members of the *B. cereus* group, particularly *Bacillus thuringiensis*, *Bacillus mycoides* and *Bacillus weihenstephanensis*, food poisoning can even be caused by these different species. Generally, symptoms caused by *B. cereus* food poisoning are regarded as mild, and therefore *B. cereus* food poisoning is probably underreported. The complexity of toxin expression in *B. cereus* still requires further studies.

See also: Food Safety and Toxicology; Food Additives; *Bacillus thuringiensis*; European Food Safety Authority (EFSA).

Further Reading

Ceuppens, S., Rajkovic, A., Heyndrickx, M., Tsilia, V., Wiele, T.V.D., Boon, N., Uyttendaele, M., 2011. Regulation of toxin production by *Bacillus cereus* and its food safety implications. Crit. Rev. Microbiol. 37 (3), 188–213.

Logan, N.A., 2011. Bacillus and relatives in foodborne illness. J. App. Micro. 112, 417–429.

Senesi, S., Ghelardi, E., 2010. Production, secretion and biological activity of *Bacillus cereus* enterotoxins. Toxins 2, 1690–1703.

Relevant Website

http://www.fda.gov/Food/FoodborneIllnessContaminants/CausesOfIllnessBadBugBook/default.htm – Bad Bug Book (second edition), Foodborne Pathogenic Microorganisms and Natural Toxins Handbook.

Bacillus thuringiensis

L Lagadic and T Caquet, INRA, UMR0985 Écologie et Santé des Écosystèmes, Équipe Écotoxicologie et Qualité des Milieux Aquatiques, Agrocampus Ouest, Rennes, France

This article is a revision of the previous edition article by Eric M. Silberhorn, volume 1, pp 204–206, © 2005, Elsevier Inc.

- Chemical Abstracts Service Registry Number: 68038-71-1
- Synonyms: Agritol, Acrobe, B 401, Agree (subsp. *aizawai*), Aquabac (subsp. *israelensis*), BTB 202, Bacillex, *Bacillus thuringiensis* berliner, Baciver (subsp. *kurstaki*), Bactimos (subsp. *israelensis*), Bactis, Bactospeine, Bactucide, Bactur, Bactura (subsp. *kurstaki*), Bakthane, Berliner (subsp. *kurstaki*), Biobest Bt, Biobit (subsp. *kurstaki*), Biotrol, Bitoksybacillin, Bitoxybacillin, Bt, Cajrab, Caswell No. 066, Caterpillar Killer, Certan (subsp. *aizawai*), Condor (subsp. *kurstaki*), Cutlass (subsp. *kurstaki*), Delfin, Dipel (subsp. *kurstaki*), DiTerra, Foil (subsp. *san diego*), Foray (subsp. *kurstaki*), Full-Bac (subsp. *kurstaki*), Gnatrol (subsp. *israelensis*), Gomelin, Guardjet, HSDB 7823, Insectobiol (subsp. *kurstaki*), Javelin (subsp. *kurstaki*), Larvatrol, Larvx (subsp. *israelensis*), Leptox, M-one, M-Peril (subsp. *kurstaki*), M-Trak (subsp. *san diego*), MEGA BT, MVP (subsp. *kurstaki*), Novabac, Novodor (subsp. *san diego*), SAN 239, Scutello DF (subsp. *kurstaki*), Selectzin, SOK-Bt, Teknar (subsp. *israelensis*), Thuricide, Thuringin, Toarrow, Trident, Vectobac (subsp. *israelensis*), Victory, Worm Attack, Xentari (subsp. *aizawai*), Zentari
- Chemical Class: Bacterium

Background

Bt is a group of strains or isolates of naturally occurring soil bacteria of the *Bacillus cereus* group that are used to control insect pests on agricultural crops, stored food crops, ornamental plants, forests, and nuisance or disease-vector insect in natural water bodies and around homes. *Bt* can be readily distinguished from other members of the *B. cereus* group by the production of large crystalline inclusions that consist of entomocidal proteins, the Crystal (Cry) and Cytolytic (Cyt) toxins, also called δ-endotoxins. Cry and Cyt toxins result from the transformation of relatively inert crystalline protoxins into cytotoxic forms at the alkaline pH conditions of insect midgut. Different strains of *Bt* have specific toxicity to particular types of insects depending on the type and number of protoxins in the crystalline inclusions that they produce. Cry toxins are highly diverse and primarily target insects in the orders *Lepidoptera* (butterflies and moths), *Diptera* (flies and mosquitoes), and *Coleoptera* (beetles and weevils); however, some Cry toxins have been reported to kill hymenopterans (wasps and bees) and nematodes. In contrast, Cyt toxins are mostly found in *Bt* strains active against *Diptera*. Most *Bt*-based insecticides are formulated mixtures of δ-endotoxin crystals and *Bt* spores. The *Bt* spores synergize the toxicity of the crystalline proteins.

Bt is considered an almost ideal agent for pest management because of its combination of insecticidal selectivity and lack of toxicity to humans, mammals, birds, fish, plants, and most aquatic organisms.

Uses

Bt has been used in spray formulations for more than 40 years, and more recently its insecticidal protein genes have been incorporated into several major crops. Due to their insecticidal activity, Cry toxins are used worldwide as bioinsecticides to control disease-vector insect and crop pest populations.

One of the most successful applications of *Bt* has been the control of lepidopteran defoliators, which are pests of coniferous forests mainly in Canada and the United States. *Bt* subsp. *israelensis* (*Bti*) is highly active against larvae of disease-vector mosquitoes like *Aedes aegypti* (vector of dengue fever), *Aedes albopictus* (vector of chikungunya), *Simulium damnosum* (vector of onchocerciasis), and certain *Anopheles* species (vectors of malaria). *Bti* formulations (WG, water-dispersible granule; DT, ready-to-use tablet) have been evaluated by the World Health Organization Pesticide Evaluation Scheme (WHOPES) and recommended as mosquito larvicides, including their use against mosquito larvae that develop in drinking-water containers. Successful application of *Bt* is highly dependent on proper timing, weather conditions, and dosage of spray applications. These factors combine to determine the probability of larvae ingesting a lethal dose.

Recently, the use of Cry toxins has increased dramatically following the introduction of *cry* genes into plants. These '*Bt* crops' have thus far proved to be an effective control strategy, and in 2004 *Bt*-maize and *Bt*-cotton were grown on 22.4 million hectares worldwide. Such widespread use, however, has led to concerns about the effect *Bt* crops may have on the environment and on human health.

Environmental Behavior, Fate, Routes, and Pathways

Bt is moderately persistent in soil with a half-life of ca. 4 months. It is rapidly inactivated in soils that have a pH below 5.1.

Bt subsp. *israelensis* is often applied directly to water for the control of mosquitoes and blackflies. It has been demonstrated that the sedimentation of *Bti* is facilitated by adsorption onto particulate material. *Bti* can persist as long as 5 months in cold water, and adsorption to particulate matter in water facilitates persistence.

Bt is relatively short-lived on foliage due to rapid photodegradation. Its half-life under normal sunlight conditions is 3.8 h. In general, *Bt* loses 50% of its insecticide activity in 1–3 days after spraying. However, high toxicity toward mosquito larvae has been found in decaying leaf litter collected in several natural mosquito breeding sites in forested areas. From the toxic fraction of the leaf litter, *B. cereus*-like bacteria were isolated and further characterized as *Bt* subsp. *israelensis* using PCR (polymerase chain reaction) amplification of specific toxin genes. The anthropogenic origin of *Bti* was demonstrated by amplified fragment length polymorphism (AFLP) profile comparisons. Nevertheless, persistence of acute toxicity several months after *Bti* spraying remains exceptional, as this was only observed once in only one out of eight sampling sites. In this particular site, *Bti* spores and toxins may be protected from degradation by the vegetal matrix.

Carcasses of mosquito larvae killed by *Bti* have been shown to allow for the complete growth cycle (germination, vegetative growth, and sporulation), thus becoming toxic themselves to scavenging mosquito larvae.

This raises the issue of the persistence, potential proliferation, and environmental accumulation of human-spread *Bti* in natural mosquito habitats. Such *Bti* environmental persistence may lengthen the exposure time of insects to this bioinsecticide, thereby increasing the risk of resistance development in target insects, and of negative impacts on non-target insects.

Persistence of *cry1Ab* gene coding for protein δ-endotoxin derived from *Bt* subsp. *kurstaki* inserted and expressed in corn was studied in surface water and sediment of rivers flowing close to corn fields. The gene persisted for more than 21 and 40 days in surface water and sediment, respectively. Field surveys revealed that the *cry1Ab* genes from transgenic corn and from naturally occurring *Bt* were persistent in aquatic environments and were detected in rivers draining farming areas. They were more abundant in the sediment than in the surface water but concentrations were always very low.

Exposure and Exposure Monitoring

The most likely routes of exposure to *Bt* for the general public are oral, dermal, and inhalation. The major direct source of human exposure is drinking-water when *Bt* subsp. *israelensis* is used for vector control in drinking-water containers or reservoirs. In addition to these routes of exposure, accidental parenteral or ocular exposures may occur in workers that apply *Bt* in the field.

Mechanism of Toxicity

Bt Cry and Cyt toxins belong to a class of bacterial toxins known as pore-forming toxins (PFT) that are secreted as water-soluble proteins undergoing conformational changes in order to insert into, or to translocate across, cell membranes of their host. The primary action of Cry toxins is to lyse midgut epithelial cells in the target insect by forming pores in the apical microvilli membrane of the cells.

Bt is ineffective against adult insects and must be eaten by feeding larvae in order to be toxic. When ingested by insect larvae, sporulated-*Bt* crystalline inclusions dissolve in the alkaline environment of insect gut, and the solubilized inactive protoxins are converted into protease resistant active Cry and Cyt toxins. Toxin activation involves N-terminal, C-terminal, and intra-molecular cleavage. The activated Cry toxins are composed of three functional domains, a seven α-helices bundle that is involved in membrane insertion (domain I), and two β-sheet domains (domains II and III) involved in receptor interactions (**Figure 1**). Once activated, Cry toxins bind to specific receptors on the brush border membrane of the midgut epithelium columnar cells before inserting into the membrane. Toxin insertion leads to the formation of lytic pores in microvilli of apical membranes. Subsequently cell lysis and disruption of the midgut epithelium release the cell content providing the spores with a germinating medium leading to a severe septicemia and insect death.

In contrast to Cry toxins, Cyt toxins do not bind to protein receptors but directly interact with membrane lipids inserting into the membrane and forming pores. Synergism between Cyt1Aa and the Cry proteins of *Bti* has been observed; by functioning as a membrane bound receptor of Cry11Aa, Cyt1Aa protein enhanced Cry11Aa membrane insertion.

Recently, it has been suggested that receptor binding of Cry toxins also activates a Mg^{2+}-dependent signaling pathway involving stimulation of G protein, adenylyl cyclase, increased cyclic AMP (cAMP) levels, and activation of protein kinase A (PKA), leading to destabilization of the cytoskeleton and ion channels, and subsequent cell death. However, this might be a secondary effect of the interaction of the toxin with the membrane rather than a direct cause of the cytolytic mechanism.

Acute and Short-Term Toxicity

Animal

To date, numerous laboratory studies have been conducted on the infectivity and toxicity of *Bt* isolates and these studies have demonstrated that the isolates of *Bt* used in commercial products are safe for mammals. In several acute oral toxicity/pathogenicity studies, no adverse effects, infectivity, or pathogenicity has been observed in laboratory animals at doses up to 4.7×10^{11} spores kg^{-1}. In acute pulmonary toxicity studies, no adverse toxic effects have been seen at doses up to 2.6×10^{7} spores kg^{-1}. Similarly, *Bt* is non-toxic and not pathogenic in acute studies that intraperitoneally administered *Bt* to mice at doses below 108 colony forming units (cfu) per animal. Repeated oral exposures for 21 days did not produce mortality or changes in weight gain in rats (1.2×10^{11} cfu) or mice (4.7×10^{10} cfu). Dermal exposures of several different *Bt* strains at levels up to 2500 mg kg^{-1} were not toxic or pathogenic to rabbits, but did produce mild irritation in some cases.

Human

A short-term study with human volunteers has not demonstrated any adverse health effects of *Bt*. Eight subjects ingested 1 g of *Bt* formulation (3×10^{9} spores g^{-1} of powder) daily for 5 days. Five of these volunteers also inhaled 100 mg of the *Bt* powder daily for 5 days. No adverse effects were observed in comprehensive medical examinations conducted before or after (4–5 weeks) exposure, and clinical chemistry data were also negative. Due to its mode of action, acute exposures to *Bt* *via* routes other than oral ingestion are not expected to produce toxicity. However, contact with *Bt* formulations in high enough concentrations may still potentially cause irritation of the skin, eyes, and respiratory tract due to the physical nature of these materials. For example, dermatitis was reported by one worker after contact with *Bt* solution.

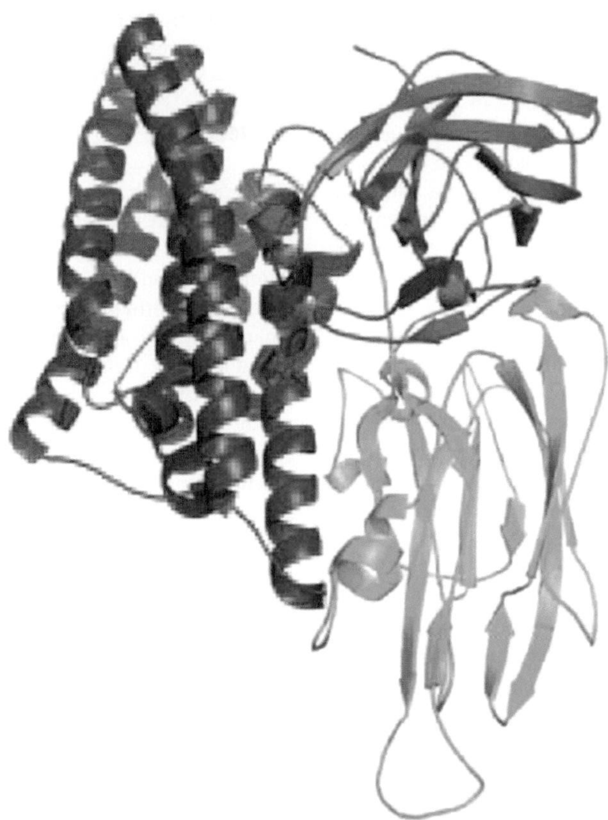

Figure 1 Crystal structure of Cry1Aa toxin. Domain I, domain II, and domain III are shown in red, green, and blue, respectively. From Pigott and Ellar, Microbiology and Molecular Biology Reviews, 71, 255–281. Copyright © 2007, American Society for Microbiology. Reproduced from Boonserm, P., P. Davis, D. J. Ellar, and J. Li. 2005. Crystal structure of the mosquito-larvicidal toxin Cry4Ba and its biological implications. J. Mol. Biol. 348: 363–382.

Chronic Toxicity

Animal

In rats, no toxicity or infectivity was associated with dietary exposure to *Bt* at a level of 4 g kg^{-1} day^{-1} for 3 months. Sheep exposed repeatedly to commercial *Bt* formulations for 60 days showed no significant clinical effects. Rats fed a *Bt* product for 2 years in the diet at 8400 mg kg^{-1} day^{-1} experienced a decrease in body weight gain (females only) during weeks 10–104 of the study, but no other significant effects.

Human

Bt microbial products have a long history (more than 40 years) of safe use. Reports of serious adverse effects in humans from the use of these products are rare and none were considered to be causally related to *Bt* itself. Two detailed epidemiology studies have been carried out on the exposure of humans to *Bt*. In a Canadian study on ground spray operators in a control program for the gypsy moth, researchers found that workers without protective clothing developed minor irritations of the skin, eyes, and respiratory tract, but no serious health problems. Symptoms were reported at two to three times the rate for the control group. These symptoms were transient and frequently occurred during the beginning of a spray run and when *Bt* spray concentrations were increased. Mean exposure values ranged from 3.0×10^3 to 5.9×10^6 *Bt* spores m^{-3} of sampled air. The exposure rates for the spray operators were up to 500 times greater than that estimated for the general population. In a passive surveillance study conducted in Oregon during 1985–86, there was only one health complaint that could be attributed to *Bt*: dermatitis and eye irritation in a spray operator who was splashed in the face and eyes with a spray solution.

Bt subsp. *israelensis* is not considered to pose a hazard to humans through drinking-water. However, it is vital that authorities can be assured that *Bti* has been prepared to the highest quality and hygienic standards under appropriate conditions that will meet the WHOPES specifications.

Ecotoxicology

To date, based upon extensive laboratory and field data, there is little evidence that commercial *Bt* formulations cause any significant ecological impacts when used for insect control. Toxicity and infectivity risks due to delta-endotoxin effects in non-target birds, freshwater fishes, freshwater aquatic invertebrates, estuarine and marine animals, arthropod predators/parasites, honey bees, annelids, and mammals are minimal to non-existent at the label use rates of registered *Bt* active ingredients. However, controversial results have been obtained in invertebrates for *Bt*-containing larvicides depending on the subspecies, type of formulation, and conditions of application.

Invertebrates

Terrestrial Insects

Field monitoring studies after application of *Bt* for control of the spruce budworm found no measurable effects on a wide variety of insects, and similar results have been found in other studies. In contrast, temporary reductions in populations of non-target *Lepidoptera* and some other susceptible insects have been documented in the field after aerial applications of *Bt*. Most *Bt* subspecies tested for toxicity to honey bees have shown minimal toxicity, but the subspecies *aizawai* has displayed high toxicity to bees. *Bt* subsp. *kurstaki* has been shown to be toxic to the beneficial parasitoid hymenoptera *Trichogramma* spp. Because of the lack of persistence of *Bt* in the environment, the effects are primarily limited to the period of use, and when *Bt* pesticides are used according to product labels the risk to bees and other beneficial insects is minimal.

Aquatic Invertebrates

Larvae of some taxa of non-target *Nematocera* such as *Chironomidae* have been shown to be susceptible to *Bti*, and there are indications that non-target organisms may be impacted by *Bti*-containing larvicides in wetlands. In a pond mesocosm study, *Bti* had a negative effect on the abundance of chironomid larvae only for application rates 1.5–2 times superior to the operational rate used for mosquito control, with differential effects according to the considered subfamily. In contrast, results from experiments performed in temporary freshwater ponds showed that *Bti* did not adversely affect the density or biomass of various invertebrate groups, nor the taxonomic richness of benthic invertebrate communities. A long-term (6 years) field study in Minnesota freshwater wetlands showed that *Bti* induced a significant decrease in the abundance of non-target invertebrates, especially *Nematocera*, associated with a reduction in insect genera richness and an increase in dominance indices. In contrast, non-*Bti*-sensitive taxa such as annelids were not affected.

However, several long-term field studies showed that *Bti* effect was generally negligible or of the same order of magnitude as those from natural factors. No effect of *Bti* was found on the abundance of insect larvae (chironomids), crustaceans, or molluscs collected in sediment samples from temperate New South Wales saltmarshes. In a 6-year survey performed in the River Dalälven floodplain (Central Sweden), no significant effect of flood-water mosquito control using aerial application of *Bti* was shown on the production of emerging insects, nor on chironomid species richness and production. In wetlands where *Bti* was aerially applied, indirect effects on predatory insects which may have resulted from food shortage due to mosquito larvae mortality were not significant. The reduction in the abundance of mosquito larvae was followed by an increase in the taxonomic richness and abundance of protozoans which are prey for mosquito larvae but also for other invertebrates such as rotifers or hydrozoans. Finally, in European Atlantic coastal wetlands, the use of *Bti*, as VectoBac® 12AS and VectoBac® WG, from 1998 to 2011, did not result in adverse effects on non-target aquatic invertebrates, but an increase in the abundance of some taxa (Hydrozoans, Crustaceans, Oligochaetes, larval Dipterans, Polychaetes) has been observed in treated areas.

Vertebrates

Bt is practically non-toxic to fish with acute LC_{50} (lethal concentration for half of an exposed group of individuals or population) values greater than 8.7×10^9 cfu l^{-1} for bluegill sunfish, rainbow trout, and the sheepshead minnow. There has been no documented evidence of fishes killed as a result of the many forestry, agriculture, and urban *Bt* spraying programs conducted in Canada and the United States over the past 30 years or more.

Bt strains are classified as practically non-toxic to birds based on acute toxicity studies conducted for the US Environmental Protection Agency as part of the pesticide registration process. In general, field studies have not shown effects on bird populations after aerial spraying of *Bt* formulations, although indirect effects on avian reproductive parameters (e.g., nesting attempts, fledgling success) have been described in some instances.

Field studies have also not shown any significant adverse effects of *Bt* products on mammals or plants exposed at typical application rates.

Resistance

Evolution of resistance in insect pests threatens the continued effectiveness of *Bt* toxins in sprays and transgenic crops. A number of insects (moths, beetles, flies, mosquitoes) have been shown to be resistant to endotoxins when selected in the laboratory. In experiments designed to select for resistance, LC_{50} increases more than 10-fold in dozens of species after a few or more than a hundred generations. High levels of resistance to *Bt* (up to 200-fold) have also been reported for field populations of a number of lepidopteran pests. In contrast, other groups of insects, such as *Diptera* and *Coleoptera*, show little changes in susceptibility after repeated exposure to *Bt*.

Resistance to individual Cry toxins appears rapidly. This was the case, in particular, for lepidopteran pests resistant to transgenic crops expressing one or a very limited number of Cry toxin genes, or for mosquitoes selected with only one or a subset of the four *Bti* toxins. However, the mix of four synergistic toxins with different modes of action remains one of the main advantages of *Bti* (and other *Bt* subspecies that express several Cry toxins) which delays the apparition and evolution of resistance. Indeed, only moderate levels of resistance to the four toxin mix have been described after long periods of treatment in natural populations or after intensive laboratory selection.

Reduced or no binding to Cry toxin receptors of the membrane of midgut epithelial cells have been identified as the main mechanisms of resistance in *Lepidoptera*. A second general mechanism of resistance is reduction or loss of proteases that convert *Bt* protoxin to activated toxin. Because *Bt* and conventional insecticides have different modes of action, they generate distinct mechanisms of resistance, so that cross-resistance is very unlikely. Similarly, selection for resistance to a given Cry toxin generally confers little or no resistance to other Cry toxins, due to the specificity of their binding sites. However, when resistance does not result from reduced binding, unexpected cross-resistance patterns to Cry toxin may occur.

See also: Biocides; Environmental Risk Assessment, Pesticides and Biocides; Pesticides; Resistance to Toxicants.

Further Reading

Boisvert, M., Boisvert, J., 2000. Effects of *Bacillus thuringiensis* var. *israelensis* on target and nontarget organisms: a review of laboratory and field experiments. Biocontrol Sci. Technol. 10, 517–561.

Bravo, A., Gill, S.S., Soberón, M., 2007. Mode of action of *Bacillus thuringiensis* Cry and Cyt toxins and their potential for insect control. Toxicon 49, 423–435.

Ferre, J., Van Rie, J., 2002. Biochemistry and genetics of insect resistance to *Bacillus thuringiensis*. Annu. Rev. Entomol. 47, 501–533.

International Programme on Chemical Safety, 1999. Environmental Health Criteria 217: Microbial Pest Control Agent *Bacillus thuringiensis*. World Health Organization, Geneva, Switzerland.

Joung, K.-B., Côté, J.-C., 2000. A Review of the Environmental Impacts of the Microbial Insecticide *Bacillus thuringiensis*. Technical Bulletin No. 29. Horticulture Research and Development Centre, Agriculture and Agri-Food, Canada.

Lacey, L.A., Siegel, J.P., 2000. Safety and ecotoxicology of entomopathogenic bacteria. In: Charles, J.-F., Delécluse, A., Nielsen-LeRoux, C. (Eds.), Entomopathogenic Bacteria: From Laboratory to Field Application. Kluwer Academic Publishers, Dordrecht, pp. 253–273.

Paris, M., Tetreau, G., Laurent, F., Lelu, M., Despres, L., David, J.P., 2011. Persistence of *Bacillus thuringiensis israelensis* (*Bti*) in the environment induces resistance to multiple *Bti* toxins in mosquitoes. Pest Manage. Sci. 67, 122–128.

Pigott, C.R., Ellar, D.J., 2007. Role of receptors in *Bacillus thuringiensis* crystal toxin activity. Microbiol. Mol. Biol. Rev. 71, 255–281.

Siegel, J.P., 2001. The mammalian safety of *Bacillus thuringiensis*-based insecticides. J. Invert. Pathol. 77, 13–21.

Tilquin, M., Paris, M., Reynaud, S., Despres, L., Ravanel, P., Geremia, R., 2008. Long lasting persistence of *Bacillus thuringiensis* subsp. *israelensis* (*Bti*) in mosquito natural habitats. PLoS ONE 3, e3432.

United States Environmental Protection Agency, 1998. Reregistration Eligibility Decision (RED) *Bacillus thuringiensis*. Office of Prevention, Pesticides and Toxic Substances, Washington, DC.

World Health Organization, 2009. *Bacillus thuringiensis israelensis* (*Bti*) in drinking-water. Background document for development of WHO Guidelines for Drinking-water Quality. WHO/HSE/WSH/09.01/8.

Relevant Websites

Extoxnet : http://extoxnet.orst.edu/pips/bacillus.htm
WHO: http://www.who.int/water_sanitation_health/gdwqrevision/thuringiensis/en/index.html
US EPA : http://www.epa.gov/oppsrrd1/REDs/0247.pdf
National Pesticide Information Center : http://npic.orst.edu/factsheets/BTgen.pdf

British Anti-Lewisite (BAL)

SP Sawant, Kimberly-Clark Worldwide, Inc., Roswell, GA, USA
HS Parihar, PCOM School of Pharmacy, Suwanee, GA, USA
HM Mehendale, University of Louisiana at Monroe, Monroe, LA, USA

This article is a revision of the previous edition article by Sharmilee P. Sawant and Harihara M. Mehendale, volume 1, pp 206–207, © 2005, Elsevier Inc.

- Name: British Anti-Lewisite (BAL)
- Chemical Abstracts Service Registry Number: 59-52-9
- Synonyms: Antoxol; Dicaptol; Dimercaprol; 2,3-Dimercaptol-1-propanol; Sulfactin
- Molecular Formula: $C_3H_8OS_2$
- Chemical Structure:

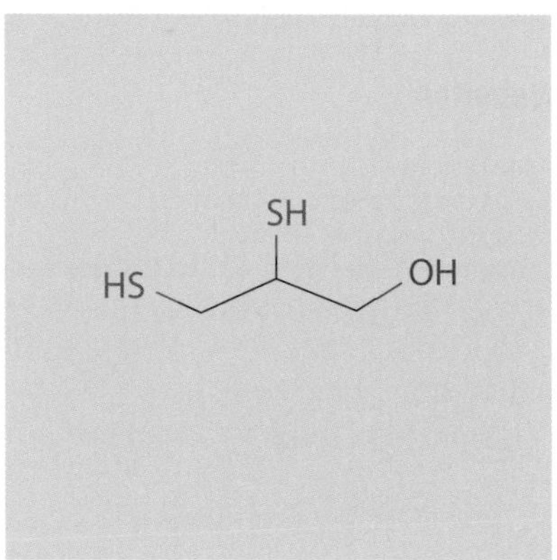

Background

British Anti-Lewisite (BAL) is a synthetic therapeutic substance developed during World War II for using as an antidote against the vesicant arsenic war gases (Lewisite). The first experiments were based on the fact that arsenic products react with sulfhydryl radicals. Among all the compounds originally tested, BAL was the most effective and the least toxic. In 1951, BAL was used by a renowned neurologist, Derek Denny-Brown, to treat patients suffering with Wilson's disease (hepatolenticular degeneration), which results from excessive copper accumulation, especially in the brain and liver. The intrinsic toxicity of BAL resulted in the development of its water-soluble and less toxic derivatives dimercaptosuccinic acid and dimercaptopropanesulfonic acid.

Chemically, BAL is called 2,3-dimercaptopropanol. It is a viscous oily liquid with the offensive odor of mercaptans. It is moderately soluble in water but highly soluble in vegetable oils. BAL is a dithiol compound highly reactive with arsenic and other heavy metal compounds. It has a higher affinity for these compounds than body lipids. Because BAL is unstable and susceptible to oxidation, there are storage difficulties as a ready-to-use preparation. BAL is administered by deep intramuscular injection (i.m.). BAL-treated individuals suffer side effects (>50%), most of which are not serious and subside with discontinuation of treatment. BAL contains two sulfhydryl groups that react to form a stable, generally nontoxic chelate with heavy metals, particularly arsenic, mercury, lead, and tin. The combined compound prevents the metal from reacting with sulfhydryl groups in physiological proteins and thereby renders them inert until they are excreted.

BAL administration is most effective when given as soon as possible after exposure to the metal. This is because it is more effective in preventing inhibition of sulfhydryl enzymes than in reactivating them. Metals that form mercaptides with essential cellular sulfhydryl groups (arsenic, gold, and mercury) are most efficiently antagonized by BAL. BAL is also used in conjunction with $CaNa_2EDTA$ to treat lead poisoning, especially when lead encephalopathy is clearly evident. Intoxication by selenites, which also oxidize sulfhydryl enzymes, is not influenced by dimercaprol.

Uses

BAL is a chelating agent used as an antidote for the treatment of metal poisoning, especially arsenic (organic and inorganic), gold salts, and inorganic mercury. BAL is more effective when given soon after toxic exposure because it is more effective in preventing inhibition of sulfhydryl enzymes than in reactivating them. BAL is also used in the treatment of Wilson's disease. The drug cannot be used in poisonings due to iron, cadmium, tellurium, selenium, vanadium, and uranium. It is contraindicated in poisonings due to elemental mercury vapor, because it can further increase the metal in the brain.

Environmental Fate and Behavior

BAL is a colorless or slightly yellowish viscous oily liquid and has a pungent odor. The molecular weight, melting point, boiling point, vapor pressure, and the octanol–water partition coefficient (log K_{ow}) are 124.23, 77 °C, 120 °C at 15 mm Hg, 4.36×10^{-3} mm Hg at 25 °C, and 0.16, respectively. The Henry's law constant is 9.39×10^{-9} atm-m^3 mol^{-1} at 25 °C. BAL is soluble in ethanol and ether, and slightly soluble in chloroform and vegetable oils. Water solubility is 8.7 g/100 ml. BAL should be protected from light and should be stored at temperatures between 2 and 10 °C in small vials.

Exposure and Exposure Monitoring

BAL is given only by i.m. injection (never intravenous (i.v.) or subcutaneous (s.c.)). Oral ingestion is only accidental or unintentional. BAL can be applied to the skin to heal local effects caused by arsenic vesicant substances.

 http://dx.doi.org/10.1016/B978-0-12-386454-3.00244-X

Toxicokinetics

Peak concentrations in blood are reported in about 30–60 min after i.m. injection of BAL. It is readily absorbed through the skin after topical application. Because it is a lipophilic drug, BAL rapidly penetrates the intracellular spaces. The highest concentrations are found in the liver, kidneys, brain, and small intestine. In animals, biological half-life is short, and metabolic degradation and renal excretions are reported within 6–24 h. The renal excretion is most often cited as its major elimination route, but there appears to be a significant contribution from its conjugation with glucuronic acid. The major portion of the drug is excreted rapidly in the urine, and part of it is eliminated in the feces (via bile). The BAL–metal complexes dissociate rapidly in the body, especially in an acid internal medium; alkalinization of the urine may prevent this dissociation and protect the kidneys from metal and BAL nephrotoxicity. If the BAL–metal complex is oxidized, the metal is released and can exert its toxic effect again; therefore, the dosage of BAL must be high enough to ensure the excess of free BAL in body fluids until the metal is completely excreted.

Mechanism of Toxicity

BAL is believed to compete with tissue sulfhydryl groups and interferes with cellular respiration. It also competes with metallic cofactors of metabolic enzyme systems and increases capillary permeability. Metabolic degradation and excretion are essentially complete within 4 h. BAL not excreted as dimercaprol–metal complex is quickly metabolized by the liver and excreted as an inactive product in the urine. Because it is a lipophilic drug, it penetrates rapidly the intracellular spaces. The highest concentrations are found in the liver, kidneys, brain, and small intestine. Due to its lipophilic characteristic, the complexes formed with mercury and other metals may be redistributed into sensitive cells in the brain following dimercaprol treatment.

Acute and Short-Term Toxicity

Animal

The LD_{50} values in rabbits and rats are in the range of 0.6–1.0 mmol kg^{-1} by i.m., i.p., or s.c. administration. In another study, the LD_{50} in rats after i.m. injection was 105 mg kg^{-1} and 100 mg kg^{-1} i.p. in mice. In animals, a lethal dose of dithiols is reported to cause convulsions and severe spasm of the abdominal muscles shortly before death. Sublethal injection of BAL to animals results in lacrimation, edema of the conjunctiva, salivation, and vomiting. With increasing doses, they develop ataxia, analgesia, tachypnea, and hyper-excitability. Nystagmus and muscle tremor develop, tonic and clonic convulsions occur at the final stages. Death occurs during coma. The most significant acute toxic effect of BAL is cardiovascular depression as indicated by a decrease in systemic and pulmonary artery pressure following i.v. injection in cats.

Human

The target organs of toxicity are kidneys, cardiovascular system, and central nervous system. The most common side effects of BAL are hypertension with tachycardia, cardiovascular collapse, convulsions, excitation, hyperglycemia, and hypoglycemia. About 50% of patients who receive high therapeutic doses (4–5 mg kg^{-1}) have minor reactions: nausea; vomiting; fatigue; restlessness; apprehension; headache; burning sensation of the lips, mouth, throat, eyes, and penis; lacrimation; salivation; tingling of extremities; a feeling of constriction in the chest muscle; diffuse pain; and muscle spasm. Large doses may cause convulsions and coma. There may be pain at the injection site. BAL may cause hemolytic anemia in individuals with a glucose-6-phosphate dehydrogenase (G6PD) deficiency. When applied locally to skin, it produces redness and swelling. It may be irritant to eyes and mucous membranes following local contact.

Chronic Toxicity

Animal

Very few chronic toxicity studies have been reported. After repeated local applications in animals, sensitization dermatitis may develop. Chronic parenteral administration of BAL is reported to increase the white blood cell count by 30%.

Human

Long-term exposure of BAL is unnecessary. There are no reports on the long-term toxic effects of BAL.

Reproductive Toxicity

Well-controlled clinical studies are not reported. BAL is classified as US Food and Drug Administration pregnancy category C (risk cannot be ruled out).

Clinical Management

There is no specific treatment, but symptomatic measures can be taken to improve the clinical course. Stop BAL immediately if adverse reactions are observed. No antidote is available. If there has been dermal exposure, wash the skin with a nonirritating soap and water. If the eyes have been exposed, irrigate them with tap water. If ingested, activated charcoal should be given. Convulsions should be treated as usual with benzodiazepines and barbiturates. If cardiovascular collapse occurs, give fluids according to the patient's hydroelectrolytic balance. Dopamine can be used, if necessary. Bicarbonate solution is useful, not only to correct acidosis but also to increase renal elimination of BAL–metal complexes, prevent their dissociation, and decrease their toxicity. Some symptoms can be relieved by administration of antihistamine. Alkalinization of urine may prevent kidney damage.

Miscellaneous

BAL is potentially nephrotoxic and hence the urine should be kept alkaline during BAL therapy since the chelate dissociates in acid medium. BAL should be used with caution or the dosage reduced in patients with oliguria. The drug should be either discontinued or used very cautiously if acute renal failure develops. BAL should be administered carefully and under strict clinical control in patients with hypertension, renal impairment, and G6PD deficiency. It is contraindicated in patient with hepatic dysfunction (except for postarsenical jaundice) and in patients with hypersensitivity to peanut oil since BAL injection is available in peanut oil.

See also: Metals.

Further Reading

Mouret, S., Wartelle, J., Emorine, S., et al., Jun 25, 2013. Topical efficacy of dimercapto-chelating agents against lewisite-induced skin lesions in SKH-1 hairless mice. Toxicol. Appl. Pharmacol. http://dx.doi.org/10.1016/j.taap.2013.06.012 pii: S0041-008X(13)00285-8. (Epub ahead of print).

Roberts, E.A., Schilsky, M.L., 2008. Diagnosis and treatment of Wilson disease: an update. Hepatology 47, 2089–2111.

Sahu, C., Pakhira, S., Sen, K., Das, A.K., 2013. A computational study of detoxification of lewisite warfare agents by British anti-lewisite: catalytic effects of water and ammonia on reaction mechanism and kinetics. J. Phys. Chem. A 117 (16), 3496–3506.

Vilensky, J.A., Redman, K., 2003. British anti-lewisite (dimercaprol): an amazing history. Ann. Emerg. Med. 41, 378–383.

Waters, L.L., Stock, C., 1945. BAL (anti-lewisite). Science 102, 601–606.

Relevant Website

http://toxnet.nlm.nih.gov – Toxnet (Toxicology Data Network): search under Toxline for BAL (British Antilewisite).

Barbiturates

F Nobay and NM Acquisto, University of Rochester, Rochester, NY, USA

Long-Acting Agents

- Representative Chemicals: Barbital (Chemical Abstracts Service Registry Number (CAS) 57-44-3), Mephobarbital (CAS 115-38-8), Phenobarbital (CAS 50-06-6)
- Synonyms:
  - Barbiturates – Courage pills, Downers, F-40s, Goof balls, Gorilla pills, Mexican yellows, Pink ladies
  - Barbital – Diethylbarbituric acid, Diethylmalonyl urea, Barbitone, DEBA
  - Mephobarbital – Methylphenobarbital, Mebaral
  - Phenobarbital – Phenylethylmalonylurea, Barbenyl, Barbiphenyl, Dormiral, Phenylbarbital, 5-Ethyl-5-phenylbarbituric acid, Solfoton
- Chemical/Pharmaceutical/Other Class: Barbituric acid derivative
- Chemical Structure:

R3 N 3 C O R5a (or S=) † O=C 2 5C R5b N C O H

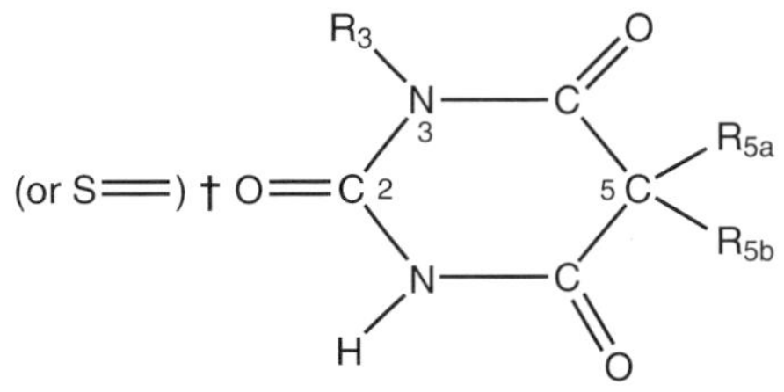

- Name: Phenobarbital
- Molecular Weight: 232.235 g mol^{-1}
- Molecular Formula: $C_{12}H_{12}N_2O_3$
- Chemical Structure:

O CH3 HN O N H O

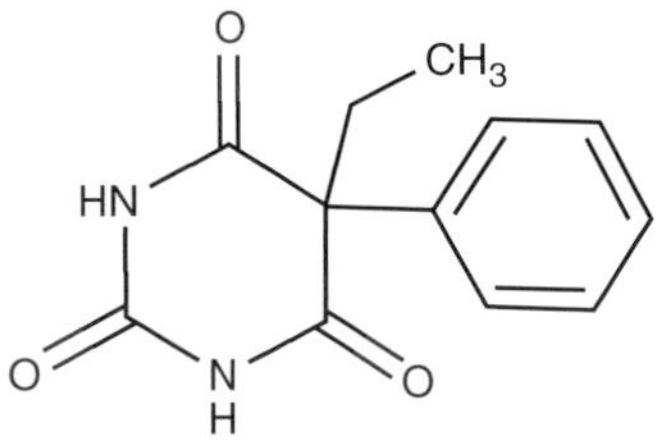

Short-Acting Agents

- Representative Chemicals: Amobarbital, Aprobarbital, Butabarbital sodium, Butalbital, Cyclobarbital, Heptabarbital, Hexobarbital, Methohexital sodium, Pentobarbital, Secobarbital sodium, Talbutal, Thiamylal, Thiopental sodium
- Chemical Abstracts Service Registry Number: 309-36-4 (Methohexital sodium)
- Synonyms:
  - Amobarbital – Amytal; $C_{11}H_{18}N_2O_3$; 5-Ethyl-5-(3-methylbutyl)-2,4,6-(1*H*,3*H*,5*H*)-pyrimidinetrione
  - Aprobarbital – Alurate; $C_{10}H_{14}N_2O_3$; 5-(1-Methylethyl)-5-(2-propenyl)-2,4,6-(1*H*,3*H*,5*H*)-pyrimidinetrione
  - Butabarbital – Butisol; Butolan; Sarisol; $C_{10}H_{15}N_2NaO_3$; 5-Ethyl-5-(1-methylpropyl)-2,4,6-(1*H*,3*H*,5*H*)-pyrimidinetrione sodium salt
  - Butalbital – Sandoptal; $C_{11}H_{16}N_2O_3$; 5-(2-Methylpropyl)-5-(2-propenyl)-2,4,6-(1*H*,3*H*,5*H*)-pyrimidinetrione
  - Cyclobarbital – $C_{12}H_{16}N_2O_3$; 5-(1-Cyclohexen-1-yl)-5-ethyl-2,4,6-(1*H*,3*H*,5*H*)-pyrimidinetrione
  - Heptabarbital – $C_{13}H_{18}N_2O_3$; 5-(1-Cyclohepten-1-yl)-5-ethyl-2,4,6-(1*H*,3*H*,5*H*)-pyrimidinetrione
  - Hexobarbital – $C_{12}H_{16}N_2O_3$; 5-(1-Cyclohexen-1-yl)-1,5-dimethyl-2,4,6-(1*H*,3*H*,5*H*)-pyrimidinetrione
  - Methohexital – Brevital; Compound 25398; $C_{14}H_{17}N_2NaO_3$; 1-Methyl-5-(1-methyl-2-pentynyl)-5-(2-propenyl)-2,4,6-(1*H*,3*H*,5*H*)-pyrimidinetrione sodium salt
  - Pentobarbital – Nembutal; $C_{11}H_{18}N_2O_3$; 5-Ethyl-5-(1 methylbutyl)-2,4,6-(1*H*,3*H*,5*H*)-pyrimidinetrione
  - Secobarbital – Seconal; $C_{12}H_{17}N_2NaO_3$; 5-(1-Methylbutyl)-5-(2-propenyl)-2,4,6-(1*H*,3*H*,5*H*)-pyrimidinetrione sodium salt
  - Talbutal – Lotusate; $C_{11}H_{16}N_2O_3$; 5-(1-Methylpropyl)-5-(2-propenyl)-2,4,6-(1*H*,3*H*,5*H*)-pyrimidinetrione
  - Thiamylal – Surital; $C_{12}H_{18}N_2O_2S$; Dihydro-5-(1-methylbutyl)-5-(2-propenyl)-2-thioxo-4,6-(1*H*,5*H*)-pyrimidinetrione
  - Thiopental – Pentothal; $C_{11}H_{17}N_2NaO_2S$; 5-Ethyldihydro-5-(1-methylbutyl)-2-thioxo-4,6-(1*H*,5*H*)-pyrimidinetrione sodium salt
- Chemical/Pharmaceutical/Other Class: Barbituric acid derivative
- Chemical Structure:

R3 N 3 C O R5a (or S=) † O=C 2 5C R5b N C H

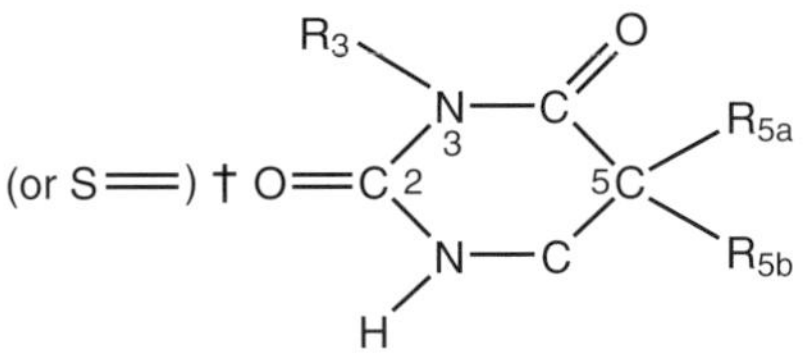

- Name: Pentobarbital
- Molecular Weight: 226.27 g mol^{-1}
- Molecular Formula: $C_{11}H_{18}N_2O_3$
- Chemical Structure:

H3C O CH3 N Na+ −O N H O CH3

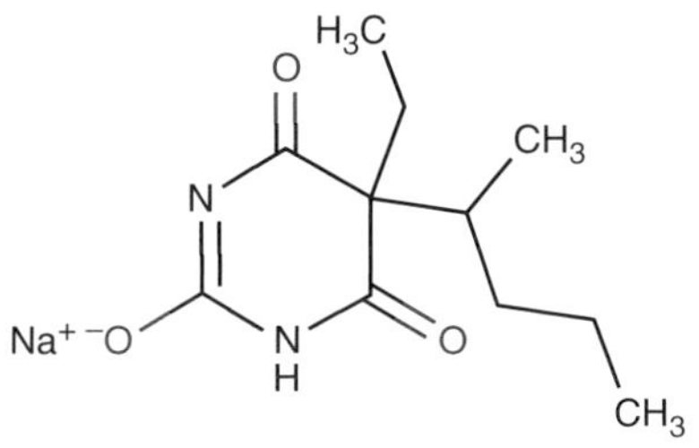

 http://dx.doi.org/10.1016/B978-0-12-386454-3.00696-5

Background

Barbituric acid was first synthesized in Germany in 1864 by Adolf von Baeyer through the condensation of urea with diethyl malonate. It was not until 1903, however, that the first therapeutic agent was discovered when Bayer chemists Emil Fischer and Joseph von Mering discovered that barbital, an analog of derivative of barbituric acid, was effective at putting dogs to sleep. It was marketed as the first barbiturate for its sedative and hypnotic effects and given the name Veronal, said to be named after Verona, Italy, the most peaceful place that von Mering knew of. Barbituric acid itself was thought to be named after Saint Barbara, the patron saint of artillerymen as on the day that von Baeyer synthesized the substance he celebrated in a tavern in which the artillery garrison was celebrating the feast of Saint Barbara. Except for certain short-acting barbiturates used for anesthesia and phenobarbital, a long-acting barbiturate used as an anticonvulsant, other drugs with better safety profiles such as the benzodiazepines have supplanted barbiturates as sedative-hypnotics.

Uses

Barbiturates are used as anesthetics for perioperative sedation as well as in the short-term treatment of insomnia, anxiety, psychosis, control of seizures, and alcohol withdrawal. These agents are also exploited in abuse settings. Abuse of barbiturates started in the 1940s as they were liberally given to military personnel stationed in the South Pacific in order to help them cope with harsh conditions. They were called 'goofballs' in this context. After World War II, many servicemen needed detoxification and treatment for barbiturate dependence upon returning to the United States. Reported barbiturate abuse peaked in the 1970s, but has since declined with the increased use of other sedatives such as benzodiazepines. Use of certain long-acting barbiturates as anticonvulsants, however, continues. Phenobarbital is currently the most commonly prescribed anticonvulsant in use worldwide. Pentobarbital has been used in the United States for lethal injection during executions. Phenobarbital is also used for the treatment of alcohol withdrawal and compares favorably to other agents including benzodiazepines.

Environmental Fate and Behavior

Short-Acting Barbiturates: Pentobarbital

Pentobarbital is water soluble. If released into air, with an estimated vapor pressure of 3×10^{-10} mmHg (25 °C), it will exist solely as in particulate phase in the atmosphere and as a particulate pentobarbital will be removed from the atmosphere by wet or dry deposition. Pentobarbital is not susceptible to photolysis from sunlight as pentobarbital does not contain chromophores that absorb wavelengths of light greater than 290 nm. If pentobarbital is released into soil, a pK_a of 7.8 indicates that it will exist partially as an anion, which does not absorb strongly to soils containing organic carbon or clays. Pentobarbital is not expected to volatilize from moist soil based upon an estimated Henry's law constant of 8.4×10^{-13} atm-cu m mol^{-1}. If released into water, pentobarbital is not expected to adsorb to suspended sediment and solids in the water based upon the estimated K_{oc}. Volatilization from water is not expected to be an important fate process based upon the estimated Henry's law constant. Pentobarbital has an estimated biological concentration factor (BCF) of 11 suggesting the potential for bioconcentration in aquatic organisms is low. Pentobarbital lacks functional groups that hydrolyze easily and hydrolysis is not expected to be an important environmental fate process.

Long-Acting Barbiturates: Phenobarbital

Phenobarbital is a very lipid soluble, long-acting barbiturate. It may be released into the environment through various waste streams, including from manufacturing, production, and sewage. If released into air, with an estimated vapor pressure of 1.4×10^{-11} mmHg (25 °C), phenobarbital will exist solely in the particulate phase in the atmosphere and will be removed solely by wet or dry deposition. Phenobarbital will be susceptible to photolysis by sunlight as it contains chromophores that absorb light at wavelengths greater than 290 nm. If released into soil, phenobarbital will have high mobility based upon an estimated K_{oc} of 59. The pK_a of phenobarbital is 7.3 indicating that it will exist partially as an anion in the environment and anions are not expected to adsorb well to soils containing organic carbon or clay. Volatilization of the neutral species from moist soil is not expected to be a significant environmental fate process as the estimated Henry's law constant is 1.7×10^{-14} atm-cu m mol^{-1}. Biodegradation is not expected to be an important environmental fate process. If released into water, phenobarbital is not expected to adsorb to suspended soils and other sediment based upon its K_{oc}. An estimated BCF of 4 suggests that the potential for bioconcentration in aquatic organisms is low and hydrolysis is not expected to be an important environmental fate since phenobarbital does not contain functional groups that will hydrolyze under environmental conditions.

Exposure Routes and Pathways

The most common route of exposure to barbiturates is ingestion of oral dosage forms. Several of these agents are also available for parenteral administration (intramuscular or intravenous) and as rectal suppositories. Barbiturates may also be released into the environment through production processes and elimination into various waste streams. Occupational exposure may occur through inhalation and dermal contact in the workplace at sites of production. In addition to ingestion of the medication, the general population may be exposed to small levels of barbiturates through ingestion of drinking water, in particular the water-soluble barbiturates such as pentobarbital.

Toxicokinetics

Long-acting barbiturates are generally absorbed more slowly from the gastrointestinal tract compared to short-acting barbiturates, which are rapidly and completely absorbed.

Sodium salts are absorbed more rapidly than the corresponding free acids by all routes of administration, but especially from liquid formulations. Furthermore, oral absorption is more rapid when ingested on an empty stomach and in the presence of alcohol. The onset of action varies from 10 to 60 min depending on the agent and formulation. For example, the onset of action for the short-acting agents is 10–15 min (oral) and 1–3 min (intravenous). This is more rapid than the long-acting agents where the onset of action is 20–60 min (oral) and approximately 5 min (intravenous).

Barbiturates are extensively distributed to all body tissues and fluids with highest concentrations achieved in the brain, liver, and kidneys. Short-acting barbiturates are generally more lipid soluble than long-acting barbiturates. This causes uptake into less vascular tissues (i.e., muscle and fat) and subsequently leads to a decline in the barbiturate plasma and brain concentration. Long-acting barbiturates are less lipid soluble, accumulate more slowly in tissue, and are excreted more readily by the kidney as an active drug. Long-acting barbiturates have an elimination half-life longer than 40 h. The apparent volume of distribution for phenobarbital is 0.5–1.0 l kg^{-1} and for most short-acting barbiturates from 0.6 to 1.9 l kg^{-1}. For long-acting barbiturates, approximately 20–45% is bound to plasma proteins enhancing the potential in the overdose setting for removal via dialysis.

All barbiturates are extensively metabolized by the hepatic microsomal enzyme system. Mephobarbital is primarily metabolized by *N*-demethylation to form phenobarbital. Phenobarbital is then metabolized to an inactive metabolite. Long-acting barbiturates induce several cytochromes in the hepatic microsomal enzyme system leading to numerous drug interactions and potential toxicity in combination with other drugs.

Phenobarbital has a long elimination half-life of about 2–6 days. Approximately 25% of a dose is eliminated unchanged in the urine with the remainder eliminated as inactive metabolites. A minimal amount of mephobarbital is eliminated unchanged in the urine. The pK_a of phenobarbital (7.24) is similar to physiologic pH. As a result, the elimination of unchanged drug is significantly influenced by changes in the urine pH and alkalinization of the urine can enhance the elimination.

Conversely, only inactive metabolites of the short-acting barbiturates are eliminated in the urine. Only aprobarbital, which is less lipid soluble, has a significant fraction (13–24%) that is eliminated unchanged in the urine. The elimination half-life of short-acting barbiturates ranges from 3 to 50 h.

Mechanism of Toxicity

Barbiturates act throughout the central nervous system (CNS) by affecting the binding of γ-aminobutyric acid (GABA), the major inhibitory neurotransmitter in the CNS. Specifically, barbiturates decrease excitability of postsynaptic membranes by binding to the GABA-A receptor and causing prolonged chloride channel opening. This allows an influx of chloride into cell membranes and subsequently hyperpolarizes the postsynaptic neuron resulting in CNS depression. It is important to note that GABA does not need to be present for barbiturates to have clinical effect; this is unlike benzodiazepines, which require GABA receptors to be present.

Intoxication with barbiturates will lead to CNS depression as well as respiratory, cardiovascular, and gastrointestinal tract depression.

Acute and Short-Term Toxicity (or Exposure)

Animal

Barbiturates agents may affect animals in the same way as humans. Lethargy, coma, shallow respirations, ataxia, hypothermia, hypotension, and depressed reflexes may occur. Some short-acting barbiturates are utilized as veterinary euthanasia agents. The treatment of overdose is similar to that in humans.

Human

The fatal or toxic dose of a barbiturate is highly variable due to patient tolerance and coingestions. The concentration of phenobarbital that can cause death is lower in patients with alcohol or other depressant drugs such as benzodiazepines. In general, the estimated potentially fatal dose of a barbiturate agent in nondependent adults ranges from 1 to 10 g or approximately 10 times the full hypnotic dose in a single ingestion. Doses of 3–5 mg kg^{-1} of most short-acting barbiturates will cause toxicity in children. Specifically, a dose of 8 mg kg^{-1} or greater of phenobarbital can cause signs and symptoms of toxicity. It is important to remember that the duration of symptoms is dependent on the half-life of the individual agent. Given the mechanism of action, barbiturate toxicity will likely produce CNS effects. These effects may include confusion, slurred speech, ataxia, diplopia, horizontal nystagmus, somnolence, and coma. Severe barbiturate toxicity may also manifest as cardiovascular depression and vasodilation, which can lead to hypotension, cardiovascular collapse, hypothermia, and multisystem organ failure. An ileus may occur due to gastrointestinal depression, which is relevant in the consideration of potential gastrointestinal decontamination. In comparison to other sedative-hypnotic drug toxicity, barbiturates have more pronounced, 'barb burns.' These are erythematous or hemorrhagic bullous skin lesions seen over areas of pressure in comatosed patients.

Hypersensitivity to barbiturates can result in a life-threatening syndrome called drug rash with eosinophilia and systemic symptoms (DRESS) that carries a mortality of 10%. It is characterized by rash, fever, organ inflammation, lymphadenopathy, and hematologic abnormalities such as eosinophilia, thrombocytopenia, and atypical lymphocytosis. DRESS syndrome may occur at any point in the treatment course with barbiturates. In those developing hypersensitivity to barbiturates, there is a potential of cross-sensitivity with other aromatic antiepileptics, such as phenytoin and carbamazepine.

Chronic Toxicity (or Exposure)

Animal

Phenobarbital is considered a carcinogen in experimental animals. Mice treated while pregnant developed a dose-related increase in the number of pups born with cleft palate (0.6% of fetuses in the 50 mg kg^{-1} diet vs 3.9% in the 150 mg kg^{-1} diet). Dogs fed amobarbital chronically developed CNS depression, slowed reaction times, and incoordination.

Human

Chronic use of high doses of barbiturates may produce psychological and physical dependence. Abrupt discontinuation of therapy may result in withdrawal signs and symptoms. Mild withdrawal may include weakness, anxiety, muscle twitching, insomnia, nausea, and vomiting. Severe withdrawal may consist of hallucinations, autonomic instability, delirium, and seizures. Severe withdrawal symptoms may be life threatening. To prevent withdrawal, those on chronic barbiturates should have the dose gradually decreased rather than abruptly discontinued. Barbiturates induce hepatic microsomal enzymes and can increase the metabolism of other medications. Concomitant medication use with drugs such as phenobarbital may require higher doses of other medications for an equivalent clinical effect. When discontinuing a CYP450 inducer, such as phenobarbital, caution needs to be taken to also decrease the dose of other agents in order to prevent toxicity.

Immunotoxicity

Hypersensitivity to barbiturates may result in a life-threatening syndrome called DRESS. For more information, refer to the Acute or Short-Term Toxicity (or Exposure) section.

Genotoxicity

Phenobarbital did not induce point mutations in various strains of *Salmonella typhimurium*. Phenobarbital has been reported to be weakly mutagenic in *Drosophila melanogaster* (with 2–3 mg (LD_{50})) to nutrient medium.

Reproductive Toxicity

Barbiturates can cause reproductive toxicity. They can cross the placenta and distribute in fetal tissue. Exposure during the first trimester of pregnancy can cause malformations and exposure during the third trimester can induce a neonatal abstinence syndrome or withdrawal following delivery. With the long-acting barbiturates in particular, the withdrawal syndrome may be delayed. With regard to teratogenicity the barbiturates used as anticonvulsants have been most frequently studied and malformations associated with anticonvulsant drug use (such as phenobarbital or the nonbarbiturate hydantoin phenytoin) during pregnancy are termed hydantoin-barbiturate embryopathy. In some studies, when phenobarbital is used with other anticonvulsants, phenytoin in particular, the rate of malformations increased from that of malformations associated with either drug alone. Understanding the risk of drug effect when used as an anticonvulsant in human reproductive toxicity studies is complicated as multifactorial genetic influences as well as maternal seizures can affect fetal development. In one review of 12 pregnant women who attempted suicide by drug overdose with barbiturates (including butobarbital, hexobarbital, and barbital), the very large doses of these barbiturates used in self-poisoning by the women were not teratogenic to the children.

Carcinogenicity

Certain barbiturates may be tumor promoting through their ability to promote hepatocellular repair following treatment of carcinogenic agents such as nitrosamines and other carcinogenic agents. Phenobarbital has been shown to be carcinogenic in animal studies and is thought to be a potential carcinogen in humans. Studies looking at barbiturates and risk for lung cancer data have not shown that the barbiturates increase the risk of cancer.

Clinical Management

Acute Toxicity

Basic and advanced life support measures should be implemented as necessary and focus on maintaining respiratory and cardiovascular support is paramount. There is no antidote for barbiturate toxicity. Gastrointestinal decontamination procedures should be used as appropriate based on the patient's level of consciousness and history of ingestion. Activated charcoal can be used to adsorb barbiturates; however, multiple-dose activated charcoal therapy (every 2–6 h for 24–48 h) has not been shown to improve patient outcomes in phenobarbital toxicity. There are no data looking at the effectiveness of multidose charcoal for treatment of overdose from other long-acting barbiturates. Given the pharmacokinetics of barbiturates, however, a second dose of activated charcoal may be indicated based on the long half-life of other agents. Hypotension should be treated with standard measures including vasopressor support. Urine alkalinization with sodium bicarbonate to obtain a urinary pH of 7.5–8 may enhance elimination of phenobarbital by 5- to 10-fold. This procedure is not effective for short-acting barbiturates since they have higher pK_a values, are more protein bound, and are primarily metabolized by the liver with very little unchanged drug excretion by the kidneys. Hemodialysis is effective for removing long-acting barbiturates but should be reserved for severe cases when standard supportive measures are inadequate. CNS stimulant agents should not be used and may increase the rate of mortality. Major complications associated with barbiturate intoxication include anoxic brain injury, aspiration pneumonia, rhabdomyolysis, and compartment syndrome.

Chronic Toxicity

The occurrence of withdrawal signs and symptoms indicates the need to reinstitute barbiturate or substitute alternative benzodiazepine therapy and gradually reduce the dose until discontinued.

See also: Anxiolytics; Neurotoxicity; Poisoning Emergencies in Humans.

Further Reading

Bankstahl, M., Bahkstahl, J.P., Loscher, W., 2013. Is switching from brand name to generic formulations of phenobarbital associated with loss of antiepileptic efficacy?: a pharmacokinetic study with two oral formulations (Luminal® vet, Phenoleptil®) in dogs. BMC Vet. Res. 9 (1), 202.

Bryczkowski, C., Geib, A.J., December 2012. Combined butalbital/acetaminophen/caffeine overdose: case files of the Robert Wood Johnson Medical School Toxicology Service. J. Med. Toxicol. 8 (4), 424–431.

Goodman, J.M., Bischel, M.D., Wagers, P.W., 1976. Barbiturate intoxication: morbidity and mortality. West. J. Med. 124, 179–186.

Hassanian-Moghaddam, H., Zarei, M.R., Kargar, M., Sarjami, S., Rasouli, M.R., 2010. Factors associated with nonbenzodiazepine antiepileptic drug intoxication: analysis of 9,809 registered cases of drug poisoning. Epilepsia 51 (6), 979–983.

Hendey, G.W., Dery, R.A., Barnes, R.L., Snowden, B., Mentler, P., 2011. A prospective, randomized, trial of phenobarbital versus benzodiazepines for acute alcohol withdrawal. Am. J. Emerg. Med. 29 (4), 382–385.

Lindberg, M.C., Cunningham, A., Lindberg, N.H., 1992. Acute phenobarbital intoxication. Am. J. Emerg. Med. 85, 803–807.

Loscher, W., Rogawski, M.A., December 2012. How theories evolved concerning the mechanisms of action of barbiturates. Epilepsia 53 (Suppl. 8), 12–25.

Prajapati, P., Sheikh, M.I., Brahmbhatt, J., 2009. Barbiturate overdose: a case report. J. Indian Med. Assoc. 107 (12), 897–898, 900.

Rosenson, J., Clements, C., Simon, B., Vieaux, J., Graffman, S., Vahidnia, F., Cisse, B., Lam, J., Alter, H., 2013. Phenobarbital for acute alcohol withdrawal: a prospective randomized double-blind placebo-controlled study. J. Emerg. Med. 44 (3), 592–598.

Saraswati, S., Alhaider, A.A., Agrawal, S.S., 2013. Anticarcinogenic effect of brucine in diethylnitrosamine initiated and phenobarbital-promoted hepatocarcinogenesis in rats. Chem. Biol. Interact. 206 (2), 214–221.

Yasiry, Z., Shorvon, S.D., 2012. How phenobarbital revolutionized epilepsy therapy: the story of phenobarbital therapy in epilepsy in the last 100 years. Epilepsia 53 (Suppl. 8), 26–39.

Relevant Websites

http://www.streetdrugs.org/html%20files/barbiturates.html – Barbiturate information at Streetdrugs.org.

http://emedicine.medscape.com/article/813155-overview – Barbiturate Toxicity including overview, clinical presentation, workup, differential diagnosis and treatment in *eMedicine*, an online Medscape resource.

http://www.deathpenaltyinfo.org/state-lethal-injection – Death Penalty Information Center with information on use of pentobarbital as injection agent.

http://www.deathpenalty.org/article.php?id=52 – Death Penalty – Lethal Injection information (pentobarbital).

http://www.emcdda.europa.eu/publications/drug-profiles/barbiturates – European Monitoring Center for Drugs and Drug Addiction (EMCDDA) Barbiturate Drug Profile.

http://www.thepoisonreview.com/2013/03/29/does-phenobarbital-add-benefit-in-treating-alcohol-withdrawal-syndrome/ – Information and Review Regarding Use of Phenobarbital in the Treatment of Alcohol Withdrawal from The Poison Review.

http://www.dpw.state.pa.us/provider/healthcaremedicalassistance/medicarepartprescription drugcoverage/listofmedicinesclassifiedasbarbituratesorbenzodiazepines/index.htm – List of Medicines Classified as Either Barbiturates or Benzodiazepines.

http://ntp.niehs.nih.gov/ – National Toxicology Program - search for Barbiturates.

http://www.erowid.org/chemicals/barbiturates/ – The Vault of Erowid Barbiturate section – Background, history, use, intoxication, additional resources.

Barium

SC Gad, Gad Consulting Services, Cary, NC, USA

- Name: Barium
- Chemical Abstracts Service Registry Number: 7440-39-3
- Valence States: +2

Background Information

Barium was discovered as an element by Carl Scheele in 1774, after which it was first isolated by Sir Humphry Davy in 1808. The abundance of barium in Earth's crust is approximately 0.05%. Barite stones found around Bologna, Italy, were some of the first exposures of humans to barium, so it was named Bolognan stone after the nearby town, and fascinated people due to its ability to phosphoresce after exposure to sunlight.

Uses

Barium is found in various alloys, paints, soap, paper, photographic chemicals, explosives, and rubber, and is used in the manufacture of ceramics and glass. Some of its compounds are used as mordants in fabric dyeing and in the preparation of phosphors. One major use is in slurry of ground barite ($ZnS + BaSO_4$) for gas and oil drilling. Barium fluorosilicate has been used as an insecticide, and some barium compounds are used as rodenticides. Medicinally, barium sulfate, being very sparingly soluble, is used as a radiopaque contrast material for X-ray diagnostic purposes and other medical imaging uses.

Environmental Fate and Behavior

Barium is a highly reactive metal that occurs naturally only in a combined state. The element is released to environmental media by both natural processes and anthropogenic sources.

Barium is released primarily to the atmosphere as a result of industrial emissions during the mining, refining, and production of barium and barium chemicals, fossil fuel combustion, and entrainment of soil and rock dust into the air. In addition, coal ash, containing widely variable amounts of barium, is also a source of airborne barium particulates. Most barium released to the environment from industrial sources is in forms that do not become widely dispersed. In the atmosphere, barium is likely to be present in particulate form. Although chemical reactions may cause changes in speciation of barium in air, the main mechanisms for the removal of barium compounds from the atmosphere are likely to be wet and dry depositions.

In aquatic media, barium is likely to precipitate out of solution as an insoluble salt (i.e., as $BaSO_4$ or $BaCO_3$). Waterborne barium may also adsorb to suspended particulate matter. Precipitation of barium sulfate salts is accelerated when rivers enter the ocean because of the high sulfate content in the ocean. Sedimentation of suspended solids removes a large portion of the barium content from surface water. Barium in sediments is found largely in the form of barium sulfate (barite). Coarse silt sediment in a turbulent environment will often grind and cleave the barium sulfate from the sediment particles, leaving a buildup of dense barites. Estimated soil–water distribution coefficients (Kd) (i.e., the ratio of the quantity of barium absorbed per gram of sorbent to the concentration of barium remaining in solution at equilibrium) range from 200 to 2800 for sediments and sandy loam soils.

As pH levels increase above 9.3 and in the presence of carbonate, barium carbonate becomes the dominant species. Barium carbonate also exhibits fast precipitation kinetics and very low solubility and in alkaline environments limits the soluble barium concentration. Barium forms salts of low solubility with arsenate, chromate, fluoride, oxalate, and phosphate ions. The chloride, hydroxide, and nitrate of barium are water soluble and are frequently detected in aqueous environments.

Exposure and Exposure Monitoring

Exposure pathways for barium primarily consist of ingestion (e.g., food and water) and inhalation. Barium is relatively abundant in nature; hence, most food contains small amounts of barium. Brazil nuts have very high barium concentrations (from 3 to 4000 ppm). It is also found in drinking water from natural deposits in certain regions. Barium is also detected in the air of most cities. The toxicity depends on the solubility of the compound.

Toxicokinetics

Soluble barium compounds are absorbed by the lungs and gastrointestinal tract and small amounts are accumulated in the skeleton. The highest concentration of barium in the body is present in the lungs. Although some barium is excreted in the urine, it is reabsorbed by the renal tubules. It is primarily excreted in feces. Accumulation occurs in the skeleton and pigmented parts of the eye.

Mechanism of Toxicity

Ingestion of toxic doses of barium affects the muscles, especially the heart. Barium has a digitalis-type effect on the heart. Ventricular fibrillation and slowed pulse rate are noted. This may be related to barium's tendency to displace potassium; the resulting potassium deficiency causes muscle weakness.

Acute and Short-Term Toxicity (or Exposure)

Animal

The LD_{50} for rats is 630 mg kg^{-1} for barium carbonate, 118 mg kg^{-1} for barium chloride, and 921 mg kg^{-1} for barium acetate.

 http://dx.doi.org/10.1016/B978-0-12-386454-3.00819-8

Human

The toxicity of barium is related to the solubility of the compound. Barium sulfate, being very sparingly soluble, is relatively nontoxic. Soluble barium salts are toxic by ingestion (e.g., acetate, chloride, nitrate, sulfide, as well as carbonate and hydroxide compounds). Ingestion results in nausea, vomiting, stomach pains, and diarrhea. Severe gastrointestinal irritation is followed by muscle twitching and then a flaccid muscular paralysis. Barium can activate catecholamines, resulting in muscle twitching and other nervous system effects. Ingestion of barium compounds can lead to gastroenteritis, hypokalemia, hypertension, cardiac arrhythmias, and skeletal muscle paralysis. Potassium infusion is used clinically to reverse many of the toxic effects, but cannot reverse the hypertensive response. Barium released during welding can decrease plasma potassium levels.

Soluble compounds also irritate skin, eyes, and mucous membranes and can be absorbed following inhalation. Barium carbonate dust is a bronchial irritant. Barium oxide dust is a dermal and nasal irritant.

Barium carbonate, a rodenticide, has an oral TD_{Lo} of less than 11 mg kg^{-1}; another rodenticide, barium chloride, has similar, though generally stronger effects. Convulsions and death from cardiac and respiratory failures can occur. Survival for more than 24 h is usually followed by complete recovery. Direct aspiration of a large amount of barium into the airway resulted in tachycardia, rapid breathing, fever, and low oxygen saturation. A family eating fish accidentally battered with barium carbonate developed nausea, vomiting, diarrhea, and abdominal pain within minutes, and the parents also developed ventricular tachycardia, flaccid paralysis of the extremities, dyspnea (mother), and respiratory failure (father). Patients were treated symptomatically and all fully recovered.

Chronic Toxicity (or Exposure)

Animal

In guinea pigs, barium caused various changes in the blood and pathological changes in bone marrow, spleen, and liver. Cardiovascular effects are evident in rats after long-term exposures. Ultrastructural changes in the kidney glomeruli were noted in rats consuming barium (1 g l^{-1}) in the drinking water for 36 weeks. Increased kidney weights were noted in female rats consuming barium (2500 ppm) in the drinking water for 15 months.

Human

Inhalation of insoluble sulfate and oxide, as dusts, produces a pneumoconiosis called baritosis, which is a relatively benign condition that is usually reversible with cessation of exposure. Cardiovascular effects are also of concern after long-term exposure in humans.

Reproductive Toxicity

Barium has been observed to have some limited reproductive affects. In the nematode *Caenorhabditis elegans*, high barium exposure resulted in vulva abnormalities and severe reductions in both reproductive capacity and speed. Testing in rats with barium chloride yielded no significant effects. Barium chloride injected into chicken yolks resulted in curled toes in 50% of surviving offspring.

Barium is not reported to be reproductively toxic in humans.

Genotoxicity

Barium chloride hydrate was positive in the mouse lymphoma assay, but negative in Ames, plate incorporation, and preincubation, as well as both the mitotic crossing over and gene conversion tests.

Barium has not been reported to be genotoxic in humans.

Carcinogenicity

In one study using barium chloride hydrate administered via drinking water, there was no evidence of carcinogenicity in either rats or mice, though the mice (both male and female) demonstrated nephropathy.

Barium has not been reported to be carcinogenic in humans.

Clinical Management

Addition of sodium sulfate as a lavage solution may precipitate the very insoluble barium sulfate. As potassium deficiency occurs in acute poisoning, serum potassium and cardiac rhythm must be monitored closely. Administration of intravenous potassium appears beneficial. As renal failure is also a concern, urinary output also must be monitored closely.

Ecotoxicology

The uptake of barium by fish and marine organisms is an important elimination mechanism. Barium levels in seawater range from 2 to 63 mg l^{-1} with a mean concentration of ~13 mg l^{-1}. Barium was found to bioconcentrate in marine plants by a factor of 1000 times the level present in the water. Bioconcentration factors in marine animals, plankton, and brown algae of 100, 120, and 260, respectively, have been reported. Relatively little information is available on the effects of barium compounds in aquatic organisms. Barium carbonate was practically nontoxic to fish (96 h LC_{50} in *Gambusia* was 410 g kg^{-1}).

Exposure Standards and Guidelines

The American Conference of Governmental Industrial Hygienists threshold limit value – time-weighted average is 0.5 mg ml^{-1} for soluble barium compounds and 10 mg ml^{-1} for barium sulfate. The permissible exposure limit is 0.5 mg m^{-3} for barium in soluble compounds. The reference dose for barium is 0.07 mg kg^{-1} day^{-1} and the tolerable daily intake (the Netherlands) is 0.02 mg kg^{-1} day^{-1}.

Miscellaneous

Brazil nuts contain more barium than other foods, with concentrations of 3000–4000 ppm.

See also: Metals.

Further Reading

Bingham, E., Cohrssen, B., 2012. Patty's Toxicology, sixth ed. John Wiley & Sons, Hoboken, NJ.

Deepthiraju, B., Varma, P.R.K., 2012. Barium toxicity – a rare presentation of fireworks ingestion. Ind. Pediatr. 49 (9), 762.

Melo, L., Alleoni, L., Carvalho, G., Azevedo, R., 2011. Cadmium and barium toxicity effects on growth and antioxidant capacity of soybean (Glycine max L.) plants, grown in two soil types with different physicochemical properties. J. Plant Nutr. Soil Sci. 174 (5), 847–859.

Nordberg, B.A., Fowler, B.A., Nordberg, M., Friberg, L.T., 2007. Handbook on the Toxicology of Metals, third ed. Elsevier, New York.

Payen, C., Dellinger, A., Pulce, C., Cirimele, V., Carbonnel, V., Kintz, P., Descotes, J., 2012. Intoxication by large amounts of barium nitrate overcome by early massive k supplementation and oral administration of magnesium sulphate. Hum. Exp. Toxicol. 30 (1), 34–37.

Relevant Websites

http://www.atsdr.cdc.gov – Agency for Toxic Substances and Disease Registry. Toxicological Profile for Barium.

http://risk.lsd.ornl.gov – Risk Assessment Information System.

http://toxnet.nlm.nih.gov/ – Toxnet homepage, search for 'barium'

Bases *see* Alkalies

Batrachotoxin

JP Dumbacher, California Academy of Sciences, San Francisco, CA, USA

- Representative Chemicals: Batrachotoxin; Homobatrachotoxin; Batrachotoxinin-A; and several other batrachotoxinin-A congeners
- Chemical Abstracts Service Registry Number: CAS 23509-16-2 (Batrachotoxin)
- Synonyms: *Phyllobates* toxin, *Pitohui* toxin, *Ifrita* toxin, and poison dart frog toxin
- Chemical/Pharmaceutical/Other Class: Steroidal alkaloid neurotoxin
- Molecular Formulas:
  - Batrachotoxin: $C_{31}H_{42}N_2O_6$
  - Homobatrachotoxin: $C_{32}H_{44}N_2O_6$
  - Batrachotoxinin-A: $C_{24}H_{35}NO_5$
- Chemical Structure:

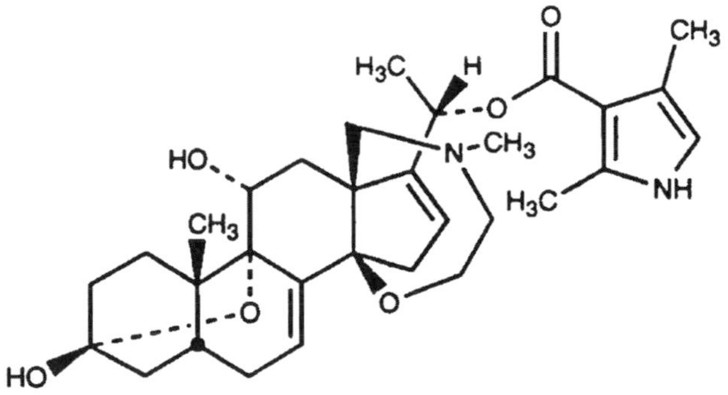

Background

Batrachotoxins are a class of steroidal alkaloid neurotoxins originally found in Colombian poison dart frogs of the genus *Phyllobates* (family Dendrobatidae). The frogs have special skin glands that store and secrete the toxins, and these glands are most densely packed on the frog's back behind the head. Evidence suggests that the frogs acquire the toxins from a dietary source; however, no potential source of these frog poisons has been identified. Of all of the so-called poison dart frogs, only three species of poison dart frogs were actually used by Native Americans for poisoning dart tips, and these 'true poison dart frogs' were all members of the genus *Phyllobates* that carry batrachotoxins as their major toxic element responsible for poisoning. More recently, batrachotoxins were found in New Guinean birds of the genus *Pitohui* and *Ifrita*. In birds, the toxins are most concentrated in the skins and feathers.

In both birds and frogs, batrachotoxins are thought to provide some protection against natural enemies. The most toxic *Phyllobates* frogs are brightly colored in comparison to other congeners, and the same is true for the most toxic *Pitohui* species. It is presumed that the bright colors act as warning or aposematic signal to visual predators. Limited experiments have shown that the toxins may be an arthropod repellent and reduce the life span of arthropod pests such as lice, and that natural predators show aversive reactions to the these toxins.

Several naturally occurring batrachotoxins have been identified from frog and bird extracts. The most common are batrachotoxin and homobatrachotoxin, which contain a pyrrole moiety. These occur in frogs in roughly equal proportions and have an LD_{50} in mice of ~2 to 3 $\mu g\,kg^{-1}$ (subcutaneous injection). Toxicity via other routes has not been well studied. The pyrrole can be manipulated in nature and in the laboratory to give the non-pyrrole form, called batrachotoxinin-A, which is about 1/500th as toxic as batrachotoxin or homobatrachotoxin. Several other congeners have been identified in nature, but the pharmacology of most of these remains unstudied. These include batrachotoxinin-A *cis*-crotonate, an allylically rearranged 16-acetate, batrachotoxinin-A 3-hydroxypentanoate, and multiple mono- and dihydroxylated derivatives.

Experiments suggest that both birds and frogs may sequester toxins from dietary sources. When brought into captivity, frogs slowly loose their toxicity, and when raised in captivity on nontoxic diets, frogs fail to produce batrachotoxins. When fed batrachotoxins in their diet, frogs readily accumulate the toxins in their skin. Although it is widely believed that ants may be the source of toxins for dendrobatid frogs, this has yet to be demonstrated for batrachotoxins in *Phyllobates* frogs. Although other frog poisons have been found in ants, no ant species has yet been found to contain batrachotoxins, and ants represent a smaller portion of the overall diet for the larger *Phyllobates* frogs than for the smaller dendrobatid frog species. In New Guinea, a small beetle (genus *Choresine*, family Melyridae) has been shown to carry significant quantities of batrachotoxins and also been shown to be eaten by toxic *Pitohui* birds. Thus, *Choresine* beetles represent a putative source of dietary toxins for the New Guinea birds. Recently, several other dendrobatid frog toxins have been found in soil mites in the family Oribatidae, and these represent a potential ultimate source of these toxins for frogs, beetles, and birds.

Toxin Uses

Batrachotoxin is an important research tool in pharmacology because of its action of holding voltage-gated sodium channels open as well as its specific effects at other ligand-binding sites. It was commonly used in ion channel and ligand research.

 http://dx.doi.org/10.1016/B978-0-12-386454-3.00998-2

Batrachotoxin has no current clinical uses for two primary reasons. First, batrachotoxin is highly toxic and dangerous to use for medical purposes. Synthetic forms with altered properties would have to be developed for clinical trials. Second, there are no commercially available sources of batrachotoxins or commercially viable synthetic pathways. Most available stocks of batrachotoxin were collected from wild-caught *Phyllobates* frogs by John Daly many years ago. Work in relevant regions of Colombia is currently difficult or impossible, so these stocks cannot be replenished. No commercially viable sources of batrachotoxin are known from New Guinea, but additional research on the ultimate source of batrachotoxins may elucidate new sources.

Human Use of Frog and Bird Secretions Containing Batrachotoxins

Very small amounts of frog secretions from *Phyllobates terribilis*, *P. bicolor*, and *P. aurotaenia* have been used by Choco and Embera Indians to poison dart tips. These poisoned darts are reportedly effective at immobilizing a variety of animals including jaguar, bear, deer, and humans. A single *P. bicolor* or *P. terribilis* frog can effectively poison 20–30 darts. Frog toxin levels are high enough that merely holding the frogs can be dangerous, and human poisonings have been reported.

In New Guinea, traditional hunters are aware that *Pitohui* and *Ifrita* birds carry neurotoxins. Toxins are more diffuse in these birds than in the frogs; however, in some populations, even a single feather, if tasted, can cause a burning sensation in the mouth that may last for several minutes to hours. Handling the birds can cause allergy-like reactions such as itchy watery eyes, running nose, and sneezing. There have been no known human deaths or serious poisonings due to bird ingestion, as it is generally recognized as inedible, and an unpleasant burning sensation sets in before much of the toxin is ingested. No anthropologists have reported local New Guineans using the toxins to immobilize prey, but bird tissues are used in some local medicinal concoctions.

Exposure Routes and Pathways

From *Phyllobates* frogs, exposure occurs through ingesting skin and flesh of the frogs. Toxin quantities can be high enough to make even handling these frogs dangerous, so presumably some absorption can occur through skin. Exposure to the toxins may occur by subcutaneous injection, such as a puncture from a poisoned dart tip. From birds, exposure can occur by eating flesh; however, even handling the birds can cause local irritation and 'allergic-like' reactions such as itchy eyes, runny nose, sneezing, and tingling around buccal membranes. These latter reactions are believed to be caused by powder or tiny feather fragments released from toxic feathers. Batrachotoxins are lipid soluble and soluble in a variety of organic solvents such as methanol, chloroform, and ethanol.

Toxicokinetics

Batrachotoxin can be absorbed through skin as well as from the gastrointestinal tract. Effects can occur within 10 min and can last for several hours to more than a day.

Mechanism of Action and Toxicity

Batrachotoxins bind specifically to voltage-gated sodium channels in nerve and muscle membranes and significantly alter channel function in four primary ways that have been documented. First, batrachotoxin significantly shifts the activation gating 30–50 mV toward hyperpolarization. Thus a batrachotoxin-bound channel will activate more readily, even at membrane resting potentials. Second, batrachotoxin eliminates or reduces both fast and slow inactivation gating, which holds the activated channels in the open conformation for hours or longer. Third, batrachotoxin can reduce single channel conductance by up to 50%. And fourth, batrachotoxin can alter the ion selectivity of the voltage-gated sodium channel.

In short, batrachotoxins activate voltage-gated sodium channels and stabilize the channel in its open conformation. This allows sodium ions to flow freely across the membrane and depolarize membrane. This causes local tingling, irritation, and numbness in peripheral nervous tissue. In higher concentrations or systemic doses, batrachotoxin will cause convulsions, paralysis, and cardiac or pulmonary failure. Because a relatively small proportion of activated channels can depolarize the membrane, batrachotoxins are highly toxic. Because batrachotoxins bind strongly to sodium channel proteins, binding is often referred to as 'irreversible,' although light exposure (resulting in local tingling or numbness) generally subsides within a few minutes to 24 h.

Acute and Short-Term Toxicity (or Exposure)

Human

Very little is known about the toxicity of batrachotoxins in humans. If it is assumed that human and mouse toxicity are roughly equivalent (at $\sim 2.5\ \mu g\ kg^{-1}$ injected subcutaneously), then a median lethal dose for a 68-kg human would be $\sim 170\ \mu g$ of batrachotoxin. Other studies show that mice are less susceptible to neurotoxins than humans, so another estimate can be based on toxicity relationships of batrachotoxin to aconitine, digitoxin, and strychnine and their toxicity in humans. Using these relationships, it is expected that a dose as small as 2–10 μg of purified batrachotoxin injected subcutaneously may be lethal to humans. Likewise, ingested amounts of as little as 120–500 μg are expected to be lethal. These are certainly rough estimates, and few, if any, human poisonings have been reported in medical literature. However, purified toxins as well as frog skin secretions should be handled with extreme care.

Only direct toxic effects on voltage-gated sodium channels have been studied. Other mechanisms of toxicity (e.g., chronic toxicity, immunotoxicity, genotoxicity, carcinogenicity, etc.) have not been investigated.

Clinical Management

No antidote is available.

See also: Animals, Poisonous and Venomous.

Further Reading

Albuquerque, E.X., Daly, J.W., Witkop, B., 1971. Batrachotoxin: chemistry and pharmacology. Science 172, 995–1002.

Catterall, W.A., 1988. Molecular pharmacology of voltage-sensitive sodium channels. ISI Atlas Sci.Pharmacol., 190–195.

Catterall, W.A., Morrow, C.S., Daly, J.W., Brown, G.B., 1981. Binding of batrachotoxinin A 20-a-benzoate to a receptor site associated with sodium channels in synaptic nerve ending particles. J. Biol. Chem. 256, 8922–8927.

Daly, J.W., Spande, T.F., 1986. Amphibian alkaloids: chemistry, pharmacology and biology. In: Pelletier (Ed.), Alkaloids: Chemical and Biological Perspectives. Wiley, New York, pp. 1–274.

Daly, J.W., Garraffo, H.M., Spande, T.F., Jaramillo, C., Rand, A.S., 1994. Dietary source for skin alkaloids of poison frogs (Dendrobatidae)? J Chem. Ecol. 20, 943–955.

Daly, J.W., Myers, C.W., Warnick, J.E., Albuquerque, E.X., 1980. Levels of batrachotoxin and lack of sensitivity to its action in poison-dart frogs (*Phyllobates*). Science 208, 1383–1385.

Daly, J.W., Secunda, S.I., Garraffo, H.M., et al., 1994. An uptake system for dietary alkaloids in poison frogs (Dendrobatidae). Toxicon 32, 657–663.

Daly, J.W., Witkop, B., Bommer, P., Biemann, K., 1965. Batrachotoxin. The active principle of the Colombian poison arrow frog, *Phyllobates* bicolor. J. Am. Chem. Soc. 87, 124–126.

Dumbacher, J.P., Beehler, B.M., Spande, T.F., Garraffo, H.M., Daly, J.W., 1992. Homobatrachotoxin in the genus *Pitohui*: chemical defense in birds? Science 258, 799–801.

Dumbacher, J.P., Spande, T., Daly, J.W., 2000. Batrachotoxin alkaloids from passerine birds: a second toxic bird genus (*Ifrita kowaldi*). Proc. Natl Acad. Sci. USA 97, 12970–12975.

Myers, C.W., Daly, J.W., Malkin, B., 1978. A dangerously toxic new frog (*Phyllobates*) used by Embera Indians of Western Columbia, with discussion of blowgun fabrication and dart poisoning. Bull. Am. Mus. Nat. Hist. 161, 307–366.

Wang, S.-Y., Mitchell, J., Tikhonov, D.B., Zhorov, B.S., Wang, G.K., 2006. How batrachotoxin modifies the sodium channel permeation pathway: computer modeling and site-directed mutagenesis. Mol. Pharmacol. 69, 788–795.

BCNU (Bischloroethyl Nitrosourea)

E Curfman and M Jiang, Indiana University School of Medicine-Fort Wayne, Fort Wayne, IN, USA
MG Soni, Soni and Associates Inc, Vero Beach, FL, USA

This article is a revision of the previous edition article by Madhusudan G. Soni, volume 1, pp 219–221, © 2005, Elsevier Inc.

- Name: BCNU (Bischloroethyl nitrosourea)
- Chemical Abstracts Service Registry Number: 154-93-8
- Synonyms: Carmustine; *N,N*-bis(2-Chloroethyl)-*N*-nitrosourea; BiCNU; Carmubris; Nitrumon; Gliadel.
- Molecular Formula: $C_5H_9Cl_2N_3O_2$
- Chemical Structure:

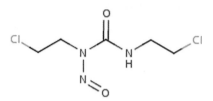

Background

Bischloroethyl nitrosourea (BCNU) is a mustard-gas-derived alkylating agent that underwent clinical trials for use as an antineoplastic agent in the mid-1960s. Intravenous BCNU received US Food and Drug Administration (FDA) approval for brain tumor treatments in 1977. Further development and trials led to the FDA approval of a BCNU-impregnated polymer wafer for use as an intracavity surgical adjunct for recurrent glioblastoma moltiforme in 1996. These wafers were again reapproved in 2003 for use in high-grade malignant glioma as an adjunct to surgery and radiation. The physical and chemical properties of BCNU are listed on **Table 1**.

Uses

BCNU has been used in human medicine as an antineoplastic agent (alone or in combination with other agents) in the treatment of Hodgkin's lymphoma, multiple myeloma, and primary or metastatic brain tumors.

Environmental Fate and Behavior

There is no information available on the environmental fate of BCNU. However, it is predicted that BCNU spontaneously decomposes due to its high reactivity. Estimates indicate that the half-life of BCNU particulates and vapor in air is 4.4 days. Though expected to be highly mobile when adsorbed to soil and suspended solids, it is likely that this adsorption may be precluded by hydrolysis. Volatilization from soil or water is not expected, and the potential for bioaccumulation is low. BCNU degrades into 2-chloroethylamine, which is not considered hazardous to the environment.

Table 1 Physical and chemical properties of BCNU

Property	*Parameters*
Molecular weight	214.049 86 g mol^{-1}
Vapor pressure	2.9×10^{-4} mm Hg at 25 °C
Melting point	31 °C
Henry's law constant	4.8×10^{-11} atm-cu m mol^{-1} at 25 °C
Log *P*	1.5
Water solubility	4.0×10^{3} mg l^{-1} at 25 °C
Other solubilities	Highly ethanol and lipid soluble

Exposure Routes and Pathways

Intravenous injection and intracavity polymer wafers are the two most common routes of exposure. Doses range from 100 to 250 mg m^{-2} body surface for courses of 2 or 3 days intravenously or an average of 61.6 mg when in wafer form. Exposure from the environment is not likely in the general public.

Toxicokinetics

In animal experiments, BCNU is rapidly absorbed, following different routes of ingestion. A few minutes after administration, no unchanged BCNU can be detected in plasma. BCNU undergoes spontaneous decomposition under physiological conditions to release both alkylating and carbamoylating entities. Hepatic microsomal enzyme oxidation systems denitrosylate BCNU to 1,3-bis(2-chloroethyl)urea, in addition to its spontaneous decomposition. Due to its high lipid solubility, BCNU is capable of crossing the blood–brain barrier and is rapidly distributed to most tissues, including brain and cerebrospinal fluid (CSF). The volume of distribution is ~0.18 l kg^{-1}. Approximately 60% of the drug appears in the urine within 96 h as degradation products, with a further 6% of the ingested BCNU removed by respiratory excretion and 1% in feces. BCNU is reported to have a biological half-life of between 15 and 30 min.

Mechanism of Toxicity

It is generally assumed that BCNU exerts its cytotoxicity through the liberation of alkylating and carbamoylating moieties. An alkylating entity, particularly chloroethyl carbonium ion, is strongly electrophilic and can alkylate a variety of biomolecules, including the purine and pyrimidine bases of DNA. BCNU causes DNA interstrand cross-linking, which is associated with cytotoxicity. The carbamoylation of lysine residues of protein can inactivate certain enzymes, thus interfering with DNA and RNA synthesis and repair processes. The inhibition of glutathione reductase by this carbamoylation further contributes to cytotoxicity.

 http://dx.doi.org/10.1016/B978-0-12-386454-3.00245-1

Acute and Short-Term Toxicity (or Exposure)

Animal

In dogs, high doses of BCNU resulted in severe bone marrow hypoplasia with delayed, reversible thrombocytopenia. The other major toxicities observed were cardiopulmonary (pulmonary edema, myocardial infarction, and pericardial hemorrhage), intestinal mucosal damage with hemorrhage, renal toxicity, and delayed hepatotoxicity. Monkeys exhibited similar toxicities, with the exception of cardiopulmonary toxicity. In rats, initially well-tolerated doses may cause death later.

Human

Various cytotoxic effects of BCNU in humans are reported. Hyperpigmentation of the skin when exposed to topical BCNU has been reported. The drug is not a vesicant, but local burning pain has been reported after intravenous administration. Nausea and vomiting occur ~2 h after injection. Flushing of the skin and conjunctiva, central nervous system toxicity, esophagitis, diarrhea, interstitial pulmonary fibrosis, and renal and hepatic toxicities have been reported. Hepatotoxicity and pulmonary toxicity may be dose limiting. Although bone marrow suppression is observed, BCNU characteristically causes an unusually delayed onset of leukopenia and thrombocytopenia. The nadir of the leukocyte and platelet counts may not reach normal levels until 6 weeks after treatment. Clinical signs associated with BCNU-induced pulmonary toxicity in humans are dyspnea, tachypnea, and a dry hacking cough. The incidence of these symptoms is between 20 and 30% and mortality varies from 24 to 80%. The onset of symptoms is usually within 3 years of treatment. There is a linear relationship between total dose received and pulmonary toxicity at doses >1000 mg m^{-2}, with 50% of patients developing pulmonary toxicity at total cumulative doses of 1500 mg m^{-2}.

Chronic Toxicity (or Exposure)

Animal

Intraperitoneal administration of BCNU three times a week for 6 months at doses of 2.5 or 5.0 mg kg^{-1} for Swiss mice and 1.5 mg kg^{-1} for Sprague–Dawley rats resulted in increases in tumor incidence in all treated animals, predominantly subcutaneous and lung neoplasms.

Human

Delayed onset of pulmonary fibrosis occurring up to 17 years after treatment has been reported in patients receiving BCNU in childhood and early adolescence (1–16 years). Pulmonary toxicity characterized by pulmonary infiltrates and/or fibrosis has been reported to occur from 9 days to 43 months after treatment with BCNU. Most of these patients were receiving prolonged therapy with total doses of BCNU greater than 1400 mg m^{-2}, but lower total doses have also been reported to result in pulmonary fibrosis. The incidence of fatal pulmonary complications is considerably higher in young children (<5 years). Renal abnormalities consisting of progressive azotemia, decrease in kidney size, and renal failure have been reported in patients who received large cumulative doses after prolonged therapy with BCNU.

Immunotoxicity

Given the leukopenic side effects of exposure, BCNU should be considered immunotoxic. Patients treated with BCNU should be expected to be moderately immunocompromised and all relevant precautions should be taken to avoid exposure to infection.

Reproductive Toxicity

BCNU can cause fetal harm in humans and animals. It has been demonstrated to be embryotoxic and teratogenic in rats and rabbits at doses nontoxic to the mother. BCNU caused testicular degeneration at intraperitoneal doses of 8 mg kg^{-1} $week^{-1}$ for 8 weeks in rats, which corresponds to a 1.3-fold relative increase in the recommended dosage for a human patient. There are no studies assessing the effect of BCNU on pregnant women. BCNU has been shown to be present in the milk of women undergoing treatment, albeit at lower concentrations than are present in the plasma. Pregnant women and women who are breastfeeding should be informed of the risks before beginning treatment with BCNU.

Genotoxicity

Multiple chromosomal aberrations and mutations resulted from BCNU treatment in mouse and rat cells *in vivo*. Various mutations have been reported in *Drosophila*, yeast, and bacteria, DNA damage has been reported in bacteria, rat cells, and human cells *in vitro*. BCNU at 5 mg kg^{-1} dosage resulted in dominant lethal mutations in rat spermatocytes, with higher doses inducing dominant lethal mutations in spermatids as well as spermatocytes.

Carcinogenicity

BCNU was mutagenic *in vitro* (Ames assay, human lymphoblast HGPRT (hypoxanthine–guanine phosphoribosyltransferase) assay) and clastogenic *in vitro* (V79 hamster cell micronucleus assay). There is sufficient evidence for the carcinogenicity of BCNU in rats. Some patients treated with BCNU have developed leukemia and bone marrow dysplasias. BCNU may be reasonably classified as a carcinogen in humans based on these findings.

Clinical Management

Most of the adverse reactions of BCNU are reversible if detected early. When such effects or reactions do occur, the drug should be reduced in dosage or discontinued and appropriate corrective measures should be taken according to the clinical judgment of the physician. Blood counts should be monitored weekly for at least 6 weeks after the dose. Baseline pulmonary function studies, hepatic functional tests, and periodic renal functional tests should be monitored. Implantation of BCNU wafers carries a significant risk of ventricular occlusion, leading to hydrocephaly due to impaired drainage of CSF. This risk may be minimized or negated by contraindicating BCNU wafers when opening of ventricles is required for surgical resection of the tumor. Furthermore, any openings larger than the diameter of a wafer should be closed to prevent migration of the wafers. Patients with implanted wafers should be monitored for seizures, intracranial infections, and brain edema. No proven antidotes have been established for BCNU overdosage.

See also: Carcinogen–DNA Adduct Formation and DNA Repair; Food and Drug Administration, US; Toxicity Testing, Mutagenicity.

Further Reading

Bartosek, I., Russo, R.G., Cattaneo, M.T., 1984. Pharmacokinetics of nitrosoureas: levels of 1,3-bis-(2-chloroethyl)-1-nitrosourea (BCNU) in organs of normal and Walker 256/B carcinoma bearing rats after i.v. bolus. Tumori 70, 491–498.

Duntze, J., Litré, C.F., Eap, C., Théret, E., Debreuve, A., et al., 2012. Implanted carmustine wafers followed by concomitant radiochemotherapy to treat newly diagnosed malignant gliomas: prospective, observational, multicenter study on 92 cases. Ann. Surg. Oncol., 2 December 2012 [Epub ahead of print].

Ewend, M.G., Brem, S., Gilbert, M., et al., 2007. Treatment of single brain metastasis with resection, intracavity carmustine polymer wafers, and radiation therapy is safe and provides excellent local control. Clin. Cancer Res. 13, 3637–3641.

Kuhnhenn, J., Kowalski, T., Steenken, S., Ostermann, K., Schlegel, U., 2012. Procarbazine, carmustine, and vincristine (PBV) for chemotherapy pre-treated patients with recurrent glioblastoma: a single-institution analysis. J. Neurooncol. 109 (2), 433–438.

Newton, H.B., 2012. Neurological complications of chemotherapy to the central nervous system. Handb. Clin. Neurol. 105, 903–916. http://dx.doi.org/10.1016/B978-0-444-53502-3.00031-8.

Sabel, M., Giese, A., 2008. Safety profile of carmustine wafers in malignant glioma: a review of controlled trials and a decade of clinical experience. Curr. Med. Res. Opin. 24 (11), 3239–3257.

Shen, Y.C., Chiu, C.F., Chow, K.C., et al., 2004. Fatal pulmonary fibrosis associated with BCNU: the relative role of platelet-derived growth factor-B, insulin-like growth factor I, transforming growth factor-β1 and cyclooxygenase-2. Bone Marrow Transplant. 34, 609–614.

Till, B.G., Madtes, D.K., 2012. BCNU-associated pneumonitis: portrait of a toxicity. Leuk. Lymphoma 53 (6), 1019–1020.

Bee *see* Hymenoptera

Behavioral Toxicity Testing *see* Toxicity Testing, Behavioral

Behavioral Toxicology

DA Cory-Slechta, University of Rochester School of Medicine, Box EHSC, Rochester, NY, USA

Introduction

Behavioral toxicology studies the effects of chemicals on behavior and also seeks to determine how such effects are caused. Behavior reflects the ultimate output of the nervous system. The impetus for such studies has come from multiple sources. Both human and experimental animal studies have been carried out to assess the behavioral consequences arising from exposures to chemicals used in the workplace as well as those dispersed in the environment. These efforts have been important in determining safe exposure and risk levels as well as in furthering our understanding of these chemicals. A second force behind many such studies has been the need to screen newly synthesized chemicals for any potential adverse behavioral effects before their introduction into use, efforts that are obviously carried out only in experimental laboratory contexts.

Human behavior is, of course, extremely diverse and complex, composed of numerous different functions, any or all of which might be perturbed by exposure to a toxicant. Thus, understanding how a chemical affects human behavior may require a determination of its effects across these different behavioral functions. Furthermore, some human behaviors require an integration of several different behavioral functions. If we think about learning in a classroom, for example, in addition to cognitive functions, sensory functions are needed to process the information presented, and motor functions are required for executing the correct response. Thus, in the event that a chemical is suspected to produce effects on cognitive functions, the possibility that such effects, instead, result indirectly from changes in sensory or motor functions must always be considered.

The entire range of behavioral functions and the tests designed to evaluate them cannot be presented here. This entry first presents the types of methods that comprise the test batteries used in animal models to screen newly developed chemicals for behavioral toxicity. While screening batteries are extremely useful in providing a preliminary assessment of adverse behavioral effects, they are less useful for elaborating the specific nature of the behavioral deficits or for yielding an understanding of their underlying behavioral and neurobiological mechanisms. For such purposes, more specific and sensitive tests of various behavioral functions are utilized. Examples of such higher order tests, in particular those related to sensory, motor, and cognitive functions, are subsequently presented in this entry and are followed by some discussion of the testing methods utilized in experimental animals to determine adverse behavioral effects of chemicals during the course of development as well as some of the test methods used in human populations.

Screening Batteries

Because a newly developed chemical may have effects on any of the numerous behavioral functions that comprise a behavioral repertoire, screening batteries must necessarily assess a wide variety of functions with sufficient sensitivity to suggest potential behavioral toxicity even in a single behavioral domain. These screening batteries are typically executed in studies using rats and mice and generally consist of two components: a functional observational battery (FOB) and a measure of motor activity (see below). FOBs include an array of measures, generally of unlearned or instinctive behaviors, designed to detect any indications of gross changes in reflexes and in gross motor or sensory function. Most FOBs are relatively easy to implement since there is typically no behavioral training or sophisticated equipment required for the measures of interest, as they are usually carried out and scored by an experienced observer. An FOB may include measures of general integrity, such as any signs of convulsions, palpebral closure, lacrimation, piloerection, salivation, and vocalizations. In addition, assessments of sensory capability based on measures such as response to a finger snap or a tail-pinch, righting reflex, and assessments of motor function, as evaluated by observations of the posture or gait of the animal, catalepsy, hindlimb foot splay, forelimb and hindlimb grip strength, and the time to begin ambulating, may be included. Finally, any signs of arousal or stress can be measured, such as ease of removal and handling, the animal's response to touch or approach, and urination and defecation. In addition, certain physiological responses, including body temperature and body weight, are sometimes measured. These evaluations are sometimes carried out in two different environments: a familiar one, such as the animal's home cage, and an unfamiliar flat surface of some type. This series of measures can be made relatively rapidly on each animal, consistent with the goal of screening of new compounds across a wide range of doses. In the event that behavioral activity of the chemical is indicated in such a screening test, more advanced and specific behavioral procedures would be required to delineate the precise nature of the behavioral impairment.

One question that has arisen with respect to the use of FOBs is whether changes in only one or two of the numerous measures taken are really indicative of neurotoxicity. For example, how is a change in two seemingly unrelated measures interpreted (e.g., vocalizations and hindlimb grip strength)? One answer that has been suggested is that neurotoxicity would be indicated by similar changes occurring within a single behavioral domain. Thus, changes in both forelimb and hindlimb grip strength would be indicative of altered motor function. Some have contended that if the toxicant under test produces body weight changes, then any changes also observed in the FOB may simply be due to 'sickness syndrome' or general malaise of the animal, not neurotoxicity. This is not necessarily a valid conclusion, however, since body weight changes may occur totally independently of any observed FOB effects. In fact, FOB changes are often reported in the absence of any body weight changes.

Motor Function

Motor function is a critical component of human behavior because it embodies the ultimate execution of a behavioral response. The feats of highly skilled athletes provide one example of incredibly refined motor performance, but even everyday functions such as walking or driving to work depend on adequate and intact motor capabilities. Motor behavior is not a unitary behavioral function, but rather one with many different components. Various motor responses entail such aspects as strength, coordination and endurance, precision and duration, frequency of occurrence, and for ambulation, gait and balance as well. Measurement of these different aspects of motor function obviously requires different procedures. As is the case for measurement of virtually all behavioral functions, the paradigms for assessing motor capabilities range from simple assessments to more complex and sensitive technologies. The former provides easily implemented but generally less specific and selective measures of function. The more advanced procedures provide measures of more specific or detailed aspects of motor function as distinct from changes in sensory or motivational processes but may require some training of the experimental subject and more sophisticated testing equipment.

Motor Activity Levels

Motor activity measures the frequency of occurrence of integrated movements and/or ambulation of the organism over some designated period of time, a behavior that generally occurs at some baseline level in mammalian species and which may be altered by exposure to a toxicant. A measure of motor activity is typically one component of a screening battery, and most studies of motor activity are carried out using rodents. Generally, the animals are placed on a horizontal surface, which could be square, rectangular, or even a maze such as a T-shaped apparatus, and the number of defined movements over a specified time period are recorded. In nonautomated versions, movements are typically recorded by an observer who, it is hoped, has no information with respect to the treatment condition (toxicant-exposed or control) of the subject which might bias the recording of data. In most automated versions, as are typically used now, the movements of the animal either interrupt a light beam or trip a switch which then records a count. In addition, behavior in such devices can be videotaped and parameters of motor activity defined and scored in a more automated manner. This can even be done with multiple animals in a single test session, with each individually identified and scored. An illustrative schematic of a videotaped scoring system appears in **Figure 1**.

Measurements of motor activity have been used to evaluate the potential central nervous system (CNS) effects of a wide variety of drugs and toxicants. One of the advantages of such measures of motor function is that no training is required of the subject. In addition, measures of motor activity can be made repeatedly across time so that the time course, including the onset and reversibility of toxicant effects, can be determined. In these types of repeated measurement experiments, moreover, an animal can serve as its own control, meaning that the experimenter looks for a change in the animal's normal pattern of motor activity after receiving the toxicant compared to the pattern observed before the treatment.

The experimenter must be cognizant of the fact that because of differences in both equipment hardware and software, different devices for measuring motor activity may not necessarily measure identical aspects of motor function or produce directly comparable outcome measures. Some devices use infrared light beams breaks to quantify responses. Differences between devices in the height of the infrared sensors used to detect vertical activity (rearing) could result in significantly different counts, for example. Such differences should also be considered in any direct comparisons of various studies of the effects of a toxicant on motor activity. Failure to do so may result in seemingly inconsistent results. Other influences must also be considered in the interpretation of changes in motor activity. For example, motor activity levels are known to be influenced by a variety of nonmotoric variables, such as time of day at which testing is carried out (rodents are nocturnal and show greater activity levels during dark hours), room lighting, and odors. As this list indicates, changes in sensory capabilities (perceived difference in the room odors or lighting) or circadian (nocturnal) rhythms could influence measures of motor activity independently of any direct toxicant-induced changes.

Motor activity may be an insensitive measure of toxicant-induced changes when it relies on relatively gross measures such as total counts per unit time. For example, in an open-field test such as shown in **Figure 1**, one might measure the

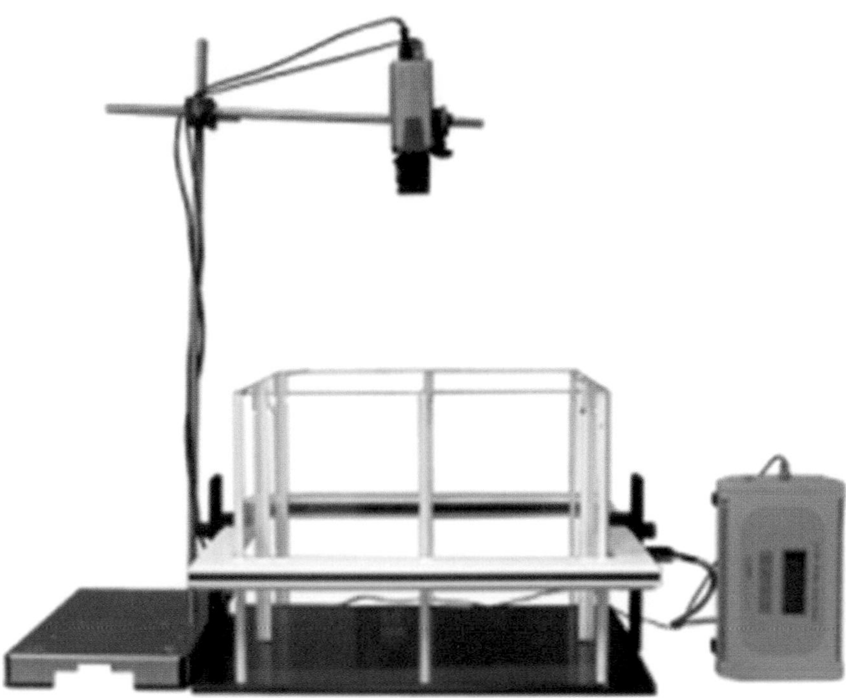

Figure 1 Open-field apparatus in which the activity of the mouse or rat is quantified over some period of time. In such a device, behavior is videotaped and subsequently scored, sometimes using automated scoring software (http://www.bioseb.com/bioseb/anglais/default/item_id=63_cat_id=_SMART%20Video%20Tracking%20System.php).

total number of squares entered into by the animal over a period of time. However, the same total number may be achieved through very different patterns of behavior. For example, the organism might show an initial period of rapid movement followed by immobility or, alternatively, cycles of high activity followed by low activity or, finally, even a continuous but moderate rate of ambulation. All three could lead to the same total number of squares entered, but the disparate patterns suggest differences in behavior that are not being captured. For such reasons, the evaluation of the time course of locomotor activity within a behavioral test session can be revealing.

Strength, Coordination, and Endurance

Weakness and fatigue are common complaints resulting from exposures to a number of different chemicals. Both simple and more complex approaches to measuring these facets of motor function are available. A simple and commonly used procedure that has the advantage of not necessarily requiring any specific training of the animal is the rotarod device shown in **Figure 2** (although pretraining can improve performance and decrease its variability). A rat or mouse is placed on a rotating cylinder, the speed of which can be manipulated (typically accelerated), and the time the animal remains on the rotating device before falling onto the plate below is recorded. Falling off more quickly may be an indication of abnormal coordination and/or endurance. As with motor activity, time spent on the rotarod can be measured repeatedly, i.e., across time, and a stable baseline performance can be generated across experimental sessions against which the impact of toxicants may be compared.

The limitations of such an approach are also evident in **Figure 2**. Mice may attempt to scramble up the dividers (see leftmost mouse in **Figure 2**); some attempt to run backward. Others begin to jump off the device and will not remain on the device regardless of being repeatedly placed back on the rotarod. As these examples indicate, the rotarod device thus measures aspects of behavior in addition to coordination and endurance, and these must obviously be considered in interpreting such data. In other words, one cannot necessarily be certain that decreased time spent on a rotarod after toxicant treatment necessarily reflects changes in endurance and coordination or, for example, whether it could reflect, increased distraction.

More advanced techniques that rely on learned behavior of animals (i.e., operant behavior) can provide controls for such nonmotoric behavioral factors and thus provide a more specific indication of changes in endurance and coordination. For example, rats can be trained to depress a lever with a specified amount of force in order to obtain a reward, for example, food delivery. The amount of force required to depress the lever can then be successively increased until the maximal force that can be exerted is reached. In addition, the force that the animal can sustain over time can also be measured as an indication of endurance. The ability to manipulate reward conditions facilitates the ability to differentiate motoric impairments from motivational deficits.

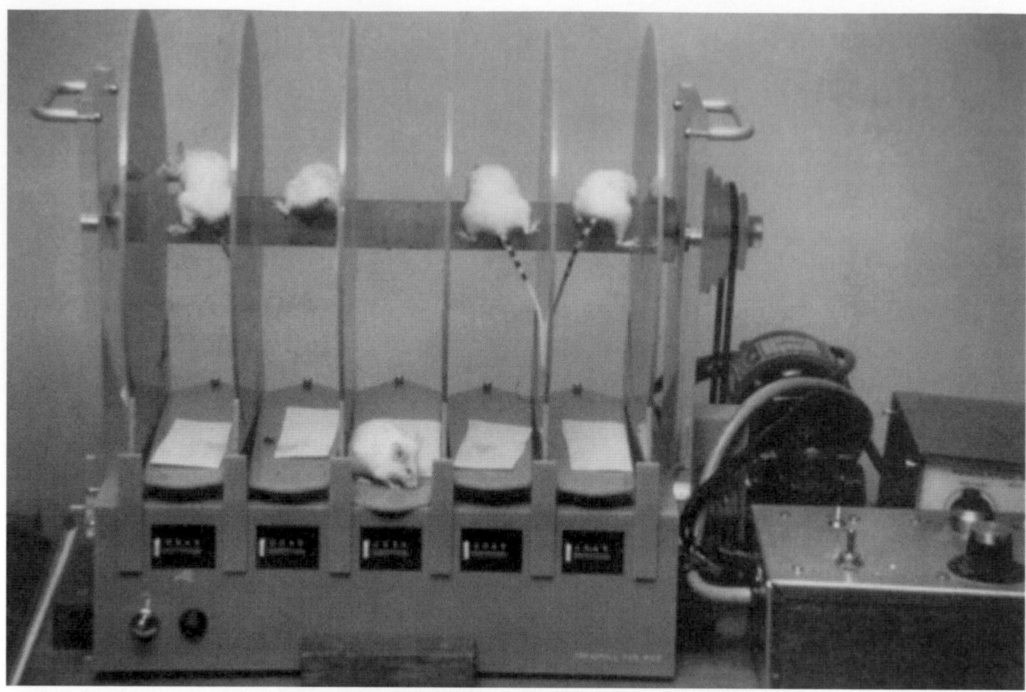

Figure 2 Illustration of the rotarod apparatus for mice. Each mouse is placed on the rotating cylinder; speed of revolution can be manipulated and time on rotarod typically constitutes the dependent variable of interest. (Reproduced from Cory-Slechta, D.A., 1989. Behavioral measures of neurotoxicity. Neurotoxicology 10, 271–296, with permission.)

Gait and Balance

Walking, running, and many other motor responses depend on intact gait and balance, and such functions may be particularly vulnerable to chemicals that affect the peripheral nervous system or cause spinal cord injury. One simple procedure that has been devised to assess postural dysfunction is known as hindlimb splay. In this procedure, the hind paws of a mouse or rat are dipped in ink and the animal is then dropped from a fixed height onto a piece of paper below as can be seen in Figure 3. An increase in the distance between the hindlimbs upon landing is indicative of damage to the peripheral nervous system with consequent effects on gait and ambulation. This approach is simple in that the rodent does not have to be specifically trained for the task, and this measurement can be made repeatedly across time without extensive equipment requirements so that time to onset and recovery of a toxicant's effects can be followed. However, hindlimb splay may not be a totally specific measure of altered motor function. Sensory disturbances, for example, might alter landing foot distance as well.

More advanced automated approaches for detection of movement abnormalities are now widely available. In a schematized version such as shown in Figure 4, a TV–microprocessor or videotaping system is utilized to record the placement of a rat's hind paws as it traverses from one rung to the next in a running wheel analogous to those offered in pet stores for rodents. Computer analysis of the recording provides a measurement of both quantitative and temporal characteristics of stepping, such as correct small steps and large steps, missteps, and the temporal parameters of these movements. In other systems, walking along an enclosed walkway or movement on a treadmill may be similarly utilized. With available software systems, an experimenter can measure with great precision how different parameters of gait differ before and after exposure to a toxicant. The animal need not be explicitly trained, and this approach provides a relatively specific measure of motor function per se. Procedures for measuring bodily sway in children have also been used in behavioral toxicology studies. In these procedures, the child stands on foam or on a hard surface under conditions of either eyes opened or closed, and the extent of the sway of his or her body is measured utilizing strain gauges.

Sensory Function

A wide range of sensory functions provide us with information about the environment. These functions include our abilities to hear, see, smell, and detect movement, vibration, and pain. Deficits in sensory function sometimes constitute some of the earliest or even the most pronounced manifestations of chemical exposures that affect the nervous system. As with the measurement of motor function, both simple and more advanced procedures are available to measure sensory function. Since almost all sensory procedures require the subject to make motor responses to indicate whether it has detected some sensory stimulus, changes in motor capabilities could conceivably be misinterpreted as sensory changes. Thus, while the simple procedures do not require any training of the subject, the experimenter must recognize that any

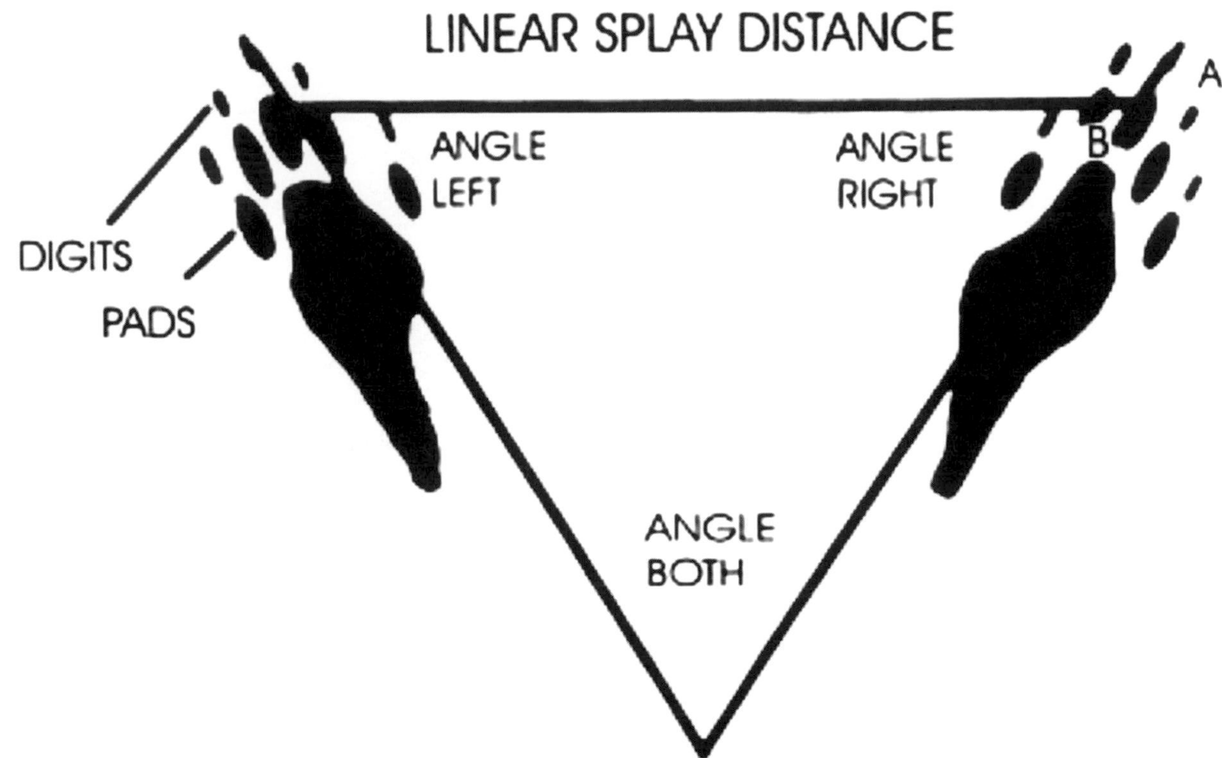

Figure 3 Illustration of the measurement of hindlimb splay: the hind paws of the mouse are dipped in ink, the animal is then dropped from a fixed height onto a piece of paper and the distance between some parameter of the hindlimbs is measured. (Reproduced from Powell, E., Anch, A.M., Dyche, J., Bloom, C., Richtert, R.R., 1999. The splay angle: a new measure for assessing neuromuscular dysfunction in rats. Physiology and Behavior 67, 819–821, with permission.)

changes measured may be due to changes in sensory function or motor function or both. While the more complex and sensitive techniques require training of the subject before it is possible to measure sensory function, they also offer the possibility of differentiating the contributions of motor abnormalities from sensory changes. The more advanced procedures can also be used across species, including rats, nonhuman primates, and humans, thus alleviating some of the questions that arise with respect to the extrapolation of findings across species.

In most procedures used to evaluate sensory function, a sensory stimulus is presented to the subject, and a response by the subject, either learned or unlearned depending on the specific procedure, then indicates whether the subject has detected that stimulus. The stimulus may vary from one presentation to the next in its important dimensions such as frequency and intensity, yielding a complete profile of sensory capabilities for that specific sensory modality. For example, in measuring hearing, tones differing in their loudness and pitch are presented in a single session so that hearing along the entire spectrum is measured.

One of the simpler experimental procedures used to test sensory function is referred to as reflex modification and is based on unlearned reflexes, in particular the startle reflex. A stimulus such as a loud noise can elicit a startle response (i.e., a startle reflex). It is also known that a stimulus presented prior to the presentation of that loud noise (a prestimulus) can measurably decrease the magnitude of the startle response. Thus, a prestimulus is 'detectable', i.e., perceived by the subject, if it decreases the magnitude of the subsequent startle response to the loud noise. The prestimulus can be varied in intensity and frequency dimensions during a testing session to produce a complete profile of sensory changes in a particular modality. For example, across the trials of a test session, the intensity and frequency of an auditory stimulus can be modified, and a threshold (e.g., the intensity for a given tone frequency that inhibits startle on 50% of its presentations) can be determined for each tone frequency, generating a classical audiogram. The advantages of reflex modification include its utility across different stimulus modalities (e.g., visual, auditory, and proprioceptive), its utility across species, and the absence of any requirement for training subjects. This approach has already been successful in revealing auditory impairments resulting from exposures to neurotoxic compounds such as trimethyltin and polychlorinated biphenyls.

One factor that must be considered in reflex modification procedures is that a less pronounced startle response could result from alterations in motor function per se rather than deficits in the subject's ability to detect the prestimulus. For this reason, it is imperative that some trials be interspersed throughout each test session in which no prestimulus is presented, only the startle stimulus. This allows the experimenter to determine whether the magnitude of the startle response

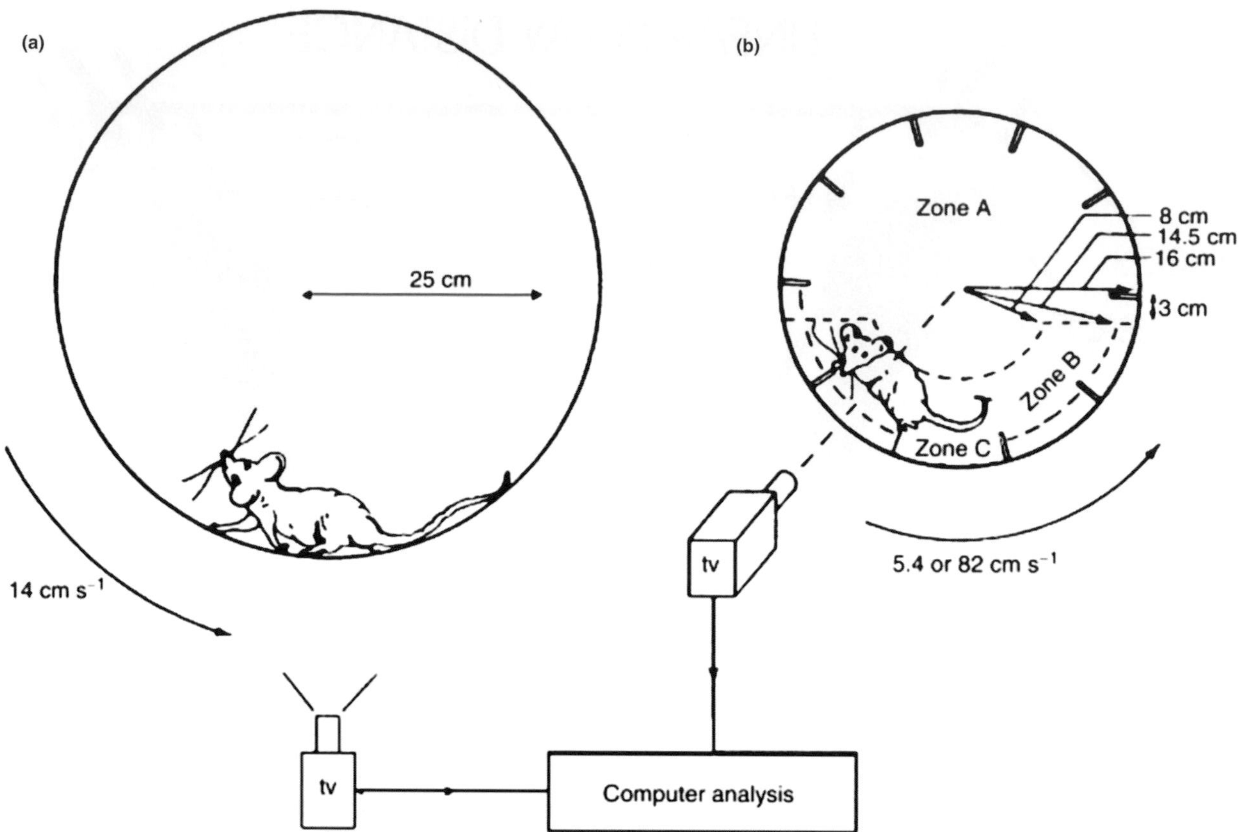

Figure 4 Automated hindlimb movement apparatus. (a) The camera can register the movements of the dyed soles of the paws of the rat from below. (b) The wheel with a transparent front facing the axially mounted color TV camera. (Reproduced from Tanger, H.J., Vanwersch, R.A.P., Wolthius, O.L., 1984. Automated quantitative analysis of coordinated locomotor behavior in rats. Journal of Neuroscience Methods 10, 237–245, with permission from Elsevier.)

remains constant across time after a chemical has been administered. If it does remain constant, then any changes in the amplitude of the startle response during prestimulus trials necessarily reflects altered sensory function. Another caution regarding this procedure is that the startle reflex itself may diminish over time. Thus, the number of trials in an experimental session must be carefully controlled.

The more advanced methods for the measurement of chemical-induced changes in sensory function are termed operant psychophysical procedures. These methods have been used in almost identical forms across a range of sensory modalities and in numerous species, including rodents (rats and guinea-pigs), chinchillas, pigeons, nonhuman primates, and humans. Additionally, they provide stable baselines across time from which chronic cumulative or progressive effects of a chemical can be assessed. **Figure 5** depicts an example of both a human and a nonhuman primate being tested for sensitivity to a vibratory stimulus presented to the left hand using operant psychophysical methods. Here, the subject is typically required to make a specified response within some designated period of time to signify that a stimulus presentation was detected. Experimental training of the subject is required before any sensory capabilities can be precisely gauged. In **Figure 5**, the subjects were required to hold down a key with the right hand when a tone sounded. If they detected a vibratory stimulus delivered to the fingertips of the left hand during the tone delivery, they released the key and received a reward. To determine how much subjects were simply guessing as to whether a vibratory stimulus was presented, some trials involved no vibratory stimulus presentation. On those trials, the subjects were rewarded for releasing the key only after the tone ended to indicate that they had detected no vibratory stimulus. As with measures of sensory function such as reflex modification, the various parameters of the sensory modality being evaluated are varied from trial to trial (e.g., intensity, magnitude, and frequency) allowing a determination of that specific sensory function along its significant dimensions. Since changes in sensory function may sometimes be quite selective (e.g., hearing loss for high-frequency tones but not low-frequency tones), the ability to map sensory changes along the entire spectrum of its significant dimensions within a single session is an important component of these methods.

There are several different variations of the methods by which stimuli are presented in the operant psychophysical procedures. In the method of constant stimuli, the subject is presented with several different values (e.g., intensities) of the stimulus in a random sequence or order across trials. The proportion of stimulus presentations detected at each intensity is then calculated, and the value yielding a 50% detection

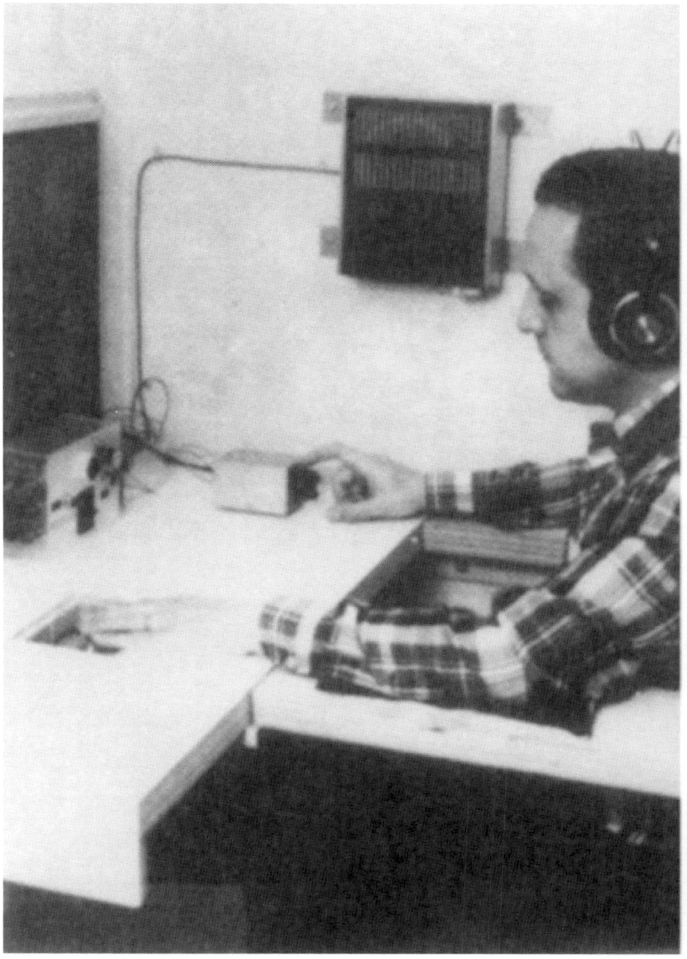

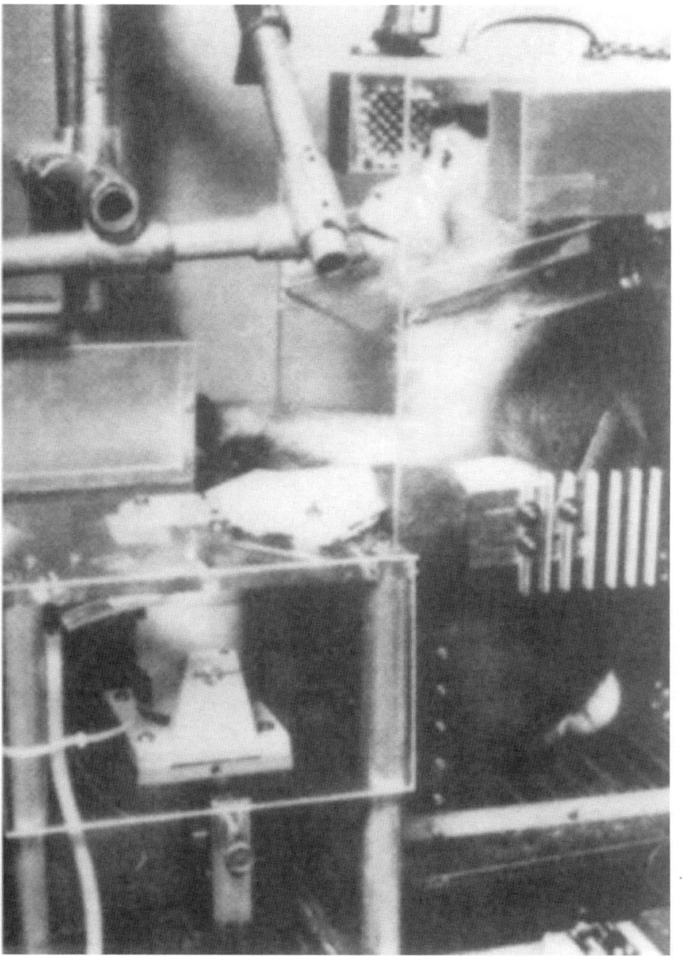

Figure 5 Photograph of a human and nonhuman primate working on the vibration sensitivity paradigm. In each case, the left hand of the subject is placed atop a device that delivers the vibratory stimulus, while the right hand holds down a telegraph key to be released when the subject detects the vibratory stimulus. A spout at the level of the monkey's mouth delivers a squirt of fruit juice for a correct response. (Reproduced from Maurissen, J.P.J., 1979. Effects of toxicants on the somatosensory system. Neurotoxicology and Teratology 1 (Suppl.), 22–31, with permission from Elsevier.)

response is deemed the threshold. The method of limits presents a series of stimulus intensities which begin either well above or well below the presumed threshold value. The stimulus value is then either progressively decreased or increased, respectively, until a change in the subject's ability to report the stimulus presentation occurs. The intensity of the stimulus at which this change in detectability occurs is designated as the threshold. In the up-and-down staircase, or titration, method of stimulus presentation, the threshold is continuously tracked by raising or lowering the stimulus intensity depending on whether the subject correctly detected the stimulus. If the subject fails to detect the stimulus, presumably because it is below the threshold for detection, the intensity is raised on the next trial; if the stimulus was detected (i.e., was above threshold), the intensity is then lowered on the next trial. In this fashion, the stimulus intensity can be titrated around the threshold value of the subject.

One of the advantages of operant psychophysical procedures over methods such as reflex modification is that stimulus presentation and subsequent responses occur on a continuous or response-dependent basis. In other words, a response of the subject is recorded, and the next stimulus is presented. In the reflex modification procedure, stimuli are presented during trials which are experimenter initiated and which are separated by a specified time interval. The continuous procedures such as used in the psychophysical approach permit the experimenter to measure the rate of responding over time and the time required to respond following stimulus presentations (latency). These measures provide the experimenter with information as to any possible motor dysfunction or motivational problems that the subject may experience as a result of chemical administration which could contribute to behavioral changes in operant psychophysical procedures. Motor dysfunction might increase the latency to respond following stimulus presentations, while an unmotivated subject might be expected to show periods of nonresponding. Armed with this information, the experimenter can better determine which behavioral changes result from true sensory loss.

Cognitive Function

One of the major concerns aroused by exposures to chemicals that affect the nervous system is their potential to adversely impact cognitive functions such as learning and memory. Such a concern certainly has precedent. Lead exposure at high levels can leave children with permanent mental retardation. Recently, it has been demonstrated that even very low levels of environmental lead exposure can produce subtle changes in cognitive processes. Pesticides are known to exert pronounced effects on cholinergic neurotransmitter systems, the very system that has been repeatedly implicated as a causative factor in Alzheimer's disease.

Learning

Learning might be defined simply as an enduring change in behavior that results from experience with changes in environmental events. As a topic of long historical interest in psychology and neuroscience, there are numerous different methods that have been applied to the study of learning ranging from the relatively simple to the more complex and advanced paradigms. Behavioral functions required by the subject for learning include the processing of sensory stimuli, the execution of motor responses, and a motivated subject. Difficulties in distinguishing the contributions of sensory, motor, and motivational deficits from learning deficits can therefore be encountered when using relatively simple learning paradigms. Some of the more complex procedures are designed to specifically differentiate such functions from learning and thus allow the experimenter to determine whether the chemical has specific effects on learning per se as distinct from changes in sensory or motor function, motivational levels, or other nonspecific behavioral alterations.

Many of the earliest studies of learning utilized rats as experimental subjects and required them to traverse mazes of various shapes and sorts, generally from a start box to a goal box where some type of food reward (reinforcement) was available. For example, in a T-maze, named because of its shape, the subject is reinforced for running from the start box at the base of the T to that arm of the T that has been designated as the correct arm and contains the goal box where food is located. The designation of which arm (stimulus) is correct may be based on side (e.g., the right side is correct), color (the arm painted black), or some other stimulus feature. Choosing the wrong arm at the choice point means no reinforcement. After entering an arm and either being reinforced or not, the animal is removed, and after a period of time (the intertrial interval), the animal is placed back in the goal box and another trial initiated. Learning under such conditions is typically measured as the number of trials required to reach a specified accuracy level or until behavior reaches a stable level of accuracy. At sufficiently high accuracy levels (considering 50% as chance), it is considered that the subject has learned to 'discriminate' between the correct and incorrect arm. The experimenter may compare two groups of rats in such an experiment: one treated with a chemical and one not treated, with the latter serving as a control group indicating 'normal' performance under the particular experimental conditions.

More complex versions of mazes soon emerged in response to the need for more difficult tasks because the T-maze was a relatively simple problem for a rodent to solve. It was thus not always adequately sensitive to effects of drugs or chemicals, particularly for measuring chronic, cumulative, or progressive effects of a chemical. Moreover, once the animal learned which was the correct arm, learning is no longer being measured, only the performance of an already learned response. Two different approaches were offered to circumvent these limitations. One was the construction of more complicated mazes, such as the Hebbs–William maze, which is actually a series of mazes. The correct route to the goal box in this device can be modified as needed by moving the various arms and boundaries into new configurations and thus requiring the subject to learn a new problem, allowing a repeated assessment of learning.

A second approach is embodied in reversal (discrimination reversal) learning. Using this approach, the correct and incorrect arms (stimuli) in the maze are reversed after the subject initially learns which is correct. For example, after the rat learns to run to the right arm of the T-maze with 90% accuracy, the discrimination is reversed, such that the left arm of the T-maze is now the rewarded arm. After criterion accuracy is achieved following this reversal, the designation of correct and incorrect stimuli may be reversed again, allowing the repeated measurement of learning over time. Eventually, however, this scheme is also learned by the subject, a phenomenon known as 'learning to learn,' such that it comes to learn each successive reversal problem with maximal efficiency (i.e., after only one or two trials).

All maze procedures have limitations that must be considered when interpreting data obtained with these methods. One related particularly to their use with rodents is that subjects leave an odor trail in the maze that can influence the behavior of rodents subsequently tested in the maze. While the experimenter can clean the maze between subjects, it must also be noted that the rodent's sense of smell is much more sensitive than humans, making it difficult to be certain that indeed no odors are still present. Another potential problem is that these nonautomated procedures obviously require interactions between the experimenter and the subject during the course of testing because the rat must be constantly retrieved from the arms and replaced in the start box. This raises the distinct possibility of both subject and experimenter bias unless the experiment can be carried out by an individual with no knowledge of any treatment (e.g., exposure to drug or chemical) of any subjects. The development of video-recording and associated software for scoring these behaviors over the past several years has assisted in minimizing some of these potential limitations.

Another limitation of simple maze methods for assessing learning is that they do not selectively measure learning. While a longer time to reach a 90% accuracy level may be observed in response to a chemical treatment, it may not necessarily be due to alterations in cognitive processing since changes in either motor performance or sensory capabilities may impact performance in the maze, altering learning independently of any real cognitive changes. Impaired motor function may increase the time taken to reach the goal box and thus delay the time to acquire reward; delay of reward itself is well known to impair learning. Further, sensory deficits may cause the subject to be unable to utilize the environmental stimuli that normally guide its path to the goal box. Motivational changes (e.g., if the reward becomes less appealing) may clearly retard the rate at which learning occurs. Changes in motor, sensory, and motivational functions as potential contributors to the observed effect may then have to be ruled out in separate additional experiments.

The water maze is a method increasingly being used in behavioral studies for evaluating learning. Used typically with rodents, the subject is placed in a large tub of water made opaque by the addition of a substance such as nonfat milk powder. Since rodents do not prefer water, the reward in this case is escaping from the water by locating a platform submerged just below the surface of the water which is not visible to the subject. Learning is measured as a decrease in the time (latency) to locate the hidden platform across successive trials. A learning deficit is suggested by a slower rate of decline in that latency or a greater number of trials to reliably locate the platform. The procedure is relatively simple and imposes no food restriction on the subject. However, despite its ostensible simplicity, it suffers from many of the same limitations as non-water-based mazes. First, although videotaping and computer scoring have minimized some such issues, the procedure is not fully automated and thus requires subject–experimenter interaction which can introduce bias into the results. Furthermore, since it is a relatively simple problem, the maze may be learned rapidly and, thus, it is of limited utility for experiments aimed at understanding the time course of a chemical's effects on learning or cumulative or progressive toxicity. This problem can be alleviated to some extent by moving the platform to a new location each time the subject has mastered the previous location. Although one might suspect that odor trails would not be a factor in a water maze, it has indeed been shown that odors are present and can be utilized by other subjects later placed in the maze. In addition, water temperature plays an important role in this task since age-related deficits in learning in the maze can be alleviated by warming up old rats between trials. Placement in the water is also a well-documented stressor for rodents and produces marked increases in stress hormones such as corticosterone.

Finally, a rat that requires a greater number of trials or exhibits a slower decrease in the time to locate the platform following chemical treatment is not necessarily exhibiting a learning deficit. Changes in motor capabilities may affect swimming performance and thus lengthen the time it takes the subject to swim to the submerged platform, even if it knows the location of the platform. This is a particular problem because swimming is a highly effortful response requiring significant endurance. It is known that subjects rely on environmental cues to find the platform; thus, changes in sensory capabilities could mean an inability of the subject to detect the necessary environmental cues, a deficit which would also increase the length of time the subject required to reach the platform. These alternative explanations must be ruled out by additional experiments before one can reasonably conclude that a cognitive impairment is present. One way to assist in addressing such potential confounds is to include an actual endurance test. Another probe frequently included to evaluate the potential influence of noncognitive motor factors is a measure of the latency to reach a visible platform; however, this may not adequately reflect total endurance, a quite different facet of motor function. Another probe used to evaluate 'memory' in this paradigm is to remove the escape platform and measure how much of the time swimming occurs in the area where it was located.

Another maze procedure frequently utilized to evaluate learning (and memory) with rodents is the radial-arm maze. The device itself consists of a central circular area from which eight arms radiate outward like the spokes of a wheel. At the end of each of the eight arms is some type of reinforcer, usually a food pellet. In essence, the subject has access to eight reinforcement deliveries, one in each of the eight arms and the accuracy and speed (efficiency), with which the subject learns to retrieve all eight reinforcer deliveries is measured. Obviously, under these conditions, the most efficient performance is to obtain all eight reinforcements without revisiting an arm from which the food has already been obtained. The measure of learning is the number of trials required for the subject to reach some specified level of efficiency in the maze. One way of further increasing task difficulty is to provide reinforcement only in a specified number of the arms (e.g., four of the eight) and to change which of the arms provides reinforcement over time or trials. The radial-arm maze obviously presents a more difficult problem to the subject than the T-maze or other simple mazes, but the possibility of interference from motor or sensory deficits produced by chemical treatment still remains. Thus, an increase in the number of trials to reach efficient performance is not necessarily indicative of a learning deficit per se with this method. By measuring the time of entry into each arm, investigators can begin to get some indication, for example, of whether changes in overall activity levels are affecting performance.

In addition to mazes, learning can be measured in Skinner boxes, also known as operant chambers, and these types of approaches have been widely used for many years across a variety of species, notably rodents, pigeons, nonhuman primates, and humans. Such chambers typically include some type of response device or devices (e.g., lever pressing or nose poking for rodents), speakers, and/or lights for presentation of auditory or visual stimuli, respectively, as well as some type of reinforcement delivery device. An operant chamber configured for a rat is shown in **Figure 6**. Discrimination paradigms are among the simplest measures of learning in operant chambers. In such procedures, a response such as a lever press is reinforced in the presence of one stimulus, i.e., the 'correct' stimulus, but not in the presence of another stimulus. Accuracy is defined as the percentage of the total responses that occur in association with the correct stimulus, and learning can be assessed as the number of experimental sessions required by the subject to achieve a criterion level of accuracy.

One distinct advantage of discrimination paradigms in the operant chamber is that behavior can occur at any time (i.e., the frequency with which it occurs is not constrained by trials as necessitated by the requirement of moving the animal from the goal box back to the start box in most maze-based methods). When responding can occur at any time, the rate or frequency of responding over time can be measured and used to gauge the possibility that motor deficits or motivational insufficiencies may contribute to any observed changes in learning accuracy. A decrease or slowdown in rate of responding would suggest such possibilities.

Other advantages of operant chamber-based procedures include the enormous flexibility they provide for behavioral assessment, the full automation they provide and the ease with which behavioral procedures can be carried out in these devices. For example, conditional discrimination problems, which are more difficult discrimination tasks, can be easily implemented in operant chambers. Matching-to-sample is one such method. In this task, the subject first makes a designated response to indicate that it is attending to a sample stimulus that is presented for a short period of time. This is followed,

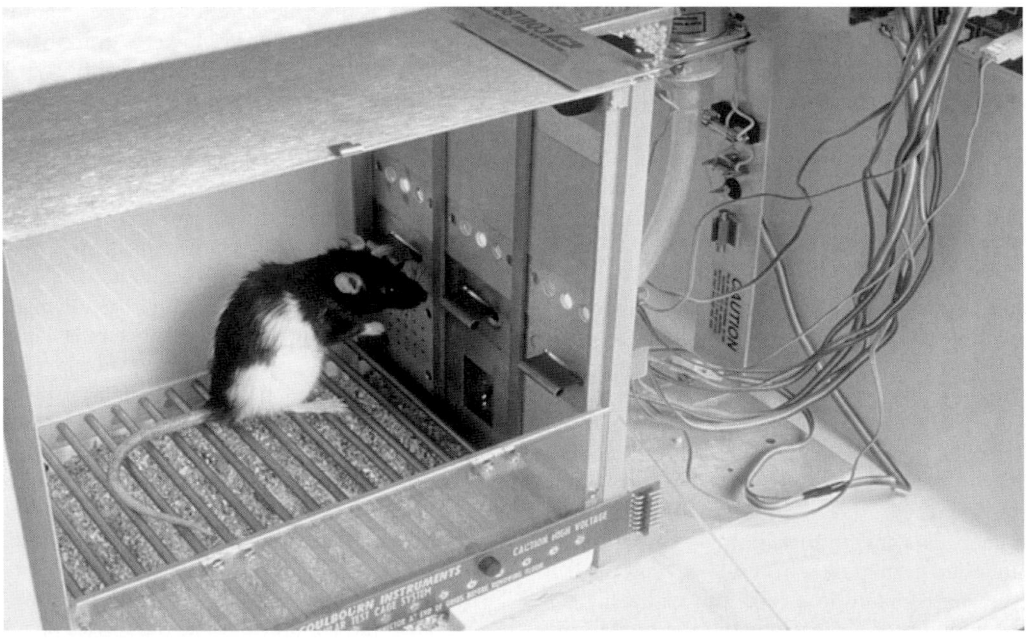

Figure 6 An operant chamber or a Skinner box for a rodent. The front wall (right) shows three response levers, with a food pellet trough situated below the middle lever. Food pellets are dispensed from a feeder located behind the front wall into the pellet trough. Above each of the levers are a set of key lights which can be illuminated with various colors and used for external or environmental stimuli. Above and to the right of the rightmost lever is a speaker through which auditory stimuli can be projected and used as external (environmental) stimuli. (Reproduced from Hayes, A.W. (Ed.), (2008). Principles and Methods of Toxicology. CRC Press, p. 1805, with permission.)

after an interval of time, by the presentation of two or more stimuli, and reinforcement is contingent upon a response to the stimulus that matches the previously observed sample stimulus. The accuracy and speed with which the subject learns to match the sample stimulus is, of course, the measure of learning. Such tasks can be used across different species by simply increasing or decreasing the number of choice stimuli or the similarity of the stimuli appropriately. Because the procedure includes an initiating response on the part of the subject to present the sample stimulus, it ensures attention to the task while also providing a measure of rate of responding, again providing information on potential motoric or motivational contributions to any deficits observed in matching accuracy.

Even the more complex matching-to-sample discrimination problems are eventually mastered by the subject in which case discrimination reversals may be implemented in which the stimuli associated with reinforcement and nonreinforcement are repeatedly switched. Eventually, however, the subjects will learn the reversal 'concept' as well, such that they come to solve each reversal problem with maximal efficiency; that is, on the basis of only one or two responses (e.g., which stimulus is correct today?).

One of the most advanced methods for the assessment of learning is the repeated learning paradigm, also called repeated acquisition, sequence acquisition, or response sequence learning. It specifically addresses the limitations discussed previously. This method actually originated for the measurement of learning in human subjects and has since been adapted for a variety of species including rats and mice. In repeated learning, the subject must complete a sequence (chain) of responses in the correct order to earn a reward, and the correct sequence changes with each successive behavioral test session. Because the procedure thus requires subjects to learn a new sequence of responses each session, learning can be measured repeatedly across time. A high rate of errors is typically evident during the early part of each test session, as the subject begins to learn the correct sequence for that specific session. The error rate gradually declines as the session progresses, and rewards for completing the correct sequence of responses are earned at an increasing rate. The ability to measure learning repeatedly across time with this task allows for the measurement of the time course of a chemical's effects (i.e., the time to onset of any learning disabilities and their potential reversibility). This is a particular advantage in situations where chemical exposure occurs in a chronic fashion.

The control for changes in sensory, motor, motivational, or other nonspecific behavioral influences as potential contributors to apparent chemical-induced learning impairments is best achieved when the repeated acquisition task is run in conjunction with a 'performance' task in what is known as a multiple schedule format. The performance task also requires the subject to emit a sequence of responses in the correct order for reward, but in the case of the performance task, the sequence of responses stays constant across behavioral test sessions. Thus, in the performance task, the subject simply performs an already learned response sequence. When used in a multiple schedule format, the repeated learning and performance components are presented alternately during the course of a behavioral test session, with a transition between them occurring either on the basis of time or on the number of rewards the subject has earned (e.g., after 15 min or 30 food deliveries switch from repeated learning to performance). Thus, during some portions of the test session, the subject is responding on the repeated acquisition task, while at other times during the session, the performance task is operative. Typically, different environmental stimuli, such as different colored lights, are used to signal to the subject whether the performance or the repeated learning task is in effect or that a transition between the two behavioral tasks is going to occur.

Both the repeated learning and the performance tasks require intact motor and sensory capabilities as well as appropriately motivated subjects. Learning per se, however, is only required during the repeated acquisition task; the performance task simply requires completion of an already learned response sequence. Thus, if a toxicant or treatment has selective effects on learning per se, impairments in accuracy should only be evident during the repeated learning components of the session. If these changes arise, however, as a result of nonspecific behavioral changes (i.e., from sensory, motor, or motivational impairments), then accuracy impairments would be expected in both the repeated learning and the performance tasks of the session since both require these behavioral capabilities. The elegance of this technique derives not only from its ability to distinguish learning effects from other types of behavioral changes but also from its ability to do so in the same subject during the same test session.

Behavior of a normal rat under these conditions is depicted in the top of **Figure 7** (labeled 0 ppm lead acetate). In this diagram, the top tracing shows correct responses, which cumulate vertically; time is represented horizontally. P indicates the performance task presentations during the session, whereas A indicates when the repeated learning task was operative. This 1-h behavioral test session began with the performance task and was followed by the repeated learning task, once again by the performance task, and finally by the repeated learning task. Illumination of lights in the operant chamber signaled to the subject that the performance task was operative, while turning out the lights signaled that the repeated learning task was in effect. Each short pip mark in the top tracing indicates where the rat earned a food delivery for correctly completing the sequence of three responses required by the operative task. The tracing below this shows the concurrent errors that occurred over the same time period.

As **Figure 7** shows, this well-trained rat exhibited a relatively high level of accuracy during the first presentation of the performance task, earning a steady rate of food rewards and making few errors. The switch to the repeated learning component (at which point the top tracing is reset to the baseline) is accompanied by an increase in errors and a decline in the number of food rewards earned per unit time, as the subject begins to learn the correct sequence of three responses required in this specific behavioral test session. Behavior during the second presentation of the performance task is again composed of a steady rate of food rewards and the occurrence of relatively few errors. The second presentation of the repeated

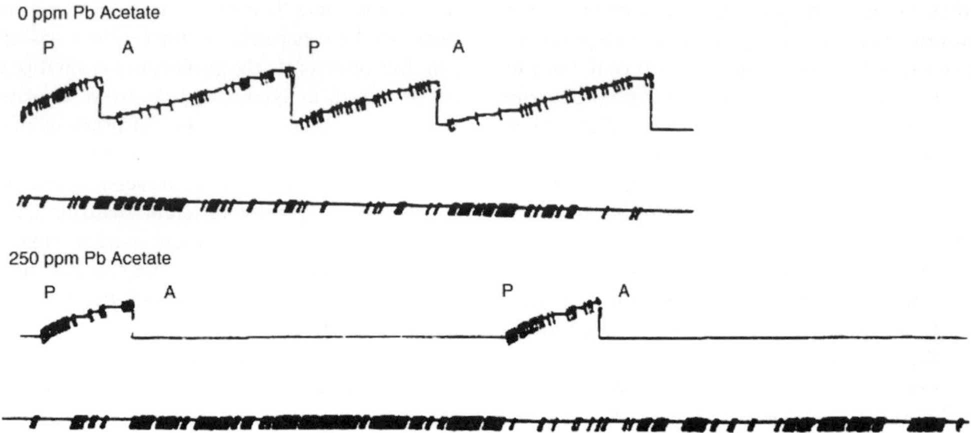

Figure 7 Behavior of a control rat (top) and a rat exposed to 250 ppm lead acetate in drinking water from weaning (bottom) on a multiple repeated acquisition (A; repeated learning) and performance (P) schedule of reinforcement. The top line of each record shows correct responses cumulating vertically with pips indicating food delivery for the completion of the correct sequence of responses; the bottom line shows errors. Time is represented horizontally. (Reproduced from J. Cohn and D. A. Cory-Slechta, unpublished data, with permission.)

learning task is marked by both a gradual increase in the rate at which food rewards were earned and a decrease in the number of errors relative to levels occurring in the first presentation of the repeated learning task, consistent with a gradual learning of the correct sequence for this session.

The bottom set of tracings (labeled 250 ppm lead acetate) shows behavior under the same conditions for a rat that has been exposed from weaning to a relatively low level of lead in drinking water. It shows, in a rather dramatic fashion, a selective effect of lead on learning processes per se, as distinct from nonspecific behavioral changes. That is, behavior during both presentations of the performance task in this behavioral test session is unimpaired in that a substantial rate of food deliveries and a minimal rate of errors occur. In contrast, there is no evidence of learning during either presentation of the repeated learning task of the schedule, in that virtually no food deliveries were obtained and a very high rate of errors was sustained. In fact, the rat continued to make errors through both presentations of the repeated learning tasks during this session. Thus, in this case, the effects of lead on accuracy were restricted to the repeated learning task of the schedule. These impairments could not have resulted from deficits in motor or sensory function or in appropriate motivation since behavior in the performance task, which also required such functions, was perfectly normal.

Although an effect of a toxicant on behavior during the repeated learning but not during the performance task of a multiple schedule is strong evidence of a chemical's selective effects on cognitive functions, there are other factors that should be taken into consideration. Some investigators subscribe to the idea that a selective effect of a chemical on learning means that its effects should be evident across a variety of learning tasks. While this notion has some validity, it should not be considered a necessary condition since, as has already been described, all learning paradigms are not equal. The extent to which different learning tasks selectively measure learning per se, as distinct from sensory, motor, or motivational influences, clearly differs, as does the possible 'contamination' of the learning measure by changes in other behavioral properties. This is not to diminish the importance of these other types of behavioral effects, be they sensory or motor, for example, since such processes are clearly essential for integrated behavioral function, including cognitive functioning. Another important consideration is that the ability to detect effects of a chemical upon learning may depend to a large extent on the degree of task difficulty. It is well established that learning tasks that are relatively easy (i.e., those resulting in relatively high levels of accuracy) will be less sensitive to disruption either by drugs or by toxicants than are tasks of greater difficulty.

Memory

Memory, or remembering, is behavioral recall (i.e., the preservation of learned behavior over time). A distinction is often made between what is referred to as short-term or working memory, occurring over relatively short delay periods, and long-term or reference memory, considered more permanent memory. Obviously, the temporal parameters associated with what is designated as short- and long-term memory are species-dependent.

The measurement of memory is typically based on the persistence of a previously learned response following some time delay; differences in recall accuracy are compared before and after delay intervals. Typically, the longer the delay, the greater the difficulty in remembering, leading to delay-dependent decreases in accuracy. An impairment of memory by a chemical accelerates the rate at which accuracy of remembering decreases with increasing delay values.

Both simple and more advanced techniques are available to evaluate memory. Again, however, many of the ostensibly simple tasks cannot easily differentiate memory deficits per se from deficits produced by changes in other behavioral functions, be they motor or sensory functions, or in level of motivation. For example, an inability to execute the response as efficiently (motor impairment) may in essence mean that the delay interval for the subject is functionally longer, thus indirectly impairing accuracy in a memory paradigm. Alternatively, a treatment that somehow increased the speed of responding could cause the subject to respond before adequately evaluating stimulus options and thus decrease accuracy independently of a real change in remembering. Here, again, the more advanced methods include the capabilities for differentiating effects of a chemical upon remembering per se from those caused by other behavioral consequences of the exposure.

One widely used simple measure of memory is passive avoidance, also known as fear conditioning. In this task, the subject, most often a rodent, is placed in a chamber that has two quite distinct compartments. The subject receives a shock in the compartment it prefers (spends most time in), engendering an association between the shock and the distinctive characteristics of that compartment. At some later time (i.e., after some delay interval), the subject is placed back into this two-compartment chamber, and memory is evaluated on the basis of the time (referred to as latency) that elapses before the subject steps back into the side of the chamber in which it previously received shock. The contention is that the longer the subject waits to enter that compartment, the better it remembers the shock it received there.

While changes in latency on this task are produced by a variety of drugs and chemical treatments, the interpretation of these changes can be problematic. If, for example, the chemical causes hyperactivity, the subject might re-enter the compartment in which it previously received shock sooner, even if it does remember its association with shock. If the treatment disrupts sensory capabilities, altering perceived distinctions between the compartments, this too may result in a more rapid re-entry into the compartment in which the subject had previously been shocked. If the administration of a chemical causes a sedative effect in the subject, rendering it less mobile, the time to re-enter the compartment in which shock was received may be increased relative to that seen in nontreated controls, but this would not be considered facilitation of memory. Again, such possible alternative interpretations must necessarily be worked out in additional experiments or with additional manipulations or probes. Importantly, and oven overlooked is the possibility that, depending upon the experimental design, chemical treatments could alter shock sensitivity and thereby modify performance since the level of shock received is a significant determinant of the extent to which fear conditioning occurs in this task.

While the more advanced procedures for memory evaluation require more extensive training of the subject, they also control for some of the possible confounds mentioned previously. There are two general types of more advanced procedures for the assessment of memory. One uses the previous responding of the subject as the event to be remembered, such as in the delayed alternation paradigm. In this procedure, the subject has access to at least two response manipulanda and is required to alternate its responses on the two for reward following a delay interval imposed between response opportunities. That is, a response such as a lever press on manipulanda A initiates a delay interval. After the delay interval ends, a response on manipulanda B produces reward. This event initiates another delay interval, after which a return to manipulanda A produces reward, and so on. Typically, a series of delay intervals are tested in each session, with the length of the delay interval varied randomly across the trials of a session and the range of delay values used being taxing for the species being tested. Responses occurring during the delay itself start the delay over again, thus increasing the time to reward. On this task, then, the subject has to remember which response manipulanda it responded on before the delay interval started in order to respond correctly after the delay. Typical behavior observed under these conditions is a decrease in remembering (accuracy) as the length of the delay interval increases. A chemically induced impairment of memory would then be manifest as a more pronounced decrease in accuracy as delay length increases than is observed under nontreatment (control) conditions.

Critical to the interpretation of any memory-related deficits with the delayed alternation task is the inclusion of a 0-s or no-delay trials. The no-delay condition requires no memory, as there is no delay between the opportunities to alternate responses. Therefore, if a treatment is impairing accuracy under the no-delay condition as well as at the various delay intervals, it is likely that the effects are due to changes in behavioral processes other than remembering. The pattern of change consistent with a selective memory impairment of a toxicant, then, is one composed of no change in accuracy at the 0-s delay, coupled with a more pronounced decrease in accuracy with increasing delay values relative to nontreated control subjects.

An example of an apparently selective impairment of memory independently of changes in other behavioral processes is shown in **Figure 8**. As can be seen, the accuracy level of a group of nontreated normal rats (solid circles) declines as the delay value increases, as expected. Corresponding data for a group of rats treated with the organic metal trimethyltin are shown in the open circles. In this group, accuracy was unaffected at the 0-s delay but decreased more rapidly than did that of normal rats as delay value lengthened.

Other methods for measurement of memory function rely on explicit discrimination tasks. The matching-to-sample task described earlier is one example. In this paradigm, a sample stimulus is presented briefly to the subject. The subject must then pick the sample stimulus when subsequently presented with multiple stimulus options (i.e., the subject must match the sample). When delay intervals are imposed between the presentation of the sample stimulus and the subsequent presentation of multiple stimuli, the task becomes a memory task. In this case, the subject must remember the sample stimulus in order to perform correctly. As in the delayed alternation procedure, delay intervals of various lengths are used, including the no-delay or zero-delay condition, and a delay function similar to that shown in **Figure 8** is expected. Many of the caveats mentioned with respect to interpreting memory effects in the delayed alternation task likewise apply

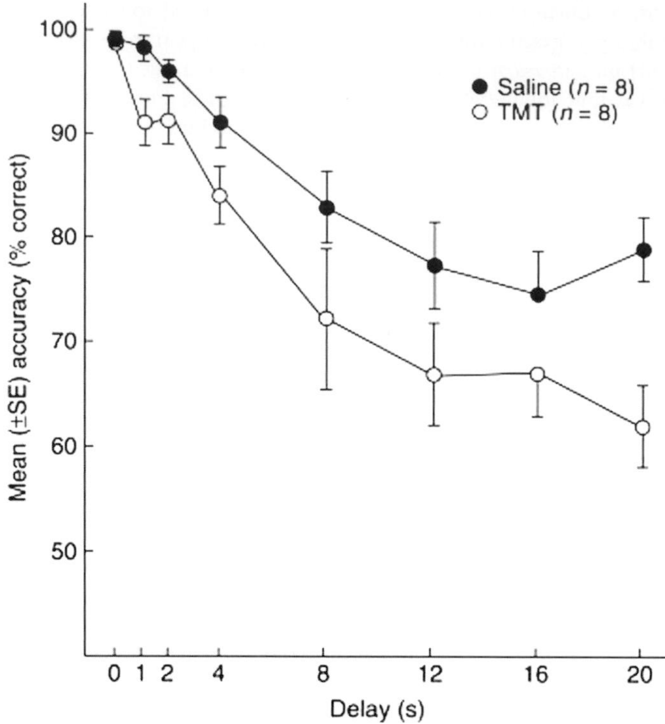

Figure 8 Effects of 7 mg kg^{-1} trimethyltin on delayed alternation performance. Lower accuracy values were evident in TMT-treated rats at all delay values, but no impairment was seen in the 0-s delay condition, consistent with a specific effect on memory function. (Reproduced from Bushnell, P.J., 1988. Effects of delay, intertrial interval, delay behavior and trimethyltin on spatial delayed response in rats. Neurotoxicology and Teratology 10, 237–244, with permission from Elsevier.)

to the delayed matching-to-sample paradigm. Separation of a chemical effect arising directly from changes in memory processes rather than from changes in motor, sensory, or motivational functions depends on the inclusion of a no-delay condition. Furthermore, as with learning paradigms, the contention that if a chemical produces a true memory deficit, it will be observed across different memory tasks must be tempered by the fact that not all memory paradigms produce an equally selective measure of memory.

Schedule-Controlled Operant Behavior

Learned voluntary behavior is a function of the consequences that follow it. If a response is followed by a reinforcing stimulus, the rate of that response subsequently increases; if followed by a punishing stimulus, or by the absence of a reinforcing stimulus, the rate of responding subsequently decreases. In addition to determining the subsequent frequency of that response, these consequence stimuli will also determine the intensity and temporal pattern with which that response will be emitted in the future.

In the real world, consequence stimuli do not necessarily follow every occurrence of the response. In fact, typically, consequences follow the response on an intermittent basis. Paychecks, for example, are typically distributed on a weekly, biweekly, or even monthly basis, not after each instance of work-related activity that occurs. The pianist plays the entire piece of music before the audience applauds. This strategy of 'intermittent' reinforcement of responding actually provides greater behavioral efficiency and economy as well as generating more robust response strength and persistence than does continuous reinforcement (reward for every occurrence of the response). A response that has been reinforced after every occurrence declines much more rapidly when reinforcement is withheld (extinction) than does one that has been reinforced on an intermittent schedule.

The term schedule of reinforcement refers to the nature of the rules governing the allocation of consequences for a particular response. Behavioral performance controlled by a schedule of reinforcement is referred to as schedule-controlled operant behavior. These schedules of reinforcement are critical because they govern the rate and pattern of responding in time which underlie other behavioral functions. For example, the rate of learning may well be influenced by the underlying schedule of reinforcement. If reinforcement of the correct response during a learning task is too infrequent, the task may not be adequately learned or not learned at all. Likewise, remembering that response, as in a memory task, may depend on the extent to which it was sufficiently reinforced (i.e., strengthened) to begin with.

Consequence stimuli can occur on the basis of time elapsing or on the basis of the number of responses that have occurred or both. In the human environment, schedules of reinforcement exhibit a remarkable complexity. For the purposes of understanding how these various reinforcement schedules or payoff schemes control the frequency and the pattern of behavior in time, simpler versions were initially studied in a laboratory context. As the understanding of simple reinforcement schedules evolved, increasingly complex schedules that more closely mimicked the human environment were elaborated and examined in laboratory experiments.

One of the important aspects of schedule-controlled behavior that deserves note is the remarkable similarity of behavior patterns generated by these schedules across a wide variety of species, even when type of response and type of consequence stimuli differ – a phenomenon of obvious importance for the issue of cross-species extrapolation because it shows the similarity and contiguity of such behavioral process across species.

Simple Schedules of Reinforcement

There are four simple schedules of reinforcement: the fixed interval (FI) and the variable interval (VI), both of which are temporally based reinforcement schedules, and the fixed ratio (FR) and the variable ratio (VR) schedules, both of which are response-based schedules. The FI and the VI schedules both stipulate that a certain amount of time must elapse from the occurrence of a previously reinforced response before a response will again produce reinforcement. On the FI schedule, that time interval remains constant (fixed) and the parameter value of the schedule indicates the length of that temporal interval (e.g., FI 1 min means that the first response occurring at least 1 min after the preceding reinforced response will result in reinforcement). On the VI schedule, the length of the interval to reward availability varies from one interval to the next, with the parameter value of the schedule indicating the average of the different interval lengths. For example, on a VI 1 min schedule, the average time between reinforcement opportunities is 1 min, but each interval may be either longer or shorter. Responses made during the interval itself, i.e., prior to its completion, on either the FI or VI schedules, have no specific consequence attached to them.

Because of the differences in the way in which they schedule reinforcement, the FI and VI control quite different rates of responding (responses per unit time) and patterns of responding, as can be seen in **Figure** 9. The FI schedule generates a characteristic 'scallop' pattern of responding, which engenders pausing, that is, little or no responding immediately after reinforcement delivery (indicated by the short pip marks), followed by a gradual increase in the rate of responding as the time of reinforcement availability again approaches. In the human environment, studying for an examination has features that are characteristic of FI performance: little or no responding early in the semester premised on the lack of any imminent reinforcement availability, but a gradual increase as the time of the examination approaches. While one might expect that the performance under such conditions would be characterized by a single response as soon as the interval ends, such a pattern would require the subject to have perfect timing capabilities. Responding at a very rapid rate as the end of the interval approaches ensures that reinforcement delivery will occur with minimal delay as soon as it is available.

The pattern of responding on the VI schedule differs from that on the FI (**Figure** 9) in that no pausing occurs after reinforcement delivery. Instead, the subject continues to respond at a steady and relatively uniform rate over time. The absence of pausing on the VI schedule is thought to reflect the lack of predictability of reinforcement. On the VI schedule, reinforcement may be available immediately after a previous reinforcement delivery since the interval length varies. Thus, pausing after reinforcement could result in a reduction in the rate or number of reinforcement deliveries. One example of VI-maintained behavior sometimes cited is that of getting a busy signal when calling someone on the telephone.

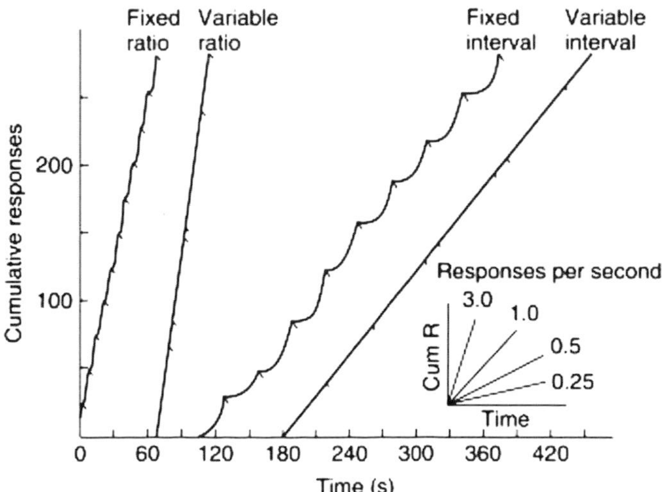

Figure 9 Schematic cumulative records of performance on the FR, VR, FI, and VI schedules of reinforcement. Responses are cumulated vertically over time. Each downward deflection of the pen represents reinforcement delivery; horizontal lines indicate pausing. (Reproduced from Seiden, L.S., Dykstra, L.A., 1977. Psychopharmacology: A Biochemical and Behavioral Approach. Van Nostrand Reinhold, New York, NY.)

The caller continues to redial and is eventually reinforced by a ringing sound on the other end. The persistent redialing reflects the variable length or interval of telephone conversations and, therefore, the unpredictability of when the line will no longer be busy.

In the other two simple reinforcement schedules, the FR and the VR, reinforcement availability is based on the number of occurrences of the designated response. On an FR schedule, the completion of the number of responses specified by the schedule parameter value is required for each reinforcement delivery. An FR 100 schedule, then, requires 100 occurrences of the designated response for reinforcement delivery. The classic examples of FR schedules are the piecework systems that operated in factories early in US history, where workers were paid for each piece or unit they produced. The FR schedule generates its own characteristic behavior pattern which consists of a pause or period of no responding after each reinforcement delivery followed by an abrupt transition to a very rapid rate of responding – a pattern known as 'break and run' and shown in **Figure 9**.

A VR schedule also requires the occurrence of a designated number of responses for reinforcement delivery, but the response requirement varies from one reinforcement delivery to the next in an unpredictable fashion. The parameter value of the schedule indicates the average response requirement. Thus, on a VR 100 schedule, the average number of responses required for reinforcement is 100, but the actual number varies unpredictably from one reinforcement delivery to the next. Perhaps the most obvious example of behavior maintained by a VR schedule is that of gambling. A slot machine may pay off on the average once every 100 plays, but the number of plays between payoffs varies in an unpredictably way; thus, one play that results in a payoff may follow immediately after a preceding payoff or may follow only after a large number of subsequent plays. The VR schedule maintains the highest rates of responding of the four simple schedules (**Figure 9**). In essence, it is characterized by a continuous high rate of responding without pausing after reinforcement deliveries.

Like the VI, the pattern of responding on the VR schedule reflects the lack of predictability of reinforcement availability. Since reinforcement availability may always be imminent, pausing would delay reinforcement. The high rates characteristic of VR and FR schedules are thought to be due to the ratio basis of reinforcement in that the faster the response requirement is completed, the faster reinforcement is available. Increases in rates of responding on interval-based schedules such as the FI and VI cannot accelerate the availability of reinforcement; one must still wait for the time interval to end and thus such increases can reflect highly inefficient behavior that is inconsistent with the normal learning of the patterning.

Complex Schedules of Reinforcement

As mentioned previously, the complexity of reinforcement schedules encountered in the human environment is much greater than those embodied in the simple schedules studied in the laboratory. Combinations and variants of the simple schedules of reinforcement produce greater approximations of this complexity. One such example is a multiple schedule of reinforcement in which component schedules alternate over the course of a behavioral test session. On a multiple FI–FR schedule, for example, the session could begin with an FI schedule in effect and would be indicated to the subject by some explicit stimulus (e.g., illumination of a red light). After some specified period of time elapsed or after the delivery of designated number of reinforcers on the FI schedule, the red light would change to a green light, and the schedule would switch to an FR. The FR schedule component would then remain in effect until a designated time had elapsed or a specified number of reinforcers had been delivered and would be followed by a switch back to the FI component, and so on. After training on this schedule, patterns of behavior characteristic of each schedule component emerge; thus, during the FI component, a scalloped pattern of responding is maintained, whereas during the FR component, break-and-run performance is exhibited. In addition, after experience on the schedule, the colored light stimuli associated with each schedule component come to exert strong control over behavior, such that performance appropriate to the schedule occurs immediately upon switching the color of the light. That is, these stimuli serve as what are termed discriminative stimuli signaling the schedule in effect.

This arrangement allows the experimenter to measure two very different types of schedule-controlled performances in the same subject during the same test session, making it a highly efficient experimental paradigm. This permits a determination as to whether a chemical may have selective effects on certain schedules (e.g., change FI performance without affecting the FR). If the compound being evaluated affects the control of the stimulus lights over responding, it might be manifest as a delay in transition to schedule-appropriate behavior whenever the light colors switched.

A mixed schedule of reinforcement is identical to a multiple schedule of reinforcement, except that there are no external stimuli provided to the subject to indicate that the operative reinforcement schedule has switched. Thus, the only indication to the subject as to 'what pays off' is the feedback it receives from its own behavior. This minimizes the extent of stimulus control over behavior relative to that of a comparable multiple schedule of reinforcement.

A chained schedule of reinforcement, like a multiple schedule of reinforcement, also has different external stimuli associated with each component of the schedule, but it requires the completion of a sequence of components for reinforcement delivery. Thus, on a chained FI–FR schedule, a red light may signal that the FI component is in effect. Completion of the FI with the first response after the interval ends produces the external stimulus (e.g., green light) associated with the FR component. Completion of the response requirement during the FR component then produces reinforcement, and the chain subsequently begins over – a course that continues throughout the behavioral session. A tandem schedule is identical to a chained schedule, but like the mixed schedule, it provides no external stimuli to signal which component schedule is in effect.

Schedules that probably most closely resemble those operative in the human environment are known as concurrent schedules of reinforcement. In the real world, we are routinely faced with a multitude of simultaneously operative schedule of reinforcement options with various schedule conditions and consequences, and we must make choices among them. The foraging (food seeking) environment of many species likewise embodies such concurrent options with differential probabilities of reinforcement among which species must make choices. Concurrent schedules provide an experimental analog of this facet of the environment and require the subject to make choices among component reinforcement schedules and reinforcers. For example, in an operant chamber such as shown in **Figure 6**, different response manipulanda might be associated with different but simultaneously available reinforcement schedule options, perhaps associated with different reinforcing events as well. In some cases, once the subject chooses one option, the alternative schedule options are no longer available for some period of time. Others allow subjects to switch back and forth between schedule options. These types of schedules allow experimenters to ask questions about how much behavior the subject is willing to emit for specified reinforcers, preferences for reinforcers and response patterns, relative magnitude of reinforcement and allocation of behavior depending on effort and reinforcement availability.

Measurement of Schedule-Controlled Behavior

The universal measure of schedule-controlled behavior is the rate of responding, which is simply the total number of responses divided by total time. While this is a useful measure of behavior, it provides no indication of other aspects of schedule-controlled behavior, such as the extent of pausing or the patterns of behavior over time. For such purposes, a more fine-grained analysis or microanalysis of performance must be undertaken.

One such measure, applicable to both FR and FI schedules, is post reinforcement pause (PRP) time, which is simply measured as the time from reinforcement delivery until the first response occurs in the next interval (FI) or ratio (FR). For the FI schedule, one may be interested in the extent to which the prototypical scalloped pattern of performance, as shown in **Figure 9**, occurs as an indication of the extent to which responding is controlled by the contingencies operative on the schedule. For this, one of two measures is utilized: the index of curvature or the quarter life. Index of curvature simply utilizes a mathematical formula to indicate how the observed scallop deviates from a straight line that would be generated by a constant rate of responding throughout the interval. Quarter life measures the time it takes for the first 25% of responses in the interval to occur.

Another measure of schedule-controlled behavior is that provided by the distribution of the times between successive responses or inter-response times (IRTs). These can be generated as a frequency distribution and have been shown to be important targets of chemical exposure. For example, lead exposure appears to affect primarily the very short IRTs on FI schedules. Many different drugs from a variety of different classes have been shown to increase the frequency of long IRTs and to decrease the frequency of short IRTs on an FI schedule – a phenomenon known as 'rate dependency' and which results in a more uniform and less scalloped pattern of responding. Rates of responding can also be calculated on schedules of reinforcement after the PRP or the IRTs longer than some designated time (pauses) have been subtracted out. This results in a 'truer' rate of responding and is known as running rate.

Behavioral Teratology

Behavioral teratology, or neurobehavioral teratology, is often referred to separately from behavioral toxicology. Behavioral teratology focuses on the behavioral impact of toxic exposures occurring prenatally or during early development. In some cases, these studies may only track the consequences of chemical exposures into early postnatal life, but in others it may be studied well into the juvenile and even adult stages of the life cycle. Because the possibility has been raised that developmental exposures may accelerate the processes of aging or contribute to neurodegenerative phenotypes, as hypothesized in fetal basis of disease models, some studies are now beginning to follow subjects throughout the lifespan. Behavioral teratology studies typically include a series of tasks designed to evaluate multiple behavioral functions. Consequently, such experiments may include assessment of the development of various reflexes, physiological processes and developmental landmarks (e.g., eye opening), performance on a FOB, motor activity, sensory capabilities, learning, and even schedule-controlled operant behavior. In addition, some such experiments may include evaluation of behaviors deemed 'species specific' (i.e., behaviors that are innate and unique to that species), such as the ontogeny of aggression, play, or vocalization in rodents.

In cases in which outcome is followed through maturity, many of the behavioral paradigms that have already been described are utilized. Assessment of behavioral changes early in life, however, may require modification of such procedures and even the development of specialized behavioral preparations. One example of such a specialized preparation which concurrently measures sensory and motor capabilities (though not independently) is that known as 'homing behavior', a behavior utilized by rodent pups to locate the nest should they wander. In this procedure, a rat pup is placed in the center of a rectangular apparatus, one side of which contains clean bedding material, whereas the other side contains bedding material from the home nest with its scent familiar to the pup. The time taken for the pup to orient or to reach the home cage bedding is then measured. Such a test is deemed apical because it requires the integration of both motor and sensory capabilities.

There are certain issues uniquely related to behavioral teratology studies that require special consideration. One is that of toxicant effects on the dam (mother). Since the behavior of the dam may ultimately influence behavior and development of the offspring, great care must be taken to determine whether any observed effects of a chemical in the offspring are direct effects of the toxicant itself or whether they arise indirectly as a result of the effect of the compound on the dam's behavior. This can be accomplished either by direct measurement of aspects of maternal behavior or be precluded through the use of fostering procedures. A cross-fostering procedure distributes the pups of treated dams to dams that are treatment free in which case there should be no chemical-induced changes in maternal behavior.

There are also issues related to statistical analyses of the data that are unique to behavioral teratology. The offspring of a given litter are not considered as individual subjects since, as members of a litter, they have all experienced factors of the fetal environment which may be unique to their dam. This means that the total number of subjects in a treatment group is really equivalent to the total number of litters represented in that group, a factor which can change the degrees of freedom in the statistical analyses.

Human Testing

Behavioral toxicological studies in humans include assessments of occupational exposure effects in adults as well as the effects of environmental exposures in both adults and children. There is frequently a good deal of overlap in the specific behavioral functions evaluated in each case, although the tests utilized must be age appropriate. However, studies in children also often include measurements of developmental profiles and landmarks that may not be relevant to studies of occupationally exposed adults. Studies in both adults and children often assess a broad variety of behavioral functions and may include tests of motor function, sensory capabilities, complex or cognitive behaviors, attentional processes, and vigilance, usually in the context of a standardized test or test battery. In the past, many such functions would be evaluated as part of a neurological or clinical examination. However, it has become increasingly clear that such examinations, meant to diagnose disease or brain damage, are neither sufficiently sensitive nor quantitative for purposes of detecting subtle effects of toxicants and ultimately for setting standards of exposure.

The test batteries commonly used in human studies have come primarily from the field of clinical neuropsychology in which human testing has predominated. Behavioral measures such as are utilized in experimental animal studies were, in the past, rarely included in human studies. This has changed, however, and will likely increase even more in the future given advances in the ease and availability of computerized testing and the obvious advantages of utilizing the same tests across species in relation to defining risks associated with chemical exposures. In part, the overall emphasis on broad testing of behavioral functions in human studies has been driven by the lack of any information on the behavioral properties of many of these chemicals and thus the attempt to further characterize their effects.

Many of the same issues raised with respect to experimental animal studies also apply to human testing and to the choices of particular tests to be utilized. There are numerous tests that can be utilized for measurement of behavioral functions in humans and questions remain as to the correct choice. One consideration related to the various tests is deemed validity and refers to the degree to which a selected test actually measures the behavioral function that it was designed to measure. For example, does a test of memory really evaluate memory function? In addition, how specifically does the test measure that function? The related issue was raised in experimental animal studies in which the possibility that changes in motor, sensory, motivational processes, etc., might contaminate a measure of memory function, and appropriate controls were included in the more advanced procedures to evaluate those possibilities.

Another important issue relates to the reliability of the test. That is, how reproducible or consistent are the test results across multiple administrations? Inadequate reliability almost guarantees that a subtle toxicant effect will not be detected against a background of scores of broad individual variability that will be present in any normal population. An issue that has not received adequate attention is the sensitivity of these tests to detect toxicant effects, a factor that is of particular importance if the test results are used in the context of setting exposure standards. If a particular test indicates effects of lead, for example, at a blood lead concentration of 40 $\mu g\ dl^{-1}$, one may wonder whether this represents the bottom limits of sensitivity of the test or the actual blood lead value at which such effects occur. In other words, could the test have detected effects at even lower levels of exposure if it had been more sensitive? A deficiency in test sensitivity could mean that exposure standards will be set at levels that are too high and will not protect the exposed populations.

A related question of relevance, particularly to tests of achievement such as the so-called intelligence tests, is standardization. This refers to the population from which the normative scores for the test were collected. This issue is often raised in the interpretation of intelligence tests for populations that are culturally and socially distinct from the populations of white middle-class English-speaking children from which normative scores for such tests have typically been derived.

Developmental Assessments

As mentioned previously, several unique considerations affect the assessment of toxicant-induced behavioral changes in children. One such consideration is the rapid development that children undergo from birth through even the preschool and early school stages. Moreover, this development is marked by wide individual differences in the rate at which it occurs and, for some facets of behavior, pronounced gender-related differences as well. An additional difficulty is that many of the behavioral processes that are of particular interest, such as complex cognitive behavior, are more difficult to evaluate at a young age. While it seems clear that children certainly have both learning and memory capabilities even from birth, preferred tests to measure such functions may require language or motor skills well beyond the capabilities represented by these early stages of development.

Because of this rapid change in the behavioral repertoire over the course of early development, the tests that are utilized in studies of children tend to differ at different ages. One test frequently utilized in the first few days after birth is the Brazelton Neonatal Behavioral Assessment Scale, which is composed of two subscales. The first taps a range of behavioral items such as habituation and responsiveness to environmental stimuli. The second primarily measures a variety of unconditioned reflexes. While the Brazelton scale is obviously limited in the extent to which it can tap cognitive functions, or define specific behavioral deficits, its utility in detecting drug-induced changes has been established.

An increasingly widely used technique for infant assessment is embodied in the Fagan Test of Infant Intelligence, which assesses visual recognition memory. In this test, an infant faces a display with two screens. On one screen, a visual stimulus is presented for a specified period of time. Subsequently, that visual stimulus is projected on one screen and, at the same time, another visual stimulus is projected onto another screen. An observer records the amount of time the infant spends gazing at each screen. Normal infants look away from the visual stimulus that they have already seen and spend more time gazing at the novel stimulus, a trait which has been shown to correlate with higher scores later in development on the Stanford–Binet intelligence test. As this indicates, the test has analogs to the novel object recognition paradigm frequently used in animal models.

A widely used test at a slightly later stage of development is the Bayley Scales of Infant Development, appropriate to children from 2 to 30 months of age. The test is composed of three subscales: motor, mental, and behavioral. Each is arranged with respect to chronological development. One of the advantages of this test is the ability to carry out repeated testing over the normed age range.

As children reach preschool and school age, the number of test choices available increases. For example, the McCarthy Scales of Children's Abilities provides an analog of an intelligence test score by combining the scores from its five subscales into a general cognitive index score. Its applicability extends from children aged 2.5–8.5 years. Like the Bayley Scales, it too allows for repeated measurement over time, which is a particular advantage for longitudinal studies; utilization of the same test instrument over time, given appropriate reliability of the instrument, provides greater assurance of the continuity and of the onset or disappearance of an effect than does the use of different instruments at different ages.

Various intelligence tests are available for preschool age children, such as the Wechsler Preschool and Primary Scale of Intelligence (WPPSI). The advantage of this particular instrument is that it represents an extension of the well-standardized and widely used Wechsler Intelligence Scale for Children (revised; WISC-R). The WISC-R is an intelligence test for children of 6 years of age or older; the WPPSI extends this age range to include children of ages 4–6.5 years. In addition, both rely on the same two subscales, verbal and performance, to measure a variety of behavioral functions, thus providing a type of continuity from the preschool to the school-aged child for repeated assessment of behavioral function.

One of the major concerns with developmental and intelligence tests such as the WISC-R and others is to be able to rule out contributions from numerous sociodemographic and other variables known to co-vary with intelligence test score. Variables that may potentially modulate intelligence include birth weight, length of gestation, maternal age, birth order, parental education, parental IQ, socioeconomic status, and quality of the home environment. Appropriate statistical controls or subject matching must be undertaken to evaluate the contributions of these variables to outcome measures.

While these developmental and intelligence tests may clearly be important to the determination of the levels and conditions of exposures to a toxicant associated with adverse behavioral function, they are less useful, as noted previously, in providing a precise delineation of the behavioral functions actually affected by a chemical. Measures such as intelligence test scores are global measures in that they rely on the integration of all behavioral functions. Even performances on subscales of these tests are jointly dependent on integrative motor, sensory, and cognitive functions. Thus, even a preferential deficit on a verbal scale, which is clearly geared toward cognitive function, may not provide a precise understanding of the nature of the behavioral deficit.

To achieve a true understanding of the behavioral processes affected by a chemical will necessarily require direct measurement of those specific functions, much as is done in the experimental animal studies described previously. Some neuropsychologists have recognized this problem and have begun to employ measures of specific behavioral functions such as learning, memory, sustained attention, and abstract thinking in an attempt to determine the source of the deficits in global intelligence test scores produced by lead exposure, for example. An alternative approach is to utilize many of the behavioral tasks already employed in experimental animal studies – tasks which are designed to evaluate specific functions and which have already been widely used across species, including humans, in other research contexts. The repeated learning paradigm actually originated in studies using human subjects and was later adapted for nonhuman primates and rodents. Procedures such as delayed matching-to-sample and operant psychophysical procedures have also been used across species with appropriate parametric modifications. These types of paradigms are increasingly available from commercial vendors and can be used in children as young as 5–6 years of age and very widely in adult populations and may play a more significant role in future developmental studies of children because they provide direct and specific measures of behavioral functions that are more difficult to differentiate in standardized tests.

Adult Assessments

Assessments of behavioral toxicity in adults frequently occur in the context of occupational exposures to chemicals. Like studies carried out in school-aged children, these evaluations have relied largely on standardized tests, including intelligence tests. They also tend to employ a broad variety of tests so that numerous behavioral functions can be tested, particularly when the effects of a toxicant are ill-defined. As such, the same considerations must be taken into account with respect to the choice of tests utilized. These include validity, reliability, and sensitivity, as well as standardization issues related to the population from which test norms were derived.

One distinction between many of the studies of behavioral toxicity in children and adults is that while the former have tended to be primarily longitudinal in nature, following the effects of toxicant exposures to children across the course of development, many occupational exposure studies are cross-sectional studies in adults that encompass only a single time point of measurement of behavioral function. This likely reflects in part the difficulties of carrying out studies in the workplace, where it may be more difficult to obtain appropriate amounts of the subjects' time for behavioral evaluation and where resistance to such experiments may be encountered from either the employer or the employee.

One of the most common inclusions in these test batteries that have been utilized in studies of occupational behavioral toxicity is the Wechsler Adult Intelligence Scale (WAIS), which is actually a battery of tests subsumed under verbal and performance subscales which, combined, provide a full-scale intelligence test score. The series of verbal tests includes information (general information questions), comprehension (interpretation test), arithmetic, similarities (between nouns), digit span (repeating sequences of digits), and vocabulary. The performance tests include digit symbol (associating digits with symbols), picture completion, block design (duplicating block patterns), picture arrangement, and object assembly. Because of the obvious overlap of behavioral functions in some of these subtests, and the consequent global and nonspecific nature of any change detected in full-scale intelligence test scores, some investigators have opted to use only selected tests from the battery to provide a shortened version of the WAIS for occupational behavioral toxicity studies.

Two different test batteries, the World Health Organization (WHO) Neurobehavioral Core Test Battery and the Neurobehavioral Evaluation System (NES), are currently among the most widely used test batteries in occupational behavioral toxicology studies. Both include components of the WAIS described previously in addition to other psychometric tests of behavioral function. The WHO Neurobehavioral Core Test Battery is a pencil-and-paper-administered test battery, whereas the NES is a computerized test battery that has been translated into several languages and in fact presents a more extensive set of tests than does the WHO in that it includes tests of psychomotor performance, cognition, memory and learning, and perceptual ability and affect.

Memory dysfunction has been a frequent complaint in populations of workers exposed to various neurotoxicants and is tapped by several different tests used in a human testing context. One of the most widely used for this purpose is the digit span that constitutes one of the WAIS subtests. As indicated earlier, this test requires the subject to recall a series of digits, and the length of the list is successively increased contingent upon the subject correctly recalling the members of the list. In some cases, words or letters are utilized instead of digits. As is the case with experimental animal studies, more complex versions of these tests have been devised and implemented. In procedures such as continuous recognition memory or memory scanning, subjects may be shown a list of digits or letters and then shown, after a delay interval, a longer list of various digits or letters and asked to recall those that were on the original list. Analogies to such tests are embodied in procedures such as the Benton Visual Recognition Test, which requires a subject to reproduce a drawing or geometrical design.

Paired associates learning is also frequently used in a memory context in occupational exposure test batteries as well as in studies with children. In these paradigms, a list of paired words is read to the subject, who must then recall the second member of the pair when the first is read after a delay. The task can be made relatively simple by using pairs which have some type of obvious relationship or made more difficult by having pairs with no apparent relationship. The test can be used in a memory context by including a delay between the experimenter's reading of the list and the subject recalling the second member of each pair. In addition, the task can be used in a repeated learning context, much as the repeated acquisition paradigm described earlier, by using new lists of paired associates after the subject masters the initial list. This particular approach has a long history of use with human subjects and has been found to be sensitive to toxicants such as lead and can be administered easily *via* a touch screen computer.

Measures of vigilance, attention, or distractibility are also frequently included in assessments of occupational behavioral toxicology. These range from very simple procedures, such as reaction time, to more complex tasks, such as simulated cockpit or tracking tasks. But even reaction time can be varied from a very simple to a highly complex procedure. In a simple reaction time task, the subject is typically presented with some type of screen on which a single visual stimulus will appear at intermittent and unpredictable intervals. The subject must respond on the single response manipulanda as soon as the stimulus appears. Complex reaction time presents the subject with multiple stimuli as well as multiple response options. For example, there may be four different stimuli, each of which is presented at random and unpredictable intervals. The appropriate response depends on which of the stimuli is presented, and the subject is asked to respond on the appropriate manipulanda as quickly as possible after detecting the stimulus. Thus, the more complex reaction time task involves not only attending to the screen to detect the stimulus presentation but also making a decision as to the correct manipulanda and then executing the response. Obviously, the number of options can be modified to fit the experimental situation.

One of the important parameters of the reaction time task is the rate at which the attention of the subject deteriorates, such that reaction time is slowed down or even that the subject misses stimulus presentations entirely. This rate of deterioration of performance will depend on many factors, one of which is the rate at which stimuli are presented to the subject and another being the length of the session during which reaction time is measured. While one might intuitively think that the slower the rate of presentation, the more rapid the rate of deterioration of performance, in fact sometimes the opposite is true. A very rapid rate of presentation of stimuli can render the subject exhausted and less alert or less motivated. With respect to session length, one typically expects to see a gradual decrement in performance as the session progresses, such that an adequately long session must be implemented to catch this function. Finally, a critical variable in reaction time studies is the prominence of the stimuli used. In fact, this parameter can be manipulated to change the sensitivity and difficulty of the task.

Reaction time tasks are by no means limited to the presentation of discrete visual stimuli. Other variants have included those in which the subject must respond to a stimulus that is different from a continuously presented array of stimuli. The so-called clock test is one example. In this procedure, the subject is instructed to respond when the hand of a clock ticks off 2 s at once rather than the typical 1 s tick; the 2 s tick is an infrequent and unpredictable occurrence. In other situations, a continuous presentation of letters or numbers may be presented and the subject instructed to respond to one particular letter or number whenever it appears.

Pursuit and tracking tests represent even more complex versions of vigilance assays. In these kinds of tasks, subjects must continuously monitor a stimulus which drifts off a home position on the dial. The situation can be made quite complex, as in flight simulators in which there may be multiple dials which must be continuously monitored and returned to the home position, with drift occurring at varying rates on each dial across time. The various vigilance tasks described previously have a long experimental history and have been shown to be sensitive to a wide variety of influences, including fatigue and various drugs and chemical exposures.

The kinds of vigilance procedures described obviously require reasonably intact motor function and are often interpreted with that in mind. However, these techniques also depend on sensory processes. In fact, assuming intact motor functions, vigilance tasks such as those described can be adapted to provide some indication of sensory function changes by modifying the saliency (intensity) of the sensory stimuli used in the paradigm. A clinical neurological examination often includes components designed to measure sensory function, but relatively speaking, these tend to be less sensitive; thus, subtle changes in sensory function might not be detected. More direct approaches to the evaluation of sensory function following occupational or environmental exposures to toxicants are provided by the types of operant psychophysical procedures elaborated previously. In fact, psychophysical procedures were developed using human subjects and only later adapted for various species of experimental animals. The psychophysical procedures clearly provide more direct and straightforward assessments of sensory detection capabilities in the absence of confounding changes in a subject's motor capabilities or motivation to respond.

Assessments of motor function are often included in the neuropsychological test batteries utilized in occupational exposure studies. Typically, these tend to be relatively simple measures of motor capabilities, probably for two reasons. The first is that the inclusion of vigilance tasks such as those described previously depends on motor coordination in addition to sensory capabilities; therefore, toxicant-induced changes in such performances may already be indicative of motor impairment. This can then be pursued by inclusion of some additional and more direct assessments of motor function in the battery. The second reason relates to logistical reasons and practicalities. Test batteries such as the WHO Neurobehavioral Core Test Battery and the NES are typically taken to the site where measurements of subjects are to be made. Thus, portability is a major consideration, and more complex assessments of motor function would incur greater equipment needs. Since the purpose of these batteries is generally to screen for adverse effects, studies providing more precise delineations of affected functions can be pursued at a later time.

Simple tests of motor function utilized are generally those such as finger tapping in which subjects are asked to tap a key or a button at as rapid a rate as possible for a designated period of time. The subjects may be asked to carry out this task with the preferred hand as well as with the alternate hand. In some cases, toe tapping has been used in addition to finger tapping. Other batteries have relied on the tests of manual dexterity that are frequently used in screening prospective applicants for some types of factory work jobs. One of the most frequently used of such tests is the Santa Ana test, which requires the subject to remove pegs from a hole and to reinsert them into the hole after turning them 180°. The measurement of interest in this case is the number of pegs that are successfully rotated within the specified time interval. The Purdue Pegboard test is likewise used in this capacity. It requires the proper orientation and placement of pins in a series of holes. Such tests have indeed successfully defined subjects occupationally exposed to chemicals from those nonexposed.

One final common inclusion in many studies of occupational behavioral toxicology and in some test batteries is assessments of symptoms experienced by those exposed to chemicals. While this might be perceived as an ostensibly simple procedure, it entails numerous potential confounds. These evaluations are typically administered *via* questionnaires. Items for the questionnaire must be carefully constructed with respect to not only the choices of items but also the wording of the text and the manner in which the response is recorded. Clearly, the motivation of the subject in answering the questions must be considered. One problem can arise when the list of symptoms includes only those that are associated with the toxicant of concern. It is necessary to include symptoms that are not associated with the particular toxicant under evaluation so that some assessment of the tendency of the subject to respond positively to all symptoms can be evaluated. Several such evaluations of subjective and mood states are available. The most widely used is the Profile of Mood States (POMS), which consists of 65 adjectives of various moods that the subject answers according to a 5-point rating scale. The POMS has been used extensively in the evaluation of the acute effects of CNS drugs and toxicants.

See also: Developmental Toxicology; Occupational Toxicology; Toxicity Testing, Developmental.

Further Reading

Annau, Z., Eccles, C.U. (Eds.), 1986. Neurobehavioral Toxicology. Johns Hopkins University Press, Baltimore, MD.

Cory-Slechta, D.A., 1994. Neurotoxicant-induced changes in schedule-controlled behavior. In: Chang, L.W. (Ed.), Principles of Neurotoxicology. Dekker, New York, pp. 313–344.

Russell, R.W., Flattau, P.E., Pope, A.M. (Eds.), 1990. Behavioral Measures of Neurotoxicity. National Academy Press, Washington, DC.

Tilson, H.A., Mitchell, C.L. (Eds.), 1992. Neurotoxicology. Raven Press, New York.

Weiss, B., Cory-Slechta, D.A., 2001. Assessment of behavioral toxicity. In: Hayes, A.W. (Ed.), Principles and Methods of Toxicology, fourth ed. Taylor & Francis, Philadelphia, pp. 1451–1528.

Weiss, B., O'Donoghue, J.L., 1994. Neurobehavioral Toxicity, Analysis and Interpretation. Raven Press, New York.

Yanai, J. (Ed.), 1984. Neurobehavioral Teratology. Elsevier, Amsterdam.

Belladonna Alkaloids

PA Prusakov, Mount Sinai Hospital, Chicago, IL, USA

This article is a revision of the previous edition article by Madhusudan G. Soni, volume 1, pp 244–245, © 2005, Elsevier Inc.

- Name: Belladonna alkaloids (atropine, scopolamine)
- Chemical Abstracts Service Registry Number: Atropine: 51-55-8; Scopolamine: 51-34-3
- Synonyms: Atropine: 1-alpha-H,5-alpha-H-Tropan-3-alpha-ol (+/−)-tropate (ester) (8CI), Scopolamine: 9-methyl-3-oxa-9-azatricyclo(3.3.1.0(sup 2,4))non-7-yl ester
- Molecular Formulas: Atropine: $C_{17}H_{23}NO_3$; Scopolamine: $C_{17}H_{21}NO_4$
- Chemical Structures:

Atropine

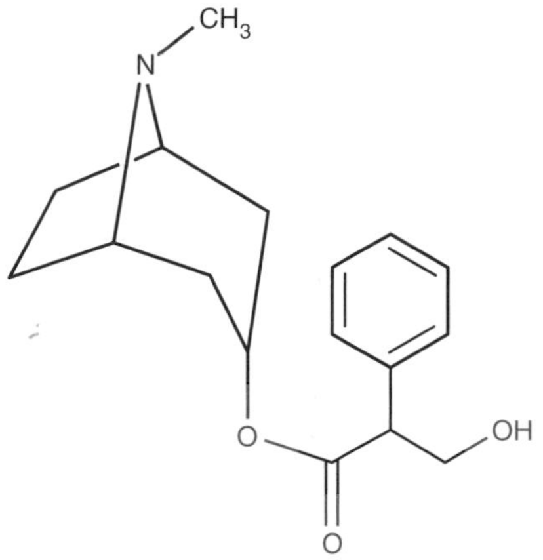

CH_3 N O OH O

Scopolamine

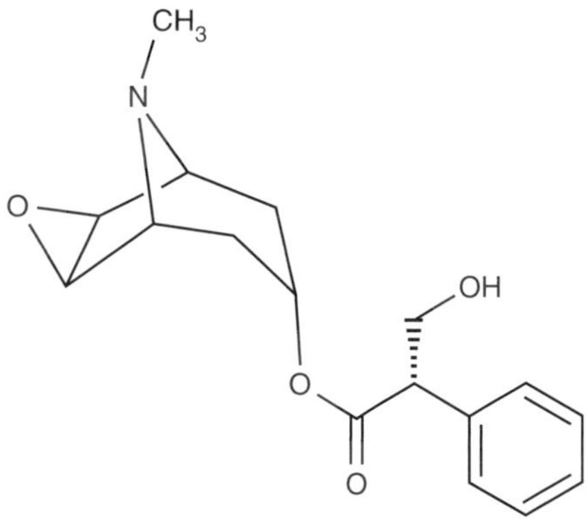

CH_3 N O OH O O

Background

Belladonna alkaloids are derived from plants belonging to Solanaceae family. *Atropa belladonna* produces berries, which may be frequently ingested erroneously. Many other plants such as *Hyoscyamus niger* (henbane), *Datura stramonium* (jimson weed), and *Brugmansia* species (angel trumpet) contain the same active ingredients, thus inducing similar effects. Belladonna alkaloids have a long history of medicinal, cosmetic, recreational, and militaristic uses. Its name, beautiful lady in Italian, was not given accidentally. Upon discovery of the plant's dilatory effects on the pupils, the plant was used for cosmetic purposes in Italy and France. Active ingredients of the plant are now commonly known as scopolamine, atropine, hyoscine, and hyoscyamine. As the popularity of the plants grew, toxic and hallucinogenic effects slowly were recognized. Militaristic uses of the plant included poisoning arrows, knives, and enemy's food supplies to weaken armies. Adolescents abuse Solanaceae family plants for their mind-altering properties. More recently, medicinal uses of the plant were discovered.

Uses

While most of the uses of belladonna alkaloids were nonmedicinal in the past, currently a majority of belladonna alkaloids and all of its derivatives are used for medical purposes. Hyoscyamine (L-atropine), atropine, and scopolamine (hyoscine) are the active ingredients of belladonna alkaloids. These agents are used for their anticholinergic, parasympatholytic effects in outpatient and inpatient settings. Medical routes of administration vary greatly based on the condition treated. Belladonna alkaloids separately and as a mixture have been used for Parkinsonism and disorders of the genitourinary system (dysmenorrhea and nocturnal enuresis). In combination with barbiturates, most commonly phenobarbital, belladonna alkaloids have been used for disorders of the gastrointestinal tract (irritable bowel syndrome, gastrointestinal ulcers, and enterocolitis).

Atropine is available as oral, intravenous, intramuscular, and ophthalmic formulations. Atropine use includes treatment of symptomatic sinus bradycardia and atrioventricular block. In different settings, atropine has been used to reduce or prevent salivation and secretions as well as an antidote for organophosphate overdose. Scopolamine is available in oral, intramuscular, intravenous, subcutaneous, and transdermal formulations. Scopolamine has been used as a sedative, antiemetic, and antisecretory medication.

Environmental Behavior, Fate, Routes, and Pathways

Despite of a wide variety of available routes of administration, accidental and intentional toxicities are generally caused by oral ingestion. Two of the most common causes of toxicity are accidental ingestion of *A. belladonna* berries and ingestion of tea made from *D. stramonium* leaves.

Exposure and Exposure Monitoring

Excessive dryness is one of the first symptoms of toxicity when excessive amounts of belladonna alkaloids have been ingested.

However, heart rate is the first parameter that should be monitored, since tachycardia is one of the most common side effects of these agents. In more severe cases, an electrocardiogram should be done to monitor the patient for arrhythmias.

Toxicokinetics

Both atropine and scopolamine are competitive antagonists of primarily M1 and M2 muscarinic cholinergic receptors. Nicotinic receptors are not affected to the degree of the muscarinic system, even at toxic levels. Atropine reaches peak levels within 60 min, but varies depending on the route of administration. Both chemicals are widely distributed throughout the body, including the brain. The volumes of distribution of atropine and scopolamine are similar and are estimated at 1.7 and 1.4 $l\,kg^{-1}$, respectively. Although, atropine's volume of distribution has been reported as high as 3.9 $l\,kg^{-1}$. Atropine levels in the urine follow first-order kinetics. The half-life of atropine has been noted to be about 2–3 h, but can be as high as 6.5 h in children. Atropine is not dialyzable although 30–50% of it is excreted in the urine. The rest of it is metabolized by the liver. Scopolamine, however, is mostly metabolized in the liver, with excretion not exceeding 10%. The half-life of scopolamine can range from 4 to 9 h.

Mechanisms of Action

Belladonna alkaloids are competitive antagonists of acetylcholine at muscarinic receptors. Affinity for receptors varies. However, the inhibition at all muscarinic receptors in exocrine glands, smooth muscle, and neurons is present. Atropine exhibits strong affinity for cardiac, gastrointestinal, and bronchial muscles. Scopolamine exhibits more potent activity on iris and ciliary body. It is more potent at reducing secretions of salivary, bronchial, and sweat glands.

Acute and Short-Term Toxicity

Doses of 10 mg of atropine or higher have been associated with symptoms of acute toxicity. Shortly after ingestion of belladonna alkaloids, several adverse effects begin to manifest. Tachycardia, dilated pupils, blurred vision, urinary retention, altered mental status, and dry and flushed skins are a few of the symptoms evident. These effects can be attributed to the rest of the anticholinergic drug class. Elderly and children are more susceptible to belladonna alkaloid toxicity and may experience more severe effects at lower doses. Coma also has been described. Several cases in Taiwan reported toxicities of belladonna alkaloids. Symptoms included dizziness, dry mouth, flushed skin, palpitation, nausea, drowsiness, tachycardia, blurred vision, mydriasis, hyperthermia, disorientation, vomiting, agitation, delirium, urine retention, hypertension, and coma. All of the patients reported experiencing adverse effects within 30 min. A more thorough case report of a middle-aged man described the progress of *A. belladonna* toxicity. Upon the ingestion of three handfuls of berries, the patient experienced disorientation, aggressiveness, and tachycardia phases, all of which came within 45 min. Patients' systolic blood pressure rose to 200 mmHg with heart rate of 130 beats per minute, flushed skin, dry mouth, and mydriasis. Symptoms persisted for 2 days. Reversal of the toxicity has been potentiated by physostigmine. In cardiac transplant patients, atropine and other anticholinergics may cause atrioventricular block, even leading up to asystole.

Without treatment, as few as 10 berries of *A. belladonna* are considered to be lethal. Animals, however, have variable bioavailability and sensitivity to these plants. Herbivores tend to have a decreased sensitivity to belladonna alkaloids. Oral intake of alkaloids in horses, rabbits, cattle, guinea pigs, and birds have minimal effects. However, horses and cattle are affected by intravenous administration at a much greater extent than rabbits, guinea pigs, and birds.

Chronic Toxicity

There are no studies specifically evaluating chronic toxicity of belladonna alkaloids. However, despite an overdose, belladonna alkaloids are not considered to be a reason for long-term concern. Chronic toxicity is likely to be secondary to adverse events from acute overdose. Induced psychosis is associated with prolonged use of anticholinergics in toxic doses.

Immunotoxicity

In patients allergic to atropine or scopolamine, a fulminant IgE antibody reaction develops. Other immunologically toxic reactions have not been described in the literature.

Reproductive and Developmental Toxicity

Atropine crosses human placenta and enters breast milk and may suppress lactation. Two animal studies have been done to specifically evaluate the teratogenicity. Prenatal exposure to atropine and other anticholinergics may induce learning deficits in pups. However, injection of doses of up to 1.5 mg of atropine into chick eggs did not produce any defects.

Genotoxicity

Belladonna alkaloids have not been evaluated in genotoxic studies. Components of belladonna alkaloids are not considered to be genotoxic.

Carcinogenicity

There are no studies in humans documenting carcinogenicity of atropine. However, tests in rats have not shown to be carcinogenic.

Clinical Management

Once the patient is suspected to have been exposed to toxic doses of belladonna alkaloids, negative response to physostigmine injection would suggest the positive diagnosis. Since physostigmine is an acetylcholinesterase inhibitor, it produces effects opposite of belladonna alkaloids. These effects would include mydriasis, lacrimation, urination, salivation, sweating, and intestinal hyperactivity, unless the patient is in acute overdose of anticholinergic agents. Activated charcoal administration and gastric lavage can be performed even if the patient has arrived to the hospital over 1 h postingestion. This is due to slowing of gastric emptying in belladonna alkaloid overdose. Physostigmine can be given at doses of 0.5–2.5 mg to adults and 0.01–0.03 mg kg^{-1} per dose, not exceeding adult doses. Physostigmine should be given over at least 5 min to reduce the potential of respiratory distress and seizures. In case of seizures, diazepam or lorazepam can be given intravenously, and rectal diazepam is an alternative. Antipyretics, fluids, and ice treatments can be used to reduce fever. Bicarbonate and lidocaine may play an important role in the treatment if the patient goes into an arrhythmia.

See also: Atropine; Anticholinergics; Cholinesterase Inhibition; Organophosphorus Compounds.

Further Reading

Adams, R.G., Verma, P., Jackson, A.J., et al., 1982. Plasma pharmacokinetics of intravenously administered atropine in normal human subjects. J. Clin. Pharm. 22, 477–481.

Berdai, M.A., Labib, S., Chetouani, K., Harandou, M., 2012. *Atropa belladonna* intoxication: a case report. Pan Afr. Med. J. 11, 72–78.

Bogan, R., Zimmermann, T., Zilker, T., Eyer, F., Thiermann, H., 2009. Plasma level of atropine after accidental ingestion of *Atropa belladonna.* Clin. Toxicol. 47 (6), 602–604.

Chang, S.S., Wu, M.L., et al., 1999. Poisoning by *Datura* leaves used as edible wild vegetables. Vet. Hum. Toxicol. 41, 242–245.3

Fang, Y.T., Chou, Y.J., Pu, C., et al., 2013. Prescription of atropine eye drops among children diagnosed with myopia in Taiwan from 2000 to 2007: a nationwide study. Eye (Lond.). http://dx.doi.org/10.1038/eye.2012.279 [Epub ahead of print].

Gilman, A.G., Rall, T.W., Nies, A.S., et al. (Eds.), 1990. Goodman and Gilman's The Pharmacological Basis of Therapeutics, eighth ed. Pergamon Press, New York, NY.

Jokanović, M., Prostran, M., 2009. Pyridinium oximes as cholinesterase reactivators. Structure-activity relationship and efficacy in the treatment of poisoning with organophosphorus compounds. Curr. Med. Chem. 16 (17), 2177–2188.

Krenzelok, E.P., 2010. Aspects of *Datura* poisoning and treatment. Clin. Toxicol. 48 (2), 104–110. http://dx.doi.org/10.3109/15563651003630672.

Pihlajamaki, K., Kanto, J., Aaltonen, L., et al., 1986. Pharmacokinetics of atropine in children. Int. J. Clin. Pharmacol. Ther. Toxicol. 24, 236–239.

Roberts, D.M., Aaron, C.K., 2007. Management of acute organophosphorus pesticide poisoning. Br. Med. J. 334 (7594), 629–634.

Skaar, D.D., OConnor, H.L., 2012. Use of the Beers criteria to identify potentially inappropriate drug use by community-dwelling older dental patients. Oral Surg. Oral Med. Oral Pathol. 113 (6), 714–721.

Worz, R., 2012. Abuse and paradoxical effects of analgesic drug mixtures. Br. J. Clin. Pharmacol. 10 (S2), 391S–393S.

Benchmark Dose

MA Rezvanfar, Tehran University of Medical Sciences, Tehran, Iran

This article is a revision of the previous edition article by Qiyu Jay Zhao, volume 1, pp 246–248, © 2005, Elsevier Inc.

Introduction

One of the main purposes of toxicology and chemical risk assessment is to identify acceptable exposure levels based on data obtained from human or experimental animal studies. These are currently developed by many organizations such as the US Environmental Protection Agency (EPA) and other international health agencies for several regulatory classes of chemicals, including industrial chemicals, food additives, pesticide residues, and environmental pollutants. In general, there is a threshold for the process of non–cancer risk assessment. In noncarcinogenic effects, protective mechanisms are induced to overcome the threat before an adverse effect is displayed. For some toxicants, there is a range of exposures up to some limited value that can be tolerated by the organism at the cellular level without any expression of adverse effects. Therefore, risk assessment of environmental contaminants aims to identify the upper bound of this tolerance range (i.e., the maximum subthreshold level). In the traditional approach of nongenotoxic agents in health risk assessment, the permissible exposure levels were based on identification of the point of departure (POD). POD is the exposure level of a chemical that serves as a starting point in the determination of guidance values and is set at doses corresponding to the no observed adverse effect level (NOAEL) or the lowest observed adverse effect level (LOAEL), when there is insufficient data to arrive at an NOAEL. The NOAEL represents the highest experimental dose for which no biologically or statistically significant adverse health effects are observed and is the key datum derived from the study of the dose–response relationship, whereas the LOAEL represents the lowest dose at which a significant adverse health effect is observed. The NOAEL is used to calculate reference doses (RfDs) for chronic oral exposure and reference concentrations (RfCs) for chronic inhalation exposure as per the US EPA. A recent alternative to using the NOAEL or LOAEL in this calculation is the use of a benchmark dose (BMD) to serve as the starting point for deriving safe doses.

Definition of BMD

The US EPA defines BMD as the exposure level that corresponds to a certain increase in the probability of an adverse response, compared with zero background exposure. This specified response change is generally referred to as the benchmark response (BMR). The lower confidence limit of the BMD (i.e., the BMDL) has been proposed to replace the NOAEL as a starting point for determination of health-based guidance values (i.e., uncertainty factors are applied to the BMDL instead of to the NOAEL; **Figure 1**). The BMDL is usually defined as the one-sided lower 95% confidence limit on the BMD (which equals the lower bound of a two-sided 90% confidence interval); it can be interpreted as the dose corresponding to a response not likely to be larger than the specified BMR (with 95% confidence). Because estimates derived by maximum likelihood methods have good statistical properties, such as asymptotic normality, maximum likelihood is often a preferred model of estimation when that assumption is reasonably close to the truth.

Characteristics of the BMD Approach

Because of several limitations and some problems associated with using the NOAEL and to move away from compulsory lethal dose 50% (LD_{50}) determination, the benchmark concept has been introduced as an alternative approach in risk assessment and has been developed and implemented by risk assessors to estimate RfDs and RfCs. The BMD concept was introduced by Crump in 1984 and has been presented as a methodological improvement in the field of risk assessment by defining a concentration between the NOAEL and LOAEL. To date, the BMD method has mostly been used by authorities, such as the US EPA and consultants in the United States; research specifically related to this approach has been performed at only a few institutions in Europe. Practical and theoretical knowledge of the method is limited.

The European Chemicals Agency stated that BMD "... can be used in parallel or as an alternative when there is no reliable NOAEL." Similar statements have been made by other organizations: the Scientific Committee of the European Food Safety Authority (EFSA) 'strongly encourage' all panels and units to adopt the BMD approach. Also the World Health Organization's International Panel for Chemical Safety (IPCS) state that BMD "... can be considered a more sophisticated or robust alternative to NOAEL." Even stronger recommendations are made by the US National Academy Committee for Acute Exposure Guidance Levels, declaring that BMD should be the 'preferred approach.' This approach can be used quite extensively in developmental and reproductive toxicity studies as

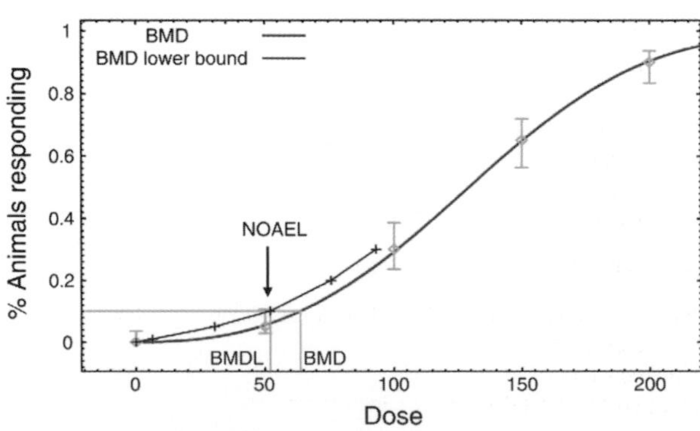

Figure 1 Example of BMD modeling results.

 http://dx.doi.org/10.1016/B978-0-12-386454-3.00588-1

Table 1 The major characteristics of BMD approach

1. The magnitude of an effect considered adverse is based on toxicology rather than statistics
2. Differences in sensitivity between two data sets may be recognized with BMD
3. BMD gives more detailed information about the dose–response relationship compared with NOAEL
4. BMD can be combined with probabilistic exposure analyses
5. BMD can be used to develop relative potency values used for risk assessment of mixtures
6. A BMD can be calculated from experiments lacking an NOAEL and there is thus no need for complementary studies
7. All doses and the slope of the curve influence the BMD; this brings extra power to the statistical evaluation compared with the NOAEL approach, which might be used to lower the number of animals used
8. The BMD is not restricted to the experimental doses; it is therefore possible to perform studies with fewer animals in some dose groups
9. In contrast to the NOAEL, the confidence interval around BMD can be calculated, giving additional information for risk managers. The incitement for increasing the number of animals will be stronger with the BMD compared with NOAEL since a narrow confidence interval (i.e., higher BMDL) will lead to a higher POD compared with the NOAEL approach, which will always be lower with increasing numbers

well as cancer risk assessment. Quantal data is ideally suited for BMD modeling.

The BMD approach was developed to better define the POD in the computation of the safe dose to overcome the shortcomings of using NOAELs or LOAELs (**Tables 1 and 2**). Using the NOAEL approach to estimate acceptable human exposure values such as RfDs and RfCs has several limitations: (1) it must be one of the tested experimental doses, so it depends on the study design and once this dose is identified, the rest of the dose–response curve is ignored; (2) it does not account for variability in the estimate of the dose–response. In essence, the NOAEL is very sensitive to sample size and there can also be high variability among experiments; (3) it does not account for the slope of the dose–response curve; and (4) it cannot be applied when there is no NOAEL, except through the application of an uncertainty factor when an LOAEL is used.

Compared with the NOAEL approach, the BMD approach provides five major advantages:

1. It is not as sensitive to dose selection. All the experimental data are used to construct the dose–response curve meaning that the BMD is based on data from the entire dose–response curve for the critical effect, rather than only from the single dose (e.g., NOAEL). Therefore, the BMD reflects the slope of the dose–response curve.
2. It is less sensitive to sample size compared with the NOAEL approach, meaning that the BMD approach treats sample size appropriately when the lower confidence limit on the BMD (i.e., BMDL) is used. For example, the smaller the sample, the larger the uncertainty associated with the BMD estimates and the lower the confidence limits (all else being equal). Therefore, data with lower statistical power result in lower BMDLs (making their use health protective), and better experiments with more statistical power are rewarded with higher BMDLs.
3. The BMDL is not constrained to being one of the experimental doses, and calculation of the BMDL allows for estimation of an NOAEL surrogate when only an LOAEL is available. In addition, the dose-independent BMDL also facilitates comparison of toxicity potencies across chemicals or end points.
4. The BMD approach can be useful when the dose spacing in a study is such that the LOAEL is much larger than the NOAEL. Thus, any good study can be used, even in the absence of an NOAEL, as long as sufficient and appropriate dose–response data are provided so that the dose corresponding to the BMR can be estimated.
5. The method represents a single methodology that can be applied to cancer and noncancer end points. It may also be possible to use fewer animals in testing.

Despite the superiority of BMD over the NOAEL, there are a number of reasons for the continued use of the NOAEL as the gold standard. The BMD method is a more advanced approach and competence in the area is limited. Many toxicologists and risk assessors are not currently conversant with BMD and find it difficult to understand. Moreover, there is no general

Table 2 Advantages and limitations of the NOAEL and BMD methods

BMD advantages	*NOAEL limitations*
Not limited to experimental doses	Highly dependent on dose selection
Less dependent on dose spacing	Highly dependent on sample size
Appropriately accounts for variability and uncertainty resulting from study quality	Does not account for variability and uncertainty in the experimental results (e.g., does not account for study quality appropriately)
Takes into account the shape of the dose–response curve and other related information	Dose–response information (e.g., shape of dose–response curve) not taken into account
Corresponds to a consistent response level and can be used to compare results across chemicals and studies	Does not correspond to consistent response levels for comparisons across studies
Flexibility in determining biologically significant rates	An LOAEL cannot be used to derive an NOAEL
BMD Limitations	**NOAEL Advantages**
Ability to estimate BMD may be limited by the format of the data presented	Can be used when data are not amenable to BMD modeling
Time consuming	Easy to derive
More complicated decision-making process	Has been the standard method for deriving a POD for decades (e.g., is familiar to most risk assessors)

agreement and international harmonization regarding the definition of BMDL and software standards. In addition, another important factor limiting the use of BMD is that critical studies are often conducted with a number of doses less than optimal for BMD analysis, therefore, with few dose groups, the chance of missing the relevant response becomes larger.

Data Requirements and Parameter Selection

The US EPA BMD guidance document discusses the computation of the confidence limit (CL) for the BMD, the fact that the method by which the CL is obtained is typically related to the data type, and the manner in which the BMD is estimated from the chosen model. Details for approaches to CLs computationally specific to particular data types (quantal, clustered, continuous, multiple outcomes) are provided in the US EPA document. A number of dose–response models have been developed for BMD analyses. The type of the model used and the necessary inputs for the model depend on the type of data to be modeled. Once potential critical effects have been selected, their adequacy for BMD modeling should be determined according to the following minimal data requirements.

1. Has the data been reported in the study in a manner that will allow it to be modeled?
2. Is there a biologically or statistically significant trend in the response?
3. Are there sufficient dose groups to support BMD modeling?
4. Are the observed dose–response relationships appropriate for BMD modeling?

For quantal data (e.g., histopathology incidence data), the incidence of the effect of interest and the total size of the group are needed, and for continuous data (e.g., liver enzyme activity), the group size, mean, and a measure of variability (i.e., standard deviation or standard error) are required. To estimate the BMD and BMDL, it is necessary to define a desired BMR. For quantal data, the BMR is defined as an incidence change from the estimated control. Usually, 10% extra risk, $[P(\text{dose}) - P(0)]/P(0)$, is used to define effective doses for comparing potencies across chemicals or end points. This response level is used because it is at or near the limit of sensitivity in most chronic bioassays. If a study has greater than usual sensitivity, then a lower BMR (5% or even 1%) can be used. For continuous data, BMR is defined as a percentage change from the estimated control mean, or as a change in a certain number of standard deviations from the control. If there is a minimal level of change in the end point (e.g., liver enzyme activity) that is generally considered to be biologically significant, then that amount of change can be used as the BMR. In the absence of end point-specific data to determine the appropriate level of response as adverse, a change in the mean equal to one control standard deviation can be used. This default approach is used because when values beyond the 98th to 99th percentile of control animals are considered abnormal, a dose that causes a shift in the average of one standard deviation results in an excess risk of approximately 10% of the animals in the abnormal range. Whenever, a BMR is chosen based on biological considerations, the US EPA recommends presenting the resulting BMDL with the BMDL estimated for the default BMR.

To make the BMD from continuous data comparable with the BMD from quantal data, the BMR for continuous data can also be expressed as incidence data. To do this, individual animal data are categorized based on a predetermined cutoff value (e.g., >10% change in organ weight). This incidence data can then be modeled as a quantal end point, with the BMR expressed in terms of an incidence change from the control. This approach is not optimal, because some information is lost in this data categorization. A better way to convert the continuous BMR to a quantal BMR is to use a hybrid approach that uses all of the information contained in the original observations. The hybrid approach fits continuous models to the continuous data. Based on the probability information in the continuous dose–response curve and a cutoff value for defining adverse response, a BMD for a specified quantal BMR (e.g., 10%) can be calculated. This result can be compared directly with other BMDs estimated from quantal data. A limitation for using the hybrid approach is that it requires definition of a background incidence of abnormality, or the specification of a level of response that can be considered the cutoff point between normal and abnormal responses. The selection of the cutoff point is often difficult.

BMD Model Evaluation

Once a particular data set is considered suitable for BMD modeling and an appropriate BMR has been chosen, a group of models (selected according to the nature of the data) is fit to the data. Good BMD model software should provide statistics for assessing model fit, including measures of global and local data fit. Guidance is available from the US EPA on evaluating the statistical fit of various models. Although statistical evaluation is critical, the use of scientific judgment remains essential when conducting dose–response modeling. An ideal data set should provide information on the shape of the dose–response curve, especially at the region close to the BMR. When this occurs, BMD estimates from various models should provide similar results as long as these models provide a comparable data fit (i.e., BMD estimates are not model dependent). In contrast, the BMD model is of limited utility if the dose spacing is such that there is no information on the shape of the dose–response curve, such as when there is 0% response in the control group, and very high (e.g., >80%) response in the low-dose group. In some cases, however, applicable models might diverge with respect to BMD estimates. Therefore, it is necessary to analyze the data and determine whether there is a reason to prefer certain models, such as there is an underlying biological basis for choosing a dose–response shape in the region of the BMR or one of the models fits the data better in the 10% response region. For some data sets, plateauing or nonmonotonicity of the response rates may occur in the high-dose region. If such plateauing drives the model fit, resulting in poor fit in the low-dose region, it may be appropriate to consider excluding the high dose(s) from the modeling. These examples are just a few of the many qualitative considerations needed to select an appropriate modeling result. The US EPA has developed a benchmark dose software (BMDS) package that provides

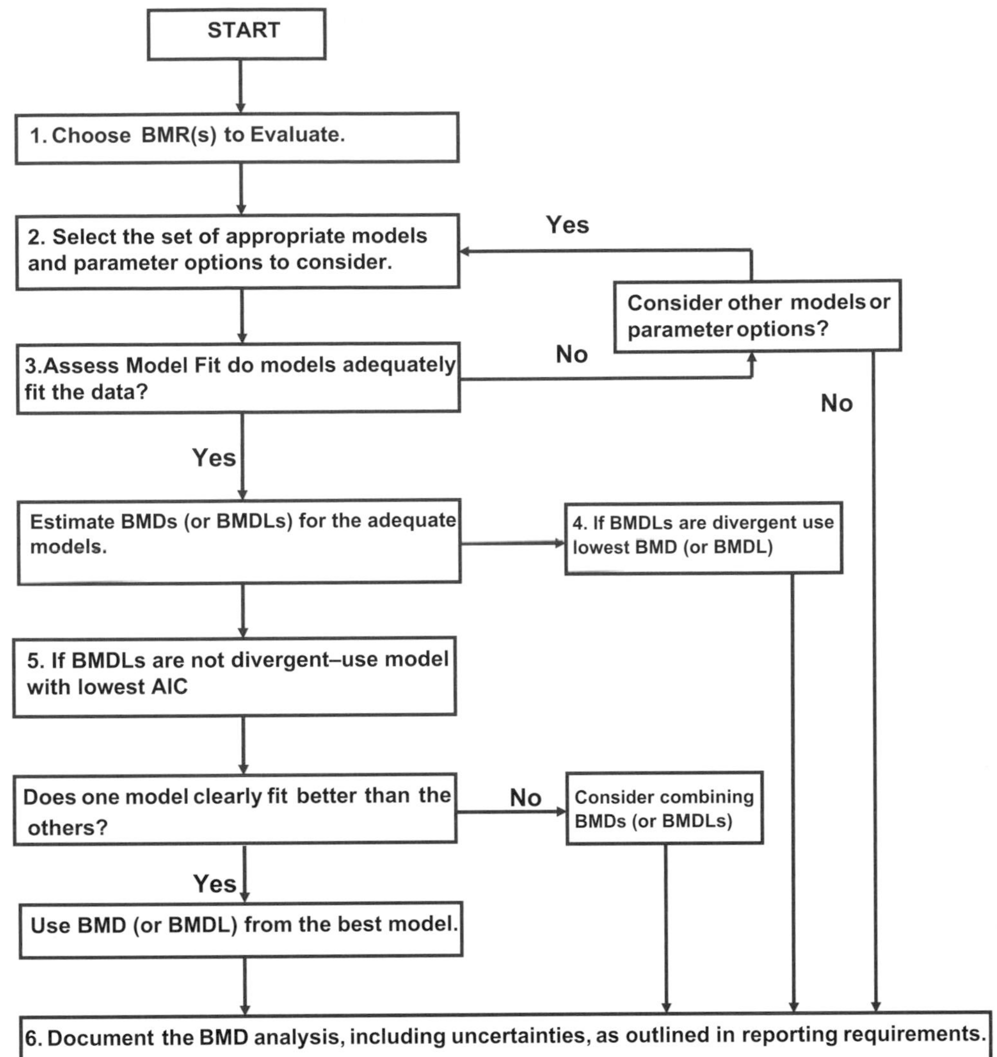

Figure 2 US EPA's BMD analysis framework.

various models for quantal, continuous, and nested data (developmental toxicity study results). Development of BMDS began in 1995 and its first prototype version was released in 1997. It underwent extensive external and public reviews in 1998–99 and quality assurance testing in 1999–2000. In September 2000, the US EPA released BMDS version 1.2 for public use and several versions have been released periodically since then. The current version of BMDS, version 2.1.1, represents more than a decade's worth of model and software development and state-of-the-science in quantitative toxicological dose–response analysis. It contains interface improvements and several new models: a ten Berge model for concentration × time ($C \times t$) analyses, a toxicodiffusion model for neurotoxicology analyses, and the new nested family of continuous exponential models. The software can be downloaded from the US EPA's Web site (http://www.epa.gov/NCEA/bmds) free of charge, and it is frequently updated. This Web site also provides support documentation, including a software user's manual and a guidance document on the interpretation and use of BMD modeling (http://www.epa.gov/ncea/pdfs/bmds/BMD-External_10_13_2000.pdf). In summary, to maintain consistency and reproducibility, the US EPA has developed a six-step process for BMD analysis (**Figure 2**). The six steps involved in the BMD analysis are (1) choosing a BMR, (2) selecting a set of models, (3) assessing model fit, (4) model selection when BMDLs are divergent, (5) model selection when BMDLs are not divergent, via Akaike's Information Criterion (AIC), a model selection criterion used to compare models belonging to different classes, and (6) data reporting.

The most important logic in favor of the BMD approach is as follows:

1. Whether the magnitude of an effect is considered adverse or not (i.e., the selection of the BMR) is determined deliberately on the basis of its toxicological relevance and not only on statistical arguments.
2. The BMD is not restricted to one of the experimental dose levels, and is therefore less dependent on dose selection and spacing.

3. A BMD can be calculated from an experiment lacking a clear NOAEL. Therefore, experiments may not have to be repeated.
4. Quantitative dose–response information is taken into account by fitting a model to all the dose–response data, so that all doses and the slope of the curve influence the calculations.
5. By using PROAST (possible risk obtained from animal studies), it is possible to analyze two related data sets at the same time (e.g., males and females), two subpopulations, or two chemicals. In this way, potential differences in sensitivity between the two data sets may be recognized. The PROAST software was developed by the Dutch National Institute for Public Health and the Environment (RIVM) in Bilthoven and is available from the RIVM web site (http://www.rivm.nl/proast).
6. The uncertainty around a BMD can be quantified by calculating the BMDL. The higher the uncertainty is, the larger the confidence interval becomes, that is, the distance between BMD and BMDL is larger as is the ratio of the two values. That means additional information for risk managers.
7. A study with more animals yields narrower CLs on the BMD and thus a higher BMDL. Therefore, the BMD approach favors good experiments with respect to study design (i.e., number of animals and spacing of dose levels).
8. The BMD approach also gives information on the dose–response relationship. For instance, if exposure exceeds the BMD, the resulting effect at that dose can be estimated from the dose–response curve.

Conclusions

With increased knowledge in research and inclusion of BMD approaches in several regulatory testing guidance documents on the health risk assessment process, it is likely that the use and acceptance of the BMD method will increase substantially in the coming years. It has been suggested that the BMD concept clearly represents a methodological improvement in the field of health risk assessment of chemicals and has clear advantages over the NOAEL approach as a tool for dose–response assessment.

See also: Risk Assessment; Safety Assessment; Dose–Response Relationship; LOAEL; NOAEL; POD; Reference Dose (rfd); Uncertainty Factors.

Further Reading

The Use of the Benchmark Dose (BMD) Approach in Health Risk Assessment. Final Report. Risk Assessment Forum, U.S. Environmental Protection Agency, Washington, DC recommendations for application in health risk assessment. Crit. Rev. Toxicol. 33, 505–542.

Davis, J.A., Gift, J.S., Zhao, Q.J., 2011. Introduction to benchmark dose methods and U.S. EPA's benchmark dose software (BMDS) version 2.1.1. Toxicol. Appl. Pharmacol. 15, 181–191.

ECHA, 2008. Guidance on Information Requirements and Chemical Safety Assessment. Chapter R.8: Characterisation of Dose (Concentration)–Response for Human Health. European Chemicals Agency, Helsinki, Finland.

EFSA, 2009. Guidance of the scientific committee in risk assessment on a request from EFSA on the use of the benchmark dose approach in risk assessment. EFSA J. 1150, 1–72.

Hodgson, E., 2010. A Textbook of Modern Toxicology, fourth ed. John Wiley & Sons, Inc., Hoboken, New Jersey.

Muri, S.D., Schlatter, J.R., Brüschweiler, B.J., 2009. The benchmark dose approach in food risk assessment: is it applicable and worthwhile? Food Chem. Toxicol. 47, 2906–2925.

Oberg, M., 2010. Benchmark dose approaches in chemical health risk assessment in relation to number and distress of laboratory animals. Regul. Toxicol. Pharmacol. 58, 451–454.

Sand, S., Victorin, K., Filipsson, A.F., 2008. The current state of knowledge on the use of the benchmark dose concept in risk assessment. J. Appl. Toxicol. 28 (4), 405–421.

Travis, K.Z., Pate, I., Welsh, Z.K., 2005. The role of the benchmark dose in a regulatory context. Regul. Toxicol. Pharmacol. 43, 280–291.

U.S. Environmental Protection Agency, 2000. Background information about the benchmark dose model used by EPA, as well as instructions for downloading and using the model http://www.epa.gov/NCEA/bmds/index.html. Additional guidance from EPA can be found at: http://www.epa.gov/ncea/pdfs/bmds/BMD-External_10_13_2000.pdf.

US EPA, 2000. Benchmark Dose Technical Guidance Document. United States Environmental Protection Agency. External Review Draft. EPA/630/R-00/001.

WHO, 2009. Principles for Modeling Dose–Response for the Risk Assessment of Chemicals. Environmental Health Criteria 239. World Health Organization, Geneva.

Relevant Websites

http://www.epa.gov/NCEA/bmds/index.html – US Environmental Protection Agency: Benchmark Dose Software.

http://cfpub.epa.gov/ncea/cfm/recordisplay.cfm?deid=20871 – US Environmental Protection Agency: Benchmark Dose Technical Guidance Document.

Benfluralin

YR Rodriguez, Phoenix, AZ, USA

- Name: Benfluralin
- Chemical Abstracts Service Registry Number: 1861-40-1
- Synonyms: Benefin, Balan, Balfin, Benafine, Benalan, Benefex
- Molecular Formula: $C_{13}H_{16}F_3N_3O_4$
- Chemical Structure:

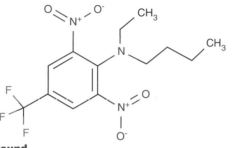

Background

Since 1970, benfluralin has been registered in the United States as a preemergent dinitroaniline herbicide. In 2004, the US Environmental Protection Agency (EPA) conducted an assessment to determine if pesticide products containing the active ingredient of benfluralin were eligible for pesticide reregistration. The criteria included meeting current human health and safety standards, and determining if the pesticide being used poses any unreasonable risks to human health and the environment. Results of the US EPA assessment were explained in the Reregistration Eligibility Decision (RED) of benfluralin. The RED document determined that pesticides with the active ingredient of benfluralin were eligible for reregistration provided certain stipulations listed in the RED document were met that included additional label requirements. Under the Federal Insecticide, Fungicide, and Rodenticide Act (FIFRA) Section 3, all new pesticides used in the United States must be registered by the Administrator of the US EPA. There are 38 products registered for benfluralin.

Uses

Benfluralin is a preemergent herbicide registered to control monocot (one cotyledon: plant embryo with single 'seed leaf') and dicot (two cotyledon: plant embryo with two 'seed leaves') weeded species in commercial and residential applications. Target species for benfluralin include Johnson grass seedlings, chickweed, lamb quarters, purslane, knotweed, clover, and barnyard grass. Benfluralin affects seed germination and prevents weed growth by inhibition of root development. Absorbed by roots, benfluralin inhibits microtubule formation by binding to tubulin, thereby disrupting cell division and leading to microfibril disorientation. Benfluralin can be used alone or formulated with other structurally related preemergent herbicides. Benfluralin has been formulated with oryzalin, isoxaben, triclopyr and/or trifluralin. Various formulated types include emulsifiable concentrate, granules, soluble concentrate/liquid, and water dispersed granules. Benfluralin is formulated as granules in 42 end-use products and one product in the form of water dispersible granules. Applications can be by broadcast (granules and fertilizer mixed) and band treatment, golf course treatment, soil incorporated treatment, and spray with ground/sprinkler irrigation systems. Agricultural usage of benfluralin is predominately on lettuce, alfalfa, clover, birdsfoot trefoil, nonbearing fruit and nut trees, and vineyards. From 2000 to 2008, the annual US agriculture consumption average of the active ingredient was an estimated 60 000 pounds. The crop responsible for the largest usage of benfluralin is lettuce, followed by alfalfa. Nonagricultural use includes turf, golf courses, ornamentals, Christmas tree plantations, fence rows/hedgerows, and rights of way. In 2007, the annual US average nonagriculture use of the active ingredient was an estimated 700 000 pounds. The primary usage of benfluralin is on commercial and residential turf. It has been reported that there is some minor benfluralin usage on tobacco, onions, broccoli, and pasture/range. There are residue tolerances for only some of these uses. Total active ingredient usage is unknown.

Environmental Fate and Behavior

Use of benfluralin as a preemergent herbicide results in a direct release into the environment. Benfluralin has an estimated Henry's law constant of 2.91×10^{-4} atm-m^{3}mol^{-1} derived from a vapor pressure of 6.6×10^{-5} mmHg. Benfluralin has a water solubility of 0.1 mg l^{-1}, an octanol/water partition coefficient of $K_{ow} = 5.29$ and a soil organic carbon–water partitioning coefficient range of $K_{oc} = 9840$ to 11 660.

Based on the Henry's law constant, volatilization of benfluralin from moist soil surfaces and water surfaces is expected. However, volatilization of benfluralin from dry soil surface is not expected. Benfluralin is typically formulated and applied to minimize volatilization. Benfluralin K_{oc} value range indicates a decreased mobility in soil. The K_{oc} value also indicates that benfluralin can be expected to adsorb to suspended solids and sediment in the water column.

Environmental degradation of benfluralin in soil occurs by oxidation (aerobic soil conditions) or reduction (anaerobic soil conditions). The rate at which benfluralin degrades in soil is based on conditions such as temperature, moisture content, and organic carbon content. Benfluralin has a moderate half-life of 22–79 days under aerobic soil conditions, suggesting a slow-degradation process. Under anaerobic soil conditions, benfluralin has a half-life of 12 days. Studies indicate any remaining benfluralin on soil surfaces can be subject to photodecomposition. The soil photolysis half-life is 12.5 days. Soil

 http://dx.doi.org/10.1016/B978-0-12-386454-3.01166-0

residual activity can range from 4 to 8 months. The aqueous photolysis half-life ranges from 5.5 to 9.9 h. Benfluralin has a short estimated half-life in air (less than 12 h), indicating persistency in air to be minimal. Major degradation products of benfluralin include 2,6-dinitro-*N*-ethyl-4-trifluoromethylbenzeneamine, *N*-(*N*-butyl)-2,6-dinitro-4-trifluoromethylbenzeneamine, and 4-nitro-2-propyl-6-trifluoromethyl-1H-benzimidazole.

Based on the K_{oc} values, benfluralin is expected to have very little mobility in soil and is not expected to leach into groundwater. However, introduction into surface water by runoff from soil treated with benfluralin is possible.

Due to a high octanol/water partition coefficient ($\log P_{ow} = 5.29$), benfluralin has the potential to bioaccumulate in aquatic organisms. Aquatic studies indicate a depuration rate of 0.54 per day for whole fish.

Exposure and Exposure Monitoring

As stated above in Uses, benfluralin is an herbicide utilized in residential and commercial applications. These applications directly release the compound into the environment. The production of benfluralin may also result in a release into the environment via various waste streams.

Occupational exposure to benfluralin may occur with inhalation and dermal contact during mixing/loading and applying. General public exposure may occur through ingestion from a contaminated drinking water source or dermal contact during and after application on home lawns and landscape ornamental plants.

Monitoring data for benfluralin is available from the US Geological Survey (GS) National Water Quality Assessment Program (NAWQA) in surface water and groundwater. Surface water monitoring has been conducted in all 50 states of the United States. Of the 29 158 surface water samples collected, 343 resulted in positive detects, with a minimum limit reporting (MLR) ranging from 0 to 0.079 $\mu g\,l^{-1}$ and a medium MLR of 0.002 $\mu g\,l^{-1}$. The maximum concentration of benfluralin in a surface water sample was 0.205 $\mu g\,l^{-1}$ which was collected in a predominately agricultural area. The USDA Pesticide Data Program database conducted a surface water source drinking water study and did not detect benfluralin in water. The detection range was from 0.002 to 0.05 $\mu g\,l^{-1}$.

USGS NAWQA groundwater monitoring has been conducted in 48 states of the United States. Of the 12 502 groundwater samples collected, 16 resulted in positive detects, with an MLR ranging from 0 to 0.09 $\mu g\,l^{-1}$ and a medium MLR of 0.01 $\mu g\,l^{-1}$. The maximum concentration of benfluralin in a groundwater sample was 0.011 $\mu g\,l^{-1}$. Benfluralin is not identified as a cause of impairment for any water body listed as impaired under the Clean Water Act section 303 (d).

Toxicokinetics

There are no data available for human absorption, distribution, metabolism, and excretion of benfluralin. In Fischer 344 rats, benfluralin is dealkylated and is excreted in the urine and feces.

Mechanism of Toxicity

Mechanism of toxicity data are limited. Liver is one known target organ. During a 3-month rat subchronic toxicity study, hepatic microsomal enzyme activity, measured by *p*-nitroanisole *O*-demethylase activity, was significantly elevated in both rat sexes. These results suggest that mixed function oxidases were induced in the livers of the rats. The rat subchronic study dose levels were the same and lower than those showing hepatocellular adenomas/carcinomas in the chronic/carcinogenicity studies. Because this chemical shows no evidence of mutagenicity in short-term genotoxicity tests, a nongenotoxic mechanism of action is likely. In plants, benfluralin inhibits microtubule formation by binding to tubulin, disrupting cell division and leading to microfibril disorientation, but whether this has any relevance to the mechanism of toxicity in mammals does not appear to have been studied.

Acute and Short-Term Toxicity

In acute studies, benfluralin has a low acute toxicity and falls into Toxicity Category IV when oral and inhalation routes of exposure are considered. In an acute oral rat study, benfluralin had an $LD_{50} > 10\,g\,kg^{-1}$. No rat died during the course of the study. Benfluralin is not a primary skin or eye irritant; however, it is classified as a dermal sensitizer and was placed in Toxicity Category III. During a guinea pig study, benfluralin was found to be a dermal sensitizer in 7 out of 12 subjects. In an acute rabbit study, benfluralin was slightly irritating to the eyes but conditions were reversible in 7 days. Based on this study, benfluralin is considered to be in the Toxicity Category III for acute eye exposure. The published human toxicity data for benfluralin are incomplete and lacking in any information about acute neurotoxicity, subchronic neurotoxicity, or immunotoxicity.

Chronic Toxicity

In long-term animal studies, benfluralin is toxic to the kidneys and liver. In a chronic female rat study, kidney and liver effects were detected at doses of 20 $mg\,kg^{-1}\,day^{-1}$. During a chronic dog study, four Beagle dogs were exposed to benefin. Liver weights were increased and an increased incidence of hepatocellular hypertrophy was observed in the high doses. Additionally, an increased incidence of hemosiderin pigment was observed in the livers at high doses and in the spleen at mid- and high-dose levels. In high-dose levels, benfluralin is toxic to the thyroid. In a chronic male rat study, dose levels as high as 136.3 $mg\,kg^{-1}\,day^{-1}$ produced thyroid toxicity.

Immunotoxicity

Benfluralin has been classified as a dermal sensitizer in guinea pigs. However, there are no confirmed human cases of allergic contact dermatitis to benfluralin. There is a case report of a 61-year-old man with allergic contact dermatitis caused by exposure to multiple pesticides. The patient was employed as a laboratory supervisor of a chemical pesticide company, performing quality testing of various herbicides and pesticide, since 1951. The individual was exposed to multiple pesticides/herbicides, including benefin, diazinon, carbaryl, prodiamine, triadimefon, chlorothalonil, dithiopyr, trifluralin, oxadiazon, mecoprop, siduron, isofenphos, and chlorpyrifos. Exposure and frequency varied from months to more than 20 years. The individual was patch tested with the North American Contact Dermatitis Group Standard Tray to manufacture-recommended, nonirritating concentrations of analytic-grade benefin and four other similar chemicals. The patient had positive reactions to benefin and two others. The case study included 12 control subjects patch tested to the same pesticides, all subjects had negative reactions. The case study investigators could not determine which herbicide was the primary sensitizer. The US EPA Office of Pesticide Programs (OPP) classifies benfluralin as a dermal sensitizer.

Reproductive and Developmental Toxicity

A two-generation rat reproduction study of benfluralin in the diet showed a decrease in live pups at the highest dose tested. A teratology study in rabbits showed no effect on fetuses at the highest dose tested that caused maternal toxicity. Benfluralin has caused reproductive effects in chronic avian studies. A chronic reproduction study using Bobwhite Quail (*Colinus virginianus*) showed developmental effects at the lowest observed adverse effect concentration (96 mg kg^{-1}) including a decrease in surviving hatchlings, decreased egg set, and a decrease in surviving hatchling weight. The LOAEC, 975 mg kg^{-1}, in the Mallard duck (*Anas platyrhynchos*) displayed an increase in the percentage of eggs that cracked. There are no available data in humans.

Genotoxicity

Mutagenicity studies indicate there is no concern for benfluralin. Studies in the *Salmonella typhimurium* gene mutation assay, mouse lymphoma cell forward gene mutation test, Chinese Hamster Ovary cell cytogenetic assay and DNA repair assay in primary rat hepatocytes were all negative.

Carcinogenicity

The Cancer Assessment Review Committee (CARC) concluded there is suggestive evidence of carcinogenicity but not sufficient to assess human carcinogenic potential. The results are based on a carcinogenicity study in $B6C3F_1$ mice. During a 2-year study of $B6C3F_1$ female mice, animals received diets containing benfluralin at dose levels of 0, 7, 42, and 224 mg kg^{-1} day^{-1}. The study resulted in a borderline statistically significant increasing trend and a borderline significant increase by pairwise comparison of the 224 mg $kg^{-1}day^{-1}$ dose group with the controls for combined liver adenomas/carcinomas only. The CARC concluded that benfluralin caused liver tumors. The International Agency for Research on Cancer (IARC) has not classified benfluralin; however, trifluralin, an analog herbicide that is sometimes formulated in conjunction with benfluralin is listed to have a carcinogen rating of III. Trifluralin has a cancer classification that suggests evidence of carcinogenicity, but is not sufficient to assess human carcinogenic potential. Chronic trifluralin studies indicate hepatocellular carcinomas in animals.

Clinical Management

There are 47 reported human cases of exposure to benfluralin in both occupational and nonoccupational settings. Three of the cases required medical attention due to skin irritation or pain and itching that required medical attention. The other exposures resulted in minor irritation or no irritation and did not require health care facility attention. In all the exposure cases hospitalization was not required. Benfluralin may be irritating to the skin and eyes. Additionally, because it has been shown to be a skin sensitizer in animal studies, decontamination steps should be taken if exposed to benfluralin. Individuals exposed should remove contaminated clothing and flush the exposed area immediately. In the event of a large accidental ingestion, activated charcoal is probably the most effective treatment. Smaller ingestion amounts will probably result in vomiting and diarrhea. There are no known human fatalities from benfluralin exposure.

Ecotoxicology

There are no acute data available in freshwater fish. In a chronic benfluralin study, rainbow trout (*Oncorhynchus mykiss*) had a no observed adverse effect concentration of 0.0019 mg l^{-1} based on reduced larval weight, length, and survival. The same study determined the LOAEC in rainbow trout (*O. mykiss*) to be 0.005 mg l^{-1}. There were no available data for acute or chronic freshwater invertebrates.

In estuarine/marine invertebrates, benfluralin is classified as very acutely toxic. In an acute study using benfluralin, Sheepshead minnow (*Cyprinodon variegatus*) had an $EC_{50} > 0.0838$ mg l^{-1}. The reported no observed effect concentration in this species is the maximum concentration tested, 0.0838 mg l^{-1}, because no sublethal effects or moralities were reported. There are no available data for chronic estuarine/marine fish studies. In acute estuarine/marine invertebrates, benfluralin is classified as very highly toxic. In an acute basis benfluralin study, Mysid shrimp (*Americamysis bahia*) had an LC_{50} of 0.043 mg l^{-1}. A flow-through acute basis benfluralin study using oysters (*Crassostrea virginica*) determined the NOEC to be 0.001 mg l^{-1}. There are no available data for chronic estuarine/marine invertebrates.

There are no acceptable data currently available for nonvascular aquatic plants. In a study for vascular aquatic plants (Duckweed, *Lemna gibba*) the EC_{50} and NOAEC are 0.036 mg l^{-1} and 0.015 mg l^{-1}, respectively. There are no acceptable data currently available for terrestrial plants.

On an acute toxicity basis, benfluralin is practically nontoxic to birds, bees, and small mammals. No sublethal effects were observed from studies using both birds and bees. In the Bobwhite Quail (*C. virginianus*) the $LD_{50} > 2000$ mg l^{-1} and in bees the $LD_{50} > 100\ \mu g\ bee^{-1}$. Benfluralin is categorized as practically nontoxic to small mammals on an acute oral basis. In a rat acute oral study, the LD_{50} was observed to be greater than $10\,000\ mg\ l^{-1}$.

Exposure Standards and Guidelines

There are established US tolerances for residues of benfluralin on alfalfa, birdsfoot trefoil, clover, lettuce, and peanuts. These tolerances are listed in 40 CFR §180.208 and are set at 0.05 ppm. There is no Codex maximum residue limit for benfluralin.

The tolerances listed in 40 CFR §180.208 have not been updated to reflect current US EPA Health Effects Division policies and are under review for the reregistration process.

No Total Maximum Daily Loads have been developed for benfluralin. Additionally, there is no Maximum Contaminant Level for benfluralin.

Noncancer occupational handler inhalation risk estimates were conducted and below the level of concern. There is a potential for occupational post application exposure to occur; however, assessments have not been completed.

See also: Pesticides; Environmental Risk Assessment, Pesticides and Biocides.

Further Reading

Benfluralin: Summary Document Registration Review: Initial Docket December 2011, Docket Number: EPA-HQ-OPP-2011-0931.

Benfluralin: Registration Review Scoping Document for Human Health Assessments, Docket Number: EPA-HQ-OPP-2011-0931-004, December 12, 2011.

Benfluralin: Registration Review – Preliminary Problem Formulation for the Environmental Fate and Ecological Risk, Drinking Water, and Endangered Species Assessments for Benfluralin, Docket Number: EPA-HQ-OPP-2011-0931-003, December 12, 2011.

Benfluralin: Hazardous Substance Data Bank: http://toxnet.nlm.nih.gov (accessed 7.03.12).

U.S. EPA RED Facts, Docket Number: EPA-738-F-04–007, July 31, 2004.

U.S. EPA Reregistration Eligibility Decision for Benfluralin, Docket Number: EPA-738-R-04–012, July 2004.

Relevant Website

http://www.epa.gov – U.S. Environmental Protection Agency

Benomyl

MA Pearson and GW Miller, Emory University, Atlanta, GA, USA

This article is a revision of the previous edition article by Jamaluddin Shaikh, volume 1, pp 248–249, © 2005, Elsevier Inc.

- Name: Benomyl
- Chemical Abstracts Service Registry Number: CAS 17804-35-2
- Synonyms: Agrocit; Fundazole; Benomyl 50W; Benlate; Fungicide D-1991; Methyl 1-(butylcarbamoyl)-2-benzimidazolylcarbamate
- Molecular Formula: $C_{14}H_{18}N_4O_3$
- Chemical Structure:

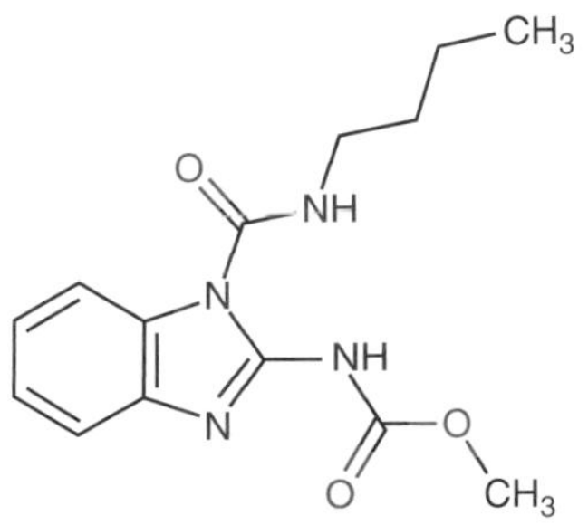

Background (Significance/History)

Benomyl, a systemic benzimidazole fungicide, was introduced by DuPont in 1968 and was one of the most widely used benzimidazoles. However, in 2001, DuPont stopped producing benomyl and canceled its registration due to the prevalent development of parasitic fungi resistance and accumulating toxicological evidence in laboratory mammals of liver abnormalities and reproductive effects. Production and use may still occur outside the United States.

Uses

Benomyl was primarily used as a fungicide against more than 190 different fungal diseases affecting fruits, nuts, vegetables, turf, and field crops. Benomyl also has an inhibitory effect on mite populations and has been used as an ascaricide. Benomyl is formulated as a wettable powder.

Environmental Fate and Behavior

Experimentally, soil tests from the site of application have shown that benomyl and its two soil metabolites did not leach or move significantly. In the field, the half-life of benomyl was 3 days; for methyl 2-benzimidazolecarbamate (MBC or carbendazim), a principal degradation product of benomyl, the half-life ranged from 51 to 83 days, depending on soil type and weather conditions. In water, benomyl is rapidly hydrolyzed to carbendazim within hours. The half-life of carbendazim is approximately 60 days. These experimental results are consistent with both the Henry's Law constant for benomyl, which is 4.93×10^{-12} atm-m^3 mol^{-1}, and its vapor pressure of 3.7×10^{-9} mm Hg.

Exposure Routes and Pathways

Probable occupational exposure routes include inhalation and dermal contact, while the general population could be exposed from ingesting food products containing benomyl.

Toxicokinetics

Benomyl is readily absorbed after oral and inhalation exposure, but poorly absorbed following dermal exposure. Benomyl is metabolized to carbendazim and butyl isocyanate (BIC). Carbendazim undergoes further hydroxylation and conjugation resulting in the principal urinary metabolites of methyl-5-hydroxy-2-benzimidazole-carbamate and 4-hydroxy-2-benzimidazole-carbamate, which are also detectable at lower percentages in feces. Benomyl and its metabolites did not accumulate in tissues following a 2-year feeding study in dogs and rats. Evidence suggests that BIC is metabolized into *S*-methyl *N*-butylthiocarbamate (MBT), and then further converted by cytochrome P450 enzymes to MBT sulfoxide (MBT-SO).

Mechanism of Toxicity

Benomyl prevents fungal proliferation by interfering with microtubule formation and has been identified as a ubiquitin–proteasome system inhibitor – carbendazim is likely responsible for both these actions. Benomyl caused aneuploidy and/or polyploidy in experimental systems *in vitro* and *in vivo*. Benomyl inhibits aldehyde dehydrogenase (ALDH) activity in liver and brain mitochondria, likely as a result of the downstream metabolite, MBT-SO, a known ALDH inhibitor.

In yeast culture treated with benomyl, alpha-synuclein aggregation and toxicity were enhanced, possibly resulting from the microtubule-disrupting properties of carbendazim. Studies of the downstream metabolites of BIC demonstrate that benomyl inhibits mouse mitochondrial ALDH *in vivo* and *in vitro* at nanomolar levels. In a recent report, benomyl also inhibited ALDH in primary mesencephalic neurons and induced dopaminergic neuronal damage. These *in vitro* studies provide potential new mechanisms through which benomyl could contribute to neurodegenerative diseases such as Parkinson's disease.

Acute and Short-Term Toxicity

Animals

The oral LD_{50} value for benomyl and carbendazim in rats and the dermal LD_{50} value of benomyl for rabbits is greater than 10 000 mg kg^{-1}. Benomyl produced temporary mild conjunctival irritation in the eyes of rats. In subchronic studies, all oral

 http://dx.doi.org/10.1016/B978-0-12-386454-3.00102-0

doses of benomyl tested (lowest dosage: 25 mg kg^{-1}) led to the premature release of germ cells (sloughing) in rats. In a separate 7-day diet study, benomyl led to a dose-dependent increase in the incidence and severity of liver changes in rats.

Humans

Benomyl may cause skin and eye irritation upon contact. Redness and edema have been reported in occupationally exposed individuals on skin not covered by clothing. Sensitization may occur, in which subsequent, low-level exposures can cause itching and a skin rash.

Chronic Toxicity

Animals

Repetitive dosing studies of benomyl indicated teratogenicity, oncogenicity, reproductive toxicity, and adverse effects on the liver. Teratogenic effects following benomyl administration during pregnancy included microphthalmia, hydrocephaly, and encephaloceles, and, in mice, skeletal and visceral anomalies were observed. Hepatotoxicity was observed in mice, rats, and dogs following long-term repetitive dosing with benomyl and/or carbendazim.

Humans

In a recent epidemiologic analysis, a 67% increased risk for Parkinson's disease was associated with estimated workplace exposure to benomyl.

Immunotoxicity

Little is known regarding the adverse effects of benomyl on the immune system.

Reproductive Toxicity

Testicular function in male rates was adversely affected by benomyl, including decreased testicular sperm counts, reduced cauda sperm reserves, decreased sperm production, increased numbers of decapitated spermatozoa, decreased testicular weight, and degeneration and atrophy of seminiferous tubules.

Genotoxicity

Benomyl induces aneuploidy, but not gene mutations. In assays using Chinese hamster lung and Chinese hamster ovary cell lines, benomyl and carbendazim are positive for numerical aberrations. An aneuploidy effect was also observed in bone-marrow micronucleus assays, with a dose-related significant increase in total micronucleated polychromatic erythrocytes and an increase in the frequency of kinetochore-positive micronuclei for benomyl.

Carcinogenicity

Increases in ovarian tumors and liver tumors in mice were observed in long-term exposure studies. A review suggested that hepatotoxicity, increased liver weights, cell proliferation, and hypertrophy precede neoplasms. There was no evidence of increased tumors in similar long-term exposure studies in rats.

Clinical Management

In the case of skin contact, remove any contaminated clothing and wash the affected skin with soap and water. If the eyes are exposed, flush the eyes with large amounts of water, lifting the upper and lower eyelids. If exposure is due to inhalation, the patient should be moved to fresh air. If the patient does not recover rapidly, medical attention should be sought. In case of ingestion, if conscious, the mouth should be rinsed with plenty of water, 250 ml of water should be consumed, and vomiting induced.

Ecotoxicology

Benomyl is slightly to highly toxic to aquatic organisms and moderately toxic to birds. Benomyl affects the growth and mortality of amphibians, reduces the abundance of duckweed, influences genetics and mortality in crustaceans, and is highly toxic to fish, especially catfish. Reduced populations of earthworms have been reported in benomyl-treated orchards, as low, chronic exposures are lethal to earthworms.

Exposure Standards and Guidelines

The acceptable daily intake is 0.03 mg kg^{-1} and the permissible exposure limit averaged over an 8-h work shift is 15 mg m^{-3} (total dust) and 5 mg m^{-3} (respirable fraction).

See also: Pesticides; Neurotoxicity; Carbamate Pesticides.

Further Reading

Fitzmaurice, A.G., Rhodese, S.L., Lullad, A., Murphyf, N.P., Lamf, H.A., et al., 2012. Aldehyde dehydrogenase inhibition as a pathogenic mechanism in Parkinson disease. Proc. Natl. Acad. Sci. USA. http://dx.doi.org/10.1073/pnas.1220399110 Published online before print.

McCarroll, N.E., Protzel, A., Ioannou, Y., Frank Stack, H.F., Jackson, M.A., et al., 2002. A survey of EPA/OPP and open literature on selected pesticide chemicals. III. Mutagenicity and carcinogenicity of benomyl and carbendazim. Mutat. Res. 512 (1), 1–35. PMID: 12220588.

Relevant Websites

http://www.epa.gov/oppsrrd1/REDs/factsheets/benomyl_fs.htm – Environmental Protection Agency's Reregistration Eligibility Decision for benomyl.

http://toxnet.nlm.nih.gov – Hazardous Substances Data Bank.

Benz[a]anthracene

JP Gray and GJ Hall, U.S. Coast Guard Academy, New London, CT, USA

This article is a revision of the previous edition article by Madhusudan G. Soni, volume 1, pp 250–251, © 2005, Elsevier Inc.

- Name: Benz[a]anthracene
- Chemical Abstracts Service Registry Number: CAS 56-55-3
- Synonyms: 1,2-Benz[a]anthracene; 1,2-Benzanthracene; 1,2-Benzanthrene; 1,2-Benzoanthracene; 2,3-Benzophenanthrene; BA; B[a]A; Benzanthracene; Benzanthrene; Benz[a]anthracene; Benzo[b]phenanthrene; Benzoanthracene; Tetraphene; Naphthanthracene
- Molecular Formula: $C_{18}H_{12}$
- Chemical Structure:

Background (Significance/History)

A procarcinogen, benz[a]anthracene is metabolized to its carcinogenic form by phase 1 and phase 2 metabolism. As with other polycyclic aromatic hydrocarbons (PAHs), the presence of the 'bay' region contributes greatly to the carcinogenicity of benz[a]anthracene metabolites. This region is sterically constrained, allowing the formation of diol epoxides, which subsequently react with intracellular molecules such as DNA.

Human exposure to benz[a]anthracene and other PAHs occurs primarily from smoking or second-hand smoke, air polluted with combustion products, or food and water polluted with combustion products.

Uses

Benz[a]anthracene is primarily used in research.

Environmental Fate and Behavior

Benz[a]anthracene is not synthesized commercially. The primary source of many PAHs in air is the combustion of wood and other fuels. PAHs released into the atmosphere may deposit onto soil or water. In surface water, PAHs can volatilize, bind to suspended particles, or accumulate in aquatic organisms. Adsorption to solid particles in the soil extended their half-life, benz[a]anthracene's half-life in Kidman sandy loam is 261 days. The vapor pressure of benz[a]anthracene is 1.9×10^{-6} mm Hg at 25 °C, and it has an atmospheric half-life of about 7.7 h due primarily to photochemical degradation.

Exposure and Exposure Monitoring

Exposure occurs primarily through the diet or smoking. Thermal processes greatly contribute to human exposure to PAHs in foods, such as grilling, roasting, and smoking. Exposure may also occur through bioaccumulation in consumed animals, such as livestock.

Toxicokinetics

Absorption, Distribution, Metabolism, and Excretion (ADME) data are derived from general data for PAHs. Oral absorption is low, but increases with lipophilicity and in the presence of oils in the gastrointestinal tract. Dermal absorption also occurs readily in the presence of lipophilic solvents. Inhalational exposure is common in smokers. PAHs are widely distributed in tissues following oral and inhalational exposure. Metabolism is widely varied, and includes the formation of epoxides, dihydrodiols, phenols, quinones, and combinations, some of which are bioactivated to become toxic products. Conjugation to glucuronides and sulfate esters occurs via phase II metabolism. Hepatobiliary excretion is the primary elimination route of PAHs in animals within 2 days of exposure.

Mechanism of Toxicity

While not toxic itself, benz[a]anthracene and other PAHs containing bay regions are carcinogenic. These compounds are metabolized by cytochrome P450 enzymes in collaboration with epoxide hydrolase to highly reactive diol epoxides. These metabolites in turn covalently bind to nucleophilic sites in DNA and other biological molecules. Benz[a]anthracene may also be metabolized to radical cations that form depurinated DNA adducts.

Acute and Short-Term Toxicity

Animal

Biochemical changes were seen in the gastrointestinal tracts of animals exposed to benz[a]anthracene. Other acute effects include increased liver weight.

Human

Humans are not exposed to benz[a]anthracene in isolation, but rather as part of a mixture of other PAHs. Hazards include eye and lung irritation, nausea, vomiting, and diarrhea. A maximum tolerated human exposure level has not been determined.

Chronic Toxicity

The major chronic toxicity risk is carcinogenesis.

Immunotoxicity

Some PAHs are immunotoxic.

Genotoxicity

Chromosomal aberrations are found in cells from workers routinely exposed to PAHs.

Carcinogenicity

Exposure to benz[a]anthracene almost never occurs in the absence of other PAHs; therefore, individual data on this compound is not available. Metabolites of benz[a]anthracene are mutagenic and carcinogenic, causing carcinogenesis in the liver and lung. Coal tar and other materials that contain benz[a]anthracene are known to be carcinogenic in humans. This compound is 'reasonably anticipated to be carcinogenic in humans' by the National Toxicology Program and is a 'probable human carcinogen' by the Environmental Protection Agency. A large number of animal studies have been performed demonstrating the carcinogenic potential of this compound.

Clinical Management

Upon exposure to any PAH, recommendations include washing contaminated skin with soap and water and flushing contaminated eyes with water or saline. Charcoal administration has been recommended but there is no evidence of its efficacy. As glutathione conjugation is one mechanism by which PAHs are metabolized, administration of *N*-acetyl cysteine was shown in rats to reduce DNA adducts formed by PAHs; however, this has not been shown in humans.

Ecotoxicology

All PAHs accumulate in the aquatic environment and may cause long-term adverse effects.

See also: Polycyclic Aromatic Hydrocarbons (PAHs).

Further Reading

Diggs, D.L., Huderson, A.C., Harris, K.L., et al., 2011. Polycyclic aromatic hydrocarbons and digestive tract cancers – a perspective. J. Environ. Sci. Health C Environ. Carcinogen. Ecotoxicol. Rev. 29, 324–357.

Ramesh, A., Walker, S.A., Hood, D.B., et al., 2004. Bioavailability and risk assessment of orally ingested polycyclic aromatic hydrocarbons. Int. J. Toxicol. 23, 301–333.

Relevant Website

http://www.atsdr.cdc.gov/toxprofiles/tp.asp?id=122&tid=25

Benzene

C Barton, Oak Ridge Institute for Science and Education, Oak Ridge, TN, USA

This article is a revision of the previous edition article by Stephen R. Clough, volume 1, pp 251–253, © 2005, Elsevier Inc.

- Name: Benzene
- Chemical Abstracts Service Registry Number: 71-43-2
- Synonyms: Cyclohexatriene, Benzol, Coal naphtha, Benzole, Phenyl hydride
- Chemical/Pharmaceutical/Other Class: Aromatic hydrocarbon
- Molecular Formula: C_6H_6
- Chemical Structure:

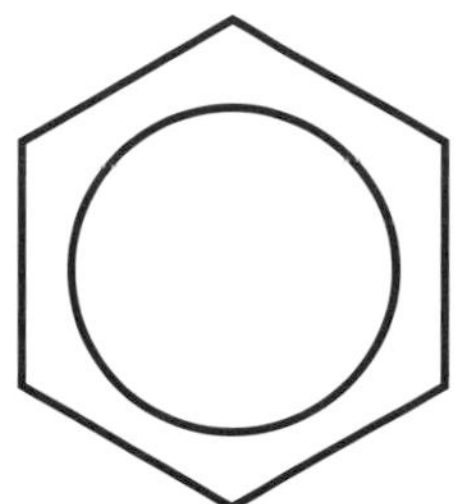

Uses

Benzene is one of the world's major commodity chemicals. Its primary use (85% of production) is as an intermediate in the production of other chemicals, predominantly styrene (for Styrofoam and other plastics), cumene (for various resins), and cyclohexane (for nylon and other synthetic fibers). Smaller amounts of benzene are used to make some types of rubbers, lubricants, dyes, drugs, synthetic detergents, insecticides, fumigants, solvents, paint removers, and gasoline. Benzene is a natural component of crude and refined petroleum. The mandatory decrease in lead alkyls in gasoline has led to an increase in the aromatic hydrocarbon content of gasoline to maintain high octane levels and antiknock properties. In the United States, gasoline typically contains less than 2% benzene by volume, but in other countries, the benzene concentration may be as high as 5%. Benzene is also a by-product of the coking process during steel production. Benzene ranks in the top 20 chemicals for production volume in the United States.

Because of its lipophilic nature, benzene is an excellent solvent. Its use in paints, thinners, inks, adhesives, and rubbers, however, is decreasing and now accounts for less than 2% of current benzene production. Benzene was also an important component of many industrial cleaning and degreasing formulations, but now has been replaced mostly by toluene, chlorinated solvents, or mineral spirits. Although benzene is no longer added in significant quantities to most commercial products, traces of it may still be present as a contaminant.

Exposure Routes and Pathways

Benzene is widespread in the environment. The major sources of benzene exposure are tobacco smoke, automobile service stations, exhaust from motor vehicles, and industrial emissions. Vapors (or gases) from products that contain benzene, such as glues, paints, furniture wax, and detergents, can also be a source of exposure.

Airborne benzene is usually produced by processes associated with chemical manufacturing or the gasoline industry, including gasoline bulk-loading and discharging facilities and combustion engines (e.g., automobiles, lawnmowers, and snowblowers). Benzene is a component of both indoor and outdoor air pollution. Benzene levels measured in ambient outdoor air have a global average of 6 $\mu g\ m^{-3}$ (range 2–9 $\mu g\ m^{-3}$). In almost all cases, benzene levels inside residences or offices are higher than levels outside and still higher in homes with attached garages and those occupied by smokers. Seasonal variations also affect benzene levels, with higher levels found in the fall and winter when buildings are less well ventilated. People living around hazardous waste sites, petroleum-refining operations, petrochemical manufacturing sites, or gas stations may be exposed to higher levels of benzene in air. In addition to being inhaled, airborne benzene is absorbed across intact skin in experimental animals. For most people, the level of exposure to benzene through food, beverages, or drinking water is not as high as their exposure through air.

Leakage from underground storage tanks and seepage from landfills or improper disposal of hazardous wastes have resulted in benzene contamination of groundwater used for drinking. Effluent from industries is also a source of groundwater contamination. In addition to being ingested, benzene in water can also be absorbed through wet skin and inhaled as it volatilizes during showering, laundering, or cooking. Typical drinking water contains less than 0.1 ppb benzene. Benzene has been detected in bottled water, liquor, and food.

Cigarette smoke is another common source of personal and environmental benzene exposure, representing about half of the benzene to which the general population is exposed. Persons who smoke one pack of cigarettes a day inhale a daily dose of approximately 1 mg of benzene, about 3–4% of the amount inhaled daily by a worker exposed at the current occupational permissible exposure limit (PEL). Nonsmokers who live with smokers and who are passively exposed to environmental tobacco smoke typically experience 50% greater exposure to benzene than do nonsmokers who live in a smoke-free environment.

Toxicokinetics

Benzene is lipid soluble and highly volatile at room temperature. As such, benzene readily crosses the alveolar membranes and is taken up by circulating blood in pulmonary vessels. Benzene is rapidly absorbed through the lungs; approximately 50% of the benzene inhaled in the air is absorbed.

Benzene can also be readily absorbed from the gastrointestinal tract. Over 90% of ingested benzene is absorbed through the gastrointestinal tract. Benzene is poorly absorbed dermally.

Absorbed benzene is rapidly distributed throughout the body and tends to accumulate in fatty tissues. Circulating benzene is preferentially taken up by lipid-rich tissues such as adipose and nervous tissue. Benzene has also been detected in the bone marrow, liver, kidneys, lungs, and spleen.

The liver serves an important function in benzene metabolism, which results in the production of several reactive metabolites. The major end products of benzene metabolism include phenol (hydroxybenzene), catechol (1,2-dihydroxybenzene), and quinol (1,4-dihydroxybenzene). These metabolic products are subsequently conjugated with inorganic sulfate and glucuronic acid before being excreted in the urine. A small fraction of the catechol derived from benzene metabolism is oxidized to hydroxyhydroquinol or transformed to muconic acids.

At low exposure levels, benzene is rapidly metabolized and excreted predominantly as conjugated urinary metabolites. At higher exposure levels, metabolic pathways appear to become saturated, and a large portion of an absorbed dose of benzene is excreted as a parent compound in exhaled air.

Mechanism of Toxicity

Benzene can be irritating to mucus membranes. Dermal exposures can defat the skin's keratin layer and can result in erythema, vesiculation, and dry, scaly dermatitis. Acute exposures to high concentrations can produce pulmonary irritation and edema, and gastrointestinal irritation (if ingested). Chronic exposure to benzene produces bone-marrow depression. Experimental evidence indicates that benzene's bone-marrow toxicity is mediated by one or more of its metabolites. For example, inhibition of benzene metabolism by administration of toluene or partial hepatectomy protects bone marrow against benzene damage. Benzene metabolites, such as 1,2-dihydroxybenzene (catechol), 1,4-dihydroxybenzene (quinol), and 1,2,4-trihydroxybenzene (hydroxyhydroquinol), have been shown to inhibit cell mitosis.

The mechanism of toxicity appears to be comprising five key events: (1) metabolism of benzene to a benzene oxide metabolite in the liver; (2) interaction of the benzene metabolite with target cells in the bone marrow; (3) formation of initiated, mutated bone-marrow target cells; (4) selective clonal proliferation of these mutated cells; and (5) formation of the neoplasm (leukemia).

There are major uncertainties to the nature of the toxic metabolites and their mechanism of toxicity. Any hypothesis of benzene toxicity must account for the role of hepatic metabolism and the selective toxicity of benzene in the bone marrow. A puzzling aspect of benzene toxicology is its lack of hepatotoxicity.

Acute and Short-Term Toxicity (or Exposure)

Animal

Benzene can cause severe eye irritation and moderate skin irritation. When given orally, benzene is moderately toxic. The oral LD_{50} in rats and mice is 3400 and 4700 mg kg^{-1}, respectively. The median lethal dose through inhalation has been evaluated in rats, mice, dogs, and cats. In these laboratory species, the LC_{50} ranges from 31 887 mg m^{-3} in mice to 170 000 mg m^{-3} in cats.

Human

The acute effects of benzene exposure generally differ markedly from the chronic effects. Acute exposure to high doses of benzene in air (at concentrations in excess of 3000 ppm) causes symptoms typical of organic solvent intoxication. Symptoms may progress from excitation, euphoria, headache, and vertigo, in mild cases, to central nervous system depression, confusion, seizures, coma, and death from respiratory failure in severe cases. The rate of recovery depends on the initial exposure time and concentration, but, following severe intoxication, the symptoms may persist for weeks.

Chronic Toxicity (or Exposure)

Animal

The effects of lifetime exposure to benzene have also been evaluated in laboratory animals. A number of animal studies have demonstrated that benzene exposure can induce bone-marrow damage, changes in circulating blood cells, developmental and reproductive effects, alterations of the immune response, and cancer. With respect to chronic toxicity, hematological changes appear to be the most sensitive indicator.

Although human epidemiological studies provide the bulk of the evidence that benzene is a human carcinogen, many experimental animal studies, both inhalation and oral, also support the evidence that exposure to benzene increases the risk of cancer in multiple organ systems, including the hematopoietic system, oral and nasal cavities, liver, forestomach, preputial gland, lung, ovary, and mammary gland.

Human

The major toxicological manifestation of chronic benzene exposure in humans is bone-marrow depression. Clinical manifestations include anemia, leucopenia, and thrombocytopenia. In severe cases, bone-marrow aplasia develops. Later stages of toxicity are manifested by pancytopenia and aplastic anemia. Death may result from aplastic anemia or from leukemia. The US Environmental Protection Agency (EPA) and International Agency for Research on Cancer classify benzene as a known human carcinogen. This classification was given to benzene in view of strong epidemiological and experimental evidence.

Epidemiologic studies and case studies provide clear evidence of a causal association between exposure to benzene and acute nonlymphocytic leukemia (ANLL) and also suggest evidence of chronic nonlymphocytic leukemia (CNLL) and chronic lymphocytic leukemia (CLL). Other neoplastic conditions that are associated with an increased risk in humans are hematologic neoplasms, blood disorders such as preleukemia and aplastic anemia, Hodgkin's lymphoma, and myelodysplastic syndrome (MDS). These human data are supported by animal studies. The experimental animal data add to the argument that exposure to benzene increases the risk of cancer in multiple species at multiple organ sites (hematopoietic, oral and nasal, liver, forestomach, preputial gland, lung, ovary, and mammary gland). It is likely that these responses are due to interactions of the metabolites of benzene with DNA. Recent evidence supports the viewpoint that there are likely multiple mechanistic pathways leading to cancer and, in particular, to leukemogenesis from exposure to benzene.

Immunotoxicity

Damage to both the humoral and cellular components of the immune system has been known to occur in humans following inhalation. This is manifested by decreased levels of antibodies, leukocytes, and B-lymphocytes. Benzene-induced immunological effects are probably a reflection of bone-marrow toxicity. Animal studies have also shown that benzene decreases circulating leukocytes and decreases the ability of lymphoid tissue to produce the mature lymphocytes necessary to form antibodies. Animals exhibited lymphoid depletion of the thymus and spleen and hyperplasia of the bone marrow. This has been demonstrated in animals exposed for acute, intermediate, or chronic periods via the inhalation route.

Reproductive Toxicity

Benzene diffuses across the placenta and is toxic to the fetus in the presence of maternal toxicity. However, benzene is not considered to be a teratogen. Data on the reproductive effects of benzene in animals have been negative. Data on the reproductive effects of occupational exposure to benzene suggest that it may impair fertility in women. However, the findings are inconclusive and limited.

Genotoxicity

Based on studies of the biochemical effects of benzene and its metabolites, four specific genotoxic mechanisms have been postulated: (1) DNA-reactive benzene metabolites forming adducts or cross-links; (2) oxidative DNA damage; (3) damage to components of the mitotic apparatus; and (4) topoisomerase II inhibition.

Animal studies using radiolabeled benzene found a low level of radiolabel in isolated DNA with no preferential binding in target tissues of neoplasia. Adducts were not identified under dosage conditions that produce neoplasms in animals. These findings suggest that DNA-adduct formation may not be a significant mechanism for benzene-induced neoplasia.

The evaluation of other genotoxicity test results revealed that benzene and its metabolites did not produce reverse mutations in *Salmonella typhimurium* but were clastogenic and aneugenic, producing micronuclei, chromosomal aberrations, sister chromatid exchanges, and DNA strand breaks.

Studies support a mode of action that involves clastogenicity rather than mutagenicity secondary to DNA-adduct formation. Although unstable DNA adducts, oxidative DNA damage, or spindle poisoning could contribute to the overall toxic effects and cannot be ruled out, the genotoxic effects produced by benzene and its metabolites are most consistent with inhibition of topoisomerase II or ribonucleotide reductase inhibition.

Carcinogenicity

The carcinogenicity of benzene has been documented in exposed workers. Epidemiological studies and case reports provide evidence of a causal relationship between occupational exposure to benzene and benzene-containing solvents and the occurrence of acute myelogenous leukemia (AML). Benzene has also been associated with ANLL in humans, and aplastic anemia may be an early indicator of developing ANLL in some cases.

The US EPA classifies benzene as a known human carcinogen (Category A carcinogen) for all routes of exposure based on convincing human evidence as well as supporting evidence from animal studies. According to EPA's Integrated Risk Information System (IRIS), "Epidemiologic studies and case studies provide clear evidence of a causal association between exposure to benzene and ANLL and also suggest evidence for CNLL and CLL. Other neoplastic conditions that are associated with an increased risk in humans are hematologic neoplasms, blood disorders such as preleukemia and aplastic anemia, Hodgkin's lymphoma, and MDS. These human data are supported by animal studies. The experimental animal data add to the argument that exposure to benzene increases the risk of cancer in multiple species at multiple organ sites (hematopoietic, oral and nasal, liver, forestomach, preputial gland, lung, ovary, and mammary gland). It is likely that these responses are due to interactions of the metabolites of benzene with DNA. Recent evidence supports the viewpoint that there are likely multiple mechanistic pathways leading to cancer and, in particular, to leukemogenesis from exposure to benzene."

The United Nations' International Agency for Research on Cancer classifies benzene as a Group 1 carcinogen (carcinogenic to humans) because there is sufficient evidence in humans for the carcinogenicity of benzene, specifically AML and ANLL.

Clinical Management

The victim should be removed from the contaminated atmosphere. Contaminated clothing should be removed and the affected area should be washed with soap and water. There is no antidote for benzene. Treatment is symptomatic and supportive. Most exposed persons recover fully. Persons who have experienced serious symptoms may need to be hospitalized. In cases of ingestion, vomiting should not be induced. Benzene or organic solvents containing benzene can cause acute hemorrhagic pneumonitis if aspirated into the lungs. Activated charcoal can be given to minimize absorption from the gastrointestinal tract. Charcoal can be given in a slurry or mixed with sorbitol or a saline cathartic. The recommended doses of activated charcoal are 30–100 g for adults, 15–30 g for children, and 1 or 2 g kg^{-1} for infants. The indicated doses can be prepared in a slurry by mixing charcoal in a diluent at a rate of 10 g charcoal per 80 ml of diluent.

Environmental Fate

Benzene enters the air, water, and soil as a result of industrial processes, emissions from burning coal and oil, tobacco smoke, gasoline exhaust, and gasoline leaks, and from natural sources, including volcanoes and forest fires. Benzene in the atmosphere chemically degrades in only a few days. Benzene released to soil or waterways is subject to volatilization, photooxidation, and biodegradation. Benzene has a short half-life in surface water because it is so volatile.

If benzene is released to soil, it will be subject to rapid volatilization near the surface. That which does not evaporate will be highly to very highly mobile in soil and may leach to groundwater. It may be subject to biodegradation in shallow, aerobic groundwater, but probably not under anaerobic conditions.

If benzene is released to water, it will be subject to rapid volatilization. It will not be expected to significantly adsorb to sediment, bioconcentrate in aquatic organisms, or hydrolyze. It may be subject to biodegradation based on a reported biodegradation half-life of 16 days in an aerobic river die-away test. In a marine ecosystem, biodegradation occurred in 2 days after an acclimation period of 2 days and 2 weeks in the summer and spring, respectively, whereas no degradation occurred in winter.

If benzene is released to the atmosphere, it will exist predominantly in the vapor phase. Gas-phase benzene will not be subject to direct photolysis but it will react with photochemically produced hydroxyl radicals with a half-life of 13.4 days, calculated using an experimental rate constant for the reaction. The reaction time in polluted atmospheres that contain nitrogen oxides or sulfur dioxide is accelerated, with the half-life being reported as 4–6 h. Products of photooxidation include phenol, nitrophenols, nitrobenzene, formic acid, and peroxyacetyl nitrate. Benzene is fairly soluble in water and is removed from the atmosphere in rain.

Ecotoxicology

With the exception of accidental spillage of petroleum products, the routine levels of environmental benzene exposure are not associated with risk to fish and wildlife. Reasons for a reduced concern of the environmental risk include (1) the lack of bioaccumulation and biomagnification, (2) the low persistence due to its high volatility from surface waters and soil, and (3) the rapid photooxidation of airborne benzene and its biodegradation in soil and water. Studies have shown that high levels of benzene are toxic to aquatic life under controlled conditions.

The US EPA ECOTOX database reports that Ceriodaphnia and Daphnia species are the most sensitive freshwater organisms following acute (48 h) exposure to benzene, with respective EC_{50} values of 130 and 400 ppb. Most organisms, however, can tolerate acute concentrations higher than this (in the 1–10 mg l^{-1} range). Following chronic exposures (4–7 day exposures), fish are relatively unaffected at concentrations up to 5 mg l^{-1} (at higher concentrations fish start to show adverse narcotic effects).

Exposure Standards and Guidelines

The odor threshold for benzene is 30 ppm, but the current American Conference of Governmental Industrial Hygienists threshold limit value considered safe for occupational exposure (8 h day^{-1}) is 0.5 ppm, with a short-term exposure limit (STEL) of 2.5 ppm. The Occupational Safety and Health Administration PEL is 1 ppm, with an STEL of 5 ppm. The National Institute for Occupational Safety and Health recommends an exposure limit (recommended exposure limit) of 0.1 ppm with an STEL of 1 ppm. EPA's maximum contaminant level for benzene in drinking water is 5 ppb. EPA classifies benzene as a Category 'A' carcinogen ('known' human carcinogen).

See also: Blood; Carcinogen–DNA Adduct Formation and DNA Repair; Solvents.

Further Reading

Galbraith, D., Gross, S.A., Paustenbach, D., 2010. Benzene and human health: a historical review and appraisal of associations with various diseases. Crit. Rev. Toxicol. 40 (Suppl. 2), 1–46.

Hays, S.M., Pyatt, D.W., Kirman, C.R., Aylward, L.L., 2012. Biomonitoring equivalents for benzene. Regul. Toxicol. Pharmcol. 62 (1), 62–73.

Zhang, L., McHale, C.M., Rothman, N., Li, G., Ji, Z., Vermeulen, R., Hubbard, A.E., Ren, X., Shen, M., Rappaport, S.M., North, M., Skibola, C.F., Yin, S., Vulpe, C., Chanock, S.J., Smith, M.T., Lan, Q., 2010. Systems biology of human benzene exposure. Chem. Biol. Interact. 184 (1–2), 86–93.

Relevant Website

http://www.atsdr.cdc.gov – Agency for Toxic Substances and Disease Registry. Toxicological Profile for Benzene.

Benzenedicarboxylic Acid, 1-2 *see* Phosphate Ester Flame Retardants

Benzidine

CV Rao, NMAM Institute of Technology, Nitte, India

- Name: Benzidine
- Chemical Abstracts Service Registry Number: 92-87-5
- Synonyms: (1,1′-Biphenyl)-4,4′-diamine; 4,4′-Bianiline; 4,4′-Biphenyldiamine; 4,4′-Biphenylenediamine; 4,4′-Diamino-1,1′-biphenyl
- Molecular Formula: $C_{12}H_{12}N_2$
- Chemical Structure:

H_2N–(biphenyl)–NH_2

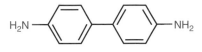

Background

Benzidine is a biphenyl amine that exists at room temperature as a crystalline grayish-yellow, white, or reddish-gray power. It is slightly soluble in cold water, more soluble in hot water, and readily soluble in less-polar solvents such as diethyl ether and ethanol. It darkens on exposure to air and light. Benzidine is a diamine, manufactured as synthetic aromatic hydrocarbon with two benzene rings covalently bonded to one another (1,1), substituted by amino group at 4,4′. Benzidine is prepared from nitrobenzene in a two-step process: nitrobenzene is converted to 1,2-diphenylhydrazine, usually using iron powder as the reducing agent, and then hydrazine is treated with mineral acids to induce a rearrangement reaction to 4,4′-benzidine. In the environment, benzidine is found in either its 'free' state (as an organic base) or as a salt (benzidine dihydrochloride or benzidine sulfate). Physical and chemical properties of benzidine are listed in Table 1.

Table 1 Physical and chemical properties of benzidine

Property	*Information*
Molecular weight	184.2[a]
Specific gravity	1.250 At 20 °C/4 °C[a]
Melting point	120 °C[a]
Boiling point	401 °C[a]
Log K_{ow}	1.34[a]
Water solubility	0.322 g l^{-1} at 25 °C[a]
Vapor pressure	8.98×10^{-7} mm Hg at 25 °C[b]
Vapor density relative to air	6.36[a]
Dissociation constant (pK_a)	4.3[a]

[a]The figures are from HSDB 2009.
[b]The figures are from ChemIDplus 2009.

In vivo, benzidine covalently binds with DNA in the liver of mice and rats. Other benzidine-induced genomic changes *in vivo* include micronuclei formation, sister chromatid exchanges, DNA strand breaks, and unscheduled DNA synthesis in cells of rodents. Upregulation of the p53 protein, a DNA damage-sensor protein, in benzidine-treated cells suggests the induction of the p53 DNA damage signaling pathway. This compound is mutagenic to plants and bacteria. Induction of bladder cancer remains the most prominent effect of benzidine. Most studies in diverse geographic locations describe benzidine exposure primarily due to working in a dyestuff industry. Data from these studies have also unequivocally demonstrated co-exposure to 2-naphthylamine along with benzidine precipitating bladder cancer in humans. Benzidine has been classified as a human carcinogen (Class A) based on sufficient evidence of carcinogenicity from studies in humans. Most humans are exposed to this compound in occupational settings, and it causes urinary-bladder cancer and bladder-cancer related deaths; the longer the exposure, the greater is the risk for developing bladder cancer.

Uses

Benzidine is used as an intermediate in the production of azo dyes, sulfur dyes, fast color salts, naphthol, and other dye compounds. However, it has not been marketed or sold in the United States since the mid-1970s, and US dye companies no longer manufacture benzidine-based dyes. However, a small amount of benzidine may still be manufactured or imported for scientific research in the United States, but in some countries it is still being manufactured. To date, more than 250 benzidine-based dyes have been reported. These dyes are primarily used for dyeing textiles, paper, and leather products.

Environmental Fate and Behavior

Industries release benzidine into the environment in the form of liquid waste and sludges. Benzidine may also be released into the environment due to spillage during transport. In air, benzidine is found bound to suspended particles or as a vapor, which may be brought back to the earth's surface by rain or gravity.

Partition Behavior in Water, Sediment, and Soil

Very small amounts of benzidine dissolve in water at moderate environmental temperatures. When released into waterways,

 http://dx.doi.org/10.1016/B978-0-12-386454-3.00249-9

it sinks to the bottom and becomes part of the bottom sludge. In soil, most benzidine is strongly attached to soil particles, so it does not easily leach into underground water from waste dumps.

Environmental Persistency (Degradation/Speciation)

Benzidine is slowly destroyed in the environment by light, certain other chemicals, and microorganisms.

Bioaccumulation and Biomagnification

Accumulation in the food chain has not been recorded so far, but it is documented that water life may take up and store very small amounts of benzidine (ATSDR 2001).

Exposure and Exposure Monitoring

Routes and Pathways

The primary routes of potential human exposure to benzidine are inhalation, ingestion, and dermal contact. The general population is not likely to be exposed to benzidine through contaminated air, water, soil, or food (ATSDR 2001).

Human Exposure

People living near a hazardous waste site are likely to get exposed to benzidine through contaminated drinking water or by breathing contaminated air or by swallowing contaminated dust and soil. Benzidine can also enter the body by passing through the skin from contaminated clothing and gloves. People working at or near a hazardous waste site may get exposed to benzidine in a similar manner (ATSDR 2001).

Toxicokinetics

Benzidine is rapidly absorbed through the skin in solid and vapor form. It is also quickly absorbed through the lungs on inhalation and from the gastrointestinal tract on consuming contaminated water and food. Generally, it will take only few hours for most of the benzidine to get into the body through the lungs and intestine. Breathing, eating, or drinking benzidine-based dyes may also expose a person to benzidine because the intestinal microflora can break down these dyes into benzidine. It is a lipophilic substance, hence easily stored in fat tissues, and it firmly binds to cell receptors. Benzidine is metabolized to aromatic amine by intestinal microflora or liver azo-reductase. The liver is the chief organ of metabolism where benzidine is converted to more reactive, toxic, and mutagenic (carcinogenic) *N*-hydroxyarylamides and *N*-hydroxylamine is considered to be a proximate carcinogen. *N*-hydroxylamides are converted to the ultimate carcinogens through conjugation with sulfuric, acetic, or glucuronic acid. *N*-acetoxyarylamines are also produced as metabolites and are highly reactive mutagens and carcinogens. Glutathione transferase plays an important role in the elimination of reactive metabolites of benzidine. Sulfonation, carboxylation, deamination, or substitution of an ethyl alcohol or an acetyl group for the hydrogen in the amino groups leads to a decrease in mutagenicity of benzidine metabolites as well as to easy elimination, primarily through urine and feces.

Mechanism of Toxicity

Benzidine is metabolized to highly toxic, reactive metabolites, such as *N*-hydroxyarylamides and *N*-hydroxyarylamines, which act as procarcinogens and are more mutagenic than parent compounds. The metabolites act as DNA adducts and bind to cell receptors. Some of the benzidine derivatives are strong mutagens. The metabolites on conjugation with sulfuric, acetic, and glucuronic acids form ultimate carcinogens. Benzidine is metabolized by cytochrome P450 enzymes (via *N*-oxidation) to form electrophilic compounds that can bind covalently to DNA. Benzidine caused mutations in bacteria and plants, but gave conflicting results in cultured rodent cells. It also caused many other types of genetic damage in various test systems, including yeast, cultured human and other mammalian cells, and rodents exposed *in vivo*. The damage included mitotic gene conversion (in yeast), micronucleus formation, DNA strand breaks, unscheduled DNA synthesis, cell transformation, chromosomal aberrations, sister chromatid exchange, and aneuploidy. Workers exposed to benzidine and or benzidine-based dyes had higher levels of chromosomal aberrations in their white bloods cells than did unexposed workers.

Chronic Toxicity

Animal

There is sufficient evidence from animal studies that benzidine is a carcinogen. When administered in the diet, benzidine-induced bladder cancer in dogs, multiple mammary carcinomas in rats, and liver cell tumors in hamsters of both sexes. When administered by the subcutaneous route to mice of both sexes, it induced malignant tumors of the Zymbal gland (ear) and hepatocellular carcinoma; hepatomas, malignant tumors of the Zymbal gland, and local sarcomas in male rats; and malignant tumors of the Zymbal gland, mammary adenocarcinomas, and amyloid leukemia in female rats. When administered by intraperitoneal injection, benzidine-induced Zymbal gland adenomas and carcinomas and malignant mammary tumors in female rats. The lethal dose in dogs is 400 mg kg^{-1} by the subcutaneous route and 200 mg kg^{-1} by the oral route. Dyes made from benzidine, such as Direct Blue 6, Direct Black 38, and Direct Brown 95 has been shown to cause cancer in animals. The Department of Health and Human Services has determined that Direct Black 38 and Direct Blue 6 cause cancer in animals, and the International Agency for Research on Cancer (IARC) has also determined that Direct Black 38, Direct Blue 6, and Direct Brown 95 cause cancer in animals.

Human

Benzidine can cause cancer in humans. This has been shown in studies of workers who were exposed for many years to levels much higher than the general population would be. An IARC study on dye industry workers reported that there is a direct correlation between the incidence of bladder cancer in the occupationally benzidine-exposed workers and the incidence of this cancer decreasing in workers after reduction in occupational exposure. Some evidences indicate that dyes made from benzidine, such as Direct Blue 6, Direct Black 38, and Direct Brown 95, may cause cancer in humans. Benzidine poisoning causes vomiting, nausea, hemolysis, liver and kidney damage, and hematuria (bloody urine). Benzidine is considered to be acutely toxic to humans by ingestion, with an estimated oral lethal dose of between 50 and 500 mg kg^{-1} for a 70 kg person. Symptoms of acute ingestion exposure include cyanosis, headache, mental confusion, nausea, and vertigo. Dermal exposure may cause skin rashes and irritation. Acetylated benzidine metabolites such as *N*-acetoxyarylamines are known to cause bladder cancer in dye industry workers.

Genotoxicity

Mutagenic potential of benzidine and its analogs was repeatedly tested using strains TA98 and TA100 in the presence and absence of Aroclor 1254-induced rat S9 mix in Ames *Salmonella*/microsome assay. 3,3′-Dichlorobenzidine-2HCl and 4,4′-dinitro-2-biphenylamine were directly mutagenic to TA98, while 4,4′-dinitro-2-biphenylamine was directly mutagenic to both TA98 and TA100 in the absence of S9 mix. 2-Aminobiphenyl, 3-aminobiphenyl, and 3,3′-5,5′-tetra-methylbenzidine were not mutagenic in either strains in the presence or absence of S9. In the presence of S9 mix, 4-aminobiphenyl, benzidine, 3, 3′-dichlorobenzidine-2HCl, 3,3′-dimethoxybenzidine, 3,3′-4, 4′-tetraaminobiphenyl, *o*-tolidine, N, N–N′, N′-tetra-methylbenzidine, and 4,4′-dinitro-2-biphenylamine were mutagenic to TA98; 4-aminobiphenyl, 3,3′-dichlorobenzidine-2HCl, 3, 3′-dimethoxybenzidine, and 4,4′-dinitro-2-biphenylamine were mutagenic to TA100. Some of the benzidine derivatives, such as 3,3,5,5-tetra-methylbenzidine, 3,3-dimethylbenzidine (*O*-tolidine), and N,N-diacetylbenzidine, were not mutagenic. Incorporation of the free radical and metal scavengers and antioxidants reduced the mutagenic responses, whereas heat-inactivated catalase and Superoxide Dismutase (SOD) had no effect. Induction of lipid peroxidation in the presence of S9 mix was observed in several instances, which suggested that benzidine derivatives induce mutations through the induction of Reactive Oxygen Species.

Human Genotoxicity

Cytogenetic effects of occupational exposure to benzidine and benzidine-based dyes (Direct Black 38 and Direct Blue 6) were studied in workers at a manufacturing plant in Bulgaria having a recognized high risk of occupational cancer. Twenty-three workers exposed for a mean of 15 years were compared with 30 controls presumed to have no exposure. A 10-fold increase in chromosomal aberrations (polyploidy) was observed in circulating lymphocytes of exposed workers when compared with controls. The highest frequency of aberrant lymphocytes was associated with the highest airborne dust concentrations of benzidine (0.42 –0.86 mg m^{-3}) or benzidine-based dyes (7.8–32.3 mg m^{-3}), with highest mean level of benzidine in urine (1.8–2.3 μg l^{-1}).

Carcinogenicity

Benzidine is confirmed to be human carcinogen (Class A). Though not universal, a synergistically elevated rate of bladder cancer in workers exposed to benzidine in cigarette smokers has been found. It is hypothesized that smokers have nearly 31-fold higher risk of developing bladder cancer compared to an 11-fold risk of developing bladder cancer among nonsmoking coworkers. This was based on a large cohort of 3322 Japanese workers exposed to benzidine and/or β-naphthylamine for 22 years and the control cohort of 13.5 years; control consisted of 177 male unexposed patients with bladder cancer. Among employees exposed to benzidine and/or β-naphthylamine, 244 workers were found to have suffered from and consequently died of cancer of genitourinary organs (primary cancer). Of these, 11 developed secondary cancers of liver, gallbladder, bile duct, large intestine, or lung. Susceptibility to bladder cancer in humans is linked to slow acetylator type of the polymorphic NAT2 (*N*-acetyl transferase gene).

Clinical Management

There is no antidote for benzidine poisoning. Since it produces reactive metabolites, administration of free radical scavengers would alleviate the toxicity. A complex of benzidine metabolites with copper and hydrochloride is known to decrease its mutagenic effects.

See also: Dyes and Colorants; Toxicity Testing, Carcinogenesis.

Further Reading

Alves de Lima, R.O., Bazo, A.P., Salvadori, D.M., et al., 2007. Mutagenic and carcinogenic potential of a textile azo dye processing plant effluent that impacts a drinking water source. Mutat. Res. 626 (1–2), 53–60.

American Conference of Governmental Industrial Hygienists TLVs and BEIs, 2008. Threshold Limit Values for Chemical Substances and Physical Agents and Biological Exposure Indices. Cincinnati, OH, p. 13.

Carreón, T., LeMasters, G.K., Ruder, A.M., Schulte, P.A., 2006. The genetic and environmental factors involved in benzidine metabolism and bladder carcinogenesis in exposed workers. Front. Biosci. 11, 2889–2902.

Ching Chen, S., Hseu, Y.C., Sung, J.C., et al., 2011. Induction of DNA damage signaling genes in benzidine-treated HepG2 cells. Environ. Mol. Mutagen. 52 (8), 664–672.

Donaldson, F.P., Nyman, M.C., 2006. Short-term interactions of aniline and benzidine with three soils in both natural and artificial matrices. Chemosphere 65 (5), 854–862.

Hemstreet, G.P., Wang, W., 2004. Genotypic and phenotypic biomarker profiles for individual risk assessment and cancer detection (lessons from bladder cancer risk assessment in symptomatic patients and workers exposed to benzidine). Front. Biosci. 9, 2671–2679.

Kobylewski, S., Jacobson, M.F., 2012. Toxicology of food dyes. Int. J. Occup. Environ. Health 18 (3), 220–246.
Letašiová, S., Medve'ová, A., Šovčíková, A., et al., 2012. Bladder cancer, a review of the environmental risk factors. Environ. Health 11 (Suppl. 1), S11. http://dx.doi.org/10.1186/1476-069X-11-S1-S11.
Makena, P., Chung, K.T., 2007. Evidence that 4-aminobiphenyl, benzidine, and benzidine congeners produce genotoxicity through reactive oxygen species. Environ. Mol. Mutagen. 48 (5), 404–413.
National Toxicology Program, 2011. Benzidine and dyes metabolized to benzidine: dyes metabolized to benzidine (benzidine dye class). Rep. Carcinog. 2011 (12), 64–66.
Ohsako, S., Deguchi, T., 1990. Cloning and expression of cDNA for polymorphic and monomorphic arylamine N-acetyltransferases from human liver. J. Biol. Chem. 265, 4630–4634.
Park, J., Shin, K.S., Kim, Y., 2010. Occupational reproductive function abnormalities and bladder cancer in Korea. J. Korean Med. Sci. 25 (Suppl.), S41–S45.
Rosenman, K.D., Reilly, M.J., 2004. Cancer mortality and incidence among a cohort of benzidine and dichlorobenzidine dye manufacturing workers. Am. J. Ind. Med. 46, 505–512.
U.S. Environmental Protection Agency's Integrated Risk Information System (IRIS), 2000. Summary on Benzidine (92-87-5). http://www.epa.gov/iris/.
Wang, C.Y., King, C.M., 2007. *N*-Acetyltransferases and the susceptibility to benzidine-induced bladder carcinogenesis. Int. J. Cancer 120 (11), 2523–2524.
Weistenhofer, W., Blaszkewicz, M., Bolt, H.M., Golka, K., 2008. *N*-acetyltransferase-2 and medical history in bladder cancer cases with a suspected occupational disease (BK 1301) in Germany. J. Toxicol. Environ. Health A 71 (13–14), 906–910.
Xiang, C.Q., Shen, C.L., Wu, Z.R., et al., 2007. Detection of mutant p53 protein in workers occupationally exposed to benzidine. J. Occup. Health 49 (4), 279–284.
Yang, M., 2011. A current global view of environmental and occupational cancers. J. Environ. Sci. Health C Environ. Carcinog. Ecotoxicol. Rev. 29 (3), 223–249.

Relevant Websites

http://www.atsdr.cdc.gov – Agency for Toxic Substances and Disease Registry. Toxicological Profile for Benzidine.

http://chem.sis.nlm.nih.gov/chemidplus – ChemIDplus Advanced – US National Library of Medicine.

http://www.nlm.nih.gov/pubs/factsheets/hsdbfs.html – HSDB (Hazardous Substances Data Bank) – US National Library of Medicine.

http://monographs.iarc.fr/index.php – IARC. Monographs on the Evaluation of the Carcinogenic Risk of Chemicals to Man. Geneva: World Health Organization, International Agency for Research on Cancer, 1972–PRESENT.

http://ntp.niehs.nih.gov/ntp/roc/twelfth/profiles/BenzidineAndDyes.pdf – NTP/NIH/NIEHS.

http://toxnet.nlm.nih.gov/cgi-bin/sis/search/a?dbs+hsdb:@term+@DOCNO+948 – TOXNET, Specialized Information Services, National Library of Medicine. Search for Benzidine.

Benzine *see* Petroleum Ether

Benzo(a)pyrene

JP Gray, U.S. Coast Guard Academy, New London, CT, USA

This article is a revision of the previous edition article by Swarupa G. Kulkarni, Harihara M. Mehendale, volume 1, pp 257–259, © 2005, Elsevier Inc.

- Name: Benzo(a)pyrene
- Chemical Abstracts Service Registry Number: 50-32-8
- Synonyms: BAP; BaP; B(*a*)P; BP; 3,4-Benzopyrene; 6,7-Benzopyrene; 3,4-Benzpyrene; 3,4-Benz(*a*)pyrene; Benzo [*d,e,f*]chrysene; and many more
- Molecular Formula: $C_{20}H_{12}$
- Chemical Structure:

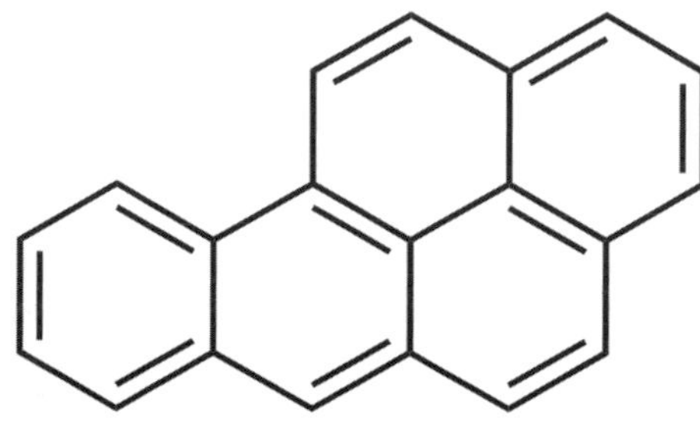

Background

Benzo(a)pyrene (BaP) is bioactivated to its carcinogenic form by phase 1 and phase 2 metabolism. As with other polycyclic aromatic hydrocarbons (PAHs), the presence of the 'bay region' contributes greatly to the carcinogenicity of BaP. This region is sterically constrained, allowing the formation of diol epoxides, which subsequently react with intracellular molecules such as DNA. Human exposure to BaP and other PAHs occurs primarily from smoking or from secondhand smoke, air polluted with combustion products, or food and water polluted with combustion products, such as those cooked over charcoal or broiled.

BaP has been extensively studied for its toxicities in children and during pregnancy. A study of pregnant active smokers showed that BaP crossed the human placenta and was bound to fetal hemoglobin at levels significantly higher than in pregnant nonsmokers.

Health concerns associated with BaP exposure for children were also evaluated. These include formation of BaP-DNA adducts, which may lead to errors in DNA replication and increased risk of cancer; increased risk of cancer associated with BaP metabolite formation; persistent effects on the development and function of the immune system; and reduced fertility in offspring during adulthood following BaP exposure during pregnancy. Concerns for BaP exposure of pregnant women and children are ambient air contamination from mobile sources (e.g., automobiles and other vehicles) and industrial sources (e.g., coke ovens, metal-processing plants); fetal exposure from maternal cigarette smoking; fetal and childhood exposure from secondhand cigarette smoke; and exposure from diet, including grilled and broiled food. Children may also have greater exposure than adults to contaminated soil in areas where BaP-contaminated soil from industrial contamination may be present, because of behavior patterns, particularly hand-to-mouth activity.

Uses

BaP is not commercially produced; it is a by-product of combustion. Its primary uses include toxicological mechanistic studies and cancer studies, as a positive control in carcinogenicity studies. There is no known commercial use for BaP.

Environmental Fate and Behavior

BaP is purposely synthesized solely for laboratory studies. The primary source of BaP and many PAHs in air is the incomplete combustion of wood, gasoline, and other fuels; in industrial settings where coal is burned; and in natural burns such as forest fires. BaP can bind to particulate matter, and inhalation is a common route of exposure. BaP is poorly water soluble, partitioning strongly to the sediment, and does not readily bioaccumulate. BaP is found in fossil fuels, crude oils, shale oils, and coal tars, and is emitted with gases and fly ash from active volcanoes. If released to air, an extrapolated vapor pressure of 5.49×10^{-9} mm Hg at 25 °C indicates BaP will exist solely in the particulate phase in the atmosphere. Particulate-phase BaP is usually removed from the atmosphere by wet or dry deposition. BaP contains chromophores that absorb at wavelengths >290 nm and therefore is expected to be susceptible to direct photolysis by sunlight; after 17 h irradiation with light >290 nm, 26.5% of BaP adsorbed onto silica gel was degraded. If released to soil, BaP is expected to have very low to no mobility based on measured soil K_{oc} values of 930–6300. Volatilization from moist soil surfaces is not expected to be an important fate process based on a Henry's Law constant of

 http://dx.doi.org/10.1016/B978-0-12-386454-3.00250-5

4.57×10^{-7} atm m^3 mol^{-1}. The stability of BaP in soil is expected to vary depending on the nature of compounds accompanying it and the nature and previous history of the soil; biodegradation half-lives of 309 and 229 days were observed in Kidman and McLaurin sandy loam soils, respectively. BaP is expected to adsorb to suspended solids and sediment based on the measured K_{OC} values, when released into water. Biodegradation of BaP is possible in aquatic systems. Volatilization from water surfaces is not expected to be an important fate process based on this compound's Henry's Law constant. Measured bioconcentration values ranging from 8.7 to 1×10^5 suggest bioconcentration in aquatic organisms can be low to very high. Hydrolysis is not expected to be an important environmental fate process since this compound lacks functional groups that hydrolyze under environmental conditions.

Exposure and Exposure Monitoring

Exposure occurs primarily through the diet or through smoking. Char grilling or broiling produces PAHs. BaP is also produced as a by-product when substances such as coal tar chemicals are burned, and is present in coal tar pitch. It can also penetrate the skin. Monitoring data indicate that the general population may be exposed to BaP via inhalation of ambient air, ingestion of food and drinking water, smoking of tobacco, and cooking processes that produce smoke.

Toxicokinetics

Absorption, Distribution, Metabolism, and Excretion (ADME) data are derived from general data for polycyclic aromatic hydrocarbons. Oral absorption is low, but increases with lipophilicity and in the presence of oils in the gastrointestinal (GI) tract. Dermal absorption also occurs readily in the presence of lipophilic solvents. Inhalational exposure is common in smokers. PAHs are widely distributed in tissues regardless of route of exposure. Metabolism is widely varied, and includes the formation of epoxides, dihydrodiols, phenols, quinones, and combinations, some of which are bioactivated to become mutagenic products. Conjugation to glucuronides and sulfate esters occurs via phase II metabolism, which are subsequently excreted. Hepatobiliary excretion is the primary elimination route of PAHs in animals within 2 days of exposure.

Specifically for BaP, following GI absorption (33% is absorbed), levels peak in the blood at 6 h after exposure. ABC transport proteins in the small intestine reabsorb BaP metabolites, which serves to attenuate further BaP absorption via competition. The liver and lung are the most susceptible to adduct formation by BaP metabolites, correlating with their high levels of cytochrome P450 enzyme activity and role in detoxification of BaP. BaP is biodistributed to body fat, other fatty tissues, placenta, and bile.

Mechanism of Toxicity

While not known to be toxic itself, BaP and other PAHs containing bay regions are carcinogenic. BaP is bioactivated via three enzymatic steps (**Figure 2**) to create a carcinogenic epoxide resistant to epoxidases. It is first metabolized by cytochrome P450 1A1 to (+) benzo(a)pyrene 7,8-oxide, next by epoxide hydrolase to (−) benzo(a)pyrene 7,8-dihydrodiol, and finally by cytochrome P450 1A1 to (+) benzo(a)pyrene 7,8-dihydrodiol-9,10-epoxide. The prototypical 'bay region' of this PAH representative facilitates DNA interaction. Other metabolites are toxic as well. The aryl hydrocarbon receptor is responsible for some BaP toxicity; knockout of AhR significantly reduced toxicity from BaP in a mouse model system (**Figure 1**).

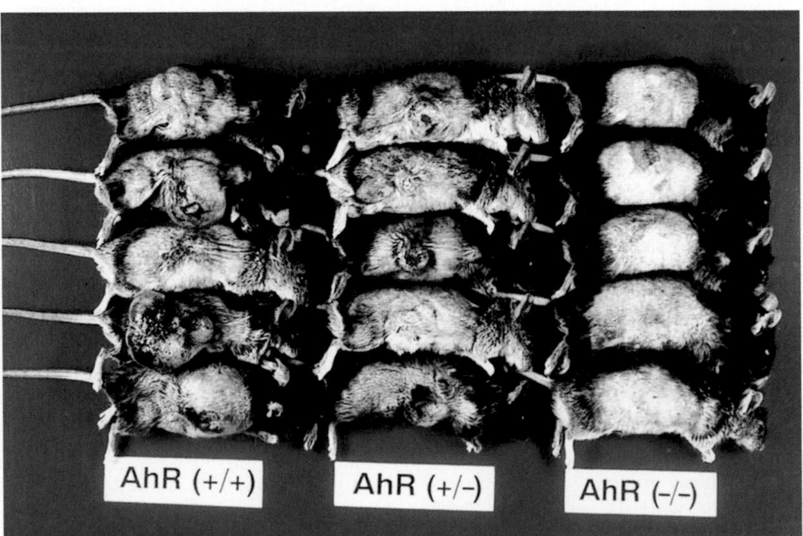

Figure 1 BaP-mediated activation of phase 1 and 2 metabolizing enzymes via activation of the AhR is required for bioactivation of BaP *in vivo*. Reproduced permission from Shimizu, Y., Nakatsuru, Y., Ichinose, M., Takahashi, Y., Kume, H., Mimura, J., Fujii-Kuriyama, Y., Ishikawa, T., 2000. Benzo[*a*]pyrene carcinogenicity is lost in mice lacking the aryl hydrocarbon receptor. Proc. Natl. Acad. Sci. U.S.A. 97 (2), 779–782.

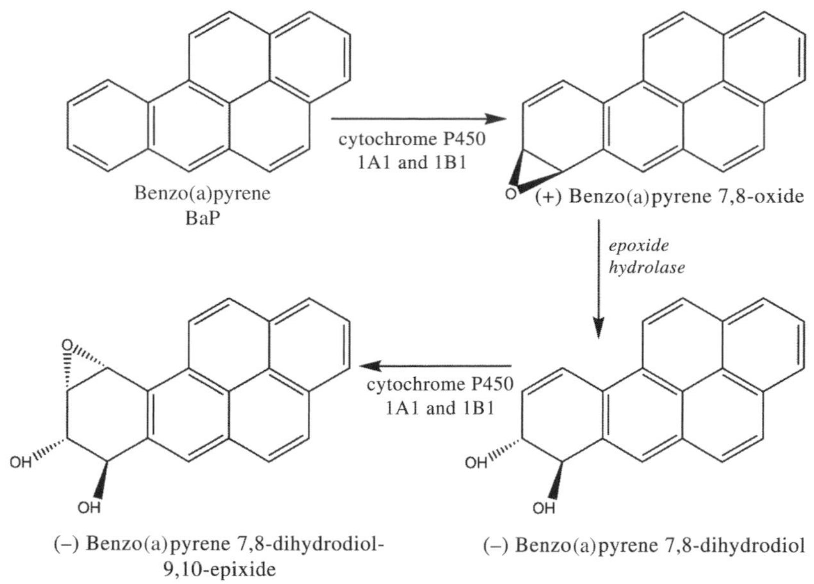

Figure 2 Bioactivation of BaP to (–) benzo(a)pyrene 7,8-dihydrodiol-9,10-epoxide.

Acute and Short-Term Toxicity

Animal

Hepatotoxicity and nephrotoxicity occur upon exposure of rats to PAHs. In experimental animal studies, BaP exposure during pregnancy resulted in increased incidence of tumors in lung, liver, ovaries, and other organs in adult offspring. BaP exposure during pregnancy resulted in increased incidence of fetal death, abnormalities (e.g., exencephaly or growth of the brain outside of the skull, and thoracoschisis or cleft in the chest wall) in offspring at birth at doses ranging from 50 to 300 mg kg^{-1}, impaired development of T lymphocytes, and decreased antibody responses. Reduced fertility during adulthood has been observed following BaP exposure during pregnancy. Formation of BaP-DNA adducts have been detected in several species and in several tissues following BaP exposure during pregnancy. LD_{50} dose in rat (subcutaneous) has been determined to be 50 mg kg^{-1}, and in mouse (intraperitoneal) about 250 mg kg^{-1}.

Human

High levels of exposure cause immune system suppression and anemia due to red blood cell damage. BaP can pass through the skin, and dermal exposure is typically due to workplace contact with coal tar. Toxicity can be increased following photoactivation by UV. In humans, BaP has been associated with chromosomal replication (DNA copying) errors and altered DNA in gametes (sperm and eggs); BaP also forms BaP-DNA adducts in fetal, child, and adult tissues. In adults, BaP exposure was associated with altered sperm morphology and decreased sperm numbers, and decreased egg numbers. At high levels of acute exposure in adults, BaP has been reported to be associated with immune system suppression and red blood cell damage, which can lead to anemia.

Chronic Toxicity

The major chronic toxicity risk is carcinogenesis. Repeated dermal exposures can result in thickening and darkening of the skin.

Immunotoxicity

Acute exposure to high levels of BaP is associated with immune system suppression and blood cell damage. BaP causes immunosuppression of the cytotoxic T cell response, mitogen-induced T cell and B cell proliferative responses, and cytokine production by human PBMCs. BaP increased susceptibility of B6C3F1 female mice to various pathogens.

Reproductive Toxicity

BaP has been shown to penetrate the placenta, and exposure to cigarette smoke, known to contain BaP, is associated with reduced fetal weight. BaP exposure *in utero* has resulted in fetal death, abnormalities, and immune system dysfunction in children. BaP exposure have been shown to influence (1) number of sperms and egg follicles; (2) fetal weights; (3) number of pups born; (4) number of resorptions; (5) lung enzymes (pyruvate kinase and lactic acid dehydrogenase) of exposed fetuses; (6) exencephaly (growth of the brain outside of the skull); and (7) thoracoschisis (cleft in the chest wall).

The ability to metabolize BaP by pregnant rodents following maternal ingestion or injection of BaP showed genetic variability. The type of Ah receptor (aryl hydrocarbon receptor, or AhR) in each strain influenced the extent of toxic effects of BaP exposure; the AhR binds aromatic hydrocarbons (compounds containing rings of carbon atoms) including BaP, and is a component of the cytochrome P450 system that metabolizes BaP and other compounds. The incidence of teratogenic effects (e.g., fetal death and decreased fetal weight) and the time of onset of aplastic anemia following BaP exposure during pregnancy via maternal ingestion varied between strains of mice that differed at the AhR locus, while numbers of tumors induced by BaP exposure did not vary. Offsprings of pregnant mice, who were injected with BaP during pregnancy, had an increased incidence of tumors, predominantly in lung, liver, and ovaries, during adulthood. Significantly, increased multiplicity of tumors (number of tumors that arose at each site) was seen in lungs of offspring exposed during pregnancy, and this effect persisted through five generations of unexposed offspring in one study. Liver tumors were found to be more common in prenatally exposed males than females.

Genotoxicity

Chromosomal aberrations are found in cells from workers routinely exposed to PAHs. BaP has consistently been shown to be positive in *in vitro* assays for point mutations in *Salmonella* and for chromosome damage in mammalian cells, in the presence of an exogenous source of metabolic activation. Indeed, it is often used as a positive control in such assays. Positive results have also been reported in a wide range of *in vivo* studies in both somatic cells (e.g., bone marrow micronucleus test) and germ cells (dominant lethal assay and cytogenetics in spermatogonial cells) using both the inhalation and oral routes. In addition, several studies have reported genotoxicity of BaP following dermal exposure. A single topical application of BaP (0.5–500 μg per mouse) to hairless mice resulted in a significant increase in micronucleated keratinocytes. In addition, male mice treated with 20 μg topical BaP at 72 h intervals exhibited increased DNA adduct formation in epidermis and lungs.

As most exposures to BaP occur as a mixture, it is important to recognize potential synergies for activation of carcinogenesis. For example, coexposure to BaP and arsenite, another carcinogen, acted synergistically to induce BaP-DNA adduct formation at levels greater than those of animals treated with BaP alone.

Carcinogenicity

Animal

BaP has been extensively studied as a prototypical member of the PAH class of toxicants. Tumors are found at the site of exposure and at distant locations, correlating well with biodistribution data showing that the chemical is rapidly transported via the blood to the liver and other parts of the body. Administration by gavage to rats, mice, and hamsters caused forestomach tumors in a dose-dependent manner from 20 ppm upward. Similar studies showed esophageal, laryngeal, and pulmonary tumors depending on the method of administration. Intraperitoneal and subcutaneous injections caused injection site tumors. BaP is considered to be both an initiator and complete carcinogen in mouse skin. The World Health Organization's International Agency for Research on Cancer concluded that there was sufficient evidence that BaP is carcinogenic (causes cancer) in experimental animals.

Human

BaP is a probable human carcinogen, based on carcinogenicity in animals. Metabolites of BaP are mutagenic and carcinogenic, causing carcinogenesis in the liver and lung. Exposure to BaP almost never occurs in the absence of other PAHs; therefore, individual data on this compound are not available. BaP and its metabolites have been detected in urine of pregnant women and children. BaP has been detected in placenta, cord blood, maternal blood, and human breast milk. BaP-DNA adducts have been detected in multiple tissues during development. The placenta can metabolize BaP, and these metabolites bound to DNA in placenta and cord blood. One study detected BaP adducts in preimplantation embryos (early in prenatal development) from couples where the father and/or mother, or even the father alone, smoked cigarettes. BaP-DNA adducts were also detected in blood of mothers and their newborn infants. Decreased birth weight and head circumference in infants at birth were significantly associated with maternal exposure to cigarette smoke during pregnancy, as measured by the combination of cotinine and BaP-DNA adduct formation concentrations in fetal cord blood together, but not with either concentration alone.

Clinical Management

There is no antidote for BaP (or PAH) exposure. Upon exposure to any polycyclic aromatic hydrocarbon, recommendations include washing contaminated skin with soap and water and flushing contaminated eyes with water or saline. Charcoal administration has been recommended but there is no evidence of its efficacy. As glutathione conjugation is one mechanism by which PAHs is metabolized, administration of *N*-acetyl cysteine was shown in rats to reduce DNA adducts formed by PAHs; however, this has not been shown in humans. Indeed, glutathione-deficient mice have increased susceptibility to transplacental BaP-induced ovarian failure and ovarian tumorigenesis. Sulforaphane, an inducer of phase II metabolic genes, and conjugated linoleic acid reduced BaP-mediated forestomach cancers in mice; these effects have not been shown in humans. Monoclonal antibodies against BaP have been shown to decrease cellular uptake of BaP in cell line models; *in vivo*, monoclonal antibodies protected against BaP-induced immunotoxicity.

Ecotoxicology

Like all polycyclic aromatic hydrocarbons, PAHs accumulate in the aquatic environment and may cause long-term adverse effects. A water-soluble fraction of Arabian crude oil was shown to cause immunotoxicity in sea bass; both naphthalene and benzo(a)pyrene were detected in contaminated fish 15 days postexposure. Killifish experimentally exposed to BaP exhibited liver injury (**Figure 3**).

Exposure Standards and Guidelines

The drinking water unit risk is 2.1×10^{-4} per $\mu g\ l^{-1}$. The US Occupational Safety and Health Administration legal

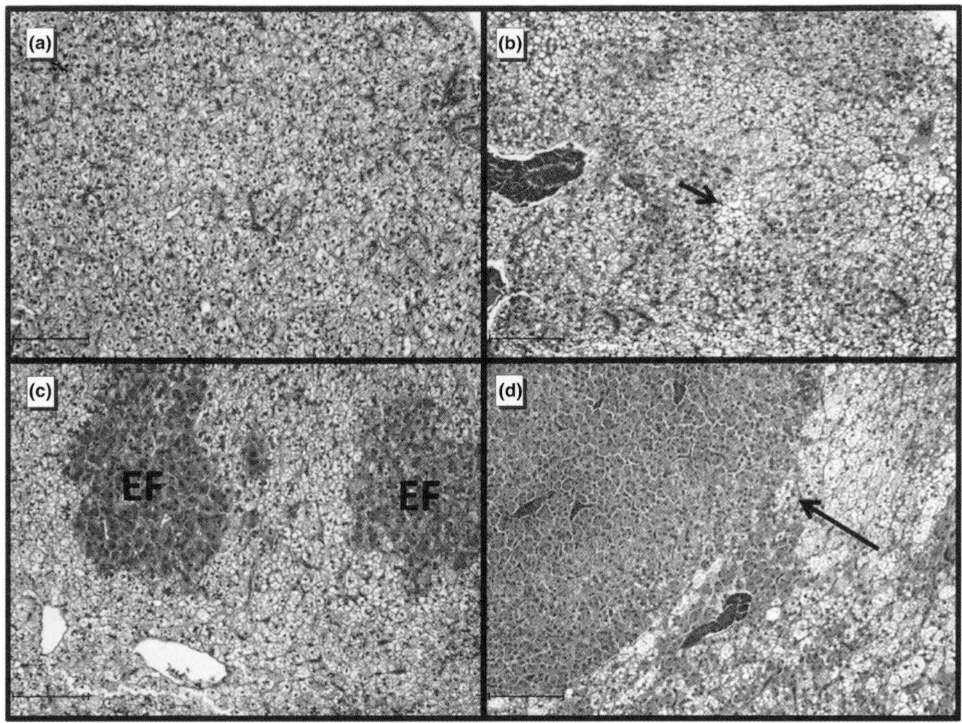

Figure 3 BaP-mediated liver damage in killifish exposed to BaP for 9 months at 400 μg l^{-1}. (a) Normal liver from DMSO vehicle control or (b–d) 400 μg l^{-1} BaP. (b) Focal steatosis in liver from a BaP-exposed killifish; arrow indicates large rounded vacuoles with smooth margins signifying lipid. (c) Eosinophilic foci (EF) in liver from a BaP-exposed killifish. (d) Hepatocellular carcinoma in liver from a BaP-exposed killifish; the arrow indicates an irregular and invasive border of the carcinoma. Bars = 100 μm. Comparative chronic liver toxicity of benzo[*a*]pyrene in two populations of the Atlantic killifish (*Fundulus heteroclitus*) with different exposure histories. Environ. Health Perspect. 118, 1376–1381. http://dx.doi.org/10.1289/ehp.0901799.

airborne permissible exposure limit is 0.2 mg m^{-3}, averaged over an 8 h work shift. The National Institute for Occupational Safety and Health recommends an airborne exposure limit of 0.1 mg m^{-3} averaged over a 10 h work shift. Although exposure by inhalation is a risk, there are currently no inhalation reference values available. The maximum contaminant level goal for BaP is zero. The US Environmental Protection Agency (EPA) has set this level of protection based on the best available science to prevent potential health problems. EPA has set an enforceable regulation for benzo(a)pyrene, called a maximum contaminant level (MCL), at 0.0002 mg l^{-1} or 200 ng l^{-1}. MCLs are set as close to the health goals as possible, considering cost, benefits, and the ability of public water systems to detect and remove contaminants using suitable treatment technologies.

See also: Polycyclic Aromatic Hydrocarbons (PAHs); Benz[a] anthracene.

Further Reading

Alexandrov, K., Rojas, M., Satarug, S., 2010. The critical DNA damage by benzo(*a*) pyrene in lung tissues of smokers and approaches to preventing its formation. Toxicol. Lett. 198 (1), 63–68.

Benford, D., Dinovi, M., Setzer, R.W., 2010. Application of the margin-of-exposure (MoE) approach to substances in food that are genotoxic and carcinogenic e.g.: benzo[*a*]pyrene and polycyclic aromatic hydrocarbons. Food Chem. Toxicol. 48 (Suppl. 1), S42–S48.

Béranger, R., Hoffmann, P., Christin-Maitre, S., Bonneterre, V., 2012. Occupational exposures to chemicals as a possible etiology in premature ovarian failure: a critical analysis of the literature. Reprod. Toxicol. 33 (3), 269–279.

Chen, Y., Huang, C., Bai, C., et al., 2013. Benzo[α]pyrene repressed DNA mismatch repair in human breast cancer cells. Toxicology 304, 167–172.

Cheng, S.Q., Xia, Y.Y., He, J.L., et al., 2013. Neurotoxic effect of subacute benzo(*a*) pyrene exposure on gene and protein expression in Sprague–Dawley rats. Environ. Toxicol. Pharmacol. 36 (2), 648–658.

Craig, Z.R., Wang, W., Flaws, J.A., 2011. Endocrine-disrupting chemicals in ovarian function: effects on steroidogenesis, metabolism and nuclear receptor signaling. Reproduction 142 (5), 633–646.

Cunningham, F.H., Fiebelkorn, S., Johnson, M., Meredith, C., 2011. A novel application of the margin of exposure approach: segregation of tobacco smoke toxicants. Food Chem. Toxicol. 49 (11), 2921–2933.

Danion, M., Le Floch, S., Lamour, F., Guyomarch, J., Quentel, C., 2011. Bioconcentration and immunotoxicity of an experimental oil spill in European sea bass (*Dicentrarchus labrax* L.). Ecotoxicol. Environ. Saf. 74 (8), 2167–2174.

Diggs, D.L., Huderson, A.C., Harris, K.L., et al., 2011. Polycyclic aromatic hydrocarbons and digestive tract cancers – a perspective. J. Environ. Sci. Health C Environ. Carcinog. Ecotoxicol. Rev. 29, 324–357.

Elamin, B.K., Callegari, E., Gramantieri, L., Sabbioni, S., Negrini, M., 2011. MicroRNA response to environmental mutagens in liver. Mutat. Res. 717 (1–2), 67–76.

Essumang, D.K., Dodoo, D.K., Adjei, J.K., 2013. Effect of smoke generation sources and smoke curing duration on the levels of polycyclic aromatic hydrocarbon (PAH) in different suites of fish. Food Chem. Toxicol. 58, 86–94.

Fujiwara, Y., Satoh, M., 11 April 2013. Protective role of Metallothionein in chemical and Radiation carcinogenesis. Curr. Pharm. Biotechnol. (Epub ahead of print).

Ikenaka, Y., Sakamoto, M., Nagata, T., et al., 2013. Effects of polycyclic aromatic hydrocarbons (PAHs) on an aquatic ecosystem: acute toxicity and community-level toxic impact tests of benzo[*a*]pyrene using lake zooplankton community. J. Toxicol. Sci. 38 (1), 131–136.

Jarvis, I.W., Bergvall, C., Bottai, M., et al., 2013. Persistent activation of DNA damage signaling in response to complex mixtures of PAHs in air particulate matter. Toxicol. Appl. Pharmacol. 266 (3), 408–418.

Lim, J., Lawson, G.W., Nakamura, B.N., Ortiz, L., Hur, J.A., Kavanagh, T.J., Luderer, U., 2013. Glutathione-deficient mice have increased sensitivity to transplacental benzo[*a*]pyrene-induced premature ovarian failure and ovarian tumorigenesis. Cancer Res. 732 (2), 908–917.

Maier, A., Schumann, B.L., Chang, X., Talaska, G., Puga, A., 2002. Arsenic co-exposure potentiates benzo[*a*]pyrene genotoxicity. Mutat. Res. 517 (1–2), 101–111.

Man, Y.B., Chow, K.L., Kang, Y., Wong, M.H., 2013. Mutagenicity and genotoxicity of Hong Kong soils contaminated by polycyclic aromatic hydrocarbons and dioxins/furans. Mutat. Res. 752 (1–2), 47–56.

Nebert, D.W., Shi, Z., Galvez-Peralta, M., Uno, S., Dragin, N., 12 June 2013. Oral benzo[*a*]pyrene: understanding pharmacokinetics, detoxication and consequences – cyp1 knockout mouse lines as a paradigm. Mol. Pharmacol.

Øvrevik, J., Refsnes, M., Holme, J.A., Schwarze, P.E., Låg, M., 2013. Mechanisms of chemokine responses by polycyclic aromatic hydrocarbons in bronchial epithelial cells: sensitization through toll-like receptor-3 priming. Toxicol. Lett. 219 (2), 125–132.

Pacheco, S.A., Torres, V.M., Louro, H., et al., 2013. Effects of occupational exposure to tobacco smoke: is there a link between environmental exposure and disease? J. Toxicol. Environ. Health A 76 (4–5), 311–327.

Pan, S., Li, D., Zhao, L., Schenkman, J.B., Rusling, J.F., 8 August 2013. Genotoxicity-related chemistry of human metabolites of benzo[ghi]perylene (B[ghi]P) investigated using electro-optical arrays and DNA/microsome biocolloid reactors with LC–MS/MS. Chem. Res. Toxicol. (Epub ahead of print).

Perumal Vijayaraman, K., Muruganantham, S., Subramanian, M., Shunmugiah, K.P., Kasi, P.D., 2012. Silymarin attenuates benzo(*a*)pyrene induced toxicity by mitigating ROS production, DNA damage and calcium mediated apoptosis in peripheral blood mononuclear cells (PBMC). Ecotoxicol. Environ. Saf. 86, 79–85.

Ramesh, A., Walker, S.A., Hood, D.B., et al., 2004. Bioavailability and risk assessment of orally ingested polycyclic aromatic hydrocarbons. Int. J. Toxicol. 23, 301–333.

Ramos, K.S., Nanez, A., 2009. Genetic regulatory networks of nephrogenesis: deregulation of WT1 splicing by benzo(*a*)pyrene. Birth Defects Res. C Embryo Today 87 (2), 192–197.

Rekhadevi, P.V., Diggs, D.L., Huderson, A.C., et al., 23 May 2013. Metabolism of the environmental toxicant benzo(*a*)pyrene by subcellular fractions of human ovary. Hum. Exp. Toxicol.

Sonkoly, E., Pivarcsi, A., 2011. MicroRNAs in inflammation and response to injuries induced by environmental pollution. Mutat. Res. 717 (1–2), 46–53.

Subashchandrabose, S.R., Megharaj, M., Venkateswarlu, K., Naidu, R., 23 April 2013. Interaction effects of polycyclic aromatic hydrocarbons and heavy metals on a soil microalga, *Chlorococcum* sp. MM11. Environ. Sci. Pollut. Res. Int.

Vega-López, A., Ayala-López, G., Posadas-Espadas, B.P., et al., 2013. Relations of oxidative stress in freshwater phytoplankton with heavy metals and polycyclic aromatic hydrocarbons. Comp. Biochem. Physiol. A Mol. Integr. Physiol. 165 (4), 498–507.

Verma, N., Pink, M., Rettenmeier, A.W., Schmitz-Spanke, S., 2013. Benzo[*a*]pyrene-mediated toxicity in primary pig bladder epithelial cells: a proteomic approach. J. Proteomics 85, 53–64.

Zaccaria, K.J., McClure, P.R., 2013. Using immunotoxicity information to improve cancer risk assessment for polycyclic aromatic hydrocarbon mixtures. Int. J. Toxicol. 32 (4), 236–250.

Relevant Websites

http://www.atsdr.cdc.gov/toxprofiles/tp.asp?id=122&tid=25 – Centers for Disease Control and Prevention.

http://www.hpa.org.uk/webc/HPAwebFile/HPAweb_C/1227169968160 – Health Protection Agency, UK.

http://nj.gov/health/eoh/rtkweb/documents/fs/0207.pdf – NJ.Gov.

http://toxnet.nlm.nih.gov/cgi-bin/sis/search/r?dbs+hsdb:@term+@rn+@rel+50-32-8 – National Library of Medicine.

http://cfpub.epa.gov/ncea/iris/index.cfm?fuseaction=iris.showQuickView&substance_nmbr=0136 – US Environmental Protection Agency.

http://www.epa.gov/iris/subst/0136.htm – US Environmental Protection Agency.

http://www.epa.gov/pbt/pubs/benzo.htm – US Environmental Protection Agency.

http://www.epa.gov/teach/chem_summ/BaP_summary.pdf – US Environmental Protection Agency.

http://water.epa.gov/drink/contaminants/basicinformation/benzo-a-pyrene.cfm – US Environmental Protection Agency.

Benzyl Alcohol

GB Corcoran, Wayne State University, Eugene Applebaum College of Pharmacy and Health Sciences, Detroit, MI, USA
SD Ray, Manchester University College of Pharmacy, Fort Wayne, IN, USA

This article is a revision of the previous edition article by Swarupa G. Kulkarni and Harihara M. Mehendale, volume 1, pp 262–264, © 2005, Elsevier Inc.

- Name: Benzyl Alcohol
- Chemical Abstracts Service Registry Number: 100-51-6
- Synonyms: Benzenemethanol; (Hydroxymethyl)benzene; Alcohol bencilico; Alpha-toluenol; Benzal alcohol; Benzenecarbinol; Benzenemethanol; Benzoyl alcohol; Benzyl alcohol (natural); Benzylicum; Hydroxytoluene; Methanol; Phenyl-; Phenolcarbinol; Phenylcarbinol; Phenylcarbinolum; Phenylmethanol; Phenylmethyl alcohol
- Molecular Formula: C_7–H_8–O
- Chemical Structure:

OH

conjunction with its comparatively modest toxicity. Products include foods, flavors, cosmetics, ointments, perfumes, and heat-sealing polyethylene films. In 1998, the Food and Drug Administration reported that benzyl alcohol was present in 322 cosmetics in 43 categories. The alcohol is classified as a High Production Volume chemical by the Environmental Protection Agency Office of Pollution Prevention and Toxics, with past US production at 10–50 million pounds per year. Yearly worldwide use as a fragrance ingredient in 2008 was estimated as 100–1000 metric tons by the International Fragrance Agency (IFRA, 2008). Benzyl alcohol finds yet other uses in photographic development for color movie films, solvent for dyestuffs, cellulose esters, casein, and waxes, chemical stock for production of benzyl esters and ethers, and an emulsion component.

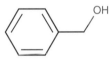

Background

As an important synthetic chemical that is also widely produced across nature at modest levels, benzyl alcohol was prepared chemically in small amounts from benzaldehyde and potassium hydroxide via the Cannizzaro reaction. It is now produced on industrial levels by treating benzyl chloride with sodium or potassium carbonate. The alcohol occurs naturally in a range of fruits and plants including honey, apricots, mushrooms, snap beans, cocoa, and cranberries as well as in the essential oils of plants like hyacinth and jasmine. In the past, as much as 60% of benzyl alcohol production was used in the textile industry as a dye assistant to render hydrophobic fibers more receptive to dyes with hydrophilic properties, with direct applications to filaments like nylon, textiles, and sheet plastics. This alcohol offers among the earliest of xenobiotic biotransformation examples to be chemically characterized in the field of pharmacology. Enzymatic oxidation to benzoic acid is followed by conjugation with glycine producing hippuric acid, which was so named because the conjugate was first isolated from horse urine.

Uses

Although available for some years as an over the counter health product, benzyl alcohol was approved in 2003 by the Food and Drug Administration as a new prescription drug for the treatment of head lice. Unlike typical pediculicides like permethrin and lindane, which act through a neurotoxic mode of action, benzyl alcohol is thought to operate via a unique mechanism involving physical pulmonary asphyxiation. The presence of benzyl alcohol in such a wide range of consumer products is explained by its bacteriostatic and antiseptic properties in

Environmental Behavior, Fate, Routes, and Pathways

Due to an abundance of useful applications across society, from industrial production to consumer products, benzyl alcohol is present in the environment and is steadily released through commercial and household waste streams. Benzyl alcohol was an early object of chemists striving for greener synthetic approaches involving mixed catalysts for oxidation. It is released into the atmosphere entirely as a vapor due to its high vapor pressure, where it is lost by degradation involving reaction with hydroxyl radicals at a half-life of about 2 days. Benzyl alcohol is expected to have quite high mobility based upon its soil to water partition coefficient, and a projected soil half-life of about 13 days.

Exposure and Exposure Monitoring

The principle routes of exposure to benzyl alcohol are through the lungs, skin, and gastrointestinal tract. It is believed that individuals encounter their most common exposure to benzyl alcohol through dermal contact with consumer products. Dermal systemic exposure has been measured for 10 of the most highly used personal care and cosmetic products, leading to an estimated total exposure of 0.042 $\mu g\ kg^{-1}\ day^{-1}$ for high-end product users. Researchers evaluating migration data recently estimated the ranges of dermal and oral exposures of children to fragrances in scented toys and concluded that maximal dermal benzyl alcohol exposure was 605 $\mu g\ kg^{-1}\ day^{-1}$. In 1979, the Joint Commission on Food Additives set acceptable dietary intake of benzoic moiety, to include all benzyl contributors including benzyl alcohol and benzyl benzoate, at 0–5 μg per kg of body weight per day (FAO/WHO, 1994). The diet, of course, is not the only route of exposure to benzyl alcohol.

 http://dx.doi.org/10.1016/B978-0-12-386454-3.00251-7

Toxicokinetics

Adults readily oxidize benzyl alcohol to benzoic acid. This is followed by the conjugation of benzoic acid with glycine in the liver to form hippuric acid. The latter is excreted in the urine. The immature metabolic capacities of infants result in limited ability to metabolize the benzyl alcohol metabolite benzoic acid to its primary excreted metabolite hippuric acid resulting in increased benzoic acid concentrations in preterm infants. These concentrations are further increased in preterm babies over term babies due to an increased ability to metabolize benzyl alcohol to benzoic acid. The relative inability to convert benzoic acid to hippuric acid may be related to glycine deficiency. Accumulation of benzoic acid in preterm infants has led to cases of severe toxicity and death.

In dogs administered 52 or 105 mg kg^{-1} iv doses of benzyl alcohol in saline, plasma half-life was about 1.5 h. Benzyl alcohol rapidly disappeared from the injection site following intramuscular administration in rats, with a disappearance half-life estimated to be less than 10 min. In nonhuman primate studies, the Rhesus monkey demonstrates high absorption (56–80%) of topically administered benzyl alcohol over 24 h, but only when the administration site is occluded. Rabbits receiving 1 g of subcutaneous benzyl alcohol eliminate 300–400 mg of hippuric acid. In humans, benzyl alcohol is readily absorbed from the gastrointestinal tract following oral ingestion. Percutaneous absorption of benzyl alcohol during its use to treat pediculosis is reported to be limited and low, although application of higher concentrations of the alcohol can result in substantial uptake. Levels of benzyl alcohol from 5 to 500 μg per 10 ml plasma are reported in uremic patients on hemodialysis. No drug interaction studies have been reported to date with benzyl alcohol.

Mechanisms of Action

When used as a treatment for head lice, benzyl alcohol is thought to operate via a unique mechanism involving physical pulmonary obstruction of respiratory spiracles by the solvent, resulting in the asphyxiation of lice. Benzyl alcohol is a local anesthetic and produces metabolic acidosis. The latter action can be attributed to direct acidification and fixed anion effects of the metabolite benzoic acid and potentially to secondary lactic acid production due to inhibition of cellular metabolism. Weak local anesthetic effects have been related to membrane fluidization.

Acute and Short-Term Toxicity

Benzyl alcohol has been studied across a large number of nonhuman species including rat, mouse, cat, dog, rabbit, and chicken. The oral LD_{50} values of benzyl alcohol in seven rat studies range from 1230 to over 3100 mg kg^{-1}. These levels of observed effects have been categorized as moderately toxic in some comparative toxicity scales. In the rat, clinical signs and symptoms of toxicity include increased respiration, piloerection, tremors, half-closed eyes, lethargy, ataxia, prostration, and ultimately coma. Depression occurs within 10–15 min, followed by death from 1 h to as late as 4 days. Signs in mice include depression with animal deaths within 18 h. Subcutaneous benzyl alcohol produces respiratory stimulation, followed by respiratory and muscular paralysis, convulsion, and central nervous system (CNS) depression. Interestingly, intravenous administration of benzyl alcohol to rat, cat, and dog produces a decrease in arterial blood pressure, which is not seen in the dog after oral administration.

The general toxicity of lower dose benzyl alcohol exposures in humans places it among Class I agents that cause reversible effects which are generally not life-threatening. Common effects are irritation and mild CNS depression. Toxic effects associated with higher exposures include vasodilatation, hypotension, convulsions, paralysis, and respiratory failure. Serious problems have occurred with this alcohol when present as a preservative in fluids administered to neonates. Benzyl alcohol was responsible for a number of deaths stemming from metabolic acidosis that progressed to respiratory distress and gasping respirations. Some infants developed CNS dysfunction, including developmental delay, convulsions, intracranial hemorrhage, and hypotension followed by cardiovascular collapse. Neonatal toxicity has been attributed to the immaturity of the benzoic acid detoxification process in premature newborns. Ocular exposure to dilute solutions of benzyl alcohol can cause slight irritation and local anesthesia. Use of benzyl alcohol in consumer products has resulted in a relatively low incidence of contact dermatitis characterized by urticaria, angioedema, erythema, and pruritus. Finally, the comparatively more favorable safety properties of benzyl alcohol have resulted in it being advocated in 2013 as a less-toxic alternative for paint stripping products containing dichloromethane. LD_{50} doses for benzyl alcohol in several rodent models are listed below:

LD_{50} Mouse sc 950 mg kg^{-1}
LD_{50} Mouse iv <0.5 ml kg^{-1} per 94% benzyl alcohol
LD_{50} Mouse oral 1360–1580 mg kg^{-1}
LD_{50} Mouse iv 324 mg kg^{-1}

LD_{50} Rat sc 1700 mg kg^{-1}
LD_{50} Rat ip >400–800 mg kg^{-1}
LD_{50} Rat oral 1230–3120 mg kg^{-1}
LC_{100} Rat inhalation 200–300 ppm per 8 h
LC_{50} Rat inhalation 74 mg l^{-1} per 4 h
LC_{50} Rat inhalation 1000 ppm per 8 h
LD_{50} Rat iv 53 mg kg^{-1}
LD_{50} Rat iv 314 mg kg^{-1}

LD_{50} Rabbit oral 1940 mg kg^{-1}
LD_{50} Rabbit dermal 2000 mg kg^{-1}

LD_{50} Guinea pig dermal <5 ml kg^{-1}
LD_{50} Guinea pig ip >400–800 mg kg^{-1}

Source: NLM-HSDB.

Chronic Toxicity

Limited signs and symptoms of chronic oral toxicity were noted for benzyl alcohol when given to rats and mice in doses of 200–400 mg kg^{-1} over 2 years (NTP, 1989). Most findings were not reliably attributable to the test article. The Environmental

Protection Agency has set the reference dose for chronic oral exposure at 0.286 mg kg^{-1} day^{-1}.

Immunotoxicity

See acute toxicity.

Reproductive and Developmental Toxicity

The effects of benzyl alcohol on fertility appear not to have been evaluated in animals or humans.

Genotoxicity

Studies have produced mainly negative but mixed outcomes. This alcohol is nonmutagenic when tested under the preincubation protocol for *Salmonella typhimurium* strains TA98, TA100, TA1535, or TA1537, both in the presence and in the absence of exogenous metabolic activation. It is also negative in the sex-linked recessive lethal assay and the replicative DNA synthesis assay in rat. Although negative in the mouse lymphoma assay with metabolic activation, benzyl alcohol is positive in this assay without metabolic activation at levels that also produce significant cell death. On the other hand, benzyl alcohol clearly increases the rate of sister chromatid exchange in Chinese hamster ovary cells in the presence but not the absence of the S9 fraction.

Carcinogenicity

The National Toxicology Program has conducted long-term carcinogenesis studies of technical-grade benzyl alcohol (99% pure). Groups of F344/N rats and B6C3F1 mice were administered the test chemical by gavage for 16 days, 13 weeks, or 2 years. Benzyl alcohol produced no evidence of carcinogenic activity in male or female F344/N rats dosed with 200 or 400 mg kg^{-1}. Male or female B6C3F1 mice dosed with 100 or 200 mg kg^{-1} for 2 years also demonstrated no evidence of carcinogenic activity.

Clinical Management

There is no proven antidote for benzyl alcohol poisoning. Treatments for significant benzyl alcohol exposure, following standard airway, breathing and circulation support as appropriate, are nonspecific and include discontinuation of the exposure, enhancement of elimination if justified, and supportive care. Management of inhalation exposure can include increased ventilation, fresh air, and rest. In cases of dermal exposure, protective gloves are recommended during removal of contaminated clothing and repeated rinsing with water. Ocular contact resulting in redness should prompt rinsing with water for several minutes, and immediate removal of contact lenses if present. Individuals who are suspected of acute benzyl alcohol ingestion and demonstrate serious symptoms including diarrhea, nausea, and/or vomiting should be promptly referred for advanced medical attention, as should those exposed via other routes. Hemodialysis may enhance the elimination of benzyl alcohol and its metabolites, and may also be a useful adjunct in correcting severe metabolic acidosis.

Exposure Standards and Guidelines

Studies characterizing safe exposure limits to benzyl alcohol are not as available as for many chemicals. One of the few published values for airborne exposure limits comes from the Occupational Alliance for Risk Science, which sets the workplace environmental exposure level (WEEL) for 8-h time-weighted average (TWA) at 10 ppm. This WEEL was developed and maintained by the American Industrial Hygiene Association until 2012. The American Conference of Governmental Industrial Hygienists has no set threshold limit value for benzyl alcohol. The Research Institute for Fragrance Materials (RIFM) classifies benzyl alcohol potency as a skin sensitizer as weak, based on animal data including a local lymph node assay value of >12 500. They report a lowest observable effect level value of 8858 μg cm^{-2}. The RIFM Expert Panel established the no expected sensitization induction level (NESIL) at 5900 μg cm^{-2}. The German Commission for the Investigation of Health Hazards of Chemical Compounds in the Work Area concluded that human and animal studies have yielded insufficient information to set a maximum workplace concentration value, placing it in Category II B. More recently, the German Working Group on Indoor Air Guidelines of the Federal Environment Agency has issued indoor air hazard guide value of 4 mg m^{-3} and a health precaution guide value of 0.4 mg m^{-3}. Florida limits the presence of benzyl alcohol in its State Drinking Water Guidelines to 2100 μg l^{-1}.

Further Reading

Api, A.M., Basketter, D.A., Cadby, P.A., et al., 2008. Dermal Sensitization Quantitative Risk Assessment for Fragrance Ingredients. Reg. Toxicol. Pharmacol. 52 (1) (special issue).

Belsito, D., Bickers, D., Bruze, M., et al., Sep 2012. RIFM Expert Panel – a toxicological and dermatological assessment of aryl alkyl alcohol simple acid ester derivatives when used as fragrance ingredients. Food Chem. Toxicol 50 (Suppl. 2), S269–S313 (Epub Mar 9 2012).

Carvalho, C.M., Menezes, P.F., Letenski, G.C., et al., 2012. *In vitro* induction of apoptosis, necrosis and genotoxicity by cosmetic preservatives: application of flow cytometry as a complementary analysis by NRU. Int. J. Cosmet. Sci. 34 (2), 176–182.

Chow, E.T., Avolio, A.M., Lee, A., Nixon, R., 2013. Frequency of positive patch test reactions to preservatives: the Australian experience. Australas. J. Dermatol. 54, 31–35.

Gerberick, G.F., Robinson, M.K., Ryan, C.A., et al., 2001. Contact allergenic potency: Correlation of human and local lymph node assay data. Am. J. Contact Dermat. 12 (3), 156–161.

IFRA (International Fragrance Association), 2008. Use Level Survey. December 2008.

Indoor air guide values for benzyl alcohol. Bundesgesundheitsblatt Gesundheitsforschung Gesundheitsschutz 53 (9), Sep 2010, 984–987. http://dx.doi.org/10.1007/s00103-010-1123-y.

LeBel, M., Ferron, L., Masson, M., Pichette, J., Carrier, C., 1988. Benzyl alcohol metabolism and elimination in neonates. Dev. Pharmacol. Ther. 11 (6), 347–356.

MacIsaac, J., Harrison, R., Krishnaswami, J., McNary, J., Suchard, J., Boysen-Osborn, M., Cierpich, H., Styles, L., Dennis Shusterman, D., 2013. Fatalities due to dichloromethane in paint strippers: a continuing problem. Am. J. Ind. Med. 56, 907–910.

Masuck, I., Hutzler, C., Luch, A., 2011. Estimation of dermal and oral exposure of children to scented toys: analysis of the migration of fragrance allergens by dynamic headspace GC-MS. J. Sep. Sci. 34 (19), 2686–2696.

Nair, B., 2001. Final report on the safety assessment of benzyl alcohol, benzoic acid, and sodium benzoate. Int. J. Toxicol. 20 (Suppl. 3), 23–50.

NTP, 1989. Toxicology and carcinogenesis studies of benzyl alcohol (CAS No. 100-51-6) in F344/N rats and B6C3F1 mice (Gavage studies). Natl. Toxicol. Program Tech. Rep. Ser. 343, 1–158.

Scognamiglio, J., Jones, L., Vitale, D., Letizia, C.S., Api, A.M., 2012. Fragrance material review on benzyl alcohol. Food Chem. Toxicol. 50 (Suppl. 2), S140–S160.

Shehab, N., Lewis, C.L., Streetman, D.D., Donn, S.M., 2009. Exposure to the pharmaceutical excipients benzyl alcohol and propylene glycol among critically ill neonates. Pediatr. Crit. Care Med. 10 (2), 256–259.

US EPA, 2008. Non-confidential production volume information submitted by companies for chemicals under the 1986–2002. Inventory Update Rule (IUR). Benzenemethanol (100-51-6). http://www.epa.gov/oppt/cdr/tools/data/2002-vol.html.

Uter, W., Johansen, J.D., Borje, A., et al., 2013. Categorization of fragrance contact allergens for prioritization of preventive measures: clinical and experimental data and consideration of structure–activity relationships. Contact Dermat.

Relevant Websites

http://ec.europa.eu/food/fs/sc/scf/out138_en.pdf – Benzyl alcohol – European Commission.

http://toxnet.nlm.nih.gov – Toxnet (Toxicology Data Network): search under Toxline for Benzyl Alcohol.

http://chem.sis.nlm.nih.gov/chemidplus – US National Library of Medicine: ChemIDplus Advanced: Search for: Benzyl Alcohol.

Benzyl Benzoate

MA Pearson and GW Miller, Emory University, Atlanta, GA, USA

This article is a revision of the previous edition article by Jamaluddin Shaikh, volume 1, pp 264–265, © 2005, Elsevier Inc.

- Name: Benzyl Benzoate
- Chemical Abstracts Service Registry Number: CAS 120-51-4
- Synonyms: Ascabin, Benylate, Benzyl alcohol benzoic ester, Scabide, Vanzoate
- Molecular Formula: $C_{14}H_{12}O_2$
- Chemical Structure:

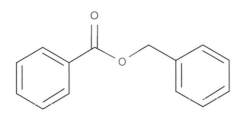

Background (Significance/History)

Benzyl benzoate occurs naturally in Peruvian and Tulu balsams as well as other essential oils. It was used in Vietnam War as a repellant for ticks and mites. Benzyl benzoate was used as an antispasmodic, but has been replaced with more effective treatments. In many poor regions, it is the first-line intervention for patients with scabies. Benzyl benzoate is used in veterinary medicine as a both scabicide and pediculicide. Benzyl benzoate is a common additive to body care, cosmetics, and food.

Uses

Benzyl benzoate is used as a plasticizer in cellulose and other polymers, a fixative in fragrances, a food additive, a solvent, a remedy for scabies, a pesticide to kill ticks, mites, and lice, and has been used as a repellent for chiggers, ticks, and mosquitoes.

Environmental Fate and Behavior

When tested in water, benzyl benzoate residues remained greater than 60% at 2 and 7 days after treatment. Benzyl benzoate appears to have a low water distribution and a high soil distribution.

Exposure Routes and Pathways

Benzyl benzoate is an active substance in Peruvian and Tulu balsams as well as other essential oils. It is also produced synthetically and is formulated as a liquid, emulsion, or lotion. Exposure to benzyl benzoate can occur via skin contact or ingestion. Migration of benzyl benzoate and other compounds from toys was derived to estimate levels of oral and dermal exposure in children from contact with the toys. Benzyl benzoate had the highest migration rate among the tested compounds and the exposure levels were maximally estimated at 22.2 mg kg^{-1} bw day^{-1}. Fetal exposure in rats following maternal exposure has also been documented.

Toxicokinetics

The dermal absorption factor of benzyl benzoate is not well documented; however, one study demonstrated that 54% of the percutaneously applied dose did penetrate human skin. After absorption, benzyl benzoate is rapidly hydrolyzed into benzoic acid. Conjugation of benzoic acid and glycine yields hippuric acid; conjugation of benzoic acid and glucuronic acid yields benzoylglucuronic acid. The formation of hippuric acid depends on the availability of glycine; when insufficient, benzoyl glucuronide is formed. Both conjugates are eliminated in urine in different ratios depending on species and dose.

Mechanism of Toxicity

Benzyl benzoate acts as a local irritant. At high levels of exposure, free benzoic acid may sequester significant amounts of acetyl coenzyme A (CoA), which could disrupt cholinergic signaling. Recent findings suggest that benzyl benzoate may have estrogenic properties.

Acute and Short-Term Toxicity

Animals

The oral LD_{50} values range from 1700 mg kg^{-1} in rats to over 22 440 mg kg^{-1} in dogs. Cats are particularly susceptible to benzyl benzoate, with an oral LD_{50} value of 2240 mg kg^{-1}. Signs of toxicity include nausea, vomiting, diarrhea, salivation, piloerection, progressive incoordination, central nervous system excitation, tremors, convulsions, progressive paralysis of hind limbs, prostration, dyspnea, and death. Rabbits treated with a lethal dermal dose died without exhibiting symptoms of systemic effects. Lethal dermal doses in cats produced excessive salivation, twitching of the treated areas, generalized tremors, muscular incoordination, paralysis of hind limbs, convulsions, and respiratory failure prior to death. In addition to the lack of benzyl benzoate sensitivity in dogs, dermally applied benzyl benzoate was nontoxic to the pig, sheep, heifer, or horse.

Humans

An evaluation of the impact of fragrance compounds on dermatitis led benzyl benzoate to be classified as a rare sensitizer. Skin reactions are the most common reaction to benzyl benzoate, usually described as nonallergic contact dermatitis. Anaphylaxis was triggered in a 16-year-old boy being treated for

 http://dx.doi.org/10.1016/B978-0-12-386454-3.00103-2

primary hypogonadism by an intramuscular injection of a depot testosterone undecanoate (Reandron 1000, Bayer: depot testosterone undecanoate with a castor oil and benzyl benzoate vehicle). Testing identified benzyl benzoate as the likely trigger for the anaphylactic reaction. Convulsions have been reported as serious reactions to benzyl benzoate, although the number of reported events was low. The death of a 7-year-old child was attributed to an overdose of the benzyl-benzoate-based scabicide in which he was bathed every other day prior to a bone marrow transplant. A retrospective study investigated the safety of both a benzyl benzoate lotion and a permethrin lotion in the treatment of scabies in pregnant women and found no significant differences in the proportion of abortions or the proportion of congenital abnormalities related to benzyl benzoate treatment, although the study had limited power to detect such differences.

Chronic Toxicity

Animals

To date, very few published studies report the chronic effects of benzyl benzoate in animals. A single report described the effects of daily doses of benzyl benzoate of 25 mg kg^{-1} bw and 100 mg kg^{-1} bw in pregnant rats. This exposure led to liver abnormalities, histopathological changes in the brain, enlargement of the intermyofibrillar area of the heart, degeneration of blood vessels in the heart, an increased rate of fetal resorption (in the higher treatment dose), increased aspartate aminotransferase, changes in vascular endothelial growth factor, and placental damage in the pregnant rats. The related fetal exposure resulted in increased weight of the fetal heart and liver, degenerated blood vessels in the heart, histopathological changes in the liver, morphological changes in the kidney, and changes in vascular endothelial growth factor. Based on these toxicological findings, it was suggested that benzyl benzoate may be potent inhibitor of angiogenesis via its effects on vascular endothelial growth factor.

Humans

To date, the chronic effects of benzyl benzoate in humans are not fully known.

Reproductive Toxicity

To date, no published studies have specifically investigated the adverse effects of benzyl benzoate on reproductive ability. However, benzyl benzoate did lead to increased fetal resorption in pregnant rats and, suggestive of endocrine system endpoints, produced estrogenic responses in MCF7 human breast cancer cells *in vitro*.

Genotoxicity

The genotoxicity of benzyl benzoate is not well established. One published study reported that at high concentrations *in vitro*, benzyl-benzoate-induced gene expression in the stably transfected ERE-CAT reporter gene and the endogenous pS2 gene in MCF7 human breast cells.

Carcinogenicity

To date, little data are available on carcinogenic properties of benzyl benzoate. Benzyl benzoate was not found to be mutagenic in a screening of tobacco smoke constituents using the Ames test.

In Vitro Toxicity Data

Benzyl benzoate increased the proliferation of estrogen-dependent MCF7 breast cancer cells over 7 days, but another report determined stimulation not to be significant after a 24-h period. Benzyl-benzoate-induced gene expression in the stably transfected ERE-CAT reporter gene and the endogenous pS2 gene in MCF7 human breast cells.

Clinical Management

In the case of skin contact, remove any contaminated clothing and wash the affected skin with soap and water. If the eyes are exposed, rinse immediately with water for at least 15 min with open eyelids. If exposure is due to inhalation, the patient should be moved to fresh air. If the patient does not recover rapidly, medical attention should be sought. In case of ingestion, do not induce vomiting. If the person is conscious, the mouth should be rinsed with plenty of water, approximately 500 ml of water should be consumed, and medical attention should be sought.

Ecotoxicology

Benzyl benzoate is relatively toxic to brine shrimp, zebra fish (LC_{50}, 3.9 mg l^{-1}), and bluegill sunfish (LC_{50}, 2.5 mg l^{-1}).

Exposure Standards and Guidelines

- Acceptable daily intake: 5 mg kg^{-1}.

See also: Pesticides; Cosmetics and Personal Care Products.

Further Reading

Charles, A.K., Darbre, P.D., 2009 Jul. Oestrogenic activity of benzyl salicylate, benzyl benzoate and butylphenylmethylpropional (Lilial) in MCF7 human breast cancer cells *in vitro*. J. Appl. Toxicol. 29 (5), 422–434. http://dx.doi.org/10.1002/jat.1429. PMID: 19338011.

Koçkaya, E.A., Kiliç, A., 2011. Developmental toxicity of benzyl benzoate in rats after maternal exposure throughout pregnancy. Environ. Toxicol. http://dx.doi.org/10.1002/tox.20771 (PMID: 21922633). Article first published online: 16 SEP 2011.

Relevant Website

http://www.fao.org/food/food-safety-quality/scientific-advice/jecfa/en/ – Food and Agriculture Organisation.

Beryllium

SC Gad, Gad Consulting Services, Cary, NC, USA

- Chemical Abstracts Service Registry Number: 7440-41-7
- Synonyms: Glucinum, Glucinium
- Valence States: 0, +2

Background

Although known through the mineral beryl, $Be_3Al_2(SiO_3)_6$, for millennia, beryllium was discovered as an element in 1797 by Louis-Nicolas Vauquelin, although it was not isolated as a metal until Friedrich Wöhler and Antoine Bussy independently succeeded in this venture independently by reacting potassium metal with beryllium chloride in a platinum crucible, yielding beryllium metal and potassium chloride. Its use in metallurgy and electrical components were largely developed in the 1920s.

Uses

Beryllium is an important industrial metal because of its material properties; that is, it is lighter than aluminum and six times stronger than steel. Often alloyed with other metals such as copper, beryllium is a key component of materials used in the aerospace and electronics industries. Beryllium has a small neutron cross-section, which makes it useful in the production of nuclear weapons and in sealed neutron sources. Specifically, beryllium is used in nuclear reactors as a neutron reflector or moderator, and in the aerospace industry in inertial guidance systems; beryllium alloys (consisting of copper or aluminum) are also used in structural material. Beryllium oxide is used as an additive in glass, ceramics, and plastics and as a catalyst in organic reactions. In the past, beryllium was widely used in the manufacture of fluorescent lights and neon signs. Alloyed with copper, aluminum, or nickel, beryllium imparts excellent electrical and thermal conductivity.

Environmental Fate and Behavior

Beryllium enters the environment principally through emissions from the combustion of fossil fuels and ore processing. Average ambient air concentrations in the United States have been measured at 0.03 ng m^{-3}, whereas median concentration in cities is 0.2 ng m^{-3}.

Insolubility of beryllium and many of its compounds can lead to long-term persistence in the environment, as particulates suspended in water until deposition in sediment, or in soils. Concentrations of beryllium in soil are found in the United States, as well as, more recently, in Brazil, Argentina, Madagascar, India, and Russia.

Long-range transport of beryllium is common in continental river systems, whereas brackish mixing zones exhibit scavenging. It is not yet known whether beryllium ceases transport in these estuarine waters and deposits in sediments, or continues to the deep ocean, although beryllium concentrations in deep ocean waters around the world are uniform.

A measured bioconcentration factor (BCF) of 19 was reported for beryllium in bluegill fish. Other investigators have reported a BCF of 100 for freshwater and marine plants, invertebrates, and fish. Chemicals with BCFs <1000 will not bioaccumulate significantly in aquatic organisms. It is possible that bottom-feeding crustaceans, such as clams and oysters, could accumulate beryllium from sediment and show higher bioconcentration than freshwater fish. No evidence for significant biomagnification of beryllium within food chains was found.

Exposure and Exposure Monitoring

The primary exposure pathway for beryllium is inhalation. Inhalation, ingestion, and dermal contact are possible exposure pathways in workplace settings. Exposure to small amounts of beryllium occurs with ingestion of some foods and drinking water. Beryllium enters the air, water, and soil as a result of natural and human activities. Emissions from burning coal and oil increase beryllium levels in air. Beryllium enters waterways from the wearing away of rocks and soil. Most of the synthetic beryllium that enters waterways comes when industry dumps wastewater and when beryllium dust in the air from industrial activities settles over water. Beryllium, as a chemical component, occurs naturally in soil; however, disposal of coal ash, incinerator ash, and industrial wastes may increase the concentration of beryllium in soil. In air, beryllium compounds are present mostly as fine dust particles. The dust eventually settles over land and water.

Toxicokinetics

Beryllium is not well absorbed by any route. Oral absorption of beryllium is <0.01% and probably only occurs in the acidic stomach environment. About half of inhaled beryllium is cleared in ~2 weeks. The remainder is cleared slowly and the residual becomes fixed in the lung (granulomata). The half-life of beryllium in rat blood is ~3 h. Beryllium is distributed to all tissues. High doses generally go to the liver and then are gradually transferred to the bone. Most beryllium concentrates in the skeleton. Beryllium is excreted in the urine; however, the fraction of administered dose excreted in urine is variable.

Mechanism of Toxicity

Beryllium compromises the immune system. Enzymes catalyzed by magnesium or calcium can be inhibited by beryllium; succinic dehydrogenase is activated. Beryllium exposure

 http://dx.doi.org/10.1016/B978-0-12-386454-3.00820-4

leads to a deficiency in lung carbon monoxide diffusing capacity. Hypercalcemia (excess of calcium in the blood) can occur.

Acute and Short-Term Toxicity (or Exposure)

Animal

The pulmonary effects of inhaled beryllium have been evaluated in a variety of laboratory animal species. Monkeys, for example, exposed to relatively high concentrations of beryllium compounds developed symptoms and histopathological findings consistent with acute beryllium disease.

Human

The major toxicological effects of beryllium are on the lung. Acute exposure to soluble beryllium compounds (e.g., fluoride, an intermediate in the ore extraction process) irritates the entire respiratory tract, may produce acute chemical pneumonitis, and can result in fatal pulmonary edema. Hypersensitivity, which appears to be mediated by the immune system, may also occur following exposure. This means that future exposure to beryllium may produce health effects at concentrations lower than those generally associated with the effect (the individual becomes much more sensitive to beryllium). The acute disease in humans is also marked by conjunctivitis, nasopharyngitis, tracheobronchitis, and dermatitis.

Chronic Toxicity (or Exposure)

Animal

Although beryllium produces cancer in more than one animal species (lung cancer in rats and monkeys; osteogenic sarcoma in rabbits), it does not appear to be teratogenic.

Human

Chronic exposure to insoluble beryllium compounds, particularly the oxides, leads to berylliosis (a chronic granulomatous disease), which begins with a cough and chest pains. In most cases, these symptoms soon lead to pulmonary dysfunction. The latency period ranges from months to 25 years. Diagnosis based on clinical, radiographic, and lung function evidence has been found to be difficult.

Other effects of beryllium exposure include enlargement of the heart (which can lead to congestive heart failure), enlargement of the liver, and kidney stones. Finger 'clubbing' is often seen with berylliosis. Skin lesions are the most common industrial exposure symptom. Three distinct skin lesions have been noted following exposure to beryllium: dermatitis, ulceration, and granulomas. There appears to be an immunological component to chronic beryllium disease, including the dermal responses.

Although available information from epidemiological studies is insufficient to confirm human carcinogenesis, the data strongly suggest beryllium is associated with cancer in humans, and it is categorized as a B1 (probable human carcinogen) by the US Environmental Protection Agency (EPA).

Immunotoxicity

Beryllium exerts several important immunotoxic effects, including induction of a beryllium-antigen specific adaptive immune response and the triggering of inflammatory and innate immune responses. Genetic susceptibility plays a role in CBD adaptive immune responses, mainly mediated through single nucleotide polymorphisms in HLA-DP and, to a lesser extent, HLA-DR. The adaptive response is characterized by influx and proliferation of CD4+ central and effector memory T cells expressing Th1 cytokines. Insights into the immunopathogenesis of CBD have implications for the understanding of other immune-mediated granulomatous disorders and for metal antigen behavior.

Reproductive Toxicity

Little data are available on the reproductive effects of beryllium. Large acute doses have had no effect on reproduction, although continued administration during pregnancy has led to death *in utero* and quickly after birth. It has also been reported that rats exposed to low levels of beryllium have an increased number of litters.

Genotoxicity

Beryllium's genotoxicity is not entirely clear, owing to weak and/or inconsistent evidence from studies, but there is sufficient evidence to consider it a weak genotoxin. *In vitro* studies indicate that beryllium induces morphological transformations in mammalian cells, but beryllium is not mutagenic in bacterial systems. There are studies that have exhibited chromosome aberrations in human lymphocytes, as well as increased sister chromatid exchange (SCE).

Carcinogenicity

The American Conference of Governmental Industrial Hygienists (ACGIH) classifies beryllium as group TLV-1 (a substance that causes cancer in humans). The DFG maintains the same classification as the ACGIH, although the group is referred to as MAK 1. Also, the IARC classifies it as group 1 (sufficient evidence for carcinogenicity in humans). US EPA classification of beryllium is as groups B1, probable human carcinogen, limited evidence from epidemiological studies, and L, meaning likely to produce cancer in humans. There are several studies suggesting that occupational exposure to beryllium, largely in the form of dust, increases incidence of lung cancer, especially in individuals after recovery from acute beryllium pneumonitis.

Clinical Management

Treatment of the acute disease includes bed rest, oxygen therapy, mechanical ventilation when needed, and corticosteroids. Chelation has been used to treat beryllium toxicity; however, no one agent is recommended over another. Aurin tricarboxylic acid has been used to protect primates from beryllium overdose, but human trials have not been conducted.

Ecotoxicology

Fish do not accumulate beryllium from water into their bodies to any great extent. A major portion of beryllium in soil does not dissolve in water but remains bound to soil, so it is not very likely to move deeper into the ground and enter groundwater. In the environment, chemical reactions can change the water-soluble beryllium compounds into insoluble forms. In some cases, water-insoluble beryllium compounds can change to soluble forms. Exposure to water-soluble beryllium compounds in the environment, in general, pose a greater threat to human health than water-insoluble forms.

No evidence was found to substantiate that biomethylation or any other environmental process results in the volatilization of beryllium into the atmosphere from water or soil.

Beryllium is extremely toxic to warm water fish in soft water. The degree of toxicity decreases with increasing water hardness. Bioconcentration of beryllium in fish to high levels is not likely because of the low uptake of beryllium from water by aquatic animals.

Other Hazards

Exposure Standards and Guidelines

The ACGIH threshold limit value, 8-h time-weighted average is 0.002 mg m^{-3} for beryllium and beryllium compounds.

Miscellaneous

Emeralds are a beryllium compound, beryl, $Be_3Al_2(SiO_3)_6$, which is colored green by the presence of trace quantities of chromium or vanadium.

See also: Metals; Respiratory Tract Toxicology.

Further Reading

Bingham, E., Cohrssen, B., Powell, C.H. (Eds.), 2001. Patty's Toxicology, fifth ed. John Wiley & Sons, Inc., New York.

Gordon, T., Bowser, D., 2003. Beryllium: genotoxicity and carcinogenicity. Mutat. Res. 533, 99–105.

Jakubowski, M., Dalezymski, C., 2009. Beryllium. In: Nordberg, G.F., Fowler, B.A., Nordberg, M., Friberg, L.T. (Eds.), Handbook on the Toxicology of Metals, third ed. Elsevier, New York, pp. 416–432.

Kreiss, K., 2011. Beryllium: a paradigm for occupational lung disease and its prevention. Occup. Environ. Med. 68 (11), 787–788.

Kriebel, D., Brain, J.D., Sprince, N.L., Kazemi, H., 1988. The pulmonary toxicity of beryllium. Am. Rev. Respir. Dis. 137, 464–473.

Muller, C., Salehi, F., Mazer, B., Bouchard, M., Adam-Poupart, A., Chevalier, G., Truchon, G., Lambert, J., Zayed, J., 2011 October. Immunotoxicity of 3 chemical forms of beryllium following inhalation exposure. Int. J. Toxicol. 30 (5), 538–545.

Nordberg, G.F., Fowler, B.A., Nordberg, M., Friberg, L.T., 2007. Handbook on the Toxicology of Metals, third ed. Associated Press, London.

Taylor, T.P., Ding, M., Ehler, D.S., et al., 2003. Beryllium in the environment: a review. J. Environ. Sci. Health A Environ. Sci. Eng. Toxic Hazard. Subst. Control 38, 439–469.

Williams, W.J., 1988. Beryllium disease. Postgrad. Med. J. 64, 511–516.

Relevant Websites

http://www.epa.gov/ttn/atw/hlthef/berylliu.html - US Environmental Protection Agency, Air Toxics website: Beryllium Compounds

http://minerals.usgs.gov/minerals/pubs/commodity/beryllium/ - US Geological Survey, Minerals Information: Beryllium

http://www.cdc.gov/niosh/topics/beryllium/ - Centers for Disease Control, Workplace Safety and Health Topics: Beryllium

http://toxnet.nlm.nih.gov/ - Toxnet homepage, search for 'beryllium'.

http://www.epa.gov/iris/toxreviews/0012tr.pdf - US Environmental Protection Agency, Toxicity review of Beryllium.

Beta-Blockers

V Dissanayake, Illinois Poison Center, Chicago, IL, USA; and University of Illinois at Chicago, Chicago, IL, USA
M Wahl, University of Illinois at Chicago, Chicago, IL, USA

This article is a revision of the previous edition article by Michael Wahl, volume 1, pp 267–269, © 2005, Elsevier Inc.

- Name: Beta-Blockers
- Synonyms: Acebutolol (Chemical Abstracts Service Registry Number (CAS) 37517-30-9), Atenolol (CAS 29122-68-7), Betaxolol (CAS 63659-19-8), Bisoprolol (CAS 66722-44-9), Carteolol (CAS 51781-21-6), Esmolol (CAS 81161-17-3), Labetalol (CAS 32780-64-6), Metoprolol (CAS 37350-58-6), Nadolol (CAS 42200-33-9), Nebivolol (CAS 38363-32-5), Penbutolol (CAS 13523-86-9), Propranolol (CAS 318-98-9), Sotalol (CAS 959-24-0), Timolol (CAS 26921-17-5)
- Chemical Structure:

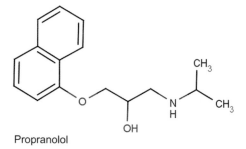

Propranolol

Background

Sir James Black synthesized the first clinically useful beta-blocker in 1958 after being inspired to find an agent that would lower heart rate in addition to blood pressure. At that time, phenoxybenzamine was the commonly utilized medication for hypertension, but the unfortunate side effect of tachycardia limited its use. Sir Black revolutionized the treatment of hypertension with his discovery, and many believe that this is the most important pharmacological contribution of the twentieth century. However, with an increasingly elderly population, beta-blockers have now become a significant cause of serious poisonings in both accidental and intentional overdoses. Liver failure and renal failure increase the risk of toxicity, making older populations more vulnerable to unintentional poisoning. It is vital that beta-blocker toxicity is considered on our list of differential diagnoses in patients presenting with hemodynamic compromise.

Uses

Beta-blockers reduce heart rate and blood pressure. Their use includes the treatment of hypertensive heart disease (essential hypertension, aortic dissection), ischemic heart disease (angina pectoris, myocardial infarction), supraventricular arrhythmias (supraventricular tachycardia, sinus tachycardia, ventricular tachycardia), structural heart disease (hypertrophic obstructive cardiomyopathy and compensated congestive heart failure), hyperadrenergic conditions (pheochromocytoma, hyperthyroidism, panic attacks, essential tremor, stage fright), glaucoma, and migraine headache.

Environmental Fate and Behavior

A few studies have examined the risk of environmental exposure of beta-blockers. It has been shown that several drugs, including beta-blockers, have been found in different water environments. Beta-blockers are susceptible to photolysis and appear to be more easily broken down in aquatic environments.

Exposure Routes and Pathways

The most common route of exposure to the beta-blockers is ingestion, including both intentional and accidental. Esmolol, labetalol, metoprolol, and propranolol are all available for parenteral administration; therefore, toxicity can occur via this additional route. Beta-blockers are also administered as ocular medications and systemic toxicity can result from administration by this seemingly innocuous route as well.

Toxicokinetics

The extent of absorption varies due to lipophilicity – the higher the lipid solubility, the more protein-bound the drug form remains in circulation. Protein-bound drugs are poorly excreted by the kidneys, and can accumulate in those with liver failure, whereas less protein-bound and less lipophilic drugs are more likely to be excreted by the kidneys. From the most lipid-soluble beta-blocker, propranolol, to the least, atenolol, oral bioavailability ranges from 25 to 100%. The rate of absorption is rapid for nonsustained release preparations. There are sustained release preparations for carvedilol, metoprolol, and propranolol, and these are more slowly absorbed and can demonstrate delayed and prolonged clinical effects following overdose. Most of the beta-blockers have hepatic metabolism of at least 50%. Atenolol, nadolol, and sotalol are principally excreted unchanged in the urine. Esmolol, although water soluble, is the most rapidly metabolized of the beta-blockers because it is metabolized by esterases in the cytosol of red blood cells. Both renal and fecal elimination occurs with beta-blockers. Elimination half-life ranges from 0.15 (esmolol) to 32 h (nebivolol).

Mechanism of Toxicity

Beta-blocker toxicity is directly related to the pharmacologic effects, including their beta-selectivity profiles. These agents

 http://dx.doi.org/10.1016/B978-0-12-386454-3.00698-9

block the effects of catecholamines such as epinephrine and norepinephrine on the beta-1 and beta-2 receptors. Beta-1 receptors are primarily located in the heart and kidneys while beta-2 receptors are primarily located in the airway and vasculature. Toxicity is most often due to antagonism of the cardiac beta-1 receptors, but varies depending on the agent's beta selectivity. For example, propranolol lacks selectivity, whereas labetalol and carvedilol are known to have both alpha-1 and beta-receptor blockade. Acebutolol, atenolol, betaxolol, bisoprolol, esmolol, metoprolol, and nebivolol are beta-1 selective antagonists. Some beta-blockers, such as pindolol or acebutolol, exhibit intrinsic sympathomimetic activity (ISA), which is due to partial agonism of the beta-receptors resulting in low levels of beta stimulation. Nebivolol has an additional feature of nitric oxide activity that results in enhancement of vasodilation and can lead to toxicity in overdose as well.

Acute and Short-Term Toxicity (or Exposure)

Human

Cardiac beta-1 stimulation results in increases in sinoatrial rate, myocardial contractility, and increased atrial, atrioventricular node, and ventricular conduction velocity. The mechanism by which this is accomplished is via a G-protein coupled second messenger system, where increased production of cyclic AMP leads to phosphorylation of calcium channels for calcium influx into the cell and myofibril contraction (**Figure 1**). Beta-2 receptors are found in the bronchioles, vasculature, intestines, uterus, pancreas, adipose tissue, and the liver. Stimulation of bronchial and vascular beta-2 receptors causes smooth muscle relaxation with resultant bronchial dilation and vasodilation. Blocking beta-2 receptors can cause contraction of bronchial smooth muscle and may result in asthma exacerbation. In overdose, acebutolol, betaxolol, carvedilol, oxprenolol, and propranolol can cause cardiac toxicity from fast sodium channel blockade that can result in QRS prolongation, seizures, and death. Pindolol has demonstrated increased sympathomimetic activity with mild tachycardia and hypertension in overdose.

Chronic Toxicity (or Exposure)

Animal

No evidence of carcinogenicity has been documented in rats at doses of atenolol up to 300 mg kg^{-1} day^{-1}. Doses of up to 200 mg kg^{-1} day^{-1} have not shown decreased fertility in rats. However, dose-related fetal resorptions were noted at doses of greater than 50 mg kg^{-1} day^{-1}. Chronic propranolol dosing at 100 mg kg^{-1} to newborn rats resulted in decreased weight gain and growth. The effects were reversible once propranolol was discontinued.

Human

The primary clinical effects observed in beta-blocker toxicity are cardiovascular in nature. Direct cardiac effects include bradycardia (sinus, atrioventricular node, ventricular), all degrees of atrioventricular block, bundle branch blocks, and asystole. Ventricular arrhythmias may occur secondary to bradycardia. Torsades de pointes has been associated with chronic toxicity from sotalol because this beta-blocker blocks delayed potassium channels responsible for repolarization and prolongs the action potential and the QT interval. Hypotension occurs and is due to decreased cardiac output and/or vasodilation. Central nervous system effects of these drugs including lethargy, coma, and seizures are secondary to the cardiovascular toxicity of lipophilic beta-blockers, such as propranolol and penbutolol. Bronchospasm can occur secondary to beta-2 blockade. Hypoglycemia and hyperkalemia can occur. Beta-blockers are also known to worsen decompensated heart failure, exacerbate peripheral vascular resistance, and blunt the warning symptoms of hypoglycemia. Beta- blockers are also known to worsen

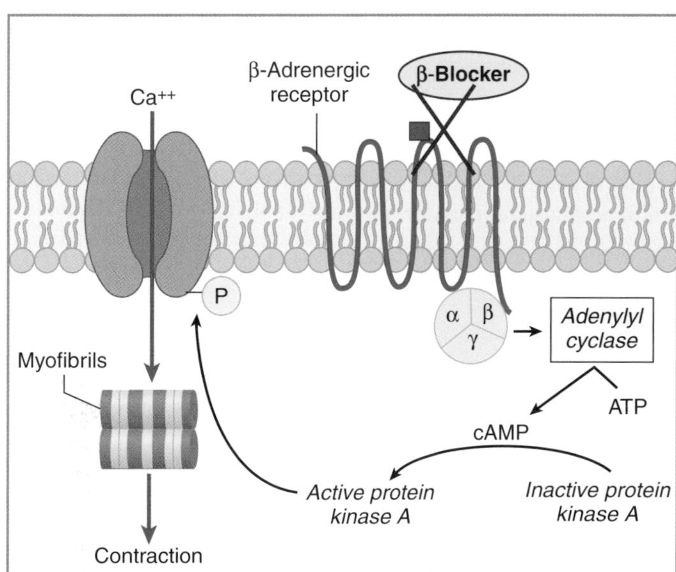

Figure 1 Mechanism of action for beta-blockers.

decompensated heart failure, exacerbate peripheral vascular resistance, and blunt the warning symptoms of hypoglycemia.

In Vitro Toxicity Data

Ames testing of propranolol by different laboratories has demonstrated equivocal results.

Immunotoxicity

There is no evidence that beta-blockers currently cause immunotoxicity. Practolol, which was withdrawn from the market in 1975, was thought to cause an oculo-mucocutaneous syndrome that resulted in a kerato-conjunctivitis, psoriasis-like skin condition and effusions of the pleura and pericardium, but this was never definitively determined.

Reproductive Toxicity

Acebutolol, pindolol, and sotalol are pregnancy category B medications when used early in pregnancy. These medications have not been found to cause harm in animal studies but have not been fully studied in pregnant humans. Category C medications have been shown to cause harm in animal studies but have not been studied in humans. Medications that have not been evaluated in animal studies also belong to this class. The following beta-blockers belong to category C: betaxolol, bisoprolol, carteolol, carvedilol, esmolol, levatol, levobunolol, metipranolol, metoprolol, nebivolol, penbutolol, propranolol, and timolol.

In late pregnancy, many consider all beta-blockers to be category D medications, but only atenolol officially belongs to category D – these medications are a risk to the fetus as confirmed in studies on pregnant women but may provide benefits that outweigh the risks as determined by the healthcare provider.

Highly protein-bound beta-blockers, such as acebutolol, atenolol, metoprolol, nadolol, and sotalol are capable of being excreted in breast milk. Atenolol and acebutolol have resulted in bradycardia, cyanosis, and hypotension in the newborn infant. One study found that the majority of beta-blockers do not result in significant levels in the breast-fed infant, except for atenolol and labetalol. It is important to consider beta-blockers with lower milk to plasma ratios for administration to nursing mothers.

Genotoxicity and Carcinogenicity

Multiple studies have been conducted on the beta-blocker class to determine potential mutagenicity, and there is no evidence that they cause genotoxicity or carcinogenicity.

Clinical Management

Advanced life-support measures should be instituted as necessary. A baseline 12-lead electrocardiogram should be obtained. Continuous cardiac and blood pressure monitoring should be initiated. Airway protection should be addressed if the patient is obtunded with signs of airway compromise.

Gastric decontamination procedures should be initiated based on the history of the ingestion and the patient's neurologic status. Consider charcoal for recent ingestions but recall that dosing should be in a 10:1 ratio (gram of charcoal per gram of medication). If the expected dose of activated charcoal is too high to administer, the patient's mental status is problematic, or it is not certain when the patient ingested the medication, charcoal should not be administered as it can easily be aspirated. Whole bowel irrigation may be useful following ingestions of sustained release preparations as long as these patients are not hemodynamically compromised.

Bradyarrhythmias and conduction disturbances should be managed with atropine and a pacemaker. Ventricular arrhythmias should be managed with class IB antiarrhythmics (e.g., lidocaine) and overdrive pacing. Class IA and IC antiarrhythmics should be avoided due to their potential to interfere with conduction. Hypotension should be managed initially with normal saline solution. If decreased cardiac output is responsible for hypotension, dobutamine, amrinone, or isoproterenol may be helpful. If systemic vascular resistance is low, vasopressors such as dopamine and norepinephrine should be administered. It is commonly difficult to determine whether a patient's clinical picture is due to beta-blocker overdose or calcium channel-blocker toxicity. Evaluating the patient's glucose level may be helpful in distinguishing the former from the latter, since calcium channel blockers inhibit insulin release and clinically demonstrate insulin resistance and hyperglycemia.

Glucagon has been effective in increasing myocardial contractility in beta-blocker toxicity. Glucagon stimulates production of cyclic adenosine monophosphate, which enhances contraction by activating sarcoplasmic reticulum calcium release. Glucagon metabolism additionally releases arachidonic acid, which also aids cardiac contractility. Initial intravenous doses of 3–5 mg have been used in adults, and if no response results, 6–10 mg (total dose) is usually administered. If there is improvement in hemodynamic parameters, an hourly infusion of the response dose of glucagon is continued. The initial pediatric dose is 50 $\mu g\ kg^{-1}$. If cardiogenic shock is resistant to traditional measures, use of insulin and glucose (to maintain euglycemia) has been successful in small numbers of patients as well as in animal models of beta-blocker toxicity. For patients who fail all other therapies, an intra-aortic balloon pump and cardiopulmonary bypass should be considered. Hemodialysis or hemoperfusion may be effective in removing acebutolol, atenolol, nadolol, and sotalol.

More recently, intravenous lipid emulsion has been found to be helpful in the crashing patient suffering from lipophilic beta-blocker toxicity. It is believed that lipid infusion is able to provide a lipid sink that retains circulating drug in the lipemic portion of blood, preventing it from causing more toxicity and allowing more time for drug metabolism. If the patient continues to do poorly after implementation of all discussed treatment strategies, it is appropriate to consider this rescue therapy for it has shown promise in experimental animal models and has been successful in the resuscitation of select human cases.

See also: Angiotensin Converting Enzyme (ACE) Inhibitors; Alpha Blockers; Digitalis Glycosides; Calcium Channel Blockers; Cardiovascular System.

Further Reading

Bailey, B., 2003. Glucagon in beta-blocker and calcium channel blocker overdoses. A systematic review. J. Toxicol. Clin. Toxicol. 41, 595–602.

Baker, J., 2005. The selectivity of beta-adrenoceptor antagonists at the human beta-1, beta-2 and beta-3 adrenoceptors. Br. J. Pharmacol. 144, 317–322.

Bers, D.M., 2008. Calcium cycling and signaling in cardiac myocytes. Annu. Rev. Physiol. 70, 23–49.

Brubacher, J.R., 2010. Beta-adrenergic antagonists. In: Nelson, L.S., Lewin, N.A., Howland, M.A., Hoffman, R.S., Goldfrank, L.R., Flomenbaum, N.E. (Eds.), Goldfrank's Toxicologic Emergencies, ninth ed. McGraw-Hill Professional, New York.

Cave, G., Harvey, M., 2009. Intravenous lipid emulsion as antidote beyond local anesthetic toxicity: a systematic review. Acad. Emerg. Med. 16, 815–824.

Dancey, D., Wulffhart, Z., McEwan, P., 1997. Sotalol-induced torsades de pointes in patients with renal failure. Can. J. Cardiol. 13, 55–58.

Descotes, J., 2004. Immunotoxicology of Drugs and Chemicals: An Experimental and Clinical Approach. Elsevier, Lyon, France, p. 90.

Doze, P., Elsinga, P.H., Vries, E.F., et al., 2000. Mutagenic activity of a fluorinated analog of the beta-adrenoceptor ligand carazolol in the Ames test. Nucl. Med. Biol. 27 (3), 315–319.

Frishman, W., Jacob, H., Eisenberg, E., Ribner, H., 1979. Clinical pharmacology of the new beta-adrenergic blocking drugs. Part 8. Self-poisoning with beta-adrenoceptor blocking agents. Recognition and management. Am. Heart J.

Frishman, W., Saunders, E., 2011. Beta-adrenergic blockers. J. Clin. Hypertens. Greenwich 13, 649–653.

Gupta, R., 2011. Transfer of drugs and xenobiotics through milk. In: Reproductive and Developmental Toxicology. Elsevier, London, pp. 65–66.

Harvey, M.G., Cave, G., 2008. Intralipid infusion ameliorates propranolol-induced hypotension in rabbits. J. Med. Toxicol. 4, 71–76.

Howland, M.A., 2010. Antidotes in depth: glucagon. In: Nelson, L.S., Lewin, N.A., Howland, M.A., Hoffman, R.S., Goldfrank, L.R., Flomenbaum, N.E. (Eds.), Goldfrank's Toxicologic Emergencies, ninth ed. McGraw-Hill Professional, New York.

Love, J.N., 1994. B-Blocker toxicity: a clinical diagnosis. Am. J. Emerg. Med. 12, 356–357.

Love, J.N., 2002. Electrocardiographic changes associated with β-blockers toxicity. Ann. Emerg. Med. 40 (6), 603–610.

Lvoff, R., Wilcken, D.E., 1972. Glucagon in heart failure and in cardiogenic shock. Circulation 45, 534–542.

Magee, L.A., Elran, E., Bull, S.B., et al., Jan 2000. Risks and benefits of beta-receptor blockers for pregnancy hypertension. Eur. J. Obstet. Gynecol. Reprod. Biol. 88 (1), 15–26.

Peterson, C.D., Leeder, J.S., Sterner, S., 1984. Glucagon therapy for B-blocker overdose. Drug Intell. Clin. Pharm. 18, 394–398.

Stapleton, M.P., 1997. Sir James Black and propranolol. The role of the basic sciences in the history of cardiovascular pharmacology. Tex. Heart Inst. J. 24 (4), 336–342.

Weinberg, G., 2007. LipidRescue™ resuscitation for cardiac toxicity. Treat. Regim.. Available from: http://lipidrescue.squarespace.com/links-to-literature/ (accessed 27.03.12.).

Weinstein, R.S., 1984. Recognition and management of poisoning with beta-adrenergic blocking agents. Ann. Emerg. Med. 13, 1123–1131.

Zimmerman, J.L., 2003. Poisonings and overdoses in the intensive care unit: general and specific management issues. Crit. Care Med. 3 (12), 2794–2801.

Relevant Websites

www.lipidrescue.org – LipidRescue™ Resuscitation.

www.nytimes.com/2010/03/23/health/23black.html – The New York Times - Dr. James Black obituary (Beta Blockers discoverer).

Beta-Propiolactone

A de Peyster, San Diego State University, San Diego, CA, USA

- Name: Beta-propiolactone
- Chemical Abstracts Service Registry Number: 57-57-8
- Synonyms: Propiolactone; 1,3-Propiolactone; 2-Oxetanone; 3-Hydroxypropionic acid lactone; 3-Propanolide
- Molecular Formula: $C_3H_4O_2$
- Chemical Structure:

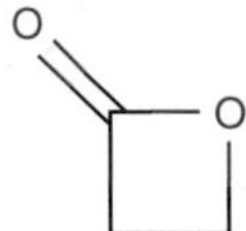

Background

Beta-propiolactone is a colorless liquid with a strong, slightly sweet odor. It may occur naturally, but no clear documentation of its occurrence in nature was found, and it must be synthesized for commercial purposes. Beta-propiolactone is unstable at room temperature but stable when stored at 5 °C in glass containers.

Its tendency to be unstable and react with other molecules in the vicinity is responsible for both its toxicity and its usefulness. Significant commercial production of beta-propiolactone took place during the late 1950s through the mid-1970s, when it was widely used in chemical synthesis in reactions with other molecules to produce new chemicals. All lactones are characterized by a ring structure consisting of two or more carbon atoms – as can be seen from its structure, beta-propiolactone has three in its ring – and a single oxygen, coupled with an adjacent ketone. The fewer the carbons in the ring, the more 'strained' is the ring structure and the more unstable and reactive its characteristics. When the ring bonds break, the beta-propiolactone molecules attach to other nearby molecules.

Beta-propiolactone has a boiling point of 162 °C and a low molecular weight (72.1). Although normally a liquid, it can also be made to vaporize. As early as the 1960s, beta-propiolactone vapor was tested along with ethylene oxide for effectiveness as a sterilizing agent for influenza virus vaccines. Its use as a sterilant was at one time extended to many other products (see Uses).

The Hazardous Substance Database notes that beta-propiolactone was first produced commercially in the United States in 1958, and the volume produced was significant through the early 1970s; for example, approximately 22 million kilograms (48.5 million pounds) were made in 1972. Production in the United States dropped to 454 kg (1000 lb) in 1975. A 2011 National Toxicology Program report states that in 2009 beta-propiolactone was produced by one European manufacturer and was available from many suppliers. No more specific data were found detailing current production, imports, exports, or annual amounts used worldwide. Beta-propiolactone has been replaced in newer chemical synthesis methods, and its use as a sterilant has also diminished considerably. As long as its use remains limited, risks to the general public will continue to be diminished significantly when compared with past decades.

Uses

Once a commercially important industrial chemical in the United States, more than 85% of the beta-propiolactone produced was used to manufacture acrylic acid and esters. Preparation of commercial acrylates involved reacting beta-propiolactone with ethylene cyanohydrin. The instability of beta-propiolactone, coupled with the discovery of other more desirable chemical synthesis methods, led to its replacement by other starting materials in newer manufacturing methods.

A variety of sources report that beta-propiolactone has also been used for disinfecting blood plasma, human and veterinary vaccines, tissue grafts, surgical instruments, enzymes, nutrient broth and milk; as a vapor-phase disinfectant in enclosed spaces; and as a sporicide against vegetative bacteria, pathogenic fungi, and viruses. It has also been used by shipboard military personnel as a disinfectant/decontaminant. It is sometimes also used in laboratory research. Because it is no longer used as a sterilant in medical procedures or in food, the potential for exposure of the general population is increasingly limited.

Environmental Fate and Behavior

It is soluble in water (370 g l^{-1} at 25 °C) and miscible in other common organic solvents including acetone, chloroform, diethyl ether, and ethanol (Log K_{ow} 0.462). Hydrolysis occurs in water where the half-life in aqueous media at 25 °C is approximately 3.5 h. If released to soil, relatively rapid hydrolysis can be expected to occur in the presence of moisture. Significant evaporation may occur from dry surfaces. With a vapor pressure of 3.4 mm Hg at 25 °C, it can also vaporize into the air as temperature rises. If released to the atmosphere, beta-propiolactone is expected to exist in the gas phase, where it may be relatively more persistent in the absence of moisture than it is in aqueous media. The half-life for the reaction with photochemically produced hydroxyl radicals was estimated to be a relatively slow rate of 45 days in the atmosphere.

Exposure Potential for Humans and the Environment

Numbers of people potentially exposed occupationally and otherwise has decreased dramatically over the past few decades. Occupations identified to be at greatest risk of potential exposure formerly included all disinfectant workers and makers of virucidal agents, acrylic plastics, and resins. Worker exposure may still occur by inhalation and dermal contact at industrial

 http://dx.doi.org/10.1016/B978-0-12-386454-3.01168-4

facilities and laboratories where beta-propiolactone is still used to inactivate viruses for research and vaccine applications. Trace amounts of beta-propiolactone and breakdown products that might still be present in vaccines and other products were also the focus of attention. Even though beta-propiolactone use has been largely discontinued as a sterilant in a number of products, the potential for exposure of the general population still exists at reduced levels and frequency. Any releases of beta-propiolactone to the environment are most likely through industrial processes and waste streams from facilities where it is still made or used. Reduced use, high instability in aqueous environments, and lack of transport, bioaccumulation, or biomagnification potential make beta-propiolactone of minimal ecotoxicity risk.

Toxicokinetics

Beta-propiolactone and its metabolites have short biological half-lives in the mammalian body. The main metabolite of beta-propiolactone is lactic acid, and its main hydrolysis product is hydracrylic acid, both of which are excreted rapidly.

An LD_{50} study using application of beta-propiolactone to the skin of guinea pigs suggested considerable absorption by that route. Skin irritation, burns, and blisters following acute dermal exposure could facilitate absorption by that route, with compromised dermal barriers allowing greater passage of substances. Finding more specific information about systemic absorption and distribution following oral or inhalation exposures was difficult; however, it seems likely that beta-propiolactone does not absorb or distribute appreciably after oral or inhalation exposures based on the fact that tissue types of tumors seen in cancer bioassays are those experiencing first contact. For example, oral/gastrointestinal exposures resulted in increased combined incidence of benign and malignant tumors of the forestomach, and cancers observed after inhalation exposure were of the nasal cavity. Toxicity to kidney and liver has been reported in animal studies, but it should be noted that this was after intravenous (IV) administration directly into the bloodstream.

Mechanism of Toxicity

Beta-propiolactone is sometimes classified as a direct-acting alkylating agent capable of attaching to DNA and forming DNA adducts. That property probably accounts for its mutagenic activity in a wide variety of *in vitro* and *in vivo* test systems using both somatic and germ cells. It can also react with amino acids of enzymes and other proteins, including blood proteins like albumin. If given by itself intravenously, it causes liver necrosis and kidney tubular damage, but if it is allowed time to react with proteins before injection, then toxicity is much reduced.

Acute and Short-Term Toxicity

Humans

Being so unstable, beta-propiolactone reacts with tissues of the body that it comes in contact with. Acute administration of beta-propiolactone as a sterilizing agent in sera has induced signs of inoculation-area skin irritation in people. Skin exposure to a 40% (or greater) solution of beta-propiolactone in water for 20 min has caused skin burns. The vapor of beta-propiolactone is unbearable to human beings at concentrations greater than 0.1 mg l^{-1} of air, a level considerably lower than workplace air standards in the United States. The immediate respiratory irritation felt upon exposure appears to be great enough to prevent most people from working in the presence of vapor concentrations that might be injurious.

Animals

In acute administration tests involving laboratory animals, beta-propiolactone has been shown to be a significant irritant to skin, eyes, the respiratory tract, and digestive system. Excessive dermal contact can even elicit blisters and burns. Scarring, erythema, and hair loss have been found on mouse skin after 1–6 administrations of 0.8–100 mg of beta-propiolactone. Permanent corneal damage has been documented in laboratory studies using rabbits exposed by the ocular route. Excessive inhalation exposure results in inflammation of the respiratory tract. Oral contact can cause stomach and mouth burns.

In rats, acute oral administration or intraperitoneal injection of beta-propiolactone caused muscular spasms, respiratory difficulty, convulsions, and death. Acute intravenous injection also caused kidney tubule damage and liver necrosis. Frequent urination, dysuria (difficulty urinating), and hematuria (blood in urine) may also accompany higher systemic doses.

Considerable testing of beta-propiolactone in acute LD_{50}/LC_{50} experiments was done in laboratory animals to establish doses deemed to be safe for humans. The IV route was tested because of the utility of this chemical as a sterilant for blood products. The IV LD_{50} ranges from 90 to 345 mg kg^{-1} in different laboratory animal species, with the following ranking seen from lowest (i.e., most sensitive species) to highest: dog = rabbit < guinea pig ≈ rat < mouse. Neither species differences nor which best represents human sensitivity appears to have been investigated further. Degradation products from the hydrolysis of beta-propiolactone have also been tested similarly for lethality (LD_{50}) and found to be as much as 5–10 times less toxic than beta-propiolactone itself.

Chronic Toxicity

Readers who may be concerned about the safety of beta-propiolactone when used to disinfect vaccines will find the following clinical studies especially interesting because of the way exposures were administered. In studies reported in the 1950s and 1960s and recounted briefly in a 2004 report to the National Academies (see Further Reading), nearly 1000 people were involved in transfusion tests where beta-propiolactone-treated plasma was being infused into human volunteers at the Henry Ford Hospital. Plasma infused had been treated with beta-propiolactone with or without ultraviolet radiation. Patients had received under 2–3 l total plasma on average. The vast majority received fewer than three administrations. Six received more than 20 administrations and a few received up to 70 transfusions. Patient follow-up ranged from 6 months to

5 years. According to this report for the National Academies, investigators reported seeing 'absolutely no chronic toxic effects.' Conclusions were based on 10 years worth of data on 2563 transfusions administered to 995 different recipients.

In related experiments using laboratory animals, marked cumulative toxicity was seen in the form of weight loss and necrosis of the liver and kidney tubules.

Reproductive Toxicity

No studies were found examining effects using standard test protocols for reproductive or developmental toxicity endpoints. Beta-propiolactone being a mutagen (see Genotoxicity), it is not too surprising that *in vivo* genotoxicity tests using mice have revealed adverse effects on rapidly dividing reproductive cells like oocytes and sperm.

Genotoxicity

Beta-propiolactone is a direct-acting alkylating agent that reacts with DNA. The genotoxicity of beta-propiolactone has been well studied *in vitro* and *in vivo*, where such testing indicates a wide range of effects. It is mutagenic in bacterial assays. In yeast, it induces mitotic gene conversion, aneuploidy, and mutations. In fruit flies (*Drosophila melanogaster*), it produces heritable translocations and sex-linked recessive lethal mutations. It induces cell transformation and gene mutations in human cells exposed *in vitro*, and cell transformation, gene mutations, chromosomal aberrations, and sister chromatid exchanges in other mammalian cells *in vitro*. When given *in vivo*, beta-propiolactone induces gene mutations in the stomach and liver in the Muta™Mouse assay; DNA strand breaks in rat liver and mouse skin keratinocytes; and chromosomal aberrations in rat bone-marrow cells. It covalently binds to mouse skin DNA and RNA. It induces chromosomal aberrations or micronuclei in oocytes, spermatids, hepatocytes, and splenocytes in mice treated *in vivo*.

Carcinogenicity

The National Toxicology Program's 2111 Report on Carcinogens considers beta-propiolactone to be reasonably anticipated to be a human carcinogen based on sufficient evidence of carcinogenicity from studies in experimental animals. It is very readily hydrolyzed to an inactive degradation product; therefore, as used in sterilization procedures, beta-propiolactone was not considered to be a carcinogen hazard. Nevertheless, the unaltered parent compound beta-propiolactone is a carcinogen, so human contact must be avoided.

The International Agency for Research on Cancer (IARC) notes that no epidemiological data are available relevant to the carcinogenicity of beta-propiolactone. There is, however, sufficient evidence in experimental animals for the carcinogenicity of beta-propiolactone. Their overall evaluation of beta-propiolactone is that it is possibly carcinogenic to humans (Group 2B). IARC also cautions that, based on results of animal studies, a single-dose exposure may be enough to pose a significant risk of cancer. A single administration of 100 mg beta-propiolactone on suckling mice 9–11 days after birth induced lymphomas and hepatomas. Single-dose exposures have also been shown to be genotoxic.

The cancer hazard designations by other authoritative groups are relatively similar, although one is worth mentioning because of the slightly different perspective. The American Conference of Governmental Industrial Hygienists (ACGIH) classifies beta-propiolactone as a confirmed animal carcinogen but with unknown relevance to humans (Group A3).

All of these designations are based on positive findings in multiple independent laboratory animal studies too numerous to detail here. Briefly, beta-propiolactone caused malignant and benign tumors in two rodent species (rats and mice) at several different tissue sites when administered by several different routes of exposure (oral, dermal, whole body inhalation, subcutaneous, IV injection, intrarectal). Tumorigenic effects in treated mature animals appeared to occur primarily around the initial site of exposure. For example, after dermal exposure, the tumors observed were benign and malignant skin tumors (papillomas, squamous cell carcinomas, keratocanthomas, melanomas, subcutaneous injection-site sarcomas, fibrosarcomas, adenocarcinomas, squamous cell carcinomas); after inhalation exposure only nasal tumors; and after oral exposure only forestomach tumors (squamous cell carcinomas). Beta-propiolactone has been ruled out as an agent causing central nervous system cancer in rats. Many more details of specific cancer types appearing in each species following these exposures can be found in the Further Reading recommended.

Clinical Management

Acute exposure to beta-propiolactone calls for the standard emergency treatment for a highly irritant chemical. This involves removing the victim from further exposure, sending for medical assistance, and initiating emergency procedures. If this is an accidental oral exposure, avoid emesis and dilute the chemical in the stomach. Contact lenses should not be worn when working with this chemical. Eye protection should be worn when working with beta-propiolactone, and an eyewash fountain should be provided within the immediate work area for emergency use. Flush exposed eyes immediately with large amounts of water for 15 min, lifting the lower and upper lids to ensure complete dilution of chemical throughout the ocular surface. If a worker is exposed over a significant amount of skin area, the US Occupational Safety and Health Administration (OSHA) requires that the victim shower with soap and water as soon as possible, unless physical injuries prevent this. Get medical attention as soon as possible.

One source suggests the possibility for chemoprevention of carcinogenic effects using sodium thiosulfate, as it may inhibit beta-propiolactone's capacity for stomach tumorigenesis (at least in animal studies) if it should be consumed accidentally. Sodium thiosulfate is an FDA-approved antidote for cyanide poisoning. There was no evidence presented in that source that the idea had actually been tested experimentally with beta-propiolactone.

Ecotoxicology

As noted, beta-propiolactone could be released to the environment accidentally or through wastewater discharges. No other relevant studies on exposures to aquatic or other wild species were found. If releases to the environment occur, it would be reasonable to expect some or all of the same irritant and genotoxic effects discussed; however, because of rapid degradation in moist environments, the potential for high level exposures is low, and long-range transport, bioaccumulation, and biomagnification are all likely to be insignificant.

Exposure Standards and Guidelines

OSHA considers beta-propiolactone to be a potential occupational carcinogen and has established no exposure limit standard. Engineering controls, work practices, and personal protective equipment are required to protect workers.

The ACGIH has recommended an airborne threshold limit value (8 h time-weighted average, TLV-TWA) of 0.5 ppm in workplace air to avoid respiratory irritant effects, and has listed beta-propiolactone as an animal carcinogen.

Similar values have been used as standards or guidelines in many countries. Australia, Belgium, Finland, France, Germany, Sweden, and Switzerland list beta-propiolactone as a probable human carcinogen.

The US Environmental Protection Agency (EPA) Clean Air Act, National Exposure Standards for Hazardous Air Pollutants, lists beta-propiolactone as a hazardous air pollutant. The EPA Toxics Release Inventory program shows beta-propiolactone as a listed substance subject to reporting requirements with a reportable quantity of 10 lb.

The World Health Organization reports that no international guideline for beta-propiolactone has been established for drinking water.

See also: Ethyl Acrylate; Ethylene Oxide.

Further Reading

International Agency for Research on Cancer (IARC), 1999. Monograph on the Evaluation of Carcinogenic Risks to Humans: Beta-Propiolactone [1017-1606], vol. 71, Pt 3. pp. 1103–1118.

National Toxicology Program (NTP), 2011. Report on Carcinogens, twelfth ed. National Toxicology Program (NTP), ResearchTriangle Park, NC.

The Center for Research Information, Inc, 2004. Health Effects of Project SHAD: Chemical Agent: Betapropriolactone [beta-propiolactone] – CAS #57-57-8. Prepared for the National Academies by Center for Research Information, Silver Spring, MD. (Contract No. IOM-2794-04-001).

Relevant Websites

http://toxnet.nlm.nih.gov/cgi-bin/sis/htmlgen?HSDB – Hazardous Substances Data Bank (HSDB). Search using chemical name or CAS number.

http://pubchem.ncbi.nlm.nih.gov – US National Library of Medicine (Pubchem): Search for beta-Propiolactone.

Bhopal Accident: Release of MIC

P Limaye, Xenometrics LLC, Stilwell, KS, USA

This article is a revision of the previous edition article by Pallavi B. Limaye and Harihara M. Mehendale, volume 1, pp 269–271, © 2005, Elsevier Inc.

Background (Significance/History)

Bhopal, the capital city of the state of Madhya Pradesh, India, is the site that witnessed probably the world's worst industrial calamity. On the night of 2 December 1984, a disastrous accident at Union Carbide plant led to the massive leakage of methyl isocyanate (MIC) gas and other related by-products. MIC was used in the production of carbaryl, an insecticide. Evidence suggests that inadvertent seepage of water into a storage tank that contained over 40 metric tons of MIC led to a violent exothermic reaction resulting in the emission of MIC and a number of other toxic decomposition by-products that could not be contained by safety valves. The exact nature and the constituents of the gas mixture are unknown. The Union Carbide plant was shutdown after the accident.

Chemical accidents take place for a variety of reasons. Some often involve explosions, massive fires, and leakage of hazardous materials. Also, mishaps can occur during the transport, storage, and industrial production of chemicals. The Bhopal plant explosion was probably the most catastrophic in the history of toxicological disasters because accidents of this nature posed a real challenge to health, environment, and industry professionals. This pesticide plant accident released a huge quantity of MIC into the atmosphere, killing nearly 4000 people within hours, and affected millions of others indefinitely. Extensive follow-up epidemiological studies continue to reveal acute and chronic, submassive to massive, pulmonary, ophthalmic, reproductive, immunologic, neurological, and hematologic toxicity among the survivors.

MIC is highly reactive. It is presumed that it can cross cellular membranes and reach distant organs, perhaps in the form of glutathione conjugate, which explains some of the systemic effects of MIC. MIC can be degraded as a result of pyrolysis and interaction with water, but none of the breakdown products can duplicate the toxicity observed in Bhopal and in animal models. MIC may be the most toxic of all isocyanates because of its very high vapor pressure relative to other isocyanates and because of its ability to exert toxic effects on numerous organ systems. A review of the health effects of the 1984 gas leak from the Union Carbide plant in Bhopal, India, shows continuing morbidity of a multisystemic nature in the exposed population. Scientific debates about the causes of the accident and the spectrum of health effects have uncovered a significant number of clinical dilemmas, faulty medical management strategies, and unsolvable public health issues. Even three decades after the disaster, numerous investigators were still reviewing human health effects that resulted from exposure to MIC. The studies were conducted during both the early and late recovery periods. Major organs affected were the eyes, respiratory tract, and skin. Although mortality declined after an initial soar upward, it remained elevated among the most severely exposed population. Studies conducted during the early recovery period focused primarily on ocular and respiratory systems. Major findings observed acute irritant effects on the eyes and respiratory tract. In follow-up studies, investigators found persistent irritant effects, including ocular lesions and respiratory impairment. Studies conducted during the late recovery period focused on the effects of various body systems including neurological, reproductive, neurobehavioral, and psychological. Early and late recovery period studies suffered from several clinical and epidemiological limitations, including study design, bias, and exposure classification, etc. Currently, long-term monitoring of the affected community persists, and exposed individuals are compared to unexposed subjects in experiments following appropriate methods of investigation that include well-designed cohort studies, case–control studies for rare conditions. Overall, a plethora of publications suggest that toxic impacts of MIC endure, concentrated in populations that live in close proximity of the disaster site.

The article is focused on the 'Bhopal tragedy' to discuss the central issues that this type of accident provokes, in terms of public health, particularly in developing countries with a highly ambitious agenda for industrial growth. Post-independent Indian government was no exception because it focused on agriculture where pesticide became an indispensable commodity. This article emphasizes the aftermath of Bhopal tragedy, some of the underlying causes, and the various health-risk related global concerns that it generated in the industrial community to devise intelligent and effective ways to avert such disasters. A combination of quantitative and qualitative information drawn from international literature on the subject is discussed.

Estimated Total Release of MIC and Estimated Individual Exposure

It has been estimated that about 40 tons of MIC escaped from the plant in a period of 1–2 h. Due to lack of planning, air monitoring for MIC was not possible, nor was it subsequently attempted. The Central Water and Air Pollution Control Board of India estimated MIC concentration to have been about 27 ppm, which is about 1400 times that of the US Occupational Safety and Health Administration workplace standard of 0.02 ppm calculated over an 8 h workday. The established limit to classify the concentration as 'immediately dangerous to life or health' is 3 ppm MIC. The American Industrial Hygiene Association's Emergency Response Planning Guideline, level 2 limit is defined as the maximum airborne concentration that nearly all persons could be exposed for up to 1 h without experiencing or developing irreversible or other serious health effects or symptoms that could impair their abilities to take protective action and is 0.5 ppm. This indicates that the MIC concentration released after the accident was ~50 times that of the acceptable limit.

 http://dx.doi.org/10.1016/B978-0-12-386454-3.00252-9

Mechanism of Toxicity

Before the accident, little was known about the MIC toxicity. Even today, mechanisms of MIC-induced toxicity are not clearly understood. It was known that MIC is a corrosive agent for the eyes, respiratory tract, and skin. Acute exposure to high vapor concentrations may cause severe pulmonary edema and injury to the alveolar walls of the lung, severe corneal damage, and death. MIC may cross the placenta and enter a developing fetus.

The Reaction

MIC production involves reacting methylamine (A) with phosgene (B) to produce methyl isocyanate (MIC). Although the actual composition of the gas cloud in the heavy presence of MIC was never determined and remains a mystery, it may have contained phosgene, hydrogen cyanide, carbon monoxide, hydrogen chloride, oxides of nitrogen, monomethyl amine, and carbon dioxide. This mixture intuitively triggered an exothermic reaction, which caused extreme suffocation to the lives in close proximity of the factory and since the gas cloud was mainly composed of materials denser than the surrounding air, it stayed close to the ground and spread very slowly with the wind current affecting rest of the population of the city.

Environmental Fate and Behavior

Because of a change in the ownership of the plant from Union Carbide to Dow Chemical, decontamination responsibility of the factory remains controversial. It is unfathomable that this industrial catastrophe has left behind tons of unused toxic chemicals that continue to contaminate the groundwater.

The decontamination of the Bhopal plant and its vicinity was a gigantic task. The German Agency for International Cooperation who earlier showed interest in removing ~347 metric tons of waste through incineration later withdrew their offer because of the Indian government's refusal to be responsible for any accident during the transport and handling of these toxic substances, and the strong opposition of German activists and environmentalists to transport and incinerate this massive amount of chemical waste in Germany. Unsubstantiated estimates suggest that between 1984 and 2012, approximately 4000–12 000 metric tons of toxic products have leached into the soil, although the extent of the spread is unknown. It is unfortunate that no efforts are being made for the removal and detoxification of the 347 metric tons of waste stocked in the former factory. Incinerating centers in India are not capable of disposing such a huge amount of waste safely.

It has been reported that waste and toxic chemicals used in manufacturing of pesticides had infiltrated the soil long before the explosion. Reports indicated that Union Carbide India, Ltd. (UCIL) had a checkered history of compliance and their internal records reveal that there were leaks in ~57 acres of basins used for storing chemical waste. Although leakage and seepage of chemicals from such complicated industrial operations are not uncommon, Union Carbide may have disregarded such warnings as temporary rectifiable problems. The evaporation basins closer to the company's compounds continue to leak, which is very alarming. Keeping public health and local environment in focus, it should be the joint responsibility of the local government and the new owner, Dow Chemical, to continuously monitor such issues to ensure all aspects of the post-disaster hazardous matters are adequately addressed and impose no risks either to the innocent lives or to the environment.

Acute and Short-Term Toxicity

Animal

The Indian Council of Agricultural Research's report indicates that a large number of cattle (~4000), as well as dogs, cats, and birds were killed due to exposure to the toxic gases released from the Bhopal plant.

Human

The gas leak had devastating effects on the exposed population. Over 200 000 residents (that comprised about one-fourth of the total population of the city of Bhopal) were exposed to MIC and other toxic gases released from the plant. Most of these residents were from the poor class and were living in the immediate surroundings of the Union carbide plant. The true estimate of human mortality remains unknown to date. Respiratory failure due to MIC inhalation was the leading cause of death. MIC caused bronchial necrosis and pulmonary edema. Within the first 24 h after the accident, around 90 000 patients were admitted in local hospitals and clinics with multiple symptoms of respiratory distress, breathlessness, choking, cough, chest pain, and hemoptysis. Acute ophthalmic effects were also reported with severe eye irritation and watering of the eyes.

Reproductive and gynecological effects were evaluated by retrospective cohort studies. An epidemiological survey conducted 9 months after the accident revealed that 43% of 865 pregnancies among exposed women suffered fetal loss, as compared to 6–10% among the general Bhopal population. The spontaneous abortion rate was highest among those exposed during their first trimester. Further studies showed a higher incidence of abnormal uterine bleeding and abnormal Pap smears amongst exposed women in the childbearing age after 105–110 days of the accident.

Few immunological toxicity studies of MIC have been reported. A study of humoral and cell-mediated immunity, in exposed subjects 2 months after exposure, found that cell-mediated immunity was suppressed, and that MIC-specific antibodies persisted for several months after the accident.

Long-Term Health Effects

Human

To this day, the Bhopal accident has claimed more than 6000 lives, and around 50 000 survivors are estimated to be suffering from long-term health effects that are termed the 'Bhopal syndrome' due to lack of information on the exact constituents of the gas cloud. The Indian Council for Medical Research established a field office named Bhopal Gas Disaster Research (BGDR) Centre immediately after the accident. In addition, the International Medical Commission on Bhopal (IMCB) was established in 1993, comprising 15 professionals from 12 different countries. BGDR and IMCB reported that after 15 years of exposure, the affected population is still suffering from multisystemic toxicities. The major long-term health effects observed are shortness of breath, chest pain, muscle/bone pain, asthma, increased spontaneous abortions, and certain psychological problems. A randomized retrospective cohort study undertaken 10 years after exposure showed the presence of persistent small airways obstruction. The lung examination carried out in the survivors several months later exhibited presence of obliterative bronchiolitis and interstitial fibrosis. Thirty nine percent of 783 patients examined showed ventilatory impairment. Taken together, these observations undoubtedly suggest that MIC continues to impact living systems even decades later.

Studies conducted well after the incidence, indicated that even the subsequent generations of the exposed population is adversely affected. These studies show a significant growth retardation in boys who were either exposed to the gases as toddlers or born to exposed parents. Interestingly, no significant effects have been observed in girls.

Prevention and Management Measures

To prevent and manage such disasters in the future, international guidelines such as United Nations Environment Program Awareness and Preparedness for Emergencies at the Local Level and Organization for Economic Cooperation and Development Guiding Principles for Chemical Accident Prevention, Preparedness, and Response have been established. Some of the important recommendations proposed by these committees are to institute Local Emergency Planning Committees that will make the community aware of the dangerous substances used locally by industries and also try to prepare the local medical personnel, emergency first responders, and municipal administrators for the management of unexpected toxic substance release into local community by an industry. These measures have been effectively undertaken in every city and township in the United States today. Unfortunately, analysis of soil/ground water samples on the former UCIL factory grounds and in the waste treatment reservoirs continue to reveal high concentrations of naphthol and naphthalene. During the tests, toxic substances exposed to the aquatic organisms were found to be lethal. The liability of cleanup efforts ultimately lies on the shoulders of the local, state, and national Indian governments regardless of who owns the property. The series of decades-long events surrounding this tragedy should serve as lesson-to-be-learned for future industrialists. The Bhopal studies exemplify the scope for biological monitoring and environmental specimen banking in chemical accidents as part of the global efforts.

Litigations

The Indian Government filed a lawsuit against the Union Carbide, which was settled out of court. In February 1989, the Supreme Court of India directed a final settlement of all Bhopal litigation in the amount of $470 million. The Government of India, UCC, and UCIL accepted the Court's direction. In 2010, Indian Supreme Court ruled again on the adequacy and finality of the settlements.

See also: Methyl Isocyanate; Carbaryl.

Further Reading

Ashraf, L., Champaneri, R., 2012. The Bhopal disaster – learning from failures and evaluating risk. Maint. Eng. 27 (3), 41–47.

Bajaj, J.S., Misra, A., Rajalakshmi, M., Madan, R., 1993. Environmental release of chemicals and reproductive ecology. Environ. Health Perspect. 101 (Suppl. 2), 125–130.

Beckett, W.S., 1998. Persistent respiratory effects in survivors of the Bhopal disaster. Thorax 53 (Suppl. 2), S43–S46.

Bessac, B.F., Jordt, S.E., 2010. Sensory detection and responses to toxic gases: mechanisms, health effects, and countermeasures. Proc. Am. Thorac. Soc. 7 (4), 269–277.

Bromet, E.J., Havenaar, J.M., 2007. Psychological and perceived health effects of the Chernobyl disaster: a 20-year review. Health Phys. 93 (5), 516–521.

Broughton, E., 2005. The Bhopal disaster and its aftermath: a review. Environ. Health 4 (1), 6.

Cordero, J.F., 1993. The epidemiology of disasters and adverse reproductive outcomes: lessons learned. Environ. Health Perspect. 101 (Suppl. 2), 131–136.

Davis, H., 2013. Making sense of disaster: towards a contextual, phase-based understanding of organizationally based acute civilian disasters. Br. J. Criminol. http://dx.doi.org/10.1093/bjc/azt003. (First published online: February 14, 2013).

Dhara, V.R., Dhara, R., 2002. The Union Carbide disaster in Bhopal: a review of health effects. Arch. Environ. Health 57 (5), 391–404.

Dhara, V.R., Gassert, T.H., 2002. The Bhopal syndrome: persistent questions about acute toxicity and management of gas victims. Int. J. Occup. Environ. Health 8 (4), 380–386.

Genuis, S.J., 2013. Chemical sensitivity: pathophysiology or pathopsychology? Clin. Ther. 35 (5), 572–577.

Lapierre, D., Moro, J. (Eds.), June 2003. Five Past Midnight in Bhopal: The Epic Story of the World's Deadliest Industrial Disaster. Warner Books. (ISBN 10: 0446530883/ISBN 13: 9780446530880).

Svendsen, E.R., Runkle, J.R., Dhara, V.R., et al., 2012. Epidemiologic methods lessons learned from environmental public health disasters: Chernobyl, the World Trade Center, Bhopal, and Graniteville, South Carolina. Int. J. Environ. Res. Public Health 9 (8), 2894–2909.

Tyagi, Y.K., Rosencranz, A., 1988. Some international law aspects of the Bhopal disaster. Soc. Sci. Med. 27 (10), 1105–1112.

Varma, D.R., Guest, I., 1993. The Bhopal accident and methyl isocyanate toxicity. J. Toxicol. Environ. Health 40 (4), 513–529.

Relevant Websites

http://sphinxsai.com/2013/conf/PDFS%20ICGSEE%202013/CT=41(815-819)ICGSEE.pdf – ChemTech - Bhopal Gas Tragedy: A Revisit to pick out some lessons we have forgotten in 28 years.

http://www.bhopal.org – The Bhopal Medical Appeal.

http://www.bhopal.com – Union Carbide - Bhopal information center.

Bifenthrin

NK Riar, University of California, Riverside, Riverside, CA, USA

Chemical Profile

- Name: Bifenthrin
- Chemical Abstracts Service Registry Number: 82657-04-3
- Synonyms: 2-Methylbiphenyl-3-ylmethyl (Z)-(1RS,3RS)-3-(2-chloro-3,3,3-trifluoroprop-1-enyl)-2,2-dimethylcyclopropanecarboxylate (IUPAC), FMC 54800, Talstar, Bifenthrine, Biphenthrin
- Molecular Formula: $C_{23}H_{22}ClF_3O_2$
- Chemical Structure:

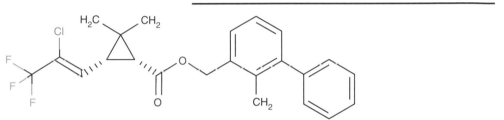

Background

Pyrethroids are synthetic derivatives of naturally occurring pyrethrin insecticides found in the extract from the flowers *Chrysanthemum cinerariaefolium*. Structurally, the six insecticidally active pyrethrins contain a cyclopropane carboxylic acid group and a cyclopentenolone group joined by an ester linkage. The major drawback of these compounds is that they are photolabile. The first-generation pyrethroids share this trait, resulting in half-lives that are in the order of hours. First-generation pyrethroids are primarily synthesized by modifying the alcohol portion of the molecule.

Later attempts at modifying the acid portion of the molecule resulted in more photostable pesticides. These can be broken down into two types: types I and II. The type II pyrethroids contain an 'α-cyano' group and are α-cyano-3-pheoxybenzyl pyrethroid esters. Type II pyrethroids are characterized by increased biological activity compared to the type I pyrethroids and can act by slightly different modes of action.

Bifenthrin is an example of a third-generation type I pyrethroid. It was first discovered and manufactured in the United States by the FMC Corporation. Bifenthrin was first registered for use by the US Environmental Protection Agency (US EPA) in 1985. The usage of bifenthrin and other pyrethroid pesticides markedly increased when the organophosphate pesticides, diazinon and chlorpyrifos, were phased out in residential applications because of concerns about toxicity to humans, especially children. There were also water quality problems associated with these organophosphate pesticides. Due to the wide variety of uses of pyrethroid pesticides and reports of low mammalian toxicity, pyrethroids naturally replaced organophosphate pesticides for many applications.

Bifenthrin contains one chiral center, giving rise to 1*R-cis*-bifenthrin and 1*S-cis*-bifenthrin. Stereoisomers have been shown to differ in insecticidal action and environmental fate and thus each must be carefully evaluated.

Uses

Bifenthrin and other pyrethroids are commonly used both in urban areas and agriculture. Major agricultural uses of bifenthrin in California include crop pest control for almonds, cotton, corn, and pistachios. It also has many urban uses in landscaping, structural pest control (termites), and in insect repellents. Bifenthrin is used in agriculture (20%), commercial projects (40%), and in homes or gardens (40%). In California, there are over 170 registered products with bifenthrin as the active ingredient.

Physical Properties, Environmental Fate, and Behavior

Bifenthrin is a viscous liquid, crystalline solid, or waxy solid with a faint, slightly sweet odor. It has a molecular weight of 422.9. At 25 °C, its vapor pressure is 1.81×10^{-7} mm Hg^{-1} and it has a Henry's law constant of 7.20×10^{-3} atm m^3 mol^{-1}. The solubility of bifenthrin in water is relatively low at 0.1 mg l^{-1}. Furthermore, the water octanol coefficient (K_{ow}) is 1×10^6 and results in bifenthrin binding to organic substrates. The soil sorption coefficients range between 1.31×10^5 and 3.02×10^5, indicating relatively tight binding to soil particles. They also tend to bind to organic particulate materials in the water column. The K_{ow} of bifenthrin may explain the bioconcentration factors (BCFs) observed in some animals, especially fish. For example, fathead minnows (*Pimephales promelas*) exposed to 0.0037 μg l^{-1} bifenthrin had BCFs of 21 000 after 127 days and 28 000 after 254 days of exposure. Hydrolysis of bifenthrin in buffered water occurs between pH 5 and 9. Photolysis studies in water and soil found that the half-lives were 408 and 96.9 days, respectively. The aerobic soil half-life was 96.3 days and the anaerobic half-life, 425 days.

Exposure and Exposure Monitoring

There is low potential for volatilization into the air; however, there is potential for airborne transport if attached to drifting soil

 http://dx.doi.org/10.1016/B978-0-12-386454-3.01169-6

particles or as a spray as in agricultural application. The major routes of exposure observed in humans are contact during application or manufacturing of the compound. Inhalation is also possible, especially during pesticide spraying.

Toxicokinetics

After a 7-day exposure in rats, most radiolabeled bifenthrin was eliminated in the urine or feces with a significant portion being converted to various metabolites. Some of the major metabolites in feces and urine include hydroxymethyl-bifenthrin, 4′-hydroxy-bifenthrin, 3′-hydroxy-hydroxymethyl-bifenthrin, 4′-hydroxy-biphenyl acid, biphenyl acid, and 4′-hydroxy-biphenyl alcohol. The main routes of biotransformation of bifenthrin have been studied in rats and include oxidation resulting in hydroxylation of the compound via NADPH-dependent cytochrome P-450 enzymes, cleavage via esterases, or abiotically through hydrolysis. Phase I reactions can also be followed by conjugation reactions resulting in the elimination of the compound.

Mechanisms of Action

Pyrethroids target the central nervous system in both target and nontarget organisms. Their main mechanism of action is interacting with voltage-gated sodium channels in neurons. This interaction results in depolarization caused by the prolonged influx of sodium ions during excitation. The extended depolarization is what leads to repetitive nerve activity that can result in hyperexcitation and death. Some pyrethroids have also been found to inhibit ATPase activity. Studies have also found that some pyrethroids interact with the aminobutyric acid receptor; however, this is normally more common only with type II pyrethroids.

Acute/Subchronic Toxicity

The oral LD_{50} of bifenthrin determined in rats was between 42.5 and 210.4 mg kg^{-1} body weight (bw) after a single dose, making it moderately toxic. The LD_{50} for dermal exposure in rats was greater than 2000 mg kg^{-1} bw. A short-term 90-day study in dogs fed bifenthrin-containing capsules determined a no observed adverse effect level (NOAEL) of 2.5 mg kg^{-1} bw and a lowest observed adverse effect level (LOAEL) (based on tremors) of 5.0 mg kg^{-1} bw per day. Similarly, a 90-day dietary study on rats found a NOAEL of 3.8 mg kg^{-1} bw and a LOAEL of 7.5 g kg^{-1} bw per day. Bifenthrin produces type I pyrethroid neurotoxic symptoms in short- and long-term animal studies. Symptoms observed include clonic convulsions, tremors, loss of coordination, staggered gait, and oral discharge.

A series of neurotoxicity studies were performed to assess both acute and subchronic neurotoxic effects. Rats given a single gavage of undiluted bifenthrin had a NOAEL of 35 mg kg^{-1} bw based on symptoms observed at the LOAEL of 75 mg kg^{-1} bw. A 90-day study on rats found a NOAEL of 2.9 mg kg^{-1} bw based on symptoms including tremors, changes in grip strength, and landing foot splay. The LOAEL in this study was 6 mg kg^{-1} bw per day. These findings support the neurotoxicity of bifenthrin.

Chronic Toxicity

An 87-week (males) or 92-week (females) study on mice observed a NOAEL and LOAEL of 7.6 and 29 mg kg^{-1} bw per day, respectively. A 24-month dietary study in rats found the NOAEL to be 2.3 mg kg^{-1} bw (males) and 3.0 mg kg^{-1} bw (females). The LOAEL was 4.7 mg kg^{-1} bw (males) and 6.1 mg kg^{-1} bw (females). The major chronic effect observed was tremors. These studies also investigated carcinogenicity of bifenthrin (see Carcinogenicity).

Immunotoxicity

No information was found on the immunotoxicity potential of bifenthrin in whole-animal systems or humans. A study investigated enantioselectivity of (*Z*)-*cis*-bifenthrin using the macrophage cell line RAW264.7. It was found that 1*S*-*cis*-bifenthrin was more toxic than the 1*R*-*cis*-bifenthrin in all concentrations assessed.

Reproductive and Developmental Toxicity

A two-generation study in rats concluded that the highest dose of 5 mg kg^{-1} bw per day showed no significant change in reproductive parameters including mating, male fertility, female fertility, and gestation indices. There was a significant increase in the incidence of tremors and marginally lower body weights at the LOAEL of 5 mg kg^{-1} bw per day in the pregnant female rats.

Two other developmental toxicity studies in both rats and rabbits found no developmental toxicity at any of the tested dose levels up to 16.3 and 8 mg kg^{-1} bw per day for rats and rabbits, respectively.

Genotoxicity

Bifenthrin was negative in several genotoxicity tests, both *in vitro* and *in vivo*. *In vitro* assays included the Ames test and Chinese hamster ovary cell assays for mutations, chromosomal aberrations, and sister chromatid exchange. *In vivo* tests included an unscheduled DNA synthesis (UDS), chromosomal aberrations, sex-linked recessive lethal assays, and a test for micronucleus formation. There was a weak positive result for a single UDS assay and a test on mouse lymphoma cells. Overall, however, bifenthrin is not considered to be genotoxic.

Carcinogenicity

In the mouse chronic toxicity study previously mentioned in the Chronic Toxicity section, the highest dose showed an increased incidence of urinary bladder tumors; however, this was not considered sufficient evidence for bifenthrin carcinogenicity in humans. The rat chronic toxicity study found no evidence of treatment-related carcinogenicity. Due mainly to limited carcinogenicity data in animals and the lack of human data, the US EPA has classified bifenthrin as a class C (possible human carcinogen).

Clinical Management

In humans, the FMC Corporation (a major bifenthrin manufacturer), received 58 bifenthrin-related emergency calls in 2002. Most calls were from people applying or having been accidentally exposed to bifenthrin. The most common complaints reported were burning or tingling of the exposed skin and eye irritation. Some FMC plant workers also reported mild paraesthesia (skin tingling) after prolonged exposure to bifenthrin. Regular medical exams found no significance deviation from baseline values for medical tests, including liver and kidney function tests.

Ecotoxicology

Due to the widespread outdoor uses of bifenthrin, there are many nontarget organisms that are exposed to the pesticide including birds, terrestrial and aquatic invertebrates, and fish. Bifenthrin was found to be only slightly acutely toxic to bobwhite quail (*Colinus virginianus*) and mallard duck (*Anas platyrynchos*) with an LD_{50} and an LC_{50} of 1800 mg kg^{-1} bw and 1280 mg kg^{-1} bw diet, respectively. Reproduction was not effected in the highest dose administered to either species. A recent study on terrestrial invertebrates observed that bifenthrin was one of two pyrethroid pesticides that reduced bee fecundity and had detrimental effects on their development rate. It was also observed that worker bees of *Apis mellifera liguistica* showed median lethal effects to bifenthrin at 16.7 mg l^{-1}. Another study investigated the toxic effects of several synthetic pyrethroids on the aquatic invertebrate *Hyalella azteca*. Bifenthrin exhibited the highest toxicity with an LC_{50} of 0.18 μg g^{-1} organic carbon in sediments. Bifenthrin has also been shown to be acutely toxic to many fish species. The 96-h LC_{50}s for rainbow trout and bluegill sunfish are 150 and 350 ng l^{-1}, respectively. Due to its toxic effects in fish and aquatic organisms, the US EPA classified bifenthrin as a restricted use pesticide in 1989.

Recent studies have discovered that exposure to pyrethroids results in estrogenic activity in some species of fish. Vitellogenin is the precursor protein to egg-yolk normally found in females. In female fish, 17-β estradiol (E2) regulates vitellogenin production in the liver. Male fish and nonsexually mature juveniles may also produce vitellogenin since they too have a receptor for E2. In this way, vitellogenin translation and production in male fish and juveniles can act as biomarkers for estrogenic exposure. Bifenthrin enantiomers were studied in male Japanese medaka where a 123-fold difference was found in vitellogenin production between the 1*S*-*cis*-bifentrhin and the 1*R*-*cis*-bifentrhin.

Exposure Standards and Guidelines

The acceptable daily intake of bifenthrin in humans as established during the joint meeting of the Food and Agricultural Organization and the World Health Organization was 0.01 mg kg^{-1} bw. There are no occupational or other specific standards for environmental exposures to bifenthrin.

See also: Permethrin; Pesticides; Pyrethrins/Pyrethroids; Cytochrome P450; Environmental Protection Agency, US.

Further Reading

Fecko, A., 1999. Environmental Fate of Bifenthrin. Environment Monitoring and Pesticide Regulatory Branch. Department of Pesticide Regulation, Sacramento, CA. 1–9.

Hougard, J., Duchon, S., Darriet, F., Zaim, M., Rogier, C., Guillet, P., 2003. Comparative performances, under laboratory conditions, of seven pyrethroid insecticides used for impregnation of mosquito nets. Bull. World Health Organ. 81, 324–333.

Johnson, M., Luukinen, B., Gervais, J., Buhl, K., Stone, D., 2010. Bifenthrin Technical Fact Sheet. National Pesticide Information Center, Oregon State University Extension Services, Corvallis, OR.

Laskowski, D.A., 2002. Physical and chemical properties of pyrethroids. Rev. Environ. Contam. Toxicol. 174, 49–170.

Martin, T., Chandre, F., Ochou, O.G., Vaissayre, M., Fournier, D., 2002. Pyrethroid resistance mechanisms in the cotton bollworm Helicoverpa armigera (Lepidoptera: Noctuidae) from West Africa. Pestic. Biochem. Physiol. 74, 17–26.

The Pesticide residues in food report form the Joint Meeting of the FAO Panel of Experts and the World Health Organization Assessment Group in 2009 provides a comprehensive summary of the toxicological studies of acute, chronic, and reproductive toxicity as well as studies on carcinogenicity, genotoxicity, and other health effects.

Pesticide Residues in Food – 2009: Toxicological Evaluations/Joint Meeting of the FAO Panel of Experts on Pesticide Residues in Food and the Environment and the WHO Core Assessment Group, Geneva, Switzerland, September 16–25, 2009.

Solliday, A., Federoff, N.E., Meléndez, J.L., 2010. Environmental Fate and Ecological Risk Assessment Problem Formulation in Support of Registration Review for Bifenthrin. U.S. EPA Office of Pesticide Programs Environmental Fate and Effects Division, June 9.

Spurlock, F., Lee, M., 2008. Synthetic pyrethroids use patterns properties and environmental effects. In: Gan, J., Spurlock, F., Hendley, P., Weston, D. (Eds.), Synthetic Pyrethroids: Occurrence and Behavior in Aquatic Environments. American Chemical Society, Washington, DC, pp. 3–25. ACS Symposium Series 991.

Vijverberg, H.P.M., van den Bercken, J., 1990. Neurotoxicological effects and the mode of action of pyrethroid insecticides. Crit. Rev. Toxicol. 21 (2), 105–126.

Wang, L.M., Liu, W., Yang, C., et al., 2007. Enantioselectivity in estrogenic potential and uptake of bifenthrin. Environ. Sci. Technol. 41, 6124–6128.

Relevant Websites

http://www.cdpr.ca.gov/docs/pur/purmain.htm – Pesticide Use Reporting, California Department of Pesticide Regulation.

http://www.epa.gov/opprd001/rup/ – US EPA Restricted Use Products Report.

Biguanides

CV Rao, NMAM Institute of Technology, Nitte, India

- Name: Biguanide
- Chemical Abstracts Service Registry Number: 56-03-1 (Metformin: 657-24-9)
- Synonyms: Imidodicarbonimidic diamide, Diguanide, Amidinoguanidine, Phenformin, Metformin, Buformin, Glucophage®
- Molecular Formula: Biguanide-$C_2H_7N_5$; Metformin-$C_4H_{11}N_5$
- Chemical Structures:

Biguanide

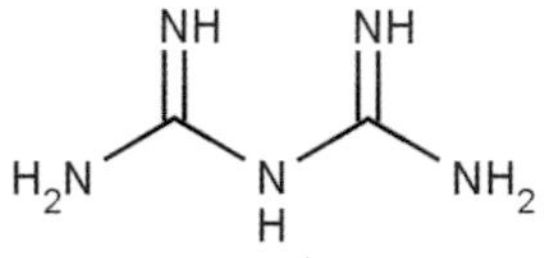

Metformin

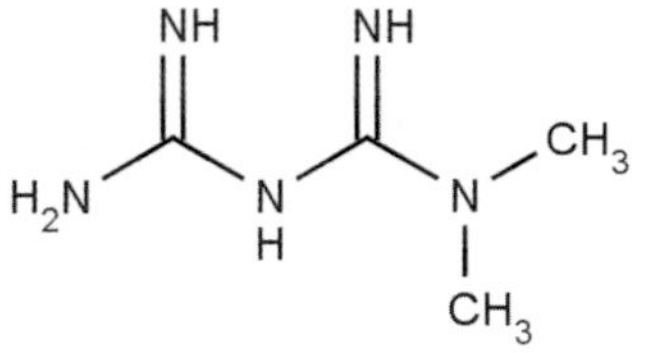

Background

French physician Jean Sterne published the first clinical trial in 1957 suggesting metformin as a treatment for diabetes. The United Kingdom introduced this drug in 1958 followed by Canada in 1972, and the United States in 1995. As of 2010, metformin was one of only two oral antidiabetics in the World Health Organization model list of essential medicines, the other being glibenclamide. Metformin is believed to enjoy the popularity of being the most widely prescribed antidiabetic drug in the world. It has been estimated that the United States alone has filled nearly a million prescriptions in 2010 for its generic formulations. Biguanides are not hypoglycemic agents; rather they promote euglycemia (antihyperglycemic). Biguanides are used both as monotherapy and in combination with other oral hypoglycemic agents to control hyperglycemia. Although very safe in most instances, the major toxicity from acute or chronic use of biguanides has been reported to be lactic acidosis. In fact, the high rate of severe lactic acidosis was the only major cause of withdrawal of phenformin from the US market in 1976.

Age (typically >60 years) is a big risk factor for lactic acidosis with the use of biguanides. Decreased cardiac, hepatic, or renal function, diabetic ketoacidosis, respiratory failure, surgery, ethanol intoxication, and fasting are additional factors that can precipitate this condition. The frequency of lactic acidosis associated with metformin therapy is much lower than the frequency associated with phenformin therapy. This is because of metformin's weak binding with mitochondrial membrane compared to phenformin. Metformin has a shorter half-life and has no hepatic metabolism, whereas phenformin has a longer half-life and undergoes hepatic transformation. Hence, patients with liver dysfunction may be at a higher risk for toxicity from phenformin. Many studies have indicated a beneficial role of metformin on specific types of liver disease, and numerous recent publications suggest that metformin may have potential as a targeted chemopreventive agent.

Metformin exhibits a multipronged attack on hyperglycemia by decreasing insulin resistance and hepatic glucose output, and by enhancing peripheral glucose uptake. The most widely acclaimed mechanisms of action include enhanced suppression of gluconeogenesis by insulin, reduced glucagon-stimulated gluconeogenesis, and increased uptake of glucose by muscle and adipose cells. The cumulative effects of these changes in diabetics are to decrease fasting and postprandial blood glucose by 20–40%, decrease hemoglobin $A1_C$, decrease body weight, decrease low density lipoprotein, and increase high density lipoprotein. Metformin is the only antidiabetic drug that has been conclusively shown to prevent the cardiovascular complications of diabetes. It is extensively prescribed because it helps reduce bad cholesterol and triglyceride levels, and is not associated with weight gain.

Uses

Biguanides are used as an oral drug for the management of mild to moderately severe noninsulin-dependent diabetes mellitus, or NIDDM, (Type II) in obese or overweight patients who are usually above 40 years of age. It is important that for the administration of this drug the disease should have adult onset. Polymeric biguanides were originally developed as a presurgery antimicrobial scrub and in 1977, it was introduced in the market for treating pools and spas as a disinfectant under the trade name Baquacil. The US Environmental Protection Agency approved this agent as the only nonhalogen sanitizer of pools and spas. Biguanide itself is combined with algaecides and hydrogen peroxide for periodic oxidation of pools and spas. Biguanides are incompatible with chlorine, ozone, detergents, and ionizers, but are compatible with water ion balancing chemicals. Biguanide in the form of polyaminopropyl biguanide serves as a disinfectant, and preservative for skin disinfection, contact lens cleaning solutions, and deodorant body sprays. Biguanides reduce the surface tension of water, which gives it a smoother feeling. They are stable in sunlight and temperature. At recommended concentrations when used in pools and spas, biguanides do not irritate the skin or eyes and do not corrode the pool equipment.

 http://dx.doi.org/10.1016/B978-0-12-386454-3.00253-0

Environmental Fate and Behavior

Biguanides, salts of biguanide, or biguanide-like compounds such as Metformin hydrochloride production and use as an antidiabetic medication may result in its release to the environment through various waste streams. Metformin hydrochloride is expected to exist in the dissociated form as metformin in the environment. If released to air, an estimated vapor pressure of 0.0034 mm Hg at 25 °C indicates metformin will exist solely in the vapor phase in the ambient atmosphere. Metformin, when in vapor phase, is expected to be degraded in the atmosphere by reaction with photochemically-produced hydroxyl radicals; the half-life for this reaction in air is estimated to be 15 min. If released to soil, metformin is expected to have high mobility based on an estimated K_{OC} of 110. Volatilization from moist soil surfaces is not expected to be an important fate process based on an estimated Henry's law constant of 7.6×10^{-16} atm-cu m mol^{-1}. The p*K*a of metformin is 12.4, indicating that this compound will primarily exist in cation form in the environment, and cations generally adsorb to organic carbon and clay more strongly than their neutral counterparts. Based on metformin's vapor pressure, it is not expected to volatilize from dry soil surfaces. Based on the estimated K_{OC} of metformin, it is not expected to adsorb to suspended solids and sediment if released into water. Volatilization from water surfaces is not expected to be an important fate process based on this compound's estimated Henry's law constant. Furthermore, a p*K*a of 12.4 indicates metformin will exist almost entirely in the ionized form at pH values of 5–9. An estimated bioconcentration factor of 3.2 suggests the potential for bioconcentration in aquatic organisms is low. Hydrolysis is not expected to be an important environmental fate process since this compound lacks functional groups that hydrolyze under environmental conditions. Occupational exposure to metformin hydrochloride may occur through inhalation and dermal contact with this compound at workplaces where metformin hydrochloride is produced or used.

Exposure and Exposure Monitoring

The exposure to this drug is through the oral route and absorption through the gastrointestinal tract. Generic metformin is available in tablet form (500, 850, or 1000 mg); the recommended regimen starts with 500 or 850 mg once daily and increases based on tolerance to 1000–2550 mg daily taken in two divided doses. There are several commercial formulations, which include Glucophage, Glumetza, Fortamet, and Riomet. Metformin is also available in extended release forms and combination formulations with several sulfonylureas, such as glipizide (Metaglip) or glyburide (Glucovance); DDP-4 inhibitors such as alogliptin (Kazano), linagliptin (Jentadueto), saxagliptin (Kombiglyze), and sitagliptin (Janumet); as well as thiazolidinediones such as pioglitazone (Actoplus) and rosiglitazone (Avandamet). Metformin is generally well tolerated, but side effects can include diarrhea, gastrointestinal upset, abdominal pain, nausea, weakness, headache, dizziness, and rash.

Toxicokinetics

Biguanide such as Metformin is absorbed (~50%) from the gastrointestinal tract. Protein binding ability of this family is very poor (~20%). However, it is distributed throughout the major organs and mainly metabolized in the liver by hydroxylation. On hydroxylation, it produces *N*-*P*-hydroxy-*B*-phenylethyl-biguanide as a metabolite. About two-thirds of the biguanide is excreted unchanged and the remaining one-third as a metabolite. Phenformin's half-life in the plasma is 7–15 h versus metformin's 1.5 h and buformin's 4–6 h. Metformin and buformin are excreted largely in an unchanged manner. The renal clearance of buformin, metformin, and phenformin are 393, 440, and 42–262 ml min^{-1}, respectively. Renal clearance was estimated to be 510 ± 120 ml min^{-1}. The plasma concentration is about 1–2 μg ml^{-1} 1–2 h after an oral dose of 500–1000 mg. Metformin barely binds to plasma proteins. The mean apparent volume of distribution ranges from 63 to 276 l kg^{-1}. Biguanides are known to show interaction with furosemide (induces diuresis), nifedipine (calcium channel blocker), and cationic drugs.

Diabetic condition does not alter metformin disposition, and apparently remains unaffected by the presence of other antidiabetic agents or the use of different formulations. Absolute oral bioavailability of metformin is 40–60%, and gastrointestinal absorption is apparently complete within 6 h of ingestion. An inverse relationship was observed between the dose ingested and the relative absorption with therapeutic doses ranging from 0.5 to 1.5 g, suggesting the involvement of an active, saturable absorption process. Metformin is rapidly distributed following absorption and does not bind to plasma proteins. No metabolites or conjugates of metformin have been identified. The absence of liver metabolism clearly differentiates the pharmacokinetics of metformin from that of other biguanides such as phenformin.

Metformin undergoes renal excretion and has a mean plasma elimination half-life after oral administration of between 4.0 and 8.7 h. This elimination is prolonged in patients with renal impairment and correlates with creatinine clearance. There are only scarce data on the relationship between plasma metformin concentrations and metabolic effects. Therapeutic levels may be 0.5–1.0 mg l^{-1} in the fasting state and 1–2 mg l^{-1} after a meal, but monitoring has little clinical value except when lactic acidosis is suspected or present.

Mechanism of Toxicity

Globally, hundreds of millions of patients are prescribed this drug annually. Metformin was discovered before the era of target-based drug discovery, and its molecular mechanism of action remains an important focus of diabetes research. Advances in our understanding of metformin's molecular targets are likely to enable target-based identification of second-generation drugs with similar properties, a development that has been a difficult task until now. Besides its potent antidiabetic properties, Metformin's potential as a targeted anticancer agent is being explored in a number of laboratories throughout the world.

A modification of the basic biguanide structure results in differences in potency, metabolism, excretion, and probably toxicity. The drug has a two-fold mechanism of action: it enhances the peripheral muscle glucose uptake and utilization, and it inhibits glucose release from the liver. Biguanides induce an increase in peripheral gluconeogenesis and a decrease in intestinal absorption of glucose, vitamin B_{12}, and bile acids. Biguanides do not usually decrease blood sugar in a normal individual unless ethanol or another hypoglycemic agent is simultaneously administered or there is severe hepatic insufficiency. Biguanide treatment to NIDDM patients having hepatic insufficiency, renal insufficiency, peripheral vascular disease, and coronary diseases is contraindicated. In contrast, Phenformin generally lowers the blood sugar level in diabetics and nutritionally starved patients. Phenformin appears initially to produce a gastric mucosal irritability, which may predispose a person to a number of gastrointestinal symptoms, including gastric hemorrhage. Phenformin may act on the cell membrane to decrease oxidative phosphorylation, produce tissue anoxia, increase peripheral glucose uptake (Pasteur Effect), and lead to lactic acidosis (accumulation of lactic acid) by inhibition of lactic acid metabolism.

The most compelling mechanism surrounding metformin's action has been activation of AMPK pathway (AMP-activated protein kinase). Activation of this enzyme leads to stimulation of hepatic fatty acid oxidation and ketogenesis, inhibition of cholesterol synthesis, lipogenesis, and triglyceride synthesis, inhibition of adipocyte lipolysis and lipogenesis, stimulation of skeletal muscle fatty acid oxidation and muscle glucose uptake, and modulation of insulin secretion by pancreatic β-cells. The notion that AMPK mediates the antihyperglycemic action of metformin has recently been challenged by genetic loss-of-function studies, thrusting the AMPK-independent effects of the drug into the spotlight for the first time in more than a decade. Key AMPK-independent effects of the drug include the mitochondrial actions that have been known for many years and which are still thought to be the primary site of action of metformin. Coupled with recent evidence of AMPK-independent effects on the counter-regulatory hormone glucagon, new paradigms of AMPK-independent drug action are beginning to take shape.

Acute and Short-Term Toxicity

Human

Although the half-life of metformin is prolonged in patients with renal impairment, no specific dosage adjustments have been recommended. Metformin fails to show its efficacy in the absence of insulin. Metformin is as effective as the sulfonylureas in treating patients with type II diabetes and has a more prominent postprandial effect than the sulfonylureas or insulin. When combined with a sulfonylurea, metformin has been shown to exert antihyperglycemic effects in addition to the sulfonylurea. Cimetidine decreases the elimination of metformin; therefore, the manufacturer recommends a reduced metformin dosage when these agents are combined.

The intestinal absorption of metformin may be primarily mediated by plasma membrane monoamine transporter (PMAT/SLC29A4), which is expressed on the luminal side of the enterocytes. However, there are no current *in vivo* data on the role of PMAT in the disposition and pharmacological effect of metformin. OCT3/SLC22A3 is also expressed in the brush border of the enterocytes and may contribute to metformin uptake. Additionally, OCT1/SLC22A1, which is expressed on the basolateral membrane and cytoplasm of the enterocytes, may facilitate transfer of metformin into the interstitial fluid. The role of OCT1 and OCT3 in intestinal transport of metformin remains to be further validated.

The hepatic uptake of metformin is primarily mediated by OCT1/SLC22A1 and OCT3/SLC22A3, which are expressed on the basolateral membrane of hepatocytes. Metformin is also a good substrate for human multidrug and toxin extrusion 1 (MATE1/SLC47A1) and MATE2-K/SLC47A2. MATE1/SLC47A1 is highly expressed in the liver, kidney, and skeletal muscle and may contribute to the excretion of metformin from both liver and kidney. However, MATE1's role in hepatic secretion has been questioned, as biliary excretion of metformin seems to be insignificant in humans. Data in Mate1 knockout mice suggest that, at least in the rodent, biliary excretion of metformin occurs. Recent drug–drug interaction studies suggest an important role of MATE1 and/or MATE2-K in metformin renal elimination. MATE2-K/SLC47A2 is predominantly expressed in the apical membrane of the renal proximal tubule cells and contributes to the renal excretion of metformin.

The uptake of metformin from circulation into renal epithelial cells is primarily facilitated by OCT2/SLC22A2, which is expressed predominantly at the basolateral membrane in the distal renal tubules. Renal excretion of metformin is mediated mainly via MATE1/SLC47A1 and MATE2-K/SLC47A2. OCT1 is also expressed on the apical and subapical domain side of both the proximal and distal tubules in kidney and may play important roles in metformin reabsorption in kidney tubules. Plasma membrane monoamine transporter (PMAT/SLC29A4) is expressed on the apical membrane of renal epithelial cells, and may play a role in renal reabsorption of metformin. However, there are no *in vivo* data yet demonstrating this role. Recently, P-gp (ABCB1) and BCRP (ABCG2) are shown to be involved in the efflux of metformin across placental apical membranes.

Chronic Toxicity

Human

Biguanides are known to cause vomiting, nausea, abdominal cramps, gastrointestinal intolerance, anorexia, epigastric fullness, photosensitivity, dyspepsia, and dysgeusia (metallic taste), confusion, and lethargy. Ethanol intake before the administration of therapeutic doses of metformin or excessive dose appears to predispose the patient to the development of lactic acidosis with a serious outcome. Despite several adverse effects, many people can tolerate phenformin; therefore, it is still sold in European and other countries worldwide. Stray cases of acute pancreatitis and megaloblastic anemia in patients going through biguanide therapy have been reported.

Monitoring vitamin B_{12} levels in patients during long-term treatment with biguanides is recommended because of the possibility of decreased vitamin absorption. Biguanides should not be prescribed to patients with diabetic coma or ketoacidosis, renal and hepatic impairment, alcohol abuse, or preexisting liver and kidney conditions.

Clinical Management

Biguanide toxicity is primarily managed by supportive means. Its elimination from the body could be enhanced by hemodialysis or enhancing excessive urination (forced diuresis). When lactic acidosis occurs in metformin-treated patients, early determination of the metformin plasma concentration appears to be the best criterion for assessing the involvement of the drug in this acute condition. After confirmation of the diagnosis, treatment should rapidly involve forced diuresis or hemodialysis, both of which favor rapid elimination of the drug. Although serious, lactic acidosis due to metformin is rare and may be minimized by strict adherence to prescribing guidelines and contraindications, particularly the presence of renal failure. Following are some ground rules that can be followed during metformin toxicity:

(1) Secure airway, breathing, and circulation. (2) For acute ingestions, administer activated charcoal: 1 g kg^{-1} (generally 50 g in adults); do not administer activated charcoal to patients with chronic toxicity. (3) For patients with profound acidosis (pH <7.10), consider sodium bicarbonate infusion (e.g., give 1–2 meq kg^{-1} IV push; then put approximately 133 meq $NaHCO_3$ in 1 l D5W, run at 250 ml h^{-1} in adults, or twice maintenance fluid infusion rate in children). For patients with profound acidosis, renal disease, or critical illness, obtain immediate nephrology consultation; hemodialysis will correct metformin-induced acid–base disturbance and slightly increase metformin clearance. Pediatric metformin toxicity should be treated in the same manner as one would treat adults. Interestingly, however, very few drug interactions have been described with metformin in healthy volunteers. Plasma levels may be reduced by guar gum and alpha-glucosidase inhibitors and increased by cimetidine, but no data are yet available in the diabetic population.

See also: Liver; Kidney.

Further Reading

Anisimov, V.N., 2013. Metformin and rapamycin are master-keys for understanding the relationship between cell senescent, aging and cancer. Aging (Albany NY) 5 (5), 337–338.

Brackett, C.C., May–June 2010. Clarifying metformin's role and risks in liver dysfunction. J. Am. Pharm. Assoc. (2003) 50 (3), 407–410.

Cone, C.J., Bachyrycz, A.M., Murata, G.H., 2010. Hepatotoxicity associated with metformin therapy in treatment of type 2 diabetes mellitus with nonalcoholic fatty liver disease. Ann. Pharmacother. 44 (10), 1655–1659.

Dell'Aglio, D.M., Perino, L.J., Kazzi, Z., et al., 2009. Acute metformin overdose: examining serum pH, lactate level, and metformin concentrations in survivors versus nonsurvivors: a systematic review of the literature. Ann. Emerg. Med. 54 (6), 818–823.

Do, M.T., Kim, H.G., Khanal, T., et al., May 21, 2013. Metformin inhibits heme oxygenase-1 expression in cancer cells through inactivation of Raf-ERK-Nrf2 signaling and AMPK-independent pathways. Toxicol. Appl. Pharmacol..

Forrester, M.B., 2008. Adult metformin ingestions reported to Texas poison control centers, 2000–2006. Hum. Exp. Toxicol. 27 (7), 575–583.

Galea, M., Jelacin, N., Bramham, K., White, I., 2007. Severe lactic acidosis and rhabdomyolysis following metformin and ramipril overdose. Br. J. Anaesth. 98 (2), 213–215.

Gambaro, V., Dell'acqua, L., Farè, F., Fidani, M., Froldi, R., Saligari, E., 2007. A case of fatal intoxication from metformin. J. Forensic Sci. 52 (4), 988–991.

Hashmi, T., September 13, 2011. Probable hepatotoxicity associated with the use of metformin in type 2 diabetes. BMJ Case Rep.. http://dx.doi.org/10.1136/bcr.04.2011.4092 pii: bcr0420114092.

Hong, Y.C., O'Boyle, C.P., Chen, I.C., Hsiao, C.T., Kuan, J.T., 2008. Metformin-associated lactic acidosis in a pregnant patient. Gynecol. Obstet. Invest. 66 (2), 138–141.

McEvoy, G.E. (Ed.), 2002. American Hospital Formulary Service Drug Information 2002. American Society of Health-System Pharmacists, Bethesda, MD, pp. 2997–3018.

Miller, R.A., Chu, Q., Jianxin Xie, J., et al., 2013. Biguanides suppress hepatic glucagon signalling by decreasing production of cyclic AMP. Nature 494, 256–260.

Nair, V., Pathi, S., Jutooru, I., Sreevalsan, S., Basha, R., Abdelrahim, M., Samudio, I., Safe, S., June 26, 2013. Metformin inhibits pancreatic cancer cell and tumor growth and downregulates Sp transcription factors. Carcinogenesis (Epub ahead of print).

Orban, J.C., Fontaine, E., Ichai, C., 2012. Metformin overdose: time to move on. Crit. Care 16 (5), 164.

Renda, F., Mura, P., Finco, G., Ferrazin, F., Pani, L., Landoni, G., 2013. Metformin-associated lactic acidosis requiring hospitalization. A national 10 year survey and a systematic literature review. Eur. Rev. Med. Pharmacol. Sci. 17 (Suppl. 1), 45–49.

Sant'anna, J.R., Yajima, J.P., Rosada, L.J., et al., June 20, 2013. Metformin's performance in in vitro and in vivo genetic toxicology studies. Exp. Biol. Med. (Maywood) (Epub ahead of print).

Soderstrom, J., Murray, L., Daly, F.F., Little, M., 2006. Toxicology case of the month: oral hypoglycaemic overdose. Emerg. Med. J. 23 (7), 565–567.

Spiller, H.A., Quadrani, D.A., 2004. Toxic effects from metformin exposure. Ann. Pharmacother. 38 (5), 776–780.

Spiller, H.A., Sawyer, T.S., 2006. Toxicology of oral antidiabetic medications. Am. J. Health Syst. Pharm. 63, 29–38.

Turkcuer, I., Erdur, B., Sari, I., Yuksel, A., Tura, P., Yuksel, S., 2009. Severe metformin intoxication treated with prolonged haemodialyses and plasma exchange. Eur. J. Emerg. Med. 16 (1), 11–13.

Vitale-Cross, L., Molinolo, A.A., Martin, D., et al., 2012. Metformin prevents the development of oral squamous cell carcinomas from carcinogen-induced premalignant lesions. Cancer Prev. Res. (Phila) 5 (4), 562–573.

Wen, Y.K., 2009. Impact of acute kidney injury on metformin-associated lactic acidosis. Int. Urol. Nephrol. 41 (4), 967–972.

Wills, B.K., Bryant, S.M., Buckley, P., Seo, B., 2010. Can acute overdose of metformin lead to lactic acidosis? Am. J. Emerg. Med. 28 (8), 857–861.

Relevant Websites

https://aapcc.s3.amazonaws.com/pdfs/annual_reports/2011_NPDS_Annual_Report.pdf – American Association of Poison Control Center Report (2011).

http://www.medscape.com/viewarticle/774596 – Lactic Acidosis Secondary to Metformin Overdose-Medscape.

http://emedicine.medscape.com/article/167027-overview – Medscpae.

http://www.medsafe.govt.nz/profs/PUarticles/5.htm – Medsafe-Australian Government.

http://livertox.nlm.nih.gov/Metformin.htm – National Institutes of Health-National Library of Medicine.

http://www.pharmgkb.org/pathway/PA165948259 – Pharmacogenomics. Knowledge. Implementation.

Bioaccumulation

K Chojnacka, Wroclaw University of Technology, Wroclaw, Poland
M Mikulewicz, Medical University of Wroclaw, Wroclaw, Poland

Introduction

Every living organism throughout life bioaccumulates various substances – both organic and inorganic. The consequences of bioaccumulation are associated with the occurrence of toxic effects and depend both on the chemical and the organism. The first step towards bioaccumulation is exposure. Different organisms accumulate chemicals by various routes, which depend on the species and living environment. The fate (metabolism) of accumulated substances, leading to their disappearance is strongly related with the type of the substance, in particular its hydrophobicity/hydrophilicity. Another issue is storage within compartments of an organism, which is also related with chemical properties of a substance. The routes of elimination are also dependent on the type of an organism.

Bioaccumulation is the phenomenon that occurs independently on our will or participation. The process occurs as a result of the presence of pollutants in the environment. The level of bioaccumulative substances (organic compounds, toxic elements) in the environment has increased in the last century as a result of industrial activity. An example is synthesis of xenobiotics – the products of heavy organic synthesis. The latter are chemicals not known to living organisms. The general mechanism of toxicity is blocking the essential cofactors in metabolic pathways. Since xenobiotics are substances not known to living organisms, the pathways of their metabolism have not emerged during evolution. Therefore, most xenobiotics are not biodegradable and accumulate in the environment.

Another example of bioaccumulative chemicals is toxic elements. Although the global amount of toxic elements remains unchanged, their mobility has increased as a result of industrial activities. Toxic elements were released from inert deposits and widely distributed in the environment, and consequently entered the biotic world.

Definitions of Bioaccumulation

Bioaccumulation (increase of chemicals concentration) is defined as the process of accumulation of chemicals in an organism over time. According to International Union of Pure and Applied Chemistry, bioaccumulation is the accumulation of a chemical in an organism due to direct uptake from the environmental matrix (bioconcentration) and uptake from food (biomagnification).

Bioaccumulation occurs only when the uptake exceeds elimination (eqn [1]).

$$\text{Bioaccumulation} = \text{Rate of uptake} - \text{Rate of elimination} \quad [1]$$

The above difference (1) depends on the chemical (physicochemical) properties and an organism.

Definitions related with bioaccumulation are provided below.

Bioaccumulation	Total amount of a substance accumulated in the body. This phenomenon is used in biomonitoring because it enables identification of bioavailability chemicals. Bioaccumulation results in adverse effects and diseases.
Biomarkers	• Measurement of biological response to chemicals determined inside an organism or its products (urine, feces, hair, feathers) indicating deviation from the normal status. • Investigation of a change in a biological response (molecular–cellular–physiological–behavioral) – which are related with exposure, toxic effects, or susceptibility.
Bioindicators	Related with organisms and the observation of their presence/absence or behavior in a given ecosystem.
Ecological indicator	A parameter informing about the structure and functioning of ecosystem.
Bioconcentration	Describes the situation when the concentration of a chemical in an organism is higher than in the environment. The extent of bioconcentration is expressed by BCF: $BCF = C_{org}/C_{env}$ [2] where C_{org} – concentration in an organism, C_{env} – concentration in the environment, BCF can be estimated from water solubility of a chemical or from octanol/water partition coefficient. Of concern are BCF >30 000.
Biomagnification	The increase of the concentration of a chemical between the trophic levels in the food web.

There are several factors (physical, chemical, biological), which influence bioaccumulation and bioavailability of chemicals. Chemicals are bioaccumulated in target tissues. Measurements of chemical content in sites of accumulation enable determination of extent of bioaccumulation. Defense mechanisms of an organism (e.g., the production of metallothionein) also can be used to measure the extent of bioaccumulation and are termed as *biomarkers of exposure*, which are used to describe bioaccumulation of chemicals in tissues. A substance present in an organism poses toxic effects (mortality, reduction of growth and reproduction, mutagenicity, carcinogenicity, sensitization) which can be described by *biomarkers of effect* (e.g., damage of DNA).

 http://dx.doi.org/10.1016/B978-0-12-386454-3.01039-3

Although biomarkers and bioindicators can deliver information about the dose of accumulated chemicals, they do not directly provide data on health or adverse effects. For this reason, tissue levels should be associated with biological effects basing on dose–response relationship. Significant is correlation between field levels of a chemical and adverse effects (if other toxins are absent). The chemical pathways depend on its hydrophilicity (readily eliminated) and hydrophobicity (persistent organic compounds, difficult to metabolize, accumulate in fat). Correlation between the extent of bioaccumulation and lipophilicity was found.

Uptake

Bioaccumulation, internal and external fate, and effects cannot occur without exposure, which is related with behavior, bioavailability, bioaccessibility, and absorption. These are influenced by several factors: size, nutrition, genetics, hormones, gender, etc. The uptake can occur from the environment (air, water, soil), either directly (from the ambient medium) or indirectly (from the food chain). The consumption of food with higher levels of chemicals poses bioaccumulation. The routes of uptake in plants in general include root (soil, water, sometimes air) and leaf (air, water) and in animals through breathing, ingesting, and dermal route.

Elimination

The final body burden is the result of absorption, distribution (tissue binding), metabolism, and excretion, the processes that are in dynamic equilibrium.

Distribution

A substance is distributed in an organism by blood and is accumulated in the body heterogeneously, which depends on tissue, species, and chemicals.

Metabolism

Metabolism is defined as the transformation of taken up substances to form different metabolites and elimination from an organism. A chemical can be metabolized which is termed biodegradation and concerns organic compounds. Metabolism of a chemical could rely on breaking to smaller molecules or mineralization to CO_2, water, and nutrients.

Storage

In animals, a chemical can be stored in different sites of an organism, for example, adipose tissue and bones.

Excretion

The routes of excretion in plants in general can be by the leaf surface and in animals by urine, feces, saliva, breast milk, sweat, and breathing.

Bioaccumulation – Mechanisms

Bioaccumulation follows the complex food webs. Species at the top of food chain have higher levels of chemicals in their tissues. It depends on feeding habits, location, and metabolic activity of species.

Bioaccumulated substance is transformed to derivatives, which can be more toxic than parent chemicals, for example, less toxic inorganic mercury is transformed to more toxic methylmercury. Bioaccumulation is dependent on the stability of binding of a chemical within cell compartments and metabolic half-life.

Bioaccumulation depends on elimination, which usually follows first-order kinetics. There are three distinctive pools distinguished: fast (a chemical disappears within weeks/days/hours/minutes), slow (within months), and unassimilated from gut (in animals; days).

Bioaccumulation in Aquatic Environment

Bioaccumulation depends on: biomass/(water volume), biomass/(concentration of a chemical), and sampling time. It is strongly depends on season of the year (temperature effect). It was found that the extent of bioaccumulation is correlated with water solubility.

Water chemistry plays an important role in the entry of chemicals into aquatic food webs: the concentration in water, initial tissue concentration in primary producers (phytoplankton, aquatic plants), higher trophic levels: ingestion of food (uptake by invertebrates and fish). Significant contribution is gill breathing of animals.

Bioaccumulation can occur by:

- the direct uptake from water. Chemicals cross cell membranes, through ion channels or pumps, passive and active transport systems (phytoplankton and algae; macrophytes present different mechanism),
- uptake through ingestion of food (invertebrates and fish). The concentration of the chemical in food and amount of consumed food influences bioaccumulation. The assimilation efficiency (the absorbed fraction) is defined as the fraction of ingested chemical that is incorporated to tissues and has not been lost by excretion or egestion. Depends on the type of ingested organism.

Bioaccumulation in Terrestrial Environment

The main route of bioaccumulation of chemicals for animals is diet. The contribution of dermal and respiratory route is lower, with the exception of dermal exposure in soil organisms. Bioaccumulation of chemicals in tissues of terrestrial animals is an order of magnitude lower than in aquatic.

Mammals and birds after a certain period of time reach dynamic equilibrium conditions (the rate of uptake equals the rate of elimination), yielding constant concentrations in tissues. Important is the length of time necessary to reach equilibrium, which depends on a chemical, species, and concentration in food. Algal cells concentrate toxic metals 2–3 orders of magnitude as compared to other organisms.

Bioaccumulation Testing

Bioaccumulation testing concerns integrated (ecosystems, food chains) and compartmentalized (individual organisms) test systems. The problems are related with individual factors that influence mathematical quantification of bioaccumulation and interpretation of the data. Size and weight influence bioaccumulation. The approach to bioaccumulation testing should include the selection of individuals of similar age, sex, weight/size, and class in comparison of bioaccumulation patterns across contamination gradients. The chemical and the matrix chosen for bioaccumulation testing are related with the level of chemical and detection limit of analytical instruments, as well as the quantity and invasiveness of available matrices.

The level of a chemical reflects an exposure but correlations between various biomarkers (invasive and noninvasive) are essential to ensure that the measured levels reflect total body burden. Bioaccumulation testing is undertaken to identify and eliminate sources of exposure, observe time trends, to prove the efficiency of law regulations, investigate relationship between the exposure and diseases or development of abnormalities, and to check the relationship between body burden and eating habits or occupational exposure. There is the need to develop standardized protocols for bioaccumulation testing (sample collection and preparation, analysis) in order to provide comparable and meaningful results.

Bioaccumulation of chemicals can be controlled by their determinations of their levels in matrices sampled from human: for example, milk or adipose tissue. This is essential for legislation purposes, in particular restrictions on use of chemicals. The concern is related with bioaccumulation of persistent and toxic chemicals from human food. Consequently, law governing manufacture and import of new substances should have determined biodegradability, for example, 8 week bioaccumulation study. If a substance is not biodegradable and is bioaccumulative, the use should be banned or restricted, for example, unless no toxicity to human in studies on mammals was proved.

Bioaccumulation of inorganic and metalloorganic compounds is usually made in static tests on fish or in sediments. For organic compounds, the ratio *n*-octanol/water is important in description of bioaccumulation potential.

- *Fish bioaccumulation tests* are usually carried out at 1/100 and 1/1000 of LC_{50} of a given chemical in a particular species. The tests can be carried out on rainbow trout or common carp and the duration is 1–2 months or until steady-state conditions are reached. Bioconcentration factor (BCF) is determined in fish tissues, preferably at the endpoint of the test. Of concern is BCF higher than 1000.
- *Sediment toxicity tests* investigate the effect of a chemical on dwelling organisms, for example, *Chironomus* and *Lumbriculus* species. These tests are undertaken for the risk assessment to predict exposure in sediments.

Bioaccumulation Models

Empirical, generalized, and mechanistic models, predictive and descriptive for chemicals and species are being elaborated. Bioaccumulation modeling is classified as: steady-state models (concentration ratios and environmental parameters; simple and predictive), hybrid models (mechanistic, steady-state; based on empirical coefficients and rate constants), and dynamic mass balance models.

Biomonitoring

Biomonitoring studies are based on determination of the extent of bioaccumulation through investigation of various biomarkers. The studies are essential to demonstrate the trends and to reduce exposure and health risks. Examples include the concentration of toxic elements in blood, serum, urine, hair, nails, breast milk, or subcutaneous fat. The chemicals, bioaccumulation of which is measured include toxic metals (Pb, Cd), metabolites of polycyclic aromatic hydrocarbons (PAH), persistent organic pollutants (POP), and volatile organic compounds (VOC).

Human biomonitoring studies showed increased bioaccumulation of metals and PAH in children and women living in industrial areas. In another biomonitoring study concerning bioaccumulation of toxic metals, the extent of bioaccumulation of Pb was higher in urban residents than in rural areas.

Using Hair to Measure Bioaccumulation of Chemicals

It is well documented that hair of mammals is a suitable accumulative indicator of bioaccumulation of metals, because significant correlations were found between hair and other tissues (liver, kidney) as well as environmental levels (soil). Hair is useful in the assessment of bioaccumulation of chemical elements from the environment. Hair is tissue formed over extended period of time, because the level of elements is one to twofold higher than in other tissues. Hair was used to investigate the adverse levels of elements to which human is exposed from various sources.

Bioaccumulation of Certain Chemicals

Organic

Organic compounds tend to accumulate in fat tissue. An example is organochlorine chemicals – the mostly endangered are marine species at the top of the oceanic food web. Birds and marine mammals accumulate these compounds from food, metabolize and eliminate (e.g., by lactation) which results in a certain body burden.

Inorganic

Toxic metals are one of the oldest known toxicants. Their bioaccumulation in human organism is of concern. Toxic metals are persistent in human environment – cannot be created nor destroyed. Anthropogenic activity resulted in increased concentration of metals in the biosphere, influenced their chemical form and increased mobility, which consequently led to their extended bioaccumulation. Bioaccumulation of toxic metals is of concern because nonessential toxic metals mimic essential metals and enter by the route through which essential elements are transported into an organism and consequently disrupt key cellular functions.

Nonessential elements are bioaccumulated because of chemical similarities (e.g., Cs^+ mimics NH_4^+, K^+): solubility, size. For instance, Cs^+ ions pass through K^+ channels in plant cells.

Organometallic compounds have lipophilic character and are accumulated either from solution or from diet. Their biomagnification depends on: lipophilicity/hydrophobicity, expressed as octanol/water partition coefficient, conditions of the aqueous phase (pH, the presence of complexing agents), and ability of elimination from an organism.

Compounds of mercury released by industry to surface waters resulted in bioaccumulation in fish. In the environment, mercury is biomethylated (e.g., in sediments) and in this form bioaccumulates. Bioaccumulation occurs progressively: from water to bacteria and plankton. Consumption of fish containing mercury, leads to dysfunction of central nervous system in human.

Practical Applications of Bioaccumulation

The phenomenon of bioaccumulation can be of practical use:

- Toxicological and ecotoxicological tests – searching for quantitative dependencies linking dose and symptoms, evaluation of threshold value – the maximum dose which produces no symptoms.
- The use of hyperaccumulating organisms is in bioremediation of polluted elements of the environment and in wastewater treatment processes. Selection toward organisms that tolerate high level of pollutants in the environment and accumulate these substances in their biomass. These are organisms that have developed some adaptive mechanisms of protection from toxic effects. An example is synthesis of specific proteins – metallothioneins, which due to high content of thiol groups, bind toxic metal ions and exclude them from the basic metabolic pathways, protecting the organism from toxic effects.
- Rule has been observed that the smaller the organism in terms of organization and size, the higher is the bioaccumulation capacity. Therefore, when using the process of bioaccumulation as a means of wastewater-treatment technology, the most beneficial use seems to be the smallest organisms – microorganisms.

Bioaccumulation from Medical Devices

As a result of the rapid development of production technology, it has become possible to insert into human body various types of medical devices. Orthopedic implants, dental implants, orthodontic miniscrews, including bridges, crowns, fixed orthodontic appliances, and many others are made of different alloys, which often contain metals considered carcinogenic, mutagenic, and allergenic: cadmium (Cd), chromium (Cr), and nickel (Ni). Medical devices are usually manufactured from stainless steel alloys, titanium alloys, and nickel–titanium alloy. Due to the prolonged presence of medical devices in the human body (e.g., orthodontic treatment – an average of 2 years, orthopedic implants – a lifetime) certain metals can bioaccumulate.

Persistent, Bioaccumulative, and Toxic Chemicals

Persistent, bioaccumulative, and toxic chemicals (PBT) are mentioned in various regulations. These compounds are toxic, persist in the environment, and bioaccumulate in food chains, consequently posing risks to human health and ecosystems. PBTs are transferred between abiotic elements of the environment (air, water, soil). These compounds differ in chemical structure and properties significantly, but are classified together for regulatory purposes. According to US EPA, PBT chemicals are classified into four categories: dioxin and dioxin-like compounds, lead compounds, mercury compounds, and PAHs. The following compounds are examples of PBT: heptachlor, polychlorinated biphenyl, toxaphene, and pentachlorobenzene. The compounds are evaluated for their persistence, bioaccumulation potential, and toxicity, according to Registration, Evaluation, Authorisation and Restriction of Chemicals regulation, Annex XIII, which distinguishes between new and existing chemicals. On the market of European Union, there are ca. 10 000 chemicals which require PBT assessment. Screening procedures for identification of PBT chemicals are being intensively elaborated. These procedures are based on the identification of the most common structural elements.

Summary and Conclusions

All living organisms throughout their lives bioaccumulate various substances such as essential macro- and microelements, toxicants, and others. The organisms have evolved metabolic pathways to protect them from excessive accumulation (e.g., routes by which accumulated substance is introduced into the cells are blocked or the substance is excreted outside).

In bioaccumulation, the accumulation of metals or organic compounds in the internal structures of the cell occurs. According to the definition, it is a process by which living organisms absorb and retain chemicals from the surrounding environment. Other definitions indicate that bioaccumulation is the accumulation of substances either directly from the medium (usually water), or from the soil (for plants), or through consumption of food (for humans and animals). A prerequisite for the occurrence of the process of bioaccumulation is the metabolic activity of cells and, therefore, bioaccumulation is considered a metabolically controlled process.

Bioaccumulation can also be understood as the absorption of chemicals by whole cells (not just through the cell wall, as in the biosorption). In unicellular organisms, toxic metal ions may enter through the transport channels, usually mistakenly, together with the essential elements (such as ions, Ca(II) or Mg(II)). In the case of plants, toxic metals may be associated with water and soil through the roots. Sometimes they are absorbed by the leaves (atmospheric deposition). The route of bioaccumulation depends on which environment is the most contaminated: water, soil, or air and on the properties of the chemical. In human, the main route is digestive system (contaminated food), but also the respiratory system (from polluted air) and through the skin (contact exposure). This has an impact on the bioaccumulation and toxicity of an organism's protective response that is activated.

Scientific reports on bioaccumulation are devoted almost exclusively on applications in environmental protection. Monitoring of environmental contamination is based on measurements of the degree of bioaccumulation of pollutants in the living organisms from the environment. The correlation between bioaccumulative capacity (concentration of chemical accumulated by the biomass) and the concentration in the environment was found. A second class of applications are processes related to the prevention of environmental pollution (e.g., industrial waste water treatment technologies) or treatment of polluted environments (e.g., bioremediation of soil by plants, so called hyperaccumulating plants). In the case of developing a new method for environmental monitoring, it is necessary to search for meaningful bioaccumulators–biomonitors. Based on analysis of the biomass and its composition, as well as on knowledge of the correlation between the concentration in the environment and biomass of bioaccumulating organism, it is possible to determine concentrations of the pollutant in the environment, and properly determine its bioavailability.

The characteristics of matrix used in biomonitoring include noninvasive sampling, which does not cause harm to an organism. An example of such a biomonitor is human hair or nails. It is also important that the concentration of a chemical in the analyzed material is on detectable level.

Bioaccumulation is the result of establishing the equilibrium between the amount of chemical taken from the environment and the amount excreted. This process depends on many factors: the availability of elements, the characteristics of the organism (species, age, health, etc.), and typical process parameters such as temperature, humidity, substrate properties, and climatic factors. Most often, these are the same factors that affect the body's metabolic functions. Therefore, the literature indicates the existence of certain difficulties in developing standardized procedures for biomonitoring and in obtaining standardized reference values. It was shown that the higher the degree of organization of a given species, more efficient is the system of protection against excessive bioaccumulation. For example, in the human body, metals are excreted to keratin materials: hair or nails, which are therefore useful in biomonitoring of prolonged exposure.

See also: Environmental Biomarkers; Biomarkers, Human Health; Biomonitoring.

Further Reading

Angerer, J., Ewers, U., Wilhelm, M., 2007. Human biomonitoring: state of the art. Int. J. Hyg. Environ. Health 210, 201–228.

Christensen, J.M., 1995. Human exposure to toxic metals: factors influencing interpretation of biomonitoring results. Sci. Total Environ. 166, 89–135.

Doğan-Sağlamtimur, N., Kumbur, H., 2010. Metals (Hg, Pb, Cu, and Zn) bioaccumulation in sediment, fish, and human scalp hair: a case study from the city of Mersin along the southern coast of Turkey. Biol. Trace Elem. Res. 136, 55–70.

Downs, S.G., Macleod, C.L., Lester, J.N., 1998. Mercury in precipitation and its relation to bioaccumulation in fish: a literature review. Water Air Soil Pollut. 108, 149–187.

Goodyear, K.L., Mcneill, S., 1999. Bioaccumulation of heavy metals by aquatic macroinvertebrates of different feeding guilds: a review. Sci. Total Environ. 229, 1–19.

Handley, J.W., 2003. Ecotoxicology. In: Knight, D.J., Thomas, M.B. (Eds.), Practical Guide to Chemical Safety Testing – Regulatory Consequences-Chemicals, Food Packaging and Medical Devices. Smithers Rapra Technology.

Ingersoll, C.G., Brunson, E.L., Dwyer, F.J., Ankley, G.T., Benoit, D.A., Norberg-King, T.J., Burton, G.A., Hoke, R.A., Landrum, P.F., Winger, P.V., 1995. Toxicity and bioaccumulation of sediment-associated contaminants using freshwater invertebrates: a review of methods and applications. Environ. Toxicol. Chem. 14, 1885–1894.

International Food Information Service, 2009. Dictionary of Food Science and Technology, second ed. International Food Information Service (IFIS Publishing).

Kouba, A., Buřič, M., Kozák, P., 2010. Bioaccumulation and effects of heavy metals in crayfish: a review. Water Air Soil Pollut. 211, 5–16.

Lin, Z.-Q., 2005. Bioaccumulation. In: Lehr, J.H., Keeley, J. (Eds.), Water Encyclopedia: Surface and Agricultural Water. John Wiley & Sons, Inc, Hoboken, NJ, pp. 34–36.

Liu, J., Goyer, R.A., Waalkes, M.P., 2008. Toxic effects of metals. In: Klaassen, C.D. (Ed.), Casarett and Doull's Toxicology – the Basic Science of Poisons, seventh ed. McGraw-Hill.

Martln-Diaz, M.L., Morales-Caselles, M.C., Jimenez-Tenorio, N., Riba, I., Delvalls, T.A., 2005. Biomarkers and bioaccumulation: two lines of evidence to assess sediment quality. In: Water Encyclopedia Surface and Agricultural Water. John Wiley & Sons, Inc, Hoboken, NJ, pp. 426–431.

Smith, J.T., Sasina, N.V., Kryshev, A.I., Belova, N.V., Kudelsky, A.V., 2009. A review and test of predictive models for the bioaccumulation of radiostrontium in fish. J. Environ. Radioact. 100, 950–954.

Turnbull, A., 1996. Chlorinated pesticides. In: Hester, R.E., Harrison, R.M. (Eds.), Chlorinated Organic Micropollutants. Royal Society of Chemistry, pp. 113–135.

van der Oost, R., Beyer, J., Vermeulen, N.P.E., 2003. Fish bioaccumulation and biomarkers in environmental risk assessment: a review. Environ. Toxicol. Phar. 13, 57–149.

Biocides

I Michalak and K Chojnacka, Institute of Inorganic Technology and Mineral Fertilizers, Wrocław University of Technology, Wrocław, Poland

This article is a revision of the previous edition article by Amy Merricle, volume 1, pp 279–280, © 2005, Elsevier Inc.

Introduction

In the European Union (EU), Regulation No. 528/2012 of the European Parliament and of the Council concerning the marketing and use of biocidal products was adopted on 22 May 2012. It will repeal and replace Directive 98/8/EC and will be applicable as of 1 September 2013. According to this regulation, "Biocidal products are necessary for the control of organisms that are harmful to human or animal health and for the control of organisms that cause damage to natural or manufactured materials. However, biocidal products can pose risks to humans, animals and the environment due to their intrinsic properties and associated use patterns."

Biocidal products are defined as active substances and preparations that contain one or more active substances, put up in the form in which they are supplied to the user, intended to destroy, deter, render harmless, prevent the action of, or otherwise exert a controlling effect on any harmful organism by chemical or biological means.

Biocide activity is affected by several factors, notably concentration, period of contact, pH, temperature, and the presence of organic matter or other interfering or enhancing materials or compounds, and the nature, numbers, location, and condition of the microorganism (bacteria, spores, yeasts and molds, protozoa). Understanding the mechanism of action of industrial biocides is important in optimizing their use and combating resistance if encountered. Biocidal action may result through physicochemical interaction with microbial target structures, specific reactions with biological molecules, or disturbance of selected metabolic or energetic processes.

According to Wiencek and Chapman (1999), biocides can function as electrophilic (electrophiles, e.g., aldehydes, carbamates, Cu, Ag, Hg, and oxidants, e.g., chlorine, bromine, ozone, peroxides) or membrane active agents (lytic, e.g., quats, phenols, alcohols, and protonophores, e.g., weak acids, parabens, pyrithiones). Electrophilic agents react with critical enzymes to inhibit growth and metabolism, with cell death occurring after several hours of contact. Membrane active agents tend to directly affect cell membranes. Biocides are known to interact with bacterial cell walls or envelopes (e.g., glutaraldehyde), produce changes in cytoplasmic membrane integrity (cationic agents), dissipate the proton motive force (organic acids and esters), inhibit membrane enzymes (thiol interactors), act as alkylating agents (ethylene oxide), cross-linking agents (aldehydes), and intercalating agents (acridines), or otherwise interact with identifiable chemical groups in the cell.

Considerable interest is being shown about how organisms circumvent biocidal activity. Bacteria are able to adapt rapidly to new environmental conditions including the presence of antimicrobial molecules and, as a consequence, resistance increases with the antimicrobial use. According to Russell (2001), bacterial insusceptibility to biocides is of two types, intrinsic and acquired. Intrinsic insusceptibility is a natural property of an organism and is shown by bacterial spores, mycobacteria, and gram-negative bacilli. Cellular impermeability is a major factor, and in some cases active efflux pumps play an important role. A special example is that of phenotypic (physiological) adaptation to intrinsic resistance found in bacteria present in biofilms. Acquired resistance arises through mutation or via the acquisition of plasmids or transposons; efflux of biocide is a major mechanism, although plasmid-mediated inactivation has also been shown to occur. An additional aspect that must be considered is the stringent response elicited in bacteria on exposure to inimical agencies.

Division of Biocides

Generally, biocides are divided into four major groups, with several subgroups.

The first group of biocides includes disinfectants and general biocidal products used for human and veterinary hygiene as well as disinfectants used in the private area, public health area, food and feed area, and disinfectants of drinking water (e.g., ethyl alcohol, iodine, citric acid, formic acid, hydrogen peroxide, sodium hypochlorite). Human hygiene biocidal products are characterized by a large number of different products and active substances. They include skin antiseptic, antimicrobial soap, hand wash for health care personnel, and sun blocks.

A second group of biocides involves preservatives. Subgroups include in-can preservatives (e.g., isothiazolinones, phenol derivatives), film preservatives (e.g., triazoles, zinc pyrithione), wood preservatives (e.g., copper compounds, boric acid) fiber, leather, rubber, and polymerized material preservatives (e.g., triclosan, quaternary ammonium compounds), masonry preservatives (e.g., sodium hypochlorite, quaternary ammonium compounds), liquid cooling and processing system preservatives (e.g., pentanedial, amines), and metalworking fluid preservatives (e.g., sodium pyrithione, quaternary ammonium compounds). Biocides prevent microorganisms from feeding on the organic plasticizer in flexible PVC formulations. Biocides stop odor, prevent color change, and help maintain polymer properties.

A third group consists of biocides with the ability to control pest. The following kinds of biocidal products are counted in this group: slimicides (e.g., 2-bromo-2-nitropropan-1,3-diol), rodenticides (e.g., aluminum phosphide), avicides (e.g., Avitrol: 4-aminopyridine), molluscicides (e.g., quaternary and polyquaternary ammonium compounds, aromatic hydrocarbons, metals and their salts), piscicides (e.g., antimycin, saponins, niclosamide), insecticides (e.g., piperonyl butoxide, permethrin), acaricides and products to control other arthropods, repellants and attractants (e.g., citronella oil, permethrin), and algicides.

 http://dx.doi.org/10.1016/B978-0-12-386454-3.00472-3

There is a demand for new, specific, more efficient, and selective biocides. Continuous screening for chemicals with high toxicity to various living organisms is needed. It became essential to control or destroy particular kinds of organisms while, at the same time, permitting other useful or non-troublesome types to remain unaffected. One of the examples of specific biocides are algicides, which are chemical substances specifically used to control or kill algae in impounded waters, lakes, ponds, reservoirs, stock tanks, and irrigation conveyance systems. Algicides can be applied as a spray directed onto floating mats of algae, sprayed or injected directly into the water column, or applied as granular crystals or pellets dispensed on the water surface. Algicides can be selective or nonselective against algae. Their selectivity depends on species, dose and timing of application, product formulation, and water chemistry.

Algicides basically fall into three groups of compounds: copper compounds (copper sulfate, copper chelates: ethanolamines, ethylene diamines, triethanolamines, triethanolamine + ethylene diamine, and copper citrate/gluconate), endothall (as the mono (*N*,*N*–dimethylalkylamine) salt), and formulations containing the active ingredient sodium carbonate peroxyhydrate. It is important to emphasize that many algicides are based on copper, which is a toxic heavy metal in the aquatic environment. It can affect nontarget species (bacteria, fish, zooplankton, other macroinvertebrates).

Algicides vary in their mechanism of action: they must come in contact with and enter algal cells. Copper-based products are believed to target specific physiological processes such as electron transport in photosystem I, cell division, and nitrogen fixation. Endothall has been shown to cause electrolyte leakage from cell membranes and may also play a role in inhibition of lipid and protein biosynthesis. Algicides containing sodium carbonate peroxyhydrate destroy algal cell membranes by forming hydroxyl free radicals.

The last group includes other biocidal products: preservatives for food or feedstock, antifouling products (e.g., thiocyanic acid, copper salt, copper oxide), and embalming and taxidermist fluids (e.g., formaldehyde, ethanol, pentanedial). It is generally known that fouling growth is prevented by the controlled release of bioactive molecules (biocides) from coatings.

Hazardous Substances in Common Biocidal Products

Biocidal products can often contain substances of concern with allergic, ecotoxic, carcinogenic, developmental neurotoxic, or endocrine-disrupting properties. For example, permethrin used as insecticide and propiconazole used as wood preservative are very toxic to aquatic organisms, may cause long-term adverse effects in the aquatic environment, are harmful by inhalation, are harmful if swallowed, and may cause sensitization by skin contact. In another example, Triclosan, which is used as in-can preservative (e.g., cosmetics), as a disinfectant, and in the treatment of textiles, is very toxic to aquatic organisms, may cause long-term adverse effects in the aquatic environment, is irritating to eyes, and is irritating to respiratory systems. Benzalkonium chloride (used, e.g., as a disinfectant for personal hygiene and in the preparation of surfaces) is highly toxic to aquatic organisms, and harmful in contact with skin.

Natural Biocides

New regulations definitely limit application of many commonly used biocides. Nowadays, it is important to replace synthetic biocides with more environmentally friendly natural products. The importance of ecological biocides is especially critical because of the REACH system introduced in the EU (Regulation (EC) No. 1907/2006 of the European Parliament and of the Council of 18 December 2006 concerning the Registration, Evaluation, Authorisation and Restriction of Chemicals.), which specifies the principles of using chemical substances in order to increase environmental safety and eliminate health hazards.

Biocides in Plant Extracts

The plant kingdom offers the largest scientific potential for these biocides. For example, volatile constituents and flavonoids of extracts of citrus fruits can be used as natural wood preservatives, which will act as defense against fungi and insects. The extracts and essential oils from different plants (e.g., *Mentha piperita*, *Thymus vulgaris*, *Citrus paradisi*, *Salvia officinalis*, *Artemisia absinthium*, *Lavandula angustifolia*), which are widely known for bacterio- and fungicidal properties, find increasingly wider application in protection of, for example, medical, sanitary, cosmetic, food and packaging products, and agriculture (plant protection). Active substances (alkaloids, flavonoids, terpenes) present in such essential oils as oils of thyme, oregano, clove, and mint are a natural source of antimicrobial properties. Algae can also act as natural biocides. Extracts of two species of green algae, filamentous *Rhizoclonium hieroglyphicum* Kiitz and a phytoplankton, *Chlorella ellipsoidea* Gerneck, were assayed against *Aedes aegypti* L., *Culex quinquefasciatus* Say, and *Culiseta incidens* (Thomson). Both fractions were found to induce significant mortality in tested mosquito species. The biological effects of extract of *Ulva fasciata* Delile (UF) and *Ulva lactuca* Linnaeus (UL) were tested against *Dysdercus cingulatus* (Fab.) third instar nymphs. Tested green algae caused dose-dependent mortality. Natural products from marine organisms can be used as replacements for the chemicals commonly used in antifouling coatings. Some seaweed species interfere with bacterial colonization on their surfaces by releasing antifouling compounds. For example, marine seaweeds *Turbinaria ornate*, *Gelidiella acerosa*, and *Jania adhaerens* could be an important source of natural antibacterial, antifouling, and anticorrosion bioactive compounds, which could be used in the protection of mild steel.

Regulations

Biocides are designed to be biologically active and toxic at least to microorganisms and often are also toxic to nontarget species. They can have toxic, carcinogenic, or endocrine-disrupting properties. Moreover, biocides are not readily biodegradable. Thus, they pose a potential hazard to the environment, particularly in cases of accidental spills and leaks. Therefore, a greater care is required in their marketing. In the European Union, the Biocidal Product Directive requires registration of active ingredients by the end of 2008.

It should be added that the Regulation (EU) No. 528/2012 incorporates the European Commission's (EC) recommendation on the definition of a nanomaterial, and requires that, where nanomaterials are used in a product, the risk to the environment and to health should be assessed separately. Labels would be required to include the name of all nanomaterials contained in biocidal products, followed by the word 'nano' in brackets. The regulation states that "approval of an active substance shall not cover nanomaterials except where explicitly mentioned."

See also: Organochlorine Insecticides; Aluminum Phosphide; Pesticides; Environmental Risk Assessment, Pesticides and Biocides.

Further Reading

Cooke, G.D., Welch, E.B., Peterson, S.A., Newroth, P.R., 1993. Restoration and Management of Lakes and Reservoirs, second ed. Lewis Publishers, Boca Raton, FL.

Elsmore, R., 2012. Biocide regulation in the EU – past, present and future. Chim. Oggi Chem. Today 30, 58–60.

Hahn, S., Schneider, K., Gartiser, S., Heger, W., Mangelsdorf, I., 2010. Consumer exposure to biocides – identification of relevant sources and evaluation of possible health effects. Environ. Health 9 (7).

Jones, G., Burch, M., 1997. Algicide and algistat use in Australia. Occasional Paper, ARMCANZ Sub-Committee on Water Resources, Canberra.

Kantida, S.R., Asha, K.R.T., Sujatha, S., 2012. Influence of bioactive compounds from seaweeds and its biocidal and corrosion inhibitory effect on mild steel. Res. J. Environ. Toxicol. 6, 101–109.

Kozlowski, R., Walentowska, J., 2008. Role of biocides from plant origin in protection of natural fibers against biodeterioration. International Conference on Flax and Other Bast Plants (ISBN #978-0-9809664-0-4).

Rasmussen, K., MacLellan, M.A.T., 2001. The control of active substances used in biocides in the European Union by means of a review regulation. Environ. Sci. Pol. 4, 137–146.

Russell, A.D., 2001. Mechanisms of bacterial insusceptibility to biocides. Am. J. Infect. Control 29, 259–261.

Russell, A.D., 2002. Antibiotic and biocide resistance in bacteria: Introduction. J. Appl. Microbiol. Symp. Suppl. 92, 1S–3S.

Senseman, S., 2007. Herbicide Handbook, ninth ed. Weed Science Society of America, Lawrence, KS.

Wiencek, K.M., Chapman, J.S., 1999. Proc., CORROSION/99, (San Antonio, TX, U.S.A.). NACE International, Houston, TX, Paper # 99308.

Relevant Websites

http://ec.europa.eu/environment/chemicals/biocides – European Commission: Environmnent: Introduction to Biocides.

http://ec.europa.eu/environment/biocides/ – Directive 98/8/EC of the European Parliament and of the Council on the placing on the market of biocidal products.

http://nanotech.lawbc.com – Nano and Other Emerging Chemical Technologies Blog: Search for Biocides.

http://www2.mst.dk/udgiv/Publications/2001/87-7944-383-4/pdf/87-7944-384-2.pdf – Danish Environmental Protection Agency. (2001). Inventory of Biocides used in Denmark.

Biocompatibility

SE Gad, Gad Consulting Services, Cary, NC, USA

Biomaterial use includes stents, intraocular lenses, wound dressings, total hip replacements, total knee replacements, tooth implants, and sutures, and can be naturally occurring or made of polymer, ceramic, or metal. It can also include submicron or nanotechnology components, *in situ* polymerizing, and bioabsorbable materials. Medical devices typically undergo a battery of safety tests before being cleared by regulatory authorities for marketing.

The biological evaluation of medical devices is performed to determine the potential toxicity resulting from contact of the component materials of the device with the body. The device materials should not produce adverse local or systemic effects, be carcinogenic, or produce adverse reproductive and developmental effects, either directly or through the release of their material constituents. Systemic testing must ensure that the benefits of the final product will outweigh any potential risks produced by device materials. Among these are tests to evaluate the biological safety, or biocompatibility, of the device, and appropriate function of the device. Guidance on how to conduct these tests is provided in standards developed by the United States or by international consensus standards bodies such as the International Organization for Standardization and their ISO 10993: Biological Evaluation of Medical Devices series.

When designing a medical device, it is important to first select appropriate materials, and then a sterilization method before searching for relative information on the materials and beginning testing. It is advisable to test individual components of a device prior to testing the complete device in case one component has toxic properties. Premarket approval (PMA) applicants often use another party's product or facility in the manufacture of their device. Many manufacturers keep data on qualified materials used in their products. This information regarding the product is pertinent to its review; the third party may choose to submit confidential information directly to the US Food and Drug Administration (FDA) in a device master file. This is not a marketing application, and additional testing or information may be necessary.

When selecting the appropriate tests for biological evaluation of a medical device, one must consider the chemical characteristics of device materials, and the nature, degree, frequency, and duration of its exposure to the body. In general, the tests include acute, subchronic, and chronic toxicity; irritation to skin, eyes, and mucosal surfaces; sensitization; hemocompatibility; genotoxicity; carcinogenicity; and effects on reproduction, including developmental effects. However, depending on varying characteristics and intended uses of devices as well as the nature of contact, these general tests may not be sufficient to demonstrate the safety of some specialized devices. Additional tests for specific target organ toxicity, such as neurotoxicity and immunotoxicity, may be necessary for some devices. Since the immune response and repair functions in the body are highly complicated, it is inadequate to describe the biocompatibility of a single material in relation to a single cell type or tissue. The specific clinical application and the materials used in the manufacture of the new device determine which tests are appropriate.

The material or device used for biocompatibility studies should contain the same colorants, fragrances, flavors, powders, lubricants, and processing chemicals as what is intended to be placed on the market. A material or device to be tested should be processed, packaged, and, if appropriate, sterilized by the same methods as the product that will be distributed. Biocompatibility studies may need to be repeated if subsequent changes are made in composition, manufacturing materials, or processing.

Some devices are made of materials that have been well characterized chemically and physically in the published literature, and have a long history of safe use. For the purposes of demonstrating the substantial equivalence of such devices to other marketed products, it may not be necessary to conduct all the tests suggested in the FDA matrix of this guidance. FDA reviewers are advised to use their scientific judgment in determining which tests are required for the demonstration of substantial equivalence under section 510(k). In such situations, the manufacturer must document the use of a particular material in a legally marketed predicate device, or a legally marketed device with comparable patient exposure.

Regulations

There are several regulatory guidances in place to guide one through biocompatibility evaluation of a medical device, and depending on which country a device is to be registered in, some variations exist. The US FDA and European Union commonly accept the ISO 10993 standards for biocompatibility. USP (US Pharmacopeia) and ASTM standards are accepted by the US FDA, are generally regarded as more stringent, and may be used by manufacturers as a marketing tool, or for specific uses. Finally, Japan's Ministry of Health, Labor, and Welfare has test criteria that are different from both the ISO 10993 and USP protocols.

ISO 10993 Biological evaluation of medical devices includes the following parts:

Part 1: Evaluation and testing within a risk management process
Part 2: Animal welfare requirements
Part 3: Tests for genotoxicity, carcinogenicity and reproductive toxicity
Part 4: Selection of tests for interactions with blood
Part 5: Tests for *in vitro* cytotoxicity
Part 6: Tests for local effects after implantation
Part 7: Ethylene oxide sterilization residuals
Part 9: Framework for identification and quantification of potential degradation products
Part 10: Tests for irritation and skin sensitization
Part 11: Tests for systemic toxicity
Part 12: Sample preparation and reference materials
Part 13: Identification and quantification of degradation products from polymeric medical devices

 http://dx.doi.org/10.1016/B978-0-12-386454-3.00821-6

Part 14: Identification and quantification of degradation products from ceramics
Part 15: Identification and quantification of degradation products from metals and alloys
Part 16: Toxicokinetic study design for degradation products and leachables
Part 17: Establishment of allowable limits for leachable substances
Part 18: Chemical characterization of materials
Part 19: Physicochemical, morphological and topographical characterization of materials
Part 20: Principles and methods for immunotoxicology testing of medical devices

The following tests are recommended:

- Cytotoxicity
- Acute systemic toxicity
- Sensitization
- Genotoxicity
- Skin irritation
- Implantation
- Intracutaneous reactivity
- Hemocompatibility

Subchronic and chronic toxicities and also carcinogenicity may also be appropriate.

For use in the United States, the blue book memorandum includes an FDA-modified matrix designating the type of testing required for various medical devices and also a flow chart entitled Biocompatibility Flow Chart for the Selection of Toxicity Tests for 510(k)s. The matrix also consists of two tables: **Table 1** – initial evaluation tests for consideration; and **Table 2** – supplementary evaluation tests for consideration. In general, the agency does not have a list of approved materials.

Some materials that have been well characterized both chemically and physically in published literature, and which have a long history of safe use, may prove themselves not to be in need of all tests, if substantial equivalence to marketed products under 510(k) is shown. In this case, the manufacturer must document the use of a particular material in a legally marketed predicate device, or a legally marketed device with comparable patient exposure.

It may be necessary to repeat biocompatibility tests when modifying a device based on the changes made. Medical device toxicity problems are most often caused by leachable or extractable toxins. Extracts of materials are often tested for biocompatibility. Section 17 of 10993 entitled Establishment of Allowable Limits of Leachable Substances gives guidance on the use of analytical data (e.g., extraction studies) to reduce biocompatibility test requirements. The extraction media should comprise a series of media with various polarities to capture results found in different solubilities. The temperature at which the extraction should be carried out varies throughout various guidelines. For *in vitro* cytotoxicity testing, complete cell-culture medium is most commonly used, with extraction performed at 37 °C for 24 h. Inexpensive nonanimal studies such as cytotoxicity and hemocompatibility tests can be used to screen device materials.

Biological control tests are recommended to determine sources of possible contamination and to ensure safety of the final product. Microbiological tests to determine the status of the final product (e.g., sterility, bacteria, contaminants, and microbial count limits) are necessary. Devices should be tested for endotoxins, as cell wall lipopolysaccharides (from Gram-negative bacteria) may be present even after sterilization. Assessment of nonspecific toxicological effects should be performed by intravenous injection of device eluate in mice.

When positive (indicative of a toxic response) biocompatibility results are reported, development discontinuation is not the only option. First it should be confirmed that no mistakes were made in the testing laboratory, including the testing of the proper article, and formulation. In addition, it should be made certain that the article was properly manufactured, cleaned, stored, and tested (e.g., the extractant used, the testing conditions, and the procedure). Finally, reproducibility of positive biocompatibility results should be confirmed. In a certain situation, where the possible benefits outweigh the risks, or when quality of life is a factor, a level of toxicity may be acceptable.

The following are special considerations that must be considered when testing devices and their component materials for safety.

Color Additives

A color additive is a dye, pigment, or other substance, whether derived from a plant, animal, mineral, or other source, which imparts a color when added to a food, drug, cosmetic, or the human body. The US Food, Drug and Cosmetic (FD&C) Act states: "Devices containing a color additive are considered unsafe, and thereby adulterated, unless a regulation is in effect listing the color additive for such use." The FD&C Act limits applicability of these color additives for devices that directly contact the body for a significant period of time (undefined by FDA). Manufacturers of devices should choose a color additive listed for use in foods, drugs, or cosmetics as a starting point, but keep in mind that these may not be appropriate for devices. The color listing regulation may permit the use of the color additives or may place limitations on its use; PMA applicants must demonstrate their safety. Color additives listed for use in medical devices are provided in 21 CFR 73 (Color additives exempt from batch certification) and 21 CFR 74 (Color additives subject to batch certification).

FDA considers the addition of color, flavor, or any chemical to a medical glove to be a significant change that should have a new 510(k) submission (21 CFR 807.81(a)(3)). The applicant should provide full characterization and chemical identity of the color, flavor, or scent additives. They may submit a 510(k) submission for a modification to an existing glove as a 'Special 510(k)'.

Color additive and flavor additive regulations are in 21 CFR parts 70 to 82 and 21 CFR part 172, Subpart F, respectively.

Combination Products

A combination product is a product consisting of two or more regulated components (drug/biologic/device, etc.) that are combined as a single entity or is a product labeled for use with a separate device or biologic where both are required to achieve the intended use, indication, or effectiveness. Intercenter

Table 1 Initial evaluation tests for consideration

Device categorization by nature of body contact (see 5.2)			*Biologic effect*							
Category	*Contact*	*Contact duration (see 5.3) A-limited (≤24 h) B-prolonged (>24 h–30 days) C-permanent (>30 days)*	*Cytotoxicity*	*Sensitization*	*Irritation of intracutaneous reactivity*	*Systemic toxicity (acute)*	*Subchronic toxicity (subacute toxicity)*	*Genotoxicity*	*Implantation*	*Hemocompatibility*
Surface device	Intact skin	A	X	X	X					
		B	X	X	X					
		C	X	X	X					
	Mucosal membrane	A	X	X	X					
		B	X	X	X	0	0		0	
		C	X	X	X	0	X	X	0	
	Breached or compromised surface	A	X	X	X	0				
		B	X	X	X	0	0		0	
		C	X	X	X	0	X	X	0	
External communicating device	Blood path, indirect	A	X	X	X	X				X
		B	X	X	X	X	0			X
		C	X	X	0	X	X	X	0	X
	Tissue/bone/dentin[a]	A	X	X	X	0				
		B	X	X	X	X	X	X	X	
		C	X	X	X	X	X	X	X	
	Circulating blood	A	X	X	X	X		0[b]		X
		B	X	X	X	X	X	X	X	X
		C	X	X	X	X	X	X	X	X
Implant device	Tissue/bone	A	X	X	X	0				
		B	X	X	X	X	X	X	X	
		C	X	X	X	X	X	X	X	
	Blood	A	X	X	X	X	X		X	X
		B	X	X	X	X	X	X	X	X
		C	X	X	X	X	X	X	X	X

X = ISO evaluation tests for consideration.
0 = These additional evaluation tests should be addressed in the submission, either by inclusion of the testing or a rationale for its omission.
[a]Tissue includes tissue fluids and subcutaneous spaces.
[b]For all devices used in extracorporeal circuits.
http://www.fda.gov/downloads/MedicalDevices/DeviceRegulationandGuidance/GuidanceDocuments/UCM348890.pdf.

Table 2 Supplementary evaluation 1142 tests for consideration

Device categorization by nature of body contact (see 5.2)		*Biologic effect*				
Category	*Contact*	*Contact duration (see 5.3) A-limited (≤24 h) B-prolonged (>24 h–30 days) C-permanent (>30 days)*	*Chronic toxicity*	*Carcinogenicity*	*Reproductive/ Developmental*	*Biodegradable*
Surface device	Intact skin	A				
		B				
		C				
	Mucosal membrane	A				
		B				
		C	0			
	Breached or compromised surface	A				
		B				
		C	0			
External communicating device	Blood path, indirect	A				
		B				
		C	0	0		
	Tissue/bone/dentin[a]	A				
		B				
		C	0	0		
	Circulating blood	A				
		B				
		C	0	0		
Implant device	Tissue/bone	A				
		B				
		C	0	0		
	Blood	A				
		B				
		C	0	0		

X = ISO evaluation tests for consideration.
0 = These additional evaluation tests should be addressed in the submission, either by inclusion of the testing or a rationale for its omission.
[a]Tissue includes tissue fluids and subcutaneous spaces.
http://www.fda.gov/downloads/MedicalDevices/DeviceRegulationandGuidance/GuidanceDocuments/UCM348890.pdf.

agreements have been made within FDA to review and oversee these categories. More information can be found at FDA website for the CBER (Center for Biologics Evaluation and Research) and CDRH (Center for Devices and Radiological Health) Intercenter agreement, and the CDER (Center for Drug Evaluation and Research) and CDRH Intercenter agreement.

In Vitro Diagnostic (IVD) Products

These are medical devices that analyze human body fluids, such as blood or urine, to provide information for the diagnosis, prevention, or treatment of a disease. Classification for these devices can be found within regulations: 21 CFR 862, 21 CFR 864, and 21 CFR 866.

Radiation-Emitting Products

Electronic product radiation means any ionizing or nonionizing electromagnetic or particulate radiation, or any sonic, infrasonic, or ultrasonic wave, that is emitted from an electronic production because of the operation of an electronic circuit in such product. If a medical device emits electronic product radiation, additional requirements apply through the Radiation Control for Health and Safety Act. Additional information concerning radiation-emitting products can be found at the FDA website.

Software

If a device contains software, the PMA submission must include documentation of software testing appropriate to the level of risk of the device. The FDA recognizes certain consensus standards of conformance when making regulatory decisions. In addition, sterility assurance is necessary, and FDA validated method for sterilization should be used and included in the PMA.

Phthalates

Within the past few decades, specific additives to some plasticizers (such as DEHP and bis-phenol-A) have been identified as toxic to animals and thus have come under scrutiny.

The impact of these formulation aids to human health has not been fully characterized. Regardless, an effort is underway to reformulate device materials without them.

Fibrosarcomas are another example of a biocompatibility measure that has been noted in animal and not yet determined if it will translate into humans. Known as the Oppenheimer effect, smooth materials with a minimum surface area, and implantation time in rats produce an increased occurrence of hard, tumorlike masses. The same material when implanted in a different configuration will not produce the same response.

Latex Testing: Testing for Skin Sensitization to Chemicals

The labeling may include special claims regarding reduced potential chemical sensitization in a 510(k), such as:

- reduced potential for sensitizing users to rubber chemical additives, or
- reduced potential for causing reaction in individuals sensitized to rubber chemical additives.

The applicant should support these claims by data from human testing. Additional guidance on testing for skin sensitization to chemicals in latex products is available in the guidance document listed in the Relevant Websites section.

See also: Foreign Body Response; Implant Studies; Medical Textiles.

Further Reading

Black, J., 1999. Biological Performance of Materials. Marcel Dekker, Inc, Boca Raton, FL.

Chu, C.C., von Fraunhofer, J.A., Greisler, H.P. (Eds.), 1997. Wound Closure Biomaterials and Devices. CRC Press, Washington, DC.

Cronin, E., 1980. Contact Dermatitis. Churchill Livingston, Edinburgh.

Dart, R.C., 2004. Medical Toxicology, third ed. Lippincott Williams & Wilkins, Philadelphia, PA.

Freitas Jr., R.A., 2003. Nanomedicine. In: Biocompatibility, vol. IIA. Landes Bioscience, Georgetown, TX.

Fries, R.C., 1998. Medical Device Quality Assurance and Regulatory Compliance. Marcel Dekker, Inc, New York.

Gad, S.C., 2009. Safety Evaluation of Medical Devices, third ed. CRC Press, Boca Raton, FL.

Gad, S.C., McCord, M.G., 2008. Safety Evaluation in the Development of Medical Devices and Combination Products, third ed. Informa, New York.

Greco, R.S., 1994. Implantation Biology. CRC Press, Boca Raton, FL.

Guelcher, S.A., Hollinger, J.O. (Eds.), 2006. An Introduction to Biomaterials. Taylor and Francis, Boca Raton, FL.

Heller, M.A., 2002. Guide to Medical Device Regulation, vol. 1 & 2. Thompson Publishing Company, Washington, DC.

Kammula, R.G., Morris, J.M., 2001. Considerations for the Biocompatibility Evaluation of Medical Devices. MDDI 23, 82–92.

Medical Device Register, 1997. Medical Economics. Hospital Marketing Services, Inc.

ODE, 1995. FDA Blue Book Memo 95-1. CDRH.

Rutner, B.D., Hoffman, A.C., Schoen, F.J., Lemons, J.E., 1996. Biomaterials Science. Academic Press, San Diego.

Silvio, L.D., 2009. Cellular Response to Biomaterials. Woodhead Publishing Limited and CRC Press, Cambridge, England.

Thompson, B.M., 1995. FDA Regulations of Medical Devices. Interpharm Press, Inc, Buffalo Grove, IL.

von Recum, A.F. (Ed.), 1998. Handbook of Biomaterials Evaluation, second ed. Taylor & Francis, Ann Arbor, MI.

Wise, D.L. (Ed.), 2000. Biomaterials and Bioengineering Handbook. Marcel Dekker, Inc, New York.

Wise, D.L., Trantolo, D.J., Altobelli, D.E., Yaszemski, M.J., Gresser, J.D., Schwartz, E.R. (Eds.), 1995. Encyclopedic Handbook of Biomaterials and Bioengineering. Marcel Dekker, New York.

Relevant Websites

http://www.fda.gov/MedicalDevices/DeviceRegulationandGuidance/GuidanceDocuments/ucm073792.htm – Premarket Notification [510(k)] Submissions for Testing for Skin Sensitization to Chemicals in Natural Rubber Products.

http://www.fda.gov – US Food and Drug Administration (FDA) website. See index pages for 'Required Biocompatibility Training and Toxicology Profiles for Evaluation of Medical Devices, Blue Book Memo, G95-1. May 1, 1995'. 'US FDA. Special Considerations. Biocompatibility.' More information can be found at the website for the CBER (Center for Biologics Evaluation and Research) and CDRH (Center for Devices and Radiological Health) Intercenter agreement, and the CDER (Center for Drug Evaluation and Research) and CDRH Intercenter agreement.

http://www.fda.gov/downloads/MedicalDevices/DeviceRegulationandGuidance/GuidanceDocuments/UCM348890.pdf – Use of International Standard ISO-10993, "Biological Evaluation of Medical Devices Part 1: Evaluation and Testing" Draft Guidance for Industry and Food and Drug Administration Staff Document issued on: April 23, 2013.

http://www.fda.gov/downloads/MedicalDevices/DeviceRegulationandGuidance/GuidanceDocuments/UCM348890.pdf – Food and Drug Administration.

Biofuels

LG Roberts and TJ Patterson, Chevron Energy Technology Company, San Ramon, CA, USA

- Name: Biofuels
- Chemical Abstracts Service Registry Number: Varied
- Synonyms for Biodiesel, Biobutanol, or Hydrotreated Renewable Fuels: Varied
- Chemical Structure: Varied

General Background and Major Types of Some Biofuels

Biofuels are a rather new type of renewable transportation fuels produced from biomass-based renewable resources such as plants, animal by-products, or microorganisms, although peanut oil was first used as a diesel fuel approximately a century ago. In order to function in existing engines, biofuels must be compatible with existing conventional petroleum fuels and engine performance requirements. Thus for many biofuels, there may be considerable similarity between the characteristic properties of a conventional fuel and its biofuel counterpart. The most common biofuel is ethanol, typically derived from corn, sugar beets, or sugar cane. Ethanol is a separate entry in the encyclopedia; readers are recommended to view the toxicological properties of ethanol there.

Biofuels may be generally grouped into the following categories: (1) those produced by fermentation into alcohols; (2) oils separated from biomass and reacted to form hydrocarbons or fatty acid methyl esters; and (3) oils processed by hydrogenation to produce hydrocarbons within the carbon range of conventional petroleum fuels.

It is important to understand that the term 'biofuels' may have various definitions by different resources, and that the feedstock biomass as well as its processing into a liquid fuel will determine the composition of the product; thus, the potential toxicity of biofuels is extremely broad. Summary information presented within the scope of this encyclopedia entry can be augmented by reference to other resources listed below. The production of biofuels is also an innovative field that is rapidly evolving, particularly in the arena of producing renewable fuels with hydrocarbon structures already found within the matrix of existing petroleum fuels. This entry focuses on biodiesel, biobutanol, and hydrocarbon renewable fuels in use today or under development and likely to be of interest in years to come.

In general, the physical and chemical properties of biofuels may be used to provide insight into health and environmental behavior. As with conventional fuels, highly volatile biofuels or biofuel constituents are expected to partition into air from water, soil surfaces, or open containers. For acute human health effects, the potential exposure from inhalation is greater for shorter-chain, highly volatile biofuel constituents than for longer-chain, oily constituents for which skin contact is more likely. Specific alcohols have varying degrees of water solubility and volatility that will determine partitioning between water and the atmosphere. Branched hydrocarbon structures may be more difficult to metabolize by soil microorganisms than normal hydrocarbons.

Uses of Biofuels

The major current uses of biofuels are as liquid transportation fuels, although use as a heating fuel may also occur. An essential consideration for use is compatibility with existing technology, both for engine design and with conventional fuel requirements. Thus, biodiesel, as should be expected by its name, is compatible with existing diesel engine (compression ignition) technology and has come into common use as a blend in petroleum-derived diesel. Biobutanol could potentially be used in gasoline engine (spark ignition) technology as a blend with petroleum gasoline. The application of hydrotreated renewable fuels would be dependent on the carbon range for the renewable fuel; for example, hydrotreated renewable fuel made up of hydrocarbons in the range of approximately 8 to 25 carbons in length could be compatible with diesel engines.

Biobutanol

- Synonyms – *n*-Butanol (CAS 71-36-3): 1-Butanol, Butan-1-ol, 1-Hydroxybutane, Butyric alcohol, Normal primary butyl alcohol; Isobutanol (CAS 78-83-1): 1-Hydroxymethylpropane, 2-Methylpropanol-1, 2-Methylpropyl alcohol

Background

Biobutanol is butanol produced by fermentation from a biomass feedstock. The production process can influence the isomer of butanol that is produced. Currently, *n*-butanol and isobutanol are the two isomers likely for use as a biofuel. Another isomer, *t*-butanol, is unlikely to be used as a fuel due to much slower environmental degradation. Biobutanol has qualities of both a fuel and an oxygenate for blends with gasoline in spark-ignition engines.

Toxicity data noted below are for butanol. As the original feedstock was often not specified in the literature, the term butanol instead of biobutanol has generally been utilized.

Environmental Fate and Behavior

Biobutanol is volatile; evaporated butanol can react in the atmosphere to form butyraldehydes. Both *n*-butanol and isobutanol are mobile in soil and may contaminate groundwater as well as volatilize from water and soil surfaces. Isobutanol and *n*-butanol are readily biodegradable; the half-life is estimated in the range of several days. As with ethanol, rapid biodegradation of biobutanol at spill sites contaminated with petroleum hydrocarbons could potentially deplete aqueous

 http://dx.doi.org/10.1016/B978-0-12-386454-3.01054-X

oxygen and result in methane production and prolonged contamination of petroleum aromatic compounds.

Exposure and Exposure Monitoring

The most likely routes of exposure to biobutanol are through contact with skin and inhalation of vapors or aerosols.

Occupational exposures to *n*-butanol and isobutanol may be measured at worksites. The odor threshold for *n*-butanol in air is 0.83 ppm; the odor threshold for isobutanol is 40 ppm. Both forms of butanol have objectionable odors described as suffocating, musty, or rancid. Systemic absorption may be estimated by analysis of urinary metabolites such as conjugates of biobutanol or the aldehyde metabolites for exposure to normal or isobutanol.

Toxicokinetics

Butanol is readily absorbed through skin, lungs, and gut, and excreted via exhalation and urine as metabolites. Percutaneous absorption rates indicate that absorption through the skin is rapid (*n*-butanol: 8.8 $\mu g\,min^{-1}\,cm^{-2}$, *in vivo* dog; 2.3 $mg\,cm^{-2}\,h^{-1}$, *in vitro* human skin assay). Within the body, *n*- and isobutanol are rapidly metabolized by alcohol and aldehyde dehydrogenases to butyric acid or isobutyric acid. The primary metabolite excreted from lungs is carbon dioxide, with conjugated metabolites, glucuronides, excreted in urine.

Mechanisms of Toxicity

Butanol is a contact irritant to eyes, the respiratory tract, and skin. Nausea and vomiting produced by ingestion may be a consequence of irritation to the gut. The mechanism of central nervous system effects due to butanol is unknown but may be similar to other alcohols thought to interfere with ion transport in cell membranes. Studies on sciatic nerve preparations from frogs suggest that the aliphatic alcohols reduce permeability constants for sodium and potassium ion channels.

Acute and Short-Term Toxicity (Animal and Human)

The acute toxicity profiles of butanol isomers are similar. Relatively low toxicity from single exposure is expected by the oral, dermal, or inhalation routes; however, *n*-butanol is classified as 'harmful' by ingestion based on oral LD_{50} values as low as 790 $mg\,kg^{-1}$ although other data suggest that the actual value should be >2000 $mg\,kg^{-1}$. The acute oral LD_{50} value for isobutanol is > 2000 $mg\,kg^{-1}$. Test data from laboratory studies point to isobutanol and *n*-butanol as irritating to skin and severe irritants to eyes, with the potential to cause irreversible eye damage. Human exposure experience indicates that butanol is irritating to eyes and the respiratory tract (nose, throat) in the range of 25–100 ppm. Both forms of biobutanol can produce signs of central nervous system depression, such as decreased alertness, headache, dizziness, and drowsiness, increasing to vertigo, confusion, coma, and death at extreme intoxication. Ingestion of butanol can also produce nausea and vomiting.

Ingestion of *n*-butanol for 13 weeks by rats produced transient neurotoxicity (hypoactivity, ataxia) at 500 $mg\,kg^{-1}\,day^{-1}$ (no observed adverse effects level, 125 $mg\,kg^{-1}\,day^{-1}$) and reduced hematocrit, hemoglobin, and red blood cell counts in the females.

Quantitative structure activity relationship (QSAR) modeling predicts that both forms of butanol are unlikely to cause allergic skin reactions.

Reproductive Toxicity

Biobutanol is unlikely to harm reproduction. Repeated exposure to isobutanol or *n*-butanol did not produce adverse effects to reproduction in rats. Exposure throughout gestation in rats indicated that isobutanol and *n*-butanol are not selective developmental toxicants; developmental effects (decreased fetal and litter weights, skeletal variations) occurred only at maternally toxic exposures for *n*-butanol (reduced maternal body weight and food consumption, narcosis).

Genetic Toxicity

Neither of the butanol isomers produced harm to genetic material in either *in vitro* or *in vivo* assays.

Carcinogenicity

Neither of the isomers of butanol are currently classified for carcinogenicity (i.e., they are identified as 'not classifiable' by the American Conference of Governmental Industrial Hygienists (ACGIH)).

QSAR modeling did not find structural alerts for carcinogenicity for isobutanol or *n*-butanol.

Clinical Management

Individuals overexposed to biobutanol by inhalation should be moved to fresh air as quickly as possible and artificial respiration should be administered if not breathing. Acute effects indicative of depression of the central nervous system may require medical treatment. Contaminated skin may be cleaned by thorough washing with soap and water, and contaminated clothing (including shoes) should be removed and laundered. Exposed eyes should be flushed thoroughly with water or saline; due to the potential for severe eye irritation, medical evaluation should be sought as soon as possible.

Ecotoxicity

Isobutanol and *n*-butanol have relatively low toxicity to aquatic ecosystems. Acute LC_{50} and EC_{50} values in freshwater fish and invertebrates are >1000 $mg\,l^{-1}$; effects on algae growth occurred only above 200 $mg\,l^{-1}$.

Other Hazards

Biobutanol is a flammable liquid (flash points 82–98 °F) that may be ignited by heat, sparks, or flames. Flashback along vapor trails near the ground or underground may occur. Equipment for handling biobutanol must be grounded, and storage should be cool and well ventilated. The spread of spilled biobutanol may be attenuated by use of vapor-suppression foam and noncombustible absorbent material.

Exposure Standards and Guidelines

The isomers of butanol have the following time-weighted-average (TWA) exposure limit recommendations from ACGIH, with the basis for the TWA in parentheses:

Isobutanol: 50 ppm (eye and skin irritation); odor threshold 43 ppm
n-Butanol: 20 ppm (eye and upper respiratory tract irritation)

Biodiesel

- Synonyms: Soy methyl ester (CAS 67784-80-9); Rapeseed methyl ester (CAS 73891-99-3); Tallow methyl ester (CAS 61788-61-2); Palm methyl ester (CAS 91051-34-2); Fatty acid methyl esters (FAME)

Background

Biodiesel is fuel made up of mono-alkyl esters of long chain fatty acids derived from biomass-based oils such as vegetable oils or animal fats. It can be produced by a transesterification reaction between the fatty acid and an alcohol, usually methanol, to produce a fatty acid alkyl ester. The distribution of carbon ranges will mirror the carbon lengths in the fatty acid feedstock. Fatty acid methyl esters (FAMEs) are described by their carbon length and number of unsaturated bonds. For example, soy oil consists largely of palmitic acid (16 carbons with no unsaturated bonds, $C_{16:0}$), stearic acid ($C_{18:0}$), oleic acid, which contains one unsaturated bond ($C_{18:1}$), linoleic acid ($C_{18:2}$), and linolenic acid ($C_{18:3}$); thus the biodiesel prepared from soy oil and methanol, soy methyl ester a.k.a. methyl soyate (CAS 67784-80-9), is primarily made up of C16 and C18 length FAMEs with a mix of saturated and unsaturated structures. **Table 1** shows the range of FAMEs that would be produced from several different biofeedstocks. When blended with conventional petroleum-derived diesel fuel, the proportion of the blend that is biodiesel is designated by a number preceded by 'B; ' i.e., B20 is a 20:80 biodiesel:diesel fuel blend.

Environmental Fate and Behavior

Biodiesel is predicted to partition primarily to the soil and, to a lesser extent, water and sediment. Shorter chain FAMEs are expected to be more mobile in soil. Biodiesel is considered readily biodegradable. Typically 80% or more will degrade in 28 days in laboratory testing. Due to faster biodegradation than petroleum diesel, biodiesel is expected to have less environmental migration than petroleum diesel; however, biodiesel may delay the biodegradation of petroleum hydrocarbons such as benzene and toluene. Biodiesel has limited volatility but some evaporation will occur; if spilled, it is lighter than water and may produce a sheen on the surface. Biodiesel is not expected to bioaccumulate as FAMEs are metabolized and excreted if uptake occurs.

Exposure and Exposure Monitoring

Due to the low volatility of biodiesel, occupational exposure monitoring may be unnecessary. The FAMEs that comprise biodiesel are metabolized to the corresponding fatty acids and methanol. As for petroleum diesel, combustion as a fuel results

Table 1 FAME composition[a] of biodiesel according to feedstock

Fatty acid methyl ester (ME)	*Soy ME*	*Canola ME*	*Palm ME*	*Tallow ME*	*Coconut ME*
6:0 Methyl hexanoate					0.4–0.5
8:0 Methyl octanoate			0.1		0.7–9.8
10:0 Methyl decanoate			0.1		0.6–9.7
12:0 Methyl dodecanoate	Trace		0.3–2.4	0.1	44.6–54.1
13:0 Methyl tridecylic			1.0		
14:0 Methyl myristate	0.1–0.3		0.5–47.5	2.1–8	13–20.6
14:1 Methyl myristoleate				0.9	
15:0 Methyl pentadanoate				0.5	
16:0 Methyl palmitate	2.3–13	1.5–6	3.5–48.8	23.3–37	6.1–10.5
16:1 Methyl palmitoleate	0.1–0.3		0.2–1.8	0.1–5	0.1
17:0 Methyl heptadecanoate	11.4		0.1	1–1.5	
17:1 Methyl heptadecenoate				0.8	
18:0 Methyl stearate	2–27.2	1–2.5	1.7–53	9.5–34.2	1–3.8
18:1 Methyl oleate	16.7–84	52–66	6–52	14–50	5–8.8
18:2 Methyl linoleate	1.6–57.1	16.1–31	5–14	1.5–50	0.4–2.7
18:3 Methyl linolenate	1.2–11	6.4–14.1	0.2–0.6	0–0.7	0.1–0.3
20:0 Methyl eicosanoate	0.2		0.3	0.2–1.2	0.1
20:1 Methyl gondoate	0.3			0.3–0.5	
22:0 Methyl behenate	0.1–0.4			0.1	
22:1 Methyl erucate	0–0.3	1–2		0.1	
24:1 Methyl nervonate	Trace				

[a]From: Coordinating Research Council, 2009. In: Hoekman, S.K.,Gertler, A., Broch, A., Robbins, C. (Eds.), CRC Project No. AVFL-17 Final Report: Investigation of Biodistillates as Potential Blendstocks for Transportation Fuels. Desert Research Institute, Reno, NV. http://www.crcao.org/reports/recentstudies2009/AVFL-17/AVFL-17%20Final%20Report%20June%202009.pdf.

in exhaust emissions, including particulates, nitrogen oxides, and polycyclic aromatic compounds.

Toxicokinetics

When ingested, FAMEs are hydrolyzed to the free fatty acids for absorption from the intestine into the blood. Further oxidation occurs to form carbon dioxide and water via breakdown into 2-carbon fragments used by the body for energy and incorporation into tissues. Radiolabeled ^{14}C-palmitate methyl ester distributed to tissue lipids in rats; retention 2 days following oral administration of methyl palmitate was lower in young rats with low body fat than mature adults. Fatty acids may be stored in fat deposits in the body. No metabolic studies were found for soy, canola, palm, tallow, or coconut methyl esters. Not all fatty acids are dietary requirements; diets consisting solely of saturated fatty acids are reported to also lead to symptoms of fatty acid deficiency in rats. Future interpretation of toxicological findings of FAMEs and fatty acids should consider nutritional confounding as a possible factor in test results.

Mechanisms of Toxicity

Biodiesel currently has little known toxicity. The oily nature of biodiesel can be a physical fouling hazard to aquatic invertebrates and water fowl if spilled into wetlands. Some fatty acids are dietary requirements; however, diets consisting solely of saturated fatty acids that are not nutritional requirements are reported to lead to symptoms of fat deficiency in rats. Interpretation of future toxicological findings of FAMEs and fatty acids should consider nutritional confounding as a possible factor in test findings. Biodiesel particulate exhaust emissions may induce proinflammatory cytokines (similar to diesel exhaust).

Acute and Short-Term Toxicity (Animal and Human)

Existing data indicate that acute exposure to biodiesel is not hazardous. Soy, sunflower, and canola methyl esters are classified as nonhazardous by the oral route (acute oral $LD_{50} > 5\ g\ kg^{-1}$), similar to petroleum diesel. Results from acute oral toxicity testing of individual FAMEs (laurate, palmitate, stearate methyl ester) also indicate that acute exposure is not hazardous. Similarly, soy methyl ester, rapeseed methyl ester, and butyl methyl ester have been tested for acute toxicity by the dermal route of exposure, without effects (dermal $LD_{50} > 2$ or $5\ g\ kg^{-1}$); however, since the acute oral toxicity values of biodiesels from various feedstocks suggest that they are nontoxic by the oral route, acute effects from exposure to skin are unlikely.

Essentially no vapors are generated from biodiesel at ambient temperature, and therefore neat (pure) biodiesel should not pose an inhalation hazard. The acute toxicity hazard of biodiesel blended into conventional petroleum diesel will be driven by the conventional fuel.

Test results with FAMEs overall suggest that the FAMEs likely to comprise biodiesel are not expected to be irritating to eyes or skin. Slight, temporary conjunctivitis was the only reported finding in eye irritancy testing. Laboratory testing with various FAMEs for skin irritation resulted in varying degrees of erythema and/or edema, with soy methyl ester being nonirritating, while methyl laurate, methyl palmitate, and methyl stearate produced irritation on rabbit skin. However, in human volunteers exposed to various carbon length ranges of FAMEs (C8–10, C12–14, C16–18), virtually no irritation occurred.

The weight of evidence for allergic skin reactions indicates that FAMEs used in biodiesel are unlikely to cause allergic skin reactions. Soy methyl ester was reported to be positive in a guinea pig skin sensitization study; however, in this study the erythema observed 24 h after exposure nearly dissipated by 48 h, which is atypical for an allergic reaction but common for mild irritation. Soy as a food product can produce allergic reactions in sensitive populations. Tallow methyl ester and methyl laurate were not sensitizing in guinea pig sensitization studies; in small-scale human testing ($n = 25$–68 subjects), both soy methyl ester and palm oil methyl ester were not skin sensitizers.

Methyl esters of fatty acids produced from edible fats and oils are approved for some uses as direct food additives or as a supplementary source of fat for animal feed (21CFR172.225; 21CFR573.640). Several of the fatty acids within the approved FAMEs are essential fatty acids. The ingestion of nonessential fatty acids appears to interfere with the absorption and/or incorporation of essential fatty acids into lipid tissues. The likelihood of fatty acid deficiency occurring through occupational exposure, or even accidental exposure, is low, given dietary ingestion. The published literature on this area is quite old; nevertheless, any future testing that involves repeated exposures should consider potential fatty acid deficiency to prevent inappropriate toxicity classifications.

Repeat-exposure subchronic toxicity testing suggests minimal toxicity from FAMEs in biodiesel. Four-week ingestion of canola, soy, or fish oil methyl esters at doses up to $500\ mg\ kg^{-1}\ day^{-1}$ produces liver hypertrophy but limited other changes (thymus weight reduction for soy methyl ester). A 12-week feeding study of methyl oleate in rats at up to $3500\ mg\ kg^{-1}\ day^{-1}$ produced only a reduction in female body weight. Male rats fed 100 mg per animal per day methyl stearate (approximately 300–$500\ mg\ kg^{-1}\ day^{-1}$) or a fat-free diet for 12 weeks had decreased body weight, while females in the study had virtually no effect.

Exhaust emissions from an engine running on soy methyl ester did not produce systemic toxicity in F344 rats exposed for 13 weeks. Exposure levels were approximately 0.04, 0.2, and 0.5 mg particulates per cubic meter; this study was conducted as part of a Tier 2 testing program under the Clean Air Act. Biologically significant effects were limited to high-exposure female rats and consisted of increased lung weight and increased alveolar macrophage content, considered to be a normal response to repeated inhalation of particulate matter.

Chronic Toxicity

No long-term testing conducted with biodiesel was found. Specific, FAMEs methyl oleate and methyl stearate, were found to decrease body weight in subchronic feeding studies in rats, but no other effects were reported. Methyl esters of higher fatty acids, including methyl esters of myristate (14:0), palmitate (16:0), stearate (18:0), oleate (18:1), and linoleate (18:2), are acceptable by the US Food and Drug Administration as a supplementary source of fat for animal feed under 21CFR573.640.

Immunotoxicity

No information on immunotoxicity was found for biodiesel. Inhalation of biodiesel exhaust in laboratory testing induced production of proinflammatory cytokines.

Reproductive Toxicity

No reproductive or developmental toxicity information was found for biodiesel. Methyl oleate was tested in a limited study design in which female rats, exposed to $100\ \text{mg kg}^{-1}\ \text{day}^{-1}$ for 12 weeks, were bred to unexposed males. There were no effects to reproductive parameters.

Several oils used as feedstocks for biodiesel have been evaluated for reproductive or developmental toxicity potential in limited testing. For tallow, a three-generation study in pigs and a one-generation study in rats failed to identify adverse effects to reproduction or offspring. In the rat study, the fatty acid profiles in fat tissues of newborn rats contained higher 14:0 and 18:0 content, reflecting the tallow composition in the diet. A screening study for developmental toxicity in rats administered palm oil at doses up to $3\ \text{ml kg}^{-1}$ (ca. $2760\ \text{mg kg}^{-1}\ \text{day}^{-1}$) resulted in prenatal mortality (resorptions), defects, and growth retardation, but the authors hypothesized that the effects may have been due to high vitamin A in the palm oil sample. Testing with palm oil for effects on sexual maturation and endocrine function, with the control group given corn oil and a second group controlling for fat content, found that vaginal opening occurred earlier in female rats given a high-fat diet. To the authors, this suggested that body weight or body fat was a factor in acceleration of vaginal patency, as there were no differences in average body weights at first estrus, no irregularities in estrous cyclicity, and no measured differences during the estrous cycles for estradiol, prolactin, or luteinizing hormone.

Biodiesel exhaust (B100 soy-derived, 0.5 mg particulates per cubic meter per day) did not cause developmental toxicity in rats. Prenatal mortality, fetal body weight, and the incidence of malformations were unaffected.

Genetic Toxicity

Biodiesel (soy methyl ester, various specific FAMEs) was not mutagenic to bacteria. The exhaust particulates of biodiesel derived from rapeseed methyl ester and soy methyl ester were found to be half as potent for mutagenicity in an Ames bacterial assay as particulates from conventional diesel fuel.

Carcinogenicity

Biodiesel has not been tested for carcinogenicity. Oleate methyl ester did not increase the number of tumor-bearing mice in a 2-year study with mice, although the total number of forestomach papillomas increased. Linoleate methyl ester was not carcinogenic when given to rats by gavage for 18 months.

Clinical Management

No clinical symptoms are predicted for acute exposure to biodiesel. Contaminated skin should be cleaned by thorough washing with soap and water, and contaminated clothing should be laundered as a precaution. Exposed eyes should be flushed thoroughly with water or saline.

Ecotoxicity

According to the US Environmental Protection Agency, petroleum oils and vegetable oils share common physical properties and can produce similar environmental effects, including coating animals and plants with oil and suffocating them by oxygen depletion, destroying food supplies.

However, substances are classified for hazards based on results in laboratory testing conducted according to regulatory guidelines that determine intrinsic chemical toxicity. Biodiesel and individual FAMEs have demonstrated negligible toxicity to aquatic species (microbe, invertebrate, fish) (LC_{50} and EC_{50} values $>1000\ \text{mg l}^{-1}$). FAMEs, like other oils, have low water solubility and should be tested for aquatic toxicity as a water-accommodated fraction (WAF); i.e., the biodiesel is blended into the aqueous medium to reach equilibrium, allowed to settle, and the aqueous phase is siphoned off for introduction into the test system. Toxicity studies with soil and sediment dwelling organisms are a data gap and relevantly based on expected environmental partitioning.

Other Hazards

Biodiesel-soaked materials may pose a risk of spontaneous combustion due to heat from oxidation of double bonds.

Hydrotreated Renewable Fuels

- Synonyms: Hydrotreated renewable jet (HRJ); hydro-esterified fatty acid jet (HEFA Jet); green diesels; renewable diesel; second-generation diesel.

Background

Hydrotreated renewable fuels are produced by processing biomass feedstocks such as animal fats, plant-based (e.g., vegetable, camelina) oils, or microbial (e.g., algae) oils with hydrogen and deoxygenation. In general, hydroprocessing produces hydrocarbons that are predominantly paraffinic alkanes, normal, branched, or cyclic, with minimal aromatic content. Fuels in various carbon ranges, for example, short hydrocarbons for blending with gasoline, longer hydrocarbons for blending with diesel, and in between for blending with jet fuel/kerosene, can be separated by distillation, as volatility decreases with increasing carbon length. Biofuels, like conventional fuels, must meet strict performance specifications. Hydrotreated renewable fuels are compositionally similar to synthetic Fischer-Tropsh (F-T) fuels. Some toxicity estimations below are based on data for F-T fuels.

Environmental Fate and Behavior

Biodegradation of spilled biofuels will be affected by various factors, including soil type, concentration of contaminants, the complexity of the chemical structures, microorganisms, and bioavailability. Short-length paraffinic hydrocarbons produced from biomass, such as pentane or isopentane, will be highly volatile and predicted to partition into the atmosphere. Midlength hydrocarbons less dense than water will form a sheen on surface waters with eventual evaporation as well as degradation by water microorganisms. Some proportion of biofuel hydrocarbons may be transported by groundwater away from the site of a spill. Simpler structures such as normal or singly branched hydrocarbons can be more quickly metabolized by microorganisms and may be considered readily biodegradable, and preferentially degraded compared to conventional petroleum fuels. Complete microbial degradation of biofuels can result in production of methane or carbon dioxide. Several potentially harmful consequences of the ready biodegradation of biofuels may occur. First, environmental contamination of hazardous constituents from preexisting petroleum fuel spills, such as benzene or toluene, may persist longer in the environment. Aerobic metabolism may occur sufficiently quickly to deplete oxygen in the water needed for biosystems, reducing or eliminating natural ecological species ('fish kill'). Methane may be produced for months after a spill, and potentially distant from the spill site. These generalizations emphasize the importance of understanding the chemical nature of each biofuel to reasonably predict environmental behavior.

Exposure and Exposure Monitoring

Occupational exposure to renewable fuels will likely occur through routine machinery and engine maintenance, fueling, and transportation. Likely routes of exposure are inhalation of volatile constituents such as smaller hydrocarbons, and dermal penetration. Although biomonitoring standards do not yet exist, potential monitoring options could include measurement of alcoholic and ketonic metabolites in urine.

Toxicokinetics

The dermal penetration of individual constituents in the carbon range for jet fuel has been shown to be low. Smaller alkanes such as nonane and undecane absorb better than longer alkanes such as tetradecane, but none absorbed as well as aromatic hydrocarbons. Inhalation of synthetic F-T jet fuel indicated deposition in bronchioles. Metabolism testing with F-T jet fuel found alcoholic and ketonic metabolites in liver, urine, and feces consistent with metabolic studies with individual alkanes.

Mechanisms of Toxicity

The hydrocarbons in hydrotreated renewable fuels, consistent with petroleum hydrocarbons, can produce hyaline droplet nephropathy in male rat kidneys due to accumulation of α-2μ-globulin, a carrier protein produced in substantial quantities in male rat livers, but in negligible amounts in female rats and humans. This mechanism is specific to male rats and considered irrelevant to human health risk assessment.

As with conventional fuels, the lipophilic nature of hydrotreated renewable fuels may cause defatting of the skin with repeated exposure.

Acute and Short-Term Toxicity (Animal and Human)

Hydrotreated renewable fuels are likely to cause little short-term toxicity by the oral and dermal routes based on comparison to F-T fuels, which were not acutely toxic. The acute inhalation LC_{50} for HRJ fuel was found to be greater than 2000 mg m^{-3}.

Low-viscosity renewable fuels may pose a risk of aspiration into the lungs if ingested, which can induce pneumonia that may be fatal.

Hydrotreated renewable fuels are likely to be irritating to the upper respiratory tract. HRJ caused respiratory depression in mice (Alarie assay), considered to represent respiratory tract irritation. HRJ was also slightly irritating to skin. Repeated inhalation exposure to HRJ for up to 2 weeks, at a maximum exposure of 2000 mg m^{-3}, produced olfactory degeneration and hyperplasia in the nasal region while inflammatory cell infiltration occurred in the bronchioles. Longer-term exposure is likely to produce hyaline droplets in male rat kidneys consistent with accumulation of α-2μ-globulin, based on comparison to F-T jet and diesel fuels. These lesions, characterized as hyaline droplet nephropathy, are attributed to accumulation of α-2μ-globulin, a carrier protein produced in substantial quantities in male rat livers, but in negligible amounts in female rats and humans. The α-2μ-globulin protein, which transports endogenous pheromones into the kidneys of male rats, also has an affinity for hydrocarbons present in petroleum and synthetic fuels. This mechanism is specific to male rats and considered irrelevant to human health risk assessment.

Symptoms of reversible central nervous system depression such as dizziness and lack of coordination are likely from high exposures to volatile hydrocarbons in hydrotreated renewable fuels. The specific mechanism of toxicity for this is unknown but other short- to medium-length hydrocarbons also produce neurotoxicity at high exposures.

Reproductive Toxicity

No studies evaluating reproductive performance or fertility are available. Inhalation of paraffinic F-T fuel did not harm sperm quality or estrous cyclicity in rats.

Genetic Toxicity

HRJ was not mutagenic in bacterial assays. Based on data from *in vitro* and *in vivo* studies with F-T jet fuel, hydrotreated renewable fuels are not expected to cause genetic toxicity; synthetic F-T jet fuel did not produce bacterial mutations, chromosomal aberrations, or micronuclei.

Clinical Management

Excessive inhalation of paraffinic biofuel hydrocarbons could result in symptoms of central nervous system depression such as dizziness, headache, drowsiness, or loss of consciousness. Overexposed individuals should be removed to fresh air.

Conventional hydrocarbon fuels and individual hydrocarbons found in conventional fuels can produce chemical pneumonitis if ingested and aspirated into the lungs. As hydroprocessed biofuels of low viscosity will contain many of the same paraffinic hydrocarbons, they should be considered aspiration hazards also and thus induction of vomiting following ingestion should be contraindicated.

Ecotoxicity

Hydrotreated renewable fuels are likely to vary in toxicity to aquatic environments with changes in composition and carbon range, based on comparison to the aquatic toxicity of F-T fuels and individual hydrocarbons. Short-chain paraffinic alkanes such as heptane and octane are very toxic to aquatic organisms, while longer chain hydrocarbons such as dodecane and hexadecane are not toxic.

Other Hazards

Paraffinic alkanes expected to be present in hydroprocessed biofuels are flammable.

Miscellaneous

Hydrotreated renewable fuels are flammable and are likely to accumulate static charge if not properly grounded.

See also: Ethanol; Diesel Fuel; Gasoline; Jet Fuels; Methanol.

Further Reading

Coordinating Research Council, 2009. In: Hoekman, S.K., Gertler, A., Broch, A., Robbins, C. (Eds.), CRC Project No. AVFL-17 Final Report: Investigation of Biodistillates as Potential Blendstocks for Transportation Fuels. Desert Research Institute, Reno, NV.

Corseuil, H.X., Monier, A.L., Gomes, A.P.N., Chiaranda, H.S., do Rosario, M., Alvarez, P.J.J., 2011. Biodegradation of soybean and castor oil biodiesel: implications on the natural attenuation of monoaromatic hydrocarbons in groundwater. Ground Water Monit. Remed., 1–8.

Gateau, P., Van Dievoet, F., Vermeersch, G., Claude, S., Staat, F., 2005. Environmentally friendly properties of vegetable oil methyl esters. J. Am. Oil Chem. Soc. 12, 308–331.

Health Canada, Fuels Assessment Section, 2012. Human Health Risk Assessment for Biodiesel Production, Distribution, and Use in Canada.

Knothe, G., 2010. Biodiesel and renewable diesel: a comparison. Prog. Energy Combust. Sci. 36, 364–373.

National Research Council, 2011. Renewable Fuel Standard: Potential Economic and Environmental Effects of US Biofuels Policy. Prepublication Copy; copyright National Academy of Sciences. The National Academies Press, Washington, DC. www.nap.edu.

Relevant Websites

http://www.apag.org/issues/methyl.htm – FAME Task Force (1997) The safety of fatty acid methyl esters.

http://www.itrcweb.org/documents/biofuels/biofuels-1.pdf – The Interstate Technology & Regulatory Council: Biofuels: Release Prevention, Environmental Behavior, and Remediation.

http://toxnet.nlm.nih.gov – Toxnet (Toxicology Data Network): search under Toxline for Biofuels.

http://toxnet.nlm.nih.gov/cgi-bin/sis/search/a?dbs+hsdb:@term+@DOCNO+5572 – National Library of Medicine Hazardous Substances Data Base: Methyl Oleate.

http://toxnet.nlm.nih.gov – Toxnet (Toxicology Data Network): search under HSDB for Isobutyl Alcohol.

http://toxnet.nlm.nih.gov – Toxnet (Toxicology Data Network): search under HSDB for N-Propanol.

http://www.dtic.mil/dtic – DTIC Online: Information for the Defense Community: Search for Biofuels.

http://itme000.louisiana.edu/assign/Solar%20Thermal%20Project/Literature/ASME%20ES%202011/ES2011-54101.pdf – Proceedings of the ASME 2011 5th International Conference on Energy Sustainability: Renewable Fuel Performance in a Legacy Military Diesel Engine.

http://www.afdc.energy.gov/afdc/ – U.S. Department of Energy Advanced Fuels and Advanced Vehicles Data Center.

http://cfpub.epa.gov/ncea/iris_drafts/recordisplay.cfm?deid=200321. www.epa.gov/iris – U.S. EPA, Integrated Risk Information System (2011) Toxicological review of n-butanol (CAS 71-36-3); EPA/635/R-11/081A.

Environmental Biomarkers

AL Miracle, Pacific Northwest National Laboratory, Richland, WA, USA

This article is a revision of the previous edition article by Lee R. Shugart, volume 1, pp 287–290, © 2005, Elsevier Inc.

Introduction

Conditions where stressors present risk in the environment are complex and varied. Different types of stressors are often found as mixtures in water, sediment, and soil, rarely occurring as single entities. Organisms are subjected to changing environmental and physiological conditions that may modulate toxicity to a chemical stressor. The environment is affected by chemical, biological, and physical stressors of both anthropogenic and natural sources that can all contribute to adverse environmental impacts. Assessing ecological or environmental toxicity is further complicated by length of exposure, dose, sex of the organism, and developmental stage. The use of metrics to monitor environmental stress provides opportunities to assess the risk of those stressors before they are manifested across large temporal or regional scales and cause irreparable damage to the environment.

The use of biomarkers to assess environmental risk is a concept rooted in human health and pharmacological toxicology. In this context, environmental biomarkers should provide quantitative measures of change in response to a specific exposure and subsequent effect. However, the use of biomarkers for environmental risk assessment has historically been limited. Biological information in the form of molecular, physiological, and organism endpoints can improve the process of environmental risk assessment. The use of these environmental biomarkers with contextual references can provide faster qualitative and quantitative chemical exposure analysis, as well as information on impacts through mechanism elucidation of toxicity and direct measures of deleterious physiological reactions. In application, environmental biomarkers have the potential to provide a more accurate representation of environmental toxicity.

Biomarkers versus Bioindicators

The term 'biomarker' has historically been used to define a broad class of biomedical measures or metrics that are used to describe or define the physiological status of a cell or organism. With the advent of more specific measurement technologies and molecular biology tools, a biomarker is generally limited to measures of response at the cellular or subcellular level. Classification of biomarkers include biomarkers of exposure, effect, and susceptibility. In contrast, the term 'bioindicator,' although sometimes used interchangeably with 'biomarker,' has been used more often to describe biological responses at the organism, population, and community levels. The application and use of a biomarker has different goals and objectives than the use of a bioindicator. For instance, biomarkers provide direct and sensitive measures of exposure to environmental stressors, but are short term and often not temporally tractable in an environmental setting. In contrast, a bioindicator is the result of an exposure or response to an environmental stressor that is manifested at higher levels of organization and may not be as sensitive, but has ecological relevance. The distinction between environmental biomarkers and bioindicators lies primarily in the management purpose that either seeks to identify exposure as an early warning to adverse consequences, or interrogation of a system that has been affected by an exposure **Figure 1**. Therefore, biomarkers are better attributed to exposure and linkage to immediate effect where bioindicators may be retrospective and difficult to connect to the initiating event.

Current Uses and Trends

Development of environmental biomarkers over the last decade has focused on discovery of measures that have strong physiological ties to specific chemical stressor exposures. The need to reduce the cost and time expended for animal toxicity testing of chemical compounds has provided an impetus for better defining environmental dose, exposure, and adverse outcome. High priority has been given to developing computational models that predict toxicity for classes of contaminants of concern. Much research involving environmental exposures and subsequent linkages to diagnostic and predictive risk assessment has made significant progress in defining candidate biomarkers that herald a cellular or organ response to an

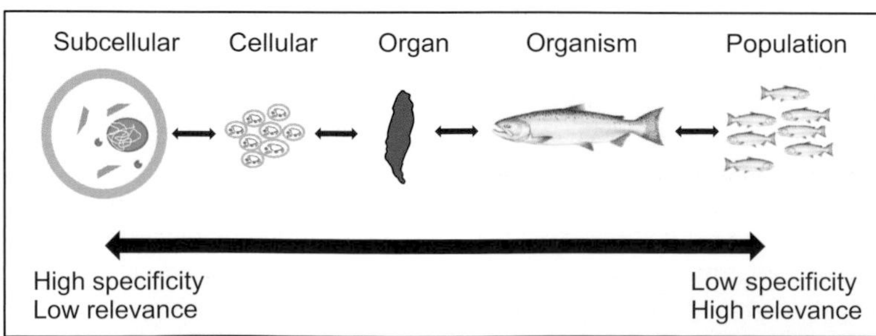

Figure 1 Conceptual linkage across levels of biological organization for ecological risk assessments.

 http://dx.doi.org/10.1016/B978-0-12-386454-3.00999-4

exposure that has a direct toxicity for growth and/or reproduction. However, the application of the computational approach to the field of environmental toxicology is still in its infancy beyond assessing human health risk.

Under ecological risk assessment guidelines, risk is traditionally assessed at the population level rather than for individual organisms (unless the organism is a threatened or endangered species). By definition, the use of biomarkers for risk assessment would not seem to meet the specific criteria for determining adverse population outcomes. The linkage between the initial molecular changes following an environmental exposure to the ultimate outcome of the organism or population has long been a gap in the field of environmental toxicology or ecotoxicology. The defining processes that affect populations are measures of growth, reproduction, and mortality. These processes are critical outcomes that, once disrupted (growth and reproduction) or enhanced (mortality), lead to noticeable changes in populations and potentially in ecosystems. Therefore, the linkage of a molecular biomarker at the subcellular or cellular level to an organism or population outcome needs to be a measure of effect or change to growth, reproduction, or mortality.

Much has been gained in the discovery of environmental biomarkers by extrapolation of concepts, molecular pathways, model organ systems, and physiological systems from the science and research of human health biomarkers. This is particularly true of the recent advances in computational and molecular tools. New concepts are evolving to define the framework needed to connect molecular interactions with adverse outcomes across the different levels of biological organization. The adverse outcome pathway is not strictly defined as a toxicity pathway in that all measures associated with a pathway or process that leads to an adverse outcome are used to predict ecological risk assessment impacts.

Current environmental risk assessment practices often have no specific information regarding the susceptibility and sensitivity of the receptor's toxicological sensitivity to a given stressor. This type of information does not exist for many environmental receptors; however, environmental biomarkers that are directed at the measure of endpoints that are likely to reflect toxicological susceptibility will help to provide this needed information.

Application for Biological Monitoring

Current limitations of environmental monitoring programs include the high cost of sampling environmental media and the low number of validated measurement endpoints. Much of the current monitoring efforts provide retrospective measures of ecosystems that are already stressed or adversely affected by a number of physical and chemical stressors. This reflects compliance monitoring in that assessing environmental risk is driven by regulations that are established for individual chemicals or actions. Such an approach has limitations in that there is poor resolution of some contaminant effects given that contaminants are present in complex environmental mixtures and causation for population endpoints is difficult to assign. This is further complicated in that some ecological receptors adapt to or compensate for exposure to environmental stressors. Even with the limitations and uncertainties, current monitoring practices have established guidelines for baseline ecological status, detection of flux, provision of feedback on process control and operations, assessment of remedial actions, and enforcement of regulations. However, a paradigm shift in ecological risk assessment from deterministic, compliance-based metrics to probabilistic, risk-based metrics is gaining traction with the recognition that a risk-based approach allows for prospective measures, allows for early warning of potential risk and adverse outcomes, and provides more targeted and informed metrics to be used for compliance.

Assessment of environmental toxicology is dependent on the understanding of how an exposure to an environmental stressor affects a given organism. Biomarkers of exposure can help to define the expected range of potential effects and guide criteria for allowable levels of a chemical stressor in environmental media. However, environmental monitoring is an integral part of assessing environmental risk from exposure to chemicals and other stressors to ecological receptors and systems. Under environmental conditions, determining how much risk a stressor poses is a complex question given the heterogeneous nature of environmental exposures that involve mixtures of chemicals from multiple sources of environmental media, and a broad range of environmental receptors.

Criteria for Use

A practical need within the field of environmental/ecological risk assessment is the ability to provide rapid, cost-effective, and specific assessments. Ideally, a diagnostic biomarker should be able to determine the causal link between environmental stressors and risk. However, it is more likely that suites of biomarkers would be used along with other environmental data to assess environmental risk and dictate what actions should be taken to remediate or monitor in a cost-effective and defensible manner. The practicability for use of environmental biomarkers in risk assessment can be generalized in the following categories:

Relevance

- Environmental biomarkers should be environmentally relevant, and accessible for measurement and attribution to a specific stressor or environmental process. An understanding of relevant environmental dose and adverse impact under complex mixture conditions needs to be considered for relevance. The specificity of the biomarker is therefore an important consideration prior to use under field conditions.

Reliability

- Biomarker measures should allow for integration of other information for validation of results. Environmental specific parameters will vary from location to location and could influence molecular responses. Biomarkers should be interpreted as an integrated biomarker response that is tied to an actionable management outcome.

Robust

- Biomarker measures should be amenable across representative environmental organisms and provide clear interpretation above inherent genetic variability, and account for organism adaptation if assessed for chronic responses. Assessment using environmental biomarkers should be performed under scenarios that best address the task. For instance, *in situ* analyses versus *ex situ* analyses provide different spatial and temporal measures.

Reproducible

- Establishment of Good Laboratory Practices or a standard of measurement and interpretation is required to assure compliance and regulation of biomarker use for environmental risk assessment. As multiple molecular tools exist that can measure each type of endpoint, clear and concise methods for sampling, storage, processing, and analysis need to be developed and instituted for comparison between analytical laboratories.

Cost-Effective

- Methods for collection of field samples, assay, and data interpretation should not be labor intensive or controversial. If environmental biomarkers meet all of the previous criteria, but are too costly for routine use in risk assessment, they are likely not going to be widely used. Molecular methods are becoming more refined and capable of high-throughput processing, and these help bring overall costs down. Likewise, the analyses or interpretation of environmental biomarkers needs to be unambiguous with criteria for acceptable ranges or values that exceed acceptable variation.

Conclusions

There is a significant need for application of environmental biomarkers for ecological risk assessment. Expanding efforts in environmental research to include molecular sciences from subcellular processes to organ, organism, and population effects will provide an understanding of exposure and outcome risk and benefits of mitigation strategies. While challenges exist with approaches to account for the problems of chemical mixtures, development of robust and relevant response biomarkers, and linkages across all levels of organization, strides to overcome these obstacles are growing. Application of cost-effective environmental biomarkers that provide critical information for assessing environmental risk under a given exposure or continued exposure will provide early warning of the potential for an adverse outcome. Thus, environmental biomarkers offer the promise of prospective risk assessment.

See also: Ecotoxicology; Environmental Risk Assessment, Aquatic; Environmental Risk Assessment, Terrestrial; Risk Assessment, Ecological.

Further Reading

Ankley, G.T., Bennett, R.S., Erickson, R.S., et al., 2010. Adverse outcome pathways: a conceptual framework to support ecotoxicology research and risk assessment. Environ. Toxicol. Chem. 29, 730–741.

Ankley, G.T., Miracle, A.L., Perkins, E., Datson, G.P. (Eds.), 2008. Toxicogenomics in Regulatory Ecotoxicology. CRC Press, Boca Raton, FL.

Bartell, S.M., 2006. Biomarkers, bioindicators, and ecological risk assessment – a brief review and evaluation. Environ. Bioindic. 1, 60–73.

Markert, B.A., Breure, A.M., Zechmeister, H.G., (Eds.), Bioindicators & Biomonitors: Principles, Concepts, and Applications, Elsevier Science Limited. Oxford, UK.

Relevant Websites

http://cfpub.epa.gov/ncea/cfm/recordisplay.cfm?deid=85844 – US Environmental Protection Agency - Environmental Assessment: Biomarkers database.

http://www.niehs.nih.gov/health/topics/science/biomarkers/index.cfm – National Institutes of Environmental Health Sciences: Biomarkers.

Biomarkers, Human Health

PCS Coelho and JP Teixeira National Institute of Health, Porto, Portugal

Introduction

In order to better protect the human health, a process of population study known as molecular epidemiology has been developed to integrate laboratory measurements with epidemiological methodologies, linking individual exposure to an important biological event. The biological component is evaluated with biological markers, also called biomarkers. Unlike their usage for many years in the medical field, they have been used only for three decades in the environmental health field.

In 2001, the World Health Organization defined biomarker as any substance, structure or process that can be measured in the body or its products and influence or predict the incidence of outcome or disease. They commonly include biochemical, molecular, genetic, immunologic, or physiologic signals of events in biologic systems. The events are represented as a continuum between an external exposure to an agent and the resulting clinical effects (**Figure 1**). Exposure to these agents can happen through contact with contaminated air, water, soil, and food and also in the occupational environment and lifestyle factors. All these routes contribute to a complex exposure situation in daily life.

Along with the concept of biomarker, comes the concept of biological monitoring or biomonitoring. In 2011, the Centers for Disease Control and Prevention defined human biomonitoring as the direct measurement of people's exposure to toxic substances in the environment by measuring the substances or their metabolites in human specimens, such as blood or urine. In other words, the assessment of human exposure via the measurement of biomarkers. Concentrations found can then be related to the internal dose and consequently investigate the possible association between these data toward the effect or back to possible source of exposure. Health risk assessment should include the measurement of actual impacts on biological endpoints from contamination in soil, surface water, groundwater, air, and sediments at various levels of biological organization.

The measurement of biomarkers in population studies requires the appropriate study design. This includes the choice of the appropriate matrix, adequate collection, shipping, and storage and also the implementation of analytical techniques that fulfill the requirements to properly execute the study.

In the last decade, great advances have been achieved in the biomarker's field, but there are still some issues/limitations that need to be taken into account in future investigations.

Classes of Biomarkers

There are different classes of biomarkers. Traditionally, these are classified as biomarkers of exposure, effect, and susceptibility (**Figure 1**). Each of which is used to answer different questions, and their accurate interpretation depends on the knowledge of the various transformations occurring in the metabolic pathways of the human body.

In 2006, the Committee on Human Biomonitoring for Environmental Toxicants of the National Research Council as defined the three categories as:

- Biomarkers of exposure: a chemical, its metabolite, or the product of an interaction between a chemical and some target molecule or cell that is measured in the human body.
- Biomarkers of effect: a measurable biochemical, physiologic, behavioral, or other alteration in an organism that, depending on the magnitude, can be recognized as associated with an established or possible health impairment or disease.
- Biomarker of susceptibility: an indicator of an inherent or acquired ability of an organism to respond to the challenge of exposure to a specific chemical substance.

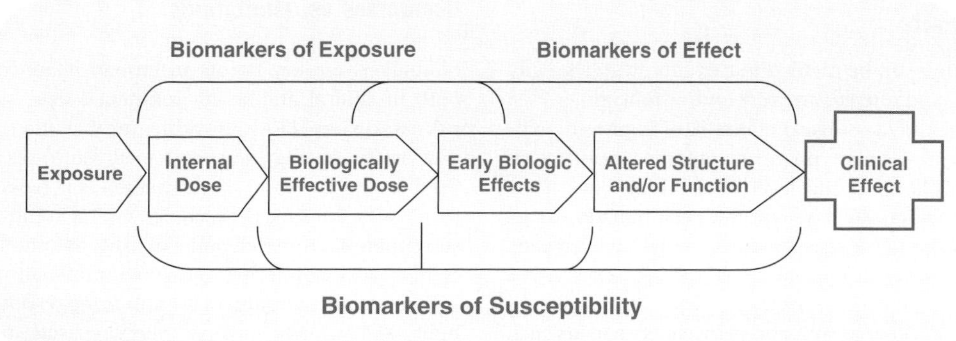

Figure 1 Simplified diagram of the three categories of biomarkers along with the biologic events taking place between exposure and clinical effect.

 http://dx.doi.org/10.1016/B978-0-12-386454-3.00365-1

Table 1 Examples of the most used biomarkers in each (sub)category. Based on the published literature review performed by Au (2007)

Biomarkers of exposure		*Biomarkers of effect*	
Internal dose	*Biologically effective dose*	*Early biologic effect*	*Altered structure and/or function*
Parent compound/metabolites	DNA/protein adducts		
		Reporter gene mutation	
		Altered gene expression	
		DNA strand breaks	
		Micronuclei	
		Chromosomal aberrations	Chromosomal aberrations
			Cancer gene mutation
Biomarkers of susceptibility			
DNA sequence variations			

In order to achieve the mechanistic understanding of the biologic effect, and therefore a better prediction of disease risk, appropriate biomarkers of each category should be used. Examples of the most commonly used biomarkers are presented in Table 1.

Biomarkers of Exposure

Biomarkers of exposure can be divided in two subcategories: internal dose and biologically effective dose.

Biomarkers of internal dose aim to determine the compound or its metabolites in tissues or body fluids such as blood, urine, breast milk, and saliva. They can also give information on other sources of exposure to that compound and the existence of genetic polymorphisms for metabolic enzymes. Biomarkers of biologically effective dose assess the interaction of compounds with molecular targets such as DNA and protein receptors (e.g., measurement of DNA and protein adducts in urine and serum). Despite the presence of these adducts being readily measured, DNA adducts have become more popular and one of the most important biomarkers of exposure as their presence may be indicative of the risk associated with the exposure.

Although biomarkers of exposure are highly relevant and specific indicators of an exposure, the information given does not necessarily translate into prediction of health consequence, and, therefore, other biomarkers need to be analyzed.

Biomarkers of Effect

Biomarkers of effect can be divided in two subcategories: early biological effects and altered structure and/or function.

Biomarkers of early biological effects have improved accuracy for exposure assessment, providing objective measures on potential health effects at the level of the individual. They include several markers such as reporter gene mutation (e.g., *HPRT*, *HLA*, *GPA*, and *TCR* gene mutation assays), altered gene expression (e.g., expression from metabolizing genes, DNA repair genes, and specific enzymes), DNA strand breaks (quantified by the comet assay), and cytogenetic markers such as micronuclei and chromosomal aberration (CA). From all the early biological effect markers, CA assay is the most widely used and best validated biomarker. The mechanisms are better understood and most environmental toxic substances have been shown to induce them. As CAs are also markers of altered structure and/or function, they are extremely useful in cancer risk assessment. Most cancer cells and developmental abnormalities present these alterations. Along with CAs, cancer gene mutations such as tumor suppressor genes and oncogenes are predictive markers for cancer morbidity and mortality.

Biomarkers of Susceptibility

The expression of all the previous described biomarkers is significantly influenced by individual factors, acquired (e.g., life styles like smoking habits and alcohol consumption), and genetic susceptibility categories.

It is well known and recognized that even under identical exposure conditions, different individuals have different responses. Therefore, some individuals are more susceptible/resistant to the exposure than others. In order to identify these variations, investigations with biomarkers of susceptibility have focused on DNA sequence variation in certain genes, such as the ones involved in chemical metabolism and DNA repair, genes related to immune function, and cell cycle control. These studies provide valuable information about the influence of such genes on specific effects of exposure(s) and response to genotoxic agents.

Usefulness vs. Limitations

Biomarkers are key factors in human health risk assessment, both in clinical and in environmental field – environmental risk assessment (ERA), providing reliable and specific information on the etiology and mechanisms of disease process, thus for disease prevention. Their usefulness is based on the ability to measure integrated exposures via all routes without being susceptible to complex and extensive assumptions or models (biological monitoring vs. environmental monitoring – **Figure 2**). In environmental monitoring, exposure models are built and usually involve applying sets of standardized assumptions about activity levels, dietary choices, behavior, routes of exposure, routes of absorption, and many other

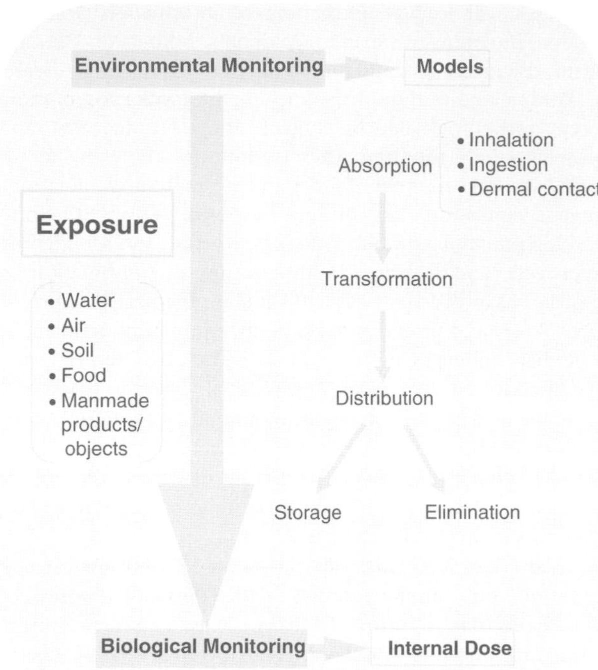

Figure 2 Sources of exposure and main pathways in environmental and biological monitoring.

factors. There is always both uncertainty and error attached to these estimations. In biological monitoring, the main concept is the measurement of the environmental contaminant in the body (internal dose). This is the amount absorbed via all routes – ingestion, inhalation, and dermal – moving through the metabolic pathways. It is transformed and either stored or eliminated. Biomarkers can help to test and validate exposure models by comparing the results obtained in environmental monitoring (exposure models) to the ones obtained in the biological monitoring (internal dose).

In the last decades, analytical techniques have become extremely sensitive and accurate allowing the detection of exceptionally low-level exposures. This is of enormous importance as most biological matrixes are complex, some of them only available in small volumes, and the majority of chemicals are present only at trace levels.

Other uses of biomarkers are related to the possibility of creating individual exposure histories when it is measured in an individual over a period of time and also the ability to evaluate the effectiveness of public health interventions like withdraw, restriction, or reformulations of chemicals. Continuous biomonitoring can determine if exposure to those chemicals actually decreased over the time period being studied.

Despite their enormous advantages, there are several issues/ limitations (**Table 2**).

One of the most important is the construction of an appropriate study design for the investigation before selecting which biomarkers should be used. To provide the linkage between exposure and disease, they must be measured in the correct matrix, and must have an adequate sample size and combination of appropriate biomarkers, using the most reliable and

Table 2 Main advantages and limitations of biomarkers

Advantages	*Limitations*
Confirm the actual amount absorbed via all routes	Many requirements to fulfill in all the process
Help to test and validate exposure models	Only few are properly validated
Detect contaminants at trace levels	Difficult to define the toxic dose
Create individual exposure trends	Sources or pathways of exposure are not defined
Verify the effectiveness of public health interventions	Reference ranges need to be established

reproducible analytical technology available. Accordingly, highly sensitive, specific, and selective multianalytical methods for the extraction, separation, and quantification must be developed. Also standardized collection, storage, and processing conditions are crucial for meaningful results. Numerous biomarkers are only used for research purpose and not clinical at the individual patient level. This is due to the fact that many lack the precision necessary for clinical utility and are often highly sensitive to poor laboratory technique.

The most common matrixes used in biomarkers research are blood, urine, expelled air, and breast milk. Other matrixes such as nails and hair have been increasingly used in recent studies as they are noninvasive and relatively easy to collect. Additionally, they can be completely self-administered, stored at room temperature, and no specific equipment is needed. Nevertheless, problems with contamination, lack of standardized procedures for collection, washing, and digestion, and with the significance of obtained results need to be solved in this field in order to validate such matrices as reliable biomarkers.

Until now, there are no reference ranges or safe ranges that describe general population exposures to contaminants for the majority of biomarkers. Also, a lack of toxicological and epidemiological information makes it often impossible to know if the exposures measured by biomarkers are below or above the toxic limit. Unless there are some studies in this field that defined the toxicity and the dose response curve for the specific contaminant, the results obtained are rather difficult to interpret.

Another important factor is that each biomarker has its own characteristics relating to sensitivity, specificity, and toxicity. Expression of some may not be highly relevant in the carcinogenic process as they represent tolerable and most possible reversible biological changes (e.g., lipid peroxidation and sister chromatid exchange). Also, most times one cannot define the toxic dose nor define sources or pathways of exposure being difficult to interpret obtained results. Choosing the appropriate biomarkers that indicate exposure to the specific agent under study and that represent biological events along the pathway from exposure to clinical effect leads to a mechanistic understanding of biological effects and consequent better prediction of disease risk.

Ethical issues are also one of the most important subjects when dealing with biological sampling. Before collecting the biological specimens, the goals of the study must be well explained, and an informed consent needs to be signed.

Research protocols demand that samples have to be anonymized by coding them. National and international regulations need to be followed when handling genetic material and banking it for long time. Communication of results to studied individuals is also a crucial subject. Only medical and/or scientific experts should have access to them and then choose the most appropriate way to analyze, interpret, and communicate them.

Future Perspectives/New Fields of Application

Nowadays, a top priority in biomarkers research is the development and validation of biomarkers linking environmental exposures to the etiology of human disease. They can then be widely used as early predictors of clinical disease enhancing health risk assessment and contributing to effective new tools for human risk assessment. Well-designed studies including clear identification of the assessment objective, rational selection of biomarkers with proper consideration of specific pathways related to specific exposures to assess individual susceptibility, and development of strategies for the evaluation of the impact of complex genetic variations on the overall pathway efficiency with reliable and efficient phenotypic assays need to be performed. Along with the validation, it is also important to perform the qualification of used biomarkers. For analytical measurements, interlaboratory comparison trials should be made. Improved modeling methods for interpreting biomonitoring data using calibrate and validate models such as pharmacokinetics are also needed.

Recently, the Council of the European Union emphasized the need to consider combined and mixed exposures of chemicals in future risk assessments. Actions like prioritizing chemicals of major concern, evaluating if there are enough tools to obtain information on internal dose biomarkers, and then modelling it both in forward and in reverse direction must be carried out.

It is also important to perform research activities including characterization of a baseline for biomarkers, application of statistical methods to assess temporal departures from that baseline, and establishment of a database of biomarker disease associations, with null and negative studies, resulting in an advance in scientific understanding and application of biomonitoring data.

Another major challenge is to establish reference ranges for the majority of biomarkers. A large amount of studies need to be conducted as mixed and often conflicting results have been obtained in studies of the distribution of biomarkers in populations environmentally and/or occupationally exposed to hazardous agents. This will allow for the development of legislation, methodology, and to support research within this area.

A vast amount of research data come from clinical trials. Biomarkers used in this field require a robust linkage or correlation with clinical endpoints. A cooperation between those working in the clinical field and in the ERA will be crucial to implement appropriate programs for health risk assessment and contribute to valuable new disease prevention policies in environmental and occupational settings.

New information available from genome-derived methods is of paramount importance. Building reliable biomarker databases will lead to integration of information from the genome programs to expand the scientific borders on etiology, health risk prediction, and prevention of environmental disease.

Further studies should also include the application of more recent technologies such as gene arrays, proteomics, and protein activity profiling. These techniques allow the monitoring of a large number of genes and the analysis of alterations in gene expression after combined exposure. This will help to develop potential new biomarkers as screening tools to identify improved candidates for biomonitoring. A combination of approaches at different levels of cellular organization, such as DNA, RNA, and proteins, could be the optimal biomarker.

Other challenges are to establish the link between exposure and health effects using a biological systems approach, changing toxicity test from using animal tests to cell-based techniques. The main goal of this field is to obtain irrefutable data showing that pathway perturbations can predict results from animal testing. Until now, no consensus was obtained on which type of cell should be used.

In the last 2 decades, an explosion in information and literature on human studies with different classes of biomarkers has occurred. Globally, one can see promising future directions in biomarkers research with several new fields of investigation and new technologies being applied.

See also: Risk Assessment, Human Health; Environmental Exposure Assessment; Biomonitoring.

Further Reading

Albertini, R., Bird, M., Doerrer, N., Needham, L., Robinson, S., Sheldon, L., Zenick, H., 2006. The use of biomonitoring data in exposure and human health risk assessment. Environ. Health Perspect. 114, 1755–1762.

Au, W.W., 2007. Usefulness of biomarkers in population studies: from exposure to susceptibility and to prediction of cancer. Int. J. Hyg. Environ. Health 210, 239–246.

Bonassi, S., Au, W., 2002. Biomarkers in molecular epidemiology studies for health risk prediction. Mutat. Res. 511, 73–86.

Bonassi, S., Neri, M., Puntoni, R., 2001. Validation of biomarkers as early predictors of disease. Mutat. Res. 480–481, 349–358.

Farmer, P., Kyrtopoulos, S., Emeny, J., 2007. State of Validation of Biomarkers of Carcinogen and Early Effects and Their Applicability to Molecular Epidemiology. Nofer Institute of Occupational Medicine, Poland.

Gil, F., Pla, A., 2001. Biomarkers as biological indicators of xenobiotic exposure. J. Appl. Toxicol. 21, 245–255.

Kyrtopoulos, S.A., 2006. Biomarkers in environmental carcinogenesis research: striving for a new momentum. Toxicol. Lett. 162, 3–15.

Needham, L.L., Calafat, A.M., Barr, D.B., 2007. Uses and issues of biomonitoring. Int. J. Hyg. Environ. Health 210, 229–238.

Owen, R., Galloway, T.S., Hagger, J.A., Jones, M.B., Depledge, M.H., 2008. Biomarkers and environmental risk assessment: guiding principles from the human health field. Mar. Pollut. Bull. 56, 613–619.

Silins, I., Hohberg, J., 2011. Combined toxic exposures and human health: biomarkers of exposure and effect. Int. J. Environ. Res. Public Health 8, 629–647.

Relevant Websites

Agency for Toxic Substances and Disease Registry – http://www.atsdr.cdc.gov/
Centers for Disease Control and Prevention – http://www.cdc.gov/
European Chemicals Agency – http://echa.europa.eu/
Environmental Cancer Risk, Nutrition and Individual Susceptibility – http://www.ecnis.org/
U.S. Environmental Protection Agency – http://www.epa.gov/
National Research Council – http://www.nationalacademies.org/nrc/
World Health Organization – http://www.who.int/

Biomonitoring

C Costa and JP Teixeira, Portuguese National Institute of Health, Porto, Portugal

This article is a revision of the previous edition article by Chris Theodorakis, volume 1, pp 294–297, © 2005, Elsevier Inc.

The increase in the usage of chemicals observed in the last centuries greatly contributed to the release of several toxic compounds to the environment. Traditionally, environmental pollution assessment is based on environmental monitoring that includes analysis of air, soil, water, sediments, and, in certain cases, living organisms. However, these measurements provide information only on the potential of chemicals to cause adverse effects in both the environment and organisms. In addition and in what concerns living organisms, this type of estimation does not consider absorbed dose or individual variability. Biomonitoring, in which living organisms, including humans, are used to assess environmental contaminant exposure and effects overcomes this disadvantage and became crucial for current knowledge on toxic mechanisms, metabolism, and chemical effects.

Regarding human health surveillance, biomonitoring was initially used in industry, but as techniques evolved and detection limits of quantitative methods decreased, biomonitoring is now widely used also for environmental surveillance (non-occupationally exposed populations). Human biomonitoring provides the opportunity to establish biological exposure index, identify populations at risk, understand dose–effect relationships, and assess cancer risk.

Biological methods involved in environmental surveillance may be divided in bioanalytics (use of biological matter for environmental analyses; biosensors, biotests) and biomonitoring (the use of biota in classical chemical analysis – early warning system; bioindicators).

According to the World Health Organization, bioindicators must be distinguished from biomonitors; while bioindicators reveal the presence or absence of a contaminant by the occurrence of typical symptoms or measurable responses, biomonitors provide information on the presence of the contaminant and provide additional information about the amount and intensity of exposure.

According to their ecological applications, bioindicators can be divided in three main categories: (1) environmental indicator – respond to environmental disturbances; (2) ecological indicator – respond to pollution, habitat fragmentation, or other stresses; and (3) biodiversity indicator – includes species richness, endemism, genetic parameters, population-specific parameters, and landscape parameters.

Different organisms can be used as bioindicators such as plants, aquatic organisms, and selected fish populations. Lower plant organisms (e.g., lichens, mosses, fungi, and algae) are commonly used to assess atmospheric depositions, soil quality, and water purity. Aquatic organisms and selected fish populations can also provide reliable information on the quality of water. One main advantage of the use of biological indicators is the direct measurement of biological availability of pollutants and time integration of the ambient pollution conditions at the site of collection.

The choice of bioindicator is essential to obtain consistent data; these must be chosen according to their sedentary life, abundance and distribution, procedure of identification and sampling, tolerance for the pollutants analyzed, population stability, and toxics accumulating capacity.

The responses of bioindicators can be monitored in a different ways; approaches include field studies or laboratory studies such as toxicity tests and bioassays. Field studies also designated as bioassessment and bioassay provide data that are fundamentally different in type, variability, and reliability. In field applications, the effect is mainly determined by using descriptive techniques, as, for example, morphological alterations.

Bioassay consists of the usage of living test-species that are directly exposed to environmental samples (e.g., soil, sediments, surface water) to measure a potential biological effect due to the presence of potential contaminants. Several toxicity bioassays have been standardized and are commercially available; these apply bacteria, microalgae, protozoa, and yeast and assess parameters such as population growth, substrate consumption, respiration, ATP luminescence, and bioluminescence inhibition. The same types of bioassays have been developed to assess genotoxicity of environmental samples. Besides the toxicity of genotoxicity endpoints, bioaccumulation of chemicals from samples may also be measured.

Occupational hazards were probably the big engine for establishment of human health biomonitoring. The need to recognize the dose of chemical reaching the worker organism and the possible consequent health effect determined the implementation of biomonitoring programs in industry.

One very important question for human biomonitoring is the relationship between the levels of environmental exposure (airborne concentration) and the biological level (absorbed dose). This information is quite complete for most industrial agents. Based on this knowledge, biological indices of exposure have been established for several compounds used in occupational context.

By now, these human biomonitoring programs have already been established in several countries and also in non-occupationally exposed populations (the United States: National Human Monitoring Program and National Biomonitoring Program; Canada: Canadian Health Measures Survey; Germany: German Environmental Surveys; and Denmark: Arctic Monitoring and Assessment Program). Human biomonitoring makes use of biomarkers that are tools that allow estimation of exposure to a toxic agent, the extent of any toxic response, and prediction of likely to response and can be categorized into biomarkers of exposure, response or toxic effect, and biomarkers of susceptibility.

At this time, the ability to quantify substances is most probably the greater one to interpret this information as several scientific disciplines must be integrated: toxicology, pharmacokinetic modeling, epidemiology, and exposure assessment.

Biomonitoring involves many issues that are crucial for correct data interpretation.

Human biomonitoring requires a suitable biological matrix of easy access in sufficient amount for routine procedures; blood and urine are the most commonly used matrices but hair, exhaled air, teeth, nails, and saliva can also be used for toxicological quantification. Understanding the toxicokinetics of the chemicals under investigation is essential to interpret the obtained results. For example, to collect urine, which is one of the most frequently used type of samples in biomonitoring programs, it is crucial to have knowledge on the toxicokinetics of the xenobiotic in order to decide whether to determine the parent compound or a metabolite and timing for sample collection.

Biomarker selection and collection of spot samples are additional points that can greatly influence the reliability of data obtained. The systematic collection of samples in different time points increases the chance to observe the different levels of chemical/metabolite dependent of exposure and toxicokinetics. Although it would be ideal to obtain robust datasets relating potential adverse effects to biomarker concentrations in human populations, assessments are available for only a few chemicals.

Recently, a new concept of biomonitoring equivalents has been established as the concentration or range of concentrations of a chemical or its metabolites in a biological medium (blood, urine, or other medium) that is consistent with an existing health-based exposure guidance value, constituting a new tool for public health surveillance.

Putting together biomonitoring information does contribute to knowledge on the effects that certain chemicals may have on the environment and human health and lead to the discussion of risk reduction strategies. These can include (1) no immediate action, (2) awareness raising, (3) controlling substance exposure, (4) banning substances, (5) increased monitoring efforts, (6) proxy monitoring, and (7) further research.

See also: Biomarkers, Human Health; Occupational Exposure Limits; Ecotoxicology; Environmental Biomarkers; Environmental Health; Environmental Toxicology.

Further Reading

Albertini, R., Bird, M., Doerrer, N., Needham, L., Robison, S., Sheldon, L., Zenick, H., 2006. The use of biomonitoring data in exposure and human health risk assessments. Environ. Health Perspect. 114 (11), 1755–1762.
Hays, S.M., Aylward, L.L., 2012. Interpreting human biomonitoring data in a public health risk context using biomonitoring equivalents. Int. J. Hyg. Environ. Health 215 (2), 145–148.
Kim, Y., Platt, U., 2007. Advanced Environmental Monitoring. Springer, The Netherlands.
Klaassen, C.D., 2008. Casarett and Doull's Toxicology – The Basic Science of Poisons, sixth ed. McGraw-Hill, USA.
National Research Council, 2006. Human Biomonitoring for Environmental Chemicals. National Academies Press, USA.
Needham, L., Calafat, A., Barr, D., 2007. Uses and issues of biomonitoring. Int. J. Hyg. Environ. Health 210, 229–238.
Paustenbach, D., Galbraith, D., 2006. Biomonitoring and biomarkers: exposure assessment will never be the same. Environ. Health Perspect. 114 (8), 1143–1149.

Relevant Websites

http://biomonitoringinfo.org – Biomonitoring Info.
http://www.cdc.gov/biomonitoring – Centers for Disease Control and Prevention: National Biomonitoring Program.
http://www.epa.gov/ncea – US Environmental Protection Agency: Environmental Assessment.

Bioremediation

M Megharaj, University of South Australia, Mawson Lakes, SA, Australia
K Venkateswarlu, Vikrama Simhapuri University, Nellore, India
R Naidu, University of South Australia, Mawson Lakes, SA, Australia

This article is a revision of the previous edition article by Lee R. Sughart, volume 1, pp 297–298, © 2005, Elsevier Inc.

Background

Global industrialization and intensive use of chemical substances such as petroleum products, solvents, pesticides, and heavy metals tend to cause pollution of soil, water, and air. Consequently, there is growing concern among the public about the risk of these contaminated environments to human and ecological health. The ever-increasing population and the rapid expansion of urban environments necessitate remediation of contaminated sites for redevelopment and beneficial use.

The traditional method of remediation that involves simply removing soil from a contaminated site to a landfill ('dig and dump') is not a sustainable solution since it only transfers the contaminant to one place to other, and poses considerable risk due to requirements for excavation, handling, and transport of hazardous materials. Bioremediation that uses living organisms, mainly microorganisms (bacteria, fungi and microalgae) or their processes to degrade or detoxify environmental contaminants, is a cost-effective and environmentally safe method to decontaminate polluted soil and water, and is emerging as an alternative to costly physicochemical remediation technologies. Certain microorganisms, especially bacteria, microalgae, and cyanobacteria, have the ability to utilize hazardous organic contaminants as sources of their carbon, energy, or other nutrients. Although bioremediation is viewed as a new technology, the use of microorganisms in waste treatment dates back at least a century. Often the contaminated sites are complex as contaminants at the sites occur in combination, often organics with inorganics, or parent chemicals with their degradation products. Successful bioremediation should therefore have an integrated approach involving disciplines such as microbiology, engineering, chemistry, ecology, and geology. The major advantage of bioremediation is that remediation achieved on site often keeps the site disruption to a minimum and eliminates the transportation costs. Another important feature of bioremediation is the detoxification or mineralization of the pollutant to CO_2, H_2O, and biomass, which involves the complete and permanent removal of contaminant, thereby eliminating the risk and long-term liability of the contaminant.

Bioremediation Approaches

Bioremediation technologies can be broadly divided into *in situ* and *ex situ* categories. The nature of microorganisms involved in these technologies could be aerobic, anaerobic, or both depending on the nature of contaminant and microorganisms. The commonly used bioremediation technologies are summarized in **Table 1**.

Ex situ treatment technologies involve physical removal of contaminated material from its original place to another area for treatment. Examples of *ex situ* technologies include bioreactors, land farming, composting, and solid-phase treatments. An *in situ* treatment technology involves treatment of the contaminated material in place. Examples of *in situ* technologies include biostimulation, bioaugmentation, and bioventing. Clearly, bioremediation has several advantages over conventional physicochemical remediation technologies (pump and treat, landfilling, etc.).

In Situ Remediation

In situ bioremediation relies on microorganisms and their activities to detoxify or destroy contaminants in place. The ability of microorganisms to break down contaminants to nontoxic or less toxic forms depends on the availability to microorganisms of nutrients, electron donors, and acceptors. Nitrogen and phosphorus are the two of the most commonly required nutrients for microbial growth, and are usually supplemented as ammonia and orthophosphate. Oxygen is the most commonly used electron acceptor in bioremediation. Under aerobic conditions, organic contaminants are transformed to CO_2, H_2O, and microbial cell mass. In the absence of O_2 many microorganisms utilize alternate electron acceptors such as nitrate, sulfate, iron, manganese, and CO_2. In few instances, the natural conditions at contaminated sites provide microorganisms able to degrade contaminants and all the essential factors (nutrients, electron acceptors, donors, etc.) required for biodegradation to take place without any human intervention – a process known as intrinsic bioremediation. In contrast to intrinsic bioremediation, engineered bioremediation provides factors for enhancing microbial growth as well as optimal conditions for microbial detoxification of contaminants.

Engineered Bioremediation

Engineered bioremediation may be a preferred option over intrinsic bioremediation if there is a need for rapid removal of a contaminant or there exists an immediate threat to ecosystems or human health. Engineered bioremediation requires less time and depends on acceleration of biodegradation process by microorganisms, thereby reducing the long-term liability associated with monitoring the site and costs.

Bioaugmentation

Bioaugmentation refers to the introduction of specialist microbes either naturally occurring or genetically modified for their exceptional ability to degrade or detoxify a specific contaminant or contaminant group in polluted soil or water.

Table 1 Summary of bioremediation treatment technologies and the target contaminants

Technology	*Matrix*	*Target contaminants*
Bioaugmentation	Soil, sludge, groundwater	Benzene, toluene, ethylbenzene, xylene (BTEX); petroleum hydrocarbons; pesticides; solvents
Biostimulation	Soil, sludge, groundwater	BTEX, petroleum hydrocarbons, pesticides, solvents
Bioventing	soil	Petroleum hydrocarbons, nonchlorinated hydrocarbons, pesticides
Intrinsic bioremediation	Soil and groundwater	Fuel hydrocarbons (BTEX), solvents
Bioreactors: Slurry based	Soil, sludge, groundwater	Explosives (TNT), hydrocarbons (BTEX), Polyaromatic hydrocarbons (PAHs), pesticides, wood preservatives
Land farming	Soil, sludge, sediment	Total petroleum hydrocarbons (TPH), pentachlorophenol (PCP), pesticides
Composting	Soil, sludge, sediment	Explosives, hydrocarbons (PAH), pesticides, PCP
Fungal remediation (white-rot fungus)	Soil	Chlorinated aromatic hydrocarbons, polychlorinated dibenzo(p)dioxins, explosives (TNT), hydrocarbons (PAHs), pesticides

Generally, microorganisms with ability to use or detoxify contaminants are isolated, cultured in the laboratory, and introduced in the contaminated sites to accelerate remediation process. *Dehalococcoides* sp. that dechlorinates trichloroethylene (TCE) to ethene was shown to have potential for bioaugmentation application in remediation of TCE-contaminated groundwater. Inoculation of microbial communities able to utilize benzene, toluene, ethylbenzene, and xylene (BTEX) isolated from BTEX-contaminated soils are efficient in bioremediation of BTEX-contaminated soils. Consortia of microorganisms containing same or different taxonomic groups (e.g., microbial mats and assemblages of bacteria–microalgae/cyanobacteria) have been efficient in bioaugmentation.

Limitations

Extensive treatability studies and site characterization may be required. The risk of contaminant leaching into groundwater due to increased mobility of contaminant has to be tackled.

Bioventing

Bioventing is a promising new technology wherein oxygen is provided to stimulate the natural *in situ* aerobic biodegradation of contaminants by existing microorganisms at the site. BTEX compounds, the common groundwater pollutants, are easily degradable by aerobic microorganisms, and hence addition of oxygen to contaminated aquifers to stimulate aerobic degradation has been considered a common bioremediation strategy. Only low air flow rates are maintained in the vadose zone in order to supply enough oxygen for sustenance of microbial activity. Oxygen is commonly provided through direct air injection into residual contamination in soil. As a result of bioventing, not only the adsorbed fuel residuals but also the volatile compounds are biodegraded since vapors move slowly through biologically active soil.

Applicability

Bioventing has been successfully used to remediate soils contaminated with petroleum hydrocarbons, nonchlorinated solvents, pesticides, wood preservatives, and other organic contaminants.

Limitations

The factors that may limit the efficacy of bioventing are (1) low permeability of soils, (2) build-up of vapors in basements within radius of influence of air injection wells, (3) extremely low moisture content, (4) monitoring of off-gases at soil surface, and (5) low temperature that in certain instances may slow remediation process.

Nitrate-Enhanced *In Situ* Bioremediation

The microbial metabolic process requires an electron donor (to oxidize a substrate) and an electron acceptor. Nitrate enhancement is yet another emerging bioremediation technology in which nitrate serves as an alternate electron acceptor for microbial activity, thereby enhancing the degradation of organic compounds. This technology utilizes circulation of nitrate throughout the contamination area of the groundwater for enhanced degradation of the contaminant.

Applicability

This technology is effective for treating BTEX-contaminated groundwater.

Limitations

The factors that may limit the effectiveness of this technology include (1) subsurface heterogeneity, (2) requirement for a groundwater circulation system so that contaminants will not escape from active zone of biodegradation, and (3) acceptability by regulators since nitrate is regulated by drinking water standards.

Cometabolic Process

Some microorganisms may not utilize the target contaminant for their growth but can transform the contaminant while utilizing another compound for growth – a process known as cometabolism. For example, methane monooxygenase, an enzyme produced during oxidation of methane by methanotrophic bacteria, can transform chlorinated solvents such as TCE. Cometabolic process is an emerging *in situ* bioremediation technology used for nonpetroleum hydrocarbons such as chlorinated solvents by involving enzymes produced during degradation of certain compounds. The key requirement for cometabolism is the presence of a suitable substrate, the metabolism of which can result in the transformation of target contaminant. Water containing methane and oxygen is injected into groundwater to enhance the methanotrophic microorganisms for degrading chlorinated organic solvents by cometabolic degradation.

Limitation

The effectiveness of cometabolic process depends on homogeneity of the subsurface since it is difficult to circulate methane solution throughout each part of the contaminated zone.

Monitored Natural Attenuation

Monitored natural attenuation (MNA) involves reliance on natural processes to attain contaminant remediation. Consideration of MNA for remediation of contaminated aquifers and groundwater systems usually requires modeling and evaluation of contaminant degradation rates, exposure pathways, impacts on sensitive receptors, and prediction of contaminant concentrations downgradient to the contaminant plume if the plume is migrating. The appropriateness of MNA is usually considered on a case-by-case basis. The evaluation of MNA is not a simple process; it involves multidisciplinary expertise and includes microbiology, chemistry, hydrogeology, and geochemistry.

Applicability

MNA has been proven successful, in particular for fuel hydrocarbons. Fuel and halogenated volatile organic compounds are generally evaluated for MNA.

Limitations

The factors that may limit the suitability and effectiveness of MNA include (1) the requirement for site-specific data for modeling, (2) not being appropriate for the sites with imminent risks, (3) the rate of contaminant migration may exceed the contaminant degradation, (4) degradation products may be more toxic and mobile, (5) longer time may be required compared to active remediation process, (6) where spills involve multiple contaminants, some of the contaminants may not be degraded in the subsurface, (7) the requirement to delineate contamination both horizontally and vertically prior to considering MNA, (8) the geochemical and hydrologic conditions that are amenable for MNA may change over a period of time and remobilize the contaminants that are stabilized, (9) requirement for removal of contaminant source prior to implementation of MNA, and (10) long-term monitoring and associated costs.

Ex Situ Remediation

Biopiles

Biopiles is a treatment technology in which excavated soils are mixed with soil amendments and placed in above-ground enclosures with a provision for aeration and a leachate collection system. It is widely used to treat petroleum hydrocarbons in excavated soils via the use of biodegradation. The treatment area is generally contained with an impermeable liner in order to minimize the risk of contaminant leaching into groundwater or to uncontaminated soil. Various nutrient and additive formulations are used to enhance the microbial activity in biopiles. Soil piles can be up to 20 feet high, although recommended height is 2–3 m, and commonly have an air distribution system placed under the soil and maintained through vacuum or by positive pressure. In order to control the runoff, evaporation, and volatilization, the biopiles are covered with a plastic sheet, which can result in increased solar heating as well. If there are volatile organic compounds (VOCs) in soil, the air leaving the soil may need to be treated to remove the VOCs prior to their discharge into the atmosphere. The operation of biopiles can require a few weeks to several months.

Applicability

Biopile treatment is proven successful for fuel hydrocarbons and nonhalogenated VOCs. Halogenated VOCs and pesticides also have been treated by this process; however, the success will vary and may not be applicable for certain compounds.

Limitations

The factors that may limit the effectiveness of biopile treatment include (1) the requirement for excavation of soils, (2) treatability tests to determine the rates of oxygenation and nutrient loads, and (3) not resulting in uniform treatment in static treatment processes compared to a process that involves periodic mixing.

Composting

Composting (windrows) is a controlled biological process where the excavated contaminated soil is mixed with bulking agents and organic amendments (wood chips, hay, manure, green waste, etc.) in a proper proportion so as to provide a proper balance of carbon and nitrogen required for maintenance of thermophilic microbial activity. During the composting process, the organic contaminants (e.g., polycyclic aromatic hydrocarbons (PAHs), 1,1,1-trichloro-2,2-bis(*p*-chlorophenyl) ethane (DDT)) are converted to innocuous stable products by microbial activities under aerobic and anaerobic conditions. The heat produced by the indigenous microorganisms during the degradation of organic materials will result in a thermophilic phase (55–65 °C) during the composting process, and this phase is crucial for proper transformation of hazardous contaminants. Higher degradation efficiencies can be attained by maintaining proper oxygenation (by windrow turning), moisture content (by irrigation), and temperature. The different designs used in composting are (1) aerated static piles wherein compost piles are aerated through blowers or vacuum pumps,

(2) in-vessel composting with mechanical agitation, wherein compost is placed in a reactor vessel and mixed and aerated, and (3) windrow composting, a more cost-effective method, in which compost is placed in long piles called windrows, and periodically mixed with mobile equipment.

Applicability

Soils and sediments with biodegradable contaminants can be treated using the composting process. There has been some evidence with pilot and full-scale projects that aerobic, thermophilic composting is able to decrease the concentration of explosives such as trinitrotoluene (TNT), RDX, HMX, and ammonium picrate to acceptable levels. Also, this process is applicable to PAHs and DDT residues.

Limitations

The limitations for the composting process include (1) requirement of a substantial space, (2) release of any uncontrolled VOCs associated with soil excavation, and (3) increase in the amount of material due to requirement for additives.

Land Farming

Land farming is a full-scale bioremediation technology wherein the excavated contaminated soil is placed onto lined beds of predetermined thickness and aerated by periodically turning over or tilled (plow depth about 4–12 in). During this process, soil conditions such as moisture content, aeration, pH, and amendments like soil bulking agents, nutrients, etc. are controlled for optimum rate of contaminant degradation. This process allows the aerobic microbial digestion to occur via aeration, and availability of nutrients and moisture.

Applicability

Land farming has been successful for treating petroleum hydrocarbons. More chlorinated or nitrated compounds are degraded slowly. It is also successful in treating diesel fuel, fuel oils, oil sludge, wood preservation wastes, coke wastes, and pesticides.

Limitations

The factors that may limit the effectiveness of land farming include (1) requirement for a large space, (2) some of the factors controlling microbiological proliferation and degradation such as rainfall and temperature are not under control and may prolong the degradation period, (3) requirement for treating volatile compounds in order to prevent off-site migration of these gases into the environment, (4) requirement for constructing a facility to collect and monitor runoff material, and (5) necessity to characterize the site for topography, erosion, climate, permeability, etc. for optimum design of the facility.

Slurry-Phase Bioreactors

Slurry-phase biological treatment involves basically creating aqueous slurry by combining the excavated contaminated soil or sediment with water and other amendments in a bioreactor under controlled conditions. The amount of water added to soil depends on the concentration of contaminant, its rate of biodegradation, and physicochemical properties of the soil itself. During the treatment process, the solids are maintained in slurry suspension in the reactor and mixed with nutrients and oxygen so that microorganisms will come in contact with soil components. Microorganisms able to degrade specific contaminants may be added if a suitable indigenous population is not present in the soil. If required, pH will be adjusted to the desirable level in the reactor vessel. Once the biodegradation is completed, the slurry can be dewatered and the treated soil is disposed of.

Applicability

Slurry-phase bioreactors have been proven successful in remediating soils and sediments contaminated with petroleum hydrocarbons, explosives, solvents, pesticides, wood preservatives, etc. Especially bioreactors are more attractive over *in situ* biological techniques for treating heterogeneous and low permeable soils, and also where quicker treatments are required.

Limitations

Some limitations for slurry-phase biotreatment include (1) the requirement for excavation of contaminated soil, (2) the amount of soil that can be added to the reactor, especially when large amount of contaminated soils are to be treated, (3) the cost associated with dewatering soil after treatment, and (4) finding a safe and acceptable method for disposal of spent wastewater.

Fungal Remediation

Fungal metabolism has been implicated in the degradation of several organic contaminants, especially hydrocarbons. One group of fungi, in particular white-rot fungus (*Phanerochaete chrysosporium*), has the ability to degrade a wide variety of organic contaminants, including PCBs, PAHs, and explosives. Lignin peroxidases, the enzymes produced by these fungi, are responsible for this extensive biodegradative ability.

Applicability

The ability of white-rot fungi to degrade chlorinated hydrocarbons, PAHs, PCBs, polychlorinated(p)dioxins, pesticides (lindane and DDT), and some azodyes has been demonstrated. Also, white-rot fungi have been shown to degrade PAHs such as benzo(a)pyrene, pyrene, fluorene, and phenanthrene, but degradation is favored under nitrogen-limited conditions and at low pH.

Limitations

The factors limiting fungal remediation include (1) their sensitivity to biological processes, (2) their inability to grow well in suspension systems, (3) the negative effect of mixing on enzyme production, (4) poor ability of fungus to attach firmly to fixed media, (5) toxicity, (6) chemical sorption, (7) competition with indigenous microbes, and (8) slow transformation ability.

Microalgal/Cyanobacterial Remediation

Microalgae and cyanobacteria, which are widespread in soil and aquatic ecosystems, detect pollution and also transform many pollutants in the environment. In soils with long-term contamination of insecticides, microalgae and cyanobacteria may serve as bioindicators of pollution. The abilities of microalgae and cyanobacteria in degrading pollutants are therefore gainfully exploited in bioremediation technologies of many polluted systems. In fact, the presence of cyanobacterial mats in the Arabian Gulf Coasts after oil pollution had received enough attention because of their potential to degrade hydrocarbons.

Limitations for Bioremediation of Soils Contaminated with Organics

Bioremediation is not without any limitations. Common disadvantages or limitations to bioremediation technologies are (1) some highly chlorinated contaminants and high molecular weight PAHs are not readily amenable to microbial degradation, and (2) microbial degradation of some chemicals may lead to the production of more toxic and mobile intermediates than the parent compound. For example, reductive dehalogenation of TCE can result in accumulation of vinyl chloride, a toxic product and a carcinogen. Thus, bioremediation is a research-intensive technology that requires a prior thorough understanding of microbial processes. Otherwise, the consequences could be more serious than the original contaminant to the ecosystem.

See also: Biotransformation; Persistent Organic Pollutants; Ecotoxicology; Chemicals of Environmental Concern; Environmental Health.

Further Reading

Alexander, M., 2001. Biodegradation and Bioremediation, second ed. Academic Press, San Diego, CA.

Juhasz, A.L., Megharaj, M., Naidu, R., 2000. Bioavailability: the major challenge (constraint) to bioremediation of organically contaminated soils. In: Wise, D., Trantolo, D.J., Cichon, E.J., Inyang, H.I., Stottmeister, U. (Eds.), Remediation Engineering of Contaminated Soils. Marcel Dekker Inc., N.Y., pp. 217–241.

Lovley, D.R., Lloyd, J.R., 2000. Microbes with a mettle for bioremediation. Nat. Biotechnol. 18, 600–601.

MacDonald, J.A., Rittman, B.E., 1994. *In situ* bioremediation: when does it work? Industrial Wastewater 2, 32–38.

Megharaj, M., Ramakrishnan, B., Venkateswarlu, K., Sethunathan, N., Naidu, R., 2011. Bioremediation approaches for organic pollutants: a critical perspective. Environ. Int. 37, 1362–1375.

Norris, R.D., Hinchee, R.E., Brown, R., et al., 1994. Handbook of Bioremediation. Lewis Publishers, Boca Raton.

Ramakrishnan, B., Megharaj, M., Venkateswarlu, K., Naidu, R., Sethunathan, N., 2010. The impacts of environmental pollutants on microalgae and cyanobacteria. Crit. Rev. Environ. Sci. Technol. 40, 694–821.

Suresh, R.S.C., Ramakrishnan, B., Megharaj, M., Venkateswarlu, K., Naidu, R., 2011. Consortia of cyanobacteria/microalgae and bacteria: biotechnological potential. Biotechnol. Adv. 29, 896–907.

Relevant Websites

http://www.bioremediationgroup.org/ – Bioremediation Discussion Group.

http://umbbd.msi.umn.edu – The University of Minnesota Biocatalysis/Biodegradation Database (UM-BBD).

http://www.lbl.gov/ERSP – US Department of Energy Office of Science, Subsurface Biogeochemical Research Program.

Biotransformation/Metabolism

JL Rourke and CJ Sinal, Dalhousie University, Halifax, NS, Canada

This article is a revision of the previous edition article by Tanya C. McCarthy and Christopher J. Sinal, volume 1, pp 299–312, © 2005, Elsevier Inc.

Introduction

Biotransformation refers to the process by which lipophilic (fat-soluble), xenobiotic (foreign), or endobiotic (endogenous) chemicals are converted in the body by enzymatic reactions to products that are more hydrophilic (water-soluble). In this context, metabolism and metabolic transformation are synonymous with biotransformation. A xenobiotic is a relatively small (molecular weight <1000), nonnutrient chemical that is foreign to the species in which metabolism occurs.

The major purpose of biotransformation is to chemically modify (metabolize) poorly excretable lipophilic compounds to more hydrophilic chemicals that are readily excreted in urine and/or bile. Without metabolism, lipophilic xenobiotics accumulate in biota, increasing the potential for toxicity. Examples of such compounds are highly halogenated polychlorinated biphenyls (PCBs) and polychlorinated dibenzofurans (tetrachlorodibenzodioxin (TCDD) and dioxins), which occur as tissue residues in humans. On the contrary, biotransformation is normally not required for xenobiotics with high water solubility because of rapid excretion in urine.

Two or more sequential enzymatic reactions are routinely required to convert lipophilic chemicals to metabolites that are efficiently excreted. R.T. Williams, a pioneer in biotransformation studies, classified these pathways as phase I (oxidation, reduction, and hydrolysis reactions) and phase II (conjugation reactions; **Table 1**). Normally, a phase I reaction precedes its phase II counterpart, but some compounds contain functional groups that are sites for direct conjugation (e.g., –OH, –COOH, and $-NH_2$). Frequently, the biological activity of a chemical decreases (called detoxication) during metabolism but this is not always the case. Both phase I and phase II reactions can function in toxication or metabolic activation processes as well, and this is a fundamental mechanism for the formation of many chemical toxicants. Multiple classes of toxic compounds, including polycyclic aromatic hydrocarbon-derived carcinogens and mutagens, are formed by cytochrome P450-dependent oxidative metabolism, the most common toxication pathway.

The highest concentration of xenobiotic metabolizing enzymes is routinely found in the liver, but epithelial cells of extrahepatic tissues, such as the lung, kidney, intestine, placenta, and eye, also have activity. Relative to liver, extrahepatic tissues do not normally play a major quantitative role in the biotransformation of foreign compounds, including drugs. Extrahepatic organs, however, can be extremely important in the metabolic activation of xenobiotics and resultant target organ toxicity because the ratio of activation to detoxication enzyme activity is frequently higher in these cells than in hepatocytes (i.e., bioactivation predominates over detoxication and results in the formation of concentrations of active metabolites that overwhelm the capacity of detoxication pathways). The contribution of intestinal flora to the *in vivo* metabolism of xenobiotics can also be significant, especially for chemicals that require anaerobic (oxygen-deficient) reduction as a quantitatively important pathway.

Table 1 Classification of major biotransformation pathways

Classification	*Enzymes*
Phase I	
Oxidation	Cytochrome P450
	Flavin-containing monooxygenase
	Alcohol dehydrogenase
	Aldehyde dehydrogenase
	Monoamine oxidase
	H_2O_2-dependent peroxidase
Reduction	Cytochrome P450
	NADPH-P450 reductase
	Carbonyl reductase
Hydrolysis	Epoxide hydrolase
	Carboxylesterase/amidase
Phase II	
Conjugation	UDP-GT
	Sulfotransferase
	GST
	Mercapturic acid biosynthesis
	Cysteine conjugate β-lyase/thiomethylase
	N-Acetyltransferase
	N-Methyltransferase
	O-Methyltransferase

Oxidation Reactions

Oxidation is the most common metabolic reaction for lipophilic xenobiotic and endobiotic compounds, in part because most mammalian tissues are well oxygenated.

Cytochrome P450 Monooxygenase System

The cytochrome P450-dependent monooxygenase system is concentrated in the endoplasmic reticulum of cells and is referred to as a microsomal enzyme system. This P450 system is composed of multiple forms or isozymes of P450 belonging, in humans, to at least 18 distinct gene families as well as the flavoprotein, reduced nicotinamide adenine dinucleotide phosphate (NADPH)-P450 reductase. This monooxygenase system has been called a universal oxidase because it catalyzes the oxidation of a multitude of lipophilic compounds including both xenobiotics (antioxidants, carcinogens, drugs, environmental pollutants, food additives, hydrocarbons, and pesticides) and endobiotics (bile acids, cholesterol, eicosanoids, fatty acids, lipid hydroperoxides, retinoids, and steroid hormones).

 http://dx.doi.org/10.1016/B978-0-12-386454-3.00007-5

With several classes of xenobiotic substrates, including chemical carcinogens such as benzo[*a*]pyrene or the mycotoxin, aflatoxin B_1, some metabolites are more toxic than the parent chemical, a process called toxication. Endogenous compounds can also be bioactivated by P450 to metabolites with greater biological activity. For example, arachidonic acid is metabolized to four isomeric epoxyeicosatrienoic acids, which have potent physiological and/or pathobiological effects in multiple tissues and cell types. Consequently, the P450 system is extremely important in toxicology (toxication and detoxication of both endogenous and exogenous substances), pharmacology (rate-limiting step in the metabolism of many drugs, drug–drug interactions, and individual qualitative and quantitative differences in drug metabolism due to genetic differences), and physiology (formation and metabolism of endobiotics that function as intercellular and/or intracellular messengers).

The multiple forms of P450 vary in their substrate selectivity and level of expression in different tissues and cell types. In lung, for example, the highest concentrations of P450 are normally found in (epithelial) Clara and alveolar type II cells but lower amounts occur in ciliated, goblet, and vascular endothelial cells as well as alveolar macrophages. The selective modulation (relative increase or decrease in concentration) of P450 isozymes in a single tissue or cell type can have pronounced effects on the metabolism of both endogenous and exogenous substances and on chemical-mediated target organ and/or cell toxicity by altering the balance between toxication and detoxication reactions.

The overall oxidation of a substrate, RH, by P450 is summarized in **Figure 1**, in which NADPH is shown as the required cofactor.

Some of the important reactions catalyzed by the P450 monooxygenase system include aliphatic hydroxylation, aromatic hydroxylation, epoxidation, heteroatom (*N*-, *O*-, and *S*-) dealkylation, nitrogen oxidation, oxidative deamination, oxidative dehalogenation, oxidative denitrification, and oxidative desulfuration. Most of these reactions result from the initial oxidation of a carbon atom, another reason that P450 is so important in the oxidative biotransformation of lipophilic chemicals. Some P450-catalyzed oxidation reactions are illustrated in **Table 2**.

The microsomal P450 system is most highly concentrated in the liver, but it is also present in many extrahepatic tissues including the lung, kidney, placenta, small intestine, skin, adrenal, testis, ovary, eye, pancreas, mammary gland, aorta wall, brain, nasal epithelial membrane, colon, salivary gland, prostate, heart, lymph node, spleen, thymus, and thyroid. A second P450 monooxygenase system, localized to mitochondria of steroid-metabolizing tissues (adrenal, ovary, and testis), is primarily involved in the oxidative biosynthesis of endogenous steroids such as cholecalciferol, cortisone, and deoxycorticosterone. In contrast to the universal oxidase properties of the microsomal system, the mitochondrial P450 system has a much higher degree of substrate specificity.

$$RH + O_2 + NADPH + H^+ \rightarrow ROH + H_2O + NADP^+$$

Figure 1 Overall reaction that occurs during the cytochrome P450-dependent oxidation of a substrate, RH.

Flavin-Containing Monooxygenases

There is also a P450-independent monooxygenase enzyme family called the flavin-containing monooxygenases (FMOs); that is, localized in the endoplasmic reticulum of virtually all nucleated mammalian cells. Six distinct genes encoding FMOs have been identified in the human genome. These enzymes contain the coenzyme flavin adenine dinucleotide (FAD) and, similar to the P450 system, also require NADPH as a cofactor. A major difference between the FMOs and the P450 is that the former do not oxidize carbon atoms. However, FMOs do oxidize many nitrogen-, sulfur-, selenium-, and phosphorus-containing xenobiotics (**Table 3**).

Since there are many drugs and environmental pollutants that contain sulfur, it is of considerable interest that FMO preferentially catalyzes the oxidation of sulfur in compounds containing both nitrogen and sulfur. Thus, FMO is an important enzyme system for the oxidation of selected classes of xenobiotics, and its spectrum complements that of the P450 system because the latter prefers oxidation of carbon atoms. Other ways in which FMO enzymes differ from many microsomal P450 isozymes include their apparent lack of induction (increased enzyme concentration) or repression (decreased enzyme concentration) by environmental factors and their more limited role in metabolic activation. Consequently, the P450 system is of greater significance in chemical toxicology.

Alcohol and Aldehyde Dehydrogenases

An extremely important metabolic pathway for alcohols and aldehydes is oxidation to aldehydes and ketones and to carboxylic acids, respectively. Mammalian liver alcohol dehydrogenases are a family of zinc-containing, cytosolic nicotinamide adenine dinucleotide $(NAD)^+$-dependent enzymes that catalyze the oxidation of primary and secondary aliphatic, arylalkyl, and cyclic alcohols. Aromatic alcohols (phenols), however, are not substrates for these enzymes. Alcohol dehydrogenases are widely distributed in mammalian tissues; the highest concentrations occur in the liver. As shown in **Figure 2**, alcohol dehydrogenases also catalyze the reverse reaction: reduction of aldehydes to primary alcohols in the presence of reduced nicotinamide adenine dinucleotide (NADH).

However, the *in vivo* reduction of aldehydes by this enzyme is not normally a quantitatively important reaction because aldehydes are rapidly oxidized to their corresponding carboxylic acid derivatives by aldehyde dehydrogenase. Alcohol dehydrogenase is a very important enzyme for the metabolism of ethanol.

Aldehyde dehydrogenases are also widely distributed in mammalian tissues; the highest concentration is in the liver. Both aliphatic and aromatic aldehydes are readily oxidized to carboxylic acids by this enzyme in the presence of NAD^+, the required cofactor (**Figure 3**).

Although this is a reversible reaction *in vitro*, the carboxylic acids formed are either converted rapidly to their ester glucuronide derivatives (a phase II reaction catalyzed by uridine diphosphate (UDP)-glucuronosyltransferase (GT); see below) or, if polar enough, are excreted unchanged. Consequently, the reverse reaction is generally not of significance *in vivo*.

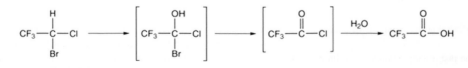

Table 2 Examples of Important Reactions Catalyzed by the Microsomal P450 Monooxygenase System

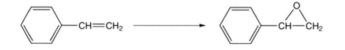

Aliphatic hydroxylation

$$C_6H_5-CH_2-CH_3 \longrightarrow C_6H_5-CH_2-CH_2(OH) + C_6H_5-CH(OH)-CH_3$$

Aromatic hydroxylation

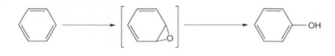

$$C_6H_6 \longrightarrow [\text{arene oxide}] \longrightarrow C_6H_5-OH$$

Epoxidation

$$C_6H_5-CH=CH_2 \longrightarrow C_6H_5-CH(-O-)CH_2$$

N-Dealkylation

$$C_6H_5-NH-CH_3 \longrightarrow [C_6H_5-NH-CH_2(OH)] \longrightarrow C_6H_5-NH_2$$

O-Dealkylation

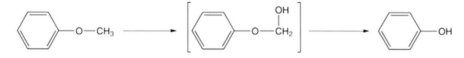

$$C_6H_5-O-CH_3 \longrightarrow [C_6H_5-O-CH_2(OH)] \longrightarrow C_6H_5-OH$$

S-Dealkylation

$$C_6H_5-S-CH_3 \longrightarrow [C_6H_5-S-CH_2(OH)] \longrightarrow C_6H_5-SH$$

Nitrogen oxidation

$$C_6H_5-NH-CH_3 \longrightarrow C_6H_5-N(OH)-CH_2$$

Oxidative deamination

$$C_6H_5-CH_2-CH(CH_3)NH_2 \longrightarrow C_6H_5-CH_2-C(CH_3)=O + NH_3$$

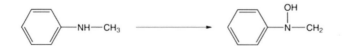

Oxidative dehalogenation

$$CF_3-CH(Br)-Cl \longrightarrow [CF_3-C(OH)(Br)-Cl] \longrightarrow [CF_3-C(=O)-Cl] \xrightarrow{H_2O} CF_3-C(=O)-OH$$

Table 2 Examples of Important Reactions Catalyzed by the Microsomal P450 Monooxygenase System—cont'd

Oxidative denitrification

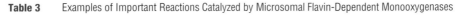

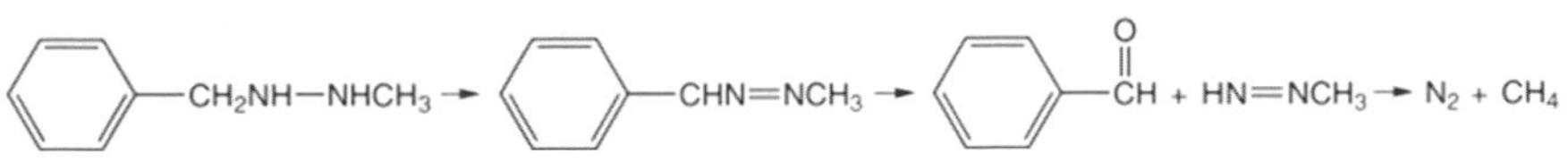

$C_6H_5-CH_2NH-NHCH_3 \rightarrow C_6H_5-CHN{=}NCH_3 \rightarrow C_6H_5-CH{=}O + HN{=}NCH_3 \rightarrow N_2 + CH_4$

Oxidative desulfuration

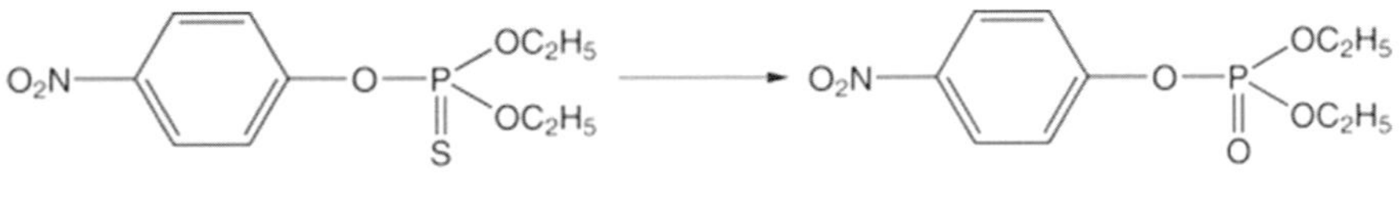

$O_2N-C_6H_4-O-P(=S)(OC_2H_5)_2 \longrightarrow O_2N-C_6H_4-O-P(=O)(OC_2H_5)_2$

Table 3 Examples of Important Reactions Catalyzed by Microsomal Flavin-Dependent Monooxygenases

Tertiary amine oxidation

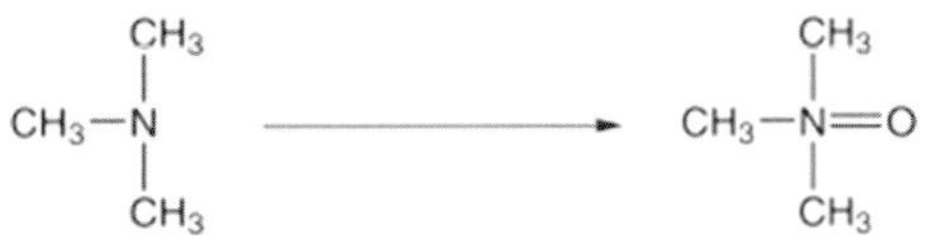

$(CH_3)_2N-CH_3 \longrightarrow (CH_3)_2N(CH_3){=}O$

Alkyldisulfide formation

$HOOC-CH(NH_2)-CH_2-SH \times 2 \longrightarrow HOOC-CH(NH_2)-CH_2-S-S-CH_2-CH(NH_2)-COOH$

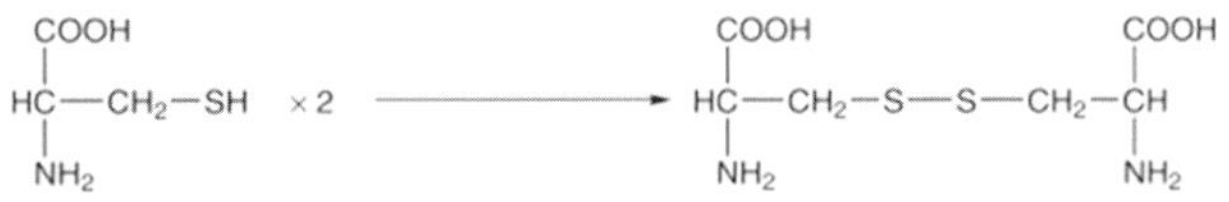

Aryldisulfide formation

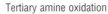

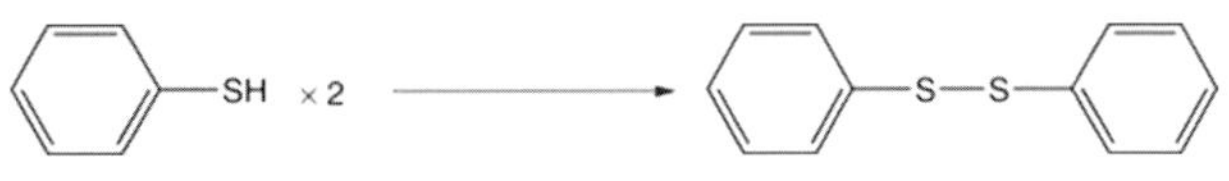

$C_6H_5-SH \times 2 \longrightarrow C_6H_5-S-S-C_6H_5$

Thioether oxidation

$C_6H_5-CH_2-S-CH_3 \longrightarrow C_6H_5-CH_2-S(=O)-CH_3 \longrightarrow C_6H_5-CH_2-S(=O)_2-CH_3$

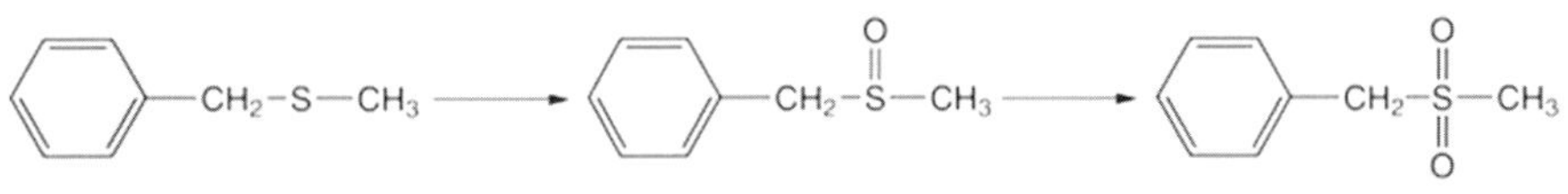

Phosphorus oxidation

$C_6H_5-S-P(=S)(OC_2H_5)(C_2H_5) \longrightarrow C_6H_5-S-P(=S)(OC_2H_5)(C_2H_5)$

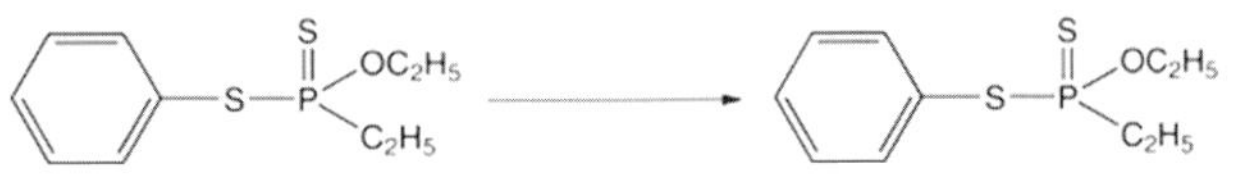

$$CH_3CH_2OH + NAD^+ \rightleftharpoons CH_3CHO + H^+ + NADH$$

Figure 2 Oxidation of ethanol and reduction of acetaldehyde by alcohol dehydrogenase and the appropriate form of NAD^+.

$$CH_3CHO + NAD^+ \rightleftharpoons CH_3COOH + H^+ + NADH$$

Figure 3 Oxidation of acetaldehyde and reduction of acetic acid by aldehyde dehydrogenase and the appropriate form of NAD^+.

Monoamine Oxidases

The monoamine oxidases are localized in the outer membrane of the mitochondria of cells and are widely distributed in most mammalian tissues; the exceptions are erythrocytes and plasma. This enzyme system catalyzes the oxidative deamination of a wide variety of xenobiotic and endobiotic (e.g., neurotransmitter) monoamines (**Figure 4**).

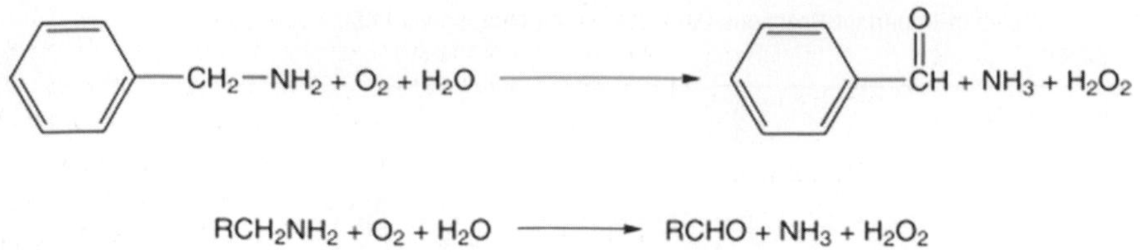

$$C_6H_5{-}CH_2{-}NH_2 + O_2 + H_2O \longrightarrow C_6H_5{-}CHO + NH_3 + H_2O_2$$

$$RCH_2NH_2 + O_2 + H_2O \longrightarrow RCHO + NH_3 + H_2O_2$$

Figure 4 Oxidation of a substituted methylamine by monoamine oxidase. R can be an alkyl (CH_3^-)or aryl ($C_6CH_5^-$) substituent.

Monoamine oxidases are flavoproteins that contain one molecule of FAD per molecule. There are two major types of monoamine oxidase (A and B), whose relative concentration varies in tissues of the same species. In general, the A form of the enzyme is more active with endogenous neurotransmitter amines (serotonin, norepinephrine, and epinephrine), whereas the B form is more active toward xenobiotic amines such as 2-phenethylamine.

H_2O_2-Dependent Peroxidases

Easily oxidized phenols and arylamines are excellent substrates for peroxidase-catalyzed one-electron oxidation reactions. These reactions are very important in toxicology because of the reactivity and toxicity of the free radicals (molecules with a highly reactive unpaired electron) formed. A well-studied example of this type is the cooxidation of xenobiotics catalyzed by the hydroperoxidase activity of prostaglandin H synthase. This enzyme, which converts arachidonic acid to prostaglandin (PG) H_2, has two distinct enzyme sites: cyclooxygenase, which oxidizes arachidonic acid to prostaglandin G_2 (PGG_2), and hydroperoxidase, which reduces PGG_2 to prostaglandin H_2 (PGH_2). PGG_2 reduction requires the donation of single electrons, which can come from a xenobiotic, and results in its conversion to a free radical. Many chemicals that are oxidized to toxic products, including acetaminophen, 2-aminofluorene, diethylstilbestrol, benzo[*a*]pyrene 7,8-dihydrodiol, and 4-phenetidine, are bioactivated to free radicals during reduction of PGG_2 to PGH_2 (**Figure 5**).

Prostaglandin H synthase activity is high in several extrahepatic sites that are targets for chemical-mediated toxicity but contain very low amounts of P450 monooxygenase activity. These include skin, kidney medulla, lung of certain species, and platelets. It is now generally accepted that prostaglandin H synthase hydroperoxidase activity is important for the metabolic activation of amines and phenols, some of which are converted to potent mutagens and carcinogens, particularly in cells deficient in P450 monooxygenase activity but high in prostaglandin synthesis activity.

Other peroxidases are also involved in bioactivation of easily oxidized compounds. Oxyhemoglobin in erythrocytes can oxidize arylamines to products that cause methemoglobinemia; chloroperoxidase and myeloperoxidase of activated polymorphonuclear leukocytes and macrophages bioactivate

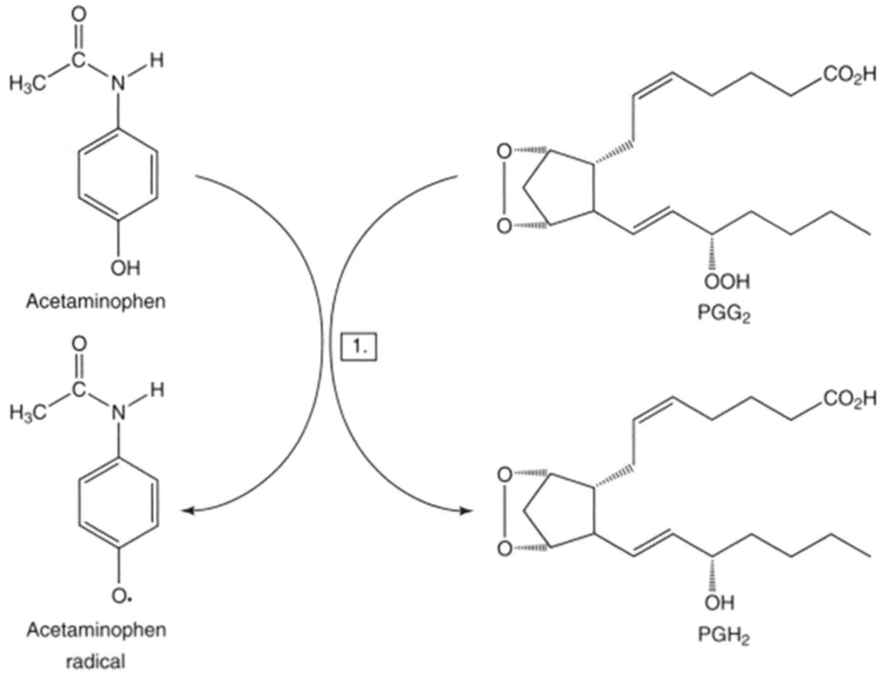

Figure 5 Conversion of acetaminophen to its reactive free radical by cooxidation mediated by the hydroperoxidase activity of 1. prostaglandin H synthase-catalyzed reduction of prostaglandin G_2 (PGG_2) to prostaglandin H_2 (PGH_2).

certain drugs including various sulfonamides by N-oxidation to reactive nitroso products that contribute to adverse drug reactions, and diethylstilbestrol, a transplacental carcinogen, is oxidized by estrogen-inducible peroxidases in the reproductive tract.

These few examples emphasize that H_2O_2-dependent peroxidases can activate aromatic alcohols (phenols) and aromatic amines to reactive free radicals, which are often very toxic.

Reduction Reactions

Several functional groups, including nitro, azo, tertiary amine *N*-oxide, aldehyde, ketone, sulfoxide, and alkyl polyhalide, are reduced by mammals *in vivo*. Toxic free radicals are often formed as intermediates during reduction. Although some of these reactions, or more accurately the initial sequence of the reactions, occur under aerobic conditions *in vitro*, anaerobic conditions are generally required for the complete reduction of xenobiotics. Those reactions that go to completion *in vivo* are either reductions of carbonyl groups or are catalyzed by the intestinal microflora. Reduction that occurs anaerobically is of much less toxicological concern due to the decreased formation of toxic oxygen-free radicals.

Cytochrome P450-Dependent Reactions

Under aerobic and anaerobic conditions, several reduction reactions can be catalyzed by the intact P450 monooxygenase system or only by its flavoprotein component, NADPH-P450 reductase.

In addition to being oxidatively metabolized, many polyhalogenated alkanes are converted by a P450-dependent, one-electron reduction pathway to a free radical intermediate and inorganic halide. The best studied example of this reaction is the reduction of carbon tetrachloride (CCl_4) to chloroform ($CHCl_3$), which occurs *in vitro* under aerobic or anaerobic conditions and *in vivo*. The trichloromethyl radical formed (CCl_3) is believed to be a major contributor to CCl_4-mediated hepatotoxicity. Halothane, trichlorofluoromethane, hexachloroethane, pentachloroethane, and dichlorodiphenyltrichloroethane (DDT) are other halogenated compounds that are substrates for this P450-dependent reductive pathway.

Several other classes of xenobiotics are also efficiently reduced by the P450 monooxygenase system under anaerobic conditions. These include tertiary amine *N*-oxides (converted to tertiary amines), hydroxylamines (primary amines), and hydrazo derivatives (primary amines).

Flavoprotein-Dependent Reactions

The first step of the NADPH-dependent reduction of aromatic nitro and azo compounds by hepatic microsomes is catalysis by NADPH-P450 reductase, which results in the formation of a free radical. In the presence of oxygen these radicals are rapidly reoxidized to the parent aromatic nitro or azo compound, concomitant with the generation of the superoxide anion radical. This futile cycling explains the toxicity of compounds, such as paraquat (**Figure** 6) or nitrofurantoin, which generate toxic superoxide under conditions in which little or no metabolism of the compound is detected. NADPH-P450 reductase is widely distributed in mammals and, consequently, these potentially toxic reactions occur in different tissues and subcellular organelles. Easily reduced compounds are readily reduced by NADPH-P450 reductase. Compounds that are more difficult to reduce, such as carbon tetrachloride, require the intact P450 monooxygenase system as a source of electrons for reduction.

Carbonyl Reductases

As mentioned previously, both alcohol and aldehyde dehydrogenases can function as reductases in the presence of NAD^+. In addition, there are a number of other carbonyl reductases that are $NADP^+$-dependent. Aldehyde reductases and carbonyl reductases are localized in the cytosol of cells, have a broad substrate specificity, have low molecular weight, and are widely distributed in extrahepatic tissues. In general, aldehyde reductases reduce only aldehydes, whereas carbonyl reductases reduce both aldehydes and ketones. Reduction of ketones can be an important metabolic pathway *in vivo*.

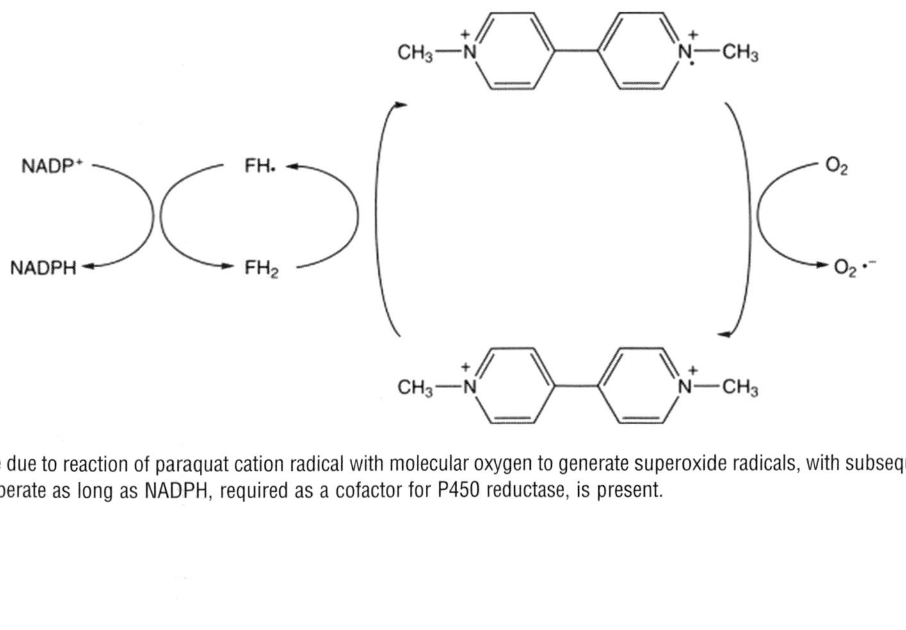

Figure 6 Futile cycle due to reaction of paraquat cation radical with molecular oxygen to generate superoxide radicals, with subsequent regeneration of paraquat. Cycle will operate as long as NADPH, required as a cofactor for P450 reductase, is present.

Hydrolysis Reactions

When certain xenobiotics, including esters and amides, are administered to animals they are hydrolyzed. Hydrolysis reactions are important for the sequential metabolism of chemicals converted to epoxides by the P450 system. These reactions are classified as phase I because they free up functional groups (e.g., $-COOH$, $-NH_2$, $-OH$, $-SH$, and $-SO_3H$) that are important sites for conjugation (phase II) reactions.

Epoxide Hydrolase

Epoxide hydrolases catalyze the hydration of epoxides to *trans*-dihydrodiols and are very important enzymes in toxication–detoxication processes. Unsaturated aliphatic and aromatic hydrocarbons are converted to epoxides (alkene and arene oxides, respectively) by P450 monooxygenase activity. Some of these electrophilic epoxides react covalently with macromolecules, such as proteins, RNA, and DNA, resulting ultimately in acute or chronic toxicity, including necrosis, mutagenesis, carcinogenesis, and teratogenesis. In most cases, the diols produced by epoxide hydrolase are much less toxic than the epoxide substrate. With some polycyclic aromatic hydrocarbons, however, the diols are precursors for potent carcinogenic and mutagenic products. For example, benzo[*a*]pyrene 7,8-dihydrodiol, formed enzymatically from benzo[*a*]pyrene 7,8-oxide (**Figure 7**), is converted to the highly toxic benzo[*a*] pyrene 7,8-dihydrodiol-9,10-oxide by the P450 system or by cooxidation by prostaglandin H synthase.

There are two distinct types of epoxide hydrolases, both widely distributed in mammalian tissues. One type is localized primarily in the endoplasmic reticulum, the second in the cytosol. The microsomal and cytosolic enzymes have different properties, including substrate selectivities. Several inducers of xenobiotic metabolizing enzymes, including phenobarbital, planar PCB congeners, and *trans*-stilbene oxide, selectively increase (induce) microsomal, but not cytosolic, epoxide hydrolase activity.

Carboxylesterases/Amidases

The term carboxylesterase refers to a wide variety of enzymes with both esterase and amidase activity. They cleave carboxylesters, carboxylamides, and carboxylthioesters, producing a carboxylic acid and an alcohol or phenol (**Figure 8**), amine, or mercaptan, respectively. There are many different esterases, some of which are important for the hydrolysis and detoxication of toxic organophosphate esters. In general, esterases are present in almost all mammalian tissues, occur as multiple isozymes, and are concentrated in the liver. The esterase activity present in plasma is normally due to the release of these enzymes from liver.

Ester or amide cleavage can result in detoxication or metabolic activation, depending on the biological and chemical properties of the acids, alcohols, or amines released during hydrolysis. For example, hydroxamic acid hydrolysis has been implicated in the formation of proximate mutagens. The functional groups that become available for reaction during hydrolysis normally undergo phase II metabolism, as discussed below.

Conjugation Reactions

Most phase II reactions markedly increase the water solubility of xenobiotics and facilitate excretion of the chemical. Exceptions are acetylation and methylation reactions.

UDP-Glucuronosyltransferases

The most common phase II reaction is the synthesis of glucuronic acid derivatives (β-D-glucuronides) of lipophilic xenobiotics and endobiotics. Alcohols, phenols, carboxylic acids, mercaptans, primary and secondary aliphatic amines, and carbamates are converted to their β-glucuronide derivatives by UDP-GT. Sixteen distinct human isozymes of UDP-GT have been identified, nine of which are encoded by a single gene. In common with the P450 monooxygenase system, UDP-GT is a microsomal enzyme, is present at highest concentrations in the liver, is expressed in many extrahepatic tissues, and is induced by exposure to different classes of compounds known to modulate P450, including phenobarbital, polycyclic aromatic hydrocarbons, planar PCB congeners, and dioxins.

UDP-GT catalyzes the translocation of glucuronic acid to a substrate from the cosubstrate UDP-α-D-glucuronic acid (UDPGA) as shown in **Figure 9**. The resulting glucuronide conjugates are excreted largely in the bile and can be hydrolyzed to their aglycone by β-glucuronidase of the intestinal microflora. The deconjugated chemical (i.e., the aglycone) can

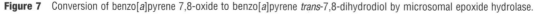

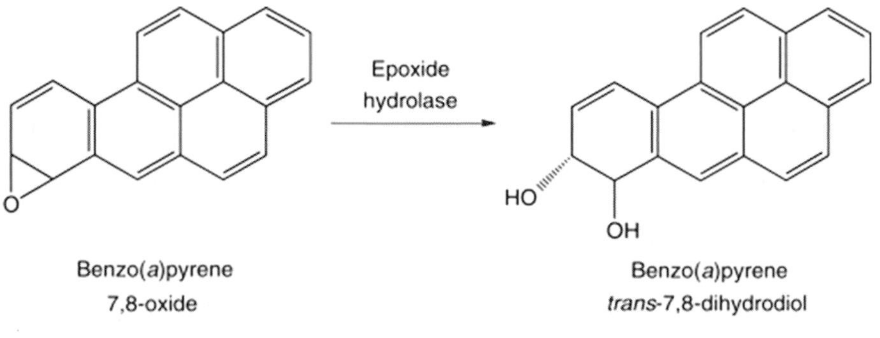

Figure 7 Conversion of benzo[*a*]pyrene 7,8-oxide to benzo[*a*]pyrene *trans*-7,8-dihydrodiol by microsomal epoxide hydrolase.

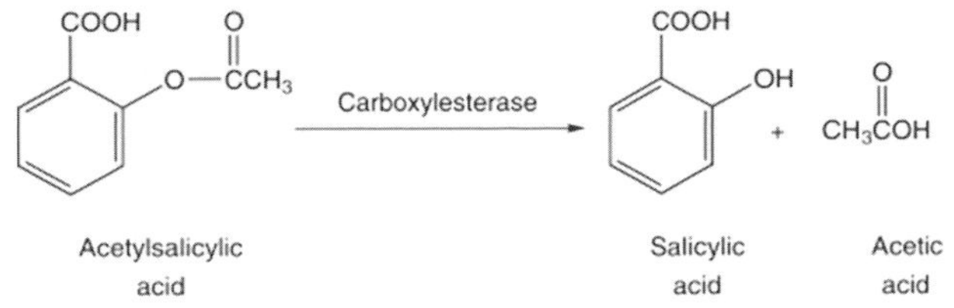

COOH O O—CCH$_3$ Carboxylesterase COOH OH + O CH$_3$COH

Acetylsalicylic acid Salicylic acid Acetic acid

Figure 8 Hydrolysis of acetylsalicylic acid (aspirin) to acetic acid and salicylic acid (a phenolic acid) by carboxylesterase activity.

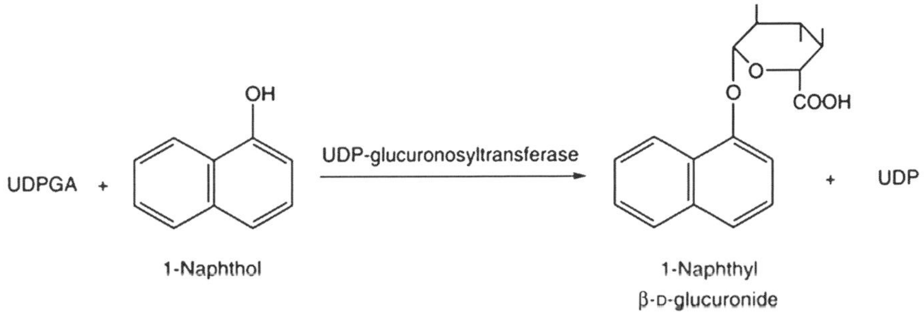

UDPGA + OH UDP-glucuronosyltransferase O COOH + UDP

1-Naphthol 1-Naphthyl β-D-glucuronide

Figure 9 Conversion of 1-naphthol to its corresponding β-D-glucuronide.

be reabsorbed and the cycle repeated. This process is called enterohepatic circulation and accounts for the prolonged excretion of some xenobiotics that are readily glucuronidated.

Certain β-glucuronides are electrophilic in nature and may also function in toxication processes. Covalent binding of the aglycone portions of several carboxylic acid (ester) glucuronides is known to occur to nucleophilic sites on serum albumin *via* transacylation reactions, for example.

Sulfotransferases

Another very common phase II reaction for phenols is conjugation with sulfate to form sulfate esters (**Figure 10**). Other substrates for this pathway include alcohols, primary and secondary amines, hydroxylamines, and sulfhydryl compounds such as thiophenols. These reactions are catalyzed by a family of cytosolic enzymes, the sulfotransferases, which require 3′-phosphoadenosine 5′-phosphosulfate (PAPS) as the cofactor.

The sulfotransferases have been divided into several groups as a result of substrate specificity determinations with purified enzymes and molecular biology studies; aryl sulfotransferases are active toward phenols, hydroxylamines, tyrosine esters, and catecholamines; alcohol sulfotransferases are active toward primary and secondary steroid alcohols; and amine sulfotransferases are active toward arylamines.

A few sulfate esters are chemically reactive and alkylate nucleophilic sites on macromolecules. This electrophilic characteristic implicates these conjugates as ultimate chemical toxicants.

Phenols, quantitatively important P450-derived metabolites of aromatic hydrocarbons, are substrates for both UDP-GT and sulfotransferases. Generally, glucuronide metabolites predominate after administration of a phenol or phenol precursor to mammals because sulfate formation is a high-affinity, low-capacity (due to sulfate depletion) system, whereas glucuronidation is a low-affinity, high-capacity system.

Glutathione *S*-Transferases

The glutathione (L-γ-glutamyl-L-cysteinylglycine; GSH) *S*-transferases (GSTs) are a multigene family of dimeric proteins found at relatively high concentrations in the cytosolic fraction of mammalian liver, as well as in a wide variety of extrahepatic tissues. Some GST isozymes are also localized in microsomes and within the mitochondrial matrix of the liver at much lower concentrations than the cytosolic enzymes.

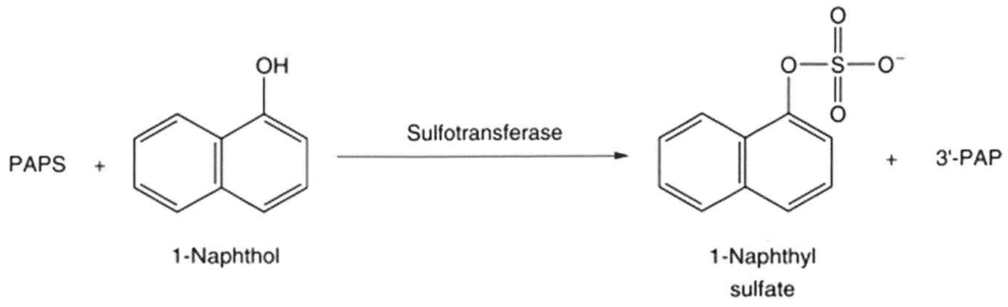

PAPS + OH Sulfotransferase O—S(=O)(=O)—O$^-$ + 3′-PAP

1-Naphthol 1-Naphthyl sulfate

Figure 10 Conversion of 1-naphthol to 1-naphthyl sulfate by sulfotransferases.

A wide variety of potentially toxic electrophilic compounds (**Figure 11**) are converted to S-substituted GSH adducts by this family of enzymes. These include aromatic compounds containing good leaving groups (halogen, sulfate, sulfonate, phosphate, and nitro). Halogens are readily displaced from aromatic compounds as long as they are activated by the presence of electron-withdrawing groups (e.g., nitro). Strained three-membered rings, such as alkene and arene oxides, and four-membered lactones are readily cleaved by GSTs. The major factor in the transferase-catalyzed reaction of these substrates with GSH is the electrophilicity of the carbon atom where the thiol attacks. Since electrophilic chemicals are frequently very toxic, the importance of the GSTs in detoxication cannot be overstated.

GSTs also catalyze a number of reactions in which an S-substituted GSH adduct is not formed or in which this adduct is oxidized glutathione. Examples of these reactions include the release of nitrate from nitrate esters and the release of cyanide from thiocyanates. Some GSTs also have glutathione peroxidase activity.

Although catalysis by GSTs is almost always associated with detoxication, a few substrates (e.g., the ethylene dihalides) are bioactivated to more toxic products by this pathway. Recent studies have also shown that glutathione conjugates are selectively accumulated in epithelial cells of the kidney where they are hydrolyzed. Those releasing metabolites that can undergo oxidation–reduction cycling result in cell-specific renal toxicity.

Mercapturic Acid Biosynthesis

A large variety of compounds, mostly xenobiotics, are excreted in urine as S-substituted *N*-acetylcysteines, also called mercapturic acids (**Figure 12**). The initial enzymatic reaction in their formation is catalyzed by the GSH *S*-transferases, as described previously. Subsequently, the glutamic acid residue is removed by γ-glutamyltranspeptidase, an enzyme with very high activity in the kidney. Next, the glycine moiety is removed by dipeptidases, which have cysteinylglycinase activity. The resulting S-substituted cysteine is converted to the corresponding mercapturic acid by *N*-acetyltransferase activity (see below).

Although mercapturic acids are normally the major thioether products of lipophilic xenobiotics found in urine of mammals, small amounts of the corresponding *S*-cysteine conjugates are also frequently excreted. All four thioether products formed during mercapturic acid biosynthesis are routinely excreted in bile.

Cysteine Conjugate β-Lyase/Thiomethylation

In addition to being acetylated to mercapturic acids, some S-substituted cysteine conjugates are also hydrolyzed. The key enzyme in this reaction sequence is cysteine conjugate β-lyase, which cleaves the cysteine adduct to a free thiol, ammonia, and pyruvate (**Figure 13**).

This enzyme is present in the cytosolic fraction of rat liver and kidney and also in the microflora of the gut. Because thiols may be toxic and are more lipophilic than their cysteine conjugate precursors, β-lyase is generally a toxication pathway.

Thiols formed by mammalian or bacterial β-lyase *in vivo* are substrates for *S*-methyltransferase (**Figure 14**), an enzyme widely distributed in mammalian tissues.

This pathway accounts for the thiomethyl metabolites formed from several classes of xenobiotics. Thiomethyl metabolites can be further oxidized by the microsomal flavin-containing monooxygenases to their corresponding sulfoxide and sulfone derivatives.

Acyl-Coenzyme A: Amino Acid *N*- Acyltransferases

Several types of xenobiotic carboxylic acids (aromatic, heteroaromatic, arylacetic, and aryloxyacetic) are conjugated with a variety of endogenous amino acids, including glycine, glutamine, or taurine, prior to excretion in mammals. An amide (peptide) bond is formed between the carboxylic acid group and the α-amino group of the amino acid during

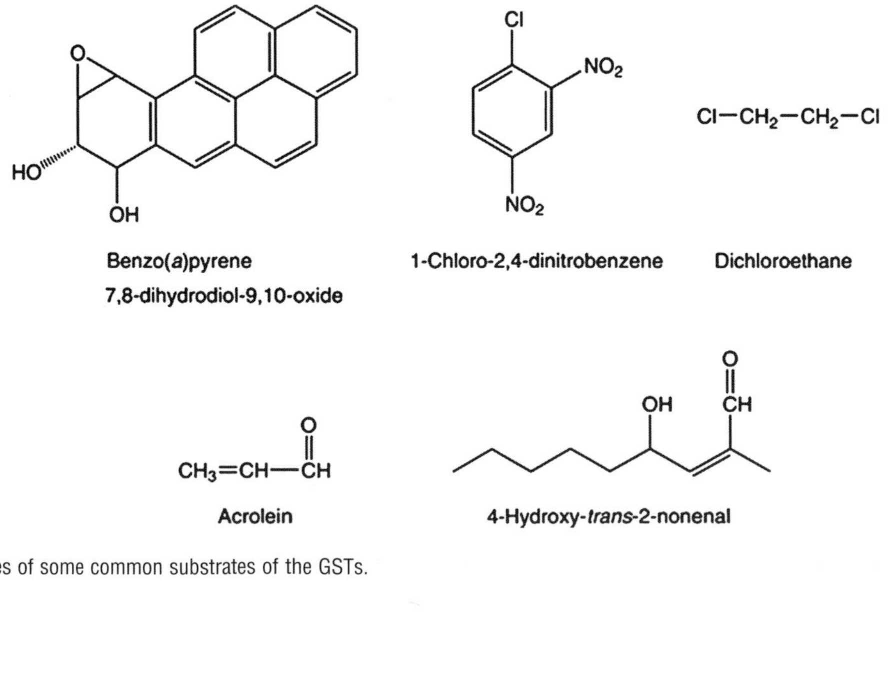

Figure 11 Structures of some common substrates of the GSTs.

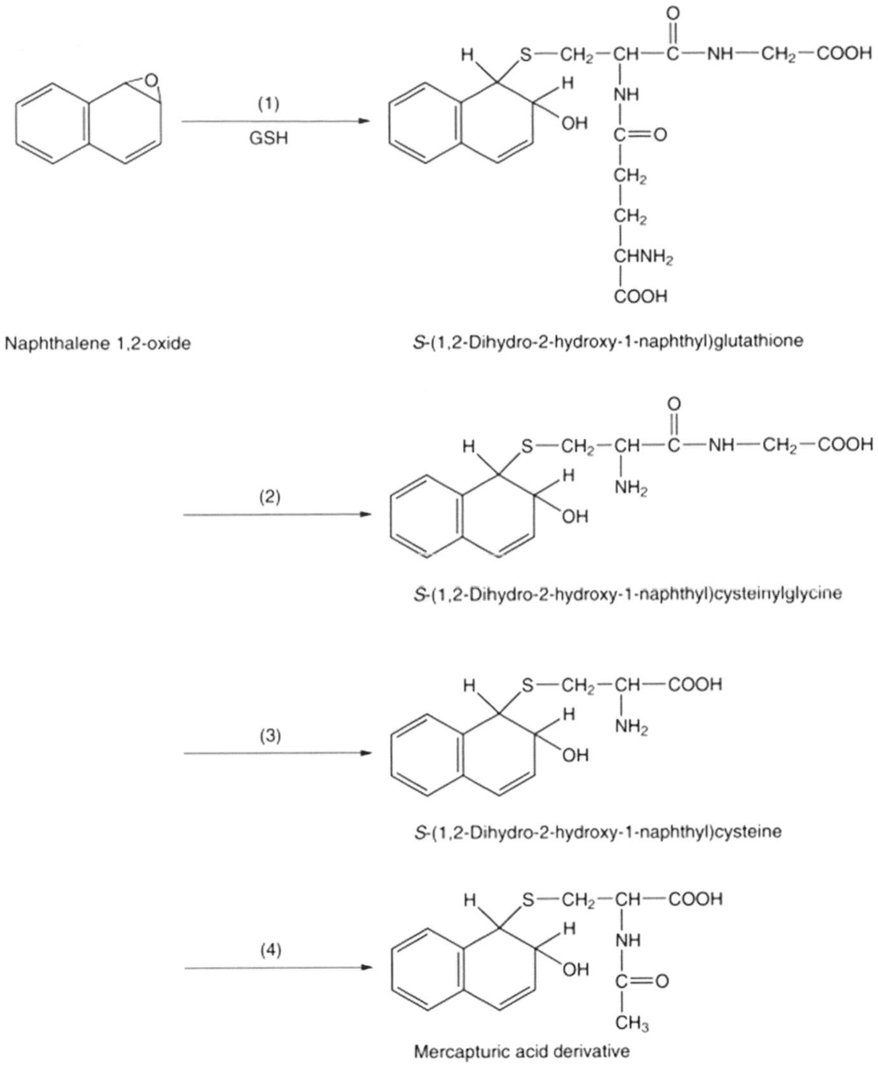

Figure 12 Mercapturic acid biosynthesis from a naphthalene 1,2-oxide. Only one of the isomers resulting from reaction of GSH with the arene oxide is shown. (1) GST, (2) γ-glutamyltranspeptidase, (3) cysteinylglycinase activity (dipeptidases), and (4) *N*-acetyltransferase.

conjugation. The reactions involved in the conversion of a carboxylic acid (e.g., benzoic acid) to its glycine derivative (hippuric acid) are illustrated in **Figure 15**.

Conversion of the carboxylic acid to its coenzyme A (CoA) ester derivative is the rate-limiting step. The enzyme that catalyzes the final reaction, acyl-CoA:amino acid *N*-acyltransferase, is localized in the mitochondria of the kidney and liver. The amino acid substrate selectivity, which varies from species to species, resides in the specific *N*-acyltransferase that catalyzes this reaction. In most mammalian species conjugation with glycine predominates.

N-Acetyltransferases

Acetylation of xenobiotic primary amine groups is a common metabolic pathway, whereas acetylation of xenobiotic hydroxyl and sulfhydryl groups is not. Primary aliphatic and aromatic amines, sulfonamides, hydrazines, and hydrazides are readily

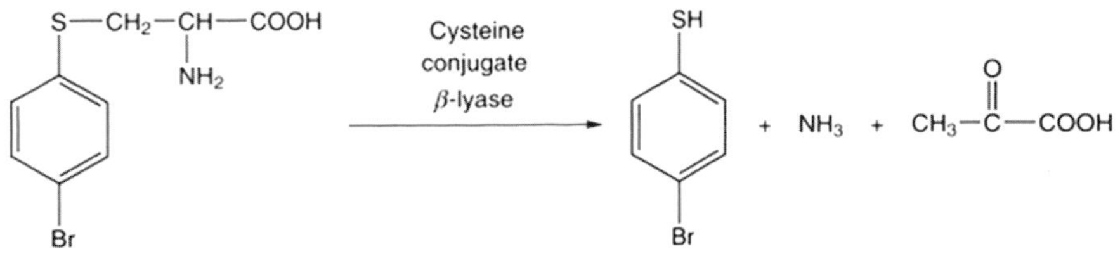

Figure 13 Hydrolysis of *S*-4-bromophenyl-L-cysteine by cysteine conjugate β-lyase.

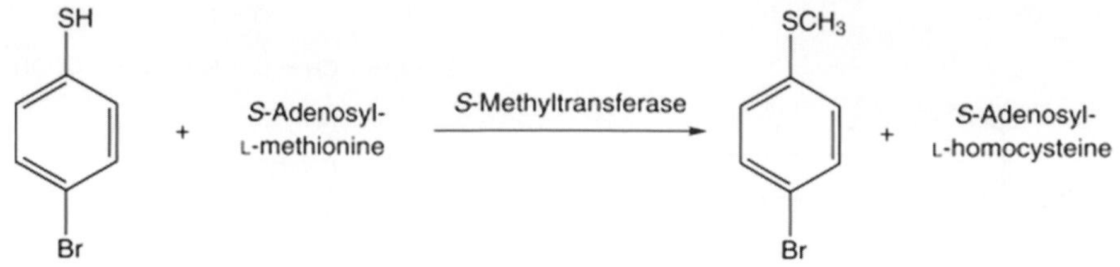

Figure 14 S-methylation of 4-bromothiophenol by *S*-methyltransferase.

N-acetylated *in vivo*, and the reaction is catalyzed by various acyl-CoA:*N*-acetyltransferases, commonly called *N*-acetyltransferases, as shown in **Figure 16**.

This family of enzymes is cytosolic and is widely distributed in a variety of mammalian tissues. There are also enzymes that hydrolyze N-substituted acetamides (i.e., amidases, as described previously) and the extent to which free versus acetylated amines are present *in vivo* depends on the relative rates of the acetylation and deacetylation reactions, on the physical and chemical properties of the two products, and whether or not the amine is metabolized by competing pathways. Some acetylated hydroxamic acids are chemically reactive and appear to be ultimate carcinogens.

N- and *O*-Methyltransferases

S-Adenosyl-L-methionine (SAM)-dependent methylation was briefly discussed under thiomethylation (see **Figure 14**). Other functional groups that are methylated by this mechanism include aliphatic and aromatic amines, N-heterocyclics, monophenols, and polyphenols. The most important enzymes involved in these methylation reactions with xenobiotics are catechol *O*-methyltransferase, histamine *N*-methyltransferase, and indolethylamine *N*-methyltransferase; each catalyzes the transfer of a methyl group from SAM to phenolic or amine substrates (*O*- and *N*-methyltransferases, respectively). Methylation is not a quantitatively important metabolic pathway for xenobiotics, but it is an important pathway in the intermediary metabolism of both N- and O-containing catechol and amine endobiotics.

Regulation of Biotransformation

The biotransformation and elimination of numerous potentially toxic xenobiotic compounds requires the concerted function of phase I and phase II enzymes. As such, exposure to elevated concentrations of xenobiotics can lead to the coordinate induction of genes encoding these enzymes. This inducibility is mediated by ligand-activated transcription factors that serve as sensors of intracellular xenobiotic concentration. Upon binding with xenobiotic compounds, these receptors interact with the regulatory region of target genes and increase the rate of gene transcription. Ultimately, this leads to an increase in the

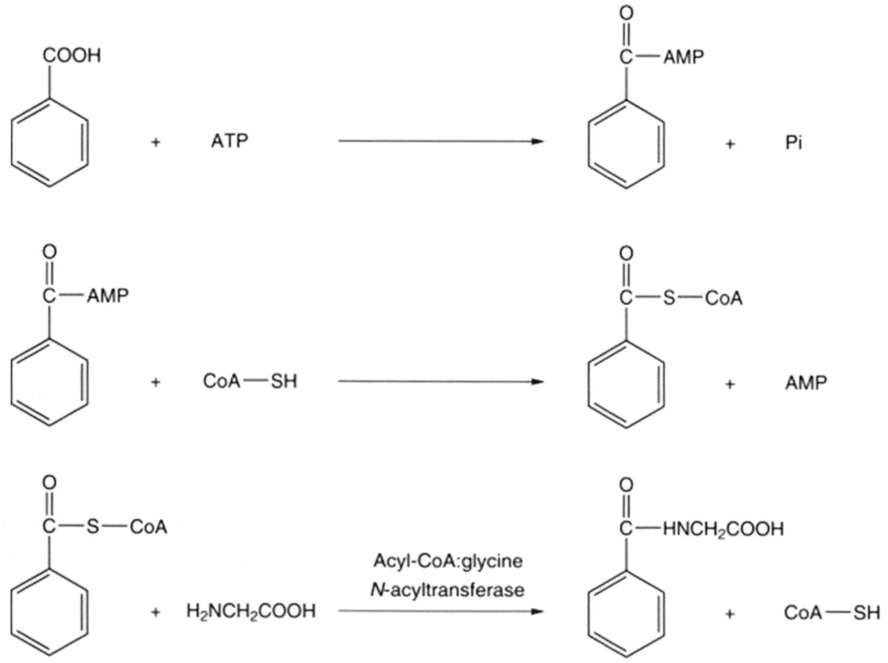

Figure 15 Metabolism of benzoic acid via its acyl-CoA derivative to hippuric acid (benzoylglycine).

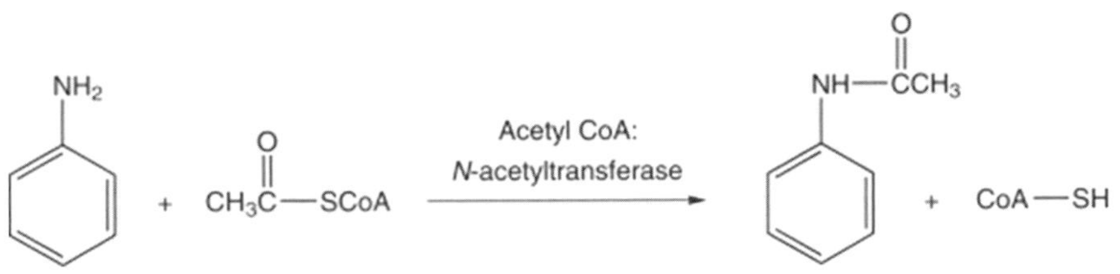

$$C_6H_5NH_2 + CH_3C(=O){-}SCoA \xrightarrow[\textit{N}\text{-acetyltransferase}]{\text{Acetyl CoA:}} C_6H_5NH{-}C(=O)CH_3 + CoA{-}SH$$

Figure 16 Acetylation of aniline by acyl-CoA:*N*-acetyltransferase activity.

amount of phase I and phase II enzymes and the rate of biotransformation of the xenobiotic substrate. This process is self-limiting as the induction in metabolism ultimately leads to a decrease in the intracellular concentration of xenobiotic and thus induction of the target gene. Examples of ligand-activated transcription factors that activate biotransformation include the aryl hydrocarbon receptor that is activated by polycyclic aromatic hydrocarbons such as the pro-carcinogen benzo[*a*]pyrene; the pregnane X receptor and the constitutive androstane receptor that are activated by a large group of structurally diverse xenobiotic and endobiotic compounds, and the peroxisome proliferator-activated receptor-alpha that is activated by a number of herbicides, industrial solvents, and plasticizers.

Variability in Biotransformation

Numerous genetic variants have been described for genes encoding phase I and phase II metabolic enzymes. These polymorphisms are heterogeneous and can be associated with a variety of genetic changes ranging from discrete changes in a single DNA base (single nucleotide polymorphisms (SNPs)) to duplications/deletions of an entire gene. Regardless of the nature of the change, all have the potential to affect the expression of the gene and/or the inherent activity of the enzyme encoded by that gene. As discussed previously, the expression of many genes encoding biotransformation enzymes is induced by exposure to xenobiotics. This, along with genetic polymorphisms, is a major reason underlying variability in biotransformation and consequently, the susceptibility of an individual to toxicity from a particular xenobiotic. Among the most highly polymorphic phase I enzymes is CYP2D6 with more than 80 genetic variants identified in humans. These polymorphisms result in four phenotypes that can be broadly classified as poor, intermediate, extensive, and ultrarapid metabolizers. Given that CYP2D6 is involved to some degree in the metabolism of 15–25% of drugs in current use, including most antidepressant drugs, numerous cardioactive compounds, and codeine, these polymorphisms have a significant clinical impact on the dosage requirements and risk for toxicities associated with these xenobiotics. Polymorphisms have also been described for genes encoding phase II enzymes. In particular, genetic variants of GST are associated with variability in xenobiotic conjugation and cancer susceptibility. For example, individuals possessing certain SNPs in the GSTP1 gene are at increased risk for toxicity and cancers on exposure to cytotoxic alkylating agents and topoisomerase inhibitors as a consequence of defective conjugation of these compounds.

Summary

A number of enzyme systems have evolved in animals and plants that effectively convert lipophilic xenobiotics to more polar compounds that are efficiently excreted. Phase I enzymes, responsible for oxidation, reduction, and/or hydrolysis, are integrated with phase II or conjugation enzymes for reactions of both types and are normally required for the formation of products polar enough to be readily excreted. The intracellular level of these enzymes, and, thus, the capacity for biotransformation, increases in a coordinate fashion in response to exposure to xenobiotic compounds. This response is achieved through changes in gene expression that are mediated by a number of ligand-activated transcription factors that serve as intracellular sensors of xenobiotic concentration. While the primary role of biotransformation is the elimination of potentially toxic xenobiotics, toxic metabolites can also be formed, primarily but not exclusively, during oxidation. When the concentration of these reactive metabolites exceeds the capacity of detoxication systems, acute (necrosis) or chronic (mutagenesis, carcinogenesis, and teratogenesis) toxicity can occur. Thus, anything that results in the reduced biotransformation of a toxic xenobiotic to an inactive metabolite, or alternatively, that increases the conversion of a relatively harmless xenobiotic to a reactive metabolite(s) increases the probability that a toxic response will occur.

See also: Carboxylesterases; Glutathione; Kidney; Liver; Pharmacokinetics.

Further Reading

Cashman, J.R., Zhang, J., 2006. Human flavin-containing monooxygenases. Annu. Rev. Pharmacol. Toxicol. 46, 65–100.

Crettol, S., Petrovic, N., Murray, M., 2010. Pharmacogenetics of phase I and phase II drug metabolism. Curr. Pharm. Des. 16, 204–219.

Hines, R.N., 2008. The ontogeny of drug metabolism enzymes and implications for adverse drug events. Pharm. Ther. 118, 250–267.

Jana, S., Mandlekar, S., 2009. Role of phase II drug metabolizing enzymes in cancer chemoprevention. Curr. Drug Metab. 10, 595–616.

Klaassen, C.D., 2008. Casarett & Doull's Toxicology: The Basic Science of Poisons, seventh ed. McGraw-Hill, New York.

Kohalmy, K., Vrzal, R., 2011. Regulation of phase II biotransformation enzymes by steroid hormones. Curr. Drug Metab. 12, 104–123.

Lewis, D.F., Ito, Y., 2010. Human CYPs involved in drug metabolism: structures, substrates and binding affinities. Expert Opin. Drug Metab. Toxicol. 6, 661–674.

Omiecinski, C.J., Vanden Heuvel, J.P., Perdew, G.H., Peters, J.M., 2011. Xenobiotic metabolism, disposition, and regulation by receptors: from biochemical phenomenon to predictors of major toxicities. Toxicol. Sci. 120 (Suppl. 1), S49–S75.

Saghir, S.A., Khan, S.A., McCoy, A.T., 2012. Ontogeny of mammalian metabolizing enzymes in humans and animals used in toxicological studies. Crit Rev Toxicol 42, 323–357.

Tolson, A.H., Wang, H., 2010. Regulation of drug-metabolizing enzymes by xenobiotic receptors: PXR and CAR. Adv. Drug Deliv. Rev. 62, 1238–1249.

Relevant Website

http://www.niehs.nih.gov/ – National Institutes of Environmental Health Sciences.

Bio Warfare and Terrorism: Toxins and Other Mid-Spectrum Agents

M Balali-Mood, Newcastle University, Newcastle Upon Tyne, UK, and Medical Toxicology Research Centre, Imam Reza Hospital, Faculty of Medicine, Mashhad University of Medical Sciences, Mashhad, Iran
M Moshiri, School of Pharmacy, Mashhad University of Medical Sciences, Mashhad, Iran
L Etemad, Pharmaceutical Research Center, Mashhad University of Medical Sciences, Mashhad, Iran

This article is a revision of the previous edition article by James M. Madsen, volume 1, pp 273–279, © 2005, Elsevier Inc.

Biological warfare is the deliberate use of disease-causing biological agents such as bacteria, virus, rickettsiae, and fungi, or their toxins, to kill or incapacitate humans, animals, or plants as an act of war. Some biological warfare agents (BWAs) can cause deterioration of material, for example, petroleum-eating bacteria. Entomological (insect) warfare is also considered as a type of BWA. BWAs can be natural or genetically modified. The effects of these types of warfare agents are not immediate, as there is an incubation period, and thus there will be a short or long time delay. The other advantages of BWAs over chemical weapons (CW) are a smaller amount of effective materials is required; BWAs are odorless and colorless. Some BWAs live and reproduce inside the host to cause incapacitating or fatal diseases. A very small quantity of BWA may be sufficient to cause morbidity and mortality. Some BWAs are highly infectious (e.g., plague and smallpox), and can be spread to a large population within a few days, causing epidemics and sometimes pandemics. In addition, specialized equipment and a huge infrastructure are not required for the production of BWAs; a very small laboratory is sufficient for their production. A small amount of pure culture is required to initiate production, which is quite easy to obtain commercially now. Some biological agents, such as anthrax and brucellosis, occur naturally in animals in certain parts of the world and can be obtained easily. Therefore, all these features as well as difficulty in detection make BWAs weapons of choice for mass destruction. Some of the rare toxins, such as saxitoxin, can be used on a very limited scale to target one or a few individuals but currently cannot be used as weapons of mass destruction. Agents that have a very short half-life or those that are subject to rapid degradation in the environment once released are, by definition, poor bioweapons. On the other hand, those with long half-lives, or those that degrade very slowly due to environmental influences such as temperature extremes, dryness, or ultraviolet radiation, would be more useful as weapons, assuming other requirements are met. Anthrax spores are one example of an ideal agent from this stand point.

Various ways of disseminating BWAs include (1) aerosol sprays, the most common delivery method; the ideal BWA particle size that would allow it to be carried for long distances by prevailing winds and inhaled deeply into the lungs of the unsuspecting victims is 1–5 μm in diameter; (2) explosive devices (artillery, missiles, detonated bombs); they are not as effective as aerosols because BWAs tend to be destroyed by the blast, typically leaving less than 5% of the agent capable of causing disease; (3) contamination of food or water; (4) absorption or injection into the skin; used for assassination, not for mass casualties.

Based on the risk to national security, these agents have been prioritized into three categories: A, B, and C.

Category A BWAs

Category A BWAs are highly toxic and have the following characteristics:

- High morbidity and mortality especially when they are used on civilian populations
- Easily disseminated or transmitted from person to person
- Highly infectious with a low dose when disseminated by aerosol, with a commensurate ability to cause large outbreaks
- Effective vaccine unavailable or available only in limited supply
- Potential to cause public and health care worker anxiety
- Pathogen or toxin easily available
- Large-scale production feasible
- Environmentally stable
- Prior research and development done on its use as a biological weapon

Anthrax, botulism, plague, smallpox, tularemia, and viral hemorrhagic fever are some of the diseases caused by category A agents.

Anthrax

Bacillus anthracis is a large, gram-positive, aerobic, encapsulated, easy spore-forming, nonmotile, rod-shaped bacillus. *B. anthracis* is considered to be the most efficient agent for large-scale biological attack, because its spore size (3–6 μm) makes it suitable for aerolization and consequently its deposition in the alveoli of human lungs. Mortality from respiratory anthrax is high. The infective dose for 50% of humans (ID_{50}), by inhalation, is estimated to be 8000–40 000 spores (about 10^{-6} g). It was used frequently in World War I, World War II, in the Soviet Union in 1979, and in Japan in 1995. Also in 2001, some letters contaminated with *B. anthracis* spores were mailed to NBC News and the offices of Senator Tom Daschle in the United States.

Edema toxin (ET) and lethal toxin (LT) are important endotoxins. ET is a calcium- and calmodulin-dependent adenylyl cyclase that distributes water hemostasis by greatly increasing the level of cAMP in the cell. ET may be responsible for infection site edema. LT is a zinc metalloprotease that cleaves members of the mitogen-activated protein kinase and induces apoptosis in macrophages.

Anthrax is a zoonotic disease and humans are infected by coming into contact with infected animals. Cutaneous, gastrointestinal, and respiratory anthrax are different forms of the disease. After penetration *via* the skin, gastrointestinal system, or respiratory system, the *B. anthracis* spores are phagocytosed by macrophages and vegetated, multiplied, and distributed. In the respiratory system, vegetated bacteria produce toxins and cause edema and hemorrhagic necrosis of the mediastinum. Bloody plural effusion, neck edema, dry cough, and stridor are consequences of the extension of the hemorrhage and necrosis into adjacent tissues.

Inhalational anthrax is typically a biphasic illness. The first phase starts 4–6 days after exposure, with malaise, low-grade fever, gastrointestinal complaints, and nonproductive cough. After a brief improvement, the second phase presents with orthopnea, stridor, dry cough, tachypnea, high fever, chills, and profound diaphoresis. Patients may have abdominal pain, hematemesis, melena, and suppurative and hemorrhagic meningitis. The end stage is characterized by delirium and coma followed by death due to cardiovascular collapse.

An enzyme-linked immunosorbent assay (ELISA) to detect IgG response to protective antigen is highly sensitive (98.6%) but it is only 80% specific. *B. anthracis*-specific nucleic acid amplification and detection by polymerase chain reaction (PCR) of sterile fluids (blood, pleural fluid) is also useful.

B. anthracis is sensitive to the fluoroquinolones, rifampin, tetracycline, vancomycin, imipenem and meropenem, chloramphenicol, clindamycin, and the aminoglycosides. But some strains of *B. anthracis* produced for BWA purposes may resist one or some of these antibiotics. A naturally occurring disease can be treated for 7–10 days. But a bioterrorism-related disease should be treated for at least 60 days because of the potential for concurrent respiratory exposure. Aggressive supportive care such as a chest tube for plural effusion and glucocorticosteroids for anthrax meningitis, substantial mediastinal, or neck edema are advocated. A vaccine (anthrax vaccine adsorbed) is currently licensed in the United States but is available only to military personnel.

Plague

Yersinia pestis is a gram-negative, nonmotile, facultatively anaerobic, non-spore-forming coccobacillus. Like anthrax, plague is a zoonosis and humans are occasionally hosts for the *Y. pestis* life cycle between rodents and fleas. It occurs by human contact with fluids from infected animals. Humans can also be infected by respiratory droplets in cases of plague pneumonia as well as animal droplets. In addition, *Y. pestis* is transmitted from rodents to humans by fleas.

Plague has some of the criteria for a high-risk BWA. It easily infects humans *via* the respiratory tract and is easily distributed. Pneumonic plague has a high attack rate and produces severe clinical disease with significant psychological stress. The three major forms of *Y. pestis* infection in humans are: classic bubonic plague, primary septicemic plague, and pneumonic plague.

Emigration of *Y. pestis* from the inoculation site to regional lymph nodes where they replicate results in necrotizing adenitis, which is characteristic of bubonic plague. The bacteria then disseminate to other organs, including lungs, spleen, and the central nervous system through secondary buboes, causing hypotension, oliguria, altered mental status, and disseminated intravascular coagulation (DIC).

Bubonic plague presents with acute febrile lymphadenitis, which develops 2–8 days after transdermal contact with fever, chills, hadache, and malaise before or simultaneously with the appearance of the bubo. Patients are febrile, tachycardic, frequently hypotensive, episodic agitated, and have tender hepatosplenomegaly. Primary septicemia is associated with metastatic infection, DIC, purpuric skin lesions (due to vasculitis and occlusion by fibrin thrombi), and acral gangrene (the likely basis of the epithet, The Black Death). Primary pneumonic plague results from inhalation of droplets containing bacilli and presents with abrupt onset of fever and flu-like symptoms 2–4 days after exposure and rapidly progresses to fulminating pneumonia and respiratory failure. This form of plague is readily transmissible by airborne droplets. Plague can be diagnosed with duplicate cultures of blood or body fluids, Gram staining of aspirated fluid from the bubo, sputum, blood, or cerebrospinal fluid, or by fluorescent antibody testing. Streptomycin is the drug of choice; however, gentamicin, doxycycline, and chloramphenicol are also effective. However, strains of bacteria that are used as BWAs may be resistant to these drugs. The pneumonic and septicemic forms have a high fatality rate despite treatment; bubonic plague is less fatal. A vaccine consisting of formaldehyde-killed bacilli had been licensed in the United States and is reserved for military and laboratory personnel and those with a high occupational risk of exposure.

Tularemia

Francisella tularensis is a small, aerobic, nonmotile, gram-negative coccobacillus. Tularemia is a zoonosis. It is transmitted by arthropod vectors among animal reservoirs, rabbits, deer, squirrels, mice, and beavers. Human infection is incidental and occurs most often *via* an insect bite or contact with contaminated animal products. It disseminates easily, has high infectivity, and the capacity to cause serious illness and death. *F. tularensis* infects patients through the skin, lungs, gastrointestinal tract, or mucous membranes, but it is not transmitted person to person. Infectivity of bacteria depends on the site of entrance; for example, 10 organisms are enough for inhalation-induced disease and 108 organisms are needed for enteral infection.

Tularemia can present with a range of manifestations from asymptomatic to rapidly progressive, fulminant, and fatal disease. It is related to inoculum size, portal of entry, host immune status, and virulence of the strain. The clinical course of untreated nonfulminant disease has been described as having three phases: 31 days of fever, 31 days of bed rest, and 31 days of disability. Six forms of the disease, with different presentations, have been described. However, they have significant overlap: ulceroglandular (21–78%), glandular (3–20%), oculoglandular (<5%), oropharyngeal (<12%), pneumonic (7–20%), and typhoidal (5–30%).

In all forms of tularemia, a history of exposure and a high clinical suspicion are essential for diagnosis. There are some nonspecific laboratory findings, such as leukocytosis and increased sedimentation rate, sterile pyuria, thrombocytopenia, hyponatremia, increased levels of aspartate aminotransferase/alanine aminotransferase, and evidence of rhabdomyolysis. The mainstay of diagnosis is serology: ELISA, microagglutinin, hemoagglutinin, and tube agglutinin assays are available. Historically, streptomycin has been the treatment for tularemia, but antibiotics such as gentamicin, ciprofloxac, tetracycline, doxycycline, or chloramphenicol, are alternative treatments. Mortality from tularemia decreases from 35% in untreated patients to 1% with treatment. A live attenuated vaccine is recommended for laboratory personnel routinely working with *F. tularensis*. The vaccine confers incomplete protection, but the disease course is milder. In BWA attacks with tularemia, exposed persons (adults and children) should receive oral doxycycline or ciprofloxacin for prophylaxis.

Botulinum Toxins

Clostridium botulinum toxins (BoNTs) are the causative agents of a diseased condition called botulism, and are produced by the bacteria *Clostridium botulinum*, a gram-positive, anaerobic spore-forming bacteria. These toxins are released on the death and lysis of the organism. BoNTs are the most poisonous substances ever known. A single gram of crystalline toxin can kill more than one million people. The toxin is 100 million times more toxic than cobra venom and 100 000 times more toxic than the most dreaded CW nerve agent, sarin. However, when humans are exposed *via* the pulmonary route, BoNTs are slightly less toxic. A recent estimate for the human lethal dose 50% (LD_{50}) by inhalation is 3 ng kg^{-1}.

BoNTs quickly degrade in the environment and are rendered nonlethal within minutes after release, although technical factors would make such dissemination difficult. BoNTs are unstable for extended periods in water and are easily destroyed by chlorination. Municipal water reservoirs are most likely safe from contamination by this toxin. BoNTs could also be released as aerosols in missiles and bombs.

There are seven antigenically distinct BoNTs (A to G). Although neurotoxins A, B, E, and F cause naturally occurring human botulism, it is assumed that all seven toxins can cause botulism in humans if the exposure level is high enough. The toxin subtype and the level of intoxication are indicated by the rapidity of the onset of symptoms, and the severity and duration of the disease.

The pulmonary tract (inhalation botulism), the gastrointestinal tract (food-borne and infant botulism), and mucous membranes of wounds (wound botulism) are three natural routes of entry of BoNTs. BoNTs can then enter the circulatory system and be transported to the neuromuscular junctions of motor neurons, the site of action. They mainly block the release of the acetylcholine, and thereby prevent transmission of nerves impulses. However, very high doses of BoNTs can block the release of other types of neurotransmitters. Neurotoxic activity of BoNTs includes three stages: binding, internalization, and enzymatic activity. The protein called synaptotagmin may be the receptor for botulinum toxin and has a role in internalization and toxicity.

The clinical hallmark of botulism is acute flaccid paralysis, which begins with bilateral cranial nerve impairment involving the muscles of the eyes, face, head, and pharynx and then descends symmetrically to involve the muscles of the thorax and the extremities. Signs and symptoms characterizing the onset of the disease include blurred vision, ambiopia, ptosis, and photophobia, followed by signs of bulbar nerve dysfunction such as dysarthria, dysphonia, and dysphagia. Its incubation period is typically 12–72 h. Death may result from respiratory failure due to upper airway occlusion caused by paralysis of the tongue or pharyngeal muscles, or diaphragm and intercostal muscles paralysis.

Classically, botulism in humans occurs as food poisoning. The symptoms appear several hours to 1 or 3 days after contaminated food is consumed. When food contaminated with bacteria or their preformed toxins is ingested, nausea, abdominal pain, vomiting, and diarrhea may often precede or accompany the neurologic signs. A confirmatory diagnosis comes from mouse bioassays demonstrating toxin in the blood or stool, neutralized by the appropriate antisera.

Inhalational botulism, the syndrome most likely to be seen on the battlefield, is rare. Accidental respiratory exposure to BoNTs occurred in a laboratory in Germany and was reported in 1962. Three laboratory workers, who had contact with BoNTs, presented (1) a mucous plug in the throat, (2) difficulty in swallowing solid food, and (3) the beginning of a cold without fever on the third day after exposure. Then, the severity of their signs increased and they complained of mental numbness and retarded ocular motion, moderately dilated pupils with slight rotary nystagmus, slurred speech, and extreme weakness.

The diagnosis of botulism under battlefield conditions might not be easy, especially in the early stages. However, the symptoms listed earlier for inhalation botulism are almost pathognomonic for botulism prior to development of respiratory failure. Some differential diagnosis such as intoxication from chemical nerve agents and neurotoxic snake bite should be considered. The absence of convulsions is the difference between botulinum intoxication and chemical nerve agent poisoning. The most likely means of laboratory diagnosis is through ELISA identification of botulinum toxin from swabs taken from the nasal mucosa within 24 h of inhalational exposure. With effective supportive therapy, mortality from botulism can be reduced to 10%.

There are two basic alternatives for prophylaxis from BoNT poisoning: active immunization using a vaccine, or passive immunotherapy using immunoglobulin. Because of the rapid action of BoNTs and that very small amounts do not cause disease, natural protection against botulism does not involve the generation of antitoxin antibodies. A licensed vaccine for botulism is not available, but pentavalent (ABCDE) botulinum toxoid (PBT) is available in the United States. PBT has been used for more than 30 years in over 3000 laboratory workers in various countries.

Category B BWAs

Category B includes a wide group of pathogenic microorganisms and toxins with varying clinical characteristics, ranging from being difficult to develop as weapons (e.g., viruses) with significant mortality to being easy to develop as weapons (e.g., bacteria). They induce clinical syndromes with minimal mortality and include pathogens with unproven risk as weapons.

Q Fever

Coxiella burneti, an obligate intracellular bacterium, is a pleomorphic, gram-negative coccobacillus. It is highly resistant to environmental stresses such as high temperature, osmotic pressure, and ultraviolet light, and can survive in the environment for a long time. Its characteristics make it suitable for a BWA. It causes Query fever (Q fever), which is a zoonosis, and its reservoirs are cattle, sheep, goats, and similar animals. Humans are infected occasionally. A single inhaled organism could infect a person. Human-to-human transmission is rare.

Clinical manifestations and the incubation period depend on the infecting dose, the characteristics of the infecting strain, and the host immune status. Q fever presents as either asymptomatic, a self-limited febrile illness, an atypical pneumonia, or hepatitis.

Atypical pneumonia, which occasionally presents as a cough, rales, or pleuritic chest pain with pleural-based opacities on radiographs, occurs in 50% of cases. This pneumonia can result in a life-threatening acute respiratory distress syndrome. Severe headache is a useful clue in the diagnosis. One-third of patients suffer from symptomatic hepatitis. Chronic forms of Q fever include endocarditis, chronic granulomatous hepatitis, aseptic meningitis, and encephalitis. Diagnosis is usually based on serologic tests, such as complement fixation, indirect fluorescent antibody, and ELISA assay, because *C. burnetii* is difficult to culture. Antibiotic therapy reduces the risk of complications and morbidity. Tetracycline, doxycycline, chloramphenicol, ciprofloxacin, ofloxacin, and hydroxychloroquine, are useful. Q-Vax, a whole cell inactivated vaccine, is available.

Staphylococal Enterotoxin (Type B)

As a potential biological weapon, aerosolized *Staphylococcus aureus* enterotoxin type B (SEB) could cause 80% or more of targeted personnel to become extremely ill within 3–12 h. SEB is stable at boiling temperature and resistant to acids and alkalis. It might take up to 12 weeks for humans to recover from SEB poisoning, and higher concentrations of SEB could even cause septic shock and death. SEB is a super antigen; it acts by stimulating cytokine release (such as interferon gamma, interleukin-6, and tumor necrosis factor) and inflammation in systemic effects. In aerosolized exposure in humans, the estimated effective dose 50% (ED_{50}) is 0.0004 $\mu g\, kg^{-1}$, whereas the estimated LD_{50} is 0.02 $mg\, kg^{-1}$.

When SEB is ingested, it is a prevalent cause of acute diarrheal illness, which is associated with histamine and leukotriene release from mast cells. It causes a self-limited syndrome that starts hours after exposure and gradually wanes within 72 h. Most of the pyrogenic toxins produce the same signs and symptoms as toxic shock syndrome: a rapid drop in blood pressure, increased temperature, and multiple organ failure.

In 16 cases of SEB exposure *via* accidental inhalation, fever up to 41 °C occurred in all victims 8–20 h after the initial exposure. Myalgia, often associated with the initial fever, and shaking chill, heralded the onset of illness. SEB inhalation could elicit nonproductive cough and inspiratory rales with dyspnea. Densities compatible with patches of pulmonary edema and Kerley lines, suggesting interstitial edema, may show on chest radiographs. Other possible manifestations include: headache, usually mild by the second day; nausea; anorexia; vomiting after prolonged paroxysms of coughing; and hepatomegaly. Ocular exposure in humans can result in purulent conjunctivitis.

In animal models exposed to aerosolized forms of SEB, initial gastrointestinal symptoms were followed by death caused by pulmonary edema on the third day. At postmortem examination in monkeys, the lungs were diffusely heavy and wet, with multifocal petechial hemorrhages and areas of atelectasis. Clear, serous-to-white, frothy fluid often drained freely from the laryngeal orifice. The small and large intestines frequently had petechial hemorrhages and mucosal erosions.

Immunological evaluation of staphylococcal enterotoxins should be possible on samples collected because of its moderate stability. These methods can detect picogram amounts of toxin in environmental samples. If actual bacterial involvement is suspected, and if cultures can be obtained, the detection of extremely minute quantities of potentially toxigenic strains is possible by using (1) PCR amplification and (2) toxin gene–specific oligonucleotide primers. In individuals exposed to a respirable aerosol, toxin can be identified in nasal swabs 12–24 h later. This may be the best approach to early diagnosis on the battlefield.

Management of SEB poisoning is conservative. Fluids, rest, and judicious use of acetaminophen or aspirin are effective for the treatment of fever, muscle aches, and arthralgias. Symptomatic therapy should be considered for gastrointestinal manifestations. Cough suppressants containing dextromethorphan or codeine should be used initially for symptomatic relief of respiratory symptoms. A wide variety of formalin-inactivated and recombinant vaccines have been tested, but none has been approved for human use. Immune protection through anti-SEB antibodies has been outlined.

Epsilon Toxin of *Clostridium perfringens*

The epsilon toxin (ETX) is produced by *Clostridium perfringensis* types B and D. It is a gram-positive, rod-shaped, anaerobic, spore-forming bacterium. The other types of *C. perfringens* (A, C, E) cause various human diseases such as gas gangrene and necrotizing enteritis. Our knowledge is largely based on experience from animal models, because the types of *C. perfringens* carrying ETX are not human pathogens. ETX is a pore-forming protein and it seems to act through alteration of the permeability of the cellular membrane causing potassium and fluid to leak from cells. ETX is used in the form of an aerosol and through poisoning water or food supplies.

Attempts to develop a recombinant vaccine against ETX are currently under way, although a formalin-inactivated vaccine exists for susceptible animals. Treatment is most likely supportive. Hyperimmune serum might be helpful if given soon after exposure. In mice, a variety of drugs, including reserpine, diazepam, apomorphine, gammabutyrolactone, phenothiazines, and butyrophenone derivatives can prevent death or delay the effects of ETX, but only if they are given before exposure. A genetically modified toxin can protect mice against lethal challenge. In natural infections with type B strains, hyperimmune serum and antibiotics may be helpful. Toxoid vaccines can prevent type B and D enterotoxemia.

Ricin Toxin

Ricin toxin (RT) is the toxic glycoprotein of the seeds from castor oil plant (*Ricinus communis*). This plant is grown worldwide. RT is relatively easily extracted from the castor bean plant and is stable in both hot and cold conditions. It is toxic when ingested, injected, or even inhaled. Although it is 1000-fold less toxic than BoNTs, the characteristics mentioned above make RT suitable for use as a biological weapon and a weapon for assassination. It is been regarded as one of the most potent poisons ($LD_{50} = 3\ \mu g\ kg^{-1}$) and can cause death within minutes of exposure.

There are several reports on the use of ricin. After World War I, it was investigated as a potential BWA in the United States. Ricin has been used for assassination rather than as a weapon of mass destruction. However, there is some evidence that ricin has been used in artillery shells in Iraq. It was found in Afghanistan following the collapse of the Taliban Government in 2001, and it is suggested that ricin was used to assassinate three members of the KGB. It was also used in a terroristic attack on the White House in February 2004.

RT (64 kDa) consists of two peptide chains, A and B, which are linked by a disulfide bound. The B-subunit binds to glycoproteins on the surface of epithelial cells, enabling the A-subunit to enter the cell *via* receptor-mediated endocytosis. The A-subunit has the ability to modify catalytically the 28S subunit of eukaryotic ribosomes to block protein synthesis. One RT molecule can inactivate 2000 ribosomes per minute, which ultimately leads to the death of the cell. RT has no selectivity for specific cells. Therefore, all types of cells are affected. Native RT, or just the ricin A- chain, is conjugated to tumor cell–specific monoclonal antibodies, leading to an antitumor effect, and a number of these compounds have undergone phase I or phase II clinical trails.

The clinical manifestations and pathological findings of ricin toxicity vary with the dose and the locus of entry. They appear within 2–24 h and death may ensue within 36–72 h after exposure. Transient leukocytosis (two- to fivefold higher than normal) appears, whether intoxication is *via* injection or oral ingestion. In oral (and parenteral) intoxication, cells in the reticuloendothelial system, such as Kupffer cells and macrophages, are particularly susceptible, because of exclusive presence of the mannose receptor.

Due to poor absorption and some enzymatic digestion, RT is less toxic by oral ingestion than by other routes. When ingested orally, the patient presents rapid (less than a few hours) onset of nausea, vomiting, and abdominal pain; followed by diarrhea, hemorrhage from the anus, anuria, cramps, dilation of the pupils, fever, thirst, sore throat, headache, vascular collapse, and shock. Death occurs on the third day or later in 6% of symptomatic patients. On autopsy, multifocal ulceration and hemorrhage in gastric mucus and mucus from the small intestine are found. Other findings include lymphoid necrosis, Kupffer cell and liver necrosis, diffuse nephritis, diffuse splenitis, and spleen necrosis.

Intravenous low-dose RT administered to cancer patients were tolerated. Intravenous injection of a lethal dose of RT, as much as 500 μg in an assassination of a man, caused immediate local pain and weakness, followed by fever, tachycardia, swollen lymph nodes in the groin after 36 h. On the second day, he suffered from vascular collapse, shock, and leukocytosis, and on the third day, when he died, atrioventricular conduction block, anuria, and hematemesis were observed. Intramuscular or subcutaneous injection of RT has resulted in severe local lymphoid necrosis, gastrointestinal hemorrhage, liver necrosis, diffuse nephritis, and diffuse splenitis.

Our knowledge on the clinical manifestations induced by inhalation of RT is based on animal studies. Diffused necrotizing pneumonia with interstitial and alveolar inflammation and edema resulted from inhalation of a lethal dose of RT. The time to presentation, clinical manifestations, and time to death are dose dependent.

Epidemiological findings, such as very severe pulmonary distress in a previously healthy population, is likely to play a role in the early diagnosis of RT. ELISA analysis of a swab sample from the nasal mucosa is a useful method for diagnosis for at least 24 h after inhalational exposure. Because it is extremely immunogenic, its antibodies can be detected in serum within 2 weeks after exposure. Because RT acts rapidly and irreversibly (directly on lung parenchyma after inhalation or is distributed quickly to vital organs after parenteral exposure), therapy after exposure is more difficult. Therefore, immunization of personnel at risk for RT exposure is important. Some new type of RT vaccines have undergone early clinical trials.

Abrin Toxin

Abrin toxin (AT) is a plant toxin and is closely related to RT in terms of its structure and chemical properties. It is obtained from the seeds of *Abrus precatorius* (commonly known as jequirity bean or rosary pea). The mechanism of AT toxicity, like RT, involves ribosome inactivating protein synthesis; it seems that AT is more potent than RT. The clinical manifestations of AT poisoning are similar to RT in nature and time, and it ends in organ failure. The principles of management of AT poisoning are similar to those for RT.

Trichothecene Mycotoxins

Trichothecene mycotoxins (TrMs) including T2 toxin are produced by a number of fungi, such as *Fusarium, Trichoderma, Myrothecium, Stachybotrys, Cephalosporium, Verticimonosporium*, etc. These toxins have been used several times, for example, in air attacks in Laos, where it was described as "yellow rain," and in Afghanistan and Cambodia. Unconfirmed reports have also implicated the use of T2 toxin in Yemen and possibly in combination with mustards during CW attacks in the Iran–Iraq War.

These mycotoxins (especially T2 toxin) have excellent potential as weapons when delivered as dusts, droplets, aerosols, or smoke from aircraft, rockets, missiles, artillery, mines, or portable sprayers. T2 toxins are about 400-fold more potent (50 ng *versus* 20 μg) than mustard in producing skin injury. TrMs at lower doses are considered to be primarily blistering agents and at higher doses can produce considerable incapacitation and death within minutes to hours.

There are some reports on natural TrM-induced diseases: (1) food-related diseases caused by the presence of a mold, *Stachybotrys atra* (*S. alternans*), on the hay fed to domestic animals in Russia, Yugoslavia, and Hungary; (2) cotton lung disease, due to inhalation of cotton dust contaminated with *Dendrochium toxicum* in Russia; and (3) red mold disease from wheat in Japan.

TrMs are cytotoxic to most eukaryotic cells by inhibition of protein and scheduled DNA synthesis. They can move bidirectionally and freely across the plasma membrane and can also bind to ribosomes and mitochondria. In addition, TrMs inhibit electron transport activity, for example, inhibition of succinic dehydrogenase activity. TrMs are lipophilic and thus are easily absorbed from intestinal or pulmonary mucous membranes. However, their absorption rate through the skin is not as fast as the mucosa. TrMs do not require metabolic activation. The liver is the major organ for their metabolism. There are some factors that might affect the severity of disease in an individual exposed to TrMs. These factors include the nutritional status of the host, liver damage, intestinal infections, route of toxin administration, and stress.

Acute TrMs exposure can result in immunosuppression; central nervous system toxicity that presents as anorexia, lassitude, and nausea; suppression of reproductive organ function; hypotension and shock. Dermal exposure to TrMs causes irritation and local cutaneous necrosis and inflammation in combination with the formation of vesicles and bullae. Individuals who were exposed to the "yellow rain" in Laos suffered from severe nausea, vomiting, burning superficial skin, discomfort, lethargy, weakness, dizziness, and loss of coordination, followed by watery to bloody diarrhea. Gradually, they presented dyspnea, coughing, sore mouth, bleeding gums, epistaxis, hematemesis, abdominal pain, and mid-chest pain. Exposed cutaneous areas can become red, tender, swollen, painful, or pruritic. Also vesicles and bullae can form; and petechiae, ecchymoses, and black, leathery areas of necrosis can appear. The potency of T2 for skin damage is 100 times more than other CW agents, even sulfur mustard. Eye contact with TrMs leads to tearing, burning sensation, and blurred vision that might last a couple of weeks.

Chronic exposure to TrMs causes a disease condition called alimentary toxic aleukia (ATA) with four different stages. ATA in man is characterized by leukopenia, agranulocytosis, necrotic angina, a hemorrhagic rash, sepsis, exhaustion of the bone marrow, bleeding from the nose, throat, and gums, and fever.

Different sizes of aerosols can involve not only the upper and lower respiratory tracts, but can also lead to secondary exposure in the gastrointestinal tract, after clearing of the tracheobronchial tree, as happened in Southeast Asia.

The following events suggest the occurrence of a biological warfare attack with TrMs:

- Clinical findings that match the symptoms and signs listed above
- High rate of attacks and fatality
- All types of dead animals
- Onset of symptoms after yellow rain or red, green, or white smoke or vapor attack

As with other BWAs and CWAs, use of masks and protective clothes, as well decontamination of the skin with soap and water, on approach to patients exposed to TrMs is important. Delayed skin washing, even up to 4–6 h after exposure, might be effective. Standardized critical care toxicology should be performed for individuals who are exposed to TrMs. Symptomatic and supportive measures for the treatment of exposure to TrMs are almost the same as for casualties of mustard gas poisoning. Upper respiratory irritation can be relieved by steam inhalation and codeine, or other cough suppressing substances. The early use of high doses of systemic glucocorticosteroids may increase survival time by decreasing the primary injury and the shock-like state. Based on animal studies; administration of activated charcoal, magnesium sulfate, selective platelet-activating factor antagonists and methylthiazolidine-4-carboxylate, which enhances the hepatic glutathione content, may be effective.

Category C BWAs

The agents classified as category C by the Centers of Disease Control and Prevention are emerging pathogens that could someday be engineered for mass exposure because of availability, ease of production and dissemination, and potential for high morbidity and mortality. Category C BWAs include hanta viruses, multidrug-resistant tuberculosis, Nipah virus, the tick-borne encephalitis viruses, the tick-borne hemorrhagic fever viruses, and yellow fever. Preparedness for category C agents requires ongoing research to improve disease detection, diagnosis, treatment, and prevention. Newly emergent pathogens for possible use as a BWA or in a terrorist attack are impossible to know in advance and require studies using new technologies.

See also: Blister Agents/Vesicants; Botulinum Toxin; Chemical Warfare; Gastrointestinal System; Ricin and Other Toxalbumins; *Staphylococcus aureus*; Sulfur Mustard; Toxicity, Acute.

Further Reading

Switala, C.A., Coren, J., Filipetto, F.A., Gaughan, J.P., Ciervo, C.A., 2011. Bioterrorism – a health emergency: do physicians believe there is a threat and are they prepared for it? American J. Disaster Med. 6 (3), 143–152. Review.

Sarkar-Tyson, M., Atkins, H.S., 2011. Antimicrobials for bacterial bioterrorism agents. Future Microbiol. 6 (6), 667–676. Review.

Dhaked, R.K., Kumar Singh, M., Singh, P., Gupta, P., 2010. Botulinum toxin: Bioweapon and magic drug. Indian J. Med. Res. 132, 489–503.

Kumar, A., Verma, A., Yadav, M., Sabri, I., Asthana, A., 2011. Biological warfare, bioterrorism and biodefence. J. Indian Acad. Forensic Med. 33, 69–73.

Vrat Kamboj, D., Goel, A.K., Singh, L., 2006. Biological warfare agents. Def. Sci. J. 56, 495–506.

Rusnak, M., Kortepeter, M., Ulrich, R., Poli, M., Boudreau, E., 2004. Laboratory exposures to Staphylococcal Enterotoxin B. Emerg. Infecti. Dis. 10, 1544–1549.

Frischknecht, F., 2003. The history of biological warfare. EMBO Reports 4, s47–s52.

Relevant Websites

Wikitox: http://curriculum.toxicology.wikispaces.net/2.4.1+Biological

Bradford: http://www.brad.ac.uk/acad/sbtwc/

http://sis.nlm.nih.gov/enviro/biologicalwarfare.html

http://www.bt.cdc.gov/bioterrorism/

http://www.cbsnews.com/8301-201_162-20128968/feds-militia-plot-involved-d.c-ricin-attack

http://fhp.osd.mil/factsheetDetail.jsp?fact=34, etc

Bis (2-Methoxyethyl) Ether

SC Gad, Gad Consulting Services, Cary, NC, USA

- Chemical Abstracts Service Registry Number: 111-96-6
- Synonyms: Diglyme, Dimethoxy diethylene glycol, Diethyl glycol dimethyl ether, 2-(2-Methoxyethoxy)-1-methoxyethane, (2-Methoxyethyl) ether
- Molecular Formula: $C_6H_{14}O_3$
- Chemical Structure:

$H_3C-O-CH_2CH_2-O-CH_2CH_2-O-CH_3$

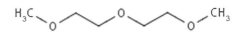

Background

Bis (2-methoxyethyl) ether, also known as diglyme, is a linear aliphatic diether widely used as a solvent and present as a clear liquid at room temperature with a mild ether odor. The compound is not known to occur in nature. It is synthesized from ethylene oxide and methanol in the presence of either acidic or basic catalysts. The reaction is based on the classic Williamson ether synthesis. It can also be produced from diethylene glycol and dimethyl sulfate. In June 2012, ECHA proposed addition of diglyme to the REACH very high concern list.

Uses

Bis (2-methoxyethyl) ether, due to being chemically inert and possessing excellent solvent properties, is mainly used as a solvent and an anhydrous reaction medium for organometallic synthesis. It is also used as a solubilizer.

Environmental Fate and Behavior

- Relevant physicochemical properties
  Freezing point = −68 °C.
  Boiling point = 162 °C.
  Log K_{ow} = −0.36.
  Solubilities: Miscible with alcohol, ether, hydrocarbon solvents; soluble in benzene; miscible in water.
  Henry's law constant = 5.23×10^{-7} atm-cu m mol^{-1} at 25 °C.
- Routes and pathways
- Partition behavior in water, sediment, and soil
  Atmospheric fate: Bis (2-methoxyethyl) ether will present as a vapor, when released to air, at a vapor pressure of 2.96 mmHg at 25 °C. The vapor phase is easily degraded in the atmosphere by reaction with photochemically produced hydroxyl radicals. The half-life for the reaction is estimated to be 22 h. Bis (2-methoxyethyl) ether does not contain chromophores that will absorb at wavelengths >290 nm and therefore is not expected to be susceptible to direct photolysis by sunlight.
  Terrestrial fate: Bis (2-methoxyethyl) ether has very high mobility in soil based on the estimated K_{oc} of 15, when released to soil. It may volatilize from dry soil surfaces based upon its vapor pressure.
  Aquatic fate: Bis (2-methoxyethyl) ether does not absorb to suspended solids and sediments when released into water. Hydrolysis is not an important environmental matter because bis (2-methoxyethyl) ether does not contain a functional group that can hydrolyze under environmental conditions.
- Environmental persistency
  Bis (2-methoxyethyl) ether is considered moderately persistent in the environment. Bis (2-methoxyethyl) ether releases into the environment are to be expected from its use as a solvent, reaction medium, and separating agent in industrial processes. Bis (2 methoxyethyl) ether is miscible in water and has a low Henry's law constant leading to a low volatility from aqueous solutions. From this and its use pattern, it is expected that the main target compartment of the chemical will be the hydrosphere.
- Long-range transport
  Bis (2-methoxyethyl) ether is easily deposited with rain and other wet deposition. From its short half-life in atmospheric reactions, long-distance transport of bis (2-methoxyethyl) ether in ambient air is assumed to be negligible.
- Bioaccumulation and biomagnification
  An estimated BCF of 3 was calculated in fish for bis (2-methoxyethyl) ether. This suggests that the potential for bioconcentration in aquatic organisms is low.

Exposure and Exposure Monitoring

- Routes and pathways
  Dermal, inhalation, and ingestion.
- Human exposure
  Occupational exposure to bis (2-methoxyethyl) ether may occur through inhalation and dermal contact with this compound at workplaces where it is being produced or used. Monitoring data indicate that the general population may be exposed to bis (2-methoxyethyl) ether via inhalation of vehicle exhaust and ingestion of contaminated drinking water.
- Environmental exposure
  Bis (2-methoxyethyl) ether production and use as a solvent and an anhydrous reaction medium for organometallic synthesis or as a solubilizer may result in its release to the environment through various waste streams.

Toxicokinetics

Multiple studies on the metabolism of bis (2-methoxyethyl) ether in experimental animals demonstrated that the compound is rapidly and completely absorbed from the gastrointestinal tract of both rats and mice. There are two principal pathways for metabolism of bis (2-methoxyethyl) ether including an oxidative dealkylation and an oxidative demethylation. Both are implicated to involve cytochrome P-450 enzyme. The oxidative dealkylation begins with the cleavage of an interior ether bond to formally give two molecules of 2-methoxyethanol, which has been extensively investigated with regard to its metabolism and toxicity. 2-Methoxyethanol is then oxidatively converted, by way of the aldehyde, to yield 2-methoxyacetic acid. This metabolite, 2-methoxyacetic acid, has shown evidence of accumulation in animals and in greater concentrations in human. In humans, its half-life was calculated to be 77 h. 2-Methoxyacetic acid has also been associated with testicular toxicity in male experimental animals and development of the conceptus in pregnant female animals. In rats, most of the 2-methoxyacetic acid is excreted in the urine but some is conjugated with glycine to produce the amide *N*-methoxyacetyl glycine. The oxidative demethylation, on the other hand, by unspecified cytochrome P-450 isozymes to give 2-(2-methoxyethoxy) ethanol, which is then oxidatively converted by way of the corresponding aldehyde to give 2-(2-methoxyethoxy)acetic acid. The major route of elimination is through the urine.

Mechanism of Toxicity

The metabolite 2-methoxyacetic acid, which is generated from 2-methroxyethanol by the reaction of alcohol dehydrogenase, may be important for the toxic effects. It can undergo activation to methoxyacetyl coenzyme A and enter the Krebs cycle or fatty acid biosynthesis. Several metabolites of 2-methoxyethanol, such as 2-methoxy-*N*-acetyl glycine, have been identified that support this pathway. Thus, 2-methoxyacetic acid may interfere with essential metabolic pathways of the cell, and it was hypothesized that this causes the testicular lesions and malformations in experimental animals.

Acute and Short-Term Toxicity

The acute oral toxicity of bis (2-methoxyethyl) ether is low. The oral LD_{50} for the rat is 5400 mg kg^{-1} bw and for the mouse 6000 mg kg^{-1} bw. Poisoning symptoms are restlessness and breathing difficulties. Necropsy of animals found dead revealed changes in lung and liver. Bis (2-methoxyethyl) ether is not a sensitizer.

Chronic Toxicity

Repeated-dose toxicity studies by the oral and/or inhalation route demonstrated that the male reproductive organs followed by the bone marrow are important target organs for high-level bis (2-methoxyethyl) ether exposure.

Reproductive Toxicity

The main targets in male animals after repeated intake of bis (2-methoxyethyl) ether are the reproductive organs. In a 2-week inhalation studies in male rats, dose-dependent decreases in weights of testes, epididymides, prostate, and seminal vesicles were observed. The testes were atrophic and damage of the spermatocytes was also observed. Experiments with mice showed morphologically altered sperm, mainly with amorphous heads, after exposure to 1000 ppm or 5580 mg l^{-1}. The positive results may be due to the effects of bis (2-methoxyethyl) ether on fertility. Bis (2-methoxyethyl) ether is also a strong teratogen. It was found to be a developmental toxicant both via inhalation and oral ingestion in rats, rabbits, and mice. It is capable of disrupting normal morphogenesis in a wide variety of tissues and organ systems. The reproductive toxicity of bis (2-methoxyethyl) ether is attributed to the minor metabolite of 2-methoxyacetic acid.

Genotoxicity

Multiple *Salmonella typhimurium* reverse mutation assays show lack of mutagenic activity in the presence or absence of metabolic activation and *in vitro* DNA damage and chromosome aberration studies have produce negative results. A study investigating the *in vivo* genotoxicity of bis (2-methoxyethyl) ether after inhalation exposure indicated a lack of genotoxic activity as evidenced by no increase in bone-marrow cell chromosome aberrations after exposures to levels of bis (2-methoxyethyl) ether that cause testicular damage.

Clinical Management

Following any route of exposure, remove from exposure or possible sources of exposure. In cases of ocular exposure, flush eye thoroughly, do not use ointment, and seek medical attention. In cases of dermal exposure, remove any contaminated clothing and wash skin with gentle soap thoroughly. Treat skin with an emollient and if irritation persists, seek medical attention. In cases of inhalation exposure, seek medical attention. If ingested, do not induce vomiting, if breathing has stopped, administer mouth to mouth resuscitation and seek medical attention. Further treatment is symptomatic.

Ecotoxicology

- Freshwater/sediment organisms toxicity
  Bis (2-methoxyethyl) ether exhibited a low toxicity to aquatic organisms.
- Marine organisms toxicity
  None known.
- Terrestrial organisms toxicity
  Due to lack of measured exposure levels, a sample risk characterization with respect to terrestrial organisms cannot be performed. However, from the use pattern of bis (2-methoxyethyl) ether, significant exposure of terrestrial organisms is not to be expected.

Other Hazards

Bis (2-methoxyethyl) ether is easily absorbed through dermal route due to its high reprotoxic potency. Therefore, all exposure of the general public to bis (2-methoxyethyl) ether should be avoided.

Exposure Standards and Guidelines

A guidance value for uptake of bis (2-methoxyethyl) ether via inhalation, a value of 0.1 ppm or $0.6\ \mathrm{mg\ l^{-1}}$ would be obtained. For the oral route, a guidance value of $0.25\ \mathrm{mg\ kg^{-1}}$ body weight would be obtained.

See also: Diethylene Glycol; Dimethyl Ether; Solvents.

Further Reading

Ferro Corporation, 2003. Diglyme. Robust Summaries & Test Plans. Submitted to U.S. EPA HPV Challenge Program. http://www.epa.gov/chemrtk/pubs/summaries/diglyme/c15023tc.htm (accessed 6.06.12).

IPCS Inchem, 2002. Diethylene Glycol Dimethyl Ether. World Health Organization. http://www.inchem.org/documents/cicads/cicads/cicad41.htm (accessed 6.06.12).

Relevant Website

http://toxnet.nlm.nih.gov – Search for Bis (2-methoxyethyl) ether.

Bis-Chloromethyl Esther *see* Chloromethyl Ether, Bis-

Bismuth

SC Gad, Gad Consulting Services, Cary, NC, USA

- Name: Bismuth
- Chemical Abstracts Service Registry Number: 7440-69-9
- Valence State: +3

Background Information

Bismuth has been used for centuries, although it is often confused with other metals with similar properties, such as tin and lead. Bismuth is one of the first elements known to man, although uses for it have been developing more recently than most others that have been known for a long time. Like water, the solid form is less dense than the liquid, known as a density anomaly.

Uses

Several bismuth compounds have been used medicinally. Some are used for gastrointestinal distress (Pepto-Bismol® contains bismuth subsalicylate). Others are used as salves and, in rare cases, for treatment of parasites. In the past, bismuth was also used to treat syphilis and malaria.

Commercially, bismuth is also used in the manufacture of permanent magnets, semiconductors, and thermoelectric materials; as a catalyst in making acrylonitrile; and as an additive to improve the machinability of steels and other metals.

Bismuth is also frequently used in cosmetics, generally nail polish and lipstick.

Environmental Fate and Behavior

In aerated water, bismuth oxidizes; however, in an anaerobic aqueous environment, bismuth is unaffected. Similarly, in the atmosphere, bismuth is unaffected unless condensation or deposition of water occurs.

Due to the inability for air and water to affect bismuth under most circumstances, bismuth tends to persist until wet or dry deposition, and therefore long-range transport is possible and likely.

Exposure and Exposure Monitoring

The primary exposure pathway for bismuth is from medicinal preparations that are administered orally or intramuscularly. For the general population, the total daily intake via food is ~5–20 mg, with much smaller amounts contributed by air and water. The cosmetic use of bismuth compounds still continues to be fairly widespread.

Toxicokinetics

Bismuth compounds are considered to be poorly to moderately absorbed following inhalation, topical application, or ingestion. Gastrointestinal absorption depends on the water solubility of bismuth salts. Citrate enhances intestinal absorption. Absorbed bismuth is distributed throughout the soft tissues and bone. The biological half-life for whole-body retention is ~5 days, but intranuclear inclusions containing bismuth seem to remain for years in the kidneys of patients treated with bismuth compounds. Peak plasma bismuth concentrations were noted within 1 h of consuming colloidal bismuth subcitrate, with none being detected by 4 h. Bismuth can accumulate, however, with repeated colloidal bismuth subcitrate exposures. Bismuth binds to plasma proteins and concentrates in the kidneys, the liver (to a lesser extent), and the skin. Bismuth can displace bound lead, thus increasing the concentration of lead in the circulatory system. Urine is the major route of excretion. For some bismuth compounds, elimination may be split equally between urine and feces.

Mechanism of Toxicity

The mechanism by which bismuth produces toxicity has not been identified. Interaction with thiol compounds has been proposed as a primary mechanism.

Acute and Short-Term Toxicity (or Exposure)

Animal

The oral rat LD_{50} for bismuth metal is $5\ g\ kg^{-1}$. Insoluble salts, for example, bismuth nitrate and bismuth trioxide, also have reported oral LD_{50} values in rats of $4–5\ g\ kg^{-1}$.

Human

Oral human LD_{Lo} is equal to $221\ mg\ kg^{-1}$. Adverse acute reactions to bismuth include acute renal failure following ingestion of excessive concentrations. Bismuth can cause nausea, vomiting, and abdominal pain within hours of exposure. Muscle cramps

 http://dx.doi.org/10.1016/B978-0-12-386454-3.00822-8

and weakness, blurred vision, and hyperreflexia may be exhibited. Liver transaminase activities may be elevated.

Chronic Toxicity (or Exposure)

Animal

In animals, bismuth interferes with the metabolism of copper and zinc, induces metallothionein, and can alter heme biosynthesis in the liver and kidney. Bismuth has not been found to be carcinogenic in animal models. Bismuth subnitrate can decrease Leydig cell density and plasma testosterone levels in rats.

Human

High-level exposure causes renal failure with degeneration and necrosis of the epithelium of the renal proximal tubules, fatty changes and necrosis of the liver, reversible dysfunction of the nervous system, skin eruptions, and gingivitis and pigmentation of the gums and intestine. Effects in humans also include reversible neurotoxic and sometimes fatal encephalopathy and bone weakness. Symptoms of bismuth poisoning include fever, weakness, pain similar to rheumatism, and diarrhea. Certain people display a rash. Bismuth salts may cause contact sensitivity. The bone and brain may also be targets for toxicity.

Reproductive Toxicity

There is currently no evidence suggesting that bismuth is a reproductively toxic material in animals or humans.

Genotoxicity

Bismuth subsalicylate (Pepto-Bismol) was negative in the Ames assay at concentrations up to 0.67 mg per plate. There have been some more recent studies with bismuth in reverse mutation or chromosome aberration that showed positive results from treatment with bismuth.

Carcinogenicity

While data on the carcinogenesis of bismuth are limited, there are studies that have shown that bismuth subcarbonate does not induce cancerous growth or affect survival rates in experimental animals.

Clinical Management

There does not appear to be an antidote of choice for bismuth toxicity in humans. Gastric lavage can be used within 1 h of exposure. Replace fluids and electrolytes. Monitor renal and liver function for several days and treat failure conventionally. The newer chelating agents, meso-2,3-dimercaptosuccinic acid and D,L-2,3-dimercapto-propane-L-sufonic acid, are being investigated experimentally as antidotes for bismuth toxicity, and the latter has been shown to be effective. In mice, D-penicillamine has proven effective.

Ecotoxicology

Little information is available on the ecotoxicity of bismuth or bismuth compounds, although data suggest that while bismuth escapes into the environment regularly, and can be solubilized by acid rain, there are no health effects on plants, animals, or humans.

Exposure Standards and Guidelines

The permissible exposure limit (PEL), threshold limit value (TLV), and recommended exposure limit for bismuth metal have not been established. The PEL for bismuth trioxide is 15 mg m^{-3}. The PEL for bismuth subsalicylate is 15 mg m^{-3}, and the TLV is 10 mg m^{-3}.

Miscellaneous

Bismuth is the most highly diamagnetic and the least effective thermal conductor among metals.

See also: Metallothionein; Metals.

Further Reading

Bingham, E., Cohrssen, B. (Eds.), 2012. Patty's Toxicology, sixth ed. John Wiley & Sons, Hoboken, NJ.

Fowler, B.A., Sexton, M.J., 2009. Bismuth. In: Nordberg, G.F., Fowler, B.A., Nordberg, M., Friberg, L.T. (Eds.), Handbook on the Toxicology of Metals, third ed. Elsevier, New York, pp. 433–445.

Pedersen, L.H., Stoltenberg, M., Ernst, E., West, M.J., 2003. Leydig cell death in rats exposed to bismuth subnitrate. J. Appl. Toxicol. Jul–Aug 23 (4), 235–238.

Reynolds, P.T., Abalos, K.C., Hopp, J., Williams, M.E., 2012. Bismuth toxicity: a rare cause of neurologic dysfunction. Int. J. Clin. Med. 3, 46–48.

Winship, K.A., 1982. Toxicity of bismuth salts. Adverse Drug React Acute Poisoning Rev 2: 103–121; J. Appl. Toxicol. 23, 235–238.

Relevant Websites

http://toxnet.nlm.nih.gov – TOXNET, Specialized Information Services, National Library of Medicine. Search for Bismuth.

http://www.intox.org – International Programme on Chemical Safety.

Bisphenol A

JE Goodman, Gradient, Cambridge, MA, USA
MK Peterson, Gradient, Seattle, WA, USA

This article is a revision of the previous edition article by Alan L. BlanKenship and Katie Loady, volume 1, pp 314–317, © 2005, Elsevier Inc.

- Bisphenol A
- Chemical Abstracts Service Registry Number: CAS 80-05-7
- Synonyms: 4,4′-(1-Methylethylidene)bisphenol; 4,4′-Bisphenol A; 4,4′-Isopropylidenediphenol; Phenol, 4,4′-(1-methylethylidene)bis-; 2,2-(4,4′-Dihydroxydiphenyl)propane
- Molecular Formula: C_{15}-H_{16}-O_2
- Chemical/Pharmaceutical/Other Class: Phenolic
- Chemical Structure:

HO–C6H4–C(CH3)2–C6H4–OH

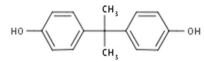

Background (Significance/History)

Bisphenol A (BPA) was first synthesized in 1891, but it was not used widely until applications in the plastic industry were identified the 1950s. One method of production is by the condensation of 2 mol of phenol with 1 mol of acetone while bubbling hydrogen chloride through the mixture. In 1953, the polycarbonate plastic manufacturing process was described using BPA as the starting material. Commercial production of polycarbonates began in 1957 in the United States and in 1958 in Europe.

Uses

BPA is one of the highest production chemicals in the world, with a total production of over 3.7 million metric tons per year. Approximately 90% of all BPA is used as an intermediate in the production of epoxy resins and polycarbonate plastics. Epoxy resins are used as food-contact surface coatings for cans (to allow high-temperature sterilization), metal jar lids, coatings and finishes, automobile parts, adhesives, aerospace applications, and as a coating for polyvinyl chloride (PVC) water pipe walls. Polycarbonate plastics are hard, shatter-proof plastics used to make numerous products, such as eyeglass lenses, water bottles, and consumer electronics. Some, but not all, dental sealants contain BPA. In addition, BPA is a component of some specialty applications, such as flame retardants, and as an antioxidant and stabilizer in the production of PVC and other plastics.

Exposure and Exposure Monitoring

Although BPA can be released into the environment during the production, processing, and use of BPA-containing materials, levels in environmental samples are generally very low or undetectable. This is because BPA has low volatility and a short half-life in the atmosphere, is rapidly biodegraded in water, and is not expected to be stable, mobile, or bioavailable from soils. Most human exposures occur *via* residues contained in food or beverages that have been in contact with polycarbonate plastic or with containers lined with epoxy resins, as these products can contain trace amounts of the original compound, and additional BPA may be generated during the breakdown of the product.

Human exposures to BPA have been estimated based on (1) levels of BPA measured in human blood and urine, (2) human and other primate pharmacokinetic data, and (3) food intake estimates. Estimates based on urine measurements and pharmacokinetic data suggest BPA intakes that range from <0.03 to $1.61\ \mu g\,kg^{-1}\,day^{-1}$, while those based on food intake studies report ranges of <0.01–$13\ \mu g\,kg^{-1}\,day^{-1}$. Food intake estimates often are based on worst-case scenarios, such as assuming infants drink milk or formula strictly out of polycarbonate bottles. Early estimates based on measured concentrations in human blood suggest exposures as high as 5–$480\ \mu g\,kg^{-1}\,day^{-1}$. This discrepancy was addressed in a robust study in which blood and urine samples were collected hourly over 24 h from 20 volunteers who ate meals enriched with canned food at the laboratory. The average urinary BPA level among volunteers was higher than estimates for 95% of the US population based on a Centers for Disease Control and Prevention study, confirming high exposures. All blood samples contained BPA levels below the limit of detection, which is consistent with the amount measured in urine and what was predicted based on prior pharmacokinetic studies, and indicates that blood measurements from prior studies were most likely inaccurate. Blood samples have been shown to be contaminated with BPA from tubing and solvents used during sample collection and processing, which could have led to the erroneously high measurements.

Toxicokinetics

The toxicokinetics of BPA have been extensively studied in rats, primates, and humans. While there are many similarities regarding how these species absorb, metabolize, and excrete this compound, there are also some significant differences that are critical to understand its potential toxicity.

Several studies have demonstrated the rapid clearance of BPA following oral administration in adult rats. The principal metabolite of BPA in the rat is BPA-monoglucuronide (BPA-glucuronide), but there are route- and dose-dependent differences in the toxicokinetics of BPA in this species. BPA administered by the oral route has reduced bioavailability and greater metabolism when compared with the subcutaneous

 http://dx.doi.org/10.1016/B978-0-12-386454-3.00366-3

route of exposure. This is consistent with the role of the liver and gut in the first-pass metabolism of BPA through the oral exposure route. Age dependency for the elimination of BPA-glucuronide was also observed with more rapid elimination of BPA-glucuronide from the plasma of neonates ($t_{1/2}$: 1.9–9.8 h) when compared with adult animals ($t_{1/2}$: 4.6–22.5 h), likely due to reduced microflora ß-glucuronidase activity in neonates and thus an absence of enterohepatic recirculation. Nearly complete metabolism of BPA to BPA-glucuronide (94–100% of the plasma radioactivity) was observed at a dose of 1 mg kg^{-1}. Unlike the parent compound, BPA-glucuronide is not a ligand for the estrogen receptor. Studies indicate that BPA does not accumulate in body fat or sex organs of either male or female test animals, but is excreted *via* the urine and feces.

Pharmacokinetic studies in adult rhesus monkeys have found that BPA is eliminated with a similar profile as rats (primarily *via* the BPA-glucuronide, with a slightly higher percentage as the sulfate conjugate), although the elimination is even more rapid *via* oral and intravenous administration ($t_{1/2}$: 2.5–3.6 h). As with rats, there is decreased bioavailability *via* the oral route due to first-pass metabolism in the gut and liver. In contrast to the age dependence observed in rats, rhesus monkey neonates did not exhibit a different metabolic profile – elimination half-lives were essentially the same as adults ($t_{1/2}$: 2.6–4.6 h). In general, for both adults and neonates, 0.1–2% of the total BPA dose was present in the unconjugated form following oral administration. It was reported that the pharmacokinetics in adult monkeys dosed at 100 μg kg^{-1} body weight was similar to that in humans.

In BPA-dosed human volunteers, BPA was cleared from human blood and urine with a half-life between 5 and 7 h ($t_{1/2}$: 5–7 h), and the applied dose was completely recovered in the urine in the glucuronide form. As with nonhuman primates, most of the BPA to which humans are exposed is metabolized in the liver and intestine and then eliminated in urine, so a very low percentage (estimated to be about 1%) reaches the general circulation, and BPA does not accumulate in the body after ingestion. Although BPA in rodents is also metabolized in the liver and intestine, enterohepatic recirculation after oral exposure (discussed above) prolongs the maintenance of BPA at low levels in systemic circulation in these animals.

Mechanism of Toxicity

Initial investigations of BPA's endocrine activity with the MCF-7 human breast cancer cell line showed that BPA binds to the estrogen receptor with a relative potency that is three to four orders of magnitude less than that of 17ß-estradiol. BPA elicited estrogenic effects (e.g., increased cell proliferation) at concentrations at or above 2 mg l^{-1}. In addition to acting as a weak estrogen mimic, BPA also competitively inhibits estrogen from binding to the estrogen receptor. Recent *in vitro* studies have confirmed that BPA acts as a weak agonist at the estrogen receptor as well as an antagonist at the androgen receptor. These studies found increased expression of estrogen receptor 1-α and androgen receptors in prostate cells treated with BPA. In addition, some studies have also found alternative receptor pathways for BPA, including activation of protein kinases *via* a membrane G-protein-coupled estrogen receptor, and high-affinity binding to the estrogen-related receptor-γ.

In vivo studies have reported a variety of endocrine-related effects for BPA. In addition to confirming estrogen-like activity and inhibition of estrogenic activity, exposure to BPA in animal models at relatively high doses has been associated with alterations in hypothalamic–pituitary function, differential modulation of ER-α protein expression, impact on brain organization *via* corticosterone-mediated actions, alteration of dopamine metabolism, and modulation of insulin secretion.

Acute Toxicity

Animal

The acute toxicity of BPA is relatively low. One to three hours after ingestion of high doses of BPA, animals exhibited atony and profuse diarrhea. Published LD_{50} values for oral exposures to laboratory mammals are 4150 mg kg^{-1} body weight in male F344 rats, 3300 mg kg^{-1} body weight in female F344 rats, 5280 mg kg^{-1} body weight in male B6C3F1 mice, 4100 mg kg^{-1} body weight in female B6C3F1 mice, 2230 mg kg^{-1} body weight in rabbits, and 4000 mg kg^{-1} body weight in guinea pigs. The LD_{50} is much lower after intraperitoneal injection, at 150 mg kg^{-1} body weight in mice.

Human

One clinical report describes photoallergic contact dermatitis to BPA, with subsequent persistent light reactivity, in a group of eight outdoor workers.

Chronic Toxicity

The estrogenic effects of BPA at high doses are well-understood and generally agreed upon by scientists, but the low-dose hypothesis purports that different hormonal effects occur at levels below which other adverse effects have been observed. The lowest level at which adverse effects have been reported in toxicity tests is 50 mg kg^{-1} day^{-1}, - to address the low-dose hypothesis, studies of BPA at doses an order of magnitude or lower (i.e., <5 mg kg^{-1} day^{-1}) are considered relevant. It should be emphasized, however, that human exposures are likely to be two to three orders of magnitude lower than this dose.

The majority of low-dose BPA studies have been conducted in rodents. Based on the toxicokinetic studies discussed above, one should consider that internal doses in these studies are higher than humans would experience based on the same exposure, and this is particularly true for non-oral exposures. In general, the studies summarized below are the most recent and/or the most reliable for determining the potential for toxic effects from BPA.

Reproductive and Developmental Toxicity

Based on hundreds of animal studies with BPA doses <5 mg kg^{-1} day^{-1}, there is an overwhelming preponderance of lack-of-effect findings compared to findings of effect over a wide variety of reproductive and developmental toxicity endpoints. The most robust reproductive and developmental BPA studies are the multigenerational studies conducted with Sprague–Dawley rats and CD-1 Swiss mice. These studies examined a wide variety of hormonally sensitive end points, a large number of animals, and a wide range of oral doses.

These studies included a two-generation reproductive study in rats, using groups of 25 males/25 females and gastric intubation doses of 0.2, 2, 20, or 200 $\mu g\,kg^{-1}\,day^{-1}$. No BPA-related effects were reported on body weight, food consumption, organ weights, surface righting reflex, negative geotaxis reflex, mid-air righting reflex, pinna detachment, incisor eruption, eye opening, testes descent, preputial separation (PPS), vaginal opening, behavior in the open field or water filled multiple T-maze, estrous cyclicity, copulation index, fertility index, number of implantations, gestation length, litter size, pup weight, pup sex ratio, pup viability, or other functional reproductive measures. The authors report several significant changes in the anogenital distance per cube root of body weight ratio at various time points and doses, but they also state that these changes were consistently small, and no continuous changes were detected.

Another of these studies was a similar multigeneration test conducted in rats. They used groups of 30 male/30 female rats, and administered BPA in diet at 0.001, 0.02, 0.3, 5, 50, and 500 $mg\,kg^{-1}\,day^{-1}$ over three generations. The authors report that mating, fertility, and gestational indices; ovarian primordial follicle counts; estrous cyclicity; precoital interval; gestational length; offspring sex ratios; postnatal survival; nipple/areolae retention in preweanling males; epididymal sperm number, motility, morphology; daily sperm production (DSP); and efficiency of DSP were all unaffected at any dose or time point. Systemic toxicity in adults was reported at 50 and 500 $mg\,kg^{-1}\,day^{-1}$, including reduced body weights and body weight gains, and reduced absolute and increased relative weanling and adult organ weights (liver, kidneys, adrenals, spleen, pituitary, and brain). A few reproductive end points were affected at 500 $mg\,kg^{-1}\,day^{-1}$, including vaginal patency and delayed PPS.

The same group of investigators also conducted a two-generation reproduction study in mice. Groups of 28 male/28 female mice were administered BPA *via* the diet at 0.003, 0.03, 0.3, 5, 50, or 600 $mg\,kg^{-1}\,day^{-1}$), and an additional group was administered 0.5 ppm 17ß-estridiol as a positive control. In adults, systemic effects were seen at 50 $mg\,kg^{-1}\,day^{-1}$ (centrilobular hepatocyte hypertrophy) as well as at 600 $mg\,kg^{-1}\,day^{-1}$ (reduced body weight, increased kidney and liver weights, centrilobular hepatocyte hypertrophy, and renal nephropathy in males). Reproductive effects observed at 600 $mg\,kg^{-1}\,day^{-1}$ included reduced F1/F2 weanling body weight, reduced weanling spleen and testes weights (with seminiferous tubule hypoplasia), slightly delayed PPS, and apparently increased the incidence of treatment-related, undescended testes. The authors indicate that many of the reproductive effects were transient, and hypothesize they were secondary to the observed systemic toxicity.

Among all other BPA low-dose animal studies, there are some that reported responses at some low doses, but no marked or consistently repeatable effects were observed for any health end point. Reported effects are not consistent between rats and mice, and there are no consistent patterns among dose groups and evaluation times. The reported effects considered together lack any common pattern consistent with a hormonal mode of action. Notably, this includes rat studies of prostate weight, so the original findings that spurred the low-dose hypothesis have not been corroborated.

Neurotoxicity

During fetal and childhood development, natural hormones can influence brain development and subsequent behavior, including sexual behavior and other social interactions. Thus, several investigators examined whether low doses of BPA during fetal development can affect subsequent behavior of pups. Early studies evaluated a number of endpoints, but their interpretation is hampered by a lack of understanding of whether results are applicable to humans. Even so, there is no consistent evidence among these studies that low doses of BPA (e.g., $<5\,mg\,kg^{-1}\,day^{-1}$) cause adverse effects on behavioral endpoints.

Because the relevance of these studies to humans is not clear, two recent studies were conducted (one by US Environmental Protection Agency (US EPA)) using robust, validated methodology to assess the effects of low doses of BPA on the developing brain. One evaluated functional and morphological effects in offspring of rat dams exposed to BPA in their diet from gestational day 0 to lactation day 21 at doses between 0.01 and 410 $mg\,kg^{-1}\,day^{-1}$ (five different dose groups; doses were evaluated during both gestation and lactation, and doses in each dose group during lactation were generally two- to threefold higher than doses during gestation). The authors observed the offspring for clinical outcomes, auditory startle, motor activity, learning and memory, brain morphometry, and brain and nervous system neuropathology; there were no significant effects on any of the parameters at the doses tested. The authors did report effects on maternal and pup weight gains at the dose group corresponding to 5.85 $mg\,kg^{-1}\,day^{-1}$ (gestation) and 13.1 $mg\,kg^{-1}\,day^{-1}$ (lactation). A similar study design was employed in the second study to evaluate sexually dimorphic behavior, puberty, fertility, and anatomy in rats, although they also included a positive control (ethinyl estradiol or EE2) in their study. Female rats were exposed *via* oral gavage at 2, 20, and 200 $\mu g\,kg^{-1}\,day^{-1}$ (or 0.05–50 $\mu g\,kg^{-1}\,day^{-1}$ of EE2) from gestation day 7 to postnatal day 18, and only female offspring were evaluated. While female offspring exposed to EE2 were reported to have multiple effects related to exposure (increased anogenital distance, accelerated age at vaginal opening, malformation of genitalia, more male-like behavior, and absence of lordosis behavior), these effects were not observed at any BPA dose levels. In summary, these studies found no evidence of neurological effects in animals exposed to low doses of BPA.

Immunotoxicity

Because there are natural interactions between hormones and the immune system, several investigators have studied whether BPA is associated with altered immune function. The data are currently insufficient for drawing conclusions about possible immunological effects at low doses such as those experienced by humans. In light of several multigenerational studies reporting no pathology indicative of immune system dysfunction at low doses, the findings reported in studies on immunological effects are unlikely to be indicative of potential human risks.

Carcinogenicity

Researchers have also examined whether BPA could be carcinogenic *via* a hormonal mode of action. BPA was first tested for carcinogenicity by the US National Toxicology Program (NTP), which concluded, "Under the conditions of this bioassay, there was no convincing evidence that BPA was carcinogenic for F344 rats or B6C3F1 mice of either sex." Rats and mice were exposed for 103 weeks, but not prenatally or during early life, in these assays.

Based on the available data, none of the prominent governmental and international organizations classify BPA as a carcinogen. NTP does not list BPA as a carcinogen in the latest (12th) edition of its Report on Carcinogens nor does the International Agency for Research on Cancer, a division of the World Health Organization. BPA is also not listed as a carcinogen in US EPA's Integrated Risk Information System, and, based on the results of the NTP study discussed above, the European Union (EU) also concludes that BPA does not have carcinogenic potential. In addition, in 2002, a panel of prominent scientists conducted a weight-of-evidence evaluation of potential BPA carcinogenicity and concluded that "BPA is not likely to be carcinogenic to humans," citing the NTP bioassay as providing "no substantive evidence to indicate that BPA is carcinogenic to rodents."

In the last decade, several non-oral BPA studies examined the association between BPA and several precursors to cancer. While some studies showed associations between BPA and these precursors, none actually reported cancer. Other studies evaluated BPA in conjunction with other chemical exposures. While some animals developed cancer in these studies, these results are not necessarily applicable to humans. Thus, these recent findings are not indicative of BPA being a human carcinogen.

Human Studies

Several human studies have evaluated the association between BPA and various health effects in humans. The health effects assessed include, for example, premature birth, miscarriages, obesity, polycystic ovarian syndrome, cancer, altered sperm and semen characteristics, and other reproductive endpoints. While some statistically significant associations have been reported, the majority of these studies have methodological limitations making their results difficult to interpret. In general, they are hypothesis-generating studies insufficient for determining causality. Several studies measured urinary BPA, which largely comprises conjugated, biologically inactive BPA. Other studies used blood measurements that were likely inaccurate because of laboratory contamination or the use of an inaccurate analytical test method. Even in studies with accurate analytical test methods, the exposures in the general population are very low and occur in such a low range (e.g., 2–3 $\mu g\,l^{-1}$ in urine) that it is difficult to discern a true effect from statistical noise (and also to determine if a dose–response relationship exists). The majority of studies were cross-sectional in nature. In these studies, BPA was measured at the same time as the health effect was assessed, so it cannot be known whether BPA was causally associated with the effect. Other studies have also shown that BPA is correlated with concentrations of other chemicals, which could confound the relationships in studies reporting effects associated with BPA. Finally, the findings of these human studies are not consistent with those in animal studies. Overall, the human studies conducted thus far are insufficient to address whether low doses of BPA are associated with health effects in humans.

Environmental Fate and Behavior

The primary sources of BPA to the environment are likely effluents and emissions from facilities that either manufacture or utilize BPA in large quantities. If released to acclimated water, biodegradation would be the dominant fate process (half-life 1–4 days). BPA may adsorb extensively to suspended solids and sediments (K_{oc} values range from 314 to 1524), and it may photolyze in the presence of sunlight. BPA is not expected to bioaccumulate significantly in aquatic organisms (bioconcentration factor 5–68), volatilize, or undergo chemical hydrolysis.

Ecotoxicology

Owing to its presence in the environment, the ecotoxicity of BPA has been evaluated for a variety of species and end points. The EU has adopted the following provisional no effect concentrations: 0.002 3 $mg\,l^{-1}$ (freshwater or marine water), 0.064 $mg\,kg^{-1}$ dry weight (freshwater or marine water sediments), and 0.030 2 $mg\,kg^{-1}$ dry weight (soil). Concentrations typically found in the environment are lower than these levels, indicating that the risk to organisms is low. Research has found that aquatic species are most sensitive to BPA's effects, and testing in these organisms is discussed in more detail below.

Generally, low BPA concentrations in environmental media indicate that the most likely scenario for ecotoxicity would result from spills or other accidental releases. Thus, acute toxicity testing data are likely the most important for evaluation of these scenarios. BPA is reported to be moderately toxic to water fleas (48-h EC_{50}s ~3.9–10.2 $mg\,l^{-1}$), Mysid shrimp (96-h LC_{50} ~1.1 $mg\,l^{-1}$; no observed effect concentration (NOEC) = 0.51 $mg\,l^{-1}$), and marine and freshwater fish (LC_{50}s in the following ranges: ~7–15 $mg\,l^{-1}$ (48 h) or ~3–10 $mg\,l^{-1}$ (96 h)).

In chronic studies, BPA induces production of vitellogenin in male fathead minnows (*Pimephales promelas*) at concentrations of 640 and 1280 $mg\,l^{-1}$ after 43 days and 160 $mg\,l^{-1}$ after 71 days. Induction of vitellogenin is a process that normally occurs only in female fish in response to estrogenic hormones during the reproductive cycle.

Overall, chronic toxicity values of BPA for freshwater organisms ranged from 160 $mg\,l^{-1}$ for the fathead minnow (*P. promelas*; based on egg hatchability) to 11 000 $mg\,l^{-1}$ for rainbow trout (*Oncorhynchus mykiss*; based on growth). Typically, chronic effects on survival, growth, and reproductive endpoints only occur at concentrations of BPA greater than 160 mg l^{-1}. Published NOECs in aquatic organisms range from 16 to 3640 mg l^{-1}. Taken together with concentrations of BPA in typical surface water samples that are less than 1 mg l^{-1}, potential risks to aquatic organisms are very low.

Exposure Standards and Guidelines

Several government and international agencies have performed human health risk assessments on BPA. Most of these risk assessments have used a no observed adverse effect level of 5 mg kg^{-1} day^{-1} derived from two multigenerational rodent studies. Thus far, all have concluded that exposure to BPA from its current uses poses no human health risks, that is, either exposure levels are far below the tolerable daily intake (TDI) or margins of safety are far above 500. US EPA published an oral reference dose of 0.05 mg kg^{-1} day^{-1}, while the European Food Safety Agency established a TDI for BPA at the same level. In 2012, the US Food and Drug Administration concluded that BPA is not harmful under the intended conditions of use.

Several of the government and international agencies that performed risk assessments on BPA have also undertaken reviews in response to claims of low-dose BPA toxicity (e.g., $\leq$5 mg kg^{-1} day^{-1}). Even though none has concluded that adverse effects reported to occur below the traditionally defined no-effect level are sufficiently plausible to constitute a health risk, several governments have initiated bans on specific uses of BPA (e.g., in children's feeding bottles in Canada and the EU, and all food contact material for children under 3 years of age in Denmark).

See also: Food Safety and Toxicology; Endocrine System; Environmental Hormone Disruptors; Estrogens V: Xenoestrogens.

Further Reading

European Food Safety Authority (EFSA), 2006. Opinion of the scientific panel on food additives, flavourings, processing aids and materials in contact with food on a request from the commission related to 2,2-bis(4-hydroxyphenyl)propane (bisphenol A): Question number EFSA-Q-2005-100. EFSA J. 428, 1–75.

Hengstler, J.G., Roth, H., Gebel, T., et al., 2011. Critical evaluation of key evidence on the human health hazards of exposure to bisphenol A. Crit. Rev. Toxicol. 41, 263–291.

Goodman, J.E., Witorsch, R.J., McConnell, E.E., et al., 2009. Weight-of-evidence evaluation of reproductive and developmental effects of low doses of bisphenol A. Crit. Rev. Toxicol. 39, 1–75.

National Toxicology Program (NTP), U.S. Department of Health and Human Services, Center for the Evaluation of Risks to Human Reproduction, Research Triangle Park, NC, 2008. Research Triangle Park, North Carolina, United States. NTP-CERHR Monograph on the Potential Human Reproductive and Developmental Effects of Bisphenol A. NIH Publication No. 08–5994.

Relevant Websites

http://www.efsa.europa.eu/ – European Food Safety Authority.

http://www.epa.gov/ – United States Environmental Protection Agency (US EPA) Integrated Risk Information System (IRIS).

http://www.niehs.nih.gov/ – National Institute of Environmental Health Sciences (NIEHS).

Black Widow Spider *see* Spiders

Bleach

K Hahn and JA Weber, Missouri Poison Center, St. Louis, MO, USA

This article is a revision of the previous edition article by Julie Weber, volume 1, pp 317–319, © 2005, Elsevier Inc.

- Chemical Name: Bleach
- Chemical Abstracts Services Registry Number: Sodium hypochlorite (CAS: 7681-52-9)
- Synonyms: Household laundry bleach (Purex®, Clorox®, Javex®, and Dazzle®); Commercial laundry bleach (caustic soda bleach); Dakin's solution; Sodium hypochlorite pentahydrate; Surgical chlorinated soda solution
- Molecular Formula: NaHClO

Background

Sodium hypochlorite is an aqueous solution produced by the mixture of chloramine gas and water. It is used as a bleaching agent and disinfectant in various settings.

Uses

Sodium hypochlorite is used in household laundry bleach; bleaching agents for pulp, fibers, and papers; antiseptics; disinfectant and cleaning products; toilet sanitizers; and deodorizers; and for water purification and as a chemical intermediate. Regular household laundry bleaches are approximately 5.25% sodium hypochlorite in water with an adjusted pH of 10.8–11.4. 'Ultra' formulations are slightly more concentrated and contain 6–8% sodium hypochlorite. Commercial laundry bleaches contain 15% sodium hypochlorite at a pH slightly over 11.

Environmental Fate and Behavior

Sodium hypochlorite solution is green to yellow with faint odor of chlorine. The solubility of the pentahydrate at 0 °C is 29.3 g per 100 ml of water. It is soluble in cold water and decomposes with hot water. It is not expected to bioaccumulate in plants or animals because it reacts with moist tissues of living systems. Sodium hypochlorite is not expected to be detected in water or soil due to its rapid reaction time and volatility.

Exposure and Exposure Monitoring

Ingestion is the most common route of exposure to sodium hypochlorite. Other modes of exposure are inhalation, dermal, ocular, and inadvertent injection.

Mechanism of Toxicity

The toxicity of hypochlorite arises from its corrosive activity on skin and mucous membranes. Corrosive burns may occur immediately upon exposure to concentrated bleach products. Most of this corrosiveness stems from the oxidizing potency of the hypochlorite itself, a capacity that is measured in terms of available chlorine. The alkalinity of some preparations may contribute substantially to the tissue injury and mucosal erosion. Sodium hypochlorite when combined with an acid or ammonia may produce chlorine or chloramine gas, respectively. An inhalation exposure to these gases may result in irritation to mucous membranes and the respiratory tract, which may manifest itself as a chemically induced pneumonitis.

Acute Toxicity

Animal

Emesis is likely to be spontaneous. Clinical signs may include salivation, emesis, abdominal pain and tenderness, hematemesis, and bleached hair. Rats given 5–15 ml kg^{-1} of an alkaline (pH 12.0) solution containing 4.5% sodium hypochlorite died within 1–3 h from severe local damage to the esophagus and stomach.

In an experimental study on rats designed to evaluate systemic effects of household bleaches (containing 4% sodium hypochlorite) on lungs, livers, kidneys, and intestines, the animals were given the hypochlorite solution via intragastric tube. After 2, 4, 6, 12, 24, and 48 h of exposure via intragastric route, there was significant congestion and some interstitial mononuclear cell infiltration seen in the lungs as well as liver and kidneys. In the same study, another group of rats were given intravenous administration of household bleach and after 4 h the same histopathological changes were observed in the lungs and other organs studied.

Human

The resulting symptoms from an exposure to sodium hypochlorite and related compounds may range from mildly irritating to corrosive depending on the volume/amount of the exposure, duration of contact, and pH and viscosity of the product. Small accidental ingestion of household bleach, containing 4–6% sodium hypochlorite, usually causes nothing more serious than orogastric irritation characterized by nausea, spontaneous emesis, sore throat, and abdominal pain. Very large ingestions, usually intentional, have caused fatal hypernatremia and hyperchloremic acidosis, and significant gastric injury. Sodium hypochlorite solutions stronger than 10% or powders may result in corrosive burns of the mouth, hypopharynx, and stomach. Prolonged dermal contact can result in irritation or burn. Inadvertent injection into the surrounding tissue during dentistry use of Dakin's solution (0.5% up to 5% sodium hypochlorite) has resulted in severe acute pain and burning sensation accompanied by immediate edema of the surrounding area. Delayed effects can include tissue necrosis, paresthesia, ecchymosis, and secondary infection. Household bleach has been advocated as a disinfectant for syringes and needles of IV drug users. There are few reports on the effects of inadvertent or intentional IV injection. Case reports of symptoms have included erythema at the injection site, vomiting, chest pain, bradycardia, and hypotension. Ocular exposure may result in irritation and lacrimation with a burning discomfort. Superficial disturbance of the corneal epithelium may occur, which recovers completely within two days. Eyelid edema has been reported, but is more common after exposure to chloramine gas. Inhalation of liberated chlorine or chloramine gas may cause respiratory tract irritation, cough, substernal chest discomfort and tightness, hoarseness, dyspnea, and wheezing. Chemical pneumonitis, acute respiratory distress syndrome, and hypoxia have developed in severe prolonged exposures.

Chronic Toxicity (or Exposure)

Animal

Bleach should not be considered a carcinogen in experimental animals. Exposure of the esophagus of rabbits and dogs to typical household bleach resulted in only minor lesions. Rats fed water with high bleach concentrations demonstrated decreased weight gain, but no other untoward signs or symptoms.

Human

Most data indicate that low-dose hypochlorite solutions (e.g., those seen in typical municipal drinking water) do not directly contribute to the development of cancer.

Carcinogenicity

Sodium hypochlorite is not considered a carcinogen. The International Agency for Research on Cancer (IARC) classifies sodium hypochlorite as Category 3, which are compounds not classifiable as human carcinogens.

Clinical Management

Basic and advanced life-support measures should be utilized as necessary. Treatment is generally symptomatic and supportive. Gastrointestinal evacuation procedures are generally contraindicated and unnecessary. If the patient is alert and able to swallow, immediately offer milk or water to drink. Stop if vomiting occurs during administration. Do not exceed 5–10 ml kg^{-1} in a child or 250 ml in an adult. Esophagoscopy is rarely needed following unintentional ingestion of small amounts of common household liquid bleach. Ingestion of commercial bleach or bleach granules may necessitate esophagoscopy to look for burns. Electrolytes should be monitored to rule out hypernatremia in a large ingestion. Administration of an acidic substance to neutralize sodium hypochlorite is contraindicated.

For inhalation exposure, remove the patient from fumes into fresh air. Establish respirations and create an artificial airway if necessary. If cough or difficulty in breathing develops and is not relieved by the fresh air, the patient should be evaluated for respiratory irritation, bronchitis, or pneumonitis in a health care facility. If significant symptoms occur, a chest X-ray may be indicated as well as pulse oximetry and arterial blood gas evaluation.

For ocular exposures to sodium hypochlorite and related agents, remove contact lenses if present. The eye(s) should be immediately irrigated with tap water or normal saline for at least 15 min. If ocular irrigation is delayed, the potential for injury is greater and the patient may have to be evaluated in a health care facility.

For dermal exposures, immediately remove contaminated clothing and flood the exposed skin with water. Gently wash the skin with soap and water.

Ecotoxicity

Sodium hypochlorite is harmful to aquatic life in very low concentrations.

Exposure Standards and Guidelines

No specific standards and guidelines set forth by the American Conference of Industrial Hygienists, the US Environmental Protection Agency, IARC, or the US National Institute for Safety and Health.

Miscellaneous

When chlorine-containing products have contaminated the dialysate of renal patients or when municipal water treated with chloramine was used in dialysis solutions, hemolysis, methemoglobinemia, shock, and cardiovascular collapse have occurred.

See also: Chlorination Byproducts; Chlorine; Clean Water Act (CWA), US; Detergent; The National Library of Medicine and Its Toxicology and Environmental Health Information Program.

Further Reading

De Torres, J.P., Strom, J.A., Jaber, B.L., Hendra, K.P., 2002. Hemodialysis-associated methemoglobinemia in acute renal failure. Am. J. Kidney Dis. 39 (6), 1307–1309.

Gernhardt, C.R., Eppendorf, K., Kozlowski, A., Brandt, M., 2004. Toxicity of concentrated sodium hypochlorite used as an endodontic irrigant. Int. Endod. J. 37, 272–280.

Hartnett, K.M., Fulginiti, L.C., Di Mondica, F., 2011. The effects of corrosive substances on human bone, teeth, hair, nails, and soft tissue. J. Forensic Sci. 56 (No. 4), 954–959.

Medina-Ramón, M., Zock, J.P., Kogevinas, M., Sunyer, J., Basagaña, X., Schwartz, J., Burge, P.S., Moore, V., Antó, J.M., 2006. Short-term respiratory effects of cleaning exposures in female domestic cleaners. Eur. Respir. J. 27, 1196–1203.

Relevant Website

http://www.nlm.nih.gov/medlineplus/ency/article/002488.htm – MedlinePlus: Sodium Hypochlorite poisoning.

Blister Agents/Vesicants

RE Jabbour and H Salem, Edgewood Chemical Biological Center, MD, USA
FR Sidell[†]

This article is a revision of the previous edition article by Harry Salem, Frederick R. Sidell, volume 1, pp 319–323, © 2005, Elsevier Inc.

- Name: *See also* Lewisite; Sulfur Mustard; Nitrogen Mustards; Arsenical Vomiting Agents; Phosgene Oxime.
- Chemical Abstracts Service Registry Number: *See also* Lewisite; Sulfur Mustard; Nitrogen Mustards; Arsenical Vomiting Agents; Phosgene Oxime.
- Synonyms: *See also* Lewisite; Sulfur Mustard; Nitrogen Mustards; Arsenical Vomiting Agents; Phosgene Oxime.
- Molecular Formula: *See also* Lewisite; Sulfur Mustard; Nitrogen Mustards; Arsenical Vomiting Agents; Phosgene Oxime.
- Chemical Structure: *See also* Lewisite; Sulfur Mustard; Nitrogen Mustards; Arsenical Vomiting Agents; Phosgene Oxime.

Background (Significance/History)

Blister agents, also known as vesicants, are chemical warfare agents that are strong cytotoxic alkylating compounds. These chemicals are used to both induce casualties and for the purpose of area denial. This class of chemical warfare agent targets the eyes, lungs, skin, mucous membranes, as well as the blood-forming organs. Blister agents/vesicants are divided into three different groups: mustards, arsenicals, and urticants. **Table 1** lists several of the known blister agents/vesicants and their classifications.

Uses

Mustard gas, also known as Levinstein mustard, was first used as a chemical warfare agent during World War I in 1917 by German forces near Ypres, Belgium. There are several documented cases of its use in warfare since its first introduction almost hundred years ago. Although it is commonly referred to as mustard gas, this term is not accurate; mustard gas is not really a gas, but rather a viscous liquid and is not likely to change into a gas immediately if released at ordinary temperatures.

Environmental Fate and Behavior

See also Lewisite; Sulfur Mustard; Nitrogen Mustards; Arsenical Vomiting Agents; Phosgene Oxime.

Exposure and Exposure Monitoring

See also Lewisite; Sulfur Mustard; Nitrogen Mustards; Arsenical Vomiting Agents; Phosgene Oxime.

Toxicokinetics

See also Lewisite; Sulfur Mustard; Nitrogen Mustards; Arsenical Vomiting Agents; Phosgene Oxime.

Mechanism of Toxicity

The action of blister agents/vesicants on cellular components results in the inhibition of mitosis with decreased tissue respiration. This inhibition leads to cellular death through either apoptosis or necrosis. Fatal injuries can occur following unprotected exposure to the eyes, airway, skin, and mucous membranes. Extensive exposures can induce systemic effects including bone marrow inhibition, as well as spleen and gastrointestinal tract damage.

Mustard Gas

Due to its stability in cool environments, mustard (H) is a greater threat in hot and humid climates as a blister agent because it will begin to vaporize. If protective measures are not taken, mustard agent can enter the body quickly either through the breathing of vapors or through skin contact with liquid or vapors. It can readily pass through clothing, subsequently coming in contact with skin. It is then absorbed through the skin and enters the circulation, which can lead to systemic effects. Mustard as well as its metabolites will exit the body through the urine within a few weeks of exposure. There is no initial pain or other symptoms immediately following contact. Most of the signs and symptoms of mustard exposure may not be apparent until the next day. At the point of contact, mustard can produce severe skin blisters or bullae occurring within several days following the initial exposure. The extent of the

Table 1 Classifications of blister agents/vesicants

Blister agent/vesicant name	*Military code*	*Blister agent/vesicant class*
Mustard	H	Mustard
Sulfur mustard	HD	Mustard
Nitrogen mustard	NH-1, NH-2, NH-3	Mustard
Sulfur mustard/agent T mixture	HT	Mustard
Lewisite	L	Arsenical
Sulfur mustard/lewisite mixture	HL	Mustard/arsenical Mixture
Phenyldichloroarsine	PD	Arsenical
Ethyldichloroarsine	ED	Arsenical
Methyldichloroarsine	MD	Arsenical
Phosgene oxime	CX	Urticant

[†] Deceased.

 http://dx.doi.org/10.1016/B978-0-12-386454-3.00590-X

injury is determined by the amount of mustard as well as the area of the body that is exposed to it. These factors will determine the clinical course of the mustard exposure injury. Areas of the body that contain moisture (e.g., eyes) or are sweaty are particularly vulnerable to mustard injury. Inhalation of mustard vapors can result in severe pulmonary injury. High-dose exposures can cause death in the near term.

The long-term consequences from mustard exposure, particularly at low doses, are unknown; however, a one-time high-dose exposure can result in chronic and recurrent lung and eye problems. Mustard agent is also a known carcinogen, and can cause lung cancer. The ability to cause birth defects in the children of exposed adults is not presently known; however, it has the potential to be teratogenic.

Sulfur Mustard

Unprotected exposure to sulfur mustard (HD) leads to signs and symptoms that are delayed and occur within hours. Dermal exposures induce erythema and blistering within 2–24 h. Ocular exposure typically induces tearing, itching, and burning accompanied by a gritty feeling in the eyes, within 4–24 h of initial exposure. Also, there may be conjunctivitis with eyelid swelling in 3–6 h with more significant ocular exposures. In severe ocular exposure cases, there is marked eyelid swelling, corneal opacity, and eye pain, all occurring in 1–2 h. Airway toxicity can occur within 12–24 h, and is marked by rhinorrhea, sneezing, coughing, nosebleeds, and hoarseness. Severe inhalation injury is marked by productive cough and shortness of breath. Gastrointestinal effects may occur if HD is ingested.

Sulfur Mustard with Agent T

Sulfur mustard with agent T (HT) is a liquid mixture of 60% HD and 40% agent T. It has a pale yellow to brown color and a garliclike odor. The toxicities and properties of HT are similar to those of H or HD, except that HT has a slightly greater vesicant property on skin compared to H or HD. It has slightly less damaging properties when passing through clothing or on ocular exposure.

Nitrogen Mustard

Nitrogen mustard (HN) actually describes three similar compounds (HN-1, HN-2, and HN-3). It is colorless when pure, but routine preparations appear pale to dark yellow. It can be odorless or have a slight fishy or soapy odor. When nitrogen mustard is vaporized and released in the air, it degrades in a matter of hours. Its properties and toxicity are similar to those of the other mustard agents mentioned above, and it is a strong blister agent/vesicant. Signs and symptoms of exposure, such as eye irritation and skin erythema, will occur sooner upon exposure to nitrogen mustard compared to an exposure to HD.

Lewisite

Lewisite (L) is a potent dichloroarsine blister agent/vesicant. Pure preparations of lewisite are colorless and odorless oily liquids, but if preparations contain impurities, they will have a fruity or geranium-like odor. As a liquid, lewisite will penetrate rubber and most fabrics. It is generally more dangerous as a liquid than as a vapor. It is unknown whether lewisite persists in the environment for an extended period of time, but it can react with water in a manner whereby its volatility and most of its blistering potency are lost. As a potent blister agent/vesicant, it has irritant effects on the eyes and respiratory system. It also has similar toxicities to the other blister agents mentioned in this article, although it exhibits less bone marrow suppression than other blister agents/vesicants. Unlike mustard agent it can cause immediate pain following initial contact. Erythema is often not present around the vesicles as with other vesicants.

Mustard and Lewisite Mixture

Mixing L with HD at the concentrations of 63 and 37% respectively produces a liquid with a low freezing point that provides a more effective weapon in colder climates at higher altitudes. It has a garlic odor and is effectively insoluble in water. It persists on the ground from 1 to 2 days under average weather conditions and can remain for 1 week or more under very cold conditions. Along with its blistering properties, it is also cytotoxic to the hematopoietic or blood-forming cells in the bone marrow. Other mixtures like mustard and phenyldichloroarsine act in a similar manner.

Phenyldichloroarsine and Other Dichloroarsines

Phenyldichloroarsine, ethyldichloroarsine, and methyldichloroarsine have similar properties and toxicities as the dichloroarsine lewisite. They may be mixed with HD similarly as can be done with lewisite and mustard mixtures. Exposures to these mixtures can confuse the diagnosis between either an arsenical or mustard injury.

Phosgene Oxime

Phosgene oxime or dichlorformoxime is classified as an urticant. It can be a liquid or colorless solid with a disagreeable odor. This acts as an irritant to skin and mucous membranes. Exposure to this chemical causes immediate severe pain on skin contact, similar to lewisite. Very low exposures can cause lacrimation. Unlike mustards and arsenicals, it is readily water soluble.

See also Lewisite; Sulfur Mustard; Nitrogen Mustards; Arsenical Vomiting Agents; Phosgene Oxime.

Acute and Short-Term Toxicity

See also Lewisite; Sulfur Mustard; Nitrogen Mustards; Arsenical Vomiting Agents; Phosgene Oxime.

Chronic Toxicity (Animal/Human)

See also Lewisite; Sulfur Mustard; Nitrogen Mustards; Arsenical Vomiting Agents, Phosgene Oxime.

Immunotoxicity

See also Lewisite; Sulfur Mustard; Nitrogen Mustards; Arsenical Vomiting Agents; Phosgene Oxime.

Reproductive Toxicity

See also Lewisite; Sulfur Mustard; Nitrogen Mustards; Arsenical Vomiting Agents; Phosgene Oxime.

Genotoxicity

See also Lewisite; Sulfur Mustard; Nitrogen Mustards; Arsenical Vomiting Agents; Phosgene Oxime.

Carcinogenicity

See also Lewisite; Sulfur Mustard; Nitrogen Mustards; Arsenical Vomiting Agents; Phosgene Oxime.

Clinical Effect

Diagnosis of a blister agent/vesicant injury, without obvious overt contamination, requires a high level of suspicion when eye, skin, and respiratory signs and symptoms become evident. The first symptoms that occur following a blister agent/vesicant exposure are eye and airway irritation. Conjunctivitis can occur after 1 h at very low nonodorous concentrations. Mild exposure results in tearing and the sensation of eye grit in 4–12 h. Severe eye lesions may occur within 2 h following heavy exposure. Lewisite and the dichloroarsines can cause gray scarring of the cornea at the point of contact. Exposure to phosgene oxime can induce severe lacrimation at even low doses.

Skin damage may not be immediately evident because the first effects may be painless until deeper skin layers are involved and blisters appear; however, the diagnosis of a chemical skin injury is readily made when the fluid-filled skin blisters or bullae appear and are recognized. There is at least a 1–12 h latent period, during which skin burning and itching may occur. Erythema or skin redness appears on exposed skin after 2–48 h. Erythema is followed by coalescing blisters on a red base. Unlike mustard, exposure to lewisite or phosgene oxime will produce immediate pain on contact and areas of erythema may recede without blister formation. Lewisite and the dichloroarsines cause a more opaque blister fluid than the mustards. These injuries tend to induce greater amounts of inflammation and affect the connective tissue as well as the vasculature. Phosgene oxime causes immediate pain and skin necrosis at the site of contact. Within 30 s, the contact area becomes blanched and is surrounded by a ring of erythema. A wheal then occurs in 30 min, and this area will turn brown within a day. Usually, an eschar will form and slough off within 1–2 weeks. Healing and resorption of uninfected blisters occur in 1–3 weeks for all vesicants. Broken blisters must be protected to minimize chances of infection and subsequent scarring of denuded skin. Currently, there is no effective medical test to determine mustard gas exposure.

Respiratory signs and symptoms from vesicant exposure can include dyspnea and rhonchi with moist rales; chest X-rays can reveal pulmonary edema. Changes consistent with chemical pneumonitis may appear after the first 24 h following exposure.

Clinical Management

The blister agents/vesicants may vary in their ability to generate local and systemic pathology; however, the general treatment principles remain the same for all vesicants. The exception is that British anti-Lewisite (BAL), also known as 2,3 dimercaptopropanol, is available for the treatment of lewisite exposure.

Mild eye lesions require little treatment other than flushing with water immediately. Steroid and antibiotic ointment can be applied to the eye. The injured eyes should not be covered with bandages. Atropine sulfate ointment should be instilled in each eye to obtain good mydriasis in all cases where there are corneal erosions, iritis, cyclitis, or marked photophobia or miosis. Blepharospasm, or eyelid spasm, is treated with atropine sulfate solution. To prevent infection, a few drops of an antibacterial ophthalmic should be instilled every 4 h. The lids must be kept separated.

Treatment of skin lesions also follows decontamination and removal of clothes. To minimize HD-induced systemic effects, decontamination should occur within 15 min after exposure. The decontaminating solutions (5% sodium hypochlorite or liquid household bleach) should be washed off quickly to prevent additional skin injury. If erythema is already present, decontamination should be performed with soap and water. Blisters should be left intact, but if broken, should be debrided to prevent secondary infection. Cleansing with tap water or saline and the application of dressings is done when needed. Mustard wounds can be treated with similar solutions used to treat burns, and infected skin wounds require antibiotics as appropriate.

In cases of lewisite skin injury, BAL ointment should be used on contaminated skin where blisters have not yet formed. Frequent BAL ointment application does cause a mild dermatitis, so it cannot be used as a protective barrier on skin not contaminated by dichloroarsines. Exposure to lewisite or dichloroarsines induces deeper skin injury compared to HD; therefore, these wounds may heal more slowly and may require skin grafting. Systemic treatment with parenteral BAL is considered when there is greater than 5% area of skin contamination (1 ft^2), which results in immediate skin blanching or erythema within 30 min after exposure or a burn the size of the palm (1% of skin area), which was not decontaminated within the first 15 min after exposure. There are two types of parenteral BAL therapies that can be used. One involves applying BAL ointment liberally onto the skin and allowing that area to remain covered. The other parenteral method is to give an intramuscular injection of 10% BAL in oil (without injecting into a blood vessel).

Inhalation of vapors from mustard or arsenical blister agents/vesicants can result in laryngeal and tracheobronchial mucosal injury. Mild injury with hoarseness and sore throat requires either no treatment or saline mist inhalation.

Moderate exposures result in hyperemia and necrosis of the bronchial epithelium, and require hospitalization to prevent secondary infection. Due to the absence of antibiotics during World War I, pneumonia was the usual cause of death following exposure to mustard agents. Severe injuries cause tracheobronchial tree casts from pseudomembrane formation. Hypoxia can occur, but subsequent bronchitis and pneumonia from infection were the chief causes of pulmonary-related deaths in World War I (2% mortality).

Blister agents/vesicants at extensive exposure can have systemic toxicity that affects not only the lungs, but also the bone marrow, lymph nodes, spleen, and endocrine systems. In these cases, complete blood counts with monitoring of granulocytes, red cells, and platelets should be performed routinely. If granulocyte depletion occurs, isolation and antibiotic prophylaxis may be necessary. Many past fatalities were due to the combination of pneumonia and bone marrow failure. Anemia and thrombocytopenia should be treated as the situation dictates. If local effects remain mild, systemic effects are not likely to be significant. In severe cases of lewisite or dichloroarsine respiratory injury, dyspnea with frothy sputum indicating pulmonary edema indicated that intramuscular BAL is necessary.

With eye injury, temporary blindness can occur, but permanent blindness is rare with vapor exposure. Blindness is more likely to occur when liquid mustard is directly splashed into the eye. With mild eye injury, recovery occurs in 1–2 weeks. More severe involvement with corneal erosions can take 2–3 months of hospital care before recovery occurs. Corneal involvement beyond erosions with opacification and ulceration (<0.1% of mustard agent casualties in World War I) takes several months for recovery, and then late relapses can still occur. In these cases blindness may ensue. Eye injuries are more severe with nitrogen mustard than with HD. The iris is frequently discolored and atrophied with nitrogen mustard exposure.

With mild blister formation, healing occurs with little scarring, but it may take months to heal while remaining painful during this time. When secondary infection occurs or in more extensive blistering, scarring can be more severe. Itching may persist after healing. Hypopigmentation or hyperpigmentation can occur as with any healing process. Deeper burns with lewisite and the dichloroarsines have similar outcomes as second- or third-degree thermal burns. Repeated exposures over time to mustards or arsenicals such as dichloroarsines can cause sensitization. Delayed healing beyond 2 months occurs with skin lesions caused by phosgene oxime.

A single low-dose exposure to mustard vapor with laryngeal and tracheobronchial mucosal effects may not lead to significant injury once healed. A cough may persist for 1 month or longer. Hoarseness usually lasts only 1–2 weeks; however, repeated or chronic low-dose exposure can lead to progressive pulmonary fibrosis, chronic bronchitis, and bronchiectasis.

**See also* Lewisite; Sulfur Mustard; Nitrogen Mustards; Arsenical Vomiting Agents; Phosgene Oxime.

Ecotoxicology

See also Lewisite; Sulfur Mustard; Nitrogen Mustards; Arsenical Vomiting Agents; Phosgene Oxime.

Other Hazards

See also Lewisite; Sulfur Mustard; Nitrogen Mustards; Arsenical Vomiting Agents; Phosgene Oxime.

Exposure Standards and Guidelines

See also Lewisite; Sulfur Mustard; Nitrogen Mustards; Arsenical Vomiting Agents; Phosgene Oxime.

Miscellaneous

See also Lewisite; Sulfur Mustard; Nitrogen Mustards; Arsenical Vomiting Agents; Phosgene Oxime.

See also: Phosgene Oxime; Arsenical Vomiting Agents; Lewisite; Sulfur Mustard; Nitrogen Mustards.

Relevant Websites

https://www.osha.gov/SLTC/emergencypreparedness/cbrnmatrix/blister.html – Chemical-Biological-Radiological-Nuclear (CBRN); Personal Protective Equipment Selection Matrix for Emergency Responders.

http://www.bt.cdc.gov – (US) Centers for Disease Control and Prevention, Agency for Toxic Substances and Disease Registry, Chemical Agents.

http://sis.nlm.nih.gov – (US) National Library of Medicine, Specialized Information Services, Chemical Warfare Agents.

Blood

M Moreno, University of Rochester Medical Center, Rochester, NY, USA
TJ Wiegand, Rochester, NY, USA

This article is a revision of the previous edition article by Gary R. Krieger, Scott Philips, volume 1, pp 323–329, © 2005, Elsevier Inc.

Introduction

Hematology is the study of pathophysiology of the cellular elements and coagulation proteins in the blood. Physicians who specialize in this field are referred to as hematologists. Hematology has several new tools available to detect abnormalities in numbers or dysfunctions. Hematologists diagnose and treat both benign and malignant blood disorders. Primary hematologic diseases are uncommon, while secondary hematologic conditions occur frequently. Thus the inquiring physician must extensively question the patients for all forms of medications, herbals, folk remedies, occupations, and family history to name a few areas that require an in-depth history.

The formed elements of the blood – red blood cells (RBCs or erythrocytes), white blood cells (myeloids), immunocytes (T and B cells), platelets (thrombocytes), and their diseases – have traditionally been the main focus of hematology. However, with the advent of increasingly sophisticated molecular investigatory tools, such as recombinant DNA technology, the appreciation of the scope and inherent complexity of the blood-forming organ has dramatically increased. The bone marrow and its formed elements can be considered as a complex organ with a total mass that is over twice as large as the liver. The cells produced by this organ provide several critical functions such as the transport of oxygen (RBCs), hemostasis (platelets), and host resistance (immunocytes and white blood cells). Generally, each step in the intricate sequence required to produce the formed elements is vulnerable to adverse effects from a wide variety of chemicals and drugs.

Bone Marrow Structure and Function

In the normal adult, the marrow is found in the central hollow segment of bones. Hematopoiesis, or the production of the formed blood elements, occurs in the bone marrow. However, in the adult, it is largely restricted to scattered clusters of hematopoietic cells in the proximal epiphyses of the long bones, skull, vertebrae, pelvis, ribs, and sternum. The hematopoietic picture in adults is quite different from that seen in either prenatal or childhood time periods. Within the first 1–5 prenatal months, the liver and spleen act as the hematopoietic organs. By the fifth prenatal month, the marrow achieves sufficient maturity to assume the dominant role in hematopoiesis. During childhood, there are high demands on the bone marrow system to produce large quantities of the formed elements; however, with increasing chronological maturity, there is less demand on the bone marrow system and the total output of the bone marrow significantly declines.

In addition to hematopoietic cells, there are other separate and distinct cells that support and augment marrow activities. Among these cells are fibroblasts, fat cells, and reticuloendothelial and endosteal cells. In aggregate, these cells are known as the bone marrow stroma. Occasionally, the term 'hematopoietic microenvironment' is also employed to differentiate these cells and supporting structure from the stem and progenitor cells. These cells are the focus of the next section, which presents an overview of the basic physiology of the blood-forming elements.

Hematopoiesis

In the average adult, between 200 and 400 billion blood cells are destroyed and replaced each day. This enormous turnover implies that new cells are constantly formed rather than simply released from a central storage area that contains all the cells necessary for an individual's lifetime. Hematopoiesis is the key concept that has been used to explain how the body can provide a lifetime worth of formed blood elements. Hematopoiesis is a process of cell amplification and differentiation in which a few stem cells give rise to increasingly more developed or differentiated progenitor cells, which in turn give rise to the formed blood elements. The earliest cell is known as the pluripotent stem cell (PSC). PSCs are uniquely responsible for the production of the formed elements throughout the lifetime of a human. Relatively, few PSCs are required since, as these cells undergo mitosis or cell division, one replacement stem cell and one committed or daughter cell are produced. This daughter cell subsequently develops and proliferates into the various formed elements. Hence, the PSCs are considered to be self-renewing because of their ability to reproduce themselves. **Figure 1** presents the overall organization and development of the bone marrow cells. This structure is quite hierarchical and resembles a company organization chart with a single chief executive officer presiding over separate divisions, which in turn develop other specialized departments or functions. Not surprisingly, each step in the organization requires both a series of growth factors and interactions with the hematopoietic microenvironment to promote and control the development of each cell type. The stimulatory or growth factors are known as poietins or colony stimulating factors (CSFs). CSFs can either be lineage-specific, i.e., they act on specific cell lines, or directly act on multipotential progenitors and stem cells. Examples of lineage-specific CSFs include (1) erythropoietin, which stimulates production of erythrocytes or RBCs; and (2) interleukin-7, which induces the growth of B- and T-lymphocyte progenitors. Direct-acting CSFs include interleukins 2–6, which act on a variety of cell lines.

Formed Elements – Erythrocytes, Myeloids, and Thrombocytes

Erythrocytes

The RBC is a biconcave disk with a diameter of ~8 μm and a life span in the circulation of ~120 days. Due to its unique shape, the RBC is twice as thick at the edges (2.4 μm) as at its

 http://dx.doi.org/10.1016/B978-0-12-386454-3.00683-7

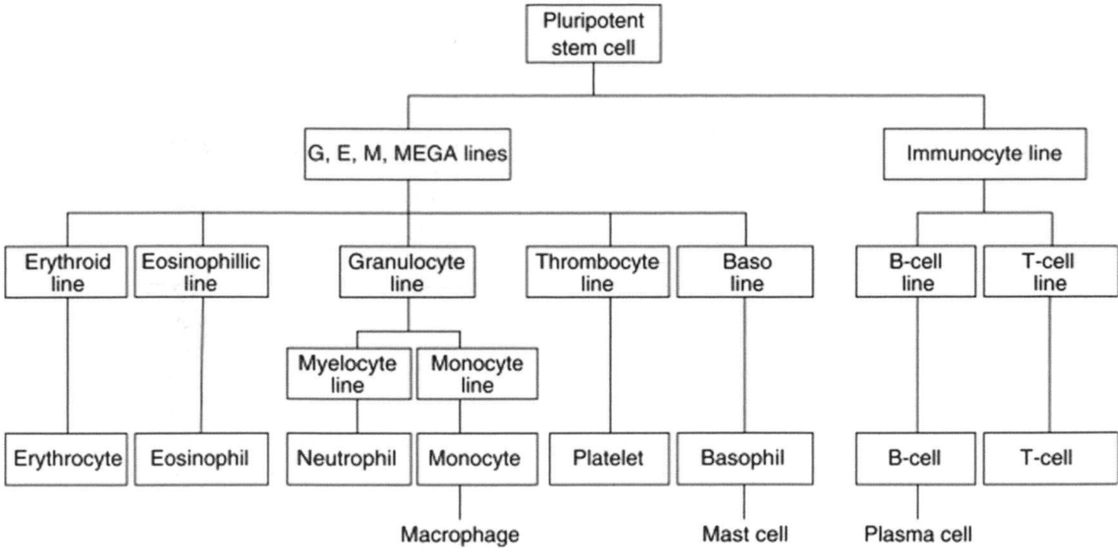

Figure 1 Bone marrow cell organization. G, Granulocyte; E, Erythrocyte; M, Monocyte; and MEGA, Megakaryocyte.

center. The explanation for this specialized geometry is not fully known; however, this shape tends to minimize intracellular diffusional distance and allows for easier passage through small blood vessels. The critical function of the RBC is transportation and delivery of oxygen to peripheral tissues. Approximately 30% of the wet weight of the RBC is composed of hemoglobin, the essential protein, which is integral to the oxygen/carbon dioxide transport and delivery system. Hemoglobin is also capable of transporting nitric oxide (NO). NO is a unique gas that can affect the ability of blood vessels to expand or contract in addition to having a role in learning and memory.

The mature RBC is formed through a series of cell divisions that progressively increase the amount of hemoglobin in the cytoplasm. Following the last division, a special cell known as a reticulocyte is formed. The reticulocyte stays in the bone marrow for 2 or 3 days before being released into the general circulation, where over a period of 24 h, it undergoes a series of transformations that results in the appearance of a mature RBC. The reticulocyte is easy to identify in laboratory tests and the reticulocyte count or index is an important parameter that can provide information about marrow function. The reticulocyte index is equal to the reticulocyte percentage multiplied by the ratio of the patient's hematocrit (packed cell volume) to a normal hematocrit.

Hemoglobin

Hemoglobin, in the normal adult, is a protein whose main function is to transport oxygen from the lungs to tissues and to transport carbon dioxide from tissues to the lungs. The hemoglobin molecule contains four separate folded peptide chains, which form a hydrophobic or water 'repelling' pocket around a heme group. The heme group is composed of a central iron atom complexed to four nitrogen atoms. Oxygen is capable of reversibly binding to the heme unit in a process known as oxygenation. The interactions among the subunits in a hemoglobin molecule are known as cooperativity. There are well-described regulators of the affinity of hemoglobin for oxygen that provide a control mechanism. The S-shaped graph of this oxyhemoglobin relationship is known as the oxyhemoglobin dissociation curve and represents the relationship between the partial pressure of oxygen (P_{O_2}) in mm of mercury (Hg) and the oxygen content per 100 ml of blood (**Figure 2**).

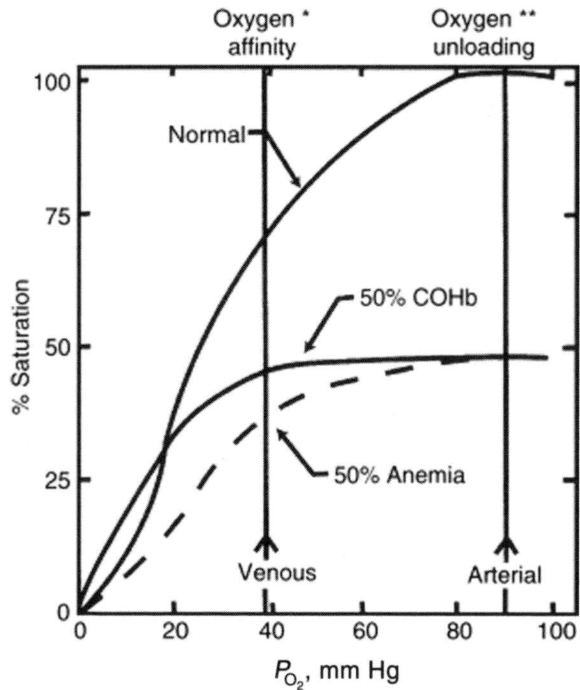

Figure 2 Oxyhemoglobin dissociation curve. *Modifiers of oxygen affinity – increase in plasma pH, decrease in temperature, decrease in 2,3-BPG. **Modifiers of oxygen unloading – decrease in plasma pH, increase in temperature, increase in 2,3-BPG.

The shape of this relationship is very important since it can be moved to the right, i.e., decreased affinity of hemoglobin for oxygen producing oxygen unloading, or to the left, i.e., increased affinity. These changes are produced by a variety of intracellular cofactors: hydrogen ion (pH), carbon dioxide, and the RBC enzyme 2,3-biphosphoglycerate (BPG). Molecules of 2,3-BPG bind to hemoglobin and decrease the affinity of the molecule for oxygen. This causes enhanced oxygen release, or unloading, and is frequently seen in situations in which the body responds to conditions of low oxygen supply. There are a wide variety of potential diseases and toxic exposures that can impact oxygenation and cooperativity and these will be discussed in subsequent sections.

Anemia

There are many other events that can produce a significant reduction in the RBC mass and a subsequent decrease in the oxygen-carrying capacity of the blood. Normally, the blood volume is maintained at a relatively constant level; hence, any process or event that causes a reduction in either RBCs or hemoglobin produces a condition known as anemia. Anemias can also shift the oxyhemoglobin dissociation curve as the body attempts to compensate for reduced oxygen-carrying capacity. In general, the etiology of anemias falls into three general categories: (1) acute or chronic blood loss from any source, (2) underproduction associated with a decreased reticulocyte count, and (3) hemolysis or destruction of RBCs associated with an increased reticulocyte count. There are a variety of laboratory tests that are useful for the evaluation of anemia; however, three of the most critical are the measurement of RBC size and shape (known as RBC indices), examination of the peripheral blood smear, and bone marrow examination. Each of these tests reveals information that can provide clues, which lead to the etiology of the anemia. In later sections, some examples of toxins (e.g., carbon monoxide, hydrogen sulfide, hydrogen cyanide) that cause anemias by altering the binding affinity for hemoglobin and oxygen will be presented.

In general, the amount of oxygen delivered to a given organ or tissue is directly related to three variables: (1) blood flow or cardiac output, (2) hemoglobin concentration, and (3) the difference in oxygen content (saturation) between arterial and venous blood. For example, the cardiac output can significantly increase in order to maintain adequate oxygenation of vital organs such as the brain and kidney at the expense of the smooth muscle. Similarly, erythropoiesis can be stimulated by erythropoietin so that the overall hemoglobin levels increase. Finally, as illustrated in **Figure 2**, oxygen unloading or delivery can be augmented by a right shift in the oxygen dissociation curve facilitated by the RBC enzyme 2,3-BPG.

The converse to anemia is known as polycythemia or erythrocytosis, which is an increase above normal in the circulating quantity of RBCs. Not surprisingly, this increase in total RBCs is usually associated with a corresponding increase in hemoglobin. There are numerous causes of polycythemia such as response to high altitude, pulmonary disease, steroids (both androgenic and glucocorticoid), stress, and smoking.

Myeloids

The myeloids or leukocytes are a highly complex and sophisticated group of cells that are primarily involved in host resistance and inflammatory response against both foreign organisms and material (e.g., chemicals and toxins). For simplicity, the leukocytes can be divided into two major groups: (1) immunocytes and (2) phagocytes. The general organizational structure and normal values are shown in **Figure 1**. These cells are thought to arise from a common PSC in the bone marrow; hence, any toxin that affects the PSC will have a potentially disastrous impact on the body's ability to respond to challenges from an external agent or foreign substance.

The immunocytes are all involved in specific types of immune response that are generally divided into two types: (1) cell-mediated, i.e., specifically sensitized T cells (derived from the thymus), which are associated with graft rejection, resistance to certain viruses, bacteria, fungi, and protozoa, and delayed-type hypersensitivity; and (2) humoral-mediated, i.e., B cells (bursa equivalent), which produce specific antibodies after the body is exposed to a specific antigen.

The phagocytes are so named because their major function is to engulf or ingest foreign organisms or material. The phagocytes include the three granulocytes known as neutrophils (54–62%), eosinophils (1–3%), and basophils (<1%) and the monocytes (3–7%). Monocytes circulate in the blood for several days until they migrate into the reticuloendothelial tissues (liver, spleen, and bone marrow), where they are known as macrophages. Macrophages are not only involved in inflammatory responses but also have a major role in the destruction and removal of old RBCs and other plasma proteins, including hemoglobin.

The phagocytes act by engulfing the foreign material/agent and produce a respiratory burst. The respiratory burst involves the production of hydrogen peroxide and other highly reactive chemicals that attack the ingested material. An inflammatory response is quite commonly produced in this situation. Glucocorticoids (steroids such as prednisone) tend to decrease the numbers of granulocytes that will be involved in an inflammatory reaction. This effect accounts for beneficial impact of these drugs when an antiinflammatory result is desired; however, there is also an increased susceptibility to infections that has been well documented.

There are several key terms and definitions that are given to absolute decreases or increases in the numbers of leukocytes. A fall in the total granulocyte count below 3000 mm^{-3} is known as granulocytopenia. Granulocytopenia is commonly associated with chemically induced bone marrow damage; however, ionizing radiation and a myriad of drugs can also produce this effect. Finally, a particularly severe form of bone marrow failure is known as aplastic anemia. Aplastic anemia is diagnosed when at least two different marrow cell lines are severely depressed as demonstrated by (1) granulocytes <500 mm^{-3}, (2) platelets <20 000 mm^{-3}, (3) reticulocyte count <1%, or (4) a bone marrow biopsy demonstrating <25% cellularity.

Granulocytosis is the opposite phenomenon of decreased cellularity and refers to elevated counts over 10 000 mm^{-3}. Stress, drugs, and some bacterial toxins can produce short-term granulocytosis; however, chemical exposure is not typically associated with mild, elevated counts. Leukemias are associated with counts over 30 000 mm^{-3} and have been associated with certain chemical exposures. This association will be presented in further detail in a subsequent section.

Thrombocytes

Platelets are produced by the fragmentation of megakaryocytes, the largest cell type in the bone marrow. Approximately one-third of the platelets are taken up by the spleen, while the other two-thirds freely circulate for 7–10 days until they are taken up by phagocytic cells. A normal platelet count is between 150 000 and 450 000 mm^{-3}. The normal platelet count is quite variable and can be affected by an individual's nutritional state or, in females, by the menstrual cycle.

Platelets are the rapid reaction troops in the situation of accidental blood loss associated with damaged blood vessels that expose collagen fibers. Normally, platelets are nonsticky; however, they rapidly and easily adhere or aggregate to exposed collagen fibers where they undergo a series of reactions that results in the formation of a thick mass known as a platelet plug. This plug acts to stop bleeding quickly; however, it must usually be reinforced with the help of the clotting system so that vascular integrity is maintained. Platelet reactions are highly sensitive and vulnerable to substances that interfere with the aggregation reaction. For example, aspirin acts in a unique fashion to inhibit the aggregation reaction and has become a useful drug in the prevention of heart attacks and strokes caused by small platelet plugs.

Any disorder or agent that injures the stem cells or prevents their proliferation can drastically affect the absolute platelet count. The minimal platelet count necessary for initial hemostasis is ~50 000 mm^{-3}. If the platelet count falls below 20 000 mm^{-3}, a condition known as thrombocytopenia exists and the affected organism is extremely vulnerable to spontaneous bleeding episodes. Usually, thrombocytopenia due to marrow failure is also associated with reduced leukocyte and RBC production since chemicals or disorders that affect the megakaryocytes also impact other stem cells. This is typically determined by examining a peripheral smear of the blood or by a hematologist's bone marrow aspiration.

The opposite phenomenon, elevated platelet count or thrombocytosis, is diagnosed when counts are greater than 400 000 mm^{-3}. There are many causes of thrombocytosis, including primary (e.g., essential thrombocytosis (ET)) and secondary (e.g., response to inflammation, acute bleeding, iron deficiency, or cancers). In ET, there are colonies of megakaryocytes in the absence of any known stimulus.

Toxic Agents and Responses

Carbon Monoxide

Carbon monoxide (CO) is an odorless, tasteless, and colorless gas that is rapidly absorbed by the lungs and attaches to hemoglobin with an affinity that is 250 times greater than oxygen. Due to this extreme differential, as CO concentrations increase, the number of available sites on the hemoglobin molecule for oxygen decreases. Normally, this reaction would cause oxygen to be more freely released so that adequate tissue oxygenation can be maintained. This would typically produce a right shift of the oxyhemoglobin dissociation curve; however, with increasing exposure to CO and formation of carboxyhemoglobin (COHgb), there is a change in the oxyhemoglobin complex, which produces a left shift in the oxygen dissociation curve (**Figure 2**). The overall effects are decreased tissue oxygenation, anaerobic metabolism, and lactic acid formation.

Exposure to CO results in a wide variety of potential adverse effects, particularly in individuals who have preexisting cardiac or lung disease. Infants, the elderly, and the developing fetus are particularly vulnerable since they have less capacity to tolerate cardiovascular compromise. An additional problem is the delayed neurological and neuropsychiatric effects that have been documented after some significant exposures. The incidence of delayed neurotoxicity is between 2 and 30%.

CO poisoning is usually diagnosed by measuring the presence of COHgb in blood. Nonsmokers have COHgb levels of <1%, whereas smokers have levels of 5–10%. Unfortunately, the measured COHgb level does not always correlate with clinical findings and symptoms; therefore, the clinician should always have a high index of suspicion and aggressively evaluate and treat exposed patients. Treatment consists of removal from the source and administration of 100% oxygen and any other basic life-support measures required. In certain circumstances, i.e., COHgb levels over 25%, the use of hyperbaric oxygen is indicated.

Hydrogen Cyanide and Hydrogen Sulfide

Both hydrogen cyanide (HCN) and hydrogen sulfide (H_2S) are metabolic poisons that act in relatively similar mechanistic ways. At the cellular level, the major energy source is adenosine triphosphate (ATP). ATP is primarily produced through a process known as oxidative phosphorylation, which involves the transfer of electrons to substances known as cytochromes. The cytochrome system can be viewed as a 'bucket brigade' that moves critical electrons in an orderly fashion so that cellular respiration is maintained. As electrons are transferred, energy is released and used to generate ATP and water. Oxygen is the final electron acceptor in the cytochrome system and can be severely affected by metabolic toxins like HCN and H_2S. These toxins ultimately act by blocking electron transfer to molecular oxygen. This blockade produces a rise in peripheral tissue partial pressure of oxygen and a decrease in the unloading gradient for oxyhemoglobin. The net effect is the production of both high levels of oxyhemoglobin in venous return blood and significant levels of lactic acid. At high exposure concentrations, cardiopulmonary compromise is rapidly produced and death ensues.

The treatment of either HCN or H_2S toxicity is based on the use of chemicals that interrupt the binding of these materials to the cytochrome oxidase system. Sodium nitrate and amyl nitrate are both used as antidotes. These substances act by overwhelming the RBC with oxidant stress and producing a somewhat less toxic material known as methemoglobin (MetHgb). MetHgb serves as a source of circulating ferric iron (Fe^{3+}), which preferentially competes for binding by cyanide or sulfide and causes the cyanide or sulfide to dissociate from the cytochrome system and move into blood in a form complexed to methemoglobin in RBCs. This less toxic material is further detoxified by the use of another drug, sodium thiosulfate, which further enhances the conversion of cyanide to the less toxic thiocyanate. The situation with H_2S is somewhat more complex since the second step use of sodium thiosulfate is not typically recommended; however, vigorous use of 100% oxygen therapy is appropriate for treating exposure to both HCN and H_2S. Cyanide toxicity can also be treated by hydroxocobalamin administration. Hydroxocobalamin is marketed under the trade name Cyanokit™ for use in cyanide poisoning. This compound complexes with the cyanide preventing the development of cellular toxicity. A standard dose is 5 g infused IV over 15 min. Additional doses depend upon response and presence of persistent toxicity. Hydroxocobalamin use is described further under the article, Cyanide.

Methemoglobin

At the molecular level, the transport of oxygen in the body is highly dependent on the maintenance of intracellular Hgb in a chemical condition known as the reduced state, or Fe^{2+}. When hemoglobin is oxidized, the Fe^{3+} state, it is known as MetHgb and is unable to bind oxygen. A small amount, <1%, of MetHgb is always found in normal RBCs. MetHgb can be chemically reduced by an enzyme system so that the body maintains adequate levels of Fe^{2+}. If MetHgb exceeds 10% of the total hemoglobin, then clinically observable changes such as dusky complexion can be detected in the affected individual. As MetHgb levels reach 35%, symptoms such as headache, fatigue, and shortness of breath are common. MetHgb levels over 80% are usually fatal.

There are many causes of MetHgb, including both hereditary and acquired. Drugs and toxins, such as nitrates, nitrites, nitroglycerine, aniline dyes, hydrazine, and hydrazones as well as sulfonamides, are associated with the production of MetHgb in certain situations. Natural substances including monomethylhydrazine-containing mushrooms such as the *Gyromitra esculenta* can also cause methemoglobinemia, as gyromitrin is similar to hydrazine in structure and function. Toxic levels of MetHgb can be treated with a compound known as methylene blue, which acts to rapidly reduce the level of circulating MetHgb.

Aplastic Anemia

Aplastic anemia is characterized by pancytopenia on peripheral smear. The criteria for severe aplastic anemia includes a bone marrow biopsy showing <50% normal cellularity in which fewer than 30% of the cells are hematopoietic and at least two of the following are present: absolute reticulocyte count <40 000 μl^{-1}, absolute neutrophil count <500 μl^{-1}, or platelet count <20 000 μl^{-1}. The major causes of acquired aplastic anemia are exposure to a wide variety of drugs, chemicals, and ionizing radiation. Many cytotoxic drugs (e.g., vinblastine, vincristine) used in the treatment of cancer to kill tumor cells can kill stem cells as well. Similarly, certain analgesics (e.g., acetaminophen, diclofenac, indomethacin, phenylbutazone) and antibiotics (e.g., chloramphenicol, mefloquine, azidothymidine, penicillin) have been associated with aplastic anemia.

Thrombocytopenia

Multiple drugs can cause thrombocytopenia (platelet count less than 150 000 μl^{-1}) via the formation of drug-dependent antiplatelet antibodies that cause platelet destruction or clearance by the reticuloendothelial system. Less common mechanisms are drug-induced bone marrow suppression or an autoimmune thrombocytopenia that is initiated by exposure to the offending drug but persists in its absence. Common drugs than can cause thrombocytopenia by antibody-mediated platelet destruction include the following: abciximab, amiodarone, carbamazepine, cimetidine, phenytoin, piperacillin, rifampin, sulfonamides, trimethoprim-sulfamethoxazole, and vancomycin. Thrombocytopenia can also occur as a result of heparin-induced thrombocytopenia (HIT). It is a form of drug-induced thrombocytopenia manifested clinically by thrombosis or skin necrosis with a clear relationship between the onset of thrombocytopenia and heparin use. Heparin and platelet factor 4 (PF4), a heparin-neutralizing protein contained in the alpha granules of platelets, can trigger an antibody response. The heparin–PF4 antibody complex attached to platelets undergo aggregation and are then removed from the circulation leading to thrombocytopenia and the generation of procoagulant platelet-derived microparticles, resulting in thrombosis. If a patient is suspected of having HIT, all sources of heparin should be discontinued immediately and the use of an alternative nonheparin anticoagulant can be recommended, unless there is a contraindication.

Hemolysis

The normal life span of a circulating erythrocyte is approximately 120 days. Any degree of reduction in this life span represents hemolysis. If hemolysis exceeds the regeneration of new erythrocytes, it results in anemia. Several chemicals or their reactive metabolites can cause hemolysis via oxidative injury (e.g., chlorates, benzocaine, methylene blue, nitrites, phenol, sulfonamides). Other chemicals can cause hemolysis in the absence of oxidant injury, for example, lead and arsine. Lead causes anemia by a combination of mechanisms, including the inhibition of several enzymes involved in heme synthesis. Toxic levels of lead above 25 $\mu g\ dl^{-1}$ can be treated with chelation therapy. The mechanism of hemolysis behind arsine toxicity involves the fixation of arsine by sulfhydryl groups of hemoglobin and impairment of membrane proteins, including Na^+–K^+–ATPase. Supportive care and cessation of exposure are the treatments of choice in most cases. In severe cases, exchange transfusion can be used.

Glucose-6-Phosphate Dehydrogenase Deficiencies

Glucose-6-phosphate dehydrogenase (G6PD) deficiency is the most common enzymatic disorder of RBCs in humans. The likelihood of developing hemolysis and the severity of disease are determined by the magnitude of the enzyme deficiency and acute hemolysis is the most common clinical presentation of previously unrecognized G6PD deficiency. Typically, hemolysis begins 1–4 days following the exposure of an offending drug (e.g., methylene blue, nitrofurantoin, primaquine, sulfamethoxazole, naphthalene). Other drugs, including, vitamin C, sulfisoxazole, and acetaminophen, are safe at therapeutic doses but can cause hemolysis in G6PD-deficient patients following an overdose. Jaundice, dark urine, and abdominal and back pain may occur. The peripheral smear can show cell fragments that have had Heinz bodies excised. Bone marrow stimulation results in reticulocytosis and an increased erythrocyte mass. More severe variants of G6PD deficiency include neonatal jaundice, kernicterus, and splenomegaly with black pigment gallstones from chronic hemolysis.

Leukemia

The leukemias are a diverse group of hematologic malignancies that arise from the malignant transformation of hematopoietic cells. These cells develop in the bone marrow and lymphoid tissue and ultimately interfere with normal cell development and immunity. Leukemias are generally divided into two groups, myeloid and lymphoid. In addition, leukemias can be further subdivided by their natural history into acute or chronic forms. The leukemias represent 3% of all malignancies and ~24 000 new cases develop in the United States every year.

The etiology of leukemia in most cases is unknown, although a combination of genetic and environmental factors is probably important. The most important environmental factors are drugs, radiation, and chemical exposures to a few selected substances. The most common form of leukemia associated with either chemicals or drugs is the acute non-lymphatic leukemias (ANLLs), which are also referred to as acute myeloid leukemias (AMLs). In ANLL, large numbers of immature hematopoietic cells develop and replace the normal cells. These abnormal cells are released into the circulation and can easily be seen on peripheral blood smears. Since these cells are quite immature, the blood does not contain adequate numbers of normally functioning mature RBCs, leukocytes, and thrombocytes. AML is an aggressive and rapidly fatal disease unless appropriate therapy is begun.

The role of chemical exposure and development of ANLL has been quite controversial. This controversy is partially due to the problems associated with accurately and appropriately classifying the various leukemias. Since the mid-1980s, the nomenclature of the ANLL subtypes was established by the French–American–British Cooperative Group also known as FAB. Older studies in the literature that do not use this classification scheme present a serious problem since there was a tendency to lump different categories together in order to achieve sufficient statistical power for epidemiological analysis. Nevertheless, there does appear to be sufficient evidence to link ANLL with certain exposures to benzene.

The association between benzene exposure and leukemia has been made since the late nineteenth century; however, the dose–response relationship and mechanistic explanation have been quite contentious. The most reliable evidence associating chronic benzene exposure with AML was presented in a retrospective National Institute for Occupational Safety and Health study of rubber hydrochloride workers in Akron, OH, from 1940 to 1949. Unfortunately, the mechanism of how benzene exposure leads to the development of AML is not known. The two most frequently discussed potential mechanisms of toxicity involve either a point mutation or a chromosomal deletion. The latter is considered more likely since neither benzene nor its metabolites are mutagenic or teratogenic.

See also: Arsine; Benzene; Carbon Monoxide; Cardiovascular System; Distribution; Heparin; Hydrogen Sulfide; Immune System; Kidney; Lead; Liver; Mushrooms, Monomethylhydrazine (MMH) - Generating; Hydrazine.

Further Reading

American Academy of Pediatrics Committee on Environmental Health, 1999. Lead. In: Handbook of Pediatric Environmental Health. American Academy of Pediatrics (AAP), Elk Grove, IL, pp. 131–143.

Arellano, M., Bernal-Mizrachi, L., Pan, L., et al., October 2011. Prognostic significance of leukopenia at the time of diagnosis in acute myeloid leukemia. Clin. Lymphoma. Myeloma Leuk. 11 (5), 427–432.

Beutler, E., 17 January 1991. Glucose-6-phosphate dehydrogenase deficiency. N. Engl. J. Med. 324 (3), 169–174.

Beutler, E., 1 December 1994. G6PD deficiency. Blood 84 (11), 3613–3636.

Beutler, E., 1 January 2008. Glucose-6-phosphate dehydrogenase deficiency: a historical perspective. Blood 111 (1), 16–24.

Blair, P.C., Thompson, M.B., Bechtold, M., Wilson, R.E., Moorman, M.P., Fowler, B.A., July 1990. Evidence for oxidative damage to red blood cells in mice induced by arsine gas. Toxicology 63 (1), 25–34.

Braunwald, E., Fauci, A.S., Kasper, D.L. (Eds.), 2001. Harrison's Principles of Internal Medicine, fifteenth ed. McGraw-Hill, New York.

Brooks, S.M., Gochfeld, M., Herzstein, J., 1995. Environmental Medicine. Mosby, St. Louis, MO.

Canfield, R.L., Henderson Jr, C.R., Cory-Slechta, D.A., Cox, C., Jusko, T.A., Lanphear, B.P., 17 April 2003. Intellectual impairment in children with blood lead concentrations below 10 microg per deciliter. N. Engl. J. Med. 348 (16), 1517–1526.

CDC, 1991. Preventing Lead Poisoning in Young Children. Department of Health and Human Services, DC, United States.

Centers for Disease Control and Prevention, 2007. Medical Management Guidelines for Arsine. Agency for Toxic Substances and Disease Registry last updated 9/24/07. Available at: http://www.atsdr.cdc.gov/MHMI/mmg169.html (accessed 05.10.07.).

Cortazzo, J.A., Lichtman, A.D., 2013. Methemoglobinemia: a review and recommendations for management. J. Cardiothorac. Vasc. Anesth. pii:S1053-0770(13) 00043–8.

Gribaldo, L., 2002. Haematotoxicology scientific basis and regulatory aspects. Altern. Lab. Anim. 30 (2), 111–113.

Lead exposure in children: prevention, detection, and management, October 2005. Pediatrics 116 (4), 1036–1046.

Murata, K., Iwata, T., Dakeishi, M., Karita, K., 2009. Lead toxicity: does the critical level of lead resulting in adverse effects differ between adults and children? J. Occup. Health 51 (1), 1–12.

Nkhoma, E.T., Poole, C., Vannappagari, V., et al., May–June 2009. The global prevalence of glucose-6-phosphate dehydrogenase deficiency: a systematic review and meta-analysis. Blood Cells Mol. Dis. 42 (3), 267–278.

Parent-Massin, D., 2001. Relevance of clonogenic assays in hematotoxicology. Cell Biol. Toxicol. 17 (2), 87–94.

Pullen-James, S., Woods, S.E., December 2006. Occupational arsine gas exposure. J. Natl. Med. Assoc. 98 (12), 1998–2001.

Rael, L.T., Ayala-Fierro, F., Carter, D.E., June 2000. The effects of sulfur, thiol, and thiol inhibitor compounds on arsine-induced toxicity in the human erythrocyte membrane. Toxicol. Sci. 55 (2), 468–477.

Smith, A., Howell, D., Patmore, R., et al., 2011. Incidence of haematological malignancy by sub-type: a report from the haematological malignancy research network. Br. J. Cancer 105, 1684.

Sullivan, J.B., Krieger, G.R. (Eds.), 1998. Hazardous Materials Toxicology. Clinical Principles of Environmental Health, second ed. Williams and Wilkins, Baltimore, MD.

Taleb, M., Ashraf, Z., Valavoor, S., Tinkel, J., 2013. Evaluation and management of acquired methemoglobinemia associated with topical benzocaine use. Am. J. Cardiovasc. Drugs 13 (5), 325–330.

Treatment guidelines for lead exposure in children, July 1995. American Academy of Pediatrics Committee on Drugs. Pediatrics 96 (1 Pt 1), 155–160.

Vardiman, J.W., Harris, N.L., Brunning, R.D., 1 October 2002. The World Health Organization (WHO) classification of the myeloid neoplasms. Blood 100 (7), 2292–2302.

Yamamoto, J.F., Goodman, M.T., 2008. Patterns of leukemia incidence in the United States by subtype and demographic characteristics, 1997–2002. Cancer Causes Control 19, 379.

Relevant Websites

http://www.atsdr.cdc.gov/csem/csem.asp?csem=7&po=0 – ATSDR (Agency for Toxic Substances and Disease Registry) webpage on lead toxicity.

http://www.cdc.gov/nceh/lead/ – CDC (US Center for Disease Control) webpage on lead toxicity.

http://www.masimo.com/pdf/whitepaper/LAB4280B.pdf – Demystifying Methemoglobinemia – White Paper. Online resource (PDF format).

http://emedicine.medscape.com/article/198759-overview – *eMedicine* online resource for approach to aplastic anemia including an overview, clinical presentation, and management.

http://emedicine.medscape.com/article/833740-overview – *eMedicine* online resource regarding arsine exposure and poisoning.

http://emedicine.medscape.com/article/200390-overview – *eMedicine* online resource regarding G6PD deficiency (glucose-6-phosphate dehydrogenase deficiency).

http://emedicine.medscape.com/article/204178-overview – *eMedicine* online resource for approach to methemoglobinemia including an overview, clinical presentation, management, and antidote use.

http://emedicine.medscape.com/article/1174752-overview – *eMedicine* online resource for approach to patient with lead exposure and poisoning including an overview, clinical presentation, and management.

http://www.g6pd.org/ – G6PD deficiency online resource from the G6PD Deficiency Association.

http://www.lls.org/diseaseinformation/leukemia/ – Leukemia and lymphoma information at the Leukemia and Lymphoma Society webpage.

http://www.haz-map.com/methem.html – Methemoglobinemia and industrial agents as cause. ACGIH (American College of Governmental Industrial Hygienists).

Blue-Green Algae *see* Algae

Boric Acid

P Lank and M Wahl, Illinois Poison Center, Chicago, IL, USA

This article is a revision of the previous edition article by Michael Wahl, volume 1, pp 329–330, © 2005, Elsevier Inc.

- Name: Boric acid
- Chemical Abstracts Service Registry Number: CAS 10043-35-3
- Synonyms: Boracic acid, Orthoboric acid, Hydrogen borate, Borofax, Three elephant, NCI-C36417
- Molecular Formula: H_3BO_3
- Chemical Structure:

OH
/
HO — B
\
OH

Boric acid

Uses

Boric acid is used as a fireproofing agent for wood, as a preservative, and as an antiseptic. It is used in the manufacture of glass, pottery, enamels, glazes, cosmetics, cements, porcelain, leather, carpets, hats, soaps, artificial gems, and in tanning, printing, dyeing, painting, and photography. It is a constituent of nickel plating baths and electric condensers, and it is used for impregnating wicks and hardening steel. In laboratory procedures, boric acid is used in the preparation of buffer solutions.

Boric acid is also used as a fungicide and as an insecticide powder. Domestic use may include its application as an insecticide for crawling insects such as roaches. In medicine, it had been widely used as a disinfectant and a constituent of baby powders, antiseptics, diaper rash ointments, eye washes, gargles, and a variety of other consumer products for its mild antiseptic property. Its routine medical use, however, has fallen out of favor because of its relatively weak antiseptic action and its potential for toxicity, although it may still be used to treat recurrent vulvovaginitis.

Background Information

Boric acid exists in natural deposits as a mineral, sassolite. It is also found in hot mineral water sources. The minerals are extracted with sulfuric acid and crystalline boric acid is separated. Borates have been used since antiquity for cleaning and as food preservatives among other things. Boric acid was first registered for use in the United States as an insecticide in 1948. It has also been used as an antiseptic and was found in numerous commercial products.

Environmental Fate and Behavior

Physicochemical Properties

Boric acid is odorless and colorless crystals or a white powder. It is soluble in water at 5.6 g per 100 ml and solubility increases as the water temperature increases. It is a weak acid (pK_a of 9.15) and exists in aqueous solutions below pH of 7 as undisocciated boric acid. The octanol–water coefficient (K_{ow}) is 0.175. The density of boric acid is 1.4. The vapor pressure at standard temperature and pressure is negligible.

Partition Behavior in Water, Sediment, and Soil

Boric acid and borate salts are present in soils throughout the earth. In soil, inorganic boron compounds can react with moisture to form various borates. Boric acid has greatest adsorption to soil at pH of 7.5–9.0. Presence of iron or aluminum oxides affect mobility. Borate concentrations are highest in seawater (averaging 4.5 mg l^{-1}), although drinking water concentrations can reach 3.28 mg l^{-1}. Boric acid and salts of borate may reach groundwater because of their high water solubility and their variable soil adsorption.

Environmental Persistency

Boric acid decomposes at temperatures above 100 °C. This produces boric anhydride. The solution of boric anhydride is a weak acid. Boric acid and borate salts are removed from soils by leaching and uptake by plants. The low volatility of boric acid and other borates results in only small amounts of these compounds being present in the earth's atmosphere. Particulates are removed through precipitation and direct deposition. Airborne borate particles have a half-life of a few days depending upon the size of the particle and conditions in the atmosphere. Boric acid and borates are not thought to degrade or transform through photolysis, oxidation, or hydrolysis in the atmosphere.

Exposure Routes and Pathways

Accidental ingestion and subcutaneous routes are the primary exposure pathways. The maximum workplace concentration is

10 mg m^{-3}. The maximum concentration in water used in fisheries is 0.1 mg l^{-1}. Boric acid can be absorbed via ingestion and inhalation or through application to damaged or abraded skin. Exposure from lavage and enema can also occur.

Toxicokinetics

Water emulsifying and hydrophobic ointments containing boric acid liberate only small amounts within 24 h compared with a near total liberation from a jelly. Boric acid is readily absorbed from the gastrointestinal tract, mucous membranes, and abraded skin. Boric acid is excreted unchanged in urine with ~50% excreted in the first 12 h and the remainder excreted over a period of a few days. The half-life of boric acid given orally is estimated to be 21 h. The fatal dose of boric acid is estimated to be 15–20 g in an adult and ~5 or 6 g in an infant, with suggested fatal serum concentrations of at least 400 μg ml^{-1} (normal range: 0–2 μg ml^{-1}).

Mechanism of Toxicity

The exact mechanism of toxicity is not known. Boric acid can inhibit production of adenosine triphosphate, a cellular form of energy.

Acute and Short-Term Toxicity (or Exposure)

Animal

Ingestion of boric acid by animals results in excessive salivation, thirst, fever, vomiting, and diarrhea. Seizures and other neurologic toxicity occur in large ingestions. The onset of toxicity and clinically apparent effects is typically within only a few hours of ingestion. The LD_{50} (oral) of boric acid in rats is 4550 mg kg^{-1}. Dogs are more sensitive to boric acid with the LD_{50} (oral) >631 mg kg^{-1}.

Human

Acute boric acid poisoning is extremely rare. In large ingestions or overdoses, gastrointestinal symptoms including nausea, vomiting, and diarrhea may occur. The diarrhea and vomitus of a patient with boric acid ingestion is characteristically described as being greenish blue. This may be followed by restlessness, delirium, headache, tremors, and generalized convulsions usually followed by weakness and coma. There is fever and tachypnea followed by Cheyne–Stokes-type respirations and respiratory arrest.

Changes on the skin include an erythematous skin eruption, with papules or vesicles appearing between the fingers and on the back of the hands initially and eventually becoming generalized enough to give a 'boiled lobster' appearance. The skin lesions may undergo bullous formation, desquamation, excoriation, and sloughing. Hypothermia often occurs.

Renal injury can occur, usually in the form of renal tubular necrosis, and can be demonstrated by the presence of oliguria, albuminuria, and eventually anuria. Signs of meningeal irritation, oliguria, and circulatory collapse may be followed by death within 5 days. Infants and young children are more susceptible to boric acid intoxication. Symptoms in extremely large doses will be similar to those seen in chronic overexposure (see below).

Chronic Toxicity (or Exposure)

Animal

Dogs and rats were able to tolerate boric acid doses of up to 350 ppm for 2 years. Larger doses of boric acid (1750 ppm) over a period of time have been shown to cause testicular damage and sterility in rats and dogs.

Human

Toxicity may occur after ingestion, injection, application to damaged skin (e.g., abrasion, burns, or diaper rash), lavage, or enema. Exposure can also occur with inhalation. Severe systemic toxicity is most likely to occur from repeated dermal application to damaged skin; this has been reported mainly in the treatment of diaper rash in young children. Symptoms include nausea, vomiting, bloody diarrhea, severe colic, and abdominal pain. Low levels of boric acid ingestion may lead to dry skin and mucous membranes, followed by the appearance of a red tongue, patchy alopecia, cracked lips, and conjunctivitis. Infertility among men is possible.

No major toxicological distinctions between boric acid and its salts are recognized in human beings.

In Vitro Toxicity Data

No mutagenic effects have been seen in *Salmonella typhi* strains TA98 and TA100 via the preincubation method.

Immunotoxicity

Exposure to boric acid through the skin can cause immune-mediated reactions including dermatitis.

Genotoxicity

No mutagenic effects have been seen in *S. typhi* strains TA98 and TA100 via the preincubation method.

Reproductive Toxicity

Developmental toxicity occurs when boric acid is given to pregnant female rats. At doses that are nontoxic to the mother, skeletal abnormalities and low birth-weights occurred in the offspring. Fetal malformations occurred in rabbits fed 250 mg kg^{-1} day^{-1} of boric acid during pregnancy.

Carcinogenicity

Boric acid is not classified as a human carcinogen by the American Conference of Governmental Industrial Hygienists.

Chronic exposure studies in rats and mice also indicate that boric acid is not carcinogenic.

Clinical Management

There is no specific antidote. Supportive care should be instituted for all patients with history of serious boric acid exposure. Substantial recent ingestions may benefit from administration of activated charcoal. Fluid and electrolyte balance, correction of acid/base disturbance, and control of seizures are essential to therapy. Case reports indicate that hemodialysis as well as forced diuresis with furosemide and very close monitoring of fluid repletion may be used to treat acute boric acid poisoning. Sodium bicarbonate may be used for any metabolic acidosis.

Ecotoxicology

Freshwater and Sediment Organism Toxicity

Boric acid has an LC_{50} of 65–88 mg l^{-1} in short-term exposure studies (24 h) for rainbow trout. Bluegill fish are the most sensitive freshwater fish to boric acid toxicity with a LD_{50} of 41 mg l^{-1} for 24-h exposures. Boric acid inhibits the growth of green algae (*Chlorella vulgaris*) at concentrations of 10.6 mg l^{-1} over a 3–4-month exposure period.

Terrestrial Organism Toxicity (Including Plants)

Boric acid acts as a poison in the stomach of insects. It also affects the nervous system and the powder is abrasive to their exoskeletons. Boric acid also acts as a herbicide; causing the desiccation of plants. While boron is an essential nutrient for the growth of plants, excessive boron, boric acid, and borate salts uptake can cause toxicity. Yellowing, splitting of the leaf and of bark, and necrosis of root tips occur when soil boron levels are excessive.

Plants take up boric acid and borate salts as undissociated boric acid through active transport when the levels of boric acid in the plants are low. Passive diffusion occurs at higher soil concentrations. Boron and its salts are transported to the leaves where water evaporates leaving the compounds behind to accumulate in the leaves. Boric acid and its salts are immobile in the phloem of plants and little moves to other parts such as stems and fruits.

While most vegetable crops are tolerant of high concentrations of boron in soil and water tubers and cereal crops are less so and citrus and nut trees are most susceptible to boron and boric acid toxicity.

Exposure Guidelines

The threshold limit value (inhalable fraction) is 2 mg m^{-3} as a time-weighted average. The short-term exposure limit for exposures that are only likely to last 15 min is 6 mg m^{-3}. The maximum workplace concentration is 10 mg m^3. The maximum concentration in water used in fisheries is 0.1 mg l^{-1}. The recommended exposure limits for exposure over a 40-h workweek are 1 mg sodium tetraborate (anhydrous) per m^3 and 5 mg boric acid per m^3.

The US Food and Drug Administration has set a reference dose (RfD) for boron compounds at 0.2 mg kg^{-1} day^{-1}. The Health Advisory level for a 10-kg child is 4 mg boron per liter for one day exposure and 0.9 mg boron per liter for a 10-day exposure. The drinking water equivalent is 7 mg boron per liter of water.

The tolerable daily intake (TDI) of boric acid as estimated by the National Academy of Sciences Food and Nutrition Board is 0.32 mg kg^{-1} day^{-1}. The TDI estimated by the World Health Organization is 0.4 mg kg^{-1} day^{-1}.

See also: TGN1412; Freons; Mouse Lymphoma Assay.

Further Reading

Bolt, H.M., Basaran, N., Duydu, Y., 2012. Human environmental and occupational exposures to boric acid: reconciliation with experimental reproductive toxicity data. J. Toxicol. Environ. Health 75 (8–10), 508–514.

Litovitz, T.L., Klein-Schwartz, W., Oderda, G.M., 1988. Clinical manifestations of toxicity in a series of 784 boric acid ingestions. Am. J. Emerg. Med. 6, 209–213.

Naderi, A.S., Palmer, B.F., 2006. Successful treatment of a rare case of boric acid overdose with hemodialysis. Am. J. Kidney Dis. 48 (6), e95–7.

Restuccio, A., Mortensen, M.E., Kelley, M., 1992. Fatal ingestion of boric acid in an adult. Am. J. Emerg. Med. 10, 545–547.

Teshima, D., Taniyama, T., Oishi, R., 2001. Usefulness of forced diuresis for acute boric acid poisoning in an adult. J. Clin. Pharm. Ther. 26, 387–390.

Teshima, D., Morishita, K., Ueda, Y., et al., 1992. Clinical management of boric acid ingestion: pharmacokinetic assessment of efficacy of hemodialysis for treatment of acute boric acid poisoning. J. Pharmacobiodyn. 15, 287–294.

Relevant Websites

http://npic.orst.edu/factsheets/borictech.html – Boric Acid Fact Sheet – including information about toxicity in animals and humans including developmental and other effects.

http://edis.ifas.ufl.edu/pi128 – University of Florida website – pesticide profile for boric acid. Includes toxicity information.

Boron

S Betharia, Manchester University College of Pharmacy, Fort Wayne, IN, USA

This article is a revision of the previous edition article by William S. Utley, volume 1, pp 331–332, © 2005, Elsevier Inc.

- Name: Boron
- Chemical Abstracts Service Registry Number: 7440-42-8
- Synonyms: Boron
- Molecular Formula: B

Background

Although boron-containing compounds have been known for thousands of years, the element in its pure form was not isolated until 1808 by Sir Humphry Davy, Joseph-Louis Gay-Lussac, and Louis-Jacques Thénard, using a reaction between boric acid and potassium. Boron was not considered to be an essential nutrient for human beings prior to 1980. In 1981, a study reported that boron stimulated bone growth in vitamin D-deficient chicks, which helped prevent bone abnormalities. Boron is now regarded as an essential trace mineral that affects the absorption, metabolism, and excretion of calcium, copper, magnesium, nitrogen, glucose, triglyceride, reactive oxygen species, and estrogen in the body.

Uses

Boron is used to harden metals and as an oxygen scavenger for copper and other metals. It is used as a reinforcing material for composites. Boron filaments are used for lightweight but high-strength building materials for aerospace structures, golf clubs, and fishing rods. Amorphous boron can produce a green flare, and is therefore useful in pyrotechnic flares. Boron is also used in the production of borosilicate glass, which is highly resistant to thermal shock. An alloy of boron, iron, and neodymium is used to create a permanent magnet, known as the neodymium magnet. These magnets are used in magnetic resonance imaging machines, cell phones, and CD and DVD players. Boron is also employed as a catalyst in olefin polymerization and alcohol dehydration. Some boron compounds are used in the production of insulating fiberglass, bleach, adhesives, bulletproof vests, and tank armor. The principal consumption pattern in the United States for boron is for the production of glass products with minor usage in the production of soaps and detergents.

In humans, boron plays an important role in keeping the bones and joints healthy, and supplements containing boron can be potentially useful in the treatment of osteoporosis and rheumatoid arthritis, especially in postmenopausal women. Boron has been found to increase collagenase and cathepsin D activity in fibroblasts, thereby modulating the turnover of extracellular matrix. Boron deficiency has been associated with decreased plasma calcium and increased urinary calcium excretion. This element has been reported to enhance the actions of estradiol on trabecular bone, promoting absorption and retention of minerals in ovariectomized rats.

Boron supplementation can increase blood hemoglobin and mean corpuscular hemoglobin levels in boron-deficient anemic subjects. Data also indicate that boron may play an important role in human brain function, alertness, hand–eye coordination, and performance in cognitive tests. An increase in steroid hormone levels (such as testosterone and estradiol) is also observed in both men and women with increased intake of boron, and is supported by the hypothesis that boron is necessary for the hydroxylation step in the formation of specific steroid hormones. This elevation of endogenous steroid hormones in subjects taking boron supplementation could make this element a potentially ergogenic safe substance for athletes. Research also suggests that boron may play a role in the immune system and inflammatory responses. Some studies have also indicated that dietary boron intake in inversely proportional to the incidence of prostate cancer.

Even though cases of boron deficiency are rare, it can impact mineral metabolism, bone integrity, cognitive function, and vitamin and steroid hormone levels. A possible role in reproduction and development is also indicated, as boron-deficient diets have been found to result in embryological defects and stunted growth in some species. Boron is supplied in significant amounts to soils by atmospheric transport from the marine environment. Deficiency problems are therefore less common in coastal areas than farther inland.

Environmental Fate and Behavior

Boron is ubiquitous in the earth's crust, and is found in most soil types in the range 2–100 ppm, and the average concentration of soil boron is estimated to be 10–20 ppm. The primary source of boron is the mineral rasorite, also called kernite. While large areas of the world are boron deficient, high concentrations are found in parts of western United States, and throughout China, Brazil, and Russia. The world's richest deposits of boron are located in a geographic region that stretches from the Mediterranean countries inland to Kazakhstan.

Vapor phase reduction can be used to obtain high-purity crystalline boron from the reaction of boron trichloride or boron tribromide with hydrogen on electrically heated filaments. Boron trioxide may also be heated with magnesium powder to obtain amorphous boron, which is an impure brownish-black powder. Boron is now available commercially at purities of 99.9999%, but is produced with difficulty, as boron tends to easily form refractory materials containing small amounts of carbon and other elements.

The low volatility of boron compounds explains why boron is not present as a vapor in the atmosphere. However, via atmospheric deposition, precipitation, or weathering of boron-containing rocks, boron can be expected to migrate to the water column. Oceans serve as major sources of boron, with an

 http://dx.doi.org/10.1016/B978-0-12-386454-3.00255-4

average concentration of 4.5 ppm. Seawater contains an average of 4.6 ppm boron, while its concentration in freshwater normally ranges from < 0.01 to 1.5 ppm, with higher concentrations in regions close to the marine coast, with poor drainage, with high concentrations of boron in soil, or with high inputs from industrial and municipal effluents.

Naturally occurring boron is present in groundwater primarily as a result of leaching from rocks and soils containing borates. Groundwater concentrations of boron range widely, from < 0.3 to > 100 ppm. Drinking water has been found to contain boron in concentrations between 0.01 and 15 ppm, with most values clearly below 0.4 ppm. These values are consistent with ranges and means observed for groundwater and surface waters, which can be explained based on two factors. First, boron concentrations in water are largely dependent on the leaching of boron from the surrounding geology and wastewater discharges, and second, conventional drinking-water treatment methods are unable to successfully remove boron.

Waterborne boron may be adsorbed by soils and sediments, making adsorption–desorption reactions to be the most significant mechanism influencing the fate of boron in water. The extent of boron adsorption depends on the pH of the water and the boron concentration in solution, with the highest adsorption taking place between pH 7.5 and 9.0. Boron is released to the environment from natural sources such as oceans, volcanoes, and geothermal steam. It cannot be destroyed, but can change its form, producing complexes with soil particles, sediments, or water.

At room temperature, elemental boron (valence 3) exists as a solid, either as pure black monoclinic crystals or as an impure yellow or brown amorphous powder. The melting point of boron is 2079 °C and its boiling/sublimation point is 2550 °C. The specific gravity of crystalline boron is 2.34, while that of the amorphous form is 2.37. Elemental boron is capable of transmitting portions of infrared light. Electrical conductivity of boron is directly proportional to temperature. Boron is capable of forming stable covalently bonded molecular networks. The energy band gap of elemental boron is 1.50–1.56 eV.

Exposure and Exposure Monitoring

The most common routes of exposure to boron for humans include consumption of private, municipal, or commercial (bottled) sources of drinking water; dietary consumption of crops and other foodstuff, including dietary supplements; inhalation of boron compounds during mining, manufacturing, and other industrial processes; and use of some consumer products such as oral care products, cosmetics, soaps, and detergents.

The presence of boron in drinking water has been previously discussed in the "Environmental Fate and Behavior" section. Food sources rich in boron include avocado, peanuts, pecans, grapes, raisins, and wine. Legumes, nuts, and avocados contain 1.0–4.5 mg boron per 100 g, while fruits and vegetables provide 0.1–0.6 mg boron in every 100 g. Meat and dairy products are poor sources, providing less than 0.6 mg boron in 100 g of source. Concentrations of boron reported in food after 1985 are thought to have higher validity due to the use of more adequate analytical methods. Mean daily intakes of boron for male and female adults have been reported to be 1.28 and 1.0 mg boron day^{-1}, respectively, while chronic intakes of as much as 40 mg day^{-1} may occur in some populations.

Workers in industries such as boron mining and processing, and manufacture of fiberglass, cosmetics, fertilizers, pesticides, and cleaning and laundry products, can be exposed to boron compounds at their workplace. Data from these exposure sites can provide a useful method to help assess the upper limits of boron exposure in humans with no concurrent adverse effects. Average boron concentrations in ambient nonoccupational air samples have been reported to be 2×10^{-5} mg boron m^{-3}. A study measuring mean dust concentrations in air samples from a borax packaging and shipping company reported 0.45–2.43 mg boron m^{-3} in the air from these workplaces.

Toxicokinetics

Boron-containing compounds can be absorbed from both the gastrointestinal and respiratory tracts, as indicated by an increase in levels of boron in the blood, tissues, or urine; or by systemic toxic effects observed in the exposed individuals or laboratory animals. While absorption through intact skin is negligible, it can occur through denuded or irritated skin. The decisive factor for the degree of liberation of boron from boron-containing topical products is the nature of the vehicle, with water-based vehicles resulting in higher boron levels achieved in blood and urine. An oral dose of boron is readily and completely (approximately 95%) absorbed in humans and appears rapidly in the blood and body tissues. Boron metabolism in the body is not energetically feasible, with 523 kJ mol^{-1} energy being required to break boron–oxygen bonds. Cessation of dietary boron results in a rapid drop in bone boron levels, with a direct relationship observed between ingestion and urinary excretion rates, which accounts for elimination of nearly 100% of the boron load. The kidneys are the primary site of homeostatic regulation of boron in the body, and at normal dietary or supplemental levels, there is no evidence for boron accumulation over time. While urine serves as the primary pathway for excretion of boron, bile, sweat, and exhaled breath constitute other routes of elimination.

Acute and Short-Term Toxicity

Direct nonsystemic effects of boron exposure are minor, and skin exposure has not been reported to cause irritant or sensitizing contact dermatitis. Respiratory exposure to dust contaminated with boron compounds has been reported to cause symptoms of acute respiratory irritation such as dryness of the mouth, nose, or throat, dry cough, sore throat, productive cough, shortness of breath, nosebleeds, and chest tightness. However, irritation does not persist for long periods after leaving the dusty area. Exposure to large amounts of boron-containing compounds over short periods of time can affect stomach, intestines, liver, kidney, and brain. Studies in animals indicate that the male reproductive organs, especially the testes, are affected if large amounts of boron are ingested for short or long periods of time. Some effects like inhibited spermiation have been found to be reversible, while focal testicular atrophy is persistent in nature after cessation of exposure. The doses of boron that produce these effects are approximately 2000 times the average level of adult exposure in the US population. Children living near boron-containing waste sites are likely to be exposed to higher than normal environmental levels of boron through breathing in boron-containing dust and eating boron-contaminated soil.

The oral LD_{50} values for boron-containing compounds has been established in the range of 400–700 mg boron kg^{-1} of body weight in mice and rats and between 250 and 350 mg boron kg^{-1} of body weight for guinea pigs, dogs, rabbits, and cats. Signs of acute toxicity in animals given single large oral doses of boron-containing compounds include depression, ataxia, kidney degeneration, testicular atrophy, convulsions, and death.

Chronic Toxicity

Chronic exposure to boron in humans can lead to anorexia, weight loss, vomiting, mild diarrhea, erythematous rash, exfoliative dermatitis, alopecia, convulsions, anemia, and kidney damage. A decrease in body weight was reported in both male and female mice exposed to boron-containing compounds for an extended period of 2 years, with a higher rate of mortality observed in male mice. In a different two-year-long study, rats exposed to boron displayed coarse hair coats, scaly tails, hunched posture, swollen and desquamated pads of the paws, abnormally long toenails, shrunken scrotum, inflamed eyelids, and bloody eye discharge. The relative weights of the testes were significantly lower, and relative weights of the brain and thyroid gland were higher, than those of controls in this study.

Reproductive Toxicity

Low birth weights, birth defects, and developmental delays have been reported in newborn animals whose mothers were orally exposed to high doses of boron-containing compounds during pregnancy. However, these doses are more than 800 times higher than the average daily intake of boron in food by adult women in the US population. Unfortunately, the human database on boron is not adequate for establishing an upper tolerable limit (UL) and there are no human data on developmental and reproductive effects comparable to those observed in animals. The current UL for boron (10 mg boron day^{-1} for adults) is based on the no observed adverse effect level (NOAEL) for decreased fetal body weight in rats following maternal exposure during pregnancy. No reproductive toxicities have been reported in males occupationally exposed to boron compounds.

Developmental Toxicity

Animal studies with boron have reported a significant reduction in fetal body weight observed in developmentally exposed rats, mice, and rabbits. Malformations consisted primarily of anomalies of the eyes, the central nervous system, the cardiovascular system, and the axial skeleton. The most common malformations were enlargement of lateral ventricles in the brain and agenesis or shortening of rib XIII.

Genotoxicity

The mutagenic activity of boron-containing compounds was found to absent in studies conducted using *Salmonella typhimurium* and mouse lymphoma assays. No induction of sister chromatid exchange, chromosomal aberrations, or gene mutations have been observed in cell transformation assays with Chinese hamster cells, mouse embryo cells, and human fibroblasts.

Carcinogenicity

The US Department of Health and Human Services, the International Agency for Research on Cancer, and the US Environmental Protection Agency (EPA) have not classified boron as a human carcinogen. While no human studies are available, one animal study found no evidence of cancer after lifetime exposure to dietary boron. No increase in tumor incidence was reported in 2-year long studies in which Sprague–Dawley rats received diets containing boron compounds.

Clinical Management

Blood and urine can be examined to determine whether excessive exposure to boron has occurred. Flushing of the eyes with water and washing skin area exposed to boron with water and soap are recommended. Inhalational exposure requires removing the subject to a ventilated area, and giving artificial respiration if required. Emesis should be induced only if the person is conscious and has recently ingested a significant quantity of boron-containing compound. It is advised that pesticides containing boron compounds should be used according to their directions and should be kept away from children. Also, household chemicals should be stored in their original labeled containers and out of reach of young children to prevent accidental poisonings.

Ecotoxicology

Boron is critical for the process of cell differentiation in growing tips of plants, and plants continue to undergo cell division without differentiation of cells under boron-deficient conditions. These plants appear stunted and deformed. Boron deficiency has been reported to result in altered cell wall properties. Studies have reported increases in the levels of actin and tubulin proteins in *Arabidopsis* roots and changes in the cytoskeletal polymerization patterns in cells of maize root apices in response to boron deficiency. Deformed flowers, reduced flowering, and improper pollination are common symptoms of boron deficiency in plants. Despite the clear and rapid effects of boron deprivation, the underlying mechanisms by which boron deficiency affects the structure and function of plasma membrane are still unknown. Boron is also involved in the process of nitrogen fixation in microorganisms and legumes, and boron deficiency leads to a lower number of developed nodules capable of fixing nitrogen in legumes.

Boron toxicity can occur in plants that are irrigated with water containing high amounts of this element, or those that are grown in soils with high boron content, usually in arid and semiarid regions characterized by low rainfall and poor drainage. Typical symptoms of boron toxicity in plants include leaf burns (necrotic patches on the margins and tips of older leaves), fruit disorders (gummy nuts, internal necrosis), and bark necrosis, depending on the plant genotype. As boron concentrations in plant roots remain low even with high boron exposure, this part of the plant is often devoid of any toxic effects. Boron toxicity can lead to decreased chlorophyll concentrations, reduced growth, and decreased CO_2 fixation.

Exposure Standards and Guidelines

Based on animal models, an NOAEL and a lowest observed adverse effect level (LOAEL) have been established at 55 and 76 mg of boron kg^{-1} day^{-1}, respectively. Risk assessments of boron indicate no significant risk of toxicity to humans at currently estimated dietary or drinking water levels of exposure. The EPA has determined that exposure to boron in drinking water at concentrations of 4 mg l^{-1} for 1 day or 0.9 mg l^{-1} for 10 days is not expected to cause no adverse effects in children. Also, the EPA has determined that a lifetime exposure to 1 mg l^{-1} boron is not expected to cause any adverse effects, and has set the RfD for boron at 0.2 mg kg^{-1} day^{-1}. The US Occupational Safety and Health Administration has limited workers' exposure to an average of 15 mg m^{-3} for boron oxide in air for an 8-h workday, 40-h workweek. The Agency for Toxic Substances and Disease Registry has derived an acute-duration inhalational minimal risk level (MRL) as 0.3 mg boron m^{-3}, an acute and intermediate duration oral MRL of 0.2 mg boron kg^{-1} day^{-1}.

The inconsistency noted for safe limits and estimated intakes reflects largely the variability of boron in human diets, with boron-poor regions providing less than 0.5 mg boron - day^{-1} and boron-rich environments providing maximal intakes of 29 mg boron day^{-1} with even higher intakes in rare instances. Evolving methods of collecting, processing, and analyzing samples and data are also cause for some variability, and even error, when determining boron in our human environment.

See also: Food Safety and Toxicology; Occupational Toxicology; Occupational Safety and Health Administration; Pollution, Soil; Pollution, Water; Reproductive System, Male.

Further Reading

Bakirdere, S., Örenay, S., Korkaz, M., 2010. Effect of boron on human health. Open Miner. Process. J. 3, 54–59.

Bolt, H.M., Başaran, N., Duydu, Y., 2012. Human environmental and occupational exposures to boric acid: reconciliation with experimental reproductive toxicity data. J. Toxicol. Environ. Health A 75 (8–10), 508–514.

Jacobs, R.T., Plattner, J.J., Keenan, M., 2011. Boron-based drugs as antiprotozoals. Curr. Opin. Infect. Dis. 24 (6), 586–592.

Meacham, S., Karakas, S., Wallace, A., Altun, F., 2010. Boron in human health: evidence for dietary recommendations and public policies. Open Miner Process J. 3, 36–53.

Nable, R.O., Bañuelos, G.S., Paull, J.G., 1997. Boron toxicity. Plant Soil 193, 181–198.

Nielson, F.H., 2008. Is boron nutritionally relevant? Nutr. Rev. 66, 183–191.

Nielsen, F.H., 2009. Micronutrients in parenteral nutrition: boron, silicon, and fluoride. Gastroenterology 137 (Suppl. 5), S55–S60.

Scialli, A.R., Bonde, J.P., Brüske-Hohlfeld, I., Culver, B.D., Li, Y., Sullivan, F.M., 2010. An overview of male reproductive studies of boron with an emphasis on studies of highly exposed Chinese workers. Reprod. Toxicol. 29 (1), 10–24.

Toxicological Profile for Boron, 2010. ATSDR. CAS #: 7440-42-8.

Botulinum Toxin

YL Leung, Musgrove Park Hospital, Taunton, Somerset, UK
SA Burr, Plymouth University Peninsula Schools of Medicine and Dentistry, Plymouth, UK

This article is a revision of the previous edition article by Fermin Barrueto Jr, volume 1, pp 332–334, © 2005, Elsevier Inc.

- Name: Botulinum toxin
- Chemical Abstracts Service Registry Number: 93384-43-1
- Synonyms: *Clostridium botulinum*, Foodborne/classic botulism, Intestinal infant botulism, Wound botulism
- Molecular Formula: Not applicable – botulism toxins contain over 1000 amino acids
- Chemical Structure: Botulinum toxin has a molecular weight of 100 000, consisting of 1300 amino acids

Background

Botulism, a disease of the nervous system in animals and humans, was first recorded in Germany in 1735 and was thought to be due to eating a tainted sausage. The name botulism comes from the German 'botulus' for sausage. Botulinum toxin (molecular weight of 100 000, consisting of 1300 amino acids) is derived from *Clostridium botulinum* – an anaerobic spore-forming gram-positive bacterium commonly found in soil. It can affect a wide range of animals, including mammals, fish, and birds. There are seven serological varieties of botulism denoted by the letters A–G. They are structurally similar but antigenically and serologically unique. Only the botulism types A, B, E, and F can cause toxicity in humans. Types C and D can cause toxicity in animals. From 1990 to 2000, the US Centers for Disease Control documented 263 individual cases from 160 foodborne botulism events in the United States; 4% of these resulted in fatality and 103 of these cases occurred in Alaska. They were due to traditional Alaska aboriginal foods, including the ingestion of raw whale fat or *muktuk*. While the numbers of cases of foodborne botulism and infant botulism are stable, the incidence of wound botulism has increased due to the use of black tar heroin. California has reported the majority of cases of wound botulism associated with tar heroin use.

Uses

The use of botulinum toxin includes medicinal (e.g., treatment of spastic conditions, hyperhidrosis), cosmetic (removal of wrinkles), or as a potential terrorism agent (e.g., via aerosolization).

Environmental Fates and Behavior

Exposures, Routes, and Pathways

Inadequately sterilized processed products (e.g., canned foods) can be contaminated with neurotoxin-producing spores, leading to potential accidental exposure by ingestion (the most common route). Poor food hygiene during food preparation has been the major causes of large outbreaks of foodborne botulism. In patients with underdeveloped intrinsic gut immunity (e.g., infants), *C. botulinum* colonization of the gastrointestinal tract can occur. Susceptibility to colonization can also occur where the normal gastrointestinal protective mechanisms are deficient (e.g., in patients who have undergone major gastric surgery whereby acid production is reduced or where bile acid formation has ceased).

Cutaneous absorption and thus toxicity do not occur if the skin is undamaged. However, an open wound or mucous membrane exposed to the bacterium increases the risk of toxicity.

Intravenous users of certain types of heroin, in particular, the poorly refined 'black tar' heroin seen in the western part of the United States, are also at risk for acquiring botulism when the intramuscular route or subcutaneous route is used or users 'miss' a vein during injection. There have been several outbreaks of injection drug use–associated botulism, primarily in California, in the United States over the past decade.

Physicochemical Properties

Clostridium botulinum is a gram-positive, rod-shaped bacterium that is prevalent in marine and soil environments around the world. Botulinum toxin is rapidly inactivated when exposed to air. Spores produced by the bacterium are heat tolerant, being able to survive short exposure (<10 min) to temperatures of up to 100 °C.

Environmental Persistence

Botulinum toxin is rapidly inactivated when exposed to air. Spores produced by the bacterium are heat tolerant, being able to survive short exposure (<10 min) to temperatures of up to 100 °C.

Exposure and Exposure Monitoring

In potential exposures to botulism, individuals should be monitored clinically for the development of symptoms and treated with antitoxin if appropriate. Stool or gastric samples (vomitus or aspirates) can be sent for detection to certified laboratories. Serum should be obtained in a red-topped tube and placed on ice for shipping. Tissue and exudates from a wound should be placed in an anaerobic environment and shipped to the appropriate laboratory.

Toxicokinetics

Botulinum toxin is the most potent toxins known. Extremely minute quantities (i.e., pictograms) are potentially lethal in

 http://dx.doi.org/10.1016/B978-0-12-386454-3.00701-6

adult humans. The incidence of poisoning from botulism is, however, low. Botulinum bacterium thrives only in optimal conditions with acidic environments (pH < 4.5), with temperatures $>10\ ^\circ C$, and under anaerobic conditions where there is no competition from other bacteria. Botulism exposure can come from infectious or noninfectious causes. Infectious causes occur in infants with colonization of an immature gastrointestinal tract, in intravenous drug users (particularly black tar heroin), and in adults with disruption of normal gastrointestinal flora (i.e., taking antibiotics or with surgeries causing 'blind loops' of bowel). Noninfectious causes can come from improperly canned foods or otherwise contaminated products (i.e., *muktuk* or whale meat exposure), through aerosolized means, or from inadvertent systemic toxicity when used for therapeutic purposes. The botulinum toxin does not cross the blood–brain barrier and affects only peripheral nerves. Human exposures are from types A, B, and E. Onset of symptoms depends on the amount of toxin ingested, absorbed in a wound, or inhaled. Pathogenesis following foodborne and inhalational toxin exposure is similar. In wound botulism, the spores grow from *C. botulinum* and the toxins are formed *in vivo*. After oral exposure, absorption from the wound, or absorption from respiratory exposure, the toxins are taken up by lymphatics and delivered to peripheral cholinergic synapses. Time to onset of symptoms can vary from a few hours to up to 8 days depending on the amount of toxin one is exposed to and the kinetics of absorption. Symptoms typically appear between 12 and 72 h after eating contaminated foods, however.

Mechanism of Toxicity

Clostridium botulinum secretes an exotoxin (of which there are seven distinctive antigenic types labeled A–G) consisting of proteinaceous heavy and light chains linked together by a disulfide bond. Human poisonings have predominantly been due to types A (vegetables), B (meat), and E (fish). The toxin inhibits acetylcholine-mediated neurotransmitter release by binding onto SNARE proteins that facilitate exocytosis of acetylcholine synaptosomes. The heavy chain directs endocytosis of the toxin into a neuron in the peripheral nervous system. The pharmacologically active zinc-dependent endopeptidase light chain then binds to the SNARE proteins (synaptobrevin, SNAP-25, syntaxin), cleaving a portion of the protein and thus destroying it. The consequence is blockage of acetylcholine release. The toxin does not cross the blood–brain barrier and affects only peripheral motor nerves.

Acute and Short-Term Toxicity

Animal

Botulism can occur in both invertebrates and vertebrates. Cases have been reported in rats, mice, frogs, toads, chickens, certain types of fish, leeches, and *Drosophila*, among other organisms.

Lactating cows appear to be very susceptible to botulinum toxicity, with an LD_{50} of 0.388 ng kg^{-1}. With toxin type C, they are 13 times more sensitive than mice.

Human

Following exposure to the toxin, there is a short incubation period of 12–72 h before symptoms present. Shorter (less than 1 h) and longer (8 days) incubation periods have, however, been reported. Botulinum toxicity typically presents symptoms in a descending fashion, from proximal to distal. Botulism initially manifests as bulbar muscle dysfunction, followed by multiple cranial nerve involvement and progressing to descending paralysis. Higher cortical function is unimpaired until hypoxia develops as a result of progressive respiratory muscle paralysis and thus respiratory failure. Muscle paralysis persists for weeks until sufficient SNARE protein is resynthesized.

Chronic Toxicity (and Exposure)

Human

Toxin type A is used for medical purposes (e.g., in the treatment of dystonia, hyperhidrosis, strabismus, and hypertonia due to neuromuscular disorders such as cerebral palsies). In the cosmetic industry, this toxin is used for the temporary removal of deep glabellar lines (wrinkles). The temporary action of botulinum type A toxin is due to the regeneration of motor end plates.

In Vitro Toxicity

Botulinum type B toxin entry into PC12 cells has been found to be mediated by synaptotagmins I and II, which act as receptor agonists for the toxin. For types A and E, this has not been found.

Immunotoxicity

The incidence of neutralizing antibody formation to botulism type A is measured by the mouse bioassay and is less than 5%. Dosage and frequency of administration are the most important factors associated with antibody formation.

Reproductive Toxicity

Botulinum toxin A is pregnancy category C. There are no adequate and well-controlled studies of botulinum toxin type A administration in pregnant women.

In a fertility and reproductive study in rats, the no observable effect limit was 4 U kg^{-1} in male rats and 8 U kg^{-1} in female rates. These doses are approximately two-thirds of the dose used in humans for botulism A or Botox (TM). When the dose was increased to 16 U in rats, lower birth weights were noticed. In rabbits, which are more sensitive to botulism, lower doses caused fetal demise and malformations.

Genotoxicity

Botulism type A was not found to be mutagenic in any *in vitro* or *in vivo* experimental models.

Carcinogenicity

Botulism type A is not thought to be carcinogenic. Studies in animals using botulism type A (Botox (TM)) have not been performed.

Clinical Management

Prompt diagnosis, antitoxin administration, and supportive management are the mainstays of treatment for a patient with botulinum toxicity. Where there has been a deliberate, unlawful release of toxin, primary responders and secondary carers should be endowed with an appropriate personal protective equipment, which includes self-contained breathing apparatus. In general, the patient is to be isolated and placed in a well-ventilated room (with its own ventilation system preferably) and a process of decontamination initiated. In cases of wound botulism, any abscesses should be debrided and appropriate antibiotic treatment initiated. Cultures from the wound and exudates should be sent for detection of botulinum toxin. Pulmonary and bulbar functions should be regularly assessed and ventilatory support provided in cases of respiratory failure. Antitoxin (containing types A, B, and E) therapy should be instituted promptly if toxicity is suspected to prevent progressive paralysis and thus complications associated with prolonged artificial ventilation in the intensive care environment. Unfortunately, the antitoxin does not reverse any damage that has already occurred, and antitoxin administration also carries the risk of hypersensitivity reactions (e.g., anaphylaxis). All suspected cases are to have samples taken and tested for botulinum toxin and the appropriate health protection agency and national poisons unit informed of confirmed cases. Full functional recovery depends on the extent and duration of neuronal damage prior to antitoxin administration.

Ecotoxicology

Clostridium species are particularly prevalent in soil and water environments. Birds such as loons are particularly sensitive to type E botulism, which has been the cause of several outbreaks of migrating birds dying related to a paralytic illness. In addition to the birds, many fish are vulnerable to this type of botulism as well. The Great Lakes region in the United States has had outbreaks of type E botulism in fish and fish-eating birds since the 1960s.

See also: Food Safety and Toxicology; Gastrointestinal System; *Clostridium perfringens*; Candidate List of Substances of Very High Concern (SVHC), REACH; Environmental Risk Assessment, Aquatic; European Food Safety Authority (EFSA); Bio Warfare and Terrorism: Toxins and Other Mid-Spectrum Agents; Nerve Agents; Poisoning Emergencies in Humans; High Temperature Cooked Meats.

Further Reading

Anderson, J., Williams, P.T., Katos, A.M., Krasna, M., Burrows, W., Hilmas, C.J., 2009. In: Gupta, R.C. (Ed.), Botulinum Toxin in Handbook of Toxicology of Chemical Warfare Agents. Academic Press, London, England, pp. 407–432.

Bossi, P., Tegnell, A., Baka, A., van Loock, F., Hendriks, J., Werner, A., Maidhof, H., Gouvras, G., 15 December 2004. Bichat guidelines for the clinical management of botulism and bioterrorism-related botulism. Euro. Surveill. 9 (12), E13–E14.

Brown, N., Desai, S., 18 July 2013. Infantile botulism: a case report and review. J. Emerg. Med. (Epub ahead of print.)

Centers for Disease Control and Prevention (CDC), 2013. Botulism associated with home-fermented tofu in two Chinese immigrants – New York City, March–April, 2012. Morb. Mortal. Wkly. Rep. 62 (26), 529–532.

Holzer, V.E., 1962. Botulism from inhalation. Med. Klin. 57, 1735–1738.

Offerman, S.R., Schaefer, M., Thundiyil, J.G., Cook, M.D., Holmes, J.F., 2009. Wound botulism in injection drug users: time to antitoxin correlates with intensive care unit length of stay. West. J. Emerg. Med. 10 (4), 251–256.

Roblot, F., Popoff, M., Carlier, J.P., Godet, C., Abbadie, P., Matthis, S., Eisendorn, A., Le Moal, G., Becq-Giraudon, B., Roblot, P., 2006. Botulism in patients who inhale cocaine: the first cases in France. Clin. Infect. Dis. 43 (5), e51–e52.

Simpson, L., 2013. The life history of a botulinum toxin molecule. Toxicon 68, 40–59.

Slovis, C.M., Jones, I.D., 1998. In: Haddon, Shannon, Winchester (Eds.), Clinical Management of Poisoning and Drug Overdose, third ed. Saunders and Co, Philadelphia, pp. 399–406.

Yuan, J., Inami, G., Mohle-Boetani, J., Vugia, D.J., 2011. Recurrent wound botulism among injection drug users in California. Clin. Infect. Dis. 52 (7), 862–866.

Zhang, J.C., Sun, L., Nie, Q.H., November 2010. Botulism, where are we now? Clin. Toxicol. 48 (9), 867–879.

Relevant Websites

http://minnesota.publicradio.org/display/web/2013/08/17/environment/loon-deaths – Botulism and Loon Deaths in Michigan, USA, August 2013 Article in Minnesota Public Radio (MPR).

http://www.cdc.gov/nczved/divisions/dfbmd/diseases/botulism/ – Centers for Disease Control General Information on Botulism.

http://www.cdc.gov/nationalsurveillance/botulism_surveillance.html – Centers for Disease Control National Botulism Surveillance Information.

http://www.bt.cdc.gov/agent/botulism/index.asp – Centers for Disease Control Site Regarding Laboratory Guidelines for the Identification of Botulism Toxin.

http://www.vdh.state.va.us/oep/pdf/BotulismGuidance.pdf – Virginia Department of Health Botulism Guidance Document.

Brodifacoum

HA Spiller, Central Ohio Poison Center, Columbus, OH, USA

- Name: Brodifacoum
- Chemical Abstracts Service Registry Number: 56073-10-0
- Synonyms: PP 581; WBA 8119; 3-(3-(4-Bromo (1,1-biphenyl)-4-yl)-1,2,3,4-tetrahydro-1-naphthalenyl)-4-hydroxy-2*H*-1-benzopyran-2-one; Talon G; Ratac; Havac
- Chemical Class: A long-acting 4-hydroxycoumarin derivative; one of the superwarfarins (also *see* Warfarin)
- Molecular Formula: $C_{31}H_{23}BrO_3$
- Chemical Structure:

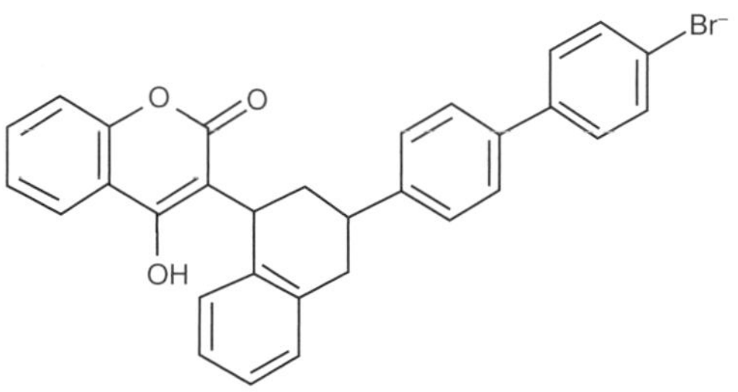

Background

Brodifacoum is a 4-hydroxycoumarin anticoagulant that acts as a vitamin K antagonist. It was registered as a pesticide in 1979 in the United States although in 2008 it was made a restricted use pesticide by the Environmental Protection Agency. This means it can only be used by certified pesticide applicators; however, the makers of D-Con which contains 0.005% brodifacoum by weight have challenged this and brodifacoum is currently available in D-Con and in various other pesticide products for the eradication of mice and rats although it is also used on larger mammals such as possums. Brodifacoum currently remains available to the general public.

Uses

Brodifacoum is used as a rodenticide (commonly 0.005% by weight).

Exposure Pathways

The most common route of exposure is oral. Transcutaneous and inhalation exposures have been implicated in workers involved in the manufacture of brodifacoum and pesticide operators.

Environmental Fate and Behavior

Relevant Physicochemical Properties

Brodifacoum is an off-white powder and is stable in solid form.

Melting point is 230 °C.

Brodifacoum is not highly flammable.

Boiling point – brodifacoum decomposes before boiling.

Solubility in water (at 20 °C) is 0.003 8 mg l^{-1}.

Solubility in acetone (at 20 °C) is 6000 mg l^{-1}.

Solubility in chloroform (at 20 °C) is 30 000 mg l^{-1}.

Octanol/water partition coefficient at pH7 (20 °C) $P = 3.16 \times 10^8$.

Vapor pressure at 25 °C (mPa) is 0.13.

Groundwater ubiquity score (GUS) leaching potential index is −1.35 indicating low leachability.

Bulk density (g/ml)/specific gravity is 1.42.

The absorption coefficient for brodifacoum $K_{oc} = 912$.

Mobility – brodifacoum has a no leaching classification.

Brodifacoum is scarcely degradable.

Bioaccumulative potential – brodifacoum has a Log P_{ow} – 100 000.

Partition Behavior in Water and Soil

Brodifacoum has a very low solubility in water and typically enters water through erosion where it is then found in the sediment. Brodifacoum concentrations are typically not measurable in water systems.

Environmental Persistency

Products that contain brodifacoum as pesticide can remain toxic for a long period of time in the environment. The rate of decay of brodifacoum depends upon the amount of rainfall. As the product that contains brodifacoum degrades over time, the brodifacoum is absorbed into the soil. Soil bacteria degrade brodifacoum over weeks to months although soil type, temperature, and the presence of microorganisms that will degrade brodifacoum all influence the time it takes to degrade.

Bioconcentration and Bioaccumulation Factors

Brodifacoum has a high potential for bioaccumulation. It is persistent and immobile in soil and fixes to organic material in water, accumulating in the sediment. It does not volatilize into the air and has low volatility from water and moist soil.

Environmental Monitoring

Brodifacoum is not used in direct application to crops or as an additive to foods. There is minimal information on concentrations of brodifacoum in air, water, and soil.

Toxicokinetics

The metabolic fate of brodifacoum in humans is not well understood. Brodifacoum is much more lipid soluble than warfarin, resulting in a larger volume of distribution. There is extensive hepatic sequestration and prolonged high liver concentrations in the rat. Brodifacoum may also undergo enterohepatic recirculation in the rat. Based on the limited data available, the elimination half-life of brodifacoum in humans ranges from 16 to 36 days. There is considerable species variation. The apparent elimination half-life in dogs is 120 days. Inducers of the cytochrome P450 system have been reported to reduce the half-life of brodifacoum in animals.

Mechanism of Toxicity

Brodifacoum, like other hydroxycoumarins, interferes with the production of vitamin K–dependent coagulation factors. Vitamin K is a cofactor for the carboxylation of specific glutamic acid groups in coagulation factors II (prothrombin), VII, IX, and X. During this step, vitamin K is oxidized to vitamin K 2,3-epoxide. The regeneration of vitamin K by vitamin K 2,3-epoxide reductase is prevented by brodifacoum. As a result, dysfunctional decarboxy-coagulation factors are produced and coagulation is impaired. Brodifacoum is over 100 times more potent than warfarin on a molar basis in rats.

Acute Toxicity

Human Toxicity

Depletion of preformed, circulating coagulation factors must occur before any anticoagulant effects are apparent. Typically, there is a delay of 24–36 h following ingestion before any effect is evident by measurement of the prothrombin time (PT). Significant toxicity from brodifacoum may be the result of large, one-time intentional ingestions. However, generally, repeated exposures over time are more likely to produce clinical toxicity. Single, small accidental ingestions in children are usually benign. Bleeding may occur virtually anywhere although cutaneous, mucosal, urinary, and gastrointestinal bleeding would be expected to be most common. Fatal intracerebral hemorrhage has been reported. Poisoning due to brodifacoum has led to prolonged periods of anticoagulation, often weeks and in some cases up to 6 months or longer. The clinical effect of brodifacoum is best monitored by following the PT and international normalized ratio (INR). Serum brodifacoum levels can be measured to confirm exposure, although there are no data to correlate serum levels and extent of toxicity. Factor activity can be assayed. An elevated serum ratio of vitamin K epoxide to vitamin K is further evidence of the presence of vitamin K reductase inhibition. While most brodifacoum exposures in humans are through oral ingestion it may also be absorbed through the skin. Irritation can occur upon contact to the eyes.

Animal Toxicity: Acute

Toxicity has been described in dogs, cats, horses, cows, pigs, sheep, goats, rats, mice, rabbits, voles, possums, Australian marsupials, chickens, ducks, and hedgehogs. Toxicity is expected in mammals, marsupial, and avian species. Owls died of hemorrhaging after feeding on rats killed with brodifacoum. Brodifacoum is very dangerous to certain bird species through secondary exposure. Birds of prey such as raptors feeding on rats and mice poisoned by brodifacoum may become poisoned in this way. The LD_{50} of brodifacoum in the Mallard is 0.26 mg kg^{-1}. Signs of poisoning occur after a latent period of 12 h to several days and may include bruising easily with occasional nose or gum bleeds; blood in stools or urine; excessive bleeding from minor cuts or abrasions; labored breathing; pale mouth and cold gums; anorexia and general weakness. Lethargy, weakness, and lack of muscular coordination may also occur. Prolonged bleeding may occur from any small wounds and extensive bruising and subcutaneous hemorrhage.

Brodifacoum lacks insecticidal properties due to differences in invertebrate physiology.

Human Toxicity: Chronic

Repeated exposures over time can lead to prolonged anticoagulation and appears to require a lower total dose than acute exposure. Clinical effects are similar to acute exposure.

Animal Toxicity: Chronic

Repeated exposures over time can lead to prolonged anticoagulation and appears to require a lower total dose than acute exposure. Clinical effects are similar to acute exposure. Brodifacoum is not readily metabolized in animals and is stored in the liver of chronically exposed animals where it remains for months.

Clinical Management

For acute, single-dose ingestions, activated charcoal should be administered. Induced emesis should be avoided in the anticoagulated individual. In large acute ingestions, the PT should be determined at 24–48 h after ingestion to assess the potential for toxicity. In the patient with clinical evidence of significant anticoagulation, extreme caution should be exercised with any invasive procedure. The airway should be protected if compromised by bleeding or hematoma formation. Volume resuscitation should be provided as indicated by clinical status. With active, uncontrolled, or life-threatening hemorrhage, fresh frozen plasma will provide preformed coagulation factors. Vitamin K_1 (phytonadion) is a specific antidote for brodifacoum toxicity. Pharmacologic doses of vitamin K allow the production of functional coagulation factors despite the presence of brodifacoum. The dose and route depend on the clinical setting. For rapid reversal, 5–25 mg should be administered intravenously no faster than 1 mg min^{-1}. Anaphylaxis has been reported with intravenous vitamin K. In children, doses of 0.6 mg kg^{-1} have been recommended in warfarin poisoning, and larger doses may be necessary with brodifacoum. Clinical effects may be seen within hours. The response and duration of a single dose is variable and depends on the severity of the intoxication. Repeat doses will be necessary. In the less emergent setting, vitamin K may be given subcutaneously or orally. The doses needed to maintain adequate coagulation status may be quite large; in some cases, doses of 100 mg day^{-1} or more orally have been reported, although typical doses are in the range of 25 mg day^{-1}. The appropriate dose is encountered typically after a period of titration of the daily dose after monitoring response to changes in the PT and INR. Oral vitamin K therapy may be necessary for weeks to months. Serial monitoring of the PT should be used to help guide therapy. Factor activity analysis may also be of use in assessing the adequacy of therapy. Phenobarbital 100–180 mg day^{-1} has been administered to adults in an attempt to induce liver microsomal enzymes and hasten metabolism of brodifacoum, but its efficacy has not been proven. Administration of phenobarbital to an adult poisoned with chlorophacinone (another long-acting hydroxycoumarin derivative) resulted in a decrease in the apparent elimination half-life from 22.8 to 5.9 days.

Ecotoxicity

Products that contain brodifacoum as pesticide can remain toxic for a long period of time in the environment. The rate of decay of brodifacoum depends upon the amount of rainfall. As the product that contains brodifacoum degrades over time the brodifacoum is absorbed into the soil. Soil bacteria degrade brodifacoum over weeks to months although soil type, temperature, and the presence of microorganisms that will degrade brodifacoum all influence the time it takes to degrade. Brodifacoum is not likely to be taken up by plants as it has a low solubility in water. Brodifacoum is very toxic to aquatic organisms and may cause long-term adverse effects in the aquatic environment. Toxic effects on fish, plankton, and other organisms have been reported. There is limited risk reported for waters as brodifacoum has a low solubility in water. Leaching from soil to water is unlikely to occur. If brodifacoum reaches water, either from pesticides thrown directly into the water or through soil erosion, it is likely to remain bound to organic material and then settle out in the sediment. When pesticides containing brodifacoum have been thrown directly into streams during eradication programs, brodifacoum residues have not been recorded in the water. In 1996 a New Zealand study assessed the effect of aerial spraying of brodifacoum during a pesticide operation on blue cod and spotties populations and found no evidence that these fish population densities were affected by the brodifacoum. In 2001 a truck spill involving 18 tons of a brodifacoum-containing pesticide (20 mg kg^{-1}) occurred in Kaikoura, New Zealand. Samples of mussels and paua were taken from the area and they were found to contain brodifacoum residues for up to 31 months. These effects were limited to a 100 m^2 area immediately around the spill site. The exposure was thought to be complicated by the effect of waves repeatedly exposing the marine life to the brodifacoum from the sea floor sediment. Typically, however, while brodifacoum is highly toxic to aquatic organisms, not enough brodifacoum will dissolve in water to cause harm to animals not specifically targeted. At a 10 mg l^{-1} dose of brodifacoum, there is no difference in the growing rate of algae and with a concentrate of 0.25% at 10 mg l^{-1} the Cl_{50} is 10 mg l^{-1} for *Daphnia*.

Genotoxicity

Brodifacoum is classified as nonmutagenic. While high concentrations (50 g ml^{-1}) inhibited mitotic activity in human lymphocytes in a study involving lymphocytes from two donors no mutagenic activity was noted.

Carcinogenicity

Brodifacoum is unlikely to be carcinogenic.

Animal Toxicity

Brodifacoum has been used as a pesticide to kill rodents including rats and mice. It has also been used to kill possums. It was the primary chemical used in several rodent eradication programs throughout the world. Treatment in animals is as for humans. The dose of vitamin K recommended for dogs and cats is 2.5–5.0 mg kg^{-1} day^{-1} for up to 4 weeks with monitoring of coagulation parameters.

Environmental Fate

In an aerobic soil, the half-life of brodifacoum is 14 days. If released into water, brodifacoum is expected to adsorb to suspended solids and sediment. Volatilization from water surfaces is not expected to be an important fate. The potential for bioconcentration in aquatic organisms is high. Brodifacoum is stable to hydrolysis in the environment. Brodifacoum is degraded by UV light when in solution.

Reproductive Toxicity

Brodifacoum ingestion in pregnancy may result in significant problems to the fetus and newborn. Problems may include embyropathy, central nervous system defects, spontaneous abortion, still birth, prematurity, and hemorrhage.

See also: Coumarins; Warfarin.

Further Reading

Bruno, G.R., Howland, M.A., McMeeking, A., Hoffman, R.S., 2000. Long-acting anticoagulant overdose: brodifacoum kinetics and optimal vitamin K dosing. Ann. Emerg. Med. 36, 262–267.

Olmos, V., Lopez, C.M., Jun–Aug 2007. Brodifacoum poisoning with toxicokinetic data. Clin. Toxicol. (Phila.) 45 (5), 487–489.

Shepherd, G., Klein-Schwartz, W., Anderson, B., 2002. Acute pediatric brodifacoum ingestions. Pediatr. Emerg. Care 18, 174–178.

Relevant Websites

http://www.abcbirds.org/abcprograms/policy/toxins/Profiles/brodifacoum.html – American Bird Conservatory – Pesticide Profile – Brodifacoum.

http://www.cdpr.ca.gov/docs/risk/toxsums/pdfs/2049.pdf – California Environmental Protection Agency Department of Pesticide Regulation Medical Toxicology Branch – Summary of Toxicology Data – Brodifacoum.

http://emedicine.medscape.com/article/818130-overview – Overview of Rodenticide Poisoning.

http://emedicine.medscape.com/article/821038-overview – Overview of Superwarfarin and Warfarin Toxicity in Particular.

Bromacil and Its Lithium Salt

TL Serex, M Battalora, KE Brugger, FX Huang, and AC Barefoot, DuPont Crop Protection, Newark, DE, USA

- Name: Bromacil and its lithium salt
- Chemical Abstracts Service Registry Number: 314-40-9 and 53404-19-6
- Synonym: 5-Bromo-3-*sec*-butyl-6-methyluracil (lithium salt); Hyvar® X; Hyvar® L; Hyvar® X-L
- Molecular Formula*: $C_9H_{12}BrN_2O_2$
- Chemical Structure*:

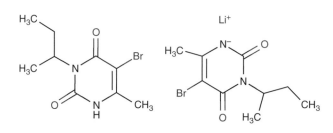

*All from ChemIDplus.

Background

Bromacil (CAS 314-40-9) belongs to a class of herbicides known as uracils, first developed by DuPont in 1962. Its herbicidal activity is due to inhibition of photosynthesis in several species of weeds and brush. Since its introduction in 1962, farmers in North and South America and Asia have used bromacil-containing herbicides for crop protection.

Uses

It is used for brush control primarily for land management purposes as it is effective on a wide range of both annual and perennial weeds. It is especially phytotoxic to perennial grasses. It is also used for selective weed control in pineapple and citrus crops.

Environmental Behavior, Fate, Routes, and Pathways

Bromacil is a nonvolatile, slightly water-soluble compound with a low octanol–water partition coefficient (K_{ow}) and a pK_a of 9. Although the lithium salt is more soluble in water than bromacil, its environmental fate is identical, since the extent of ionization of bromacil, that is, the ratio of unionized bromacil to its anionic form, will be controlled by the pH and buffering capacity of the terrestrial or aquatic system to which it is applied. The physicochemical properties are reflected in the environmental fate properties. Bromacil is weakly absorbed to soil and is considered highly mobile. The low K_{ow} indicates that bromacil will not bioaccumulate. Bromacil is stable in water over the pH range of 5–9, and photolyzes through both direct and indirect mechanisms in surface water with a half-life of 4–7 days at pH 9. In soil under aerobic conditions in the laboratory, bromacil degrades slowly forming several metabolites as a result of microbial activity. In anaerobic environments, bromacil may degrade very rapidly through a debromination reaction. In field dissipation studies, bromacil half-lives of 124–1155 days were observed.

Bromacil has been detected in groundwater, particularly in vulnerable areas with shallow surficial aquifers, high recharge, and sandy soils of low organic matter. While bromacil's environmental fate properties indicate that it may be transported off-site through runoff, it is detected in surface water infrequently and at low concentrations.

Exposure and Exposure Monitoring

At the label recommended use rates, there is expected to be very little exposure to the pesticide applicator. Additionally, very little exposure due to residues in commodities is expected. Residue measurements for bromacil in citrus and pineapple crops have largely resulted in nondetectable residue levels.

Toxicokinetics

Bromacil was absorbed readily from the gastrointestinal tract following oral administration in rats, with peak blood levels (t_{max}) measured at 1 and 2 h for males and females, respectively. It was extensively metabolized (primarily by hydroxylation at the 6-methyl position and on the sec-butyl moiety), and rapidly excreted via the urine. The hydroxylated metabolites were eliminated as glucuronide conjugates. Radiolabel was found in all tissues examined, but there was no evidence of accumulation and an estimated elimination half-life of about 13 h was determined for both sexes. The major metabolite of bromacil in the urine of rats was 5-bromo-6-hydroxymethyl-3-*sec*-butyluracil.

Mechanisms of Action

The herbicidal activity of bromacil and other uracils is due to inhibition of photosynthesis in several species of weeds and brush. The uracil herbicides translocate only apoplastically (capable of only upward movement). Movement is upward with the transpiration stream (water moving through the plant from the soil and evaporating into the atmosphere at the leaf surfaces).

Acute and Short-Term Toxicity

Bromacil is considered to be moderately toxic by the oral route. The oral LD_{50} value for bromacil is 550 mg kg^{-1} in female rats. For the lithium salt, the oral LD_{50} value is 3927 and 1414 mg kg^{-1} for males and females, respectively. The dermal

 http://dx.doi.org/10.1016/B978-0-12-386454-3.01104-0

LD_{50} value in rabbits is > 5000 mg kg^{-1} and the inhalation LC_{50} value is >5.6 mg l^{-1} in a 4-h acute inhalation toxicity study with male and female rats. Neither bromacil nor its lithium salt is considered to present a dermal sensitization hazard based on results in guinea pig studies. Bromacil and its lithium salts are considered mild eye irritants. Skin irritation was not observed in a dermal irritation study with bromacil, however, the lithium salt was determined to be a moderate skin irritant based on studies in rabbits. Bromacil and other uracil compounds are herbicides; therefore, their pesticidal mode of action is designed to target physiological processes unique to plants and not designed to interact with the nervous system as is the case for some insecticides. An evaluation of the acute and repeated dose data available for bromacil as well as other uracil compounds supports the conclusion that this class of herbicides does not possess the potential to be neurotoxic.

Chronic Toxicity

The most sensitive effect in the long-term feeding studies in rats, mice, and dogs was decreased body weight gain. At the high dose, body weight gains were consistently decreased compared to controls over the course of 2 years in male and female rats at 2500 ppm. Thyroid effects were observed at higher doses in males and females. While there was not a statistically significant increase in thyroid tumors in males by pairwise comparison with controls, there was a suggested increase by trend analysis (see below). Liver effects were observed in mice which included hepatocellular hypertrophy, single cell and centrilobular vacuolation and necrosis, and hepatocellular lysis with red blood cell accumulation. A marginal increase in tumors was observed in the livers of male mice in the high-dose (871 mg kg^{-1} bw day^{-1}) group where significant liver toxicity was also observed (see below).

Immunotoxicity

No specific immunotoxicity studies have been performed with bromacil or its lithium salt.

Reproductive and Developmental Toxicity

There was no evidence of increased pre- or postnatal susceptibility to bromacil based on the results of developmental toxicity studies in rats and rabbits. A two-generation reproductive toxicity study in rats has been conducted and no impact on fertility was observed in this study. Therefore, bromacil is not considered to be a reproductive or developmental toxicant.

Genotoxicity

A full battery of *in vitro* studies with bromacil has been conducted in bacterial and in mammalian cells. Additionally, an *in vivo* genetic toxicity study in mice was also performed. Results from most of these studies were negative. Therefore, the weight of evidence indicates bromacil is not considered to present a genotoxic hazard.

Carcinogenicity

As described above, in rats, there was not a statistically significant increase in tumors by pairwise comparison. However, there was a possible indication of a test substance-related increase in thyroid tumors when analyzed for trend, since there was a marginal increase in this tumor type at the highest dose tested (103–118 mg kg^{-1} bw day^{-1}). Other factors could have impacted this marginal increase, since there were also body weight decreases at this dose and survival was significantly increased. In this regard, overall body weight gain at the highest dose was decreased by 22% in males. A slight increase in liver tumors was also observed in male mice at the highest dose tested (871 mg kg^{-1} bw day^{-1}); however, they occurred under the following circumstances: (1) the increased incidence of liver tumors was observed in only one sex and species at the highest dose only, the majority of liver tumors were observed at the end of the study; (2) tumor incidence was only slightly higher than historical controls and was only significant when benign and malignant tumors were combined; (3) liver tumors are common in this strain (CD-1) of mouse with a wide range of historical control values; (4) single-celled liver necrosis also occurred in males at this dose level which was accompanied by decreased body weight gain (↓ 14% over 18 months, ↓ 21% over the first 26 weeks); and (5) bromacil is not genotoxic. In view of the fact that tumors were only observed at high doses in rats and mice, where body weight gain was depressed by more than 10%, it is clear that these tumors only occur in cases of excessive toxicity and are of questionable relevance to humans.

Ecotoxicology

Bromacil is practically nontoxic to birds (Northern bobwhite oral LD_{50} > 2250 mg kg^{-1} bw). It is nontoxic in bees (contact 48-h LD_{50} = 193.3 μg bee^{-1}). Bromacil is slightly to practically nontoxic to fish and aquatic invertebrates. The rainbow trout 96-h LC_{50} = 36 mg l^{-1}, bluegill sunfish 96-h LC_{50} = 123 mg l^{-1}, and sheepshead minnow 96-h LC_{50} = 162 mg l^{-1}. The *Daphnia* 48-h LC_{50} = 121 mg l^{-1}, oyster larvae 96-h EC_{50} = 130 mg l^{-1}, and mysid shrimp 48-h EC_{50} = 12.9 mg l^{-1}. Bromacil does not bioaccumulate. Bromacil is toxic to green algae (*Selenastrum* EC_{50} = 6.8 μg l^{-1}) and terrestrial plants. For seedling emergence, oilseed rape is the most sensitive dicot (EC_{25} = 0.0156 lb ai A^{-1}) and wheat is the most sensitive monocot (EC_{25} = 0.0731 lb ai A^{-1}). For vegetative vigor, cucumber is the most sensitive dicot (ER_{25} = 0.0106 lb ai A^{-1}) and soybean is the most sensitive monocot (EC_{25} = 0.0184 lb ai A^{-1}).

Exposure Standards and Guidelines

The United States Environmental Protection Agency (US EPA) has established tolerances for residues of agricultural uses of bromacil that include a soil treatment on citrus and a preemergent, postemergent, or postharvest application to pineapple. The tolerances for residues on these crops at 0.1 ppm are published in the 40 Code of Federal Regulations (CFR). There are no tolerances established for secondary residues of bromacil in/on livestock commodities. There are no registered uses of the lithium salt form on food crops.

The US EPA has set a chronic reference dose of $0.1\ mg\ kg^{-1}\ bw\ day^{-1}$ based on the chronic toxicity study in rats where the most sensitive effect observed was decreased body weight gain with a lowest observed effect level identified as $103\ mg\ kg^{-1}$ and a total uncertainty factor of 100X applied to achieve a chronic dietary exposure limit for all populations.

See also: Herbicides.

Further Reading

Bucha, H.C., Cupery, W.E., Harrod, J.E., Loux, H.M., Ellis, L.M., 1962. Substituted uracil herbicides. Science 137, 537–538.

EPA, 1996. Reregistration eligibility decision (RED), Bromacil.

EPA, 2012. Memorandum, Bromacil and its Lithium Salt: Human Health Assessment Scoping Document in Support of Registration Review (EPA-HQ-OPP-2012-0445). Case Number 0041.

Tomlin, C.D.S., 2006. The Pesticide Manual, fourteenth ed. Bromacil, British Crop Protection Council (BCPC), Hampshire, UK, pp. 112–113.

Relevant Website

http://www.epa.gov – US Environmental Protection Agency: search for Bromacil.

Bromadiolone

S Ramasahayam, Oklahoma State University, Stillwater, OK, USA

This article is a revision of the previous edition article by K. S. Rao, volume 1, pp 338–340, © 2005, Elsevier Inc.

- Name: Bromadiolone
- Chemical Abstracts Service Registry Number: 28772-56-7
- Synonym: 3-[3-(4′-Bromo [1,1′-biphenyl]-4-yl)-3-hydroxy-1-phenylpropyl]-4-hydroxy-2H-1-benzopyran-2-one
- Chemical Formula: $C_{30}H_{23}BrO_4$
- Chemical Structure:

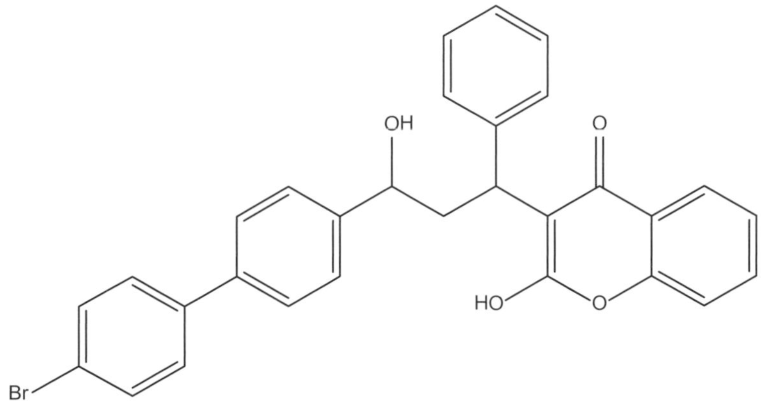

Background

Bromadiolone is used to control rodents around buildings, inside transport vehicles and sewers. It is often formulated as meal bait, rat and mouse bait ready-to-use place packs, paraffinized pellets and blocks.

Uses

Bromadiolone is a potent anticoagulant rodenticide. It is a second-generation anticoagulant of the hydroxy-4-coumarin used for the control of commensal rats and mice, including those resistant to warfarin and first-generation anticoagulants, voles, and water voles. Bromadiolone products can be applied only indoors in nonurban areas. Bromadiolone is applied in baits and bait packs at the rate of 16 oz per 15 ft interval for controlling commensal rats and 2 oz of bait per 8 ft interval for house mice.

Environmental Fate and Behavior, Partition, Pathways, Degradation, and Bioaccumulation

Bromadiolone is a white-yellow powdered solid with a melting point of 198 °C. The solubility in water is 19 mg l^{-1} at 25 °C. The solubilities in organic solvents such as ethyl acetate, acetone, chloroform, ethanol, and hexane are 25.0, 22.3, 10.1, 8.2, and 0.2 gm l^{-1}, respectively. The octanol–water partition coefficient (log K_{ow}) is 4.27. The Henry's law constant is 8.99×10^{-7} pa-m^3 mol^{-1}.

Bromadiolone may be released into the environment through various waste streams and its use.

If released to air, it will exist in the particulate phase in the ambient atmosphere and will be removed by dry and wet deposition. In soil, it is not persistent under aerobic conditions (half-life is 14 days) and is usually immobile except in soils of low organic matter and clay, such as sand.

When released to water, it adsorbs to suspended solids and sediment. Bromadiolone is stable to hydrolysis at pH 5, 7, and 9. Two major degradates, [1,3-diphenyl-5(4′-bromobiphenyl) pentane-1-ol] and [1,3-diphenyl-5(4′-bromobiphenyl) pentane-1,5-diol], are detected in the aerobic soil metabolism study.

Bromadiolone is bioaccumulated in edible and nonedible tissues in bluegill sunfish at the bioaccumulation concentration factors of 160X and 1658X. It was also detected in birds.

Exposure and Exposure Monitoring

Routes, Pathways, and Human Exposures

National Institute for Occupational Safety and Health (NIOSH Survey 1981–83) has statistically estimated that 96 workers are potentially exposed to bromadiolone in the United States. The general population may be exposed to the chemical through occupational settings as well as its use. Exposures occur via dermal or inhalation routes. Since bromadiolone is a nonfood use pesticide, it is unlikely that there will be any exposure through food sources or through water contamination.

No environmental monitoring studies are reported.

 http://dx.doi.org/10.1016/B978-0-12-386454-3.00367-5

Toxicokinetics

Oral administration of bromadiolone in rodents resulted in a significant retention in the liver for a very long time. In addition, it was also detected in kidney and plasma. The half-life for the decline in the liver concentration of the chemical after 28 days of dosing was found to be 17 days. The major route of elimination is through feces after biliary excretion; smaller amounts can also be excreted via urine.

Mechanism of Toxicity

Bromadiolone belongs to second generation of long-acting anticoagulant rodenticide. It acts by interfering with the prothrombin synthesis by blocking the regeneration of vitamin K dependant proteins in the liver and thereby disrupting the clotting mechanisms and increasing the tendency to hemorrhages and subsequent death.

Acute and Short-Term Toxicity (Animal/Human) (To Include Irritation and Corrosivity)

Available data indicate that bromadiolone is very toxic. The acute oral LD_{50} in rats was reported to be in between 0.56 and 0.84 mg kg^{-1} (Environmental Protection Agency (EPA) Toxicity Category I). The acute dermal LD_{50} in rabbits was 1.71 mg kg^{-1} (EPA Toxicity Category I). The LC_{50} for acute inhalation toxicity in rats was 0.43 μg l^{-1} (EPA Toxicity Category I). Eye irritation with conjunctivitis and iritis were observed in rabbits' eye irritation test (EPA Toxicity Category III). Bromadiolone was found to be minimally irritating in the rabbit dermal irritation test (EPA Toxicity Category IV). Humans exposed to this chemical may develop hematoma, hematuria, blood in feces or excessive bleeding from minor cuts, gum bleeding, gastrointestinal bleeding, abdominal or back pain, hemarthrosis, epistaxis, cerebrovascular accidents, and massive hemorrhage (internal bleeding) resulting in a shock.

Chronic Toxicity (Animal/Human)

Beagle dogs administered with bromadiolone gelatin capsules for 90 days at the highest dose, 100 μg kg^{-1}, exhibited respiratory difficulties, pale mucosa, hypothermia, atonia, bloody urine, hematomas, hematuria, and external hemorrhage. Given the exclusively nonfood uses of bromadiolone, not many chronic studies were reported.

Reproductive and Developmental Toxicity

Pregnant rats receiving bromadiolone at different doses, showed increased incidence of vaginal bleeding, hypotonicity, pale eyes, and deaths at the highest dose: 70 μg kg^{-1} per day. There was no evidence of embryotoxicity or developmental toxicity.

Genotoxicity

There was no evidence of mutagenic effect of bromadiolone neither *in vitro* nor *in vivo* studies.

Carcinogenicity

Due to the nonfood use of this chemical, no cancer studies were reported.

Clinical Management

In case of contact with bromadiolone, a complete blood history and physical examination should be stressed. People with a history of blood disorders and bleeding are at a higher risk from exposure.

Ecotoxicology

Freshwater/Sediment Organisms Toxicity

The 96-h acute toxicity studies indicated that bromadiolone is moderately toxic to fish, including rainbow trout (*Oncorhynchus mykiss*, $LC_{50} = 0.24$ ppm) and bluegill sunfish (*Lepomis macrochirus*, $LC_{50} = 3$ ppm). This chemical is moderately to highly toxic to fresh water invertebrate waterflea (*Daphnia magna*) with an EC_{50} in the range of 0.1–10 ppm.

Terrestrial Organisms Toxicity

Birds

Bromadiolone is moderately toxic to birds with an LD_{50} of 50–500 mg kg^{-1} in acute toxicity studies. It is highly to very highly toxic in subacute avian (LC_{50} <50–500 ppm) dietary toxicity studies.

No data are identified on marine organisms, terrestrial invertebrates, and plants.

Other Hazards

Information for bromadiolone is still not complete, especially in regards to hazards not covered in the above text.

Exposure Standards and Guidelines

Since it is a nonfood pesticide, dietary risk assessment was not performed.

See also: Small Animal Toxicoses - Rodenticides; Anticoagulant Rodenticide Toxicity.

Further Reading

US Environmental Protection Agency, 1998. Registration Eligibility Decision (RED): Rodenticide Cluster. Office of Prevention, Pesticides and Toxic Substances, Washington, DC. http://www.epa.gov.

Relevant Website

http://toxnet.nlm.nih.gov – Toxnet (Toxicology Data Network): search under HSDB for Bromadiolone.

Bromethalin

AJ García-Fernández and IM Navas, University of Murcia, Murcia, Spain

- Name: Bromethalin
- Chemical Abstract Service Registry Number: 63333-35-7
- Synonyms: Bromethaline; 4,6-Dinitro-*N*-methyl-*N*-(2,4,6-tribromophenyl)-alpha,alpha,alpha-trifluoro-o-toluidine; Benzenamine, *N*-methyl-2,4-dinitro-*N*-(2,4,6-tribromophenyl)-6-(trifluoromethyl)-(9CI); *N*-Methyl-2,4-dinitro-*N*-(2,4,6-tribromophenyl)-6-(trifluoromethyl)benzenamine; alpha, alpha, alpha-Trifluoro-*N*-methyl-4,6-dinitro-*N*-(2,4,6-tribromophenyl)-o-toluidine; (IUPAC = 2,4,6-Tribromo-*N*-methyl-*N*-(2,4-dinitro-6-trifluoromethylphenyl)aniline)
- Molecular Formula*: $C_{14}H_7Br_3F_3N_3O_4$
- Chemical Structure*:

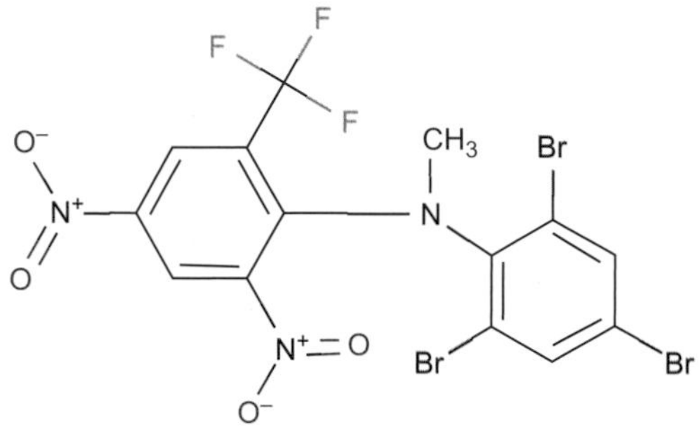

F F F O⁻ N⁺ O CH3 N Br N⁺ O O⁻ Br Br

*All from ChemIDplus

Background

Bromethalin was discovered in the mid-1980s by investigators at Lilly Research Laboratories, and it became readily available to replace the anticoagulant rodenticides when some rodents developed resistance. It is the active ingredient of some rodenticides marketed in 0.005% or 0.01% formulations, which are commercially available as baits (pellets, bars, place packs, grain, or meal). It has been marketed under the trade names Vengeance®, Assault®, and Trounce®. Bromethalin baits are frequently similar to other rodent baits in color and appearance, and bromethalin has also commonly been involved in accidental poisoning of companion animals. Bromethalin does not induce bait shyness. The WHO Recommended Classification of Pesticides by Hazard identifies bromethalin (technical grade) as Class IA (extremely hazardous).

In the United States, federal regulations require that bromethalin rodenticide products should be applied out of reach of children, domestic animals, pets, and nontarget wildlife, or in bait stations. Bait stations must be resistant to destruction by dogs and by children under 6 years of age.

Uses

Bromethalin is the active ingredient of several commercial baits registered for the control of rats, mice, and moles. Its use is restricted in and around buildings (residential, commercial, industrial, and agricultural premises), sewers, alleys in urban areas, and transportation and cargo vehicles. Bromethalin baits used for mole control are placed in residential lawns, ornamental gardens, recreation areas, golf courses, nurseries, and other nonagricultural areas. Several commercial baits are registered under different formulation types, including pellets, blocks, tablets, and packages containing granular bait, and it has also been registered as impregnated material that mimic grubs and worms for mole control. All registered products of bromethalin are baits that contain only bromethalin as an active ingredient, and therefore risk assessments for mixtures of active ingredients have not been carried out.

Environmental Fate and Behavior

Bromethalin is a pale, odorless, crystalline solid compound in the diphenylamine family. It is soluble in many organic solvents but essentially insoluble in water with a melting point of 150.5 °C and a molecular weight of 577.9 g mol^{-1}. Bromethalin is stable to hydrolysis in aqueous buffered solutions at pH between 5 and 9 when incubated at 25 °C in the dark for 30 days. Regarding aerobic soil metabolism, bromethalin has been found to be slowly biodegraded, with a half-life of 178 days for the parent compound, and desnitrobromethalin as the main compound, which comprises 43% of the applied material. Although this degradate is also persistent, its mobility is unknown. It is expected to be relatively stable to microbial/chemical degradation in the soil. Concentration of volatiles is very low (lesser than 5%) and unknown degradates are about 4%.

Because the only use of bromethalin is in bait for rodent and mole control, no potential for spray drift exists, and exposure from volatilization is expected to be minimal. Based on an estimated Henry's law constant of 4.0×10^{-9} atm m^{-3} mol^{-1} and based upon a vapor pressure of 9.7×10^{-8} mm Hg, volatilization from both moist and dry soil surfaces, and also from water surfaces, is not expected to be an important fate process. As a consequence of its outdoor use, leaching from the baits exposed to rainwater and runoff could be expected. However, the extremely low application rate, the hydrophobic nature of the bromethalin (water solubility lesser than 0.01 mg l^{-1}), and its high K_{oc} value (>55 000 ml g^{-1}) make leaching unlikely and indicate that bromethalin is expected to be immobile in soil. Similarly, in aquatic ecosystems, bromethalin is expected to adsorb to sediments and suspended solids.

It has been suggested that its bioconcentration factor (BCF) is 7400, calculated from an estimated log K_{ow} of 7.7. This BCF suggests that the potential for bioconcentration in aquatic organisms is very high, provided the compound is not physically altered after released into the environment.

Exposure and Exposure Monitoring

Occupational exposure can occur through inhalation and dermal contact at workplaces during production, formulation,

 http://dx.doi.org/10.1016/B978-0-12-386454-3.00473-5

application, and disposal of bromethalin. Exposure in workplaces would occur only as a result of accidents. Similarly, data indicate that the general population may be exposed to bromethalin via dermal contact with consumer products containing bromethalin. The major concern is about potential accidental oral and inhalation exposures as consequence of loading and application of bromethalin at bait stations when they are handled for rodent control. Children and pets are most likely to be accidentally exposed.

Exposure assessment of terrestrial species to bromethalin as consequence of application of baits is possible by assuming species directly consumed several types of baits. Bromethalin must be contained in protected bait stations or located in areas inaccessible to nontarget wildlife, where primary exposure of birds is expected to be minimal. However, exposure of small mammals that feed on the bait should also be evaluated. There is not any method to evaluate the secondary exposure in animals that prey other animals which have ingested bromethalin. In spite of this, field studies and wildlife monitoring studies have not identified bromethalin as a widespread contaminant in wildlife samples. No data are available on exposure to plants and insects.

There are no monitoring data for bromethalin in surface water. Although bromethalin is very toxic to aquatic organisms, based on the use pattern and its environmental chemistry data, concentrations of bromethalin in both freshwater and saltwater marshes are expected to be negligible.

Toxicokinetics

After ingestion, bromethalin is rapidly absorbed from the gastrointestinal tract, reaching the highest plasma concentration within 4 h. Experimental studies in rats demonstrated that bromethalin rapidly undergoes *N*-demethylation by mixed-function oxygenases in the hepatic microsomes forming desmethylbromethalin, its major toxic metabolite. Possible interspecific differences on metabolism of bromethalin should be taken into account. It has been demonstrated that some species, such as guinea pigs, are more resistant to bromethalin toxicosis due to its low hepatic *N*-demethylase activity. Both bromethalin and its metabolite are readily distributed throughout the body, reaching their highest concentrations in adipose tissue, although chemical residues are also detected in other organs such as liver, kidney, and brain. Due to its high lipophilicity, bromethalin has affinity for fat and brain, where it achieves the highest concentrations. It can also be detected in plasma due to it is slow excretion from the body, with a plasma excretion half-life of approximately 6 days. Excretion of bromethalin is mainly through bile (5–25% of an oral dose), and reabsorption of bromethalin by enterohepatic recirculation is suspected. Excretion via urine is minimal (less than 3%).

Mechanism of Toxicity

Unlike anticoagulant and cholecalciferol-based rodenticides, bromethalin and its primary metabolite are uncouplers of mitochondrial oxidative phosphorylation, being that desmethylbromethalin (major metabolite) is about two to three times more potent than bromethalin. Uncoupling of this reaction may result in a lack of ATP and diminished Na^+, K^+-ATPase-dependent ion channel pump activity, which in turn leads to intracellular sodium retention and a loss of ability to maintain osmotic control, and the cells swell with water. Because signs of bromethalin toxicosis are most pronounced in the central nervous system (CNS), it is considered as a potent neurotoxicant. The outcome is cerebral edema, elevated cerebrospinal fluid pressure, and vacuolization of myelin, and eventually leading to respiratory failure because of lack of nerve impulse transmission to the lungs. Exposure to bromethalin at levels that do not cause acute respiratory failure are enough to provoke intramyelinic edema and spongy degeneration of white matter of the brain, spinal cord, and optic nerve. As a result, alterations in CNS involve damage to nerve axons, inhibition of neural transmission, and paralysis, convulsions, and, ultimately, death.

Acute and Short-Term Toxicity

Animal

The oral LD_{50} value of bromethalin in dogs is 3.7 mg kg^{-1}, and in wild birds and monkeys is ~ 5 mg kg^{-1}. Rats (LD_{50} = 2 mg kg^{-1}) and mainly cats (LD_{50} = 0.54 mg kg^{-1}) are more sensitive to toxic effects of bromethalin ingestion. Quails and rabbits are more resistant than these species, with an LD_{50} higher than 11 mg kg^{-1} in both cases. However, the most resistant species studied is the guinea pig with an LD_{50} of bromethalin greater than 1000 mg kg^{-1}, probably because this species is not able to metabolize bromethalin to its more active metabolite (desmethylbromethalin). The oral LD_{50} values of technical bromethalin are always greater than those reported for pure compound (LD_{50} in rat is 9.1–10.7 mg kg^{-1}). Regarding dermal toxicity tests, no dermal irritation has been described with either the technical compound or the compound in baits. The dermal LD_{50} of technical bromethalin in rabbits was reported to be 2000 mg kg^{-1}. Bromethalin is slightly irritating to the eyes in rabbits and does not cause dermal sensitization in the guinea pig. Bromethalin induces a marked respiratory distress in poisoned animals. Inhalation toxicity tests reported an LC_{50} for the rat of 0.024 mg l^{-1}.

Clinical signs in poisoned animals usually develop within 10–24 h after ingestion; however, animals ingesting a supralethal dose will show signs of toxicity within 2 h postingestion. Dogs exposed to a single oral dose above the LD_{50} (3.7 mg kg^{-1}) develop a neurotoxic syndrome characterized by hyperexcitability, tremors, hyperthermia, running fits, hyperesthesia, seizures sound- or light-induced, depression, prostration, and death within a few days. Although the ingestion of high doses occasionally occur, the ingestion of doses of bromethalin lower than minimum lethal dose (2.5 mg kg^{-1}) but greater than the minimum toxic dose (1.7 mg kg^{-1}) is more probable. In these cases, a more delayed onset of signs is expected, with the first symptoms appearing within several days after ingestion and progressing within 1 or 2 weeks. In these circumstances, poisoned dogs and cats develop signs of a paralytic syndrome beginning with hindlimb ataxia, paresis with associated decreased conscious proprioception of the hindlimbs, and loss of deep pain. Other occasional clinical signs include vomiting, anorexia, nystagmus, loss of bark, anisocoria, opisthotonos, seizures, Schiff-Sherrington syndrome, and coma. Marked respiratory distress has been observed in poisoned animals, and it could be the cause of death. Signs may persist several weeks and up to 1 or 2 months in animals recovering from bromethalin poisoning.

The greater sensitivity of cats to bromethalin induces a paralytic syndrome regardless of the dose ingested. Cats show similar signs to those reported in dogs, but they may also show abdominal distention due to ileus and inability to urinate due to an increased urethral tone as a consequence of upper motor neuron bladder paralysis. Finally, cats may show a decerebrate posture.

Lesions are mainly confined to the CNS, with mild cerebral edema being the most frequently observed sign. Diffuse white matter spongiosis, mild microgliosis, and vacuolization of the optic nerve are the histologic lesions most commonly seen.

Human

Children are potentially at highest risk because of their small body size and their attraction by the brightly colored baits. For this reason, children and pets could swallow the poison if it is placed within their reach and/or if the bait is not in a tamper-resistant station.

Reports of toxicity in humans have not been widely documented, and the most relevant available information is on poisoned animals and experimental studies both *in vivo* and *in vitro*. Bromethalin is very toxic when swallowed and inhaled, and highly toxic when absorbed through skin. Irritation of eyes or skin is not expected due to dermal contact based on studies in rodents. However, some fatal cases have been described, such as a 21-year-old man who died after ingesting 17 mg (0.33 mg kg^{-1}) of bromethalin. An overdose of bromethalin can cause headache, personality changes, confusion, tremors, seizures, coma, and marked respiratory depression in humans. Increased cerebrospinal fluid pressure, cerebral edema, and death have been reported after overdose with bromethalin.

Chronic Toxicity

Animal

Sprague-Dawley rats (10 per sex and group) daily exposed to technical bromethalin to oral doses from 0 to 125 μg kg^{-1} per day over 3 months were pathologically evaluated based on spongy degeneration (leukoencephalomyelopathy) in white fiber tracts of the brain, cerebellum, brain stem, pons, thoracic spinal cord, and optic nerves of males. The no-observed-effect level (NOEL) and lowest observed effect level (LOEL) were set at 25 and 125 μg kg^{-1} per day, respectively. Paralysis was the clinical sign most frequently observed. No histopathological findings were observed in other tissues.

In another 90-day study, dogs were orally dosed by gavage at levels from 0 to 200 μg kg^{-1} per day with technical bromethalin. The NOEL was set at 25 μg kg^{-1} per day, and the LOEL was set at 125 μg kg^{-1} per day, based on spongy degeneration observed in nervous tissue. Dogs exposed at the high dose showed neurotoxic symptoms such as salivation, hypoactivity, trembling, hyperesthesia, myoclonia, groaning, and prostration before death.

Human

Chronic toxicity in human might result in numbness, headache, mild confusion, and incoordination.

Reproductive Toxicity

The most interesting experimental studies about reproductive toxicity have been carried out in pregnant rats and rabbits exposed daily to bromethalin for a period of 10–12 days during gestation.

The first study was carried out using Harlan-Wistar rats (25 rats/group) orally gavaged on gestation days 6–15 at a dosing volume of 5 ml kg^{-1} with 0, 0.1, 0.3, or 0.5 mg kg^{-1} day^{-1} technical bromethalin. The NOEL for developmental toxicity was 0.5 mg kg^{-1} day^{-1} (high dose tested, HDT), and the NOEL and LOEL for maternal toxicity were 0.3 and 0.5 mg kg^{-1} day^{-1}, respectively. In 10 of the 25 high-dose females clinical signs were seen, including hind leg weakness or paralysis, decreased muscle tone, poor grooming, ventral soiling, chromodacryorrhea, decreased and labored respiration, and hypothermia. Four of them died during gestation (days 12, 16, 17, and 17). During the dosing period, high-dose females suffered a 30% decrease in weight gain, and during the postdosing period the decrease in weight gain was about 12%. For the entire gestation period the decrease in weight gain was 14% in comparison to controls. It has been considered that these decreased weight gains are dose related. No teratogenic effects have been described.

The second study used Dutch Belted rabbits (15 rabbits/group) that were orally gavaged at a volume of 1 ml kg^{-1} with bromethalin at doses of 0, 0.10, 0.25, or 0.50 mg kg^{-1} day^{-1} during gestation days 6–18. The NOEL for developmental toxicity is 0.5 mg kg^{-1} day^{-1} (HDT). The NOEL for maternal toxicity is 0.10 mg kg^{-1} day^{-1}. Five high-dose females show clinical signs that included nasal discharge, loss of muscle tone, weakness, decreased respiration, coolness, and prostration. Two of them died during gestation (days 16 and 21) and they had respiratory infections, one had pneumonia and the other had an acute upper respiratory tract infection. Abortion was observed in two high-dose females, in one middose female, and in one low-dose female. Finally, mid- and high-dose females had decreased weight gains during the dosing period. All mentioned clinical signs, abortions, decreased weight gains, and deaths were considered compound related. No teratogenic effects were observed.

Genotoxicity

In mutagenicity studies using *Salmonella typhimurium*, no indications of an increased number of revertants at the histidine locus in any of the strains used have been described. Similarly, in *in vivo* assays there was no evidence of induced mutagenicity response. There is no information available in GENETOX or CTD.

Carcinogenicity

There is no information available in Chemical Carcinogenesis Information or Carcinogenic Potency Database.

Clinical Management

Because no specific antidote for this compound has been developed, treatment of intoxication is usually symptomatic and supportive, but special attention must be paid to CNS effects and observation for potential seizures. In acute poisoning, the treatment is initially directed to reducing gastrointestinal absorption, i.e., emesis and gastric lavage. Because bromethalin is rapidly absorbed, emesis must be induced as soon as possible after ingestion and even within 2 h postingestion. Emetics should be avoided when the patient is displaying dyspnea, hypoxia, seizures, CNS depression, or abnormal pharyngeal reflexes. Because the enterohepatic recirculation of bromethalin after its biliary excretion has been demonstrated, repeated oral administration of activated charcoal powder should be given every 4–8 h for 3 days by gastric tube, in combination with sorbitol or sodium sulfate.

Cerebral edema and elevated intracranial pressure have to be controlled. Administration of a diuretic such as mannitol or furosemide in combination with dexamethasone has been successfully used for these purposes.

Careful maintenance of the hydration status is critical and must be controlled. Finally, benzodiazepine (i.e., diazepam or lorazepam) to control tremors and/or phenobarbital or propofol to abolish seizures can be used.

In case of inhalation exposure, the patient must be moved to fresh air and the respiratory distress must be monitored. Administration of oxygen and assisted ventilation should be used if required. In case of bronchospasm, inhaled beta-2 agonist and oral or parenteral corticosteroids must be prescribed.

Ecotoxicology

In laboratory tests, bromethalin is highly to very toxic to aquatic organisms, however, due to its extremely low solubility in water, a remarkable exposure of aquatic organisms through current use of baits containing bromethalin is not expected. The 48 h EC_{50} values in *Daphnia magna* were between 1.98 and 5.10 $\mu g\,l^{-1}$. The 96 h LC_{50} values in bluegill (*Lepomis macrochirus*) and rainbow trout (*Oncorhynchus mykiss*) were 598.0 and 38.0 $\mu g\,l^{-1}$, respectively.

Regarding terrestrial vertebrates, acute oral toxicity of bromethalin has been assessed in northern bobwhite quail (*Colinus virginianus*) with a single dose, obtaining different LD_{50} values depending on the vehicle used to administrate bromethalin orally. When the ingredient was ingested in a polyethylene glycol vehicle, the LD_{50} value was 4.56 (3.6–5.8) $mg\,kg^{-1}$ body weight (bw). However, when the ingredient was ingested in an acacia vehicle, the LD_{50} value was 11.0 (9.3–13.1) $mg\,kg^{-1}$ bw. The first study was chosen to classify bromethalin toxicity, and therefore, according to the US Environmental Protection Agency (EPA) classification system, toxicity data categorized bromethalin as *very highly toxic* to birds and mammals on an acute oral basis (oral $LD_{50} < 10\ mg\,kg^{-1}$).

Another study on northern bobwhite quail (*C. virginianus*) was conducted to assess subacute dietary toxicity after 8 days of exposure. The LC_{50} value obtained was 210 ppm, which classified bromethalin as *highly toxic* to birds on a dietary basis according to US EPA classification (dietary $LC_{50} = 50$–500 ppm).

No avian reproduction and chronic exposure data are available for bromethalin.

No data are available to assess toxicity and risk of bromethalin to terrestrial plants. Neither are there data on toxicity to terrestrial invertebrates; however, the US EPA considers that the mode of action of bromethaline demonstrated in vertebrates should also be considered relevant to invertebrates. Therefore, without data, the US EPA assumes that bromethalin is likely highly toxic to terrestrial invertebrates as it is to vertebrates.

Based on a study in dogs, it has been suggested that bromethalin poses less secondary risk to wildlife than anticoagulant rodenticides. However, there is a lack of data to fully characterize this risk.

Other Hazards

Rodenticide products containing bromethalin are not flammable or reactive as formulated.

Exposure Standards and Guidelines

There are no occupational exposure guidelines for this compound.

Miscellaneous

Use of rubber gloves is recommended when handling rodent baits containing this compound.

See also: Biocides; Pesticides; Neurotoxicity; Federal Insecticide, Fungicide, and Rodenticide Act, US; Environmental Risk Assessment, Pesticides and Biocides.

Further Reading

Cherry, L.D., Gunnoe, M.D., Van Lier, R.B.L., 1982. The metabolism of bromethalin and its effects on oxidative phosphorylation and cerebrospinal fluid pressure. Toxicologist 2, 108.

Dorman, D.C., 2001. Bromethalin. In: Peterson, M.E., Talcott, P.A. (Eds.), Small Animal Toxicology. Sanders, Philadelphia, PA, pp. 435–444.

Dorman, D.C., Parker, A.J., Buck, W.B., 1990. Bromethalin toxicosis in the dog. Part I: clinical effects. J. Am. Anim. Hosp. Assoc. 26, 589–594.

Dorman, D.C., Parker, A.J., Dye, J.A., et al., 1990. Bromethalin neurotoxicosis in the cat. Prog. Vet. Neurol. 1, 189–196.

Dorman, D.C., Zachary, J.F., Buck, W.B., 1992. Neuropathologic findings of bromethalin toxicosis in cats. Vet. Pathol. 20, 139–144.

Dunayer, E., 2003. Bromethalin: the other rodenticide. Vet. Med. 9, 732–736.

Krieger, R. (Ed.), 2001. Handbook of Pesticide Toxicology, second ed., vol. 2. Academic Press, San Diego, CA,, p. 1240.

Lyman, W.J., Rosenblatt, D.H., Reehl, W.J., 1990. Handbook of Chemical Property Estimation Methods: Environmental Behavior of Organic Compounds. American Chemical Society, Washington, DC, pp. 4–5.

Silberhorn, E.M., 2005. Bromethalin. In: Wexler, P., Anderson, B., de Peyster, A., Gad, S., Hakkinen, P.J., Kamrim, M., Locey, B., Mehendale, H., Pope, C., Shugart, L. (Eds.), Encyclopedia of Toxicology, second ed. Academic Press, Hardbound.

Tomlin, C.D.S. (Ed.), 1997. The Pesticide Manual World Compendium, eleventh ed. British Crop Protection Council, Surrey, England, p. 143.
USEPA (U.S. Environmental Protection Agency), 1998. Reregistration Eligibility Decision (RED) Rodenticide Cluster. EPA738-R-98–007. Office of Prevention, Pesticides and Toxic Substances, Washington, DC. Available at: http://www.epa.gov.
USEPA (U.S. Environmental Protection Agency), 2004. Potential Risks of Nine Rodenticides to Birds and Nontarget Mammals: A Comparative Approach. Environmental Fate and Effects Division. Office of Pesticide Programs, Washington, DC, pp. 1–225. Available at: http://wwwepa.gov..
USEPA (U.S. Environmental Protection Agency), 2011. Risks of bromethalin Use to Federally Threatened Alameda whipsnake (*Masticophis lateralis euryxanthus*) and the Federally Endangered Salt Marsh Harvest Mouse (*Reithrodontomys raviventris*). Environmental Fate and Effects Division. Office of Pesticide Programs, Washington, DC, pp. 1–88. Available at: http://wwwepa.gov..
van Lier, R.B.L., Cherry, L.D., 1988. The toxicity and mechanism of action of bromethalin: a new single-feeding rodenticide. Fundam. Appl. Toxicol. 11, 664–672.
WHO (World Health Organization), 2010. The WHO Recommended Classification of Pesticides by Hazard and Guidelines to Classification: 2009. International Programme on Chemical Safety. WHO Library, Geneva, pp. 1–78.

Relevant Websites

http://www.inchem.org/ – Chemical Safety Information from Intergovernmental Organizations.
http://toxnet.nlm.nih.gov/cgi-bin/sis/htmlgen?HSDB – Hazardous Substances Data Bank.
http://ntp.niehs.nih.gov – National Toxicology Program (United States Department of Health and Human Services).
http://www.pesticideinfo.org/ – The Pesticide Action Network (PAN) Pesticide Database.
http://www.epa.gov/ – United States Environmental Protection Agency (EPA).
http://chem.sis.nlm.nih.gov/chemidplus – United States National Library of Medicine – ChemIDplus Advanced.

Bromine

D Brown, Manchester University College of Pharmacy, Fort Wayne, IN, USA

This article is a revision of the previous edition article by Sanjay Chanda and Harihara M. Mehendale, volume 1, pp 342–344, © 2005, Elsevier Inc.

- Name of Chemical: Bromine
- Chemical Abstracts Service Registry Number: 7726-95-6
- Synonyms: Brom, Brome, Broom, Dibromine
- Molecular Formula: Br_2

Background

Bromine, or dibromine, Br_2, is the elemental form of bromine, Br. Free bromine does not occur in nature; instead, bromine is usually found in the form of mineral halide salts. At ambient temperature, bromine is a fuming, red-brown liquid that is corrosive and toxic, and has a highly offensive and suffocating odor. Bromine has the unique distinction of being one of only two (mercury being the other) elements that are in liquid form under standard conditions. The chemical properties of bromine fall in between those of chlorine and iodine, and its compounds are similar to those of the other halogens.

Bromine, in its liquid and vapor forms, is highly corrosive and toxic to human tissues. The corrosiveness of bromine is due to the strongly oxidizing hydrobromous acid (HOBr) that is formed from reaction with water in the aqueous environment of living organisms. High levels of various bromide salts are toxic, particularly to the thyroid and the central nervous system.

Uses

Elemental bromine is used in industrial settings mainly for the production of bromine-containing organic compounds. These substances are used as flame retardants, insecticides, fuming agents, emulsifiers, dyes, agrichemicals, and pharmaceuticals, and bromine was used as an additive to leaded gasoline.

Additionally, bromine is used in the reduction of mercury emissions from coal-fired power plants, in the maintenance of swimming pools and spas, and as a sensitizing agent in daguerreotype plates. Bromine is also used extensively in organic synthesis.

Environmental Fate, Behavior, Routes, and Pathways

Bromine is a dense, mobile, fuming, reddish-brown liquid at room temperature. It has a highly unpleasant odor resembling that of chlorine. Bromine is slightly soluble in water and highly soluble in many organic solvents, including carbon disulfide, carbon tetrachloride, acetic acid, and aliphatic alcohols.

Bromine is not thought to persist in the environment. Due to bromine's high reactivity with other elements, the inorganic salts of bromide pose little or no risk of poisoning. The greatest risk of exposure is to workers during bromine recovery when bromine is applied in the synthesis of bromine-containing compounds. Professions with the highest risk of exposure include drug and dye manufacturing, gold extraction, organic chemical manufacturing, petroleum refinement, and photographic chemical production.

Exposure and Exposure Monitoring

Bromine has been shown to enter the body via inhalation of vapors, dermal contact, and ingestion.

Some preliminary studies have reported monitoring workers' exposure to bromine by measuring serum bromide levels.

Toxicokinetics

The effects of bromine on biological systems are difficult to separate from those of bromine-containing compounds and its metabolites due to the high reactivity of bromine. Because of this high reactivity, bromine does not persist in organisms, but rather is converted to bromide. Bromide has been shown to accumulate in living tissues and displace endogenous halides.

Mechanism of Toxicity

When bromine encounters the aqueous environment of living organisms, it reacts with water to produce hydrobromic acid and hydrobromous acid, according to the following reaction:

$$Br_2 + H_2O \rightarrow HBr + HOBr$$

Both of these reaction products are highly detrimental to living tissue: HBr is a strong acid and causes burns, and HOBr is a very potent oxidizing agent. The pK_a of HOBr is 8.7 and hence passes unencumbered into most cells. Once inside the cytoplasm, the hypobromite ion is capable of oxidizing proteins and various other biomolecules, interfering with cellular process such as ATP formation. Additionally, stable compounds containing bromine-nitrogen bonds are formed.

Increased concentrations of bromide ions have been shown to have adverse health effects. High levels of bromide have been associated with neurotoxicity. Bromide has also been shown to interfere with the whole-body metabolism of iodide by decreasing iodide levels in thyroid and skin and enhancing iodide excretion by the kidneys. The resulting depletion of iodide by bromide has various effects on metabolism and can result in thyroid goiters.

Acute and Short-Term Toxicity

Animal

Toxicity in animals is similar to that in humans. The LC_{50} value of bromine in mice is 3100 and 4160 mg kg^{-1} in rabbits.

Human

The respiratory system, eyes, and central nervous system are the major sites of affected by bromine. Bromine is extremely irritating to the skin, eyes, and mucous membranes of the upper respiratory tract. Severe burns of the eye may result from liquid or concentrated vapor exposure. Liquid bromine splashed on the skin may cause vesicles, blisters, and slow-healing ulcers. Inhalation of bromine is corrosive to the mucous membranes of the nasopharynx and upper respiratory tract, producing brownish discoloration of the tongue and buccal mucosa, a characteristic odor of breath, edema and spasm of the glottis, asthmatic bronchitis, and possible pulmonary edema, which may be delayed until several hours after exposure. Additionally, a measles-like rash may occur.

Exposure to high levels of bromine may lead to death due to choking caused by edema of the glottis and pulmonary edema. Exposure to low levels of bromine results in cough, copious mucous secretion, nose bleeding, respiratory difficulty, vertigo, and headache. These symptoms are usually followed by nausea, diarrhea, abdominal distress, hoarseness, and asthmatic-type respiratory difficulty.

Chronic Toxicity

Animal

Pulmonary edema, pneumonia, diarrhea, and rashes may be delayed complications of severe exposures.

Human

Repeated or prolonged exposure to bromine results in toxicity to mucosal membranes, the liver, kidneys, cardiovascular system, central nervous system, and thyroid. Chronic eye irritation and severe skin irritation have been observed following prolonged exposure to mist. Prolonged exposure to mist may also produce respiratory tract irritation leading to frequent bronchial infections.

Carcinogenicity

There is no evidence suggesting that bromine is a carcinogen.

Clinical Management

Exposure should be terminated as soon as possible by removing the victim to fresh air. The eyes and mouth should be washed with copious amounts of water. A 15–20 min wash may be necessary. Skin should be washed with soap. Contaminated clothing and jewelry should be removed and isolated. Contact lenses should be removed to avoid prolonged contact of the chemical with the eye. When the chemical has been swallowed, large quantities of milk should be given; if milk is not available, water should be given. Emetics should not be given. If breathing has stopped, artificial respiration should be administered. If breathing is difficult, oxygen should be given.

Exposure Standards and Guidelines

Many organizations have set exposure limits of 0.1 ppm.

See also: Alkyl Halides; Carbon Tetrabromide; Chlorine; Ethyl Bromide; Methyl Bromide.

Further Reading

DiGangi, J., Blum, A., Bergman, A., et al., 2010. San Antonio Statement on brominated and chlorinated flame retardants. Environ. Health Perspect. 118 (12), A516–A518.

Erickson, P.R., Grandbois, M., Arnold, W.A., McNeill, K., August 7, 2012. Photochemical formation of brominated dioxins and other products of concern from hydroxylated polybrominated diphenyl ethers (OH-PBDEs). Environ. Sci. Technol. 46 (15), 8174–8180.

Lai, Y., Lu, M., Gao, X., et al., 2011. New evidence for toxicity of polybrominated diphenyl ethers: DNA adduct formation from quinone metabolites. Environ. Sci. Technol. 45 (24), 10720–10727.

Louwen, J.N., Stedeford, T., 2011. Computational assessment of the environmental fate, bioaccumulation, and toxicity potential of brominated benzylpolystyrene. Toxicol. Mech. Methods 21 (3), 183–192.

Makarovsky, I., Markel, G., Hoffman, A., et al., 2007. Bromine–the red cloud approaching. Isr. Med. Assoc. J. 9 (9), 677–679.

Nájera-Martínez, M., García-Latorre, E.A., Reyes-Maldonado, E., et al., 2012. Halomethane-induced cytotoxicity and cell proliferation in human lung MRC-5 fibroblasts and NL20-TA epithelial cells. Inhal. Toxicol. 24 (11), 762–773.

Pavelka, S., 2004. Metabolism of bromide its interference with the metabolism of iodine. Physiol. Res. 53, S81–S90.

Price, J.A., Rogers, J.V., Wendling, M.Q., et al., 2011. Temporal effects in porcine skin following bromine vapor exposure. Cutan. Ocul. Toxicol. 30 (3), 187–197.

Rattley, M., May 22, 2012. Ambiguous bromine. Nat. Chem. 4 (6), 512.

Seiler, H.G., Segal, A., 1988. Handbook on the Toxicity of Inorganic Compounds. Dekker, New York.

Shannon, M., 1998. Bromine and iodine compounds. In: Haddad, L., Shannon, M., Winchester, J. (Eds.), Clinical Management of Poisoning and Drug Overdose, third ed. Saunders, Philadelphia, pp. 803–812.

Smyth, A.M., Thompson, S.L., de Foy, B., et al., 2013. Sources of metals and bromine-containing particles in Milwaukee. Atmos. Environ. 73, 124–130.

Relevant Websites

http://www.inchem.org/documents/pims/chemical/pim080.htm – International Programme on Chemical Safety: INCHEM: Bromine.

http://www.osha.gov/dts/chemicalsampling/data/CH_221800.html – United States Department of Labor: Occupational Safety & Health Administration - Bromine.

Bromobenzene

MA Bryant, Manchester University, North Manchester, IN, USA

This article is a revision of the previous edition article by William S. Utley, volume 1, pp 344–345, © 2005, Elsevier Inc.

- Name: Bromobenzene
- Chemical Abstracts Service Registry Number: 108-86-1
- Synonyms: Phenyl bromide
- Molecular Formula: C_5H_5Br
- Chemical Structure:

Uses

Bromobenzene is a colorless, flammable liquid with a density greater than water and with an aromatic odor. It is synthesized by the reaction of bromide with benzene in the presence of iron powder. It is used for organic synthesis, particularly in the production of the intermediate phenylmagnesium bromide. Bromobenzene is an additive to motor oils and used as a crystallizing solvent. Bromobenzene is used as an ingredient in the manufacture of phencyclidine, a recreational drug.

Environmental Fate and Behavior

Bromobenzene will volatilize from dry surfaces, due to its vapor pressure of 4.18 mm Hg at 25 °C, and therefore will exist as a vapor in the environment. Bromobenzene will undergo little hydrolysis in water and little biodegradation by aquatic microorganisms. Bromobenzene is not expected to adsorb to sediment from water due to its soil sorption constant (K_{oc}) of 150 and water solubility of 446 mg l^{-1}. It is also expected to have a high mobility in soil and volatilize easily from moist surfaces due to its Henry's law constant of 2.47×10^{-3} atm m^3 mol^{-1} at 25 °C. Bioconcentration factors range from low values of 8.8 in carp to moderately high values of 190 in algae.

Toxicokinetics

Bromobenzene is readily absorbed by the gastrointestinal tract following ingestion. Bromobenzene is also absorbed by the lungs after inhalation. Distribution of bromobenzene and its metabolites is spread throughout the body with the highest concentrations found in adipose tissues soon after absorption.

Bromobenzene is initially converted into epoxide derivatives by CYP isozymes, specifically cytochrome P-450. Subsequently, the major metabolic pathway in rat liver is the conjugation of the 3,4-epoxide derivative with glutathione (GSH) (either spontaneously or via glutathione-S-transferases), followed by excretion as mercapturic acids. Approximately 70% of bromobenzene in the form of mercapturic acids have been recovered within 8 h of ingestion in rats. Catechol, quinone, phenol, and dihydrodiol (or bromophenol) metabolites have also been detected in urine excretion from animals. While the liver is capable of producing all the various metabolites of bromobenzene, lung and kidney tissues have been shown to produce limited amounts of some metabolites.

Mechanism of Toxicity

Liver toxicity is due to reactive metabolites of bromobenzene, such as the epoxide and quinone derivatives, and not due to bromobenzene itself. Reactive metabolites can covalently bind with hepatocellular macromolecules or organelles and may cause decreased hepatocyte oxygen uptake and ATP levels, altered Ca^{2+} homeostasis, and reduced cytosolic and mitochondrial GSH levels. Increased toxicity is associated more so with the 3,4-epoxide metabolic intermediate rather than the 2,3-epoxide. Hepatic centrilobular necrosis has been observed after the depletion of GSH reserves. For instance, rats that have been administered bromobenzene and diethyl maleate (which depletes GSH) developed extensive liver necrosis, while rats that were administered bromobenzene and cysteine (a GSH precursor) exhibited no necrosis. Also, conjugation of quinone derivatives with GSH can lead to reactive metabolites that can cause toxicity in the kidney.

Acute and Short-Term Toxicity

Exposure may cause irritation to skin and eyes. Ingestion causes gastrointestinal irritation with nausea, vomiting, and diarrhea and may lead to liver damage. The probably lethal dose is between 50 and 500 mg kg^{-1} (between one teaspoon and 1 ounce for 70 kg (150 lb) person). Animal studies reveal that acute exposure to bromobenzene targets most severely the liver, and to a much lesser extent the kidney and lungs. Reduced hepatic GSH, moderate periportal and midzonal hydropic changes, increased serum liver enzyme levels, and hepatic centrilobular necrosis have been observed. Higher doses are required to observe effects in the kidneys (decreased GSH levels, increased blood urea nitrogen (BUN) levels, and severe tubular necrosis) and lungs (increased lactate dehydrogenase (LDH) levels and bronchiolar damage). Oral LD_{50} values ranging from 1700 mg kg^{-1} for guinea pigs to 3300 mg kg^{-1} for rats have been reported. Bromobenzene is used to produce drug-induced liver injury in animals.

Chronic Toxicity

The liver and kidney are the only organs affected by longer-term exposure to bromobenzene. Bromobenzene inhalation studies were conducted on rats and mice for 13 weeks with doses ranging from 64.2 to 1926 $mg\,m^{-3}$ for 6 h per day for 5 days per week. Increased incidence of cytomegaly in the liver was observed in female mice at the highest vapor concentration. Mild renal histopathology was also observed in male rats at the highest concentration. In another study, rats and mice were administered oral doses of bromobenzene by gavage in corn oil at concentrations ranging from 50 to 600 $mg\,kg^{-1}$ per day for 90 days. Hepatocellular necrosis was observed at oral doses of 400 and 600 $mg\,kg^{-1}$ in rats and mice (600 $mg\,kg^{-1}$ in female mice) and hepatocellular cytomegaly was observed at doses of 200 $mg\,kg^{-1}$ and higher in rats and mice ($>$400 $mg\,kg^{-1}$ in female rats). Kidney lesions were observed at the highest oral dose in rats and mice.

Genotoxicity

Very few mutagenic effects have been observed for bromobenzene, such as positive clastogenic and mutagenic results in mammalian cell cultures and whole-animal studies. The Ames assay showed negative mutagenic results and inconsistent cytogenic effects *in vitro* with mammalian cells. However, bromobenzene exhibited binding to RNA, and to a lesser extent to proteins and DNA, in liver, kidney, and lung tissues. Bromobenzene is $>$20-fold more reactive in binding to rat liver DNA than benzene, a known carcinogen and more reactive than 1,2-dichloroethane, a probable carcinogen.

Carcinogenicity

At present, there is inadequate information to determine the carcinogenic potential of bromobenzene in humans.

Ecotoxicology

Bromobenzene has been shown to be toxic to bacteria, algae, cladoceran, and fish cells with EC_{50} values at $\sim$1 mM (0.2 $g\,l^{-1}$) with 24-h exposure.

Exposure Standards and Guidelines

No exposure limits have been set.

See also: Cytochrome P450; Chlorobenzene; Benzene; 1,1-Dichloroethane; 1,2-Dichloroethylene.

Further Reading

Dodd, D.E., Pluta, L.J., Sochaski, M.A., Banas, D.A., Thomas, R.S., 9 Mar 2012. Subchronic hepatotoxicity evaluation of bromobenzene in Fischer 344 rats. J. Appl. Toxicol. [Epub ahead of print].

EPA, 2009. Toxicological Review of Bromobenzene (CAS RN: 108-86-1): In Support of Summary Information on the Integrated Risk Information System. U.S. Environmental Protection Agency. www.epa.gov/iris EPA/635/R-07/002F.

Kiyosawa, N., Manabe, S., Sanbuissho, A., Yamoto, T., 2010. Gene set-level network analysis using a toxicogenomics database. Genomics 96 (1), 39–49.

Koen, Y.M., Hajovsky, H., Liu, K., Williams, T.D., Galeva, N.A., Staudinger, J.L., Hanzlik, R.P., 2012. Liver protein targets of hepatotoxic 4-bromophenol metabolites. Chem. Res. Toxicol. 25 (8), 1777–1786.

Minami, K., Saito, T., Narahara, M., Tomita, H., Kato, H., Sugiyama, H., Katoh, M., Nakajima, M., Yokoi, 2005. Relationship between hepatic gene expression profiles and hepatotoxicity in five typical hepatotoxicant-administered rats. Toxicol. Sci. 87 (1), 296–305.

Rappaporta, S.M., Kimb, S., Lanc, Q., et al., 2010. Human benzene metabolism following occupational and environmental exposures. Chem. Biol. Interact. 184, 189–195.

Stierum, R., Heijne, W., Kienhuis, A., van Ommen, B., Groten, J., 2005. Toxicogenomics concepts and applications to study hepatic effects of food additives and chemicals. Toxicol. Appl. Pharmacol. 207 (Suppl. 2), 179–188.

Van Vleet, T.R., Schnellmann, R.G., 2003. Toxic nephropathy: environmental chemicals. Semin. Nephrol. 23 (5), 500–508.

Zurita, J.L., Jos, A., del Peso, A., Salguero, M., López-Artíguez, M., Repetto, G., 2007. Ecotoxicological assessment of bromobenzene using a test battery with five model systems. Food Chem. Toxicol. 45 (4), 575–584.

Relevant Websites

www.epa.gov/iris – Environmental Protection Agency Integerated Risk Information System (EPA IRIS).

toxnet.nlm.nih.gov – National Library of Medicine (NLM) Hazardous Substances Data Bank (HSDB) Database Toxicology Data Network (Toxnet).

Bromoform

MA Bryant, Manchester University, North Manchester, IN, USA

This article is a revision of the previous edition article by William S. Utley, volume 1, pp 345–347, © 2005, Elsevier Inc.

- Name: Bromoform
- Chemical Abstracts Service Registry Number: 75-25-2
- Synonyms: Methyl tribromide, Tribromomethane
- Molecular Formula: $CHBr_3$
- Chemical Structure

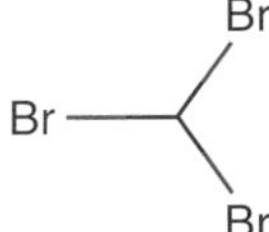

Uses

Bromoform is a colorless to yellow liquid with a density about three times that of water. It has an odor and sweetish taste similar to chloroform and is not combustible. It has been used as a degreasing solvent, in chemical synthesis, and in fire extinguishers, and is no longer used as a sedative for children with whooping cough. Currently, bromoform is produced only in small amounts for use in laboratories and in geological and electronics testing.

Environmental Fate and Behavior

Bromoform is not found as a liquid in the environment because it is expected to volatilize from dry soil surfaces due to its vapor pressure of 5.40 mm Hg at 25 °C. It is also expected to volatilize from moist or wet surfaces because Henry's law constant is 5.4×10^{-4} atm m^3 mol^{-1}. Bromoform is expected to have high mobility in soil due to its K_{oc} value of ~120. This low K_{oc} value implies that bromoform will have only a little tendency to adsorb to soil or sediment from water sources. Bromoform does not hydrolyze in water. Bromoform undergoes limited biodegradation under aerobic conditions but is readily biodegraded in the presence of methane-producing bacteria under anaerobic conditions. Bromoform exhibits a low bioconcentration factor of 14, and little bioconcentration in aquatic organisms is expected.

Exposure

Bromoform is used in various industries such as aircraft and chemical, which may result in the introduction of bromoform into the environment through waste streams. It is also a by-product of the reaction of chlorine disinfectant compounds on drinking water containing small amounts of bromine-containing compounds, which suggests that the most common route of human exposure is drinking water or during swimming or showering. Reported concentrations of bromoform in drinking water, if detected at all, are usually below ~10 μg l^{-1}.

Toxicokinetics

Absorption of bromoform occurs through oral and dermal exposure and inhalation. Effects of exposure have been reported on the liver, kidneys, lungs, and central nervous system, indicating wide distribution through the body. Tissue–air coefficients determined for human tissues indicate a tendency for bromoform to accumulate in blood and tissues with high lipid content, although one study reported no increased concentration in adipose tissues after absorption.

Bromoform is most likely converted to tribromomethanol by cytochrome P-450, which in turn decomposes to dibromocarbonyl, a highly reactive species. Dibromocarbonyl can react with glutathione and ultimately produce carbon dioxide and bromide, although carbon monoxide can also be produced in smaller amounts. Radical species have also been observed as metabolism intermediates. In rats, bromoform administered orally in corn oil by gavage was exhaled as unchanged bromoform (67%) and carbon dioxide (4%) within 8 h, with 2% excreted in urine and 2% retained in tissues. In mice, a greater amount was exhaled as carbon dioxide (40%) and only 6% exhaled as bromoform within 8 h, with 12% retention in tissues and 5% excretion.

Mechanism of Toxicity

Although the mechanism of toxicity of bromoform is not completely understood, the structural similarity of bromoform to chloroform, which has been extensively investigated, suggests that mechanisms of toxicity are similar. Mice exposed to chloroform by inhalation along with a cytochrome P-450 inhibitor, which inhibits metabolism of trihalomethanes, were completely protected from hepatic and renal toxicity observed in mice exposed to chloroform only. Studies of bromodichloromethane also showed a dependence of toxicity effects on metabolism intermediates.

Acute and Short-Term Toxicity

Inhalation of bromoform has been reported to result in irritation of the nose and throat of humans and can cause lacrimation. Acute doses have been reported to cause central nervous system depression and death in dogs. LD_{50} values are reported to be 1150 mg kg^{-1} for female rats and 1400 mg kg^{-1} for male rats and mice for oral doses, and about 400 mg kg^{-1} for rats for intraperitoneal doses.

Chronic Toxicity (Animal/Human)

Studies of rats exposed to bromoform for 2 years showed hepatocellular necrosis at a dose of 200 mg kg^{-1} (5 days per week), hepatocellular damage at a dose of 720 mg kg^{-1} day^{-1}, and a decrease in serum glucose levels at a dose of $\geq$40 mg kg^{-1} day^{-1}.

Reproductive Toxicity

Mice exposed by gavage to doses from 50 to 200 mg kg^{-1} day^{-1} exhibited a significant decrease in postnatal survival at the 200 mg kg^{-1} day^{-1} dose level. Other studies report little or no effects on pregnant rats at doses up to 200 mg kg^{-1} day^{-1}.

Genotoxicity

Conflicting results have been reported on the potential of bromoform to induce gene mutations. Both positive and negative Ames assay results have been reported for different *Salmonella* strains. Similar mixed results have been reported for a variety of mammalian and nonmammalian cells. For example, an increase in chromosome aberrations was observed in rats given five daily gavage doses or a single intraperitoneal dose, but not in mice given an intraperitoneal dose.

Carcinogenicity

Bromoform has been classified by the U.S. Environmental Protection Agency as a probable human carcinogen based on the increased incidence of neoplastic lesions found in the large intestines of rats after oral administration. Surface adenomas in the lungs of mice given intraperitoneal administration of bromoform were also reported. Also, bromoform is structurally similar to other possible or probable carcinogenic halogen-containing compounds.

Ecotoxicology

Reported LC_{50} values have ranged from about 20 000 μg l^{-1} for sheepshead minnow (96 h exposure) to about 50 000 μg l^{-1} for water flea (*Daphnia magna*, 24 h exposure).

Exposure Standards and Guidelines

In 2005, the World Health Organization derived a guideline for drinking-water quality for bromoform of 100 μg l^{-1} assuming a 60 kg adult drinking 2 l of water a day. The American Conference of Industrial Hygienists has established an 8 h time-weighted average (TWA) threshold limit value of 0.5 ppm (5 mg m^{-3}). The U.S. Occupational Safety and Health Administration has derived TWA permissible exposure level of 0.5 ppm (5 mg m^{-3}) for bromoform, noting that there is a danger of cutaneous absorption.

See also: Chloroform; Cytochrome P450; Chlorination Byproducts; Trihalomethanes.

Further Reading

ATSDR, 2005. Toxicological Review of Bromoform and Dibromochloromethane. Agency for Toxic Substances and Disease Registry. www.atsdr.cdc.gov/toxprofiles.

Kavcar, P., Odabasi, M., Kitis, M., Inal, F., Sofuoglu, S.C., 2006. Occurrence, oral exposure and risk assessment of volatile organic compounds in drinking water for Izmir. Water Res. 40 (17), 3219–3230.

Lourencetti, C., Grimalt, J.O., Marcoa, E., Fernandez, P., Font-Rivera, L., Villanueva, C.M., et al., 2012. Trihalomethanes in chlorine and bromine disinfected swimming pools: air–water distributions and human exposure. Environ. Int. 45, 59–67.

Panyakapo, M., Soontornchai, S., Paopuree, P., 2008. Cancer risk assessment from exposure to trihalomethanes in tap water and swimming pool water. J. Environ. Sci. (China) 20 (3), 372–378.

Rockett, L., Ewence, A., Gardner, M., Young, W., Rumsby, P., 2010. A review of the current knowledge on dermal and inhalation toxicity of regulated THMS. Drinking Water Inspectorate. WRc Ref: UC7907.06 DWI Ref: 70/2/230.

Valcke, M., Krishnan, K., 2011. Evaluation of the impact of the exposure route on the human kinetic adjustment factor. Regul. Toxicol. Pharmacol. 59 (2), 258–269.

Relevant Websites

www.epa.gov/iris – Environmental Protection Agency Integerated Risk Information System (EPA IRIS).

toxnet.nlm.nih.gov – National Library of Medicine (NLM) Hazardous Substances Data Bank (HSDB) Database Toxicology Data Network (Toxnet).

Bromotrichloromethane

MC Korrapati, Medical University of South Carolina, Charleston, SC, USA

This article is a revision of the previous edition article by Midhun C. Korrapati and Harihara M. Mehendale, volume 1, pp 347–349, © 2005, Elsevier Inc.

- Name: Bromotrichloromethane
- Chemical Abstracts Service Registry Number: 75-62-7
- Synonyms: EINECS 200-886-0, Carbon bromotrichloride, Trichlorobromomethane
- Molecular Formula: $BrCCl_3$
- Chemical Structure:

Br
Cl Cl
Cl

Background

Bromotrichloromethane ($BrCCl_3$) is practically insoluble in water, but it is soluble in all proportions in alcohol and ether, and miscible with many organic liquids. Uncatalyzed addition of bromotrichloromethane to ethylene can lead to violent explosion. It is frequently used in organic synthesis and as a flame retardant. The general population may be exposed to bromotrichloromethane via ingestion of food and drinking water. Bromotrichloromethane has been identified as a volatile compound in both bacon and pork. Production of bromotrichloromethane has been banned in the United States, and therefore occupational exposure would only occur when using $BrCCl_3$ for organic synthesis. The acute lethal dose in humans is 500–5000 mg kg^{-1}. Inhalation of 20 000 ppm for 60 min will result in surgical anesthesia and possibly death. Based on effects in monkeys and rats, this compound may induce coma and possibly death in humans exposed to 20 000 ppm for 60 min; 10 000 ppm for 30 min will provoke marked incoordination; 2000 ppm for 5 min may produce disturbance of equilibrium. $BrCCl_3$ exposure to cells can cause destruction of CYP450 (drug-metabolizing enzymes), making cells resistant to toxicity. This compound is considered a prolific inducer of lipid peroxidation as measured by MDA (malondialdehyde production) and 4-HNE (4-hydroxynonenal concentration).

Uses

Although bromotrichloromethane is no longer produced in the United States, it is still used in organic syntheses of various compounds.

Environmental Fate/Exposure Summary

Bromotrichloromethane is no longer produced in the United States. However, its use during organic syntheses may result in its release to the environment. If released to the atmosphere, bromotrichloromethane is expected to exist solely as a vapor in the ambient atmosphere. Vapor-phase bromotrichloromethane slowly degrades in the atmosphere by reaction with photochemically produced hydroxyl radicals; the half-life for this reaction in air is estimated to be greater than 44 years. Photolysis occurs based on bromotrichloromethane's structural similarity to other halogenated methane compounds but not at an environmentally important rate. In soil, bromotrichloromethane is expected to have low mobility based on an estimated K_{oc} of 567. The potential for volatilization of bromotrichloromethane from dry soil surfaces may exist based on this compound's vapor pressure. Bromotrichloromethane may volatilize from moist soil surfaces based on an estimated Henry's Law constant of 3.7×10^{-4} atm-cu m mol^{-1} at 25 °C. Volatilization from water surfaces is expected based on the estimated Henry's Law constant for this compound. Estimated volatilization half-lives from a model river and model lake are 7.4 h and 6.6 days, respectively. An estimated bioconcentration factor of 49 suggests the potential for bioconcentration in aquatic organisms is moderate. Biodegradation of bromotrichloromethane in the environment is expected to be slow because of its highly halogenated structure. Occupational exposure to bromotrichloromethane may occur through inhalation or dermal contact with this compound in workplaces where it is produced or used. The general population may be exposed to bromotrichloromethane via ingestion of food and drinking water.

Exposure Routes and Pathways

It is used in organic syntheses and may result in its release into the environment directly to the atmosphere. The most common exposure route to bromotrichloromethane is through inhalation or dermal contact in workplaces where it is produced or used.

Toxicokinetics

Bromotrichloromethane is readily absorbed from the lungs and rapidly reaches equilibrium with levels in blood and expired air approximately proportional to the exposure concentration. At high concentrations, kinetic processes like metabolism or excretion may become saturated, limiting the rate of uptake. It is metabolized by conjugation with glutathione to yield *S*-methylglutathione, *S*-methyl cysteine, and other sulfur-containing compounds.

Mechanism of Toxicity

With the loss of bromide ion, mediated by cytochrome P450 enzyme in the liver, the trichlorocarbon free radical is

 http://dx.doi.org/10.1016/B978-0-12-386454-3.00259-1

responsible for lipid peroxidation, which is the predominant mechanism of hepatotoxicity. $BrCCl_3$, when metabolized *in vitro* and *in vivo*, produces phosgene ($COCl_2$) and trichloromethyl free radicals that ultimately cause massive lipid peroxidation and depletion of cellular glutathione. Both these events contribute to toxicity. Activation of membrane phospholipase A2 has also been considered as another prime suspect contributing to toxic outcomes. It is also known to cause cerebellar degeneration in rodents. It is cytotoxic to the sperm in the testes at the time of exposure. Renal tumors are induced in male mice due to depletion of glutathione, increased lipid peroxidation, and DNA lesions.

Acute and Short-Term Toxicity (or Exposure)

Animal

Inhalation of bromotrichloromethane by rats increased total lipids in liver and stimulated hepatic lipid peroxidation. After intragastric administration, liver steatosis was observed. Rats injected with 0.26 mmol bromotrichloromethane died after massive accumulation of neutral lipids and necrosis of the liver.

Human

Bromotrichloromethane causes irritation and reddening of eyes. Prolonged or repeated exposure may cause cataracts and severe, permanent damage to the eyes. Bromotrichloromethane causes rash, blistering, and allergic reactions upon dermal contact; it may also cause nasal, gastrointestinal, and lung irritation.

Inhalation of vapors may cause drowsiness and dizziness, which may be accompanied by narcosis, reduced alertness, loss of reflexes, lack of coordination, and vertigo. Acute intoxication by halogenated aliphatic hydrocarbons appears to take place over two stages. Signs of a reversible narcosis are evident in the first stage, and in the second stage signs of injury to organs may become evident; a single organ alone is (almost) never involved. Depression of the central nervous system is the most outstanding effect of most halogenated aliphatic hydrocarbons. Inebriation and excitation, passing into narcosis, is a typical reaction. In the case of iodized and brominated compounds, exposure effects cannot be described by simple central nervous system depression produced by other halogenated aliphatic hydrocarbons. Headache, nausea, ataxia (loss of muscle coordination), tremors, speech difficulties, visual disturbances, convulsions, paralysis, delirium, mania, and apathy are all evidence of additional effects.

Chronic Toxicity (or Exposure)

Animal

Bromotrichloromethane, when tested for its mutagenic activity, gave positive results for the Ames test.

Human

Rated D (not classifiable as human carcinogen) in the US Environmental Protection Agency's Integrated Risk Information System (IRIS). Chronic intoxication with ionic bromides, historically, has resulted from medical use of bromides but not from environmental or occupational exposure; depression, hallucinosis, and schizophrenic forms of psychosis can be seen in the absence of other signs of intoxication. Bromides may also induce sedation, irritability, agitation, delirium, memory loss, confusion, disorientation, forgetfulness (aphasias), dysarthria, weakness, fatigue, vertigo, stupor, coma, decreased appetite, nausea and vomiting, diarrhea, hallucinations, an acne like rash on the face, legs, and trunk known as bronchoderma, and a profuse discharge from the nostrils (coryza). Ataxia and generalized hyperreflexia have also been observed. Correlation of neurologic symptoms with blood levels of bromide is inaccurate. The use of substances such as brompheniramine as antihistamines largely reflects current usage of bromides; ionic bromides have been largely withdrawn from therapeutic use due to their toxicity. Several cases of fetal abnormalities have been described in mothers who took large doses of bromides during pregnancy.

Long-term exposure to $BrCCl_3$-like respiratory irritants may result in disease of the airways involving difficult breathing and related systemic problems. Some evidence links repeated or long-term occupational exposure to cumulative health effects involving organs or biochemical systems. There is some evidence that human exposure to the material may result in developmental toxicity, although evidences were derived from animal studies. Marked maternal toxicity were absent (secondary nonspecific consequences of the other toxic effects).

In Vitro Toxicity Data

In the *in vitro* test with FAF-cells of Chinese hamsters, only bromochloromethane produced an increase of the sister chromatid exchange frequency.

Clinical Management

Administration of vitamin E and cadmium acetate was shown to be protective against bromotrichloromethane toxicity by free radical scavenging and chelating properties of vitamin E and cadmium acetate, respectively. If orally exposed, administer activated charcoal as slurry (240 ml water per 30 g charcoal; usual dose: 25–100 g in adults/adolescents, 25–50 g in children 1–12 years), and 1 g kg^{-1} in infants less than 1 year old. If a potentially life-threatening amount of poison was ingested, consider activated charcoal soon after ingestion (generally within 1 h). Protect airway by placement in the head downleft lateral decubitus position or by endotracheal intubation. Control any seizures first. Eye exposures should be dealt with prolonged irrigation with water. Inhalation exposed patients should be removed from the contaminated area and provided fresh air as soon as possible.

Environmental Fate

Terrestrial Fate

Bromotrichloromethane is expected to have low mobility in soil. The potential for volatilization of bromotrichloromethane from dry soil surfaces may exist based on a measured vapor pressure of 39 mm Hg at 25 °C. Based on the highly halogenated structure of bromotrichloromethane, biodegradation in soil is expected to be slow.

Aquatic Fate

Bromotrichloromethane is expected to adsorb to suspended solids and sediment in water. Volatilization from water surfaces is expected. The potential for bioconcentration in aquatic organisms is moderate. Based on the highly halogenated structure of bromotrichloromethane, biodegradation in water is expected to be slow.

Atmospheric Fate

According to a model of gas/particle partitioning of semivolatile organic compounds in the atmosphere, bromotrichloromethane, which has a measured vapor pressure of 39 mm Hg at 25 °C, is expected to exist solely as a vapor in the ambient atmosphere. Based on bromotrichloromethane's structural similarity to bromotrifluoromethane, it is expected to slowly degrade in the atmosphere by reaction with photochemically produced hydroxyl radicals; the half-life for bromotrichloromethane's reaction in air is estimated to be greater than 44 years. Photolysis may occur based on bromotrichloromethane's structural similarity to other halogenated methane compounds, but not at an environmentally relevant rate.

Ecotoxicology

Bioconcentration of bromotrichloromethane in aquatic organisms is moderate. Aquatic toxic effects to aquatic organisms are not reported as such.

Exposure Standards and Guidelines

According to the US Occupational Safety and Health Administration, the threshold limit value–time-weighted average (TLV–TWA) limit for bromotrichloromethane is 8 h at TWA 200 ppm. Excursions in worker exposure levels may exceed three times the TLV–TWA for no more than a total of 30 min during a workday, and under no circumstances should they exceed five times the TLV–TWA.

See also: Ames Test; Carcinogen Classification Schemes; Glutathione; Lipid Peroxidation; Carbon Tetrachloride; Bromine.

Further Reading

Azri-Meehan, S., Mata, H.P., Gandolfi, A.J., Brendel, K., 1994. The interactive toxicity of CHCl3 and BrCCl3 in precision-cut rat liver slices. Fundam. Appl. Toxicol. 22 (2), 172–177.

Danni, O., Aragno, M., Tamagno, E., Ugazio, G., 1992. In vivo studies on halogen compound interactions. IV. Interaction among different halogen derivatives with and without synergistic action on liver toxicity. Res. Commun. Chem. Pathol. Pharmacol. 76 (3), 355–366.

Faroon, O.M., Henry, R.W., Soni, M.G., Mehendale, H.M., 1991. Potentiation of BrCCl3 hepatotoxicity by chlordecone: biochemical and ultrastructural study. Toxicol. Appl. Pharmacol. 110 (2), 185–197.

Glende Jr., E.A., Recknagel, R.O., 1992. Phospholipase A2 activation and cell injury in isolated rat hepatocytes exposed to bromotrichloromethane, chloroform, and 1,1-dichloroethylene as compared to effects of carbon tetrachloride. Toxicol. Appl. Pharmacol. 113 (1), 159–162.

Jochmann, C., Klee, S., Ungemach, F.R., Younes, M., 1994. The role of glutathione and protein thiols in CBrCl3-induced cytotoxicity in isolated rat hepatocytes. Pharmacol. Toxicol. 75 (1), 7–16.

Lowrey, K., 1981. Destruction of liver microsomal calcium pump activity by carbon tetrachloride and bromotrichloromethane. Biochem. Pharmacol. 30, 135.

Mehendale, H.M., 1991. Role of hepatocellular regeneration and hepatolobular healing in the final outcome of liver injury. A two-stage model of toxicity. Biochem. Pharmacol. 42 (6), 1155–1162.

Müller, K., Grune, T., Klee, S., Jochmann, C., Ungemach, F., Siems, W., 1993. Trichlorobromomethane-induced changes of purine nucleotides in hepatocytes. Biochem. Mol. Biol. Int. 31 (3), 405–412.

Pirlich, M., Müller, C., Sandig, G., et al., 2002. Increased proteolysis after single-dose exposure with hepatotoxins in HepG2 cells. Free Radic. Biol. Med. 33 (2), 283–291.

Sano, M., Kawabata, H., Tomita, I., Yoshioka, H., Hu, M.L., 1994. Potentiation of oxidative damage to rat red blood cells by the concurrent presence of *t*-butyl hydroperoxide and bromotrichloromethane. J. Toxicol. Environ. Health 43 (3), 339–350.

Tyson, C.A., Hawk-Prather, K., Story, D.L., Gould, D.H., 1983. Correlations of in vitro and in vivo hepatotoxicity for five haloalkanes. Toxicol. Appl. Pharmacol. 70 (2), 289–302.

Waller, R.L., Recknagel, R.O., 1982. Evaluation of a role for phosgene production in the hepatotoxic mechanism of action of carbon tetrachloride and bromotrichloromethane. Toxicol. Appl. Pharmacol. 66 (2), 172–181.

Relevant Websites

http://toxnet.nlm.nih.gov/cgi-bin/sis/search/r?dbs+hsdb:@term+@rn+@rel+75-62-7 – National Library of Medicine-National Institutes of Health-Hazardous Substances Data Bank.

http://datasheets.scbt.com/sc-252520.pdf – Santa Cruz Biotechnology.

Brown Recluse Spider *see* Spiders

Busulfan

M Janes, La Jolla, CA, USA

- Chemical Abstracts Service Registry Number: 55-98-1
- Synonyms: 1,4-Bis(methanesulfonoxy)butane, Leucosulfan, Myleran, Mylosulfan
- Chemical Formula: C_6–H_{14}–O_6–S_2
- Chemical Structure:

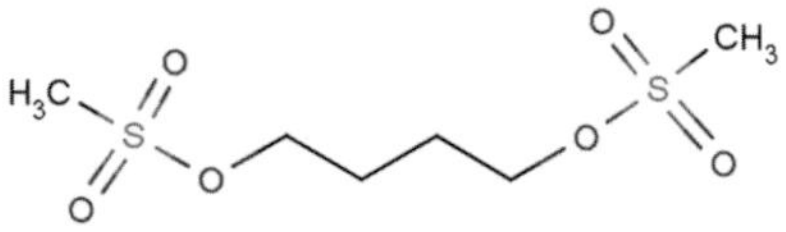

Background

Busulfan was noted to have strong antitumor activity in the 1950s. Because of this, GlaxoSmithKline developed the compound, launching Myleran in 1954 for the treatment of chronic myelogenous leukemia (CML) in the United States. Following the discovery, clinical development, and approval of imatinib (a drug that targets the aberrant fusion product of a chromosomal aberration in CML that initiates and drives the disease) in the late 1990s, busulfan's use as an anti-chemotherapeutic agent has been displaced. Today, busulfan is used primarily as a component of a preparative conditioning regimen prior to either allogeneic or autologous hematopoietic stem cell transplantation (HSCT) in patients who have been diagnosed with CML.

Uses

Busulfan is a cytotoxic alkylating chemotherapeutic agent that is extensively used as preparative conditioning regimen prior to allogeneic HSCT for hematologic malignancies. Busulfan has been widely used in the treatment of CML and other hematologic malignancies and myelodysplastic disorders. The principal effect of busulfan is myelosuppression and myeloablation when used at the recommended dosage. Currently, busulfan is indicated for use in combination with cyclophosphamide to destroy cancer cells and make room for new bone marrow to grow prior to a bone marrow or peripheral blood progenitor cell replacement procedure. As a component of a conditioning regimen for HSCT, busulfan also suppresses the immune system so that the patient does not reject the new bone marrow.

Mechanism of Action

Busulfan is a bifunctional alkylating agent that consists of two methanesulfonate groups attached at opposite ends of a four-carbon alkyl chain. In aqueous media, busulfan hydrolyzes to release the methanesulfonate groups to produce reactive carbonium ions that can alkylate DNA. DNA damage is believed to be the major mechanism of toxicity of busulfan. Busulfan is therefore considered a mutagen and a clastogen. Busulfan induces a G2 cell cycle block and apoptosis in rapidly proliferating cells, in particular in hematopoietic cells of the myelogranulocytic lineage.

Toxicokinetics

In all studies, busulfan toxicity occurs in a dose-dependent manner.

Exposure and Exposure Monitoring

Exposure to this compound therapeutically is by the oral route when formulated in pills (Myleran). Busulfan is also formulated to be used as an injection for intravenous administration (Busulfex). Variation in exposure is often observed for oral busulfan resulting in substantial risk of over- or undertreatment. The intravenous formulation has been reported to reduce exposure variability based on improved absorption pharmacokinetic parameters. Patients typically receive $0.8\ \text{mg kg}^{-1}$ busulfan every 6 h in a total of 16 doses over 4 days. At steady state, this schedule achieves a maximum concentration (C_{max}) and target area under the curve (AUC) value of $1200\ \mu\text{M min}^{-1}$ (range $550–1673\ \mu\text{M min}^{-1}$, 20% coefficient of variation). As described above, busulfan is often combined with cyclophosphamide as a BuCy regimen, in which after the 4-day busulfan infusion, cyclophosphamide is administered for 2 days ($60\ \text{mg kg}^{-1}$ daily). The HSCT is typically performed after 1 day of rest. Using this schedule, all patients experience myeloablation with a median time of neutropenia of 4 days.

Acute and Short-Term Toxicity

Busulfan lowers white blood cell counts, most profoundly in the weeks after the drug is given. This can increase the chance of getting an infection. Busulfan may also lower platelet counts in the weeks after it is given, which can increase the risk of bleeding. Busulfan may lower red blood cell counts, which can cause shortness of breath, or make the patient feel weak or

 http://dx.doi.org/10.1016/B978-0-12-386454-3.00008-7

tired. Exposure to busulfan may be accompanied by nausea and vomiting. Seizures have been reported 1–3 days after treatment/exposure; therefore, patients are often premedicated with phenytoin before busulfan administration. In *in vitro* laboratory tests, busulfan caused mutations in bacteria and insect cell cultures, and induced chromosomal aberrations in rat, mouse, and human cells.

Chronic Toxicity

Ovarian suppression and amenorrhea commonly occurred in premenopausal women receiving chronic low-dose busulfan for CML treatment. Pulmonary toxicity has been reported in patients receiving chronic low-dose busulfan therapy for CML. High plasma concentrations have been associated with an increased risk of developing hepatic venoocclusive disease.

Immunotoxicity

The most common serious consequence of busulfan exposure at the recommended dose and schedule is profound myelosuppression. Severe bone marrow depression accompanied by granulocytopenia, thrombocytopenia, anemia, or combination thereof have been reported.

Reproductive Toxicity

Busulfan may cause fetal harm when administered to pregnant women. Sterility, azoospermia, and testicular atrophy have been reported in male patients. Pronounced adverse effects on reproductive glands, germ cells, and fertility are observed in exposed animals. Busulfan induces sterility in male rats and hamsters and depletes oocytes of female rats.

Carcinogenicity

Busulfan is a presumed human carcinogen. Administration of busulfan (at 30% of the total dose equivalent) has been shown to increase the incidence of thymic and ovarian tumors in mice. Four cases of acute leukemia occurred among a study of 243 patients using busulfan as adjuvant therapy following resection of lung cancer. Clinical appearance of leukemia was observed 5–8 years after oral busulfan treatment.

Clinical Management

Following any exposure, hematologic status should be closely monitored and vigorous supportive measures should be instituted as medically indicated. There is one report that busulfan is dialyzable, thus dialysis should be considered in the case of overdose. Busulfan is metabolized by conjugation with glutathione, thus administration of glutathione may be considered in the case of overdose.

Ecotoxicology

Busulfan is a white crystalline powder that is relatively insoluble in water (at 0.1 $g\,l^{-1}$). In pill form, busulfan is supplied as white, film-coated, round biconvex tablets containing 2 mg busulfan (Myleran). Some pharmaceutical agents and their metabolites are often detected in environmental samples and therefore pose significant concerns for wildlife; however, busulfan is so far of little regulatory concern to the US Environmental Protection Agency.

See also: Alkylating Agents; Blood; Cancer Chemotherapeutic Agents; Carcinogen–DNA Adduct Formation and DNA Repair; Immune System.

Further Reading

Ciurea, S.O., Andersson, B.S., 2009. Busulfan in hematopoietic stem cell transplantation. Biol. Blood Marrow Transplant. 15, 523–536.

Nath, C.E., Shaw, P.J., 2007. Busulphan in blood and marrow transplantation: dose, route, frequency, and role of therapeutic drug monitoring. Curr. Clin. Pharmacol. 2, 75–91.

Relevant Websites

http://www.cancer.org/Treatment/TreatmentsandSideEffects/GuidetoCancerDrugs/busulfan – American Cancer Society - Busulfan.

http://www.busulfex.com/ – Otsuka information sheet on IV BUSULFEX.

Butadiene, 1,3-

RJ Parod, BASF Corporation, Wyandotte, MI, USA

- Chemical Abstracts Service Registry Number: 106-99-0
- Synonyms: Biethylene, Bivinyl, Buta-1,3-diene, Butadiene monomer, Vinylethylene
- Molecular Formula: C_4H_6
- Chemical Structure:

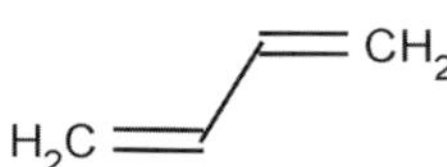

Background

Butadiene is produced during the combustion of organic matter. Significant amounts of butadiene are released to the environment from both natural and anthropogenic sources such as forest fires, gasoline and diesel engine exhaust, and wood space heating. It is also a component of cigarette smoke. Industrially, butadiene is most commonly produced as a coproduct of ethylene manufacture in which hydrocarbon feedstocks are cracked with steam and butadiene is removed from the resulting crude C_4 stream by liquid–liquid extraction with solvents.

Uses

Butadiene is a reactive monomer used in the production of synthetic rubber (60%) and plastics. Styrene–butadiene rubber, polybutadiene rubber, adiponitrile, styrene–butadiene latex, acrylonitrile–butadiene–styrene resins, and nitrile rubber are used in the manufacture of tires, nylon products, plastic bottles and food wraps, molded rubber goods, latex adhesives, carpet backing and pads, shoe soles, and medical devices. There are no direct consumer uses of butadiene and unreacted monomer is not expected to be present in polymers and plastics made from butadiene.

Environmental Fate and Behavior

Butadiene is a gas under normal environmental conditions with limited water solubility (735 $mg\,l^{-1}$ at 25 °C). Butadiene released to the atmosphere will remain there with very small amounts being distributed to water and soil. In air, butadiene will be removed by reaction with photochemically produced hydroxyl radicals (5.6-h half-life), nitrate radicals (15-h half-life), and ozone (1.5-day half-life). When released to water, butadiene will be removed by volatilization to air (Henry's law constant of 7460 $Pa\,m^3\,mol^{-1}$), biodegradation (aerobic half-life of 15 days), and reaction with singlet oxygen. Based on its estimated organic carbon partition coefficient (K_{oc} of 288), butadiene will not exhibit significant adsorption to soil or suspended particulate matter; its biodegradation half-life in soil is estimated to be 30 days. Due to volatilization to air and degradation in soil, butadiene is not expected to leach to groundwater. As butadiene is readily metabolized, it is not expected to pose a significant bioaccumulation hazard.

Exposure and Exposure Monitoring

Butadiene is a heavier than air under normal environmental conditions. In the workplace, the most significant route of exposure to butadiene is inhalation during its production and use. Potentially significant exposures to butadiene are likely limited to the industrial setting. Workplace concentrations have declined since the late 1970s (<10 ppm) to the current date (<1 ppm). Typical levels of butadiene in rural (0.01 ppb) and urban (0.4–1 ppb) air as well as the residual butadiene monomer content in consumer products are low and unlikely to pose a significant health threat to the general public.

Toxicokinetics

Butadiene is readily absorbed through the respiratory tract. Dermal absorption is anticipated to be limited due to the volatility of liquid butadiene. Once absorbed, butadiene is rapidly distributed throughout the body. A tissue distribution study in rats indicates that the highest concentration of butadiene is located in the peripheral fat; lower concentrations are observed in the liver, brain, spleen, and kidney. Based on a radiolabel study in mice, most of the absorbed butadiene is exhaled as the parent compound, with a lesser amount exhaled as CO_2. Smaller amounts of butadiene and/or its metabolites are detected in urine and feces, with most of the label being eliminated from the carcass within 65 h. The bulk of the butadiene body burden (77–99%) in rodents is eliminated with a half-life of 2–10 h.

Metabolism of butadiene is qualitatively similar across species, although there are significant quantitative differences in the amounts of metabolites formed. Butadiene is rapidly metabolized via enzyme systems located in the liver, lung, nasal mucosa, and possibly bone marrow. Initially, most of the absorbed butadiene is converted to the reactive monoepoxide metabolite 1,2-epoxy-3-butene (EB) by cytochrome P450 monooxygenase, an enzyme that also metabolizes EB to a reactive diepoxide, 1,2,3,4-diepoxybutane (DEB). EB can also be detoxified to 3-butene-1,2-diol (B-diol) by epoxide hydrolase. B-diol (via cytochrome P450) and DEB (via epoxide hydrolase) can be metabolized to another monoepoxide, 3,4-epoxybutane-1,2-diol (EBD). At similar exposure

 http://dx.doi.org/10.1016/B978-0-12-386454-3.00368-7

concentrations, the concentration of butadiene metabolites in mouse blood is about three-fold higher in rat blood and >10-fold higher in monkey blood. All three epoxides can be inactivated by conjugation with glutathione via glutathione S-transferase and by hydrolysis via epoxide hydrolase. Glutathione conjugation predominates in mice followed by rats and then humans; conversely, hydrolysis via epoxide hydrolase predominates in humans followed by rats and then mice. The three epoxides also form unique conjugates with the N-terminal valine of hemoglobin. These epoxide-hemoglobin adducts are used as biomarkers of butadiene exposure and to assess the relative importance of the different metabolic pathways in individual species. The activation/inactivation profiles of these three enzyme systems are species-specific resulting in DEB tissue levels in mice that are higher than those found in similarly exposed rats (30-fold) and humans (100-fold).

Mechanism of Toxicity

The carcinogenic potential of butadiene in rodents is thought to reflect the metabolism of butadiene to DNA-reactive metabolites resulting in genetic alterations in proto-oncogenes and/or tumor suppressor genes. Mechanistic data suggest that the higher carcinogenic potency of butadiene in mice versus rats is primarily due to the higher body burden in mice of DEB, considered the most mutagenic butadiene metabolite (see Genotoxicity). This is supported by the observations that carcinogenicity tests with EB were equivocal, while DEB was carcinogenic in mice and rats when administered via multiple routes of exposure. Although the mechanism by which butadiene causes noncancer effects is not well understood, there is strong evidence that ovarian atrophy in mice, the most sensitive noncancer endpoint, is mediated by DEB.

Acute and Short-Term Toxicity

Animal

Acute inhalation studies have shown that butadiene exhibits low toxicity in animals. Butadiene is a relatively weak central nervous system (CNS) depressant. Mice exposed to butadiene for 6–12 min exhibited excitement and narcosis (200 000 ppm), light narcosis (150 000 ppm), and no effects (100 000 ppm). Deep anesthesia was produced in rabbits exposed to 200 000–250 000 ppm butadiene for 8–10 min; death due to respiratory paralysis occurred within 25–35 min at 250 000 ppm. Butadiene exhibits low toxicity in rodents with 2- and 4-h LC_{50} values >100 000 ppm.

Human

Exposures of industrial workers to butadiene concentrations of 2000–8000 ppm have been reported to cause eye, skin, and nasal irritation. High butadiene levels (150 000–250 000 ppm) may cause CNS depression as evidenced by blurred vision, drowsiness, fatigue, bradycardia, and hypotension. However, explosion is probably the greater health hazard as butadiene levels approach these concentrations. The mildly aromatic odor of butadiene, which can be detected at ≥1 ppm, serves as a good warning aid. Dermal contact with liquid butadiene may produce frostbite due to cooling caused by the rapid evaporation of butadiene from the skin.

Chronic Toxicity

As described in other sections, the chronic toxicity of butadiene observed in animals and humans is generally limited to reproductive toxicity and carcinogenicity.

Immunotoxicity

There are limited chronic data in animals and humans. Subchronic exposures (weeks–months) of mice to butadiene (62.5–1250 ppm) have been reported to alter stem cell development and depress cell-mediated immunity as well as the cellularity and weight of some lymphoid organs. The biological significance of these findings is unknown.

Reproductive Toxicity

Mice are more sensitive than rats to the reproductive toxicity caused by inhalation of butadiene. In mice, ovarian atrophy was induced in a dose-dependent fashion at lifetime exposures >6.25 or at 1000 ppm after a 13-week exposure. Degenerative changes in the testes of mice were observed only after lifetime exposures to butadiene at >200 ppm. No effects on the reproductive organs were seen in rats receiving a lifetime exposure up to 8000 ppm butadiene. Under its Integrated Risk Information System (IRIS) program, US Environmental Protection Agency (EPA) used the data on ovarian atrophy in the lifetime mouse study and a combined uncertainty factor of 1000 to derive a chronic inhalation reference concentration for the general population of 0.9 ppb. The value of 1000 is inconsistent with the selection of uncertainty factors in subsequent IRIS assessments on other chemicals and may be overly conservative given species differences in tissue levels of DEB, the metabolite recognized by US EPA as the likely reproductive toxicant.

In prenatal developmental toxicity studies, mice and rats were exposed by inhalation to butadiene at concentrations of 40, 200, and 1000 ppm for 6 h day^{-1} during gestational days 6–15. In mice, maternal toxicity (decreased body weight gain) and fetal toxicity (growth retardation, decreased placental weights, and increased morphological variations) were seen at 200 and 1000 ppm; the maternal and fetal no-observed-adverse-effect concentrations (NOAECs) were 40 ppm. In rats, maternal toxicity (decreased body weight gain) was seen at 1000 ppm, while developmental effects were not observed at any concentration; the NOAECs for maternal and fetal toxicity were 200 and 1000 ppm, respectively. Based on limited available data, there is no conclusive evidence that butadiene is fetotoxic or teratogenic at concentrations below those toxic to the mother.

Genotoxicity

Animal

Butadiene, in the presence of metabolic activation, and its epoxide metabolites (EB, DEB, and EBD) are genotoxic in a variety of *in vitro* and *in vivo* test systems. While all three epoxides can react with DNA, their mutagenic potencies are very different (DEB $\gg$ EB > EBD). The potency of the diepoxide (DEB) is likely related to its ability to form macromolecular crosslinks. Mutagenicity is detected *in vivo* in mice at a lower butadiene concentration (3 ppm) than that of rats (62.5 ppm). The fact that internal DEB levels at these concentrations as measured by DEB-hemoglobin adducts are comparable suggests that DEB is the primary mutagenic metabolite at these concentrations. Butadiene is clastogenic in mice but not rats.

Human

Studies of mutations in peripheral blood lymphocytes of workers exposed to butadiene have produced mixed results. In positive studies of butadiene monomer and styrene–butadiene rubber workers, high butadiene exposures resulted in a higher mutation frequency than low exposures. Follow-up studies of these worker populations reported similar results. However, the new exposure measurements in these follow-up studies no longer supported the previous high/low exposure classifications, and there was no apparent association between individual mutation frequency values and butadiene exposures within the assigned groups. In one of these studies, it was observed that workers employed for 11–39 years had a twofold greater mutation frequency than workers employed for 1–10 years. Although other confounders cannot be excluded, the study authors interpreted these results to reflect a cleaner work environment and the persistence of lymphocyte mutations generated when exposure levels were higher. There have also been several studies reporting that lymphocyte mutations are not increased in butadiene-exposed workers. The two epidemiological studies with the most comprehensive exposure measurements showed that gene mutations do not occur in workers exposed to time-weighted average (TWA) butadiene concentrations of 0.8 and 2.0 ppm.

Carcinogenicity

Animal

Lifetime studies in rats and mice indicate that the inhalation of butadiene increases the incidence of tumors at various sites, with mice being significantly more susceptible to the tumorigenic effect of butadiene than rats. In mice, tumors were induced at lifetime exposures of 6.25–1250 ppm or in as little as 13 weeks at 625 ppm. In rats, tumors were observed primarily at 8000 ppm and typically only in organs where tumors develop spontaneously.

Human

It is not known if butadiene itself poses a carcinogenic risk in humans. A large well-conducted epidemiological study reported an increase in mortality from leukemia among workers in the styrene–butadiene rubber industry and that the increase was associated with cumulative butadiene exposure. The risk of leukemia remained but was attenuated after controlling for exposures to styrene and other potential confounding agents. However, these results were not consistent with those of three smaller studies of adequate statistical power in butadiene monomer workers. Under its IRIS program, the US EPA has classified butadiene as carcinogenic to humans by inhalation and used the data on leukemia in styrene–butadiene workers to derive an inhalation unit risk for cancer of 8×10^{-5} $(\text{ppb})^{-1}$.

Clinical Management

There is no antidote for butadiene toxicity. The primary toxicity of butadiene is CNS depression at high concentrations. Treatment involves removal from exposure and support of respiratory function.

Ecotoxicology

Due to its volatility and explosivity, data on the toxicity of butadiene to aquatic organisms are generally limited quantitative structure–activity relationship modeling estimates. For freshwater and saltwater fish (96-h LC_{50}) and invertebrates (48-h EC_{50}), acute toxicity values generally range between 20 and 50 mg l^{-1}; chronic no-observed-effect concentration (NOEC) values for these species are about 10-fold lower. Butadiene is predicted to be slightly more toxic to algae based on its acute (96-h $EC_{50} = 11\ \text{mg l}^{-1}$) and chronic ($\text{NOEC} = 4\ \text{mg l}^{-1}$) toxicity values and modestly less toxic to earthworms (14-day $LC_{50} = 93\ \text{mg kg}^{-1}$ soil). Predicted values are more conservative (i.e., lower) than the limited experimental values obtained with structurally similar compounds.

Other Hazards

Butadiene is a highly flammable gas at standard temperature and pressure. In air, butadiene will form explosive peroxides that are sensitive to shock or heating above 27 °C and will explode upon contact with aluminum tetrahydroborate. Butadiene has lower and upper explosive limits of 2% and 12% by volume in air, respectively.

Exposure Standards and Guidelines

International Occupational Exposure Limits (OELs) for butadiene generally range from 0.5 to 15 ppm as an 8-h TWA, with 2 ppm being the TWA OEL established by the American Conference of Governmental Industrial Hygienists. US Occupational Safety and Health Administration lists a permissible exposure limit of 1 ppm for butadiene (TWA) with a 15 min short-term exposure limit of 5 ppm. National Institute of Occupational Safety and Health indicates that 2000 ppm butadiene is immediately dangerous to life or health. Butadiene is classified as a human carcinogen by the International Agency for Research on Cancer and the US National Toxicology Program.

See also: American College of Toxicology; ACGIH® (American Conference of Governmental Industrial Hygienists); Risk Assessment, Human Health; Toxicity Testing, Aquatic; Toxicity Testing, Carcinogenesis; Toxicity Testing, Developmental; Toxicity Testing, Mutagenicity; Toxicity Testing, Reproductive; Toxicity, Acute; Toxicity, Subchronic and Chronic; Pharmacokinetics; Uncertainty Factors.

Further Reading

Albertini, R.J., Carson, M.L., Kirman, C.R., Gargas, M.L., 2010. 1,3-Butadiene: II. Genotoxicity profile. Crit. Rev. Toxicol. 40 (Suppl. 1), 12–73.

Kirman, C.R., Albertini, R.J., Gargas, M.L., 2010. 1,3-Butadiene: III: assessing carcinogenic modes of action. Crit. Rev. Toxicol. 40 (Suppl. 1), 74–93.

Kirman, C.R., Albertini, R.J., Sweeney, L.M., Gargas, M.L., 2010. 1,3-Butadiene: I. Review of the metabolism and the implications to human health risk assessment. Crit. Rev. Toxicol. 40 (Suppl. 1), 1–11.

Swenberg, J.A., Bordeerat, N.K., Boysen, G., Carro, S., Georgieva, NI., et al., 2011. 1,3-Butadiene: biomarkers and application to risk assessment. Chem-Biol. Interact. 192, 150–154.

Relevant Websites

http://www.atsdr.cdc.gov – Agency for Toxic Substances and Disease Registry. Toxicological Profile for 1,3-Butadiene

http://apps.echa.europa.eu/registered/registered-sub.aspx – European Chemicals Agency. Information on Buta-1,3-diene

http://www.epa.gov/iris/index.html – US EPA IRIS. 1,3-Butadiene

http://www.iarc.fr/ – International Agency for Research on Cancer. 1,3-Butadiene.

Butane

MA Kamrin

- Chemical Abstracts Service Registry Number: 1069-97-8
- Synonyms: *n*-Butane; Butyl hydride; Methylethylmethane; Liquefied petroleum gas
- Chemical Formula: $CH_3(CH_2)_2CH_3$
- Chemical Structure:

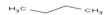

Background

Butane is a widely used compound, most commonly as a fuel in lighters, torches, and stoves. Although it is an asphyxiant when inhaled in large amounts, it has been used in smaller amounts by those looking for substances that can produce altered mental states. Such abuse of butane has resulted in a number of deaths from what is known as Sudden Sniffing Death Syndrome.

Uses

Butane is used as a fuel in lighters, small blow torches, and camping stoves. It is also used in calibrating instruments and as a food additive. In addition, it is a raw material for organic synthesis.

Environmental Fate and Behavior

Routes and Pathways

Butane is relatively nonpersistent in the environment and has a low leaching potential. It is moderately volatile from water and it does not bioaccumulate.

Physicochemical Properties

Butane's Log K_{ow} is 2.89 and its estimated Henry's law constant is 9.47×10^{-1} atm m^3 mol^{-1} at 25 C.

Exposure Routes and Pathways

Since butane is a gas, the major routes of exposure are inhalation and contact with skin and eyes. It is a widely used substance of abuse by inhalation.

Mechanism of Toxicity

Gaseous butane acts as a simple asphyxiant, which means that it causes toxicity by displacing oxygen and preventing it from reaching important tissues and organs. In its liquid state, it causes frostbite due to rapid cooling on evaporation.

Acute and Short-Term Toxicity

Animal

An LC_{50} of 658 g m^{-3}, for a 4-h inhalation exposure, has been established in rats.

Human

Because of its asphyxiant properties, high doses of inhaled butane can affect the central nervous system and lead to a variety of symptoms. These include euphoria, excitation, vomiting, confusion, hallucinations, drowsiness, and coma. Skin contact with liquid butane can cause frostbite.

Clinical Management

The affected person should be removed from exposure and provided fresh air. Symptomatic and supportive treatment should be administered. This may include support of both cardiovascular and respiratory systems.

Environmental Fate

Butane is relatively nonpersistent in the environment and has a low leaching potential. It is moderately volatile from water and it does not bioaccumulate.

Other Hazards

Butane poses severe fire and explosion hazards. It should be stored and used distant from any ignition sources.

Exposure Standards and Guidelines

The American Conference of Governmental Industrial Hygienists time-weighted average (TWA) for butane is 800 ppm (1900 mg m^3) and the TWA for liquefied petroleum gas is 1000 ppm (1800 mg m^3).

See also: Drugs of Abuse.

Further Reading

European Chemicals Bureau (ECB) (2000) IUCLID Data Sheet on Butane (Pure). Ispra, Italy.

International Program on Chemical Safety (1998) Butane. INCHEM Poisons Information Monograph 945. Geneva, Switzerland.

Relevant Website

http://www.inchem.org B Chemical Safety Information from Intergovernmental Organization.

 http://dx.doi.org/10.1016/B978-0-12-386454-3.00369-9

Butter Yellow

KN Thakore, California Department of Public Health, Richmond, CA, USA

- Name: Butter yellow
- Chemical Abstracts Service Registry Number: 60-11-7
- Synonyms: *p*-Dimethylaminoazobenzene (DAB); *N*,*N*-Dimethyl-4-(phenylazo) benzenamine; Methyl yellow; C.I. solvent yellow 2; C.I. 11020.
- Molecular Formula: $C_{14}H_{15}N_3$
- Chemical Structure:

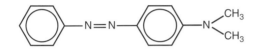

Uses

Butter yellow was largely used as a food coloring agent. It was also used for the determination of free hydrochloric acid in gastric juice, for the spot test identification of peroxidized fats, as a pH indicator, and as a laboratory reagent.

Environmental Fate and Behavior

Butter yellow exists as a stable crystalline material at normal temperature and pressure. It is insoluble in water, but soluble in organic solvents such as alcohol, chloroform, ether, petroleum ether, mineral acids, oils, and pyridine. Its octanol/water partition coefficient is 4.58, vapor pressure is 3.3×10^{-7} mm Hg; and Henry's law constant is 7.1×10^{-9} atm-m^3 mol^{-1}.

Butter yellow may be released into the environment as a result of its manufacture and use in the consumer products. It may bind to the soil and when released into water, may bioconcentrate in aquatic organisms, or may be adsorbed into the sediment. If released in the atmosphere, it may undergo direct photolysis.

Exposure and Exposure Monitoring

Exposure through inhalation and dermal routes is very common.

Toxicokinetics

The potential routes of human exposure to butter yellow are inhalation, dermal, and ingestion. Biotransformation involves reduction by cytochrome P450 dependent enzymes followed by cleavage of the azo group, demethylation, ring hydroxylation, *N*-hydroxylation, *N*-acetylation, and *O*-conjugation of metabolites in liver. The metabolites can bind to macromolecules such as proteins and nucleic acids. When [^{14}C-dimethyl]-aminoazobenzene was fed to rats, most of the radioactivity was found in expired carbon dioxide. In rats, 50–60% of administered butter yellow is excreted in urine in the form of sulfates or glucuronides of *N*-acetylated metabolites.

Mechanism of Toxicity

Butter yellow is metabolized *in vivo* to a reactive form that covalently binds to cellular macromolecules, such as proteins and DNA, and causes toxicity. Agents that interfere with this covalent binding can modulate its toxicity.

Acute and Short-Term Toxicity

Animal

Intravenous administration of butter yellow is toxic. It is moderately toxic by other routes such as oral, intraperitoneal, intramuscular, and subcutaneous. It is an antihypertensive agent. The oral and intraperitoneal LD_{50} values in the rat are 200 and 230 mg kg^{-1}, respectively. The oral and intraperitoneal LD_{50} values in the mouse are 300 and 230 mg kg^{-1}, respectively.

Human

Butter yellow is known to cause occupational contact dermatitis in factory workers who handle it. The target organs for toxicity are skin, liver, and bladder. Overexposure to butter yellow can potentially cause symptoms such as enlarged liver, hepatic and renal dysfunction, contact dermatitis, coughing, wheezing, difficulty in breathing, bloody sputum, bronchial secretions, frequent urination, hematuria, and dysuria.

Chronic Toxicity

Animal

There is sufficient evidence of carcinogenicity in animals. It is carcinogenic by various routes in the rat and mouse (liver carcinoma). It causes carcinoma of the bladder and lungs, if ingested. Diet can influence its carcinogenic activity. Its activated form is shown to be mutagenic and teratogenic.

Human

On the basis of animal carcinogenic data, butter yellow is suspected to be human carcinogen both by the US Occupational Safety and Health Administration (OSHA) and the National Toxicology Program (NTP). Mutation effect in human is also reported.

Reproductive Toxicity

Butter yellow can cause adverse reproductive effects.

 http://dx.doi.org/10.1016/B978-0-12-386454-3.00260-8

Genotoxicity

Butter yellow induces unscheduled DNA synthesis in HeLa human cervical cancer cells. It is mutagenic in *Salmonella typhimurium* TA100 and TA98.

Carcinogenicity

Butter yellow is suspected to be a human carcinogen by the US OSHA and NTP. It has been linked with gall bladder cancer.

Clinical Management

In case of contact, the eyes and skin should be flushed with water for 15–20 min. In the case of inhalation exposure, the victim should be moved to fresh air, and oxygen and artificial respiration should be administered, if necessary. If the patient is in cardiac arrest, cardiopulmonary resuscitation should be given. Life-support measures should be continued until medical assistance has arrived. In the case of an unconscious or convulsing person, liquids should not be administered and vomiting should not be induced.

Ecotoxicology

It may bind to the soil. It may bioconcentrate in aquatic organisms, adsorb to sediment, and be subject to direct photolysis.

Other Hazards

Butter yellow when heated to decompose emits toxic fumes of nitrous oxides.

Exposure Standards and Guidelines

Engineering controls, standard work practices, and personal protective equipment, including respirators, should be employed to prevent worker exposure to butter yellow. After use, the clothing and equipment should be placed in an impervious container for decontamination or disposal. Preemployment and periodic medical examination should focus on liver function.

See also: Dimethylaminoazobenzene; Food Safety and Toxicology; Butylated Hydroxyanisole; Butylated Hydroxytoluene; Food and Drug Administration, US; Food Additives.

Further Reading

International Agency for Research on Cancer (IARC), 1987. para-Dimethylaminoazobenzene. In: IARC Monographs. Overall Evaluation of Carcinogenicity: An Update of IARC Monographs, vols. 1–42. (Suppl. 7). IARC, Lyon, France, p. 62.

Lenga, R.E., 1988. Butter yellow. In: Lenga, R.E. (Ed.), The Sigma Aldrich Library of Chemical Safety Data, second ed. vol. 2. Sigma Aldrich Co, U.S.A., p. 2464.

Lewis, R.J., 2012. 4-Dimethylaminoazobenzene. In: Lewis, R.J. (Ed.), Sax's Dangerous Properties of Industrial Materials, twelth ed. vol. III. John Wiley & Sons, Inc, New York, pp. 1672–1673.

Mishra, V., Mishra, M., Ansari, K.M., Chaudhari, B.P., Khanna, R., Das, M., 2012. Edible oil adulterants, argemone oil and butter yellow, as aetiological factors for gall bladder cancer. Eur. J. Cancer 48 (13), 2075–2085.

National Toxicology Program (NTP), 2011. 4-Dimethylaminoazobenzene. In: National Toxicology Program (Ed.), Report on Carcinogens, twelfth ed. US Department of Health and Human Services, Public Health Service, Research Triangle Park, NC, pp. 167–168.

Woo, Y.T., Lai, D.Y., 2012. Aromatic amino and nitro-amino compounds and their halogenated derivatives. In: Bingham, E., Cohrssen, B. (Eds.), Patty's Toxicology, sixth ed. vol. 2 John Wiley & Sons, Inc, New York, pp. 682–683.

Relevant Websites

http://chem.sis.nlm.nih.gov/chemidplus – US National Library of Medicine: ChemIDplus Advanced: Search for: 4-(dimethylamino)azobenzene.

http://toxnet.nlm.nih.gov – Toxnet (Toxicology Data Network): search under 4-(dimethylamino)azobenzene.

http://www.cdc.gov/niosh/npg/npgd0220.html – Centers for Disease Control and Prevention - NIOSH Pocket Guide to Chemical Hazards: 4-Dimethylaminoazobenzene.

http://scorecard.goodguide.com/4-Dimethylaminoazobenzene – Pollution information site.

http://www.epa.gov/ttn/uatw/hlthef/di-benze.html – US Environmental Protection Agency: Technology Transfer Network - Air Toxics Web Site. 4-Dimethylaminoazobenzene.

Button Batteries

T Litovitz, Washington, DC, USA

Background

Button batteries pose a human health hazard when ingested or placed in the ear, nose, or vagina. In recent years, outcomes of button battery ingestion have worsened substantially, related to the increasing use of the 20 mm diameter lithium coin cell (also called lithium button batteries) as a power source for household products. About 3500 button battery ingestions are reported to US poison centers annually, representing a fraction of cases that actually occur since it is likely that many cases are never reported. Although battery ingestion frequency has not shown a consistent upward or downward trend, from 1985 to 2010 there was a nearly sevenfold increase in severity, measured as the percentage of button battery ingestions with life-threatening, debilitating, or lethal outcomes. Lithium coin cells, at 3 V rather than the 1.5 V of traditional button cells, can cause severe complications if lodged in the esophagus for just 2 h. Furthermore, lithium coin cells are most commonly available with a 20 mm diameter, a size intermediate between a penny and a nickel and likely to lodge in the esophagus of a small child. These 20 mm lithium cells can be recognized by their imprint code, with the prefix CR (or BR) followed by 2032, 2025, or 2016, where the 20 refers to the diameter in millimeters and the final 2 digits refer to the height in tenths of a millimeter.

Uses

Button batteries are ubiquitous. They are used as a power source for hearing aids, games and toys, watches, cameras, calculators, media players, remote controls, key fobs, digital thermometers, lighted jewelry, musical or talking books, singing greeting cards, phones, monitors, medical equipment including medication pumps, garage door openers, penlights, clocks, dog collars, flameless candles, flashing or musical shoes or other fashion accessories, musical instruments, baby monitors, and a variety of other household products. Most button cells range in diameter from 5.8 to 23 mm, with four sizes accounting for 95% of ingested cells including 11.6 mm, 7.9 mm, 20 mm, and 5.8 mm (in decreasing frequency order). The chemistry of ingested button cells, in decreasing frequency order, is either manganese dioxide (alkaline), zinc-air, lithium, or silver oxide. Since the 1996 enactment of the US Mercury-Containing and Rechargeable Battery Management Act, mercuric oxide button batteries are no longer marketed; other types of button cells do not contain clinically significant amounts of mercury.

Exposure Routes and Pathways

Button cell ingestions are most commonly unintentional, with peak incidence in the very young (<4 years) and the elderly. Children younger than 6 years were involved in 62.5% of button cell ingestions and 15.9% involved adults 60 years or older. In young children, batteries were most often obtained directly from a product (61.8%), were found loose or sitting out (29.8%), or obtained directly from the battery packaging (8.2%). In contrast, adults most often ingested batteries that were loose or sitting out (80.8%) or swallowed batteries within a hearing aid (12.1%). Batteries were ingested because they were mistaken for pills in 15.5% of ingestions, an ingestion scenario predominant in patients 50 years of age or older. Batteries in the nose, ear, or vagina also cause severe tissue damage.

Toxicokinetics

Battery passage through the gut occurs in less than 72 h in 64% of patients, in less than 96 h in 74% of patients, and in less than 14 days in 96% of patients. Transit times in excess of a year have been reported without adverse effects.

Mechanism of Toxicity

Button batteries are composed of two wafer-like plates separated by an electrolyte-soaked fabric. In nonlithium button cells, the electrolyte is generally an alkaline solution, typically up to 45% sodium or potassium hydroxide. Lithium cells contain a mildly irritating organic electrolyte. The battery contents are housed in a steel can with a plastic grommet separating the positive and negative battery poles.

Injury from button batteries is due to local corrosive effects rather than systemic poisoning. The major mechanism of injury occurs when batteries are lodged in one place and generate an external electrolytic current that flows through and hydrolyzes adjacent tissue fluids or surface mucous, producing hydroxide at the battery's negative pole. The injury that follows is similar to a localized alkaline injury. Button batteries other than lithium cells may also leak an alkaline electrolyte, adding to the damage created by locally generated hydroxide. Although considered a possible minor contributing factor, pressure necrosis alone, for example, from a fully discharged battery, does not produce significant damage. With lithium cells, leakage cannot contribute to the injury as they contain no alkaline electrolyte, but due to the greater voltage and capacitance, lithium cells generate more hydroxide, more rapidly, than other button cells. Furthermore, the implication of lithium cells in the most severe cases confirms that it is local hydroxide generation rather than leakage that causes most of the damage. Although sensitivity may manifest as a rash following ingestion of nickel-plated button cells, heavy metal poisoning from leakage of battery contents is not expected, and symptomatic cases of heavy metal poisoning have not been reported.

Since hydroxide is generated at the negative battery pole, the anatomic position and orientation of an ingested cell predicts the injury that will develop, with the most severe complications (burns, perforations, fistulas) anticipated adjacent to the negative pole. The three Ns mnemonic, negative-narrow-necrotic, reminds clinicians that the negative battery pole,

 http://dx.doi.org/10.1016/B978-0-12-386454-3.00017-8

identified as the narrow side on lateral chest radiographs, causes the most necrotic damage.

Acute and Short-Term Toxicity (or Exposure)

Human

While most battery ingestions are benign, batteries lodged in the esophagus, auditory canal, or nasal cavity may have devastating consequences. A major (life-threatening or debilitating) or lethal outcome has been observed in 12.6% of children younger than 6 years who ingested 20–25 mm diameter button batteries. Esophageal batteries cause serious injury in just 2 h, providing a narrow opportunity for removal. Unfortunately, ingestions are often not witnessed (92% of fatal ingestions and 56% of major outcome cases), and subsequent clinical effects may be slow to emerge and may be nonspecific. Adding to the diagnostic challenge, about 36% of esophageal battery ingestions are initially asymptomatic.

Complications of lodged esophageal batteries include ulceration, esophageal perforation, tracheoesophageal fistulas, aortoesophageal fistulas, esophageal strictures, vocal cord paralysis from recurrent laryngeal nerve damage, mediastinitis, tracheal stenosis or tracheomalacia, spondylodiscitis, pneumo- or hemothorax, and pulmonary abscesses. Serious complications are often delayed, with tracheoesophageal fistulas becoming symptomatic up to 9 days after battery removal, aortoesophageal fistulas evident up to 27 days after battery removal, strictures delayed by weeks to months, and spondylodiscitis presenting nearly 6 weeks after battery removal. Eighteen fatalities have been reported, most involving exsanguination following fistulization into a major vessel, usually the aorta. Batteries in the ear or nose may also be associated with severe injury including perforation or destruction of the tympanic membrane, destruction of the ossicle, hearing impairment, nasal septal perforation, saddle deformity of the nose, destruction of the nasal turbinates, facial nerve paralysis, chondritis, or atrophic rhinitis.

Chronic Toxicity (or Exposure)

Human

Patients with prolonged impaction of a button battery in the esophagus, ear, or nose experience the same complications that are described above under acute toxicity. Since patients with caustic injury to the esophagus are known to experience a substantially increased risk of developing esophageal cancer, it is assumed that patients with significant battery-induced esophageal injury are at a similarly increased risk. But in the majority of button battery ingestions, gastrointestinal transit is rapid, leakage of battery components is minimal, and mucosal damage minor, thus there is little concern about development of long-term systemic effects, immunotoxicity, reproductive impairment, or cancer.

Clinical Management

The initial clinical management of battery ingestions focuses on ensuring that esophageal lodgment has not occurred. Following ingestion, patients should avoid eating or drinking until an esophageal position is excluded. The imprint code (or diameter) of the ingested battery (or a companion or replacement cell) should be determined quickly, if possible, and the National Battery Ingestion Hotline consulted at +1 202 625 3333 for assistance with battery identification and treatment. Since symptoms may be absent or delayed, an initial radiograph must be obtained immediately to locate the battery in all patients 12 years of age or younger. Older patients require immediate radiography only if a large cell was ingested (>12 mm diameter or unknown diameter), a magnet was coingested, symptoms develop, the patient has preexisting esophageal disease, or the patient is unreliable or not mentally competent.

Batteries lodged in the esophagus must be removed immediately as serious burns can occur in just 2 h. Endoscopic removal is preferred over retrieval by balloon catheter or magnetized tube as direct visualization of tissue injury guides subsequent treatment. The endoscopist should note the position of the battery, direction the negative pole faces, and areas with the deepest injury. If esophageal mucosal injury is present, patients must be observed for delayed complications and managed with serial imaging, stool guaiacs, and esophageal rest as indicated by the severity of the injury. All patients with significant esophageal burns should be hospitalized and monitored carefully for delayed complications (esophageal perforation, tracheoesophageal fistula, aortoesophageal fistula). While oral feeding is withheld from the most severely injured patients, those with less severe injuries may have their diet advanced very slowly following imaging to confirm that an esophageal perforation is not present, avoiding progression beyond soft foods for about 4 weeks until the patient is beyond the usual window for development of fistulas. In cases with significant esophageal injury anatomically adjacent to major vessels, clinicians must carefully monitor for the likely fatal complication of fistulization into a vessel, pursuing aggressive imaging, cardiovascular surgical evaluation, and extended observation for patients at risk.

Batteries located beyond the esophagus can be left to pass spontaneously unless a magnet was coingested or the patient develops symptoms. These patients are managed at home, with regular diet and activity. Battery passage can be confirmed by inspecting stools; radiography to confirm passage may be done if passage is not documented in 10–14 days. Young children (<6 years) who ingest button cells with a diameter of 15 mm or greater should undergo radiography again 4 days after ingestion (or sooner if symptoms develop) to confirm passage from the stomach, and these batteries should be removed endoscopically if they fail to progress beyond the pylorus within this time frame. Any patient with a battery in the stomach should be monitored for symptoms and endoscopic removal pursued if even minor symptoms develop, unless these are attributable to another cause. Symptomatic patients with batteries beyond the reach of the endoscope will require surgical removal for occult or visible bleeding, persistent or severe abdominal pain, vomiting, signs of an acute abdomen and/or fever, or profoundly decreased appetite.

Batteries in the nose or ear should be removed promptly to avoid development of significant damage to adjacent structures.

Ecotoxicology

Although button batteries now contain clinically insignificant amounts or no mercury, and zinc from button batteries has virtually no migration from soil to waterways where it might be toxic to fish, there remains a consumer-driven push for battery recycling. With batteries, special attention must be focused on safe recycling practices. Since used or dead batteries usually contain some residual charge, there is a potential for short circuit and heat generation when battery terminals contact each other. Transportation regulations require protection against short circuit for both new and used batteries, requiring batteries to be individually protected rather than loose in a large container. For recycled batteries, this protection is most commonly achieved by placing tape over at least one terminal. Most importantly, any battery recycling program must avoid increasing the risk of pediatric ingestion and must include strategies to keep loose or discarded button batteries out of the reach of children.

See also: Alkalies.

Further Reading

Kavanagh, K.T., Litovitz, T.L., 1986. Miniature battery foreign bodies in auditory and nasal cavities: A report of nine cases. JAMA 255, 1470–1472.

Litovitz, T., Schmitz, B.F., 1992. Ingestion of cylindrical and button batteries: An analysis of 2,382 cases. Pediatrics 89, 747–757.

Litovitz, T., Whitaker, N., Clark, L., 2010. Preventing battery ingestions: An analysis of 8648 cases. Pediatrics 125, 1178–1185.

Litovitz, T., Whitaker, N., Clark, L., White, N.C., Marsolek, M., 2010. Emerging battery ingestion hazard: Clinical implications. Pediatrics 125, 1168–1177.

Yamashita, M., Saito, S., Koyama, K., Hattori, H., Ogata, T., 1987. Esophageal electrochemical burn by button-type alkaline batteries in dogs. Vet. Hum. Toxicol. 29, 226–230.

Yoshikawa, T., Asai, S., Takekawa, Y., 1997. Experimental investigation of battery-induced esophageal burn injury in rabbits. Crit. Care Med. 25, 2039–2044.

Relevant Websites

For updated information on button battery ingestions, the reader is referred to the National Capital Poison Center's National Battery Ingestion Hotline website.

www.poison.org/battery/tips.asp – Battery ingestion and injury prevention tips.

www.poison.org/battery/stats.asp – Battery ingestion statistics.

www.poison.org/battery/guideline.asp – Battery ingestion triage and treatment guidelines.

www.poison.org/battery – General information on the button battery ingestion hazard.

www.poison.org/battery/mechanism.asp – Mechanism of battery injury.

Butyl Acrylate

RJ Parod, BASF Corporation, Wyandotte, MI, USA

- Chemical Abstracts Service Registry Number: 141-32-2
- Synonyms: 2-Propenoic acid, butyl ester; Acrylic acid, *n*-butyl ester; Butyl 2-propenoate
- Molecular Formula: $C_7H_{12}O_2$
- Chemical Structure:

$H_2C{=}CH{-}C({=}O){-}O{-}CH_2CH_2CH_2{-}CH_3$

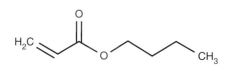

Background

Butyl acrylate is a chemical intermediate manufactured and processed almost entirely within closed systems to produce homopolymers and copolymers with little remaining monomer (<0.1 wt%). Butyl acrylate readily polymerizes under the influence of heat and light and typically contains inhibitors to prevent spontaneous polymerization during storage, which must be under air because oxygen is required for the stabilizer to function effectively. Due to its flash point of 37 °C, the storage temperature for butyl acrylate must not exceed 35 °C.

Uses

Butyl acrylate monomer is used to make acrylic resins as well as emulsion (water-based) polymers. Water-based butyl acrylate polymers are used in architectural (e.g., latex paint) and paper coatings, adhesives and sealants, and leather and textile finishes. Butyl acrylate is also a useful feedstock for chemical syntheses because it readily undergoes addition reactions with a wide variety of organic and inorganic compounds.

Environmental Fate and Behavior

Butyl acrylate is a liquid (5 hPa at ~ 20 °C) under normal environmental conditions. At equilibrium in the environment, butyl acrylate will partition primarily to air (95%) with the balance to water (5%). In air, butyl acrylate will be removed by reaction with photochemically produced hydroxyl radicals (28 h half-life) and ozone (6.5 days half-life). In water, butyl acrylate is relatively stable to hydrolysis at acidic and neutral pHs (half-life ≥ 1100 days) but will slowly volatilize to air (Henry's law constant of 21.9 $Pa\,m^{-3}\,mol^{-1}$ at 25 °C) or be biodegraded (58–90% removal in 28 days). Based on its relatively low octanol–water partition coefficient ($\log K_{ow}$ of 2.38) and rapid metabolism in biological systems, butyl acrylate does not pose a significant bioaccumulation hazard.

Exposure and Exposure Monitoring

Exposures to butyl acrylate monomer are most likely to occur in an occupational environment via inhalation and skin contact. However, the closed systems used during manufacture and transportation will limit worker exposures to those that may occur during routine process maintenance, periodic plumbing leaks, and the collection of quality control samples. Under these conditions, exposures are further limited by the use of industrial hygiene controls and personal protective equipment. The acrid odor of butyl acrylate, which can be detected at 0.035 ppm, also serves to limit exposure. Studies of monomer production workers have indicated that mean exposures to butyl acrylate are typically <1 ppm. Although peak air levels exceeding an 8 h TWA OEL of 2 ppm have been reported, these exposures typically occur during specialized activities (e.g., sampling, equipment maintenance, waste disposal) when workers are wearing personal protective equipment (PPE) that limits their exposure. The general population does not receive a significant exposure to butyl acrylate due to low concentrations of residual monomer in consumer products.

Toxicokinetics

Data in rats dosed with radiolabeled butyl acrylate indicate it is readily absorbed from the gastrointestinal tract. During the first 24 h postoral exposure, most of the butyl acrylate is metabolized by carboxylesterase to acrylic acid and *n*-butanol, which undergo further metabolism to CO_2 (75%); a smaller butyl acrylate fraction is conjugated with glutathione and excreted in the urine as mercapturic acids (10%). Only minor dose fractions appear in the feces (2%) and as volatiles (1%). Following intravenous administration, butyl acrylate is also rapidly metabolized and excreted in a similar pattern; but there is a slight shift in the metabolic profile to less CO_2 production and more glutathione conjugation suggesting a first-pass effect after oral exposure. From 24 h to 72 h postoral or post-intravenous exposure, radiolabel levels in the major organs remain relatively constant due to its apparent incorporation into tissue biomolecules.

Mechanism of Toxicity

The toxic mode of action for butyl acrylate is unknown. However, the parent compound may play a significant role since with other acrylates pretreatment of rats with a carboxylesterase inhibitor enhances the respiratory irritation and lethality associated with inhalation exposures. The enhanced toxicity could be a direct effect of the acrylate on surrounding tissues and/or a secondary effect due to its increased conjugation with glutathione that occurs under these conditions, which in turn can result in toxicity due to the depletion of local glutathione stores.

 http://dx.doi.org/10.1016/B978-0-12-386454-3.01108-8

Acute and Short-Term Toxicity

Toxicological studies in animals indicate that butyl acrylate exposures do not generally result in systemic toxicity at sublethal doses. The acute oral and dermal LD_{50} values are 3150 mg kg^{-1} (rat) and 2000–3024 mg kg^{-1} (rabbit, occlusive), respectively. The 4 h LC_{50} for butyl acrylate vapor is 19 650 ppm (rat). Butyl acrylate toxicity in both animals and humans is largely limited to irritant effects, and their sequelae, at the site of application. Butyl acrylate can produce an allergic contact dermatitis that may cross-react with other acrylic esters.

Chronic Toxicity

In a 13-week inhalation study, rats were exposed to butyl acrylate concentrations of 0, 21, 108, 211, or 546 ppm for 6 h day^{-1}, 5 days a week. At 108 ppm, histological changes in the nasal mucosa and olfactory epithelium were noted. At 211 ppm, butyl acrylate caused eye and nasal irritation, changes in clinical chemistry and organ weights, and a significant decrease in body weight; 77% mortality occurred at 546 ppm. The 13 week NOAEC was 21 ppm for local irritation and 108 ppm for systemic toxicity; these results were used by the ACGIH to derive its 8 h TWA TLV for butyl acrylate of 2 ppm. In a 2-year inhalation study, rats were exposed to butyl acrylate concentrations of 0, 15, 45, or 135 ppm for 6 h day^{-1}, 5 days a week. Histological changes in the nasal mucosa were noted at 15 ppm; ocular toxicity (epithelial stippling and cloudiness of the cornea) occurred at 135 ppm, which was the NOAEC for systemic toxicity. In a 13-week study, rats were exposed to butyl acrylate in drinking water at concentrations (1500 mg l^{-1}) approaching its solubility limit in water (1700 mg l^{-1} at 20 °C). The NOAELs corresponded to the highest doses tested, 84 mg kg^{-1} day^{-1} in males and 111 mg kg^{-1} day^{-1} in females. These NOAELs are consistent with NOAEC for systemic toxicity of 108 ppm butyl acrylate ($\sim$ 70 mg kg^{-1} day^{-1}) when the latter is expressed in the same units, assuming 100% pulmonary absorption.

Reproductive Toxicity

Although a guideline reproductive toxicity study with butyl acrylate has not been performed, several lines of evidence indicate butyl acrylate is not a reproductive toxin. First, in the 13-week inhalation study with butyl acrylate described above, adverse effects on male and female sex organs were not observed upon microscopic examination at any concentration. The only effect noted was an increase in relative testes weight, which occurred at the high concentration (546 ppm) along with significant decrements in body weight and death. Second, in a two-generation reproduction study with a chemical surrogate (methyl acrylate), rats were exposed to 0, 5, 25, and 75 ppm methyl acrylate vapor for 6 h day^{-1}, 7 days a week. Parental body weights and feed consumption were decreased at 75 ppm, and nasal lesions were seen histologically at 25 and 75 ppm. Reproduction function and pup survival were not affected at any concentration, although pup body weights at 75 ppm were decreased on postnatal days 14–28. The parental and pup effects were likely secondary to the stress associated with nasal irritation.

In developmental toxicity studies, fetal effects were noted only in the presence of maternal toxicity. When pregnant rats were exposed to butyl acrylate at vapor concentrations of 0, 25, 135, or 250 ppm on days 6–15 of gestation, the two highest doses produced decrements in maternal body weight gain, irritation to the nose and eyes, and embryo lethality as evidenced by a dose-dependent increase in postimplantation loss. No signs of teratogenicity were observed at any concentration. In another study, pregnant rats were exposed to butyl acrylate at vapor concentrations of 0, 100, 200, or 300 ppm on days 6–20 of gestation. Maternal body weight gain was significantly reduced at all experimental concentrations. Developmental toxicity was limited to reductions in fetal body weight at the two highest concentrations. Fetal malformations were not observed at any concentration. Results from both inhalation studies indicate that the NOAELs for maternal toxicity, developmental toxicity, and teratogenicity were 25, 100, and $\geq$300 ppm butyl acrylate, respectively. In a developmental gavage study, pregnant mice were exposed to butyl acrylate in cottonseed oil on gestation days 6–15 at doses of 0, 100, 1000, 1500, 2000, 2500, 3000, or 4000 mg kg^{-1} day^{-1}. No dams survived the highest dose, and occasional mortality was observed at doses $\geq$1000 mg kg^{-1} day^{-1}. Fetal body weights were significantly reduced at doses $\geq$1500 mg kg^{-1} day^{-1}, and doses $\geq$2500 mg kg^{-1} day^{-1} resulted in embryo lethality as well as external and skeletal malformations. The NOAELs for maternal toxicity, developmental toxicity, and teratogenicity were 100, 1000 , and 2000 mg kg^{-1} day^{-1}, respectively.

The absence of effects on reproductive function in animals at parentally toxic exposures combined with the occurrence of fetotoxicity only in the presence of maternal toxicity suggests that butyl acrylate does not pose a significant reproductive and developmental hazard to humans.

Genotoxicity

Data on the *in vitro* mutagenicity (*Salmonella* reverse mutation assay) as well as the induction of micronuclei and unscheduled DNA synthesis in Syrian hamster fibroblasts are negative. Two *in vivo* cytogenetic assays were conducted by exposing animals for 6 h day^{-1} for 4 days to butyl acrylate at vapor concentrations of 820 ppm (rats) and 817 ppm (hamsters). Despite clear signs of toxicity (e.g., dyspnea, bloody discharges from eyes and nose, body weight decrements, death), chromosomal damage in bone marrow cells from either species or sex was not observed.

Carcinogenicity

In a 2-year inhalation study, tumor incidences were not increased in rats exposed for 6 h day^{-1}, 5 days a week to butyl acrylate at concentrations of 0, 5, 15, or 45 ppm (months 1–3) and 0, 15, 45, or 135 ppm (months 4–24). Butyl acrylate (1% in acetone) was also not carcinogenic when applied to the skin of mice 3 days a week for a lifetime at a dose of $\sim$8 mg kg^{-1} day^{-1}. In the absence of relevant epidemiological data, IARC used the results from both bioassays as well as other studies to determine that butyl acrylate was not classifiable as to its carcinogenicity in humans (Group 3).

Clinical Management

Clinical management involves removal from exposure and treatment of symptoms.

Ecotoxicology

Butyl acrylate is acutely toxic to aquatic organisms. In a series of studies with analytically measured concentrations, butyl acrylate exhibited 96 h LC_{50} values of 5.2 mg l^{-1} in freshwater fish (*Oncorhynchus mykiss*, flow-through) and 2.1 mg l^{-1} in marine fish (*Cyprinodon variegatus*, flow-through), a 48 h EC_{50} (mobility) of 8.2 mg l^{-1} in freshwater invertebrates (*Daphnia magna*, flow-through), and an 96 h EC_{50} (cell number) of 2.6 mg l^{-1} in freshwater algae (*Pseudokirchneriella subcapitata*, static). In a 21-day semi-static study in *D. magna*, the measured NOEC values were 0.136 mg l^{-1} (reproduction) and 0.457 mg l^{-1} (growth); the LOEC values were 0.457 mg l^{-1} (reproduction) and 1.23 mg l^{-1} (growth). Butyl acrylate is not anticipated to have a significant effect on soil microflora since the 28 day EC_{50} (glucose-induced respiration rate) for a chemical surrogate (methyl acrylate) was >1000 mg kg^{-1} dry soil, the highest concentration tested.

Other Hazards

Butyl acrylate is flammable with lower and upper explosive limits of 1.1% and 7.8% by volume in air, respectively.

Exposure Standards and Guidelines

OELs recommended by the ACGIH (TLV) and Germany (MAK) are an 8 h TWA of 2 ppm butyl acrylate; NIOSH lists a recommended exposure limit (REL) of 10 ppm as a 10 h TWA. The ACGIH notes that its TLV may not necessarily protect susceptible workers from the induction of sensitization or the elicitation of an allergic reaction in previously sensitized individuals.

See also: Acrylic Acid; ACGIH® (American Conference of Governmental Industrial Hygienists); Ames Test; Carboxylesterases; Chromosome Aberrations; Developmental Toxicology; Dose–Response Relationship; Aquatic Ecotoxicology; Ecotoxicology, Aquatic Invertebrates; Environmental Exposure Assessment; Environmental Protection Agency, US; Gastrointestinal System; Genetic Toxicology; Glutathione; International Agency for Research on Cancer; LD_{50}/LC_{50} (Lethal Dosage 50/Lethal Concentration 50); Mechanisms of Toxicity; Methyl Acrylate; Mode of Action; National Institute for Occupational Safety and Health; The National Toxicology Program; Occupational Exposure Limits; Occupational Safety and Health Administration; Respiratory Tract Toxicology; Risk Assessment, Human Health; Toxicity Testing, Aquatic; Toxicity Testing, Carcinogenesis; Toxicity Testing, Developmental; Toxicity Testing, Mutagenicity; Toxicity Testing, Reproductive; Toxicity, Acute; Toxicity, Subchronic and Chronic; Pharmacokinetics.

Further Reading

Dearman, R.J., Betts, C.J., Farr, C., McLaughlin, J., Berdasco, N., Wiench, K., Kimber, I., 2007. Comparative analysis of skin sensitization potency of acrylates (methyl acrylate, ethyl acrylate, butyl acrylate, and ethylhexyl acrylate) using the local lymph node assay. Contact Dermat. 57, 242–247.

Engelhardt, G., Klimisch, H.-J., 1983. *n*-Butyl acrylate: cytogenetic investigations in the bone marrow of Chinese hamsters and rats, after 4-day inhalation. Fund. Appl. Toxicol. 3, 640–641.

Merkle, J., Klimisch, H.-J., 1983. *n*-Butyl acrylate: prenatal inhalation toxicity in the rat. Fund. Appl. Toxicol. 3, 443–447.

Murphy, S.R., Davies, J.H., 1993. Butyl acrylate health effects overview. In: Tyler, T.R., Murphy, S.R., Hunt, E.K. (Eds.), Health Effect Assessments of the Basic Acrylates. CRC Press, Boca Raton, pp. 83–100.

Reininghaus, W., Koestner, A., Klimisch, H.J., 1991. Chronic toxicity and oncogenicity of inhaled methyl acrylate and *n*-butyl acrylate in Sprague-Dawley rats. Food Chem. Toxicol. 29, 329–339.

Saillenfait, A.M., Bonnet, P., Gallissot, F., Protois, J.C., Peltier, A., et al., 1999. Relative developmental toxicities of acrylates in rats following inhalation exposure. Toxicol. Sci. 48, 240–254.

Sanders, J.M., Burka, L.T., Matthews, H.B., 1988. Metabolism and disposition of *n*-butyl acrylate in male Fischer rats. Drug Metab. Dispos. 16, 429–434.

Staples, C.A., Murphy, S.R., McLaughlin, J.E., Leung, H.-W., Cascieri, T.C., Farr, C.H., 2000. Determination of selected fate and aquatic toxicity characteristics of acrylic acid and a series of acrylic esters. Chemosphere 40, 29–38.

Wiegand, H.J., Schiffmann, D., Henschler, D., 1989. Non-genotoxicity of acrylic acid and *n*-butyl acrylate in a mammalian cell system (SHE cells). Arch. Toxicol. 63, 250–251.

Relevant Websites

http://monographs.iarc.fr/ENG/Monographs/vol71/mono71-14.pdf – IARC Monograph on *n*-Butyl Acrylate.

http://webnet.oecd.org/Hpv/UI/Search.aspx – OECD Existing Chemicals Database: Search for Butyl acrylate.

Butylated Hydroxyanisole

KN Thakore, California Department of Public Health, Richmond, CA, USA

- Name: Butylated hydroxyanisole
- Chemical Abstracts Service Registry Number: 25013-16-5
- Synonyms: (1,1-Dimethylethyl)-4-methoxyphenol; 2(3)-*t*-Butyl-4-hydroxyanisole; BHA; Anthracine 12
- Molecular Formula: $C_{11}H_{16}O_2$
- Chemical Structure:

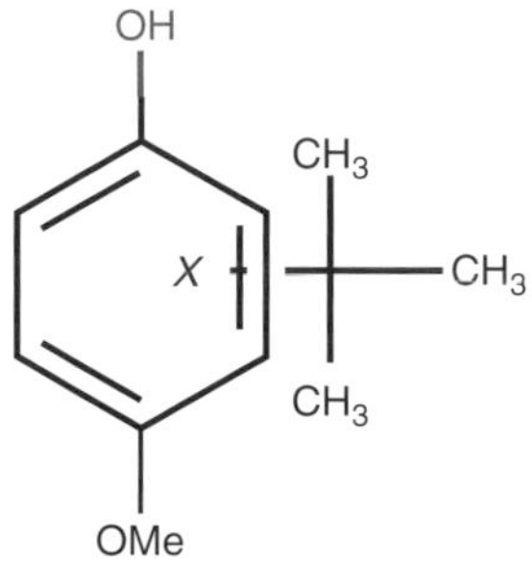

Uses

Butylated hydroxyanisole (BHA) is used as an antioxidant and food preservative; it is also used in cosmetics, pharmaceuticals, and rubber and petroleum products.

Environmental Fate and Behavior

BHA is a white or slightly yellow, waxy solid with a characteristic odor. It is insoluble in water, but soluble in fats, oils, and solvents like petroleum ether, chloroform, and alcohol. Its octanol/water partition coefficient is 3.50; vapor pressure is 2.48×10^{-3} mm Hg at 25 °C; and Henry's law constant is 1.17×10^{-6} atm-m^3 mol^{-1}.

BHA is released into the environment through waste streams. It has low soil mobility and volatilizes slowly from water. It may bioconcentrate in aquatic organisms, adsorb to sediment, and be subject to direct photolysis.

Exposure and Exposure Monitoring

Human exposure to BHA can occur by ingestion and skin application.

Toxicokinetics

BHA is absorbed rapidly via the oral route in both experimental animals and humans. It is distributed to various organs such as liver, lungs, and gastrointestinal tract. The major metabolic pathways are conjugation (phase II) reactions, whereas oxidative metabolism (*O*-demethylation) is a minor pathway. BHA is metabolized to its main metabolites 4-*O*-conjugates, *O*-sulfates, and *O*-glucuronides. The metabolites are rapidly excreted through urine with no long-term tissue storage. When human volunteers were given a single oral dose of ^{14}C-labeled BHA (0.5 mg kg^{-1} body weight), 60–70% of the radioactivity was excreted in the urine within 2 days and 80–86.5% by day 11. After administration of a single dose of 1000 mg BHA to New Zealand white rabbits, 46% of the dose was excreted in the urine as glucuronides, 9% as ethereal sulfates, and 6% as free phenols. Excretion of glucuronides was inversely dose dependent.

Mechanism of Toxicity

The metabolites of BHA can bind to cellular macromolecules, such as proteins and DNA, and cause toxicity.

Acute and Short-Term Toxicity

Animal

In rat, the oral and intraperitoneal LD_{50} values are 2000 and 881 mg kg^{-1}, respectively. In mouse, the oral LD_{50} value is 1100 mg kg^{-1}, whereas in rabbit the value is 2100 mg kg^{-1}.

Human

Exposure to BHA through inhalation, dermal or oral route, is harmful. It is irritating to the eyes, skin, mucous membranes, and upper respiratory tract. Prolonged or repeated exposure may cause allergic reactions in certain sensitive individuals. The target organs for toxicity are liver, lungs, and forestomach.

Chronic Toxicity

Animal

BHA induces benign and malignant tumors of the forestomach in rats and hamsters by administration through diet.

Human

BHA may cause cancer.

Reproductive Toxicity

It is toxic to the reproductive system and embryo in rats but not toxic to rabbits, pigs, or rhesus monkeys.

Genotoxicity

It is not mutagenic to *Salmonella typhimurium*, *Drosophila melanogaster*, or Chinese hamster cells *in vitro* and does not cause chromosomal effects.

 http://dx.doi.org/10.1016/B978-0-12-386454-3.00262-1

Clinical Management

In case of contact, eyes and skin should be flushed with water for 15–20 min. In case of inhalation exposure, the victim should be moved to fresh air and oxygen and artificial respiration should be administered, if necessary. Cardiopulmonary resuscitation should be administered, if the patient is in cardiac arrest. Life-support measures should be continued until medical assistance has arrived. An unconscious or convulsing person should not be given liquids or induced to vomit.

Other Hazards

When heated to decompose, it emits acrid and irritating fumes to cause inhalation exposure.

Exposure Standards and Guidelines

BHA and its residues are exempted from the requirement of a tolerance when used as an antioxidant in accordance with good agricultural practice. This way it can be used as inert (or occasionally active) ingredients in pesticide formulations applied to growing crops or to raw agricultural commodities after harvest. BHA is also used as a chemical preservative in food for human consumption, animal drugs, animal feeds, and related products. It is generally recognized as safe by the US Food and Drug Administration when used in accordance with good manufacturing or feeding practice. Approximately 50 countries reportedly permit the use of BHA as a food additive. Engineering controls, standard work practices, and personal protective equipment, including respirators are employed to prevent worker exposure to BHA. After use, the clothing and equipment should be placed in an impervious container for decontamination or disposal.

See also: Food Safety and Toxicology; Butter Yellow; Butylated Hydroxytoluene; Food and Drug Administration, US; Food Additives; Generally Recognized as Safe (GRAS).

Further Reading

Fujisawa, S., Atsumi, T., Kadoma, Y., Sakagami, H., 2002. Antioxidant and prooxidant action of eugenol-related compounds and their cytotoxicity. Toxicology 177 (1), 39–54.

Gangolli, S., 2007. Butylated hydroxyanisole. In: Gangolli, S. (Ed.), The Dictionary of Substances and Their Effects, second ed. vol. 1. Royal Society of Chemistry, Cambridge, UK, pp. 803–806.

International Agency for Research on Cancer (IARC), 1986. Butylated hydroxyanisole. In: IARC Monographs. Some Naturally Occurring and Synthetic Food Components, Furocoumarins and Ultraviolet Radiation vol. 40. IARC, Lyon, France, pp. 123–124.

Lenga, R.E., 1988. Butylated hydroxyanisole. In: Lenga, R.E. (Ed.), The Sigma Aldrich Library of Chemical Safety Data, second ed. vol.1. Sigma Aldrich Co, USA, p. 618.

Lewis, R.J., 2012. Butylated hydroxyanisole. In: Lewis, R.J. (Ed.), Sax's Dangerous Properties of Industrial Materials, twelth ed. vol. II. John Wiley & Sons, Inc, New York, p. 751.

Mehlman, M.A., 2012. Ethers. In: Bingham, E., Cohrssen, B. (Eds.), Patty's Toxicology, sixth ed. vol. 3. John Wiley & Sons, Inc, New York, pp. 630–632.

National Toxicology Program (NTP), 2011. Butylated hydroxyanisole. In: National Toxicology Program (Ed.), Report on Carcinogens, twelfth ed. US Department of Health and Human Services, Public Health Service, Research Triangle Park, NC, pp. 78–79.

Vandghanooni, S., Forouharmehr, A., Eskandani, M., Barzegari, A., Kafil, V., Kashanian, S., Ezzati Nazhad Dolatabadi, J., 2013. Cytotoxicity and DNA fragmentation properties of butylated hydroxyanisole. DNA Cell Biol. 32 (3), 98–103.

Williams, G.M., Iatropoulos, M.J., Whysner, J., 1999. Safety assessment of butylated hydroxyanisole and butylated hydroxytoluene as antioxidant food additives. Food Chem. Toxicol. 37 (9–10), 1027–1038.

Relevant Websites

http://chem.sis.nlm.nih.gov/chemidplus/Butylated hydroxyanisole – ChemIDplus Advanced.

http://toxnet.nlm.nih.gov/Butylated hydroxyanisole – HSDB database.

Butylated Hydroxytoluene

KN Thakore, California Department of Public Health, Richmond, CA, USA

- Name: Butylated hydroxytoluene
- Chemical Abstracts Service Registry Number: 128-37-0
- Synonyms: 2,6-Bis(1,1-dimethylethyl)-4-methylphenol; 2,6-Di-*t*-butyl-*p*-cresol; BHT; Anthracine 8
- Molecular Formula: $C_{15}H_{24}O$
- Chemical Structure:

H_3C CH_3 OH H_3C CH_3 H_3C CH_3 CH_3

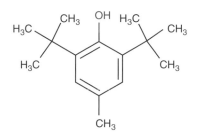

Uses

Butylated hydroxytoluene (BHT) is used as an antioxidant for food, animal feed; it is used in petroleum products, synthetic rubbers, plastics, animal and vegetable oils, and soaps. It is also used as an antiskinning agent in paints and inks.

Environmental Fate and Behavior

BHT is a white crystalline solid. It is insoluble in water and alkalies; but soluble in most common organic solvents such as alcohol and ether. Its melting point is 70 °C, boiling point is 265 °C, flash point is 127 °C, and specific gravity is 1.048 at 20 °C.

Exposure and Exposure Monitoring

Exposure through inhalation dermal and oral routes, is very common.

Toxicokinetics

In male and female BALB/c mice, a single intragastric dose was widely distributed to various tissues within 30 min, primarily to the small intestine, stomach, liver, kidneys, and lungs. Oxidative metabolism is the major route for degradation, which involves oxidation of the ring methyl group, predominantly in rat, rabbit, and monkey, and oxidation of the *t*-butyl groups in humans. The major metabolites are 3,5-di-*t*-butyl-4-hydroxybenzoic acid, both free and as a glucuronide, and *S*-(3,5-di-*t*-butyl-4-hydroxybenzyl)-*N*-acetylcysteine. More over, BHT-quinone methide (2,6-di-*t*-butyl-4-methylene-2,5-cyclohexadienone), a reactive metabolite, has been identified in the liver and bile of rats. Metabolites produced in mice are similar to those produced in rats, except that the major biotransformation in mice was by oxidation of *t*-methyl group. BHT is cleared less rapidly from most species due to enterohepatic circulation. The major metabolites of BHT in rat urine are 3,5-di-*t*-butyl-4-hydroxybenzoic acid (BHT acid; III), both free (90% of the dose) and as a glucuronide (15%), and *S*-(3,5-di-*t*-butyl-4-hydroxybenzyl)-*N*-acetylcysteine. The ester glucuronide and mercapturic acid were major metabolites in rat bile, while free BHT acid was the main component in the feces. In addition, 1,2-bis(3,5-di-*t*-butyl-4-hydroxyphenyl) ethane has been identified in rat bile. In BALB/c mice, 75% of a single oral dose was excreted in the urine during the first 24 h; this was followed by a slower phase during which an additional 10% was excreted over the next 4 days. The total amount found in the feces was less than 1%. Female rats have greater urinary excretion of BHT than male rats, whereas male BALB/c mice excreted BHT more rapidly than females.

Mechanism of Toxicity

The metabolites of BHT can bind to cellular macromolecules, such as proteins and DNA, and cause toxicity.

Acute and Short-Term Toxicity

Animal

Exposure through both intraperitoneal and intravenous routes in animals is poisonous. However, it is moderately toxic by ingestion. The oral LD_{50} values in rat and mouse are 890 and 1040 mg kg^{-1}, respectively. In mouse, the intraperitoneal and subcutaneous LD_{50} values are 138 and 650 mg kg^{-1}, respectively. In the guinea pig, the oral LD_{50} value is 10 700 mg kg^{-1}.

Human

Exposure to BHT through inhalation, dermal, and oral routes is harmful. It causes irritation of the eyes, skin, mucous membranes, and upper respiratory tract. Prolonged or repeated contact can damage the eyes and cause nausea, dizziness, and headache.

Chronic Toxicity

Animal

BHT is known to produce reproductive effects in experimental animals. There is limited evidence of carcinogenicity of BHT. However, it induces liver tumors in long-term experiments.

Human

It does not represent a relevant mutagenic/genotoxic risk to humans.

 http://dx.doi.org/10.1016/B978-0-12-386454-3.00263-3

Genotoxicity

In vitro studies on bacterial, yeast, and various mammalian cell lines, and primary hepatocytes demonstrate the absence of interactions with or damage to DNA.

Carcinogenicity

Carcinogenicity of BHT to humans has not been evaluated. BHT is a possible carcinogen with the target organ being the lungs.

Clinical Management

In case of contact, eyes and skin should be flushed with water for 15–20 min. In case of inhalation exposure, the victim should be moved to fresh air and oxygen and artificial respiration should be administered, if necessary. Cardiopulmonary resuscitation should be administered if the patient is in cardiac arrest. Life-support measures should be continued until medical assistance has arrived. An unconscious or convulsing person should not be given liquids or induced to vomit.

Other Hazards

BHT is combustible when exposed to heat or flame and can emit acrid smoke and fumes. It can react with oxidizing materials.

Exposure Standards and Guidelines

BHT and its residues used as inert antioxidant ingredients in pesticide formulation for application to animals are exempted from the requirement of a tolerance when used in accordance with good agricultural practice. BHT used as a chemical preservative in food for human consumption, in animal drugs, feeds, and related products is Generally Recognized as Safe by the US Food and Drug Administration when used in accordance with good manufacturing or feeding practice. Approximately 40 countries reportedly permit the use of BHT as a direct or indirect food additive. Engineering controls, standard work practices, and personal protective equipment, including respirators, are employed to prevent worker exposure to BHT. After use, the clothing and equipment should be placed in an impervious container for decontamination or disposal. The American Conference of Governmental Industrial Hygienists recommends that occupational exposure to airborne BHT not exceed 2 mg m^{-3} (threshold limit value) as an 8 h time-weighted average.

See also: Food Safety and Toxicology; Butter Yellow; Butylated Hydroxyanisole; Food and Drug Administration, US; Food Additives; Generally Recognized as Safe (GRAS).

Further Reading

American Conference of Governmental Industrial Hygienists (ACGIH), 2011. Butylated hydroxytoluene. In: ACGIH (Ed.), ACGIH Threshold Limit Values and Biological Exposure Indices, seventh ed. Cincinnati, OH, pp. 1–4.

Gangolli, S., 2007. Butylated hydroxytoluene. In: Gangolli, S. (Ed.), The Dictionary of Substances and Their Effects, second ed. vol. 1. Royal Society of Chemistry, Cambridge, UK, pp. 806–809.

International Agency for Research on Cancer (IARC), 1986. Butylated hydroxytoluene In: IARC Monographs. Some Naturally Occurring and Synthetic Food Components, Furocoumarins and Ultraviolet Radiation, vol. 40. IARC, Lyon, France, pp. 161–163.

Lenga, R.E., 1988. Butylated hydroxytoluene. In: Lenga, R.E. (Ed.), The Sigma Aldrich Library of Chemical Safety Data, second ed. vol. 1. Sigma Aldrich Co, U.S.A., p. 1101.

Lewis, R.J., 2012. Butylated hydroxytoluene. In: Lewis, R.J. (Ed.), Sax's Dangerous Properties of Industrial Materials, twelfth ed. vol. II. John Wiley & Sons, Inc, New York, pp. 536–537.

Stierum, R., Heijne, W., Kienhuis, A., van Ommen, B., Groten, J., 2005. Toxicogenomics concepts and applications to study hepatic effects of food additives and chemicals. Toxicol. Appl. Pharmacol. 207 (Suppl. 2), 179–188.

Williams, G.M., Iatropoulos, M.J., Whysner, J., 1999. Safety assessment of butylated hydroxyanisole and butylated hydroxytoluene as antioxidant food additives. Food Chem. Toxicol. 37 (9–10), 1027–1038.

Relevant Websites

http://chem.sis.nlm.nih.gov/chemidplus/Butylated hydroxytoluene – ChemIDplus Advanced.

http://toxnet.nlm.nih.gov/Butylated hydroxytoluene – HSDB database.

http://www.cdc.gov/niosh/Butylated hydroxytoluene – NIOSH Pocket Guide.

http://scorecard.goodguide.com/Butylated hydroxytoluene – Pollution information site.

Butyl Ether

H Robles, Irvine, CA, USA

- Chemical Abstracts Service Registry Number: 142-96-1
- Synonyms: Dibutyl ether, 1-Butoxybutane, Dibutyl oxide, Di-*n*-butyl ether, *n*-Dibutyl ether
- Chemical Formula: $C_8H_{18}O$
- Chemical Structure:

H_3C–CH_2–CH_2–CH_2–O–CH_2–CH_2–CH_2–CH_3

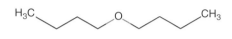

Uses

Butyl ether is used mainly as a solvent for organic materials such as resins, oils, hydrocarbons, esters, gums, and alkaloids. It is also used as an extracting agent in metal separation, as a reacting medium in organic synthesis processes, and as a solvent in teaching, research and analytical laboratories.

Environmental Fate and Behavior

Production of butyl ether and its use as an extracting agent and a solvent may result in its release to the environment through various waste streams. If released to air, a vapor pressure of 6.0 mmHg at 25 °C indicates that butyl ether will exist solely as a vapor in the ambient atmosphere. Vapor-phase butyl ether reacts in the atmosphere with hydroxyl radicals; the half-life for this reaction in air has been estimated to be 13 h. Direct photolysis is not expected to be an important removal process since aliphatic ethers do not absorb light in the environmental spectrum. If released to soil, butyl ether is expected to have high mobility based on its estimated adsorption coefficient (K_{oc}) of 51. Volatilization from moist soil surfaces may be an important fate process based on its reported Henry's law constant of 6.0×10^{-3} atm m^3 mol^{-1}. Butyl ether is expected to volatilize from dry soil surfaces based on its reported vapor pressure. If released into water, butyl ether is not expected to adsorb to suspended solids and sediment in water based on its K_{oc}. Aqueous screening studies indicate biodegradation may be an important fate process in both soil and water; for example, butyl ether reached 3–4% of its theoretical biological oxygen demand (BOD) over 4 weeks using an activated sludge seed. Volatilization from water surfaces is expected to occur based on this compound's estimated Henry's law constant. Estimated volatilization half-lives for a model river and model lake have been reported to be 3.5 h and 4.6 days, respectively. Bioconcentration factors (BCFs) ranging from 30 to 114 in carp suggest that bioconcentration in aquatic organisms is moderate to high. Butyl ether is not expected to undergo hydrolysis in the environment due to the lack of hydrolyzable functional groups.

Exposure and Exposure Monitoring

Exposure to butyl ether can occur through inhalation of vapor or mist, dermal contact, or oral ingestion of liquid butyl ether. Oral ingestion of butyl ether has been practiced to produce an alcohol-like euphoria. Occupational exposure to butyl ether may occur through inhalation and dermal contact with this compound at workplaces where butyl ether is produced or used. The general population may be exposed to butyl ether through the use of consumer products, such as latex paints, containing this compound.

Toxicokinetics

Butyl ether is rapidly adsorbed and eliminated from the body. Butyl ether can cause irritation to the skin, mucus membranes, eyes, and respiratory and gastrointestinal tracts. Systematically, butyl ether causes central nervous system depression and transient liver changes.

Mechanism of Toxicity

Butyl ether has the ability to dissolve lipids. As a result, it causes irritation and pain on contact with the eyes and nasal mucosa. It also causes dermal irritation and dermatitis on contact with the skin. Damage caused by butyl ether appears to be scattered loss of epithelial cells due to solution of phospholipid cell membranes. At the central nervous system (CNS) level, butyl ether, like other volatile organic solvents, depresses the CNS by dissolving in the lipid membrane of the cells and disrupting the lipid matrix. These effects are known as membrane fluidization. At the molecular level, membrane fluidization disrupts solute gradient homeostasis, which is essential for cell function.

Acute and Short-Term

Signs and symptoms of excessive exposure to dibutyl ether resemble those of ethanol intoxication except that symptoms are seen shortly after exposure and the effects are short lived. Typical symptoms include dizziness, giddiness, headache, euphoria, and CNS depression. Chronic, repeated dermal exposure may cause dermal irritation, defatting of skin, and dermatitis. Excessive consumption of dibutyl ether as an intoxicating agent has been reported to produce ether jags, respiratory depression, and death.

Butyl ether is moderately toxic by the oral route. The oral lethal dose 50% (LD_{50}) in rats has been reported to range from 3200 to 7400 mg kg^{-1}. The inhalation lethal concentration 50% (LC_{50}) also in rats has been found to be 4000 ppm in air for 4 h. The skin LD_{50} in rabbits is reported to be about 10,000 mg kg^{-1}.

 http://dx.doi.org/10.1016/B978-0-12-386454-3.00009-9

Chronic Toxicity

In humans, chronic, repeated dermal exposure may cause dermal irritation, defatting of skin, and dermatitis. Excessive consumption of butyl ether as an intoxicating agent has been reported to produce ether jags, respiratory depression, and death.

Reproductive Toxicity

Butyl ether is known to cross the placental barrier. Thus, butyl ether concentrations in fetal blood is likely to be the same as that seen in maternal blood.

Clinical Management

Given the CNS and respiratory depression properties of butyl ether, treatment is directed at maintaining respiration and treating irritation at the site of exposure. Patients should be monitored for respiratory distress and apnea, hyperglycemia, as well as hepatic and renal dysfunction.

Ecotoxicology

The LC_{50} in sheephead minnows (*Cyprinodon variegatus*) aged 14–28 days is above 430 ppm after exposure for 24, 48, 72, and 96 h.

The LC_{50} in fathead minnows (*Pimephales promelas*) was measured to be 32.5 $mg\,l^{-1}$ after exposure for 96 h in a flow-through bioassay.

The LC_{50} in 1-day old water fleas (*Daphnia magna*) was measured to be 32.0 $mg\,l^{-1}$ after exposure for 24 h and 26.0 $mg\,l^{-1}$ for exposure for 48 h.

Other Hazards

Butyl ether is highly flammable and is easily ignited by heat, sparks, or flames. Vapors may form explosive mixtures with air.

See also: Ethanol.

Further Reading

Sax, N.I., Lewis, R.J. (Eds.), 1989. Dangerous Properties of Industrial Materials, seventh ed. Van Nostrand Reinhold, New York.

Relevant Website

http://toxnet.nlm.nih.gov – National Library of Medicine (NLM) Hazardous Substances Database (HSDB): search for butyl ether

Butyl Nitrite

KN Thakore, California Department of Public Health, Richmond, CA, USA

- Name: Butyl nitrite
- Chemical Abstracts Service Registry Number: 544-16-1
- Synonyms: *N*-butyl nitrite; NCI-C56553; Nitrous acid; *n*-Butyl ester
- Molecular Formula: $C_4H_9NO_2$
- Chemical Structure:

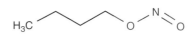

Butyl nitrite (CAS RN 544-16-1)

Uses

Butyl nitrite is used in the manufacture of rare earth azides. It is used as a recreational drug due its vasodilator property.

Environmental Fate and Behavior

It is an extremely flammable, insoluble liquid with vapor pressure of 62 mm Hg and boiling point of 75 °C.

Exposure and Exposure Monitoring

Exposure to butyl nitrite through both oral and intraperitoneal routes is poisonous. However, it is mildly toxic by inhalation route. Toxic effects of this compound are listed in **Table 1**.

Toxicokinetics

Exposure of rats to butyl nitrite in air for 5 min period causes an uptake of about 44%. After absorption, it is transformed and distributed rapidly to various parts of the body, including muscles and circulatory system. There are several likely metabolites of butyl nitrite *in vivo* namely butyl alcohol, nitrite ion, nitrate ion, nitrosothiols, and possibly other nitroso compounds. The metabolites can bind to hemoglobin, glutathione, and other plasma proteins. Metabolites such as nitrite ions can be eliminated in exhaled air.

Mechanism of Toxicity

Butyl nitrite causes rapid *S*-nitrosyl glutathione formation and simultaneously reduces protein thiols, followed by marked adenosine triphosphate depletion. It also causes lipid peroxidation. It produces methemoglobinemia in which oxidized hemoglobin has no oxygen carrying capacity. Also, in the clinical state of methemoglobinemia, the unaltered hemoglobin shows an increased affinity for oxygen that results in symptoms of tissue hypoxia. Cyanosis occurs when methemoglobin levels are greater than 10%. Levels above 70% are potentially lethal.

Acute and Short-Term Toxicity

Animal

In experimental mice, butyl nitrite is metabolized in liver to butyl alcohol that produces hepatotoxicity. The oral LD_{50} values in rat and mouse are 83 and 171 mg kg^{-1}, respectively. The intraperitoneal LD_{50} value in mouse is 158 mg kg^{-1}. The LC_{50} values in rat and mouse are 420 ppm per 4 h and 567 ppm per hour, respectively.

Human

Butyl nitrite is harmful if swallowed, inhaled, or absorbed through skin. It causes irritation of eyes, skin, mucous membranes, and the upper respiratory tract. Overexposure by ingestion can cause methemoglobinemia, lowering of blood

Table 1 Toxic effects of *n*-butyl nitrite in humans and experimental animals

Organism	*Test type*	*Route*	*Reported dose (normalized dose)*	*Effect*
Man	TDLo	Oral	153 mg kg^{-1} (153 mg kg^{-1})	Blood: methemoglobinemia–carboxyhemoglobin
Mouse	LC_{50}	Inhalation	567 ppm per h (567 ppm)	Lungs, thorax, or respiration: cyanosis Behavioral: changes in motor activity (specific assay) Kidney, ureter, and bladder: urine volume increased
Mouse	LD_{50}	Intraperitoneal	158 mg kg^{-1} (158 mg kg^{-1})	Liver: other changes
Mouse	LD_{50}	Oral	171 mg kg^{-1} (171 mg kg^{-1})	Blood: methemoglobinemia–carboxyhemoglobin Liver: other changes
Rat	LC_{50}	Inhalation	420ppm per 4 h (420ppm)	Behavioral: excitement, altered sleep time (including change in righting reflex) Lungs, thorax, or respiration: cyanosis
Rat	LD_{50}	Oral	83 mg kg^{-1} (83 mg kg^{-1})	Behavioral: rigidity Behavioral: ataxia Lungs, thorax, or respiration: dyspnea

Source: ChemIDPlus: http://chem.sis.nlm.nih.gov/chemidplus/jsp/common/Toxicity.jsp.

 http://dx.doi.org/10.1016/B978-0-12-386454-3.00261-X

pressure by vasodilatation, headache, pulse throbbing, and weakness. It causes behavioral changes such as altered sleep time, excitement, motor activity, ataxia, and rigidity. It can also cause dyspnea, cyanosis, and changes in liver and kidneys. It is immunosuppressive for human lymphocytes *in vitro*.

Chronic Toxicity

Butyl nitrite has not been tested for cancer and reproductive effects as well as for other long-term effects. It is metabolized *in vivo* to *N*-nitroso compounds that can initiate tumor development.

Genotoxicity

Solutions of isobutyl nitrite have been shown to be more mutagenic than sodium nitrite in Ames assay.

Clinical Management

Methylene blue (antidote), alone or in combination with oxygen is indicated as a treatment in nitrite induced methemoglobinemia. Poison control centers must be contacted immediately for advice. In case of contact, affected eyes and skin should be flushed with water for 15–20 min. If inhaled, the affected person should be moved to fresh air, and oxygen and artificial respiration should be administered, if necessary. If the patient is in cardiac arrest, cardiopulmonary resuscitation should be administered. Life-support measures should be continued until medical assistance has arrived. In the case of an unconscious or convulsing person, liquids should not be administered and vomiting should not be induced.

Other Hazards

Butyl nitrite is an extremely flammable liquid. When heated to decomposition, it emits toxic fumes of nitrogen oxides.

Exposure Standards and Guidelines

Engineering controls, standard work practices, and personal protective equipment, including respirators are employed to prevent worker exposure to butyl nitrite. After use, the clothing and equipment should be placed in an impervious container for decontamination or disposal.

See also: Nitrite Inhalants; Food and Drug Administration, US; Nitrites; Nitrosamines; Drugs of Abuse.

Further Reading

Fechter, L.D., Richard, C.L., Mungekar, M., Gomez, J., Strathern, D., 1989. Disruption of auditory function by acute administration of a "room odorizer" containing butyl nitrite in rats. Fundam. Appl. Toxicol. 12 (1), 56–61.

Ford, J.B., Sutter, M.E., Owen, K.P., Albertson, T.E., 2013. Volatile substance misuse: an updated review of toxicity and treatment. Clin. Rev. Allergy Immunol. May 7, 2013. (Epub ahead of print.)

Gunja, N., 2012. Teenage toxins: recreational poisoning in the adolescent. J. Paediatr. Child Health 48 (7), 560–566.

Lenga, R.E., 1988. Butyl nitrite. In: Lenga, R.E. (Ed.), The Sigma Aldrich Library of Chemical Safety Data, second ed., vol. 1. Sigma Aldrich Co, USA, p. 642.

Lewis, R.J., 2012. Butyl nitrite. In: Lewis, R.J. (Ed.), Sax's Dangerous Properties of Industrial Materials, twelth ed., vol. 2. John Wiley & Sons, Inc, New York, p. 780.

Maickel, R.P., 1988. The fate and toxicity of butyl nitrites. NIDA Res. Monogr. 83, 15–27.

Mirvish, S.S., Williamson, J., Babcook, D., Chen, S.C., 1993. Mutagenicity of iso-butyl nitrite vapor in the Ames test and some relevant chemical properties, including the reaction of iso-butyl nitrite with phosphate. Environ. Mol. Mutagen. 21 (3), 247–252.

National Institute on Drug Abuse (NIDA), 1988. Health hazards of nitrite inhalantsHaverkos, H.W., Dougherty, J.A. (Eds.), NIDA Research Monograph Series: Health Hazards of Nitrite Inhalants, vol. 83. U.S. Department of Health and Human Services, National Institute of Health, Bethesda, MD, pp. 1–112.

Ovesen, J.L., 2012. Aliphatic nitro, nitrate, and nitrite compounds. In: Bingham, E., Cohrssen, B. (Eds.), Patty's Toxicology, sixth ed., vol. 2. John Wiley & Sons, Inc, New York, p. 394.

Relevant Websites

http://scorecard.goodguide.com/ – Butyl Nitrite: Pollution information site.
http://chem.sis.nlm.nih.gov/chemidplus/ – *n*-Butyl Nitrite-ChemIDplus Advanced.
http://www.drugabuse.gov/ – Nitrite Inhalants: 'National Institute on Drug Abuse.

Butylamines

JM McKee, Arcadis-US, Brighton, MI, USA

Background

Butylamines are organic amines of butane. There are four isomeric forms of butylamine. All forms of butylamine appear as a flammable colorless liquid with a fishy, ammonia-like odor. The isomers are as follows:

- Isobutylamine (Chemical Abstract Service Registry Number (CASRN) 78-81-9)
  Synonyms: Monoisobutylamine; Valamine; 1-Amino-2-methylpropane; 2-Methylpropylamine; 3-Methyl-2-propylamine; IBA; 2-Methyl-1-aminopropane; 2-Methyl-1-propanamine; UN 1214; i-Butylamine; 2-Methylpropanamine (**Figure 1**)

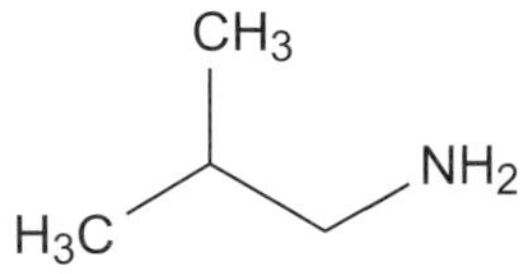

Figure 1 Isobutylamine.

- *n*-Butylamine (CASRN 109-73-9)
  Synonyms: Butylamine; Mono-*n*-butylamine; Monobutylamine; Norvalamine; 1-Aminobutane; 1-Butylamine; Butylamine, *n*; *N*-Butylamin; 1-Amino-butaan; 1-Aminobutan; 1-Butanaminen-butilamina; *n*-Butilamina; Monobutilamina; UN 1125; Aminobutane; Norralamine; Tutane; Butanamine (**Figure 2**)

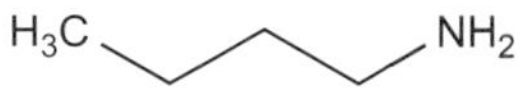

Figure 2 *n*-Butylamine.

- *sec*-Butylamine (CASRN 135-98-8)
  Synonyms: Butafume; Propylamine, 1-Methyl-; Tutane; 1-Methylpropanamine; 1-Methylpropylamine; 2-Aminobutane; 2-AB; 2-Butylamine; *sec*-Butanamine; Deccotane; Frucote; 2-Aminobutane base; (*Rs*)-2-aminobutane; (*Rs*)-*sec*-butylamine; Secondary butylamine; CSC 2-Aminobutane (**Figure 3**)

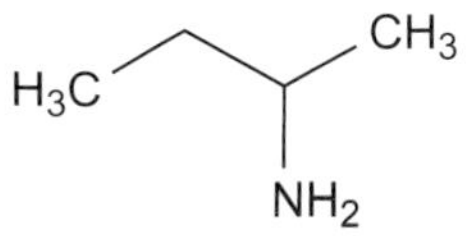

Figure 3 *sec*-Butylamine.

- *tert*-Butylamine (CASRN 75-64-9)
  Synonyms: Trimethylaminomethane; 1,1-Dimethylethylamine; 2-Amino-2-methylpropane; 2-Aminoisobutane; 2-Methyl-2-aminopropane; 2-Methyl-2-propylamine; 2-Methyl-2-propanamine; *t*-Butylamine; Butylamine, *tert*; Butylamine, tertiary (**Figure 4**)

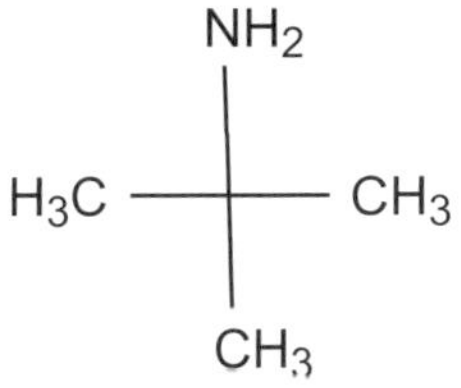

Figure 4 *tert*-Butylamine.

Uses

Butylamines are used as intermediates in the manufacture of textiles, plasticizers, rubber chemicals, dyes, tanning agents, pharmaceuticals, emulsifying agents, agrochemicals, antioxidants, UV absorbers, and lubricating oil additives. Butylamines are used as additives for seafood, alcoholic beverages, ice cream, chocolate, candy, and baked goods. They also occur naturally in some plants, foods, tobacco, and animal waste. *sec*-Butylamine was formerly used as a fungicide in the United States, England, and Australia.

Environmental Fate and Behavior

Relevant Physicochemical Properties

- Isobutylamine
  Molecular weight: 73.14
  Log octanol/water partition coefficient: 0.73
  Solubility in water: 1×10^{6} mg l^{-1} (25 °C)
  Henry's law constant: 1.4×10^{-5} atm m^{3} mol^{-1} (25 °C)
- *n*-Butylamine
  Molecular weight: 73.14
  Log octanol/water partition coefficient: 0.97
  Solubility in water: 1×10^{6} mg l^{-1} (25 °C)
  Henry's law constant: 1.74×10^{-5} atm m^{3} mol^{-1} (25 °C)
- *sec*-Butylamine
  Molecular weight: 73.14
  Log octanol/water partition coefficient: 0.74
  Solubility in water: 1.12×10^{5} mg l^{-1} (25 °C)
  Henry's law constant: 1.5×10^{-4} atm m^{3} mol^{-1} (25 °C)
- *tert*-Butylamine
  Molecular weight: 73.14.
  Log octanol/water partition coefficient: 0.40.
  Solubility in water: 1×10^{6} mg l^{-1} (25 °C)
  Henry's law constant: 3.6×10^{-5} atm m^{3} mol^{-1} (25 °C)

 http://dx.doi.org/10.1016/B978-0-12-386454-3.00474-7

Partition Behavior in Water, Sediment, and Soil

Butylamines exist primarily in the cation form in the environment, resulting in reduced potential for volatilization from water surfaces and the surface of moist soil. Butylamines are not expected to adsorb significantly to suspended solids and sediment in water. When released into the soil, butylamines are expected to be highly mobile. Some volatilization from dry soil is expected.

Environmental Persistence

In water, butylamines may biodegrade to a moderate extent. Hydrolysis is not expected to be an important environmental fate process since butylamines lack functional groups that hydrolyze under environmental conditions. The half-life in water is between 1 and 10 days.

Studies indicate that butylamines in soil will readily biodegrade, both through aerobic and anaerobic processes.

When released into the air, butylamines will exist solely as a vapor and are expected to be readily degraded by reaction with photochemically produced hydroxyl radicals. The half-life is expected to approximately 9–33 h. Butylamines are not susceptible to direct photolysis by sunlight.

Long-Range Transport

Long-range transport in the atmosphere is not expected due to abiotic degradation. Butylamines may be transported in groundwater.

Bioaccumulation and Biomagnification

Butylamines have an estimated bioconcentration factor of 2.59–4.14 in the embryo of *Danio rerio* (zebra fish), suggesting that the potential for bioconcentration in aquatic organisms is relatively low.

Exposure and Exposure Monitoring

Routes and Pathways

The use of butylamine as a chemical intermediate may result in occupational exposure as well as exposure to residues released in waste streams. Most exposure in the general population is from diet and tobacco use.

Butylamines can be absorbed through oral, dermal, and inhalation routes, as well as causing damage at the point of contact (i.e., skin, eyes, lungs, and gastrointestinal tract).

Human Exposure

Occupational exposure to butylamines may occur through inhalation and dermal contact where these chemicals are produced or used. The US National Institute for Occupational Safety and Health estimates that, in the United States, approximately 413 workers are potentially exposed to *n*-butylamine and 4354 to *tert*-butylamine.

Isobutylamine is present in Italian wines (0.06–0.23 ppm), cheeses (0.2 ppm), freeze-dried coffee (1 ppm), cocoa (6 ppm), cod (0.3 ppm), as well as tobacco products, German wine, American beef, Valencia oranges, and California lemons. *n*-Butylamine occurs naturally in kale (7 ppm), pickles, cucumbers in aromatic vinegar (0.6 ppm), pickled cucumbers (5.3 ppm), Tilsiter cheese (3.7 ppm), brown bread (1.1 ppm), mulberry leaves, fish and seafood, and beef. Residues of *sec*-butylamine have been detected in citrus fruits (0.88–7.65 ppm), pears (11.2–11.6 ppm), and apples (2.75–3.61 ppm) when used as a postharvest fungicide.

Isobutylamine and *n*-butylamine have been detected in amniotic fluid and in human breast milk during the first several weeks after parturition.

Environmental Exposure

Isobutylamine and *sec*-butylamine have been detected in soil. *n*-Butylamine was detected at one location in the River Elbe (1.5 ppb). A shallow sediment core sample collected from Chesapeake Bay, Maryland, had *sec*-butylamine at a concentration of 0.05 μM. Isobutylamine has been detected in various species of marine algae. *n*-Butylamine and *sec*-butylamine have been found to be volatile components of cattle feed lots, probably from the decomposition of manure.

Toxicokinetics

Butylamines are well absorbed from the gut and respiratory tract and are readily absorbed into the blood. Residues have been found in muscle, liver, fat, and kidney in a cow feeding study. Butylamines are expected to be deaminated by monoamine oxidase and diamine oxidase (histaminase) and excreted in the urine. *n*-Butylamine was readily metabolized to acetoacetic acid in the guinea pig.

Mechanism of Toxicity

Butylamines are strongly alkali and they are potent skin, eye, and mucous membrane irritants. Contact may cause minor irritation to severe tissue damage. Butylamines may be neutralized in the stomach by hydrochloride.

Cellular changes caused by butylamines may include hyperplasia, squamous metaplasia, and necrosis. Butylamines also retard the internalization of transferrin bound to transferrin receptors on the plasma membrane of reticulocytes, retard the externalization of internalized transferrin, and block the transport into the cytosol of iron released from transferrin. Amines may cause a selective blockade of lysosomal degradation of protein.

It is believed that the fungistatic action of *sec*-butylamine may be due to effects on the pyruvate dehydrogenase system.

Acute and Short-Term Toxicity

Animal

Signs of toxicity observed after single oral doses of butylamines include sedation, ataxia, nasal discharge, gasping, labored breathing, increased reflex excitability, increased pulse rate, dyspnea, convulsions, cyanosis, and salivation followed by convulsions and death due to pulmonary edema. Oral LD_{50}s in rats were reported to be 224–228 mg kg^{-1} for isobutylamine, 152–500 mg kg^{-1} for *n*-butylamine, 147–157 mg kg^{-1} for *sec*-butylamine, and 78–82 mg kg^{-1} for *tert*-butylamine. The inhalation LC_{50} for *n*-butylamine was reported at 3000–5000 ppm in rats and 800 mg cu m^{-1} for 2 h in mice; death was due to pulmonary edema.

Severe skin irritation with necrosis has been reported after dermal contact in rabbits and guinea pigs. The *n*-butylamine LD_{50} by dermal exposure was reported to be 850 mg kg^{-1} in rabbits and 370 mg kg^{-1} in guinea pigs. The dermal LD_{50} for *sec*-butylamine was reported to be 2500 mg kg^{-1} in rabbits. Butylamines are severely damaging to the eyes when directly applied; however, the vapor is only mildly irritating to the eyes.

Intravenous and intragastric administration of *sec*-butylamine carbonate in dogs resulted in elevated blood pressure, heart rate, and respiration. The primary acute response was similar to other amines, producing a standard sympathomimetic response.

Human

Butylamines are primary irritants to the skin, eyes, and mucous membranes, and direct contact with liquid or vapor may cause severe irritation, blistering, burns, erythema, and tissue necrosis. Contact with the eye may result in loss of vision.

Vapors may be irritating to the respiratory tract at concentrations greater than 5 ppm. Concentrations of 5–10 ppm have resulted in headache and facial flushing. Concentrations greater than 25 ppm are difficult to tolerate for even short periods of time, and concentrations greater than 300 ppm may immediately threaten life. Symptoms of exposure include lacrimation, runny nose, scratchy throat, facial flushing, increased pulse and respiratory rate, and shortness of breath. Exposure to high concentrations can result in cyanosis, hyperactive reflexes, pulmonary edema, convulsions, and coma.

Ingestion of butylamines has induced within 3 h after exposure to vapors, and desquamation of the facial skin with burning and itching may follow in 3 days. Exposure to vapors may also cause nausea and salivation at 40 mg kg^{-1} in humans, and sufficiently high concentrations may cause irritation to the mouth, throat, and gastrointestinal tract with vomiting and possibly death. Isobutylamine has been found to be a cardiac depressant and convulsant in humans.

Skin absorption may cause damage at the site of contact, as well as nausea, vomiting, and shock.

Chronic Toxicity

Animal

No effects were reported from *sec*-butylamine exposure in a 2-year feeding study in rats and dogs exposed to 2500 ppm in the diet. Inhaled *n*-butylamine produced concentration-dependent nasal epithelial hyperplasia and squamous metaplasia, inflammation, and necrosis in rats, with a no observable adverse effects level (NOAEL) of less than 17 ppm. Chronic exposure to skin and mucous membranes at sufficiently high levels may cause inflammation, hyperplasia, metaplasia, and necrosis due to chronic inflammation. Other effects noted in the literature include inhibition of iron uptake in rabbit reticulocytes (*n*-butylamine) and effects on protein degradation and synthesis in isolated rat hepatocytes.

Human

Repeated exposure to levels greater than 1–5 ppm may cause bronchitis with cough, phlegm, and/or shortness of breath. Workers with daily exposures of 5 to 10 ppm of *n*-butylamine may experience nose, throat, and eye irritation and headaches. Individuals with chronic respiratory, skin, or eye disease are at increased risk from *n*-butylamine exposure. Chronic exposure to irritating levels of butylamines can cause symptoms and/or increase the severity of symptoms in people with preexisting conditions.

Immunotoxicity

No data on the immunotoxicity of butylamines are available.

Reproductive Toxicity

Ingestion of butylamines has been shown to affect the reproductive process and cause harm to the fetus. Reported effects from oral exposure to *n*-butylamine in rats include reduced maternal feed consumption, increased early post-implantation losses, reduced fetal and placental weight, retarded skeletal development, and malformations. One hundred milligrams per kilogram was the NOAEL for prenatal developmental toxicity in this study. The authors hypothesized that the neutralization of *n*-butylamine by hydrochloride in the stomach converts it from a strong alkali into *n*-butylamine hydrochloride, a weak acid/base which is fetotoxic. A *sec*-butylamine rat feeding study resulted in normal reproduction, fertility, gestation, viability, and lactation indices; however, a reduction of growth was noted throughout the study at the high dietary level. Additional studies with rats and rabbits have resulted in reduced fetal weights at higher dose levels.

Inhalation exposure to *n*-butylamine produced maternal effects in rats, but no embryo/fetoxicity or effects on morphology were reported. The developmental NOAEL was 152 ppm in this study.

Genotoxicity

All four butylamines tested negative in the Ames test with *Salmonella typhimurium* with and without metabolic activation. In a mouse micronucleus assay, *n*-butylamine hydrochloride did not have any clastogenic effect, and there were no indications of any impairment of chromosome distribution in the course mitosis.

Carcinogenicity

Butylamine was an equivocal animal carcinogen by the intraperitoneal route in mice, and inhaled *n*-butylamine produced concentration-dependent nasal epithelial hyperplasia and squamous metaplasia in rats.

One area of concern is the possibility that aliphatic amines may react with nitrate or nitrite *in vivo* to form nitroso compounds, many of which are known to be potent carcinogens in animals; however, the potential for this to occur in primary amines is low.

Clinical Management

The degree of injury should be considered when determining initial treatment. Exposed skin and eyes should be immediately irrigated with copious amounts of tepid water. The extent of damage to the eye may not be fully evident until 48–72 h after exposure.

After inhalation exposure, the victim should be moved to fresh air and monitored for respiratory distress. One hundred percent of humidified supplemental oxygen with assisted ventilation should be administered as required. If coughing or breathing difficulties are noted, the patient should be evaluated for irritation, bronchitis, or pneumonitis, including chest X-rays and determination of blood gasses. The symptoms of pulmonary edema often do not become manifest until a few hours have passed and they are aggravated by physical effort. Rest and medical observation is therefore essential. If pulmonary edema is present, positive end expiratory pressure ventilation and steroids should be considered.

For ingestion exposures, copious amounts of water should be given to dilute stomach contents. Because of the potential for gastrointestinal tract irritation or burns, do not induce emesis. Significant esophageal or gastrointestinal tract irritation or burns may occur following ingestion. The possible benefit of early removal of some ingested material by cautious gastric lavage must be weighed against potential complications of bleeding or perforation.

Ecotoxicology

Freshwater/Sediment Organisms

- Isobutylamine
  - *D. rerio* (zebra fish, embryo) $LC_{50} = 1267\ \mu mol\ l^{-1}$ for 48 h
  - *Semotilus atromaculatus* (creek chub) $LC_{100} = 820\ \mu mol\ l^{-1}$ for 24 h
- *n*-Butylamine
  - *Leuciscus idus* (ide) $LC_{50} = 171\ mg\ l^{-1}$ for 96 h
  - *Lepomis macrochirus* (bluegill) $LC_{50} = 32\ mg\ l^{-1}$ for 96 h
  - *Menidia beryllina* (inland silverside) $LC_{50} = 24\ mg\ l^{-1}$ for 96 h
  - *Oryzias latipes* (medaka) $LC_{50} = 1000\ mg\ l^{-1}$ for 24 and 48 h
  - *Pimephales promelas* (fathead minnow) $EC_{50} = 268\ mg\ l^{-1}$ for 96 h (loss of schooling behavior, hyperactivity, increased respiration, loss of equilibrium); $LC_{50} = 268\ mg\ l^{-1}$ for 96 h
  - *Artemia salina* (brine shrimp) $LC_{50} = 30–70\ mg\ l^{-1}$ for 24 h
  - *Daphnia magna* (water flea) $EC_{50} = 100\ mg\ l^{-1}$ for 24 and 48 h (intoxication, immobilization); $LC_{50} = 75\ mg\ l^{-1}$ for 24 h
  - *Anabaena subcylindrica* (blue-green algae) $EC_{50} = 1.8 \times 10^{-8}\ \mu g\ cell^{-1}$ for 3 h (decreased photosynthesis, oxygen production)
- *sec*-Butylamine
  - *L. idus* (ide) $LC_{50} = 46–68\ mg\ l^{-1}$ for 96 h
  - *Tetrahymena pyriformis* (ciliate) $EC_{50} = 25\ mg\ l^{-1}$ for 12 or 36 h (general growth)
- *tert*-Butylamine
  - *Oncorhynchus mykiss* (rainbow trout) $LC_{50} = 28–270\ mg\ l^{-1}$ for 4 days
  - *Pseudokirchneriella subcapitata* (green algae) $EC_{50} = 16\ mg\ l^{-1}$ for 96 h (general growth)

Marine Organisms

No data available.

Terrestrial Organisms

- *n*-Butylamine
  - *Aedes aegypti* (yellow-fever mosquito) $LC_{50} = 0.024\ \mu g\ l^{-1}$ for 4 h
  - *Lactuca sativa* (lettuce) $EC_{50} = 7.9\ mol\ m^{-3}$ for 3 days

Other Hazards

Butylamines form explosive mixtures with air. The lower explosive limit of *n*-butylamine is 1.7% and the upper explosive limit is 9.8%. Butylamines may accumulate static electrical charges, which can cause ignition of its vapors. The vapors are heavier than air and may travel to a source of ignition and flash back.

Butylamines are weak bases which can react with strong oxidizers and acids, causing a fire and explosion hazard. Contact with strong acids will cause spattering. Butylamines are incompatible with organic anhydrides, isocyanates, vinyl acetate, acrylates, substituted allyls, alkylene oxides, epichlorohydrin, ketones, aldehydes, alcohols, glycols, phenols, cresols, and caprolactum solution. They can explode on contact with perchloryl fluoride and 2,2-dibromo-1,3-dimethylcyclopropanoic acid. Butylamines corrode some metals in the presence of moisture and will degrade some forms of plastics, rubber, and coatings.

When heated to decomposition, butylamines emit toxic oxides of nitrogen as well as carbon monoxide, carbon dioxide, and ammonia.

Exposure Standards and Guidelines

Isobutylamine (**Table 1**).

Table 1 Exposure standards and guidelines for isobutylamine

Organization	Standard
Occupational Exposure Limit – Austria	MAK 5 ppm (15 mg m^{-3}), skin, Jan. 1999
Occupational Exposure Limit – Denmark	Time-weighted average 5 ppm (15 mg m^{-3}), skin, Jan. 1999
Occupational Exposure Limit – Germany	MAK 5 ppm (15 mg m^{-3}), skin, Jan. 1999
Occupational Exposure Limit – Switzerland	MAK-week 5 ppm (15 mg m^{-3}), short-term exposure limit 25 ppm (75 mg m^{-3}), Jan. 1999

Reference: National Institute for Occupational Safety and Health (NIOSH) (2004). Isobutylamine. Registry of Toxic Effects of Chemical Substances (RTECS). Retrieved 8/31/2011. http://www.skcgulfcoast.com/nioshdbs/rtecs/np970fe0.htm.

n-Butylamine (Table 2).

Table 2 Exposure standards and guidelines for *n*-butylamine

Organization	Standard
Mine Safety and Health Administration (MSHA) STANDARD	Air-ceiling concentration 5 ppm (15 mg m^{-3}) (skin), 1971
Occupational Safety and Health Administration (OSHA) Permissible Exposure Limit (General Industry)	Ceiling concentration 5 ppm (15 mg m^{-3}) (skin), 1994
Occupational Safety and Health Administration (OSHA) Permissible Exposure Limit (Construction)	Ceiling concentration 5 ppm (15 mg m^{-3}) (skin), 1994
Occupational Safety and Health Administration (OSHA) Permissible Exposure Limit (Shipyards)	Ceiling concentration 5 ppm (15 mg m^{-3}) (skin), 1993
Occupational Safety and Health Administration (OSHA) Permissible Exposure Limit (Federal Contractors)	Ceiling concentration 5 ppm (15 mg m^{-3}) (skin), 1994
Occupational Exposure Limit – Australia	Time-weighted average 5 ppm (15 mg m^{-3}), skin, Jan. 1999
Occupational Exposure Limit – Austria	MAK 5 ppm (15 mg m^{-3}), skin, Jan. 1993
Occupational Exposure Limit – Belgium	Short-term exposure limit 5 ppm (15 mg m^{-3}), skin, Jan. 1993
Occupational Exposure Limit – Denmark	Time-weighted average 5 ppm (15 mg m^{-3}), skin, Jan. 1999
Occupational Exposure Limit – Finland	Short-term exposure limit 5 ppm (15 mg m^{-3}), skin, Jan. 1999
Occupational Exposure Limit – France	VLE 5 ppm (15 mg m^{-3}), skin, Jan. 1999
Occupational Exposure Limit – Germany	MAK 5 ppm (15 mg m^{-3}), skin, Jan. 1999
Occupational Exposure Limit – Japan	Occupational Exposure Limit (continuous) 5 ppm (15 mg m^{-3}), Jan. 1999
Occupational Exposure Limit – The Netherlands	MAC-continuous 15 mg m^{-3}, skin, 2003
Occupational Exposure Limit – Norway	Time-weighted average 5 ppm (15 mg m^{-3}), Jan. 1999
Occupational Exposure Limit – The Philippines	Time-weighted average 5 ppm (15 mg m^{-3}), skin, Jan. 1993
Occupational Exposure Limit – Russia	Short-term exposure limit 5 ppm (10 mg m^{-3}), skin, Jan. 1993
Occupational Exposure Limit – Sweden	Ceiling 5 ppm (15 mg m^{-3}), skin, Jan. 1999
Occupational Exposure Limit – Switzerland	MAK-week 5 ppm (15 mg m^{-3}), short-term exposure limit 25 ppm (75 mg m^{-3}), skin, Jan. 1999
Occupational Exposure Limit – Thailand	Time-weighted average 5 ppm (15 mg m^{-3}), Jan. 1993
Occupational Exposure Limit – Turkey	Time-weighted average 5 ppm (15 mg m^{-3}), skin, Jan. 1993
Occupational Exposure Limit – United Kingdom	Short-term exposure limit 5 ppm (15 mg m^{-3}), skin, Sep. 2000
Occupational Exposure Limit in Argentina, Bulgaria, Colombia, Jordan, Korea	American Conference of Governmental Industrial Hygienists (ACGIH) Threshold Limit Value; ceiling concentration 5 ppm (skin)
Occupational Exposure Limit in New Zealand, Singapore, Vietnam	American Conference of Governmental Industrial Hygienists (ACGIH) Threshold Limit Value ceiling concentration 5 ppm (skin)

Reference: National Institute for Occupational Safety and Health (NIOSH) (2004). Butylamine. Registry of Toxic Effects of Chemical Substances (RTECS). Retrieved 8/31/2011. http://www.emedco.info/rtecs/eo2d6518.htm.

sec-Butylamine (Table 3).

Table 3 Exposure standards and guidelines for *sec*-butylamine

Organization	Standard
Occupational Exposure Limit – Austria	MAK 5 ppm (15 mg m^{-3}), skin, Jan. 1999
Occupational Exposure Limit – Denmark	Time-weighted average 5 ppm (15 mg m^{-3}), skin, Jan. 1999
Occupational Exposure Limit – Germany	MAK 5 ppm (15 mg m^{-3}), skin, Jan. 1999
Occupational Exposure Limit – Norway	Time-weighted average 5 ppm (15 mg m^{-3}), Jan. 1999
Occupational Exposure Limit – Switzerland	MAK-week 5 ppm (15 mg m^{-3}), short-term exposure limit 25 ppm (75 mg m^{-3}), Jan. 1999

Reference: National Institute for Occupational Safety and Health (NIOSH) (2004). *sec*-Butylamine. Registry of Toxic Effects of Chemical Substances (RTECS). Retrieved 8/31/2011. http://www.skcgulfcoast.com/nioshdbs/rtecs/eo32bc48.htm.

Miscellaneous

Butylamines are clear, colorless liquids. The odor is described as fishlike and ammonia-like. Odor may be detected at concentrations as low as 0.12 ppm, is noticeable at 2 ppm, moderately strong at 2–5 ppm, and strong at 5–10 ppm.

Butylamines have an almost unlimited shelf life in unopened, original containers if protected from heat and properly stored in a protected storage area.

See also: Corrosives; Eye Irritancy Testing.

Further Reading

American Conference of Governmental Industrial Hygienists, 2001. *n*-Butylamine. In: Documentation of the Threshold Limit Values and Biological Exposure Indices. Cincinnati, OH.

Clayton, G.D., Clayton, F.E. (Eds.), 1994. Patty's Industrial Hygiene and Toxicology, Vol. II., Part B, fourth ed. John Wiley & Sons Inc, New York, NY, pp. 1121–1124.

Joint FAO/WHO Meeting on Pesticide Residues, 1975. *sec*-Butylamine. WHO Pesticide Residue Series 5. http://www.inchem.org/documents/jmpr/jmpmono/v075pr07.htm.

National Institute for Occupational Safety and Health, 1981. Occupational safety and health guideline for butylamine. Occupational Health Guidelines for Chemical Hazards. http://www.cdc.gov/niosh/docs/81-123/pdfs/0079-rev.pdf DHHS (NIOSH) Publication Number 81-123.

National Institute for Occupational Safety and Health (NIOSH), 2004. Isobutylamine. Registry of Toxic Effects of Chemical Substances (RTECS). Retrieved 8/31/2011. http://www.skcgulfcoast.com/nioshdbs/rtecs/np970fe0.htm.

National Institute for Occupational Safety and Health (NIOSH), 2004. Butylamine. Registry of Toxic Effects of Chemical Substances (RTECS). Retrieved 8/31/2011. http://www.emedco.info/rtecs/eo2d6518.htm.

National Institute for Occupational Safety and Health (NIOSH) (2004). *sec*-Butylamine. Registry of Toxic Effects of Chemical Substances (RTECS). Retrieved 8/31/2011. http://www.skcgulfcoast.com/nioshdbs/rtecs/eo32bc48.htm.

Butyraldehyde

SJ Klein, Manchester University, North Manchester, IN, USA

This article is a revision of the previous edition article by Sanjay Chanda and Harihara M. Mehendale, volume 1, pp 367–368, © 2005, Elsevier Inc.

- Name: Butyraldehyde
- Chemical Abstracts Service Registry Number: CAS 123-72-8
- Synonyms: Butyraldehyde; Butal; Butaldehyde; Butyl aldehyde; *n*-Butyl aldehyde; Butyral; *n*-Butyraldehyde; Butyric aldehyde; Butyrylaldehyde; *n*-Butanal; Butanaldehyde
- Chemical/Pharmaceutical/Other Class: Aliphatic aldehyde
- Molecular Formula: C_4H_8O
- Chemical Structure:

Uses

Butanal is used in the manufacture of rubber accelerators, synthetic resins, solvents, and plasticizers. *n*-Butyraldehyde is used as an intermediate in the manufacturing of plasticizers, alcohols, solvents, and polymers (such as 2-ethylhexanol, *n*-butanol, trimethylolpropane, *n*-butyric acid, polyvinyl butyral, and methyl amyl ketone). It is also used as an intermediate to make pharmaceuticals, agrochemicals, antioxidants, rubber accelerators, textile auxiliaries, perfumery, and flavors. It has no therapeutic use at the present time.

Background Information

n-Butyraldehyde is a clear, mobile, flammable, liquid with a pungent odor. It is miscible with all common solvents, for example, alcohols, ketones, aldehydes, ethers, glycols, and aromatic and aliphatic hydrocarbons, but is only sparingly soluble in water.

Environment Fate and Behavior

Routes and Pathways

Primary exposure is from vapor. Butyraldehyde's vapor pressure of 111.4 mm Hg at 51 °C indicates that it will evaporate rapidly from surfaces. Butanal is highly mobile with a K_{oc} value of 72. The Henry's Law constant has been measured at 1.15×10^{-4} atm-m^3 mol^{-1}.

Partition Behavior in Water, Sediment, and Soil

Terrestrial Fate

The primary degradation process in soil is expected to be biodegradation. A number of biological screening studies have demonstrated that butyraldehyde is readily biodegradable.

Aquatic Fate

The major environmental fate processes for butyraldehyde in water are biodegradation and volatilization. A number of biological screening studies have demonstrated that butyraldehyde is readily biodegradable. Volatilization half-lives of 9 h and 4.1 days have been estimated for a model river (1-m deep) and a model pond, respectively. Aquatic hydrolysis, adsorption to sediment, and bioconcentration are not expected to be important fate processes.

Environmental Persistency

Reaction of butanal vapor with hydroxyl radicals in the atmosphere is quite fast, with a half-life of 16 h. The reaction with nitrate radical in the atmosphere is somewhat slower, with a half-life of 2.9 days. Butanal can also directly absorb solar radiation to degrade into smaller compounds. During intense smog pollution episodes, the natural formation rate of butyraldehyde can exceed the degradation rate. The detection of butyraldehyde in cloud and fog water indicates that physical removal from air can occur through wet deposition.

Bioaccumulation

Based on the Henry's Law constant value and the volatility, butanal is not expected to bioaccumulate.

Exposure and Exposure Monitoring

Routes and Pathways

Butanal is a liquid at room temperature, with a relatively low vapor pressure. Limited contact could occur by exposure to butanal vapors. Butanal has appreciable solubility in water; therefore, exposure would be expected to be primarily through ingestion of or through skin contact with the compound or a solution of the compound.

Human Exposure

Butyraldehyde is destructive to mucosal membranes and upper respiratory tract. Inhalation may be fatal due to pulmonary edema, as well as edema of the larynx and bronchi.

Environmental Exposure

General exposure is from dermal contact or inhalation in workplace environments where butyraldehyde is used.

Toxicokinetics

Butanal is readily metabolized to carbon dioxide by conversion to butyryl CoA and subsequent metabolism via the pathways of

 http://dx.doi.org/10.1016/B978-0-12-386454-3.00264-5

short-chain fatty acid oxidation. Detoxication by reaction with glutathione also occurs. Clearance is rapid and complete.

Mechanism of Toxicity

Butanal does not possess high acute toxicity but is a potent irritant of the skin, eyes, and upper respiratory tract. The mechanism of toxicity probably involves direct reaction between the active aldehyde group and cellular components.

Acute and Short-Term Toxicity (or Exposure)

Animal

The oral LD_{50} value for rat is 5.9 g kg^{-1}, whereas the LC_{50} is 60 000 ppm (30 min exposure). Acute exposures to butanal vapors induce inflammation of the alveolar and bronchial regions of the lung, with death due to pulmonary edema. Severe irritation of the eyes and nose is noted. Relatively high levels of butanal in the drinking water of mice for 50 days produced abnormal sperm morphology. Exposure of rodents to low concentrations of butanal allowed rapid recovery after exposure is ceased. Skin irritation to rabbits has been determined to be 3560 mg kg^{-1}. Beagles were exposed to butanal vapors in various concentrations that resulted in goblet cell hyperplasia within the nasal mucosa at concentrations of 125–500 ppm, and squamous metaplasia of the nasal tissues at 2000 ppm.

Human

Butanal has low acute toxicity. Exposure to a large dose may have a temporary narcotic effect. Exposure to low concentrations of butanal vapors produces irritation of the eyes, nose, and throat. The compound has an unpleasant odor. Impurities (butyric acid) may be present that make the smell even more objectionable. Health effects attributed to chronic exposure to low doses of butanal vapors have not been described. Dermatitis may be expected after prolonged and repeated exposures to solutions containing butanal.

Reproductive Toxicity

No information on human reproductive toxicity is available. In male mice, an intraperitoneal injection of 30 mg kg^{-1} or 0.2 mg l^{-1} for 50 days in drinking water resulted in chromosomal and meiotic anomalies in all stages of spermatogenesis.

Genotoxicity

Standard assay test with several strains of *Salmonella typhimurium* were found to be negative, indicating that butyraldehyde is not genotoxic. However, when butyraldehyde is injected intraperitoneally in mice there arose chromosomal abnormalities during spermatogenesis. Exposure to butanal in the presence of copper (II) chloride causes strand breakage in PM2 DNA.

Clinical Management

Support should be given to the patient until butanal has been cleared from the body, which occurs in a relatively short time. Recovery is uneventful.

Ecotoxicology

Freshwater/Sediment Organisms Toxicity

Pseudokirchneriella subcapitata (green algae) showed decreased photosynthesis with exposure to concentrations of 1480 μg l^{-1} for 48 h.

Marine Organisms Toxicity

Daphnia magna (water flea) in conditions of freshwater, 20–22 °C, pH 7.6–7.7, exposure to a concentration of 340 000 μg l^{-1} for 24 h resulted in intoxication and immobilization. In *Pimephales promelas* (fathead minnow), an LC_{50} of 13 400 μg l^{-1} over 96 h was measured in freshwater, 24.1 °C, pH 7.7, and dissolved oxygen 6.8 mg l^{-1}.

Terrestrial Organisms Toxicity

Inhalation at levels above 6000 ppm caused bronchial and alveolar edema in rats. Dermal and eye exposures in rodent are moderately to severely irritating. Butyraldehyde has been shown to be a vasodepressor in dogs.

Exposure Standards and Guidelines

Workplace environmental exposure level: 8 h time-weighted average (25 ppm).

See also: Butyric Acid; Crotonaldehyde.

Further Reading

Becker, T.W., Krieger, G., Witte, I., 1996. DNA single and double strand breaks induced by aliphatic and aromatic aldehydes in combination with copper (II). Free Radic. Res. 24, 325–332.

Martelli, A., et al, 1994. Cytotoxic and genotoxic effects of five n-alkanals in primary cultures of rat and human hepatocytes. 323, 121–126.

National Toxicology Program, February 1999. NTP toxicology and carcinogenesis studies of isobutyraldehyde (CAS No. 78-84-2) in F344/N rats and B6C3F1 mice (inhalation studies). Natl. Toxicol. Program Tech. Rep. Ser. 472, 1–242.

Poirier, M., Fournier, M., Brousseau, P., Morin, A., 2002. Effects of volatile aromatics, aldehydes, and phenols in tobacco smoke on viability and proliferation of mouse lymphocytes. J. Toxicol. Environ. Health A 65, 1437–1451.

Relevant Websites

http://www.epa.gov – Butyraldehyde Fact Sheet (from the US EPA's OPPT) (EPA 749-F-95–005a), 1994.

http://toxnet.nlm.nih.gov – Toxnet (Toxicology Data Network): search for Butyraldehyde, n-.

Butyric Acid

G Karimi and M Vahabzadeh, Medical Toxicology Research Center and Pharmacy School,
Mashhad University of Medical Sciences, Mashhad, Iran

This article is a revision of the previous edition article by James Deyo, volume 1, pp 368–370, © 2005, Elsevier Inc.

- Chemical Abstracts Service Registry Number: 107-92-6
- Synonyms: 1-Butyric acid, 1-Propanecarboxylic acid, 4-02-00-00779 (Beilstein Handbook Reference), AI3-15306, BRN 0906770, Butanic acid, Butanoic acid, Buttersaeure (German), Butyrate, CCRIS 6552, EINECS 203-532-3, Ethylacetic acid, FEMA No. 2221, HSDB 940, Kyselina maselna (Czech), NSC 8415, Propylformic acid, UNII-40UIR9Q29H, *n*-Butanoic acid, *n*-Butyric acid
- Molecular Formula: $C_4H_8O_2$
- Chemical Structure:

O

OH

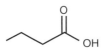

Background

Butyric acid (Chemical Abstracts Service Registry Number 107-92-6) is a four-carbon acid with an unpleasant and obnoxious odor, with a butter-fat taste. It is a clear and colorless oily liquid and occurs in butter and animal fat as the glycerol ester. *n*-Butyric acid is manufactured in enclosed, continuous equipment by the catalyzed air oxidation of butyraldehyde. It can be produced *via* fermentation of organic materials by anaerobic bacteria in the large intestine, and remains a major energy supply for colonic cells. Butyric acid is involved in a range of processes in the body such as native immunity, induction of apoptosis, and regulation of water and electrolytes. It is an important metabolite in the breakdown of carbohydrates, fats, and proteins and is mainly used as an industrial intermediate and food additive.

Uses

Butyric acid is used in the manufacture of cellulose acetate butyrate (CAB) plastics. CAB sheets are used for thermoformed signs, blister packaging, and in goggles and face shields. Molded CAB is used to make pen barrels, eyeglass frames, and screwdriver handles. CAB is a component in acrylic enamel used in automotive manufacturing coatings. Some butyric acid is used to make butyroperoxides and herbicides. It is also used as an intermediate for pharmaceuticals, emulsifiers, and disinfectants, as a leather tanning agent, and a sweetening agent in gasoline. It is used in the synthesis of butyrate ester perfumes and in the manufacture of esters, some of which serve as the bases of artificial flavoring ingredients in certain liquors, soda-water syrups, and candies. It is also used as a food additive in butter, cheese, butterscotch, caramel, and fruit and nut flavors. Butyric acid is classified as a generally considered as safe (GRAS) material by the US Food and Drug Administration (US FDA). Butyric acid is also used in the preservation of high moisture wheat grains to prevent fungal deterioration. In therapeutics, butyric acid is used as a histamine antagonist. Due to its powerful odor, it has also been used as an additive in fishing bait. The antiangiogenic and antineoplastic activities of the butyric acid prodrugs, AN-7 and AN-9, were demonstrated *in vitro* by inhibition of proliferation and vascular tube formation, enhanced apoptosis, and inhibition of 22Rv-1 cell migration. The inhibition of tumor growth and metastasis and the low toxicity of AN-7 and AN-9 have been demonstrated in preclinical studies and clinical trials. Generally, prodrugs of butyric acid rapidly penetrate into cancer cells where they hydrolyze to butyric acid and aldehyde. The most active prodrugs in this family of acyloxyalkyl esters are the ones that release formaldehyde and they possess anticancer properties superior to those elicited by the homologous prodrugs that release acetaldehyde. The potential use of butyric acid prodrugs for the treatment of neoplastic diseases and β-globin disorders has been suggested.

Environmental Fate and Behavior

Butyric acid is miscible with ethanol, water, and ether, and is slightly soluble in carbon tetrachloride. It has the following physical properties: melting point −7.9 °C; boiling point 163.5 °C; molecular weight 88.1; flash point 72 °C; autoignition temperature 443 °C; pH 4 (acidic); pK_a 4.82 at 25 °C; critical temperature 342.05 °C; critical pressure 4.06 MPa; stable under normal conditions of use and storage; vapor pressure 1.65 mmHg; octanol/water partition coefficient, log K_{ow} 0.79; viscosity 1.426 mPa s at 25 °C; Henry's law constant 5.35×10^{-7} atm m^3 mol^{-1} at 25 °C. In addition, a Henry's law constant of 3.4×10^{-6} atm m^3 mol^{-1} has been calculated for *n*-butyric acid from its physical properties, using a vapor pressure of 2.2 hPa (1.65 mmHg) at 25 °C, an aqueous solubility of 56 200 mg l^{-1} and molecular weight of 88.11 g mol^{-1}.

n-Butyric acid is not expected to accumulate in organisms or adsorb onto soil or sediment, given its low bioconcentration factor (BCF) (2.3–3.16 l kg^{-1} wet weight) calculated from a log K_{ow} of 0.79 and measured soil partition coefficient (14.7–27.6 l kg^{-1} dry weight). Based on a classification scheme, an estimated K_{oc} value of 64, determined from a log K_{ow} of 0.79 and a regression-derived equation, and experimental values of 19.1, 27.6, and 14.7 in mud, muddy sand, and sand, respectively, indicate that *n*-butanoic acid is expected to have very high to high mobility in soil. The pK_a of *n*-butanoic acid is 4.82, indicating that this compound exists primarily in the anion form in the environment and anions generally do not adsorb more strongly to soils containing organic carbon and clay than their neutral counterparts. Volatilization of butyric acid from moist

 http://dx.doi.org/10.1016/B978-0-12-386454-3.00591-1

soil surfaces is expected to be slow given a Henry's law constant of 5.35×10^{-7} atm m^3 mol^{-1}. *n*-Butanoic acid is expected to volatilize from dry soil surfaces based on a vapor pressure of 1.65 mmHg. Using Henry's law constant and an estimation method, volatilization half-lives for a model river and model lake were 64 and 471 days, respectively. According to a classification scheme, an estimated BCF of 3.2, from a log K_{ow} of 0.79 and a regression-derived equation, suggests the potential for bioconcentration in aquatic organisms is low. *n*-Butanoic acid is expected to exist solely as a vapor in the ambient atmosphere. Vapor-phase butyric acid is degraded in the atmosphere by reaction with photochemically produced hydroxyl radicals; the half-life for this reaction in air is estimated to be 7 days, calculated from its rate constant of 2.40×10^{-12} cm^3 mol^{-1} s^{-1} at 25 °C. *n*-Butanoic acid does not contain chromophores that absorb at wavelengths more than 290 nm and therefore is not expected to be susceptible to direct photolysis by sunlight.

Butyric acid is not environmentally persistent as it is biodegradable in aqueous media, volatilizes from surface waters at a moderate rate, and readily undergoes photodegradation in the atmosphere. *n*-Butanoic acid may be susceptible to biodegradation in terrestrial and aquatic environments based on the observed degradation of 72% after 5 h when incubated with activated sludge. At an initial concentration of 100 mg l^{-1}, *n*-butanoic acid displayed a 72% theoretical biological oxygen demand (BODT) after 5 h when incubated with activated sludge. *n*-Butanoic acid at an initial concentration of 5 ppm displayed a BODT of 76.6% in freshwater and 72.4% in seawater after 5 days. *n*-Butanoic acid had a BODT of 17.4, 23.8, 26.2, and 27.7% after 6, 12, 18, and 24 h, respectively, when incubated with an activated sludge seed at an initial concentration of 500 ppm. In a screening study, the BODT of *n*-butanoic acid was 46, 48, and 58% after 2, 10, and 30 days, respectively, using a sewage seed. In a screening study using a sewage seed, *n*-butanoic acid had a 5-day BODT of 72–78% and a 20-day BODT of 92–99%.

Butyric acid must be separated from strong oxidants, strong bases, food, and feedstuffs for long-range transport (UN Hazard Class 8; UN Packing Group III; stable during transport). It should be stored in a cool, dry, well-ventilated location, away from any area where fire hazard may be acute. Outside or detached storage is preferred, separate from oxidizing materials, heat, oxidizers, and sunlight.

n-Butyric acid is not likely to bioaccumulate.

Exposure and Exposure Monitoring

n-Butanoic acid is present in butter as an ester (4–5%). It occurs as a glyceride in animal milk fats. Butyric acid has been found in essential oils of Citronella Ceylon, *Eucalyptus globulus*, *Araucaria cunninghamii*, *Lippia scaberrima*, *Monarda fistulosa*, Cajeput, *Heracleum giganteum*, lavender, *Hedeoma pulegioides*, valerian, nutmeg, hops, *Pastinaca sativa*, and Spanish anise. It has also been identified in strawberry aroma. *n*-Butanoic acid is found in vegetable oils and in animal fluids, such as sweat, tissue fluids, and milk fat. Free *n*-butanoic acid is an important metabolite in the breakdown of carbohydrates, fats, and proteins. *n*-Butanoic acid may arise from natural fermentative processes occurring in sediment. It has also been detected as a volatile flavor component in the fruit of dalieb, a deciduous palm. *n*-Butanoic acid was the principal metabolite in a growth medium containing an aquatic actinomycete streptomyces species and represented the greatest potential as an odorous water pollutant under natural conditions.

Most of the *n*-butyric acid released to the environment partitions primarily into water and soil (37.2 and 57.0%, respectively), with most remaining in the air (5.67%) and little (<0.1%) in sediment. *n*-Butyric acid is found naturally in vegetable oils and in animal fluids, such as sweat, tissue fluids, and milk fat.

Monitoring data indicate that the general population may be exposed to *n*-butanoic acid *via* inhalation of ambient air, ingestion of food and drinking water, and dermal contact with this compound and other products containing *n*-butanoic acid. Target organs are the respiratory system, skin, and the eyes. Direct administration onto the skin or into the stomach results in corrosion of the epithelial surfaces. Industrial processes with risk of exposure are fur dressing and dyeing, leather tanning and processing, and painting (pigments, binders, and biocides). National Institute for Occupational Safety and Health has statistically estimated that 11 600 workers (3391 of these were female) are potentially exposed to *n*-butanoic acid in the United States. Occupational exposure to *n*-butanoic acid may occur through inhalation and dermal contact with this compound at workplaces where *n*-butanoic acid is produced or used. *n*-Butanoic acid has been detected as an emission during the welding of steel coated with protective paints.

n-Butyric acid is regulated in the United States as a hazardous substance under the Comprehensive Environmental Response, Compensation and Liability Act, under which its reportable quantity (when there is an environmental release) is 2270 kg. *n*-Butyric acid is regulated under the Clean Air Act as a volatile organic chemical and therefore actions are taken to minimize equipment leaks in the synthetic organic chemical manufacturing industry. Exposure to *n*-butyric acid by the general population arises from its artificial and natural presence in the environment. It may be released to the environment as a fugitive emission during its production and use, and in motor vehicle exhaust. *n*-Butyric acid is not used in consumer products, but consumers ingest food that contains naturally occurring *n*-butyric acid. Thus, environmental exposure to *n*-butyric acid is limited.

Toxicokinetics

Butyric acid is rapidly metabolized in the liver to acetic acid and ketone bodies (acetone, acetoacetate, β-hydroxybutyrate). In humans, the butyric acid elimination curve can be divided into two parts corresponding to two half-lives: for the first (0.5 min), the slope suggests accelerated excretion; for the second (13.7 min), a slow plateau is observed.

Mechanism of Toxicity

The most probable mechanism of toxicity is the formation of an acid proteinate following exposure to high concentrations. Such complexes result in an inhibition of protein function and disruption of cellular homeostasis. Butyric acid induces apoptosis by production of ceramide and reactive oxygen species in the mitochondria followed by activation of JNK in mitogen activated protein (MAP) kinase cascades. Butyric acid has two contrasting functional roles. As a product of fermentation within the human colon, it serves as the most important energy source for normal colorectal epithelium. It also promotes differentiation of cultured malignant cells. A switch from aerobic to anaerobic metabolism accompanies neoplastic transformation in the colorectum. The separate functional roles for *n*-butyrate may reflect the different metabolic activities of normal and neoplastic tissues. Deficiency of *n*-butyrate, coupled with the increased energy requirements of neoplastic tissue, may promote the switch to anaerobic metabolism. *n*-Butyrate was previously found to increase epidermal growth factor receptor binding in primary cultures of rat hepatocytes. It was shown that butyrate and dexamethasone synergistically modulate the surface expression of epidermal growth factor receptors. The butyrate-induced enhancement of high-affinity epidermal growth factor binding was slight in the absence of glucocorticoid, but was strongly and dose-dependently amplified by dexamethasone. Butyrate counteracted the inhibition by insulin of the dexamethasone-induced increase in epidermal growth factor binding. The results indicate that the glucocorticoid has a permissive effect on a butyrate-sensitive process that determines the surface expression of the high-affinity class of epidermal growth factor receptors.

Acute and Short-Term Toxicity

Animal

Data on laboratory animals suggest that *n*-butyric acid is only slightly acutely toxic with an oral lethal dose 50% (LD_{50}) value in rats ranging from 2940 to 8790 mg kg^{-1}, an intraperitoneal or subcutaneous LD_{50} value of 3180 mg kg^{-1} in mice, an inhalation lethal concentration 50% (LC_{50}) of 440 mg l^{-1} in rabbits, an oral LD_{50} value of 2 mg kg^{-1} (2000 mg kg^{-1}) in rabbits, and a dermal LD_{50} value of 530 mg kg^{-1} in rabbits. Butyric acid is a moderately strong irritant to skin and may induce severe eye irritation. After a 90-min exposure to a butyric acid aerosol (40 mg l^{-1}), rabbits displayed increased lethargy and dyspnea. Signs of bronchial and capillary dilation and emphysema were evident on necropsy. In another study, no lethality was reported when rats were exposed for 8 h to air saturated with butyric acid vapor. Severe corneal burns were produced in rabbits by an excess of a 5% aqueous solution of butyric acid (unspecified volume). Large intravenous doses of butyric acid (sodium salt) caused temporary central nervous system (CNS) depression in rabbits (1.6 g kg^{-1}) and dogs (0.86 g kg^{-1}); similar effects were reported after subcutaneous administration of the acid to cats. Intravenous application of butyrate (continuous infusion 2.5 ml min^{-1}, 0.02 mM kg^{-1} min^{-1} for 10 min) produced an abrupt and substantial increase in mean plasma insulin concentration in lambs. It is also a moderately strong skin and eye irritant in guinea pigs.

Human

Acute exposure to butyric acid induces irritation or burns following contact with skin or eyes, or if inhaled. Such effects occur in a concentration-dependent manner. Inhalation of the spray may contribute to severe respiratory symptoms including shortness of breath, coughing, or choking. Signs and symptoms due to inhalation of butyric acid are sore throat, cough, burning sensation, shortness of breath, labored breathing. Symptoms may be delayed. Signs and symptoms due to dermal contact are pain, redness, blisters, and skin burns. Signs and symptoms due to eye contact are pain, redness, severe deep burns, and loss of vision. Signs and symptoms due to ingestion are burning sensation, abdominal pain, shock, or collapse.

Chronic Toxicity

Animal

Repeated inhalation or oral exposure to moderate to high doses of *n*-butyl acetate and *n*-butanol is well tolerated in animals. These molecules are readily and rapidly metabolized to *n*-butyric acid. The no observed effect level (NOEL) for repeated-dose oral exposure to *n*-butanol was 125 mg kg^{-1} day^{-1}. In a 90-day inhalation study in rats with *n*-butyl acetate, an NOEL of 500 ppm was reported for systemic effects, and an NOEL of 3000 ppm (highest dose tested) was reported for postexposure neurotoxicity based on functional observational battery end points, quantitative motor activity, neuropathy, and scheduled, controlled operant behavior end points. Rats (number not specified) fed diets containing butyric acid at concentrations of 25% for up to 35 weeks barely maintained their weight, and histology on four rats revealed papillomatosis and hyperkeratosis of gastric tissues.

Human

Butyric acid is a GRAS food additive for chronic consumption when used in accordance with good manufacturing practice. Chronic exposure also occurs through endogenous production as *n*-butyric acid is an important metabolite in the breakdown of carbohydrates, fats, and proteins, and is produced in the human colon by fermentation. *n*-Butyric acid is present in butter as an ester (4–5%). However, it is toxic to the lungs, the nervous system, and mucous membranes. Frequent and prolonged exposure can lead to target organ damage.

Immunotoxicity

Prolonged exposure (of unspecified duration) of mice, rats, and rabbits to an atmospheric concentration of 0.1–0.2 mg l^{-1} butyric acid caused a massive increase in circulating lymphocytes and neutrophils, attributed to the irritant nature of the compound.

Reproductive Toxicity

Results of inhalation studies conducted on *n*-butanol and *n*-butyl acetate were negative for inducing reproductive and developmental toxicity. The NOEL for female reproductive toxicity was 6000 ppm for *n*-butanol and 1500 ppm for *n*-butyl acetate. In a 90-day repeated-dose inhalation toxicity study with butyl acetate, the NOEL for male reproductive toxicity was 3000 ppm. For developmental toxicity, an NOEL of 3500 ppm was observed with *n*-butanol and an NOEL of 1500 ppm (the highest exposure tested) was seen in both rats and rabbits following exposure to *n*-butyl acetate. Sprague–Dawley rats were administered butyric acid in corn oil by gavage on gestation days 6–15 at dose levels of 100 or 133 mg kg^{-1} day^{-1}. The dams were allowed to deliver, and their litters were examined on postnatal day 6. Maternal mortality was high (20 and 47% for the groups on 100 and 133 mg kg^{-1} day^{-1}, respectively), and maternal body weight gain was markedly depressed. Rales and dyspnea were reported for most treated animals. No evidence of effects on progeny were reported. In a frog embryo teratogenesis assay, it was found that butyric acid caused malformations in 50% of surviving offspring at a concentration of 400 mg l^{-1}. Malformations included microcephaly, eye defects, edema, and gut defects.

Genotoxicity

n-Butyric acid is not genotoxic. No clastogenic effects were seen in Chinese hamster fibroblast cells at concentrations up to 1 mg ml^{-1}. Butyric acid did not induce mutations at concentrations up to 10 mg per plate in an Ames *Salmonella typhimurium* test with strains TA 92, TA 94, TA 98, TA 100, TA 1535, and TA 1537 with or without a liver homogenate from rats pretreated with the polychlorinated biphenyl KC-400.

Carcinogenicity

n-Butyric acid is not a carcinogen.

Clinical Management

First Aid

Exposure should be terminated as soon as possible by the removal of the victim to fresh air. Call the emergency medical service. Give artificial respiration if the victim is not breathing. Do not use mouth-to-mouth resuscitation if the victim ingested or inhaled the substance; give artificial respiration with the aid of a pocket mask equipped with a one-way valve or other proper respiratory medical device. Administer oxygen if breathing is difficult. Remove and isolate contaminated clothing and shoes. In case of contact with the substance, immediately flush the skin or eyes with running water for at least 20 min. For minor skin contact, avoid spreading material on unaffected skin. Keep the victim warm and quiet. Effects of exposure (inhalation, ingestion, or skin contact) to the substance may be delayed. Ensure that medical personnel are aware of the material(s) involved and take precautions to protect themselves.

Medical Treatment

1. Oral exposure
   - Dilution: Immediately dilute with 120–240 ml) of water or milk (not to exceed 120 ml in a child). Because of potential gastrointestinal tract irritation, do not induce emesis.
   - Gastric lavage: Consider after ingestion of a potentially life-threatening amount of poison if it can be performed soon after ingestion (generally within 1 h). Protect the airway by placing the patient in the head down, left lateral decubitus position or by endotracheal intubation. Control any seizures first. Contraindications: loss of airway protective reflexes or decreased level of consciousness in unintubated patients; following ingestion of corrosives; hydrocarbons (high aspiration potential); patients at risk of hemorrhage or gastrointestinal perforation; and trivial or nontoxic ingestion.
   - Activated charcoal: Administer charcoal as a slurry (240 ml water/30 g charcoal). Usual dose: 25–100 g in adults/adolescents, 25–50 g in children (1–12 years), and 1 g kg^{-1} in infants less than 1 year old.
2. Inhalation exposure
   - Move patient to fresh air. Monitor for respiratory distress. If cough or difficult breathing develops, evaluate for respiratory tract irritation, bronchitis, or pneumonitis. Administer oxygen and assist ventilation as required. Treat bronchospasms with inhaled beta-2 agonist and oral or parenteral corticosteroids.
3. Eye exposure
   - Decontamination: Irrigate exposed eyes with copious amounts of water at room temperature for at least 15 min. If irritation, pain, swelling, lacrimation, or photophobia persist, the patient should be seen in a health care facility.
4. Dermal exposure
   - Decontamination: Remove contaminated clothing and wash exposed area thoroughly with soap and water. A physician may need to examine the area if irritation or pain persists.

Advanced Treatment

Consider orotracheal or nasotracheal intubation for airway control in the patient who is unconscious, has severe pulmonary edema, or is in severe respiratory distress. Early intubation, at the first sign of upper airway obstruction, may be necessary. Positive-pressure ventilation techniques with a bag valve mask device may be beneficial. Consider drug therapy for pulmonary edema. Consider administering a beta agonist such as albuterol for severe bronchospasm. Monitor cardiac rhythm and treat arrhythmias as necessary. Start intravenous administration of dextrose 5% in water (D5W) slow replacement protocol 'to keep open,' minimal flow rate. Use 0.9% saline or lactated Ringer solution if signs of hypovolemia are present. For hypotension with signs of hypovolemia, administer fluid cautiously. Consider vasopressors if the patient is hypotensive with a normal fluid volume. Watch for signs of fluid overload. Use proparacaine hydrochloride to assist eye irrigation.

Ecotoxicology

In freshwater or freshwater sediment, *n*-butyric acid is hazardous to aquatic life in high concentrations. The biological oxygen demand is 1.150 mg l^{-1} after 5 days and 1450 mg l^{-1} after 20 days. The LC_{50} for *Daphnia magna* (water flea) is 2750 mg l^{-1} after 24 h and 61 mg l^{-1} after 48 h; conditions of bioassay not specified.

The substance is harmful to marine aquatic organisms. Based on data from *n*-butyric acid and analogous compounds, it can be concluded that the toxicity of *n*-butyric acid (in unbuffered test systems) to fish, invertebrates, and green algae is expected to range between 22.7 and 77 mg l^{-1}. The LC_{50} for *Lepomis macrochirus* (Bluegill sunfish) is 5000 mg l^{-1} after 24 h (conditions of bioassay not specified; sodium salt).

With regard to the toxicity to terrestrial organisms (soil microorganisms, plants, terrestrial invertebrates, terrestrial vertebrates), nematodes either exposed to vapors of butyric acid or incubated in sand treated with butyric acid for 7 days showed a considerable reduction in number. Concentrations of 0.1 and 1 M of butyric acid significantly reduced the plant parasitic and fungivorous nematodes. A positive relationship was observed between the LC_{50} of butyric acid and the ratios of nematode surface area to volume for plant parasitic nematodes; a negative correlation in bacterivorous, entomogenous, and fungivorous nematodes was found.

Butyric acid forms carbon dioxide, carbon monoxide, and irritating fumes during combustion. Explosive vapor/air mixtures of butyric acid may be formed at temperatures above 72 °C.

Exposure Standards and Guidelines

Workplace exposure to *n*-butyric acid during manufacture and its use as an intermediate is limited by the use of closed processes, the use of protective clothing, and by the compound's limited volatility. Occupational Safety and Health Administration permissible exposure limit is not applicable; threshold limit value is also not applicable.

Butyric acid is designated as a hazardous substance under section 311(b) (A) of the Federal Water Pollution Control Act and further regulated by the Clean Water Act Amendments of 1977 and 1978. These regulations apply to discharges of this substance. This designation includes any isomers and hydrates, as well as any solutions and mixtures containing this substance. The US FDA requirements state that *n*-butyric acid used as a synthetic flavoring substance or adjuvant in animal drugs, feeds, and related products is generally recognized as safe when used in accordance with good manufacturing or feeding practice.

Miscellaneous

Analytical laboratory methods involve gas chromatography. Butyric acid treatment may result in sensitization of multiple intracellular signal transduction pathways including apoptotic signaling pathways and the p38 MAP kinase pathway.

See also: Butyraldehyde; Butyronitrile; Ethionine.

Further Reading

Blank-Porat, D., Gruss-Fischer, T., Tarasenko, N., Malik, Z., Nudelman, A., Rephaeli, A., 2007. The anticancer prodrugs of butyric acid AN-7 and AN-9, possess antiangiogenic properties. Cancer Lett. 256, 39–48.

Browning, M., Dawson, C., Alm, S.R., Gorrës, J.H., Amador, J.A., 2004. Differential effects of butyric acid on nematodes from four trophic groups. Appl. Soil Ecol. 27, 47–54.

Ochiai, K., Kurita-Ochiai, T., 2009. Effects of Butyric acid on the periodontal tissue. Jap. Dental Sci. Rev. 45, 75–82.

Spina, L., Cavallaro, F., Fardowza, N.I., Lagoussis, P., Bona, D., Ciscato, C., 2007. Butyric acid: pharmacological aspects and routes of administration. Dig. Liver Dis. Suppl. 1, 7–11.

Relevant Websites

http://chem.sis.nlm.nih.gov/chemidplus/
http://nlquery.epa.gov/epasearch/epasearch
http://www.osha.gov/dts/chemicalsampling/data/CH_223885.html
http://www.inchem.org/documents/icsc/icsc/eics1334.htm

Butyronitrile

C Pope, Oklahoma State University, Stillwater, OK, USA

Background

Butyronitrile is an aliphatic nitrile. Cyanide can be released through biological degradation processes to elicit toxicity.

- Molecular Formula: C_4H_7N
- Chemical Structure:

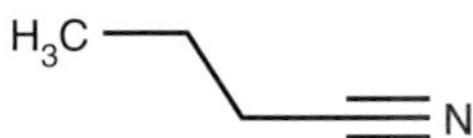

Uses

Butyronitrile is used as a process solvent and chemical intermediate.

Environmental Fate and Behavior

When heated to decomposition, nitriles may release cyanide. Butyronitriles can undergo microbial degradation, including transformation to cyanide and butyramide. Butyronitrile does not significantly hydrolyze at environmentally relevant pHs.

Butyronitrile use in chemical and pharmaceutical industry can lead to environmental contamination. It will exist as a vapor in the atmosphere, with degradation via photochemical products (hydroxyl radicals) and a half-life of approximately 1 month. In soil, butyronitrile is mobile ($K_{ow} = 46$). It can volatilize from wet or dry soil and from surface water. Butyronitrile can undergo microbial degradation to carboxylates and ammonium. In water, butyronitrile has little potential to adsorb to suspended particulates or sediment. Butyronitrile has little potential for bioconcentration or bioaccumulation.

Exposure and Exposure Monitoring

Dermal and inhalation routes are primary exposure pathways in occupational settings.

Toxicokinetics

Toxicokinetic data are available for the related chemical, propionitrile. When administered as a ^{14}C radioisotope in rats, 93% of the compound was recovered. Most radioactivity was eliminated in air or urine within 24 h. About 27% was recovered as a volatile organic material within 0.5 h of gavage exposure. By 3 h, either carbon dioxide or cyanide exhalation was estimated at 38–49% of the total. At 24 h, recovery in the urine was 0.8–6%. Less than 2% was found in liver and kidneys at 72 h after dosing. It was concluded that propionitrile and related alkyl nitriles are rapidly absorbed from the gastrointestinal tract and eliminated through expired air as the parent compound, CO_2 or cyanide.

Mechanism of Toxicity

The acute toxicity of butyronitrile and related alkyl nitriles is thought to be due to release of cyanide through metabolism of the parent compound. Signs of acute butyronitrile intoxication including dyspnea, ataxia, and convulsions are similar to those noted with acute cyanide intoxication. The onset and duration suggest that these nitriles require metabolism to elicit toxicity. Cyanide and thiocyanate have both been found in urine and blood after butyronitrile exposure. Butyronitrile toxicity is antagonized by sodium thiosulfate and sodium nitrite and blockade of hepatic metabolism. All of these support the hypothesis that cyanide is the ultimate toxicant following butyronitrile exposure.

Acute and Short-Term Toxicity

Animal

The oral LD_{50} values in rats for all butyronitriles are from 40 to 270 mg kg^{-1}. Inhalation LD_{50} values (1–4 h exposure) were from 1000 to 1465 ppm. Dermal LD_{50} values of *n*-butyronitrile and isobutyronitrile in rabbits were 239–389 mg kg^{-1}. Butyronitrile is a mild eye and skin irritant. Aliphatic nitriles including butyronitrile were shown to affect embryonic development *in utero* and in culture, apparently through liberation of cyanide.

Human

Skin and eye irritation can occur. With severe intoxication, characteristic signs of cyanide toxicity can be elicited. Headache, dizziness, weakness, exhaustion, confusion, convulsions, dyspnea, abdominal pain, nausea, and vomiting are possible.

Chronic Toxicity

Animal

In a developmental toxicity study, rats exposed to 50, 100, or 200 ppm butyronitrile for 6 h a day during gestation showed no teratogenic effects but did exhibit decreased fetal weights at the highest dosage. As noted above, some data indicate potential for disruption of embryonic development with exposures to aliphatic nitriles. Repeated exposures to propionitrile led to neurotoxicity (ataxia, tremors, and convulsions) at high dosage levels. Dyspnea, nasal, and ocular discharge, increased salivation, reduced motor activity, and alopecia were

 http://dx.doi.org/10.1016/B978-0-12-386454-3.00104-4

observed. Significant reduction in red blood cells and hemoglobin and increases in spleen weights were also noted.

Human

Little is known regarding chronic effects of butyronitrile exposure in humans.

Immunotoxicity

There is little information on immunotoxic effects of butyronitrile or other alkyl nitriles.

Reproductive Toxicity

Butyronitrile and other alkyl nitriles have little evidence of reproductive toxicity potential.

Genotoxicity

Butyronitriles were generally negative in *in vitro* mutagenicity and cytogenetic assays.

Carcinogenicity

Butyronitrile is not classified as a known, possible, probable, anticipated, or potential carcinogen.

Clinical Management

For mild signs of intoxication (nausea, dizziness, and drowsiness) with blood cyanide concentrations $<2\ \mathrm{mg\,l^{-1}}$, give oxygen and bed rest. With more severe intoxication exhibiting short-lived periods of unconsciousness, convulsions, vomiting, and/or cyanosis and with blood cyanide concentrations of 2–3 $\mathrm{mg\,l^{-1}}$, provide 100% oxygen for not more than 24 h and observe in intensive care area. Give 50 ml of 25% sodium thiosulfate solution (1.5 g) intravenously over 10 min.

Ecotoxicology

Concentrations near 100 $\mathrm{mg\,l^{-1}}$ (96-h static) of both isobutyronitrile and *n*-butyronitrile were without effect on fathead minnows. Daphnia treated with 94.3 $\mathrm{mg\,l^{-1}}$ isobutyronitrile showed no abnormal behavior or movement changes. The same concentration of *n*-butyronitrile resulted in 1/20 daphnids becoming immobile at 48 h, but this was not considered treatment related. According to the U.S. Environmental Protection Agency (EPA) assessment criteria, these values correspond to a 'low concern level.'

Exposure Standards and Guidelines

The time-weighted average (TWA) for butyronitrile is 8 ppm. No permissible exposure limit or reference concentration is available.

See also: Cyanide; Solvents.

Further Reading

Grogan, J., DeVito, S.C., Pearlman, R.S., Korzekwa, K.R., 1992. Modeling cyanide release from nitriles: prediction of cytochrome P450 mediated acute nitrile toxicity. Chem. Res. Toxicol. 5, 548–552.

Saillenfait, A.M., Sabaté, J.P., 2000. Comparative developmental toxicities of aliphatic nitriles: *in vivo* and *in vitro* observations. Toxicol. Appl. Pharmacol. 163, 149–163.

Relevant Websites

http://www.cdc.gov/niosh/pdfs/78-212b.pdf.
http://www.cdc.gov/niosh/npg/npgd0086.html.
http://www.epa.gov/hpv/pubs/summaries/alkyntrl/c14860.pdf.

Butyrophenones

J Chilakapati, Alcon Laboratories, Fort Worth, TX, USA
HM Mehendale, University of Louisiana at Monroe, Monroe, LA, USA

- Name: Butyrophenones
- Chemical Abstracts Service Registry Numbers: Butyrophenone: 495-40-9; Haloperidol: 52-86-8; Droperidol: 548-73-2; Melperone: 3575-80-2; Domperidone: 57808-66-9
- Synonyms: Butyrophenone: 1-Phenyl-1-butanone; Haloperidol: ((4-[4-(4-Chlorophenyl)-4-hydroxy-1-piperidyl]-1-(4-fluorophenyl)-butan-1-one); Droperidol: 1-(1-(3-(*p*-Fluorobenzoyl)propyl)-1,2,3,6-tetrahydro-4-pyridyl)-2-benzimidazolinone; Melperone: 1-(4-Fluorophenyl)-4-(4-methyl-1-piperidyl)butan-1-one; Domperidone: 2H-Benzimidazol-2-one, 5-chloro-1-(1-(3-(2,3-dihydro-2-oxo-1H-benzimidazol-1-yl)propyl)-4-piperidinyl)-1,3-dihydro-
- Molecular Formula: Butyrephenone: $C_6H_5COCH_2CH_2CH_3$ (molecular weight 148.3); Haloperidol: $C_{21}H_{23}ClFNO_2$ (molecular weight 375.9); Droperidol: $C_{22}H_{22}FN_3O_2$ (molecular weight 379.43); Melperone: $C_{16}H_{22}FNO \cdot HCl$ (molecular weight 263.35); Domperidone: $C_{22}H_{24}ClN_5O_2$ (molecular weight 425.911)
- Chemical Structures:

Butyrophenone (CASRN: 495-40-9)

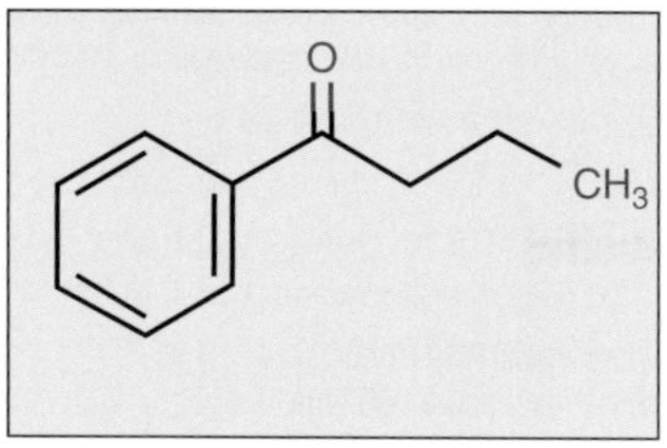

Haloperidol (CASRN: 52-86-8)

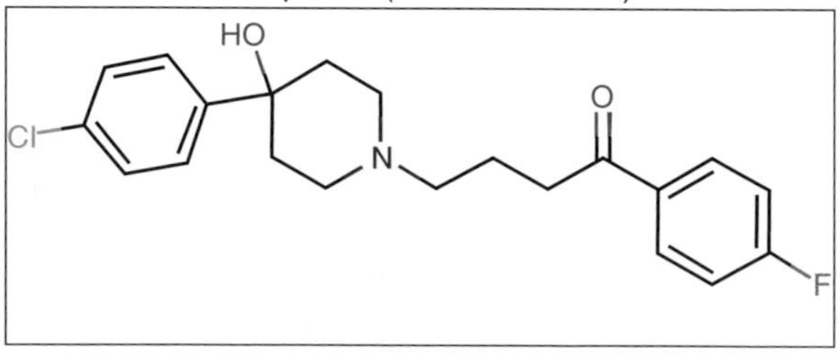

Droperidol (CASRN: 548-73-2)

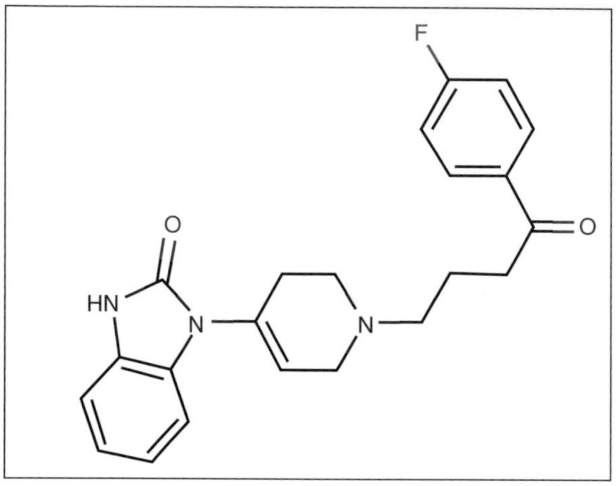

Melperone (CASRN: 3575-80-2)

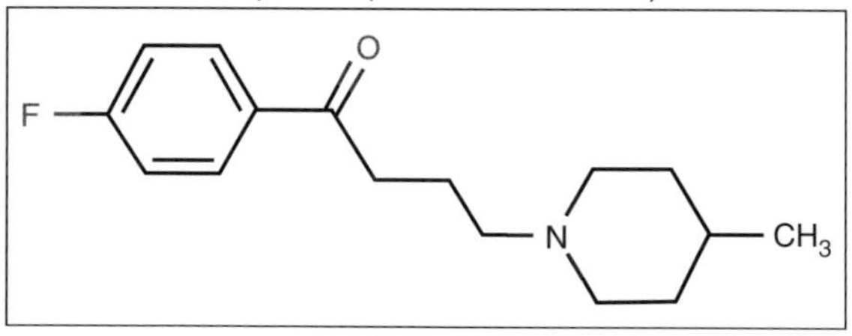

Domperidone (CASRN: 57808-66-9)

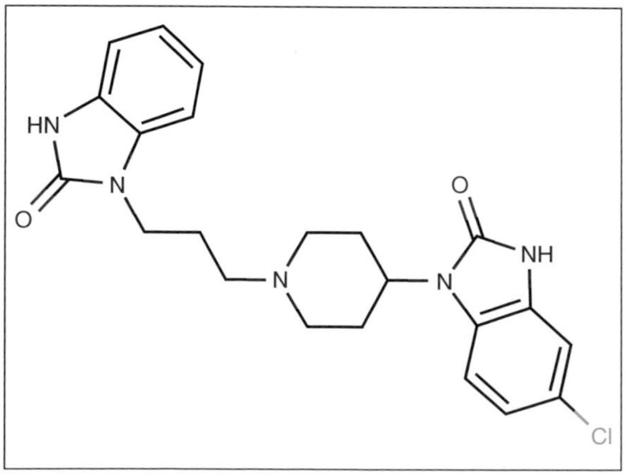

 http://dx.doi.org/10.1016/B978-0-12-386454-3.00265-7

Background

Haloperidol is a synthetic product (approved for use in the United States in 1967), and is one of the first of the butyrophenone series of major tranquilizers. Besides its use in psychotic disorders such as schizophrenia and mania, it is indicated for the control of tics and vocal utterances of Tourette's disorder in children and adults. It is also used in the management of Gilles de La Tourette's syndrome and intractable hiccup. It is also used as an antiemetic, and for the treatment of severe behavior problems in children of combative, explosive hyperexcitability. The main features of severe overdosage are extrapyramidal reactions, hypotension, respiratory difficulty, and impairment of consciousness. Haloperidol acts mainly as a dopamine antagonist. Consciousness may be depressed, progressing to coma; paradoxically, some patients manifest confusion, excitement, and restlessness. Tremor or muscle twitching, muscle spasm, rigidity, and convulsions are seen. Extrapyramidal signs can include dystonia, sometimes severe enough to impair swallowing or breathing; torticollis; oculogyric crises; and opisthotonos. The pupils may be constricted or dilated. Hypotension and tachycardia are common. Sometimes there can be cardiac arrhythmias, including ventricular fibrillation, conduction defects, and cardiac arrest.

Severe dystonic reactions have followed the use of haloperidol, particularly in children and adolescents. It should therefore be used with extreme care in children. Haloperidol may also cause severe neurotoxic reactions in patients with hyperthyroidism and in patients receiving lithium. Haloperidol is contraindicated in severe toxic central nervous system depression or comatose states from any cause and individuals who are hypersensitive to this drug or have Parkinson's disease. The decanoate ester of haloperidol is very slowly absorbed from the site of injection and is therefore suitable for depot injection. It is gradually released into the bloodstream where it is rapidly hydrolyzed to haloperidol.

Drug Interactions

The use of alcohol with this drug should be avoided due to possible additive effects and hypotension.

Lithium

Treatment with lithium plus haloperidol for encephalopathic syndrome (characterized by weakness, lethargy, fever, tremulousness and confusion, extrapyramidal symptoms, leukocytosis, elevated serum enzymes, blood urea nitrogen (BUN), and fasting blood sugar (FBS)) patients resulted in irreversible brain damage in a few patients. Although a causal relationship between these events and the concomitant administration of lithium and haloperidol has not been established, patients receiving such combination therapy should be monitored closely for early evidence of neurological toxicity and treatment discontinued promptly if such signs appear.

Beta-Blockers

Severe hypotension or pulmonary arrest may be a consequence of the haloperidol and beta-blocker combination.

Methyldopa

When used with methyldopa, haloperidol causes dementia, psychomotor retardation, memory impairment, and inability to concentrate.

Indomethacin

Main adverse effects: Severe drowsiness and confusion. In general, the symptoms of overdose would be an exaggeration of known pharmacological effects and adverse reactions. Anticholinergic side effects and sedation occur less often than with aliphatic phenothiazines, but extrapyramidal reactions are more common. Administration of antidopaminergic and anticholinergics may worsen or bring forward the onset of extrapyramidal effects. This drug can produce idiosyncratic reaction, e.g., drowsiness. When used with indomethacin, haloperidol causes severe drowsiness and confusion. Other interacting drugs are levodopa, quinidine, tricyclic antidepressants, epinephrine, and amphetamines.

Uses

Butyrophenones (compounds with a functional ketone group) are used to treat psychoses including schizophrenia, organic psychosis, paranoid syndrome, acute idiopathic psychotic illnesses, and the manic phase of manic depressive illness. Other uses include treatment of aggressive behavior, delirium, acute anxiety, nausea and vomiting, pain, organic brain syndrome, and Tourette's syndrome.

Environmental Fate and Behavior

Haloperidol's production and use as an antidyskinetic and an antipsychotic may result in its release to the environment through various waste streams. If released to air, an estimated vapor pressure of 4.85×10^{-11} mmHg at 25 °C indicates haloperidol will exist solely in the particulate phase in the ambient atmosphere. Particulate-phase haloperidol will be removed from the atmosphere by wet and dry deposition. If released to soil, haloperidol is expected to have no mobility based on an estimated K_{oc} of 5200. Volatilization from moist soil surfaces is not expected to be an important fate process based on an estimated Henry's law constant of 2.3×10^{-14} atm m^3 mol^{-1}. The pK_a of haloperidol is 8.66, indicating that this compound will exist primarily in the protonated form in the environment, and cations generally adsorb more strongly to organic carbon and clay than their neutral counterparts. If released into water, haloperidol is expected to adsorb to suspended solids and sediment based on the estimated K_{oc}. Volatilization from water surfaces is not expected to be an important fate process based on this compound's estimated Henry's law constant. Haloperidol will exist almost entirely in the ionized form at pH values of 5–9, and therefore volatilization from water surfaces is not expected to be an important fate process. An estimated bioconcentration factor of 59 suggests the potential for bioconcentration in aquatic organisms is moderate. Hydrolysis is not expected to be an important environmental fate process since this compound lacks functional groups that hydrolyze under environmental conditions. Occupational exposure to haloperidol may occur through dermal contact with this compound at workplaces where haloperidol is produced or used. Users of haloperidol can be exposed through intravenous injection or oral consumption (tablets and liquid).

Pharmacokinetics and Toxicokinetics

Haloperidol is well absorbed orally with a bioavailability of 60–65% due to first-pass hepatic metabolism. It has a reversible oxidation/reduction metabolic pathway: it is metabolized via reduction to reduced haloperidol, which is biologically inactive. Both agents are rapidly absorbed after intramuscular injection, peaking within 10 min. Butyrophenones are metabolized in the liver to inactive metabolites. Concentrations of butyrophenones are found in the liver, in the central nervous system, and throughout the body. Haloperidol is 92% protein bound. Up to 15% haloperidol is eliminated through the bile. The elimination half-life is 14–41 h. The half-life of droperidol is 2 h; 10% is recovered unchanged in the urine. The apparent volume of distribution is about 20 l kg^{-1}, consistent with the high lipophilicity of the drug. Haloperidol circulates in blood bound predominantly (90–94%) to plasma proteins.

Although the exact metabolic fate has not been clearly established, it appears that haloperidol is principally metabolized in the liver by oxidative *N*-dealkylation of the piperidine nitrogen to form fluorophenylcarbonic acids and piperidine metabolites (which appear to be inactive), and by reduction of the butyrophenone carbonyl to the carbinol, forming hydroxyhaloperidol. Few studies suggest that the reduced metabolite, hydroxyhaloperidol, has some pharmacologic activity, although its activity appears to be less than that of haloperidol. Several metabolites have been identified: *p*-fluorophenaceturic acid, beta-*p*-fluorobenzoylpropionic acid, and several unidentified acids in urinary metabolites in rats.

Primary biotransformation enzymes of haloperidol are cytochrome P450 (CYP), carbonyl reductase, and uridine diphosphoglucose glucuronosyltransferase. The greatest proportion of the intrinsic hepatic clearance of haloperidol is by glucuronidation, followed by the reduction of haloperidol to reduced haloperidol and by CYP-mediated oxidation (CYP3A4 appears to be the major isoform responsible for the metabolism of haloperidol in humans). The intrinsic clearances of the back-oxidation of reduced haloperidol to the parent compound, oxidative *N*-dealkylation, and pyridinium formation are of the same order of magnitude, suggesting that the same enzyme system is responsible for the three reactions. Large variation in the catalytic activity was observed in the CYP-mediated reactions, whereas there appeared to be only small variations in the glucuronidation and carbonyl reduction pathways. Haloperidol is a substrate of CYP3A4 and an inhibitor, as well as a stimulator, of CYP2D6.

In vivo pharmacogenetic studies have indicated that the metabolism and disposition of haloperidol may be regulated by genetically determined polymorphic CYP2D6 activity. However, these findings appear to contradict those from studies *in vitro* with human liver microsomes and from studies of drug interactions *in vivo*. Interethnic and pharmacogenetic differences in haloperidol metabolism may explain these observations. There is wide intersubject variation in plasma concentration of haloperidol and its therapeutic effects.

Pharmacodynamics

Dopamine receptors currently are classified as D1 (stimulate adenylate cyclase) and D2 (inhibit adenylate cyclase). Neuroleptic drugs block both D1 and D2 receptors, but the significance of the ratio remains unclear. The therapeutic dose of neuroleptic drug appears to correlate with its affinity for brain dopamine D2 receptors. Neuroleptic drugs also block a number of other receptors, including H1 and H2 histamine, alpha-1 and alpha-2 adrenergic, muscarinic and serotoninergic receptors.

Toxicity

Human data

There have been three cases of sudden death after taking 20–140 mg daily for 1–4 days. Children: A 29-month-old girl and an 11-month-old boy who divided 265 mg of haloperidol between them developed lethargy, hypothermia, hyperreflexia, neuromuscular rigidity, unsteady gait, and intention tremors. Although disturbances such as galactorrhea, amenorrhea, gynecomastia, and impotence have been reported, the clinical significance of elevated serum prolactin levels is unknown for most patients.

Mechanism of Toxicity

Butyrophenones work primarily by blocking dopamine-mediated synaptic neurotransmission by binding to dopamine receptors. In addition to significant antidopaminergic action, butyrophenones also possess anticholinergic, α-adrenergic blockade, and quinidine-like effects. The antiemetic mechanism of droperidol is believed to involve direct suppression of the chemoemetic trigger zone.

The mechanism by which haloperidol causes serum aminotransferase elevation is not known, but is likely due to production of a toxic intermediate by its metabolism. Haloperidol is extensively metabolized by the liver via sulfoxidation and oxidation, partially via CYP3A4. Some instances of serum aminotransferase elevations occurring on haloperidol therapy may be due to nonalcoholic fatty liver disease caused by weight gain that occurs in at least one-quarter of treated patients, generally during the first 1–2 years of therapy.

Although the exact metabolic fate of droperidol is not clearly established, the drug is metabolized in the liver. The butyrophenone moiety of droperidol is metabolized to *p*-fluorophenylacetic acid, which is then conjugated with glycine. The nitrogenous moiety of droperidol appears to be metabolized to benzimidazolone and *p*-hydroxypiperidine.

Acute and Short-Term Toxicity (or Exposure)

Animal

Signs of toxicity reported in animals have included sedation, dullness, photosensitivity, weakness, anorexia, fever, icterus, colic, anemia, and hemoglobinuria. Treatment consists of gastric decontamination and aggressive supportive care.

Human

Clinical signs of toxicity most commonly include extrapyramidal effects, somnolence, coma, respiratory depression, cardiac dysrhythmias, hypotension, and sedation. Neuroleptic malignant syndrome has been reported after therapeutic use and acute intoxication. The most commonly reported dystonic reactions include akathisias, stiff neck, stiff or protruding tongue, and tremor. Children appear to be more sensitive than adults to the extrapyramidal effects of butyrophenones with facial grimacing and oculogyric crisis noted. Anticholinergic effects, including dry mouth, blurred vision, and tachycardia, may occur. Other cardiac effects include prolonged QT interval and mild hypotension. Hypokalemia has also been noted. Since haloperidol may lower the seizure threshold, the drug should be used with caution in patients receiving anticonvulsant agents and in those with a history of seizures of electroencephalographic abnormalities. Possible sequelae include neuroleptic malignant syndrome and acute renal failure. Adverse reactions following therapeutic use include sedation, dysphoria, anorexia, nausea, vomiting, constipation, diarrhea, and dyspepsia.

Chronic Toxicity (or Exposure)

Animal

Rats chronically treated with haloperidol (1.5 mg kg^{-1} i.p.) significantly developed vacuous chewing movements and tongue protrusions.

Human

Chronic poisoning by ingestion may induce neurological syndromes, the most severe of which are parkinsonism, akathisia, and tardive dyskinesia, a syndrome that is characterized by rhythmical, involuntary movements of the tongue, face, mouth, or jaw (e.g., protrusion of tongue, puffing of cheeks, puckering of mouth, chewing movements). Sometimes these may be accompanied by involuntary movements of extremities.

Reproductive Toxicity

These agents are contraindicated in humans during late pregnancy because of dystonic reaction in the neonate. Infants should not be nursed during drug treatment. There are no well-controlled studies with haloperidol in pregnant women. There are reports, however, of cases of limb malformations observed following maternal use of haloperidol along with other drugs that have suspected teratogenic potential during the first trimester of pregnancy (causal relationships not established in these cases). Since such experience does not exclude the possibility of fetal damage due to haloperidol, this drug should be used during pregnancy or in women likely to become pregnant only if the benefit clearly justifies a potential risk to the fetus.

Carcinogenicity

Carcinogenicity studies using oral haloperidol were conducted in Wistar rats and in albino Swiss mice. In the rat study, survival was less than optimal in all dose groups, reducing the number of rats at risk for developing tumors. However, although a relatively greater number of rats survived to the end of the study in high-dose male and female groups, these animals did not have a greater incidence of tumors than control animals. Therefore, although not optimal, this study does suggest the absence of haloperidol-related increase in the incidence of neoplasia in rats. In female mice, there was a statistically significant increase in mammary gland neoplasia and total tumor incidence; there was a statistically significant increase in pituitary gland neoplasia. In male mice, no statistically significant differences in incidence of total tumors or specific tumor types were noted. Neuroleptic drugs elevate prolactin levels; the elevation persists during chronic administration. Teratogenicity: Rodents given haloperidol by oral or parenteral routes showed an increase in incidence of resorption, reduced fertility, delayed delivery, and pup mortality. No teratogenic effect has been reported in rats, rabbits, or dogs at dosages within this range, but cleft palate has been observed in mice.

Mutagenicity

No mutagenic potential of haloperidol was found in the Ames *Salmonella* microsomal activation assay.

Clinical Management

All basic and advanced life-support measures should be implemented. Gastric decontamination should be performed. Butyrophenones are readily absorbed by activated charcoal. Emesis should not be induced. Aggressive supportive care should be instituted. Dystonic reactions respond well to intravenous benztropine or diphenhydramine. Oral therapy with diphenhydramine or benztropine should be continued for 2 days to prevent recurrence of the dystonic reaction. For patients suffering from neuroleptic malignant syndrome, a potentially fatal condition associated with the administration of antipsychotic drugs, dantrolene sodium and bromocriptine have been used in conjunction with cooling and other supportive measures. Arrhythmias should be treated with lidocaine or phenytoin. Diazepam is the drug of choice for seizures; phenytoin is used to prevent recurrence. Hemodialysis and hemoperfusion have not been shown to be effective.

Exposure Routes and Pathways

Haloperidol is available both in an injectable form and in oral dosage form. The principal exposure pathway is intentional ingestion by adults or accidental ingestion by small children. Pharmacists, physicians, and nurses dispensing or administering haloperidol could be exposed through dermal contact. Droperidol is available only as an injectable drug. The most common route of exposure is an accidental injection.

See also: Anxiolytics; Neurotoxicity.

Further Reading

Altunkaynak, B.Z., Ozbek, E., Unal, B., et al., 2012. Chronic treatment of haloperidol induces pathological changes in striatal neurons of guinea pigs: a light and electron microscopical study. Drug Chem. Toxicol. 35 (4), 406–411.

de Oliveira, G.V., Gomes, P.X., de Araújo, F.Y., et al., 2013. Prevention of haloperidol-induced alterations in brain acetylcholinesterase activity by vitamins B co-administration in a rodent model of tardive dyskinesia. Metab. Brain Dis. 28 (1), 53–59.

Declercq, T., Petrovic, M., Azermai, M., et al., 2013. Withdrawal versus continuation of chronic antipsychotic drugs for behavioural and psychological symptoms in older people with dementia. Cochrane Database Syst. Rev. 3, CD007726. http://dx.doi.org/10.1002/14651858.CD007726.pub2.

Gajre, M.P., Jain, D., Jadhav, A., November–December 2012. Accidental haloperidol poisoning in children. Indian J. Pharmacol. 44 (6), 803–804.

Ikemura, M., Nakagawa, Y., Shinone, K., Inoue, H., Nata, M., 2012. The blood concentration and organ distribution of haloperidol at therapeutic and toxic doses in severe fatty liver disease. Leg Med. (Tokyo) 14 (3), 147–153.

Larry, D., Ripault, M.P., 2013. Hepatotoxicity of psychotropic drugs and drugs of abuse. In: Kaplowitz, N., DeLeve, L.D. (Eds.), Drug-Induced Liver Disease, third ed. Elsevier, Amsterdam, pp. 443–6226.

Molleston, J.P., Fontana, R.J., Lopez, M.J., et al., 2011. Characteristics of idiosyncratic drug-induced liver injury in children: results from the DILIN prospective study. J. Pediatr. Gastroenterol. Nutr. 53 (2), 182–189.

Richards, J.R., Schneir, A.B., 2003. Droperidol in the emergency department: is it safe? J. Emerg. Med. 24 (4), 441–447.

Spiller, H.A., Hays, H.L., Aleguas Jr., A., 2013. Overdose of drugs for attention-deficit hyperactivity disorder: clinical presentation, mechanisms of toxicity, and management. CNS Drugs 27 (7), 531–543.

Xu, H., Yang, H.J., Rose, G.M., 2012. Chronic haloperidol-induced spatial memory deficits accompany the upregulation of D(1) and D(2) receptors in the caudate putamen of C57BL/6 mouse. Life Sci. 91 (9–10), 322–328.

Relevant Websites

http://www.drugs.com/pro/haldol.html – Drugs.com.

http://www.genome.jp/kegg-bin/show_pathway?map07031 – KEGG Pathway metabolism.

http://emedicine.medscape.com/article/815881-overview#a0199 – Medscape.

http://dailymed.nlm.nih.gov/dailymed/search.cfm?startswith=DOMPERIDONE – National Library of Medicine.

http://livertox.nlm.nih.gov/Haloperidol.htm – National Library of Medicine.

http://toxnet.nlm.nih.gov – Toxnet (Toxicology Data Network): search for Butyrophenones.

http://pubchem.ncbi.nlm.nih.gov/summary/summary.cgi?sid=134222172 – US National Library of Medicine (Pubchem): Melperone.

BZ (3-Quinuclidinyl Benzilate): Psychotomimetic Agent

RE Jabbour and H Salem, RDECOM, Edgewood Chemical Biological Center, MD, USA

This article is a revision of the previous edition article by Harry Salem, volume 1, pp 373–374, © 2005, Elsevier Inc.

- Name: BZ
- Chemical Abstracts Service Registry Number: 6581-06-2
- Synonyms: 3-Quinuclidinyl benzilate (3-QNB-BZ); 1-Azabicyclo(2.2.2)octan-3-ol, benzilate (9CI); Benzene acetic acid, alpha-hydroxy-alpha-phenyl-, 1-azabicyclo (2.2.2)oct-3-yl ester (9CI); Benzilic acid, 3-quinuclidinyl ester; 3-Chinuclidylbenzilate; 3-(2,2-Diphenyl-2-hydroxyethanoyloxy)-quinuclidine; Quinuclidinyl benzilate (QNB-BZ); Agent Buzz; Agent 15
- Molecular Formula: $C_{21}H_{23}NO_3$
- Chemical Structure:

HO
O
N
O

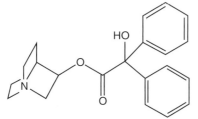

Background (Significance/History)

The 3-quinuclidinyl benzilate (3-QNB) was first discovered by Hoffmann-La Roche in 1951 during research investigation that involved development of antispasmodic agents, resembling atropine, for treating gastrointestinal conditions. Soon after, the US Army investigated 3-QNB under the name of EA2277 agent and was standardized for use in chemical munitions in 1961 under the name agent of BZ. The United States declared complete destruction of its stockpile of BZ by 1989. Moreover, Agent 15 is speculated either to be identical to BZ or a closely related derivative, and has similar physicochemical properties as BZ. In 1998, Agent 15 was speculated to be stockpiled by Iraq but later on intelligence reports did not find any conclusive evidence for such claim[1]. The BZ is a glycolate anticholinergic chemical related to atropine, scopolamine, and, hyoscyamine. It is odorless, nonirritating, and is stable in most solvents. It has a half-life of 3–4 weeks in moist air and is extremely persistent in soil, water, and most surfaces. BZ has a slow onset and a long duration-of-action. The rate of BZ action climaxed after 9.5 h of exposure and the duration-of-action could last up to 96 h. Moreover, most of the causalities of BZ exposure will require physical restraint and continuous monitoring to prevent self-injury and paranoia symptoms during recovery[2]. Recent speculation about the usage of Agent 15 in Syrian civil war had been reported but no confirmation findings had been established[3].

Uses

BZ is a nonlethal chemical warfare agent that following a delayed onset is incapacitating and causes severe hallucinations. US Army intended to use BZ in critical point situations such as special operation, incapacitating adversaries during raid, and overcoming fortified field positions. Medically, BZ is used as a muscarinic receptor antagonist.

Environmental Fate and Behavior

QNB-BZ or Agent 15 has been tested on different surfaces by the US Army Medical Research Institute of Chemical Defense and the overall conclusion was that QNB-BZ persists as a parent molecule for an extended period of time reaching 72 h[4].

Environmental Persistency (Degradation/Speciation)

BZ persistent was measured on different surfaces and media. The study included soil, water, aerosol (wind tunnel), glass, granite, water, pavement, etc. BZ has half-life of 3–4 weeks in moist air. Quinuclidinyl benzoate hydrolyzes to quinuclidine and benzylic acid; the hydrolysis rate at 25 °C and pH 6.8–8.10 was 0.000 377–0.008 9 per hour[5].

Exposure and Exposure Monitoring

Exposure to BZ agent is through inhalation of aerosolized solid or BZ dissolved in a solvent such as propylene glycol, dimethyl sulfoxide, and other solvents. Exposure can also occur through the skin and via the gastrointestinal tract.

Toxicokinetics

BZ is a competitive inhibitor of muscarinic receptors associated with the parasympathetic nervous system that innervates the eyes, heart, respiratory system, skin, gastrointestinal tract, and bladder. The sweat glands, innervated by the sympathetic nervous system, are also modulated by muscarinic receptors. By any route of exposure, the onset of action is approximately 1 h, with peak effects occurring 8 h postexposure. Signs and symptoms gradually subside over 2–4 days. Most of the absorbed BZ is excreted via the kidney.

Mechanism of Toxicity

BZ acts by blocking the action of acetylcholine on the central and peripheral nervous systems. It is a tertiary amine and crosses the blood–brain barrier. BZ on acute exposure increases both heart and respiratory rates, dilates the pupils, and causes paralysis of the eye muscles necessary for near focusing. It also causes dry mouth and skin, elevates body temperature, impairs coordination, and causes flushing of the skin, hallucinations, stupor, forgetfulness, and confusion.

 http://dx.doi.org/10.1016/B978-0-12-386454-3.00592-3

Within 15 min to 4 h following exposure, the principal effects are dizziness, involuntary muscle movements, near vision difficulty, and total incapacitation. From 6 to 10 h after exposure, the effects are psychotropic and full recovery is expected after 4 days.

The peripheral nervous system effects are considered as understimulation of the end organs. This decreased stimulation of eccrine and apocrine sweat glands in the skin results in dry skin and a dry mouth, and is considered 'dry as a bone.' The reduction in the ability to dispel heat by evaporative cooling decreases sweating, and the compensatory cutaneous vasodilation causes the skin to become warm or 'hot as a hare' and 'red as a beet.' This is similar to the atropine flush. The decreased heat loss also results in an increased core temperature.

The peripheral effects described above usually precede the central nervous system (CNS) effects and have been summarized by the mnemonic 'dry as a bone, hot as hares, red as a beet, and blind as a bat.'

The CNS effects of BZ and Agent 15 result in dose-dependent 'mad as a hatter' mental changes. These effects fluctuate between a conscious state and delirium that range from drowsiness to coma. Disorientation, decreased social restraints, inappropriate behavior, and decreased short-term memory are common. Speech becomes slurred and indistinct.

The human estimated incapacitation ICt_{50} is reported to be 100 mg min m^{-3} and the LCt_{50} to be 200 000 mg min m^{-3}.

Acute and Short-Term Toxicity (Animal/Human)

Acute Human Toxicity

Very limited data are available regarding lethality in humans following the exposure to BZ agent. Limited data on human exposure to BZ have been reported by the Board on Environmental Studies and Toxicology, National Research Council[6]. Briefly, four subjects were exposed to varying concentrations ranging from 0.5–8 μg kg^{-1} and for 8 days. The result of this study showed that the exposure subjects did not show any unexpected symptoms beyond the common BZ symptoms of high blood pressure, hallucination, and disorientation. Also, there are reported human toxicity estimates for the nitrogen mustard compound. The toxicity data collected by Natural Resources Defense Council (NRDC) study showed that the body parts affected by the exposure were directly related to the type of nitrogen mustard vapor and to the concentration level. Overall, nitrogen mustards have a relative potency of HN3 > HN1 > HN2 and concentration increases inflict erythema on the neck, upper back, and auxiliary folds.

Acute Animal Toxicity

As shown in **Table 1**, the acute animal toxicity of exposure to BZ has been measured in mice, rats, guinea pigs, rabbits, and dogs. The research showed that the LD_{50} is 18–25 mg kg^{-1} and it was determined that the parent molecule of BZ is extremely toxic as compared to its hydrolysis products, i.e., benzylic acid and 3-quinuclidinyl. The symptoms of exposure to high dose of BZ were shown in increased heart rate, large cases of death, and impaired performance.

Table 1 Acute toxicity

Species	*LCt_{50} (mg min m^{-3})*	*IV LD_{50} (mg kg^{-1})*
Mouse	12 000	14.1
Rats	64 000	14.0
Guinea pigs	123 000	10.0
Rabbits	32 000	10.0
Dogs	25 000	9.6

Subchronic and Chronic Toxicity (Animal/Human)

Although the chronic toxicity in human is not well studied, the animal testing result could be extrapolated to predict human response to chronic exposure to BZ. The reported results on animal testing in dogs show that chronic and subchronic exposure to BZ for 40–50 days at 100 μg kg^{-1} affected the gastrointestinal tract causing ulceration and bloody stool. Moreover, there was a slight decrease in the weight of kidney and liver upon chronic exposure to BZ.

Immunotoxicity

Animal studies had been reported on the effect of BZ on the immunotoxicity of the studied rats. In this study, acute exposure of rats to BZ showed a decrease in nonspecific resistance of the organism to various infections. Also, it reduces the antibody production mainly to T-dependent antigens. A decrease in the antibody-dependent cell-mediated cytotoxicity, and BZ exposure suppressed the formation of delayed type hypersensitivity.

Genotoxicity

No human genotoxicity data were identified for BZ, but the details for potential genotoxicity effect could potentially resemble those observed with exposure to Atropine containing compounds.

Ecotoxicology

BZ in aerosolized form tends to persist for 3–4 weeks and in liquid and aquatic environment BZ does not hydrolyze easily and persist in water and estuary. As for solid surface the BZ is very stable in soil, concrete, glass, and on other solid surfaces as the parent molecule. BZ hydrolyze upon heat and in aqueous solution into benzylic acid and 3-quinuclidinyl by-product, both are less toxic than BZ.

Clinical Management

The clinical effects from exposure to BZ through ingestion or inhalation could be observed as early as 30 min or as late as 20 h, with a common range of 0.5–4 h and a mean of 2 h. Skin exposure to BZ release could show clinical effect as late as 36 h. The duration-of-effect is typically 72–96 h and is dose dependent, with mild effect persisting in some cases for several days.

The clinical course from BZ poisoning can be divided into the following four stages:

- First phase (0–4 h after exposure), often results in parasympathetic blockade and mild CNS effects.
- Second phase (4–20 h after exposure), stupor with ataxia and hyperthermia.
- Third phase (20–96 h after exposure), full-blown delirium is seen but with periodic and frequent fluctuations.
- Fourth phase (>96 h after exposure), paranoia, deep sleep, reawakening, crawling or climbing automatisms, and eventual reorientation.

The common signs and symptoms of exposure to BZ are varied and include restlessness, dizziness, failure to obey orders, erratic behavior, stumbling, tachycardia, blurred vision, pupillary dilation, slurred speech, hallucinations, inappropriate smiling or laughter, elevated blood pressure, stomach cramps and vomiting, and euphoria. Patients who lack anticholinergic peripheral nervous system (PNS) signs could also experience panic attack after BZ exposure.

Medical Management

The initial medical management of exposed patients to BZ should include decontamination of skin and clothing, confiscation of weapons and related items, and observation. Physical restraint is essential for patients having erratic behavior that could endanger the patients and medical staff. Moreover, patients exposed to BZ could develop hyperthermia due to the nature of surrounding environment (hot, humid, or dehydrated conditions) and overexposure to BZ could lead to comatose with serious cardiac arrest and electrolyte disturbance and imbalance.

Since BZ decreases the level of acetylcholine throughout the body, specific antidotal therapy is required. The antidotal therapy involves administering carbamate anticholinesterase physostigmine to raise acetylcholine concentration level in the body. In patients with BZ poisoning affecting their CNS, physostigmine is used to inhibit postsynaptic activities of BZ. The effectiveness of oral administration of physostigmine is maximized after 4 h from BZ exposure. Intramuscular or intravenous (IV) administration had been used but their duration-of-action is limited to 1 h and frequent redosing is required. Course treatment by physostigmine should be implemented for BZ poisoning to avoid relapse of symptoms. IV administration of physostigmine is not desired due to the delicate requirements of its administration that could lead to nerve agent like bradycardia in slow infusion or arrhythmias and convulsion in rapid one. It is not recommended to administer physostigmine by IV for causalities with cardiorespiratory compromise, acid–base imbalance, and seizure disorder history.

Other Hazards: Exposure Standards and Guidelines

The exposure associated with BZ agent has been reported by Ketchum (1963). Probit analysis for exposures associated with various total response indices (TRIs), which is calculated as (2 × Performance Index + 21 2 × Heart Rate Index + Blood Pressure Index) ÷ 5, was reported by Ketchum using Probit analysis that is correlated with TRI indices as shown in **Table 2** below.

Table 2 Probit analysis for response criteria for inhalation exposure to BZ

Response criteria (TRI score)	*Sample size*	*ED_{50} (mg min m^{-3})*	*95% Conf. limits (mg min m^{-3})*
4.0	36	90.5	66.2–123.6
5.0	36	124.8	102.8–151.5
6.0	36	134.8	110.3–164.7
7.0	36	183.1	132.9–252.0

Miscellaneous

Although there is a limited experiment performed to determine the effect of BZ exposure on human, however the scarce number of human subject exposed to the agent provides an adequate description of the incapacitating effect of BZ. Moreover, the inhalation data for BZ exposure are lacking when compared to data for other exposure routes. The data for animal exposure to BZ are sufficient to provide assessment on its lethality but lack certainty in wide range of exposure time.

See also: Atropine.

Further Reading

2005. Army, Marine Corp., Navy, Air Force Report, Potential Military Chemical/biological Agents and Compounds, Technical Report FM 3–11.9, MCRP 3-37.1B, NTRP 3-11.32, AFTTP(I) 3-2.55, II-37-II-43.

Clark, D.N., 1989. Review of Reactions of Chemical Agents in Water. Battelle Columbus, Columbus, OH. AD A 213 287. pp.72.

Fitzgerald, B.B., Costa, L.G., 1993. Modulation of muscarinic receptors and acetylcholinesterase activity in lymphocytes and in brain areas following repeated organophosphate exposure in rats. Fundam. Appl. Toxicol. 20, 210–216.

Ketchum, J.S., 1963. The Human Assessment of BZ. CRDL Tech. Memorandum 20–29. Human Investigations Facility, Directorate of Medical Research, U.S. Army Chemical Research and Development Laboratories, Edgewood Arsenal, Maryland (Unclassified, Limited Distribution).

Ketchum, J.S., Sidell, F.R., 1997. Incapacitating agents. In: Sidell, F.R., Takafuji, E.T., Franz, D.R. (Eds.), Medical Aspects of Chemical and Biological Warfare. Office of the Surgeon General, Dept. of the Army, United States of America, Falls Church, VA.

Richards, J.R., Schneir, A.B., 2003. Droperidol in the emergency department: is it safe? J. Emerg. Med. 24 (4), 441–447.

United States Army Field Manual FM 3-10B, Employment of Chemical Agents, 1966, pp. 4–5, 47.

USACHPPM (U.S. Army Center for Health Promotion and Preventive Medicine), 2004. Acute Toxicity Estimation and Operational Risk Management of Chemical Warfare Agent Exposures. USACHPPM Report No. 47-EM-5863–04. USACHPPM, Aberdeen Proving Ground, MD.

Relevant Websites

https://www.cia.gov/library/reports/general-reports-1/gulfwar/cwagents/index.htm – Central Intelligence Agency, Report. April 2002.

http://www.nap.edu/catalog.php?record_id=9527 – National Research Council.

http://www.reuters.com/article/2013/01/16/us-syria-usa-chemical-idUSBRE90F00P20130116 – Reuters: News story on chemical weapons use in Syria.

http://www.bt.cdc.gov – US Centers for Disease Control and Prevention, Agency for Toxic Substances and Disease Registry, Chemical Agents.

http://sis.nlm.nih.gov – US National Library of Medicine, Specialized Information Services, Chemical Warfare Agents.

C

Cadmium

SC Gad, Gad Consulting Services, Cary, NC, USA

- Name: Cadmium
- Chemical Abstracts Service Registry Number: 7440-43-9
- Valence State: +2 is the only natural state

Background

Discovered in 1817 as an impurity in calamine (zinc carbonate) by Friedrich Stromeyer and Karl Samuel Leberecht Hermann while working independently, cadmium exists in abundance of ~0.1 ppm in the Earth's crust.

Uses

Cadmium is primarily used for electroplating and galvanizing other metals because it is relatively resistant to corrosion. It is also used in electrical contacts, in soldering alloys, in nickel–cadmium storage batteries, in television phosphors, and as a stabilizer for polyvinyl chloride. Given its brilliant orange color, it has been used extensively as a pigment in paints, plasters, and plastics. Cadmium is also a by-product of zinc, lead, and copper mining and smelting. It is also frequently used in jewelry and toys as a cheap metal alternative.

Environmental Fate and Behavior

As indicated in the Exposure and Exposure Monitoring section, cadmium is widely distributed in the environment from a variety of natural and anthropogenic sources. Cadmium emitted into the air is often found bound to small particulates and can travel with these particulates over long distances. As a result, cadmium can remain in the atmosphere for long periods of time until it is deposited by gravitational settling or in rain and snow. Cadmium tends to be more mobile in water than other heavy metals although it will complex with humic substances and can precipitate out under certain conditions. Cadmium can bioaccumulate in aquatic organisms; the degree of accumulation is associated with the pH and humic content of the water. It can also bioaccumulate in plants and in the animals that feed on these plants; for example, cattle and wildlife. However, terrestrial bioaccumulation is much lower than that in water and cadmium concentrations at the top of the terrestrial food chain are not much higher than those at the lower end of the chain.

Exposure and Exposure Monitoring

Due to the wide use of cadmium-based products, cadmium is widely distributed in the environment. The cadmium content in soil and water has been increasing as a result of disposal of cadmium-contaminated waste and the use of cadmium-containing fertilizers (particularly on cereal crops). Commercial sludge, contaminated with cadmium, has been used to fertilize agricultural fields. Cadmium concentrations in urban air are quite low, because of regulation of industrial air emissions. Lead and zinc smelters and waste incineration account for the majority of cadmium present in ambient air.

Ingestion and inhalation are the primary routes of exposure to cadmium. Dermal contact is not a significant route of exposure. Exposure to cadmium via foodstuffs is common, since plants and animals accumulate cadmium from soil or water, especially fish and crustaceans. Cigarette smoke is a major source of cadmium exposure via inhalation.

Toxicokinetics

Absorption of cadmium in the gastrointestinal tract is ~4–7% in adults; absorption is probably higher in children. Diets low in calcium, iron, and protein enhance cadmium absorption. Zinc is an antagonist to cadmium (decreases cadmium absorption). Cadmium absorption by the lungs is dependent on particle size and the solubility of the cadmium compound, but is generally between 15 and 30%. Dermal absorption of cadmium is insignificant.

Cadmium is a classic cumulative poison that accumulates in the kidneys over a lifetime. It is transported in the blood by erythrocytes and by albumin, and it is stored mainly in the liver and kidneys as metallothionein (50–75% of the body burden). Cadmium binds to many proteins at the sulfate and carbonyl sites. The half-life of cadmium in these two organs may be as long as 30 years. The correlation between years of exposure and blood levels does not appear to be significant. Cadmium also accumulates in the bones and the placenta of pregnant women.

Urine is the most important excretion mechanism in humans. Urine concentration of cadmium increases with age and following kidney damage. Cadmium found on examination of hair is generally due to external contamination rather than internal absorption and distribution to the hair.

 http://dx.doi.org/10.1016/B978-0-12-386454-3.00823-X

Mechanism of Toxicity

Cadmium inhibits plasma membrane calcium channels and Ca^{2+}-ATPases. It also inhibits repair of DNA damaged by various chemicals, an effect which is believed to be associated with the induction of tumors. Although cadmium forms a metallothionein, the preformed cadmium metallothionein is nephrotoxic (toxic to the kidneys); it is suggested that effects occur when, at some stage in the kidney, the cadmium is dissociated from the metallothionein. In Itai-Itai disease (see Human under Chronic Toxicity section), patients were found to have chromosome abnormalities.

Cadmium has an affinity for sulfhydryl groups, and hence can inhibit enzymes; however, cells treated with cadmium showed proliferation of peroxisomes, which contain catalase, an enzyme. It appears that cadmium at first inhibits catalase activity and then, after a time, enhances that activity. In addition, cadmium inhibits enzymes involved in gluconeogenesis (the generation of glycogen for energy production from non-carbohydrate precursors). It also inhibits oxidative phosphorylation (energy production) and depresses trypsin inhibitor capacity.

Acute and Short-Term Toxicity (or Exposure)

Animal

Cardiac effects (electrical and biochemical changes in the myocardium) were observed in rats exposed to cadmium in drinking water.

Human

Acute toxicity may result from ingestion of relatively high concentrations of cadmium from contaminated food or beverages (e.g., 16 $mg\,l^{-1}$ cadmium in a beverage). Cadmium exhibits local irritant effects on the gastrointestinal tract such as nausea, vomiting, diarrhea, abdominal pain, chills, and a choking sensation. The effects of acute toxicity are apparent immediately. Pulmonary edema and chemical pneumonitis may also occur after acute exposure.

Inhalation of cadmium fumes produces local irritant effects and may result in chemical pneumonitis and pulmonary edema, possibly resulting in death.

Chronic Toxicity (or Exposure)

Animal

Animal studies have shown cadmium to be a teratogen and a reproductive toxin; however, the results of mutagenesis experiments are equivocal. Cadmium produced local sarcomas in a number of rodent species when the metal, sulfide, oxide, or salts were administered subcutaneously. Intramuscular injection of cadmium powder and cadmium sulfate also produced local sarcomas. Injection of cadmium chloride into the ventral prostate resulted in a low incidence of prostatic carcinoma. Exposure via inhalation of cadmium chloride produced a dose-dependent increase in lung carcinomas in rats.

Human

Chronic exposure to cadmium through any route will have adverse effects on the heart, lungs, bones, gonads, and especially the kidneys. The principal long-term effects of low-level cadmium exposure are generally chronic obstructive pulmonary disease, emphysema, and chronic renal tubular disease. Cardiovascular and skeletal effects are also possible. The initial symptoms of chronic inhalation exposure are those associated with metal fume fever (e.g., fever, headache, chest pain, sore throat, coughing, and rhinitis). Metal fume fever is most often associated with inhalation of zinc oxide but may occur following exposure to other metals such as cadmium. Although inconclusive, there is evidence that the cadmium burden in the body can lead to hypertension.

Since cadmium can displace zinc, its accumulation in the testes can suppress testicular function. Evidence obtained in the past several years appears to relate cadmium to prostate cancer in young men who work with cadmium. Additional investigation, such as epidemiological studies with a larger cohort, needs to be performed to investigate this apparent association of cadmium with prostate cancer.

Skeletal changes due to cadmium accumulation are probably related to calcium loss, which can be influenced by diet and hormonal status. These skeletal changes include osteomalacia (softening of bone resulting from loss of minerals) and pseudofractures. In Japan, people who ate fish contaminated with cadmium experienced skeletal changes, especially in their backs. This very painful effect was called the 'Itai-Itai' ('ouch-ouch') disease. Postmenopausal women with low calcium and vitamin D intake were apparently most susceptible.

Since the kidneys are the main depot for cadmium, they are of the greatest concern for cadmium toxicity. Cadmium interferes with the proximal tubule's reabsorption function. This leads to abnormal actions of uric acid, calcium, and phosphorus. Aminoaciduria (amino acids in the urine) and glucosuria (glucose in the urine) result; in later stages, proteinuria (protein in the urine) results. When this happens, it is assumed that there is a marked decrease in glomerular filtration. Long-term exposure to cadmium leads to anemia, which may result from cadmium interfering with iron absorption.

Cadmium metallothionein has also been studied extensively. This metalloprotein is high in the amino acid cysteine ($\sim$30%) and is devoid of aromatic amino acids. Metallothionein itself may function to help detoxify cadmium. For some experimental tumors, cadmium appears to be anticarcinogenic (e.g., it reduces the induction of tumors). While cadmium is not genotoxic, International Food Additives Council classifies it as a human carcinogen.

Immunotoxicity

Cadmium adversely affects (suppresses) the immune system, and can induce increased spleen cellularity, as well as a decrease in bone marrow cellularity accompanied by an increase in cell size distribution in bone marrow, demonstrating an increased affect on immature B cells.

Reproductive Toxicity

Studies in animals have shown a small range of reproductive affects of cadmium. Generally, reproductively toxic effects are seen in males at lower doses than in females, with necrosis of the testicles and atrophy of the seminiferous tubular epithelium being among the more common. In females, cadmium had induced hemorrhagic effects in the ovaries, and in the pups, decreased body weights and malformations have been seen.

There are currently conflicting study results on the affect of cadmium on human reproduction, and it cannot as such be classified for its reproductive toxicity.

Genotoxicity

There are studies which have shown chromosome aberrations *in vivo* and *in vitro* in both eukaryotes and mammalian cells, including human lymphocytes.

Carcinogenicity

Cadmium has been given similar classifications as to its carcinogenicity by different organizations, with the American Conference of Governmental Industrial Hygienists (ACGIH) giving an A2, a suspected human carcinogen. The US Environmental Protection Agency's Integrated Risk Information System has given a B1, a probable human carcinogen. Cadmium's International Agency for Research on Cancer monograph states that there is sufficient evidence to consider cadmium a human carcinogen, although animal data are limited and inconclusive.

Clinical Management

For treatment of oral poisoning, administration of syrup of ipecac is indicated, followed by gastric lavage. The chelating agent calcium ethylenediaminetetraacetic acid (EDTA) (calcium disodium salt of EDTA) is indicated for acute exposure if administered shortly after cadmium exposure before new metallothionein is synthesized. British anti-Lewisite (BAL; 2,3-dimercaptopropanol) is contraindicated as it may enhance kidney toxicity. Newer dimercapto compounds dimercaptosuccinic acid and dimercaptopropane sulfonate are being evaluated as are derivatives of dithiocarbamates. Delayed pulmonary edema may result from inhaled cadmium dusts; therefore, supportive measures are indicated.

The apparent affinity for zinc metallothionein may someday be found to be useful as an antidote for cadmium toxicity. Antagonists to cadmium toxicity include a pretreatment with selenium and zinc. It is believed that this pretreatment allows cadmium to displace zinc in the zinc metallothionein.

Ecotoxicology

Commercial runoff and use of fertilizers are major anthropogenic sources of environmental cadmium. Rivers can transmit cadmium long distances before it settles into sediment, increasing the area potentially affected by cadmium toxicity. Cadmium has been seen to both bioaccumulate and biomagnify, especially in crustacean populations and at higher trophic levels in this chain. Cadmium has a tendency to accumulate in the leaves of plants and therefore is seen more in leafy vegetable crops than in fruits or nuts.

Other Hazards

The frequency with which cadmium is used industrially causes a high number of workers to be potentially exposed to the toxic metal. This problem became clear in the 1950s and 1960s and was largely addressed by necessitating the use of fume hoods in the workplace, although toxic exposure is still possible.

More recent problems with exposure to cadmium have developed in the form of cheap jewelry and toys. This is increasingly problematic in that many of the products in question are often appealing to children who have a lesser resistance. Also, due to the length of time needed for clearance of cadmium, early-life exposures can elicit problems for many years afterward. Since public awareness for the dangers of lead poisoning has grown in recent years, manufacturers often replace lead with cadmium in their products, and legislation to match the lead scare has not yet been implemented. Even in California, which has the most stringent laws about component materials of goods, there are frequent events in which products are labeled as adhering to laws and when tested are not within acceptable bounds for lead, cadmium, as well as other substances.

Exposure Standards and Guidelines

ACGIH lists cadmium as a suspected human carcinogen. The ACGIH threshold limit value–time-weighted average (TLV–TWA) is 0.01 $mg\,m^{-3}$ for elemental cadmium and inorganic compounds as total dust/particulate. The ACGIH TLV–TWA for the respirable fraction of cadmium particulate is 0.002 $mg\,m^{-3}$.

See also: Cardiovascular System; Kidney; Metallothionein; Metals; Pollution, Air in Encyclopedia of Toxicology; Pollution, Soil; Pollution, Water; Respiratory Tract Toxicology; Sensory Organs.

Further Reading

Bingham, E., Cohrssen, B., 2012. Patty's Toxicology. John Wiley and Sons, Hoboken, NJ.

Fowler, B.A., 2009. Monitoring of human populations for early markers of cadmium toxicity: a review. Toxicol. Appl. Pharmacol. 238 (3), 294–300.

Guney, M., Zagury, G.J., 2012. Heavy metals in toys and low-cost jewelry: a critical review of U.S. and Canadian legislations and recommendations for testing. Environ. Sci. Technol. 46 (8), 4265–4274.

Hartwig, A., 2010. Mechanisms in cadmium-induced carcinogenicity: recent insights. Biometals 23 (5), 951–960.

Nawrot, T.S., Staessen, J.A., Roels, H.A., Munters, E., Cuypers, A., Richart, T., Ruttens, A., Smeets, K., Clijsters, H., Vangronsveld, J., 2010. Cadmium exposure in the population: from health risks to strategies of prevention. Biometals 23 (5), 769–782.

Nordberg, G.F., Nogawa, K., Nordberg, M., Friberg, L.J., 2009. Cadmium. In: Nordberg, G.F., B.A., Fowler, B.A., Nordberg, M., Friberg, L.T. (Eds.), Handbook on the Toxicology of Metals, third ed. Elsevier, New York, pp. 407–415.

Romero-Puertas, M.C., Ortega-Galisteo, A.P., Rodriguez-Serrano, M., Sandalio, L.M., 2012. Metal Toxicity in Plants: Perception, Signaling and Remediation. Insights into Cadmium Toxicity: Reactive Oxygen and Nitrogen Species Function.
Satarug, S., Baker, J.R., Urbenjapol, S., et al., 2003. A global perspective on cadmium pollution and toxicity in nonoccupationally exposed population. Toxicol. Lett. 137 (1–2), 65–83.
Sigel, A., Sigel, H., Sigel, K.O. (Eds.), 2012. Cadmium: from toxicity to essentiality. Metal Ions in Life Sciences, vol. 11. Springer Verlag, Dordrecht.
Verougstraete, V., Lison, D., Hotz, P., 2003. Cadmium, lung and prostate cancer: a systematic review of recent epidemiological data. J. Toxicol. Environ. Health B Crit. Rev. 6 (3), 227–255.
Waalkes, M.P., 2003. Cadmium carcinogenesis. Mutat. Res. 533 (1–2), 107–120.
Wang, B., Li, Y., Shao, C., Tan, Y., Cai, L., 2012. Cadmium and its epigenetic effects. Curr. Med. Chem. 19 (16), 2611–2620.

Relevant Websites

http://www.atsdr.cdc.gov – Agency for Toxic Substances and Disease Registry. Toxicological Profile for cadmium.
http://toxnet.nlm.nih.gov – Toxnet Homepage; Search for 'Cadmium.'

Caffeine

CP Holstege, University of Virginia School of Medicine, Charlottesville, VA, USA
E Holstege, Calvin College, Grand Rapids, MI, USA

This article is a revision of the previous edition article by Christopher P. Holstege, volume 1, pp 377–379, © 2005, Elsevier Inc.

- Name: Caffeine
- Chemical Abstracts Service Registry Number: 58-08-2
- Synonyms: 1,3,7-Trimethylxanthine; Guaranine; Methyltheobromine; Theine; and Mateine
- Molecular Formula: $C_8H_{10}N_4O_2$
- Chemical Structure:

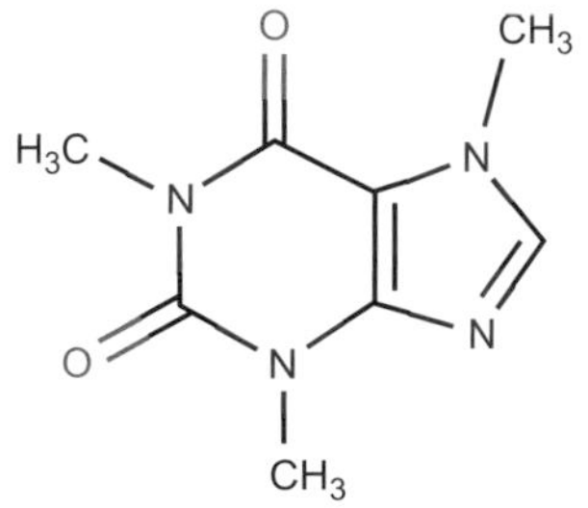

Background

Caffeine is one of the world's most widely ingested chemicals. Caffeine is found within the seeds, leaves, and fruit of numerous plants. It is consumed in common beverages, such as coffee and tea. It was first isolated from coffee in 1819 by the German chemist Friedlieb Ferdinand Runge. Caffeine comes from the French word for coffee (café). Beverages containing caffeine have been ingested since ancient times. The first use of coffee beans occurred in Ethiopia as far back as the ninth century.

Uses

Caffeine is used as a central nervous system (CNS) stimulant, anorexiant, and diuretic, and in a number of analgesic and cold medication compounds. It is also used in the treatment of spinal headaches and has been used as a respiratory stimulant in preterm infants.

Environmental Fate and Behavior

Caffeine's production and widespread use as an additive to food and as a stimulant may result in release to the environment through waste systems. It has an estimated vapor pressure of 7.3×10^{-9} mmHg (25 °C), which indicates that it will exist as particulate in the atmosphere. Caffeine is not susceptible to photolysis and if released into soil it has a high mobility based on the K_{oc} of 22.

Partition Behavior in Water, Sediment, and Soil

Caffeine is highly mobile in soil. It has an estimated K_{oc} of 22. It will exist as primarily a cation in the environment and will not volatilize from water or moist soil. It will generally absorb to organic clays and carbons. When caffeine is released into water it does not absorb to sediment.

Physicochemical Properties

Sublimation point 178 °C
Melting point 238 °C
Density 1.23 g cm^{-3}
pK_a dissociation constant 10.4 at 40 °C
Log P (octanol–water) coefficient −0.07
Water solubility 2.17 g per 100 ml
Vapor pressure 15 mmHg at 89 °C and 7.3×10^{-9} (25 °C)
Henry's law constant 1.9×10^{-19}
Atmospheric OH rate constant 1.52×10^{-10} cm^3 molecule s^{-1}

Environmental Persistency (Degradation/Speciation)

Using *Scirpus validus*, the uptake, accumulation, and translocation of caffeine in hydroponic conditions were investigated. The plants were cultivated using Hoagland's nutrient solution with a concentration of caffeine ranging from 0.5 to 2.0 mg l^{-1}. In this study, 15–19% of caffeine was lost from the solution after 3 and 7 days from biodegradation. Caffeine is not susceptible to photolysis from sunlight.

Bioaccumulation

Plant uptake of caffeine was studied using *S. validus* plants cultivated using Hoagland's nutrient solution with a caffeine concentration ranging from 0.5 to 2.0 mg l^{-1}. Uptake was significant and caffeine was detected in both roots and shoots of the plant. Root concentrations of caffeine were 0.1–6.1 μg g^{-1} and shoot concentrations for caffeine were 6.4–13.7 μg g^{-1}. The bioaccumulation factors (BAFs) for the

 http://dx.doi.org/10.1016/B978-0-12-386454-3.00703-X

roots ranged from 0.2 to 3.1, while the BAFs for shoots ranged from 3.2 to 16.9. Translocation from roots to shoots were the primary mechanism for the accumulation of caffeine in the shoots. An estimated bioconcentration factor of 3 suggests that bioconcentration in aquatic organisms is negligible. Caffeine has an estimated half-life of 0.8 days based on river infiltration.

Exposure and Exposure Monitoring

Ingestion is the most common route of exposure. Caffeine is consumed in wide variety of beverages, such as coffee, tea, and soda. It is found alone or in combination with other pharmaceutical products. It is also available for injection. A wide variety of sports supplements and natural products also contain caffeine. The widely marketed energy drinks such as Red Bull, Rock Star, Amped, and others contain caffeine, and some of these products contain multiple sources of caffeine, including herbal sources such as guarana, kola nut, and other sources.

Toxicokinetics

Caffeine is rapidly absorbed after an oral dose, with peak levels reached within 1–2 h at therapeutic doses. Onset of clinical effects occurs within 60 min. In adults, caffeine is extensively metabolized by the liver, primarily by *N*-demethylation. It is excreted in the urine primarily as 1-methyluric acid and 1-methylxanthine. Theophylline (1,3-dimethylxanthine) is a minor product of caffeine metabolism in adults (<1%). After massive caffeine overdoses, serum levels of theophylline are measurable. The elimination half-life of caffeine is 3–6 h at therapeutic doses. The half-life is shorter in smokers and is prolonged by oral contraceptives, cimetidine, in late pregnancy and in overdose. The half-life of caffeine is much longer in infants and does not approximate that seen in adults until 6 months of age. The half-life of caffeine may exceed 100 h in preterm infants. Only 1–10% of caffeine appears unchanged in the urine in adults. Neonates may excrete up to 85% of caffeine unchanged.

Mechanism of Toxicity

Caffeine can have profound effects on the cardiovascular system. At least four mechanisms have been proposed for the pro-arrhythmic potential of caffeine in overdose. First, caffeine increases circulating catecholamines. Second, caffeine inhibits phosphodiesterase. Increased circulating catecholamines after caffeine overdose increase β1-receptor stimulation. Stimulation of β1-receptors increases intracellular cAMP by G protein stimulation of adenylate cyclase. The activity of cAMP is prolonged due to its decreased metabolism as phosphodiesterase is inhibited by caffeine. Subsequently, β1-receptor effects are exaggerated and tachydysrhythmias are induced. Third, caffeine increases myocardial intracellular calcium. Caffeine both induces release of calcium from the sarcoplasmic reticulum and blocks calcium's reuptake into the sarcoplasmic reticulum. This resulting increase in cytosolic calcium may provoke dysrhythmias. Fourth, caffeine blocks cardiac adenosine receptors, which have been shown to be antiarrhythmic.

The hypotension that has been noted with overdoses of caffeine is due primarily to two mechanisms. First, caffeine-induced tachydysrhythmias lead to inadequate filling of the heart and subsequent decrease in cardiac output. Second, caffeine augments β2-effects and causes subsequent vasodilation with resulting hypotension.

Caffeine in overdose also acts as a nonselective antagonist of neuronal adenosine receptors that may lead to seizures. Caffeine is also a mild diuretic, and it stimulates gastric acid secretion, respiration, and lipolysis.

Acute and Short-Term Toxicity

Human Toxicity: Acute

Acute toxicity manifests primarily in the CNS, cardiovascular system, and gastrointestinal system. CNS signs include restlessness, tremor, nervousness, headache, insomnia, tinnitus, confusion, delirium, psychosis, and seizures. Cardiac manifestations of overdose include sinus tachycardia, various dysrhythmias, asystole, and cardiovascular collapse. Other findings include tachypnea, nausea, vomiting, hematemesis, diarrhea, and fever. Case reports also include rhabdomyolysis and pulmonary edema. Laboratory findings include metabolic acidosis, respiratory alkalosis, ketosis, hypokalemia, and hyperglycemia. The estimated lethal dose in adults is 150–200 mg kg^{-1}, whereas doses of 10–15 mg kg^{-1} may produce early signs of toxicity. Serum levels greater than 30 μg ml^{-1} have been associated with adverse symptoms. Levels exceeding 80 μg ml^{-1} have been associated with death, although levels as high as 405 μg ml^{-1} have been reported in survivors.

Animal Toxicity: Acute

Some animals such as dogs and birds are at much higher risk for toxicity from caffeine than humans. This is in part due to a limited ability to metabolize caffeine compared to humans. In addition to dogs and birds, caffeine also has much greater effect on certain mollusks, insects, and spiders. Otherwise, animal toxicity is similar to human toxicity. Dehydration and hyperthermia may occur.

Chronic Toxicity: Human

No definite association has been demonstrated between habitual caffeine use and hypertension, myocardial infarction, carcinogenicity, or teratogenicity. Abrupt cessation of chronic caffeine ingestion may cause withdrawal headaches. Regular or chronic caffeine users have tolerance to some of the acute effects of caffeine, including a tolerance to the diuretic and pressor effects of caffeine. This tolerance also extends to the autonomic effects, including tachycardia, but not to the CNS stimulation from caffeine.

Chronic Toxicity: Animal

Toxicity in animals is similar to that found in humans.

Reproductive Toxicity

Evidence that caffeine is a reproductive toxin is limited; however, some authorities recommend that pregnant women limit consumption of coffee or caffeinated beverages to two cups per day or less. The American Congress of Obstetricians and Gynecologists have found that caffeine is safe up to 200 mg day^{-1} when consumed during pregnancy. The UK Food Standards Agency has also recommended that pregnant women limit caffeine intake to 200 mg day^{-1}. There is evidence that some of the hormonal changes that occur during pregnancy will lead to decreased metabolism and subsequent clearance of caffeine, resulting in a much longer duration of effects (up to 15 h during the third trimester). Moderate consumption of caffeine (<150 mg of caffeine per day) has not been associated with premature delivery or low birth weight.

Carcinogenicity

There is inadequate evidence that caffeine is carcinogenic in humans or animals. Caffeine is not classified as a carcinogen in humans. Rats and Mice Cancer Test summary identified no positive target sites in The Carcinogenic Potency Project for caffeine.

Clinical Management

In patients presenting with caffeine toxicity, the airway should be patent and adequate ventilation ensured. If necessary, endotracheal intubation should be performed. The patient should be placed on continuous cardiac monitoring with pulse oximetry. The initial treatment of hypotension consists of intravenous fluids. If hypotension persists, then pressors such as phenylephrine and vasopressin may be considered. Frequent neurological checks should be made. Gastrointestinal decontamination should be considered only after initial supportive care has been provided and airway control has been ensured. Activated charcoal (1 g kg^{-1}) may be administered, but vomiting may make retention difficult. Beta-blocking agents have been used to treat caffeine tachydysrhythmias; however, one report described cardiovascular collapse following administration. Standard therapy for seizures should be employed. Monitoring should be performed for fluid and electrolyte imbalances.

Various techniques to enhanced elimination of caffeine have been reported in the literature. Multidose activated charcoal has been advocated both to prevent further absorption of drug and to enhance elimination by gut dialysis. Hemodialysis has been reported in the literature for the treatment of caffeine toxicity. The mean plasma protein binding of caffeine (36%), the molecular size (194), and the volume of distribution (0.6–0.8 l kg^{-1}) make hemodialysis a possible modality to enhance elimination of caffeine. There have also been cases of severe caffeine toxicity treated with peritoneal dialysis, but this modality is less efficient at drug clearance than hemodialysis.

Ecotoxicology

Freshwater/Sediment Organisms Toxicity

Caffeine is not listed as having a Pesticide Action Network (PAN) Ground Water Contaminant Rating.

Marine Organism Toxicity

Caffeine is recognized as a contaminant of aquatic systems. Concentrations are typically very low (from ng l^{-1} to μg l^{-1}). Mussels (*Mytilus californianus*) exposed to 0.05, 0.2, and 0.5 μg l^{-1} of caffeine for 10, 20, and 30 days were compared to controls and found to have significant elevations of stress protein (Hsp70 – a marker of cellular stress) in the 0.5 μg l^{-1} treatment. Mollusks have higher sensitivity to toxicity of caffeine than other organisms.

Exposure Standards and Guidelines

A threshold limit value has not been established for caffeine. Other exposure standards and guidelines have not been set for caffeine. Caffeine is classified as generally recognized as safe in humans by the US Food and Drug Administration (FDA); however, the FDA restricts beverages to containing less than 0.02% caffeine.

See also: Poisoning Emergencies in Humans; Theophylline.

Further Reading

Bigard, A.Z., 2010. Risks of energy drinks in youths. Arch. Pediatr. 17 (11), 1625–1631.

Centers for Disease Control and Prevention (CDC), 2012. Energy drink consumption and its association with sleep problems among U.S. service members on a combat deployment – Afghanistan, 2010. Morb. Mortal. Wkly Rep. 61 (44), 895–898.

Holstege, C.P., Hunter, Y., Baer, A.B., et al., 2003. Massive caffeine overdose requiring vasopressin infusion and hemodialysis. J. Toxicol. Clin. Toxicol. 41, 1003–1007.

Higdon, J.V., Frei, B., 2006. Coffee and health: a review of recent human research. Crit. Rev. Food Sci. Nutr. 46, 101–123.

Poussel, M., Kimmoun, A., Levy, B., Gambier, N., Dudek, F., Puskarczyk, E., Poussel, J.F., Chenuel, B., 2013. Fatal cardiac arrhythmia following voluntary caffeine overdose in an amateur body-builder athlete. Int. J. Cardiol. 166 (3), e41–e42.

Zhang, D.Q., Hua, T., Gersberg, R.M., Zhu, J., Na, W.J., Tan, S.K., 2013. Fate of caffeine in mesocosms wetland planted with *Scirpus validus*. Chemosphere 90 (4), 1568–1572.

Relevant Websites

http://www.energyfiend.com/the-caffeine-database – Caffeine Content of Drinks Found on This Website.

http://emedicine.medscape.com/article/821863-overview – Caffeine Toxicity on eMedicine by Medscape.

http://www.foodnavigator-usa.com/Regulation/Caution-recommended-when-adding-caffeine-to-new-foods – Discussion Regarding Caffeine as Additive to Food and Beverages and the GRAS Opinion by the FDA Regarding Caffeine.

Calcium Channel Blockers

SC Gad, Gad Consulting Services, Cary, NC, USA

- Name: Calcium Channel Blockers
- Chemical Abstracts Service Registry Number: Varies
- Molecular Formula: Varies
- Chemical Structure: Varies
- Representative Compounds: Amlodipine (Norvasc; CASRN 88150-42-9); Diltiazem (Cardizem LA, Tiazac; CASRN 33286-22-5); Felodipine (Plendil; CASRN 72509-76-3); Isradipine (Dynacirc CR; CASRN 88977-22-4); Nicardipine (Cardene SR; CASRN 55985-32-5); Nifedipine (Adalat CC, Procardia; CASRN 21829-25-4); Nimodipine (Nimot op; CASRN 66085-59-4); Nisoldipine (Sular; CASRN 63675-72-9); Verapamil (Verelan, Covera HS, Calan; CASRN 56949-77-0)
- Chemical/Pharmaceutical/Other Class: Class IV antiarrhythmic agents; Antihypertensive agents; Vasodilatory agents; Tocolytic agents

Background Information

Calcium channel blockers (also referred to as calcium channel antagonists) inhibit the slow voltage-dependent L-type calcium channel found on cardiac myocytes and in peripheral vascular smooth muscle cells. During the 1950s, Bernard Katz (Biophysics Department, University College London) and his colleagues Paul Fatt and Bernard Ginsborg found (by accident) that contraction of crustacean muscle fibers in response to electrical stimuli persisted even in the absence of sodium ions. It was subsequently discovered that Ca^{2+} was acting as a charge carrier during excitation–contraction coupling of muscle cells. In 1962, Hass and Hartfelder reported that the calcium antagonist verapamil caused coronary vasodilation, but unlike other vasodilatory agents (e.g., nitroglycerin) it also possessed negative chronotropic (reduction in heart rate) and inotropic (reduction in force of myocardial contraction) effects. The study of calcium ion channels and the role of the calcium ion in cardiovascular pharmacology became an area of intense research and led to the development of great cardiovascular drugs.

Calcium channel blockers are a structurally diverse group of chemicals and are categorized according to their physiological effects. The dihydropyridine calcium channel blockers (amlodipine besylate (Norvasc), felodipine (Plendil), isradipine (Dynacirc), nifedipine (Adalat, Procardia), nicardipine (Cardene), and nimodipine (Nimot op)) are selective primarily toward the peripheral vascular smooth muscle cells with relatively little effect on the cardiac myocardium. They cause peripheral arterial vasodilation with little or no direct effect on cardiac myocyte conduction or contractility, thus making them useful in the treatment of hypertension. An indirect increase in heart rate (reflex tachycardia) can occur after administration of dihydropyridine calcium channel blockers if they are administered too rapidly or at too great of a dose. In this case, a sudden fall in blood pressure occurs and triggers a compensatory reflex increase in heart rate (baroreceptor response).

In contrast, the nondihydropyridine calcium channel blockers (verapamil (Isoptin, Calan), diltiazem (Cardizem)) exhibit greatest selectivity toward cardiac myocytes, thus causing negative inotropic (decreased myocardial force of contraction), chronotropic (decreased heart rate), and dromotropic (decreased conduction speed through the AV node of the heart) effects with little or no effect on the peripheral vasculature. Nondihyropyridine calcium channel blockers are useful in the treatment of angina; however, they can cause disturbances in cardiac conduction that can lead to the development of Bradyarrhythmia. They may also aggravate preexisting left ventricular heart failure.

Uses

Calcium channel blockers are used in the management of angina pectoris, hypertension, supraventricular arrhythmias, subarachnoid hemorrhage, and pulmonary hypertension, and for the prevention of migraine. They are recommended for the treatment of angina in patients with certain coexisting medical conditions such as asthma, chronic obstructive pulmonary disease, mild peripheral vascular disease, and severe peripheral vascular disease with rest ischemia. Calcium channel blockers may be used to inhibit uterine contractions to delay delivery during preterm labor (tocolytic therapy). They are sometimes used in the treatment of Raynaud's disease.

Environmental Fate and Behavior

Calcium channel blockers in general have low vapor pressures; it is unlikely that they would exist as particulates in the atmosphere. They tend to become adsorbed to organic particles (sludge, sediment) in waste treatment facilities. Some of the calcium channel blockers (e.g., nifedipine) are subject to direct photolysis by sunlight and decompose rapidly. Volatilization from water or moist or dry soil is not considered to be an important fate. The potential for bioconcentration in aquatic organisms is low. They are susceptible to oxidative metabolism by humans as well as microorganisms.

Exposure and Exposure Monitoring

Ingestion is the most common route for both accidental and intentional exposures. Occupational exposure may occur through inhalation, dermal, or ocular routes to dust generated at the workplace where the drug is manufactured. Verapamil, diltiazem, and nicardipine are available for parenteral administration, and toxicity can occur via the parenteral route. Plasma levels of the calcium channel blockers can be monitored by HPLC analysis.

 http://dx.doi.org/10.1016/B978-0-12-386454-3.00824-1

Toxicokinetics

Following oral administration of calcium channel blockers, absorption is rapid and almost complete (80–100%); however, their ultimate bioavailability is limited and variable (15–94%) following oral administration due to a significant first-pass metabolism by the liver. Metabolism in the liver occurs via the cytochrome P450 microsomal enzyme system (CYP3A4) and produces highly water-soluble, inactive metabolites that are excreted primarily in the urine. Only small amounts (0–10%) are excreted unchanged in the urine. Protein binding is high and ranges from 70 to 99%. The volumes of distribution for some calcium channel blockers are as follows: verapamil, $5\,l\,kg^{-1}$; diltiazem, $3.1\,l\,kg^{-1}$; nifedipine, $0.78\,l\,kg^{-1}$; and nicardipine, $1.1\,l\,kg^{-1}$. The relatively low values for volume of distribution (<10 l) indicates that the drug is mainly confined to the intravascular fluid (in this case, highly bound to the plasma protein albumin). Peak plasma concentrations typically occur within 0.5–2 h after oral administration of conventional capsules to patients with normal renal and hepatic function. The half-life after administration of extended-release tablets is about 7 h. The presence of food in the gastrointestinal tract appears to decrease the rate but not the extent of metabolism. Elimination half-life ranges from 1 h (nimodipine) to 50 h (amlodipine). Coadministration of an inhibitor of CYP3A (e.g., quinidine, verapamil) causes an increased exposure to calcium channel blockers by competing for metabolism. Increased exposure to calcium channel blocking agents occurs in patients with compromised hepatic function due to decreased hepatic metabolism. Calcium channel blocker clearance is thought to be decreased and exposure increased in the elderly due to a decline in renal function with age.

Mechanism of Toxicity

Calcium channel blockers inhibit the flux of extracellular calcium ions across the cell membranes of myocardial cells and vascular smooth muscle cells. They interfere with electrical conduction through the atrioventricular node, cause a decrease in myocardial contractility, and cause vasodilation. Calcium channel blockers also interfere with pancreatic release of insulin by blocking L-type calcium ion channels in the pancreatic beta-cells.

The interference with electrical conduction through the atrioventricular node is caused by interference with the influx of calcium in phase II of the action potential and is manifested by bradycardia, lengthening of the PR interval (PR is the time between P and R waves in a corrected electrocardiogram), QRS widening (QRS is a combination of three of the waves (Q, R, and S) seen in a standard electrocardiogram), and QTc prolongation (QTc is the time between the beginning of the Q wave and the end of the T wave in an electrocardiogram corrected for heart rate).

Myocardial contractility is dependent on calcium influx into the cell, which in turn results in increased release of calcium inside the cell from the sarcoplasmic reticulum. The overall effect of this calcium influx and release is the bridging of actin and myosin and subsequent myocardial contraction. The negative inotropic effect of the calcium blockers is due to interference with this process.

Vasoconstriction occurs when calcium activates vascular myosin kinase, which in turn allows for phosphorylation of myosin and subsequent bridging with actin. Administration of calcium channel blockers interferes with this process and produces vasodilation. Dihydropyridine calcium channel blockers have a high vascular selectivity – they are potent vasodilators with little or no effect on cardiac contractility. They are useful in the treatment of hypertension but are not used to treat angina because their blood pressure lowering effects can lead to reflex cardiac stimulation (increase in heart rate and strength of contraction, thus increasing the myocardial oxygen demand). The nondihydropyridine calcium channel blocker verapamil is selective toward the myocardium and is useful for the treatment of angina (reduces myocardial oxygen demand and combats coronary vasospasm). Diltiazem is a nondihydropyridine calcium channel blocker that has both cardiac depressant and vasodilatory effects; it reduces arterial pressure but is less likely to cause reflex tachycardia than the dihydropyridines.

Acute and Short-Term Toxicity (or Exposure)

Animal

Some examples of the acute oral median lethal dose (LD_{50} values) for dihydropyridine calcium channel blockers include nifedipine (1022, 310, and $504\,mg\,kg^{-1}$ in rats, mice, and rabbits, respectively), amlodipine ($37\,mg\,kg^{-1}$, mouse), and felodipine (1050 and $2250–2390\,mg\,kg^{-1}$, rat). The oral LD_{50} for some nondihydropyridine calcium channel blockers include verapamil (108 and $163\,mg\,kg^{-1}$, rat and mouse, respectively) and diltiazem ($508\,mg\,kg^{-1}$, mouse).

Human

In a manufacturing setting, calcium channel blocking agents can cause irritation to the eyes, respiratory system, and skin.

The most common side effects reported after administration of calcium channel blockers include constipation, nausea, headache, rash, edema (legs), hypotension, drowsiness, dizziness, and sexual dysfunction. Hepatotoxicity and overgrowth of the gingiva have also been reported. The nondihydropyridine calcium channel blockers (verapamil, diltiazem) can exacerbate preexisting heart failure due to their negative chronic and inotropic effects on the heart.

Many of the clinical side effects associated with calcium channel blockers are primarily cardiovascular in nature. Due to their interference with conduction, the calcium channel blockers can cause a variety of dysrhythmias (sinus bradycardia, atrioventricular block, junctional rhythms, pulseless electrical activity, and asystole). Profound hypotension can occur following calcium channel blocker poisoning (due to their vasodilatory properties). Renal failure secondary to decreased renal perfusion may occur. The neurologic toxicities of the calcium channel blockers are most likely secondary to their cardiovascular effects. The most common neurologic effects are lethargy and coma. Seizure activity has also been observed after calcium channel blocker overdose. Metabolic effects associated with calcium channel blocker overdose include metabolic acidosis, hyperglycemia, and hypokalemia. Hyperkalemia has also been reported.

The nondihydropyridine calcium channel blockers (verapamil, diltiazem) decrease the metabolism of certain co-administered drugs (e.g., carbamazepine, simvastatin, atorvastatin, and lovastatin), causing an increase in exposure and potential toxicity. Consumption of grapefruit juice up to 2 h before or 4 h after administration of calcium channel blockers can cause an increase in their plasma levels and potential toxicity.

Immunotoxicity

Calcium channel blockers exhibit immunosuppressant properties that are independent of their cardiovascular effects. They have been shown to be beneficial to patients who have undergone solid organ transplant procedures (reduced immune-mediated organ rejection).

Reproductive and Developmental Toxicity

Nifedipine (dihydropyridine) was associated with a reduction in fertility in rats. It was considered to be teratogenic in rats and rabbits (digital anomalies, rib deformities, cleft palate), and embryotoxic and fetotoxic (stunted fetuses) in rats, mice, rabbits, and monkeys. Nifedipine prolonged pregnancy and caused a reduction in neonatal survival (rats).

Amlodipine (dihydropyridine) exhibited no signs of teratogenicity or embryo/fetal toxicity when administered orally to pregnant rats and rabbits during the period of organogenesis. However, litter size was decreased (~ 50%) and the number of intrauterine deaths was increased in rats dosed with amlodipine prior to and throughout mating and gestation. Amlodipine prolonged gestation and the duration of labor.

Oral administration of isradipine (dihydropyridine) was associated with decreased maternal weight gain (rats and rabbits) and an increase in fetal resorptions (rabbit). There was no evidence of embryotoxicity at doses that were not maternally toxic and no evidence of teratogenicity. Peri- and postnatal administration of isradipine to rats resulted in decreased maternal weight gain and reduced birth weight and survival of the pups. Fertility in male and female rats was unaffected.

Oral administration of felodipine (dihydropyridine) to rats had no effect on fertility parameters but did cause teratogenic effects (digital anomalies) in both rats and monkeys. Felodipine prolonged parturition, made labor more difficult, and caused an increased frequency of fetal and early postnatal deaths. There was no effect on fertility in rats. A dose-related increase in mammary size occurred in rabbits administered felodipine.

Oral administration of nimodipine (dihydropyridine) to rabbits was teratogenic and produced stunted fetuses. In rats, nimodipine produced embryotoxicity but no signs of teratogenicity and had no effect on fertility.

Intravenous administration of nicardipine (dihydropyridine) was embryotoxic (rats, rabbits) but not teratogenic. Oral administration of nicardipine was neither embryotoxic nor teratogenic but did cause dystocia, decreased birth weights, and decreased neonatal survival. Fertility was not affected in mice or rats.

Oral administration of verapamil (nondihydropyridine) to female rats did not impair fertility. Verapamil was nonteratogenic in rats and rabbits; however, embryotoxicity and retarded fetal growth and development were observed.

Diltiazem (nondihydropyridine) was evaluated in mice, rats, and rabbits and caused embryotoxicity, fetotoxicity, and skeletal abnormalities in the offspring. In perinatal and postnatal studies there was evidence of an increased number of stillbirths.

The dihydropyridines nifedipine, nicardipine and felodipine and the nondihydropyridines verapamil and diltiazem are excreted in breast milk. It is not known if amlodipine or isradipine are excreted in breast milk.

Genotoxicity

Dihydropyridine and nondihydropyridine calcium channel blockers have not exhibited mutagenic and/or clastogenic effects.

Carcinogenicity

In general, nondihydropyridine as well dihydropyridine calcium channel blocking agents were not associated with carcinogenic effects after lifetime oral administration to mice and/or rats. However, the dihydropyridine calcium channel blocking agents did cause an increased incidence of benign Leydig cell tumors and testicular hyperplasia, thought to be secondary to an effect on circulating gonadotropin levels. In addition, rats fed nicardipine in the diet for 2 years developed increased thyroid hyperplasia and neoplasia, thought to be secondary to decreased circulating thyroxin levels and chronic stimulation of the thyroid gland. This effect was not observed in mice, dogs, and humans.

Clinical Management

Advanced supportive care is a primary component of patient management. Emergent intubation and assisted ventilation are often necessary in these patients. Pulse oximetry should be utilized to assess respiratory status. Extensive cardiovascular monitoring is also necessary. Arterial blood gases, serum electrolytes, and glucose measurements should be obtained. Serum concentrations of specific calcium channel blockers are difficult to obtain and have limited clinical utility. Syrup of ipecac-induced emesis is contraindicated due to the rapid decreases in level of consciousness that may occur as well as emesis-induced vasovagal effects. Gastric lavage and activated charcoal can be used if warranted by the history of the ingestion and the patient's neurologic status. Whole bowel irrigation along with activated charcoal should be utilized in ingestions involving sustained-release products. Calcium salts are often administered as antidotes for calcium channel blocker toxicity, although they have been used with limited success. Calcium chloride is preferred over calcium gluconate since it contains more elemental calcium on a milligram per milligram basis. Doses of up to 4 g of calcium have been recommended in this setting.

Glucagon, which has been used in b-adrenergic blocker toxicity, has been recommended in calcium blocker toxicity. This agent has positive inotropic properties due to activation of cyclic adenosine monophosphate. It has limited beneficial effects in calcium channel blocker toxicity. Control of heart rate and rhythm presents a significant challenge in this patient population. Transcutaneous pacemakers should be utilized to stabilize rate and enhance atrioventricular conduction. A vagolytic, atropine, has also been used to increase heart rate. It has limited effect since it primarily affects the sinoatrial node. The negative inotropic effects of these agents must also be treated aggressively. Positive inotropic agents such as dopamine, dobutamine, amrinone, and isoproterenol can be utilized to increase contractility. Isoproterenol should be used with caution due to its vasodilatory properties. Vasopressors such as dopamine, epinephrine, and norepinephrine may be effective. Cardiopulmonary bypass has been used experimentally to treat patients with calcium channel blocker toxicity who do not respond to traditional therapy. Sodium bicarbonate should be administered to treat acidosis.

Seizure activity should be initially treated with benzodiazepines. If benzodiazepines are not effective, phenytoin and barbiturates can be administered. Insulin replacement may be necessary to correct hyperglycemia.

See also: Cardiovascular System.

Further Reading

Brunton, L., Ehabner, B., Knollman, B., 2011. The Pharmacological Basis of Therapeutics, twelfth ed. McGraw Hill Medical, New York.

Chitwood, K.K., Heim-Duthoy, K., 1993. Immunosuppresive properties of calcium channel blockers. Pharmacotherapy 13 (5), 447–454.

Dipiro, R.T., Talbert, R.L., Matzhe, G., Yee, G.C., 2011. Pharmacotherapy, eighth ed. McGraw-Hill, New York.

Eisenberg, M.J., et al., 2004. Calcium channel blockers: an update. Am. J. Med. 116 (1), 35–43.

Nabel, E.G., Eatman, K.H., Fox, D.D., et al., 2011. ACP Medicine. Dekker, New York.

Relevant Websites

http://www.cvpharmacology.com/vasodilator/CCB.htm – Klabunde, R.E. (2008) Cardiovascular Pharmacology Concepts - Calcium Channel Blockers (CCBs).

http://www.ncbi.nlm.nih.gov/pubmed/15520904 – Mears D (2004) Regulation of insulin secretion in islets of Langerhans by Ca(2+) channels. J. Membr Biol. 200(2):57–66.

http://www.medicinenet.com/calcium_channel_blockers/article.htm – Ogbru, O. Calcium channel blockers (CCBs).

http://www.ncbi.nlm.nih.gov/books/NBK6465/ – Tsien RW, Barrett CF. A Brief History of Calcium Channel Discovery.

Calomel

KN Thakore, California Department of Public Health, Richmond, CA, USA

- Name: Calomel
- Chemical Abstracts Service Registry Number: 10112-91-1
- Synonyms: Mercurous chloride; Mercury(I) chloride; Dimercury dichloride; Calotab; Calogreen
- Molecular Formula: Cl_2Hg_2
- Chemical Structure:

Cl–Hg–Hg–Cl

Uses

Calomel is used as a laboratory reagent, as a fungicide, and as a depolarizer in dry batteries.

Environmental Fate and Behavior

Calomel decomposes gradually in the presence of sunlight. It slowly decomposes to mercury and mercuric chloride under aqueous conditions.

Exposure and Exposure Monitoring

The primary routes of entry are dermal, inhalation, and oral. Calomel is found in the environmental and occupational settings, such as in mercury mining operations, battery plants, and chemical laboratories. It is also present in some consumer products like paints and dyes, photography, perfumes, and cosmetics. Exposure to calomel through oral and dermal routes is poisonous.

Toxicokinetics

Following inhalation, 70–80% of metallic vapor is retained and absorbed. Absorption through the gastrointestinal tract is only less than 10%. In the body, it is oxidized to mercuric mercury, which binds to reduced sulfhydryl groups. It is deposited in the kidney following exposure to both metallic and mercuric mercury. In addition to other organs, it passes into the brain and fetus. The metabolite is eliminated mainly in urine and feces; it is also excreted in milk. In humans, inorganic mercury compounds have two elimination half-lives: one lasts for days or weeks and the other much longer.

Mechanism of Toxicity

Calomel can generate reactive oxygen species and deplete glutathione levels. Both genotoxic and nongenotoxic mechanisms may contribute to renal carcinogenic effect of mercury.

Acute and Short-Term Toxicity

Animal

In animals, intense exposure causes lung damage, intestinal and renal tubular necrosis, immunosuppression, and possible cytogenetic effects. The oral LD_{50} values in rat and mouse are 210 and 180 mg kg^{-1}, respectively. In mice, the intraperitoneal LD_{50} value is 10 mg kg^{-1}.

Human

Exposure to calomel by inhalation and oral routes is harmful and may be fatal. When swallowed, it causes central nervous system depression; and when inhaled, it causes tightness and pain in the chest, coughing, and breathing difficulties. Ocular and dermal exposures cause irritation of the eyes and skin. In case of chronic exposure, mercury builds up in the brain, liver, and kidneys and causes headache, shakes, loose teeth, loss of appetite, skin ulceration, and impaired memory. Mercury concentration in urine, blood, and plasma is useful for biological monitoring.

Chronic Toxicity

Animal

There is limited evidence for carcinogenicity. Calomel causes renal adenoma and adenocarcinoma in male mice and female rats.

Human

There is inadequate evidence for carcinogenicity.

Genotoxicity

It was positive with sister chromatid exchange in *in vitro* assay.

Clinical Management

In case of contact, eyes and skin should be flushed with water for 15–20 min. If inhaled, the victim should be removed to fresh air and oxygen and artificial respiration should be administered, if necessary. If the patient is in cardiac arrest, cardiopulmonary resuscitation should be provided. These life-support measures should be continued until medical assistance has arrived. An unconscious or convulsing person should not be given liquids or induced to vomit.

Other Hazards

Calomel is a poison by ingestion. When heated to decompose, it emits very toxic fumes of Cl^- and Hg.

 http://dx.doi.org/10.1016/B978-0-12-386454-3.00266-9

Exposure Standards and Guidelines

Engineering controls, standard work practices, and personal protective equipment, including respirators are employed to prevent worker exposure to calomel. After use, the clothing and equipment should be placed in an impervious container for decontamination or disposal.

See also: Dimethylmercury; Mercury Tragedies: Incidents and Effects; Mercuric Chloride ($HgCl_2$); Federal Insecticide, Fungicide, and Rodenticide Act, US; Mercury; Methylmercury.

Further Reading

Gangolli, S., 2007. Calomel. In: Gangolli, S. (Ed.), The Dictionary of Substances and Their Effects, second ed., vol. 2. Royal Society of Chemistry, Cambridge, UK, pp. 75–76.

Grandjean, P., Yorifuji, T., 2012. Mercury. In: Bingham, E., Cohrssen, B. (Eds.), Patty's Toxicology, sixth ed., vol. 1. John Wiley & Sons, Inc, New York, pp. 213–228.

Gray, J.E., Plumlee, G.S., Morman, S.A., et al., 2010. In vitro studies evaluating leaching of mercury from mine waste calcine using simulated human body fluids. Environ. Sci. Technol. 44 (12), 4782–4788.

International Agency for Research on Cancer (IARC), 1993. Mercury. In: IARC Monographs (Ed.), Beryllium, Cadmium, Mercury, and Exposure in the Glass Manufacturing Industry, vol. 58. IARC, Lyon, France, pp. 239–345.

Lewis, R.J., 2012. Mercury Chloride. In: Lewis, R.J. (Ed.), Sax's Dangerous Properties of Industrial Materials, twelth ed., vol. IV. John Wiley & Sons, Inc, New York, p. 2648.

Relevant Websites

http://chem.sis.nlm.nih.gov/chemidplus/Calomel – ChemIDplus Advanced.

http://www.epa.gov/ttnatw01/112nmerc/volume5.pdf/Mercury – EPA Mercury Report.

http://scorecard.goodguide.com/Mercury – Pollution information site.

http://www.who.int/ipcs/publications/cicad/en/cicad50.pdf/Mercury – WHO Mercury Report.

Camphor

HL Rivera and F Barrueto, University of Maryland School of Medicine, Baltimore, MD, USA

This article is a revision of the previous edition article by Fermin Barrueto Jr., volume 1, pp 382–383, © 2005, Elsevier Inc.

- Name: Camphor
- Chemical Abstracts Service Registry Numbers: CAS 464-48-2 and CAS 464-49-3 (optical isomers); CAS 21368-68-3 (racemic mixture)
- Synonyms: Campho-phenique, Musterole, Ben-Gay children's vaporizing rub, Vicks Vaporub, Alcanfor
- Molecular Formula: $C_{10}H_{16}O$
- Chemical Structure:

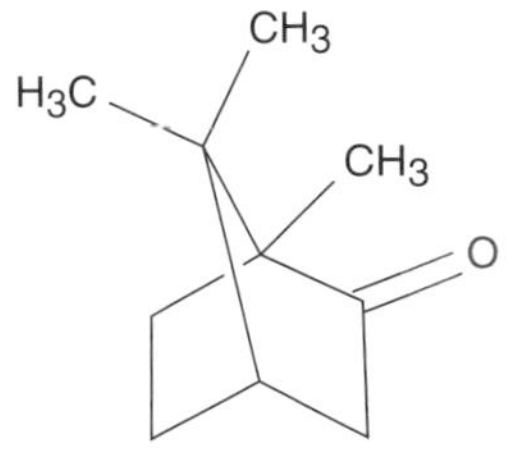

Background

Camphor is a white or transparent, waxy substance found in the wood of the camphor laurel and other trees found in Asia and Borneo. It is also produced synthetically from the oil of turpentine. It has been used for centuries for its medicinal features, in religious rituals, and in cooking. It is no longer used as pesticide. In 1982, the US Food and Drug Administration restricted commercial products intended for medicinal use to contain <11% camphor.

Uses

Industrial uses of camphor include its use as a plasticizer. Camphor is also used as a repellant for certain insects, in particular moths, and it has been used historically as an ingredient in foods and beverages in particular in liquors and sweet dishes. Camphor is still used as a flavoring for certain foods in India and other parts of Asia. Medicinally, camphor is employed externally as a rubefacient, a mild analgesic, an antipruritic, and a counterirritant in commercially available products that contain 1–10% camphor.

Environmental Fate and Behavior

Camphor is a white or transparent, waxy or crystalline substance with a strong aromatic odor. The boiling point is 204 °C and melting point is 176–180 °C. Camphor sublimates at room temperature and standard atmospheric pressure. Camphor has a specific gravity of 0.99, relative vapor density of 5.2, and vapor pressure of 20 Pa at 20 °C. Its solubility in water is 0.125 g per 100 ml water at 25 °C and it is soluble in ethanol, ethyl ether, turpentine, and essential oils.

Camphor vaporizes easily and is degraded in the atmosphere by reaction with photochemically produced hydroxyl radicals; the half-life for this reaction in air is estimated to be 1.6 days. If released to soil, camphor is expected to have moderate mobility, based on an estimated K_{oc} of 470. Volatilization from moist soil surfaces is expected to be an important fate process, based on an estimated Henry's Law constant of 8.1×10^{-5} atm-m^3 mol^{-1}. Camphor may volatilize from dry soil surfaces based on its vapor pressure. If released into water, camphor may adsorb to suspended solids and sediment, based on the estimated K_{oc}. Biodegradation is not expected to be an important environmental fate process in water or soil, based on its persistence in water. Estimated volatilization half-lives for a model river and model lake are 10 h and 9 days, respectively.

Exposure and Exposure Monitoring

Ingestion of mothballs, Vicks® VapoRub®, and camphorated oils is the most common route of intentional and unintentional exposures to camphor. Ocular exposures may also occur, as can transdermal and inhalational exposure.

Toxicokinetics

In liquid form, camphor is absorbed rapidly through the skin, mucous membranes, and gastrointestinal tract. Symptoms may appear within 5–90 min following oral ingestion. The absorption is highly dependent on the presence of food and other chemicals. Camphor is metabolized to campherols (2-hydroxycamphor and 3-hydroxycamphor), which is conjugated with glucuronic acid in the liver. It is unclear whether camphor toxicity is attributed to the parent compound, a metabolite, or both. Camphor-related metabolites are fat soluble. Thus, significant concentrations may accumulate in fatty tissue. However, camphor is distributed widely in all tissues. Measurable serum levels are apparent within minutes after ingestion of 0.5–1.0 g. The volume of distribution is 2–4 l kg^{-1}. The glucuronide form is excreted in the urine. The half-life of a 200-mg dose is 167 min.

Mechanism of Toxicity

Camphor is a central nervous system (CNS) stimulant with effects that range from mild CNS excitation to generalized seizures. Camphor is highly lipid soluble and easily crosses the blood–brain barrier. The action of camphor has been postulated to be intraneuronal on the oxidation cycle at a phase above the cytochrome *b* level of the cytochrome oxidase system; though its precise mechanism has not been elucidated. It is primarily a neurotoxin with a chemical structure that allows easy penetration of the blood–brain barrier. Camphor also has irritant properties to skin and mucosa and ingestion of large amounts causes vomiting and diarrhea.

Acute and Short-Term Toxicity (or Exposure)

Animal

Animal toxicity is similar to human toxicity. Mouse intraperitoneal LD_{50} is 3000 mg kg^{-1}. The lowest estimated lethal dose (LD_{Lo}) in rats (intraperitoneal) is 900 mg kg^{-1}, mouse (subcutaneous) is 2200 mg kg^{-1}, and the dog (oral) is 800 mg kg^{-1}.

Human

Upon ingestion, an initial burning sensation may be noted in the mouth and throat. Spontaneous nausea and vomiting may occur within minutes after ingestion. Confusion, vertigo, restlessness, delirium, hallucinations, tremors, and convulsions are all directly related to CNS involvement and may be predictors of serious toxicity. More severe intoxications may result in hepatic failure. Death may be caused by respiratory depression or may follow status epilepticus. Camphor should be considered an eye irritant. In adults, ingestion of 50–500 mg kg^{-1} is thought to be lethal. A dose of 2 g generally causes systemic toxicity in adults. In infants, the LD_{Lo} is estimated to be 70 mg kg^{-1}. Ingestion of toxic amounts causes gastrointestinal irritation and nausea, vomiting and diarrhea occur after ingestion. Camphor is absorbed from all exposure routes.

Chronic Toxicity (or Exposure)

Animal

Chronic camphor dosing in a mouse model has led to development of neuronal necrosis.

Human

Chronic ingestion of camphor may produce toxicity similar to that of an acute ingestion but in a more insidious fashion. Liver failure is a more pronounced clinical manifestation. A syndrome similar to Reyes syndrome has been noted after chronic exposure in humans.

Immunotoxicity

Camphor is not thought to be immunotoxic.

Reproductive Toxicity

D-Camphor showed no evidence of teratogenicity when orally administered to pregnant rats up to 1000 mg kg^{-1} by weight per day and to pregnant rabbits at doses up to 681 mg kg^{-1} by weight per day during the fetal period of organogenesis.

Camphor is not listed as a developmental or reproductive toxin in the CA Prop 65 Developmental Toxins, the US Toxic Release Inventory (TRI) Developmental Toxins, the CA Prop 65 Female or Male Reproductive Toxins or the US TRI Reproductive Toxins.

Genotoxicity

Camphor is not mutagenic with the Ames test.

Carcinogenicity

Camphor is not thought to be carcinogenic in humans. Carcinogenicity tests have been negative. Camphor is neither listed as an International Agency for Research on Cancer (IARC) carcinogen nor listed in the California Prop 65 list of known carcinogens.

Clinical Management

Basic and advanced life support measures should be used as necessary. Gastrointestinal decontamination procedures are marginally effective and should not be considered because of the high probability of seizures. Oils, alcohols, and other lipophilic substances enhance intestinal absorption and are contraindicated. Ocular exposures necessitate flushing with a gentle system of tepid water for a minimum of 15 min. If signs of irritation persist, an ophthalmic consultation is required. The seizure activity is often singular, self-limiting, and responsive to benzodiazepines or other GABAergic agents such as barbiturates or propofol. Patients who remain asymptomatic after 4 h can be observed safely at home.

Ecotoxicology

No effect is coded for fish under aquatic toxicity in the pesticide action network (PAN) Pesticides Database – Chemicals camphor entry. Camphor is acutely toxic to aquatic insects and certain terrestrial insects. No chronic toxicity data is available for honeybees in the PAN Pesticides Database camphor entry.

Exposure Standards and Guidelines

The National Institute for Occupational Safety and Health immediately dangerous to life or health concentration: 200 mg m^{-3}.

The Occupational Safety and Health Administration permissible exposure limit: 2 mg m^{-3} time-weighted average (TWA).

American Conference of Governmental Industrial Hygienists threshold limit value: 2 ppm, 12 mg m^{-3} TWA; 3 ppm, 19 mg m^{-3} short-term exposure limit.

See also: Poisoning Emergencies in Humans; Plants, Poisonous (Humans).

Further Reading

Khine, H., Weiss, D., Graber, N., et al., 2009. A cluster of children with seizures caused by camphor poisoning. Pediatrics 123, 1269–1272.

Leuschner, J., 1997. Reproductive toxicity studies of D-camphor in rats and rabbits. Arzneimittelforschung 47 (2), 124–128.

Manoguerra, A.S., Erdman, A.R., Wax, P.M., et al., 2006. Camphor poisoning: an evidence-based practice guideline for out-of-hospital management. Clin. Toxicol. 44, 357–370.

Zuccarini, P., Soldani, G., 2009. Camphor: benefits and risks of a widely used natural product. Acta Biol. Szeged. 53 (2), 77–82.

Relevant Websites

http://www.botanical.com/botanical/mgmh/c/campho13.html – Botanical.com Information on Camphor in Particular Related to Botanical Sources and Uses.

http://www.cdc.gov/niosh/idlh/76222.html – Centers for Disease Control and Prevention (CDC) NIOSH Publications and Products – Camphor – Documentation for Immediately Dangerous to Life or Health Concentrations.

http://www.inchem.org/documents/pims/pharm/camphor.htm – IPCS INCHEM Homepage – Camphor.

https://www.osha.gov/dts/chemicalsampling/data/CH_224600.html – United States Department of Labor Occupational Safety and Health Administration Chemical Information – Camphor.

Cancer *see* Carcinogenesis

Cancer Chemotherapeutic Agents

GL Finch, Drug Safety Research and Development, Worldwide Research and Development, Pfizer Inc., Groton, CT, USA
LA Burns-Naas, Drug Safety Evaluation Gilead Sciences, Inc., Foster City, CA, USA

This article is a revision of the previous edition article by David S. Fisher, volume 1, pp 384–401, © 2005, Elsevier Inc.

Introduction and Historical Perspective

Cancer is a general term used to describe 100 or more malignant neoplasms that invade tissues from which the cancer derives and that may also metastasize to distant sites and grow there. The defining characteristic of the cancer cell is rapid, poorly controlled, or uncontrolled proliferation and multiple genetic alterations. A tumor is a circumscribed noninflammatory growth arising from existing tissue but growing independently of the normal rate or structural development of such tissue and serving no physiological function. When the growth of tumors at the initial location becomes clinically detectable, this is referred to as a primary tumor. Tumors may be malignant or benign. Benign tumors do not invade or metastasize. Metastasis refers to the ability of cancer cells to travel from the site of the initial primary tumor to other tissues and grow to form a secondary tumor.

A chemotherapy drug is a chemical agent used to treat diseases. The term may be applied to a drug used to treat infection, but more frequently is used to refer to drugs used to treat cancer. The term, cancer chemotherapy, is used more generally by some to include biological and/or immunomodulatory agents that are used to treat cancer while others prefer to use the more specific terms biotherapy, cancer biotherapy, immunotherapy, or biologic therapy of cancer.

Historically, the only useful treatment for tumors was surgical removal. With the development of cellular and tissue pathology in the mid-nineteenth century, malignant tumors could be identified without demonstrating distant metastases, and malignancies of the blood were identified and called leukemia. In 1865, the German physician Lissauer used potassium arsenite (Fowler's solution) by chance and found that it restored to health two near moribund patients with chronic myeloid leukemia. This was the first chemical agent effective in the treatment of a malignant disease and it continued to be used for 70 years. Recently, arsenic trioxide has been used as an effective drug for treating acute promyelocytic leukemia (APL).

After Roentgen discovered X-rays in 1895, they were used for many medical purposes and were found to be effective in shrinking Hodgkin's disease tumors and the enlarged spleens of patients with chronic leukemias with a resultant drop in their high white cell counts, results similar to those produced by potassium arsenite. Paul Ehrlich used organic arsenicals in his search for a 'magic bullet' to cure syphilis. Other investigators were frustrated by their inability to find effective agents to treat cancers because they did not understand the biology of cancer and the search was largely abandoned for many decades.

Modern Chemotherapy

The development of effective antibacterial agents, for example, sulfanilamide and penicillin in the 1930s, aroused interest in chemical and biological agents in the treatment of cancer. During World War II, a number of investigators studied the effects of chemical warfare agents that might be used by adversaries. Nitrogen mustard, then known by the wartime code name HN2, was extensively studied in the laboratory and in mice and rabbits before the first near moribund patient with lymphoma was treated in December 1942 at the New Haven Hospital affiliated with the Yale School of Medicine.

The treatment resulted in a dramatic regression of disease and the era of cancer chemotherapy began. Several books relate the story that the use of nitrogen mustard as a chemotherapeutic agent was suggested by the serendipitous finding of marrow and lymphoid hypoplasia in seamen exposed to mustard gas following the sinking of a ship in Bari Harbor, Italy, containing chemical warfare agents. That event is well documented but it occurred in December 1943, 1 year after the Yale human trials.

Nitrogen mustard will hereafter be referred to by its generic name, mechlorethamine, and generic names will be used for all drugs.

As a therapeutic agent, mechlorethamine has many toxic effects. Acutely, it causes nausea and vomiting, skin blistering, and ulceration. After a week or two, it causes leukopenia, lymphopenia, anemia, thrombocytopenia, diarrhea, oral ulcers, and hyperuricemia. It can cause sterility and after a few years, leukemia. The most susceptible tissues are those with rapidly dividing cell populations, including bone marrow, lymphoid tissues, and gastrointestinal (GI) epithelium. The therapeutic index (TI) of mechlorethamine and most of the cytotoxic chemotherapy drugs is low, meaning that the therapeutic dose is very close to the toxic dose.

Both the benefits and toxicities of mechlorethamine stimulated a worldwide search for new antineoplastic agents. In the United States, the National Cancer Institute (NCI) was established in 1937 and was evaluating plant extracts for anticancer activity. In 1955, the NCI established the Cancer Chemotherapy National Service Center to systematically screen drugs *in vitro* and *in vivo*. Shortly after World War II, investigations into a second approach to drug therapy of cancer began with research showing folic acid seemed to promote the proliferation of acute lymphoblastic leukemia (ALL) cells. Folic acid analogues, including amethopterin (now known as

 http://dx.doi.org/10.1016/B978-0-12-386454-3.00079-8

methotrexate), could block the function of folate-requiring enzymes and were subsequently shown in 1948 to induce remission in children with ALL. This led to investigations into other antimetabolites. Yet another advance occurred in the mid-1960s when it was recognized that just as for antibiotics, treatment with combinations of drugs, each with differing mechanisms of action, could produce increased efficacy over that achieved with single agents alone.

Over the past half century, a growing understanding of the biology and metabolism of proliferating cells has led to the development of over 100 active anticancer drugs that have been Food and Drug Administration (FDA) approved and marketed, and many more are in the pipeline. The various classes of agents generally have similar or related toxicities, because the mechanism of action that is successful in injuring or eliminating the cancer cell is usually the same mechanism of action that injures or destroys the normal cell leading to the adverse toxic effects. Drugs in the same therapeutic class also have some dissimilar and unique toxicities. The goal is to develop drugs that are able to differentially damage or kill neoplastic cells and spare benign cells. An increased understanding of the molecular and genetic mechanisms operative in cell signaling showed that many of the signaling networks were significantly altered in cancer states, and pointed the way to more targeted development of anticancer drugs such as the tyrosine kinase inhibitors and monoclonal antibodies. And in the area of solid tumor therapy, the recognition that rapidly dividing cancer cell populations need a rich supply of blood-supplied oxygen and nutrients led to the development of antiangiogenesis approaches in which neovascularization of the tumor could be suppressed to essentially 'starve' the tumor.

Other modern developments in chemotherapy have focused on drug delivery advancements. For example, polyethylene glycol, a relatively high molecular weight polymer, can be complexed with chemotherapeutic drugs. This is referred to a 'pegylation.' This modification extends circulating half-lives (prolongs time the active drug remains in the body's circulation) and leads to increased dosing intervals. Another approach involves the encapsulation of chemotherapeutic drugs into liposomes, which are artificially prepared vesicles filled with drugs and surrounded by phospholipids. Liposomes can be prepared in a range of sizes and with varying characteristics. An example of an approved product is liposomal doxorubicin, used in combination therapy with cyclophosphamide in metastatic breast cancer.

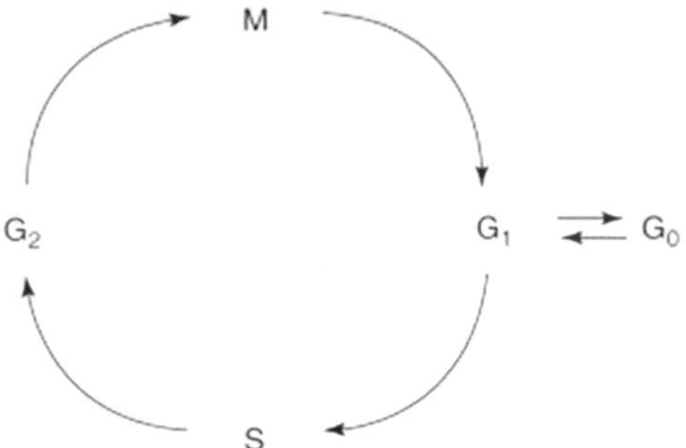

Figure 1 Phases of the cell cycle. G_0, resting phase (nonproliferation of cells); G_1, pre-DNA synthetic phase (12 h to a few days); S, DNA synthesis (usually 2–4 h); G_2, post-DNA synthesis (2–4 h; cells are tetraploid in this stage); and M, mitosis (1–2 h).

Table 1 Cell cycle phase-specific drugs

S phase dependent	*M phase dependent*	*G_2 phase dependent*	*G_1 phase dependent*
Antimetabolites	Docetaxel	Bleomycin	Asparaginase
Capecitabine	Etoposide	Irinotecan	
Cytarabine	Paclitaxel	Mitoxantrone	
Doxorubicin	Podophyllotoxins	Topotecan	
Floxuridine	Taxanes		
Fludarabine	Teniposide		
Gemcitabine	Vinblastine		
Hydroxyurea	Vinca alkaloids[a]		
Mercaptopurine	Vincristine		
Methotrexate	Vinorelbine		
Pemetrexed			
Procarbazine			
Thioguanine			

[a]Have greatest effect in S phase and possibly late G_2 phase; cell blockade or death, however, occurs in early mitosis.

Cell Kinetics and the Cell Cycle

The rate of growth of a tumor is a reflection of the proportion of actively dividing cells (the growth fraction), the length of the cell cycle (doubling time), and the rate of cell loss. Acute leukemias, some lymphomas, germ cell tumors, Wilms' tumor, neuroblastoma, and choriocarcinoma are characterized by a rapid growth fraction as demonstrated by tritiated thymidine uptake and turnover studies. Most solid cancers are not characterized by rapid growth. For example, breast, lung, and colon cancer cells may take up to 100 days to double their population. The growth and division of normal and neoplastic cells occur in a sequence of events called the cell cycle. The cell cycle is divided into several different phases (**Figure 1**). Many of the antineoplastic drugs have been and many continue to be classified based on whether their activity is cell cycle specific or nonspecific. Alkylating agents are nonspecific. Other classes, such as antimetabolites, vinca alkaloids, taxanes, podophyllotoxins, are cell cycle specific (**Table 1**).

Synthesis of RNA and protein occurs during the G_1 phase. When cells are in G_1 for prolonged periods of time, they are often said to be in a resting phase, referred to as G_0. Synthesis of DNA occurs during the S phase. During G_2, DNA synthesis halts, and RNA and protein synthesis continue. The final steps of chromosome replication and segregation occur during the mitotic or M phase. The cell undergoes cell division and produces two daughter cells. The rate of RNA and protein synthesis slows during this phase as the genetic material is transferred into the daughter cells.

Also located within the cell cycle of normal cells are checkpoints. These are biochemically designated systems that can be activated during the cell cycle process. They prevent the cell from moving forward from one phase to the next if adverse genetic conditions have occurred in the previous phase. Many cancer cells have lost these checkpoints. Drugs that exert their cytotoxic effects during a specific phase of the cell cycle (i.e., phase-specific agents) are usually not effective against cells that are predominantly in a dormant phase (G_0). In contrast, nonphase-specific agents are theoretically more likely to be effective against a tumor population that is not in a state of rapid division.

General Classes of Anticancer Drugs

Anticancer drugs are generally categorized by their mechanism of action or the means by which the therapy was derived and includes alkylating agents, antimetabolites, natural products, hormonal agents, antiangiogenics, biotherapeutics, and miscellaneous agents. This section discusses the antineoplastic drugs in groups related to these properties. The Anatomic Therapeutic Chemical (ATC) Classification System divides drugs into different groups depending on the organ system upon which they act and/or their therapeutic and chemical characteristics. Subcodes often designate specific agents. The ATC system is controlled by the World Health Organization and was first published in 1976.

Alkylating Agents

Alkylating agents (ATC code L01A) are highly reactive compounds that easily attach to DNA and cellular proteins. The primary mode of action for most alkylating drugs is via cross-linking of DNA strands. They can be classified as either monofunctional alkylating agents, implying reactions with only one strand of DNA, or bifunctional alkylating agents, which cross-link two strands of DNA. Replication of DNA and transcription of RNA are prevented by these cross-links.

Many alkylating agents have been developed (**Table 2**). Although these drugs have similar mechanisms of action, there are major differences in spectrum of activity, pharmacokinetic parameters, and toxicity. Alkylating agents play a significant role in the treatment of lymphoma, Hodgkin's disease, breast cancer, multiple myeloma, and other malignancies. In addition to conventional chemotherapy, the linear dose–response curve of alkylating agents expands their role for incorporation into transplant regimens.

The major clinical toxicities of most of the alkylating agents are similar to those of mechloramine, primarily bone marrow depression (including anemia, leukopenia, and thrombocytopenia) and nausea and vomiting. As noted above, alkylating agents generally have low TIs, because they target all dividing cells. Individual drugs have additional toxicities. Chlorambucil, mechlorethamine, melphalan, and procarbazine can cause gonadal dysfunction and occasionally, late leukemias. Busulfan, carmustine, chlorambucil, and lomustine can cause pulmonary fibrosis. Cyclophosphamide and ifosfamide can cause hemorrhagic cystitis and in a small percent of patients, bladder cancer. Cisplatin, carmustine, lomustine, and streptozocin can cause renal damage. Carboplatin and cisplatin can cause ototoxicity and peripheral neuropathy. Procarbazine is a weak monoamine oxidase inhibitor. It can cause hypertensive reactions if used concurrently with sympathomimetic agents, tricyclic antidepressants, foods with high tyramine content, and with the narcotic meperidine.

Table 2 Alkylating agents

Classical alkylators	Aziridine, chlorambucil, cyclophosphamide, estramustine, ifosfamide, mechlorethamine, melphalan, nitrogen mustards, thiotepa
Platinum complexes	Carboplatin, cisplatin, oxaliplatin
Nonclassical alkylators	Altretamine, dacarbazine, procarbazine

Antimetabolites

The interest in antibacterial chemotherapy and its mechanisms of action had direct consequences for antineoplastic drug development. An antimetabolite is a substance that interferes with the normal metabolic processes within cells. After sulfanilamide was found to be an antimetabolite of para-minobenzoic acid, an essential growth factor for streptococci, the group at Lederle Laboratories synthesized antimetabolites of folic acid – first aminopterin and later amethopterin now known generically as methotrexate. As noted above, 1948, Farber and the Harvard Children's Hospital group used these antimetabolites to induce remission of ALL in children. This led to further studies of anticancer drugs based on the biochemistry and metabolism of cancer cells. In 1954, Hitchings and Elion at the Burroughs Wellcome laboratories developed the antipurine drugs, 6-mercaptopurine and 6-thioguanine, for leukemias. In 1957, Heidelberger and his group at the McArdle Institute at the University of Wisconsin introduced the first antipurine, 5-fluorouracil, for GI tumors. Additional antimetabolites have been developed (**Table 3**). Despite the fact this class of chemotherapeutic agents has been in use for decades, they are generally effective and still in wide clinical use.

Antimetabolites interfere with the synthesis of DNA, RNA, and ultimately proteins. They exert their effects largely in the synthetic (S) phase of the cell cycle. Some antimetabolites are structural analogs of normal metabolites essential for cell growth and replication. This property allows some of them to be incorporated into DNA and/or RNA so that a false message is transmitted. Other antimetabolites inhibit enzymes that are necessary for the synthesis of essential compounds. One drug can sometimes interfere with multiple cell processes. For example, Azacitidine (VIDAZA, Mylosar) is a pyrimidine nucleoside analogue of cytidine. Azacitidine is incorporated into DNA, where it reversibly inhibits DNA methyltransferase, thereby blocking DNA methylation. Hypomethylation of DNA by azacitidine may activate tumor suppressor genes silenced by hypermethylation, resulting in an antitumor effect. This agent is also incorporated into RNA, thereby disrupting normal RNA function and impairing tRNA cytosine-5-methyltransferase activity.

Table 3 Antimetabolites

Class	*Drug examples*
Folate analogs	Methotrexate, pemetrexed, trimetrexate
Purine analogs	Cladribine, fludarabine, mercaptopurine, pentostatin, thioguanine
Pyrimidine analogs	Azacitidine, capecitabine, cytarabine, floxuridine, fluorouracil, gemcitabine
Ribonuclease reductase inhibitor	Hydroxyurea

The action and toxicity of the antimetabolites are significantly modified by the duration of exposure as well as the dose. Prolonged infusions or prolongation of absorption by pegylation or incorporation into liposomes can change both the response and the toxicity. Since this is a large subject to cover in any detail, it will suffice to note here that some of the anticancer antibiotics and biotherapy drugs discussed below are also available in pegylated or liposomal forms.

The toxicity of antimetabolites is, as expected, due to their incorporation into the metabolism of normal cells, which is nearly identical to that of the malignant cells that they were designed to injure. The normal cells injured most severely are the rapidly proliferating cells of the bone marrow, the lymphoid system, and the GI epithelium. Thus, the common toxicities are bone marrow depression, nausea and vomiting, diarrhea, and mucositis. Cytarabine and pentostatin can also cause conjunctivitis. Capecitabine and prolonged use of fluorouracil or cytarabine can cause cerebellar ataxia and the hand-foot syndrome, that is, palmar–plantar erythrodysesthesia or acral erythema. Pentostatin and high-dose methotrexate can cause renal toxicity. Azacitidine can cause rapid heartbeat, chest pain, and difficulty breathing or swallowing.

Natural Products

The natural products may be divided into six primary groups (**Table 4**): campothecin analogs, epipodophyllotoxins, antitumor antibiotics, microtubule agents, enzymes, and metals. Plant alkaloids and terpenoids have the ATC category L01C. The first three act primarily on the topoisomerases, and topoisomerases have ATC code L01CB and L01XX. Topoisomerases are enzymes that break and reseal DNA strands. The plant alkaloid campothecin and its analogs (topotecan and irinotecan) are nonclassic enzyme inhibitors of topoisomerase I. These agents are no longer referred to as inhibitors but are instead classified as topoisomerase I targeting agents or topoisomerase I poisons. The epipodophyllotoxins (etoposide and teniposide) and the antitumor antibiotics (dactinomycin, daunorubicin, doxorubicin, epirubicin, idarubicin, mitoxantrone, and valrubicin; these have ATC code L01D) are inhibitors of topoisomerase II. The drugs form a stable complex by binding to DNA and topoisomerase enzymes, resulting in DNA damage that interferes with replication and transcription.

Mitotic Inhibitors

A group of mitotic inhibitors (vinblastine, vincristine, and vinorelbine) exert their cytotoxic effects by binding to tubulin. This inhibits formation of microtubules, causing metaphase arrest. Their mechanism of action and metabolism are similar, but the antitumor spectrum, dose and clinical toxicities of vinblastine, vincristine, and vinorelbine are very different. Paclitaxel and docetaxel are also mitotic inhibitors. However, they differ from the vinca alkaloids by enhancing microtubule formation. As a result, a stable and nonfunctional microtubule is produced. Vinca alkaloids have the ATC code L01CA, podophyllotoxin has ATC code L01CB, and the taxanes have ATC code L01CD.

Table 4 Natural products

Class	*Drug examples*
Camptothecin analogs	Irinotecan, topotecan
Epipodophyllotoxins	Etoposide, teniposide
Antitumor antibiotics	Bleomycin
Microtubule agents	Docetaxel, paclitaxel, vinblastine, vincristine, vinorelbine
Enzymes	Asparaginase, pegasparaginase
Metals	Arsenic trioxide, gallium nitrate, platinum

The major toxicities of these four groups are bone marrow depression, nausea and vomiting, mucositis, and diarrhea. Daunorubicin, doxorubicin, epirubicin, idarubicin, and, to a lesser extent, mitoxantrone cause cardiac toxicity. Mitomycin and bleomycin cause pulmonary fibrosis. Paclitaxel and vincristine cause peripheral neuropathy, and paclitaxel (or its vehicle) can cause anaphylaxis. Dactinomycin, daunorubicin, docetaxel, doxorubicin, epirubicin, etoposide, idarubicin, mitoxantrone, mitomycin, paclitaxel, teniposide, and vinblastine all cause alopecia to varying degrees. Etoposide and topotecan can cause leukemia.

Enzymes

L-Asparaginase is an enzyme product that acts primarily by inhibiting protein synthesis by depriving tumor cells of the amino acid asparagine. Cells that have the ability to form their own asparagine, such as many normal cells, are not affected by L-asparaginase.

L-Asparaginase is a foreign protein, is antigenic, and can cause serious hypersensitivity reactions. Included in this category are the long-acting pegylated asparaginase and Erwinia-derived asparaginase, both similar in mechanism to L-asparaginase.

Metals

At one time, gallium nitrate was used for the treatment of hypercalcemia and bladder cancer, but it causes nausea, vomiting, and renal toxicity and has been largely replaced by superior drugs. Arsenic trioxide has been available for a century and was sometimes used instead of potassium arsenite for the treatment of chronic myeloid leukemia. Both arsenicals were abandoned for this purpose after superior agents became available. Arsenic trioxide was recently reintroduced into cancer chemotherapy by the Chinese. Its efficacy for inducing remissions in APL has been confirmed in Europe and the United States. Its major toxicities are nausea, vomiting, abdominal pain, diarrhea, pruritis, headache, dermatitis, hyperpigmentation, some skin exfoliation, and some bone marrow depression. 'Retinoic acid syndrome' (RAS) occurs in $\sim$30% of patients treated and is characterized by high fever, dyspnea, respiratory distress, pulmonary infiltrates, and pericardial and/or pleural effusions. Some patients have required intubation and mechanical ventilation. Initiation of corticosteroid treatment at the first sign of dyspnea is advised and then maintained until symptoms resolve.

Platinum-containing compounds (ATC code L01XA), most notably cisplatin and to a lesser extent carboplatin and oxaliplatin, have been used to treat various types of cancers including sarcomas, some carcinomas, lymphomas, and germ cell tumors. These platinum complexes react and cross-link DNA, and can have a variety of side effects that can limit their use. Nephrotoxicity is a dose-limiting side effect and may be related to the generation of reactive oxygen species; maintenance of adequate hydration and diuresis is used to reduce damage. Cisplatin causes nausea and vomiting, which may be managed with prophylactic antiemetics. Ototoxicity may be severe, and there is no effective treatment against this side effect.

Hormonal Agents

The palliation of breast and prostate cancer by means of endocrine manipulation is an effective and relatively nontoxic therapy. Toward the end of the nineteenth century, it was noted that the ovaries influenced mammary physiology. In 1896, Beatson, an English surgeon, removed the ovaries in some premenopausal women with breast cancer and reported striking palliation in a few. This was the first use of cancer therapy that involved hormonal manipulation although the term hormone and the concept of a humoral regulator were not developed until 1902. Subsequent studies of oophorectomy showed temporary improvement in one-third of premenopausal patients, and it is still used in some selected patients although it causes a prompt menopause with all its side effects.

In 1941, Huggins, Stevens, and Hodges showed that bilateral orchiectomy could lead to shrinkage of prostatic cancer and its metastases and relieved the pain of bone metastases in many patients. This approach is still used, although less frequently since the availability of medical alternatives. As expected, orchiectomy leads to impotence, loss of libido, gynecomastia, softening of the skin and beard, fatigue, loss of muscle tone, changes in personality, decreased bone mineral density, and hot flashes. In recent years, long-acting gonadotropin-releasing hormone (GnRH) analogs also known as leuteinizing-hormone releasing hormone analogs alone or in combination with androgen antagonists have offered an alternative therapy with equal efficacy and more control and reversibility of the side effects with intermittent therapy. These drugs are listed in **Table 5**.

Hormonal management of breast cancer used to depend on androgens, estrogens, and progestins. In recent years, they have been largely replaced by estrogen antagonists, aromatase inhibitors, and GnRH antagonists. These new groups of agents have the side effects one would expect from estrogen deprivation, such as hot flashes, decreased energy, a variable decrease in bone mineral density, variable nausea, and in some cases an increased incidence of thromboembolic phenomena.

Corticosteroids are widely used throughout medical practice. In cancer therapy, prednisone and dexamethasone are the most frequently used. They have a lytic effect on lymphoma and myeloma cells, reduce the edema associated with brain metastases, reduce immunological and allergic reactions, and exert an antiemetic effect alone and with 5-HT_3 blockers. The many side effects of corticosteroids are often the consequence of the desired effect on the disease process being treated also impacting the normal tissues adversely. These toxicities are well known as they are seen throughout clinical medicine.

Table 5 Hormonal agents

Class	*Drug examples*
Estrogen receptor agonists	Diethylstilbestrol, estradiol, polyestradiol phosphate
Estrogen receptor antagonists	Raloxifene, tamoxifen, toremifene
Progestins	Medroxyprogesterone, megestrol
Androgen receptor agonists	Fluoxymesterone, testosterone
Androgen receptor antagonists	Abiraterone, bicalutamide, flutamide
Antiandrogens	Ketoconazole, nilutamide
Aromatase inhibitors	Aminoglutethimide, anastrozole, exemestane, letrozole
GnRH antagonists	Abarelix, goserelin, leuprolide, triptorelin pamoate
Corticosteroids	Dexamethasone, prednisone

Signal Transduction Inhibitors

Signal transduction inhibitors target regulatory molecules that govern the fundamental processes of cell growth, differentiation, and survival. Most cancers have aberrant signal transduction elements (and often more than one), so they are logical targets for therapeutic intervention. Targets for signal transduction inhibitors can include cell surface receptors (e.g., epidermal growth factor receptor (EGFR)) and intracellular biochemical molecules (e.g., kinases such as Src, PI3K, and Raf). **Table 6** lists some signal transduction inhibitors.

Imatinib mesylate inhibits the Bcr-Abl tyrosine kinase and can induce apoptosis (programmed cell death) and inhibit further proliferation of the cell lines that are positive for Bcr-Abl. It was the first tyrosine kinase inhibitor approved. These cell lines are prominent in Philadelphia chromosome-positive chronic myeloid leukemia and in GI stromal tumors. In many cases, the initial responses have been very good. Dasatinib and nilotinib are also inhibitors of the Bcr-Abl tyrosine kinase. Toxicity of these three agents is primarily associated with GI distress (nausea, vomiting, diarrhea) and all promote fluid retention and may cause hepatotoxicity. Additionally, dasatinib may cause pleural effusions and nilotinib has been associated with QT prolongation.

Gefitnib is an inhibitor of the EGFR, a transmembrane receptor tyrosine kinase (RTK) essential for the growth and

Table 6 Signal transduction inhibitors

Agent	*Major molecular target(s)*
Axitinib	VEGFR1–3, PDGFR, c-kit
Cetuximab	EGFR
Crizotinib	Anaplastic lymphoma kinase (EML4-ALK mutation) and c-met
Dasatinib	Bcr-abl, Src
Erlotinib	EGFR
Everolimus	m-TOR
Gefitinib	EGFR
Imatinib	Bcr-abl, PDGFR, c-kit
Lapatinib	EGFR, HER2/neu
Nilotinib	Bcr-ab, c-kit, lck
Panitumumab	EGFR
Pazopanib	VEGFR1-3, PDGFR, c-kit
Sorafenib	VEGFR, PDGFR, Raf
Sunitinib	Multi-TKR
Temsirolimus	m-TOR
Trastuzumab	HER2/neu
Vemurafinib	Mutant (*V600E*) *B-Raf*

differentiation of epithelial cells. The EGFR is located in varying amounts in tumor cells of the colon, lung, head, and neck. Gefitinib is FDA approved for the treatment of nonsmall cell lung cancer, and is being investigated for activity in other malignancies. Erlotinib is also an inhibitor of the EGFR tyrosine kinase and like gefitinib binds to the kinase domain of the receptor and inhibits its enzymatic function. Erlotinib is FDA-approved as a second- or third-line treatment of advanced nonsmall-cell lung cancer. The most common side effects of both gefitinib and erlotinib are mild to moderate acniform rash (not allergic), diarrhea, anorexia, and fatigue.

There are also more specific inhibitors of the EGFR family. Lapatinib is an inhibitor of a specific form of EGFR known as EGFR2 or HER2, also known as the protooncogene, neu (e.g., HER2/neu). Overexpression of HER2/neu has been correlated with more aggressive breast cancers. It is approved for use in HER2-amplified, trastuzumab-resistant breast cancer (in combination with capecitabine). Like erlotinib and gefitinib, it binds to the kinase domain and inhibits activity. Lapatinib also inhibits a truncated form of the EGFR2 (HER2) receptor. The primary adverse effects are GI distress (nausea, vomiting, diarrhea) and hand–foot syndrome. It has also been associated with hepatotoxicity.

In addition to targeting cell-surface RTKs, many signal transduction inhibitors work at various places in the myriad of biochemical pathways involved in transducing signals from the cell surface to the nucleus.

Rapamycin (sirolimus) is an immunosuppressive drug that was used in the functional characterization of the mammalian target of rapamycin (mTOR), an unusual kinase coordinating growth factor and nutrient availability with cell growth and proliferation. Several rapamycin-related compounds – known as rapalogs – are now approved for use as anticancer agents.

Everolimus is an mTOR inhibitor approved for use in advanced pancreatic neuroendocrine tumors, second- or third-line advanced renal cell carcinoma, and subependymal giant cell astrocytoma associated with tuberous sclerosis. Temsirolimus is the first mTOR inhibitor approved for use in advanced renal cell carcinoma. The most common adverse effects reported for mTOR inhibitors are mouth ulcers, rash, diarrhea, fatigue, and increased incidence of common infections.

Vemurafenib interferes with the Raf/MEK/ERK pathway in individuals with melanoma who have a specific mutation in the *B-Raf* gene (*V600E*). Because it also acts on cells which possess normal *B-Raf*, it may cause a paradoxical enhancement of proliferation (tumor promotion) in those cells. In clinical trials, this was observed as an increase in basal cell carcinomas. Nonclinical reports suggest the potential to be a tumor promoter in other epithelial tissue (e.g., esophagus, bladder) but this has not been reported in humans to date.

Other signal transduction inhibitors (cetuximab, panitumumab, pazopanib, sunitinib, sorafinib, trastuzumab) are considered in sections below as they share a common chemotherapeutic mechanism – antiangiogenesis.

Antiangiogenesis Agents

Angiogenesis inhibitors are drugs that inhibit the growth of new blood vessels. As tumors grow, they need new blood vessels (neovascularization) to provide systemically delivered nutrients to permit rapid growth. The concept underlying antiangiogenesis approaches is that if neovascularization can be inhibited, the tumor will 'starve.' A number of endogenous molecules have some antiangiogenic activity, and several exogenous antiangiogenesis drugs have been developed. The primary target for these drugs has been vascular endothelial growth factor (VEGF), a signaling protein that may be overexpressed in a variety of cancers.

Bevacizumab is an anti-VEGF-A monoclonal antibody (mAb) that binds VEGF and prevents VEGF from interacting with its receptors on the surface of endothelial cells. It is approved for treatment of a variety of tumors. Side effects may include hypertension, proteinuria, a slight increase in bleeding, and impaired surgical wound healing in patients undergoing surgery during bevacizumab treatment. In a small number of patients, potentially life-threatening effects such as arterial thrombotic events (blood clots), GI perforation, and hemoptysis (coughing up of blood or bloody mucus from respiratory tract) have been observed.

Small molecule antiangiogenic drugs include sorafenib, a Raf kinase and VEGF receptor kinase inhibitor; and sunitinib and pazopanib, both multitargeted RTK inhibitors. Adverse events associated with sorafenib include skin rash, hand–foot skin reactions, diarrhea, and hypertension. Sorafenib has also been implicated in the development of reversible posterior leukoencephalopathy syndrome and reversible erythrocytosis. Sunitinib is generally well tolerated; common adverse effects include fatigue, diarrhea, nausea, anorexia, hypertension, a yellow skin discoloration, hand–foot skin reaction, and stomatitis. More serious adverse events occurring in $\leq$10% of patients include hypertension, fatigue, asthenia, diarrhea, and chemotherapy-induced acral erythema. Most adverse events can be managed through supportive care, dose interruption, or dose reduction. The most common adverse reactions for pazopanib include GI distress (nausea, vomiting, diarrhea), hypertension, depigmentaiton of hair, and myelosuppression. Severe and fatal hepatotoxicity was observed in clinical trials.

Another drug having antiangiogenic activity is thalidomide; although its exact mechanism of action is not known, its activity is thought to require enzymatic activation. This drug is discussed in the Miscellaneous Agents section below.

Biotherapeutic Agents

A significant amount of drug development work has occurred in this class of agents within the last two decades. The immune system is responsible for protecting the body from bacteria, viruses, and cancer, and in general it has been hypothesized that an increase in immunologic function may lead to increased immunosurveillance of tumor cells through recognition of tumor-specific antigens. Early work with nonspecific stimulators of the immune system failed to demonstrate any reliable benefit. More recent investigations of immunological responses have increased our knowledge of tumor biology and coupled with recombinant DNA technology have led to the development of the biologic response modifiers and monoclonal antibody targeting agents that are effective as targeted cancer treatment options (**Table 7**). More treatment options are in the pipeline.

Interferons were originally isolated from human leukocytes as antiviral agents, but the interferon alpha-2 used today in

Table 7 Biotherapeutic agents

Agent	*Molecular targets*
Aldesleukin	Interleukin-2
Alemtuzumab	CD52
Bevacizumab	VEGF-A
Brentuximab vedotin	CD30
Cetuximab	EGFR
Denosumab	RANKL
Gemtuzumab ozogamicin	CD33
Ibritumomab tiuxetan	CD20
Interferon alpha-2	Interferon alpha-2
Ipilimumab	CTLA4
Ofatumumab	CD20
Panitumumab	EGFR
Rituximab	CD20
Tositumomab	CD20
Trastuzumab	HER2/neu

cancer therapy is a recombinant product. It is used primarily in the treatment of Hairy cell leukemia, the Kaposi sarcoma of acquired immunodeficiency syndrome (AIDS), melanoma, and renal cell carcinoma. The major toxicity is a flu-like syndrome with fever, chills, rigors, and myalgias. Long-term toxicities include profound fatigue, confusion, neurologic side effects, and depression, sometimes severe enough to lead to suicide.

Interleukins (ILs) are a family of cytokines, substances secreted by T-cells (lymphocytes), monocytes, macrophages, and other cells. Recombinant IL-2, known generically as aldesleukin, is effective in the therapy of a small percent of patients with renal cell carcinoma and melanoma, sometimes with very gratifying results. Its toxicity is dose-, route-, and time dependent. At its worst, high-dose intravenous prolonged infusions cause fever, fluid retention, hypotension, respiratory distress, capillary-leak syndrome, suppression of hematopoiesis, nephrotoxicity, and hepatotoxicity.

Therapeutic monoclonal antibodies (ATC code L01XC) were made possible by the development of the hybridoma methodology in the 1980s. Hybridomas are hybrid cells produced by the fusion of an antibody-producing lymphocyte with a tumor cell and used to culture continuously a specific monoclonal antibody. Monoclonal antibodies are classified and named based on their derivation. Murine monoclonal antibodies, among the first developed, have the suffix ending 'momab,' are cleared relatively quickly from the body, and have a greater chance of inducing a human antimouse antibody (HAMA) reaction. Chimeric antibodies are a human–mouse antibody mixture; they possess the suffix ending 'imab' and are more efficient and effective at destroying cells via complement-dependent cytotoxicity (CDC) and antibody-dependent cell-mediated cytotoxicity (ADCC). Chimeric antibodies circulate longer in the human body and are less likely to invoke an HAMA reaction. Humanized and fully human monoclonal antibodies, developed later, possess the suffix ending 'umab' and are less likely to be cleared quickly or to induce an antidrug antibody response.

Monoclonal antibody therapy is based on the ability to target markers and bind to cell membrane antigens with great specificity. Many times the enhanced specificity demonstrated toward the tumor antigens allows normal cells to be protected against harmful effects, unlike conventional chemotherapy. There are several mechanisms by which monoclonal antibodies destroy or prevent further replication of malignant cells. Some monoclonal antibodies utilize tumor immunology and components of the host natural defense mechanism to exert their desired effect. For example, monoclonal antibodies can utilize tumor effector cells to promote tumor cell lysis or have the ability to directly modulate tumor function. Effector cells such as natural killer cells and monocytes/macrophages express Fc-gamma receptors that can interact with the Fc domain of immunoglobulin G (IgG)-based antibodies, and this interaction can in some cases lead to enhanced tumor cell killing through ADCC. Different IgG subclasses have a greater ability to induce ADCC activity. Some mAbs may also recruit the complement cascade system to kill target cells through CDC.

A common toxicity of monoclonal antibodies is the potential to produce a side effect referred to as an infusion-related symptom complex. The probability of this reaction occurring increases in patients with a large tumor burden. This reaction is generally observed with the first or second dose of the monoclonal antibody; however, it is important to note that mild to severe latent reactions have occurred. The symptom complex is characterized by a rapid release of cytokines leading to one or more of the following: fever, chills, rigors, dyspnea, bronchospasm, headache, hypotension, rash, nausea, throat tightness, flushing, and urticaria. This reaction can range from very mild symptoms to a severe and/or fatal reaction. It is vital to assess each patient on an individual basis due to the variability of reactions. The management of infusion-related reactions begins with stopping the infusion, assessing the patient, and administering hypersensitivity medications as needed (e.g., diphenhydramine, meperidine, H2 blockers, corticosteroids, and epinephrine). Once patient symptoms have resolved, many patients can have the infusion restarted at a slower rate, under clinical observation.

In the last two decades, selected monoclonal antibodies have become a routine part of care for certain malignancies. Rituximab, a chimeric monoclonal antibody used against CD 20 positive B-cell non-Hodgkin's lymphoma, is now utilized in combination with the CHOP regimen (cyclophosphamide, doxorubicin, vincristine, and prednisone). Trastuzumab, a humanized monoclonal antibody, is a weekly maintenance therapy for HER2/neu-positive metastatic breast cancer patients.

A recent novel approach taken by the mAb ipilimumab is to block the downregulating signaling of the cytotoxic T-lymphocyte antigen type 4 (CTLA4) pathway. When CTLA4 receptors are bound by ipilimumab, the resulting downstream pathway is blocked, resulting in sustained T-cell activation and antitumor activity. This drug was approved in 2011 for use in melanoma therapy, and in addition CTLA4 blockade is being investigated in combination with other approaches to enhance tumor recognition by the immune system. The term immune-related adverse events (irAE) has been used to describe the unique constellation of adverse reactions that may occur with the use of drugs of this class. Effects are generally observed in the GI tract (diarrhea, sometimes severe with associated weakness, electrolyte imbalance, and weight loss; and colitis, potentially leading to obstruction and/or perforation), skin (rash; may be pruritic, erythematous, and blanching), and liver (hepatotoxicity). Other irAEs with infrequent occurrence include hypophysitis, uveitis, lymphadenopathy, pancreatitis, and neuropathies.

A unique and promising new class of biotherapeutic agents seeks to employ the best of the small molecule chemotherapeutic agents and the monoclonal antibodies. Antibody-drug conjugates (ADCs) comprise a recombinant antibody covalently bound via a small linker to a cytotoxic drug (also called the payload). As described in this article, many cytotoxic drugs have a narrow therapeutic window which limits efficacy and can result in severe side effects and thus due to their lack of selectivity plasma concentrations needed for superior antitumor response cannot be achieved. ADCs are designed to minimize the systemic toxicity of the free cytotoxic drug and to augment the existing antitumor activity of the monoclonal antibody. The first ADC to be approved was Mylotarg (gemtuzumab ozogamicin; 2001) for the treatment of acute myelogenous leukemia. Mylotarg targets CD33 and exerts its cytotoxic action through conjugation to calicheamycin. Primary toxicities include myelosuppression and in about 30–40% of treated patients, hepatotoxic effects (hyperbilirubinemia and enzyme elevations) and in some, hepatic veno-occlusive disease. The drug has since been removed from the market in the United States due to limited efficacy, but is still available in certain other countries. The only other ADC currently approved for use in oncology is Adcetris (brentuximab vedotin; 2011) for the treatment of relapsed and refractory Hodgkin lymphoma and anaplastic large cell lymphoma. This ADC targets CD30 on tumor cells and uses an auristatin (tubulin inhibitor) as the cytotoxic payload. To date, in clinical trials the primary adverse effect associated with Adcetris were myelosuppression and peripheral sensory neuropathy. A potential increased risk for the development of progressive multifocal leukoencephalopathy has also recently been noted.

Retinoids

Retinoids are differentiation agents related to or derivative of vitamin A. They bind to a cellular protein that facilitates their transfer from the cytoplasm to the nucleus where they are believed to increase DNA, RNA, and protein synthesis and to affect cellular mitosis. Alitretinoin is dispensed as a gel, which is applied topically to treat the skin lesions of Kaposi's sarcoma secondary to AIDS. Except for mild skin irritation and a rash, it has no significant toxicity. Betarotene is used in the treatment of refractory cutaneous T-cell lymphoma (CTCL) and the treatment of AIDS-related Kaposi's sarcoma. It may cause headache, rash, bone marrow depression, and photosensitivity.

Isotretinoin is widely used for the treatment of severe disfiguring acne. It is being evaluated for the treatment of head and neck cancer, CTCL, and neuroblastoma and as a prevention agent for myelodysplastic syndromes. Isotretinoin is teratogenic, and fetal abnormalities can result if used during pregnancy, particularly in the first trimester. Its toxicities include bone pain, myalgia, arthralgia, nausea, vomiting, headache, cheilitis, and elevated serum lipids. Although depression is uncommon, it has been associated with suicides, especially in teenage patients receiving it for the treatment of acne.

Tretinoin is better known as all-transretinoic acid. It is a derivative of vitamin A and binds to a chromosomal receptor that is near the chromosomal lesion that is associated with APL. Differentiation of APL cells occurs after administration of tretinoin and remissions occur but the treatment is not curative and must be followed with cytotoxic chemotherapy for consolidation. Tretinoin is teratogenic and should not be used during pregnancy. General toxicity can also be severe and includes headache, xerosis, pruritis, arthralgia, myalgia, cheilitis, hypertriglyceridemia, and RAS which were described in relation to arsenic trioxide. It may be that the APL contributes to the drug effect in causing RAS. In either case, corticosteroid therapy with dexamethasone can control it.

Miscellaneous Agents

Several agents fall outside the general classes discussed above. Denileukin diftitox is a fusion protein that combines portions of the IL-2 molecule with the diphtheria toxin to destroy cells with the IL-2 receptor by inhibition of protein synthesis. It is used primarily in CTCL in patients whose disease expresses the CD 25 component of the IL-2 receptor. Its major toxicity is hypersensitivity reactions and the vascular leak syndrome.

Mitotane is an adrenal cytotoxic agent for the treatment of adrenocortical cancer. It has been suggested that it damages the mitochondria of adrenocortical cells. The major toxicity is nausea and vomiting and central nervous system effects like lethargy, somnolence, dizziness, and vertigo.

Octreotide is a long-acting somatostatin analog that inhibits the secretion of serotonin, vasoactive intestinal peptide, gastrin, motilin, insulin, glucagons, secretin, and pancreatic polypeptide. It is used for the control of symptoms in patients with carcinoid and vasoactive intestinal peptide-secreting tumors (VIPomas). Its major toxicity is nausea and vomiting.

Thalidomide is best known as a drug that caused an international medical disaster. In 1957, it was marketed in Europe as a hypnotic, particularly for use by pregnant women. After a short period, it became apparent there was an increased incidence of a relatively rare birth defect, phocomelia, in which the hands and feet are attached close to the body resembling flipper of a seal or develop only as limb buds with no digits. It soon reached epidemic proportions, and retrospective epidemiologic research firmly established the causative agent to be thalidomide taken early in the course of pregnancy. Thalidomide was not licensed in the United States and was withdrawn from the European market in 1961. There were some cases in the United States in children born to women on investigational studies. In 1962, the Food Drug and Cosmetic Act was amended to give the FDA more authority in requiring evidence of both efficacy and relative safety before marketing new drugs.

In 1998, the FDA approved the marketing of thalidomide for erythema nodosum leprosy. Subsequently, it has demonstrated activity against multiple myeloma, myelodysplastic syndrome, AIDS wasting syndrome, melanoma, and renal cell carcinoma.

To prevent severe birth defects and possible death of the newborn child, when thalidomide is used in women of childbearing age or in sexually active men (due to levels of thalidomide in semen), adherence to strict guidelines adopted by the

FDA is required. The specific guidelines fall under the term 'S.T.E.P.S. program' or 'System for Thalidomide Education and Prescribing Safety.' All prescribers (physicians) and distributors (pharmacists, etc.) must register and adhere to these guidelines. Other toxicities include headache, dizziness, rash, pruritis, drowsiness, somnolence, peripheral neuropathy, leukopenia, and venous thrombosis.

Like the vaccines for infectious disease that we are most familiar with, cancer vaccines are designed to enhance the immune system's ability to protect itself from the adverse effects posed by damaged or abnormal cells such as transformed (cancer) cells. Also like infectious disease vaccines, cancer vaccines may be prophylactic (preventative), but they may also be therapeutic and actually treat cancer. To date, the FDA has approved two preventative cancer vaccines. The first cancer vaccine was approved in 1981 and was developed against hepatitis B virus, a virus which can cause liver cancer after chronic infection. The newest prophylactive cancer vaccines (Gardasil and Cervarix) were developed against the two serotypes of human papillomavirus, which are considered to be responsible for approximately 70% of all cervical cancers worldwide.

Therapeutic cancer vaccines have proven extremely difficult to develop, likely because cancer cells develop mechanisms to evade the immune system. Effectiveness, therefore, relies on the ability to have a response that is not only highly specific to the cancer cell (and not 'normal' cells) but which is robust enough to be able to overcome the defense mechanism of the cancer cells. To date, only a single therapeutic vaccine has been approved (sipuleucel-T; 2010) and is for some men with metastatic prostate cancer. The vaccine was designed to stimulate an immune response to prostatic acid phosphatase (PAP), an antigen that is found on most prostate cancer cells. Approval was granted based on an increase of approximately 4 months in the survival of men with a certain type of metastatic prostate cancer. Sipuleucel-T is quite different from other vaccines in that each vaccine is unique to the patient. White blood cells are isolated from the individual by leukophoresis, cultured with a PAP that has been conjugated to the granulocyte–monocyte colony-stimulating factor (CSF), which stimulates the immune system as well as enhancing the presentation of the antigen to the white cells. The patient's cells are then transfused back into him. This is repeated two more times.

Combination Cancer Chemotherapy

Just as combination antibiotic chemotherapy has been found to be more efficacious in the treatment of tuberculosis and serious gram-negative sepsis, as compared to single antibiotics, in a similar fashion, combination anticancer chemotherapy has been achieving better results than single agents in many of the tumors tested. Possible exceptions include some of the more sensitive neoplasms such as gestational trophoblastic tumors and African Burkitt's lymphoma where a single agent is often curative. Still, combination regimens seem to have higher response rates and longer durations of disease-free survival in many instances when compared to single agents.

It is best to select drugs with different mechanisms of cell destruction. One can combine an alkylating agent to kill cells in G_0 or any other phase of the cycle, an antimetabolite to kill rapidly developing tumors in M phase, and a corticosteroid or other hormone to control cell growth without definitive cell kill. These agents with differing mechanisms reduce the chances of cell resistance. Tumor angiogenesis is a very complex process, and effective therapy likely requires a combinatorial approach. A number of studies have shown that the use of antiangiogenic agents in combination with chemotherapy or radiotherapy results in additive or synergistic effects.

While combination chemotherapy and high-dose therapy (with or without stem-cell transplantation) can increase cancer response rates, they generally increase toxicity significantly and sometimes in unanticipated ways when drugs interact with each other. Hence, the toxicity of each combination chemotherapy protocol and each high-dose therapy protocol must be considered individually.

Management of Organ System Toxicity

It has been previously emphasized that cancer chemotherapy involves a process of differential and selective toxicity. Agents are used that injure neoplastic cells and normal cells and the goal is to damage the neoplastic cells irreversibly and allow the normal cells and tissues to recover sooner. In addition, it is important to ameliorate the unpleasant side effects and to support the patient. A few major classes of toxicity are discussed in this section.

Bone Marrow Suppression

All elements of the bone marrow are injured by cytotoxic drugs.

Neutrophils are depressed first because they renew their population every day. Neutropenia is defined as an absolute neutrophil count (ANC) 500 cells μl^{-1}. Patients with an ANC of less than 100 cells μl^{-1} or those with prolonged neutropenia (more than 7 days) are at significantly high risk for serious infection. That risk can be reduced with prophylactic antibiotics and the administration of CSFs. Current evidence does not support the routine use of CSFs (filgrastim, pegfilgrastim, and sargramostim) in afebrile neutropenic patients unless the patient is at high risk because of bone marrow compromise or comorbidity, for example, previous radiation to large areas of bone marrow, recurrent febrile neutropenia with similar dose chemotherapy, extensive prior chemotherapy, or active tissue infection. The exceptions to this guideline include administration of trimethoprim–sulfamethoxazole for immunosuppressed patients at risk for *Pneumocystis carinii* pneumonitis and antifungal therapy (with fluconazole) and antiviral therapy (with acyclovir or gancyclovir) for prophylaxis of patients undergoing allogeneic stem-cell transplantation. The development of fever (a single temperature of 101 °F or 38.3 °C or persistent temperature greater than or equal to 100.4 °F or 38 °C) in a neutropenic patient represents an urgent clinical problem requiring a prompt infectious agent assessment and intervention with appropriate antibiotics. Leukocyte transfusions are seldom, if ever, indicted.

Thrombocytopenia (platelet count of less than 10 000 μl^{-1} is a frequent consequence of cytotoxic chemotherapy. A moderate risk of bleeding exists when the platelet count falls to less than 50 000 μl^{-1} and a major risk is associated with platelet counts

Table 8 Summary highlights of American Society of Clinical Oncology's (ASCO) clinical practice guidelines for platelet transfusions[a]

Indication	*Guideline*
Platelet product	Use random donor pooled platelets unless histocompatible platelets are needed, then use single donor platelets
Prophylactic platelet transfusion: acute leukemia and hematopoietic cell transplant	A threshold of 10 000 μl^{-1} is recommended for asymptomatic patients. Transfusions at levels above this threshold are indicated for patients with complicating clinical conditions
Prophylactic transfusions: solid tumors	A threshold of 20 000 μl^{-1} is recommended for patients with bladder cancer receiving aggressive therapy and those with necrotic tumors. For all others, a threshold of 10 000 μl^{-1} is recommended
Surgical or invasion procedures	A platelet count of 40 000–50 000 μl^{-1} is deemed sufficiently safe to perform invasive procedures in the absence of coagulation problems
Prevention of alloimmunization with leukoreduced blood products	Recommended for patients with AML from time of diagnosis; consider for all other patients

[a]Source: Shiffer, C,A., Anderson, K.C., Bennet, C.L. et al. 2001. Platelet transfusion for patients with cancer: clinical practice guidelines of the American Society of Clinical Oncology. J. Clini. Oncol. 19, 1519–1538.

less than 10 000 μl^{-1}. Adequate coagulation can be further compromised by drugs that interfere with platelet function, like aspirin, nonsteroidal antiinflammatory drugs, ginkgo biloba, and anticoagulants like warfarin and heparin. Platelet transfusions can reduce or eliminate fatal consequences in patients at high risk because of thrombocytopenia. Generally accepted guidelines for platelet transfusions are summarized in **Table 8**. An infrequently used approach is to stimulate the production of platelets before administering chemotherapy by the administration of oprelvekin, a recombinant IL-11. This drug stimulates megakaryocytopoiesis and thrombopoiesis and platelet increases are observed 5–9 days after initiation of treatment.

Anemia is associated with cancer and may be multifactorial. It may be due to bleeding, hemolysis, or bone marrow suppression secondary to the malignancy or it may be due to chemotherapy. Treatment for an acute need is generally by red cell transfusion. For chronic anemia in patients due to cancer chemotherapy who are not hemolyzing and not iron deficient, epoetin alpha or the long-acting darbepoetin alpha can raise hemoglobin levels and relieve some of the fatigue of malignancy.

Nausea, Vomiting, and Antiemetic Therapy

There are three patterns of nausea and vomiting associated with chemotherapy: acute, delayed, and anticipatory. Acute occurs within the first 24 h of treatment, delayed occurs or is a continuation beyond 24 h, and anticipatory is the experience of nausea or vomiting before receiving another chemotherapy treatment. It is a conditioned or learned response to previous effects from therapy. It may be prevented by minimizing the adverse effects of the first and subsequent treatments. The incidence and severity of nausea and vomiting are related to the emetogenic potential of the drug (**Table 9**), dose, route of administration, schedule, infusion rate, time of day drug is given, patient characteristics, and combination of drugs. It is easier to prevent nausea and vomiting than to treat. Hence, antiemetics are given shortly before chemotherapy administration. In general, one should use aggressive antiemetic therapy for chemotherapy naïve patients, give an adequate duration of coverage for the predicted risk period and select the appropriate agents and dosing according to the emetic potential of the chemotherapy. While **Table 9** is a good guide, combination chemotherapy will frequently move the potential antiemetic effect higher, that is, one group to the left.

Therapy for nausea and vomiting is directed at blocking the effect on the chemoreceptor trigger zone of the brain and the receptors in the GI tract. For low-risk emetogenic chemotherapy, dexamethasone, metoclopromide, or prochlorperazine are most useful. A psychotropic agent like lorazepam may be helpful if one suspects a degree of apprehension. There are other antiemetics available (e.g., butyrophenones and the cannabinoids), but they are of low therapeutic efficacy and are not recommended as first-line therapy. For moderate or high-risk emetogenic therapy, a 5-HT_3 antagonist (dolasetron, ganisetron, ondansetron, and palonosetron) with dexamethasone is recommended. For delayed emesis due to moderately emetogenic

Table 9 Emetic potential of chemotherapy drugs as single agents

Very high (>90%)	*High (60–90%)*	*Moderate (30–60%)*	*Low (10–30%)*
Carmustine[a]	Azacitidine	Altretamine	Cytarabine
Cisplatin	Carboplatin	Daunorubicin	Docetaxel
Cyclophosphamide[a]	Carmustine	Doxorubicin	Etoposide
Cytarabine[a]	Cyclophosphamide	Epirubicin	5-Fluorouracil
Mechlorethamine	Dacarbazine	Idarubicin	Gemcitabline
Melphalan[a]	Dactinomycin	Ifosfamide	Irinotecan
Streptozocin	Lomustine	Mitomycin	Paclitaxel
		Mitoxantrone	Thiotepa
		Oxaliplatin	Topotecan
		Plicamycin	
		Procarbazine	

[a]High dose.

chemotherapy, a single dose of the long-acting palonosetron (with dexamethasone) may be more effective than the other 5-HT_3 inhibitors. For both acute and delayed emesis due to highly emetogenic drugs, aprepitant plus a 5-HT_3 inhibitor plus dexamethasone is the current treatment of choice. For breakthrough emesis despite optimal prophylactic pretreatment, an agent from another pharmaceutical class may be added and antiemetic doses increased.

Renal and Bladder Toxicity

Major risk factors for renal toxicity in cancer patients include nephrotoxic chemotherapy drugs, age, nutritional status, concurrent use of other nephrotoxic drugs (e.g., aminoglycoside antibiotics), and preexisting renal dysfunction. Drugs with a high risk for renal toxicity include cisplatin, ifosfamide, methotrexate (high dose), mitomycin, and streptozocin. Carboplatin is significantly less nephrotoxic than cisplatin, but if administered in high doses (e.g., in stem-cell transplantation), or given with other nephrotoxic drugs, it has the potential to contribute to renal damage. Before using a renal toxic chemotherapy agent, renal function should be evaluated with a serum creatinine or creatinine clearance as a guide to the need for dose reduction or omission.

Hemorrhagic cystitis and an increased incidence of bladder cancer are associated with the use of ifosfamide and cyclophosphamide. Contact of the bladder wall with their toxic metabolites, primarily acrolein, produces mucosal erythema, inflammation, ulceration, necrosis, diffuse small-vessel hemorrhage, oozing, and a reduced bladder capacity. Symptoms include hematuria (microscopic or gross) and dysuria. The uroprotective agent 2-mercaptoethane sulfonate sodium (mesna) acts by binding to acrolein to result in a nontoxic thioether. The use of adequate mesna and hydration with ifosfamide or high-dose cyclophosphamide significantly reduces the incidence of bladder toxicity.

Cardiopulmonary Toxicity

Chemotherapy drugs can directly or indirectly cause acute pneumonitis (bleomycin, carmustine, gemcitabine, methotrexate, mitomycin, procarbazine, and vinca alkaloids); pulmonary fibrosis (bleomycin, carmustine, cyclophosphamide, methotrexate, and mitomycin); hypersensitivity pneumonitis (bleomycin, methotrexate, and procarbazine); and noncardiogenic pulmonary edema (cytarabine, cyclophosphamide, methotrexate, mitomycin, and teniposide). Docetaxel is associated with fluid retention, which may result in pulmonary edema or pleural effusion. Some of these conditions respond to corticosteroid therapy but some cases of pulmonary fibrosis are fatal.

Cardiomyopathy is the most common chemotherapy-associated cardiac toxicity. Myocardial ischemia, pericarditis, arrhythmias, miscellaneous electrocardiogram changes, and angina occur much less frequently. The anthracyclines (daunorubicin, doxorubicin, epirubicin, and idarubicin) have the highest consistent risk for cardiomyopathy, which is cumulative dose related. There is evidence that high-dose cyclophosphamide, mitoxantrone, and fluorouracil also pose an increased risk of cardiac damage. The concurrent use of traztuzumab with an anthracycline and cyclophosphamide is associated with a risk of cardiac dysfunction, but the consequences of sequential use are not yet known.

Management of chemotherapy-induced cardiac dysfunction is conventional therapy for heart failure. Because of the limited value of this intervention in the face of existing cardiac disease, prevention of cardiac toxicity is important. This can be done by limiting the cumulative total dose, giving it more slowly, and using dexrazoxane, an intracellular iron-chelating agent that prevents iron from combining with anthracyclines to form free oxygen radicals. Dexrazoxane is initiated after two-thirds of the cumulative toxic dose is administered (i.e., at 300 mg m^{-2} for doxorubicin). Long-term follow-up is indicated because congestive heart failure may develop several years after therapy is completed.

Dermatological and Neurological Toxicity

Chemotherapy drugs can cause a variety of dermatological conditions including rashes, pruritis, swelling, hyperkeratosis, urticaria, exfoliation, photosensitivity, flushing, nail changes, and pigmentation. Extravasation of some agents, especially carmustine, dactinomycin, daunorubicin, doxorubicin, epirubicin, idarubicin, mechlorethamine, mitomycin, and the vinca alkaloids, can lead to tissue necrosis, ulceration, and sloughing. To reduce the incidence of extravasation, central venous catheters are frequently used to administer these drugs. Skin is also a target of toxicity with therapies such as CTLA4 blockade; rashes may be pruritic, erythematous, and blanching.

Encephalopathy, peripheral neuropathy, cerebellar syndromes, autonomic neuropathy, and cranial nerve toxicity represent the range of neurological complications associated with cancer chemotherapy. Dose, route of administration, age of the patient, hepatic and renal function, prior and/or concomitant use of other neurotoxic drugs, and the concurrent use of cranial or central nervous system radiotherapy can each influence the incidence rate and severity of neurologic symptoms associated with selected chemotherapy drugs.

The management of the dermatological and neurological toxicities secondary to chemotherapy drugs is essentially the same as those due to other causes. Tables of drugs and their specific subtypes of these toxicities and fuller discussions of them are available in the references listed in Further Reading. They also include discussions of other toxicities including mucositis, diarrhea, constipation, hypercalcemia, headache, depression, anxiety, fatigue, anorexia, weight loss, impotence, sterility, premature menopause, pregnancy risks, and teratogenicity.

See also: Androgens; Arsenic; BCNU (Bischloroethyl Nitrosourea); Blood; Busulfan; Carcinogenesis; Cisplatin; Corticosteroids; Cyclophosphamide; Gallium; Mitomycin C; Nitrogen Mustards; Platinum; Tamoxifen.

Further Reading

Abeloff, M.D., Armitage, J.O., Niederhuber, J.E., Kastan, M.B., McKenna, W.G. (Eds.), 2008. Clinical Oncology, fourth ed. Elsevier Churchill, Philadelphia, PA.

Berger, A., Portenoy, R.K., Weissman, D.E. (Eds.), 2002. Principles and Practice of Palliative Care and Supportive Oncology, second ed. Lippincott Williams and Wilkins, Philadelphia, PA.

Chabner, B.A., Longo, D.L. (Eds.), 2001. Cancer Chemotherapy and Biotherapy, third ed. Lippincott Williams and Wilkins, Philadelphia, PA.

DeVita Jr., V.T., Lawrence, T.S., Rosenberg, S.A., 2011. Cancer, ninth ed. Lippincott Williams and Wilkins, Philadelphia, PA.

Fischer, D.S., Knobf, M.T., Durivage, H.J., Beaulieu, N.J., 2003. The Cancer Chemotherapy Handbook, sixth ed. Mosby, Philadelphia, PA.

Kaehler, K.C., Piel, S., Livingstone, E., et al., 2010. Update on immunologic therapy with anti-CTLA-4 antibodies in melanoma: identification of clinical and biological response patterns, immune-related adverse events, and their management. Semin. Oncol. 37, 485–498.

Mansi, L., Thiery-Vuillemin, A., Nguyen, T., et al., 2010. Safety profile of new anti-cancer drugs. Exp. Opin. Drug Saf. 9 (2), 301–317.

Rosenberg, S.A. (Ed.), 2000. Principles and Practice of the Biological Therapy of Cancer, third ed. Lippincott Williams and Wilkins, Philadelphia, PA.

Relevant Websites

http://www.cancer.gov/cancertopics/druginfo/alphalist – Drug listing pages for the National Cancer Institute.

http://www.nccn.org/professionals/physician_gls/f_guidelines.asp?button=I+Agree – National Comprehensive Cancer Network provides regularly-updated guidance for physicians.

Cancer Potency Factor

FF Farris and SD Ray, Manchester University, Fort Wayne, IN, USA

Introduction

Cancer potency factor (CPF), or cancer slope factor (CSF), is a parameter that arises during the quantitative risk assessment of chemicals or agents being evaluated as carcinogens. It represents a measure of cancer risk from a lifetime exposure to an agent and is typically expressed in units of proportion of a population affected per milligram of substance per kilograms of body weight per day (expressed in units of reciprocal dose ($\text{mg kg}^{-1}\ \text{day}^{-1})^{-1}$). Cancer potency is measured as the slope of the straight line generated during linear extrapolation of the low-dose region on the dose–response curve of the agent.

Quantitative risk assessment is a scientific process by which the relationship between levels of exposure to a noxious agent and the lifetime incidence rates of an undesirable consequence is determined. In toxicology, the process has evolved into one that typically involves four distinct steps: hazard identification, dose–response assessment, exposure assessment, and risk characterization. The first step, hazard identification, attempts to answer the question: Does the chemical or agent involved pose a potential risk? In cancer risk assessment, the question would be more specifically: Does the chemical or agent in question act as a potential carcinogen? Once it has been established that the agent possesses a particular hazard, the second step of the risk assessment process (dose–response assessment) explores the relationship between the dose of the agent and the onset of adverse effects (e.g., tumors). Exposure assessment, the third step of the risk assessment process, involves estimating the extent to which a given population may be exposed to the hazard. Finally, risk characterization involves integrating the first three steps, thereby establishing whether a population is potentially at risk. A second goal of the risk characterization step is to establish exposure levels, such as acceptable daily intakes, which are considered safe for the population. It is in the process of dose–response assessment that the CPF is generated.

Dose–Response Assessment

As noted earlier, a primary goal of dose–response assessment is to understand the relationship between the level of exposure (plotted along the abscissa) to a potential hazard and the onset of effects or degree of response (plotted along the ordinate). In simple terms, the goal is to describe, in quantitative terms, the shape of the dose–response curve. Traditionally, dose–response relationships in toxicology have been described as one of two general forms – the threshold model and the linear no-threshold (LNT) model. The threshold model is widely considered the standard model in pharmacology and toxicology, with two exceptions. In the areas of mutagenesis/carcinogenesis and radiation biology, the LNT has been the dominant model. Both the threshold and LNT models are monotonic; that is, there is no reversal in the direction of the path of the dependent variable as the independent variable increases in value. The threshold model assumes, as its name implies, that there is a true threshold dose, below which no effect is observed – neither harmful nor beneficial. For such a model, the response profile of the experimental population follows that of the control or baseline population until the threshold dose is reached. Thereafter, the profile diverges unidirectionally from that of the control with increasing dose. The LNT model assumes that there is no threshold for effect. In other words, a response is possible for any dose greater than zero, but the effect always diverges unidirectionally and linearly from the baseline effect as the dose increases. In recent years, a third model, the hormetic model, has gained increasing popularity as a potential replacement for the threshold and LNT models. In contrast to the threshold and LNT models, the hormetic model is nonmonotonic (the dependent variable changes in more than one direction with a unidirectional change in the independent variable). Hormesis is a type of biphasic dose–response phenomenon, in which the stimulatory or inhibitory effects observed at low dose are reversed at higher doses. Irrespective of the overall nature of the dose–response relationship, dose–response assessment is performed in two steps. First, the portion of the curve for which experimental data are available is assessed. This is then followed by extrapolation to lower exposures to the extent that is necessary.

Assessment of Experimentally Determined Data

The first step of dose–response assessment is evaluation of data that fall within the range of observations. Ideally, epidemiological data would be used to determine the dose–response relationship for human exposures. Unfortunately, human epidemiological data are often limited, and insufficient exposure data makes it difficult to discern the shape of the curve. Analysis of such data by linear models is often appropriate. When such models fit the data poorly, linear-quadratic or Hill models are often used as alternatives.

In the absence of adequate human data, information collected from animal studies is generally used. The advantage of animal data is that it is often abundant and may provide a rich source of information relating to the mode of action of tumor formation. The disadvantage of animal data is that it typically requires dose and interspecies extrapolations.

If there is sufficient data (human or animal) to ascertain the mode of action of the carcinogen and to support parameter estimation, toxicodynamic modeling may be used to characterize the observed data. These models can provide insight into the relationship between tumor development and key precursor events but the effort involved in their development can be extensive. When a toxicodynamic model is not available, or the purpose of the assessment does not warrant or justify the development of such a model, empirical curve-fitting of the data may be used. Unfortunately, several pitfalls may be associated with this approach. Many different curve-fitting models

 http://dx.doi.org/10.1016/B978-0-12-386454-3.00448-6

are available, and they may lead to ultimately different final results. In the absence of any detailed understanding of the origin of the differences between the results, it is often difficult or impossible to make a reasoned judgment about which result is most appropriate.

Point of Departure

Analysis of the observed data is used as the source for estimation of the value known as the point of departure (POD). The POD is an estimated dose (expressed in human-equivalent terms) near the lower end of the observed range of values that is used as the staring point for subsequent analysis and extrapolation of the dose–response curve at low-dose levels. When low-dose extrapolation is linear, the POD is used to calculate the *slope factor* or *potency* (CPF) of the carcinogen. In situations where nonlinear extrapolation is warranted, the POD is used in the calculation of the *reference dose* or *reference concentration*.

The precise value for the POD is often open to some interpretation. Ideally, the POD represents the lowest value on the dose–response curve that is justified by the experimental data without significant extrapolation to lower doses. If the POD is positioned either too high (above some data points) or too low (well below any observed data points) uncertainty or bias can be introduced into analysis of the low-level data. In the absence of appropriate data, the POD is routinely calculated by means of benchmark dose modeling. Using this approach, the POD is set as the lower 95% confidence limit on a dose associated with an estimated 10% increased tumor incidence or a 10% increase in a nontumor response causally related to the carcinogenicity (ED_{10}).

The significance of the POD is that it represents the point from which low-dose extrapolation begins. For this reason, its placement can markedly influence the estimated value of the CPF.

Extrapolation to Lower Doses and Calculation of CPF

The purpose of low-dose extrapolation is to incorporate as much information as possible in the assessment for doses that are relevant to human exposure. Since many, if not most, exposures to carcinogens are presumed to occur at doses below those for which epidemiological or experimental data have been reported, the low-dose extrapolation represents an important region for assessment. The first step in completing assessment of the low-dose region of the dose–response curve is to decide on how extrapolation between the POD and zero dose will be modeled as linear or nonlinear.

Genotoxic (mutagenic and carcinogenic) agents are assumed to follow the LNT dose–response model. This means that a single genotoxic event is assumed to give rise to the formation of a mutation and initiate the onset of tumor formation. These agents are assumed to have a zero-dose threshold and to induce tumor formation in proportion to exposure, especially at low doses. On this basis, linear extrapolation would be used for agents that are DNA-reactive and by that have direct mutagenic activity.

Linear extrapolation is also appropriate when the mode of action is unknown but there is evidence that there is an approximate linear relationship between exposure and the carcinogenic process. Linear extrapolation is also the default approach and is used when there is no knowledge of information relating to the mode of action of the carcinogen. Linear extrapolation from the POD to zero dose yields a straight line, the slope of which defines the parameter known as the CPF, the CSF, or simply cancer potency. This is diagrammatically represented in **Figure 1**. The value of the CPF represents an upper-bound estimate of risk per increment of dose that can be used to estimate risk probabilities for different environmentally relevant exposure levels. Slope factors should always be accompanied by a weight-of-evidence classification to indicate the strength of the evidence that the agent is a human carcinogen.

Because the LNT model assumes there is no safe dose for carcinogens, a risk that would be considered acceptable must be estimated. This is a probability that a lifetime exposure to a chemical or agent will lead to an excess cancer risk of a specified amount. To determine the excess lifetime cancer risk for exposure to an agent, the exposure dose is multiplied by the potency factor. For example, if a population is exposed to 0.0005 mg kg^{-1} day^{-1} of a carcinogen for a lifetime, and the potency factor for the agent is 0.005 mg kg^{-1} day^{-1}, the excess lifetime cancer risk for exposure to this agent is expressed in eqn [1].

$$\text{Risk} = \text{Dose}\cdot\text{CPF} = (0.0005\ \text{mg kg}^{-1}\ \text{day}^{-1})\,(0.005\ \text{mg kg}^{-1}\ \text{day}^{-1})^{-1} = 2.5\times10^{-6} \quad [1]$$

According to this calculation, 2.5 people out of 1 million exposed to a daily dose of 0.0005 mg kg^{-1} day^{-1} of the agent for a lifetime can be expected to develop cancer.

As noted earlier, the slope factor is usually expressed in units of reciprocal dose (mg kg^{-1} day^{-1}) but toxicology values for carcinogens can be expressed in several ways. If data are sufficient, slope factors listed in the Environmental Protection

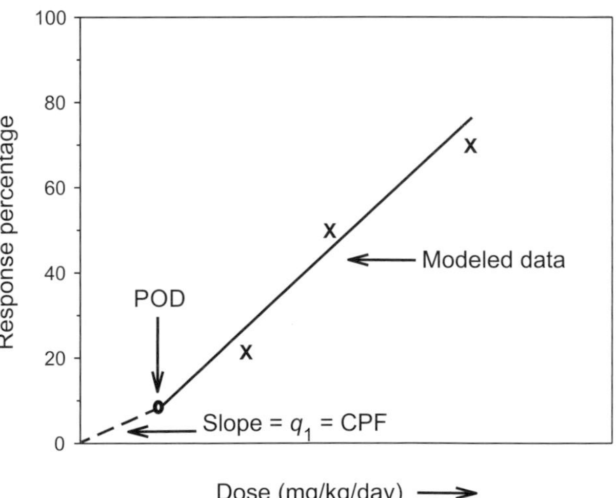

Figure 1 Dose–response modeling of no-threshold dose data. The straight line in the upper portion of the graph (solid line) represents modeling of data within the observational range and extrapolated to the point of departure (POD). The line (dotted) connecting the POD to the zero-dose point represents low-dose linear extrapolation. The slope of this line represents either the cancer potency factor (CPF) or the parameter q_1.

Agency's Integrated Risk Information System are based on absorbed (or administered) dose. Values can also be expressed in terms of risk per unit concentration of the agent in the particular medium where human contact occurs. These measures are called unit risks and express the slope in terms of $\mu g\, l^{-1}$ if lifetime exposure is from drinking water or as ppm if exposure is from air. When the slope factor for inhalation is expressed in units of ppm, it is sometimes referred to as the inhalation unit risk. Unit risk estimates often assume a standard rate of intake ($2\, l\, day^{-1}$ for water and $20\, m^3$ for air) and a standard body weight (70 kg). The respective equations for water eqn [2] and air eqn [3] unit risk calculations are shown below:

$$\text{Water unit risk} = \text{Risk per } \mu g\, l^{-1} = (\text{slope factor})(1/70\text{ kg})(2\, l\, \text{day}^{-1})(10^{-3}) \quad [2]$$

$$\text{Air unit risk} = \text{Risk per } \mu g\, m^{-3} = (\text{slope factor})(1/70\text{ kg})(20\, m^3\, \text{day}^{-1})(10^{-3}) \quad [3]$$

The 10^{-3} term in the earlier equations are necessary to convert between mg (slope factor is given in $(mg\, kg^{-1}\, day^{-1})^{-1}$) and μg (unit risk is expressed in μg).

If adequate information is available, a method preferred to linear approach used earlier is to develop a toxicodynamic model of the carcinogen's mode of action and use this for low-dose extrapolation. One such model is the multistage model constructed based on multistage carcinogenesis and the absence of a carcinogenic threshold. Equation [4] represents the multistage model, estimating the probability of developing cancer from exposures equivalent to a daily dose d:

$$P(d) = 1 - e^{-(q_0 + q_1 d + q_2 d^2 + \ldots + q_k d^k)} \quad [4]$$

where $P(d)$ is the probability of risk of cancer, d is the dose, and k, q_0, q_1, ... q_k are constants that can be estimated by fitting the polynomial to data. For the low-dose range of interest, the equation reduces to approximately the linear term $(q_1 d)$ of the exponent and the constant q_1 (cancer potency) represents the 95% upper confidence limit of the slope factor. Accordingly, the model defines cancer risk as:

$$\text{Cancer risk} = \text{Dose} \cdot q_1 \quad [5]$$

When there is sufficient information to conclude that the mode of action of the agent being assessed is not linear at low doses, nonlinear extrapolation may be warranted. If it is found that the data support a nonlinear mode of action but there is also evidence of mutagenicity, the assessment may require special attention.

See also: Radiation Toxicology, Ionizing and Nonionizing; Carcinogen Classification Schemes; Carcinogenesis; Hazard Identification; Hormesis; Regulation, Toxicology and; Risk Characterization; Risk Assessment, Human Health; Risk Assessment, Uncertainty; Benchmark Dose; Epidemiology; Toxicity Testing, Carcinogenesis; Toxicity Testing, Mutagenicity; Dose–Response Relationship.

Further Reading

California EPA, May 2009. Technical Support Document for Cancer Potency Factors: Methodologies for Derivation, Listing of Available Values, and Adjustments to Allow for Early Life Stage Exposures. California Environmental Protection Agency, Office of Environmental Health Hazard Assessment, Air Toxicology and Epidemiology Branch.

Ecobichon, D.J., 1997. Risk assessment. In: Ecobichon, D.J. (Ed.), The Basis of Toxicity Testing, second ed. CRC Press, Boca Raton, pp. 191–210.

Knafla, A., Petrovic, S., Richardson, M., Campbell, J., Rowat, C., 2011. Development and application of a skin cancer slope factor for exposures to benzo[a]pyrene in soil. Regul. Toxicol. Pharmacol. 59, 101–110.

Theodore, L., Dupont, R.R., 2012. Environmental Health and Hazard Risk Assessment: Principles and Calculations. CRC Press, Boca Raton.

US EPA, March 2005. Guidelines for Carcinogen Risk Assessment. EPA/630/P-03/001F. US Environmental Protection Agency, Risk Assessment Forum, Washington DC.

Candidate List of Substances of Very High Concern (SVHC), REACH

MJ Ramos-Peralonso, Green Planet Environmental Consulting, Madrid, Spain

Background

REACH (Registration, Evaluation, Authorisation, (and Restriction), of Chemicals) is the European Union (EU) regulation adopted to improve the protection of human health and the environment from the risks that can be posed by chemicals, while enhancing the competitiveness of the EU chemicals industry. It also promotes alternative methods for the hazard assessment of substances in order to reduce the number of tests on animals.

Certain substances that may have serious and often irreversible effects on human health and the environment can be identified as Substances of Very High Concern (SVHC). An important objective of the new European Regulation REACH is to encourage and in certain cases to ensure that substances of high concern are eventually replaced by less dangerous substances or technologies where suitable economically and technically viable alternatives are available.

This objective is achieved through the authorization process, the 'A' of REACH, imposing special controls and conditions for substances with some intrinsic properties that lead to particular concern.

The 'Candidate' and the 'Authorization' lists

Under the REACH Regulation, an EU Member State, or the European Chemicals Agency (ECHA) following a request from the European Commission may propose a substance to be identified as a SVHC. If the substance meets the hazard-based criteria, it is included in the 'Candidate List.'

Substances identified as of Very High Concern are first included in the 'Candidate List,' this is the first step of the Authorization Process, and impose some obligations to industry, but not yet a formal request for authorization prior to manufacturing, import, or use.

The Candidate List is the basis for further actions by authorities. It is considered a stepping-stone/portal to authorization (i.e., leading to eventual inclusion of the substance into Annex XIV, following the prioritization steps). It is a tool to gather information on uses in articles through a specific notification process and, where necessary, to require registration or initiate restriction measures. In addition, the Candidate List can have other effects through increased information awareness. In fact, the listing in the Candidate List is a way to provide information on SVHC in articles (to recipients and consumers) and to promote their replacement by alternative substances/technologies or articles.

Following the identification as SVHC and inclusion in the Candidate List, a substance may be prioritized and then included in the Authorization List (which is Annex XIV of the REACH Regulation). Substances that are included in Annex XIV are subject to authorization. This means that after a fixed date, set in Annex XIV at the moment of the inclusion of the substances, they may not be used or placed on the EU market without an authorization; they may, however, continue to be manufactured in the EU for export without authorization. If an SVHC is placed on the Authorization List companies which want to market or use this substance are required to send an application requesting the authorization for specified uses, and the European Commission, taking into account the opinions of the ECHA Committees, would decide if the authorization should be granted or refused. The decision to grant or refuse an authorization is taken by the European Commission in consultation with the EU Member States under a comitology procedure. The authorization decision is subject to a review period and may also be subject to conditions. The presence of the substance listed in Annex XIV in articles manufactured outside the EU and placed on the market in the EU is not affected by the Authorization Process.

REACH Criteria for the Identification of SVHC

The intrinsic properties which a substance must have to be identified as SVHC are listed in Article 57 of REACH. These criteria cover three main groups:

- CMR substances: Substances meeting the criteria for classification as carcinogenic, mutagenic, or toxic for reproduction category 1A or 1B in accordance with the Classification, Labeling, and Packaging (CLP) Regulation (EC) No. 1272/2008, which implements in the EU the United Nations Global Harmonized System for Classification and Labeling.
- Substances which are Persistent, Bioaccumulative, and Toxic (PBT) or very Persistent and very Bioaccumulative (vPvB) according to the criteria established under Annex XIII of REACH.
- Substances identified on a case-by-case basis, for which there is scientific evidence of probable serious effects that cause an equivalent level of concern as with CMR or PBT/vPvB substances. REACH mentions specifically endocrine disruptors, but other health and environmental concerns may be considered.

The SVHC Identification Process

The Authorization Process can be triggered by a Member State that submits an Annex XV dossier to ECHA or by the preparation of an Annex XV dossier by ECHA at the request of the European Commission. This dossier must identify which of the properties listed as criteria for SVHC identification are applicable. In case of substances that are subject to an harmonized classification for the relevant criteria in accordance with the CLP Regulation, the dossier may be limited to a reference to that CLP entry if appropriate. For all the other cases, the dossier must justify that the intrinsic properties of

 http://dx.doi.org/10.1016/B978-0-12-386454-3.00547-9

the substance meet one of the conditions in Article 57. In addition, it is recommended that the dossier includes any available information on uses, emissions, and exposures to facilitate the scientific process leading to ECHAs recommendation for inclusion in Annex XIV.

Prior to the submission of an Annex XV proposal, it is highly recommended to request ECHA to include the substance in the 'Registry of Intentions.' The aim of the public registry of intentions is to allow interested parties to be aware of the substances for which the authorities intend to submit Annex XV dossiers and therefore facilitates timely preparation of the interested parties for commenting later in the process. A second aim is to avoid duplication of work and encourage cooperation between Member States when preparing Annex XV dossiers. The registry allows to check if another EU Authority has in the past worked on an Annex XV dossier for a specific substance or is currently preparing an Annex XV dossier on the substance.

After the formal submission, there is a public consultation. Anyone can comment or add further information related to the use, exposure, alternatives, and risks of a proposed substance. Those most likely to be interested are companies, organizations representing industry or civil society, individual citizens, as well as public authorities. Comments are welcomed from the EU or beyond. The public consultation lasts for 45 days. The dossier is also submitted to the Member States who have the right to comment within 60 days.

If no comments are received, the substance is included in the Candidate List. If there is any comment, the dossier, the comments, and the responses from the submitting party are referred to the Member State Committee, which has 30 days to reach a unanimous agreement. If unanimity is reached, the substance is included in the Candidate List. If no unanimous agreement is reached, the Commission has 3 months to prepare a decision, which must be adopted under a comitology procedure.

The ECHA decisions including substances in the Candidate List are published in the ECHA website. The information includes the substance identity with the EC number and CAS number, and the reason for inclusion. Additional supporting information is also presented. This includes a document with relevant information supporting the ECHA decision and the IUCLID 5 Substance Datasets, which are partly pre-filled substance data sets in IUCLID 5.3 format. IUCLID 5 data sets are provided as a support for importers or producers of articles preparing notifications for substances in articles. Information on conditions applicable to the classification of the substance is also provided.

Obligations Resulting from Inclusion in the Candidate List

The inclusion of substances in the Candidate List may create specific obligations for manufacturers, importers, and even downstream users. These obligations refer not only to the listed substances on their own or in mixtures but also to their presence in articles.

For substances marketed on their own the main obligation starts on the date of inclusion, obliging EU and European Economic Area (EEA) suppliers of substances on the Candidate List to provide their customers with a safety data sheet.

For substances marketed as components in mixtures, the main obligation also starts on the date of inclusion, but its implementation depends on the request from their clients. EU and EEA suppliers of mixtures not classified as dangerous have to provide the recipients, at their request, with a safety data sheet if the mixture contains at least one substance on the Candidate List and the individual concentration of this substance in the mixture is $\geq 0.1\%$ (w/w) for nongaseous mixtures if the substance is PBT or vPvB.

Nevertheless, the most relevant obligations are for substances in articles, these obligations include requirements regarding the transfer of information through the supply chain and to consumers. Producers or importers of articles have additional obligations regarding notification to ECHA.

EU or EEA suppliers of articles which contain substances on the Candidate List in a concentration above 0.1% (w/w) have to provide sufficient information to allow safe use of the article to their customers. In addition and upon request from a consumer, they must provide within 45 days of the receipt of the request, sufficient information to allow safe use of the article by the consumer. This information must contain as a minimum the name of the substance.

In addition, EU and EEA producers or importers of articles have to notify ECHA if their article contains a substance on the Candidate List. This obligation applies if the substance is present in those articles in quantities totaling over 1 ton per producer or importer per year and if the substance is present in those articles above a concentration of 0.1% (w/w).

The notifications have to be submitted no later than 6 months after the inclusion. A notification is not required when the substance has already been registered for that use or when the producer or importer of an article can exclude exposure of humans and the environment during the use and disposal of the article. In such cases, the producer or importer shall however supply appropriate instructions to the recipient of the article.

ECHA published in their website the received notifications. However, the real value of this information for consumers is very limited if no additional information is provided for facilitating the consumers to have educated decisions regarding the use of articles containing SVHC.

From the Candidate List to the Authorization List

ECHA regularly submit to the European Commission recommendations of substances identified as SVHC that should be subject to authorization. To this end, ECHA prioritizes the substances from the Candidate List to determine which ones should be included in the Authorization List (Annex XIV). The prioritization is based on the available information on intrinsic properties, uses, and volumes of the substances on the EU market, using a tiered approach.

Tier I considers the three prioritization criteria related to (1) the intrinsic properties of a Candidate List substance, (2) the nature of its uses, and (3) its volume supplied to uses in the scope of the Authorization.

The inherent properties of substances on the Candidate List are scored with respect to the extent of their persistency, liability to bioaccumulate, and toxicity (PBT-ness) or their potency to elicit health effects (threshold versus nonthreshold mode of action) as follows:

Inherent properties	*Score*
PBT and vPvB or PBT with T nonthreshold C or M	4
PBT or vPvB properties	3
C or M properties (without effect threshold)	1
C, M, or R properties (with effect threshold)	0

This scoring considers that priority shall normally be given to substances with PBT or vPvB properties but also reflects differences in the characteristics of the hazard potential of each substance.

Wide-dispersive uses are characterized by use(s) of a substance on its own, in a preparation or in an article at many places (sites) that may result in not insignificant releases and exposure to a considerable part of the population (workers, consumers, general public) and/or the environment. The scoring is done using the following equation:

$$\text{Wide-Dispersive Use} = \text{Site-\#}^{*}\text{Release}$$

where Site-# is a number between 0 and 3 related to the number of point sources or number of sites from which a substance is being released, and Release is a number between 0 and 3 indicating the potential for releases to the environment, for worker exposure, and for consumer exposure in all steps of the life cycle.

The annual volume supplied in the EU to uses not exempted from the authorization requirement is used for scoring the volume criteria as follows:

Volume on EU market	*Score*
No volume on EU market in the scope of authorization	0
Low (<10 ton year^{-1})	1
Relatively low (10–100 ton year^{-1})	3
Relatively high (100–1000 ton year^{-1})	5
High (1000–10 000 ton year^{-1})	7
Very high (>10 000 ton year^{-1})	9

The total score is calculated by a weighted sum method, with relative weights representing 18, 41, and 41% for the hazard, dispersive use, and volume criteria, respectively.

In Tier II, the regulatory effectiveness and coherence-related considerations are taken into account for finally concluding as to whether the substance considered should be recommended for inclusion in Annex XIV. This second tier was introduced because situations may occur where inclusion in Annex XIV will require regulatory efforts but most likely will not result in benefits for human health or the environment, or where authorization may hamper the use of other risk management instruments while not contributing significantly to achieving the risk reduction.

The ECHA draft recommendation is then subjected to a public consultation. Anyone can comment on the proposed recommendation. In particular, comments may address uses which should be exempted from the authorization requirement. Comments are welcomed from the EU or beyond. The public consultation lasts for 3 months.

ECHA takes into account the comments for updating the draft recommendation. The comments are considered by the Member State Committee to draft its opinion, which is the basis for the Commission Decision to include the substance in the Authorization List which is Annex XIV of REACH.

The Authorization List and the Authorization Process

The Authorization List includes the names and identifiers (EC and CAS numbers), the intrinsic properties justifying the inclusion, the excepted uses and review periods if needed, and two key dates:

- The sunset date is the date from which the placing on the market and the use of the substance shall be prohibited unless an authorization is granted.
- The latest application date is the date by which applications must be received if the applicant wishes to continue to use the substance or place it on the market for certain uses after the sunset date(s); these continued uses shall be allowed after the sunset date until a decision on the application for authorization is taken.

The placing on the market and use of SVHC included in the Authorization List require an authorization. A manufacturer, an importer, or a downstream user can apply for an authorization. Applications for authorization are submitted to ECHA. The application will include a chemical safety report, an analysis of the possible alternatives, and a plan to substitute the substance if suitable alternatives are available. It may also include a socioeconomic analysis. The application for Authorization Process includes an 8-week period of public consultation. Anyone can comment on the uses of the substance related to the application, in particular to provide information on alternative substances or technologies.

At the end of the Authorization Process, which includes a public consultation and the development of opinions by ECHA's Committees on Risk Assessment and Socioeconomic Analysis, the European Commission decides on the granting or refusing of authorizations.

Authorizations will be granted if the applicant can demonstrate that the risk from the use of the substance is adequately controlled. If not, an authorization may still be granted when it is proven that the socioeconomic benefits of using the substance outweigh the risks and there are no suitable alternative substances or technologies.

Holders of an authorization must comply with the requirements of the decision and include the authorization number on the label before they place the substance or the mixture containing the substance on the market. Downstream users of an authorized substance must also comply with the decision and notify to ECHA the use of the substance within 3 months of the first supply of the substance. ECHA keep a register of these notifications and give access to the Competent Authorities of the Member States.

All authorization decisions define a time-limited review period. Holders of authorizations must submit a review report at least 18 months before this review period ends. In addition, an authorization may be reviewed at any time if the circumstances of the authorized use change so as to affect the risks or the socioeconomic impact or if new information on alternatives becomes available.

See also: REACH; Risk Management.

Further Reading

ECHA, 2009. Workshop on the Candidate List and Authorisation as Risk Management Instruments. ECHA-09-R-02-EN. http://echa.europa.eu/documents/10162/13639/authorisation_workshop_proceedings_20090121_en.pdf.

ECHA, 2010. General Approach for Prioritisation of Substances of Very High Concern (SVHCs) for Inclusion in the List of Substances Subject to Authorisation. http://echa.europa.eu/documents/10162/13640/axiv_prioritysetting_general_approach_20100701_en.pdf.

ECHA, 2011. Guidance on the Preparation of an Application for Authorization. ECHA-11-G-01-EN. http://echa.europa.eu/documents/10162/13637/authorisation_application_en.pdf.

European Commission DG Environment, 2011. Assessing the Health and Environmental Impacts in the Context of Socio-economic Analysis under REACH. ENV.D.1/SER/2009/0085r. http://ec.europa.eu/environment/chemicals/reach/pdf/REACH SEA Part 1_Final publ.pdf and. http://ec.europa.eu/environment/chemicals/reach/pdf/REACH%20SEA%20Part%202%20LogicFrame%20Final%20publ.pdf.

REACH Regulation: Regulation (EC) No 1907/2006 of The European Parliament and of the Council of 18 December 2006 concerning the Registration, Evaluation, Authorisation and Restriction of Chemicals (REACH), establishing a European Chemicals Agency, amending Directive 1999/45/EC and repealing Council Regulation (EEC) No 793/93 and Commission Regulation (EC) No 1488/94 as well as Council Directive 76/769/EEC and Commission Directives 91/155/EEC, 93/67/EEC, 93/105/EC and 2000/21/EC

Relevant Websites

http://echa.europa.eu/web/guest/addressing-chemicals-of-concern/authorisation – ECHA, European Chemicals Agency: Authorisation site.

http://ec.europa.eu/environment/chemicals/reach/reach_intro.htm – European Commission DG Environment, REACH web page.

http://ec.europa.eu/enterprise/sectors/chemicals/reach/index_en.htm – European Commission DG Enterprise and Industry, REACH web page.

Cannabinoids

J Chilakapati, Alcon Research Ltd, Fort Worth, TX, USA
FF Farris, Manchester University College of Pharmacy, Fort Wayne, IN, USA

This article is a revision of the previous edition article by Jaya Chilakapati and Harihara M. Mehendale, volume 1, pp 405–407, © 2005, Elsevier Inc.

- Name: Cannabinoids
- Chemical Abstracts Service Registry Number: Cannabinoids are a class of compounds; no individual number has been assigned
- Chemical Structures:

Phytocannabinoids
Δ^9-Tetrahydrocannabinol (THC)

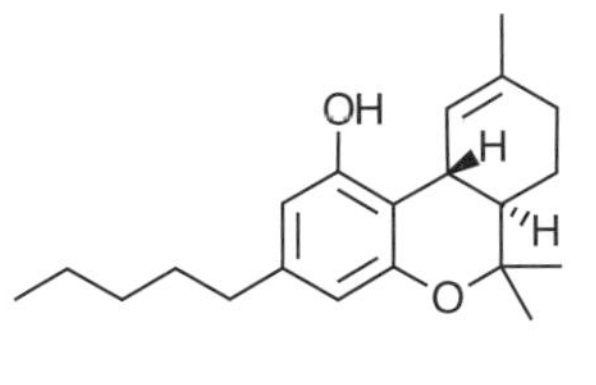

Endocannabinoids
Arachidonoylethanolamide (AEA, anandamide)

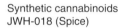

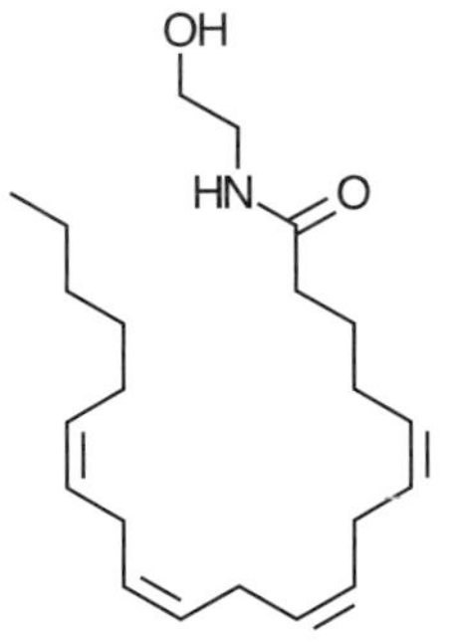

Synthetic cannabinoids
JWH-018 (Spice)

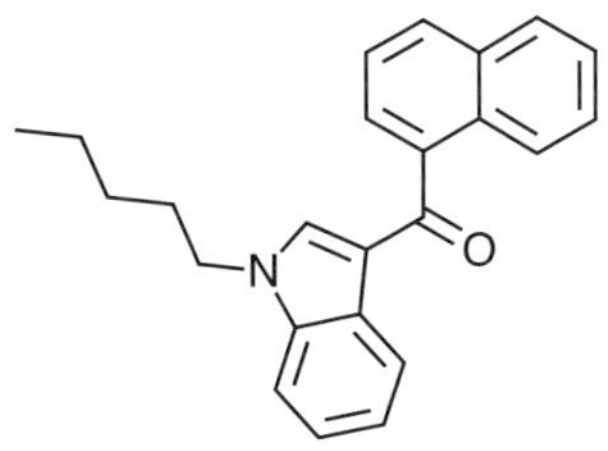

Background

The first cannabinoids to be discovered were those derived from *Cannabis sativa*, the hemp plant. Collectively, these agents are known as phytocannabinoids and, to date, more than 60 have been identified and structurally characterized. The most potent psychoactive agents derived from cannabis is Δ^9-tetrahydrocannabinol (THC). Other plant-derived cannabinoids include cannabinol (CBN) and cannabidiol (CBD). *Cannabis sativa* is the plant from which marijuana (leaves, stems, seeds) is derived. The most potent form of this plant's extracts is hash oil, a liquid. The dried resins are referred to as 'hashish.' The dried flowering tops and leaves are smoked as a cigarette, known as a 'joint' or a 'reefer.' This plant has been used for several thousands of years both recreationally and medicinally. Pharmacological experiments with these, and other phytocannabinoids, were first performed in the 1940s and 1950s, although the term marijuana became popular in the 1930s; it was originally a slang word for the medicinal part of cannabis smoked by Mexican soldiers. As it was discovered that pharmacological activity of the phytocannabinoids is highly dependent on chemical structure, it became more clearly evident that activity was associated with receptor binding.

Cannabinoids are a structurally diverse family of compounds with a large number of biological targets. Based on their origins, cannabinoids can be classified into three groups: phytocannabinoids, endocannabinoids, and synthetic cannabinoids. Phytocannabinoids are present in the stalks, leaves, flowers, and seeds of the plant, and also in the resin secreted by the female plant. A 'joint' made out of skunkweed, netherweed, and other potent subspecies of *C. sativa* may contain ~150 mg of THC, or 300 mg if laced with hashish oil. Endocannabinoids are produced within the body and serve as intercellular lipid messengers. It is believed that these are synthesized on demand rather than made and stored for later use. Synthetic cannabinoid receptor agonists are a large family of chemically unrelated structures that act as Δ^9-THC but are more effective.

Cannabinoid receptors were discovered in the late 1980s. At present, there are two known types of cannabinoid receptors, CB_1 and CB_2. Both CB_1 and CB_2 receptors are G-protein coupled receptors but they differ significantly in their anatomical distribution and their pharmacological effects. Cannabinoid type 1 receptors (CB_1) are expressed mainly in the brain, spinal cord, and peripheral nervous system but are also found in organs and tissues, including endocrine glands and parts of the reproductive, urinary, and gastrointestinal tracts. CB_1 receptors are absent in the medulla oblongata, the part of the brainstem responsible for respiratory and cardiovascular functions, which may account for cannabis-related acute fatalities. CB_1 receptors appear to be responsible for the euphoric and anticonvulsive effects of cannabis. CB_2 receptors are expressed primarily in the immune system, or in immune-derived cells such as leukocytes. CB_2 receptors possibly influence the release of cytokines and therefore are believed to be responsible for the anti-inflammatory and therapeutic effects of cannabis. Because activation of the CB_2 receptor does not cause psychological

 http://dx.doi.org/10.1016/B978-0-12-386454-3.00267-0

effects, selective agonists have become increasingly investigated for their therapeutic effects.

Since cannabis smoke contains many of the same components as tobacco smoke, there are valid concerns about the adverse pulmonary effects of smoked cannabis. Investigators found that occasional and low-cumulative cannabis use is not associated with adverse effects on pulmonary function. Several European countries and the United States have placed restrictions or banned the use and sale of spice drugs due to the dangerous effects and abuse potential of the drugs. The US Drug Enforcement Administration has temporarily designated five of these chemicals (JWH-018, JWH-073, JWH-200, CP-47,497, and cannabicyclohexanol) as Schedule I substances.

Withdrawal symptoms, e.g., irritability, insomnia with sleep electroencephalogram disturbance, restlessness, hot flashes, and, rarely, nausea and cramping, have been observed. However, these symptoms appear to be mild compared with withdrawal symptoms associated with opiates or benzodiazepines, and the symptoms usually dissipate after a few days. Although cannabinoids are considered by some to be addictive drugs, their addictive potential is considerably lower than that of other prescribed agents or substances of abuse. The brain develops a tolerance to cannabinoids. Short-term memory is impaired even after small doses in both naive and experienced users. The deficits appear to be in acquisition of memory, which may result from an attentional deficit, combined with the inability to filter out irrelevant information and the intrusion of extraneous thoughts.

Uses

Δ^9-THC and some synthetic analogs are used therapeutically, for example, for nausea and vomiting produced by antineoplastic chemotherapy, analgesic, anticonvulsant for epilepsy, anti inflammatory agent, appetite stimulant for patients with AIDS, as well as treatment for conditions such as asthma and glaucoma. Synthetic cannabinoids used therapeutically include Dronabinol®, Nabilone®, and Levonamtradol®. The newest clinically available cannabinoid, Sativex®, is an equal mixture of Δ^9-THC and a plant-derived cannabinoid lacking psychotropic effects known as cannabidiol.

Environmental Fate and Behavior

The use of cannabinoids as antiemetics, appetite stimulants, and illicit-use drugs may result in their release to the environment through various waste streams. *Cannabis sativa* is an annual herb, and phytocannabinoids within this plant may be released to air. For example, THC has an estimated vapor pressure of 4.6×10^{-8} mmHg at 25 °C, indicating that it will exist in both the vapor and particulate phases in the atmosphere. Vapor-phase Δ^9-THC will be degraded in the atmosphere within a few hours by reaction with photochemically produced hydroxyl radicals. Particulate-phase Δ^9-THC will be removed from the atmosphere by wet or dry deposition. If released to soil, phytocannabinoids are likely to have little or no mobility. If released into water, they are expected to adsorb to suspended solids and sediment base. Volatilization from water surfaces is expected. The potential for bioconcentration in aquatic organisms is very high, provided the compound is not metabolized by the organism. Occupational exposure to cannabinoids may occur through inhalation and dermal contact. Limited monitoring data indicate that the general population may be exposed to Δ^9-THC via inhalation, ingestion, and dermal contact with contaminated air and water. The general population may also be exposed via passive inhalation of marijuana smoke both from the illicit substance as well as through administration of pharmaceutical products.

Exposure Routes and Pathways

The usual route of administration for medical purposes is oral. The commonest routes of abuse can be primarily via inhalation, not excluding all other routes.

Toxicokinetics

About 50% of the THC in a joint of herbal cannabis is inhaled in the mainstream smoke; nearly all of this is absorbed through the lungs. It rapidly enters the bloodstream, and reaches the brain within minutes. Effects are perceptible within seconds and fully apparent in a few minutes. Bioavailability after oral ingestion is much less; blood concentrations reached are 25–30% of those obtained by smoking the same dose, partly because of first-pass metabolism in the liver. The onset of effect is delayed (0.5–2 h) but the duration is prolonged because of continued slow absorption from the gut. Once absorbed, THC and other cannabinoids are rapidly distributed to all other tissues at rates dependent on the blood flow. Because they are extremely lipid soluble, cannabinoids accumulate in fatty tissues, reaching peak concentrations in 4–5 days. They are then slowly released back into other body compartments, including the brain. Because of the sequestration in fat, the tissue elimination half-life of THC is ~7 days, and complete elimination of a single dose may take up to 30 days. Clearly, with repeated dosage, high levels of cannabinoids can accumulate in the body and continue to reach the brain. Within the brain, THC and other cannabinoids are differentially distributed. High concentrations are reached in neocortical, limbic, sensory, and motor areas.

Cannabinoids are metabolized in the liver. A major metabolite is 11-hydroxy-THC, which is possibly more potent than THC itself and may be responsible for some of the effects of cannabis. More than 20 other metabolites are known, some of which are psychoactive and all of which have long half-lives of several days. The metabolites are partly excreted in the urine (25%) but mainly into the gut (65%) from which they are reabsorbed, further prolonging their actions. Because of the pharmacokinetic characteristics of cannabinoids – both the sequestration in fat and the presence of active metabolites – there is a very poor relationship between plasma or urine concentrations and degree of cannabinoid-induced intoxication.

Mechanism of Toxicity

The most potent cannabinoid, THC, was isolated in the 1960s. Nearly 3 decades later, in the early 1990s, the specific cannabinoid receptors were discovered, CB_1 (or Cnr1) and CB_2 (or Cnr2). Cannabinoids exert their effect by interaction with specific endogenous cannabinoid receptors. Neuronal cannabinoid receptors are termed CB_1 receptors and have been found in rat, guinea pig, dog, monkey, pig, and human brains and peripheral nerves. A second cannabinoid receptor, the CB_2 receptor, was identified in macrophages in the spleen and is also present in other immune cells. The highest densities are found in the frontal cerebral cortex (higher functioning), hippocampus (memory, cognition), basal ganglion and cerebellum (movement), and striatum (brain reward). Other brain regions in which the CB_1 receptors are found include areas responsible for anxiety, pain, sensory perception, motor coordination, and endocrine function. This distribution is consistent with the clinical effects elicited by cannabinoids.

The discovery of cannabinoid receptors naturally stimulated a search for an endogenous ligand with which the receptors naturally interact. The CB_2 receptor, on the other hand, is located peripherally. Specifically, it is involved in the immune system (splenic macrophages, T and B lymphocytes), peripheral nerves, and the vas deferens. The two main endocannabinoids discovered were anandamide (arachidonoyl ethanolamine) and 2-arachidonoyl glycerol. Anandamide (named after the Sanskrit word for bliss, *ananda*) was isolated from the pig brain. It was found to be chemically different from plant cannabinoids: it is a derivative of the fatty acid arachidonic acid (arachidonyl ethanolamide) related to the prostaglandins. It has a high affinity for CB_1 receptors and mimics most of the actions of THC. Both the CB_1 and CB_2 receptors inhibit adenylate cyclase and stimulate potassium channels. As a result, the CR_1 receptors inhibit the release of several neurotransmitters, including acetylcholine, glutamate, norepinephrine, dopamine, serotonin, and gamma-aminobutyric acid (GABA). CR_2 receptor signaling is involved in immune and inflammatory reactions.

At the biochemical level, THC is metabolized via the hepatic cytochrome P450 (CYP) system. THC is metabolized into an active compound, 11-hydroxy-THC (11-OH-THC), which is further metabolized into inactive forms. The elimination half-life of THC can range from 2 to 57 h following intravenous use and inhalation. The half-life of 11-OH-THC, the active metabolite of THC, is 12–36 h. Intravenous use or inhalation results in 15% excretion in the urine and 25–35% in the feces. Within 5 days, nearly 90% of THC is eliminated from the body.

Acute and Short-Term Toxicity (or Exposure)

Animal

With THC, the oral LD_{50} in mice is 482 mg kg^{-1}, the rat oral LD_{50} is 666 mg kg^{-1}, and the intravenous LD_{50} is 29 mg kg^{-1}. Δ^9-THC and other cannabinoids with psychoactive effects in humans have particularly unusual effects on the overt behavior of dogs. At dose levels that elicit blood concentrations of THC similar to those found in regular human marijuana users, THC markedly disrupts the menstrual cycle in the rhesus monkey. Naturally occurring cannabinoids, unique to the plant *C. sativa* and constituting 15% of the cannabis by weight, have been implicated as immunomodulatory. Δ^9-THC has been studied to characterize its immunosuppressive properties, and studies have shown that it suppresses both humoral and cell-mediated immunity in experimental animals.

Human

Absorption of the cannabis product chiefly depends on the route of exposure. For example, onset of action is extremely rapid (within minutes) via smoking; it results in 10–35% absorption of the available THC and peak plasma concentrations occur within 8 min. The second commonest route is via ingestion, and onset occurs within 1–3 h (highly unpredictable); 5–20% is absorbed due to stomach acid content and metabolism; peak plasma levels occur 2–6 h after ingestion. In contrast, synthetic forms include (1) dronabinol (Marinol) – 10% absorption, peak concentration 2–3 h after ingestion; and (2) nabilone (Cesanet) – up to 90% absorption; peak concentration in 2 h after ingestion.

High levels of intoxication are associated with decreased motor coordination, muscle strength, and hand steadiness. Lethargy, sedation, poor concentration ability, slurred speech, ataxia, and an increase in reaction time may also occur. High doses of Δ^9-THC can induce frank hallucinations, delusions, and paranoid feelings. Thinking becomes confused and disorganized; depersonalization and altered time sense are accentuated. Anxiety reaching panic proportions may replace euphoria, often as a result of the feeling that the drug-induced state will never end.

The most consistent effects on the cardiovascular system are an increase in heart rate, an increase in systolic blood pressure while supine, decreased blood pressure while standing, and a marked reddening of the conjunctivae.

Chronic Toxicity (or Exposure)

Animal

Under the conditions of 2-year gavage studies, there was no evidence of carcinogenic activity of 1-*trans*-Δ^9-tetrahydrocannabinol in male or female F344/N rats administered 12.5, 25, or 50 mg kg^{-1}. There was equivocal evidence of carcinogenic activity of THC in male and female B6C3F1 mice based on the increased incidences of thyroid gland follicular cell adenomas in rats treated with 125 mg THC per kg.

Human

Chronic use can be associated with subtle impairment in cognitive function, which is dependent on dose and duration of use. At present, most of the available data indicate that these cognitive deficits are reversible after more than a week of abstinence. Chronic use may be associated with the induction of 'amotivational syndrome' and loss of memory. Endocrine effects have been reported following chronic use, including impairment of gonadotropin secretion, follicle-stimulating hormone (FSH), and luteinizing hormone (LH); reduction in testosterone levels; and direct effects on cytochrome P450 of the Leydig cells with inhibition of testosterone synthesis. Abrupt discontinuation of chronic THC use has resulted in a mild abstinence syndrome, consisting of agitation, apprehension, and aggressiveness, as well as tremulousness, insomnia, and diaphoresis, and the development of common migraine headaches.

THC produces euphoria, or a 'high,' including feelings of intoxication and detachment, relaxation, altered perception of time and distance, intensified sensory experiences, laughter, talkativeness, decreased anxiety, decreased alertness, and depression. These effects depend on the dose, expectations of the user, mode of administration, social environment, and personality. This is primarily because THC triggers dopaminergic neurons in the ventral tegmental area of the brain, a region known to mediate the reinforcing (rewarding) effects. This dopaminergic drive is thought to underlie the reinforcing and addicting properties of this drug. Dysphoric reactions to cannabis are not uncommon, especially in naive users. THC effects may include severe anxiety or panic, unpleasant somatic sensations, delirium, mania, or paranoia. Anxiety and panic are the most common reactions; they are of sudden onset during or shortly after smoking, or they can appear more gradually 1–2 h after an oral dose. These anxiety/panic reactions usually resolve without intervention. Flashbacks occasionally occur in which the original drug experience (usually dysphoria) is relived weeks or months after use.

Pulmonary Toxicity

Transient bronchodilation is the most prominent effect after an acute exposure. Heavy smokers or chronic users experience increased cough, sputum production, and wheezing. These complaints are augmented by concurrent tobacco use. A gradual decline in respiratory function is greater among marijuana smokers compared to tobacco smokers. Marijuana cigarettes contain the same components as tobacco smoke, including bronchial irritants, tumor initiators (mutagens), and tumor promoters, in addition to nicotine. Estimates based on smoking had revealed that the amount of tar in a marijuana cigarette is three times higher compared to a tobacco cigarette, with one-third greater deposition in the respiratory tract. Bronchitis, squamous metaplasia of the tracheobronchial epithelium, and emphysema are the commonest features among chronic users. Several case reports strongly suggest a link between cannabis smoking and cancer of the aerodigestive system, including the oropharynx and tongue, nasal and sinus epithelium, and larynx. Most illegally obtained marijuana is believed to be contaminated with *Aspergillus* species (a producer of carcinogenic aflatoxin), which can cause invasive pulmonary aspergillosis in immunocompromised users.

Immunotoxicity

Agonists of the CB_2 receptors act as immune modulators, reducing the release of inflammatory cytokines. They are also known to produce anti-inflammatory effects. It has been repeatedly shown that cannabis use can impair the immune system's ability to fight off microbial and viral infections. Use of cannabis-containing products may compromise lung macrophage functions, including phagocytosis, migration, and cytokine production, in a dose-dependent manner. This has been demonstrated in limited human *in vitro* studies. Although human T and B lymphocytes contain cannabinoid receptors, no conclusive effects have been reported on the use of cannabis and the clinical effects related to the presence of these receptors.

Neurotoxicity

A strong correlation exists between cannabis use and mental health. Adolescent abusers commonly suffer one or more comorbid health or behavioral problems. Several studies have demonstrated marijuana abuse to coexist with attention deficit hyperactivity disorder, other learning disabilities, depression, and anxiety. Cohort and well-designed cross-sectional studies suggest a modest association between early, regular, or heavy cannabis use and depression. An association exists between cannabis use and schizophrenia. Several well-controlled studies with well-defined samples looked at cannabis use and psychosis and concluded an overall twofold increase in the relative risk for developing schizophrenia, although it was not determined whether cannabis use is necessary or sufficient to cause schizophrenia. Cannabis use is believed to worsen schizophrenic psychotic symptoms.

Cardiovascular Toxicity

A sudden 20–100% rise in heart rate is very common with naïve user, lasting up to 2–3 h.

Peripheral vasodilatation causes postural hypotension, which may lead to dizziness or syncope.

Cardiac output increases by as much as 30%. In addition, the cardiac oxygen demand is also increased. Tolerance to these effects can develop within a few days of use. Naive users can experience angina. In addition, users with preexisting coronary artery disease or cerebrovascular disease may experience myocardial infarctions, congestive heart failure, and strokes. Chronic users may experience a combination of all these effects prior to onset of persistent cardiac anomalies.

Reproductive Toxicity

Acute and chronic administration of cannabinoids, including THC, CBN, and CBD, has been reported to decrease sexual functioning in both male and female rodents and primates. THC alters the normal ovulatory cycle. Some studies suggest that cannabinoids decrease serum testosterone, FSH, and LH levels in males, and also cause morphologic abnormalities in sperm. In females, cannabinoid administration has been reported to suppress the cyclic surge of LH and ovulation. High-dose THC in animals causes a drop in testosterone levels, decreased sperm production, and compromised sperm motility and viability.

A reduction of birth weight in animals is very common with cannabis administration during pregnancy. However, studies are equivocal in humans. No evidence exists that cannabis increases the risk of birth defects. A growing body of evidence suggests permanent, though subtle, effects on memory, informational processing, and executive functions in the offspring of women who use cannabis during pregnancy. Children younger than 1 week of age born to mothers who used cannabis during pregnancy had increased incidence of tremors and staring. Children of chronic users (>5 joints per week) were found to have lower verbal and memory scores at age 2 years. A few studies have demonstrated a possible increased risk of nonlymphoblastic leukemia, rhabdomyosarcoma, and astrocytoma in children whose mothers reported using cannabis during their pregnancies.

Genotoxicity

Phytocannabinoids are not genotoxic. Relatively little data are available regarding the genotoxicity of other cannabinoids.

Carcinogenicity

There is mixed evidence on the effects of THC and other cannabinoids on cancers: in some *in vitro* and *in vivo* studies, THC and some synthetic cannabinoids have had antineoplastic effects, but in other studies THC seems to impair the immune response to cancer.

Clinical Management

The consumption of illicit substances is on the rise despite tireless efforts to control drug abuse, and it is considered a serious threat to the health and well-being of our communities. Hospitalization is required very often for the treatment of the direct toxic effects of the drugs as well as for injuries sustained while under their influence. Although poisoning with 'traditional' substances of abuse such as opioids, cocaine, and cannabis still predominate in terms of numbers, the availability and use of new psychoactive substances are on the rise. Activated charcoal is administered as slurry. Depressive, hallucinatory, or psychotic reactions should be treated by placing the patient in a quiet area, providing reassurance that no permanent effects will occur. Benzodiazepines are preferred drugs for treatment of extreme agitation. When psychotic phenomena predominate, haloperidol 5 mg i.m. is recommended. The patient should be kept well hydrated.

Ecotoxicology

There is limited data relating to the ecotoxicology of cannabinoids. However, considering their widespread use, it is likely that they are present in wastewaters and enter the environment either as the parent molecules or metabolites. This is an area that needs additional work.

Exposure Standards and Guidelines

The average THC potency of cannabis has increased due to cultivation of improved biotechnology-based plant breeding in the last two decades. Marijuana cigarettes in the past contained approximately10 mg of THC, but recent versions contain approximately 60–150 mg. Because the effects of THC are dose-dependent, modern cannabis users may experience greater morbidity than their predecessors. Cannabis is available in the following forms: Marijuana is a combination of the *C. sativa* flowering tops and leaves. The THC content is 0.5–5%. Several preparations are as follows: (1) Bhang – dried leaves and tops; (2) Ganja – leaves and tops with a higher resin content, which results in greater potency; (3) Hashish is dried resin collected from the flowering tops. The THC concentration is 2–20% in hash oil, a liquid extract that contains up to 15% THC. Sinsemilla is unpollinated flowering tops derived from the female cannabis plant in which THC content is as high as 20%, and in Dutch hemp (netherweed) has a THC concentration as high as 20%.

US Food and Drug Administration requirements: tetrahydrocannabinol is a chemical derivative of cannabis (marijuana), named in section 502(d) of the Federal Food, Drug, and Cosmetic Act, and is thereby designated as habit forming.

Commercially available cannabinoids such as Dronabinol® and Nabilone® are approved drugs for the treatment of cancer-related side effects. Cannabinoids may have benefits in the treatment of cancer-related side effects.

See also: Benzodiazepines; Marijuana; Tobacco.

Further Reading

Albertson, T.E., 7 July 2013. Recreational drugs of abuse. Clin. Rev. Allergy Immunol. (Epub ahead of print).

Ashton, J.C., 2012. Synthetic cannabinoids as drugs of abuse. Curr. Drug Abuse Rev. 5 (2), 158–168.

Brown, I., Cascio, M.G., Rotondo, D., et al., 2013. Cannabinoids and omega-3/6 endocannabinoids as cell death and anticancer modulators. Prog. Lipid Res. 52 (1), 80–109.

Centers for Disease Control and Prevention (CDC), 2013. Acute kidney injury associated with synthetic cannabinoid use – multiple states, 2012. Morb. Mortal. Wkly Rep. 62 (6), 93–98.

Choi, H., Heo, S., Choe, S., et al., 2013. Simultaneous analysis of synthetic cannabinoids in the materials seized during drug trafficking using GC–MS. Anal. Bioanal. Chem. 405 (12), 3937–3944.

Donovan, J., Grundy, D., October 2012. Endocannabinoid modulation of jejunal afferent responses to LPS. Neurogastroenterol. Motil. 24 (10), 956–e465.

Fernández-Ruiz, J., Moreno-Martet, M., Rodríguez-Cueto, C., et al., August 2011. The "new" marijuana. Br. J. Pharmacol. 163 (7), 1365–1378.

Foster, A.J., Prime, L.H., Gustafsson, F., et al., 12 December 2012. Bioactivation of the cannabinoid receptor antagonist rimonabant to a cytotoxic iminium ion metabolite. Chem. Res. Toxicol. (Epub ahead of print).

Gunderson, E.W., Haughey, H.M., Ait-Daoud, N., et al., 2012. "Spice" and "K2" herbal highs: a case series and systematic review of the clinical effects and biopsychosocial implications of synthetic cannabinoid use in humans. Am. J. Addict. 21 (4), 320–326.

Hermanns-Clausen, M., Kneisel, S., Szabo, B., Auwärter, V., 2013. Acute toxicity due to the confirmed consumption of synthetic cannabinoids: clinical and laboratory findings. Addiction 108 (3), 534–544.

Howlett, A.C., Breivogel, C.S., Childers, S.R., et al., 2004. Cannabinoid physiology and pharmacology: 30 years of progress. Neuropharmacology 47, 345–358.

Lopes, C.F., de Angelis, B.B., Prudente, H.M., et al., 2012. Concomitant consumption of marijuana, alcohol and tobacco in oral squamous cell carcinoma development and progression: recent advances and challenges. Arch. Oral Biol. 57 (8), 1026–1033.

McGuinness, T.M., Newell, D., August 2012. Risky recreation: synthetic cannabinoids have dangerous effects. J. Psychosoc. Nurs. Ment. Health Serv. 50 (8), 16–18.

Meyer, M.R., Peters, F.T., 2012. Analytical toxicology of emerging drugs of abuse – an update. Ther. Drug Monit. 34 (6), 615–621.

Rajasekaran, M., Brents, L.K., Franks, L.N., et al., 2013. Human metabolites of synthetic cannabinoids JWH-018 and JWH-073 bind with high affinity and act as potent agonists at cannabinoid type-2 receptors. Toxicol. Appl. Pharmacol. 269 (2), 100–108.

Resuehr, D., Glore, D.R., Taylor, H.S., Bruner-Tran, K.L., Osteen, K.G., 2012. Progesterone-dependent regulation of endometrial cannabinoid receptor type 1 (CB1-R) expression is disrupted in women with endometriosis and in isolated stromal cells exposed to 2,3,7,8-tetrachlorodibenzo-*p*-dioxin (TCDD). Fertil. Steril. 98 (4), 948.e1–956.e1.

Rosenbaum, C.D., Carreiro, S.P., Babu, K.M., 2012. Here today, gone tomorrow…and back again? A review of herbal marijuana alternatives (K2, Spice), synthetic cathinones (bath salts), kratom, Salvia divinorum, methoxetamine, and piperazines. J. Med. Toxicol. 8 (1), 15–32.

Sagredo, O., González, S., Aroyo, I., et al., 2009. Cannabinoid CB2 receptor agonists protect the striatum against malonate toxicity: relevance for Huntington's disease. Glia 57 (11), 1154–1167.

Seely, K.A., Lapoint, J., Moran, J.H., Fattore, L., 2012. Spice drugs are more than harmless herbal blends: a review of the pharmacology and toxicology of synthetic cannabinoids. Prog. Neuropsychopharmacol. Biol. Psychiatry 39 (2), 234–243.

Sekiguchi, K., Kanazu, T., Takeuchi, M., Hasegawa, H., Yamaguchi, Y., 13 June 2013. Non-clinical evaluation of the metabolism, pharmacokinetics and excretion of S-777469, a new cannabinoid receptor 2 selective agonist. Xenobiotica (Epub ahead of print).

Spano, M.S., Fattore, L., Cadeddu, F., Fratta, W., Fadda, P., 2013. Chronic cannabinoid exposure reduces phencyclidine-induced schizophrenia-like positive symptoms in adult rats. Psychopharmacology (Berl.) 225 (3), 531–542.

Tofighi, B., Lee, J.D., 2012. Internet highs – seizures after consumption of synthetic cannabinoids purchased online. J. Addict. Med. 6 (3), 240–241.

Tomlinson, L., Tirmenstein, M.A., Janovitz, E.B., et al., October 2012. Cannabinoid receptor antagonist-induced striated muscle toxicity and ethylmalonic–adipic aciduria in beagle dogs. Toxicol. Sci. 129 (2), 268–279.

Vardakou, I., Pistos, C., Spiliopoulou, Ch, et al., 2010. Spice drugs as a new trend: mode of action, identification and legislation. Toxicol. Lett. 197 (3), 157–162.

Wells, D.L., Ott, C.A., 2012. Prospects for cannabinoid therapies in basal ganglia disorders. Ann. Pharmacother. 45 (3), 414–417.

Wiebelhaus, J.M., Poklis, J.L., Poklis, A., et al., 2012. Inhalation exposure to smoke from synthetic "marijuana" produces potent cannabimimetic effects in mice. Drug Alcohol Depend. 126 (3), 316–323.

Wiegand, T.J., Wax, P.M., Schwartz, T., et al., 2012. The toxicology investigators consortium case Registry – the 2011 experience. Toxicology investigators consortium case registry investigators. J. Med. Toxicol. 8 (4), 360–377.

Winstock, A.R., Barratt, M.J., 2013. The 12-month prevalence and nature of adverse experiences resulting in emergency medical presentations associated with the use of synthetic cannabinoid products. Hum. Psychopharmacol. 28 (4), 390–393.

Wong, G.T., Irwin, M.G., 2013. Poisoning with illicit substances: toxicology for the anaesthetist. Anaesthesia 68 (Suppl. 1), 117–124.

Wood, D.M., Dargan, P.I., 2012. Novel psychoactive substances: how to understand the acute toxicity associated with the use of these substances. Ther. Drug Monit. 34 (4), 363–367.

Yen, M., Ewald, M.B., 2012. Toxicity of weight loss agents. J. Med. Toxicol. 8 (2), 145–152.

Relevant Websites

http://https//aapcc.s3.amazonaws.com/pdfs/annual_reports/2011_NPDS_Annual_Report.pdf – American Association of Poison Control Centers, Annual Report 2011.

http://www.drugtext.org/Cannabis-marijuana-hashisch/review-on-clinical-studies-with-cannabis-and-cannabinoids-2005-2009.html – Drug Text: University of Leiden Publication.

http://emedicine.medscape.com/article/833828-overview – Emedicine.

http://www.cancer.gov/cancertopics/pdq/cam/cannabis/healthprofessional/page1 – National Cancer Institue.

http://rstb.royalsocietypublishing.org/content/367/1607/3326.abstract?sid=20cf2c23-e4fd-49e3-9398-ec8be2e00226 – Philosophical Transactions of the Royal Society: B. Biological Sciences.

Cannabis *see* Cannabinoids; Marijuana

Captafol

P Raman, Northeast Ohio Medical University, Rootstown, OH, USA

- Name: Captafol
- Chemical Abstracts Service Registry Number: 2425-06-1
- Synonyms: 3a,4,7,7a-Tetrahydro-2-[(1,1,2,2-tetrachloroethyl)thio]-1*H*-isoindole-1,3(2*H*)-dione; Folcid; Difolatan
- Molecular Formula: $C_{10}H_9Cl_4NO_2S$
- Chemical Structure:

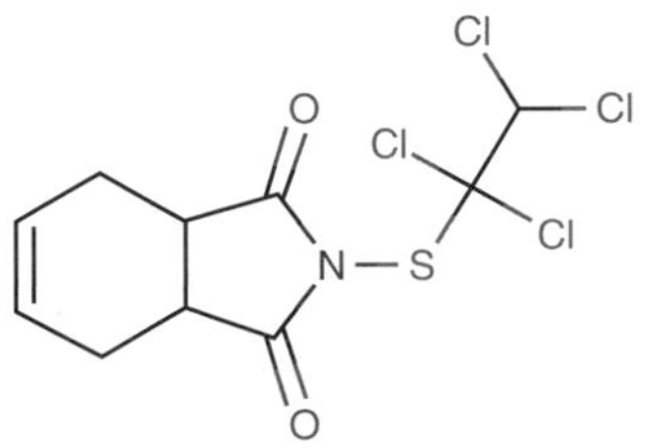

Background

Captafol is colorless to pale yellow in color with a distinct odor. It has a molecular weight of 349.1, water solubility of 1.4 mg l^{-1} at 20 °C, and melting point of 160–162 °C. Some common trade names of products containing captafol include Crisfolatan, Difolatan, Difosan, Folcid, Haipen, Kenofol, Pillar-tan, and Sanspor. Captafol is a nonsystemic antifungal chemical extensively used to control foliage and fruit diseases of tomatoes, coffee berry disease, potato blight, and tapping panel disease of rubber trees. Both the lumber and timber industries have used this compound for years to prevent growth of wood rot fungi in logs and wood products. Captafol was shown to be hepatotoxic and to induce potentially pre-neoplastic glutathione *S*-transferase placental form positive (GST-P+) foci in the liver of male F344 rats in both the initiation and promotion phases of studies of tumor development. In addition, promotion with captafol increased the incidences of hyperplasia of the forestomach and adenoma of the small intestine, thyroid follicular-cell adenoma, and the expression of a marker of cell proliferation (proliferating-cell nuclear antigen) in the kidneys in F344 rats. In addition to direct genotoxic activity, several epigenetic mechanisms depleted cellular thiol groups (nonprotein and protein), inhibited DNA replication enzymes (DNA topoisomerases and polymerases), DNA synthesis, RNA synthesis, and induced CYPP450 mono-oxygenases, suggesting underlying causes of pathogenesis of tumor formation.

Uses

Captafol is a widely used broad-spectrum contact fungicide belonging to the class of sulfanilamides. It is effective for the control of a wide variety of fungal diseases in plants and is widely used outside the United States to control foliage and fruit diseases on apples, citrus, tomato, cranberry, sweet corn, barley, wheat, and several other plants. Captafol is also extensively used as a seed protectant in cotton, peanuts, and rice. It is also used to reduce losses from wood rot fungi in logs and wood products. Mixed formulations of this compound include (captafol +) triadimefon; ethirimol; folpet; halacrinate; propiconazole; and pyrazophos. Captafol is compatible with most plant-protection products, with the exception of alkaline preparations and formulating materials.

Environmental Fate and Behavior

Captafol is not persistent in the environment. Captafol is stable under ordinary environmental conditions and rapidly degrades in soil, the rate of degradation being a function of soil type and pesticide concentration. It does not leach from basic soils and is unlikely to contaminate groundwater. Captafol sprayed on most crops has a half-life of less than 5 days. Captafol and/or its metabolites and degradation products are readily absorbed by roots and shoots of plants. If released to air, an extrapolated vapor pressure of 8.27×10^{-9} mm Hg at 25 °C indicates captafol will exist solely in the particulate phase in the ambient atmosphere. Particulate-phase captafol will be removed from the atmosphere by wet and dry deposition. If released to soil, captafol is expected to have slight mobility based on K_{oc} values of 2073 and 2120. Volatilization from moist soil surfaces is not expected to be an important fate process based on a Henry's Law constant of 2.7×10^{-9} atm-cu m mol^{-1}. In a laboratory setting, the biodegradation half-life of captafol in three soils was found in the range of 23–55 days. The overall half-life of captafol in soil is about 11 days, independent of soil type or initial concentration. If released into water, captafol is expected to adsorb to suspended solids and sediment based on the K_{oc}. Volatilization from water surfaces is not expected to be an important fate process based on this compound's estimated Henry's Law constant. An estimated bioconcentration factor of 170 suggests the potential for bioconcentration in aquatic organisms is high, provided the compound is not altered physically or chemically after being released to the

 http://dx.doi.org/10.1016/B978-0-12-386454-3.00268-2

environment. The half-lives for the hydrolysis of Difolatan at pH 3.0, 7.0, and 8.0 were 77.8, 6.54, and 0.72 h, respectively. Hydrolysis is likely to be the predominant pathway of degradation in the aquatic environment.

Exposure Routes and Pathways

Dermal and ocular exposures are the most common routes of exposure to captafol. Contact dermatitis has been reported after exposure to captafol. During occupational exposure, captafol has been reported to cause severe irritation of the respiratory tract, eye damage, and other systemic effects. Oral ingestion of captafol is unlikely to cause acute poisoning.

Toxicokinetics

Captafol is poorly absorbed from the gastrointestinal tract. The liver and the gastrointestinal tract are the primary sites of metabolism of captafol. It is eliminated via urine, feces, and exhaled air. The major single metabolite, tetrahydrophthalimide (THPI), was detected in blood, urine, and feces, but most of the activity in the blood and urine was in the form of more water-soluble metabolites. Following oral administration in animals, captafol is hydrolyzed to THPI and dichloroacetic acid. THPI is degraded to tetrahydrophthalimidic acid and further to phthalic acid and ammonia.

Mechanism of Toxicity

The primary toxicity following captafol exposure probably occurs through a hypersensitivity mechanism. Most experiments suggest captafol to be DNA active.

Acute and Short-Term Toxicity (or Exposure)

Animal

The acute oral LD_{50} of captafol has been reported to be 6780 mg kg^{-1} in male rats and 6330 mg kg^{-1} in female rats. The rabbit dermal LD_{50} is reported to be 15 400 mg kg^{-1}, showing moderate dermal irritation at 72 h with severe dermal sensitization. Another test for captafol-induced eye irritation in rabbit showed corneal opacity and iris and conjunctival irritation, all symptoms being present for 21 days. Captafol was reported to be teratogenic and to cause fetal developmental abnormalities at very high (maternally toxic) doses in hamsters. Teratogenicity studies in rabbits indicated a teratogenic no observed effect level (NOEL) >50 mg kg^{-1} day^{-1} and a fetotoxic NOEL of 16.5 mg kg^{-1} day^{-1}. Captafol was, however, found to have no effect on embryonic development in rabbits and monkeys. Further, most animal feeding studies have shown that most of the captafol is excreted unchanged and the major metabolite is tetrahydrophthalimide. When rats, dogs, and monkeys were fed $(14)^{C}$-captafol, almost 80% was excreted within 36 h, mainly in the urine, and none via expired carbon dioxide. Most of the small amount in the feces was unmetabolized and probably unabsorbed. Unmetabolized captafol was undetectable in most biological fluids and tissues. Several teratology studies have been conducted in many mammalian species, including nonhuman primates, which concluded low to no teratogenic potential after administering captafol throughout organogenesis.

Human

The primary symptoms of captafol exposure reported in humans include contact dermatitis and conjunctivitis. The reaction may be severe and may include stomatitis and painful bronchitis. Persons with a skin rash following exposure to captafol were found to have systemic as well as dermal disorders. Hypertension was reported in patients with marked edema. Other findings following captafol exposure include protein and urobilinogen in the urine, depression of liver function, anemia, and depression of blood cholinesterase activity. Acute oral or dermal exposure to captafol rarely results in severe toxicity. However, due to a higher level of toxicity in animal models following intraperitoneal exposure, parenteral exposure may present a greater hazard potential. Captafol has been classified as a group 2A probable human carcinogen.

Exposed individuals include farm and timber workers; workers involved in formulation and dispensing pesticides; agricultural spray workers and crop harvesters during disease vector control periods. Inhalation of captafol as spray mists or powders has been reported in an occupational setting. The acute oral toxicity is low. Skin, eyes, and respiratory tract are targets for local irritation and sensitization. Ingestion of large quantities of captafol has caused vomiting and diarrhea. Respiratory sensitization and conjunctivitis are known to have occurred. Systemic disorders including hypertension and hepatic and renal disturbances, usually paralleling the degree of dermatitis, have been reported following captafol exposure. Wheezing due to bronchospasm, contact dermatitis, and vomiting and diarrhea are the features of exposure to captafol by inhalation, skin contact, and ingestion, respectively. Chronic exposure can cause hypertension, depression of liver function, dermatitis, conjunctivitis, and anemia.

Chronic Toxicity (or Exposure)

Animal

Rats exposed to captafol at dietary levels of 1500 and 5000 ppm demonstrated growth depression, some liver and kidney changes, and an increased mortality. Following exposure to 300 or 100 mg kg^{-1} of captafol, dogs suffered frequent vomiting and diarrhea during the first 4 weeks and were observed to be slightly anemic and deficient in growth during a 2 year study. Dogs at dosages of 30 mg kg^{-1} or greater developed both absolute and relative increases in the weights of the liver and kidney. Oral administration in mice produced a high incidence of adenocarcinomas of the small intestine, vascular tumors of the heart, and spleen and hepatocellular carcinomas. In a 2-year rat-feeding study, a dose-related increased incidence of neoplastic nodules in the liver of females was reported. The US Environmental Protection Agency (EPA) reported a NOEL for nononcogenic effects at 56 ppm based on a chronic toxicity study in rats. There is sufficient evidence in experimental animals for carcinogenicity of captafol.

Human

Captafol is also known to be a skin sensitizer and has been reported to cause both allergic and contact dermatitis in humans. Breakdown products may contribute to the skin irritation and sensitization associated with captafol.

Genotoxicity

Captafol is an alkylating agent and has produced genotoxic effects in a variety of systems. Short-term *in vitro* and *in vivo* genotoxicity studies support mutagenicity as a mechanism of carcinogenesis. Captafol caused mutations in *Salmonella typhimurium* (base-pair mutations) and *Escherichia coli* and in nonmammalian *in vivo* systems (*Aspergillus nidulans* and *Drosophila melanogaster*). Captafol caused DNA single-strand breaks, sister chromatid exchange, chromosomal aberrations, micronucleus formation, polyploidy (in one of two studies), mitotic spindle disturbances, and cell transformation in *in vitro* studies that employed cell lines from rodents and other mammals. In human cells *in vitro*, it caused DNA single-strand breaks, sister chromatid exchange, micronucleus formation, and chromosomal aberrations. In rodents exposed *in vivo*, captafol caused DNA strand breaks, micronucleus formation, and dominant lethal mutations in rats but did not cause mutations in the host-mediated assay in rats or dominant lethal mutations in albino mice.

Carcinogenicity

There is sufficient evidence in experimental animals for the carcinogenicity of captafol. However, the task force for evaluation found captafol to be active in a wide range of tests for genetic and related effects, including the generally insensitive *in vivo* assay for dominant lethal mutation. Based on the above observation, captafol was labeled as probable human carcinogen (Group 2A) by the International Agency for Research on Cancer, whereas US EPA categorized this compound as Group 2B: probable human carcinogen, and the American Conference of Governmental Industrial Hygienists (ACGIH) recognized it as not classifiable as a human carcinogen.

Clinical Management

Exposed eyes and skin should be flushed with copious amounts of water. In case of an inhalation exposure, the patient should be monitored for respiratory distress. Artificial ventilation may be provided and symptomatic treatment may be administered as necessary.

Ecotoxicology

Avian toxicity for captafol is low, the LD_{50} being greater than 2510 ppm. However, high levels of exposure can cause reproductive impairment. Captafol is characterized as being very highly toxic to both cold-water and warm-water fish, 96 h LC_{50} being 0.027–0.50 and 0.045–0.230 mg l^{-1} in rainbow trout and bluegill sunfish, respectively. It is considered only moderately to very highly toxic to freshwater invertebrates. Captafol is considered nontoxic to bees. Most of captafol's release to the environment occurred through various waste streams and its use as a fungicide on crops. If released to air, an extrapolated vapor pressure of 8.27×10^{-9} mm Hg at 25 °C indicates captafol will exist solely in the particulate phase in the ambient atmosphere. Particulate-phase captafol will be removed from the atmosphere by wet and dry deposition. If released to soil, captafol is expected to have slight mobility based on K_{oc} values of 2073 and 2120. Volatilization from moist soil surfaces is not expected to be an important fate process based on a Henry's Law constant of 2.7×10^{-9} atm-cu m mol^{-1}.

Exposure Standards and Guidelines

Captafol is a general use pesticide with a toxicity classification of IV (relatively nontoxic). It is classified as a restricted use pesticide in the United States. It is no longer sold in the United States. The US Occupational Safety and Health Administration threshold limit value for captafol is reported to be 0.1 mg m^{-3}. Captafol is a restricted use fungicide and as of 2010, the use of captafol on food crops has been banned.

ACGIH Threshold Limit Value: 0.1 mg m^{-3} time-weighted average (TWA) (skin); Appendix A4 (Not Classifiable as a Human Carcinogen).

National Institute for Occupational Safety and Health Recommended Exposure Limit: 0.1 mg m^{-3} TWA (skin) potential carcinogen.

See also: Pesticides.

Further Reading

BCPC, 2006. Captafol. In: Tomlin, C.D.S. (Ed.), The Pesticide Manual, fourteenth ed. British Crop Protection Council, Hampshire, UK, pp. 140–141.

Cushman, J.R., Street, J.C., 1991. Contact sensitivity to captafol in BALB/c mice. Contact Dermat. 24 (5), 363–365.

Dalvi, R.R., Mutinga, M.L., 1990. Comparative studies of the effects on liver and liver microsomal drug-metabolizing enzyme system by the fungicides captan, captafol and folpet in rats. Pharmacol. Toxicol. 66 (3), 231–233.

Ito, N., Hagiwara, A., Tamano, S., Futacuchi, M., Imaida, K., Shirai, T., 1996. Effects of pesticide mixtures at the acceptable daily intake levels on rat carcinogenesis. Food Chem. Toxicol. 34 (11–12), 1091–1096.

Kennedy Jr., G.L., Arnold, D.W., Keplinger, M.L., 1975. Mutagenicity studies with captan, captafol, folpet and thalidomide. Food Cosmet. Toxicol. 13 (1), 55–61.

National Toxicology Program, June 2008. Final report on carcinogens background document for captafol. Rep. Carcinog. Backgr. Doc. 8-5974 (i–xvi), 1–99.

National Toxicology Program, 2011. Captafol. Rep. Carcinog. 12, 83–86.

Nazir, A., Saxena, D.K., Kar Chowdhuri, D., 2003. Induction of hsp70 in transgenic *Drosophila*: biomarker of exposure against phthalimide group of chemicals. Biochim. Biophys. Acta 1621 (2), 218–225.

Rahden-Staron, I., 2002. The inhibitory effect of the fungicides captan and captafol on eukaryotic topoisomerases in vitro and lack of recombinagenic activity in the wing spot test of *Drosophila melanogaster*. Mutat. Res. 518 (2), 205–213.

Robbiano, L., Baroni, D., Carrozzino, R., Mereto, E., Brambilla, G., November 15, 2004. DNA damage and micronuclei induced in rat and human kidney cells by six chemicals carcinogenic to the rat kidney. Toxicology 204 (2–3), 187–195.

Tamano, S., Kurata, Y., Kawabe, M., et al., 1990. Carcinogenicity of captafol in F344/DuCrj rats. Jpn. J. Cancer Res. 81 (12), 1222–1231.

Tamano, S., Kurata, Y., Shibata, M., Tanaka, H., Ogiso, T., Ito, N., 1991. 13-Week oral toxicity study of captafol in F344/DuCrj rats. Fundam. Appl. Toxicol. 17 (2), 390–398.

Tamano, S., Kawabe, M., Sano, M., Masui, T., Ito, N., 1993. Subchronic oral toxicity study of captafol in B6C3F1 mice. J. Toxicol. Environ. Health 38 (1), 69–75.

Whyatt, R.M., Barr, D.B., Camann, D.E., et al., 2003. Contemporary-use pesticides in personal air samples during pregnancy and blood samples at delivery among urban minority mothers and newborns. Environ. Health Perspect. 111 (5), 749–756.

Zang, X., Wang, J., Wang, O., et al., 2008. Analysis of captan, folpet, and captafol in apples by dispersive liquid–liquid microextraction combined with gas chromatography. Anal. Bioanal. Chem. 392 (4), 749–754.

Relevant Websites

http://pmep.cce.cornell.edu/profiles/extoxnet/24d-captan/Captafol-ext.html – Cornell University.

http://ntp.niehs.nih.gov/ntp/roc/twelfth/profiles/Captafol.pdf – National Toxicology Program.

http://ull.chemistry.uakron.edu/erd – The Chemical Database - The Department of Chemistry at the University of Akron.

Captan

X Song, Merck & Co., Inc., West Point, PA, USA

- Chemical Abstracts Service Registry Number: 133-06-2
- Synonyms: 3a,4,7,7a-Tetrahydro-2-[(trichloromethyl)thio]-1H-isoindole-1,3(2H)-dione; 1,2,3,6-Tetrahydro-*N*-(trichlor omethylthio) phthalimide; Captano (Italy); Captane (France); Captex; Hexacap; Kaptan; Orthocide®; Vancide 89®
- Chemical Class: Phthalimide
- Chemical Structure:

N–S–CCl_3

Background

Captan was first registered in 1951 and was widely employed for many antifungal uses. Its use has been limited over the years, mostly based on cancer risks.

Uses

Captan is a broad-spectrum, nonsystemic fungicide. It is used as a seed treatment for numerous food and feed crops, and has foliar uses on many crops, including apples, almonds, and strawberries. Since 1989, however, most applications of captan on food crops in the United States have been limited.

Environmental Fate and Behavior

The half-life of captan is 1–10 days in a soil environment, and hours to days in water depending on acidities and temperatures. Captan is not mobile in soil but can significantly evaporate from the soil surface. It is quickly degraded in neutral water.

Exposures and Exposure Monitoring

Exposure to captan can occur through dermal, oral, or inhalation routes during the manufacture or application of captan, or consumption of agricultural products with captan residue.

Toxicokinetics

Animal studies showed that captan is readily excreted after either oral or intraperitoneal dosing. Metabolism is similar between males and females. Twenty-four hours after treatment, approximately 75% of captan is eliminated in urine and 6.5% in feces in rats. Nearly all is eliminated by 36 h. A small portion of captan given orally was metabolized into thiozolidine-2-thione-4-carboxylic acid, a salt of dithiobis (methanesulfonic acid) and the disulfide monoxide derivative of dithiobis (methanesulfonic acid). The major metabolic site is the gastrointestinal tract.

Mechanism of Toxicity

Liver enzymes were modulated after repeated captan exposure at relatively high dosage. Evidence suggested that captan caused the breakdown of the inner membrane of mitochondria. *In vitro* studies showed that captan caused swelling of mitochondria in rat liver and loss of intracellular potassium of human erythrocytes. Captan inhibits mitochondrial function nonspecifically, involving uncoupling of oxidative phosphorylation.

Acute and Short-Term Toxicity

Animal

Generally, captan has been found to have low toxicity to laboratory animals after an oral dose. An oral LD_{50} value of greater than 5000 mg kg^{-1} was reported in rats. Intraperitoneal LD_{50} values of 40 and 35 mg kg^{-1} were reported in male and female rats, respectively. Oral LD_{50} values of 7840 and 7000 mg kg^{-1} were reported for male and female mice whereas intraperitoneal LD_{50} values of 518 and 462 mg kg^{-1} were found in male and female mice, respectively. A dermal LD_{50} value of greater than 2000 mg kg^{-1} was found in rabbits. Captan given at a dietary level of 10 000 ppm for 54 weeks caused marked growth depression in both male and female rats. Captan fed at 5000 ppm for 2 years (about 50 mg kg^{-1} day^{-1}) produced growth depression in female but not in male rats. Testicular atrophy was observed at autopsy in some animals fed with captan at 10 000 ppm. No significant changes in organ weights, hematology, and gross and histological morphology were found.

Human

Sensitivity, e.g., dermatitis, to captan exposure was observed. Eye irritation potentially exists but is minimal. Captan, however, is generally well tolerated.

Chronic Toxicity

Effects in laboratory animals following chronic exposures of captan included inappetence, decreased body weight, decreased organ weight, and death.

 http://dx.doi.org/10.1016/B978-0-12-386454-3.00105-6

Reproductive Toxicity

Captan was reported to cause fetal mortality in pregnant mice that inhaled captan at high doses. Captan is unlikely, however, to cause reproductive toxicity in humans with usual exposures. Captan was not reported to cause reproductive toxicity in humans.

Genotoxicity

Captan has been determined by the US Environmental Protection Agency (EPA) to be nonmutagenic or to have very low mutagenicity in animals, although captan was found mutagenic in some *in vitro* tests.

Carcinogenicity

In chronic studies, captan causes cancer in rats and mice. Captan is classified as B2, a probable human carcinogen, by the US EPA. Captan is considered by the US National Institute for Occupational Safety and Health (NIOSH) to be a potential occupational carcinogen.

Clinical Management

Intoxication after acute captan exposure is unlikely. Treatment is needed if symptoms occur.

Ecotoxicity

Captan is very toxic to fish. The US EPA has concluded, however, that the potential aquatic effects of captan would be minor since there are no aquatic applications of captan. Honeybees are sensitive to captan while birds are relatively tolerant to this fungicide. Captan does not substantially accumulate in living tissues.

Exposure Standards

The US EPA chronic reference dose for captan is $0.13\ mg\ kg^{-1}\ day^{-1}$, and the accepted dietary intake established by European Food Safety Authority is $0.1\ mg\ kg^{-1}\ day^{-1}$. The US Occupational Safety and Health (OSHA) permissible exposure limit (PEL) time-weighted average (TWA) of $5\ mg\ m^{-3}$ is still enforced in some states in the United States. The NIOSH recommended exposure limit is a 10-h TWA of $5\ mg\ m^{-3}$.

See also: Fungicide; Pesticides.

Further Reading

Arce, G.T., Gordon, E.B., Cohen, S.M., Singh, P., 2010. Genetic toxicology of folpet and captan. Crit. Rev. Toxicol. 40, 546–574.

Cohen, S.M., Gordon, E.B., Singh, P., Arce, G.T., Nyska, A., 2010. Carcinogenic mode of action of folpet in mice and evaluation of its relevance to humans. Crit. Rev. Toxicol. 40, 531–545.

Gordon, E.B., 2001. Captan and folpet. In: Krieger, R. (Ed.), Handbook of Pesticide Toxicology, second ed. Academic Press, San Diego, CA, pp. 1711–1742.

Relevant Websites

http://extoxnet.orst.edu – Extension Toxicology Network, Oregon State University.

http://www.epa.gov/iris/subst/0018.htm – US Environmental Protection Agency.

http://www.epa.gov/oppsrrd1/REDs/0120red.pdf – US Environmental Protection Agency.

Carbamate Pesticides

RC Gupta, Murray State University, Breathitt Veterinary Center, Hopkinsville, KY, USA

This article is a revision of the previous edition article by Stephanie Padilla, volume 1, pp 410–412, © 2005, Elsevier Inc.

Chemical Structure and Uses

The carbamate compounds are subdivided into three main groups: carbamates, thiocarbamates, and dithiocarbamates (see basic structures in **Figure 1**). *N*-methylcarbamates are usually used as insecticides, such as bendiocarb, carbaryl, carbofuran, methomyl, oxamyl, propoxur, and many others. Currently, carbaryl and propoxur are the only two carbamates that are also recommended for the control of ectoparasites on animals. Some of the carbamates, such as aldicarb, carbofuran, and propoxur, are commonly encountered in malicious poisonings in dogs and mammalian and avian wildlife. Derivatives of carbamic acid (asulam, barban, chloropropham, chlorbupham, karbutilate, and phenmedipham), thiocarbamic acid (butylate, cycloate, diallate, EPTC, molinate, and triallate), and dithiocarbamic acid (metham sodium) are used as herbicides. Fungicides of this group include ferbam, mancozeb, maneb, and thiram. When used properly, carbamate pesticides offer enormous benefits to society, as they preserve and increase agricultural production, as well as protect human and animal health from insect-vector-mediated diseases. However, overexposure of humans and animals to these pesticides can result in everything from minor health effects to even death.

Historical Background

During the mid-nineteenth century, the first carbamate compound physostigmine (eserine alkaloid) was extracted from the Calabar beans (ordeal poison) of a perennial plant *Physostigma venenosum* commonly found in tropical West Africa. It was not until the 1960s and 1970s that dozens of carbamates (esters of carbamic acid) were synthesized for pesticidal use. Carbaryl was the first carbamate to be used as an insecticide. The knowledge of autonomic pharmacology, especially the cholinergic system, enabled us to synthesize more potent carbamates and also to understand their mechanism of toxicity.

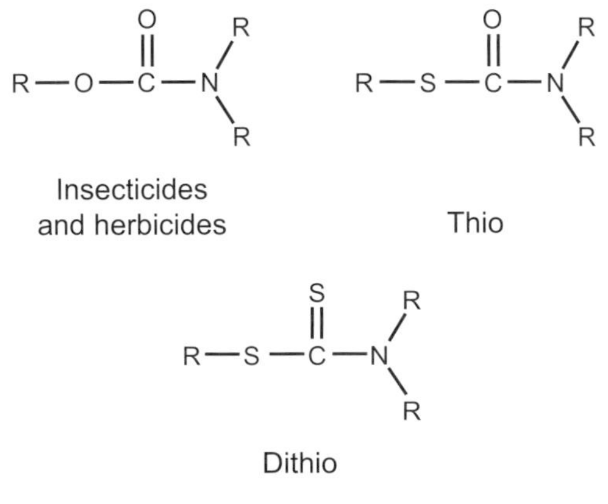

R—O—C(=O)—N(R)R

Insecticides and herbicides

R—S—C(=O)—N(R)R

Thio

R—S—C(=S)—N(R)R

Dithio

Figure 1 General formulas for carbamates.

Aldicarb was synthesized to mimic the chemical structure of acetylcholine (ACh). Currently, aldicarb has the maximal potential for mammalian toxicity and is commonly marketed globally under the trade name Temik®. Although thousands of carbamates have been synthesized, not more than two dozen compounds have been used practically as insecticides and ectoparasiticides. Currently, the carbamate insecticides are more popular worldwide, because they are safe and very little residue persists in the environment and mammalian system compared with organochlorines and organophosphates.

Since the 1940s, derivatives of carbamic acid, including ethylene bisdithiocarbamates (EBDCs), have been widely used as fungicides throughout the world. Common examples of this group of fungicides include mancozeb, maneb, metiram, nabam, and zineb. In general, thiocarbamates and dithiocarbamates are of low mammalian toxicity because they do not inhibit acetylcholinesterase (AChE) activity, and therefore pose less risk when compared with *N*-methylcarbamate insecticides.

Exposure Routes

The majority of carbamates are easily absorbed following oral, respiratory, and parenteral exposure. Carbamates can also be absorbed through the skin, although the absorption rate appears to be relatively slow. It is established that following absorption, these pesticides are well distributed in tissues throughout the body. Being lipophilic, maximum levels of these compounds are usually found in the adipose tissue and the brain. Carbamates are usually metabolized in the liver to less toxic or nontoxic metabolites. However, some of the metabolites of carbamates are quite toxic. For example, the two major metabolites of carbofuran (3-hydroxycarbofuran and 3-ketocarbofuran) have a significant impact on the overall toxicity of carbofuran. This is partly because these metabolites are toxic and they are trapped in enterohepatic circulation. Because of the extensive metabolism of carbamates in the body, rarely are parental carbamates detected in the urine. Also, only a few metabolites are detected in the urine that can be used as biomarkers of carbamate exposure. In essence, *N*-methylcarbamate insecticides are readily absorbed, widely distributed, and extensively metabolized before being excreted in the urine and/or bile. Residues of some carbamates and their metabolites can be detected in the milk.

Carbamic acid derivative fungicides, such as EBDCs, are readily absorbed, rapidly metabolized, and excreted within 24 h through urine and feces, with no evidence of long-term bioaccumulation.

Mechanism of Toxicity

Acute clinical signs of *N*-methylcarbamate insecticides toxicity are primarily associated with the inhibition of acetylcholinesterase (AChE) at synapses in the brain and neuromuscular junctions in skeletal muscles. Of course, these insecticides can also bind to many other enzymes, receptors, and proteins. Carbamates inhibit AChE activity by carbamylation, and as a result, acetylcholine (ACh) accumulates at the nerve endings of all cholinergic nerves and causes an overstimulation of electrical activity. Inhibition of AChE >70% leads to a toxic-level accumulation of ACh at cholinergic junctions (e.g., central nervous system, neuromuscular junction, autonomic preganglionic and parasympathetic postganglionic synapses, and the sympathetic innervation of the adrenal and sweat glands). Carbamates interact with AChE in the same manner as the natural substrate ACh, except the rates of hydrolysis and reactivation of AChE (decarbamylation) appear to be drastically slower than for the hydrolysis of the acetylated enzyme. The turnover time for ACh is of the order of 150 μs, whereas the carbamylated enzyme $t^1/_2$ for hydrolysis is substantially slower (~15–30 min). Accumulated ACh overstimulates muscarinic receptors (mAChRs) and nicotinic receptors (nAChRs), and consequently the symptoms of hyper cholinergic preponderance are seen. Evidence also suggests that some carbamates, such as aldicarb, bendiocarb, physostigmine, and propoxur, directly interact with ACh receptors.

Some carbamate insecticides induce a variety of toxic effects through noncholinergic mechanisms. Evidence of non-cholinergic mechanisms was presented by the involvement of glutamate release, causing activation of *N*-methyl-D-aspartate (NMDA) receptors. In addition, the adenosinergic, gamma-aminobutyric acid (GABAergic), and monoaminergic systems may also be involved in the seizures and lethality associated with carbamates. Carbamate-induced neuronal cell death is a consequence of a series of extracellular and intracellular events leading to the intracellular accumulation of Ca^{2+} ions and the generation of free radicals. Excessive free radical production causes oxidative/nitrosative stress, to which the brain is especially vulnerable. These events result in mitochondrial damage and dysfunction, neuronal energetic dysfunction, and neurodegeneration and neuronal death.

Thiocarbamates and dithiocarbamates are of low mammalian toxicity and have received less attention, and consequently their mechanisms of action are less understood. Among thiocarbamate herbicides, molinate and diallate are of concern because these two compounds are relatively more toxic. Molinate decreases aldehyde dehydrogenase, an enzyme important in the catabolism of many neurotransmitters, which may account for its central and peripheral neurotoxicity in several species. Metabolites of molinate can also interfere with testicular esterases, inhibiting testosterone production and leading to reproductive toxicity in laboratory animals.

Fungicides such as mancozeb, maneb, and metiram produce toxicity in the thyroid. These compounds inhibit the synthesis of thyroid hormones thyroxine (T4) and triiodothyronine (T3), leading to elevated levels of thyroid-stimulating hormone (TSH) via feedback stimulation of the hypothalamus and pituitary. Continuous and prolonged elevation of TSH levels results in hypertrophy and hyperplasia of the thyroid follicular cells, leading to development of follicular nodular hyperplasia, adenoma, and/or carcinoma.

Acute Toxicity

Depending on the dose, frequency, and length of exposure, carbamate insecticides can produce minor health effects, such as mild discomfort or chest pain, or effects as serious as convulsions, seizures, coma, and death. By employing *in vivo* and *in vitro* models, AChE inhibiting carbamates are known to produce a variety of toxicologic effects on the central nervous system, peripheral nervous system, musculoskeletal, cardiovascular, ocular, immunologic, reproductive, and other body systems, in addition to oxidative stress, apoptosis, endocrine disruption, and carcinogenesis. Based on acute toxicity, some of the carbamate compounds, such as aldicarb, carbofuran, oxamyl, methomyl, and many others are extremely toxic to mammalian and avian species.

In general, onset of clinical signs appears within less than an hour. Symptoms of acute poisoning with carbamate insecticides result from overstimulation of both muscarinic and nicotinic ACh receptors because of accumulation of ACh resulting from AChE inactivation. The muscarinic symptoms include hypersalivation, excessive tracheobronchial secretions, gastrointestinal cramps, lacrimation, dacryorrhea, nausea, excessive sweating, urinary incontinence, diarrhea, miosis, and bradycardia. The nicotinic receptor-associated effects include muscle fasciculations, tremors, muscle weakness, flaccid paralysis, blurred vision, vomiting, and paralysis of respiratory muscles. Exposure to high doses of a carbamate can lead to symptoms of CNS origin, including restlessness, tremors, convulsions, partial or generalized seizures, mental disturbance, incoordination, cyanosis, and coma. Finally, death ensues within a few hours because of cardiac and respiratory failure. Clinical signs of acute poisoning usually resolve within a few hours of exposure, but some symptoms of a neuropsychological nature appear to persist for a longer period. The surviving patient may exhibit symptoms such as schizoid reactions, paranoid delusions, poor sleep because of hallucinations and nightmares, and deficits in memory and attention.

Signs and symptoms of thiocarbamate toxicity include anorexia, squinting, hypersalivation, lacrimation, piloerection, dyspnea, ataxia, hypothermia, incoordination, depression, paresis, muscular fibrillation, convulsions, and death. Thiobencarb has been shown to cause toxic neuropathies in neonatal and adult rats. Diallate poisoning is reported in many species with signs and symptoms of anorexia, ataxia, muscular contractions, exhaustion, and prostration. The cat appears to be the most sensitive species.

Intermediate Syndrome

In the late 1980s, intermediate syndrome (IMS) was reported for the first time in human patients who were poisoned with large quantities of OP insecticides. Recently, a carbamate insecticide carbofuran was demonstrated to cause IMS in patients accidentally or intentionally exposed to large doses of this insecticide. Clinically, IMS is characterized by acute paralysis and weakness in several cranial motor nerves, neck flexors and facial, extraocular, palatal, nuchal, proximal limb, and respiratory muscles 24–96 h after poisoning. Generalized weakness, depressed deep tendon reflexes, ptosis, and diplopia are also evident. From mechanisms and treatment viewpoints, IMS is better characterized for OPs than carbamates, because recovery is much faster with carbamates. IMS with OPs involves depressed AChE, expressed nAChR mRNA, and increased oxidative stress. But the central mechanism seems to be the defect(s) at the neuromuscular endplate and postsynaptic level involving nAChRs. It can be hypothesized that carbamate-induced IMS may involve similar mechanisms as described for OPs.

Chronic Toxicity

Interestingly, carbamates do not cause peripheral neuropathy, as do some organophosphates (OPs). This is because carbamates may inhibit neurotoxic esterase activity (the 'first step' in the precipitation of the neuropathy), but do not 'age' (the definitive step in precipitation of the neuropathic response). Also, tolerance development has been known for OPs following chronic exposure for almost half a century, but to date no tolerance development is reported for any carbamate insecticides.

In addition to inhibition of AChE activity, carbamates have been reported to cause skin and eye irritation, hemopoietic alterations, degeneration of the liver, kidneys, and testes, as well as functional and histopathologic changes in the nervous system after long-term, high-dose exposures. Moreover, some carbamates are known to produce reproductive and teratogenic effects. Fetuses of mothers dosed with a carbamate have been reported to exhibit increased mortality and decreased weight gain. Men chronically exposed to carbofuran have semen of low quality, as the spermatozoa and spermatids are found to be multinucleated. Carbamates are also considered embryotoxic, fetotoxic, teratogenic, mutagenic, and carcinogenic.

Chronic studies with thiophanate (a methyl-benzimidazole carbamate) fungicide caused an increase in liver weight in rats, and increased thyroid weights in rats and dogs. The major concern with EBDC pesticides (including maneb and metiram) is that their major metabolite, ethylene thiourea (ETU), is goitrogenic. ETU is known to interfere with thyroid peroxidase. In a 2-year chronic study in rats, ETU produced thyroid follicular hyperplasia at $\geq$50 ppm and malignant thyroid neoplasia at $\geq$250 ppm. ETU is also known to cause hepatocellular adenomas, anterior pituitary adenomas, and reproductive and developmental abnormalities. Mancozeb can produce small effects on thyroid morphology and a depression of iodine uptake.

Interaction with Other Anticholinesterase Pesticides

Carbamate and OP insecticides are often used in combination, with the objective of achieving synergistic interaction and controlling a wide range of insects, including those that are resistant. Therefore, exposure of the environment as well as humans and animals to multiple pesticides is inevitable. Under such circumstances, exposure to a single AChE-inhibiting insecticide is at the subtoxic level, but simultaneous exposure to more than one can sometimes lead to devastating health effects because of an additive or potentiating interaction. Studies based on laboratory animals have revealed potentiating toxicity following simultaneous exposure to OPs (P=S type) and *N*-methylcarbamate insecticides. Thus, predicting and avoiding such interactions in nontarget species are the challenges that we face today.

Biomarkers and Biomonitoring

Biomonitoring data are useful for a variety of applications, from exposure assessment to risk assessment. Because carbamates are unstable compounds, their metabolites are also considered to be determined in serum/plasma, blood, and urine to estimate the exposure levels of carbamates. Carbamates that are commonly encountered in poisonings include aldicarb, bendiocarb, benomyl, carbaryl, carbofuran, carbosulfan, methomyl, pirimicarb, and propoxur. Major metabolites of carbaryl (1-naphthol, 2-naphthol, and/or 4-hydroxycarbarylglucuronide), carbofuran (3-hydroxycarbofuran and 3-ketocarbofuran), and propoxur (2-isopropoxyphenol) are also analyzed in addition to the parent compounds in case of carbamate poisoning. Carbamates and their metabolites are also measured in saliva for pharmacokinetics and dosimetry. Recently, liquid chromatography–mass spectrometry has been employed to identify novel biomarkers of AChE-inhibiting pesticide exposure by detecting their adducts on serine of butyrylcholinesterase and tyrosine of albumin. Both scientific and regulatory communities have recognized that erythrocytes-AChE inhibition is a sensitive biomarker of exposure to carbamates and OPs, because it serves as a sensitive surrogate endpoint for the inhibition of brain-AChE. However, AChE inhibition measurement cannot ascribe to a specific pesticide exposure event.

Human Risk

Risks to humans are significant from overexposure to *N*-methylcarbamate insecticides, whereas risks are minimal from thiocarbamate and dithiocarbamate herbicides and fungicides. It needs to be pointed out that the cumulative risks from food, water, and residential exposure to *N*-methylcarbamates normally do not exceed the Environmental Protection Agency's level of concern.

Clinical Management

Humans and animals acutely poisoned with carbamate insecticides usually show the signs and symptoms of hypercholinergic preponderance, such as salivation, lacrimation, diarrhea, nausea, tremors, miosis, bradycardia, headache, confusion, and sometimes death. Dogs exposed to large doses of a carbamate insecticide in a malicious intent usually die. Both in humans and dogs, signs and symptoms are reported within minutes of exposure and can last for hours. However, because of reversibility of the inhibition of AChE, recovery is usually apparent within 24 h, depending on the dose of the carbamate and severity of poisoning. Metabolites of carbamates in the urine and inhibition of erythrocytes-AChE activity can be used for biological monitoring. In acute poisoning cases, atropine sulfate is recommended with a full dose. It should be repeated at half a dose on hourly intervals, until all hypersecretory signs completely subside. Oximes are typically contraindicated. Supportive therapy is highly recommended.

Ecotoxicology

When applied directly to the soil, many carbamates can cause significant reduction in microflora and worms. Bees are especially sensitive to some carbamate pesticides. Some of the carbamate insecticides, such as aldicarb, carbofuran, and propoxur are deadly toxic to both mammalian and avian wildlife. Morbidity and mortality have been noted in wildlife even when some carbamates were used at the recommended levels. Deaths in many nontarget species have been reported as a result of malicious intent or secondary poisoning.

Environmental Fate

In general, carbamates are degraded into metabolites of lesser toxicity, and they have very little impact in terms of environmental persistence. Carbamates can be degraded by microorganisms, soil, water, light, and animals. These compounds do not bioaccumulate in the food chain or environment. Of course, groundwater can have carbamate residue for an extended period of time. There are serious concerns about EBDC-based fungicides that produce a toxic metabolite ethylene thiourea (ETU) in the environment.

Future Directions

In every aspect, carbamates have received less attention compared with organophosphates, because carbamates produce toxicity by a similar mechanism and the toxic effects are reversible. Evidently, one area that needs attention is the clinical management of carbamates' poisoning, because atropine is inadequate to cover the entire spectrum of toxicity.

See also: Aldicarb; Benomyl; Carbaryl; Carbofuran; Cholinesterase Inhibition; Dithiocarbamates; Methomyl; Propoxur.

Further Reading

Gupta, R.C., 2004. Brain regional heterogeneity and toxicological mechanisms of organophosphates and carbamates. Toxicol. Mech. Meth. 14, 103–143.

Gupta, R.C., 2006. In: Gupta, R.C. (Ed.), Toxicology of Organophosphate and Carbamate Compounds. Academic Press/Elsevier, Amsterdam, pp. 1–763.

Gupta, R.C., Crissman, J.W., 2012. Agricultural chemicals. In: Haschek-Hock, W.M., Rousseaux, C.G., Wallig, M.A. (Eds.), Handbook of Toxicologic Pathology, third ed. Elsevier, Amsterdam, in press.

Gupta, R.C., Milatovic, D., 2012a. Organophosphates and carbamates. In: Gupta, R.C. (Ed.), Veterinary Toxicology: Basic and Clinical Principles. Academic Press/Elsevier, pp. 573–585.

Gupta, R.C., Milatovic, D., 2012b. Toxicity of organophosphates and carbamates. In: Marrs, T.C. (Ed.), Mammalian Toxicology of Insecticides. RSC Publications, Cambridge, pp. 104–126.

Jokanovic, M., 2010. Medical treatment of poisoning by organophosphates and carbamates. In: Satoh, T., Gupta, R.C. (Eds.), Anticholinesterase Pesticides: Metabolism, Neurotoxicity, and Epidemiology. John Wiley and Sons, Hoboken, pp. 583–597.

Satoh, T., Gupta, R.C., 2010. In: Satoh, T., Gupta, R.C. (Eds.), Anticholinesterase Pesticides: Metabolism, Neurotoxicity, and Epidemiology. John Wiley and Sons, Hoboken, pp. 1–625.

Carbamazepine

JCY Lo, San Diego, CA, USA

This article is a revision of the previous edition article by Henry A. Spiller, volume 1, pp 413–414, © 2005, Elsevier Inc.

- Name: Carbamazepine
- Chemical Abstracts Service Registry Number: 298-46-4
- Synonyms: CBZ; 5*H*-dibenz(b,f)-azepine-5-carboxamide; Tegretol
- Molecular Formula: $C_{15}H_{12}N_2O$
- Chemical Structure: $NCONH_2$

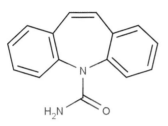

Background

Carbamazepine is a synthetic iminostilbene derivative structurally similar to imipramine, a tricyclic antidepressant. While unrelated structurally, carbamazepine shares a similar therapeutic action with phenytoin. Carbamazepine was first discovered in 1953 by Swiss chemist Walter Schindler. Throughout the 1960s, antimuscarinic was used and marketed for trigeminal neuralgia and as an anticonvulsant. By the 1970s, it was being used as a mood stabilizer for patients with bipolar disorder.

Uses

Carbamazepine is used in the treatment of epilepsy and trigeminal neuralgia. Unlabeled uses include treatment of postherpetic pain syndrome, neurogenic diabetes insipidus, bipolar disorder, alcohol withdrawal, and cocaine dependence.

Environmental Fate and Behavior

Environmental exposure occurs via direct release into water or via vaporization into the air. It is susceptible to photolysis and is thought to have a half-life of roughly 63 days in lake water *in vitro*. However, when dissolved and exposed to direct photolysis, it has a half-life of approximately 1 day.

Exposure Routes and Pathways

The exposure pathway for carbamazepine is exclusively oral (ingestion of tablets or suspension).

Toxicokinetics

Carbamazepine is slowly and incompletely absorbed during therapeutic use. With large ingestions, absorption may be delayed and unpredictable, producing peak levels from 4 to 72 h after the overdose. The absorption phase in an overdose is highly variable because of carbamazepine's poor solubility, ability to significantly decrease gut motility, and to form pharmacobezoars. One of the primary metabolites of carbamazepine is carbamazepine-10,11-epoxide (CBZE), which also has anticonvulsant activity. A minor pathway results in iminostilbene formation. Further hydrolysis and conjugation produce six other known metabolites including 10,11-dihydroxycarbamazepine. Protein binding is 75% for carbamazepine and 50% for CBZE. However, the percentage of protein binding may decrease in massive overdose due to saturable binding sites. The volume of distribution is 0.8–1.9 $l\ kg^{-1}$. The hydrolyzed and conjugated metabolites are eliminated through the kidneys, with only 1.2% free carbamazepine being found in the urine and 28% is eliminated unchanged in the feces. Carbamazepine induces drug-metabolizing enzymes so that drug half-life is reduced in chronic use. The half-life in healthy adults ranges from 18–65 h in a single dose to 8–17 h during chronic administration. In newborns and children, the half-life is below 9 h.

Mechanism of Toxicity

Carbamazepine is both an important anticonvulsant in therapeutic doses and a powerful proconvulsant in overdose. The therapeutic anticonvulsant mechanism is primarily related to blockade of presynaptic voltage-gated sodium channels. Blockade of the sodium channels is believed to inhibit the release of synaptic glutamate and possibly other neurotransmitters. Carbamazepine is also a powerful inhibitor of the muscarinic and nicotinic acetylcholine receptors, *N*-methyl-D-aspartate (NMDA) receptors, and the central nervous system (CNS) adenosine receptors. In addition, carbamazepine is structurally related to the cyclic antidepressant imipramine and in massive overdose, it may affect cardiac sodium channels.

Acute and Short-Term Toxicity (or Exposure)

Animal

Carbamazepine is not commonly used in animals. Limited information on toxicity exits. Tachyarrhythmias, hypotension, and seizures have been seen.

Human

The primary and common toxic event involves the CNS. Cardiac conduction delays and ventricular arrhythmias can be seen but are infrequent. Sinus tachycardia and hypotension are more commonly seen. In the few deaths directly attributable to carbamazepine toxicity, ventricular dysrhythmias have been

 http://dx.doi.org/10.1016/B978-0-12-386454-3.00705-3

the terminal event. Coma, seizures, and respiratory depression are commonly seen in adults at levels greater than 40 mg ml^{-1} (170 mmol l^{-1}). Status epilepticus has been reported. The incidence of serious toxicity is similar in adults and children. However, serum levels are less predictive in children. Therefore, coma, seizures, and apnea may be seen at lower serum levels than in adults. Other manifestations of neurological toxicity are nystagmus, ataxia, choreoathetoid movements, encephalopathy, absence of corneal reflexes, decreased deep tendon reflexes, urinary retention, and dystonias. A cyclic clinical course can be seen, with a waxing and waning of symptoms. This may be due to the presence of a pharmacobezoar in the gut or more commonly due to a decrease in gastrointestinal motility produced by the prominent anticholinergic effects of carbamazepine.

Chronic Toxicity (or Exposure)

Animal

Male albino rats given injections of carbamazepine over 3 months demonstrated decreased prostate weight and decreased sperm motility. These changes did not affect fertility.

Human

Idiopathic hepatotoxicity has been reported as a rare manifestation of chronic therapy and is not dose related. Hyponatremia is a common adverse effect associated with carbamazepine exposure. Increased antidiuretic hormone secretion and increased aquaporin 2 expression are proposed mechanism. Hypersensitivity syndrome, or drug rash with eosinophilia and systemic symptoms, and Stevens–Johnson syndrome/toxic epidermal necrolysis (SJS/TEN) have been described with carbamazepine administration.

In vitro toxicity studies of carbamazepine on rat cerebellar granule cells have shown inhibition of NMDA-stimulated calcium entry in a rapid and reversible manner. These findings occurred in therapeutic concentrations of carbamazepine, which may help explain the antiseizure activity of carbamazepine. It is believed that the toxic cerebellar effects of carbamazepine may be due to this mechanism.

Immunotoxicity

Isolated cases of transient hypogammaglobulinemia have been reported with carbamazepine administration. IgG, IgA, and IgM were not found to be significantly reduced in patients treated with carbamazepine in comparison to control subjects who did not receive carbamazepine. An increase in cytotoxic activity of natural killer cells was noted in patients treated with carbamazepine.

Carbamazepine has been associated with a potentially fatal idiosyncratic reaction known at antiepileptic hypersensitivity syndrome. This is characterized by eosinophilia, fever, rash, coagualopathy, and hepatotoxicity.

Pancytopenia has also been reported with carbamazepine including neutropenia and agranulocytosis.

Reproductive Toxicity

Animal

Rats born to mothers chronically fed carbamazepine during gestation demonstrated challenges with maintaining balance and had more difficulty lifting their hind legs than controls. Mice born to mothers who received intraperitoneal administration of carbamazepine demonstrated eye malformation.

Human

Carbamazepine is highly teratogenic. Neural tube defects are associated with carbamazepine exposure during pregnancy and can lead to spina bifida. Carbamazepine is pregnancy category D.

Genotoxicity

Animal

High dose carbamazepine resulted in increased number of mutations per *Drosophila* wing.

Human

Associations have been shown for carbamazepine and human leukocyte antigen (HLA)-B*1502 and HLA-A*3101-induced cutaneous adverse drug reactions. HLA-B*1502 is present in certain Asian populations who are predisposed to SJS/TEN.

Carcinogenicity

High-dose (25 mg kg^{-1} day^{-1}) carbamazepine administration for more than 2 years caused hepatocellular tumors in female rats and benign interstitial tumors of the testes in male rats.

Clinical Management

Basic and advanced life-support measures should be utilized as necessary. Gastrointestinal decontamination procedures should be used as appropriate. Activated charcoal effectively binds carbamazepine. Multiple-dose activated charcoal (0.5 g kg^{-1} every 4 h) has been shown to decrease the half-life of carbamazepine. Generally, supportive measures are all that is required in carbamazepine overdose. Seizures initially should be managed with diazepam or lorazepam. However, persistent seizures may require advancement to phenobarbital or pentobarbital. Ventricular arrhythmias should be managed with lidocaine. Patients that present with widening of the QRS complex can be given sodium bicarbonate in 50 meq boluses.

The presence of persistently high serum levels or fluctuating elevated serum levels may suggest the presence of a pharmacobezoar in the gut. Removal should be attempted, in the presence of an active bowel, with whole bowel irrigation using a polyethylene glycol–electrolyte solution. Hemodialysis and charcoal hemoperfusion have been used in carbamazepine overdose.

Ecotoxicology

Carbamazepine is not expected to produce acute ecotoxicological effects.

Other Hazards

Carbamazepine is an inducer of CYP 3A4. Coadministration of carbamazepine and contraceptive drugs may result in decreased level of contraceptive drugs and permit ovulation.

See also: Diazepam; Lidocaine; Polyethylene Glycol.

Further Reading

Bridge, T.A., Norton, R.L., Robertson, W.O., 1994. Pediatric carbamazepine overdoses. Pediatr. Emerg. Care 10, 260–263.

Donner, E., Kosjek, T., Qualmann, S., Kusk, K.O., Heath, E., Revitt, D.M., Ledin, A., Andersen, H.R., January 15, 2013. Ecotoxicity of carbamazepine and its UV photolysis transformation products. Sci. Total Environ. 443, 870–876.

Kasarskis, E.J., Kuo, C.S., Berger, R., 1992. Carbamazepine-induced cardiac dysfunction: characterization of two distinct clinical syndromes. Arch. Intern. Med. 152, 186–191.

Spiller, H.A., 2001. Management of carbamazepine overdose. Pediatr. Emerg. Care 17, 452–456.

van den Brandhof, E.J., Montforts, M., November 2010. Fish embryo toxicity of carbamazepine, diclofenac and metoprolol. Ecotoxicol. Environ. Saf. 73 (8), 1862–1866.

Carbaryl

SE Koshlukova and NR Reed, California Environmental Protection Agency, Sacramento, CA, USA

This article is a revision of the previous edition article by Paul R. Harp, volume 1, pp 414–416, © 2005, Elsevier Inc.

Background

Carbaryl is an *N*-methyl carbamate manufactured as an insecticide and molluscicide. Its most prominent toxicity to insects and mammals is associated with binding and inhibition of the enzyme acetylcholinesterase (AChE).

First sold in 1959, carbaryl is used worldwide to control agricultural and structural pests, and mosquitos. In the late 1990s, it was one of the top selling pesticides for agriculture, turf management, residential pet, and lawn. Over the last decade, concerns regarding human and ecological risks have limited its use. Carbaryl was phased out in the United Kingdom by 1998. It was phased out by 2007 under the Council Directive 91/414/EEC and currently not authorized for use in the European Union. In the United States, about 80% of products were canceled, and many agricultural and residential uses were restricted by 2005. Use limitations were imposed in Australia in 2007.

Chemical Profile

- Chemical Abstracts Service Registry Number: 63-25-2
- Chemical Name: Naphthalen-1-yl *N*-methylcarbamate
- Synonyms: Carbaril; CARBARYL; Sevin; 1-Naphthalenol, methylcarbamate; 1-Naphthyl *N*-methylcarbamate; Caprolin; Carbatox; Carbavur; Carpolin; Carylderm
- Chemical Class: Carbamate; Insecticide, Acaricide, Molluscicide
- Chemical Structure: (from PubChem) http://pubchem.ncbi.nlm.nih.gov/image/structurefly.cgi?cid=6129&width=400&height=400

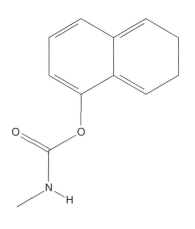

- Molecular Formula: $C_{12}H_{11}NO_2$
- Molecular Weight: 201.22 g mol^{-1}
- Density: 1.23 g cm^{-3} at 25 °C
- Vapor Pressure: 0.000 001 4 mmHg at 25 °C
- Boiling Point: Decomposes before boiling point
- Melting Point: 145 °C
- Flash Point: 183.8–202 °C
- Conversion Factor: 1 ppm = 0.82 mg m^{-3}
- Appearance: Colorless to light tan crystals, white or gray solid
- Odor: Odorless

Uses

Carbaryl is a widely used *N*-methyl carbamate insecticide. In the United States, about 3.9 million pounds were sold for over 400 uses during 1992–2001. Half of this amount was used non-agriculturally. Since 2003, more than two-thirds of all registered carbaryl products were canceled, including the extensively used liquid broadcast formulations for residential lawns and pet flea control. Nevertheless, carbaryl is still among the most widely applied pesticides in the United States for many types of fruits and vegetables, grain crops, cut flowers, nursery and ornamentals, turf, green houses, golf courses, and oyster beds. Non-agriculturally, carbaryl is used on residential sites, gardens, ornamentals, and turf grass. Although phased out in the European Union, carbaryl continues to be used in Australia, the United States, Canada, and developing countries.

Environmental Fate and Behavior

Carbaryl is soluble in organic solvents (e.g., dimethyl formamide, acetone) and is moderately soluble in water (32 mg l^{-1} solubility at 20 °C). The calculated Henry's law constant of 0.000000003 atm m^3 mol^{-1} indicates that surface water volatilization is unlikely an important fate process. The estimated half-life for reacting with airborne photochemically generated hydroxyl radicals is 12.6 h. Photolysis produces naphthoquinone products.

Carbaryl undergoes abiotic hydrolysis, photodegradation, and biotic degradation in soil and water. Depending on soil type and climate, its soil persistence varies from 13 days to 2 years. Half-lives in canal and river waters vary from 4 to 30 days, hydrolysis rate is greater with increasing temperature and alkalinity. Carbaryl can persist for years under acidic environments. The estimated log K_{oc} of 1.87–2.46 indicates moderate adsorption to soil and the potential for groundwater leaching.

1-Naphthol, the major degradate of carbaryl, is less persistent and mobile than the parent compound. Its soil persistence is 12–14 days, and further transforms to phenolic radicals and CO_2. Based on the measured log K_{ow} of 1.6–2.4, carbaryl is not expected to bioaccumulate in aquatic and terrestrial food chains.

 http://dx.doi.org/10.1016/B978-0-12-386454-3.00107-X

Exposure and Exposure Monitoring

Exposure to carbaryl occurs through ingesting residues in food, inhaling vapors, and skin contact. Before 2004, residential exposure was widespread. Carbaryl was the most frequently detected pesticide in indoor and outdoor air in the United States and Canada. It has also been found in house dust in association with its agricultural use. Today, there are fewer potential residential exposure scenarios because of the numerous product cancellations. Exposure to the general public occurs mainly via the diet, ambient air, and during pest control operations in home and recreation areas. Workers' exposures are mainly dermal and inhalation from handling or re-entering treated fields.

Maximum Residue Levels (MRL) of carbaryl (or 'Tolerances' in the United States) are established for more than 100 food commodities. These are the highest levels allowable in or on these commodities. At a given exposure concentration, children generally have higher body burden owing to their higher intake (inhalation volume, amount of food intake) or contact on a per body weight basis.

Toxicokinetics

The oral absorption of carbaryl is 96–100% in rats, mice, and humans. In rats, peak blood concentrations of carbaryl and its metabolites are reached within 15–30 min after dosing. The dermal absorption estimated from recovery of urinary metabolites is 13–34% in rats and 45% in humans. Inhalation absorption is indicated by the inhibition of ChE activities.

Carbaryl is extensively metabolized by the liver cytochrome P450 enzymes (CYP). The main routes of metabolism are similar in humans, rats, mice, guinea pigs, monkeys, and sheep. Hydrolysis results in 1-naphthol, CO_2, and methylamine, whereas alkyl oxidation forms *N*-hydroxymethylcarbaryl. Hydroxylation produces 5-hydroxycarbaryl, 4-hydroxycarbaryl, 5-6-dihydro-5-6-dihydroxycarbaryl, and 3,4-dihydro-3,4-dihydroxycarbatyl, via epoxide intermediates.

In animals, the highest levels of carbaryl and its major metabolite 1-naphthol are found in the kidney, blood, liver, and brain; the oxidation product *N*-hydroxymethylcarbaryl is detected in brain only. Carbaryl binds to plasma proteins (e.g., albumin). In rats and mice, transplacental transfer is evidenced by fetal plasma and brain ChE inhibition and the presence of carbaryl in the fetal eye, liver, and brain.

Carbaryl is mainly eliminated through urine, in which 68–74% of a single oral dose is found within 24 h. About 2–11% is excreted in the bile/feces. Enterohepatic circulation is significant. The major metabolites in excreta are 1-naphthol, 5-hydroxycarbaryl, glucuronide, and sulfate conjugates. Urinary 1-naphthol is commonly used in human biomonitoring studies. A shift in the urinary metabolite pattern, with increases in the hydroxylated compounds derived from epoxide intermediates, is observed in rats and mice at high doses of carbaryl, which caused severe toxicity and tumors in chronic dietary studies. Carbaryl's potential for tumor formation is discussed in the Carcinogenicity section.

Mechanism of Toxicity

Like other *N*-methyl carbamates, the mechanism of carbaryl toxicity is related to its binding and inhibition of serine hydrolase AChE. AChE hydrolyzes the neurotransmitter acetylcholine, thereby terminating its synaptic action. AChE inhibition increases the availability of acetylcholine at the neural synapse, leading to cholinergic overstimulation, autonomic, and neuromuscular dysfunction, and at higher levels, resulting in coma and death. AChE is also a target of the organophosphorus insecticides.

N-methyl carbamates and the organophosphates differ in their interaction with the cholinesterase (ChE) enzyme. Generally, the carbamylated ChE is more labile and dissociates quickly, within minutes to hours. The fast ChE recovery and the significant metabolic clearance within 24 h account for the relatively short-lived neurotoxicity of carbaryl. Carbaryl also inhibits other esterases, including butyrylcholinesterase and neuropathy target esterase. Butyrylcholinesterase may function as a molecular scavenger for anticholinesterase compounds in the blood or substitute for AChE, where it is low. Neuropathy target esterase may be involved in the delayed neurotoxicity syndrome.

Other non-ChE actions may influence the overall toxicity of carbaryl. The potential targets include macromolecule synthesis, chromatin protein, mitotic spindle formation, neurotransmitter receptors, aryl hydrocarbon receptor (AhR), and serotonin and catecholamine metabolism. Carbaryl induces hepatic CYPs. The toxicities of carbaryl major metabolites are not associated with ChE inhibition. The mechanism is unknown for 1-naphthol, which induces the same mitotic abnormalities as carbaryl. Hydroxycarbaryl and dihydro-dihydroxycarbaryl are implicated in tumor induction in mice and rats based on their possible formation via epoxide intermediates.

Acute and Short-Term Toxicity

Animal

Carbaryl is classified by USEPA as a moderate oral toxicant (Category II). The acute oral LD_{50} is 108–840 mg kg^{-1} for rats, mice, rabbits, guinea pigs, dogs, cats, and deer. The dermal LD_{50} in rats and rabbits is >2000 mg kg^{-1} day^{-1}. The 4-h inhalation LC_{50} in rats is >0.9 mg l^{-1}. Carbaryl is a category IV skin and eye irritant (slight conjunctival irritation).

The main target of short-term oral toxicity is the nervous system. Cholinergic syndromes from overstimulation of the muscarinic and nicotinic receptors include hypersalivation, respiratory distress, miosis, muscular twitches, tremors, ataxia, diarrhea, and vomiting. Other nonlethal effects are hematological and liver enzyme changes, alterations in brain enzymes and neurotransmitter levels, changes in catecholamine metabolism, renal effects, hypothermia, and body weight decreases. No delayed neuropathy was observed in hens receiving a 300–560 ng kg^{-1} ip dose of carbaryl.

Young animals are twofold more sensitive to ChE inhibition than adults. Applying the Benchmark Dose (BMD) analysis, USEPA established a BMDL (lower bound of BMD) at 1.1 mg kg^{-1} day^{-1} for 10% brain ChE inhibition in postnatal day (PND) 11 pups after a single oral exposure.

Human

Human deaths occurred from intentional ingestion of carbaryl. Pulmonary edema was reported in a case with about 5700 mg kg^{-1}. Initial signs involved tremors, disturbed vision, and severely inhibited RBC ChE. Postmortem, carbaryl was detected in the gastrointestinal tract, blood, liver, kidney, and urine. Nonlethal effects include CNS, cardiovascular, and respiratory systems.

Common clinical signs of cholinergic toxicity in humans are lacrimation, salivation, tremors, nausea, miosis, and muscle incoordination. Abdominal pain, profuse sweating, lassitude, and vomiting occurred after a single oral dose of 2.8–5.5 mg kg^{-1}. Rash, burning, skin irritation, and depressed plasma ChE levels are reported in workers following dermal contact or after spraying carbaryl. Unlike in animals, limited human data indicate that carbaryl has irritant properties. In studies of male adults, the acute Lowest Observable Effect Level (LOEL) for plasma and RBC ChE inhibition is 2 mg kg^{-1}.

A large number of human adult nonoccupational poisonings are reported. Carbaryl cases were twice as likely as other pesticides to show major medical crisis (life-threatening, significant disability) and require hospitalization or involve critical care unit. This pattern was not seen among occupational settings, suggesting heightened hazards of handling by nonprofessionals.

Chronic Toxicity

Animal

Nonlethal LOELs included 12–15 mg kg^{-1} day^{-1} for thyroid follicular and liver hepatocellular hypertrophy in rats, and globular deposits in the bladder epithelium in mice, 10–31 mg kg^{-1} day^{-1} for decreased pupil size, reduced rearing activity, tremors, lacrimation and salivation in rats and dogs, 24 mg kg^{-1} day^{-1} for increased liver weight in rats, 30–79 mg kg^{-1} day^{-1} for decreases in body weight, body weight gains and food consumption in dogs and rats, 145–350 mg kg^{-1} day^{-1} for progressive nephropathy and opaque eyes in mice, and bladder epithelial hyperplasia, pelvic urothelial hyperplasia, cataracts, degeneration of sciatic nerve and muscle, chromodacryorrhea, and alopecia in rats.

Human

Studies with human volunteers ingesting carbaryl for 6 weeks reported abdominal changes and difficulty in sleeping at the LOEL of 0.13 mg kg^{-1} day^{-1}. Case report suggested possible effects of chronic neurological or psychological problems. Effects of sperm morphological abnormalities and increased risk for multiple tumors are discussed under Reproductive and Developmental Toxicity and Carcinogenicity sections.

Immunotoxicity

Carbaryl given as a single or repeated doses at 1.5–200 mg kg^{-1} day^{-1} impaired the humoral immune response in mice, decreased the phagocytic activity of leukocytes and antibody formation, and disrupted the ability of the immune system to combat *Erysipelothrix rhusiopathiae* and *Staphylococcus* infections in rats and rabbits. Carbaryl enhanced the replication of varicella zoster virus in human lung cells.

Reproductive and Developmental Toxicity

Animal

The reproductive and developmental toxicity of carbaryl has been studied in more than 10 mammalian species. Fetal growth retardation and malformations were observed in the presence of maternal toxicity when pregnant rats received carbaryl up to 30 mg kg^{-1} day^{-1} orally on GD 6–20 or pregnant rabbits received up to 150 mg kg^{-1} day^{-1} on GD 6–29. Carbaryl caused severe malformations in pups of pregnant dogs or pigs at 5–50 mg kg^{-1} day^{-1}.

In two-generation studies, rats fed with 4.7–111 mg kg^{-1} day^{-1} carbaryl mated normally and exhibited normal pregnancy. Parental body weights and food consumption were impacted only at the high dose. However, decreased pup survival LOEL was 24 mg kg^{-1} day^{-1}. Decreased sperm motility and count occurred after 90 days of oral dosing at as low as 50 mg kg^{-1} day^{-1}.

Developmental neurotoxicity studies in rats showed evidence of increased susceptibility of the developing organisms. Gestational and early postnatal exposure to 10 mg kg^{-1} day^{-1} carbaryl produced changes in brain structures (decreased cerebellar length in pups, thickened cerebral cortex of the offspring later in life). The less severe maternal toxicity included decreased body weight gain, pinpoint pupils, tremors, gait abnormalities, and plasma, RBC, and brain ChE inhibition.

Human

Collective results from several epidemiological studies suggest toxicity to the human reproductive system. A study with farm families in Canada indicated an increased risk of miscarriages following carbaryl usage by males. In the United States and China, carbaryl-exposed factory workers showed decreased sperm count, sperm abnormality, and sperm chromosomal aberrations. An association with various indicators of sperm toxicity (decreased motility and concentrations, DNA damage) were reported when urinary 1-naphthol is used as the biomarker for exposure.

Genotoxicity

Carbaryl tested negative in reverse mutation tests in multiple strains of *Salmonella* and in Chinese hamster ovary cell/hypoxanthine-guanine phosphoribosyl-transferase (CHO/HGPRT) forward mutation assay. Carbaryl caused chromosomal aberrations in an *in vitro* assay with CHO cells in the presence of metabolic activation but is negative in an *in vivo* micronucleus assay in both male and female mice. No unscheduled DNA synthesis was found in a rat hepatocyte assay. The Joint FAO/WHO Meeting on Pesticide Residues (JMPR) concluded in 1996 that carbaryl is not genotoxic.

Carcinogenicity

Carbaryl carcinogenicity is evident in 2-year dietary inclusion studies with rats and mice. Neoplastic lesions in Sprague-Dawley rats at the highest tested level of 7500 ppm included urinary bladder transitional cell papilloma and carcinoma in males and females, kidney transitional cell carcinoma, and thyroid adenoma and carcinoma in males, and liver adenoma in females. Neoplastic lesions in CD-1 mice included vascular hemangioma and hemangiosarcoma in the males at all dose groups (100–8000 ppm) and in the females at 8000 ppm. Additional lesions at 8000 ppm included kidney tubular cell adenoma and carcinoma in the males and hepatocellular adenoma, carcinoma, and hepatoblastoma in the females. In both studies, excess toxicity occurred at the highest tested dose. In 2002, USEPA classified carbaryl as a Group C carcinogen – 'Likely to be carcinogenic in humans' based on increased hemangiosarcomas in male mice. The human equivalent upper bound potency slope is 8.75×10^{-4} per (mg kg^{-1} day^{-1}).

Several epidemiological investigations in Canada and the United States during the past two decades showed associations between carbaryl exposure and non-Hodgkin's lymphoma, cutaneous melanoma, and prostate cancer.

Clinical Management

The muscarinic signs of carbaryl poisoning are antagonized by atropine, which blocks acetylcholine but only at muscarinic receptors. Oximes, widely used to treat nicotinic effects of organophosphates, are ineffective or even harmful in carbaryl poisoning. Benzodiazepines and barbiturates are used to control carbaryl-induced seizures.

Ecotoxicology

Carbaryl is highly toxic to estuarine/marine invertebrates and other aquatic species, including Atlantic salmon. The 96-h LC_{50} for shrimp species is 5.7 ppb. The 48-h LC_{50} for *Daphnia magna* and stonefly species ranges from 1.7 to 26 ppb. The acute LC_{50} for fish varies widely, e.g., 0.25–0.69 ppm for Atlantic salmon and lake trout, 1.2–20 ppm for rainbow trout, fathead minnow, and black bullhead. The chronic No Observed Adverse Effect Concentration (NOAEC) for reproduction is 1.5 ppb for *Daphnia magna* and 0.21 ppm for fathead minnow.

Carbaryl is highly toxic to honey bees with an acute LC_{50} of 1 ppb. The acute toxicity to birds varies (e.g., LD_{50} of 707 mg kg^{-1} for pheasant, >2500 for mallard duck). Chronic reproductive toxicity includes decreased number of eggs and fertility at the Lowest Observable Adverse Effect Concentration (LOAEC) of 600 ppm. The NOAEC for reproduction is 300 ppm for mallard duck. Toxicities to mammals are presented in the Acute and Chronic Toxicity sections.

Based on estimated risk quotients in 2003, USEPA concluded high risk of carbaryl to aquatic invertebrate species, fish, and all-sized mammals from a single outdoor application, and prolonged risk for birds, aquatic species, and all-sized mammals from multiple applications.

Other Hazards

Age is a modifying factor for the acute toxicity of carbaryl owing to low level of carboxylesterases in the young for detoxification. Concomitant exposure to other *N*-methyl carbamates with similar mechanism of action may result in cumulative toxicity. Nutritional factors influence the toxicity of carbaryl. Rats fed high protein diets showed higher toxicity than those given ordinary diet (LD_{50} of 67 and 575 mg kg^{-1} day^{-1}, respectively), possibly because of decreased metabolism. Carbaryl metabolism is inhibited by other environmental chemicals (e.g., fipronil and chlorpyrifos) that are substrates of common CYPs (CYP3A4, CYP2B6) and share biotransformation pathways. *In vitro*, toxicity is increased by agents that inhibit liver metabolic enzymes. In contrast, acute toxicity in mice is decreased by CYP inducers (e.g., phenobarbital) or compounds that accelerate carbaryl urinary excretion (e.g., chlordane).

Exposure Standards and Guidelines

American Conference of Governmental Industrial Hygienists (ACGIH) – Threshold Limit Value (TLV): 0.5 mg m^{-3} Time Weighted Average (TWA), inhalable fraction and vapor; (skin) (A4 – not classifiable as a human carcinogen).

National Institute for Occupational Safety and Health (NIOSH) – Recommended Exposure Limit (REL): 5 mg m^{-3} TWA.

Occupational Safety and Health Administration (OSHA) – Permissible Exposure Limit (PEL): 5 mg m^{-3} TWA.

NIOSH Immediately Dangerous to Life or Health Concentration (IDLH): 100 mg m^{-3}.

USEPA – Population Adjusted Dose (PAD) (oral): 0.01 mg kg^{-1} day^{-1} (acute).

See also: Behavioral Toxicology; Developmental Toxicology; Toxicity Testing, Developmental; Carbamate Pesticides; Carbaryl; Carboxylesterases; Cholinesterase Inhibition; Common Mechanism of Toxicity in Pesticides; Neurotoxicity; Organophosphorus Compounds; Pesticides; Cytochrome P450; National Institute for Occupational Safety and Health; Carcinogen Classification Schemes; Federal Insecticide, Fungicide, and Rodenticide Act, US; Genetic Toxicology; International Agency for Research on Cancer; Regulation, Toxicology and; Toxicity Testing, Reproductive; Risk Assessment, Human Health; Occupational Exposure Limits; Ecotoxicology; ACGIH® (American Conference of Governmental Industrial Hygienists); Food Quality Protection Act; Children's Environmental Health; Epidemiology; Environmental Fate and Behavior.

Further Reading

ACGIH, 2008. Carbaryl: TLV® Chemical Substances 7th Edition Documentation. ACGIH®. Publication #7DOC-104. American Conference of Governmental Industrial Hygienists, Cincinnati, OH.

DPR, 2010. Carbary. Dietary Risk Characterization Document. California Environmental Protection Agency. Department of Pesticide Regulation, Medical Toxicology Branch, Sacramento, CA. www.cdpr.ca.gov/docs/risk/rcd/carbaryl.pdf.

Gunasekara, A.S., et al., 2008. Environmental fate and toxicology of carbaryl. Rev. Environ. Contam. Toxicol. 196, 95–121.

National Institute for Occupational Safety and Health (NIOSH), 2007. Pocket Guide to Chemical Hazards. DHHS (NIOSH) Publication No. 2005-149. September 2007. Department of Health and Human Services, Centers for Disease Control and Prevention. http://www.cdc.gov/niosh/docs/2005-149/pdfs/2005-149.pdf.

USEPA, 2008. Amended Reregistration Eligibility Decision (RED) for Carbaryl. United States Environmental Protection Agency, Washington, D.C. http://www.epa.gov/pesticides/reregistration/REDs/carbaryl-red-amended.pdf.

Relevant Websites

http://toxnet.nlm.nih.gov – Hazardous Substance Data Bank.
http://npic.orst.edu – National Pesticide Information Center.
http://www.epa.gov – United States Environmental Protection Agency.
http://www.osha.gov – United States Occupational Safety and Health Administration.

Carbofuran

X Song, Merck & Co., Inc., West Point, PA, USA

- Chemical Abstracts Service Registry Number: 1563-66-2
- Synonyms: 2,3-dihydro-2,2-dimethyl-7-benzofuranyl *N*-methylcarbamate; Brifur®; Crisfuran®; Curaterr®; Furadan®; Pillarfuran®; Yaltox®; FMC 10242; Bay 70143; Chinufur; Niagra NIA-10242; OMS 864; NIOSH/RTECS FB 9450000; NA 2757; STCC 4921525
- Chemical Class: *N*-methyl carbamate insecticide, acaricide, and nematocide
- Chemical Structure:

OOCNHCH$_3$ … O … CH$_3$ / CH$_3$

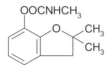

Background

Effective 1 September 1994, all granular formulations of carbofuran have been banned by the US Environmental Protection Agency (EPA), with five minor-use exceptions. The phaseout started on 1 September 1991. Before then, the primary application of carbofuran was in granular formulations. Not related to human health concerns, the ban has been established to protect birds, as birds died when they ingested carbofuran granules, which resemble grain seeds in size and shape, or when predatory or scavenging birds ingested smaller birds or mammals that had consumed carbofuran pellets. The ban does not apply to liquid formulations of carbofuran.

Uses

Carbofuran is used as an agricultural insecticide on tobacco, corn, alfalfa, and other field crops.

Environmental Fate and Behavior

Carbofuran has a high potential for groundwater contamination because of its solubility in water and relatively long half-life in soil. Carbofuran is mobile in soil, where it is degraded by chemical hydrolysis and microbial metabolism. Carbofuran also breaks down in sunlight. In water, carbofuran is degraded by chemical hydrolysis, photodegradation, and microbial metabolism. Carbofuran does not accumulate in aquatic systems, volatilize from water, or adsorb to sediment or suspended particles. The half-life of carbofuran is approximately 4 days or more when applied to crops.

Exposures and Exposure Monitoring

Exposure may occur via the dermal, inhalation, and oral routes. Dermal exposure can be evaluated with Tegaderm patches placed on the skin. Hand and wrist exposure can be measured in the hand rinse and on wrist patches. Inhalation exposure can be measured with an air sampler using polyurethane foam as the adsorbent. Urine samples collected at 24-h intervals after exposure can be measured for carbofuran. Exposure in blood can be estimated by analyzing acetylcholinesterase (AChE), pseudocholinesterase (ChE), and several other blood parameters.

Toxicokinetics

Carbofuran is absorbed by the oral, inhalation, and dermal routes. It is poorly absorbed through intact skin. Approximately 75% of absorbed carbofuran is protein bound. Carbofuran is metabolized to yield 3-hydroxycarbofuran and 3-ketocarbofuran via oxidation, and to yield 3-hydroxy-7-phenol, 3-keto-7-phenol, and 7-phenol via hydrolysis. Most metabolites form glucuronide or sulfate conjugates, which are excreted in the urine. The half-life in rat is 20 min for the parent compound and 64 min for 3-hydroxycarbofuran metabolite.

Mechanism of Toxicity

Carbofuran is a reversible inhibitor of acetylcholinesterase. Inhibition of acetylcholinesterase activity leads to an increase in acetylcholine at the nerve synapse resulting in excessive cholinergic stimulation. Following intravenous injection of 50 $\mu g\ kg^{-1}$ in rats, blood acetylcholinesterase activity was depressed by 83% in 2 min. With oral exposure, acetylcholinesterase activity was depressed by 37% within 15 min of ingestion. Recovery of acetylcholinesterase activity parallels carbofuran elimination.

Acute and Short-Term Toxicity

Animal

The oral LD_{50} values are 5.3–13.2 mg kg^{-1} in rats, 2.0 mg kg^{-1} in mice, 19 mg kg^{-1} in dogs, and 420 mg Kg^{-1} in wild bird species. The dermal LD_{50} values are >1000 mg kg^{-1} in rats, >2000 mg kg^{-1} in rabbits, and 100 mg kg^{-1} in wild bird species. The inhalation LC_{50} values are 85 mg m^{-3} in rats and 52 mg m^{-3} in dogs.

Human

Exposure to carbofuran may lead to cholinergic crisis with signs and symptoms including increased salivation, lacrimation, urinary incontinence, diarrhea, gastrointestinal cramping, and emesis (SLUDGE syndrome). The syndrome may be indistinguishable from that seen after organophosphate poisoning. Seizures, coma, diaphoresis, muscle weakness and fasciculation, bradycardia, and tachycardia may occur. Death may result from severe bronchoconstriction and/or respiratory paralysis.

 http://dx.doi.org/10.1016/B978-0-12-386454-3.00108-1

Chronic Toxicity

The no-effect levels in chronic feeding studies are 20 ppm in dogs and 25 ppm in rats. At 50 ppm chronically in the diet, significant decreases in cholinesterase activity were seen in dogs and rats. Chronic administration of 10 or 25 ppm of carbofuran in the diet for 180 days had no cumulative effect in rats. Chronic exposure to carbofuran may cause the same symptoms as an acute exposure. In addition, consumption of carbofuran at high levels well above the EPA Lifetime Health Advisory level over a long period of time was reported to cause adverse effects in the testes and uterus of test animals.

Immunotoxicity

Very limited investigations have been conducted to evaluate the immunotoxicity of carbofuran. Carbofuran was reported to suppress T-cell-mediated immune responses by the suppression of T-cell responsiveness.

Reproductive Toxicity

Daily feeding of 100 ppm of carbofuran to pregnant rats substantially decreased the ability of pups to survive.

Genotoxicity

No mutagenic effects have been found in laboratory animals or in Ames test. Genetic changes were reported in algae.

Carcinogenicity

Carbofuran is unlikely a carcinogen to humans.

Clinical Management

Rescuers and medical personnel must take precautions to avoid becoming contaminated themselves during rescue and emergency treatment. Victims should be removed from the toxic environment and 100% humidified supplemental oxygen should be administered with assisted ventilation as required. Patients with significant bronchorrhagia, pulmonary edema, convulsions, or coma may require endotracheal intubation and airway suctioning. Exposed skin and eyes should be flushed with copious amounts of water. Measures to decrease absorption may be beneficial soon after ingestion, but induced emesis should be avoided because of the potential for early development of coma or seizures. Atropine is antidotal for muscarinic symptoms and should be given in an initial dose of 2 mg and repeated every 15–30 min as required. The endpoint for atropinization is normalization of vital signs and drying of pulmonary secretions, not pupillary dilatation.

Administration of 2-PAM chloride (Protopam and pralidoxime) is generally not recommended in carbamate poisoning because it has been shown to interfere with the efficacy of atropine. It was reported that the condition of a patient suffering from carbaryl-related poisoning deteriorated rapidly after the administration of 2-PAM. Seizure control with diazepam, phenobarbital, or phenytoin may be required. Cardiovascular support and intensive supportive care may be required in serious cases.

Ecotoxicity

Carbofuran is very toxic to birds, trout, Coho salmon, perch, bluegills, and catfish. It may be teratogenic to frogs.

Exposure Standards

The US EPA has concluded that dietary, worker, and ecological risks are unacceptable for all uses of carbofuran, and has revoked all tolerances.

See also: Carbamate Pesticides; Pesticides; Cholinesterase Inhibition; Neurotoxicity.

Further Reading

Ecobichon, D.J., 2000. Carbamates. In: Spencer, P.S., Schaumburg, H.H. (Eds.), Experimental and Clinical Neurotoxicology, second ed. Oxford University Press, New York, pp. 289–298.

Gupta, R.A., 2006. Toxicology of Organophosphate and Carbamate Compounds. Elsevier, Amsterdam.

Hussain, M., Yoshida, K., Atiemo, M., Johnston, D., 1990. Occupational exposure of grain farmers to carbofuran. Arch. Environ. Contam. Toxicol. 19 (2), 197–204.

Relevant Websites

http://extoxnet.orst.edu – Extension Toxicology Network, Oregon State University.

http://www.epa.gov/pesticides/reregistration/carbofuran/ – US EPA Pesticide Chemical Search - Carbofuran.

Carbon Dioxide

S Goel, Supernus Pharmaceuticals, Inc., Rockville, MD, USA
D Agarwal, SB Physiotherapy and Rehabilitation Center, Mawana, Uttar Pradesh, India

This article is a revision of the previous edition article by Swarupa G. Kulkarni and Harihara M. Mehendale, volume 1, pp 419–420, © 2005, Elsevier Inc.

- Name: Carbon dioxide
- Chemical Abstracts Service Registry Number: 124-38-9
- Synonyms: Carbon oxide, Carbonic dioxide, Carbonice, carbonic acid gas, dry ice
- Molecular Formula: CO_2
- Chemical Structure:

$$O=C=O$$

Background

Carbon dioxide (CO_2) is a naturally occurring colorless and odorless gas. It has a boiling point of −70 °C (sublimes), vapor density of 1.53, and is slightly soluble in water. The atmospheric concentration in preindustrial times was 0.028% and in May 2013 was 0.04% recorded at Mauna Loa, Hawaii, USA. It is essential for the survival of most living organisms and cycles in the ecosystem, through respiration (aerobic and anaerobic), photosynthesis, and combustion. Carbon dioxide plays an important role in the regulation of earth's temperature, and is one of the greenhouse gases.

Uses

Carbon dioxide is used in the synthesis of urea, for organic synthesis, in the manufacture of dry ice and aspirin. It is also used in soft drinks, welding, fire extinguishers, and aerosol propellants. CO_2 is often used as a pesticide to store grains (at 60% concentration), respiratory stimulant, anesthetic, and euthanizing agent. It is essential in *in vitro* cell culture environment at 5%, where it dissolves in the culture media to form bicarbonate (HCO_3^-) and acts as a buffer to help maintain the pH of CO_2. Industries that use carbon dioxide include fire extinguishing; processing, preserving, and freezing of food; metal working; livestock slaughtering; oil and gas recovery; and foundries. It is also used to produce harmless smoke or fumes on a stage, chill golf ball centers before winding, and fumigate rice.

Environmental Fate and Behavior

The CO_2 cycle is part of carbon cycle in the ecosystem. Carbon dioxide cycles in the environment (atmospheric air and surface water) through respiration (aerobic and anaerobic), photosynthesis, decomposition, and release from earth's carbon sinks (fossil fuels – coal, petroleum, methane; and calcium carbonate rocks) during combustion. In water, dissolved CO_2 reacts with calcium to form calcium carbonate and precipitates to the ocean floor. Few examples of most common reactions in the CO_2 and carbon cycles in animals, plants, and the environment are presented below. Most of these reactions either use or produce energy.

Aerobic Metabolism: Glucose ($C_6H_{12}O_6$) + Oxygen (O_2) ↔ Carbon Dioxide (CO_2) + Water (H_2O).

Reaction in the Water (including body fluids): Carbon Dioxide (CO_2) + Water (H_2O) ↔ Carbonic Acid (H_2CO_3) and Carbonic Acid (H_2CO_3) ↔ Proton (H^+) + Bicarbonate (HCO_3^-).

Reaction in Water in Oceans: Calcium Carbonate + Carbon Dioxide (CO_2) + Water (H_2O) ↔ Calcium ion (Ca^{2+}) + Bicarbonate (HCO_3^-).

Anaerobic Decomposition: Carbon Dioxide (CO_2) + Hydrogen (H_2) ↔ Methane (CH_4) + Water (H_2O).

Combustion: Methane (CH_4) + Oxygen (O_2) ↔ Carbon Dioxide (CO_2) + Water (H_2O).

Carbon dioxide is transported over long distances across the globe in air by winds and in water with ocean currents, polluting the environment in distant places from its source of origin. The general concerns about greenhouse gases and climate changes are well known, through our ability to model the climate. However, the timing and magnitude of these effects are uncertain. The major greenhouse gases are CO_2 and methane, which together represent 92% of all US greenhouse gas emissions (CO_2 accounts for 82%). There is a clear trend of increasing concentrations of greenhouse gases in the atmosphere. The impact of further increases in concentrations of these gases will lead to ever-increasing warming of the climate, leading to a serious impact on human health and the environment. Many scientists believe that these impacts could include an increase in severe weather events such as hurricanes and floods, sea level rise, and increase in heat waves. These weather changes would trigger an increase in heat strokes, which may cause a migration of tree and plant species, and initiate the penetration of airborne diseases in areas that do not currently experience these. Little attention has also been directed to investigating the possibility that escalating levels of CO_2 may serve as a selection pressure altering the genetic diversity of plant populations.

Exposure and Exposure Monitoring

The major route of exposure to external CO_2 is inhalation and dermal (cornea of eye). However, large quantity of CO_2 is released within the body during aerobic metabolism of carbohydrates to generate energy, and contributes to CO_2 poisoning during hypoxia or anoxia. Physiologically, slightly elevated CO_2 gives sensation of suffocation and dizziness. Numerous air CO_2 monitoring devices with sensitivities of 20–50 ppm are available at a cost ranging from US$100–1000. These devices use nondispersive infrared or chemical sensors.

In hospitals, devices such as, radiometers are used to measure partial pressure of CO_2 in blood. Transcutaneous and nasal air monitoring devices are available to measure CO_2 through the skin and expired air, respectively.

Mechanism of Toxicity

Carbon dioxide is an asphyxiant, means it causes toxicity by displacing oxygen from the breathing atmosphere primarily in enclosed spaces or in open spaces due to sudden release of massive amounts of CO_2 (for example, forests fire or natural emission during a volcanic eruption) and results in hypoxia. The human body produces about 12 000–13 000 mmols per day of CO_2 and is excreted primarily via lungs. The CO_2 concentration in plasma is maintained within a narrow range of 40 ± 5 mm Hg (4.7–6 KPa). At plasma concentration of 22.5 mm Hg (3 KPa) or less death can occur within few minutes. The cause of death in breathing high concentration of CO_2 is due to CO_2 poisoning, that results in rapid decrease in blood pH (respiratory acidosis, $<$pH 7.35), central nervous system (CNS) depression, arrhythmias, and death and not hypoxia.

Low concentrations of CO_2 in the air, or insufficient time for CO_2 in blood to exchange with oxygen (O_2) in air such as in the situations of hyperventilation, can lead to an increase in blood pH (respiratory alkalosis, $>$pH 7.45). The reaction of CO_2 with water in the body is catalyzed by the enzyme carbonic anhydrases (or carbonate dehydratases), which leads to formation of carbonic acid, followed by dissociation into protons (H^+) and bicarbonate (HCO_3^-). Carbonic acid is buffered in the cell primarily by hemoglobin and proteins, which have limited capacity.

Acute and Short-Term Toxicity

Animal

Extremely high concentrations (40%) have resulted in death. At lethal concentrations effects have been seen in the CNS, lungs, liver, kidneys, and the myocardium in rats. Dogs exposed to 50% CO_2 for 90 min or 80% for several minutes died from respiratory or cardiac failure.

Human

Carbon dioxide is a simple asphyxiant that displaces oxygen from the breathing atmosphere resulting in hypoxia. Four stages have been described (depending on the arterial oxygen saturation): (1) indifferent stage, 90% oxygen saturation; (2) compensatory stage, 82–90% oxygen saturation; (3) disturbance stage, 64–82% oxygen saturation; and (4) critical stage, 60–70% oxygen saturation or less.

Following exposure to asphyxiants, cardiovascular effects like tachycardia, arrhythmias, and ischemia are common. Carbon dioxide exerts a direct toxic effect to the heart, resulting in diminished contractile force. It is also a vasodilator and the most potent cerebrovascular dilator known. Respiratory effects like hyperventilation, cyanosis, and pulmonary edema are also not uncommon. Various neurologic effects like dizziness, headaches, sleepiness, and mental confusion can occur. Prolonged hypoxia may result in unconsciousness; seizures may be seen during serious cases of asphyxia. Gastrointestinal effects, like nausea and vomiting, may occur, but usually resolve within 24–48 h following termination of exposure. Decreased vision and increased intraocular pressure may be seen with inhalation of 10% CO_2. Combined respiratory and metabolic acidosis was seen in a serious exposure to dry ice. The Lake Nyos disaster in West Africa during August 1986 has been postulated to have resulted from the release of CO_2 from rising cold deepwater producing a deadly cloud of gas killing humans and livestock, alike. Cough, headache, fever, malaise, limb swelling, and unconsciousness were noted in the victims. Inhalation of CO_2 is teratogenic and has caused both male and female adverse reproductive effects in rodents. Increased fetal movements have been noted in humans following inhalation with 5% CO_2 in air. Carbon dioxide build up and resulting acidosis is considered to be involved in corneal complications such as ulcerative keratitis, neovascularization, epithelial microcysts, and endothelial polymegathism of eye in people using extended wear contact lenses for prolonged periods.

The lowest lethal concentration (inhalation) for humans is 100 000 ppm for 1 min. Carbon dioxide concentrations of 20–30% can cause convulsions and coma within a minute. Unconsciousness may occur when inhaling a concentration of 12% for 8–23 min. Inhalation of 6–10% causes dyspnea, headache, dizziness, sweating, and restlessness. Submarine personnel exposed continuously at 30 000 ppm CO_2 were only slightly affected, provided oxygen content of the air was maintained at normal concentrations (minimal content 18% by volume); when the oxygen content was reduced to 15–17%, the crew complained of ill effects. Signs of intoxication were produced by a 30 min exposure at 50 000 ppm. Several healthy submarine volunteers when exposed at 1% carbon dioxide for 22 days, serum calcium and urinary output of phosphorus fell progressively throughout the exposure period, indicating onset of mild metabolic stress.

Chronic Toxicity

Animal

Changes in body weight, nutrient metabolism, adrenal cortical activity, and blood chemistry were observed in guinea pigs following inhalation of 1.5% for up to 91 days. Rats on chronic exposure have had reversible tissue changes in the CNS, lungs, liver, kidneys, and muscle tissue of the heart.

Human

Carbon dioxide is an important component of the body and is not expected to have a chronic toxicity. However, long-term exposures to levels as low as 0.5–1%, while being generally well tolerated, can alter the acid–base and calcium–phosphorus balance resulting in metabolic acidosis and increased calcium deposits in soft tissues. Long-term exposures in the range of 1–2% can stress the adrenal cortex because of constant respiratory stimuli and this level of exposure is considered dangerous after several hours. Exposure to 2% for several hours produces headache, breathing difficulty, and exertion with deepened respiration. Fatalities have occurred with prolonged exposure to 15–30% CO_2.

Immunotoxicity

In aqueous media, the CO_2 reacts with both the reactive oxygen and nitrogen species. This reaction is protective and reduces oxidative damage. However, in biological membranes CO_2 contributes to nitration of protein and oxidative damage. Hence, CO_2 stimulates and suppresses functions of immune system. The ambient pCO_2 modulates oxidant generation and interleukin-8 secretion in neutrophils.

Genotoxicity and Carcinogenicity

Carbon dioxide is not genotoxic or carcinogenic.

Clinical Management

Victims should be moved immediately from the toxic atmosphere and receive 100% humidified supplemental oxygen with assisted ventilation as required. Patients with severe or prolonged exposure should be carefully evaluated for neurologic sequel and provided with supportive treatment. Seizures may be controlled by administration of diazepam. If seizures cannot be controlled with diazepam or recur, phenytoin or phenobarbital should be administered. Rewarming has been indicated for frostbite. On ocular exposure, the eyes should be thoroughly rinsed for at least 15 min.

Exposure Standards and Guidelines

The American Conference of Governmental Industrial Hygienists (ACGIH) threshold limit value – time-weighted average (TLV – TWA) is 5000 ppm and the ACGIH short-term exposure limit (STEL) is 30 000 ppm; the Occupational Safety and Health Administration (OSHA) permissible exposure limit (PEL) – TWA is 500 ppm (transitional limit) and 10 000 ppm (final rule limit), and the OSHA PEL – STEL is 30 000 ppm; the National Institute for Occupational Safety and Health recommended exposure limit is 10 000 ppm (TWA). Currently, there has been a debate on the 'social cost of carbon emissions,' which includes CO_2. A significant effort is being made to rationalize the risks and benefits of reducing carbon in the atmosphere based on 'the best available science.' It is believed that this effort may contribute to minimizing chronic toxic effects of CO_2, among other components of carbon.

Ecotoxicology

The concentration of CO_2 has been increasing in the air, from preindustrial concentration of 0.028 to 0.035% in 1995 and recently in May 2013 registered at 0.040%. The increased CO_2 in air is leading to change in the pH of fresh and marine water. This is altering the soluble mineral contents and impacting the nutrient imbalance. Coral reefs have been found to be damaged by change in water pH, because the carbonic acid in water dissolves calcium carbonate backbones of the coral reef. The increased CO_2 in the atmosphere is causing weather changes, which would trigger an increase in heat strokes, which may cause a migration of tree and plant species, and initiate the penetration of airborne diseases in areas that do not currently experience these. Little attention has also been directed to investigating the possibility that escalating levels of CO_2 may serve as a selection pressure altering the genetic diversity of the global flora and fauna.

Miscellaneous

Carbon dioxide is a colorless and odorless gas. It has a molecular weight of 44.01 and specific gravity of 1.52 normal temperature and pressure relative to air. Certain reactive metals, hydrides, moist cesium monoxide, lithium acetylene diammino can ignite in the presence of CO_2. Additionally, mixtures of peroxides of sodium, aluminum, and magnesium upon exposure to CO_2 may explode.

Further Reading

Bonanno, J.A., Polse, K.A., 1987. Corneal acidosis during contact lens wear: effects of hypoxia and CO_2. Invest. Ophthalmol. Vis. Sci. 29, 1514–1520.

Briffa, M., de la Haye, K., Munday, P.L., 2012. High CO_2 and marine animal behaviour: potential mechanisms and ecological consequences. Mar. Pollut. Bull. 64 (8), 1519–1528.

Briva, A., Lecuona, E., Sznajder, J.I., 2010. Permissive and non-permissive hypercapnia: mechanisms of action and consequences of high carbon dioxide levels. Arch. Bronconeumol. 46, 378–382.

Chen, X., Gallar, J., Pozo, M.A., Baeza, M., Belmonte, C., 1995. CO_2 stimulation of the cornea: a comparison between human sensation and nerve activity in polymodal nociceptive afferents of the cat. Eur. J. Neurosci. 7, 1154–1163.

Colasanti, A., Esquivel, G., Schruers, K.J., Griez, E.J., 2012. On the psychotropic effects of carbon dioxide. Curr. Pharm. Des. 18 (35), 5627–5637.

Garner, M., Attwood, A., Baldwin, D.S., Munafò, M.R., 2012. Inhalation of 7.5% carbon dioxide increases alerting and orienting attention network function. Psychopharmacology (Berl) 223 (1), 67–73.

Guais, A., Brand, G., Jacquot, L., et al., 2011. Toxicity of carbon dioxide: a review. Chem. Res. Toxicol. 24 (12), 2061–2070.

Koch, A.E., Koch, I., Kowalski, J., et al., 2013. Physical exercise might influence the risk of oxygen-induced acute neurotoxicity. Undersea Hyperb. Med. 40 (2), 155–163.

Kohut, R., 2003. The long-term effects of carbon dioxide on natural systems: issues and research needs. Environ. Int. 29, 171–180.

Rupp, W.R., Thierauf, A., Nadjem, H., Vogt, S., 2013. Suicide by carbon dioxide. Forensic Sci. Int. http://dx.doi.org/10.1016/j.forsciint.2013.05.013 pii: S0379-0738(13)00283-1. (Epub ahead of print).

Varlet, V., Smith, F., de Froidmont, S., et al., 2013. Innovative method for carbon dioxide determination in human postmortem cardiac gas samples using headspace-gas chromatography-mass spectrometry and stable labeled isotope as internal standard. Anal. Chim. Acta 784, 42–46.

Ziska, L.H., Bunce, J.A., Shimono, H., et al., 2012. Food security and climate change: on the potential to adapt global crop production by active selection to rising atmospheric carbon dioxide. Proc. Biol. Sci. 279 (1745), 4097–4105.

Zwiers, F.W., Weaver, A.J., 2000. Climate change: the causes of 20th century warming. Science 290, 2081–2083.

Relevant Websites

http://www.cdc.gov/niosh/idlh/124389.html – Centers for Disease Control and Prevention: NIOSH Publications and Products. Documentation for Immediately Dangerous To Life or Health Concentrations (IDLHs): Carbon Dioxide.

http://toxnet.nlm.nih.gov/cgi-bin/sis/htmlgen?HSDB – National Library of Medicine, TOXNET, Hazardous Substance Data Bank, Search term 'Carbon Dioxide'.

http://online.wsj.com/article/SB10001424127887323566804578551672709633396.html?mod=WSJ_hps_sections_opinion – The "Social Cost of Carbon" Gambit (2013) Review and Outlook, Wall Street Journal, June 27, 2013.

http://hpd.nlm.nih.gov/cgi-bin/household/search?queryx=124-38-9&tbl=TblChemicals&prodcat=all – US DHHS-Household Product database.

Carbon Disulfide

M Abdollahi, Tehran University of Medical Sciences, Tehran, Iran
A Hosseini, Razi Drug Research Center, Tehran University of Medical Sciences, Tehran, Iran

This article is a revision of the previous edition article by Christopher H. Day, volume 1, pp 420–423, © 2005, Elsevier Inc.

- Name: Carbon disulfide
- Chemical Abstracts Service Registry Number: 75-15-0, Other Registry Number: 355120-85-3
- Synonyms: 4-03-00-00395, AI3-08935, BRN 1098293, CCRIS 5570, Carbon bisulfide, Carbon bisulphide, Carbon disulfide, Carbon disulphide, Carbone (sulfure de), Carbonio (solfuro di), Caswell No. 162, Dithiocarbonic anhydride, EINECS 200-843-6, EPA Pesticide Chemical Code 016401, HSDB 52, Kohlendisulfid (schwefelkohlenstoff), Koolstofdisulfide (zwavelkoolstof), NCI-C04591, RCRA waste number P022, Schwefelkohlenstoff, Solfuro di carbonio, Sulfure de carbone, Sulphocarbonic anhydride, Sulphuret of carbon, UN 1131, UNII-S54S8B99E8, Weeviltox, Wegla dwusiarczek.
- Molecular Formula: CS_2
- Structure:

$$S{=}C{=}S$$

Background (Significance/History)

For many years, carbon disulfide was manufactured by the reaction of charcoal with sulfur vapor at temperatures of 750–1000 °C, but by the mid-twentieth century, especially in the United States, the process was superseded by the reaction of natural gas (principally methane) with sulfur.

Uses

The principal industrial uses of carbon disulfide include the manufacturing of cellophane film, viscose rayon, xanthogenates, carbon tetrachloride, and electronic vacuum tubes.

Carbon disulfide is used for fumigation in airtight flat storages, airtight storage warehouses, bins, grain elevators, shipholds, barges, and cereal mills. It is also used as an insecticide for the fumigation of grains, in fresh fruit conservation, nursery stock, and as a soil disinfectant against insects and nematodes. Carbon disulfide is a solvent for selenium, phosphorus, sulfur, iodine, bromine, fats, resins, and rubber. It is also used in the purification of single-walled carbon nanotubes.

Environmental Fate and Behavior

Routes and Pathways Relevant to Its Physicochemical Properties (e.g., Solubility, P_{ow}, and Henry Constant)

Carbon disulfide is a clear, colorless or faintly yellow, mobile liquid at room temperature, and has an 'ether-like' odor. It is highly flammable and volatile. It has a solubility of 2160 mg l^{-1} in water at 25 °C, and is very slightly soluble in water, as well as in alcohol, benzene, ether, chloroform, carbon tetrachloride, and oils. If released to air, an estimated vapor pressure of 359 mmHg at 25 °C indicates that carbon disulfide will exist solely as a vapor in the ambient atmosphere and may potentially volatilize from dry soil surfaces given its vapor pressure. Based on the estimated Henry's law constant of 1.44×10^{-2} atm-m^3 mol^{-1} at 24 °C for carbon disulfide, volatilization is expected to occur from moist soil surfaces and rapidly from water surfaces. Other physical properties include an octanol/water partition coefficient as log P_{ow} of 1.84, a boiling point of 46 °C, and a melting point of −111 °C.

Partition Behavior in Water, Sediment, and Soil

An estimated K_{oc} (soil organic-water partitioning coefficient) value of 1.94 suggests that carbon disulfide is expected to have moderate mobility in soil. Experiments have shown that the rate of adsorption was greater in moist soil, but only when the soil was unsterilized. Further experiments suggest that this 'adsorption' in moist soils can be the result of microbial action. Based on the estimated K_{oc}, if carbon disulfide is released into water, it is not expected to adsorb to suspended solids and sediment in the water column.

Environmental Persistency (Degradation/Speciation)

Vapor-phase carbon disulfide is expected to degrade in the atmosphere by reaction with photochemically produced hydroxyl radicals, and the estimated half-life for this reaction in air is 5.5 days. Carbon disulfide has a weak UV adsorption band at 317 nm, indicating that this substance has a potential for direct photolysis. Photolysis is not intended to be a relevant loss mechanism for the chemical. Carbon disulfide in alkaline solutions hydrolyzes slowly to hydrogen disulfide and carbon dioxide. The half-life for hydrolysis at pH 9 is ~1.1 years, and it is stable in oxygenated seawater for >10 days.

Long-Range Transport

In terrestrial systems, the K_{oc} value of 1.94 suggests that carbon disulfide has moderate mobility in soil.

Bioaccumulation and Biomagnification

An estimated bioconcentration factor (BCF) of <6.1 and <60 for carbon disulfide indicates that bioconcentration in aquatic organisms is low to moderate.

Exposure and Exposure Monitoring

Routes and Pathways (Including Environmental Release)

Carbon disulfide's production and use as a chemical intermediate and a solvent may result in its release to the environment

 http://dx.doi.org/10.1016/B978-0-12-386454-3.00475-9

through various waste streams, but use as an insecticide resulted in its direct release to the environment. Carbon disulfide is a natural product of anaerobic biodegradation and can be released into the atmosphere from landmasses and oceans as well as geothermal sources. Coastal and marshland areas of high biological activity and ocean appear to be major sources of carbon disulfide.

Human Exposure

Human exposure to carbon disulfide is mostly occupational via inhalation and dermal contact with the vapor or dermal contact with the liquid of this compound at workplaces in which carbon disulfide is produced or used. Inhalation is the principal route of carbon disulfide absorption, and workers engaged in any process using carbon disulfide may be exposed to some degree, but only workers in the viscose rayon industry are exposed to high concentrations. For the general population, exposure to carbon disulfide is likely to happen via inhalation of ambient air, ingestion of vegetables and fruits, or other food products containing carbon disulfide.

Environmental Exposure (Monitoring Data in Air, Water, Sediment, Soil, and Biota)

Carbon disulfide has little potential to exert effects in air. Carbon disulfide released into water is expected to volatilize and its rate of biodegradation in water is negligible compared with its rate of volatilization from surface water. Owing to its low affinity for absorption to organic substances, very little carbon disulfide is likely to partition to or remain in sediment. Because of its relatively low log K_{ow} value (2.14) and rapid metabolism in most animals, carbon disulfide is expected to have little or no tendency to bioaccumulate or biomagnify in biota.

Toxicokinetics

Carbon disulfide is extensively and rapidly absorbed via inhalation, oral, and dermal routes and then is distributed throughout the body. Because of carbon disulfide's lipophilic nature, most of its distribution is in organs such as the brain and liver, where it is metabolized to thiocarbamates. Carbon disulfide can reach fetuses through the placenta or babies by way of mother's milk. Carbon disulfide is metabolized by cytochrome P450 to an unstable oxygen intermediate that either hydrolyzes to form atomic sulfur and monothiocarbonate or spontaneously degrades to atomic sulfur and carbonyl sulfide.

Carbonyl sulfide is converted to monothiocarbonate and then degrades to carbonyl sulfide or carbon dioxide and hydrogen sulfide. In humans, unlike animals, oxidation of sulfur to inorganic sulfate is not significant in the metabolism of carbon disulfide. Carbon disulfide combines readily with the amine groups of amino acids to produce dithiocarbamates. Dithiocarbamates are the common metabolites formed in humans and animals that contribute in part to the neurotoxic effects of carbon disulfide. The kidneys are the primary route of excretion of carbon disulfide metabolites. Conjugation of carbonyl sulfide or carbon disulfide with endogenous glutathione results in the formation of 2-oxythiazolidine-4-carboxylic acid and thiozolidine-2-thione 4-carboxylic acid, respectively, which are excreted in the urine. The unmetabolized and unchanged carbon disulfide is excreted in the breath, and small amounts ($<1\%$) may be detected in the urine.

Mechanism of Toxicity

Carbon disulfide reacts with a variety of important nucleophilic compounds in the body (e.g., pyridoxamine, cerebral monoamine oxidases, dopamine carboxylases, amino acids, biogenic amines, and sugars). Acute CNS toxicity and peripheral neurotoxicity caused by carbon disulfide may result from formation of dithiocarbamates. Carbon disulfide may react with macromolecules of enzymes, structural proteins, polypeptides, and nucleic acids. Chelation of zinc- or copper-containing enzymes by carbon disulfide metabolites has been proposed as one of the mechanisms by which carbon disulfide induces neurotoxicity. Carbon disulfide alters the metabolism of vitamin B_6 and nicotinic acid and causes vitamin B deficiency. It is an inhibitor of brain monoamine oxidase that leads to impairment of catecholamine metabolism. Carbon disulfide affects liver enzymes, particularly those related to lipid metabolism, which finally results in higher serum cholesterol. Carbon disulfide also interacts with microsomal drug metabolism through deactivation of cytochrome P450.

Acute and Short-Term Toxicity

Animal

The inhalation LC_{50} for carbon disulfide in rat and mouse is 25 g m^{-3} and 10 g m^{-3} per 2 h, respectively. Liver toxicity was found in animals exposed by inhalation to very high concentrations of carbon disulfide. The oral LD_{50} for carbon disulfide in rat and mouse is 1200 mg kg^{-1} and 2780 mg kg^{-1}, respectively. In rabbits carbon disulfide causes severe irritation to skin and eyes.

Human

Inhalation exposure to very high concentrations of carbon disulfide during an accidental occupational release can cause unconsciousness. Carbon disulfide irritates the skin, eyes, and respiratory tract. Acute pulmonary exposure to this substance results in psychiatric disturbances, central nervous system depression, coma, and respiratory paralysis. Exposure of 200 to 500 ppm may cause death. Acute inhalation exposure to carbon disulfide causes typical symptoms of narcosis, with facial flushing and sometimes a state of euphoria, tremor, and dazed behavior. The postnarcotic effects include headache, nausea, vomiting, tendency to excitability, and spasms. It seems that exposures resulting in deep narcosis can lead to death from respiratory paralysis. Swallowing the liquid may cause aspiration into the lungs and cause chemical pneumonitis. In several studies, ingestion of approximately 18 g of carbon disulfide caused neurological signs, cyanosis, hypothermia, and peripheral vascular collapse, followed by death resulting from central nervous system depression and respiratory paralysis within a few hours.

Chronic Toxicity

Animal

Animal studies have found an association between inhalation chronic exposure to carbon disulfide and toxic effects on the nervous system such as swelling, degeneration, and loss of protecting nerve fibers. Chronic inhalation exposure can affect the liver, blood, and kidneys of animals. No clear evidence of carcinogenicity and genotoxicity has been reported in long-term studies with animals. In experimental animals, carbon disulfide at high concentrations is embryotoxic and fetotoxic, and it is teratogenic at exposure levels toxic to the dam.

Human

Repeated or prolonged contact of carbon disulfide with skin may cause dermatitis. Occupational studies have indicated that chronic exposure to carbon disulfide can cause eye problems such as degeneration of the retina or hemorrhage of blood vessels. Headaches, muscle pain, and general fatigue have been observed in workers chronically exposed to carbon disulfide in the air. Long-term exposure to this substance is toxic to the kidneys and liver, and may also have toxic effects on the cardiovascular and nervous systems, resulting in coronary heart disease and severe neurobehavioral effects, polyneuritis, and psychoses.

Immunotoxicity

There is no evidence on immunotoxicity of carbon disulfide in animals or humans.

Reproductive Toxicity

Developmental effects, including visceral and skeletal malformations, fetal loss (resorptions), embryotoxicity, and behavioral and functional disturbances have been observed in animal studies across a wide inhalation and oral exposure range. Developmental effects may occur at lower doses than all other adverse effects. Carbon disulfide and its metabolites also cross the placenta and localize in the target organs of the fetus (blood, brain, liver, and eyes). Reproductive effects such as menstrual disturbances in women and decreased sperm count and libido in men have been found from occupational settings involving inhalation exposure to carbon disulfide. Therefore, carbon disulfide has been classified in pregnancy risk group B.

Genotoxicity

Genotoxicity studies of carbon disulfide on *Salmonella typhimurium*, *Drosophila*, human fibroblasts, and cultures of human and rat blood leukocytes have been done, but results are not yet conclusive and further investigations are needed.

Carcinogenicity

Available data are inadequate to consider carbon disulfide as a carcinogen. Only a few studies have been conducted on carcinogenicity of carbon disulfide; thus, the US Environmental Protection Agency (EPA) has considered carbon disulfide a Group D carcinogen, meaning 'inadequate evidence to classify as a carcinogen.'

Clinical Management

In inhalation exposure, the patient should be removed from exposure to the contaminated area. In dermal exposure, remove contaminated clothing and wash with copious amounts of water. In eye exposure, irrigate thoroughly with water. Similar to all acute exposures, maintain a clear airway, give oxygen, and assist respiration if necessary. After recent ingestion of carbon disulfide, induction of vomiting is not recommended, but gastric lavage with activated charcoal is fine. There is no specific antidote for carbon disulfide.

Ecotoxicology

Freshwater/Sediment Organism Toxicity

Carbon disulfide has moderate acute toxicity to aquatic organisms, and acute toxicity values range between >1 and $100\ \text{mg l}^{-1}$. LC_{50} values for carbon disulfide in fish are 3.0–$5.8\ \text{mg l}^{-1}$. This material is moderately toxic to *Daphnia magna* and guppies, and slightly toxic to green algae. It is practically nontoxic to mosquitofish and bacteria.

Terrestrial Organism Toxicity (Soil Microorganisms, Plants, Terrestrial Invertebrates, and Terrestrial Vertebrates)

No data are available in the literature for terrestrial organism toxicity. Oral LD_{50} ($3188\ \text{mg kg}^{-1}$) in the rat suggests that carbon disulfide would not be acutely toxic to terrestrial animals except in very high concentrations. Studies in laboratory animals suggest that this material at expected environmental levels would not cause developmental/reproductive effects on terrestrial species.

Other Hazards

Other effects of carbon disulfide include changes in circulating levels of thyroid hormones, gonadotropins, or adrenal and/or testicular hormones and increase in the incidence of diabetes or reduction of glucose tolerance.

Exposure Standards and Guidelines

Based on OSHA standards, the permissible exposure limit: 8-h TWA: 2 ppm; acceptable ceiling concentration: 30 ppm;

acceptable maximum peak above the acceptable ceiling concentration for an 8-h shift, concentration: 100 ppm, maximum duration: 30 min. Threshold limit values: 8-h TWA: 1 ppm, skin. Based on NIOSH recommendations, recommended exposure limit: 10-h TWA: 1 ppm (3 mg m^{-3}), skin; 15 min short-term exposure limit: 10 ppm (30 mg m^{-3}), skin. Immediately dangerous to life or health: 500 ppm. Emergency response planning guidelines (ERPGs) for up to 1-h exposure: ERPG (1) 1 ppm (no more than mild, transient effects); ERPG (2) 50 ppm (without serious, adverse effects); and ERPG (3) 500 ppm (not life threatening).

Miscellaneous

Miscellaneous applications include direct uses of carbon disulfide for the cold vulcanization of rubber, as a flame lubricant in cutting glass, and for generating petroleum catalysts, optical glass, paints, enamels, varnishes, paint removers, tallow, explosives, and so on.

See also: Occupational Toxicology; Toxicity, Acute; Toxicity, Subchronic and Chronic; Neurotoxicity; Organochlorine Insecticides; Volatile Organic Compounds; Solvents.

Further Reading

Gelbke, H.P., Göen, T., Mäurer, M., Sulsky, S.I., April 2005. A review of health effects of carbon disulfide in viscose industry and a proposal for an occupational exposure limit. The Reconsideration of Registrations of Products Containing Carbon Disulfide and their Associated Labels. Australian Pesticides & Veterinary Medicines Authority.

Holleman, A.F., Wiberg, E., 2001. Inorganic Chemistry. Academic Press, San Diego. ISBN 0-12-352651-5.

Rutchik, J.S., 18 Jan. 2002. Organic solvents. Medscape. 27 Oct. 2004. In: Seidman, R.J., et al. (Eds.), eMedicine. http://emedicine.com/neuro/topic285.htm#section~treatment.

Relevant Websites

http://toxnet.nlm.nih.gov – Toxicology Data Network, US National Library of Medicine
http://www.inchem.org – IPCS International Program on Chemical Safety
http://chem.sis.nlm.nih.gov/chemidplus

Carbon Monoxide

CM Stork, Upstate Medical University, Syracuse, NY, USA

This article is a revision of the previous edition article by Christine M. Stork, volume 1, pp 423–425, © 2005, Elsevier Inc.

- Name: Carbon monoxide
- Chemical Abstracts Service Registry Number: 630-08-0
- Synonyms: Carbonic oxide, Carbon oxide
- Molecular Formula: CO
- Chemical Structure: C≡O

Background

Carbon monoxide (CO) is historically known as a deadly gas to humans. Although produced in small amounts in the human body, toxicity occurs predominately after inhalation of preformed CO. Exposure to CO can occur in occupational settings, in tobacco smoke, and in home settings whenever there is incomplete combustion of carbon-containing materials in an unventilated setting.

Uses

CO is used in industries as a feedstock for the production of methanol, acrylates, phosgene, and ethylene. It is also used in metallurgy applications and in industrial fuels. It is also recently being studied in preclinical stages for medicinal use. A major source of CO is the incomplete combustion of carbon-containing materials.

Environmental Fate and Behavior

Routes and Pathways

The physical and chemical properties of CO suggest that its atmospheric removal occurs primarily by reaction with hydroxyl radicals. Atmospheric reactions involving CO can produce ozone in the troposphere. CO emitted into the atmosphere each year is removed by reactions with hydroxyl radicals, by soils, and by diffusion into the stratosphere. There is evidence of long-range transport of CO.

Exposure and Exposure Monitoring

Exposure to this colorless, odorless gas occurs primarily though inhalation. CO exposure associated with the paint stripper methylene chloride is unique in that methylene chloride is biologically metabolized to CO *in vivo*. Dermal, oral, and inhalation exposure to methylene chloride can cause CO poisoning.

Aside from tobacco smoke, the most important sources of CO exposure for most individuals are the emissions created by internal combustion engines of vehicles and in household and occupational locations where combustion occurs. Specific sources of exposure include the burning of wood, charcoal, natural gas, or propane for heating and cooking, and propane-powered indoor equipment such as forklifts and ice rink resurfacers.

Average levels of CO in homes without gas stoves vary from 0.5 to 5 ppm. Levels near properly adjusted gas stoves are often 5–15 ppm, and those near poorly adjusted stoves may be 30 ppm or higher. CO exposures occur in a variety of occupational settings. The number of persons occupationally exposed to CO in the working environment is greater than for any other physical or chemical agent. The smoke of a cigarette contains approximately 14 mg of CO. The smoke of cigars ranges from approximately 38 mg for little cigars to almost 100 mg for large and premium cigars. CO in secondhand tobacco smoke has led to levels of CO as high as 50 ppm.

Global concentrations of CO range from 60 to 140 $\mu g\ m^{-3}$ (50 to 120 ppb). Levels are higher in the Northern Hemisphere than in the Southern Hemisphere. In remote areas of the Southern Hemisphere, background CO concentrations average around 0.05 mg m^{-3} (0.04 ppm), primarily as a result of natural processes. Environmental CO concentrations also fluctuate seasonally. Higher levels occur in the winter than in the summer.

Toxicokinetics

Absorption of inhaled CO occurs in the gas exchange region of the respiratory tract following inhalation. After absorption, methylene chloride is metabolized in the liver to CO. Most CO distributes reversibly to hemoglobin (Hb) in red blood cells; smaller amounts remain in solution or bind to myoglobin and cellular cytochromes. The distribution of the CO molecule by Hb is a function of the alveolar partial pressures of CO and oxygen, and the concentrations of CO and oxygen in blood. CO's affinity for Hb is 200–250 times greater than that of oxygen.

After binding to Hb to displace oxygen and form carboxyhemoglobin (COHb), CO is distributed rapidly throughout the body, where it produces asphyxia. The majority of the body burden exists as COHb, bound to Hb of red blood cells, while 10% is present in extravascular and other sites.

Carbon monoxide is predominately eliminated via the lungs. COHb is completely dissociable from Hb, and is liberated and expired. Higher concentrations of oxygen and hyperbaric oxygen hasten CO excretion. Small amounts are oxidized to carbon dioxide.

Mechanism of Toxicity

CO has varied effects on multiple enzymatic reactions and processes. Most easily seen and measured via co-oximetry is its high affinity and binding to Hb. This results in an overall lack of oxygen carrying capacity along with a shift of the oxygen dissociation curve to the left so that even available oxyhemoglobin is less able to offload oxygen to tissue sites. This,

 http://dx.doi.org/10.1016/B978-0-12-386454-3.00706-5

coupled with CO's ability to bind to and arrest cellular metabolism, results in global hypoxemia. The overall lack of tissue perfusion and energy production results in metabolic lactic acidosis.

CO also has the ability to bind to other globins, most importantly myoglobin. Significant myoglobin binding results in lack of tissue oxygenation to heart and myocardial damage.

The final high-risk organ system affected after CO exposure is the central nervous system. CO has the ability to cause delayed neuropsychiatric sequelae in addition to the acute effects seen as a result of hypoxemia. This is thought to be due to delayed lipid peroxidation achieved through the displacement of nitric oxide. A reperfusion-like injury occurs in these cases.

Acute and Short-Term Toxicity (or Exposure)

Animal

Animals display similar toxicity to humans when exposed to CO. Organ systems with large oxygen demands are affected initially and most profoundly.

Human

The effects of acute exposures to CO are well documented. They result from hypoxic action exerted on the tissues, and among the earliest and most prominent effects are central nervous system disorders, such as headache and lightheadedness. At blood COHb levels approaching 30–40%, dizziness, incoordination, nausea, vomiting, and loss of consciousness may result. At still higher levels (440% blood saturation), cardiovascular collapse, seizures, coma, and death may occur – usually attributed to cardiac dysrhythmias. Some studies have indicated that relatively small increments in COHb levels may produce adverse cardiovascular effects, such as myocardial ischemia. Delayed neurological sequelae most likely involve lesions of the white matter. Severe tissue damage occurring during acute CO poisoning is due to one or more of the following: (1) ischemia resulting from the formation of COHb, (2) inhibition of oxygen release from oxyhemoglobin, (3) inhibition of cellular cytochrome function (e.g., cytochrome oxidases), and (4) metabolic acidosis.

Chronic Toxicity (or Exposure)

Animal

Chronic, low-level CO exposures produce decreased birth weights, cardiomegaly, electrocardiograph changes, and disruptions of cognitive function in several animal models. Rabbits exposed to CO for 11 weeks demonstrated plaque formation in cardiac vessels indistinguishable from those seen from atherosclerotic heart disease.

Human

Humans are exposed to low levels of CO every day from automobile traffic, from smoking, from being close to those who are cooking or heating with natural gas, or through occupational means. Toxicity is dose dependent. At doses that produce COHb concentrations of 10%, no symptoms were evident in studies of humans, even during vigorous exercise. Higher doses produce more pronounced, yet at times latent effects.

Immunotoxicity

Epidemiological studies, animal studies, and *in vitro* studies suggest a potential for CO to exert effects on the immune system.

Reproductive Toxicity

Epidemiologic evidence suggests that humans exposed to even moderate doses of CO during pregnancy have lower birthweight children and have offspring who are at higher risk for sudden infant death syndrome. The absorption and elimination of CO are slower in the fetal circulation than in the maternal circulation. Thus, the fetus may experience toxicity when the mother is at a low CO level with no effects. Fetal deaths have been reported in cases of maternal CO poisoning during pregnancy.

Genotoxicity

There is limited evidence of genotoxicity of CO in bacteria and in rodents.

Carcinogenicity

Carbon monoxide has not been assessed for carcinogenicity using animal models. The International Agency for Research on Cancer, the US National Toxicology Program, and the US Environmental Protection Agency have not classified CO for human carcinogenicity.

Clinical Management

Careful attention to airway, breathing, and circulation is imperative in the treatment of CO-poisoned patients. The victim should be removed from exposure and assisted in breathing as necessary. Methylene chloride should be washed well off the skin and the victim removed from the area to avoid continued absorption. Administration of 100% oxygen using a non-rebreather in any CO-poisoned patient will decrease the half-life of blood COHb from approximately 6 h to less than 100 min.

All patients with significant exposure to CO should receive an early electrocardiogram, and patients complaining of chest pain should have cardiac indices, including troponin and creatinine kinase and the mb fraction measured. Patients older than 36 years having high CO levels or having sustained a significant neurologic insult are at higher risk for delayed neurologic sequelae. The use of hyperbaric oxygen at 2.8 atm should be considered in these patients to hasten elimination of CO and to provide neurologic protection. The potential effectiveness of hyperbaric oxygen therapy declines as the time from exposure termination is extended and is best offered within the first 6 h.

Exposure Standards and Guidelines

The current US Occupational Safety and Health Administration permissible exposure limit for CO is 50 ppm parts of air (55 mg m^{-3}) as an 8 h time-weighted average (TWA) concentration.

The National Institute for Occupational Safety and Health (NIOSH) has established a recommended exposure limit for CO of 35 ppm (40 mg m^{-3}) as an 8 h TWA and 200 ppm (229 mg m^{-3}) as a ceiling. The NIOSH limit is based on the risk of cardiovascular effects.

The American Conference of Governmental Industrial Hygienists (ACGIH) has assigned CO a threshold limit value of 25 ppm (29 mg m^{-3}) as a TWA for a normal 8 h workday and a 40 h workweek. The ACGIH limit is based on the risk of elevated COHb levels.

The World Health Organization has set air quality guidelines for CO based on effects other than cancer of 100 mg m^{-3} (87 ppm) for a 15 min exposure, of 60 mg m^{-3} (52 ppm) for a 30 min exposure, of 30 mg m^{-3} (26 ppm) for a 1 h exposure, and of 10 mg m^{-3} (9 ppm) for an 8 h exposure.

See also: Blood; Combustion Toxicology; Methanol; Phosgene; Carbon Tetrabromide.

Further Reading

Annane, D., Chadda, K., Gajdos, P., et al., 2011. Hyperbaric oxygen therapy for acute domestic carbon monoxide poisoning: two randomized controlled trials. Intensive Care Med. 37, 486–492.

Buckley, N.A., Juurlink, D.N., Isbister, G., et al., 2011. Hyperbaric oxygen for carbon monoxide poisoning. Cochrane Database of Syst. Rev. (4). Art. No.: CD002041.

Thom, S.R., Taber, R.L., Mendiguren II, , 1995. Delayed neuropsychologic sequelae after carbon monoxide poisoning: prevention by treatment with hyperbaric oxygen. Ann. Emerg. Med. 25, 474–480.

Weaver, L.K., 2009. Carbon monoxide poisoning. N. Engl. J. Med. 360, 1217–1225.

Weaver, L.K., 2011. Hyperbaric oxygen in the critically ill. Crit. Care Med. 39, 1784–1791.

Relevant Websites

http://www.epa.gov – An Introduction to Indoor Air Quality (IAQ). Carbon Monoxide (CO).

http://www.inchem.org – Environmental Health Criteria (Number 213) for Carbon Monoxide (Second ed.) (from IPCS INCHEM).

http://www.atsdr.cdc.gov – Toxicological Profile for Carbon Monoxide.

Carbon Tetrabromide

KN Thakore, California Department of Public Health, Richmond, CA, USA

This article is a revision of the previous edition article by Kashyap N. Thakore and Harihara M. Mehendale, volume 1, pp 425–426, © 2005, Elsevier Inc.

- Name: Carbon tetrabromide
- Chemical Abstracts Service Registry Number: 558-13-4
- Synonyms: Carbon bromide; Methane, tetrabromide; Tetrabromomethane
- Molecular Formula: CBr_4
- Chemical Structure:

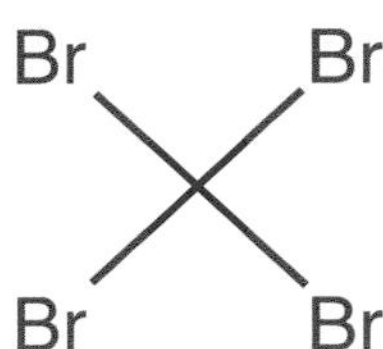

Background

Carbon tetrabromide is considered a highly toxic chemical, may be fatal if inhaled, swallowed, or absorbed through skin. It is metabolized *in vitro* to produce carbon monoxide but the *in vivo* significance has not been established. Under anaerobic reducing conditions it forms complexes with ferrous cytochrome P450. Carbon monoxide is detected as a metabolic product of the interaction. Carbon tetrabromide's production and use in organic syntheses may result in its release to the environment through various waste streams. Carbon tetrabromide has been isolated from red algae, *Asparagopsis toxiformis,* found in the ocean near Hawaii. It was detected in water from treated chlorinated seawater used for drinking at oil platforms. Occupational exposure to carbon tetrabromide may occur through inhalation and dermal contact with this compound at workplaces where it is produced or used. The general population may be exposed to carbon tetrabromide via ingestion of drinking water. Acute exposures to high concentrations may cause upper respiratory tract irritation and injury to lungs, liver (hepatotoxicity) and kidneys (nephrotoxicity). Chronic exposure effects at very low levels will be almost entirely limited to liver injury. It is a potent lachrymator even at low exposure concentrations. Although carbon tetrabromide may release bromine ions during metabolism, clinical bromism is not expected to occur.

Uses

Carbon tetrabromide is used as an industrial solvent.

Environmental Fate and Behavior

Carbon tetrabromide is a colorless nonflammable solid at room temperature. It is insoluble in water, but soluble in several organic solvents such as alcohol, ether, and chloroform. Its specific gravity is 3.42, melting point is 90 °C, boiling point is 189 °C, and vapor pressure is 0.72 torr at 25 °C. Production and use of carbon tetrabromide may result in its release in the environment through various hazardous waste streams. Carbon tetrabromide is expected to have very high mobility in soil and volatilizes slowly from dry soil surface. Its biodegradation is expected to be slow and to exist solely as a vapor in the ambient atmosphere. It is not expected to adsorb to suspended solids and sediment in the water column. Its potential for bioconcentration in aquatic organisms is moderate.

Exposure and Exposure Monitoring

Exposure to carbon tetrabromide occurs primarily through dermal, inhalation, and oral routes.

Toxicokinetics

Carbon tetrabromide is metabolized by rat liver microsomes to electrophilic and potentially toxic metabolites, which cause primary effects on the kidneys. The electrophilic bromine derivatives formed can be excreted as such in urine.

Mechanism of Toxicity

Carbon tetrabromide inhibits protein synthesis and causes lipid peroxidation, both of which may be involved in cell injury or death mediated by free radicals.

Acute and Short-Term Toxicity

Animal

Exposure to carbon tetrabromide through dermal and oral route is toxic. It causes kidney toxicity and is narcotic at high concentrations. In mouse, the subcutaneous and intravenous LD_{50} values are 298 and 56 mg kg^{-1}, respectively.

Human

Exposure to carbon tetrabromide through inhalation, ingestion, and dermal routes is harmful to health. It causes irritation to eyes, skin, mucous membranes, and the upper respiratory tract.

Chronic Toxicity

No data are available to assess the mutagenic, carcinogenic, and teratogenic potential of this agent.

Clinical Management

In case of contact, eyes and skin should be flushed with water for 15–20 min. If inhaled, the victim should be removed to fresh air and oxygen and artificial respiration should be administered, if necessary. If the patient is in cardiac arrest, cardiopulmonary resuscitation should be performed. These life support measures should be continued until medical assistance has arrived. An unconscious or convulsing person should not be given liquids or induced to vomit.

Other Hazards

When heated to decompose, carbon tetrabromide emits toxic fumes of Br^-. It is not flammable, but has hazardous reactivity, when mixed with metals like lithium.

Exposure Standards and Guidelines

Engineering controls, standard work practices, and personal protective equipment, including respirators are employed to prevent workers' exposure to carbon tetrabromide. After use, the clothing and equipment should be placed in an impervious container for decontamination or disposal. The American Conference of Governmental Industrial Hygienists threshold limit value for carbon tetrabromide is 0.1 ppm. National Institute for Occupational Safety and Health Recommendations are as follows:

1. Recommended exposure limit: 10 h time-weighted avg: 0.1 ppm (1.4 mg m^{-3}).
2. Recommended exposure limit: 15 min short-term exposure limit: 0.3 ppm (4 mg m^{-3}).

See also: Methyl Bromide; Neurotoxicity; Bromine; Bromoform; Bromotrichloromethane; Volatile Organic Compounds; Solvents.

Further Reading

Agarwal, A.K., Berndt, W.O., Mehendale, H.M., 1983. Possible nephrotoxic effect of carbon tetrabromide and its interaction with chlordecone. Toxicol. Lett. 17 (1–2), 57–62.

American Conference of Governmental Industrial Hygienists (ACGIH), 2011. Carbon tetrabromide. In: ACGIH (Ed.), ACGIH Threshold Limit Values and Biological Exposure Indices, seventh ed. ACGIH, Cincinnati, OH, pp. 1–2.

Fraga, C.G., Leibovitz, B.E., Tappel, A.L., 1987. Halogenated compounds as inducers of lipid peroxidation in tissue slices. Free Radic. Biol. Med. 3 (2), 119–123.

Gangolli, S., 2007. Carbon tetrabromide. In: Gangolli, S. (Ed.), The Dictionary of Substances and Their Effects, second ed., vol. 2. Royal Society of Chemistry, Cambridge, UK, pp. 136–137.

Lenga, R.E., 1988. Carbon tetrabromide. In: Lenga, R.E. (Ed.), The Sigma Aldrich Library of Chemical Safety Data, second ed., vol. 1. Aldrich Chemical Co, Milwaukee, WI, p. 686.

Lewis, R.J., 2012. Carbon tetrabromide. In: Lewis, R.J. (Ed.), Sax's Dangerous Properties of Industrial Materials, twelth ed. vol. 2. John Wiley & Sons, Inc, New York, pp. 872–873.

Reid, J.B., Muianga, C.V., 2012. Halogenated One-Carbon Compounds. In: Bingham, E., Cohrssen, B. (Eds.), Patty's Toxicology, sixth ed. vol. 3. John Wiley & Sons, Inc, New York, pp. 47–49.

Salehzadeh, O., Watkins, S.P., 2011. Effect of carbon tetrabromide on the morphology of GaAs nanowires. Nanotechnology 22 (16), 165603.

Relevant Websites

http://www.cdc.gov/niosh/ – Carbon Tetrabromide.

http://scorecard.goodguide.com/ – Carbon Tetrabromide.

http://toxnet.nlm.nih.gov/cgi-bin/sis/search/a?dbs+hsdb:@term+@DOCNO+2032 – Carbon Tetrabromide.

http://pubchem.ncbi.nlm.nih.gov/summary/summary.cgi?sid=162548087#x332 – PubChem.

Carbon Tetrachloride

E del Río, L Rojo, and E Vilanova, Universidad Miguel Hernández de Elche, Elche, Spain

This article is a revision of the previous edition article by Thomas R. Parker, Robert Howd and Heriberto Robles, volume 1, pp 426–428, © 2005, Elsevier Inc.

- Name: Carbon tetrachloride
- Chemical Abstracts Service Registry Number: 56-23-5
- Synonyms: Methane tetrachloride, Carbon tetrachloride, Carbon chloride, Benzinoform, Carbona
- Molecular Formula: CCl_4
- Chemical Structure:

Cl
Cl—C—Cl
Cl

Background

Carbon tetrachloride is a manufactured chemical and does not occur naturally in the environment. It is produced by chlorination of a variety of low molecular weight hydrocarbons such as carbon disulfide, methane, ethane, propane, or ethylene dichloride and also by thermal chlorination of methyl chloride. Carbon tetrachloride is a precursor for chlorofluorocarbon (CFC) gases that have been used as aerosol propellant. A decrease in this use is occurring due to the agreement reached in the Montreal Protocol for the reduction of environmental concentrations of ozone-depleting chemicals, including carbon tetrachloride. Carbon tetrachloride classification according to the Globally Harmonized System of Classification and Labeling of Chemicals (CLP/GHS) is shown in **Table 1**.

Uses

The main use of carbon tetrachloride has been in CFCs production. However, since the mid-1970s this use started to decrease in order to reduce the harm that many refrigerant fluids and aerosol propellants produce on the ozone layer. It has been used as a solvent for fats, oils, waxes, lacquers, and resins, as a fire extinguisher, as a degreasing agent in industry and dry cleaning establishments, and as a spot remover in household. Until 1986, carbon tetrachloride was used as a pesticide to eliminate insects in grain. Carbon tetrachloride has been used in medicine: administered orally for the treatment of intestinal worms and as an anesthetic. Currently, due to its toxic effects the uses are limited to as solvent and intermediate chemical under controlled conditions and for laboratory and analytical uses.

Environmental Fate and Behavior

Routes and Pathways

Most of the carbon tetrachloride produced is released to the atmosphere. In the atmosphere, photodegradation by shorter wavelength ultraviolet radiation appears to be the primary removal process although it is very stable in the environment remaining in the air for several years before breaking down, so a significant global transport is expected. The estimated half-life of atmospheric carbon tetrachloride is 30–100 years. Small amounts can be released to the water but due to the relatively high rate of volatilization from water, carbon tetrachloride tends to evaporate in a short time. It is stable to hydrolysis in water. Most of the amount released to soil evaporates rapidly due to its high vapor pressure but a small proportion could remain associated to the soil organic matter. Carbon tetrachloride is mobile in most soils depending on the organic carbon content and can reach groundwater where it remains for long periods before it is broken down to other chemicals.

Relevant Physicochemical Properties

Carbon tetrachloride is a colorless, clear, and heavy liquid (density = 1.5940) with sweetish and aromatic odor. It is

Table 1 Carbon tetrachloride classification according to the globally harmonized system of classification and labeling of chemicals

Hazard class and category code(s)	*Hazard statement code(s) and meaning*	*Pictogram signal word code(s)*
Acute toxicity 3	H331 toxic if inhaled	GHS08
Acute toxicity 3	H311 toxic in contact with skin	Dgr
Acute toxicity 3	H301 toxic if swallowed	
Carc. 2	H351 suspected of causing cancer	GHS06
STOT RE 1	H372 causes damage to organs through prolonged or repeated exposure	
Aquatic chronic 3	H412 harmful to aquatic life with long lasting effects	
Ozone	EUH059 hazardous to the ozone layer	

Source: ESIS. Annex VI. Table 3.1 in "Regulation (EC) No 1272/2008 of the European Parliament and of the Council of 16 December 2008 on classification, labelling and packaging of substances and mixtures, amending and repealing Directives 67/548/EEC and 1999/45/EC, and amending Regulation (EC) No 1907/2006 (Text with EEA relevance)," Official Journal of the European Union, L 353/, 31.12.2008. Available in http://eur-lex.europa.eu/Notice.do?val=486098:cs&lang=en&list=485811:cs,486098:cs,485673:cs,496044:cs,601402:cs,&pos=2&page=4&nbl=35&pgs=10&hwords (accesses 15 November 2013).

Table 2 Physical properties of carbon tetrachloride

Physical property	*Value*	*Units*
Melting point	−2.30E + 01	°C
Boiling point	76.8	°C
Log P_w (octanol–water)	2.83	
Water solubility at 25 °C	793	mg l^{-1}
Vapor pressure at 25 °C	115	mm Hg
Henry's law constant at 25 °C	0.0276	atm m^3 mol^{-1}
Atmospheric OH rate constant at 25 °C	1.20E − 16	cm^3 (molecule s)$^{-1}$

Source: http://apps.echa.europa.eu/registered/data/dossiers/DISS-9d8c7535-6286-5b49-e044-00144f67d249/DISS-9d8c7535-6286-5b49-e044-00144f67d249_DISS-9d8c7535-6286-5b49-e044-00144f67d249.html.

ethereal and somewhat resembles that of chloroform. It evaporates readily. It is nonflammable. The chemical structure is a tetrahedron with bond angles of 109.50°. Some physicochemical properties are summarized in **Table 2**.

Exposure and Exposure Monitoring

Routes and Pathways (Including Environmental Release)

Exposure could happen by breathing carbon tetrachloride present in the air, eating or drinking contaminated water, or by skin contact with contaminated soil. Damage from exposure may be influenced by many factors such as the dose, duration, exposure pathway, other chemicals exposure, age, sex, diet, family traits, lifestyle, and health state.

Human Exposure

Although carbon tetrachloride is mainly for laboratory and analytical uses, it could be released to the environment.

Carbon tetrachloride is relatively stable; contributing to its accumulation in the atmosphere and the groundwater, so the general population is exposed to background levels. Exposure to concentrations higher than the 'background' levels is restricted to occur near point sources such as industries that produce or use carbon tetrachloride or waste contaminated sites. For the general population, the main routes of exposure are the inhalation of contaminated air or volatilization of contaminated water during showering or bathing and the ingestion of contaminated drinking water, being skin contact with contaminated soil a minor route of exposure. The average daily intake of carbon tetrachloride for the general population is estimated to be 0.1 μg per kg of body weight. The estimated average daily amount that the general population may drink in water is 0.01 μg per kg of body weight.

Environmental Exposure (Monitoring Data in Air, Water, Sediment, Soil, and Biota)

Background levels of carbon tetrachloride found in air, water, and soil are represented in **Table 3**.

Toxicokinetics

Carbon tetrachloride is rapidly absorbed through the gastrointestinal and respiratory tract and the skin. After absorption, CCl_4 is distributed to different organs or tissues, especially those with high lipid concentration as liver, kidney, lung, brain, spinal cord, fat, heart, muscle, adrenals, blood, and spleen. Animal studies reflect that maximal tissue concentrations are achieved faster by oral exposure than by inhalation. Indeed, independent of the exposure route the maximal tissue concentration is reached slower in fat than in other tissues and apart from fat it is similarly distributed in all tissues except in liver where the maximal levels are higher and reached more quickly. It is metabolized primarily by the liver, but also by other organs containing CYP450 enzymes as the kidney and lung. Firstly, carbon tetrachloride is metabolized by CYP450 to chloride ion and a biologically active trichloromethyl radical. This radical can then suffer dimerization to hexachloroethane, reduction to chloroform, or bind to cellular macromolecules. An alternative metabolic pathway produces carbon monoxide and, via phosgene formation, carbon dioxide. Carbon tetrachloride is quickly excreted; the unmetabolized compound and the volatile metabolites are excreted in exhaled air whereas the nonvolatile metabolites are eliminated in feces and in small amounts, in urine.

Acute and Short-Term Toxicity (Animal/Human)

The acute effects of carbon tetrachloride in humans as a result of oral or inhalation exposure are similar. Some reported effects are gastrointestinal toxicity (nausea, vomiting, diarrhea, and abdominal pain), neurotoxicity (drowsiness, headache, dizziness, coma, or seizures), hepatic effects (liver enlargement, elevations in alanine aminotransferase or aspartate aminotransferase and bilirubin levels, liver granular degeneration), renal effects (oliguria and increases in blood urea nitrogen), and pulmonary lesions (lung congestion, edema, bronchopneumonia, and alveolar epithelial proliferation) as

Table 3 Background levels of carbon tetrachloride in air, water, and soil

Environment	*Value*
Air	0.1 ppb
Air cities	0.2–0.6 ppb
Drinking water supplies	<0.5 ppb
Water or soil of the waste sites	50–1000 ppb

Source: ATSDR, 2005. Toxicological Profile for Carbon Tetrachloride. Available in http://www.atsdr.cdc.gov/toxprofiles/tp.asp?id=196&tid=35.

a secondary effect of renal failure. Only one case of carbon tetrachloride dermal exposure in humans has been reported and the acute health effects reported are polyneuritis (weakness, pain in the limbs, and loss or reduction of some reflexes) and weight loss.

Acute toxicity studies in animals subjected to oral exposure show liver toxicity as the primary target; renal damage also appears but higher doses are needed. Indeed, effects in the lungs have also been observed. However, acute effects in animals to inhalation exposure suggest the central nervous system and the liver as the primary targets; main acute effects in short-term exposures appear to be hepatotoxicity and to a lesser extent nephrotoxicity. In addition, comparative studies in animals of liver toxicity caused by oral or inhalation exposure show worse effects in oral exposure.

Carbon tetrachloride is classified for acute toxicity category 3 for inhalation, dermal, and oral exposure according to the Global Harmonized System (**Table 1**).

Chronic Toxicity (Animal/Human)

The liver is the major target organ in both humans and animals exposed orally or by inhalation. Hepatic carcinogenicity has also been reported in rats and mice exposed orally or by inhalation to carbon tetrachloride. Also, the kidney is a sensitive target organ following inhalation exposure to carbon tetrachloride. Carbon tetrachloride has been classified for repeated toxicity as STOT RE 1 H372 (cause of damage to organs through prolonged or repeated exposure) according to the Global Harmonized System (**Table 1**).

Immunotoxicity

Immunological effects of carbon tetrachloride have been evaluated in mice and rats exposed by parenteral, oral, and inhalation routes. The toxic effects of carbon tetrachloride are generally attributed to reactive products of metabolism. The first step of carbon tetrachloride metabolism results in the production of the trichloromethyl radical. In the presence of molecular oxygen, the trichloromethyl radical forms reactive trichloromethyl peroxy radical that can induce lipid peroxidation. The immunological effects were secondary to hepatotoxicity and the process of hepatic repair. Just like observed after administration of other hepatotoxic chemicals, the regenerative process includes hepatic synthesis acting on liver cells to induce mitosis. Results of available studies indicate that carbon tetrachloride produces adverse effects on T-cell-dependent immunity at doses that are hepatotoxic. Also hepatotrophic factors on peripheral organs, notably on the spleen, were found. Experiments suggest that the immune effects of tetrachloride carbon are the induction of suppression of T-cells function.

Reproductive Toxicity

No human studies on the reproductive toxicity after inhalation, oral, and dermal exposure to carbon tetrachloride have been published. There is evidence of transfer of carbon tetrachloride through breast milk from mother to newborn; however, the real infant exposure levels would be very low. No studies on developmental effects in humans after inhalation exposure to carbon tetrachloride have been published. Studies in animals subjected to repeated inhalation exposure to carbon tetrachloride show some reproductive effects like decrease in fertility, testicular degeneration, deposition of ceroid in the ovaries, and increase in testicular weight. The most comprehensive studies of inhalation exposure suggest that developmental effects of carbon tetrachloride occur at concentrations toxic to the mother and at exposure concentrations higher than those associated with liver and kidney toxicity. A study on rats detected both maternal and developmental toxicity at a lowest observed adverse effect level of 334 ppm by inhalation exposure to carbon tetrachloride, where significant reductions in fetal body weight and crown-rump length were observed.

There are no conclusive studies about reproductive toxicity in animals orally exposed to carbon tetrachloride either because the doses received by the experimental animals are unknown or because it is difficult to determine whether the effects are directly caused by carbon tetrachloride or are secondary to maternal toxicity. However, in general, studies of reproductive performance in animals found no evidence of reproductive or maternal effects. Teratogenic effects in rats following maternal oral exposure to carbon tetrachloride have not been reported. Studies of developmental toxicity in animals orally exposed to carbon tetrachloride have showed an increase in prenatal loss but not malformations in the surviving litters with carbon tetrachloride exposure.

Genotoxicity

Carbon tetrachloride has been extensively studied for its genotoxic and mutagenic effects. More than 100 studies *in vivo* on mammalian systems, mammalian cells, or in submammalian systems, such yeast and bacteria, report genotoxicity results. Genotoxic effects have been observed in a consisted and close relationship with cytotoxic, lipid perforation, or oxidative DNA damage. Intragenic or point mutations have been shown to play a determining role in chemical carcinogenesis. There is also some evidence of DNA breakage and fragmentation of treated mice and rats' livers. A change in the expression of specific genes occurs in the target organ. There is no evidence of unscheduled synthesis of DNA in the livers of rats or mice treated with CCl_4 when tested under conditions of significant hepatotoxicity.

Carcinogenicity

The primary targets for carbon tetrachloride toxicity are liver and kidney. In experiments with mice and rats, inductions of hepatomas and hepatocellular carcinomas have been proved. The doses inducing hepatic tumors were higher than those inducing cell toxicity. It is likely that the carcinogenicity is secondary to its hepatotoxic effects.

Carbon tetrachloride is classified by International Agency for Research on Cancer as being possibly carcinogenic to humans (Group 2B): there is sufficient evidence that carbon tetrachloride is carcinogenic in laboratory animals, but inadequate evidence in humans. Carbon tetrachloride has been classified as carcinogen category 2 with hazard statement H351 (suspected of causing cancer) according to the Global Harmonized System (**Table 1**).

Clinical Management

The simplest method to detect levels of carbon tetrachloride in highly exposed populations is the measurement of exhaled air. Tests in other tissues and blood are not routine by applied because of its complexity. Anyway, these tests do not predict future damage or harmful effects and taking into account that the tetrachloride leaves the body quickly are effective only if exposure has occurred in the last days.

In case of accidental exposure or poisoning, the victim should be removed from the contaminated environment and provided with appropriate first-aid measures and medical treatment. Care should be taken to provide fresh and clean air and if necessary, to maintain respiration by giving humidified oxygen through assisted ventilation. Contaminated clothing should be removed and the affected area should be washed with abundant water. Eyes exposed to the liquid should be irrigated with plentiful water for several minutes (if it is possible remove the contact lenses). In case of ingestion, rinse the mouth and drink a couple of glasses of water. Additional treatment will be provided if liver and kidney damage is evident.

Ecotoxicology

The limited available information suggests that carbon tetrachloride has a moderated to low toxicity to aquatic organisms, with acute LC_{50} values in fish and crustaceans in the range of 25–35 mg l^{-1} and chronic no effect concentrations (NOECs) around 1 mg l^{-1}.

Other Hazards

Chemical dangers: on contact with hot surfaces or flames this substance decomposes forming toxic and corrosive fumes (hydrogen chloride ICSC0163, chlorine fumes, phosgene ICSC0126 ICSC0007) and reacts with certain metals such as aluminum, magnesium, and zinc, causing fire and explosion.

Exposure Standards and Guidelines

WHO guideline value for drinking water is 0.004 mg l^{-1}. The guideline value is lower than the range of values associated with upper-bound lifetime excess cancer risk of 10^{-4}, 10^{-5}, and 10^{-6}. Occurrence in concentrations of drinking water is less than 5 μg l^{-1}. Acceptable daily intake value is 1.4 mg kg^{-1} of body weight, based on a no observed adverse effect level of 1 mg kg^{-1} of body weight per day of hepatotoxic effects in a 12-week oral gavage study in rats. Guideline values and guideline derivation are shown in **Table 4**.

Table 4 Exposure standards and guideline values in drinking water is 0.004 mg l^{-1}

Guideline derivation	*Value*
Allocation to water	10% of ADI
Weight	60 kg adult
Consumption	2 l day^{-1}
Limit of detection	0.1–0.3 μg l^{-1} by GCMS

Source: WHO/SDE/WSH/03.04/82. WHO Guidelines for Drinking-Water Quality. Chemical Hazards in Drinking-Water – Carbon Tetrachloride. http://www.who.int/water_sanitation_health/dwq/chemicals/carbontetrachloride/en/.

The main route of exposure in occupational population is the inhalation of contaminated air. Workers of companies producing carbon tetrachloride are those most exposed to higher concentrations of the compound. Employees who do the production, formulation, handling, and application are the population with potential high exposures. Occupational Safety and Health Administration has set a maximum concentration limit in workplace air of 10 ppm for 8-h workday over 40-h workweek. In Europe, the daily exposure levels regulated is 0.1 ppm for the same working conditions. Workers exposed to 20–125 ppm concentrations in air ranging for intermediate durations experience neurological effects. Current regulations restrict the acceptable concentration of carbon tetrachloride in workplace air to 2 ppm, but this is still much higher than commonly encountered in the environment. Other potentially exposed populations are persons living near hazardous waste sites.

See also: Common Mechanism of Toxicity in Pesticides; Aerosols; Volatile Organic Compounds; Ethane; Methane; Propane; The Globally Harmonized System for Classification and Labeling of the GHS; Hazardous Waste; Carbon Disulfide; Ozone; Solvents.

Further Reading

IPCS, 1999. Carbon Tetrachloride. World Health Organization, International Programme on Chemical Safety, Geneva (Environmental Health Criteria 208) http://www.inchem.org/.

Manibusan, M.K., Odin, M., Eastmond, D.A., July–September 2007. Postulated carbon tetrachloride mode of action: a review. J. Environ. Sci. Health C Environ. Carcinog. Ecotoxicol. Rev. 25 (3), 185–209.

WHO, 2003. Carbon Tetrachloride in Drinking-Water. Background Document for Preparation of WHO Guidelines for Drinking-Water Quality. World Health Organization, Geneva. http://www.inchem.org/documents/ehc/ehc/ehc208.htm.

WHO/SDE/WSH/03.04/82. WHO Guidelines for Drinking-Water Quality. Chemical Hazards in Drinking-Water – Carbon Tetrachloride. http://www.who.int/water_sanitation_health/dwq/chemicals/carbontetrachloride/en/.

Relevant Websites

http://www.atsdr.cdc.gov – Agency for Toxic Substances and Disease Registry. Toxicological Profile for Carbon Tetrachloride, March 2010.

http://chem.sis.nlm.nih.gov/chemidplus – ChemIDplus.

http://echa.europa.eu/web/guest/information-on-chemicals/registered-substances – European Chemicals Agency (ECHA): Registered Substances.

http://esis.jrc.ec.europa.eu – European Chemical Substances Information System.

http://www.cdc.gov – NIOSH International Chemical Safety Cards.

http://ehp.niehs.nih.gov – NTP Tenth Report on Carcinogens (12/02).

Carbonyl Sulfide

MP Míguez-Santiyán and F Soler-Rodríguez, Avda. de la Universidad s/n, Cáceres, Spain

This article is a revision of the previous edition article by Amy Merricle, volume 1, pp 428–432, © 2005, Elsevier Inc.

- Name: Carbonyl sulfide
- Chemical Abstracts Service Registry Number: 463-58-1
- Synonyms: Carbon monoxide monosulfide, Carbon oxide sulfide, Carbon oxysulfide, Oxycarbon sulfide
- Molecular Formula: COS
- Chemical Structure:

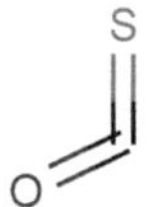

Uses

Carbonyl sulfide (COS) is a colorless, odorless (when pure) relatively stable gas with a boiling point of −50 °C.

There are limited commercial uses of COS. It is produced only in small quantities and used for small-scale experimental purposes and as an intermediate in the synthesis of organic sulfur compounds, thiocarbamate herbicides, and alkyl carbonates. Pesticide manufacturers are believed to be the largest users of COS. Similar to CS_2, research conducted by the Stored Grain Research Laboratory at the Australia's Commonwealth Scientific and Industrial Research Organisation (CSIRO) has shown COS to be an effective soil and grain fumigant for controlling insects on crops such as wheat, barley, oats, and peas, although it is not currently approved for this commercial use.

The use of COS as a fumigant for durable commodities and structures was patented worldwide in 1992 by CSIRO Australia. COS has the potential to replace methyl bromide, being phased out due to its ozone depletion properties, in several of its applications for durable commodities and also to be used as an alternative to phosphine when there is a significant problem with insect resistance.

Commercial sources of COS have been reported to contain significant quantities of H_2S, even where otherwise of high purity (>97.5%). This is an important consideration when interpreting studies that have not specifically reported an analysis of the COS used.

Environmental Fate and Behavior

Most of the releases of COS to the environment are to air, where it is believed to have a long residence time. Its half-life in the atmosphere is estimated to be approximately 2 years. It may be degraded in the atmosphere via a reaction with photochemically produced hydroxyl radicals or oxygen, direct photolysis, and other unknown processes related to the sulfur cycle. Sulfur dioxide, a greenhouse gas, is ultimately produced from these reactions. COS is relatively unreactive in the troposphere, but direct photolysis may occur in the stratosphere. Also, plants and soil microorganisms have been reported to remove COS directly from the atmosphere. Plants are not expected to store COS.

COS is extremely mobile in soils. If released to soil, it will volatilize quickly to the atmosphere ($K_{oc} = 88$). It has a high solubility in water and will not readily adsorb to soil particles, sediment, or suspended organic matter. Therefore, COS is expected to volatilize rapidly from soil and water or, depending on volume, concentration, and site-specific characteristics (e.g., soil type, depth to groundwater, temperature, and humidity), may be able to move rapidly through the ground and impact groundwater. COS may be hydrolyzed in water to form H_2S and CO_2.

COS is also actively taken up by some plants and converted to CS_2; that is, the atmospheric pathways are reversed, and soils may act as both a net source and a net sink for COS depending on the concentration of COS and the characteristics of the soil. COS is therefore accurately described as a naturally occurring and widely distributed chemical found or produced in the air, soils, live and decomposing vegetation, and food.

Exposure and Exposure Monitoring

Exposure occurs predominantly by the inhalation route, as most COS released to the environment is released to the air. Occupational exposure may occur through inhalation or dermal contact during its production and use. The general population is exposed primarily from inhalation to ambient air. An estimated two-thirds of total COS release worldwide is attributed to natural sources. It is released from natural sources such as deciduous and coniferous trees (mainly roots and shoots), oceans, volcanoes, salt marshes, soils, manure, compost, and microorganisms. COS can also be formed in the atmosphere through the chemical reaction of gas-phase CS_2, and photochemically produced hydroxyl radicals. Ambient COS levels have been determined to be about 0.5 ppb.

Industrial sources of atmospheric release include automobile exhaust, coal-fired power plants, biomass combustion, fish processing, combustion of refuse and plastics, petroleum manufacture, and manufacture of synthetic fibers, starch, and rubber. Recent evidence from a study of 350-year-old Antarctic ice cores shows that the atmospheric levels of COS have increased over this time period, which is attributed to human industrial activity.

COS can be discharged to surface waters in the wastewater of viscose rayon plants. Drinking water normally does not contain COS. It is not expected to bioaccumulate in fish or other aquatic organisms; therefore, fish consumption is not considered a relevant route of exposure to this substance.

COS as volatile sulfur compound is a component of food flavors. COS has been identified in cheese, horseradish, and brassica vegetables. Naturally occurring levels of COS in grain,

 http://dx.doi.org/10.1016/B978-0-12-386454-3.00477-2

legumes and oil seeds vary between 0.02 and 1 mg kg^{-1}. Cigarette smoke has been shown to contain COS.

A preliminary study of purgeable organic compounds in breast milk detected COS in one of eight breast milk samples from nursing mothers living in urban centers in Pennsylvania, New Jersey, and Louisiana, suggesting the potential for exposure to breastfed infants. COS has been measured in normal human breath, and disease processes increase the level of COS exhaled.

Toxicokinetics

COS is absorbed primarily in the lungs via the inhalation route, but can also be absorbed through the gastrointestinal tract and through the skin. COS is known to be absorbed into the blood, but transport and distribution are not fully understood. Studies of its metabolism using rat liver microsomes have demonstrated that is a metabolic intermediate in the formation of CO_2. Its metabolism is mediated by the microsomal cytochrome P450 monooxygenase system and is NADPH-dependent. COS is oxidized to atomic sulfur and carbon dioxide. The oxidative metabolism of COS is a potential cause of toxicity due to the formation of highly reactive sulfur atoms. The atomic sulfur liberated in these reactions can be covalently bound to macromolecules or be oxidized to sulfate and excreted in urine. The primary route of COS metabolism in mammals is through carbonic anhydrase, present in the cytosol of cells and in erythrocytes, to monothiocarbamate, which is spontaneously degraded to CO_2 and H_2S, which may be oxidized to sulfate or other still unknown metabolites. Monothiocarbamate can enter the urea cycle, forming thiourea, which is excreted in urine.

Mechanism of Toxicity

Toxicity from exposure to COS is likely the result of its decomposition to CO_2 and H_2S. H_2S inhibits respiration at the cellular level, causing methemoglobinemia, which inhibits the cytochrome oxidase system, causing cytotoxic anoxia. In one study, rats treated with acetazolamide, an inhibitor of carbonic anhydrase, showed lower blood levels of H_2S following exposure to COS and exhibited decreased toxicity. H_2S is believed to be primarily responsible for many of the reported adverse effects associated with exposure to COS.

COS reacts readily with ammonia and primary amines to form ammonium thiocarbamate and amine salts of monothiocarbamic acid, respectively. Reaction with two primary amines may result in the formation of H_2S and linking of the two amines via a carbonyl group reaction, suggesting considerable potential for protein cross-linking by COS *in vivo*, and this has been proposed as a mechanism to explain occupational neuropathy observed with CS_2, and predicted for COS.

Acute and Short-Term Toxicity

Animal

The considerable number of inhalation studies available for COS were all conducted using whole body exposures. The acute inhalational dose–response curve for COS is steep, in terms of both concentration and duration of exposure. Four hour LC_{50} values for rats of approximately 1100 ppm have been reported. Repeated exposure to subacutely toxic doses showed little cumulative toxicity. The LC_{50} in mice appears to be similar to that in rats. Some interspecies variability is seen in the acute inhalational toxicity studies.

Exposure to COS in animals produces serious nervous system effects, with narcotic effects and acute respiratory failure at high concentrations. Rats exposed to COS via inhalation for 4 h showed hypoactivity, lacrimation, breathing difficulties, cyanosis, bleeding from the nose, convulsions, tremors, and behavioral abnormalities such as circling.

In a 2-week inhalation study, results showed COS toxicity for the high dose group (450 ppm), but only after at least 6 days of exposure. A diminished weight in females and signs of central nervous system (CNS) dysfunction (ataxia, head tilting, circling, pivoting, prostrate and arched back postures, tremors, loss of muscle control, convulsions, and bulging and dilated eyes) were observed. Depressed red cell counts, slight depression in mean corpuscular volume, and methemoglobinemia were present in both sexes.

Rats exposed to 200, 300, and 400 ppm of COS for 6 h day^{-1}, 5 days a week, over 12 weeks showed no significant differences in body weight; although reductions in several serum chemistry parameters were noted in exposed males relative to control animals, the effects did not appear exposure related. COS targeted specific neuroanatomical sites in the auditory system, suggesting that decreases in cytochrome oxidase in exposed rats may be involved in the pathogenesis of neuronal injury. These studies demonstrate that this environmental air contaminant has the potential to cause a wide spectrum of brain lesions that are dependent on the degree and duration of exposure.

When Fischer 344 rats were exposed to 0 or 500 ppm COS for 1–10 days, 6 h day^{-1}, important gene expression changes occurring in the posterior colliculi after 1 or 2 days of COS exposure that were predictive of the upregulation of genes associated with DNA damage, apoptosis, and vascular mediators. These gene expression findings could be predictive of later CNS lesions caused by COS exposure.

COS is acutely toxic to rats, with an LD_{50} of 22.5 mg kg^{-1}, i.p.

Human

COS appears to elicit similar symptoms of poisoning as those seen from exposure to H_2S, although it produces less prominent initial warning signs, such as local irritation to the skin, eyes, and respiratory tract. Exposure to COS may cause central and peripheral nervous system damage, damage to the respiratory tract, and ocular effects. COS exposure has also been associated with cardiovascular disease. Breathing high concentrations of COS (greater than 1000 ppm) over a short time period may cause sudden collapse and unconsciousness, convulsions, coma, and fatal central respiratory paralysis. At low to moderately high vapor concentrations, COS can cause burning or redness of the eyes, painful conjunctivitis, photophobia, corneal opacity, headache, nausea, dizziness, confusion, cardiac arrhythmia, and pain and weakness in the extremities. Direct skin contact with COS vapors may produce skin irritation and pain. Prolonged or repeated exposure to the skin may cause dermatitis. Gastrointestinal effects include profuse salivation, nausea, vomiting, and diarrhea. CNS effects include giddiness, headache, vertigo, amnesia, confusion, and unconsciousness. Recovery is eventually complete in most nonfatal cases.

Increased concentration of COS in exhaled breath is an early marker for acute rejection of lung transplants, which involves inflammatory processes associated with the production of reactive oxygen species. Elevated COS levels in exhaled breath are also a marker for liver disease, resulting in hepatocellular injury, but not for bile duct-related diseases, where conversely COS concentrations are markedly reduced. Inflammatory processes or damage to the normal antioxidant mechanisms associated with hepatocellular injury are possible causes for the increased COS production in liver disease. Thus, COS is unquestionably produced endogenously in humans and other mammals as demonstrated by levels in exhaled breath in normal subjects.

The available evidence suggests that COS at sublethal concentrations may be at most a slight eye and respiratory irritant but is unlikely to be a skin irritant.

Chronic Toxicity

Animal

No information was identified on the chronic reproductive, developmental, or carcinogenic effects of COS in animals. However, COS is the oxidation product of S_2C, which has been shown by the US National Institutes of Health to be positive in the strain A mouse lung tumor bioassay. Significant increases in the incidence (tumor-bearing mouse) and frequency (tumors per mouse of lung adenomas) were observed in A/J mice.

Human

Chronic exposure to low concentrations of COS may cause damage or irritation to the respiratory tract, including symptoms of rhinitis, pharyngitis, bronchitis, and pneumonitis, and may cause pulmonary edema, or eye irritation with painful conjunctivitis, photophobia, lacrimation, and corneal opacity. Recovery depends on the length of exposure and the dose. Residual effects during recovery may include coughing, slow pulse, and amnesia.

No information regarding the potential carcinogenicity or the developmental or reproductive toxicity of COS in humans was identified. The US Environmental Protection Agency (EPA) and the International Agency for Research on Cancer have not classified COS with respect to potential carcinogenicity.

COS is neither genotoxic nor a developmental toxicant but does reversibly impair male fertility. Prolonged, repeated exposure to COS is likely to present similar neurotoxicity hazards to that of the structurally and toxicologically related compound CS_2.

Genotoxicity

The US National Toxicology Program found that COS produced a weak positive response in the *Salmonella* mutagenicity test. No further information regarding this test was identified.

Clinical Management

Following inhalation exposure, the victim should be moved to fresh air immediately. If the victim is not breathing, artificial respiration or cardiopulmonary resuscitation should be given, if necessary. If breathing is labored, the victim should be given oxygen. In case of ocular or dermal contact, the skin or eyes should be flushed with running water immediately. Soap and water may be used for washing exposed skin. If COS is accidentally ingested, medical treatment should be sought immediately. Vomiting should not be induced. Further treatment is symptomatic. Rescuers must prevent exposure by wearing a self-contained breathing apparatus to rescue the victim. Acute or chronic respiratory conditions may be aggravated by overexposure to this gas.

Ecotoxicology

COS is not expected to bioaccumulate in fish or other aquatic organisms since an estimated bioconcentration factor of 11 was calculated in fish. The US EPA reported that quantitative structure–activity relationship estimates of acute toxicity for fish, daphnid, and algae are greater than 1000 $mg\,l^{-1}$.

Other Hazards

COS is a flammable gas, and may be explosive or spontaneously flammable in air under the right conditions. Vapors may ignite at distant ignition sources and flash back. When exposed to fire, humidity, or strong alkalis, COS may form the toxic decomposition products CO and H_2S gas. In the presence of strong oxidizers, COS presents a fire or explosion hazard. COS has a vapor density of 2.1 and is therefore heavier than air. Cylinders or tank cars containing COS may rupture violently or rocket under fire conditions.

The National Fire Protection Agency flammable limits are as follows: lower – 12% by volume, upper – 29% by volume, and explosive limits are 12–29%.

Miscellaneous

The Clean Air Act Amendments of 1990 list COS as a hazardous air pollutant generally known or suspected to cause serious health effects. COS is also regulated under the Comprehensive Environmental Response, Compensation, and Liability Act, the Superfund Amendments and Reauthorization Act, and Section 4 of the Toxic Substances Control Act.

See also: Carbon Disulfide; Hydrogen Sulfide; Pollution, Air in Encyclopedia of Toxicology.

Further Reading

Bartholomaeus, A.R., Haritos, V.S., 2005. Review of the toxicology of carbonyl sulfide, a new grain fumigant. Food Chem. Toxicol. 43 (12), 1687–1701.

Chengelis, C.P., Neal, R.A., 1980. Studies of carbonyl sulfide toxicity: metabolism by carbonic anhydrase. Toxicol. Appl. Pharmacol. 55 (1), 198–202.

Monsanto Agricultural Company, 1990. TSCA 8(e) submission. Acute Inhalation Toxicity of Carbon Oxysulfide to Sprague–Dawley Rats, ML-82-213. OTS0540051.

Monsanto Agricultural Company, 1992. TSCA 8(e) submission. Two Week Study of COS Administered by Inhalation to Rats, ML-83-029. OTS0534820.

Morgan, D.L., Little, P.B., Herr, D.W., et al., 2004. Neurotoxicity of carbonyl sulfide in F344 rats following inhalation exposure for up to 12 weeks. Toxicol. Appl. Pharmacol. 200 (2), 131–145.

Morrison, J.P., Ton, T.V., Collins, J.B., et al., 2009. Gene expression studies reveal that DNA damage, vascular perturbation, and inflammation contribute to the pathogenesis of carbonyl sulfide neurotoxicity. Toxicol. Pathol. 37 (4), 502–511.

Sills, R.C., Harry, G.J., Valentine, W.M., Morgan, D.L., 2005. Interdisciplinary neurotoxicity inhalation studies: carbon disulfide and carbonyl sulfide research in F344 rats. Toxicol. Appl. Pharmacol. 207, 245–250.

Wright, E.J., 2003. Carbonyl sulfide (COS) as a fumigant for stored products: progress in research and commercialization. In: Wright, E.J., Webb, M.C., Highley, E. (Eds.), Stored Grain in Australia 2003; Proceedings of the 3rd Australian Postharvest Technical Conference. ACT, CSIRO Entomology, Canberra, pp. 224–229.

Relevant Websites

http://toxnet.nlm.nih.gov – TOXNET, Toxicology Data Network, National Library of Medicine.

http://ofmpub.epa.gov/sor_internet/registry/substreg/home/overview/home.do – U.S. Environmental Protection Agency – Substance Registry System.

http://www.epa.gov/iris/subst/index.html – U.S. Environmental Protection Agency – Integrated Risk Information System (IRIS).

Carboxylesterases

B Yan, University of Rhode Island, Kingston, RI, USA

This article is a revision of the previous edition article by Ramesh C. Gupta, volume 1, pp 432–435, © 2005, Elsevier Inc.

Background

Carboxylesterases (CESs) hydrolyze chemicals containing a functional group such as a carboxylic acid ester, amide, and thioester. In addition to catalyzing hydrolysis, some CESs catalyze synthetic and transesterification reactions. Hydrolysis by CESs has been studied for more than half a century. These enzymes were historically categorized as nonspecific esterases. The nomenclature system has since undergone several major changes. Early classification was based on the substrate specificity. This approach soon became unsatisfactory because these enzymes have broad and overlapping substrate specificities. Classification was later made based on isoelectrophoretic points. This approach, although more definitive in terms of linking to individual CESs, was unsatisfactory because the same CESs may have different isoelectrophoretic points due to protein aggregation or differences in glycosylation. In addition, it is difficult to make a direct connection between the catalytic function (substrate specificity) and a CES based on its isoelectrophoretic point.

Currently, classification of CESs is based on sequence identity of CES proteins. In this system, all mammalian CESs (e.g., human and rodents) are taken into consideration. Members in the same family have a sequence identity of 60% or higher, otherwise, a different family is assigned. According to this method, five families are created: CES1, CES2, CES3, CES4, and CES5. Human CESs use gene symbol CES, whereas rodent CESs use ces as the symbol. Many transcript isoforms of human CESs have been identified due to gene duplications, alternative splicing, and difference in the use of transcription-starting sites. Nevertheless, rodents have many more distinct CES genes than humans. Mice have 20, rats have 15, and humans have only 8. In humans, the CES1 family has three members, commonly referred to as CES1A1, CES1A2, and CES1A3. CES1A2 is an alternative form of CES1A3, thus humans may express CES1A2 or CES1A3 but not both.

Tissue Distribution

CESs are present in a wide range of tissues and cells. However, the expression level varies markedly depending on a CES and also a tissue. Among all organs, the liver expresses the highest level of CESs. Of all cellular organelles, the endoplasmic reticulum contains the most abundant CES activity. High levels of CESs are also present in the gastrointestinal, respiratory, and urinary tracks as well as in the skin. Rodents, compared with humans, have much higher CES activity in the blood. Three human CESs are catalytically characterized including CES1, CES2, and CES3. All of them are highly expressed in the liver. Overall, CES1 has the broadest tissue presence, whereas CES3 has the most restricted tissue expression. CES2 is highly expressed in the intestine and kidney, suggesting that CES2 plays a dominant role in xenobiotic elimination, whereas CES1, probably CES3 as well, is involved in the metabolism of both endo- and xenobiotics.

Regulated Expression

The expression of CESs is affected by many factors such as age, hormones, and xenobiotics. In both humans and rodents, the expression of CESs is developmentally regulated. The levels of CESs are low at birth but rapidly increase during the early period of the postnatal stage. In humans, it appears that the developmental regulation consists of a neonatal surge followed by an incremental increase throughout the entire adolescence. CESs, like many other enzymes, are induced by endogenous factors and xenobiotics. However, the induction is minimal or moderate at the most, presumably due to high levels of basal expression (adults). Phenobarbital, an antiepileptic, induces both rodent and human CESs in primary hepatocytes and/or *in vivo*. Recently, several antioxidants have been shown to induce human CESs in hepatoma cell lines. The induction is achieved largely by transactivation. Multiple transcription factors are implicated to support the induction including the pregnane X receptor, the constitutive androstane receptor, the glucocorticoid receptor, and nuclear factor (erythroid-derived 2)-like 2.

On the other hand, the expression of CESs is suppressed by disease mediators and xenobiotics. Interleukin-6, a proinflammatory cytokine, has been shown to suppress the expression of human CESs. Lipopolysaccharides, potent stimulants of proinflammatory cytokine production, decrease the expression of mouse CESs by as much as 70%. The suppression of CESs has profound cellular consequences. For example, pretreatment with interleukin-6 significantly decreases the hydrolysis of the antiplatelet agent clopidogrel accompanied by marked increases in the cytotoxicity. Some xenobiotics cause opposite effects in the expression between human and rodent CESs. Glucocorticoid dexamethasone, for example, causes moderate induction of human CESs but profoundly suppresses the expression of their rodent cess.

Activators and Inhibitors

Like many other enzyme systems, the activity of CESs can be enhanced or inhibited. While the inhibition has been extensively studied, little information is known on the activation. Several chemicals such as pinacolone and pinacolyl alcohol have been shown to increase the hydrolytic activity of CESs. Enhancement has been observed *in vitro* and *in vivo* with pinacolone and pinacolyl alcohol. These chemicals are metabolites of soman, a potent and irreversible inhibitor of serine enzymes including CESs. The precise mechanism

 http://dx.doi.org/10.1016/B978-0-12-386454-3.00109-3

remains to be elucidated for enhanced hydrolytic activity. Interestingly, the commonly used solvent acetone also enhances hydrolytic activity of CESs, pointing to a possible mechanism of improving the accessibility of enzymes to a substrate.

In contrast to activation, several types of inhibitors are well characterized. Ester compounds hydrolyzed by the same CESs may function as competitive inhibitors toward each other. For example, clopidogrel and oseltamivir are substrates of CES1 with the former being kinetically favorable. As a result, clopidogrel inhibits the hydrolysis of oseltamivir by as much as 90% when the same concentrations are used. The first-pass hydrolysis accounts for 90% of total oseltamivir activation, presumably due to the initial high concentration in the liver. Coadministration of clopidogrel likely inhibits the first-pass activation of oseltamivir.

The second type of inhibition is achieved by chemicals that irreversibly modify the active-site serine residues, the so-called serine enzyme inhibitors. As described below, organophosphorus pesticides are potent inhibitors of CESs. In addition, several irreversible inhibitors of serine enzymes are characterized including phenylmethylsulfonyl fluoride and inorganic salts such as sodium fluoride. While these inhibitors generally act nonspecifically among serine enzymes, the IC_{50} values can vary markedly from one CES to another. For example, rat ces hydrolase A is ~1000 times more sensitive than hydrolase B based on the IC_{50} values (100 nM *vs* 100 μM). Two classes of compounds, with a potential of clinical use, are well characterized for the inhibition of CESs. Benzil derivatives belong to one of the classes and trifluoromethyl ketone–containing analogs belong to the other. These compounds inhibit catalysis of CESs by acting on the active-site serine residue. Although they are called transitional analog inhibitors, the inhibition is reversible. Among trifluoromethyl ketone compounds, thioether analogs are more potent than their sulfinyl or sulfonyl counterparts.

Detoxification of Organophosphorus, Carbamate, and Pyrethroid Pesticides

CESs are established to play critical roles in detoxifying organophosphorus, carbamate, and pyrethroid pesticides. These compounds constitute more than 80% of total insecticides on the global use including agriculture, residential setting, parasite eradication, and public facility. As described below, CESs detoxify these pesticides through distinct mechanisms. These mechanisms likely operate in a manner of addition or synergy toward the metabolic fate of pesticides. As a result, CESs-based detoxification represents a major target for toxicological interactions, particularly between organophosphates and carbamates or pyrethroids.

Detoxification of most organophosphates by CESs is achieved by an inhibition-based scavenging mechanism. Organophosphates induce toxicity largely by targeting serine enzymes, particularly acetylcholinesterase (AChE), a vital enzyme that terminates neurotransmission of acetylcholine. CESs are structurally related to AChE. Importantly, like AChE, CESs use a catalytic triad for hydrolysis and a serine residue acts as the nucleophile in the triad. As a result, CESs interact with organophosphates similarly as AChE. As shown in **Figure 1**, organophosphates contain a leaving group 'X.' Upon interacting with AChE or a CES, this leaving group is displaced by the enzyme through the active-site serine residue, resulting in the formation of phosphorylated enzyme complex. The phosphorylated enzyme can undergo spontaneous reactivation (very slow) or a so-called aging process (permanent inhibition). In support of the role of CESs in the detoxification of organophosphates, CES activity is inversely correlated with the sensitivity to organophosphorus poisons, and intravenous administration of purified CESs affords considerable protection against the toxicity of organophosphorus-type compounds such as soman, sarin, and paraoxon. In addition, repeated low dosing regimens of organophosphates induce tolerance accompanied by increased recovery of CES activity. While AChE is the primary target, particularly during the induction of acute toxicity, organophosphates induce toxicity by targeting other proteins such as the neuropathy target esterase (NTE).

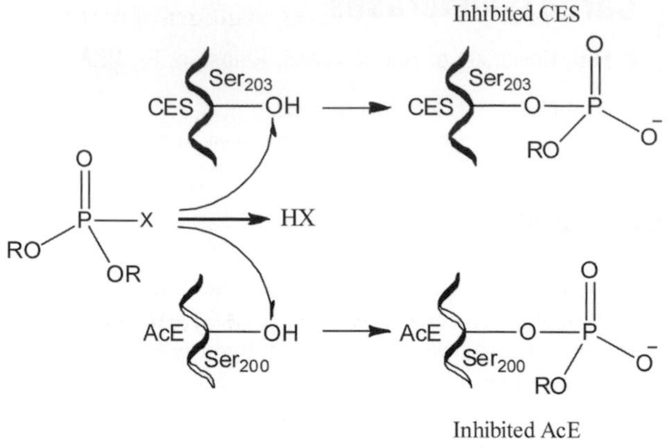

Inhibited CES

Inhibited AcE

Figure 1 Inhibition of CES and AChE by organophosphates.

In addition to the scavenging mechanism, CESs detoxify organophosphorus compounds through the action of hydrolysis as well. For example, malathion is organophosphorothioate and contains a P=S instead of a P=O bond seen in organophosphates (**Figure 2**). Oxidative desulfuration of malathion results in the formation of the corresponding oxon, an organophosphate. On the other hand, malathion contains two carboxylic acid ester bonds, thus undergoes hydrolysis by CESs as well. Hydrolysis of malathion prevents oxidative desulfuration, thus represents detoxification (inactivation). Therefore, the relative activity between desulfuration

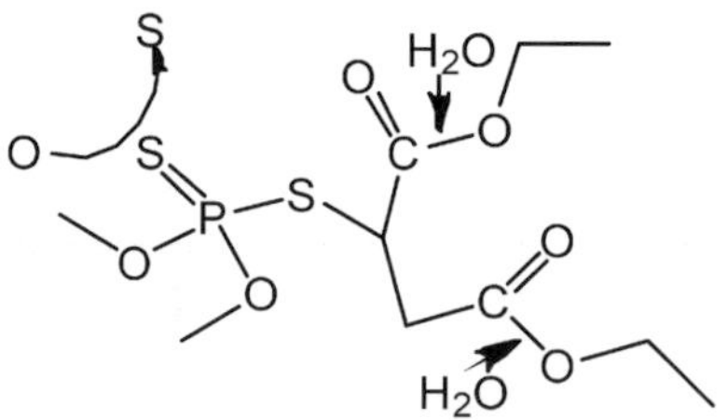

Figure 2 Hydrolytic and desulfuration sites of malathion.

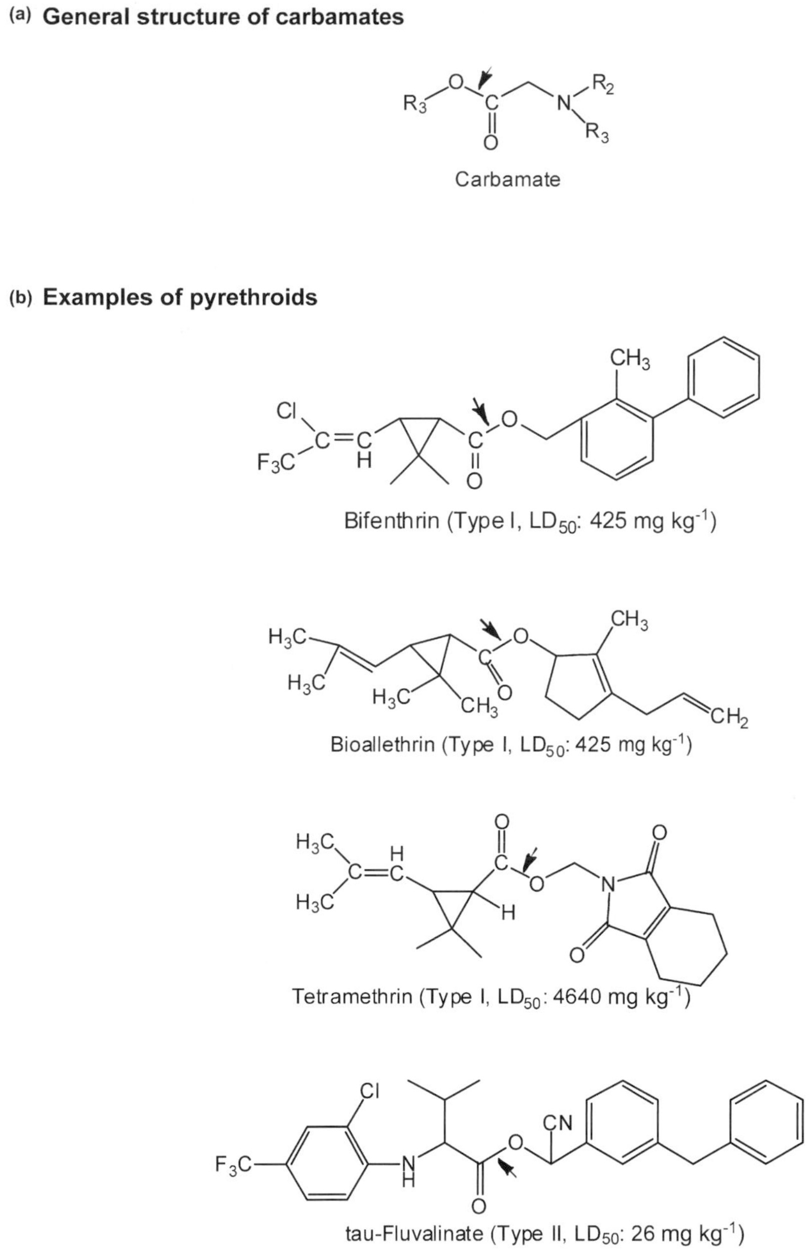

(a) General structure of carbamates

(b) Examples of pyrethroids

Figure 3 (a) General structure of carbamates and (b) examples of pyrethroids.

and hydrolysis is a major toxicological determinant of malathion.

In contrast, CESs detoxify carbamates and pyrethroids primarily through the action of hydrolysis. Both types of pesticides are esters (**Figure 3**), thus substrates of CESs. It is generally accepted that these pesticides are less accumulative in the environment and less toxic to mammalian species. Therefore, they are currently mainstream pesticides. Based on the presence of a cyano moiety (**Figure 3(b)**), pyrethroids are divided into Types I and II. Type I pyrethroids lack a cyano moiety in the α-position, whereas those with the cyano group belong to Type II pyrethroids. Introduction of the cyano moiety drastically increases the insecticidal activity as well as lethal potency in rodents. The magnitude of hydrolysis likely determines the overall toxicity of pyrethroids, particularly the lethal potency. The median lethal dose (LD_{50}) values for these compounds in rats range from 26 mg kg^{-1} (tau-fluvalinate) to 4640 mg kg^{-1} (tetramethrin). Consistent with such a large difference in the LD_{50} values, tetramethrin is hydrolyzed nine times as fast as tau-fluvalinate by human liver microsomes. These findings suggest that these pyrethroids are hydrolyzed comparably in both humans and rats. While the hydrolytic rates are generally correlated with their LD_{50} values, there are notable exceptions. For example, bioallethrin is hydrolyzed eight times as fast as bifenthrin (**Figure 3**), however, bifenthrin is less toxic than bioallethrin based on the LD_{50} values in rats (545 *vs* 425 mg kg^{-1}, **Figure 3(b)**). It is likely that bifenthrin is effectively hydrolyzed by rat cess. Alternatively, other metabolic pathways such as oxidation contribute significantly to the detoxification of bifenthrin in rats. In support of the critical role of CES in detoxifying pyrethroids, neonatal rats express only 10–15% of hepatic CESs of adult rats, and exhibit a 16-fold greater sensitivity to pyrethroid deltamethrin. In addition, the relative insensitivity of adult rats to pyrethroids is attenuated by pretreatment with tri-*o*-tolyl phosphate, an organophosphate with potent inhibitory activity on CESs. Therefore, it is hypothesized that organophosphates synergistically enhance the toxicity of pyrethroids.

Bioactivation through Hydrolytic, Transesterification, and Synthetic Activity

While hydrolysis is generally considered detoxification, in some cases, hydrolysis produces metabolites with increased cytotoxicity. For example, hydrolysis of oseltamivir, an anti-influenza agent, produces oseltamivir carboxylate. This hydrolytic metabolite exerts the antiviral activity but also shows much higher cytotoxic effect. In addition to hydrolysis, transesterification and synthetic activities of certain CESs are associated with the production of toxic intermediators (**Figure 4**). In the presence of ethyl alcohol, cocaine is converted into ethylcocaine by CESs. Likewise, ethyl alcohol is conjugated with fatty acids by CESs to form fatty acid ethyl esters. Both ethylcocaine and fatty acid ethyl esters represent toxic species of ethyl alcohol.

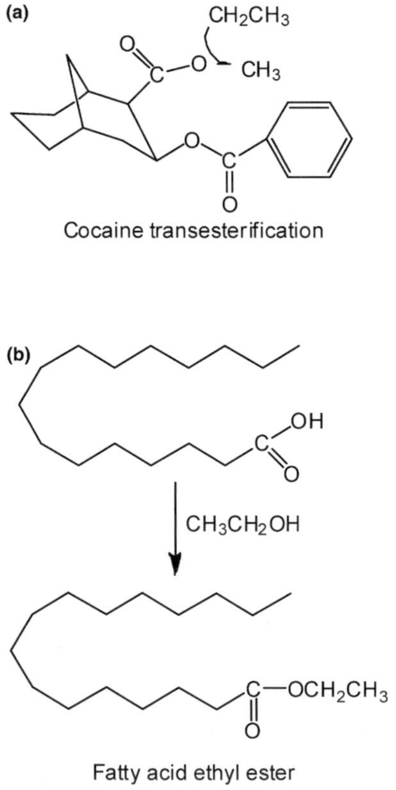

Figure 4 Transesterification of cocaine (a) and fatty acid ethyl ester synthesis in the presence of ethyl alcohol (b).

Comparison between Human and Animal CESs

Human and animal CESs share many similarities. First, humans and animals express multiple forms. Secondly, the highest CES activity is present in liver among these species. Thirdly, the expression of CESs is developmentally regulated. On the other hand, there are notable differences, particularly in tissue distribution, regulation, and species-specific hydrolysis. Rodents but not humans, for example, have high levels of serum CESs. The synthetic glucocorticoid dexamethasone exerts opposing effect on the regulation of several major rat and human CESs. The local anesthetic procaine is hydrolyzed much faster by rat microsomes than their human counterparts. Finally, rodents express twice or even triple the number of CESs as humans. These differences raise concerns regarding the relevance of animal models to human situation.

See also: Biotransformation; Developmental Toxicology; A-esterase; Chlorpyrifos; Cholinesterase Inhibition; Deltamethrin; Malathion; Organophosphorus Compounds; Permethrin; Pesticides; Cytochrome P450; Ethanol; Toxicology; Liver; Sarin (GB); Cocaine; Phthalates.

Further Reading

Anand, S.S., Kim, K.B., Padilla, S., et al., 2006. Ontogeny of hepatic and plasma metabolism of deltamethrin in vitro: role in age-dependent acute neurotoxicity. Drug Metab. Dispos. 34, 389–397.

EPA 2008. http://www.epa.gov/pesticides/reregistration/status_page_r.htm.

Holmes, R., Wright, M., Laulederkind, S., et al., 2010. Recommended nomenclature for five mammalian carboxylesterase gene families: human, mouse and rat genes and proteins. Mamm. Genome 21, 427–441.

Jokanović, M., Kosanović, M., Brkić, D., Vukomanović, P., 2011. Organophosphate induced delayed polyneuropathy in man: an overview. Clin. Neurol. Neurosur. 113, 7–10.

Jokanović, M., Kosanovic, M., Maksimovic, M., 1996. Interaction of organophosphorus compounds with carboxylesterases in the rat. Arch. Toxicol. 70, 444–450.

Satoh, T., Hosakawa, M., 2006. The mammalian carboxylesterases: from molecules to functions. Annu. Rev. Pharmacol. Toxicol. 38, 257–288.

Shi, D., Yang, J., Yang, D., et al., 2006. Anti-influenza prodrug oseltamivir is activated by carboxylesterase HCE1 and the activation is inhibited by anti-platelet agent clopidogrel. J. Pharmacol. Exp. Ther. 319, 1477–1484.

Shi, D., Yang, J., Yang, D., You, L., Yan, B., 2008. Dexamethasone suppresses the expression of multiple rat carboxylesterases through transcriptional repression: evidence for an involvement of the glucocorticoid receptor. Toxicology 254, 97–105.

Shi, D., Yang, D., Prinssen, E.P., Brian, E., Davies, B.E., Yan, B., 2011. Surge in expression of carboxylesterase-1 during the post-natal stage enables a rapid gain of the capacity to activate the anti-influenza prodrug oseltamivir. J. Infect. Dis. 203, 937–942.

Wheelock, C.E., Shan, G., Ottea, J., 2005. Overview of carboxylesterases and their role in the metabolism of insecticides. J. Pestic. Sci. 30, 75–83.

Yang, D., Pearce, R., Wang, X., Gaedigk, R., Wan, Y.J., Yan, B., 2009. Human carboxylesterases HCE1 and HCE2: ontogenic expression, inter-individual variability and differential hydrolysis of oseltamivir, aspirin, deltamethrin and permethrin. Biochem. Pharmacol. 77, 238–247.

Yang, J., Shi, D., Yang, D., Song, X., Yan, B., 2007. Interleukin-6 alters the cellular responsiveness to clopidogrel, irinotecan, and oseltamivir by suppressing the expression of carboxylesterases HCE1 and HCE2. Mol. Pharmacol. 72, 686–694.

Carcinogen Classification Schemes

MA Kamrin

Introduction

Several classification schemes have been developed for ranking the relative hazards to humans associated with chemicals that, by one or more criteria, may be considered to be potential carcinogens. The classification schemes are based on scientific judgments that typically take into account all the data available from *in vivo* animal bioassays, *in vitro* tests for genetic toxicity, human epidemiology, and structural relationships with other known carcinogens. Classification of a chemical as a carcinogen involves the consideration of many different factors. Classification schemes provide guidance on evaluating and weighting the available evidence and placing chemicals into defined categories that can be used to communicate the implications for risk. Factors usually taken into consideration in interpreting the results of an animal bioassay include the following:

- Adequacy of experimental design and conduct.
- Statistical significance of any increase in tumor incidence.
- Presence or absence of a dose–response relationship and correct dose selection.
- Nature of tumors (benign or malignant) and relevance of tumor type to humans.
- Historical control data (incidence and variability) for tumor type.
- Common (spontaneous) versus uncommon tumors.
- Number of organs/tissues with tumors.
- Mechanistic information.

While there has been an attempt, under UN auspices, to develop a common global scheme for classifying chemicals, it relies on voluntary compliance and agencies in the United States and abroad have been slow to adopt this scheme. The classification categories for carcinogens under this scheme, the Globally Harmonized System (GHS), will be described so it can be compared to the schemes that are now in place.

At present, the most commonly used classification schemes are those developed by United States Environmental Protection Agency (US EPA) and by the International Agency for Research on Cancer (IARC). The US EPA classification schemes are used for the regulation of chemicals under those laws it administers; for example, Federal Insecticide, Fungicide and Rodenticide Act, and Toxic Substances Control Act as well as by many state regulatory agencies. The IARC Carcinogen Classification scheme is commonly used in the European Community and is considered in certain US regulations and laws (e.g., Occupational Safety and Health Administration (OSHA) Hazard Communication Standard).

Other respected carcinogenic classification schemes include those developed by the UN – known as the GHS, European Commission Scientific Committee on Occupational Exposure Limits (EC SCOEL), the German Commission for the Investigation of Health Hazards of Chemical Compounds in the Work Area (MAK Commission), and a number of US organizations including National Institute of Occupational Safety and Health (NIOSH), OSHA, National Toxicology Program (NTP), and American Conference of Government Industrial Hygienists (ACGIH). Each of these schemes is described in the following sections. It should be emphasized that these classification systems are constantly evolving and that changes may occur over time.

UN GHS Carcinogen Classifications

While there has been an attempt, under UN auspices, to develop a common global classification scheme, it relies on voluntary compliance and agencies in the United States and abroad have been slow to adopt this scheme. The classification scheme for carcinogens under this scheme, the Globally Harmonized System of Classification and Labeling of Chemicals (GHS), will be described so it can be compared to the schemes that are now in place.

Category 1: Known or presumed human carcinogens. The placing of a substance in Category 1 is done on the basis of epidemiological and/or animal data. An individual substance may be further distinguished.

Category 1A: Known to have carcinogenic potential for humans; the placing of a substance is largely based on human evidence.

Category 1B: Presumed to have carcinogenic potential for humans; the placing of a substance is largely based on animal evidence.

Based on the strength of evidence together with additional considerations, such evidence may be derived from human studies that establish a causal relationship between human exposure to a substance and development of cancer (known human carcinogen). Alternatively, evidence may be derived from animal experiments for which there is sufficient evidence to demonstrate animal carcinogenicity (presumed human carcinogen). In addition, on a case-by-case basis, scientific judgment may warrant a decision of presumed human carcinogenicity derived from studies showing limited evidence of carcinogenicity in humans together with limited evidence of carcinogenicity in experimental animals.

Category 2: Suspected human carcinogen – The placing of a substance in Category 2 is done on the basis of evidence obtained from human and/or animal studies, but which is not sufficiently convincing to place the substance in Category 1. Based on the strength of evidence together with additional considerations, such evidence may be from either limited evidence of carcinogenicity in human studies or limited evidence of carcinogenicity in animal studies.

US EPA Carcinogen Classifications

The US EPA originally promulgated its carcinogen classification approach in 1986 in its Guidelines for Carcinogens Risk Assessment. However, in 2005, the EPA published a new set of

 http://dx.doi.org/10.1016/B978-0-12-386454-3.00370-5

Guidelines for Carcinogen Risk Assessment designed to replace the 1986 version. This, in effect, established two different classification systems that both are now in effect. The new guidelines apply only to those compounds that have been newly evaluated or reevaluated since 2005. As a result, carcinogen classifications for some compounds are based on the old system and the new approach is applied to others. Thus, both classification schemes will be described in detail.

Classification Based on the 1986 Guidelines for Carcinogen Risk Assessment

The US EPA 1986 'total-weight-of-evidence' scheme classifies potential carcinogens into five groups, A–E that indicate the likelihood that they are human carcinogens. These groups are described below.

Group A: Human carcinogen – This is reserved for chemicals where there exists clear epidemiological evidence indicating an association between exposure to the chemical and cancer.

Group B: Probable human carcinogen – This group is divided into two subgroups, B1 and B2.

Group B1 indicates that there is 'sufficient' evidence to indicate that the material is an animal carcinogen and that there is 'limited' evidence of effects in humans.

Group B2 indicates that although there is sufficient evidence in animals, the total weight of evidence for effects in humans is weaker or inadequate.

Group C: Possible human carcinogen – classification in this group indicates limited, often marginal evidence of carcinogenicity in animals and no evidence of any effects in humans.

Group D: Not classifiable as to human carcinogenicity – This group is used for chemicals for which no data are available.

Group E: Evidence of noncarcinogenicity for humans – this group is used for chemicals that show no evidence of any carcinogenicity in at least two adequately conducted animal tests with different species.

Classification Based on the 2005 Guidelines for Carcinogen Risk Assessment

The descriptors of the 2005 Guidelines substitute for the letter designations of the 1986 Guidelines. They also reflect a change in approach since the descriptors do not stand-alone but instead are incorporated into a narrative that places the descriptors within a discussion of factors that have affected the choice of descriptor. The descriptors are as follows.

Carcinogenic to Humans

This descriptor indicates strong evidence of human carcinogenicity. It covers different combinations of evidence.

- This descriptor is appropriate when there is convincing epidemiologic evidence of a causal association between human exposure and cancer.
- Exceptionally, this descriptor may be equally appropriate with a lesser weight of epidemiologic evidence that is strengthened by other lines of evidence. It can be used when all of the following conditions are met: (1) there is strong evidence of an association between human exposures and either the cancer or the key precursor events of the agent's mode of action but not enough for a causal association, (2) there is extensive evidence of carcinogenicity in animals, (3) the mode(s) of carcinogenic action and associated key precursor events have been identified in animals, and (4) there is strong evidence that the key precursor events that precede the cancer response in animals are anticipated to occur in humans and progress to tumors, based on available biological information. In this case, the narrative includes a summary of both the experimental and the epidemiologic information on mode of action and also an indication of the relative weight that each source of information carries, for example, based on human information, based on limited human and extensive animal experiments.

Likely to Be Carcinogenic to Humans

This descriptor is appropriate when the weight of the evidence is adequate to demonstrate carcinogenic potential to humans but does not reach the weight of evidence for the descriptor 'Carcinogenic to Humans.' Adequate evidence consistent with this descriptor covers a broad spectrum. As stated previously, the use of the term 'likely' as a weight of evidence descriptor does not correspond to a quantifiable probability. The examples below are meant to represent the broad range of data combinations that are covered by this descriptor; they are illustrative and provide neither a checklist nor a limitation for the data that might support the use of this descriptor. Moreover, additional information, for example, on mode of action, might change the choice of the descriptor. Supporting data for this descriptor may include the following:

- An agent demonstrating a plausible (but not definitively causal) association between human exposure and cancer, in most cases with some supporting biological, experimental evidence, though not necessarily carcinogenicity data from animal experiments;
- An agent that has tested positive in animal experiments in more than one species, sex, strain, site, or exposure route, with or without evidence of carcinogenicity in humans;
- A positive tumor study that raises additional biological concerns beyond that of a statistically significant result, for example, a high degree of malignancy, or an early age at onset;
- A rare animal tumor response in a single experiment that is assumed to be relevant to humans; or
- A positive tumor study that is strengthened by other lines of evidence, for example, either plausible (but not definitively causal) association between human exposure and cancer or evidence that the agent or an important metabolite causes events generally known to be associated with tumor formation (such as DNA reactivity or effects on cell growth control) likely to be related to the tumor response in this case.

Suggestive Evidence of Carcinogenic Potential

This descriptor of the database is appropriate when the weight of evidence is suggestive of carcinogenicity; a concern for potential carcinogenic effects in humans is raised, but the data are judged not sufficient for a stronger conclusion.

This descriptor covers a spectrum of evidence associated with varying levels of concern for carcinogenicity, ranging from a positive cancer result in the only study on an agent to a single positive cancer result in an extensive database that includes negative studies in other species. Depending on the extent of the database, additional studies may or may not provide further insights. Some examples include:

- a small, and possibly not statistically significant, increase in tumor incidence observed in a single animal or human study that does not reach the weight of evidence for the descriptor 'Likely to Be Carcinogenic to Humans.' The study generally would not be contradicted by other studies of equal quality in the same population group or experimental system;
- a small increase in a tumor with a high background rate in that sex and strain, when there is some but insufficient evidence that the observed tumors may be due to intrinsic factors that cause background tumors and not due to the agent being assessed. (When there is a high background rate of a specific tumor in animals of a particular sex and strain, then there may be biological factors operating independently of the agent being assessed that could be responsible for the development of the observed tumors.) In this case, the reasons for determining that the tumors are not due to the agent are explained;
- evidence of a positive response in a study whose power, design, or conduct limits the ability to draw a confident conclusion (but does not make the study fatally flawed), but where the carcinogenic potential is strengthened by other lines of evidence (such as structure–activity relationships); or
- a statistically significant increase at one dose only, but no significant response at the other doses and no overall trend.

Inadequate Information to Assess Carcinogenic Potential

This descriptor of the database is appropriate when available data are judged inadequate for applying one of the other descriptors. Additional studies generally would be expected to provide further insights. Some examples include:

- little or no pertinent information;
- conflicting evidence, that is, some studies provide evidence of carcinogenicity but other studies of equal quality in the same sex and strain are negative. Differing results, that is, positive results in some studies and negative results in one or more different experimental systems, do not constitute *conflicting evidence* as the term is used here. Depending on the overall weight of evidence, differing results can be considered either suggestive evidence or likely evidence; or
- negative results that are not sufficiently robust for the descriptor, 'Not Likely to Be Carcinogenic to Humans.'

Not Likely to Be Carcinogenic to Humans

This descriptor is appropriate when the available data are considered robust for deciding that there is no basis for human hazard concern. In some instances, there can be positive results in experimental animals when there is strong, consistent evidence that each mode of action in experimental animals does not operate in humans. In other cases, there can be convincing evidence in both humans and animals that the agent is not carcinogenic. The judgment may be based on data such as:

- animal evidence that demonstrates lack of carcinogenic effect in both sexes in well-designed and well-conducted studies in at least two appropriate animal species (in the absence of other animal or human data suggesting a potential for cancer effects);
- convincing and extensive experimental evidence showing that the only carcinogenic effects observed in animals are not relevant to humans;
- convincing evidence that carcinogenic effects are not likely by a particular exposure route; or
- convincing evidence that carcinogenic effects are not likely below a defined dose range.

A descriptor of 'not likely' applies only to the circumstances supported by the data. For example, an agent may be 'Not Likely to Be Carcinogenic' by one route but not necessarily by another. In those cases that have positive animal experiment(s) but the results are judged to be not relevant to humans, the narrative discusses why the results are not relevant.

Multiple Descriptors

More than one descriptor can be used when an agent's effects differ by dose or exposure route. For example, an agent may be 'Carcinogenic to Humans' by one exposure route but 'Not Likely to Be Carcinogenic' by a route by which it is not absorbed. Also, an agent could be 'Likely to Be Carcinogenic' above a specified dose but 'Not Likely to Be Carcinogenic' below that dose because a key event in tumor formation does not occur below that dose.

IARC Carcinogen Classifications

IARC is a department of the World Health Organization. The overall classification scheme developed by IARC is similar to that promulgated by the US EPA in its 1986 Guidelines (this US EPA scheme was initially developed based on an IARC scheme). Chemicals are classified into four groups with respect to their potential to cause cancer in humans. The classification reflects the strength of the evidence available from animal studies, epidemiology, and other relevant data. The IARC groups are outlined below.

Group 1: The agent is carcinogenic to humans – this group is reserved for those chemicals or agents where there is 'sufficient evidence' of carcinogenicity in humans.

Group 2: The agent is probably carcinogenic to humans – this group, like the US EPA Group B, is divided into two subgroups, Groups 2A and 2B, depending on the strength of the evidence available.

Groups 2A and 2B indicate that the agent is 'probably' or 'possibly' carcinogenic to humans, respectively.

Group 3: The agent is not classifiable as to its carcinogenicity to humans – this group is used for chemicals that do not fall into any of the other groups.

Group 4: The agent is probably not carcinogenic to humans – this group is used for compounds where there exists evidence suggesting an absence of carcinogenic potential in humans.

NTP Carcinogen Classifications

The NTP is responsible for preparing Reports on Carcinogens. The Reports on Carcinogens are mandated by Public Law 95-662 and are for informational purposes only. The listing of a substance in the annual report does not by itself establish that such a substance presents a risk to persons in their daily lives. Clause (I) in subparagraph (4) (A) of Section 301 (b) of the Public Health Service Act requires that a report be published which contains a list of all substances (1) 'which are either known to be carcinogens or may reasonably be anticipated to be carcinogens,' and (2) to which a significant number of persons residing in the United States are exposed.

As of the 2011 update, for the purpose of Biennial Report on Carcinogens, the classification scheme is outlined below.

Known to Be Human Carcinogen

There is sufficient evidence of carcinogenicity from studies in humans, which indicates a causal relationship between exposure to the agent, substance, or mixture, and human cancer.

Reasonably Anticipated to Be Human Carcinogen

There is limited evidence of carcinogenicity from studies in humans, which indicates that causal interpretation is credible, but that alternative explanations, such as chance, bias, or confounding factors, could not adequately be excluded, or there is sufficient evidence of carcinogenicity from studies in experimental animals, which indicates there is an increased incidence of malignant and/or a combination of malignant and benign tumors (1) in multiple species or at multiple tissue sites, or (2) by multiple routes of exposure, or (3) to an unusual degree with regard to incidence, site, or type of tumor, or age at onset, or there is less than sufficient evidence of carcinogenicity in humans or laboratory animals; however, the agent, substance, or mixture belongs to a well-defined, structurally related class of substances whose members are listed in a previous Report on Carcinogens as either known to be a human carcinogen or reasonably anticipated to be a human carcinogen, or there is convincing relevant information that the agent acts through mechanisms indicating it would likely cause cancer in humans.

Conclusions regarding carcinogenicity in humans or experimental animals are based on scientific judgment, with consideration given to all relevant information. Relevant information includes, but is not limited to, dose–response, route of exposure, chemical structure, metabolism, pharmacokinetics, sensitive subpopulations, genetic effects, or other data relating to mechanism of action or factors that may be unique to a given substance. For example, there may be substances for which there is evidence of carcinogenicity in laboratory animals, but there are compelling data indicating that the agent acts through mechanisms which do not operate in humans and would therefore not reasonably be anticipated to cause cancer in humans.

OSHA Carcinogen Classifications

The Occupational Safety and Health Act of 1970 provides the establishment of workplace standards for toxic materials or harmful physical agents which most adequately assures, to the extent feasible, on the basis of the best available evidence, that no employee will suffer material impairment of health or functional capacity even if such employee has regular exposure to the hazard dealt with by such standard for the period of his or her working life.

Potential occupational carcinogens regulated under OSHA are classified into two main categories based on the nature and extent of the available scientific evidence: Category I potential carcinogens and Category II potential carcinogens.

Category I Potential Carcinogens

A substance shall be identified, classified, and regulated as a Category I potential carcinogen if, upon scientific evaluation, the secretary determines that the substance meets the definition of a potential occupational carcinogen in (1) humans or (2) a single mammalian species in a long-term bioassay in which the results are in concordance with some other scientifically evaluated evidence of a potential carcinogenic hazard, or (3) a single mammalian species in an adequately conducted long-term bioassay, in appropriate circumstances in which the secretary determines the requirement for concordance is not necessary. Evidence of concordance is any of the following: positive results from independent testing in the same or other species, positive results in short-term tests, or induction of tumors at injection or implantation.

Category II Potential Carcinogens

A substance shall be identified, classified, and regulated as a Category II potential carcinogen if, upon scientific evaluation, the secretary determines that (1) the substance meets the criteria set forth for Category I, but the evidence is found by the secretary to be only 'suggestive'; or (2) the substance meets the criteria set forth for Category I in a single mammalian species without evidence of concordance.

NIOSH Carcinogen Classifications

Acting under the authority of the Occupational Safety and Health Act of 1970 (Public Law 91-596), the NIOSH develops and periodically revises recommended exposure limits (RELs) for hazardous substances or conditions in the workplace. These recommendations are then published and transmitted to OSHA for use in promulgating legal standards. NIOSH may identify numerous chemicals that it believes should be treated as occupational carcinogens even though OSHA has not yet identified them as such. Generally, where OSHA has adopted the NIOSH recommendations as OSHA standards, the OSHA permissible exposure limits (PELs) and NIOSH RELs are equal. In cases in which the NIOSH recommendations have not been formally adopted by OSHA, the NIOSH RELs may be different from the OSHA PELs. The NIOSH classification scheme is one of the simplest carcinogen classification schemes; it combines all carcinogens into one category. Within this single category, NIOSH narratively describes the site of the cancer and whether the effect was seen in humans or animals. In determining carcinogenicity, NIOSH uses a classification scheme outlined in 29 CFR 1990.103, which states in part: Potential occupational carcinogen means any substance, or combination or mixture of substances, which causes an increased incidence of benign and/ or malignant neoplasms or a substantial decrease in the latency period between exposure and onset of neoplasms in humans or in one or more experimental mammalian species as the result of any oral, respiratory, or dermal exposure, or any other exposure which results in the induction of tumors at a site other than the site of administration. This definition also includes any substance which is metabolized into one or more potential occupational carcinogens by mammals.

The NIOSH thresholds for carcinogens were not designed to be protective of 100% of the population. NIOSH usually recommends that occupational exposures to carcinogens be limited to the lowest feasible concentration.

ACGIH Carcinogen Classifications

ACGIH classifies substances associated with industrial processes that are recognized to have carcinogenic or cocarcinogenic potential. In general, the stated classification is intended to provide a practical guideline for the industrial hygiene professional to assist in control of exposures in the workplace. The classification and threshold limit values (TLVs) are not mandated by federal or state regulations, although the ACGIH classifications and values may be considered when standards are adopted by the regulatory agencies. Currently, five categories of carcinogens have been designated by the TLV Committee to recognize the qualitative differences in research results or other data. These five categories are outlined below.

A1: Confirmed human carcinogen – The agent is carcinogenic to humans based on the weight of evidence from epidemiologic studies of exposed humans and/or convincing clinical evidence in exposed humans.

A2: Suspected human carcinogen – The agent is carcinogenic in experimental animals at dose levels, by route(s) of administration, at site(s), of histologic types(s), or by mechanism(s) that are considered relevant to worker exposure. Available epidemiologic studies are conflicting or insufficient to confirm an increased risk of cancer in exposed humans.

A3: Animal carcinogen – The agent is carcinogenic in experimental animals at a relatively high dose, by route(s) of administration, at site(s), of histologic types(s), or by mechanism(s) that are not considered relevant to worker exposure. Available epidemiologic studies do not confirm an increased risk of cancer in exposed humans. Available evidence suggests that the agent is not likely to cause cancer in humans except under uncommon or unlikely routes or levels of exposure.

A4: Not classifiable as a human carcinogen – There are inadequate data on which to classify the agent in terms of its carcinogenicity in humans and/or animals.

A5: Not suspected as a human carcinogen – The agent is not suspected to be a human carcinogen on the basis of properly conducted epidemiologic studies in humans. These studies have sufficiently long follow-up, reliable exposure histories, sufficiently high dose, and adequate statistical power to conclude that exposure to the agent does not convey a significant risk of cancer to humans. Evidence suggesting a lack of carcinogenicity in experimental animals will be considered if it is supported by other relevant data. Substances for which no human or experimental animal carcinogenic data have been reported are assigned no carcinogen designation by the ACGIH.

European Commission SCOEL Carcinogen Classifications

SCOEL has developed a system of carcinogen classifications to support decisions about the occupational exposure limits (OELs) for chemicals in the workplace. A key distinction in this system is whether the chemical is genotoxic or not. The categories are as follows:

Group A: Nonthreshold genotoxic carcinogens – for low-dose risk assessment the linear nonthreshold (LNT) model appears appropriate.

Group B: Genotoxic carcinogens for which the existence of a threshold cannot be sufficiently supported at present. In these cases, the LNT model may be used as a default assumption, based on the scientific uncertainty.

Group C: Genotoxic carcinogens for which a practical threshold is supported.

Group D: Nongenotoxic carcinogens and non-DNA-reactive carcinogens; for these compounds a true (perfect) threshold is associated with a clearly founded NOAEL.

Health-based OELs are derived by SCOEL for carcinogens of Groups C and D. If dataset allows, SCOEL might perform a risk assessment for carcinogens and/or mutagens placed in Categories A and B.

German MAK Carcinogen Classifications

Maximale Arbeitsplatzkonzentrationen (MAKs) are the maximum concentrations of a chemical substance allowed in the workplace. They are daily 8-h time-weighted average values and apply to healthy adults. These are established by the MAK Commission and the following carcinogen classifications are used in the derivation of MAK values:

Category 1: Substances that cause cancer in man and can be assumed to contribute to cancer risk. Epidemiological studies provide adequate evidence of a positive correlation between the exposure of humans and the occurrence of cancer. Limited epidemiological data can be substantiated by evidence that the substance causes cancer by a mode of action that is relevant to man.

Category 2: Substances that are considered to be carcinogenic for man because sufficient data from long-term animal studies or limited evidence from animal studies substantiated by evidence from epidemiological studies indicate that they can contribute to cancer risk. Limited data from animal studies can be supported by evidence that the substance causes cancer by a mode of action that is relevant to man and by results of *in vitro* tests and short-term animal studies.

Category 3: Substances that cause concern that they could be carcinogenic for man but cannot be assessed conclusively because of lack of data. The classification in Category 3 is provisional.

Category 3A: Substances for which the criteria for classification in Category 4 or 5 are fulfilled but for which the database is insufficient for the establishment of a MAK value.

Category 3B: Substances for which *in vitro* or animal studies have yielded evidence of carcinogenic effects that is not sufficient for classification of the substance in one of the other categories. Further studies are required before a final decision can be made. A MAK or Biological Tolerance Value (BAT) can be established provided no genotoxic effects have been detected.

Category 4: Substances with carcinogenic potential for which a nongenotoxic mode of action is of prime importance and genotoxic effects play no or at most a minor part provided the MAK and BAT values are observed. Under these conditions, no contribution to human cancer risk is expected. The classification is supported especially by evidence that, for example, increases in cellular proliferation, inhibition of apoptosis, or disturbances in cellular differentiation are important in the mode of action. The classification and the MAK and BAT values take into consideration the manifold mechanisms contributing to carcinogenesis and their characteristic dose–time–response relationships.

Category 5: Substances with carcinogenic and genotoxic effects that are considered to contribute very slightly to human cancer risk provided the MAK and BAT values are observed. The classification is supported by information on the mode of action, dose-dependence, and toxicokinetic data pertinent to species comparison.

See also: ACGIH® (American Conference of Governmental Industrial Hygienists); Carcinogenesis; Dose–Response Relationship; Epidemiology; Federal Insecticide, Fungicide, and Rodenticide Act, US; The Globally Harmonized System for Classification and Labeling of the GHS; International Agency for Research on Cancer; Levels of Effect in Toxicology Assessment; National Institute for Occupational Safety and Health; The National Toxicology Program; Occupational Safety and Health Act, US; Occupational Safety and Health Administration; Risk Assessment, Human Health; Toxic Substances Control Act; Toxicity Testing, Carcinogenesis.

Further Reading

American Conference of Governmental Industrial Hygienists, 2001. Documentation of the Threshold Limit Values and Biological Exposure Indices, seventh ed. ACGIH, Cincinnati, OH.

Bolt, H.M., Huici-Montagud, A., 2008. Strategy of the scientific committee on occupational exposure limits (SCOEL) in the derivation of occupational exposure limits for carcinogens and mutagens. Arch. Toxicol. 82 (1), 61–64.

Greim, H., Reuter, U., 2001. Classification of carcinogenic chemicals in the work area by the German MAK Commission: Current examples for the new categories. Toxicology 166 (1–2), 11–23.

National Institute for Occupational Safety and Health, 2010. NIOSH Pocket Guide to Chemical Hazards. US Department of Health and Human Services, Public Health Service, Washington, DC.

National Toxicology Program, 2011. Report on Carcinogens, twelfeth ed. United States Department of Health and Human Services, Public Health Service, National Toxicology Program, Research Triangle Park, NC.

Occupational Safety and Health Administration, 1996. Identification, Classification, and Regulation of Potential Occupational Carcinogens. Subtitle B – Regulations Relating to Labor, Chapter XVII. Title 29 Code of Federal Regulations (CFR) (1990). Occupational Safety and Health Administration, Washington, DC.

US EPA, 1986. Guidelines for Carcinogen Risk Assessment. Risk Assessment Forum, EPA/630/R-00/004, Washington, DC.

US EPA, 2005. Guidelines for Carcinogen Risk Assessment. Risk Assessment Forum, EPA/630/P-03/001B, Washington, DC.

Relevant Websites

http://www.acgih.org – American Conference of Governmental Industrial Hygienists.

http://osha.gov/dsg/hazcom/ghs.html – Guide to Globally Harmonized System of Classification and Labeling of Chemicals.

http://www.iarc.fr – International Agency for Research on Cancer.

http://www.cdc.gov – National Institute for Occupational Safety and Health.

http://ntp-server.niehs.nih.gov – National Toxicology Program.

http://www.osha.gov – Occupational Safety and Health Administration.

http://www.epa.gov – US Environmental Protection Agency.

http://www.mak-collection.com – Wiley Online Library: The MAK Collection for Occupational Health and Safety.

Carcinogen–DNA Adduct Formation and DNA Repair

A Weston, National Institute for Occupational Safety and Health, Centers for Disease Control and Prevention, Morgantown, WV, USA
MC Poirier, National Cancer Institute, National Institutes of Health, Bethesda, MD, USA

Carcinogen–DNA Adducts

Importance of DNA Adduct Formation and DNA Repair in the Process of Carcinogenesis

Carcinogen–DNA adducts of exogenous and endogenous genotoxic chemical carcinogens may induce errors in DNA sequence (mutations). Subsequent transcription on a damaged template may result in formation of abnormal proteins or the loss of a protein. DNA adduct formation and mutagenesis are considered to bring about changes in gene expression that produce clonal expansions of cells lacking in growth control (tumors). A substantial period of time is required after DNA damage occurs for a tumor to become evident, however; DNA damage alone is not sufficient for tumorigenesis, since other events must also take place. DNA adduct levels, measured at any point in time, reflect tissue-specific rates of damage processing that include DNA adduct formation and removal (DNA repair), DNA adduct instability, tissue turnover, and other events. In experimental model systems, dose–response associations have been observed for DNA adduct formation, mutagenesis, and tumorigenesis. Reductions in tumor incidences have been observed when DNA adduct levels have been lowered, either by DNA repair processes or by administration of chemopreventive agents that inhibit DNA adduct formation with no change in carcinogen dose.

Biotransformation of Carcinogenic Chemicals to Species That Modify DNA

Exogenous carcinogenic chemicals that form DNA adducts can bind to DNA directly if they are highly reactive. Examples are the nitrosoureas, some nitrosamines, ethylene oxide, and ozone. However, most carcinogenic chemicals are inert and require biotransformation or metabolic activation, a process by which families of enzymes convert a fraction of the initial dose to highly reactive intermediate metabolites able to bind covalently to DNA. Exogenous carcinogens that require metabolic activation in order to bind to DNA include plant and fungal products (aflatoxins, ochratoxins, hydrazines); pyrolysis products from cooking (heterocyclic amines, polycyclic aromatic hydrocarbons (PAHs)); industrial combustion products (aromatic amines, PAHs, nitro-PAHs, benzene, vinyl chloride, nitrosamines, ethylene oxide); urban pollution contaminants (PAHs, nitro-PAHs, aromatic amines); and components of tobacco (tobacco-specific nitrosamines) and tobacco smoke (PAHs, nitrosamines, aromatic amines, and many others). Most of the carcinogenic chemicals that bind to DNA not only induce specific covalent DNA adducts, but also increase the burden of oxidative damage; some examples will be discussed below.

The PAHs, including benzo[*a*]pyrene (BP), classified by the International Agency for Research on Cancer as a human carcinogen (IARC, 2010), are composed of variable numbers of fused benzene rings and are chemically unreactive, as well as very sparingly soluble in water. PAHs are ubiquitous environmental contaminants that are commonly formed as products of partial combustion of organic material, and are found in cigarette smoke, automobile exhaust, exhaust from many industrial processes, indoor air (especially during the winter months), charred meats, and elsewhere. PAHs are metabolized, and several pathways exist for formation of covalent DNA adducts. In the most well-known and possibly the most important pathway, PAHs are converted to simple arene oxides by cytochrome P450, hydrated through the action of epoxide hydrolase, and subjected again to epoxidation (cytochrome P450) to form unstable dihydrodiol epoxides. These unstable metabolites spontaneously convert to positively charged, highly reactive free radicals (carbocations, the ultimate carcinogenic forms), which can bind covalently to DNA. The structure of the major stable adduct of BP with DNA, r7,t8,t9-trihydroxy-*c*-10-(N^2-deoxyguanosyl)-7,8,9,10-tetrahydro-benzo[*a*]pyrene (BPdG), is illustrated in **Figure 1(a)**. Additional examples of DNA adducts relevant to human exposures are presented in **Figure 1**, which shows aromatic amines (**Figure 1(b) and 1(c)**), a heterocyclic amine **Figure 1(d)**), a fungal mycotoxin (**Figure 1(e)**), methylated (alkylated) adducts (**Figure 1(f) and 1(g)**), and a hydroxyl adduct resulting from oxyradical attack (**Figure 1(h)**).

Aromatic amines, such as 4-aminobiphenyl (4-ABP) and 2-acetylaminofluorene (2-AAF), are found in tobacco smoke and industrial exhaust, and are considered to play a role in the etiology of human bladder cancer. They are characterized by the presence of benzene rings and an exocyclic nitrogen. Activation of the aromatic amine 2-AAF proceeds by *N*-oxidation with sulfotransferase catalysis, resulting in the formation of acetylated (**Figure 1(b)**) and non-acetylated (**Figure 1(c)**) guanine adducts.

The heterocyclic amines, an example of which is 2-amino-1-methyl-6-phenylimidazo[4,5-*b*]pyridine (PhIP), are formed from the pyrolysis of amino acids, creatinine, and glucose, which occurs during cooking of meat and fish. Consequently, they are known collectively as food mutagens. Their metabolism, which is similar to that of the aromatic amines, involves cytochrome P450-induced *N*-hydroxylation, with and without enzymic *O*-esterification, followed by direct reaction with DNA (**Figure 1(e)**).

The fungal mycotoxins, including aflatoxin B_1 derived from *Aspergillus* molds and fumonisin derived from *Fusarium* molds, contaminate cereals, grains, and nuts. Ingestion of these compounds is highly correlated with subsequent incidence of liver cancer. Aflatoxins are heterocyclic, contain several endocyclic oxygen molecules, and are activated by simple cytochrome P450-driven epoxidation. The major aflatoxin B_1-guanine adduct is shown in **Figure 1(d)**.

Guanine can be readily alkylated by methyl and ethyl additions at the O6 and N7 positions. The O^6- methylated guanine adduct is shown in **Figure 1(e)**, and the N^7- methylated guanine adduct is shown in **Figure 1(g)**. Such adducts may be formed endogenously or induced by a wide variety of chemicals. Of

 http://dx.doi.org/10.1016/B978-0-12-386454-3.00593-5

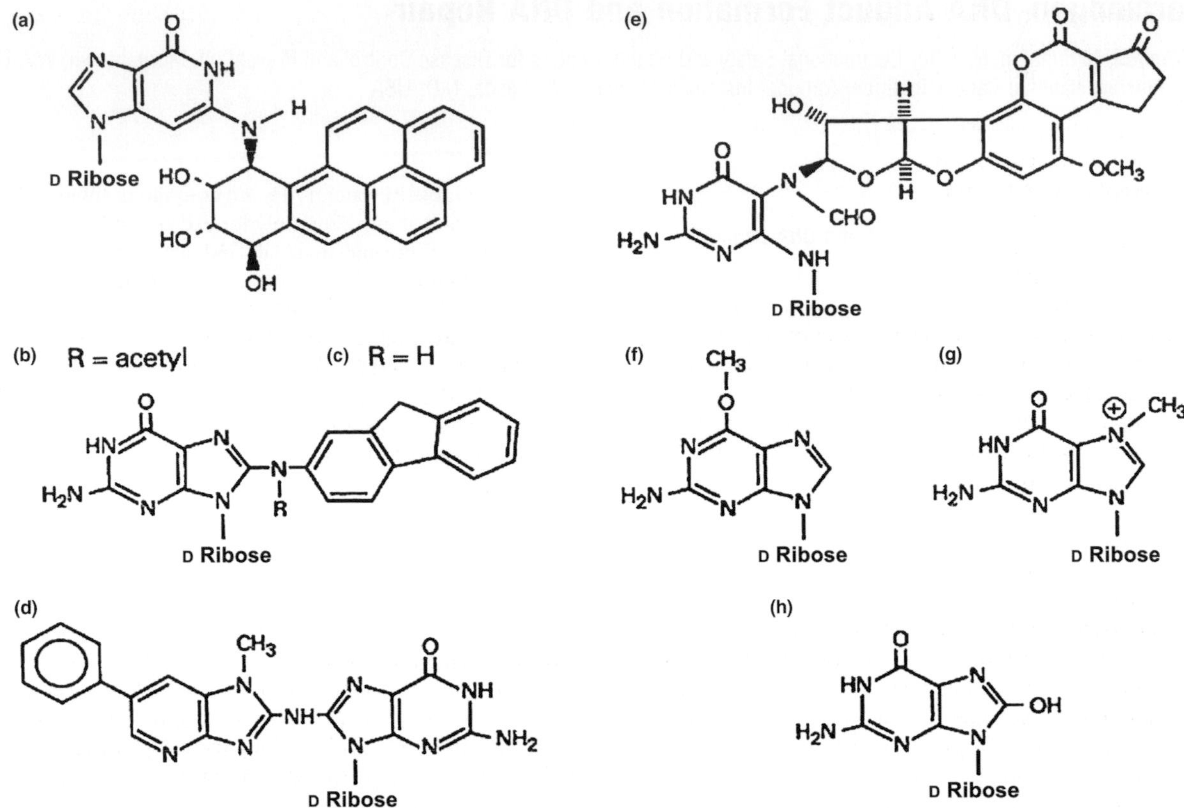

Figure 1 Molecular structures of carcinogen–DNA adducts, (a) (7R)-N^2-(10-{7β, 8α, 9α-trihydroxy-7,8,9,10-tetrahydro-benzo[*a*]pyrene}-yl)-deoxyguanosine, formed when benzo[a]pyrene-7,8-diol 9,10-epoxide reacts with the exocyclic amino group of deoxyguanosine; (b) *N*-(deoxyguanosin-8-yl)-2-(acetylamino)fluorene, formed when *N*-hydroxylacetylaminofluorene reacts with the C8-position of the imidazole ring; (c) *N*-(deoxyguanosin-8-yl)-2-(amino)fluorene, formed when *N*-hydroxylaminofluorene reacts with the C8-position of the pyrimidine ring structure; (d) *N*-(deoxyguanosin-8-yl)-2-amino-1-methyl-6-phenylimidazo-[4,5-*b*]-pyridine, formed when the *N*-hydroxylamine metabolite of 2-amino-1-methyl-6-phenylimidazo-[4,5-*b*]-pyridine (PhIP), a glutamic acid pyrolyzate, reacts with deoxyguanosine; (e) Ring-opened form of *N*-(deoxyguanosin-7-yl)-9-hydroxyaflatoxin B_1, formed following reaction of the 8,9-epoxide metabolite of aflatoxin B_1 at the N^7-methyl position of deoxyguanosine; (f) O^6-methyldeoxyguanosine, formed when an alkyl radical (CH_3^+), derived from an alkylating agent, reacts at the O^6-methyl-position of deoxyguanosine; (g) N^7-methyldeoxyguanosine, formed when an alkyl radical (CH_3^+), derived from an alkylating agent, reacts at the N^7-methyl-position of deoxyguanosine; (h) 8-Hydroxydeoxyguanosine, formed through exogenous or endogenous oxyradical (H_2O_2, $^{\cdot}OH$, $O_2^{\cdot-}$) damage at the C8-position of deoxyguanosine.

particular interest are the methylated adducts formed by some chemotherapeutic agents, including procarbazine, dacarbazine, methyl-methane sulfonate, carmustine, and others.

Oxyradicals (reactive oxygen species) may be formed by exposure to exogenous chemicals and by various endogenous processes. There are many species of oxyradical-damaged DNA, but among the most common is the mutagenic 8-hydroxydeoxyguanosine adduct (**Figure 1(h)**). Endogenous oxyradical exposures, which include $O_2^{\cdot}$ (superoxide anion) and H_2O_2 (hydrogen peroxide), frequently occur because of leakage from the mitochondria during oxidative phosphorylation. Other endogenous sources of oxyradicals include reactions of $O_2^{\cdot}$ with Fe^{3+} or nitric oxide (NO) to form unstable intermediates, which are powerful direct-acting oxidants and major factors in inflammation. Exposure to organic peroxides, catechol, hydroxyquinone, and 4-nitroquinoline-*N*-oxide, among others, leads to oxyradical damage. Moreover, cells can be stimulated to produce peroxisomes by treatment with certain drugs and plasticizers. The role of endogenous oxyradical DNA damage in chemical carcinogenesis is currently unclear, although the mutagenic potential of these adducts has been amply demonstrated in experimental systems.

Measurement of Carcinogen–DNA Adducts as Human Exposure Dosimeters

The long-term goal of DNA adduct biomonitoring is the development of a human biomarker that is directly correlated with cancer risk, and that can be followed during the process of cancer prevention/intervention. Exponential expansion of this field over the past 40 years has been made possible by the development of highly sensitive methods for the detection of DNA adducts in human tissues. The most widely used methods include immunoassays, gas chromatography/mass spectrometry (GC/MS), immunohistochemistry, fluorescence and phosphorescence spectroscopy, and ^{32}P-postlabeling. Detection limits for quantitative assays are typically in the range of 1 adduct in 10^9 nucleotides. Accelerator mass spectrometry, a highly sophisticated method, has a detection limit of ~1 adduct in 10^{12} nucleotides. However, accelerator mass spectrometry is less accessible and requires administration of minute quantities of C^{13}-labeled carcinogenic chemicals to human subjects, which does not always meet the approval of institutional review boards.

Recent developments in approaches to chemical derivatization have facilitated various novel permutations of GC/MS, and the resulting increase in sensitivity has allowed direct assay of human DNA samples, with specific characterization of DNA adducts. In contrast, most commonly used techniques lack a high level of specificity, and chemical characterization is typically not possible without some purification steps. Because humans are exposed to complex mixtures of chemical carcinogens, human DNA is considered to contain adducts induced by many xenobiotics. In addition to GC/MS, the combination of preparative methods (e.g., immunoaffinity chromatography, high-performance liquid chromatography), with immunoassays, ^{32}P-postlabeling assays, or synchronous fluorescence spectrometry, has made possible the identification of specific DNA adduct structures and/or the identification of chemical classes of DNA adducts.

The majority of studies designed to monitor DNA adducts in human tissues fall into the category of exposure documentation, and many involve environmental and occupational exposures to agents for which precise dosimetry is difficult or impossible. These types of studies have shown that formation of DNA adducts is widespread in the human population, supporting the notion that DNA adduct formation, after carcinogen exposure, is essential for tumorigenesis. It has been possible to show decreases in DNA adduct levels in groups of human subjects removed from exposure by virtue of location or season, showing qualitative or relative dosimetry before and after high exposure. Quantitative dosimetry for human DNA adduct formation has been possible with medicinal (cisplatin, procarbazine, dacarbazine, 8-methoxypsoralen) and dietary (aflatoxin, PAH) exposures, where dosimetry can be established with reasonable accuracy.

Human DNA Adduct Determination as an Indicator of Cancer Risk

In addition to documentation of exposure, a major goal of carcinogen–DNA adduct dosimetry in humans is to define a relationship between DNA adduct formation and cancer risk. This goal has been achieved in increasing numbers of case-control studies and prospective studies, some of which have nested case-control cohorts. **Table 1** shows a variety of studies, most measuring DNA adducts in human blood, but some using target tissues (e.g., liver, breast). In these studies, which are reviewed in Poirier (Discovery Medicine, 2012), the risks for cancer, measured as odds ratios (OR) or relative risk (RR), were increased two- to nine-fold among (the approximately 25% of) individuals with the highest DNA adduct levels, compared to those with the lowest DNA adduct levels. While epidemiological investigations elucidating the relationship between DNA adduct levels and cancer risk will likely continue to be carried out for many years, results of published studies support the notion that cancer risk is highest for subgroups of individuals with the highest levels of DNA adducts in blood or in any organ of interest. In addition, OR or RR values for cancer in such studies are of similar magnitude whether based on 'bulky' DNA adducts measured by ^{32}P-postlabeling, which measures a broad spectrum of DNA adducts but cannot characterize them chemically, or on carcinogen class-specific PAH–DNA or aromatic amine–DNA adducts measured by immunoassay (**Table 1**). The moderate increases in cancer risk associated with the highest DNA adduct levels suggest that DNA damage is an early essential event in tumorigenesis.

Table 1 Association between DNA adduct level and cancer risk in humans

DNA adduct measurement method	*Organ for cancer*	*Organ for DNA adduct measurement*	*Carcinogen: source of DNA adduct*	*Cancer risk estimate for[a,b] subgroup with the highest DNA adduct levels*
BPDE-DNA ELISA[c]	Colon	Blood	PAHs	2.8
BPDE-DNA ELISA	Lung	Blood	PAHs	7.7
BPDE-DNA IHC[d]	Liver	Liver	PAHs	4.4
PHIP-DNA IHC	Breast	Breast	PhIP	4.0
4-ABP-DNA IHC	Liver	Liver	4-ABP	6.5
HPLC[e] of AFB_1-dG[f]	Liver	Urine	Aflatoxin B_1	9.1
^{32}P-Postlabeling[g]	Bladder	Blood	'Bulky'	4.1
^{32}P-Postlabeling	Colon	Blood	'Bulky'	2.3
	Stomach	Blood	'Bulky'	2.2
^{32}P-Postlabeling	Lung	Blood	'Bulky'	1.6 Current smokers
^{32}P-Postlabeling	Lung	Blood	'Bulky'	2.0 Current smokers
^{32}P-Postlabeling	Lung	Blood	'Bulky'	3.0 Current smokers

[a]RR = Relative Risk or OR = Odds Ratio.
[b]Studies referred to in Poirier, M.C., 2012. Chemical-induced DNA damage and human cancer risk. Discov. Med. 14, 283–288.
[c]ELISA = Enzyme-Linked Immunosorbent Assay.
[d]IHC = Immunohistochemistry.
[e]HPLC = High-performance liquid chromatography.
[f]AFB_1-dG = ring opened form of *N*-(deoxyguanosin-7-yl)-9-hydroxyaflatoxin B_1.
[g]'Bulky' DNA adducts isolated by ^{32}P-postlabelling are typically stable, high-molecular-weight ($\geq$150 kDa) DNA adducts that are formed from PAHs, aromatic amines, nitroaromatics, hormones, aflatoxins, and/or other hydrophobic DNA-binding agents, which can be extracted by butanol and separated by chromatography. The technique measures overall DNA binding, but does not allow for chemical characterization of individual DNA adducts unless additional purification and separation is applied.

DNA Repair

Multiple metabolic pathways have evolved to reverse DNA damage through removal of the lesions and restoration of the DNA sequence. Typically such mechanisms are complex, involving multiple proteins acting in concert. Most DNA repair protein complexes comprise a damage sensor, a damage eliminator that also removes some normal nucleotides, a polymerase to replace the excised nucleotides, and a ligase to close strand gaps. More than 150 DNA repair genes are now known, and some contribute to more than one DNA repair pathway. Essentially, mechanisms of DNA repair can be separated into six categories: direct DNA repair (DR), nucleotide excision repair (NER), base excision repair (BER), mismatch repair (MMR), homologous recombination repair (HRR), and nonhomologous end-joining (NHEJ). With the exception of NHEJ, these mechanisms are summarized in **Figures 2** and **3**. All types of DNA damage may lead to permanent changes in DNA sequence, and some defects in DNA repair genes have been associated with disease conditions, for example, cancer, progeria, Cockayne syndrome, retinal dystrophy, thalassemia, xeroderma pigmentosum, and birth defects (**Table 2**).

Direct DNA Repair

Unlike most of the DNA repair mechanisms, DR (**Figure 2(a)**) is driven by a suicide enzyme mechanism. The best example is O^6-alkylguanine-DNA alkyltransferase (AGT), which removes an alkyl group from an alkylated deoxyguanosine (e.g., O^6-methyldeoxyguanosine, **Figure 1(f)**) to a cysteine residue in its own active site (Cys145). The alkylated AGT is quickly degraded through processing in the ubiquitination pathway. There is no need for patch synthesis or ligation in this pathway, and one alkyl-adduct consumes one molecule of enzyme. Other examples of alkyltransferases include O^6-ethyldeoxyguanosine and O^6-benzyldeoxyguanosine alkyltransferase.

Excision Repair (NER and BER)

There are two types of excision repair, NER and BER (**Figure 2(b) and 2(c)**). Both processes require multiple enzymes that act sequentially or in concert as a molecular complex. Excision repair is characterized by strand scission, degradation of the segment of the DNA strand containing the damage, 5′ to 3′ synthesis of a new DNA patch using the undamaged strand as a template, and ligation of the free end. The difference between NER and BER relates to the proteins involved, the types of adducts that are repaired, and the size of the patch removed.

In NER, sensory proteins (coded for by *XPA*, *XPC*, and *XPE*) recognize bulky adducts that distort the DNA helix. Typical examples include those arising from the metabolic activation of PAHs (e.g., benzo[*a*]pyrene, **Figure 1(a)**), aromatic amines (e.g., 2-AAF, **Figure 1(b)**), and heterocyclic amines (e.g., PhIP, **Figure 1(d)**). Endonucleases (XPF, XPG, ERCC1, or FEN) then degrade up to 30 base pairs of DNA. A patch is synthesized by a polymerase (pol δ or pol ε) and the gap is sealed by a ligase (DNA Ligases I–IV; DNA Ligase III complexes with the excision repair protein ERCC1 in NER). Depending on where in the DNA the repair occurs, there are two types of NER: global genomic repair (GGR) and transcription coupled repair (TCR). GGR is not restricted and uses recognition or sensory proteins to localize DNA lesions. TCR is restricted to transcribed strands of transcriptionally active genes; this process does not need sensory proteins, but recognizes DNA lesions where an RNA molecule has been stalled by the presence of a lesion. In GGR and TCR, the patch size is large (15–30 nucleotides).

In BER, the removal of a small segment of DNA containing an adduct is initiated by a glycosylase. In this case, the recognized damage consists of small adducts (methylpurines or 8-oxoguanosine, **Figure 1(f), 1(g), and 1(h)**). The action of the glycosylase to remove the damaged base is accomplished by the 8-oxoguanosine DNA glycosylase I, or the 3-methylpurine glycosylase, producing an apurinic/apyrimidinic (AP) site. The AP endonuclease then cleaves the 5′ phosphodiester bond and recruits pol δ or pol ε, which, when complexed with replication factor C, a DNA polymerase, and proliferating cell nuclear antigen (PCNA), cuts away a 2–10 nucleotide flap and repairs the gap. The flap is removed by FEN1 and the patch is ligated by Ligase I. This mechanism is known as a long-patch BER. In an alternative pathway, a glycosylase (an AP lyase) removes the damaged base and the phosphodiester bond 3′ of the AP site is cleaved. In this case, pol1 β complexes with Ligase III and XRCC1 to fill a single nucleotide gap. This latter mechanism is known as a short-patch BER.

Mismatch Repair

Mismatches in DNA are repaired by MMR (**Figure 2(d)**), a highly conserved function that exists in *Escherichia coli*. DNA mismatches are recognized by MutS, following which MutL joins to form a complex. The presence of this complex further recruits MutH that binds to an unmethylated GATC sequence. The DNA is distorted by the binding of MutL to MutH to form a loop, and an exonuclease proceeds to remove the nucleotides from the GATC site to just beyond the mismatch. The action of a polymerase and a ligase resynthesizes the daughter strand on the original template and closes the gap.

Formation of nucleotide mismatches occurs as a result of glycosylation. For example, the deamination of cytosine can result in mispairing thymidine with guanosine. In addition, post-replication DNA 'repair,' which is a DNA damage tolerance mechanism, always results in insertion of adenosine, and mismatches can occur during DNA replication. Therefore, DNA mismatches can be either transitions (purine–purine or pyrimidine–pyrimidine: G–T or A–C) or transversions (purine–pyrimidine or pyrimidine–purine: A–A, G–G, A–G or C–C, T–T, C–T). To repair these mismatches, a multiprotein complex is needed to recognize both the mismatch and the closest unmethylated GATC recognition sequence in a hemimethylated segment of DNA. In humans, the multiprotein complexes that recognize mismatches are either MSH1–MSH2–MSH6–PMS1 or MSH1–MSH2–MSH6–PMS2, and these human complexes correspond to the Mut gene complexes in *E. coli*. The entire segment of unmethylated or daughter strand DNA is eroded by an exonuclease (e.g., *ExoI*), and PCNA is recruited to support the action of a polymerase (e.g., pol δ or pol ε). DNA Ligase I then complexes with the polymerase to complete the repair.

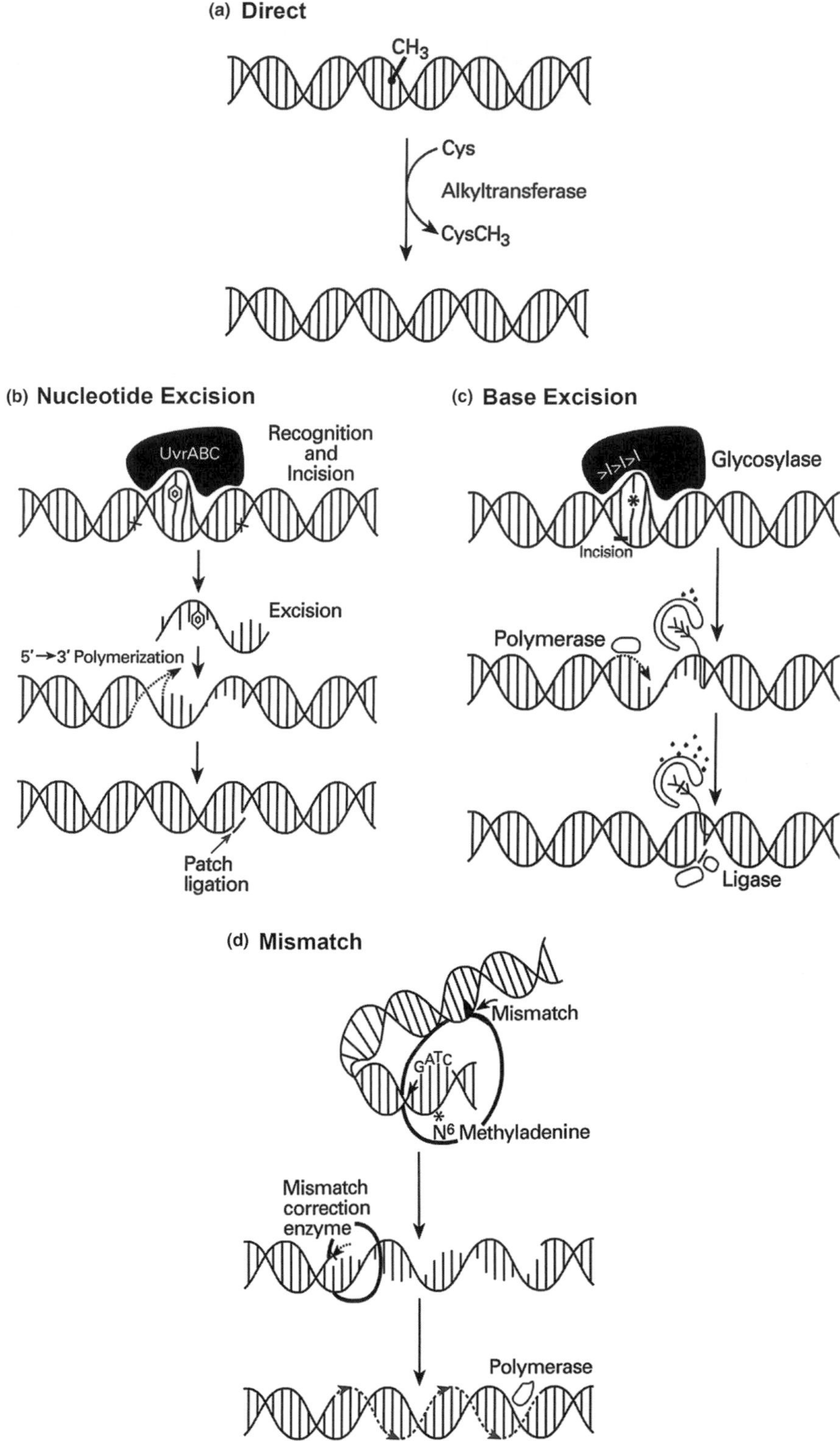

Figure 2 Mechanisms of DNA repair: (a) DR, where an alkyltransferase acts as a suicide enzyme; (b) NER, where XP proteins recognize bulky adduct damage, an endonuclease degrades up to 30 nucleotides around the lesion, a polymerase reconstructs the DNA and a ligase closes the gap; (c) BER, where a glycosylase recognizes the lesion and recruits an endonuclease that removes a small section of DNA including the damage, and again a polymerase and a ligase act to close the gap; (d) MMR, where a protein complex binds to the mismatched base pair and the closest hemi-methylated GATC an exonuclease degrades, the non-methylated daughter DNA strand including the mismatch and a polymerase and a ligase act to close the gap.

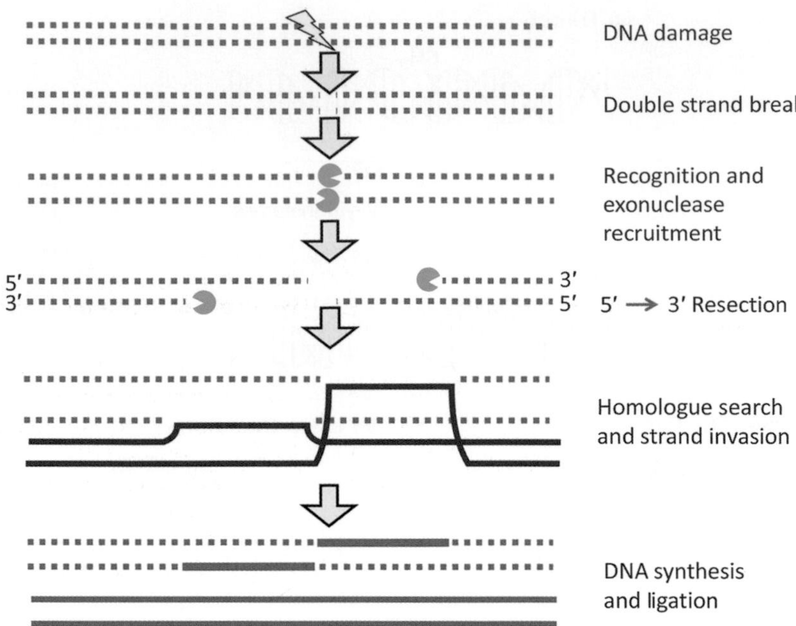

Figure 3 Scheme for HRR showing repair of double-strand breaks. Following recognition, an endonuclease is recruited that degrades the DNA in the 5′ to 3′ direction on both strands. DNA sequences that are homologous to the degraded segments are paired with the gaps in a process of strand invasion. The homologous search provides a template for resynthesis of the DNA segment that was removed, and a ligase completes the process.

Homologous Recombination Repair

HRR is a mechanism by which new haplotypes can arise from exchange of DNA sequence information between homologous, but not necessarily identical, chromosomes (**Figure 3**). It also provides a mechanism for the repair of double-strand breaks (DSBs) in DNA, where an intact DNA molecule is used as a template for the repair process. DSBs can result from exposure to ionizing radiation, antibiotics, oxidative damage, or a mechanical stressor (such as that occurring when a topoisomerase, responsible for regulation of helical winding during replication, encounters a bulky DNA adduct).

HRR occurs during the S phase or G2 phase of cell cycle. The first step in HRR is recognition of the lesion by *ataxia telangectasia* mutated (ATM), RAD3-related ATM, and DNA kinases (e.g., Chk2). Triggered by this recognition, an MRN complex forms on either side of the break. This consists of a nibrin (NBS1), a chromosomal structural protein (e.g., Rad50), and an exonuclease (Mre11). In the next step, 5′ to 3′ recission of both DNA strands occurs to allow pairing with homologous sequences. Rad51 (paralogs: RAD51B, C, D) facilitates invasion of homologous double-stranded DNA, which permits polymerization using an undamaged strand as a template. Completion of this process can occur in one of two ways. In the first model, four DNA strands come together to form Holliday junctions, which can be resolved by the actions of an exonuclease and a ligase. This mechanism presents opportunity for chromosomal crossover events. In the second model, only noncrossover products are formed because there is disengagement of the Holliday junctions, an annealing of one of the invading sequences, and gap filling of the damaged homolog.

Nonhomologous End-joining

Nonhomologous end-joining is another DNA repair mechanism that resolves DSBs. Since it relies on no sequence homology or short overhangs at DSBs, it is an error-prone process. Unlike HRR, which is active in the S and G_2 phases, NHEJ is active in all phases of cell cycle, but is most important in the G_1 phase. NHEJ is essentially a three-step process consisting of end binding and tethering, end processing, and ligation. The ATM kinase begins the process by recruiting and phosphorylating histone H2X so that it becomes H2AX, which then relaxes the DNA structure. The heterodimer Ku70–Ku80 complex, encoded by XRCC5 and XRCC6, appears to be the damage detector, with one molecule binding to each side of the DSB. DNA protein kinases bind to the Ku heterodimer and connect by bridge domains aligning the ends of the DSB. This provides a scaffold for the XRCC4 and Ligase IV to repair the DSBs. NHEJ is also an important mechanism for V(D)J recombination that leads to immunoglobulin diversity (so named because it involves variable and diverse joining of genes).

Diseases and Conditions Associated with Defects in DNA Repair Genes

For each of the six major DNA repair mechanisms, there is at least one known human disease/syndrome resulting from defects in DNA repair genes (**Table 2**). Xeroderma pigmentosum (XP) was first described in the latter part of the nineteenth century (named in 1874 by Hebra and Karposi), defective DNA repair was implicated as its cause in the late 1960s (Cleaver, 2008). Multiple XP genes have now been cloned and sequenced, revealing the underlying molecular basis of disease.

Table 2 Expanded[a] list of DNA repair defects and associated disease or pathology

	Disease category		
DNA repair mechanism	*Gene symbol*	*Gene function*	*Pathology or cancer*
Cancer susceptibility			
Direct DNA repair	AGT ATT	Suicide enzymes[b]	Low levels of alkylases result in susceptibility to cancer; high levels interfere with some chemotherapeutic agents
Nucleotide excision	ERCC1	Damage	Cerebro-oculo-facio-skeletal recognition syndrome; carcinogenesis
	BRCA1	Directs p53	Breast and ovarian cancer transcription
	RB1	Cell-cycle restriction	Retinoblastoma, breast cancer, osteosarcoma progression
Mismatch	MLH1	Damage	HNPCC2[c], glioma recognition
	MLH2	DNA binding	HNPCC1, ovarian cancer
	MSH3	MutS homolog	Endometrial cancer
	MSH6	Sliding clamp	Endometrial cancer, HNPCC1
	PMS1	Damage	HNPCC3 recognition
	PMS2	Repair initiation	HNPCC4, glioblastoma
Double-strand breaks	BRCA2	Regulates Rad51	Breast and pancreatic cancer
Homologous recombination	RAD54	Helicase	Non-Hodgkin's lymphoma, breast and colon cancer
General	hOgg1	Glycosylase	Cancer susceptibility
	TP53 (NER, DSBs)	Cell cycle control	Li–Fraumeni syndrome cancer susceptibility
Xeroderma pigmentosum			
Nucleotide excision	XPB and D	Helicases	Skin lesions
	XPG	Endonuclease	Acute sun sensitivity
	XPC (and BER)	Exonuclease	Mental retardation, sensitive skin, microcephaly
	DDB1 and 2	Binds DNA damage	Skin sensitivity
	XPA, C and E	Damage sensors	Skin and neurologic problems, skin, tongue, lip cancers
Other syndromes			
Nucleotide excision			
Cockayne	(CBS)	ATPase	Cutaneous, ocular, neurologic, and somatic abnormalities; short stature, deafness, mental retardation, early death
Juberg-Marsidi	(ATRX)	Helicase	Thalassemia/mental retardation
Strand breaks			
Nijmegan	(NBS1)	Nibrin, cell cycle regulation	Microcephaly; mental retardation immunodeficiency, slow growth; radiation sensitivity, malignancy
Ataxia-telangiectasia	(ATM)	Phosphorylation	Neurologic deficiencies, no muscular coordination, leukemia lymphoma, malignancy
	MRE11	Exonuclease	DNA damage sensitivity, genomic instability; telomere shortening, aberrant meiosis; SCID[d]
	PRKDC	Ser/Thr kinase	SCID
	Bloom's BLM	Helicase	Lymphatic and malignancies, Fanconi anemia
	FANCA-G	Protein control	Multiple congenital malformations Pancytopenia, short telomeres
	Werner WRN	Helicase exonuclease	Premature senility, short stature cataracts, loss of muscle and connective tissue, malignancy
	RecQ4	Helicase	Osteosarcoma, premature aging

AGT=O^6-alkyl-*G*-Alkytransferase; ATT=O^4-alkyl-*T*-alkyltransferase.
[a]Expanded to other DNA repair genes beyond those listed in the text.
[b]One alkyltransferase molecule accepts one methylated adduction product from the DNA.
[c]HNPCC, hereditary nonpolyposis colorectal cancer.
[d]Severe combined immunodeficiency.

More recently, multiple genes related to colon cancer susceptibility have been shown to be missing or have DNA sequence mutations. Some of these defects are inherited, but others acquire mutations or deletions. This latter molecular mechanism, originally described as the 'Mutator Phenotype,' was first advanced by Loeb in 1974 (Loeb, 1989). The mutator phenotype implies the rapid acquisition of mutations during tumor development, which led to the concept of tumor suppressor genes. The concept of tumor suppressor genes was further refined to encompass 'caretaker genes,' 'gatekeeper genes,' and 'landscaper genes.' The genes involved in heredity nonpolyposis colorectal cancer are examples of caretaker genes (Kinzler and Vogelstein, 1998, and **Table 2**).

Summary

Human chemical carcinogens are frequently inert or poorly reactive, and generally they require activation by enzymes before they can exert their biological effects. Principal enzymes involved in this process belong to the cytochrome p450 superfamily. Activated or unstable chemical species then bind covalently with electrophilic molecules, for example, DNA and proteins. This process in turn can lead to DNA sequence mutations. However, DNA damage resulting from chemical carcinogen exposure may be mitigated by the DNA repair process. With the exposition of the human genome, it is expected that the elucidation of the molecular basis of DNA repair, and diseases associated with defects in the genes that control DNA repair, will move forward in the future.

Disclaimer

The findings/conclusions in this article are those of the authors and do not necessarily represent the views of the National Institute for Occupational Safety and Health or the National Cancer Institute.

See also: Aminobiphenyl, 4-; Coal Tar; Radon; Uranium; Cancer Chemotherapeutic Agents; The Exposome; Persistent Organic Pollutants; Aflatoxin; Apoptosis; Benz[a]anthracene; Benzo(a) pyrene; Chrysene; Coke Oven Emissions; Cytochrome P450; Dibenz[*a,h*]anthracene; National Institute for Occupational Safety and Health; Oxidative Stress; Biomarkers, Human Healthealth; Carcinogenesis; Diesel Exhaust; Genetic Toxicology; International Agency for Research on Cancer; Toxicology; Mixtures, Toxicology, and Risk Assessment; Risk Assessment, Human Health; Pollution, Air in Encyclopedia of Toxicology; Pollution, Soil; Pollution, Water; Levels of Effect in Toxicology Assessment; Polycyclic Aromatic Amines; Polycyclic Aromatic Hydrocarbons (PAHs); Tobacco; Toxicology Testing, Carcinogenicity; Toxicology Testing, Mutagenicity; Environmental Biomarkers; Biomonitoring; Environmental Toxicology; Heterocyclic Amines; UVA; UVB.

Further Reading

Cleaver, J.E., 2008. Historical aspects of xeroderma pigmentosum and nucleotide excision repair. Adv. Exp. Med. Sci. 637, 1–9.

Gyorffy, E., Anna, L., Kovacs, K., Rudnai, P., Schoket, B., 2008. Correlation between biomarkers of human exposure to genotoxins with focus on carcinogen-DNA adducts. Mutagenesis 23, 1–18.

International Agency for Research on Cancer, 2010. IARC Monographs on the Evaluation of Carcinogenic Risks to Humans. In: Some Non-heterocyclic Polycyclic Hydrocarbons and Some Related Exposures, vol. 92. IARC, Lyon, France, p 394, 565–584.

Kasparek, T.R., Humphrey, T.C., 2011. DNA double-strand break repair pathways, chromosomal rearrangements and cancer. Semin. Cell. Dev. Biol. 22, 866–897.

Kinzler, K.W., Vogelstein, B., 1998. Landscaping the cancer terrain. Science 280, 1036–1037.

Kraemer, K.H., Patronas, N.J., Schiffmann, R., Brooks, B.P., Tamura, D., DiGiovanna, J.J., 2007. Xeroderma pigmentosum, trichothiodystrophy and Cockayne syndrome: a complex genotype-phenotype relationship. Neuroscience 145, 1388–1396.

Li, J., Bhat, A., Xiao, W., 2011. Regulation of nucleotide excision repair through ubiquination. Acta Biochim. Biophys. Sin. 43, 919–929.

Loeb, L.A., 1994. Human cancers express mutator phenotypes: origin, consequences and targeting. Nat. Rev. Cancer 11, 450–457.

Pegg, A.E., 2011. Multifaceted roles of alkyltransferases and related proteins in DNA repair, DNA damage, resistance to chemotherapy, and research tools. Chem. Res. Toxicol. 24, 618–639.

Poirier, M.C., 2012. Chemical-induced DNA damage and human cancer risk. Discov. Med. 14, 283–288.

Rezazadeh, S., 2012. RecQ helicases; at the crossroad of genome replication, repair, and recombination. Mol. Biol. Rep. 39, 4527–4543.

Weston, A., Harris, C.C., 2010. Chemical carcinogenesis. In: Holland, J.F., Frei, E., Bast, R. (Eds.), Cancer Medicine, eighth ed. B.C. Decker Inc, Hamilton, ON, Canada, pp. 225–236.

Carcinogenesis

MC Botelho and JP Teixeira, National Institute of Health, Porto, Portugal
PA Oliveira, University of Trás-os-Montes e Alto Douro, Vila Real, Portugal

This article is a revision of the previous edition article by David E. Malarkey and Robert R. Maronpot, volume 1, pp 445–466, © 2005, Elsevier Inc.

Overview

Cancer, or neoplasia, which occurs in one of every four individuals and results in the death of one of every four individuals in the United States and Europe, is a complex disease with multiple causes. Many intrinsic and extrinsic factors influence the development of cancer. Intrinsic or host factors include age, sex, genetic constitution, immune system function, metabolism, hormone levels, and nutritional status. Extrinsic factors include substances eaten, drunk, or smoked; workplace and environmental (air, water, and soil) exposures; natural and medical radiation exposure; sexual behavior; and elements of lifestyle such as social and cultural environment, personal behavior, and habits. Intrinsic and extrinsic factors can interact with one another to influence the development of cancer. Because of the physical and emotional suffering associated with cancer and the immense cost to the nation in lost production and income and medical and research expenditures, considerable effort continues to be exerted to understand this complex disease so that strategies can be developed to decrease or prevent its occurrence. Current regulatory guidelines have been crafted to reduce the probability of developing cancer by lowering human exposure to agents identified as potentially capable of causing cancer.

During the past 40 years of cancer research, much information has been generated indicating that cancer is a multistep, progressive disease. Support for this contention is derived from research on epidemiology and population genetics, morphological and clinical study of neoplasms, as well as experimental investigations in animals. Structural studies of biopsy and autopsy tissue samples from humans and necropsy samples from animals, particularly experimental animal models of carcinogenesis, have provided important information about this multistep process at the phenotypic level. More recently, molecular biological analyses have confirmed the principles that neoplasms arise from the clonal expansion of a single cell and that during its evolution into a neoplastic mass, it accumulates nonlethal genetic damage, particularly in genes that regulate growth and DNA repair processes. The process of carcinogenesis may take months in experimental laboratory animals and years in humans. Identification of this process early in its evolution enhances the likelihood that intervention strategies such as surgical removal of a benign neoplasm may result in termination of the disease and clinical cure. By the time a neoplasm has progressed to the malignant stage and spread throughout the body, even heroic radiation and chemotherapy combined with surgery are unlikely to result in clinical cure. The process of carcinogenesis may be depicted schematically as in **Figure 1** with the various steps along the pathway from normalcy to malignancy characterized by morphological and/or clinical features. It is here that the disciplines of clinical oncology, molecular biology, and pathology are utilized to define the location of the specific neoplasm in this progressive cascade.

Nomenclature of Cancer (Neoplasia)

The nomenclature associated with the study of cancer is frequently confusing because a given term often has a relatively

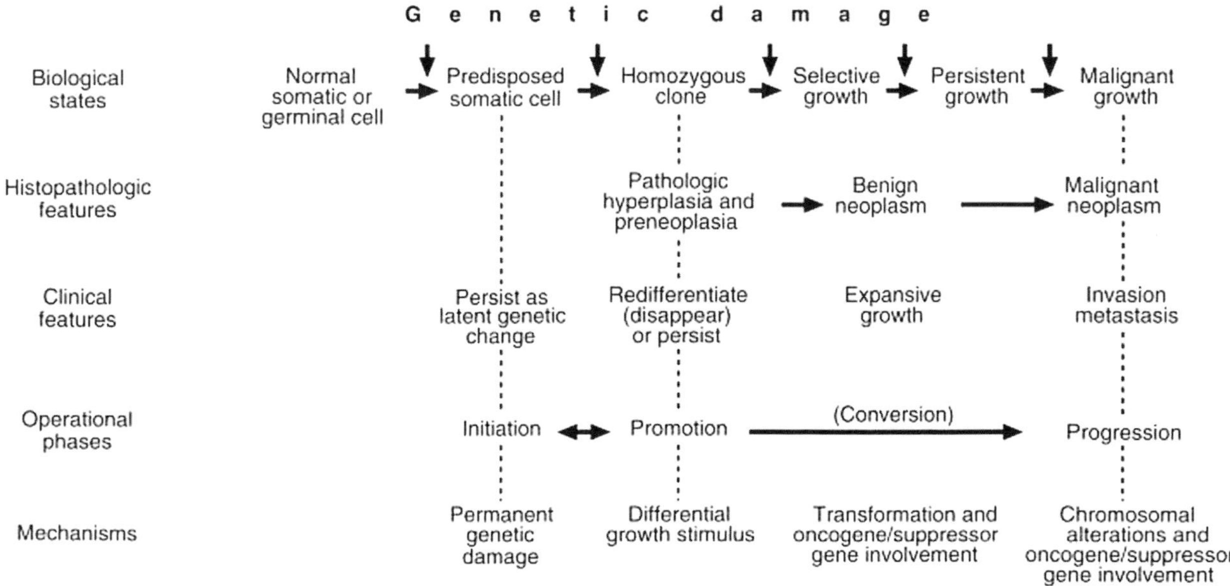

Figure 1 Process of carcinogenesis depicted schematically showing the postulate pathway in which accumulation of genetic damage leads to malignant neoplasia.

 http://dx.doi.org/10.1016/B978-0-12-386454-3.00371-7

narrow as well as a considerably broader definition based on common usage. Carcinogenesis, for example, is narrowly defined as the production of carcinoma but is more commonly used in the broadest possible sense to indicate generation of neoplasms that are new and typically abnormal growths, generally uncontrolled, and becoming progressively more serious with time. Neoplasia, meaning 'new growth' and often used synonymously with carcinogenesis, refers to the process of development of neoplasms. Two important terms that relate to the clinical behavior and growth characteristics of neoplasms are (1) benign and (2) malignant, characteristic features of which are listed in **Table 1**. Basically, benign neoplasms are slow-growing, localized growths frequently amenable to surgical removal with a low probability of recurrence. Malignant neoplasms have a more aggressive growth, are locally invasive, sometimes metastasize (spread to distant sites), and are difficult to remove surgically.

Two terms that have both a narrow and a broad definition are (1) tumor and (2) cancer. Tumor broadly refers to any tissue enlargement or swelling; however, it is often used synonymously with the term neoplasm. A cancer generally refers to a malignant neoplasm. Unfortunately, the layperson and the professional frequently use tumor and cancer interchangeably alike without qualifying whether it is a benign or malignant process. In other words, if it is said that an individual has a tumor, that individual may have a benign neoplasm (most often the case) but could have a malignant neoplasm if the term 'tumor' is being used loosely. If an individual is said to have a cancer, that usually means the individual has a malignant neoplasm but, here again, loose use of the term 'cancer' might include any neoplasm, including a benign one. Scientists contribute to the confusion by sometimes indicating that an agent may cause cancer, meaning either benign or malignant neoplasia. Alternatively, they may indicate that an agent is tumorigenic, which could mean that it causes tumors but frequently means that it may also cause malignant neoplasms (cancers). Common and uncritical usage of these terms is so ingrained that attempts to standardize nomenclature have been largely unsuccessful. The least ambiguous terms are 'benign neoplasm' and 'malignant neoplasm.'

Most neoplasms are classified and named based on (1) the cell or tissue of origin and (2) benign or malignant growth characteristics. There are two basic cell types from which neoplasms may originate: mesenchymal cells and epithelial cells (**Figure 2**). Mesenchymal pertains to mesenchyme (embryonic connective tissue in the mesoderm) from which adult tissues such as connective tissue, blood and lymphatic vessels, and muscles and bones are formed. Epithelial cells line the internal and external surfaces of the body and form many of the major organs such as liver and lungs. Most epithelial tissues are derived from the embryonic germ layers referred to as entoderm and ectoderm.

There are general guidelines used in naming neoplasms. A benign epithelial neoplasm originating within a glandular tissue is called an 'adenoma,' having the prefix 'adeno' to designate that the origin is one of many glandular tissues and the suffix 'oma' to indicate a swelling or tissue enlargement. One or more qualifiers may be added to the name to indicate the tissue of origin and various morphological features as in hepatocellular (liver cell) adenoma, thyroid follicular (forming follicles) adenoma, or renal (kidney) tubular cell adenoma. An adenoma with morphological features resembling fingerlike or warty projections would be called a papillary adenoma; with cystic spaces, a cystadenoma; with both of these features, a papillary cystadenoma. Benign mesenchymal neoplasms also utilize the 'oma' suffix in their name, as in meningioma, hemangioma, and fibroma. The prefix for mesenchymal neoplasms usually identifies the specific tissue of origin such as meninges (meningioma), blood vessels (hemangioma), or fibrous connective tissue (fibroma). Nomenclature for several benign neoplasms is presented in **Table 2**.

Malignant epithelial neoplasms are typically called 'carcinomas' and qualified by histogenetic origin. Thus, malignant skin neoplasms are called epidermal carcinomas if they arise in the superficial layers or epidermis of the skin. If they are composed predominantly of squamous cells, they are called squamous cell carcinomas; if chiefly basal cells, basal cell carcinomas. Malignant mesenchymal neoplasms are called 'sarcomas.' Examples of the latter include fibrosarcoma, a malignant neoplasm of the connective tissue; osteosarcoma,

Table 1 Comparative features of benign and malignant neoplasms

Effect	*Benign*	*Malignant*
General effect on host	Little; not generally lethal	Will usually kill the host if not treated
Injury to host	Usually negligible but may compress or obstruct vital tissue	Can kill the host by destruction of vital tissue
Growth rate	Slow	Rapid (but slower than tissue repair); growth escapes, normal control mechanisms
Extent of growth	Encapsulated; remains localized at site of origin	Infiltrates or invades and spreads to distant sited
Mode of growth	Typically grows by expansion and displaces surrounding tissues	Invades and destroys surrounding tissues
Microscopic features	Cells and structures formed by cells resemble normal tissues; may be encapsulated	Anaplastic, dysplastic, and pleomorphic; may be associated with hemorrhage, necrosis, and inflammation
Cytologic features	Mitoses rare; nucleus normal in staining and shape; nucleolus not conspicuous	Mitoses may be numerous and abnormal; nucleus often enlarged, irregular in shape, and hyperchromatic; nucleolus hyperchromatic and enlarged
Radiation sensitivity	Radiation sensitivity similar to that of normal tissues; rarely treated with radiation	Radiation sensitivity increased in approximate proportion to the degree of malignancy; frequently treated with radiation

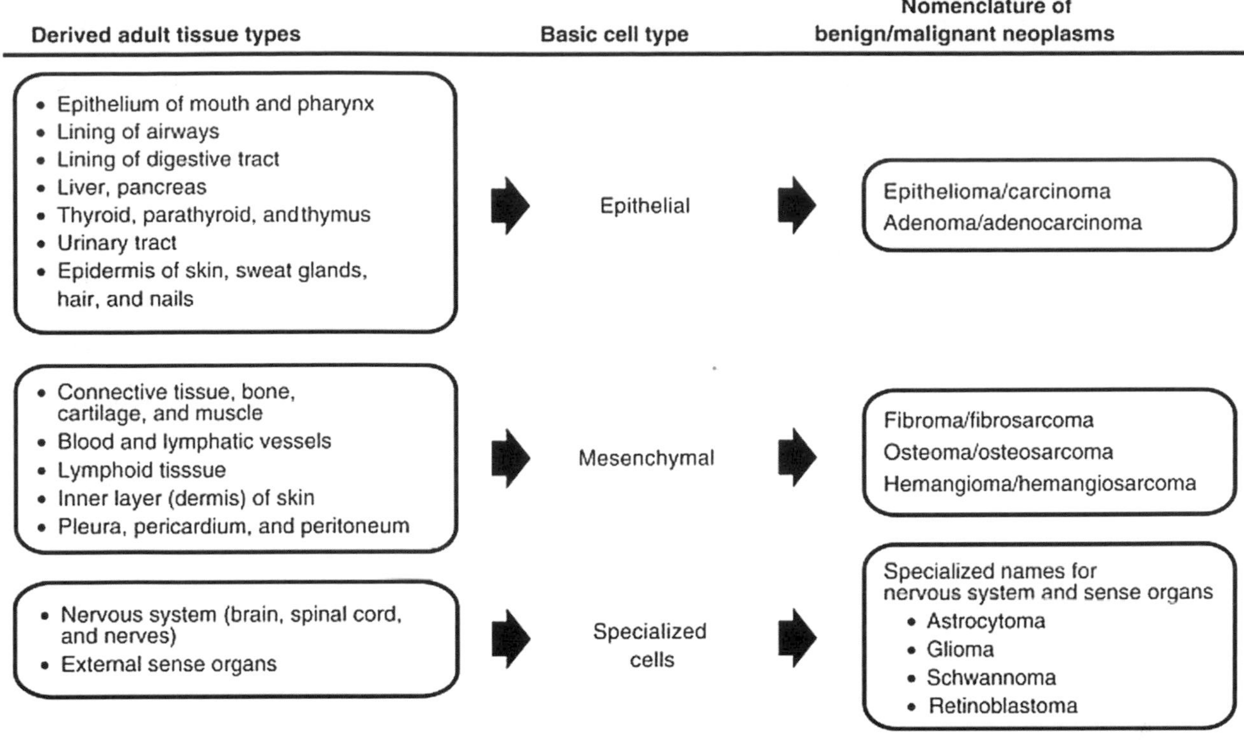

Derived adult tissue types
Basic cell type
Nomenclature of benign/malignant neoplasms
• Epithelium of mouth and pharynx
• Lining of airways
• Lining of digestive tract
• Liver, pancreas
• Thyroid, parathyroid, and thymus
• Urinary tract
• Epidermis of skin, sweat glands, hair, and nails
Epithelial
Epithelioma/carcinoma
Adenoma/adenocarcinoma
• Connective tissue, bone, cartilage, and muscle
• Blood and lymphatic vessels
• Lymphoid tisssue
• Inner layer (dermis) of skin
• Pleura, pericardium, and peritoneum
Mesenchymal
Fibroma/fibrosarcoma
Osteoma/osteosarcoma
Hemangioma/hemangiosarcoma
• Nervous system (brain, spinal cord, and nerves)
• External sense organs
Specialized cells
Specialized names for nervous system and sense organs
• Astrocytoma
• Glioma
• Schwannoma
• Retinoblastoma

Figure 2 Tissue types associated with neoplasm names.

a malignant bone neoplasm; and leiomyosarcoma, a malignant neoplasm of the smooth muscle tissue. The nomenclature for several malignant neoplasms is presented in **Table 2**.

Much of the general confusion surrounding the nomenclature of neoplasms results from numerous exceptions and permutations in the general histogenetic and clinical guidelines for naming neoplasms. Many of these exceptions are deeply ingrained in traditional pathology practice, and attempts at standardization have been largely unsuccessful. Examples are thymoma, lymphoma, melanoma, and neuroblastoma – neoplasms that are generally regarded as malignant despite their benign-sounding names and should more properly be called malignant thymoma or thymic sarcoma, malignant lymphoma or lymphosarcoma, malignant melanoma or melanosarcoma, and malignant neuroblastoma, respectively. Other neoplasms are named for their physical attributes such as pheochromocytoma (dark-colored neoplasms typically arising in the adrenal medulla). In addition, some neoplasms were originally named for the person first describing the lesion, and examples such as Hodgkin's disease of lymphoid tissue and Wilms' kidney tumor have persisted to this day. Neoplasms composed of mixtures of cells are named accordingly; examples include fibroadenoma, adenosquamous carcinoma, and carcinosarcoma. To complicate matters further, there are several tissue alterations that are not neoplasms but have names suggesting that they are: hamartomas (a disorganized aggregate of normal tissue components thought to represent faulty differentiation during embryonic development) and choristomas (focal collections of normal tissue found at an abnormal site such as islands of pancreatic cells in the wall of the stomach). There are also instances in which a neoplasm is histologically considered malignant but clinically benign, such as in basal cell carcinoma of the skin. In addition, localized overgrowths of normal tissue components such as skin tags and vocal cord polyps are clinically recognized as tumors but are not truly neoplastic.

Tissue Changes Associated with Carcinogenesis

Quantitative – Hyperplasia and Preneoplasia

Proliferative lesions, which may be classified morphologically as hyperplasia, preneoplasia, benign neoplasia, or malignant neoplasia, represent a continuum of change with considerable overlap rather than discrete morphologic entities (**Figure 3**). The definitive classification of a given lesion as preneoplasia, benign neoplasia, or malignant neoplasia represents a judgment based on the experience of the diagnostic pathologist and familiarity with the species and tissue in question. These lesions are recognized by their microscopic appearance and effect on surrounding tissues and typically are a localized proliferation or hyperplasia of a specific cell type. Most neoplasms are believed to be derived from the clonal proliferation of a single initiated cell. Usually at some point early in the clonal expansion, the differentially proliferating cells become phenotypically distinguishable from the surrounding normal tissue. Although such lesions may not yet have sufficient characteristics to qualify as neoplasms, their recognition early in the process of carcinogenesis has led many to regard them as 'preneoplastic.'

There is considerable confusion regarding the significance of hyperplasia in the neoplastic process. Hyperplasia is an increase

Table 2 Selected nomenclature of neoplasia

Tissue	*Benign neoplasia*	*Malignant neoplasia*
Epithelium		
Squamous	Squamous cell papilloma	Squamous cell carcinoma
Transitional	Transitional cell papilloma	Transition cell carcinoma
Glandular		
Liver cell	Hepatocellular adenoma	Hepatocellular carcinoma
Islet cell	Islet cell adenoma	Islet cell adenocarcinoma
Connective tissue		
Adult fibrous	Fibroma	Fibrosarcoma
Embryonic	Myxoma	Myxosarcoma
Cartilage	Chondroma	Chondrosarcoma
Bone	Osteoma	Osteosarcoma
Fat	Lipoma	Liposarcoma
Muscle		
Smooth	Leiomyoma	Leiomyosarcoma
Skeletal	Rhabdomyoma	Rhabdomyosarcoma
Cardiac	Rhabdomyoma	Rhabdomyosarcoma
Endothelium		
Lymph	Lymphangioma	Lymphangiosarcoma
Blood	Hemangioma	Hemangiosarcoma
Lymphoreticular		
Thymus	Not recognized	Thymoma
Lymph nodes	Not recognized	Lymphosarcoma (malignant lymphoma)
Hematopoietic		
Bone marrow	Not recognized	Leukemia
Neural tissue		
Nerve sheath	Neurilemmoma	Neurilemmosarcoma
Astrocytes	Not recognized	Astrocytoma

Note: -oma, swelling; sarc-, malignant neoplasm of mesenchymal origin; carcin-, malignant neoplasm of epithelial origin.

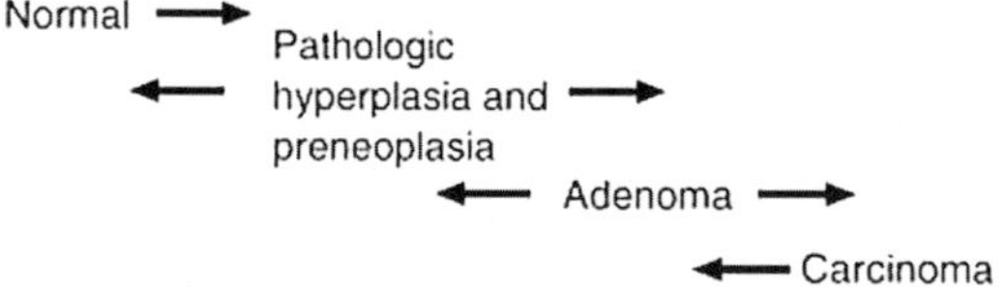

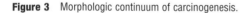

Figure 3 Morphologic continuum of carcinogenesis.

in the number of cells per unit of tissue, typically limited in amount and terminating when the stimulus that evoked it is removed. Different cell types have varying capacities to undergo hyperplasia in response to physiological or pathological stimuli. One of the most difficult judgments, even for the experienced pathologist, is whether an observed hyperplasia is part of the process of cancer development or merely an adaptive or physiologic response not likely to progress to neoplasia. The tissue affected, whether the hyperplasia is diffuse or nodular, the age of the affected individual, the proximate cause of the hyperplastic response, and the growth pattern of the hyperplastic tissues influence this judgment.

Preneoplasia refers to an increase in proliferative lesions that lead to the development of a tumor (an absolute increase in the number of cells in a tissue). Although not all neoplasms exhibit a preneoplastic change recognizable by the pathologist, in those instances in which presumptive alterations are observed, their occurrence documents that there is a response to tissue insult. Examples of presumptive preneoplastic lesions are presented in **Table 3**. In those experimental models of carcinogenesis in which preneoplasia is observed, it precedes the occurrence of benign neoplasia. An important feature of preneoplastic lesions is their propensity for reversibility. In some instances, a preneoplastic lesion represents the clonal expansion of a cell that has sustained genetic damage so that benign neoplasms arise within the preneoplastic lesion, presumably when one of the preneoplastic cells sustains additional genetic damage, giving it a growth advantage. In other situations, the antecedent change is a localized polyclonal cellular proliferation historically associated with subsequent development of a neoplasm in the same tissue. A classical example is alcoholic cirrhosis, which in the case of chronic alcohol abuse, leads to multiple, polyclonal areas of liver cell hyperplasia and an increased risk for the development of hepatocellular neoplasia. In both preneoplasia and certain forms of hyperplasia, the antecedent lesions typically have a higher rate of cell proliferation than the surrounding normal cells and, thus, these cells are at increased risk to sustain additional genetic damage and progress to the next stage in the carcinogenic process.

A benign neoplasm is generally a localized expansive growth that compresses adjacent normal tissue but is usually not immediately life threatening unless it physically interferes with normal function, for example, by blocking the intestinal tract or compressing vital areas in the brain. Controversy regarding the significance of benign neoplasia with respect to the development of malignancy is similar to that associated

Table 3 Examples of presumptive preneoplastic lesions

Tissue	*Presumptive preneoplastic lesion*
Mammary gland	Hyperplastic alveolar nodules
	Atypical epithelial hyperplasia
	Lobular hyperplasia
	Intraductal hyperplasia
	Hyperplastic terminal duct
Liver	Foci of cellular alteration
	Hepatocellular hyperplasia
	Oval cell proliferation
	Cholangiofibrosis
Kidney	Atypical tubular dilation
	Atypical tubular hyperplasia
Skin	Increase in dark basal keratinocytes
	Focal hyperplasia/hyperkeratosis
Pancreas	Foci of acinar cell alteration
	Hyperplastic nodules
	Atypical acinar cell nodules
Colon	Aberrant crypt foci
Bladder cancer	Nodular hyperplasia

with preneoplastic lesions. A benign neoplasm, the clonal expansion of cells that have sustained some degree of genetic damage, is further along the spectrum of changes that precede the development of malignant neoplasia. In experimental carcinogenesis animal models, malignant neoplasia is not infrequently observed arising from or within a benign neoplasm. Features of benign neoplasms are listed in **Table 1**.

Malignant neoplasms are rapidly growing, locally invasive tissue proliferations that destroy surrounding tissues and are thus life threatening. They also have the malicious feature of spreading to distant sites in the body via the blood and lymphatic system. Although malignancy develops with greater frequency in association with (1) pathologic hyperplasia and preneoplasia, (2) qualitative alterations in cells, and (3) benign neoplasia than in association with normal tissues, these changes are not necessary precursors to malignancy. *In situ* carcinomas are malignant neoplasms that originate without evidence of antecedent benign tissue alteration. When precursor lesions are present prior to or concomitant with malignant neoplasia, it is probable that the malignancy is a consequence of the same or similar factors that produced the precursor lesions. Characteristics of malignant neoplasms are listed in **Table 1**.

Qualitative – Metaplasia, Dysplasia, and Anaplasia

In addition to quantitative increases in certain cells, several qualitative cytological features help allow the morphologic classification of the spectrum of proliferative lesions that may be observed in the process of carcinogenesis. Three frequently used qualitative cytological features are metaplasia, dysplasia, and anaplasia.

Metaplasia is the reversible substitution of one type of fully differentiated cell for another within a given tissue. A classic example is the replacement of the normal ciliated columnar epithelial cells in the respiratory tract airways by squamous epithelium (**Figure 4**) in situations in which there is chronic irritation from certain components of inhaled tobacco smoke. While the squamous epithelium is believed to provide functional protection against the irritant properties of the smoke, the loss of the ciliated columnar epithelium results in the reduction of functional capacity of the lungs to clear particulates from respiratory tract. When the irritation is removed, the squamous epithelium is replaced by normal ciliated columnar epithelium.

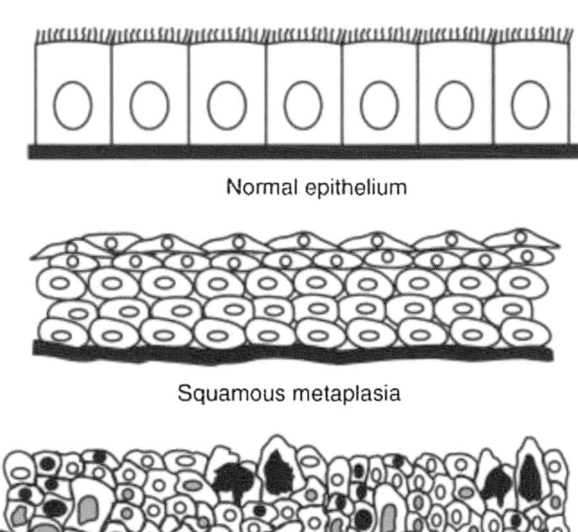

Figure 4 Qualitative changes in epithelial tissues.

Dysplasia is defined as abnormal growth of a tissue with respect to shape, size, and organization of component cells. Normal cell-to-cell orientations are disorganized or disrupted, and the cells themselves vary in size and shape (**Figure 4**). When present, dysplasia may be associated with chronic irritation, occur with metaplasia, and be seen in neoplastic transformation. It is a change that is a hallmark of increased risk for development of neoplasia. Like metaplasia, dysplasia is a potentially reversible tissue alteration. It is also considered in some circumstances as a preneoplastic change.

Anaplasia is a qualitative alteration of cellular differentiation. Anaplastic cells are typically undifferentiated and may bear little, if any, resemblance to mature cells. This feature is considered a hallmark of malignancy.

Staging and Grading of Cancers

In human oncology, the experience from collective years of observation of the outcome of many cancers has strengthened the predicitivity of histological grades and clinical staging in prognostication. The purpose of grading and staging a neoplasm is to predict its biological behavior and to help establish an appropriate therapeutic regimen. Grading is a subjective evaluation of morphologic characteristics based on the extent of cellular anaplasia and the degree of proliferation evident from microscopic evaluation. Generally, neoplasms with a high degree of anaplasia, associated specific morphologic patterns of growth, and evidence of numerous mitoses, some of which may be abnormal, are given a high grade of malignancy. Most grading schemes categorize neoplasms into one of three or four grades of increasing malignancy.

Staging of a cancer, which is independent of grading, is an index of the extent to which a cancer has spread in the body. It also provides information regarding the patient's clinical prognosis, and usually influences the choice of appropriate therapy more than grading. Criteria used for staging neoplasms include the size of the primary neoplasm, the degree to which there is invasion of surrounding normal tissues, whether the cancer has spread to local lymph nodes, and the presence of spread to distant sites in the body. Thus, it is apparent that staging will have a large influence on the therapeutic approach. A small and localized breast cancer would most likely be treated by surgical excision and possibly radiation therapy, whereas a large, infiltrative breast cancer would more likely be treated by mastectomy. If the cancer has spread to lymph nodes or distant sites, more aggressive therapy is implemented.

The ultimate fate of cells or proliferative tissue masses is influenced by the amount of sustained genetic damage. Cells with minimal DNA damage may persist in a latent form, indistinguishable from surrounding normal cells. If such a latent cell sustains additional damage even long after the initial insult, it may then progress further along the pathway to malignancy (see **Figure 1**). As additional genetic damage occurs, the altered cell population expands and eventually leads to irreversible uncontrolled growth that may or may not be corrected by aggressive medical intervention.

Molecular Basis of Cancer

Multistep Genetic Model of Carcinogenesis

Genetically, the multistage process involves the activation of growth-enhancing proto-oncogenes, inactivation of the recessive growth-inhibitory tumor suppressor genes, as well as epigenetic events that alter gene expression and processes such as those involved in cell death, DNA repair, and methylation (**Table 4**). Cancer cells frequently contain mutations in multiple genes as well as large chromosomal abnormalities. Since their discovery ~25 years ago, more than 100 proto-oncogenes and ~15 tumor suppressor genes have been identified. Proto-oncogenes were first discovered in cancer-causing animal viruses that carried them. Intense study of these viruses, particularly by Varmus and Bishop in the 1970s, resulted in the discovery that endogenous animal genes had been picked up by virus ancestors and incorporated into the viral genome. Soon thereafter a number of these proto-oncogenes were identified in both the animal and human genome and later found to play a role in cancer development.

A widely accepted multistep model of carcinogenesis proposed by Fearon and Vogelstein in 1990 serves as the framework for studies in carcinogenesis (**Figure 5**). By studying multiple benign and malignant colonic neoplasms from individuals with multiple tumors, they found that benign neoplasms harbored mutations in genes such as APC, *ras*, and p53, and that there were frequently multiple mutations per neoplasm, particularly of the malignant neoplasms. The model describes a progressive acquisition of mutations, and it is believed the total accumulation of mutations (at least five to seven) rather than the order is important in the carcinogenic process. New evidence has been published to further refine this model. Recently, it has been proposed that some neoplasms are dependent on the continued activation or overexpression of a particular oncogene for maintaining malignant behavior. Others have found that some neoplasms are 'hypersensitive' to the inhibitory effects of specific tumor suppressor genes. These findings suggest that the multistage process of carcinogenesis is not simply a summation of individual effects of cancer genes but that some individual cancer genes can override the others (referred to by some as the 'Achilles heel of cancer'), and they offer new strategies for the prevention and therapy of cancer.

Table 4 Genetic and epigenetic events involved in cancer development

Proto-oncogenes (growth-enhancing)	
Growth factors	PDGF-B, FGF, sis
Growth factor receptors	EGFR, CSF
Signal transduction	*ras, abl*
Nuclear regulatory proteins	*myc, fos*
Cell cycle regulators	Cyclins and cdks
Tumor suppressor genes (growth-inhibiting)	
Cell surface molecules	TGF-βR
Regulate signal transduction	NF1
DNA repair, cell cycle	p53, Rb, BRCA1
Apoptosis genes	Bcl-2, Bcl-x, Bax, bad, Bcl-xS
DNA repair genes	HNPCC, XP
Epigenetic events	Methylation

Oncogenes

Among the estimated 25 000 genes in the mammalian genome, there are about 100 genes that are classified as oncogenes because activation of these genes appears to be an essential event for the development of many, if not all, cancers. In fact, oncogenes were first discovered by studying genetic alterations in cancers. The term oncogene activation indicates a quantitative or qualitative alteration in the expression or function of the oncogene. The term oncogene is unfortunate since the unaltered (nonactivated) oncogene (usually referred to as a proto-oncogene) actually serves an essential function in the mammalian genome. That proto-oncogenes are highly conserved in evolution is evidenced by structurally and functionally similar genes in yeast, earthworms, animals, and humans. The highly conserved nature of proto-oncogenes is believed to be related to their essential function in normal tissue growth and differentiation. Since their normal function is to control how a tissue grows and develops, it is apparent that, if they do not function appropriately, abnormal growth and development may occur. When a primary manifestation of such abnormal growth was observed to be neoplasia, these proto-oncogenes were named oncogenes. This nomenclature has persisted despite the ultimate discovery that the unaltered forms of these genes are normal components of the genome.

The appearance (phenotype) and function of a tissue is a consequence of which genes are actively producing their programmed product, typically a protein, which in turn affects the structure and function of the cells comprising a given tissue. All somatic cells in the body inherit a complete complement of maternal and paternal genes. The reason that some cells form liver and produce products such as albumin while other cells form kidney tubules that function to excrete substances from the body is a consequence of which genes are expressed in those cells. In liver cells, several critical genes that are important in kidney function are not expressed and vice versa. Specific gene expression and its effect on tissue phenotype and function are modulated by several intrinsic and extrinsic factors (**Figure 6**). Since a primary function of many oncogenes is to control cell growth, proliferation, and differentiation, inappropriate expression of these genes would be expected to influence abnormally tissue proliferation and growth. Oncogene activation is a consequence of inappropriate or excessive expression of a proto-oncogene.

Oncogenes can be activated by several different mechanisms (e.g., retroviral transduction, chromosomal translocation, gene amplification, point mutation, promoter/enhancer insertion, or decreased methylation of promoters). Once activated, an oncogene will be either inappropriately expressed (e.g., production of an altered message and protein) or overexpressed (e.g., production of too much of a normal message and protein). Either situation may contribute to the

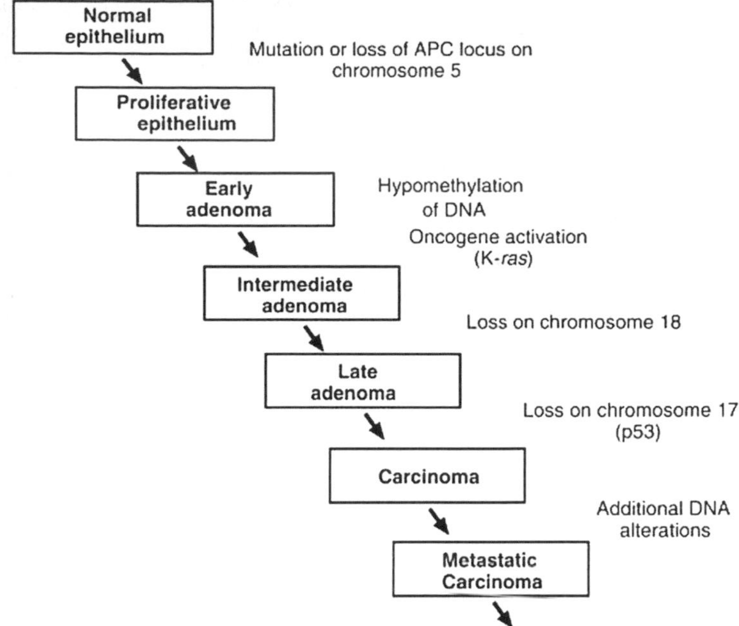

Figure 5 Multistep aspects of human colon carcinogenesis.

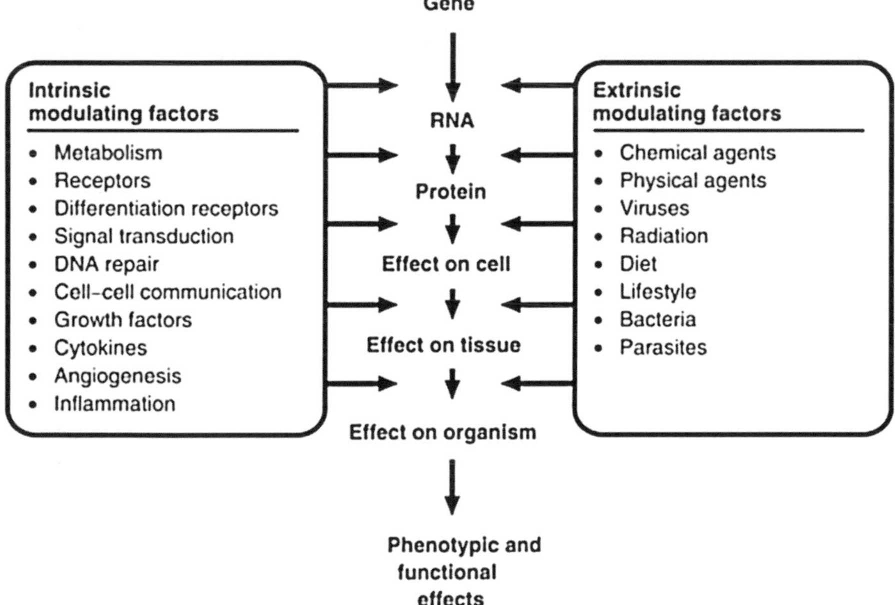

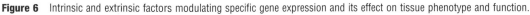

Figure 6 Intrinsic and extrinsic factors modulating specific gene expression and its effect on tissue phenotype and function.

neoplastic process by influencing cellular proliferation and differentiation. Examples of activated or amplified oncogenes detected in human and animal neoplasms are listed in **Tables 5** and **6**, respectively. For some cancers, the frequency of oncogene activation is relatively high, while for other cancers, the activation of known oncogenes is uncommon. Identification of specific alterations in oncogenes in certain cancers represents a first step in determining the molecular basis of cancer and could eventually lead to the development of molecular intervention and therapeutic strategies. Experimental evidence indicates that oncogene activation can be an early critical event in carcinogenesis, and experimental studies with known chemical carcinogens show that they produce specific alterations in certain oncogenes, reflecting the manner in which the carcinogen chemically affects DNA.

Tumor Suppressor Genes

Tumor suppressor genes, originally called antioncogenes, function to suppress the development of cancerous growth.

Table 5 Examples of human neoplasms associated with activated or amplified oncogenes

Oncogene	*Type of human neoplasia*
H-RAS	Squamous cell carcinoma
	Urinary bladder carcinoma
	Lung carcinoma
	Acute myelogenous leukemia
K-RAS	Lung adenocarcinoma
	Colon carcinoma
	Ovarian carcinoma
	Gastric carcinoma
	Renal cell carcinoma
	Acute myelogenous leukemia
	Pancreatic ductal adenocarcinoma
N-RAS	Acute myelogenous leukemia
	Chronic myelogenous leukemia
ABL	Chronic myelogenous leukemia
$ERBB_2$	Breast carcinoma
	Salivary gland adenocarcinoma
MYC	Small cell carcinoma of the lung
	Burkitt's lymphoma
N-MYC	Neuroblastoma

Table 6 Examples of animals neoplasms associated with activated oncogenes

Oncogene	*Type of animal neoplasia*
H-ras	Hepatocellular adenoma and carcinoma
	Harderian gland adenoma
	Mammary carcinoma
	Skin squamous cell carcinoma
K-ras	Lung adenoma and adenocarcinoma
	Pancreatic carcinoma
	Hepatocellular carcinoma
N-ras	Leukemia
	Lymphosarcoma
Raf	Fibrosarcoma
neu ($erbB_2$)	Neuroblastoma
Abl	Lymphosarcoma
C-myc	Leukemia
	Lymphosarcoma

While oncogenes must be activated to be effective, tumor suppressor genes must be inactivated or lost for cancer to develop. It has been shown that loss or mutation of both paternal and maternal copies, that is, in both alleles, of a tumor suppressor gene must occur to ablate their effect of suppressing cancer formation. A well-known and extensively studied tumor suppressor gene is the retinoblastoma gene (*RB-1*). In hereditary retinoblastoma, an affected child is born with deletions of portions of one allele of chromosome 13 containing the *RB-1* gene. If a second event leading to a loss or alteration of the remaining *RB-1* allele occurs while retinal cells are undergoing growth during development, the ocular neoplasm retinoblastoma, frequently present in both eyes, will occur early in life. Loss or alteration of both copies of this tumor suppressor gene is sufficient to cause retinoblastoma. Although named for the disease in which it was discovered, alterations in the *RB-1* gene have been detected in breast, lung, prostate, and bone cancers.

Acquisition of Mutations

The rate of mutation has been intensely studied in the carcinogenic process. Mutations in cellular DNA can arise during normal cell replication by infidelity in DNA replication (mispairing) as well as by chromosomal deletions, amplifications, or rearrangements. Considering mispairing in nucleotide bases alone, it is estimated that spontaneous mispairing during normal cell replication can occur with a frequency of $\sim 1.4 \times 10^{-10}$ nucleotide bases per cell division. Since there are $\sim 10^{16}$ cell divisions per human lifespan and 2×10^9 nucleotide base pairs per genome, a total of 2.8×10^{15} mispairings could occur in a lifetime $((1.4 \times 10^{-10}) \times (2 \times 10^9) \times 10^{16})$. If each mispair led to a mutation that resulted in a cancer, a typical human would have billions of cancers in one average lifetime. Since such estimates of cancer frequency are clearly in excess of what is observed, it is necessary to postulate that events in addition to a single mutation are necessary for most cancers to occur and that many mispairings are repaired or fatal to the cell. There are efficient mechanisms to repair DNA damage, thereby precluding successive accumulation of critical mutations. Cell proliferation is also critical for 'fixing' DNA damage since, without production of daughter cells from a damaged mother cell, there would be no inheritance of DNA damage. The cell has relatively efficient mechanisms to repair damage provided there is time prior to cell division. If a tissue is proliferating rapidly, cell division could occur before the cell has time to mend damaged DNA. While all of the above underscore the importance of cell proliferation in carcinogenesis, neoplasia does not occur exclusively or necessarily at higher frequency in tissues that have a rapid intrinsic rate of cell proliferation. Consequently, other important mechanistic factors influence the complex process of carcinogenesis.

In 1994, Loeb et al. proposed that neoplastic cells likely have a higher mutation rate than normal cells ($\sim 2 \times 10^{-7}$ per gene per cell division) and thereby increase the likelihood of neoplastic cells acquiring further mutations conducive to neoplastic growth features. This is referred to as the 'mutator phenotype' (**Figure 7**). It suggests that early mutation in stability genes (i.e., DNA repair, mismatch repair, DNA replication, or chromosome maintenance) will lead to the mutator phenotype and further mutations contribute to the subsequent invasive and metastatic properties of the neoplastic growth. Others argue that the mutation rate is similar between neoplastic and normal cells and that it is the higher rate of cell proliferation in neoplasms that gives them more opportunity to accumulate mutations. The healthy debates continue to feed our quest to prevent and cure the neoplastic process.

Growth Factors, Hormones, and Signal Transduction

While alterations in cellular DNA are critical in carcinogenesis, some cancer-causing agents, particularly those that are not genotoxic, play a major role in cancer development by indirectly influencing gene expression and growth control by altering signal transduction. While the pivotal role of hormones in the orchestration of tissue growth and

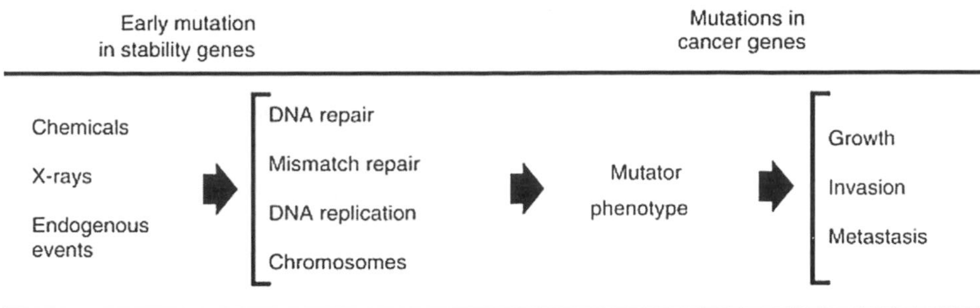

Figure 7 Mutator phenotype model.

development has been appreciated for decades, the recent discovery of polypeptide growth factors has added to our knowledge of the complex constellation of control mechanisms that affect normal cellular growth. Both hormones and growth factors bind to specific cellular receptors and thereby trigger a cascade of intracellular reactions that seem to be associated ultimately with cellular proliferation. This cascade of intracellular reactions is sometimes referred to as signal transduction, the process whereby a stimulus external to the cell triggers a cascade of intracellular biochemical reactions that ultimately lead to expression of specific genes. A simplified depiction of the interaction of hormones and growth factors with cellular signal transduction is presented in **Figure 8**. This concept is perhaps best exemplified by the process whereby a normal hormone stimulates a tissue to grow. An example is breast development and milk production in response to the hormone prolactin. In this example, prolactin binds to a specific prolactin receptor on the external surface of the cell, which, in turn, triggers a biochemical change inside the cell membrane via molecules that are attached to the external receptor and pass through the cell membrane. This in turn triggers a long chain of biochemical reactions ultimately resulting in a signal to specific genes in the cellular DNA so that they become active. The specific genes, in this example, initiate a program that causes breast cells to divide and secrete milk. The signal transduction pathways in mammalian cells are highly interactive with numerous positive (signal-sending) and negative (signal-blocking) feedback loops. An appropriate balance between the positive and negative feedback loops is necessary for the proper functional response to the initial stimulus.

Some forms of cancer development are believed to be facilitated by perturbations in one or more places in the signal transduction pathway. Thus, exposure to certain agents may potentially affect the balance of positive and negative feedback loops in the signal transduction pathway and make cells more

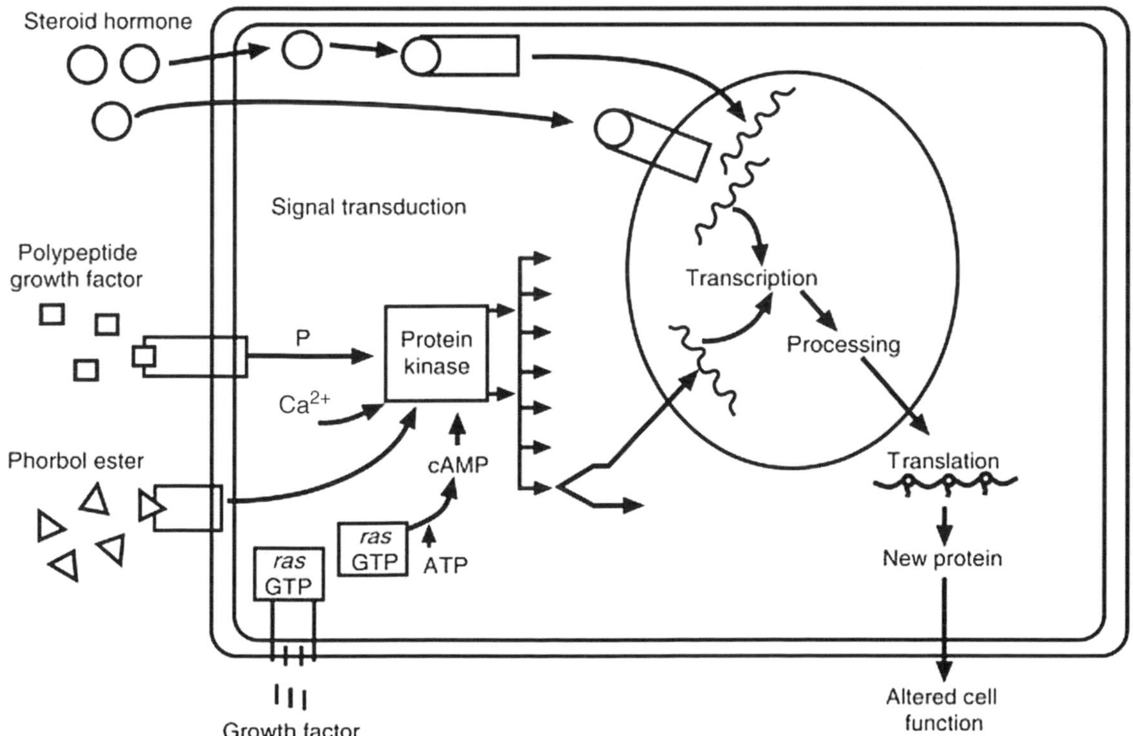

Figure 8 Simplified depiction of the interaction of hormones and growth factors with cellular signal transduction.

susceptible to stimuli that promote growth. An example is the nongenotoxic skin tumor promoter phorbol ester, which activates protein kinase C, a multifunctional element in the signal transduction pathway that mediates many critical cellular regulatory processes. Treatment of initiated mouse skin with phorbol ester activates protein kinase C, resulting in the development of benign and malignant skin neoplasms. The complexity and pivotal importance of the signal transduction pathways help explain why multiple types of agents influence carcinogenesis, why multiple steps are involved in the carcinogenic process, and why different cancers are so heterogeneous. Signal transduction involves shifts in intracellular ion fluxes for elements such as sodium, potassium, and calcium. It also often involves activation of protein kinase C, an enzyme that phosphorylates many proteins that may be important in producing a mitogenic response. Part of the signal transduction cascade involves increased expression of cyclic adenosine monophosphate, now recognized as a mitogenic signal, and increased expression of one or more cellular proto-oncogenes. Current research results demonstrate that increasing numbers of proto-oncogenes and growth factors are integral parts of the signal transduction pathway and, when altered, influence development of cancer by subverting signal transduction.

Telomeres and Telomerase

Telomerase activation appears to be a critical component of the immortalization process in neoplastic cells, and it may provide the basis for new therapeutic targets. Telomeres are specialized structures at the ends of chromosomes, and telomerase is the enzyme that maintains the length of the telomeres. During each round of cell division, there is a loss of a small number of nucleotides, causing progressive erosion of genetic material at the end of each chromosome. As the normal cell divides, the telomeres shorten and telomerase is inactive. After a certain number of divisions, the shortened telomeres signal the cell to cease dividing and the cells become 'senescent' or perhaps will die by apoptosis. Germ cells and some neoplastic cells have sustained function of the telomerase enzyme, which helps maintain lengthening of the telomeres and promote continued replication. Tumors having an increased telomerase activity suggest a direct effect, but it is only part of the story. For example, p53 is activated by telomerase and in the absence of p53 these cells fail to undergo apoptosis and go on to proliferate.

Heredity and Cancer: Family Cancer Syndromes

That certain cancers occur in greater frequency within families represents primary empirical evidence for susceptibility based on some hereditary element. Some genetic predispositions exist for cancers of unknown etiology, while interactions between genetic susceptibility and environmental factors are probably responsible for a large proportion of human cancers. Hereditary predispositions include DNA repair deficiencies, inability to detoxify carcinogens, and germline loss or mutations of critical genes. Examples of genetic predispositions to cancer are listed in **Table 7** and include neurofibromatosis, retinoblastoma, breast cancer, and adenomatosis of the colon. In many of these instances, one event in the carcinogenic process is believed to be an inherited germline mutation in the DNA. Another inherited anomaly, an inability to repair ultraviolet light-induced DNA damage in individuals with the condition xeroderma pigmentosum, is associated with sensitivity to sunlight and a high incidence of skin neoplasia. However, the majority of genetic damage associated with carcinogenesis is acquired either *in utero* or from environmental and/or lifestyle factors to which individuals are exposed. Even for those individuals with a hereditary predisposition to neoplasia, additional DNA damage is necessary to lead ultimately to its development. Environmental factors that may increase the risk of cancer development in genetically predisposed individuals include exposure to radiation and agents that stimulate cellular proliferation. Experimental systems in which to study genetic susceptibility to cancer are critically needed to assess the role of gene–environmental interaction in the development of human cancer.

Table 7 Examples of genetic predisposition to cancer development in humans

Genetic predisposition	*Associated cancer*
Germline deletion on chromosome 13	Retinoblastoma Osteosarcoma
Germline deletion on chromosome 11	Renal nephroblastoma (Wilms' tumor) Hepatoblastoma Rhabdomyosarcoma Adrenal carcinoma
Germline mutation in BRCA1 or BRCA2	Breast or ovarian cancer
Li–Fraumeni syndrome	Soft tissue sarcomas in children Breast cancer in mother
Von Hippel–Lindau disease	Hemangiomas in the brain and retina
Von Recklinghausen's disease	Fibrosarcoma Neuroma Pheochromocytoma
Familial dysplastic nevi	Malignant melanoma
Xeroderma pigmentosa-defective ability to repair damaged DNA	Cutaneous squamous cell carcinoma
Ataxia-telangiectasia	Leukemia Malignant lymphoma Stomach carcinoma
Familial adenomatous polyposis	Colon adenocarcinoma

For some cancers in genetically predisposed individuals, the data are consistent with an association between malignant neoplasia and biallelic genetic alteration, and this is supported by studies of tumor suppressor genes, which prevent the development of neoplasia. Alteration or loss of a single tumor suppressor gene allele is usually insufficient to permit the development of neoplasia. In other words, the remaining functional tumor suppressor gene copy is sufficient to prevent the development of neoplasia; if it is lost or altered, however, neoplasia can develop. This situation occurs in hereditary childhood retinoblastoma, a malignant neoplasm of the retinal cells of the eye. Susceptible individuals inherit a partial loss of one copy (one allele) of chromosome 13, where the retinoblastoma tumor suppressor gene (*RB-1*) is located, and acquire an alteration or loss of the remaining *RB-1* allele during early development. The affected child subsequently develops retinoblastoma, often within the first 2 years of life.

The Immune System and Cancer

The proper functioning of the immune system is evidenced by recovery from common childhood diseases such as mumps and chicken pox. A properly functioning immune system recognizes the foreignness of the agents responsible for these diseases, responds to the infection, eliminates the foreign agents, and confers long-term immunity to subsequent infection by the same or similar agents. It has been proposed that cancer cells are recognized as foreign and that the immune system functions to eliminate such cells from the body before they are transformed into large, malignant neoplasms. This process involves elaboration of antibodies that bind to the cancer cells and activate a process whereby the cancer cells are killed. In addition, specific cells of the immune system, such as cytotoxic T lymphocytes, natural killer cells, and macrophages, have a mechanism for recognizing foreign cells and eliminating them from the body. The process of immune surveillance and removal of cancer cells is facilitated when the cancer cells express surface antigens that are recognized as foreign. Exposure to agents that depress the normal functioning of the immune system can lead indirectly to neoplasia by permitting early persistence and development of recently emergent cancer cells. Once a neoplasm has reached a critical size and growth rate, it may not be possible for even a properly functional immune system to effectively eliminate the neoplastic cells. The pharmacologic manipulation of the immune system can ameliorate cancer patients. This is the case of immunotherapy, a good example is the use of BCG (Bacillus Calmette Guerin) in bladder cancer patients.

Operational Phases and Theoretical Aspects of Carcinogenesis

In addition to being complex, the process of carcinogenesis is typically prolonged, requiring a significant portion of the lifespan to become clinically apparent. While perturbations in cellular DNA are essential to carcinogenesis, they alone are not sufficient to cause cancer in all cases. Thus, in some experimental situations, a few minutes of exposure to a carcinogen is sufficient to result ultimately in cancer, whereas in other situations, exposure to the same carcinogen will not result in cancer unless there is additional experimental manipulation. Smokers illustrate this principle since many, but not all, ultimately develop lung cancer. In other experimental studies, simultaneous administration of a carcinogen and a second agent may enhance, reduce, or block the carcinogenic process depending on the agent employed. These and other carcinogenesis studies have elucidated some of the mechanisms and factors that influence carcinogenesis, delimited some of the specific stages in the multistep process, and continually reminded us of the complexity of this disease process.

Multistep experimental models of carcinogenesis are useful in defining events in the neoplastic process; provide the foundations for current operational descriptions and hypotheses of the biological mechanisms of carcinogenesis (see **Figure 1**); are available for many organ systems including the skin, liver, urinary bladder, lung, intestine, mammary gland, and pancreas; and frequently are derived from studies of the effects of chemical agents on laboratory animals. The operational phases of carcinogenesis include initiation, promotion, and progression.

Initiation

During the initiation phase of chemical carcinogenesis, a chemical agent or carcinogen interacts with a cell to produce an irreversible change that may ultimately be manifested by a capacity for autonomous growth. The initiated cell appears normal, and the capacity for autonomous growth may remain latent for weeks, months, or years. Initiation implies alteration of the affected cell's DNA at one or more sites, a mutational event that is by definition hereditary. Direct-acting carcinogens interact directly with cellular DNA to produce the damage while indirect-acting carcinogens must be metabolized by the cell to produce a chemical species that interacts with cellular DNA. The majority of damaged cells have the ability to repair the damaged DNA over a period of days or weeks; however, if a cell undergoes cell division with its attendant DNA replication prior to repair of the DNA damage, the DNA alteration becomes 'fixed,' is no longer reparable, and is inherited by all subsequent daughter cells. The operational phase of initiation is relatively short and may occur within hours or days. In contrast, the progression of an initiated cell to a fully malignant neoplasm is a prolonged process requiring months in animals and years in humans. Based on a large body of evidence that most initiators are mutagenic or genotoxic, a battery of short-term mutagenicity tests in bacteria and cell culture systems has evolved to identify chemicals with genotoxic properties. Once identified, such chemicals should be rigorously regulated to prevent human exposure. This approach is considered prudent because of the irreversible and hereditary nature of the changes that occur during initiation. Indeed, it is generally believed that even a single molecule of a mutagenic substance is potentially sufficient to damage DNA irreversibly. Thus, for practical purposes, there is no threshold or safe level of exposure to a mutagenic agent. Salient features of initiation are listed in **Table 8**.

Initiators interact with host cellular macromolecules and nucleic acids in specific patterns. The majority of known initiators have both initiating and promoting (see below) activity and can thus induce neoplasms rapidly and in high yield when there is repeated or high-level exposure. When given at sufficiently low single doses, an initiated cell requires subsequent promotion for the development of any neoplasia. Thus, the dose of an initiator is a critical determinant of its carcinogenic potential.

Promotion

Promotion is classically considered that portion of the multistep carcinogenic process in which specific agents, known as promoters, enhance the development of neoplasms by providing initiated cells with a selective growth advantage over the surrounding normal cells. The characteristic features of promotion are listed in **Table 8**. By definition, a promoter is given at some time after chemically induced or fortuitous initiation, and

Table 8 Salient features of initiation and promotion of neoplasia

Initiators/initiation

- Effect is irreversible
- Only one exposure may suffice
- Multiple exposures may be additive
- Cannot identify initiated cells
- Agents are considered carcinogens
- Agents are usually mutagenic
- No measurable threshold dose
- Must be administered before the promoter
- Does not result in neoplasia unless promoter is subsequently applied
- Number of initiated cells dependent on dose of initiator

Promoters/promotion

- Nonadditive
- Agents not capable of initiation
- Modulated by diet, hormones, environment, and other factors
- Measurable threshold dose
- Measurable maximal response
- Agents not considered carcinogens but may be cocarcinogens
- Must be administered after the initiator
- Agents are usually not mutagenic
- Prolonged exposure is usually required
- Progression

the experimental doses of promoting agent are insufficient to produce cancer without prior initiation. When classical promoters are administered at sufficiently high doses and for prolonged intervals, neoplasia can occur without evidence of prior initiation. Under these conditions, a promoting agent must be considered a complete carcinogen unless fortuitous initiation from background radiation, dietary contaminants, environmental toxins, etc., is believed to have occurred. However, under experimental conditions commonly employed in short- and medium-term initiation–promotion experiments, neoplasia does not typically occur in animals that are not previously initiated.

The temporal sequence of promoter administration is critical to the operational definition of promotion. The agent must be administered after initiation and cause enhancement of the neoplastic process to be considered a promoter. If an agent is given simultaneously with an initiator and results in enhancement of development of neoplasms, it is regarded as a cocarcinogen rather than a promoter. While some promoters are cocarcinogenic (e.g., phorbol esters), not all promoters (e.g., phenobarbital and phenol) possess cocarcinogenicity and, conversely, not all cocarcinogens are promoters. Under these same conditions of simultaneous administration, a diminution in the neoplasm response is considered evidence of anticarcinogenic activity. Several rodent liver tumor promoters, which are active when administered after a variety of initiators, prevent or delay the development of liver neoplasms when added to diets along with an active carcinogen. Finally, reversing the order of administration by giving a known promoter prior to an initiator may prevent the expression of carcinogenic activity on the part of the initiator.

While upper and lower thresholds have been demonstrated experimentally for promoters, some consider that, in an absolute sense, it is statistically impossible to prove or disprove the existence of thresholds for promoters for much the same reasons that this cannot be done for initiators. One can never be certain that an apparent no-effect level would, indeed, be without effect if a sufficiently large enough number of animals were used. Promoters include agents such as drugs, plant products, and hormones that do not directly interact with host cellular DNA (are not genotoxic) but somehow influence the expression of genetic information encoded in the cellular DNA. Experimental evidence suggests that regulation of gene expression is unique to the nature of the promoting agent administered. Some promoters are believed to produce their effect by interaction with receptors in the cell membrane, cytoplasm, or nucleus (e.g., hormones, dioxin, phorbol ester, and polychlorinated biphenyls). Alternatively, promoting agents may exert their effect through their molecular orientation at cellular interfaces. Other promoters may selectively stimulate DNA synthesis and enhance cell proliferation in initiated cells, thereby giving them a selective growth advantage over surrounding normal cells.

Promoters appear to have a relatively high tissue specificity. Thus, phenobarbital functions as a promoter for rodent liver neoplasia but not urinary bladder neoplasia. Saccharin, on the other hand, promotes urinary bladder neoplasia but not liver neoplasia in the rat. Similarly, 12-*o*-tetradecanoylphorbol-13-acetate (phorbol ester) is a potent skin and forestomach neoplasm promoter in the laboratory rodent but has no appreciable activity in the liver. Other agents, such as the antioxidants 3-*t*-butyl-4-methoxyphenol and 2,6-di-*t*-butyl-4-methoxyphenol, may act as promoters in one organ and antipromoters in another and have no effect in a third organ. Thus, the practical definition of a promoter must include the designation of the susceptible tissue.

Tumor promotion may be modulated by several factors such as age, sex, diet, and hormone balance. The correlation of increased rates of breast cancer in women following a 'Western' lifestyle has implicated meat and fat consumption as playing an important role in breast cancer development. Experimental demonstration of the role of a high-fat diet in the promotion of mammary cancer in rats exposed to the mammary carcinogen dimethylbenzanthracene has been documented. Similarly, bile acids, as modulated by fat consumption, are known promoters of rat liver carcinogenesis and human colorectal cancer. Age- and sex-associated modulations in hormonal levels of estrogens, progesterone, and androgens have been implicated as potential promoters of breast cancer on the basis of epidemiological studies in humans. Experimental studies have repeatedly shown that these hormones, in addition to pituitary prolactin, serve to promote mammary cancer in rats initiated with mammary carcinogens.

Progression

Progression is that part of the multistep neoplastic process associated with the development of an initiated cell into a biologically malignant cell population. In common usage, progression is frequently used to signify the stages whereby a benign proliferation becomes malignant or, alternatively, where a neoplasm develops from a low grade to a high grade of malignancy. During progression, neoplasms show increased invasiveness; develop the ability to metastasize; and then biochemical, metabolic, and morphologic characteristics are altered.

Expression of tumor cell heterogeneity, an important characteristic of tumor progression, includes production of antigenic and protein product variants, ability to elaborate angiogenesis factors, emergence of chromosomal variants, development of metastatic capability, alterations in metabolism, and a decrease in sensitivity to radiation. The development of intraneoplastic diversity may result from increasing genetic damage. Alternatively, the heterogeneity observed in tumor progression may be generated by epigenetic, regulatory mechanisms that are a part of the process of promotion. More than likely, genetic and nongenetic events subsequent to initiation operate in a nonmutually exclusive manner during progression, possibly in an ordered cascade of latter events superimposed upon earlier events.

The most plausible mechanism of progression invokes the notion that, during the process of tumor growth, there is a selection that favors enhanced growth of a subpopulation of the neoplastic cells. In support of this mechanism is increased phenotypic heterogeneity observed in malignant but not benign neoplastic proliferations. Presumably, a variety of subpopulations arises, and it is only a matter of time before the emergence of a subpopulation with more malignant biological characteristics or at least an accelerated growth advantage. This can be observed occasionally during experimental hepatocarcinogenesis when a phenotypically distinguishable carcinoma can be observed arising within an existing adenoma.

Distinction between tumor promotion and tumor progression is not readily discernible in the routine histopathologic evaluation of neoplasms and may be somewhat academic because promotion may be considered part of the process of progression. In both situations, the critical event is accentuated growth. What is believed to distinguish progression from promotion is the presence of structural genomic alterations in the former and their absence in the latter. Both structural genomic changes and biochemical changes associated with tumor progression cannot be defined by conventional histopathology. Established and emerging technologies centered on histochemistry, immunocytochemistry, *in situ* hybridization, identification of activated oncogenes, loss of tumor suppressor genes, gene expression, proteomic and metabolomic profiling, and discovery offer promise to distinguish various stages of progression in the evolution from benign to malignant neoplasms.

Exogenous Factors Influencing Carcinogenesis

Important exogenous factors that contribute to induction of cancer include natural and synthetic chemicals, environmental exposures to ultraviolet and medical radiation, diet and lifestyle, and infectious agents such as viruses, parasites, and bacteria. Evidence for a causal association between exogenous factors and neoplasia is derived from studies of epidemiology, occupationally common cancers, and animal models.

Chemical and Physical Agents and Lifestyle Factors

Many chemicals that cause cancer interact directly with and alter DNA or are metabolized to chemical derivatives capable of doing so. Exposure to carcinogens can occur in certain occupational settings. Associations of human hepatic angiosarcomas with workplace exposure to vinyl chloride, pulmonary mesotheliomas with exposure to asbestos fibers, and leukemia with benzene are well-known examples. Exposure to other carcinogenic agents may occur in the diet or as a consequence of certain lifestyle practices such as cigarette smoking associated with pulmonary cancer and high animal fat diets linked to breast and colon cancer. Strong associations have been made between exposure of light-skinned individuals to ultraviolet radiation and skin cancer. Exposure to occupational ionizing radiation, X-rays, and medical use of radioisotopes has also been associated with human neoplasia. Examples include leukemias in radiologists and atom bomb victims, lung cancer in uranium mineworkers, and thyroid and breast cancer following diagnostic or therapeutic use of radiation, and bladder cancer in paint industry workers.

Infectious Agents and Inflammation

Viral, parasitic, and bacterial infections have been linked to cancer (**Table 9**). DNA viruses such as Epstein–Barr, hepatitis B, hepatitis C, papillomaviruses, and Kaposi sarcoma herpes virus

Table 9 Viruses and parasites causally related to or strongly associated with animal and human neoplasia

Virus	*Type of neoplasm*	*Species*
DNA viruses		
Myxoma	Myxoma Myxomatosis	Rabbit Rabbit
Herpes	Lymphosarcoma	Chicken Money Rabbit
Herpes simplex 2	Cervical carcinoma	Human
Papillomaviruses	Papillomas	Cow Rabbit Horse Dog
Human papillomavirus	Warts Epidermoid carcinoma Cervical carcinoma	Human
Woodchuck hepatitis virus	Hepatocellular carcinoma	Woodchuck
Hepatitis B virus	Hepatocellular carcinoma	Human
Epstein–Barr		
Hepatitis B & C		
Papillomaviruses		
T-cell leukemia virus type I		
RNA retroviruses		
Human T cell leukemia virus (HTLV-I and -II)	T cell lymphoma	Human
Avian erythroblastosis virus	Leukemia Sarcoma	Chicken
Abelson leukemia virus	Leukemia	Mouse
Hervey sarcoma virus	Sarcoma Leukemia	Rat
Feline sarcoma virus	Sarcoma	Cat
Parasites		
Schistosoma haematobium	Bladder	Human
Opisthorchis viverrini	Cholangiocarcinoma	Human

and RNA viruses such as human T-cell leukemia virus type I and human immunodeficiency virus have been implicated in causing cancer in humans and are listed as 'known-to-cause-cancer' in humans by the International Agency for Research on Cancer (IARC). In man, the liver fluke, *Opisthorchis viverrini*, is associated with the development of cholangiocarcinomas of the liver and the blood fluke, *Schistosoma haematobium*, with carcinoma of the urinary bladder. There is evidence that chronic *Helicobacter pylori* infection of the stomach in humans not only is related to gastrointestinal ulcers, but also may be linked to gastric carcinoma or lymphoma development.

For oncogenic viruses, the viral or host genes generally drive the neoplastic process while with some agents there appears to be an association of chronic inflammation and nitric oxide (NO) production in the development of cancer. When DNA viruses infect cells, the viral DNA inserts itself wholly or partially into the genome of the infected cell. It appears that such integration of viral DNA into the mammalian genome is sometimes sufficient to cause neoplastic transformation of the infected cell, which is accompanied by the production of new proteins essential for the neoplastic process. RNA viruses associated with neoplasia are chiefly represented by the retroviruses. RNA viruses possess an enzyme called reverse transcriptase, which is capable of forming a DNA copy of the viral RNA when the virus infects a host cell. This DNA ultimately inserts itself into the host genome in much the same way as DNA viruses do, possibly resulting in the development of neoplasia.

The role of inflammation in cancer development is being intensely studied. There are a number of chronic inflammatory conditions, infectious and noninfectious, in humans and animals associated with an increasing risk of cancer, and there are many investigators examining the role of NO and oxygen radical damage to DNA or other cellular processes such as cell proliferation and apoptosis. NO induces p53, prevents apoptosis in cells such as endothelium, promotes angiogenesis, and inhibits DNA-repair activities – all processes that might provide a selective advantage to neoplastic cell growth.

Identification of Carcinogenic Agents

There are two methods utilized to identify potential human carcinogens, the most direct of which is based on retrospective epidemiological studies in human populations using existing historical records associated with known cases of neoplasia. These records include death certificates where cause of death is indicated; hospital records; responses to questionnaires that document environmental or work-associated exposure to potential carcinogenic agents; and studies of neoplasia in culturally, ethnically, or religiously distinctive human populations. Association of cigarette mesotheliomas and exposure to chemicals and bladder cancer was the result of such retrospective epidemiological work. Prospective epidemiological studies identify a given population of individuals who agree to be monitored for several years to permit identification of potential carcinogenic factors associated with neoplasms that may occur.

Another method used to identify potential human carcinogens involves testing known chemicals and agents in experimental animals. Such tests have been referred to as animal bioassays and are typically conducted using rats and mice exposed to high doses of the suspect agent for a large portion (typically 2 years) of their lifespan. If such agents are observed to produce neoplasia in the experimental animals, the agent is regarded as a potential human carcinogen. In countries throughout the world, legal requirements mandate that all new chemical agents and drugs be tested in animal bioassays to determine whether they cause cancer in the test animals. Additionally, since the mid-1960s in the United States, the National Cancer Institute and currently the National Toxicology Program have collectively conducted animal bioassays on more than 500 chemical agents to assess their potential to cause cancer.

Interpretation of results from human epidemiological studies and animal bioassays to identify carcinogenic agents has often proved difficult and controversial. Humans are rarely exposed to only one potential cancer-causing agent in their lifetime, and the amount and duration of that exposure may be difficult or impossible to quantify rigorously. Many years may intervene between exposure to a potential carcinogen and ultimate development of neoplasia, making accurate assessment of cause and effect almost impossible. Despite such limitations, epidemiological studies that clearly show an association between a given chemical exposure or lifestyle habit with an enhanced rate of a specific cancer are regarded as the most relevant method for identification of human carcinogens. While animal bioassays have proved useful for the identification of agents that can cause cancer in the laboratory rodent, they only identify an agent as potentially hazardous to human health. Additional facts and factors must be considered in classifying such an agent as a likely human carcinogen.

The current approach for assessing the scientific relevance of either epidemiological or animal bioassay results to human health risk involves a 'weight-of-evidence' procedure in which national and international panels of expert scientists from several disciplines examine all available information on the suspect agent in making their assessment. Included in this analysis are the strength of the epidemiological evidence, the dose–response curve of the animal response, comparative species metabolism and ability to extrapolate between species, likely mechanism of cancer induction for the agent in question, the genotoxicity of the agent, the amount of the agent in the environment, and the number of people potentially exposed to the agent. Based on this type of analysis, so far 88 agents have been classified as known human carcinogens by the IARC (some of which are in **Table 10**) and 64 more agents have been designated as probable human carcinogens. The 10th US Health and Human Services *Annual Report on Carcinogens* lists 49 known human carcinogens and 174 substances that are reasonably anticipated to be human carcinogens.

Molecular Epidemiology of Cancer

The molecular epidemiology of cancer is the study of molecular alterations, primarily mutations, in investigating the causative agents of cancer as well as identifying individual cancer risk. The possibility of identifying cancer-causing agents based on the occurrence of predictable molecular alterations that are

Table 10 Some selected agents or mixtures for which there is sufficient evidence of carcinogenicity in humans

Organic compounds
2-Napthylamine
4-Aminobiphenyl
Aflatoxin B_1
Analgesics containing phenacetin
Azathioprine
Benzene
Benzidine
Betel quid with tobacco
Bis(chloromethyl)ether
Chlorambucil
Chlornaphazine
Chloromethyl methyl ether
Cyclophosphamide
Diethylstilbestrol
Melphalan
Methyl-CCNU
MOPP (and other combined therapies)
Mustard gas
Myleran
Thiotepa
Tobacco products and tobacco smoke
Treosulfan
Vinyl chloride
Soots, tars, and oils
Coal tar pitches
Coal tars
Mineral oils, untreated and mildly treated
Shale oils
Soots
Hormones
Diethylstilbestrol
Estrogens
Oral contraceptives
Metals
Arsenic compounds
Chromium compounds
Nickel and nickel compounds
Fibers
Asbestos
Erionite
Talc-containing asbestos fibers
Other
8-Methoxypsoralen + UV radiation

found in the neoplasm is intriguing. It is based on the hypothesis that there are carcinogen-specific patterns of mutations that reflect direct interactions of carcinogens with cancer genes. For example, lung and colon cancers from people who smoke tend to have a specific mutation in the *ras* oncogene or p53 tumor suppressor gene (i.e., mostly a G–T nucleotide base substitution) and that this mutation is likely due to the direct interaction of the carcinogen in smoke benzo(*a*)pyrene with DNA. Such chemical-specific mutational profiles (or 'molecular signatures') have been used to support a causal association between particular genetic events in tumors and a specific carcinogen such as neoplasms associated with exposure to radon, aflatoxin B1, vinyl chloride, and the nitrosamines (**Tables 11** and **12**). The strongest evidence for linkage between a cancer-causing agent and a specific type of neoplasm is that of the CC–TT double base changes observed in skin neoplasms of humans and animals. This mutation is consistent with the predicted UV-induced damage of dipyrimidine dimers. In liver tumors from persons living in geographic areas with a high exposure to aflatoxin B1, there is a frequent mutation at the third nucleotide pair of codon 249 in the p53 gene, suggesting the mutation is chemical specific and imparts a specific growth or survival advantage to the mutated liver cells.

Animal studies have confirmed that there are certainly chemical-specific mutational profiles in neoplasms; however, there are many examples where the mutational profile varies by strain (**Table 13**), species, dose, or dosing regiment. For example, diethylnitrosamine, a strong, cross-species hepatocarcinogen, will induce liver neoplasms in mice, rats, and rainbow trout, but the frequency and type of *ras* mutation in the neoplasm vary widely, and the mutations are not simply a reflection of direct DNA interaction (**Table 14**). In some studies, *in vitro* mutation assays were poor predictors of liver tumor mutation profiles in the mouse. In this complex process, carcinogens might also be influencing events such as DNA repair, oxidative DNA damage, methylation, cell death, proliferation, and/or a hypermutable state.

Molecular epidemiologic studies aimed at identifying an individual's risk of developing cancer have found that persons

Table 11 Molecular signatures of malignant human cancers

Exposure	*Neoplasm type*	*Predominant mutation (nucleotide base changes)*
Cigarette smoke	Lung carcinoma	K-*ras*, codons 12 and 13 (G–T)
	Colon	K-*ras*, codons 12 and 13
	Lung carcinoma	p53, multiple codons (G–T)
Radon	Lung carcinoma	p53, codon 249 (G–T)
Aflatoxin B_1	Hepatocellular carcinoma	p53, codon 249 (G–T)
Ultraviolet light	Skin carcinoma	p53, dipyrimidine sites (CC–TT)
Vinyl chloride	Hepatic angiosarcoma	p53, codon 249 (A–T)
	Hepatocellular carcinoma	K-*ras*, codons 12 and 13 (G–A)

Table 12 Molecular signatures of malignant rodent cancers

Exposure	*Neoplasm type (species)*	*Predominant mutation (nucleotide base changes)*
Methylnitrosourea	Mammary carcinoma (R)	K-*ras*, codon 12 (G–C)
Aflatoxin B_1	Lung carcinomas (M)	K-*ras*, codon 12 (G–C)
Diethylnitrosamine	HCC (M)	H-*ras*, codon 61 (A–G)
Ultraviolet light	Skin carcinoma (M)	p53, dipyrimidine sites (CC–TT)
Vinyl chloride	HCC (R)	H-*ras*, codon 61 (A–T)

HCC, hepatocellular carcinoma; M, mouse; R, rat.

Table 13 Sensitivity to liver tumor development and H-*ras* codon 61 mutations in spontaneous hepatocellular tumors of various strains of mice

Sensitivity	*Strain*	*Frequency*		*Codon 61 mutation (normal = CAA)* AAA	CGA	CTA
High	C3H	23/89	(26%)	17	3′	3
Intermediate	B6C3F1	183/333	(56%)[a]	106	50	21
	CD-1	9/36	(25%)	8	1	0
Low	C57BL	5/34	(15%)[a]	0	1	4

[a]Occasional mutations in other codons of H- and K-*ras*.
Adapted from Maronpot, R.R., Fox, T., Malarkey, D.E., Goldsworthy, T.L., 1995. Mutations in the *ras* proto-oncogene: clues to etiology and molecular pathogenesis of mouse liver tumors. Toxicology 101, 125–156.

Table 14 Species and strain comparisons of mutational profiles induced by diethylnitrosamine (DEN)

Animal	*Frequency of* ras *mutations*		*Type*	*Nucleotide base substitutions* C–A	A–G	A–T	A–C	G–A
CD-1 mouse	13/25	(52%)	H- and N-*ras*	12	1	0	0	0
C3H mouse	54/114	(26%)	H-*ras*	28	24	2	0	0
B6C3F1 mouse	63/239	(26%)	H-*ras*	16	32	15	0	0
C57BL mouse	2/59	(2%)	H-*ras*	0	1	0	1	0
F344 rat	0/19	(0%)	K-*ras*	0	0	0	0	0
Rainbow trout	6/7	(86%)	K-*ras*	0	0	0	0	6

Data adapted partly from Maronpot, R.R., Fox, T., Malarkey, D.E., Goldworthy, T.L., 1995. Mutations in the *ras* proto-oncogene: clues to etiology and molecular pathogenesis of mouse liver tumors. Toxicology 101, 125–156.

with germline mutations in cancer genes (i.e., BRCA1 or BRCA2) or variations (polymorphisms) of carcinogen-metabolizing enzyme activities (i.e., cytochrome P450s or glutathione-S-transferases) or DNA repair capacities can be at increased risk of developing neoplasia in their lifetime. High-throughput analyses to examine single nucleotide polymorphisms (SNPs) are being used to search for biomarkers of cancer risk in individuals, and some of this information is being used to help people take preventive measures to decrease their risk of developing cancer.

Summary and Conclusions

All of life is a balancing act of good versus evil and production versus destruction. Similar balancing factors are evident in carcinogenesis where regulatory mechanisms for tissue proliferation are balanced against those for cellular differentiation. It is well established that carcinogenesis requires the accumulation of multiple alterations in the genome of the affected (cancer) cells. At the genetic level, two opposing classes of genes, oncogenes, and tumor suppressor genes, have been implicated in the carcinogenic process. In addition, the development of cancer is influenced by host factors such as age, sex, diet, nutrition, general health status, and inherited predispositions for cancer and by complex positive and negative intracellular signaling mechanisms. Treatment of cancer is based on our understanding of the mechanistic underpinnings of the carcinogenic process and attempts to shift the balance of critical factors in favor of patient survival. The probability of developing cancer is directly proportional to the intensity, route, and duration of exposure to cancer-causing factors as well as genetic susceptibility. Public health strategies are based on the premise that reduction or prevention of exposure to cancer-causing factors will decrease the incidence of cancer.

See also: Carcinogen Classification Schemes; Carcinogen–DNA Adduct Formation and DNA Repair; Cell Proliferation; Chromosome Aberrations; Epidemiology; Immune System; International Agency for Research on Cancer; Mechanisms of Toxicity; Molecular Toxicology: Recombinant DNA Technology; Mouse Lymphoma Assay; Radiation Toxicology, Ionizing and Nonionizing; Skin; Toxicity Testing, Carcinogenesis.

Further Reading

Benigni, R., April 2012. Alternatives to the carcinogenicity bioassay for toxicity prediction: are we there yet? Expert Opin. Drug Metab. Toxicol. 8 (4), 407–417.
Columbano, A., Feo, F., Pani, P. (Eds.), 1991. Chemical Carcinogenesis 2: Modulating Factors. Springer, New York.
Doktorova, T.Y., Pauwels, M., Vinken, M., Vanhaecke, T., Rogiers, V., February 2012. Opportunities for an alternative integrating testing strategy for carcinogen hazard assessment? Crit. Rev. Toxicol. 42 (2), 91–106.
Grice, H.C., Ciminera, J.L. (Eds.), 1988. Carcinogenicity: The Design, Analysis, and Interpretation of Long-Term Animal Studies. Springer-Verlag, New York.
Hsu, C.-H., Stedeford, T. (Eds.), 2010. Cancer Risk Assessment: Chemical Carcinogenesis, Hazard Evaluation, and Risk Quantification. John Wiley & Sons, Inc., New Jersey.
Monk, D., 2010. Deciphering the cancer imprintome. Brief. Funct. Genomics. 9, 329–939.
Nowsheen, S., Aziz, K., Kryston, T.B., Ferguson, N.F., Georgakilas, A., 1 July 2012. The interplay between inflammation and oxidative stress in carcinogenesis. Curr. Mol. Med. 12 (6), 672–680.
Oliveira, P.A., Colaço, A., Chaves, R., Guedes-Pinto, H., De-La-Cruz, P.L.F., Lopes, C., 2007. Chemical carcinogenesis. An. Acad. Bras. Cienc. 79, 593–616.

Pavanello, S., Lotti, M., April 2012. Biological monitoring of carcinogens: current status and perspectives. Arch. Toxicol. 86 (4), 535–541.

Penning, T.M. (Ed.), 2011. Chemical Carcinogenesis. Springer Science + Business Media, New York.

Peters, J.M., Shah, Y.M., Gonzalez, F.J., 9 February 2012. The role of peroxisome proliferator-activated receptors in carcinogenesis and chemoprevention. Nat. Rev. Cancer 12 (3), 181–195.

Sharma, S., Kelly, T.K., Jones, P.A., 2010. Epigenetics in cancer. Carcinogenesis 31, 27–36.

Simic, M.G., Grossman, L., Upton, A.C. (Eds.), 1986. Mechanisms of DNA Damage and Repair: Implications for Carcinogenesis and Risk Assessment. Plenum Press, New York.

Wallace, T.A., Martin, D.N., Ambs, S., 2011. Interactions among genes, tumor biology and the environment in cancer health disparities: examining the evidence on a national and global scale. Carcinogenesis 32, 1107–1121.

Waters, M.D., Jackson, M., Lea, I., 2010. Characterizing and predicting carcinogenicity and mode of action using conventional and toxicogenomics methods. Mutat. Res. 705, 184–200.

Relevant Website

http://monographs.iarc.fr/ – Important Monograph Series.

Carcinogenicity Toxicity Testing *see* Toxicity Testing, Carcinogenesis

Cardiovascular System

PA Stapleton, TL Knuckles, VC Minarchick, G Gautam, and TR Nurkiewicz, West Virginia University School of Medicine, Morgantown, WV, USA

This article is a revision of the previous edition article by Arthur Penn and Gleeson Murphy, volume 1, pp 467–485, © 2005, Elsevier Inc.

The central tenet of toxicology was stated by the sixteenth-century physician Paracelsus: "All substances are poisons. There is none that is not a poison. The right dose differentiates a poison and a remedy." This tenet has withstood the repeated tests of science and time; and over 500 years later, firmly remains the foundation for all toxicological considerations. The scope of this article encompasses the toxicities of several classes of chemicals on the cardiovascular system (CVS). These include drugs (therapeutic, and those commonly abused), pesticides, organic and inorganic chemicals, metals, pollutants, and complex mixtures (e.g., combustion exhaust, cigarette smoke, etc.).

The CVS consists of the heart and the vasculature (arteries, arterioles, capillaries, venules, and veins). The lymphatics, while a critical component for normal cardiovascular function, are commonly not included in CVS discussions for a variety of reasons (as it is a parallel system focused on interstitial fluids). Therefore, this article focuses on the heart and vasculature because they are either the primary targets, or the major site of effect/consequence after exposure to the toxicants described herein. It begins by defining cardiovascular homeostasis, followed by cardiac anatomy and physiology. Next are examples of toxicants that can alter ion movement, muscle function, and thus, cardiac output. The second part of the article begins with a description of the anatomy and physiology of vasculature, followed by examples of specific toxicants. A list of cardiotoxic agents and their mechanisms of toxicity is presented in **Table 1**. A listing of vasculotoxic agents and related compounds is presented in **Table 2**. Neither the contents of this article nor the material in the tables is intended to be exhaustive or fully inclusive. The agents noted here serve as common or representative cardiotoxic and vasculotoxic agents. There are detailed articles in specialty texts that discuss these and other agents more fully. A brief bibliography as well as mention of some websites with excellent graphics of the CVS are presented at the end of this article. As with all of these compounds, it is important to keep in mind that the toxicological manifestation associated with these agents must not overshadow the therapeutic benefit.

Cardiovascular Homeostasis

Homeostasis is the regulation of an internal environment in order to maintain stability. The preeminent French physiologist Claude Bernard introduced the notion that the blood (and lymph fluid), which bathe all mammalian tissues, constitute the *milieu interne* or internal milieu of the greater organism. The CVS functions primarily to transport nutrients (oxygen, glucose) and wastes (carbon dioxide) to and from (respectively) all tissues in the body. Equally important CVS functions include cellular communication/feedback, temperature regulation, fluid and ion balance, and host defense. Hence, cardiovascular homeostasis refers to the regulation of these collective functions, which serve to maintain the internal milieu; thereby, maintaining the stability of the organism. It is these functions that are directly and indirectly impacted by exposure to various toxicants. Therefore, an understanding of the impacted components or tissues is necessary first if we are to comprehend the consequences of toxicant exposure on human health.

The Heart

The Heart as a Pump

To maintain cardiac homeostasis, blood must flow continuously throughout the body. Blood flow is proportional to blood pressure. Blood pressure is generated by heart muscle contractions, or pumping. The mammalian heart (**Figure 1**) is a dual pump (left and right) that normally operates through a tightly controlled conduction of electrical impulses that ultimately produce cardiac contractions in a continuous rhythm. This creates two independent circuits: the pulmonary and systemic circuits. Each pump consists of two connecting chambers – an atrium and a ventricle – which contract in sequence to provide pressure (or force) via their concerted pumping action. The atria function primarily as reservoirs for blood between contractions, whereas the ventricles are responsible for pumping the blood through the circuits, have thick muscular walls, and are located beneath the thinner-walled atria. The atria also force the last volume of blood into the ventricle necessary for more efficient pumping. In a normal cardiac cycle, the atria contract first, and the ventricles contract second (while the atria relax). To ensure one-way flow during alternating contractions, the heart is equipped with specialized valves. The atrioventricular (AV) valves prevent backflow of blood into the atria during ventricular contraction (systole), and the aortic/pulmonary (semilunar) valves prevent backflow of blood into the ventricles during ventricular relaxation (diastole). During systole, the two ventricles develop

 http://dx.doi.org/10.1016/B978-0-12-386454-3.00985-4

Table 1 General mechanisms of cardiotoxicity; and cardiotoxicity of key pharmaceutical agents, naturally occurring substances used as pharmaceuticals, and selected industrial agents (Arrhythmic – a drug or substance that alters the natural rhythm of the heart; inotropic – toxicants that increase (positive) or decrease (negative) the force of heart muscle contraction; chronotropic – toxicants that increase (positive) or decrease (negative) the number of beats per minute of the heart; and blockade – substances that inhibit receptor function)

Mechanism	*Cellular perturbations*	*Organ manifestations*
General mechanisms of cardiotoxicity		
Interference with ion homeostasis		
Inhibition of Na^+/K^+ ATPase	↑ $[Ca^{2+}]_i$	Positive inotropic effect
	↓ Conduction velocity	Proarrhythmic
Na^+ channel blockade	↓ Na^+ channel activity	Proarrhythmic
	↓ Conduction velocity	
K^+ channel blockade	↓ K^+ channel activity	Proarrhythmic
	↓ Repolarization	
	↑ Action potential duration	
Ca^{2+} channel blockade	↓ L-type Ca^{2+} channel activity	Negative inotropic effect Negative chronotropic effect
	↓ Ca^{2+}-induced-Ca^{2+} release	Bradycardia
	↓ AV conduction	
Altered coronary blood flow		
Coronary vasoconstriction or obstruction	Ischemia (ATP depletion, intracellular acidosis)	Myocardial infarction Cardiac myocyte death Cardiac remodeling
Ischemia/reperfusion injury	Oxidative stress, ↑ $[Ca^{2+}]_i$ intracellular pH change	Cardiac myocyte death
Oxidative stress	Lipid peroxidation DNA damage Mitochondrial dysfunction, Altered $[Ca^{2+}]_i$ homeostasis	Cardiac myocyte death
Organellar dysfunction		
Sarcolemmal injury	Altered membrane integrity	Cardiac myocyte death
Sarcoplasmic reticulum dysfunction	Altered $[Ca^{2+}]_i$ homeostasis	Cardiac myocyte death
Mitochondrial injury	ATP depletion Cytochrome *c* release Altered mitochondrial $[Ca^{2+}]_i$ homeostasis	Cardiac myocyte death
Apoptosis	Cellular shrinkage Sarcolemmal blebbing Chromatin condensation Redistribution of membrane phospholipids DNA fragmentation	Cardiac myocyte death
Oncosis	Cellular swelling Sarcolemmal blebbing Chromatin clumping Mitochondrial swelling	Cardiac myocyte death
Agents	*Cardiotoxic manifestations*	Proposed mechanisms of cardiotoxicity

pressure and eject blood into the pulmonary artery and aorta. At this time the AV valves are closed and the semilunar valves are open. The semilunar valves are closed and the AV valves are open during diastole. The right atrium receives blood flowing from the systemic venous system via the superior and inferior vena cava. This blood initially passes passively through the right AV orifice directly into the right ventricle. An atrial contraction then propels a small volume of additional blood into the right ventricle (mentioned above). A ventricular contraction closes the AV valve allowing blood now to be propelled past the pulmonary valve into the pulmonary circuit. As blood flows through the pulmonary vasculature, carbon dioxide in the venous-return blood is exchanged for oxygen (gas exchange occurs down concentration gradients via passive diffusion) so that the blood pumped through the next (systemic) circuit to the rest of the body will be properly oxygenated. The left atrium receives freshly oxygenated blood from the pulmonary vasculature via the pulmonary vein. Again, blood traverses the AV orifice until an atrial contraction provides complete filling of the ventricle and closes the AV valve. The strong contraction of the thick-muscled left ventricle now opens the aortic valve, allowing blood to flow into the systemic circulation (under high pressure) via the aorta. In the absence of injury and/or disease, the heart is a very efficient, durable, and reliable pump. In the 80-year life span of a person, and at a contraction rate of 72 beats per minute, a heart will beat ~3 000 000 000 times. Two major features of the heart contribute to its unique characteristics: the nature of the heart muscle and the specialized electrical conduction system of the heart.

Table 2 Cardiotoxicity of key pharmaceutical agents

A. Cardiotoxic agents			
Agents	*Sources*	*Prominent cardiac effects*	*Physiological endpoints*
Ethanol		Decreased conductivity	Hypertension
		Altered $[Ca^{2+}]_i$ balance	Cardiomyopathy
		Oxidative stress	Ventricular tachycardia
		Mitochondrial injury	Decreased energy production, heart failure
Antiarrhythmic drugs			
Adenosine		K^+ Hyperpolarization	Cardiac arrest
		Decreased refractory period	Atrial arrhythmia
Class I (disopyramide, encainide, flecainide, lidocaine, mexiletine, moricizine, phenytoin, procainamide, propafenone, quinidine, tocainide)		Na^+ channel blockade	Arrhythmia
Class II (acebutolol, esmolol, propranolol, sotalol)		β-adrenergic receptor blockade	Bradycardia, cardiac arrest
Class III (amiodarone, bretylium, dofetilide, ibutilide, quinidine, sotalol)		K^+ channel blockade	Arrhythmia
		QTc interval prolongation	Ventricular tachycardia
Class IV (diltiazem, verapamil)		Ca^{2+} channel blockade	Bradycardia
			Weakened ventricular contraction
			Arrhythmia
Inotropic drugs and related agents			
Cardiac glycosides (digoxin, digitoxin)		Inhibition of Na^+, K^+-ATPase, increased $[Ca^{2+}]_i$	Arrhythmia
Ca^{2+} sensitizing agents (adibendan, levosimendan, pimobendan)		Increased Ca^{2+} sensitivity, inhibition of phosphodiesterase	Decreased ventricular filling during relaxation, arrhythmia
Catecholamines (dobutamine, epinephrine, isoproterenol, norepinephrine)		β_1-adrenergic receptor activation	Tachycardia
		Coronary vasoconstriction	Ischemia, myocardial infarction (MI)
		Mitochondrial dysfunction	Decreased energy production, heart failure
		Increased $[Ca^{2+}]_i$	Arrhythmia
		Oxidative stress	Heart failure
		Apoptosis	Heart failure
Bronchodilators (albuterol, bitolterol, fenoterol, formeterol, metaproterenol, pirbuterol, procaterol, salmeterol, terbutaline)		Nonselective activation of β_1-adrenergic receptors	Tachycardia (acute)
			Heart failure (chronic)
Appetite suppressants (amphetamines, fenfluramine, phentermine)		Increased serotonin?	Tachycardia, pulmonary hypertension
		Na^+ channel blockade?	Arrhythmia
			Valvular insufficiency
Antineoplastic drugs			
Anthracyclines (daunorubicin, doxorubicin, epirubicin)		Altered $[Ca^{2+}]_i$ balance	Decreased cardiac output
		Oxidative stress	Heart failure
		Mitochondrial injury	Cardiomyopathy
		Apoptosis	Heart failure
5-Fluorouracil		Coronary vasospasm?	Arrhythmia
Cyclophosphamide	4-Hydroxycyclophosphamid (metabolite)	Altered ion balance	Arrhythmia
			Heart failure
Antibacterial drugs			
Aminoglycosides (amikacin, gentamicin, kanamycin, netilmicin, streptomycin, tobramycin)		Decreased $[Ca^{2+}]_i$	Weakened ventricular contraction
Macrolides (azithromycin, clarithromycin, dirithromycin, erythromycin)		K^+ channel blockade	Arrhythmia
		QTc interval prolongation	Ventricular tachycardia
Fluoroquinolones (grepafloxacin, moxifloxacin, sparfloxacin)		K^+ channel blockade	Arrhythmia
		QTc interval prolongation	Ventricular tachycardia
Tetracycline		Decreased $[Ca^{2+}]_i$	Weakened ventricular contraction
Chloramphenicol		Decreased $[Ca^{2+}]_i$	Weakened ventricular contraction

Table 2 Cardiotoxicity of key pharmaceutical agents—cont'd

A. Cardiotoxic agents			
Agents	*Sources*	*Prominent cardiac effects*	*Physiological endpoints*
Antifungal drugs			
Amphotericin B		Ca^{2+} channel blockage? Na^{+} channel blockade? Increased membrane permeability?	Weakened ventricular contraction Arrhythmia
Flucytosine	5-Fluorouracil metabolite	Coronary vasospasm?	Arrhythmia, cardiac arrest
Antiviral drugs			
Nucleotide analog reverse transcriptase inhibitors (stavudine, zalcitabine, zidovudine)		Mitochondrial injury Inhibition of mitochondrial DNA polymerase and synthesis Inhibition of mitochondrial ATP synthesis	Cardiomyopathy Decreased energy production, heart failure Decreased energy production, heart failure
Centrally acting drugs			
Tricyclic antidepressants (amitriptyline, desipramine, doxepin, imipramine, protriptyline)		Altered ion balance (Ca^{2+}, K^{+}, Na^{+}) QTc interval prolongation	Arrhythmia, cardiac arrest Ventricular tachycardia
Selective serotonin reuptake inhibitors (fluoxetine, citalopram)		Ca^{2+} channel blockade Na^{+} channel blockade QTc interval prolongation	Bradycardia, arrhythmia Arrhythmia Ventricular tachycardia
Phenothiazine antipsychotic drugs (chlorpromazine, thioridazine)		Ca^{2+} channel blockade? QTc interval prolongation	Tachycardia, weakened ventricular contraction Ventricular tachycardia
Other antipsychotic drugs (clozapine)		QTc interval prolongation	Ventricular tachycardia Myocarditis
General inhalational anesthetics (enflurane, desflurane, halothane, isoflurane, methoxyflurane, sevoflurane)		Ca^{2+} channel blockade Altered Ca^{2+} balance, β-adrenergic receptor sensitization	Weakened ventricular contraction Decreased cardiac output Arrhythmia
Other general anesthetics (propofol)		Ca^{2+} channel blockade Altered Ca^{2+} balance, β-adrenergic receptor sensitization	Weakened ventricular contraction Decreased cardiac output Arrhythmia
Local anesthetics			
Cocaine		Na^{+} channel blockade Sympathomimetic effects Coronary vasospasm Altered Ca^{2+} balance Mitochondrial injury Oxidative stress Apoptosis	Arrhythmia Tachycardia, strengthened ventricular contraction, and increased blood pressure Ischemia, MI Decreased cardiac output Cardiomyopathy Heart failure
Other local anesthetics (bupivacaine, etidocaine, lidocaine, procainamide)		Na^{+} channel blockade	Arrhythmia Cardiac arrest Bradycardia
Antihistamines			
Astemizole, terfenadine		K^{+} channel blockade QTc interval prolongation	Arrhythmia Ventricular tachycardia
Immunosuppressants			
Rapamycin, tacrolimus		Altered Ca^{2+} balance	Decreased cardiac output Heart failure
Miscellaneous drugs			
Cisapride		K^{+} channel blockade QTc interval prolongation	Arrhythmia Ventricular tachycardia
Methylxanthines (theophylline)		Altered Ca^{2+} balance, Inhibition of phosphodiesterase	Increased cardiac output Tachycardia Arrhythmia
Sildenafil		Inhibition of phosphodiesterase	Arrhythmia
Radiocontrast agents (diatrizoatemeglumine, iohexol)		Apoptosis	Heart failure Arrhythmia Cardiac arrest

(*Continued*)

Table 2 Cardiotoxicity of key pharmaceutical agents—cont'd

A. Cardiotoxic agents			
Agents	*Sources*	*Prominent cardiac effects*	*Physiological endpoints*
Naturally occurring substances			
Interleukin-2 (Aldesleukin)		Increased nitric oxide synthase expression	Weakened ventricular contraction
Interferon-γ (Actimmune)		Increased nitric oxide synthase expression	Cardiomyopathy
		Altered ion balance	Arrhythmia
Selected industrial agents			
Solvents			
Toluene (paint products)		Decreased parasympathetic activity Increased adrenergic sensitivity Altered ion balance	Arrhythmia
Halogenated hydrocarbons			
Carbon tetrachloride Chloroform Chloropentafluoroethane		Decreased parasympathetic activity Increased adrenergic sensitivity Altered ion balance	Arrhythmia Weakened ventricular contraction Decreased cardiac output Arrhythmia
1,2-Dibromotetra-fluoromethane Dichlorodifluoromethane *cis*-dichloroethylene *trans*-dichloroethylene Dichlortetrafluorethane Difluoroethane Ethyl bromide Ethyl chloride Fluorocarbon 502 Heptafluoro-1-iodo-propane 1,2-Hexafluoroethane Isopropyl chloride Methyl bromide Methyl chloride Methylene chloride Monochlorodifluoroethane Monochlorodifluoromethane Octafluorcyclobutane Propyl chloride 1,1,1-trichloroethane Trichloroethane Trichloroethylene Trichlorofluoromethane Trichloromonofluoroethylene Trichlorotrifluoroethane Trifluoroiodomethane Trifluorobromomethane		Altered coronary blood flow	Ischemia/MI
Ketones			
e.g., Acetone, methyl ethyl ketone		Decreased parasympathetic activity Increased adrenergic sensitivity Altered ion balance	Arrhythmia Arrhythmia
Heavy metals			
Cadmium, cobalt, lead		Metal ions are taken up by the cell leading to altered cellular structure Altered Ca^{2+} balance	Weakened ventricular contraction Arrhythmia Cardiac hypertrophy
(Barium, lanthanum, manganese, nickel)		Ca^{2+} channel blockade	Arrhythmia

Table 2 Cardiotoxicity of key pharmaceutical agents—cont'd

B. Vasculotoxic agents			
Agents	*Sources*	*Prominent Vascular Effects*	*Physiological Endpoints*
Industrial and environmental agents			
Allylamine	Acrolein and hydrogen peroxide	Smooth muscle cell injury and resultant proliferation	Atherosclerosis
β-Aminopropionitrile		Damage to connective tissue	Aortic lesion, atherosclerosis, aneurysm
Boron		Increase in microvascular permeability	Pulmonary edema, hemorrhage
Butadiene	Synthetic precursor	Blood vessel tumors	Ischemia, cancer
Carbamylhydrazine		Tumors of pulmonary blood vessels	Cancer
Carbon disulfide	Fumigant/solvent	Endothelial injury	Impaired vision, blindness, blood clot, ischemia, MI Atherosclerosis
Chlorophenoxy herbicides		Cell membrane damage, vasodilation, oxidative stress	Hypotension, cardiomyopathy
Dimethylnitrosamine		Impaired q venous blood flow	Impaired venous return, hemorrhage, necrosis
Dinitrotoluenes	Synthetic precursor	Hemoglobin methylation	Decreased O_2 carrying capacity, hypotension
		Vascular smooth muscle cell proliferation	Atherosclerosis
Glycerol		Vasoconstriction	Acute renal failure
Hydrogen fluoride		Edema	Pulmonary edema, hemorrhage
Paraquat		Platelet activation	Cerebral/pulmonary blood clots
Pyrrolidine alkaloids		Damage to endothelial and smooth muscle cells	Pulmonary hypertension, venous occlusion
Organophosphate pesticides		Reduced enzyme function	Atherosclerosis
Vinyl chloride		Blood vessel tumors	Cancer, portal hypertension
Gases			
Carbon monoxide	Environmental	Endothelial damage, clot formation, edema	Blood clots, atherosclerosis, ischemia, MI
Nitric oxide		Endothelial permeability, edema	Pulmonary edema
Oxygen		Vasoconstriction, increased permeability, edema	Impaired vision, blindness
Ozone		Arterial lesion in the lung, intimal thickening	Pulmonary edema, atherosclerosis
Therapeutic agents and related compounds			
Antibiotics/antimitotics			
Cyclophosphamide	4-Hydroxycyclophosphamid (metabolite)	Endothelial damage	Pulmonary fibrosis
5-Fluorodeoxyuridine		Hemorrhage; clot formation	Blood clots, hypotension, ischemia
Gentamicin		Vasoconstriction	Renal failure
Vasoactive agents			
Amphetamine		Blood vessel inflammation	Ischemia, stroke, MI
Dihydroergotamine		Vasospasm	Ischemia, stroke, MI
Ergonovine		Vasospasm	Angina
Ergotamine		Vasospasm	Gangrene
Epinephrine		Vasoconstriction	Localized ischemia
Histamine		Vasospasm, endothelial damage	Ischemia, angina
Methysergide		Intimal proliferation, vascular occlusion	Coronary artery disease
Nicotine	Tobacco	Systemic endothelial and smooth muscle cell dysfunction	Hypertension, atherosclerosis, aneurysm
Nitrites and nitrates		Reduced smooth muscle responsiveness	Ischemia, hypertension
Norepinephrine		Vasospasm, endothelial damage	Ischemia, angina
Metabolic affectors			
Alloxan		Vascular damage, occlusion, loss of blood vessel number	Impaired vision, blindness
Chloroquine		Vascular damage, occlusion, loss of blood vessel number	Impaired vision, blindness

(*Continued*)

Table 2 Cardiotoxicity of key pharmaceutical agents—cont'd

B. Vasculotoxic agents			
Agents	*Sources*	*Prominent Vascular Effects*	*Physiological Endpoints*
Fructose		Vascular damage, occlusion, loss of blood vessel number	Impaired vision, blindness
Iodoacetates		Vascular damage, occlusion, loss of blood vessel number	Impaired vision, blindness
Anticoagulants			
Warfarin		Edema	Hemorrhage
Clopidorgrel bisulfate (plavix)		Clot formation	Blood clot, embolism, ischemia
Radiocontrast dyes			
Metrizamide; metrizoate		Coagulation; cell death	Blood clots, kidney failure
Cyanoacrylate adhesives			
2-Cyano-acrylate-*n*-butyl		Cell adhesion	Blood clots
Miscellaneous			
Aminorex fumarate		Intimal and medial thickening	Pulmonary hypertension
Oral contraceptives		Clot formation	Blood clots, ischemia, stroke, MI
Penicillamine		Vascular lesion	Kidney failure
Talc and other silicates		Clot formation	Blood clots
Tetradecylsulfate Na		Clot formation	Deep-vein thrombosis, pulmonary embolism
Nonsteroidal antiinflammatories (NSAIDs)			
Cyclooxygenase-2 inhibitors (Vioxx and Celebrex)		Platelet aggregation, clot formation	Embolism, ischemia, MI
Aspirin		Inhibition of platelet aggregation	Hemorrhage

Cardiac Muscle

There are three distinct types of muscle tissue in vertebrates: striated, smooth, and cardiac. Striated, or skeletal muscle is attached, at least at one end, to the skeleton via tendons. This muscle type is often referred to as the voluntary muscle, as it can be consciously controlled by the somatic nervous system. Smooth muscle is usually arranged in sheets or layers in tubular systems, such as arteries and veins (see section Blood Vessels), the gastrointestinal and respiratory tracts, and the genitourinary tracts. The activities of the smooth muscles are not under conscious control; rather they are coordinated by the autonomic (involuntary) nervous system. The cardiac muscle comprises the bulk of the heart wall proper; and small amounts are found in the superior vena cava and pulmonary vein. The cardiac muscle is not under conscious control; it has an automaticity center which is influenced by the autonomic nervous system (see section Impulse Conduction). In the heart, cardiac muscle cells are joined in a network of fibers and are connected by gap junctions, which facilitate the conduction of electrical impulses through the cardiac muscle network. This is referred to as a functional syncytium. In addition to cardiac myocytes, there are specialized cardiac conducting cells that initiate, attenuate, or accelerate the electrical impulses for coordinated contraction of the cardiac network. Proportionally speaking, cardiac myocytes make up ~99% of the contracting heart mass, whereas the conducting cells make up ~1%. Despite their small percentage, numerous toxicants have robust effects on these conducting cells, and this results in significant myocyte dysfunction that can result in fatalities.

Impulse Conduction

The specialized electrical conduction system of the heart allows for the synchronous contraction of the left and right sides of the heart and the sequential contraction of the atria and ventricles (**Figure 1(b)**). Electrical impulses most quickly arise in the spontaneously firing cells of the sinoatrial (SA) node commonly called the 'pacemaker.' The SA node is located at the junction of the superior vena cava and the right atrium. A wave of depolarization (see below) originating at the SA node is conducted first to the cells of the right atrium, then to the cells of both atria, finally converging on a second group of specialized cells – the cells of the AV node. These cells act as a conduit for the original impulse from the SA node to the AV node, which lies at the junction of the median wall of the right atrium and the septum separating the two ventricles. From the AV node, the impulse wave next passes into the ventricular conduction system – the bundle of His and Purkinje fibers – located within the ventricular septum, which allows for the depolarization of ventricular muscle.

If a microelectrode is inserted into a resting muscle or nerve cell (termed 'excitable tissue'), an electrical potential difference will be recorded across the membrane of that cell. In the case of cardiac muscle cells, this resting potential is −90 mV (intracellular relative to extracellular). In other words, the cell membrane is electrically polarized with the inward facing surface of the membrane having a net negative charge with respect to the outer facing surface of the membrane. This polarity is maintained primarily by the presence of extracellular positively charged ions and intracellular negatively charged proteins. The flux of ions through active (requiring

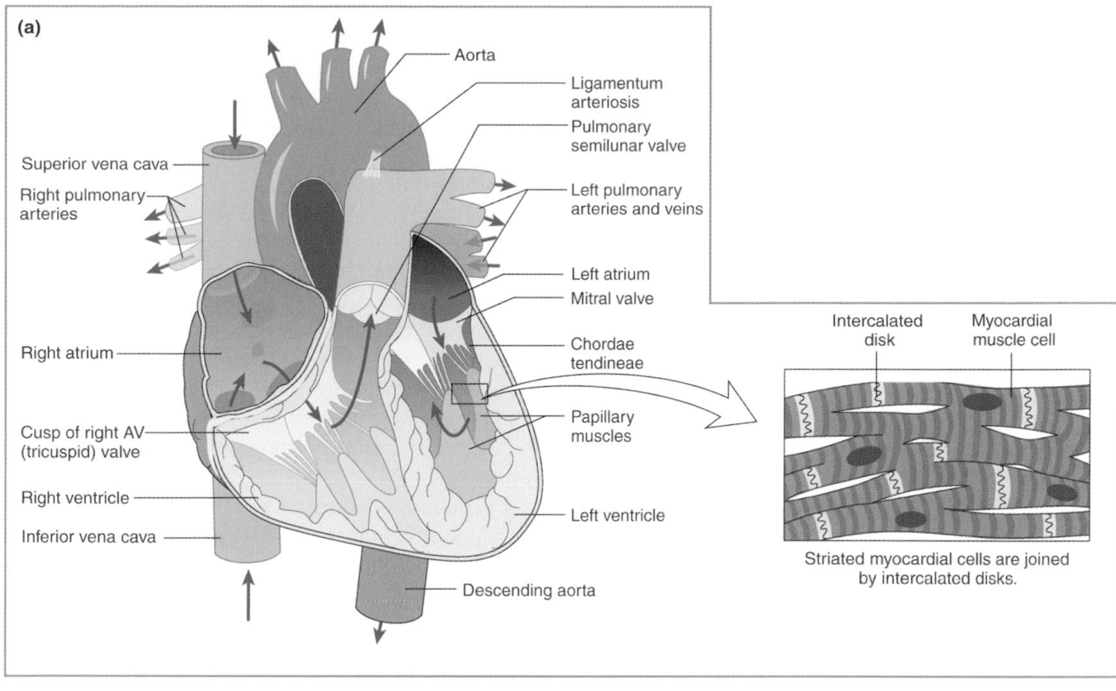

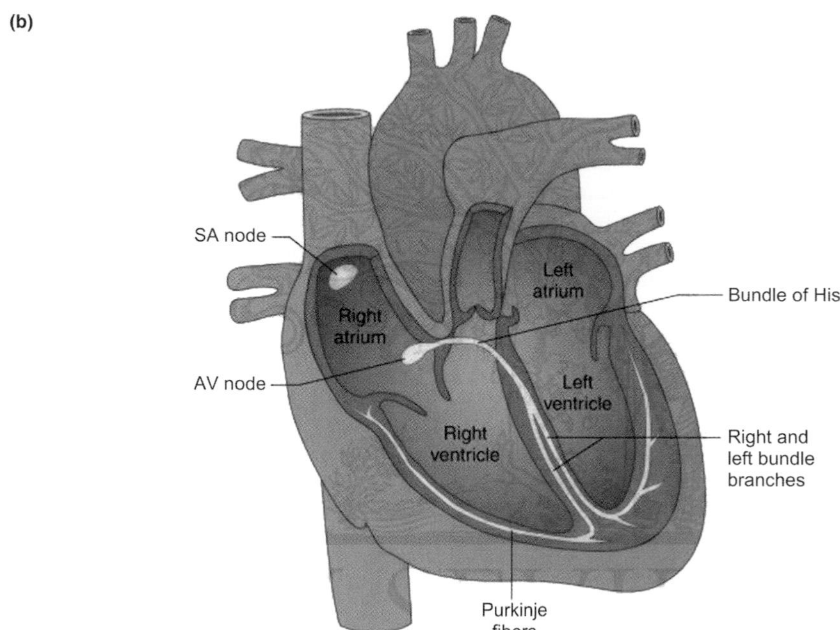

Figure 1 (a) Anatomy of the heart. Reproduced from Robert G. Carroll. The Heart. Elsevier's Intergrated Physiology 66. http://www.elsevierimages.com/image/33151.htm (b) Conduction system of the heart. Reproduced from Goldman, L., Ausiello, D. Electrocardiography. Cecil Medicine, 23rd Edition. 230. http://www.elsevierimages.com/image/25955.htm.

cellular energy) and passive (concentration-driven) processes is responsible for changes in electrical potential. In the resting cardiac muscle cell, the concentration of potassium ions (K^+) is higher inside the cell than outside, while sodium ions (Na^+) are at a much higher concentration outside the cell than inside. Cellular energy is required to maintain the appropriate resting state distributions of the different ions across the cell membrane. In the case of K^+ and Na^+ ions, there is a cell membrane pump, which requires energy derived from the hydrolysis of the terminal phosphate group from adenosine triphosphate (ATP). The associated enzyme responsible for this hydrolysis is the Na^+–K^+ ATPase. When an electrical stimulus is received by a cardiac muscle cell, voltage-gated channels in the cell membrane open allowing Na^+ to diffuse down its concentration and electrical gradients into the cell. This influx of positive charge causes the cell membrane to become 'depolarized' (i.e., to have less negative charge). As depolarization proceeds, the membrane may reach the threshold potential (−70 mV for most cardiac muscle cells). Any further depolarization results in a phenomenon known as the action potential, which completely depolarizes the cell. At the peak of the action potential, the inside of the cell actually becomes positive relative to the outside (+30 mV). The cell membrane then repolarizes relatively slowly and reaches the −90 mV resting potential before it can respond to another electrical impulse. The wave of depolarization moves very rapidly across the membrane of an individual cardiac muscle cell. In addition, the wave of action potentials is propagated to adjacent cells via the specialized gap junctions. This propagation allows for the complete depolarization of most cells in the network, thus initiating the contraction of the heart muscle as a group.

Cardiac muscle cells predominantly display a fast response action potential (**Figure 2**), and cells in the atria and ventricles exhibit a rapid conduction velocity due to the gap junctions. The depolarization–action potential–repolarization process is divided into five phases. Phase 0 begins when the threshold potential has been reached. At this time, many 'fast' Na^+ channels in the cell membrane open allowing an inrush of Na^+ ions to initiate the action potential. At the end of phase 0, the cell is completely depolarized. Toward the end of phase 1 and the start of phase 2, the Na^+ influx begins to decrease, as does the membrane potential. During the relatively long (200–300 ms) phase 2 plateau, calcium (Ca^{2+}) and Na^+ ions enter through 'slow' membrane channels. Movement of ions through these 'slow' channels only takes place after the membrane potential has dropped to approximately −55 mV, that is, after the 'fast' Na^+ ion current has ceased. While these 'slow' inward currents occur, there is also a slow outward movement of K^+ ions which keeps the plateau relatively steady. The Ca^{2+} influx of phase 2 triggers the process known as excitation–contraction coupling, in which the myosin thick filaments slide past the thin actin filaments in the contractile unit of the muscle known as the sarcomere. This process requires energy and involves activation of a myosin ATPase that hydrolyzes ATP. The released energy is utilized to form cross-bridges between the actin and myosin molecules. Both the velocity and the force of contraction are dependent on the amount of Ca^{2+} ions that reaches the site of contraction. Within the resting muscle cell, Ca^{2+} is sequestered in a compartment called the sarcoplasmic reticulum. During the action potential, Ca^{2+} and Na^+ ions that enter the cell cause depolarization of the sarcoplasmic reticulum membrane, resulting in the release of large amounts of Ca^{2+}, which are needed for effective contraction of the sarcomere. Between contractions, Ca^{2+} is once again sequestered in the sarcoplasmic reticulum so that the actin–myosin interaction is not overly prolonged. During the long duration of the plateau phase, a new action potential cannot be initiated because the 'fast' Na^+ channels are inactivated or refractory to further electrical stimulation. During phase 3, membrane permeability to K^+ increases and the 'slow' Ca^{2+} and Na^+ channels become inactive. The ensuing efflux of K^+ ions allows for repolarization of the membrane until the normal resting potential is reached (phase 4).

In contrast, conduction velocity is slow in muscle fibers at the SA and AV nodes. Unlike the majority of cardiac muscle cells, these pacemaker cells have an unstable resting potential (approximately −60 mV) due to a cell membrane alteration that allows Na^+ ions to leak into the cell without a concurrent K^+ ion efflux. This Na^+ leakage reduces the membrane potential allowing even more Na^+ ions to move into the cell. In addition to the inward Na^+ movement, there is also an inward Ca^{2+} flow which causes the pacemaker cells to have a more positive resting potential. Finally, the cell produces an action potential at approximately −40 mV. This phenomenon is called spontaneous diastolic depolarization. The overall effect is that pacemaker cells initiate waves of depolarization that move across the heart causing the muscle to contract. As noted previously, this phenomenon occurs ~72 times per minute (more or less depending on autonomic nervous system stimulation, periods of stress, or physical activity). The SA node is responsible for this rate as it depolarizes the fastest. The other nodes and components of the cardiac conduction may also drive depolarizations, only slowly. The purpose of this redundancy is to ensure pacemaker activity in the heart (to support cardiac homeostasis). The waves of electrical activity may be

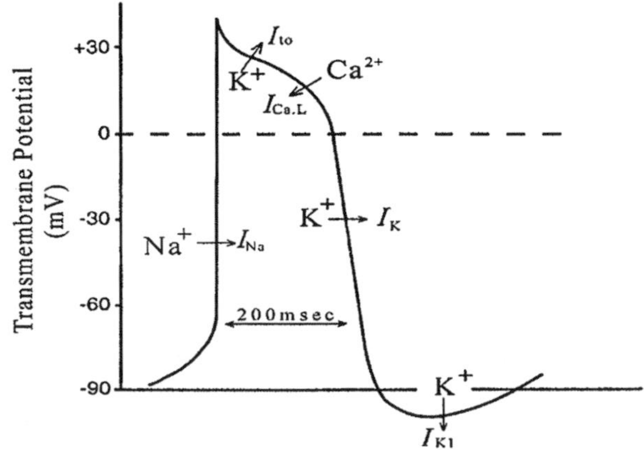

Figure 2 The principal ionic movements during the different phases of the action potential in a cardiac muscle cell. Reprinted with permission from Raffaele De Canterina, et al., 2003. Antiarrhythmic effects of omega-3 fatty acids: from epidemiology to bedside. Am. Heart J. 146 (3), 240–430. http://www.sciencedirect.com/science/article/pii/S0002870303003272

recorded in an electrocardiogram (ECG), which displays the net electrical changes relative to where the recording electrodes are placed on the surface of the body.

Intrinsic Modulators of Cardiac Activity

The heart responds constantly to hormonal and nervous system signals. Sympathetic nervous system terminals releasing norepinephrine are found in cardiac cells of the atria and ventricles. This allows for reflex regulation of heart muscle contractility. Sympathetic innervation is also present to the SA node and AV junction, where norepinephrine release acts to increase heart rate (enhanced phase 4 depolarization) and also to increase conduction velocity by reducing the AV junction impedance to conduction. Sympathetic innervation also occurs down to the resistance arterioles functionally increasing total peripheral resistance upon stimulation. Parasympathetic innervation is provided by cranial nerve 10, the vagus nerve, to the SA node and the AV junction. These fibers release acetylcholine, which slows SA node activity (decreasing the rate of phase 4 depolarization) and decreases conduction throughout the AV junction.

A practical example of normal nervous system regulation of cardiovascular activity is the processes of blood pressure regulation via baroreceptors located in the aortic arch and carotid arteries. Baroreceptors sense mechanical deformation when these arterial walls stretch and relax. These receptors send impulses to the cardiovascular regulatory sensors in the medulla (nucleus tractus solitarii) where dual reflex impulses are generated that reduce sympathetic signaling and increase parasympathetic outflow (vagus nerve) that ultimately decrease heart rate contractility, peripheral vascular resistance, and venous return. This results in a decreased blood pressure. Conversely, a decrease in blood pressure will decrease vagal stimulation in favor of sympathetic input. The sympathetic reflex is characterized by increases in heart rate, myocardial contractility, venous return, peripheral vascular resistance, and cardiac output. In addition, the sympathetic response can be produced by the release of naturally occurring catecholamines (epinephrine and norepinephrine) from the medulla of the adrenal gland.

Pathologic Changes in the Heart

The major pathologic changes that occur in the heart are associated with effects on heart rate, contractility of heart muscle, or electrical conduction. Regarding heart rate changes, an arrhythmia, as the name indicates, is a loss of rhythm and here refers to an irregularity of the heartbeat. Two of the more common forms are tachycardia, which is an abnormally rapid heartbeat, and fibrillation, which is a rapid twitching of the muscle fibrils. Either of these can occur in the atria or the ventricles. Agents that alter ion levels and fluxes and alter aspects of impulse transmission can produce arrhythmias. The most common site of arrhythmic impulse generation is the SA node. If depolarization after an action potential is accelerated or delayed anywhere within the heart, an aberrant action potential can be triggered and result in an arrhythmia.

Still other pathologic changes are associated with effects on the force of contraction. The heart muscle exhibits a higher rate of oxygen consumption and a greater energy requirement than many other tissues. Thus, impaired contraction can result from interference with any of the major cycles critical for proper energy metabolism or from processes that interfere with delivery or utilization of the optimum levels of oxygen. For example, if blood flow through the coronary arteries is occluded, as occurs during atherosclerosis, compromising blood flow and leading to a decreased delivery of oxygen to the heart muscle. This decrease in blood flow, reducing vital nutrient delivery, is termed ischemia. When the heart becomes ischemic, a patient may feel significant discomfort as heart or chest pain, termed angina. When this occurs acutely and to the point of cell (cardiac myocyte) death, a myocardial infarction (MI) may result, leading to devitalization of a segment of the heart musculature. Even if death does not occur, there will likely be a decrease in the force or efficiency of contraction of the heart muscle. 'Recreational' use of psychoactive drugs (e.g., amphetamines, cocaine) can result in profound and sudden cardiovascular responses including increases in blood pressure and heart rate due to acute catecholamine release in response to the drugs. These effects can be life threatening in individuals with underlying, and possibly previously unknown, cardiovascular problems including coronary artery disease, high blood pressure, or cerebrovascular disease.

Cells with high-energy requirements, such as cardiomyocytes, have large numbers of organelles called mitochondria, which produce and supply ATP. Enzymes are organic catalysts that interact with specific substrate molecules to help speed up chemical reactions. The ATPases are enzymes that catalyze the hydrolysis of ATP with its attendant release of energy, which is made available for cellular processes. The myosin ATPase involved in muscle contraction was mentioned above and ATPases involved in the energy-driven pumping of ions including Na^+, K^+, and Ca^{2+} were mentioned above and are noted again below. During oxidative metabolism of organic substrates, the process of electron transport to molecular oxygen in mitochondria is coupled to oxidative phosphorylation, which yields ATP. Some poisons and anticancer drugs, such as cyanide and doxorubicin, interfere with electron transport and/or uncouple phosphorylation. This causes a direct decrease in the amount of energy available to the heart muscle and results in reduced contractility.

As noted above, the inward Ca^{2+} ion movement is vital for the contraction of the cardiac muscle. This inward movement is blocked by Ca^{2+} antagonists, such as cobalt and barium, and is stimulated by catecholamines. Increased Ca^{2+} influx leads to increases in the intracellular level of cyclic adenosine monophosphate (AMP), a compound that helps mediate numerous metabolic responses within cells. This, in turn, leads to increased availability of Ca^{2+} ions for interaction with the contractile proteins. The same effect can be achieved by increased levels of free Ca^{2+} ions outside of the cells or increased levels of cyclic AMP within cells, as is seen with the vasodilating drug papaverine. Another mechanism for increasing intracellular Ca^{2+} levels in cardiac cells involves the cardiac glycoside drugs, for example, digitalis from the foxglove plant. This drug inhibits the ATPase that pumps Na^+ ions out of cells. This results in elevation of Na^+ ion levels inside the cell, which in turn leads to increases in intracellular Ca^{2+} ion levels and therefore increased rate and strength of contraction.

Toxins that increase the permeability of the cardiac muscle cell membrane to the Na^+ ion, for example, the marine compound, ciguatoxin or the Columbian frog poison active agent, batrachotoxin, have a similar effect. On the contrary, agents that decrease membrane permeability to Na^+ ions will depress myocardial contractility. Included here are a diverse group of compounds including tetrodotoxin, from the Japanese pufferfish; the shellfish-derived poison, saxitoxin; and polyethylene glycol, the active ingredient in many antifreeze preparations. Local anesthetics such as lidocaine and procaine depress the fast inward Na^+ ion current, the slow Ca^{2+} ion inward current, and the K^+ ion outward current. They tend to slow the heart rate and the force of contraction; thus, they are commonly used as antiarrhythmic drugs.

There are compounds that interfere with the regular activity of Ca^{2+} ions in cardiac cells, either by replacing them (as is the case with a number of heavy metals) or by altering the flux of Ca^{2+} ions across the cell membrane. Among metals, lanthanum, manganese, and nickel all block Ca^{2+} channels in the cell membrane. Both barium and cobalt ions antagonize endogenous Ca^{2+} ion levels and tend to shorten the action potential. Lead ions have multiple effects, including displacement of Ca^{2+} and interference with Ca^{2+} ion availability, energy metabolism, and ATP synthesis in heart muscle cells. Among organic chemicals, the opium derivative, papaverine, also blocks slow Ca^{2+} ion channels. Cardiotoxins such as cobra venom and bacterial endotoxins both interfere with Ca^{2+} ATPase activity; but endotoxin also depresses Ca^{2+} uptake by heart muscle cells.

Drugs prescribed to alleviate one set of medical problems can have striking and sometimes fatal effects on the cardiac system. Antipsychotics derived from phenothiazine, including chlorpromazine, depress myocardial contractility and cardiac output. Chlorpromazine can also impair cardiac reflex mechanisms and cause a focal myocardial necrosis. Cyclophosphamide, an anticancer agent, also causes myocardial necrosis as well as changes in ECG patterns. Another anticancer agent, doxorubicin, can produce cardiomyopathies with subsequent congestive heart failure. Severe dysrhythmias and some cases of sudden death have been reported. Overdoses of the tricyclic antidepressants, for example, amitryptaline, can result in severe cardiotoxicity, probably due to anticholinergic activity. At high doses, the antidepressant imipramine will depress contractility, lower heart rate, and depress cardiac output. Cardiac arrest may also occur. Some antibiotics, including gentamycin and neomycin, depress Ca^{2+} ion uptake and therefore reduce contractility of the cardiac muscle. Although the sympathetic system transmitters, the catecholamines, are essential for maintenance of normal myocardial contractility, it has been long recognized that when administered at higher than normal levels for extended periods of time, they can lead to severe myocardial necrosis.

In addition to inducing direct cardiac toxicity, many drugs increase the time between depolarization and repolarization of the left and right ventricles. This increase in time is referred to as QT interval prolongation (time from the start of the Q wave to the end of the T wave on an ECG) (**Figure 3**). Common classes of drugs that induce QT interval prolongation are the tricyclic antidepressants, fluoroquinolones among others (**Table 1**). QT interval prolongation is a sensitive biomarker for risk of developing a fatal arrhythmia, torsades de pointes (a.k.a. polymorphic tachycardia). In addition to being a measurement for risk of developing sudden cardiac death, QT prolongation, has been used as an important screening tool for the evaluation of pharmaceutical drugs in development.

Profound cardiotoxic responses can result from inhalation of a number of halogenated alkanes. These are low molecular weight hydrocarbons with some or all of the hydrogen atoms being substituted by halogens, usually chlorine or fluorine. These agents depress heart rate, contractility, and electrical conduction. The effects are generally more pronounced as the number of halogen atoms increases. Some of these compounds have the additional and profound effect of sensitizing cardiac muscle cells to catecholamines. In humans without preexisting cardiac disease, the effects of most of these compounds are reversible, although chronic exposure may cause some irreversible damage. As would be expected, the older halogenated hydrocarbon anesthetics such as halothane and enflurane had similar effects.

In contrast, low-pressure fluorocarbons, such as trichlorofluoromethane, can be particularly toxic. In most cases, the levels generally encountered in the environment are too low to have any major lasting effect and even at relatively high levels (up to 15%) fatalities are rarely recorded. However, at levels much above this, for example, over 20%, tragic results can ensue. Among people who inhale these agents from closed bags to 'get high,' fatalities can result because the levels of these agents in the bags can reach 35–40%.

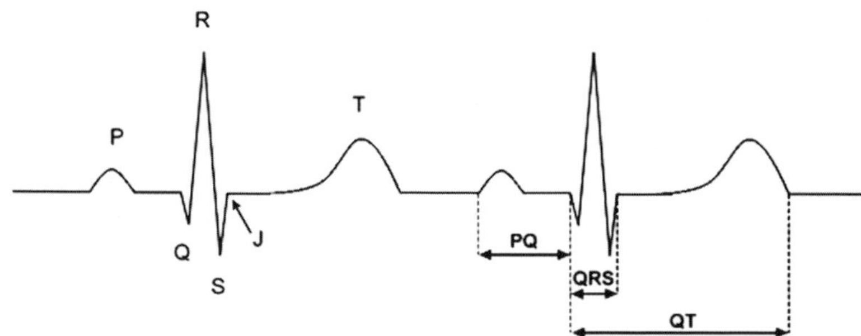

Figure 3 EKG schematic. Reproduced from Farkas, A., et al., 2004. How to measure electrocardiographic QT interval in the anaesthetized rabbit. J. Pharm.Toxicol. Methods 50 (3), 175–185. http://www.sciencedirect.com/science/article/pii/S0002870303003272

Agents Causing Morphologic Changes

A number of cardiotoxic compounds have been listed to this point, including some that interfere with Na^+/K^+ ATPases; increase Na^+ or Ca^{2+} influx; or depress myocardial function by replacing Ca^{2+}, decreasing Na^+ permeability, or altering contractility. These agents produce toxic responses in the heart muscle often resulting in death, but do so without causing any major morphologic changes in the heart. Other cardiotoxic compounds produce characteristic morphologic lesions in the heart muscle. There are a few basic types of such pathologic alterations, such as toxic myocarditis and MI. Chemicals, which produce toxic myocarditis cause cell damage and, ultimately, cell death. Whether or not they produce damage acutely or chronically is generally a function of the toxicant dose. The acute myocarditis is characterized by edema (accumulation of excess fluid), inflammatory cell responses, and multiple regions of cardiac cell death. However, the inflammatory response will be attenuated or may be absent if the toxic agent suppresses the immune system, for example, drugs given to prevent rejection of transplanted organs.

MI in the heart arises from a sudden insufficiency or local arrest of the blood supply to the heart that can result in necrosis of a region of the heart. In advanced arteriosclerosis, occlusion of the major arteries supplying the heart muscle with blood can result in an MI. Even in the absence of arteriosclerosis, MIs can result, for example, from amphetamine abuse, which produces severe inflammations of critical arteries (i.e., an arteritis). Intravenous drug use can cause infective endocarditis (an inflammation of the internal lining of the heart), which can lead to vessel occlusion with an embolus, thus resulting in an MI. Cocaine abuse can result in ventricular tachycardia (i.e., rapid heartbeat) and fibrillation, MI, and sudden death. At higher doses, cocaine can increase the levels of catecholamines, ultimately resulting in increased Ca^{2+} ion activity, accelerated heartbeat, arrhythmias, etc. Chemicals that antagonize Ca^{2+} ion movement through Ca^{2+}-specific membrane channels prevent the ventricular arrhythmias induced by cocaine. Gross MI can result from toxic exposures to carbon monoxide, nitrates, ergot derivatives, and some potent anticancer drugs (see above).

Media attention and Food and Drug Administration (FDA) guidelines have focused on the cardiovascular effects of appetite-suppressant drugs and nutraceuticals or herbal medicines. In 1997, the antiobesity drugs fenfluramine and dexfenfluramine were withdrawn from the United States sales market due to convincing correlations made between drug usage and cardiac valvular abnormalities. Since then, the deleterious morphologic effects of these drugs have been described as valvular encasement and/or endocardial fibrosis. These lesions can have life-threatening consequences, including progressive aortic valvular regurgitation. The mechanism underlying the pathogenesis of these lesions remains unclear. There appears to be a correlation with increased serotonin levels in the blood and endocardial fibrosis; thus, there is speculation that these drugs may increase serotonin levels or may increase sensitivity of tissues to serotonin. In addition, the dietary supplement ephedra (ma huang) has been implicated in cases of MI due to coronary artery vasoconstriction and sudden cardiac death; thus, in 2004, the FDA issued a warning about ephedra with a ban on its sale and use in the United States.

Another type of gross morphologic lesion in the heart muscle is hypersensitivity myocarditis. This is an inflammatory response that is the most common type of heart disease associated with therapeutic drug use. There are five primary clinical criteria for diagnosis of this condition: (1) previous use of the drug(s) without deleterious incidents; (2) no apparent relationship between the size of the drug dose and the hypersensitivity response; (3) clinical symptoms consistent with responses to allergens or infectious disease agents; (4) independent confirmation of immunologic responses; and (5) persistence of the symptoms as long as drug use is continued. Histologically, there is infiltration of the heart muscle with numerous types of white blood cells and this is associated with local regions of lysis of the cardiac muscle cells. However, gross fibrosis and extensive regions of myocardial necrosis are usually absent. Among the drugs that have been reported to elicit this response are the antibiotics penicillin, streptomycin, ampicillin, tetracycline, and sulfadiazine.

The Blood Vessels

The second part of the CVS is composed of the blood vessels, which are an extensive series of tubular conduits of varying diameters. All but the narrowest of these vessels have a complex wall structure (see below). One major group of vessels, the arteries, distributes blood under various degrees of pressure to all parts of the body. A second major group of vessels, the veins, returns the blood to the heart. With the exception of the pulmonary artery, which brings blood from the heart to the lungs, the arteries carry blood that is more oxygenated than the blood in their venous counterparts. The large- and medium-sized arteries and veins share the same general structure, although the thicknesses of specific cell layers as well as the cell density within layers can vary considerably.

Blood Flow

Despite the system's vital function of transporting blood throughout the body, it would be overly simplistic to view the vascular system as merely a series of pipes of varying diameter. When the left ventricle contracts to deliver blood to the aorta, the largest artery in the body, not only is the blood pressure generated at contraction relatively high, but it is also maintained at a moderately high pressure between contractions of the heart. If the arteries were a set of rigid pipes, the pressure in the artery system would fall to zero between contractions. The fact that this does not occur is due chiefly to the presence of numerous elastic layers (composed of the protein elastin) in the largest arteries. As the heart contracts, the blood pumped into these large arteries causes the elastin in the walls to stretch. Following contraction, the semilunar valves close (see description of valves above) and the walls of the elastic arteries contract passively to maintain pressure within the system until the ventricles fill and contract once again. Overall, this expansion and passive contraction is termed vascular compliance. There are large, elastic arteries, which function primarily to maintain the pressure within the arterial system during diastole, the resting phase of heart contraction. This allows for steady flow to downstream capillaries, despite the inconsistent pressure highs (systole) and lows (diastole) at each heartbeat. There are also muscular arteries, which function primarily to distribute the blood throughout the body to organs and tissues, each of which may require different amounts of blood. To help ensure that appropriate volumes of blood are delivered on demand, the size of the lumen (the space through which the blood flows) of the muscular arteries must be regulated quickly and reliably. Any delay or interruption to this arteriole regulation or delivery would be termed vascular dysfunction and could lead to tissue or organ damage downstream. This is accomplished systemically via innervation by sympathetic fibers of the autonomic nervous system and by local vasoactive chemical signals at the tissue level.

Because capillary walls are thin (to permit diffusion) the blood that is delivered to them must be delivered under reduced pressure. This is accomplished by the arterioles, which combine relatively muscular walls with a narrow lumen. The arterial blood pressure is a function of cardiac output and the total peripheral vascular resistance, which is primarily a function of the degree of normal tension (tone) of the smooth muscle cells in the arteriolar walls. Arteriolar tone is a unitless value with 100% tone representing complete vessel closure/constriction, and 0% representing a maximally dilated vessel. Broadly speaking, arterioles typically maintain a partial state of tone (~40–60%) to be able to maintain tissue homeostasis, by constricting or dilating as needed. Tone is under the influence of many intrinsic and extrinsic factors such as the autonomic nervous system (almost exclusively sympathetic activity), circulating hormones (catecholamines), tissue metabolic state (oxygen and carbon dioxide), temperature, and physical forces (blood flow shear stress). If tone increases above the normal range and remains so for extended periods of time, hypertension (high blood pressure) can result.

From the capillaries, blood flows first into the narrowest members of the venous system, the collecting venules, and then into the muscular venules, whose diameter is approximately twice as large and whose walls contain one or two layers of smooth muscle cells. Blood then flows into progressively larger veins, first to the small and then to the medium-sized veins. Veins that are located deep within tissue tend to have thinner, less muscular walls than do superficial veins. The final set of veins to receive blood before it is delivered back to the heart are the inferior and superior vena cava. The outermost cellular layer in these veins is considerably thicker and the innermost layer is considerably thinner than those of the aorta, the first artery leaving the heart. Another difference between arteries and veins is that the latter have a more extensive vasa vasorum, an arterial blood supply to the vessel wall. Since venous blood is relatively poorly oxygenated, veins require supplemental oxygenation supplied by the vasa vasorum. Because venous blood is under low pressure, the vasa vasorum can penetrate closer to the innermost layer of the vein without being occluded by compressive pressures in the wall.

Pathological Changes

Approximately 90% of the pathologic alterations seen in veins are associated with one of three conditions: deep-vein thrombosis, which often appears following acute MI, thrombotic strokes and/or major surgery; varicose veins, which usually arise secondary to sustained increases of venous pressure; and superficial thrombophlebitis, which occurs in humans with varicose veins as well as in some females after pregnancy. A few venotoxic responses to exogenous (i.e., from outside the body) agents are noted below; however, the great majority of vasculotoxic agents have their effects on the arteries. Therefore, only a description of the artery wall structure is presented below along with listings and selected descriptions of agents that damage the arteries. The majority of these vasculotoxic agents affect vascular compliance or arteriole regulation, resulting in an inappropriate distribution of blood flow. There are many normal physiological processes, which also effect vascular compliance and may compound toxicological exposure, including aging, hypertension, and atherosclerosis. Additionally, exposure to toxicological agents (e.g., carbon disulfide or methysergide; see **Table 2** for additional examples) may compound existing disease or hasten disease progression.

Artery Wall Structure

There are three principal layers (tunics) that have been identified in the wall of large- and medium-sized arteries (**Figure 4**). The outermost layer, the tunica adventitia, is composed of connective tissue cells as well as extensive deposits of the proteins collagen and elastin. The adventitia in muscular arteries is approximately one-half the thickness of the middle layer, the media. In muscular arteries, the media is composed primarily of layers of smooth muscle cells. The principal extracellular protein component is elastin. In elastic arteries the tunica media also predominates, but in this case there are many layers of elastin with smooth muscle cells between the layers. The media is separated from the adventitia by a prominent elastic layer, the external elastic lamina. The adventitia of elastic arteries is thinner than that of muscular arteries. In large arteries, a vasa vasorum will also be present. The innermost layer of the artery wall is the tunica intima, which is separated from the media by the internal elastic lamina. In photomicrographs, the inner elastic lamina appears fenestrated (pores that allow cells or otherwise nonpermeable materials to exit the vascular lumen). This may serve as a relatively low-resistance pathway for migration of smooth muscle cells into the intima from the media, a process thought to be involved in the development of atherosclerotic plaques (see below). A single layer of endothelial cells (see below) borders the intima at the lumenal surface.

The media is the most heterogeneous in composition and the most variable in size of the three major coats of the artery. The predominant cell type in the media is the smooth muscle cell. Although some subtle differences in both appearance and behavior have been noted between smooth muscle cells in the intima versus those in the media, it is still not clear whether this is due to the presence of more than one type of smooth muscle cell, or to differing microenvironments in these two adjacent regions of the artery wall.

Atherosclerosis is a major cause of death in most industrial societies. The characteristic lesion of this disease, the

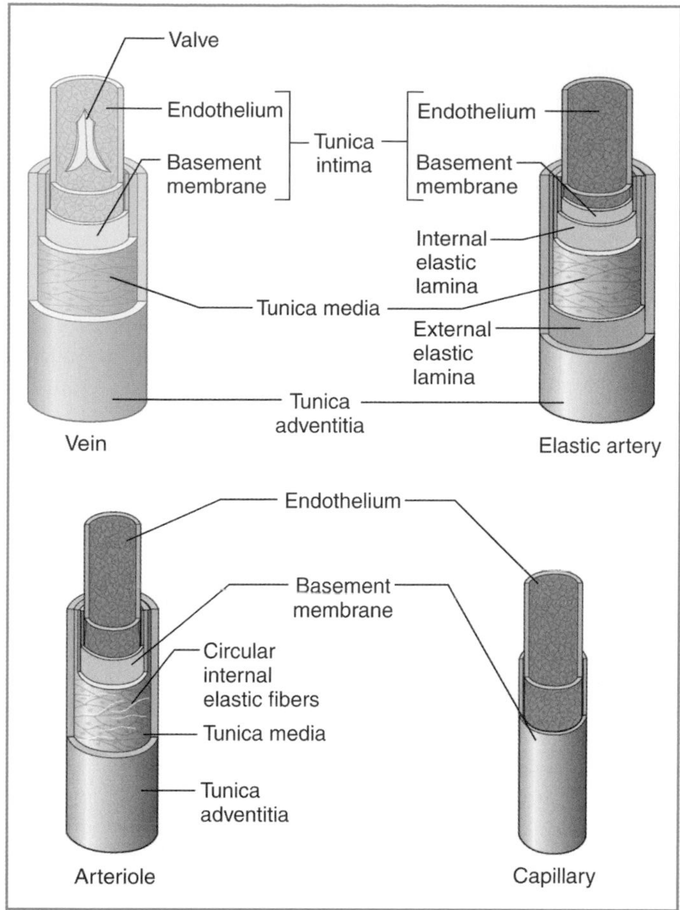

Figure 4 Comparison of typical artery and typical vein. Reprinted with permission from Cotran, R., Kumar. V., Collins. T. (Eds.), 1999. Robbins Pathologic Basic of Disease, sixth ed. Saunders, Philadelphia, PA; Carroll, R.G. Vascular System. Elsevier's Integrated Physiol. 78. http://www.elsevierimages.com/image/33161.htm.

atherosclerotic plaque, is found in the intima of large- and medium-sized arteries, thereby thickening the vessel, effecting vascular compliance, and the ability to efficiently distribute blood. An additional problem with advanced plaques is that thrombus formation is likely to occur in regions of plaque rupture. The combination of the two events can lead to partial or even total occlusion of major arteries. If this occurs in one or more of the coronary arteries, a serious or even fatal MI may result. A discussion of arteriosclerosis and exogenous agents that can modulate this condition is presented below.

There are a large variety of compounds that evoke toxic responses within the arterial intima, several of which will be discussed below. These compounds are of interest not only because of their cardiovascular side effects but also by gaining an understanding of the mechanism(s) whereby these agents act in living organisms, new insights into the complexities of the arterial intima may be revealed. Currently, heart disease and stroke are the leading causes of death in the United States and they account for nearly 900 000 deaths per year. These deaths can be contributed to many factors including both cardiotoxic and vasculotoxic agents; however, the major (and largely unavoidable) vasculotoxic agent that is associated with these diseases is tobacco smoke, which will be discussed later.

Endothelial Damage

Maintenance of the integrity of the single layer of endothelial cells that lines all of the vascular system is critical for normal vessel function. The intact endothelium is a dynamic system. It acts as a permeability barrier, preventing access of blood-borne contaminants to intimal cells. The intact endothelium also prevents adherence of white blood cells and thrombi; produces and secretes a wide range of growth regulatory molecules; and maintains vascular tone by releasing molecules that modulate dilation and constriction of blood vessels crucial for the appropriate distribution of blood. Endothelial injury or dysfunction is often considered a first-step of atherosclerosis. Endothelial cells are capable of oxidizing low-density lipoprotein (LDL), which is primarily responsible for transporting cholesterol through the blood to tissues. Oxidized LDL can injure the endothelium directly, produce molecules that allow specific types of white blood cells to adhere to the endothelial surface, and attract inflammatory cells to the inner surface of the artery. Presently, the prevailing view is that these events are critical to the early stages of atherosclerotic plaque formation. Since the structural and metabolic integrity of endothelial cells is vital to normal arterial function, and agents causing damage to endothelial cells might be present in the blood at any time, there must be efficient processes available to repair the endothelium and maintain its integrity should it become damaged.

Blood vessels of similar anatomical structure have distinct responses to chemical stress depending on the organ system with which they are associated. This may be due to subtle differences at the cellular and subcellular levels between similar cells and/or to local responses to different stimuli, for example, due to specific hormone receptors or patterns of innervation. Consider the blood–brain barrier, which prevents many potentially toxic blood-borne agents from reaching the brain. If the metabolic status of the endothelial cells in vessels at the brain level is altered, one result can be a disruption of the tight junctions between the endothelial cells, with a resulting increase in permeability. As a result, the brain, which normally is shielded from a number of toxic agents, may now be exposed to them. Lack of oxygen or markedly reduced local blood flow (ischemia) will lead to swelling of the endothelial cells and a widening of the junctions. Chemicals, including alcohols and surfactants, that solubilize lipids, which are an important component of cell membranes, can also impair the barrier. Lead ions interact with sulfhydryl (–SH) groups that are critical to the functioning of many endothelial cell enzymes and structural proteins. Lead ions thus produce damage to the endothelial cells in blood vessels supplying the brain well before the typically recognized damage to nervous system cells is recognized. Chemicals that raise osmotic pressure, such as solutions of high salt or the alcohol, mannitol, can cause endothelial cells to shrink, thereby causing the tight junctions between the cells to separate.

The liver is the organ largely responsible for detoxification of xenobiotic (foreign biological) chemicals and partly, as a consequence, is also constantly at risk for damage by toxic chemicals. One such chemical, the carcinogen dimethylnitrosamine, first induces the proliferation of endothelial cells, followed by increased formation of vascular connective tissue, and, ultimately, total venous occlusion. Plant toxins of the pyrrolizidine alkaloid family, including monocrotaline, can produce identical effects. Monocrotaline, which enters the body in a nontoxic form, is metabolized to its toxic form(s) by the liver. In addition to liver damage, this agent causes structural remodeling of blood vessels in the lung and a resultant increase in pulmonary arterial pressure. This effect is similar to the chronic pulmonary hypertension from which many people suffer.

Metals

A number of metals that cause kidney damage act on arteries supplying blood to this organ. Elevated levels of cadmium are associated with hypertension, at least in animal studies. Cadmium has also been implicated in thickening of the wall of arterioles and deposition of fibrotic tissue in capillaries in the testes as well as the kidneys. Agents that chelate cadmium can reverse many of these effects, as can elevation of body levels of zinc. It appears that cadmium and zinc are antagonistic and that maintenance of a cadmium/zinc ratio within fairly well defined limits may be important in preventing cadmium-associated vessel wall changes.

Three other metal ions that have been implicated in damage to vessel walls are mercury, chromium, and arsenic. Mercury, which interferes with protein –SH groups, may cause vasoconstriction of preglomerular vessels in the kidney.

Arsenic, though an unlikely contributor to blood vessel damage on a worldwide level, represents a striking example of how local environmental alterations can have profound effects on a large portion of a population. On the southwest coast of Taiwan, the artesian well water consumed by the local population has high levels of arsenic and about one out of every 100 people suffer from blackfoot disease. In late stages of this disease, extremities can become gangrenous, leading to spontaneous or surgical amputation of extremities. People suffering from this disease exhibit much higher levels of both peripheral vascular disease and cardiovascular disease. The mechanism of the action of arsenic on the blood vessels remains unclear.

Primary Amines

Cardiotoxicity of primary amines (epinephrine, norepinephrine, isoproterenol) was noted earlier, and has been recognized for nearly 100 years. The vascular toxicity of these and related compounds has also recently been recognized. The effects seem to focus on medial cells of the artery wall, rather than on adventitial or endothelial cells. Early changes include loss of medial cells, mineralization, and loss of elastic fibers. Later there is a compensatory proliferation of intimal cells. The vascular toxicity of two related compounds is particularly striking. One of these compounds, allylamine, will be discussed in the end of this article. The second is β-aminoproprionitrile (β-APN), which is the active agent in the toxic sweet pea, *Lathyrus odoratus*. Consumption of flour derived from this plant results in lathyrism, a condition often seen in children and young adults residing in Algeria, Ethiopia, and parts of India. Sudden death can result because of rupture of aortic aneurysms, which are ballooned and weakened segments of the artery wall. The toxicity of β-APN has been related to its inhibition of an enzyme which normally cross-links collagen and elastin in large elastic arteries, including the aorta, thereby strengthening them.

Atherosclerosis and Arteriosclerosis

Atherosclerosis is a physiological term to describe the progressive thickening of the arteries that compromises lumen size (thus decreasing the open area available for appropriate blood flow). Whereas arteriosclerosis (literally 'artery hardening') is the general term used to describe stiffening that can occur for a variety of reasons in arteries of all sizes. From a clinical perspective, the atherosclerotic plaque or lesion is of greatest interest (**Figure 5**). It is the principal lesion associated

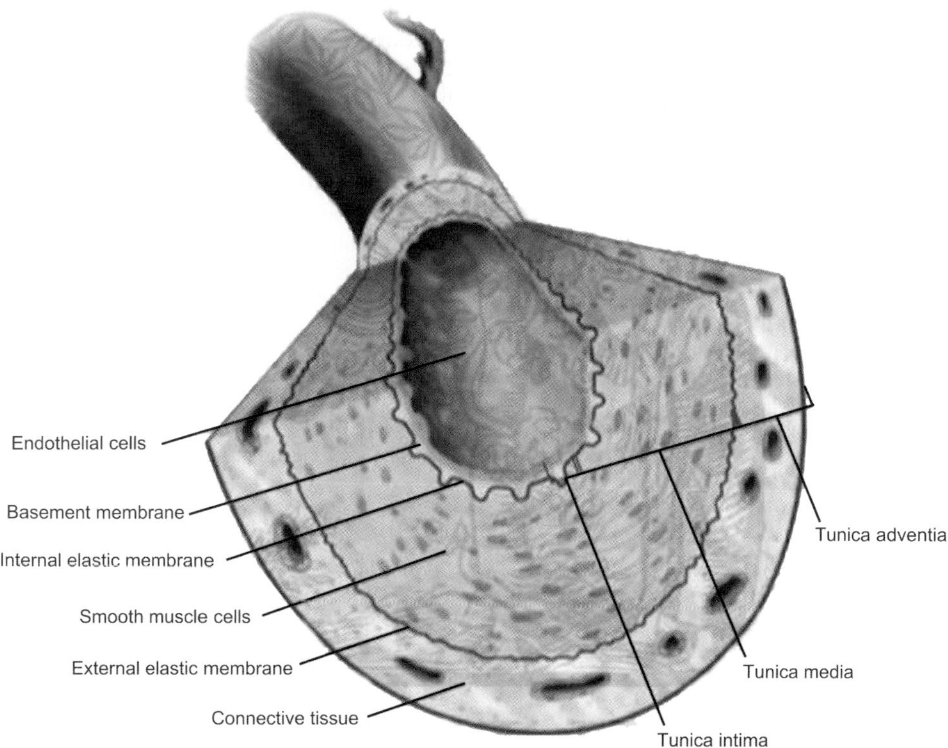

Figure 5 Diagrammatic representation of the main components of the vascular wall. Reprinted with permission from Cotran, R., Kumar, V., and Collins, T. (Eds.), 1999. Robbins Pathologic Basis of Disease, sixth ed. Saunders, Philadelphia, PA; Mulroney, S.E., Myers, A.K. The peripheral circulation. Netter's Essential Physiol. 126. http://www.netterimages.com/image/21407.htm.

with human thrombosis leading to myocardial and cerebral infarction, which are the primary causes of death in the United States, Canada, Europe, and Japan. Plaque development is complex, involving processes as diverse as cell proliferation, cell death, synthesis and deposition of a variety of extracellular macromolecules (e.g., collagens, elastin, proteoglycans), lipid accumulation, and mineralization. The plaque typically appears in the arterial intima with a variety of associated cell types, including smooth muscle cells, macrophages, lymphocytes, platelets, and endothelial cells. From a mechanical perspective, the thickening leading to the eventual hardening of the arteries (arteriosclerosis) decreases their elasticity, which directly compromises vascular compliance, and results in an increased cardiac workload (for each beat), ineffective vascular pressure regulation, and altered blood flow distribution. Plaque formation has been classified both as a problem of proliferation and one of degeneration, as well as an inflammatory process, a response to injury, and a process related to benign tumor formation. There is considerable clinical and experimental evidence that supports each of these views.

Although in most cases atherosclerosis does not become manifest as a clinically serious condition until well into middle age or beyond, it is a disease that begins early in life. Autopsy studies on US soldiers killed during the Korean War revealed that many already had arterial deposits characteristic of the early stages of atherosclerosis. More recent studies on children through people in the third decade of life have confirmed and expanded these findings. The good news is that while there are genetic factors which may predispose an individual to develop atherosclerosis, there is considerable evidence that individual choices and lifestyle decisions can play a large role in preventing, or at least mitigating, the early onset of clinical symptoms of this disease. Further, results from a limited number of laboratory animal studies suggest that it may even be possible to reverse the clinical course of the disease.

Since aging is inevitable, there are three areas where lifestyle modification can have profound effects on moderating development of clinically significant atherosclerosis. In addition to exercise, the two areas most amenable to change are diet and smoking. There is strong epidemiological evidence associating elevated levels of serum cholesterol with increasing risk of atherosclerosis and subsequent heart attacks. As noted above, LDL is primarily responsible for transporting cholesterol and its esters through the bloodstream to the tissues. Oxidized LDL can damage vessel wall cells, including endothelial cells. Oxidized LDL can act as and also generate a chemoattractant, which attracts monocytes to the endothelial surface and possibly helps mediate passage of monocytes across the endothelium where they may differentiate into tissue macrophages. Monocyte-derived macrophages act as scavengers to help remove harmful molecules such as oxidized LDL. When normal control mechanisms are dysfunctional, macrophages filled with oxidized LDL can become foam cells, which are critical to the formation of early stage atherosclerotic plaques. Studies on experimental animals as well as humans have shown that reduction in levels of plasma cholesterol and LDL can lead to significant widening of the arterial lumen. There is evidence that probucol, a drug originally used for its plasma cholesterol-lowering capability, may function primarily as an antioxidant protecting the integrity of LDL.

Relaxation of blood vessels appears to be at least partially under the control of endothelial cells and their secreted products, especially endothelium-derived relaxation factor (more specifically, nitric oxide). Oxidized LDL directly inhibits the endothelial cell-associated vessel relaxation. The generation of increased reactive oxygen species in association with elevated levels of blood cholesterol has also been reported. One of these reactive oxygen species, superoxide (O_2^-), may interact with nitric oxide within the artery wall, preventing endothelium-dependent vasodilation. In addition, a common product of the reaction between nitric oxide and superoxide is peroxynitrite ($ONOO^-$). This highly reactive molecule may act to stimulate lipoprotein oxidation, which, as noted above, is regarded as an early step in the development of atherosclerotic plaques.

Oxidants arise from two sources. The first, which is internal, is related to various metabolic processes, including respiration, phagocytic activity to destroy bacteria- and/or virus-infected cells, and, paradoxically, attempts to detoxify foreign substances. In the process of carrying out the latter activity, toxic oxidant by-products can be produced. The second source is external. While the potential protective effects of dietary components and supplements, for example, vitamins, are still being debated, it is reasonable to conclude that decreasing exposure to oxidants from external sources would be beneficial not only in reducing chances of premature atherosclerosis, but also of other diseases, including cancer. By far the most common, avoidable, and dangerous source of external oxidants is cigarette smoke, which is considered a principal contributor to one-quarter of all heart disease cases, one-third of all cancers, and ~440 000 premature deaths in the United States every year. As economies of developing countries expand and as cigarette smoking becomes more popular throughout the world, health problems associated with cigarette smoking will increase rapidly.

Cigarette Smoke

Cigarette smoke is composed of active smoke, the smoke coming from the mouth end of the cigarette and breathed in by the smoker; and passive smoke (second-hand smoke; environmental tobacco smoke) which is composed mostly of the smoke coming off the burning end of the cigarette plus a small percentage of exhaled smoke. Active and passive smoke contain many constituents in common, but often in strikingly different concentrations. Among the more than 4000 different chemicals that have been identified in cigarette smoke, prominent candidates that have been considered as vasculotoxic agents include carbon monoxide and various carcinogens. In addition to interfering with transport of well-oxygenated blood, carbon monoxide may cause endothelial cell damage directly, although the mechanism is not clear. Another major class of potential, vasculotoxins in cigarette smoke is the carcinogens. Most of these are found in the tar condensate fraction of cigarette smoke. Some, including benzo(*a*)pyrene, are well-known carcinogens that are found in other environmentally prominent substances including coal tar derivatives, charcoal-broiled meat, and automobile exhaust. Other smoke carcinogens include the nitrosamines, some of which are tobacco-specific. Both benzo(*a*)pyrene and the parent nitrosamines require metabolic activation to become carcinogenic. The enzymes involved in these processes are members of the cytochrome P-450 system. During the course of detoxifying these agents so that they ultimately can be excreted readily, one or more toxic and possibly carcinogenic metabolites may be generated. Compounds such as benzo(*a*)pyrene induce the appearance of the cytochrome P-450 system enzymes, and smokers are constantly exposed to the P-450 inducers. Generation of endothelial cell-damaging agents during the metabolism of benzo(*a*)pyrene derived from cigarette smoke has been shown to be a possible mechanism to explain the initiation of atherosclerotic plaques. Oxidants derived from cigarette smoke can damage lipids, an important constituent of cell membranes, as well as cellular macromolecules, including DNA. There is some evidence that cigarette smoke may cause damage to artery wall cell DNA in animal models; however, if such damage does occur it would provide independent support for the view that DNA alterations are characteristic of atherosclerotic plaques in animal models of the disease as well as in humans. In related experimental animal studies, the chemical allylamine caused both myocardial lesions and vascular fibrosis. Allylamine toxicity is thought to be mediated via metabolism of this compound to the reactive aldehyde, acrolein, which is also a prominent component of cigarette smoke. Studies with cultured artery wall cells indicate that the primary arterial effect of allylamine is on the smooth muscle cells. Proliferation of intimal smooth muscle cells in response to allylamine exposure results in activation of a specific cellular DNA sequence, the H-ras oncogene, which is implicated in the development of certain forms of cancer. This lends further support to the contention that there may be molecular similarities between the development of the lesions of atherosclerosis and of cancer.

One of the problems researchers have faced in identifying specific health-threatening components of cigarette smoke is that while at moderate to high concentrations many of these agents can be toxic, in many cases the individual concentrations of these factors in cigarette smoke are likely too low to be able to account individually for the toxic and disease-promoting effects of cigarette smoke. The US Environmental Protection Agency sidestepped this problem in 1992 by declaring environmental tobacco smoke, with its thousands of components, to be a human class A carcinogen. The American Heart Association has classified environmental tobacco smoke as an environmental poison and as a major preventable cause of cardiovascular disease. Regarding environmental tobacco smoke, estimates provide evidence that as many as 69 000 excess heart disease deaths annually in the United States can be attributed directly to involuntary exposure to cigarette smoke. In support of these estimates, a number of laboratories have reported that inhalation of sidestream cigarette smoke accelerates arteriosclerosis in different experimental model systems of the disease. Since epidemiological and autopsy evidence strongly support the view that atherosclerosis begins as early as childhood, the experimental results with environmental tobacco smoke suggest that involuntary exposure of children to tobacco smoke may accelerate plaque development. The insidious nature of involuntary exposure to environmental tobacco smoke is further emphasized by recent findings in a mouse model of atherosclerosis. Male mice exposed only *in utero* to environmental tobacco smoke develop accelerated atherosclerosis as adults, even in the absence of a high fat diet. In the United States, where studies show that many children are less active physically and have poorer diets than children growing up a few of generations ago, involuntary exposure to second-hand smoke may well represent a major additional risk factor for the development of atherosclerosis. Fortunately, extensive epidemiologic evidence from both cancer and heart disease studies indicates that as the time since cessation of smoking increases, the chances of dying prematurely from either disease decrease. Thus, the vasculotoxic effects of cigarette smoke, both active and passive, may be largely reversible.

Nicotine

Tobacco smoke has been associated with various cardiovascular diseases. However, the use and dependency on tobacco products stems from a need to reach a level of nicotine that is consistent with the user's addiction. The introduction of nicotine cannot be thought of as benign and the use of nicotine (e.g., e-cigarettes, nicotine patch, nicotine gum, nasal sprays, inhalers, lozenges, or smokeless tobacco products) should also be considered to have negative cardiovascular health consequences, though the extent of these health consequences is currently unclear. Acutely, nicotine can stimulate the release of catecholamines through activation of the sympathetic nervous system, thereby increasing blood pressure and heart rate; while chronic use has been shown to have multiple cellular targets that alter cardiac and vascular molecular pathways promoting hypertension, cardiovascular disease, and altering cardiac rhythm. Nicotine has also been implicated in abdominal aortic aneurysm both through indirect mechanisms (e.g., hypertension) and direct alterations leading to vascular smooth muscle cell damage and aortic remodeling. Taken together, the movement of patients from tobacco use to nicotine replacement therapies, but more importantly nicotine cessation, should be considered paramount to prevent the cardiovascular effects associated with nicotine use.

Conclusion

Through hundreds of years, and countless agents, studies and trials, the fundamental principle of toxicology remains the balance between a poison and a remedy. That is, the difference between an untoward outcome and positive therapeutic application of compounds must be considered. This article is not meant to associate a 'good' or 'bad,' but to open awareness to all toxicological considerations, and encourage special consideration for cardiovascular impacts.

See also: Amphetamines; Arsenic; Batrachotoxin; Blood; Chemicals of Environmental Concern; Chromium; Cocaine; *hERG* (Human Ether-a-Go-Go Related Gene); Mercury; Tetrodotoxin; Tobacco.

Further Reading

Acosta, D., 2001. Cardiovascular Toxicology. Target Organ Toxicology Series, third ed. CRC Press.

Bishop, S., Kerns, W., 1997. Cardiovascular toxicology. In: Sipes, I.G., McQueen, C.A., Gandolfi, A.J. (Eds.), Comprehensive Toxicology, vol. 6. Elsevier, New York, pp. 1–4.

Glass, C., Witzum, J., 2001. Atherosclerosis: The road ahead. Cell 104, 503–516.

James Kang, Y. (Ed.), 2004. Cardiovascular Toxicology: The First Journal on Cardiovascular Toxicities of Drugs, Novel Therapies and Environmental Pollutants. Humana Press, New Jersey. http://www.humanpress.com.

Libby, P., 2003. Vascular biology of atherosclerosis: overview and state of the art. Am. J. Cardiol. 91 (3A), 3A–6A.

Ramos, K.S., Melchert, R.B., Chacon, E., Acosta Jr, D., 2001. Toxic responses of the heart and vascular systems. In: Klassen, C. (Ed.), Casarett and Doull's Toxicology, the Basic Science of Poisons, sixth ed. McGraw-Hill, New York, pp. 597–651.

Relevant Website

http://www.fleshandbones.com – is a website to the biomedical sciences including anatomy, physiology, pharmacology, and general medicine. Among this website's features is an 'Imagebank' containing color images that can be downloaded.

Catecholamines

S Othumpangat, National Institute for Occupational Safety and Health, Morgantown, WV, USA

This article is a revision of the previous edition article by Zhengwei Cai, volume 1, pp 487–489, © 2005, Elsevier Inc.

Description

Catecholamine is the name of a group of compounds that contain a catechol nucleus (a benzene ring with two adjacent hydroxyl substituents) and an amine group. This group includes the mammalian neurotransmitters or hormones, such as dopamine, norepinephrine, and epinephrine, and non-mammalian compounds such as octopamine. Each compound has its own synonyms.

- Name: Dopamine
- Chemical Abstracts Service Registry Number: 51-61-6
- Synonyms: Pyrocatechol; 4-(2-Aminoethyl) pyrocatechol; 3-Hydroxytyramine; 3,4-Dihydroxyphenethylamine; 4-(2-Aminoethyl)-1,2-benzenediol; Dopastat
- Molecular Formula: $C_8H_{11}NO_2$
- Name: Epinephrine
- Chemical Abstracts Service Registry Number: 51-43-4
- Synonyms: Benzyl alcohol, Adrenalin, Epirenamine, Methylaminoethanolcatechol, Vasotonin
- Molecular Formula: $C_9H_{13}NO_3$
- Name: Norepinephrine
- Chemical Abstracts Service Registry Number: 51-41-2
- Synonyms: 4-(2-Amino-1-hydroxyethyl)-1,2-benzenediol; α-(Aminomethyl)-3,4-dihydroxybenzyl alcohol; 2-Amino-1-(3,4-dihydroxyphenyl)ethanol; 1-(3,4-Dihydroxyphenyl-2-aminoethanol; Noradrenaline.
- Molecular Formula: $C_8H_{11}NO_3$
- Chemical Structures:

Dopamine

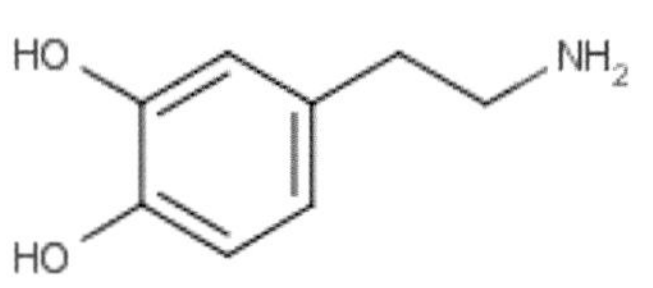

HO, HO, NH_2

Epinephrine

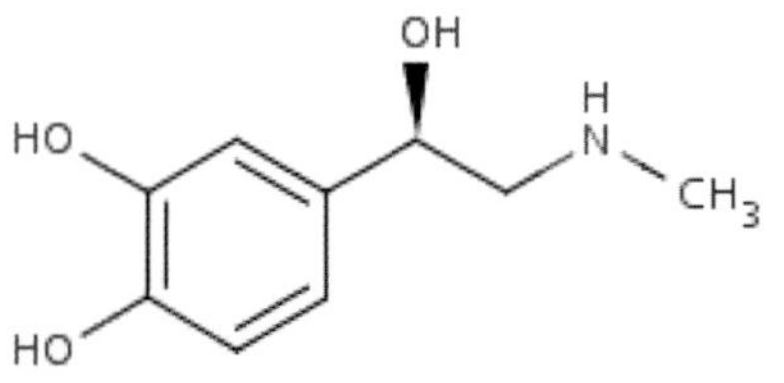

OH, HO, HO, H, N, CH_3

Norepinephrine

HO, HO, OH, NH_2

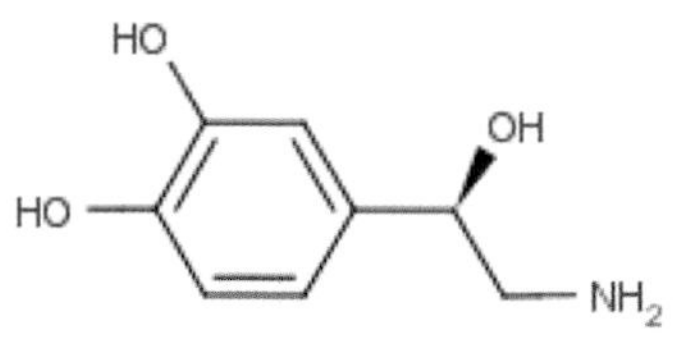

Background

Catecholamines are endogenous neurotransmitters or hormones. Dopamine and norepinephrine are in the monoamine class. Catecholamines are synthesized in the brain, the adrenal medulla, and by some sympathetic nerve fibers. The biosynthesis of catecholamines begins with the hydroxylation of tyrosine by tyrosine hydroxylase to form L-dopa, which is decarboxylated by aromatic amino acid decarboxylase to form dopamine. Catecholamines are formed from dopamine by the enzyme dopamine beta-hydroxylase, and epinephrine is formed from norepinephrine by enzyme phenylethanolamine *N*-methyltransferase. Parkinson's disease is one of the most common neurodegenerative disorders and is characterized by the selective loss of dopaminergic neurons in the substantia nigra. Dopamine is widely distributed throughout the CNS and is involved in the control of movement. Dopamine is synthesized from the amino acid tyrosine. This amino acid is abundant in meats, dairy products, and soy. Tyrosine undergoes a series of enzymatic modifications to yield dopamine. The amount of dopamine that can be made is limited by the activity of the first enzyme in the synthesis chain – tyrosine hydroxylase. Cells that use dopamine as a neurotransmitter are referred to as dopaminergic. Norepinephrine is an important neurotransmitter in both the CNS and the sympathetic part of the autonomic nervous system. The hormone epinephrine acts together with the sympathetic nervous system to initiate the body's quick response to stressful stimuli.

Uses

Catecholamines are sympathomimetic drugs. Dopamine and norepinephrine are used as vasopressors (antihypotensives). Catecholamines are water-soluble and are 50%-bound to plasma proteins, and are always seen in the circulating blood. Epinephrine stimulates both the alpha- and beta-adrenergic systems, causes systemic vasoconstriction and gastrointestinal relaxation, stimulates the heart, and dilates bronchi and cerebral vessels. It is also used as a vasoconstrictor, cardiac stimulant, or bronchodilator to counter allergic reaction, anesthesia, and cardiac arrest. Epinephrine is used to treat severe allergic (anaphylactic) reactions because it can prevent or minimize the effects of histamine. It is also an antiglaucoma agent.

Environmental Fate and Behavior

Routes and Pathways

Catecholamines are mostly administered by intravenous injection or infusion. They have a very short half-life when circulating in the blood and are easily soluble in water. Epinephrine is available in nebulized racemic dosage form for inhalation.

 http://dx.doi.org/10.1016/B978-0-12-386454-3.00271-2

Intoxication from catecholamine usually results from iatrogenic overdoses, accidental intravenous administration, and the injection of solution intended for nebulization. High concentrations of dopamine present inside of a cell than there are vesicles to store it in, oxidative stress can occur and cause damage or death to the cell. It is thought that dopamine overload causes biochemical damage to cellular mitochondria, that provide the cell with all of the energy it requires to function, resulting in death of the cell. Catecholamines produced circulatory changes that reversed propofol anesthesia in animal models.

Toxicokinetics

Epinephrine is well absorbed after oral administration but is rapidly inactivated in the gut mucosa. When catecholamines were intravenously injected or infused, the onset of drug effect is rapid (within 5 min for dopamine and 3–10 min for epinephrine) and the duration of drug effect is short (10 min for dopamine, 1 or 2 min for norepinephrine, and 15 min to hours for epinephrine depending on route of administration). Exogenous catecholamines in the circulation are rapidly and efficiently taken up by adrenergic neurons. Catecholamines are metabolized by monoamine oxidase, which is localized largely in the outer membrane of neuronal mitochondria, and by catechol-O-methyl transferase, which is found in the cytoplasm of most animal tissues, particularly the kidneys and the liver.

The primary metabolites of dopamine are homovanillic acid and dihydroxyphenylacetic acid (75%) and norepinephrine (25%). The primary metabolites of epinephrine and norepinephrine are vanillylmandelic acid and 3-methoxy-4-hydroxyphenethyleneglycol. Catecholamine metabolites and their conjugates are excreted in urine.

Mechanism of Toxicity

Catecholamines are sympathomimetic drugs. These drugs increase heart rate and cardiac output and may produce cardiac arrhythmias. Administration of norepinephrine also results in increased peripheral vascular resistance. Both effects may cause serious systemic hypertension, which may cause cerebral hemorrhage. Reduced hepatic and renal blood flow may cause tissue ischemia, increase glycolysis, and serum lactic acidosis. In very high doses, a paranoid state may be induced. Recent studies have demonstrated that norepinephrine may enhance or inhibit immune function under certain conditions. Increased levels of catecholamines can also increase fat lipolysis and reduce adipogenesis.

Production of reactive oxygen species and formation of quinone during the metabolism of dopamine are involved in dopamine toxicity. Numerous *in vitro* and *in vivo* studies concerning dopamine-induced neurotoxicity have been reported in recent decades. The reactive oxygen species generated in the enzymatic oxidation or auto-oxidation of excess dopamine-induced neuronal damage and apoptotic cell death. Dopamine and its metabolites containing two hydroxyl residues exert cytotoxicity in dopaminergic neuronal cells mainly due to the generation of highly reactive dopamine quinones which are dopaminergic neuron-specific cytotoxic molecules. Dopamine quinones may irreversibly alter protein function through the formation of 5-cysteinyl-catechols on the proteins. The formation of dopamine quinone-alpha-synuclein consequently increases cytotoxic protofibrils and the covalent modification of tyrosine hydroxylase by dopamine quinones. The melanin-synthetic enzyme tyrosinase in the brain may rapidly oxidize excess amounts of cytosolic dopamine and prevent slowly progressive cell damage by auto-oxidation of dopamine, thus maintaining dopamine levels.

Acute and Short-Term Toxicity

Animal

Overdose of catecholamines may result in animal death. In test animals, there is evidence that death is the result of respiratory arrest caused by hypertension following overdose of epinephrine.

Human

At high infusion rates of dopamine, ventricular arrhythmias, and hypertension may occur. Nausea, vomiting, and angina pectoris are occasionally seen. Gangrene of the extremities may occur in patients with profound shock given large doses of dopamine for long periods of time. Norepinephrine may cause dose-related hypertension (sometimes indicated by headache), reflex bradycardia, increased peripheral vascular resistance, and decreased cardiac output. High doses of norepinephrine (in excess of 8–12 mg of base per min) cause intense vasoconstriction, which results in 'normal' blood pressure but decreased tissue perfusion. Local necrosis may result from perivascular infiltration and angina, mesenteric ischemia, and peripheral ischemia. Epinephrine may cause dose-related restlessness, anxiety, tremor, cardiac arrhythmias, palpitation, hypertension, weakness, dizziness, and headache. A sharp rise in blood pressure from over-dosage of epinephrine may cause cerebral hemorrhage and pulmonary edema. High catecholamine levels in blood are also associated with stress, due to psychological or environmental stressors.

Chronic Toxicity

Human

Prolonged use and repeated injection of epinephrine may lead to tolerance and local necrosis. Prolonged use of norepinephrine may cause edema, hemorrhage, focal myocarditis, necrosis of the intestine, or hepatic and renal necrosis. It may also cause plasma volume depletion, which may result in perpetuation of the shock state or recurrence of hypotension when the drug is discontinued. High levels of catecholamines may be also due to the low levels of monoamine oxidase A (MAO-A). MAO-A is one of the enzymes responsible for degradation of these neurotransmitters, and thus balance the levels of catecholamines.

Clinical Management

Basic and advanced life-support measures should be utilized as necessary. Treatment is directed at ameliorating tachycardias, shock, cardiac arrhythmias, systemic hypertension, pulmonary edema, and lactic acidosis. In the case of severe toxicity, administration of a rapidly acting α-adrenergic blocking drug such as phentolamine may be considered. Glutathione is a scavenger for dopamine oxidation intermediates and it may provide complete protection against dopamine-mediated toxicity.

Ecotoxicology

Toxicity of catecholamines in a ciliated protozoan *Tetrahymena pyriformis* has been reported in a recent study. Catecholamines exhibited moderate acute toxicity to the protozoans. Dopamine showed toxic potential Effective Concentrations (EC_{10}) of 0.63 ppm in *T. pyriformis* and a higher concentration of dopamine inhibited the synthesis of adrenalin in these protozoans.

Disclaimer

The findings and conclusions in this report are those of the author and do not necessarily represent the views of the National Institute for Occupational Safety and Health, Center for Disease control and Prevention.

See also: Mode of Action; Occupational Exposure Limits; Monoamine Oxidase Inhibitors; Estrogens II: Catechol Estrogens.

Further Reading

Asanuma, M., Miyazaki, I., Ogawa, N., 2003. Dopamine- or L-DOPA-induced neurotoxicity: the role of dopamine quinone formation and tyrosinase in a model of Parkinson's disease. Neurotox. Res. 5 (3), 165–176.

Behonick, G.S., Novak, M.J., Nealley, E.W., Baskin, S.I., 2001. Toxicology update: the cardiotoxicity of the oxidative stress metabolites of catecholamines (aminochromes). J. Appl. Toxicol. 21 (Suppl. 1), S15–S22.

Madden, K.S., 2003. Catecholamines, sympathetic innervation, and immunity. Brain Behav. Immun. 17, S5–S10.

Stokes, A.H., Hastings, T.G., Vrana, K.E., 1999. Cytotoxic and genotoxic potential of dopamine. J. Neurosci. Res. 55, 659–665.

Ud-Daula, A., Pfister, G., Schramm, K., 2008. Growth inhibition and biodegradation of catecholamines in the ciliated protozoan *Tetrahymena pyriformis*. J. Environ. Sci. Health A 43, 1610–1617.

Wang, Q., Zhang, M., Ning, G., Gu, W., Su, T., Xu, M., Li, B., Wang, W., 2011. Brown adipose tissue in humans is activated by elevated plasma catecholamines levels and is inversely related to central obesity. PLoS ONE 6 (6), e21006.

Worstman, J., 2002. Role of epinephrine in acute stress. Endocrinol. Metab. Clin. North Am. 31, 79–106.

CCA-Treated Wood

C Barton, Oak Ridge Institute for Science and Education, Oak Ridge, TN, USA

This article is a revision of the previous edition article by C. Charles Barton and Thomas T. Newton, volume 1, pp 489–490, © 2005, Elsevier Inc.

- Name: CCA-treated wood
- Chemical Abstracts Service Registry Number: None
- Synonyms: None
- Molecular Formula: None
- Chemical Structure: None

Chromated copper arsenate (CCA) is a chemical mixture registered by the US Environmental Protection Agency (EPA) for use as a wood preservative. It has been demonstrated to protect wood from dry rot, fungi, molds, termites, and other pests that can threaten the integrity of wood products. CCA-treated wood (also known as pressure-treated wood) is most commonly used in outdoor settings. Over 90% of all outdoor wooden structures are made with CCA-treated lumber. Around the home, CCA-treated wood is commonly used for decks, walkways, fences, gazebos, boat docks, and playground equipment. Other common uses of CCA-treated wood include highway noise barriers, signposts, utility poles, and retaining walls.

Untreated wood generally deteriorates within 3–5 years, depending on its exposure to soil and environmental conditions. CCA-treated wood, on the other hand, is relatively strong and long lasting and maintains its integrity in conditions under which untreated wood would quickly degrade. CCA-treated wood products often retain their structural integrity 10–20 times longer than untreated woods.

In the pressure-treatment process, lumber is loaded into a horizontal cylinder. The cylinder door is sealed, and a liquid solution containing CCA is pumped in. The pressure in the cylinder is then raised, forcing the CCA into the wood. At the end of the process, the excess treatment solution is pumped back to a storage tank for reuse. The CCA solution is toxic. Therefore, it can be applied only by EPA-certified operators. However, wood that has been treated with CCA is not classified as hazardous because the CCA 'fixes' to the wood in a way that makes the chemical insoluble and somewhat leach resistant. Thus, CCA-treated wood is not considered to be a health risk unless burned in fireplaces or woodstoves.

The arsenic penetrates deeply into the wood and remains there for a long time. However, some of the chemical may migrate from treated wood into surrounding soil over time and may also be dislodged from the wood surface upon contact with skin. The amount and rate at which arsenic leaches, however, vary considerably depending on numerous factors, such as local climate, acidity of rain and soil, age of the wood product, and how much CCA was applied. Interestingly, leaching occurs more with newer structures and decreases with time.

Since excessive exposure to arsenic can be hazardous to health, precautions should be taken to decrease exposure. Applying a sealant on a regular basis (e.g., one reapplication every other year depending upon wear and weathering) should prevent the migration of arsenic from the wood. One should wash hands thoroughly after contact with treated wood, especially prior to eating and drinking; and ensure that food does not come into direct contact with any treated wood. Furthermore, workers should take certain precautions: wear gloves when handling wood, wear goggles and dust-mask when sawing and sanding, always wash hands before eating, and never burn CCA-treated wood.

During an 8 year investigation, the EPA examined the safety of using and handling CCA-treated wood. None of the EPA's investigations produced any findings showing increased risks of cancer or other toxic effects on humans handling CCA-treated wood. In 1985, the EPA concluded that the benefits of CCA-treated wood far outweighed any risks. The EPA established modest use precautions, which the treating industry agreed to disseminate in a voluntary consumer-awareness program.

The actual exposure levels to arsenic in CCA are considered to be minuscule. In 1990, the Consumer Product Safety Commission (CPSC) measured dislodgeable arsenic in eight samples of CCA-treated wood. In five of the samples, the amount was undetectable. Two other samples yielded small quantities of arsenic. The eighth sample, which yielded the greatest amount of arsenic, was rough-sawn lumber, a material classified by the wood-treatment industry as not acceptable for playground equipment. The CPSC concluded that the amounts of arsenic that people may be exposed to are below the level that may cause a health concern, and deemed it safe.

Plants grown in soil touched by CCA-treated wood have the same minuscule exposure levels. For decades, CCA-treated wood has been used commercially near crops in the form of tomato stakes, vineyard supports, banana props, and mushroom trays. No problems have ever been recorded that indicate that the preservative migrates into plants and causes any health effects.

On 12 February 2002, the EPA announced a voluntary decision by industry to move away from using CCA to treat wood used in residential settings. This transition affects virtually all residential uses of wood treated with CCA, including wood used in play-structures, decks, picnic tables, landscaping timbers, residential fencing, patios, and walkways/boardwalks. Effective from 31 December 2003, no wood treater or manufacturer may treat wood with CCA for most residential uses. This decision will facilitate the transition in both the manufacturing and retail sectors to wood preservatives that do not contain arsenic, as well as other alternatives, such as naturally resistant woods and plastic alternatives. The EPA does not believe there is any reason to remove or replace CCA-treated structures, including decks and playground equipment. Furthermore, the EPA is not recommending surrounding soils be removed or replaced. Also, CCA-treated wood can be disposed of with regular municipal trash (i.e., municipal solid waste, not yard waste).

See also: Wood Dusts; Arsenic.

Further Reading

Chang, F.C., Wang, Y.N., Chen, P.J., Ko, C.H., Factors affecting chelating extraction of Cr, Cu, and As from CCA-treated wood. J. Environ. Manag. 122, 42–46.

Chirenje, T., Ma, L., Clark, C., Reeves, M., 2003. Cu, Cr and As distribution in soils adjacent to pressure-treated decks, fences and poles. Environ. Pollut. 124, 407–417.

Choi, Y.S., Kim, J.J., Kim, M.J., et al., 2013. Optimization of bioleaching conditions for metal removal from CCA-treated wood by using an unknown *Polyporales* sp. KUC8959. J. Environ. Manag. 121, 6–12.

Hemond, H.F., Solo-Gabriele, H.M., 2004. Children's exposure to arsenic from CCA-treated, wooden decks and playground structures. Risk Anal. 24 (1), 51–64.

Hingston, J., Collins, C., Murphy, R., Lester, J., 2001. Leaching of chromated copper arsenate wood preservatives: a review. Environ. Pollut. 111, 53–66.

Hu, L., Greer, J.B., Solo-Gabriele, H., et al., 2013. Arsenic toxicity in the human nerve cell line SK-N-SH in the presence of chromium and copper. Chemosphere 91 (8), 1082–1087.

Kartal, S.N., Imamura, Y., 2005. Removal of copper, chromium, and arsenic from CCA-treated wood onto chitin and chitosan. Bioresour. Technol. 96 (3), 389–392.

Katz, S.A., Salem, H., 2005. Chemistry and toxicology of building timbers pressure-treated with chromated copper arsenate: a review. J. Appl. Toxicol. 25, 1–7.

Lew, K., Acker, J.P., Gabos, S., Le, X.C., 2010. Biomonitoring of arsenic in urine and saliva of children playing on playgrounds constructed from chromated copper arsenate-treated wood. Environ. Sci. Technol. 44 (10), 3986–3991.

Relevant Websites

http://www.cpsc.gov/phth/ccafact.html – CPSC Fact Sheet.

http://www.epa.gov/oppad001/reregistration/cca/ – EPA registration for CCA.

https://www.soils.org/publications/sh/abstracts/54/2/sh12-12-0032 – Soil Science Society of America.

http://www.woodpreservativescience.org/index.shtml – Wood Preservative Science Council.

Cell Cycle

N Yang, Manchester University, Fort Wayne, IN, USA
AM Sheridan

This article is a revision of the previous edition article by Vishal S. Vaidya, Alice Sheridan and Harihara M. Mehendale, volume 1, pp 490–494, © 2005, Elsevier Inc.

Introduction

The cell cycle is the orderly progression of cells through specific stages during which DNA is replicated and distributed to two daughter cells, resulting in cell proliferation. Precise regulation of the passage of cells through this cycle is necessary to ensure the maintenance of DNA integrity through multiple generations. Cell cycle regulation also ensures that cell proliferation occurs only under defined conditions in response to growth factors and in the presence of a suitable environment. Loss of cell cycle regulation is a characteristic of cancer.

The cell cycle comprises four stages, which are called G1, S, G2, and M phases (**Figure 1**). S (for DNA synthesis) is the stage in which DNA is duplicated. M (for mitosis) is the stage in which the cell divides. G1 (for gap 1) is the stage immediately prior to S during which the cell prepares for DNA synthesis. G2 (for gap 2) is the stage preceding M during which the cell prepares for cell division. Two major points of regulation are at the transitions between G1 and S phases, and between G2 and M phases. The progression of cells through late G1/S requires the presence of growth factors. A restriction point in late G1 marks the point at which cycle progression becomes growth factor independent. Cells that are actively proliferating progress from M phase back to G1 where preparations for DNA synthesis immediately start anew. Cells that are not actively proliferating are said to be quiescent and are in G0 phase. The entry of cells from G0 into the cell cycle is also a closely regulated step and requires an extracellular stimulus or growth factor. We describe below the critical proteins that have been identified to date that regulate G1/S and G2/M transitions. We emphasize that the cell cycle paradigm is rapidly evolving and expanding and that this description is likely incomplete.

Cyclins and Cyclin-Dependent Kinases

Numerous proteins have been identified that stringently regulate the passage of cells at G1/S and G2/M phase transitions. Conserved serine/threonine kinases, called cyclin-dependent kinases (cdks), phosphorylate and activate specific regulatory proteins that drive cell cycle progression. The activity of cdk is controlled at three levels. First, cdks are activated by their interaction with proteins, called cyclins. Cyclins are proteins with very short half-lives of less than 30–60 min. Whereas the cdks are constitutively expressed throughout the cell cycle, the level of the cyclins varies throughout. Cyclin levels are controlled by both regulated synthesis and ubiquitin-mediated proteolysis. Specific cyclin–cdk complexes function at different cell cycle phases.

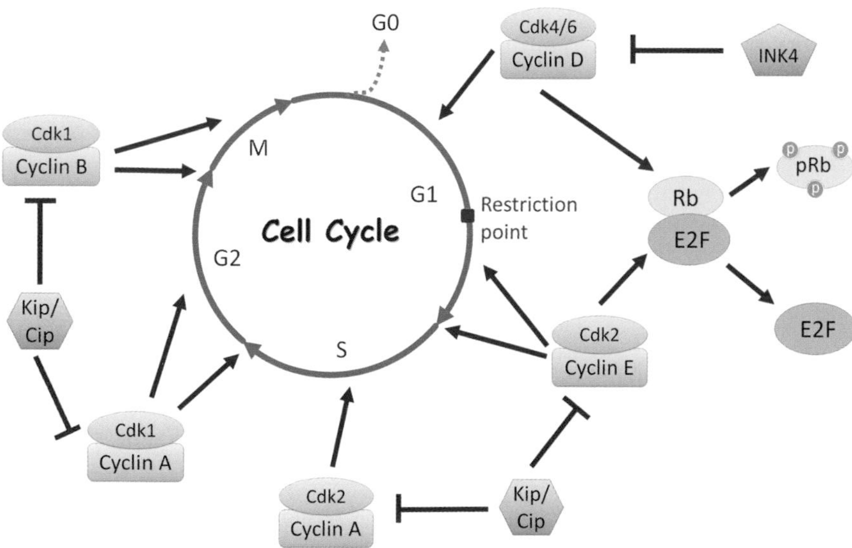

Figure 1 Overview of the different phases of the cell cycle. Quiescent cells are in G0 phase and reenter the cell cycle at G1, during which cells prepare for DNA synthesis. After passing the restriction point in late G1, cells are committed to enter the S phase, during which DNA replication occurs. Cells in G2 phase prepare for mitosis (M phase). Cell cycle progression is controlled by various positive and negative cell cycle regulatory proteins, including cyclins (A, B, D, E); cyclin-dependent kinases (cdk 1, 2, 4, 6); cdk inhibitors (INK4 and Kip/Cip); and retinoblastoma (Rb).

 http://dx.doi.org/10.1016/B978-0-12-386454-3.00273-6

Formation of the heterodimers cyclin D/cdk4, cyclin D/cdk6, and cyclin E/cdk2 is necessary for entry into and progression through G1. The induction of cyclin D family members is provoked by an extracellular signal or growth factor and initiates the entry of quiescent cells from G0 into G1. Cyclin D/cdk heterodimers phosphorylate and inactivate retinoblastoma protein (pRb), causing the release and activation of the E2F family of transcription factors. This family of transcription factors drives transcription of genes necessary for the G1/S transition, including cyclin E. Cyclin E/cdk2 also phosphorylates pRb but unlike cyclin D heterodimers, its activity is mitogen independent. Both cyclin E/cdk2 and cyclin A/cdk2 drive entry and progression through S phase via the phosphorylation of non-Rb proteins that initiate DNA synthesis. Cyclins A and B form complexes with cdk1 (also called cdc2) and are called the mitotic cyclins since these complexes regulate mitosis. Cyclin B/cdk1 controls the G2/M transition. Cyclin B is synthesized as the cell progresses through G2. Upon binding of cyclin B to cdk1, the activated heterodimer phosphorylates proteins that are involved in mitosis.

Activity of the cyclin/cdk complexes is also regulated by phosphorylation/dephosphorylation by cdk activating kinases (CAKs) and phosphatases. A third level of regulation is achieved by control of protein levels of cdk inhibitors. Cdk inhibitors are proteins that accumulate in response to multiple environmental stimuli, including DNA damage, hypoxia, cell–cell contact, and cytokines, and inhibit the activity of cyclin/cdk heterodimers. The cdk inhibitors include two classes of proteins. The INK4 proteins, which include p16INK4a, p15INK4b, p18INK4c, and p19INK4d, specifically inhibit the activity of cdk4 and cdk6 by competitive inhibition of cyclin D binding to the monomeric kinases. Mutations and deletions of the p16INK4a gene and inactivation by hypermethylation have been shown to play a role in tumorigenesis in many different types of tumors.

The Kip/Cip proteins include three structurally related proteins, p21, p27, and p57. In contrast to the INK4 proteins, the Kip/Cip proteins inhibit most cyclin/cdk heterodimers. Specific Kip/Cip proteins are induced by upstream events. p21 is induced in response to DNA damage and specifically inhibits cyclin E/cdk2. Protein levels of p27 are highest in quiescent cells and induce G1 arrest in response to conditions that typically result in cell quiescence such as growth factor deprivation or contact inhibition. Both the INK4 and the Kip/Cip proteins inhibit the phosphorylation and inactivation of pRb.

Recent genetic studies using knockout mouse models indicate that Cdk2, Cdk4, or Cdk6 singular knockout mouse embryos are viable and only Cdk1 knockout mice are embryonic lethal. Cdk4 and Cdk6 are not required for organogenesis and cell cycle except for some endocrine and hematopoietic cells. Cdk2 is not needed for the mitotic cell cycle. Those studies suggest the compensatory role of various Cdks.

Retinoblastoma

The retinoblastoma gene (Rb) was the first tumor suppressor to be identified. Rb mutations were first shown to be causal in familial and sporadic retinoblastoma, a rare tumor of the eye, but have since been associated with many other tumors, including osteosarcoma, small cell lung cancer, and prostate and breast cancer. In addition, mutations in the upstream Rb signaling pathway that result in the functional inactivation of the Rb gene product, pRb, are found in virtually all malignancies.

Three Rb homologs have been described, including $p110^{Rb}$ (or Rb), $p107^{Rb}$ (or p107), and $p130^{Rb}$ (or p130). All Rb homologs are characterized by a 'pocket' domain, which is highly conserved and necessary for pRb's tumor suppressor function. All the Rb homologs bind viral oncoproteins as well as E2F family members. Binding of viral oncoproteins disrupts the pocket domain of pRb and impairs pRb's tumor suppressor function. All pRb homologs cause G1 arrest.

The primary role of pRb is the inhibition of transcription of genes that mediate passage across the G1/S transition. There are two mechanisms by which pRb inhibit transcription. First, pRb binds to and inhibits the E2F family of transcription factors. The binding characteristics of the homologs vary slightly, whereas pRb binds preferentially to E2F1–4, p107 and p130 bind preferentially to E2F4 and E2F5. Phosphorylation of pRb regulates its interaction with E2F. The phosphorylation status of pRb fluctuates throughout the cell cycle. Hypophosphorylated pRb is active and binds to E2F family members thus sequestering E2F and inhibiting its transcriptional activity. Hyperphosphorylated pRb is inactive and releases E2F, which results in the transcription of genes that allow the cell to progress to S phase. Upon release from pRb, E2F binds to DP-1 or DP-2, and the resulting heterodimer activates genes necessary for DNA replication. The mechanism by which pRb inhibits E2F transcriptional activity is still debated, but it may be via the recruitment of chromatin remodeling enzymes such as histone deacetylases (HDACs) that directly repress transcription by removing acetyl groups from chromatin, which causes the chromatin to be less accessible to transcription factors. The role of the pRb-bound HDAC may be to counteract the activity of the E2F-bound acetyltransferase protein, p300/CBP, which transfers acetyl groups to chromatin and enhances transcriptional activity. In addition to its inactivation of E2F resulting in a decrease in transcription of E2F-responsive genes, the complex of pRb and E2F actively represses transcription, which may also be via the recruitment of HDACs to the promoter regions.

The regulation of pRb activity is complex. There are 16 possible sites for cdk-mediated phosphorylation, and data suggest that phosphorylation at each different site regulates a distinct pRb function. pRb is phosphorylated by multiple cyclin/cdk complexes. Cyclin D/cdk4/6 initiates phosphorylation in early G1 and cyclin E/cdk2 hyperphosphorylates pRb in late G1. Cyclin A/cdk2 maintains phosphorylation of pRb throughout S phase.

pRb may perform other roles in addition to regulation of G1/S including the regulation of apoptosis. A decrease in functional pRb results in the activation of p53-induced apoptosis, which appears to be mediated via the release of E2F1. Free E2F1 activates transcription of ARF (alternate reading frame of the p16INK4a locus), which inhibits a protein called mdm-2 ubiquitin ligase (mdm-2). Mdm-2 targets proteins for ubiquitin-mediated proteolysis. Since mdm-2 initiates the degradation of p53, its inhibition results in an increase in p53 and a corresponding increase in apoptosis. Thus, a decrease in functional pRb, which could otherwise result in unchecked cell proliferation, triggers an apoptotic response. A decrease in functional pRb also creates a selection pressure for p53 mutations, since only cells that have mutated dysfunctional p53 survive. Not surprisingly, p53 mutations are often found to coexist with Rb mutations in malignant tumors.

Checkpoints

Checkpoints are surveillance mechanisms comprising numerous genes that detect DNA damage and induce either cell cycle arrest and DNA repair mechanisms, or, in the presence of extensive DNA damage, apoptosis. The data elucidating this surveillance network are very incomplete but have been advanced significantly since the isolation of the mutation that is associated with ataxia telangiectasia (AT). AT is a rare pediatric disease that is associated with immune deficiency and an increased susceptibility to cancer. Prior to the isolation of the AT mutation, it had long been observed that stimuli that induce DNA damage delay progression through the cell cycle. For years, this phenomenon was assumed to be the passive response of the cell as a direct result of the DNA damage itself. By contrast, cells that harbor the AT mutation demonstrate a marked decrease in cell cycle arrest after DNA damaging radiation. These data suggested that an active system exists in normal cells that retard cell cycle progression in the presence of DNA damage. The checkpoint surveillance system comprises sensor proteins (proteins that detect DNA damage and initiate a signaling cascade); transducers (modifying enzymes such as kinases that relay the signal to effector proteins); and effectors (downstream target proteins that, upon activation by modifying enzymes, cause cycle arrest). Of these proteins, the least is known about sensor proteins, although several candidate genes have been suggested. The effector proteins include kinase inhibitors such as p21, or cyclin/cdk heterodimers that are either activated or inhibited to cause cycle arrest. Major transducer proteins include p53, ATM (AT-mutated protein kinase), and ATR (ATM and Rad3-related protein kinase).

P53 is a transcription factor that activates the transcription of genes that cause cell cycle arrest at either G1/S or G2 phase. In addition, p53 activates genes that initiate DNA repair and cause apoptosis. Mutations of p53 are commonly described in association with human tumors. The result of p53 activation is cell type-specific and depends on the type and severity of injury. P53-induced G1 cell cycle arrest is mediated via the induction of p21 and p16. p53 has a very short half-life and is generally undetectable in healthy cells. In the presence of DNA damage induced by either ultraviolet or γ-irradiation, p53 is activated by posttranscriptional modifications, including phosphorylation and acetylation, that either enhance its stability or alter its affinity for binding proteins. ATM and its related protein, ATR, phosphorylate p53, which decreases its binding to mdm-2. A decrease in the interaction between p53 and mdm-2 causes a decrease in ubiquitin-mediated proteolysis of p53 and a resulting increase in p53 protein levels. As described previously, ARF also activates p53 via the inactivation of mdm-2. In addition to phosphorylation, the acetylation status of p53 also determines its stability. P53 is acetylated and stabilized by p300/CBP, which increases apoptosis. The recently described NAD-dependent deacetylase protein SIRT1 removes acetyl groups from p53 and decreases apoptosis.

ATM and ATR are closely related phosphoinositide 3-kinases that are activated by DNA damage. Upon activation, ATM phosphorylates and activates multiple proteins in addition to p53, including mdm-2 and a serine/threonine kinase called Chk-2. Activated Chk-2 phosphorylating p53. ATR phosphorylates many but not all of the same substrates as ATM. ATR phosphorylates and activates Chk-1, which also phosphorylates p53.

p53, ATM, and ATR also contribute to G2 arrest. Upon activation, cdk1 initiates mitosis. cdk1 is activated via its interaction with cyclin B and via dephosphorylation by cdc25C phosphatase. Upon phosphorylation by ATM and ATR, Chk-2 and Chk-1 phosphorylate and inhibit cdc25C, which prevents the activation of cdk1. P53 activates transcription of two genes that inhibit cdk1 activity, including GADD45 and 14-3-3s. GADD45 disrupts the cyclin B/cdk1 heterodimer. The protein product of 14-3-3s sequesters cdc25C, which prevents the dephosphorylation of cdk1.

In the face of overwhelming DNA damage, checkpoints, in particular p53, induce cell death by apoptosis rather than cell cycle arrest. Apoptosis, or programmed cell death, is an evolutionarily conserved, energy-requiring mechanism by which unwanted or irreparably damaged cells are removed from the organism. Apoptosis is a fundamental component of both normal embryogenesis and adult homeostasis. Apoptosis is also a physiologic response to diverse toxic stimuli, including viral infection, DNA damage induced by irradiation or reactive oxygen species, hypoxia, growth factor deficiency, or genetic aberration. Apoptosis is carried out by caspases, which are proteases that contain a cysteine nucleophile and cleave proteins whose sequence contains specific motifs that include an aspartic acid residue. Upstream or initiator caspases are activated by the binding of an extracellular ligand to a death receptor. Death receptors are members of the tumor necrosis superfamily and are characterized by an intracellular death domain. An important example of a death receptor is CD95, or fas, which binds fas ligand. Upon binding of a ligand, the death receptor binds to intracellular adapter proteins. Adapter proteins bind to initiator caspases 2, 8, or 10, which provokes their autocleavage and activation. Initiator caspases activate downstream effector or executioner caspases, such as caspase 3, 6, or 7, or proapoptotic BCL-2 proteins. The BCL-2 family includes proteins that contain BCL-2 homology domains. These domains allow for heterodimerization by which BCL-2 proteins activate other family members. BCL-2 proteins modulate the intrinsic apoptotic pathway and may have either pro- or anti-apoptotic effects. Proapoptotic BCL-2 proteins increase mitochondrial membrane permeability, which allows for the release of cytochrome *c*. Cytochrome *c* release from mitochondria results in dimerization of an adapter protein called Apaf-1 (apoptotic protease activating factor), which

Table 1 Summary of some toxicants that are known to influence specific cell cycle events

Compound	*Cell cycle stage*	*Specific mechanism*	*References*
Acetaminophen	G1/S border	It causes G1/S arrest by inhibiting DNA synthesis.	Wiger, R., et al., 1997. Pharmacol. Toxicol. 81, 285.
Alcohol	G2/M transition	It results in cell cycle arrest at the G2/M transition by activating CHK-2.	Clemens, D.L, et al., 2011. Alcohol 45, 785.
Anti-diabetetic drugs			
Insulin	G1, S phases	It stimulates cell proliferation by increasing cyclin D/E.	Chappell, J., et al., 2001. J. Biol. Chem. 276, 38023.
Metformin	G0, G1 phases	It blocks the cell cycle in G0–G1 phases by decreasing cyclin D, Cdk4/6.	Kato, K., et al., 2012. Mol. Cancer Ther. 11, 549.
Ciglitazone	G2, M phases	It induces G2/M arrest by increasing p53, p27 and decreasing cyclin B1.	Plissonnier, M.L., et al., 2011. PLoS One, e28354.
Chemotherapy agents			
Cisplatin	All phases	As an alkylating agent, it causes cell arrest at various phases due to dosage and cell types.	Basu, A., et al., 2010. J. Nucleic Acids. Article ID 201367.
Dexamethasone	G1 phase	It induces G1 arrest by inhibiting cyclin D, E2F, and increasing p21.	Greenberg, A.K., et al., 2002. Am. J. Respir Cell Mol. Biol. 27, 320.
Etoposide	S, G2 phases	As a specific topoisomerase II inhibitor, it arrests cells in late S and G2 phase.	Fearnhead, H.O., et al., 1994. Biochem. Pharmacol. 48, 1073.
Hydroxyurea	G1, S border	As a specific inhibitor of DNA synthesis, it blocks cells at G1/S border.	Kim, J.H., et al., 1967. Cancer Res. 27, 1301.
Paclitaxel	M phase	It stabilizes microtubules and causes M phase arrest.	Carlier, M.F., et al., 1983. Biochemistry 22, 4814.
Metals			
Water soluble (Cd^{2+}, Hg^{2+}, Co^{2+}, Cu^{2+}, Ni^{2+}, Zn^{2+}, Pb^{2+}) Water insoluble (As, Ni)	S phase	Toxic metals induce an S-phase-specific cell cycle block by their selective interaction with DNA metabolism.	Costa, M., et al., 1982. Res. Commun. Chem. Pathol. Pharmacol. 38, 405.
Prozac (or fluoxetine)	G0, G1 phase	As an antidepressant drug, it arrests cells at G0/G1 phase by accumulating p21 and p27.	Krishnan, A., et al., 2008. Biochem. Pharmacol. 75, 1924.
Sulindac	G0, G1 phase	As an anti-inflammatory drug, it causes cells to accumulate in the G0/G1 phase by increasing p53 and p21.	Jung, B., et al., 2005. Cancer Lett. 219, 15.

binds procaspase 9, resulting in its cleavage and activation. Caspase 9 activates the downstream effectors, caspase 3, 6, or 7. Antiapoptotic proteins in the BCL-2 family inhibit the proapoptotic members and prevent the increase in mitochondrial membrane permeability. The downstream effector caspases target multiple proteins for degradation, including enzymes, nuclear structural proteins such as lamins, cytoskeletal proteins such as actin, proteins critical for cell–cell interaction such as β-catenin, and DNA repair enzymes.

p53 activates multiple genes that are involved in apoptosis, including genes that encode proteins that function via receptor-mediated signaling and those which encode proteins that modulate downstream effectors. p53-activated IGF-BP3 inhibits binding of IGF-1 to the IGF-1 receptor, which can induce apoptosis. p53 activates transcription of the death receptor ligands fas/CD95 and the death receptor KILLER/DR5. p53 also induces the proapoptotic BCL-2 protein bax as well as other proteins that enhance cytochrome *c* release from mitochondria, including p53, AIP1, PUMA, and Noxa. Apoptosis may also be induced via an increase in oxidative stress generated by multiple p53-induced genes that are homologous to NADPH-quinone oxidoreductase.

Importantly, no singular p53-activated gene product has been conclusively shown to initiate apoptosis. It appears that many p53-induced proapoptotic genes need to be activated concurrently in order for apoptosis to occur. It is not clear which variables determine whether p53 induces cell cycle arrest or apoptosis. The decision between p53-induced cell cycle arrest and apoptosis may be dependent on the protein levels of p53 and the cell type. Higher levels of p53 induce apoptosis and lower levels cause cell cycle arrest. Certain cell types, such as T lymphocytes, are especially sensitive to apoptosis whereas fibroblasts are more likely to undergo cell cycle arrest. Whereas p53 induces arrest or senescence in normal cells, p53 activation usually causes apoptosis in transformed cells. The reason for the enhanced sensitivity to p53-induced apoptosis in transformed cells may be related to the deregulation of E2F due to the inactivation of pRb. Cycle arrest induced by p21 may protect the cell from apoptosis. Other factors that may predispose the cell toward p53-induced apoptosis include alterations in the bax/bcl-2 ratio, concurrent absence of growth factors, and a greater intensity of stress. Posttranslational modifications may also determine p53 promoter specificity, which may play a major role in determining whether p53 expression results in cell cycle arrest or apoptosis.

Clinical Application

The normal regulation of the cell cycle plays an important role in tissue repair and inflammation. All tissues may be stratified by proliferative capability into three categories including labile, quiescent, or permanently nondividing cells.

Labile cells are continuously dividing and include surface epithelial cells such as stratified squamous epithelial cells of the skin and columnar epithelial cells of the gastrointestinal tract.

Quiescent cells are nondividing under normal circumstances but can be induced to reenter the cell cycle by exposure to growth factors. Quiescent cells include parenchymal cells of the liver, kidney, and pancreas and mesenchymal cells such as fibroblasts. The cytokine-induced reentry of quiescent cells into G1 phase is an important component of the inflammatory response, which has been well characterized in the kidney. Glomerular mesangial cells proliferate in many models of glomerular disease, including lupus nephritis and diabetes. The proliferation of mesangial cells occurs in response to cytokines such as platelet-derived growth factor and basic fibroblast growth factor. Inhibition of mesangial cell proliferation may abrogate the glomerulosclerosis or the glomerular scarring that occurs as a result of inflammation.

Permanently nondividing cells have lost all capacity for proliferation and include nerve cells and cardiac muscle cells.

The deregulation of the cell cycle resulting in unchecked cell proliferation is a hallmark of cancer. All human cancers are characterized by defects of restriction point control, checkpoints, DNA repair, or apoptosis. Defects of restriction point control allow for uncontrolled proliferation and result in loss of terminal differentiation. Although cdks are seldom mutated in human cancers, many human tumors harbor mutations or epigenetic changes in upstream factors of cdks, including INK4, Cip/Kip, Cyclin D, and Cyclin E, and downstream targets of cdks, mainly Rb. Therefore, cdks have been considered as therapeutic targets for many years. Another important target for cancer therapy is p53 because mutations of p53 are the most common mutations associated with cancer and occur in almost 50% of all human cancers.

Conclusion

The regulation of the cell cycle plays an important role in normal tissue repair and regeneration. Loss of cell cycle regulation is a chief characteristic of cancer. Cell cycle regulation involves numerous signaling pathways that determine whether cells will proliferate, remain quiescent, arrest, or undergo apoptosis. It has been established that both carcinogenic and non-carcinogenic toxicants can considerably alter cell cycle specific events. **Table 1** represents list of agents that can influence cell cycle specific events. Many drug- or chemical-induced alterations are reversible and many are irreversible; it all depends whether the cell cycle regulatory events are altered/influenced by parent compounds, their metabolites, and their biological reactive intermediates. While enormous progress has been made in the elucidation of these signaling pathways, our understanding of cell cycle regulation remains incomplete. Further studies may allow better understanding of diseases that result from deregulation of these pathways.

See also: Cell Proliferation; Apoptosis.

Further Reading

Abouzeid, A.H., Torchilin, V.P., 2013. The role of cell cycle in the efficiency and activity of cancer nanomedicines. Expert Opin. Drug Deliv. 10 (6), 775–786.

Becker, W., 2012. Emerging role of DYRK family protein kinases as regulators of protein stability in cell cycle control. Cell Cycle 11 (18), 3389–3394.

Bock, J.M., Menon, S.G., Sinclair, L.L., et al., 2007. Celecoxib toxicity is cell cycle phase specific. Cancer Res. 67 (8), 3801–3808.
Boehme, K.A., Blattner, C., 2009. Regulation of p53–insights into a complex process. Crit. Rev. Biochem. Mol. Biol. 44 (6), 367–392.
Fabian, G., Farago, N., Feher, L.Z., et al., 2011. High-density real-time PCR-based in vivo toxicogenomic screen to predict organ-specific toxicity. Int. J. Mol. Sci. 12 (9), 6116–6134.
Filipič, M., 2012. Mechanisms of cadmium induced genomic instability. Mutat. Res. 733 (1–2), 69–77.
Griffin, S.V., Pichler, R., Wada, T., et al., 2003. The role of cell cycle proteins in glomerular disease. Semin. Nephrol. 23, 569–582.
Kehe, K., Balszuweit, F., Steinritz, D., Thiermann, H., 2009. Molecular toxicology of sulfur mustard-induced cutaneous inflammation and blistering. Toxicology 263 (1), 12–19.
Kim, Y.J., Woo, H.D., Kim, B.M., et al., 2009. Risk assessment of hydroquinone: differential responses of cell growth and lethality correlated to hydroquinone concentration. J. Toxicol. Environ. Health A 72 (21–22), 1272–1278.
Könczöl, M., Weiss, A., Stangenberg, E., et al., 2013. Cell-cycle changes and oxidative stress response to magnetite in A549 human lung cells. Chem. Res. Toxicol. [Epub ahead of print].
Malumbres, M., Barbacid, M., 2009. Cell cycle, CDKs and cancer: a changing paradigm. Nat. Rev. Cancer 9, 153–166.
Marlowe, J.L., Puga, A., 2005. Aryl hydrocarbon receptor, cell cycle regulation, toxicity, and tumorigenesis. J. Cell Biochem. 96 (6), 1174–1184.
Orlando, D.A., Lin, C.Y., Bernard, A., et al., 2008. Global control of cell-cycle transcription by coupled CDK and network oscillators. Nature 453, 944–947.
Ray, S.D., Kamendulis, L.M., Gurule, M.W., et al., 1993. Ca^{2+} antagonists inhibit DNA fragmentation and toxic cell death induced by acetaminophen. FASEB J. 7 (5), 453–463.
Sartiani, L., Stillitano, F., Luceri, C., et al., 2010. Prenatal exposure to carbon monoxide delays postnatal cardiac maturation. Lab. Invest. 90 (11), 1582–1593.
Serrano, L., Martínez-Redondo, P., Marazuela-Duque, A., et al., 2013. The tumor suppressor SirT2 regulates cell cycle progression and genome stability by modulating the mitotic deposition of H4K20 methylation. Genes Dev. 27, 639–653.
Stevens, S.K., Strehle, A.P., Miller, R.L., et al., 2013. The anticancer ruthenium complex KP1019 induces DNA damage, leading to cell cycle delay and cell death in *Saccharomyces cerevisiae*. Mol. Pharmacol. 83 (1), 225–234.
Valdiglesias, V., Costa, C., Sharma, V., et al., 2013. Comparative study on effects of two different types of titanium dioxide nanoparticles on human neuronal cells. Food Chem. Toxicol. 57C, 352–361.
Vitale, I., Jemaà, M., Galluzzi, L., et al., 2013. Cytofluorometric assessment of cell cycle progression. Cell Senescence. Methods Mol. Biol. 965, 93–120.
Wang, Y.T., Tzeng, D.W., Wang, C.Y., et al., 2013. APE1/Ref-1 prevents oxidative inactivation of ERK for G1-to-S progression following lead acetate exposure. Toxicology 305, 120–129.

Cell Phones

S Saeidnia and M Abdollahi, Tehran University of Medical Sciences, Tehran, Iran

Cell phones emit radio frequency (RF) radiation. Although governments have deemed that RF radiation is safe, there is no sufficient data available from research projects to support that claim. In 2011, the World Health Organization (WHO), International Agency for Research on Cancer recommended that electromagnetic radiation from mobile phones and other wireless devices may be a causative agent for 'possible human carcinogen,' 2B.

Mobile phones or cell phones cause a novel, ubiquitous, and quickly growing exposure worldwide as they have two-way microwave radios that also emit low levels of electromagnetic radiation. Children are increasingly employing cell phones, since 'Family Plans' encourage parents to buy mobile phones for their children in order to simply access their children.

Since children are probably more sensitive to the adverse effects of exposure to mobile phones, the risk of brain cancer should be elevated in young users. Many manufacturers and expert scientists advise prevention by taking the simple precaution of 'distance' to minimize exposures to the brain and body.

Radiation Effects

Several organs and tissues may be targeted by radiation of cell phones, and specific concerns have been raised for the brain, skin, and reproductive system organs. Recently, a group of researchers concentrated on the possible side effects of radiation from the mobile phone base transceiver stations (BTS). They intended to find out the psychological and psychobiological reactions of the residents who were living close to mobile phone BTS antenna, in Isfahan, Iran. The researchers demonstrated that almost all the side symptoms such as nausea, headache, dizziness, irritability, sleep disturbance, memory loss, and lowering of libido have been significantly increased in the inhabitants who were living near BTS, closer than 300 m, in comparison to those living far from the antenna (>300 m).

Immune System Effects

The fast and increasing application of cell phones in recent years leads to enhanced consideration in relation to the possible immune effects of the exposure to RF/microwave frequency (MW) radiation. In the literature, the impacts of weak RF/MW fields, including cell phone radiation, on various immune functions have been discussed. There is much evidence that clearly reveals that alterations in both the number and (or) the activity of immunocompetent cells may occur. For instance, a number of lymphocyte functions might be enhanced or weakened within a single experiment based on exposure to similar intensities of MW radiation. Generally, short-term exposure to low MW radiation can temporarily stimulate particular humoral and cellular immune responses, while prolonged irradiation inhibits the same functions.

Cytotoxicity and Genotoxicity

Most recently, the cytotoxicity and genotoxicity of plutonium-239 alpha particles and GSM 900 modulated mobile phone (model Sony Ericsson K550i) radiation were compared in a study on the *Allium cepa* test designed to evaluate the cytotoxicity and genotoxicity of RF electromagnetic fields. The authors revealed that the mobile phone radiation had a time-dependent enhancement of the mitotic index and its frequency, chromosome abnormalities, and micronucleus frequency. Such results should make us aware of potential dangers and possible side effects that could result from long-term exposure to mobile phones. Of course, this concern is growing rapidly since it is reported that the number of students who employ cell phones increases daily.

Reproductive Effects

Epidemiological studies suggest that cell phones may be a causative factor affecting the quality of semen by reducing sperm motility (but not sperm counts), viability, and morphology. Although there are consistent results, further studies are necessary to show the probable association between cell phone radiation and male reproductive system impacts. To address the concern that carrying a cell phone influences the reproductive system (like the testes), one group of researchers conducted a study to investigate the effects of a 1.95 GHz electromagnetic field on testicular function in male Sprague–Dawley rats. Their findings indicated that the number of sperm in the testis and epididymis did not decrease in the electromagnetic field exposed groups. Further, there were no abnormalities observed for sperm motility or morphology, and the histological appearance of seminiferous tubules, including the stage of the spermatogenic cycle, was normal. In spite of their consistent results, large multifactorial studies are essential to determine the possible association between cell phone radiation and male reproductive systems.

Effects of Prolonged Exposure

Most papers conclude that a reasonable suspicion of mobile phone risk to human health exists after prolonged, intermittent exposures. The regular and long-term application of microwave devices (including mobile phone, microwave oven) can affect biological systems, especially the brain. Moreover, it is suggested that increased reactive oxygen species play a predominant role by increasing the impact of microwave radiation, which may cause neurodegenerative diseases and brain cancer. However, some results differ. For instance, in Taiwan, a 10 year observational study revealed that the intensive rate of cell phone use is not relative to the incidence rate or on the mortality of malignant brain tumors in that country, and also there was no significant association between the morbidity/mortality of malignant brain tumors and cell phone applications. Moreover, in a large prospective study, it was reported that cell phone usage might not be related to the enhanced incidence of glioma, meningioma, or noncentral nervous system cancers.

An influential report in 2009 published by 40 independent scientists and physicians from 14 diverse countries was entitled "Cell-phones and Brain Tumors: 15 Reasons for Concern, Science, Spin and the Truth Behind Interphone." The researchers discussed that a risk of brain tumors from cell phone use is possible, and that children have enhanced risks compared to adults for brain tumors.

Various research groups have explored an enhanced risk of some low-incidence brain cancers among users who were exposed for a long time and known as heavy users. Actually, there is no approved etiological link between cell phone use and cancer initiation. But children are known to be at a greater risk because of being in earlier stages of neural development. The problem is that data from children have not been incorporated in many investigations until very recently. It is apparent that further documentation and evidence are essential to statistically or anecdotally define the relationship between cell phone use and brain cancer. Taken together, it is safer to use precaution and encourage users to decrease their exposure to electromagnetic frequencies from cell phones. For instance, using a hands-free device or limiting the application of cell phones for conversations is recommended.

Cell Phones as E-Waste

Electronic waste is one of the fastest growing ecotoxicological problems in the world because many electronics contain both toxic metals and toxic organics. Most scientists believe that exposure to such dangerous wastes poses serious health risks, particularly to pregnant women and children. Moreover, the WHO reveals that even small amounts of lead, cadmium, and mercury (which can be found in old phones) is able to generate irreversible neurological damage and threaten the development of a child. Electronic waste is quickly flooding Asia, especially China, and it inevitably results in a large volume of toxic components to the environment if not handled properly.

The important question is to what extent can toxicants leach from the cell phone waste or their components into water? Also which class of toxicants (metals or hydrophobic organics) is responsible for toxicity? A recent toxicological assessment with C18 and ethylenediamine tetra acetic acid addition revealed that metals were responsible for the observed toxicity from leachates of cell phones. The findings indicated that electronic waste is able to leach toxic components even in short-term leaching with pure water. Lithium is employed in the batteries of cell phones and possesses the greatest effect on metal depletion, causing remarkable environmental and health impacts. In addition, lithium can be incorporated in the food chain from soils via flora to humans. For detailed toxicity of lithium and electronic wastes in human and animals, please *see* Lithium and Electronic Waste and further readings.

See also: Electronic Waste; Lithium.

Further Reading

Benson, V.S., Pirie, K., Schüz, J., et al., 2013. Mobile phone use and risk of brain neoplasms and other cancers: prospective study, million women study collaborators. Int. J. Epidemiol. 42, 792–802.

Davis, D.L., Kesari, S., Soskolne, C.L., et al., 2013. Swedish review strengthens grounds for concluding that radiation from cellular and cordless phones is a probable human carcinogen. Pathophysiology 20, 123–129.

Hardell, L., Carlberg, M., Hansson Mild, K., 2011. Pooled analysis of case-control studies on malignant brain tumours and the use of mobile and cordless phones including living and deceased subjects. Int. J. Oncol. 38, 1465–1474.

Hsu, M.H., Syed-Abdul, S., Scholl, J., et al., 2013. The incidence rate and mortality of malignant brain tumors after 10 years of intensive cell phone use in Taiwan. Eur. J. Cancer Prev. 2013 (Epub ahead of print); PMID: 22, 596–598.

Kesari, K.K., Siddiqui, M.H., Meena, R., et al., 2013. Cell phone radiation exposure on brain and associated biological systems. Indian J. Exp. Biol. 51, 187–200.

Mostafalou, S., Abdollahi, M., 2013. Environmental pollution by mercury and related health concerns: renotice of a silent threat. Arh. Hig. Rada. Toksikol. 64 (1), 179–181.

Pesnya, D.S., Romanovsky, A.V., 2012. Comparison of cytotoxic and genotoxic effects of plutonium-239 alpha particles and mobile phone GSM 900 radiation in the *Allium cepa* test. Mutat. Res. 750, 27–33.

Roberts, H., Tate, B., 2010. Nickel allergy presenting as mobile phone contact dermatitis. Australas. J. Dermatol. 51, 23–25.

Shahbazi-Gahrouei, D., Karbalae, M., Moradi, H.A., et al., 2013. Health effects of living near mobile phone base transceiver station (BTS) antennae: a report from Isfahan, Iran. Electromagn. Biol. Med. 2013. http://dx.doi.org/10.3109/15368378.2013.801352.

Szmigielski, S., 2013. Reaction of the immune system to low-level RF/MW exposures. Sci. Total Environ. 454–455, 393–400.

Relevant Websites

http://www.cancer.gov/cancertopics/factsheet/Risk/cellphones – National Cancer Institute Cell Phones and Cancer Risk Fact Sheet (accessed 29.08.13.).

http://www.fountainmagazine.com/Issue/detail/the-cell-phone-brain-cancer-controversy – The Fountain on Life, Knowledge and Belief.

http://www.nytimes.com/2013/05/05/opinion/sunday/where-do-old-cellphones-go-to-die.html?_r=0 – The New York Times, Sunday Review.

Cell Proliferation

N Yang and SD Ray, Manchester University, Fort Wayne, IN, USA
K Krafts, University of Minnesota, Minneapolis, MN, USA

This article is a revision of the previous edition article by Sanjay Chanda and Harihara M. Mehendale, volume 1, pp 495–498, © 2005, Elsevier Inc.

Introduction

Unicellular organisms like yeasts, bacteria, or protozoa have a strong selective pressure to grow and divide as rapidly as possible. The rate of cell division in these cases is limited only by the rate at which nutrients can be taken from the medium and converted into cellular materials.

Multicellular organisms, in contrast, are made up of many different types of cells performing a variety of functions. The primary drive is the survival of the organism as a whole rather than the survival or proliferation of a single individual type of cell. Therefore, different cells proliferate at different times, depending on the changing needs of the organism.

Some tissues contain cells that, once terminally differentiated, are incapable of reentering the cell cycle. These tissues are called nondividing tissues; an example is neural tissue. Other tissues, such as liver tissue, contain cells that normally reside outside the cell cycle, but which can be stimulated to proliferate when necessary. These tissues are called stable tissues. A third type of tissue, termed continuously dividing tissue, is continuously being replaced due to frequent cell sloughing or cell death. Skin and bone marrow are examples of this type of cell. Replacement in these tissues is accomplished through native stem cell populations.

For multicellular organisms to survive, some cells must refrain from dividing even when nutrients are plentiful. In tissues capable of cell proliferation (stable and continuously dividing tissues), when the need arises for new cells, as in the case of tissue injury, cells are replaced either by cell division or by replenishment from stem cell reserves.

Division Cycle of Cells

Adult multicellular animals must produce millions of new cells in order to replace dead cells. Cells undertake the process of division by progressing through a highly regulated process known as the cell cycle (**Figure 1**), the end product being a duplication of the contents of the mother cell into two daughter cells. In an adult animal, most cells are stable cells, and reside in the G0 (gap) phase of cell cycle. When division is necessary, cells that are capable of doing so enter the G1 phase of the cell cycle. In most cells the DNA in the nucleus is replicated during only a limited portion of the cell cycle called the S (synthesis) phase of the cell cycle.

After the S phase, the cells enter a second gap phase called the G2 phase. Finally, in the M (mitosis) phase, the contents of the nucleus condense to form visible chromosomes, which through an elaborately orchestrated series of movements are pulled apart into two equal sets. The cell itself then splits into two daughter cells. Upon loss of tissues due to injury, or due to normal cell sloughing, the division cycle of cells is stimulated in tissue- or organ-specific fashion so that the lost tissues can be replaced promptly to restore tissue function. The phases of cell division and the transitions between the phases are orchestrated by an intricate series of signaling mechanisms. When the lost tissue is replaced, the cells return to the normal resting state, thereby reestablishing the cellular, organ, and tissue homeostatic mechanisms.

Genetic Control of Cell Structure and Function during and after Embryonic Development

Multicellular animals are clones of cells descended from a single original cell, the fertilized egg. The cells in the body, as a rule, are genetically alike. However, they are phenotypically different; some are muscle cells, others neurons, still others hepatocytes, and so on. The different cell types are arranged into precisely organized tissues and organs, and the entire structure has a well-defined shape. All of these features are determined by the DNA sequence of the genome, which is reproduced in every cell. Each cell must act according to the same genetic instructions, but it must interpret them with due regard to time and circumstance so as to play a proper part in multicellular organization.

The development of vertebrates can be divided into three phases. In the first phase, the fertilized egg divides into many smaller cells that become organized into epithelium. Following a complex series of gastrulation and neurulation movements, a rudimentary gut cavity and neural tube are formed. In the second or organogenesis phase, the various organs, such as limbs, eyes, and heart, are formed. In the third

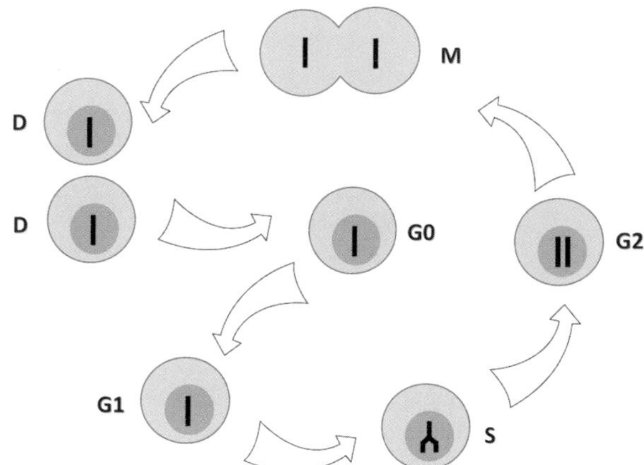

Figure 1 In adult organisms normally cells are in resting phase (G0) of the cell division cycle. Upon appropriate stimulus the cells enter the division cycle, which is characterized by G1, S, G2, and M phases. After division, the daughter cells (D) may either reenter the division cycle or enter the resting phase, depending on the stimulus.

 http://dx.doi.org/10.1016/B978-0-12-386454-3.00274-8

phase, the generated structures grow to their adult size. These phases are not sharply distinct but overlap considerably in time.

Terminal Differentiation and Cell Division

After embryonic development, cells in the normal adult human body divide at very different rates. Some, such as neurons and skeletal muscle cells, do not divide at all; others, such as liver cells, normally divide once every year or two; and certain epithelial cells in the gut divide more than twice a day so as to provide constant renewal of the gut lining. Most cells in the vertebrates fall somewhere between these extremes: they are able to divide, but normally do so infrequently. Almost all the variation in division rate lies in the time cells spend between mitosis and the S phase; slowly dividing cells remain arrested after mitosis for weeks or even years. By contrast, the time taken for a cell to progress from the beginning of S phase through mitosis is brief (typically 12–24 h in mammals) and remarkably constant, irrespective of the interval from one division to the next.

The time cells spend in a nonproliferative state (G0 in the cell cycle) varies according to both the cell type and the circumstances under which division is stimulated. Hepatocytes, for example, exist mostly in a resting state unless liver damage provokes proliferation. In contrast, uterine lining cells enter the cell cycle for a few days each month. A fraction of all hematopoietic precursors are always dividing to compensate for normal cell loss; this fraction increases after an episode of blood loss. Delicately adjusted and highly specific controls govern the proliferation of each class of cells in the body in each situation.

Role of Growth Factors and Cytokines in Cell Division

When put into an artificial culture medium completely devoid of serum, vertebrate cells normally do not pass through the G1/S restriction point, even though all the requisite nutrients are present in the medium. Rather, they halt their progress through the cell cycle. In order to complete the cycle of cell growth and division, cells require highly specific growth factors and cytokines, usually present in very small concentrations (10^{-9}–10^{-11} mol l^{-1}) in the serum. Different cells require different combinations of growth factors and cytokines. Some directly stimulate cell division and are called complete mitogens. Others control cell division by directly inhibiting cell cycle progression; these are called growth inhibitors. Yet others cause cell cycle progression in an indirect way and are called growth triggers. **Table 1** provides examples of growth factors and cytokines involved in cell division along with their particular functions.

Growth factors and cytokines often interact with cell-surface receptors in order to carry out their particular functions. For example, epidermal growth factor (EGF) binds to a receptor tyrosine kinase (RTK) (a cell-surface molecule present on many different kinds of cells). This triggers phosphorylation of tyrosine residues and dimerization of the receptors. An adaptor protein called Grb2 (growth factor receptor-bound protein 2) is then recruited to promote the formation of Ras-GTP. Active Ras-GTP binds to and activates a protein kinase termed Raf. Raf further phosphorylates and activates MEK (MAP kinase kinase). The downstream target is MAP kinase (MAPK). Active MAPK phosphorylates various proteins, including transcription factors that regulate the expression of cell cycle proteins to induce cell proliferation.

Cell Senescence and Reluctance to Divide

Most normal mammalian cells show a striking inability to proliferate indefinitely. Fibroblasts taken from a normal human fetus, for example, undergo approximately 50 population doublings when cultured in a standard growth medium. Toward the end of this time, proliferation slows down and after spending some time in a quiescent state, the cells die. Similar cells taken from a 40-year-old person stop dividing after approximately 40 doublings, while cells from an 80-year-old stop after approximately 30 doublings. Fibroblasts from animals with shorter life spans stop after a smaller number of division cycles in culture. Because of the

Table 1 Example of growth factors and cytokines known to regulate cell proliferation

Factor	*Representative functions*
Platelet-derived growth factor (PDGF)	Stimulates proliferation of connective tissue cells and neuroglial cells
Epidermal growth factor (EGF)	Stimulates proliferation of many cell types
Insulin like growth factors I and II (IGF-I and -II)	Work with PDGF and EGF to stimulate fat cell proliferation
Fibroblast growth factor (FGF)	Stimulates proliferation of many cell types including fibroblasts, endothelial cells, and myoblasts
Interleukin-2 (IL-2)	Stimulates proliferation of T lymphocytes
Transforming growth factor β (TGF-β)	Inhibits cell cycle progression of different cell types
Interleukin-1 (IL-1)	Inhibits proliferation of hepatocytes and other cells types
Hepatocyte proliferation inhibitor	Inhibits hepatocyte proliferation
Nerve growth factor (NGF)	Promotes axon growth and survival of sympathetic and some sensory and CNS neurons
Hematopoietic cell growth factors (IL-3, GM-CSF, M-CSF, G-CSF, and erythropoietin)	Promote division of different blood cells and various other types of cells

correspondence with aging of the body as a whole, this phenomenon is called cell senescence.

According to one theory, cell senescence is the result of a catastrophic accumulation of self-propagating errors in a cell's biosynthetic machinery. An alternative theory suggests that cell senescence is the result of a mechanism that has evolved to protect us from cancer by limiting the growth of tumors. It has been reported that telomeres play an essential role in chromosome capping affecting the cell proliferation. Telomere DNA undergoes progressive shortening of 50 and 200 bp per round of DNA replication. And then, telomere dysfunction leads to disruption of the telomere structure, resulting in end-to-end chromosome fusions and genomic instability. It can activate DNA damage-induced pathways that trigger cell cycle arrest or apoptosis.

Cell Proliferation as a Compensatory Response to Toxic Tissue Injury

Human beings are exposed to numerous toxic insults every day. Fortunately, the body has several defense mechanisms to combat toxicants. Some toxicants are prevented from entering the body by virtue of their particle size. Toxicants that do enter the body are metabolized or conjugated in an attempt to safely carry out their excretion.

When these first lines of defense are overcome, toxic substances may cause severe cell injury or even cell death. At this point, the tissue may respond by stimulating its healthy cells to divide and restore tissue structure and function. The ability of the tissue to undergo repair depends on the type of tissue damaged and the extent of the damage. Damage occurring in tissues that are unable to proliferate (for example, cardiac muscle) will not result in replacement of parenchymal cells, and a scar will take place of the dead cells. Likewise, damage that disrupts the supporting structure of the tissue – the basement membrane scaffolding upon which the cells reside – will likewise involve scarring rather than complete resolution to the normal, pre-damaged state. The process of tissue repair stops at a precise, preordained point. For example, liver regeneration ends when the functional mass of the liver is restored.

At low to moderate doses of a particular toxicant, the process functions well, and repair is usually adequate. At high doses of a toxicant, however, the ability of the cells to progress through the cell cycle is inhibited, leading to two consequences. First, dead cells are not replaced, which may lead to organ failure and death. Second, in the absence of compensatory cell division, which normally serves to contain the toxic injury, tissue injury can progress in an unrestrained manner. The ability of cells to enter and progress through the cell cycle following toxic injury decreases with age, a finding which explains, in part, why an 80-year-old person may be more susceptible to the same dose of a toxicant as a 40-year-old. **Table 2** shows a list of drugs and chemicals that affect cell proliferation in a variety of model systems.

Stem Cells and Terminally Differentiated Cells

Many of the tissues in the body undergoing constant renewal, such as skin and the lining of the intestine, accomplish this task by means of a small population of tissue stem cells. The defining properties of a stem cell are (1) the ability to divide virtually without limit throughout the lifetime of the organism and (2) the ability to divide symmetrically (leading to two terminally differentiated cells) or asymmetrically (giving rise to one stem cell and one terminally differentiated cell).

Stem cells are required wherever there is a recurring need to replace nondividing, terminally differentiated cells. Some terminally differentiated cells, such as mature mammalian red blood cells and the cells in the outermost layer of the skin, lack a cell nucleus and are therefore unable to divide. Others contain cytoplasmic structures (such as the myofibrils of striated muscle cells) that hinder cell duplication. And in some terminally differentiated cells, the chemistry of differentiation may simply be incompatible with cell division.

The job of the stem cell is not to carry out the function of the differentiated cell, but rather to produce the cells that will carry out those functions. Stem cells that give rise to only one type of differentiated cell are called unipotent; these are capable of differentiating along only one lineage. Also, adult stem cells in many differentiated undamaged tissues are typically unipotent and give rise to just one cell type under normal conditions. Additionally, a small number of cell types are called oligopotent. These stem cells have the ability to differentiate into just a few types of cells. A lymphoid stem cell is an example of an oligopotent stem cell. These stem cells cannot develop into any type of blood cell as bone marrow stem cells can. They give rise to only blood cells of the lymphatic system, such as T cells. Cells that give rise to many cell types are called pluripotent or totipotent. Yet, there is another type of stem cell that is called multipotent. These cells are progenitor cells that have the genetic potential to differentiate into multiple, but limited cell types.

Cell Proliferation and Cancer

Cells within a tissue exert an inhibitory effect on each other's growth. This restraining force is called social control of cell division, and it is mediated by a set of genes called social control genes. A cell that acquires a DNA mutation that disrupts this social restraint will divide without regard to the needs of the organism as a whole, and its progeny may become tumor cells.

Approximately 10^{16} cell divisions take place in a human body in the course of a lifetime. Even in an environment that is free of mutagens, mutations occur spontaneously at an estimated rate of about 10^{-6} mutations per gene per cell division, a value set by fundamental limitations on the accuracy of DNA replication and repair. Thus, in an average person's lifetime, every single gene is likely to have undergone mutations on about 10^{10} separate occasions.

Some mutated genes – if not repaired by the cell's DNA repair mechanisms – are involved in the regulation of cell division. Consequently, the affected cell, now lacking the normal 'brakes' on cell growth, may continuously progress through the cell cycle. To transform into a malignant cell, however, a cell must acquire not just one but a number of DNA mutations to escape the multiple controls on cell division. Further mutations endow the cell with the capacity for invasion

Table 2 Summary of some toxicants that may affect cell proliferation

Compound	*Origin*	*Specific mechanism*	*Source reference*
Natural food toxicants			
Ochratoxin A	Fungi	Induces cell proliferation by activating Cyclin-D and Cox-2.	Kumar R., et al., 2013. Carcinogenesis. 34:647.
Citrinin	Fungi	Inhibits cell proliferation by increasing p53 and p21.	Chang C.H., et al., 2011. Toxicol. Sci. 119:84.
Okadaic acid	Algae	Inhibits cell proliferation by inducing c-*Myc*.	Zhang L., et al., 2007. Cancer Res. 67:10198.
Glucosinolates	Plants	Inhibits cell proliferation by G2/M arrest.	Liang H et al., 2008. J. Nat. Prod. 71:1911.
Psoralen	Plants	Inhibits cell proliferation by BMP signaling.	Tang D.Z., et al., 2011. Biochem. Biophys. Res. Commun. 405:256.
Pyrrolizidine alkaloid	Plants	Inhibits cell proliferation by activating p38.	Ji L.L., et al., 2002. Toxicon. 40:1685.
Environmental toxicants			
Nonmetals (As, S)	Soils, air	Inhibit cell proliferation by DNA damage.	Wu J.Z., et al., 2006. Eur. J. Pharm. Sci. 29:35.
Metals (Cd^{2+}, Hg^{2+}, Pb^{2+})	Water	Inhibit cell proliferation by their interaction with DNA metabolism.	Costa M., et al., 1982. Res. Commun. Chem. Pathol. Pharmacol. 38:405.
1,3-Butadiene	Rubber, plastics	Increases cell proliferation by DNA modification.	Melnick R.L., et al., 2001. Chem. Biol. Interact. 135:27.
Polycyclic aromatic hydrocarbons (PAHs)	Tobacco smoke	Increases cell proliferation by increasing ER.	Plísková M., et al., 2005. Toxicol. Sci. 83:246.
Dichlorodiphenyl-trichloroethane (DDT)	Pesticides	Increases cell proliferation by chromosomal alterations.	Uppala P.T., et al., 2005. Environ. Mol. Mutagen. 46:43.
Polychlorinated biphenyls (PCBs)	Pesticides	Induces cell proliferation of collecting ducts in kidneys.	Chaudhuri L., et al., 2010. Free Radic. Biol. Med. 49:40.
Lithium	Nephrogenic diabetes insipidus	Induces cell proliferation in the liver.	Gao Y., et al., 2013. Am. J. Physiol. Renal. Physiol. July 24 2013. (Epub ahead of print)
Dimethylnitrosamine	Food and environment	Inhibits cell proliferation in the liver	Syed, I., et al., 2012. Mol. Cell. Biochem. 365(1–2): 351–361.
Doxorubicin + caffeine	Anticancer drug	Increases in hematopoietic cell proliferation	Motegi, T., et al., 2013. Res. Vet. Sci., July 18 2013. pii: S0034-5288(13) 00210-5. doi: 10.1016/j.rvsc.2013.06.011. (Epub ahead of print)
TCDD	Environmental toxin		National Toxicology Program. Natl. Toxicol. Program Tech. Rep. Ser. November 2010; (558):1–206.

and metastasis. Statistically, it is estimated that somewhere between three and seven independent random events, each of low probability, are typically required to turn a normal cell into a cancer cell; the smaller numbers apply to leukemia and the larger numbers to carcinomas.

Proto-oncogenes are normal genes encoding proteins involved in cell proliferation. Like any gene, a proto-oncogene may undergo mutation. When a mutation in a proto-oncogene confers a gain of function, the new mutant gene (now called an oncogene) will dramatically stimulate cell division. Tumor suppressor genes, in contrast, are normal genes that encode proteins that inhibit cell proliferation. If a tumor suppressor gene is mutated in such a way as to inactivate the gene, this removal of inhibition may make the cell grow continuously. Mutations may be spontaneous, or they may result from exposure to chemical carcinogens or radiation. Mutations in tumor suppressor genes generally need to occur on both alleles for a tumor to arise, whereas most proto-oncogenes need only one mutated allele (one oncogene) to contribute to malignancy.

Importance of Understanding the Mechanisms in Control of Cell Proliferation

An understanding of the mechanisms in control of cell proliferation is critical in the development of new tissue restoration therapies. Current clinical treatments for patients with drug overdoses or chemical poisoning are aimed primarily at preventing additional injury, either by blocking further formation of toxic metabolites or by increasing clearance of the toxin from the body. While these strategies are useful, the survival of the tissue – and sometimes the patient – is heavily dependent on tissue repair, the success of which is in turn contingent on the ability of cells to proliferate.

In cases of toxic exposure in which tissue repair is delayed, either due to the massivity of the exposure or to a delay in treatment, organ loss and even death may occur because the damage compromises the regenerating ability of the cells, thereby paving the way for unrestrained progression of injury. If cellular regeneration after massive tissue damage could be actively stimulated, it might be possible to prevent organ loss and death.

Animal experiments provide concrete examples of how modification of tissue repair can directly influence survival. Animals given ordinarily lethal doses of toxins are able to survive – even when there is massive liver injury – when tissue repair in the liver is stimulated. Conversely, animals receiving otherwise nonlethal doses of toxins develop liver failure and die if cell division (and therefore tissue repair) is blocked by antimitotic agents.

Perhaps carefully induced suppression of pathways involved in cell death and stimulation of pathways involved in cell division could stop the progression of toxic injury and restore organ structure and function. With the advent of gene therapy, specific genes could, one day, be delivered directly to the damaged organ to induce expression/suppression of the appropriate factors needed for recovery. Although this may require time, with technological advances this route of therapy appears to be doable.

See also: Cell Cycle.

Further Reading

Alberts, B., Johnson, A., Lewis, J., Raff, M. (Eds.), 2007. Molecular Biology of the Cell, fifth ed. Garland, New York.

Chanda, S., Mehendale, H.M., 1996. Hepatic cell division and tissue repair: a key to survival after liver injury. Mol. Med. Today 2, 82–89.

Gallagher, E.J., LeRoith, D., 2011. Diabetes, cancer, and metformin: connections of metabolism and cell proliferation. Ann. N. Y. Acad. Sci. 1243, 54–68.

González-Mariscal, L., Lechuga, S., Garay, E., 2007. Role of tight junctions in cell proliferation and cancer. Prog. Histochem. Cytochem. 42, 1–57.

Lodish, H., Berk, A., Kaiser, C.A., et al. (Eds.), 2007. Molecular Cell Biology, sixth ed. Scientific American Books (Distributed by Freeman New York), New York.

Mehendale, H.M., 1995. Injury and repair as opposing forces in risk assessment. Toxicol. Lett. 82–83, 891–899.

Reinehr, R., Häussinger, D., 2009. Epidermal growth factor receptor signaling in liver cell proliferation and apoptosis. Biol. Chem. 390, 1033–1037.

Centipedes

HH Lin and TJ Wiegand, University of Rochester Medical Center, Rochester, NY, USA

This article is a revision of the previous edition article by Elizabeth J. Scharman, volume 1, p 499, © 2005, Elsevier Inc.

Background

Centipedes are nocturnal multisegmented elongated arthropods known for the distinct feature of having a pair of legs for each body segment except for the last. The first pair of legs on the cranial segment is, in actuality, modified into a pincerlike apparatus, known as forcipules, used to inject venom into prey. The last segment contains a pair of filamentous caudal appendages that despite popular belief play no role in envenomation. There are over 3000 species, varying in size from 1 to 30 cm with body segments numbering from 15 to more than 100. Centipedes are divided into four orders; Geophiulomorpha (soil centipedes), Lithobiomorpha (rock or garden centipedes), Scolopendromorpha (tropical or giant centipedes), and Scutigeromorpha (house or feather centipedes) of which only two, Scolopendromorpha and Scutigeromorpha, are of medical significance. Because the majority of centipede envenomations results in minor symptoms alone, treatment consists mainly of symptomatic alleviation. Centipedes are most commonly found in tropical and subtropical regions but can be found worldwide on all six inhabited continents.

Exposure Routes and Pathways

A venom gland is found at the base of the forcipules, which act as fangs. Upon penetration into the human skin by the forcipules, venom passes through the ducts of the forcipules and is injected into the bite site, causing local envenomation. Distal extremities such as hands and feet are common sites of envenomation. There has been one case report in the literature of an accidental ingestion resulting in symptomatic presentation.

Mechanism of Toxicity

Much is still unknown regarding the components that make up centipede venom but considerable work has been done surrounding the venom of *Scolopendra* spp. Centipede venom is a complex mixture of lipid toxin, similar to scorpion venom, thus facilitating local cellular penetration and absorption. Known components include polysaccharides, lipoproteins, various enzymes including proteinases and esterases, amino acid naphthylamidase, alkaline phosphatase, 5-hydroxytryptamine, histamine, and a cardiotoxic agent known as toxin-S. Toxin-S is a large heat-labile acid that has been shown to increase capillary permeability, induce vasoconstriction, and act as a cardiodepressant. In addition, there is an identified presence of a smooth muscle contractile agent that has muscarinic activity as well. It is thought that the digestive enzymes and toxin-S serve as a primary predatory function of the venom, whereas pain mediators such as 5-hydroxytryptamine and histamine serve as a secondary defensive function of the venom.

Acute and Short-Term Toxicity (or Exposure)

Animal

Acute toxicity of centipede extract has been demonstrated in animal models. One study demonstrated cardiac arrest in a toad shortly after being injected with an extract made from *Scolopendra morsitans*. The effect was prevented by giving atropine. Though the underlying mechanism is not clearly understood, it is thought to be associated with the muscarinic activity agent present in centipede venom.

Human

The majority of acute centipede envenomations produce minor localized symptoms that are self-limiting and generally resolve spontaneously within 48 h. Localized symptoms around envenomation sites include burning pain, edema, erythema, bullae formation, ecchymosis, paresthesia, delayed itchiness, lymphangitis, and lymphadenopathy. Occasionally, the bite wound is complicated by necrosis and gangrene but this is thought to be secondary to wound infection and not a property of envenomation. A minority of acute centipede envenomations produce minor systemic symptoms including chest pain, palpitations, headache, dizziness, and vomiting. It is thought that the severity of symptoms correlates with the size of the centipede.

There have been several case reports of acute centipede envenomations resulting in acute myocardial infarction or acute coronary ischemia. In one case, a previously healthy 22-year-old male with no cardiac risk factors developed severe retrosternal chest pain radiating to his left arm, diaphoresis, nausea, and vomiting 2 h after being bitten by a *Scolopendra* sp. The patient presented to the emergency department where electrocardiogram, echocardiogram, and cardiac marker levels revealed an anterior wall myocardial infarction 14 h after envenomation. An emergent coronary angiography revealed entirely normal coronary arteries. All abnormal findings with the electrocardiogram, echocardiogram, and cardiac marker levels had resolved 3 days after admission. Another case report described a 20-year-old male who presented to the emergency department with severe chest pain and electrocardiogram findings suggestive of an inferolateral myocardial infarction approximately 24 h after being bitten by a suspected *Scolopendra* sp. The exact pathophysiology has not yet been identified but the suspected mechanism is thought to be an acute release of inflammatory mediators causing increased capillary permeability, hypotension, and coronary artery spasm that may result in an acute myocardial infarction.

Rare but severe presentations of centipede envenomations have been documented in the literature. In one case, a 46-year-old female in the southwestern United States was bitten on the right foot by *Scolopendra heros*. She went on to develop necrosis of the peroneal muscles, rhabdomyolysis, acute renal failure, and massive edema of the leg, requiring fasciotomy to relieve

 http://dx.doi.org/10.1016/B978-0-12-386454-3.00707-7

increased compartmental pressures within the leg. Another case documented eosinophilic cellulitis or Wells syndrome associated with the bite of an unidentified centipede. An Israeli female bitten on the neck was unable to turn her head, most likely secondary to muscle spasm. There have been no reported deaths associated with centipede envenomation within the United States. In the early twentieth century, there was a reported case of a 7-year-old female in the Philippines who died after being bitten on the head by a *Scolopendra subspinipes*.

In the one reported case of symptomatic ingestion, a 6-month-old Australian infant accidentally ingested a centipede identified as *Scutigera* sp. and proceeded to develop pallor, hypotonia, vomiting, and lethargy. The symptoms were thought to be secondary to the systemic absorption of venom. The child fully recovered after approximately 48 h. A prospective study of centipede exposures identified three cases of ingestions that resulted in no adverse effects or symptoms.

Chronic Toxicity or Exposure

Animal

Chronic exposure of centipede extract has been demonstrated as an antihyperlipidemic agent in animal models. One study isolated the substance centipede acidic protein (CAP) from an alcohol extract comprising powdered dried *Scolopendra subspinipes mutilans* and injected it into rodent models. Rodents that received CAP were shown to have lower levels of triglycerides, cholesterol, and low-density lipoprotein when compared to control models injected with saline.

Human

In a death associated with *Scolopendra* spp. envenomation, a 21-year-old Thai female had been exposed to repeated envenomations. She had been envenomated on three separate occasions, each resulting in a local urticarial reaction, 9 months prior to her death. Upon her fourth envenomation, she presented with chest discomfort, hypotension, tachypnea, and a generalized urticarial rash. Despite aggressive medical intervention, she decompensated into respiratory failure and died from cardiovascular collapse and acute respiratory distress syndrome. The mechanism was thought to be secondary to an allergic reaction. It is theorized that there is similarity between centipede and hymenoptera venom allergies suggesting that chronic or repeated envenomations in an individual with a centipede venom allergy may result in life-threatening allergic reactions that may not have been seen with prior envenomations.

Clinical Management

As the majority of centipede envenomations produce minor and self-limiting symptoms, the mainstay of treatment is supportive care and symptomatic relief. Appropriate wound care and cleaning should be performed along with the administration of tetanus prophylaxis. The use of antibiotics should be reserved for recognized wound infections. The use of ice packs, hot water immersion, and analgesics have all been shown to alleviate pain from centipede envenomations. The mechanism of analgesia produced from hot water immersion is not yet identified but it is thought to be secondary to the denaturing of the heat-labile toxin. Severe pain may also be treated with injection of local anesthetic around the envenomation site.

Miscellaneous

Millipedes

Like centipedes, millipedes are also multisegmented elongated arthropods. Millipedes differ from centipedes in that they do not possess venom-injecting apparatuses and the majority of their body segments have two pairs of legs per segment instead of one. Though millipedes do not bite, they can secrete and spray noxious chemicals that upon exposure can act as skin and eye irritants. Like centipedes, millipedes are also commonly found in the southern United States.

See also: Animal Models; Animals, Poisonous and Venomous; Cardiovascular System; Hymenoptera; Immune System; Lipid Modifying Drugs; Scorpions; Spiders.

Further Reading

Balit, C.R., Harvey, M.S., Waldock, J.M., Isbister, G.K., 2004. Prospective study of centipede bites in Australia. J. Toxicol. Clin. Toxicol. 42 (1), 41–48.

Barnett, P.L., 1991. Centipede ingestion by a six-month-old infant: toxic side effects. Pediatr. Emerg. Care 7 (4), 229–230.

Bush, S.P., King, B.O., Norris, R.L., Stockwell, S.A., 2001. Centipede envenomation. Wilderness Environ. Med. 12 (2), 93–99.

Chaou, C.H., Chen, C.K., Chen, J.C., Chiu, T.F., Lin, C.C., 2009. Comparisons of ice packs, hot water immersion, and analgesia injection for the treatment of centipede envenomations in Taiwan. Clin. Toxicol. 47 (7), 659–662.

Cherniack, E.P., 2011. Bugs as drugs, part two: worms, leeches, scorpions, snails, ticks, centipedes, and spiders. Altern. Med. Rev. 16 (1), 50–58.

Friedman, I.S., Phelps, R.G., Baral, J., Sapadin, A.N., 1998. Wells' syndrome triggered by centipede bite. Int. J. Dermatolo. 37 (8), 602–605.

Fung, H.T., Lam, S.K., Wong, O.F., 2011. Centipede bite victims: a review of patients presenting to two emergency departments in Hong Kong. Hong Kong Med. J. 17 (5), 381–385.

Lersloompleephunt, N., Eakthunyasakul, S., Sittipunt, C., et al., 2003. Severe hypotension and adult respiratory distress syndrome (ARDS) following centipede bite. In: Proceedings of the 5th Asia-Pacific Congress on Animal, Plant and Microbial Toxins. International Society on Toxinology, Thailand.

Logan, J.L., Ogden, D.A., 1985. Rhabdomyolysis and acute renal failure following the bite of the giant desert centipede *Scolopendra heros*. West. J. Med. 142 (4), 549–550.

Pineda, E.V., 1923. A fatal case of centipede bite. J. Med. Assoc. 3, 59–61.

Senthilkumaran, S., Meenakshisundaram, R., Michaels, A.D., 2011. Acute ST-segment elevation myocardial infarction from a centipede bite. J. Cardiovasc. Dis. Res. 2 (4), 244–246.

Yildiz, A., Biçeroglu, S., Yakut, N., Bilir, C., Akdemir, R., Akilli, A., 2006. Acute myocardial infarction in a young man caused by centipede sting. Emerg. Med. J. 23 (4), e30.

Relevant Websites

http://soilbugs.massey.ac.nz/chilopoda.php – Massey University – Images and information regarding centipedes.

http://emedicine.medscape.com/article/769448-overview – Medscape *eMedicine* – Information regarding clinical presentation and management of centipede envenomations.

http://www.caes.uga.edu/publications/pubDetail.cfm?pk_id=6198 – The University of Georgia College of Agricultural and Environmental Sciences website related to centipede and millipedes.

http://www.ipm.ucdavis.edu/PMG/PESTNOTES/pn7472.html – University of California Davis – Images and information regarding centipedes and millipedes.

Cephalosporins

SC Gad, Gad Consulting Services, Cary, NC, USA

- Name: Cephalosporins
- Chemical/Pharmaceutical/Other Class: β-Lactam antibiotics (as are penicillins)
- Example Compounds: Cefaclor, Cefadroxil, Cefamandole, Cefazolin, Cefepidime, Cefoperazone, Cefotaxime, Cefoxitin, Ceftriaxone, Cephalexin, Cephalothin, Cephradine, Cephaprin, Cefmetazole, Cefonicid, Ceforanide, Cefotetan, Cefprozil, Loracarbef, Cefperazone, Cefpodoxime, Cefixime, Ceftazidime, Ceftizoxime, Moxalactarn

Background Information

The cephalosporins have sustained their position as a very significant class of antibiotics worldwide for many years, comprising over one-half of the available β-lactam antibiotics. Initially, cephalosporin compounds produced by the fungal organism *Cephalosporium acremonium* were isolated in the early 1940s from fungus in sewage seawater in Cagliari, Sardinia, after it was observed that a natural pattern of periodic clearing of microbes was taking place from a local harbor area. Filtrates from *C. acremonium* cultures were found to have antimicrobial activity against infections in animals and humans, including the injection of filtrates into 'boils' and other cutaneous infections. The initial work later expanded to result in the discovery of cephalosporin C, the structural nucleus for cephalosporin compound development over the next four decades. Ongoing research and development have led to several additional cephalosporin antibiotics that have been released since the 1960s, with 24 unique, yet structurally similar compounds currently available for clinical use in the United States. The first three generations of cephalosporin antibiotics include both parenterally (i.e., intravenously or injection) and orally administered agents. The fourth-generation compound, cefepidime, is available for parenteral administration.

Uses

Cephalosporins (a class of β-lactam antibiotics) induce their antimicrobial effect by inhibiting the integration of bacterial peptidoglycan. Individual peptidoglycan units are synthesized in the cytoplasm of the bacterial cell and are transported across the cytoplasmic membrane where they are inserted by peptidase enzymes into a cross-linked lattice that forms the structural support of the bacterial cell wall. The peptidase enzymes present in the outer cytoplasmic membrane are referred to as penicillin-binding proteins and represent the target sites for antibacterial action of cephalosporins and other β-lactam antibiotics. Cephalosporins are active *in vitro* against many gram-positive aerobic bacteria and some gram-negative aerobic bacteria. There are substantial differences among the cephalosporins in their spectra of activity as well as levels of activity against susceptible bacteria. Later-generation cephalosporins also are used in the later stages of livestock husbandry for adding weight.

Environmental Fate and Behavior

The environmental behavior of most of the cephalosporin compounds is quite similar. In the atmosphere, most are expected to exist solely in the particulate phase, and are removed via wet or dry deposition. In aquatic environments, due to their anionic nature, they are not expected to volatize, and they adsorb slowly. Cephalosporins are highly mobile in soils, with low adsorption. Data suggest that even with water treatment, some of these compounds will persist. They may be susceptible to photolyzation.

Exposure and Exposure Monitoring

The routes of exposure to cephalosporins are commonly oral, intravenous, or intramuscular. Accidental ingestion of oral dosage forms by children is the most common poisoning exposure. There are some workers who may be exposed to cephalosporins, primarily those involved in the production of drug forms.

Toxicokinetics

Cephalosporins are generally well absorbed following administration, with bioavailability being greater than 75%. Many of these compounds are not stable in the acid environment of the stomach; therefore, only a limited number are useful for oral administration. The distribution is limited to the extracellular fluid space, with volumes of distribution for most ranging from 0.25 to 0.5 $l\,kg^{-1}$. Protein binding is primarily to albumin. Most cephalosporins are widely distributed to tissues and fluids, including pleural fluid, synovial fluid, and bone. Some of the third-generation compounds have good distribution to the cerebrospinal fluid. The metabolites possess antibacterial activity. The cephalosporins and their metabolites are rapidly excreted by the kidneys by glomerular filtration and/or tubular secretion. Serum half-lives of these compounds range from 0.4 to 10.9 h. Patients with immature renal systems or with renal compromise are at risk for toxicity due to decreased elimination. Cefamandole, cefmetazole, cefmenoxime, cefoperazone, and moxalactam have been associated with coagulopathies due to inhibition of platelet aggregation and prolongation of bleeding time.

Mechanism of Toxicity

Hematologic when given in higher doses, cephalosporins bind to cell membrane proteins and act as haptens. High-dose treatments can induce a hemolytic anemia. They can also prolong bleeding times by reducing platelet adhesion and activation.

 http://dx.doi.org/10.1016/B978-0-12-386454-3.00825-3

Many cephalosporins are substrates for the organic anion transport system in the proximal tubules and can accumulate in the kidney, competing for and inhibiting the transport system, leading to renal necrosis. Nephrotoxicity, with potency ranging from mild to high (cephaloridine), can cause renal tubule injury. There is great variability in the potential for renal toxicity among different members of the family of compounds. Renal toxic members deplete glutathione levels in the renal cortex. There is evidence that this nephrotoxicity is due to action of the drugs on mitochondria.

Chronic Toxicity (or Exposure)

Animal

The extent of renal accumulation and effect is species dependent (rabbit > guinea pig > rat). There is also great variability in toxicity between different compounds.

Human

Like penicillins, cephalosporins are a relatively nontoxic group of antibiotics. The primary adverse effect reported is hypersensitivity, a rare event. Cross-allergenicity and sensitization with penicillins may occur and is of concern, though allergic responses to cephalosporins are less likely than to penicillins. Toxicity is unlikely in children less than 6 years of age who acutely ingest less than 250 mg kg^{-1}. Nephrotoxicity is a possible, but rare, occurrence with acute ingestion. Coagulopathies have been reported following chronic intravenous use of certain cephalosporins. At higher concentrations, cephalosporins cause renal tubular injury, characterized by decreased glomerular filtration rate, glucosuria, enzymuria, and proteinuria.

Immunotoxicity

Lymphocyte response may be inhibited by some of the cephalosporin class. There are also effects on interleukin-2 function and production. Additional testing will be required to make a positive determination on the immunotoxic affects of cephalosporins, and there will be variability, possibly wide, among the members of the class. Hypersensitivity does occur.

Reproductive and Developmental Toxicity

- *Cefotan*: Has adverse effects on the testes of prepubertal rats. Subcutaneous administration of 500 mg kg^{-1} day^{-1} (~8–16 times the usual adult human dose) on days 6–35 of life (thought to be developmentally analogous to late childhood and prepuberty in humans) resulted in reduced testicular weight and seminiferous tubule degeneration in 10 of 10 animals. Affected cells included spermatogonia and spermatocytes; Sertoli and Leydig cells were unaffected. Incidence of severity of lesions was dose dependent; at 120 mg kg^{-1} day^{-1} (B2–4 times the usual human dose) only 1 of 10 treated animals was affected, and the degree of degeneration was mild. Similar lesions were observed in experiments of comparable design with other methylthiotetrazole-containing antibiotics, and impaired fertility has been reported, particularly at high dose levels. No testicular effects were observed in 7-week-old rats treated with up to 1000 mg kg^{-1} day^{-1} subcutaneously for 5 weeks, or in infant dogs (3 weeks old) that received up to 300 mg kg^{-1} day^{-1} intravenously for 5 weeks. Pregnancy category B: Reproduction studies have been performed in rats and monkeys at doses up to 20 times the human dose and have revealed no evidence of impaired fertility or harm to the fetus due to cefotetan.
- *Cefixime*: In rats, fertility and reproductive performance were not affected by cefixime at doses up to 125 times the adult therapeutic dose. Pregnancy category B: Reproduction studies have been performed in mice and rats at doses up to 400 times the human dose and have revealed no evidence of harm to the fetus due to cefixine.
- *Cefoperazone*: Produced no impairment of fertility and had no effects on general reproductive performance or fetal development when administered subcutaneously at daily doses up to 500–1000 mg kg^{-1} prior to and during mating, and to pregnant female rats during gestation. These doses are 10–20 times the estimated usual single clinical dose. Cefoperazone had adverse effects on the testes of prepubertal rats at all doses tested. Subcutaneous administration of 1000 mg kg^{-1} day^{-1} (~16 times the average adult human dose) resulted in reduced testicular weight, arrested spermatogenesis, reduced germinal cell population, and vacuolation of Sertoli cell cytoplasm. The severity of lesions was dose dependent in the 100–1000 mg kg^{-1} day^{-1} range; the low dose caused a minor decrease in spermatocytes. This effect has not been observed in adult rats. Historically, the lesions were reversible at all but the highest dosage levels. However, these studies did not evaluate subsequent development of reproductive function in the rats. Pregnancy category B: Reproduction studies have been performed in mice, rats, and monkeys at doses up to 10 times the human dose and have revealed no evidence of impaired fertility or harm to the fetus due to cefoperazone.

Genotoxicity

- *Cefixime*: SUPRAX did not cause point mutations in bacteria or mammalian cells, DNA damage, or chromosome damage *in vitro* and did not exhibit clastogenic potential *in vivo* in the mouse micronucleus test.
- *Cefoperazone*: The maximum duration of cefoperazone animal toxicity studies is 6 months. In none of the *in vivo* or *in vitro* genetic toxicology studies did cefoperazone show any mutagenic potential at either the chromosomal or subchromosomal level.

Carcinogenicity

Studies have yet to be undertaken for the carcinogenicity of cephalosporins in animals or humans. Cephalosporins are not listed by regulatory agencies.

Clinical Management

If a toxic or unknown amount of a cephalosporin has been ingested, gastric decontamination and the administration of activated charcoal are usually all that is needed. In the symptomatic patient, evaluation of renal function and electrolytes may be necessary. Chronic exposure usually requires discontinuation of the drug and supportive care. Anaphylaxis should be treated with epinephrine and/or diphenhydramine.

Ecotoxicology

Cephalosporins have a low bioconcentration factor, and are not expected to bioconcentrate or bioaccumulate to any serious degree. They are not expected to significantly impact species outside of the bactericidal activity they are in use for.

Other Hazards

When heated to decomposition, many of the cephalosporins will emit much more toxic fumes.

Exposure Standards and Guidelines

Exposure guidelines have yet to be set by regulatory agencies.

See also: Hemocompatibility; Kidney.

Further Reading

Ballantyne, B., Marrs, T., Syversen, T., 2009. General and Applied Toxicology, third ed. Macmillan References Ltd, New York, pp. 1138–1140, 686–687.
Dancer, S.J., 2001. The problem with cephalosporins. J. Antimicrob. Chemother. 48, 463–478.
Del Rosso, J.Q., 2003. Cephalosporins in dermatology. Clin. Dermatol. 21, 24–32.
Greenberg, M.L., Hendrickson, R.G., Muller, A.A., 2003. Occupational exposure to cephalosporins leading to clostridium difficile infection. J. Toxicol. Clin. Toxicol. 41, 205–206.
Karalis, V., Tsantili-Kakoulidou, A., Macheras, P., 2003. Quantitative structure–pharmacokinetic relationships for disposition parameters of cephalosporins. Eur. J. Pharm. Sci. 20, 115–123.
Walsh, C., 2003. Antibiotics. ASM Press, Washington DC.

Relevant Websites

http://medical-dictionary.thefreedictionary.com – Search for 'Cephalosporins'.
http://www.drugs.com – Search for 'Cephalosporins'.
http://accessmedicine.com/ – Search for 'Cephalosporins'.

CERCLA; Revised as the Superfund Amendments Reauthorization Act (SARA)

RW Kapp, Jr., BioTox, Monroe Township, NJ, USA

Background

Until the 1970s, citizens were mostly unaware of how the indiscriminate dumping of chemical wastes might affect public health and the environment. The common practice in years past was to simply abandon waste chemicals on properties and in landfills with no consideration for their ultimate fate. This resulted in thousands of uncontrolled and abandoned hazardous waste sites throughout the nation. Although the Environmental Protection Agency (EPA) had been created in 1970, there were no specific provisions to deal with this ever-growing environmental problem. The Clean Water Act (1977), the Resource Conservation and Recovery Act – RCRA (1976), the Water Pollution Control Act (1972), and the Rivers and Harbors Act (1899) set the stage for more comprehensive legislation. However, in the late 1970s, three events occurred that brought to a head the fact that abandoned hazardous waste could prove to be a serious threat to any community. One was the discovery that some 21 000 t of toxic waste had been buried in the abandoned Love Canal in the early 1950s. The town of Niagara Falls bought the land and built an elementary school directly over the dump which opened in 1954. There was a rash of diseases and birth defects over the next few years which were brought to light in newspaper articles beginning in 1976. The events at Love Canal, New York, resulted in a state of emergency being declared in August 1978 by the State of New York Department of Health. The EPA reviewed the situation in 1979 and found residents exhibited a 'disturbingly high rate of miscarriages. Love Canal can now be added to a growing list of environmental disasters involving toxics, ranging from industrial workers stricken by nervous disorders and cancers to the discovery of toxic materials in the milk of nursing mothers.' Another unregulated hazardous waste site that had been in operation since the early 1960s was found near Louisville, Kentucky, which was named 'Valley of the Drums' after almost 20 000 empty waste-containing drums from numerous local businesses were found at the 23-acre site. A third incident materialized in Times Beach, Missouri, where it was discovered that dioxin waste from a facility that had manufactured Agent Orange during the Vietnam War had been sprayed on dirt roads in the town from 1972 to 1976. In late 1979, an investigation by the Centers for Disease Control and Prevention revealed the situation which immediately made national headlines. The confluence of these three specific events and other factors led to intense citizen concern over the magnitude of toxic waste. In response to this concern, Congress established The Comprehensive Environmental Response, Compensation, and Liability Act (CERCLA) to locate, investigate, and clean up the worst sites nationwide.

Overview of CERCLA (Superfund)

On 11 December 1980, Congress passed the CERCLA (also known as the Superfund). This law empowered the EPA and state authorities to investigate and respond to the release of waste and hazardous materials into the environment such as was found at the Love Canal, New York, Louisville, Kentucky, and Times Beach, Missouri. The Office of Emergency and Remedial Response at the EPA administers the program in cooperation with states and tribal governments. This legislation essentially created a tax on the chemical and petroleum industries and provided broad Federal authority to respond directly to chemical releases or potential releases of hazardous substances that are deemed threatening to public health or the environment. The taxes collected from inception through 1986 totaled $1.6 billion. CERCLA also established the National Priorities List (NPL) which is the list of national priorities among the known releases or anticipated releases of hazardous substances throughout the United States and its territories. The NPL is intended primarily to guide the EPA in determining which sites warrant further investigation.

The legislation was amended on 17 October 1986 with the enactment of the Superfund Amendments and Reauthorization Act (SARA). One of the critical changes provided in the SARA was to increase the fund from $1.6 to $8.5 billion and called on the US EPA to make changes to the Hazard Ranking System (HRS) to more accurately note the level of danger of sites to be placed on the NPL. HRS is a numerically based screening system that uses information from initial, limited preliminary investigations and the site inspection to assess the relative potential of sites to pose a threat to human health or the environment. In addition, SARA stressed the importance of permanent remedies and innovative treatment technologies in cleaning up hazardous waste sites; required Superfund actions to consider the standards and requirements found in other state and federal environmental laws and regulations; provided new enforcement authorities and settlement tools; increased state involvement in every phase of the Superfund program; increased the focus on human health problems posed by hazardous waste sites; and encouraged greater citizen participation in making decisions on how sites should be cleaned up. Finally, the NPL must be revised and republished every 2 years and informally reviewed annually.

The term 'Superfund' is derived from the fund of money that is collected by EPA to investigate sites and to pay for cleanups where no responsible parties can be determined. The legislation also provided for studies and the use of new technologies.

There are four basic components to the CERCLA/Superfund Legislation:

1. The legislation set up an information gathering and analysis system that enables federal, state, and tribal governments to designate chemical dumpsites and develop priorities for cleaning them up. The EPA administrator issues regulations that, in the administrator's opinion, identify 'hazardous' or 'toxic' substances. The owners and operators of sites containing any listed chemical must notify the EPA of the amount and types of identified wastes their sites contain. This information assists the EPA in developing the NPL to plan responses.

2. The legislation also gave the EPA the authority to respond to toxic substance emergencies where immediate short-term response is deemed necessary for the public welfare.
3. The legislation further established a Hazardous Substance Trust Fund to pay for removing wastes and for remedial actions associated with the cleanup where no responsible parties can be determined.
4. The legislation holds responsible persons and companies liable for toxic wastes cleanup and restitution costs. Unfortunately, the legislation was not clear on this point and not all federal courts have applied the same standards to determine parent corporation liability for CERCLA infractions.

Site Cleanups – Remediations and Removals

- Remediations are conducted according to the National Contingency Plan (NCP) are refer to permanent cleanups.
- Removals are cleanups other than permanent – i.e., emergency or temporary cleanups.
- EPA generally takes remedial actions only at sites listed on the NPL.
- EPA assigns responsibility by looking at all potentially responsible parties (PRPs) including current owners/operators, previous owners/operators, facilities that generated the waste, and transporters that delivered the waste.
- 'Strict' liability is defined as parties that are responsible regardless of how careful they were in their practice of disposing of the waste.
- 'Joint and several' liability is defined as any one PRP that is potentially liable for all costs of the cleanup no matter how much of the total contamination is directly due to their disposal activities.
- General remediation process is specified under the Superfund's NCP as follows:
  - Emergency removal to address immediate environmental problems.
  - A remedial investigation/feasibility study to determine cleanup approaches.
  - A Record of Decision to document the approach EPA has selected for cleanup.
  - The design, construction, operation, and maintenance of the final cleanup.
  - In addition, the cleanup process is required to meet all other environmental requirements during its operation. These are referred to as relevant and appropriate requirements.

New Releases

The CERCLA hazardous substance release reporting regulations (40 CFR Part 302) are to minimize environmental releases of current manufacturing processes. A designated person at the facility must report the release of any hazardous material when it exceeds the reportable quantity to the National Response Center (NRC). The hazardous substances and reportable quantities are defined and listed in 40 CFR § 302.4.

The NRC telephone number is 1-800-424-8802.

US EPA's RCRA/Superfund/UST Hotline to answer questions regarding guidance for the Superfund Program: 1-800-424-9346.

As of 15 March 2012, there were 1302 sites listed on the National Priority List, 62 proposed new sites, and 359 sites have been remediated and removed from the original list.

See also: Love Canal; Times Beach; Valley of the Drums; National Environmental Policy Act, USA; Pollution Prevention Act, United States; Resource Conservation and Recovery Act (USA).

Further Reading

EPA, October 1992. CERCLA/Superfund Orientation Manual. Document No. EPA/542/R-92/005. Available online: http://www.epa.gov/superfund/policy/remedy/pdfs/542r-92005-s.pdf.

Switzer, C.S., Gray, P.L., 2008. Basic Practice Series: CERCLA – Comprehensive Environmental Response, Compensation, and Liability Act (Superfund), second ed. American Bar Association, Chicago, IL.

Relevant Websites

http://www.epa.gov/; http://www.law.cornell.edu/lii/get_the_law

Cerium

SC Gad, Gad Consulting Services, Cary, NC, USA

This article is a revision of the previous edition article by Shayne C. Gad, volume 1, pp 502–503, © 2005, Elsevier Inc.

- Name: Cerium
- Chemical Abstracts Service Registry Number: 7440-45-1
- Synonyms: Cerium, EINECS 231-154-9, UNII-30K4522N6T
- Molecular Formula: Ce^{3+}, Ce^{4+}

Background Information

Cerium is a rare earth metal and the most abundant member of the lanthanide series discovered by Jons J. Berzelius and W. von Hisinger in 1803 in Sweden. Berzelius and Hisinger discovered the new element in a rare reddish-brown mineral now known as cerite, a cerium–lanthanide silicate. Although they could not isolate the pure metal, they found that cerium had two oxidation states: trivalent state (Ce^{3+}, cerous, usually orange-red) and the tetravalent state (Ce^{4+}, ceric, usually colorless). Cerium is the only material known to have a solid-state critical point.

Uses

Cerium is used in metallurgy as a stabilizer in alloys and in welding electrodes; in glass as a polishing agent, decolorizer, and to render glass opaque to near-ultraviolet radiation. It is also used in ceramics and as a catalyst. Cerium is used as a component of some diesel fuel additives, and may be added to residual fuel oils to improve combustion. Cerium is found in portable rechargeable batteries.

Environmental Fate and Behavior

Although cerium is a rare earth element, it is relatively abundant in the earth's crust. It makes up about 0.0046% of the Earth's crust by weight and ranks 25th in occurrence at an average distribution of 20–60 ppm. Cerium is a malleable, soft, ductile, iron-gray metal, slightly harder than lead. It is very reactive and readily tarnishes in the air. Cerium oxidizes slowly in cold water and rapidly in hot water. It dissolves in acids. Cerium can burn when heated or scratched with a knife.

Cerium is not expected to exist in elemental form in the environment since it is a reactive metal. Cerium is dumped in the environment in many different places, mainly by petrol-producing industries. It can also enter the environment when household equipment is thrown away. Cerium compounds exist solely in particulate form if release into air and not expected to volatilize. Water-soluble cerium compounds usually have a pK_a of 8.5, which indicates that the hydrated Ce^{3+} ion will remain in solution at environmental pHs of 4–9. The ion is expected to hydrolyze and polymerize at environmental pH and may precipitate out of solution. Thus, cerium will gradually accumulate in soils and water, which eventually leads to increasing concentrations in humans, animals, and soil particles.

Exposure and Exposure Monitoring

Inhalation, dermal, and oral are the possible exposure routes. Exposure to commercially used cerium compounds is most likely through exposure to cerium oxide.

Toxicokinetics

Cerium is poorly absorbed by the intestine following oral exposure in animals, except for water-soluble cerium compounds and cerium oxide. As poorly soluble particles, cerium oxide may dissolve slowly from the lung into systemic circulation and is observed in the liver, skeleton, and tracheobronchial lymph nodes. Cerium has also been observed to be localized in the cell, particularly in the lysosomes, where it is concentrated and precipitated in an insoluble form in association with phosphorus. As an element, cerium is neither created nor destroyed within the body. The particular cerium compounds, such as cerium chloride and cerium oxide, may be altered as a result of various chemical reactions within the body, particularly dissolution. Following inhalation exposure, the initial rapid elimination of insoluble cerium from the body is due primarily to transport up to the respiratory tract via the mucociliary escalator and eventual swallowing of the material. Initial short-term clearance rates range from 35 to 95% of initial cerium body burden, depending on the species tested and length of clearance time investigated. Elimination of orally administered soluble cerium has been shown to be age dependent in animals. The cerium may remain in the intestinal cells, may not be available systemically, and may eventually be eliminated in the feces. Cerium is capable of crossing the placenta and entering the fetal circulation in mice, but the amounts found in the uterus and placenta were generally less than 5% of the maternal body burden and decreased rapidly with increased time after exposure.

Mechanism of Toxicity

Cerium resembles aluminum in its biologic and chemical properties. Cerium and cerium compounds have low to moderate toxicity unless the associated anions are toxic. Intratracheally administered nanoparticles tend to accumulate in liver and cause damage there.

 http://dx.doi.org/10.1016/B978-0-12-386454-3.00826-5

Acute and Short-Term Toxicity (or Exposure)

Animal

The LD_{50} values reported in rats ranged from 4 to 50 mg kg^{-1} for cerium nitrate with female rats being more sensitive than males. After peritoneal injection, the LD_{50} of cerium nitrate was 470 mg kg^{-1} in female mice and 290 mg kg^{-1} in female rats; the LD_{50} of cerium chloride was 353 mg kg^{-1} in mice and 103 mg kg^{-1} in guinea pigs. The oral toxicity of cerium nitrate was much lower (LD_{50} of 4200 mg kg^{-1} in female rats and 1178 mg kg^{-1} in female mice) than after intravenous or intraperitoneal administration. The LD_{50} of ingested cerium oxide could not be determined in rats when delivered at a dose of 1000 or 5000 mg kg^{-1}. An LD_{50} of 622 mg kg^{-1} has been reported for cerium oxide ingested by mice. The LC_{50} after inhalation of cerium oxide in rats was greater than 50 mg m^{-3}. The primary targets after inhalation of cerium are the lung and the associated lymph nodes; other organs could be affected via clearance through the blood. Studies of cerium injected systemically have shown that, once in the circulation, cerium can cause liver toxicity with a no observed adverse-effect level of 1 mg kg^{-1} after a single intravenous injection and a lowest observed adverse effect level (LOAEL) of 2 mg kg^{-1} for effects on liver detoxifying enzymes. Effects on other organs where cerium can accumulate (such as spleen, bones, and kidney) have not been studied. A single-dose study on the effects of in utero intravenous administration reported reduced weight in newborn mouse pups, with an LOAEL of 80 mg kg^{-1}. Cerium has been found to depress certain behaviors in mice administered this chemical, and cerium administered to pregnant mice on day 7 or 12 of gestation or 2 days postpartum caused significant decreases in open-field activity of offspring. Fetal growth was impaired, as evidenced by weight decreases of 7–19%. The potential carcinogenicity of cerium-containing particles has not been studied in conventional rodent bioassays; *in vivo* mutagenicity studies have been negative.

Human

Cerium can increase blood coagulation rate and produce gastrointestinal effects. Inhalation can lead to polycythemia.

Chronic Toxicity (or Exposure)

Animal

An animal inhalation study involved exposure of rats to cerium oxide particles substantially larger than those in diesel emission. The exposure concentrations ranged between 5 and 500 mg m^{-3} for 13 weeks. Effects observed included lung discoloration, enlargement of lymph nodes, and increased lung and spleen weight at all concentrations.

Human

Case reports of workers occupationally exposed to rare earth metals (including cerium) describe a condition termed rare earth pneumoconiosis with pathologic features including interstitial fibrosis, granulomatosis, and bilateral nodular chest x-ray infiltrates. Although the disease sometimes is associated with accumulation of cerium in particles, the role of cerium in this complex disease is unclear relative to other metals or gases to which workers may also have been exposed.

Immunotoxicity

No relevant human or animal data are available regarding immunotoxicity in cerium or cerium compounds.

Reproductive Toxicity

A cross-fostering design was employed to separate effects of prenatal and postnatal exposure following a single subcutaneous dose of cerium citrate (80 mg kg^{-1}) in pregnant female mice. Analysis revealed that neonatal weight was reduced both in offspring exposed to cerium *in utero* and in the offspring of mothers receiving cerium during lactation. Cerium also appeared to affect maternal-offspring interaction: Pups exposed prenatally to cerium were retrieved in less time than control pups.

Genotoxicity

In vitro mutagenicity studies have been negative. Other cerium compounds, such as cerium chloride observed no induction DNA damage in two strains of *Bacillus subtilis* by using rec-assay, but cerium nitrate was reported to induce chromosomal breaks and reduce the mitotic index in rat bone marrow *in vivo*, and cerium sulfate was reported to cause differential destaining of chromosomal segments in plants.

No information was located regarding genotoxic effects of cerium and cerium compounds in humans.

Carcinogenicity

Data regarding the carcinogenicity of cerium compounds in humans or experimental animals are unavailable. In accordance with US Environmental Protection Agency, cerium and cerium compounds are classified as "inadequate information to assess the carcinogenic potential" in humans.

Clinical Management

Treatments are addressed symptomatically.

Ecotoxicity

Toxicity to aquatic species is dependent upon the particle size.

Exposure Standards and Guidelines

No standards have been recommended for elemental cerium, cerium compounds, or any other lanthanides because either suitable data for setting a standard, such as inhalation studies or studies on these compounds are lacking. However, because of the accumulating evidence of induction of fibrosis with the lanthanides and their expanding use, the exposure should probably be limited to 1 mg m^{-3}.

See also: Aluminum; Metals.

Further Reading

Arvela, P., Kraul, H., Stenback, F., Pelkonen, O., 1991. The cerium-induced liver injury and oxidative drug metabolism in DBA/2 and C57BL/6 mice. Toxicology 69, 1–9.

Berry, J.P., Meignan, M., Escaig, F., Galle, P., 1988. Inhaled soluble aerosols insolubilised by lysosomes of alveolar cells. Application to some toxic compounds; electron microprobe and ion microprobe studies. Toxicology 14, 127–139.

Binghma, E., Cohrssen, B., Powell, C.H., 2001. Patty's Toxicology, fifth ed. A Wiley-Interscience Publication, New York.

Biswas, A., Gaiser, B.K., Jepson, M.A., Lead, J.R., Rosenkranz, P., Stone, V., 2011. Effects of silver and Cerium dioxide micro- and nano-sized particles on Daphni. J. Environ. Monit. 5, 1227–1235.

Nalabotu, S.K., Kolli, M.B., Triest, W.E., Ma, J.Y., Manne, N.D.P.K., 2011. Intratracheal instillation of cerium oxide nanoparticles induces hepatic toxicity. Nanomedicine 6, 2327–2335.

Relevant Websites

http://www.healtheffects.org – Evaluation of Human Health Risk from Cerium Added to Diesel Fuel. Health Effects Institute Communication 9 (August 2001).

http://www.chemicool.com/elements/cerium.html – "Cerium." Chemicool Periodic Table. Chemicool.com. (June 2011)

Cesium

SC Gad, Gad Consulting Services, Cary, NC, USA
T Pham, Charlotte, NC, USA

This article is a revision of the previous print edition article by Shayne C. Gad, volume 1, pp 503–504, © 2005, Elsevier Inc.

- Name: Cesium
- Chemical Abstracts Service Registry Number: 7440-46-2
- Synonyms: *Cesium*
- Molecular Formula: Cs^+

Background Information

Cesium was discovered in 1860 by Robert Bunsen and Gustav Kirchoff. It is used in the most accurate atomic clocks. Cesium melts at 28.41 °C (just below body temperature) and occurs in Earth's crust at 2.6 ppm. Cesium is the rarest of the naturally occurring alkali metals as the isotope ^{133}Cs. Its compounds are correspondingly rare. Granites contain about 1 ppm cesium and sedimentary rocks contain approximately 4 ppm cesium. The most common commercial source of cesium is pollucite, which contains between 5 and 32% cesium oxide. Radioactive forms of cesium (^{134}Cs and ^{137}Cs) can also be found in the environment. They are produced during nuclear fission, and are used in cancer treatment.

Uses

Cesium is used in photovoltaic cells, vacuum tubes, scintillation counters, and atomic clocks.

Environmental Fate and Behavior

Appearance: silvery white, soft, ductile metal; liquid (slightly above room temperature).

Boiling point: 685 °C.

Solubility: soluble in liquid ammonia.

Naturally occurring cesium can enter the environment mostly from the erosion and weathering of rocks and minerals. The production and use of cesium compounds may also result in their release to the environment through various waste streams. However, there are relatively few commercial uses for cesium compounds, such as cesium radioactive isotopes (^{134}Cs and ^{137}Cs), and they have been released into the environment by human activities such as the atmospheric testing of nuclear weapons (1945–80) and leakages at nuclear power plants. Cesium compounds can travel long distances in the air before being brought back to the earth by rainfall and gravitational settling. If released to water, cesium compounds are deposited on land and water via wet and dry deposition. These deposited-cesium particles may be resuspended into the atmosphere from soil and dust. If released to soil, cesium compounds have low mobility and do not migrate below 40 cm in depth. The majority of cesium ions are retained in the upper 20 cm of the soil surface. Clay and zeolite minerals strongly bind cesium cations irreversibly. Soils rich in organic matter also adsorb cesium ions. However, cesium compounds are readily exchangeable and highly available for plant uptake in these soils. If released into water, cesium compounds are very water soluble and exist primarily as cesium cations. Because most cesium compounds are ionic, they will not volatilize from water surfaces. Most cesium compounds released to water adsorb to suspended solids in the water column and ultimately they are deposited in sediments. Cesium compounds bioconcentrate and have been shown to bioaccumulate in both terrestrial and aquatic food chains. The half-life of ^{134}Cs is ~2 years and that of ^{137}Cs is ~30 years.

Exposure and Exposure Monitoring

Occupational exposure to cesium compounds occurs primarily through inhalation and dermal contact at workplaces in which pollucite is mined or cesium compounds are manufactured or used. General population exposure to cesium occurs by ingestion of food and drinking water, inhalation of ambient air, and dermal contact with cesium compounds in soil. Current exposure of the general population of the United States to radioactive cesium-134 and cesium-137 is expected to be low because atmospheric testing of nuclear weapons has been discontinued for many years.

Toxicokinetics

Stable and radioactive cesium can be taken into the body by ingestion of food, water, or inhalation. Once absorbed, cesium behaves in a manner similar to potassium and distributes uniformly throughout the body as cations, becoming incorporated into intracellular fluids. Gastrointestinal absorption from food or water is the principal source of internally deposited cesium in the general population. Essentially all cesium that is ingested is absorbed into the bloodstream through the intestines. Cesium tends to concentrate in muscles because of their relatively large mass. Like potassium, cesium is excreted from the body fairly quickly. In an adult, 10% is excreted with a biological half-life of 2 days, and the rest leaves the body with a biological half-life of 110 days. Clearance from the body is somewhat quicker for children and adolescents. This means that if someone is exposed to radioactive cesium and the sources of exposure are removed, much of the cesium will readily clear the body along the normal pathways for potassium excretion within several months. Urinary excretion is the major route of elimination of cesium.

The metabolism and tissue distribution of cesium-137 were studied in rats injected intraperitoneally and sacrificed

 http://dx.doi.org/10.1016/B978-0-12-386454-3.00827-7

1–300 days postinjection. In a chronic study, rats were administered cesium-137 in their drinking water daily. In the acute study, with the exception of the brain, muscle, and total animal, all tissues showed retention curves resolvable into three exponential components with half-lives of 1.5–2, 5–8, and 15–17 days. Retention in muscles was resolvable into a two-exponential function with half-lives of 8 and 16 days. In the chronic study, the highest equilibrium cesium-137 concentrations, 10% of the average daily intake per gram, occurred in the muscle. The authors concluded that the muscle should be considered as the formal critical organ for cesium-137.

Mechanism of Toxicity

Stable cesium was shown to affect various central nervous system functions, mainly involving displacing potassium, with which it competes for transport through the potassium channel, and it can also activate sodium pump and subsequent transport into the cell across membranes. Thus, this resulted in potassium deficiency.

Radioactive isotopes of cesium, such as ^{134}Cs and ^{137}Cs, are a greater health concern than stable cesium. These radioactive isotopes of cesium are formed during nuclear fission. Both ^{134}Cs and ^{137}Cs emit beta and gamma radiations. Beta radiation travels short distances and can penetrate the skin and superficial body tissues, whereas gamma radiation can travel great distances and penetrate the entire body. Both beta and gamma radiations may induce tissue damage and disruption of cellular function.

Acute and Short-Term Toxicity (or Exposure)

Animal

Animal studies indicated that stable cesium and its salts have relatively low toxicity, with acute oral LD_{50} values for rats and mice in the range 800–2000 mg kg^{-1}, with the exception of cesium hydroxide, which is more toxic than cesium iodide or cesium chloride and has an intraperitoneal LD_{50} of 89 mg kg^{-1}. Stable cesium is found to be a primary skin and eye irritant in rabbits and cutaneous sensitizer in pigs. Cesium can induce cardiac arrhythmias.

Human

Cesium has been reported to cause hyperirritability and muscle spasms. The symptoms of cesium toxicity include fatigue, muscle weakness, palpitations, and cardiac arrhythmia. Human data for cesium hydroxide are unavailable.

Chronic Toxicity (or Exposure)

At very high exposure doses to radionuclides of ^{134}Cs and ^{137}Cs, the beta and gamma radiations can cause adverse effects, such as radiation syndrome (vomiting, nausea, and diarrhea) erythema, ulceration, tissue necrosis, neurological signs, chromosomal abnormalities, compromised immune function, and death.

Immunotoxicity

No data were located regarding immunological effects in animals or humans following acute- or chronic-duration oral exposure to stable cesium.

Reproductive Toxicity

Exposure to radioisotopes of cesium may result in reduced fertility in males, as evidence by reduced concentration of spermatozoa in men who were exposed externally and internally to ^{137}CsCl for about 1 month before testing. Reduced fertility, including sterility, was also reported in male mice exposed to gamma radiation from ^{137}Cs. Developmental effects such as reduced postnatal body weight, impaired motor activity, morphological changes in the brain, reduced head size, and retarded odontogenesis and palatal closure had been reported in rats that were exposed to radioactive cesium sources (^{137}Cs) *in utero*.

Genotoxicity

Chromosome damage has been induced by cesium chloride in the bone marrow cells of mice given a single oral dose and human blood cells in culture. The chloride was not mutagenic in an Ames bacterial test, but caused DNA damage in bacteria, as did carbonate, sulfate, and nitrate.

Carcinogenicity

Animal studies indicate an increased risk of cancer following external and internal exposure to relatively high doses of radiation from ^{137}Cs sources, but not from the nonradioactive element itself. An increased lifetime incidence of mammary tumors was noted in female rats that were acutely exposed to whole-body radiation. Intravenous injection of ^{137}CsCl in dogs resulted in long-term increased risk of all cancers combined in males and females. However, studies of increased cancer risk specifically associated with exposure to humans to radioactive cesium isotopes were not found.

Clinical Management

Prussian blue is administered by a duodenal tube to act as a chelating agent, which binds to cesium chemically and reduces the biological half-life to 30 days.

Ecotoxicology

Toxic effects to aquatic organisms by pH shift.

Natural soil cesium concentrations are generally low but are nontoxic to plants. Consequently, cesium is not readily available for uptake by vegetation through their roots. However, radiocesium can enter plants upon falling onto the surface of leaves.

Other Hazards

Radioactive cesium is much more dangerous. This is caused by radioactivity and not the cesium itself.

Exposure Standards and Guidelines

The National Institute for Occupational Safety and Health (NIOSH) recommended a limit of 2 mg m^{-3} of cesium hydroxide as an average for a 10-h workday, 40-h workweek.

The EPA has established a maximum contaminant level of 4 mg per year for beta particles and photon radioactivity for synthetic radionuclides (including radioactive cesium).

Miscellaneous

Radioactive decay is a way of decreasing the amount of ^{134}Cs and ^{137}Cs in the environment.

See also: Lithium; Metals; Potassium; Sodium.

Further Reading

ATSDR, 2011. Toxic Substance Portal, Cesium. Agency for Toxic Substances & Disease Registry (ATSDR), Atlanta, GA.

Ballou, J.E., Thompson, R.C., 1958. The metabolism of cesium-137 in the rat: comparison of acute and chronic administration experiments. Health Phys. 1, 85–89.

Bingham, E., Cohressen, B., Powell, C.H., 2001. Patty's Toxicology, fifth ed. Wiley Interscience, New York.

Cochran, K.W., Doull, J., Mazur, M., DuBois, K.P., 1950. Acute toxicity of zirconium, columbium, strontium, lanthanum, cesium, tantalum and yttrium. Arch. Ind. Hyg. Occup. Med. 1, 637–650.

Johnson, G.T., Lewis, T.R., Wagner, W.D., 1975. Acute toxicity of cesium and rubidium compounds. Toxicol. Appl. Pharmacol. 32, 239–245.

Nordberg, G.F., Fowler, B.A., Nordberg, M., Friberg, L.T., 2007. Handbook on the Toxicology of Metals, third ed. Academic Press, MA.

Relevant Website

http://www.epa.gov – Cesium. US Environmental Protection Agency.

Channel Blockers *see* Calcium Channel Blockers

Charcoal

M Abdollahi, Tehran University of Medical Sciences, Tehran, Iran
A Hosseini, Iran University of Medical Sciences, Tehran, Iran

This article is a revision of the previous edition article by William S. Utley, volume 1, p 505, © 2005, Elsevier Inc.

- Name: Charcoal
- Chemical Abstracts Service Registry Number: 16291-96-6, Other registry number: 1333-85-3.
- Synonyms: Charcoal, Charcoal, activated, Charcoal, except activated, Charcoal briquettes, EINECS 240-383-3, HSDB 2017, Swine fly ash, UNII-2P3VWU3H10, Whetlerite.
- Molecular Formula: Unspecified
- Chemical Structure:

C
(v0)

Background (Significance/History)

The first use of charcoal comes from the black pigment used in European cave paintings around 32 000 years ago. It is possible that the earliest use of charcoal as a fuel in the smelting of copper began over 7000 years ago. The first definite evidence of human involvement with charcoal as a fuel goes back to 5500 years ago in the Middle East and Southern Europe, when the Egyptians, who were expert metal workers, discovered the smelting of iron using charcoal.

Uses

Charcoal has been used since the earliest times for several of purposes, including medicine and art, but by far its most important use has been as a metallurgical, cooking, industrial, and automotive fuel. Charcoal is used as a conventional fuel where an intense heat is wanted. Charcoal was also used historically as a source of carbon black in chemical reactions by grinding it up. In this form charcoal was a constituent of formulas for mixtures such as gunpowder and was important to early chemists. Due to its high surface area, charcoal can be used as a catalyst, a filter, or an adsorbent.

Other uses of charcoal include in:

- the decolorizing of sugar
- water and air purification
- waste treatment
- solvent recovery
- removal of jet fumes from airports
- removal of sulfur dioxide from stack gases and 'clean' rooms
- deodorant
- catalyst in natural-gas purification
- brewing
- chromium electroplating
- air conditioning.

Environmental Fate and Behavior

Relevant Physiochemical Properties

Charcoal is an odorless, tasteless, fine black powder or black porous solid. It is typically encountered as course granules or powder. It is insoluble in water and also in organic solvents. Other physical properties include specific gravity: 0.08 to 0.5; heat of combustion: 14 100 Btu/lb = 7830 cal g^{-1} = $3.28 \times 10 + 5$ J kg^{-1}; boiling point: 4200 °C.

Partition Behavior in Water, Sediment, and Soil

The presence of charcoal in a compound elevates the K_{oc} value, resulting in reduction of mobility of compounds through the sediment and soil.

Environmental Persistency (Degradation/Speciation)

Charcoal is stable under ambient environmental conditions.

Bioaccumulation and Biomagnification

Hazardous short-term degradation products of charcoal are not likely. Charcoal and its products of degradation are not toxic. Special remarks on the products of biodegradation are not available.

Toxicokinetics

Activated charcoal is neither absorbed in the gastrointestinal (GI) tract nor metabolized and excreted in the feces. The

 http://dx.doi.org/10.1016/B978-0-12-386454-3.00685-0

adsorptive capacity of activated charcoal may be decreased by concurrent use of iso-osmolar electrolyte solution and polyethylene glycol for whole-bowel irrigation. The adsorptive efficacy of activated charcoal may also be decreased by the emesis induced by ipecac syrup. In general, activated charcoal can reduce the absorption of and therapeutic response to other orally administered drugs; therefore medications other than those used for GI decontamination or antidotes for ingested toxins should not be taken orally within at least 2 h of administration of activated charcoal. When concomitant drug therapy is needed, drugs can be given parenterally.

Mechanism of Toxicity and Clinical Use in Gastrointestinal Decontamination

Due to its large surface area, charcoal exerts its effects by absorbing a wide variety of drugs and chemicals. After the toxic substance attaches to the surface of the charcoal and because charcoal is not absorbed, it stays inside the GI tract, being eliminated in the feces along with the charcoal. In single-dose therapy, activated charcoal adsorbs the toxic substance ingested, and thus inhibits GI absorption and prevents or reduces toxicity. When used repeatedly, as in multiple-dose therapy, activated charcoal also creates and maintains a concentration gradient across the wall of the GI tract that facilitates passive diffusion of the toxic substance from the blood stream into the GI tract lumen, where it is adsorbed onto the charcoal and thus prevented from reabsorption. In this process, activated charcoal interrupts the enterohepatic or enteroenteric cycle or recirculation and increases the rate of elimination of the toxic substance from the body. Use of multiple-dose charcoal in this manner is also called GI (gut) dialysis.

Acute and Short-Term Toxicity (to Include Irritation and Corrosivity)

Animal

Special remarks on toxicity of charcoal to animals are not available and no LD_{50} has been reported.

Human

Acute exposure to charcoal irritates skin, eyes, GI, and the respiratory tract. Redness, swelling, and pain may occur with dermal exposure. Stinging pain, watering of eyes, inflammation of eyelids, and conjunctivitis may happen with eye exposure. Aspiration pneumonitis, decreased GI transit time, vomiting, GI obstruction, constipation, pulmonary fibrosis and subsequent emphysema, intestinal perforation, charcoal deposits in the esophageal and gastric mucosa, and ulceration of rectal mucosa are possible if charcoal is ingested. Cough, tachypnea, wheezing, rapid irregular breathing, headache, fatigue, mental confusion, nausea, and vomiting may occur after inhalation. Burning charcoal in a fireplace or in a grill may be hazardous as carbon monoxide (CO) is produced. CO is a tasteless, odorless, invisible gas that is toxic when inhaled in significant amounts. Symptoms of CO poisoning include headaches, confusion, dizziness, nausea, and, at high concentrations, loss of consciousness and death.

Chronic Toxicity

Animal

Special remarks on charcoal toxicity to animals are not available.

Human

Chronic exposure to charcoal may damage mucous membranes and lungs. Chronic skin exposure can result in dryness, rashes, and clogging of hair follicles, rendering them black. Chronic inhalation can cause accumulation of carbon particles in the lungs. Chronic exposure to coal causes a pneumoconiosis called coal workers pneumoconiosis or black lung disease. No evidence has been found for the equivalent with occupational exposure to charcoal.

Immunotoxicity

There is no evidence on immunotoxicity of charcoal in animals or human.

Reproductive Toxicity

There is no evidence that charcoal causes reproductive or developmental problems.

Genotoxicity

No genotoxicity was reported.

Carcinogenicity

Charcoal is not listed as a potential carcinogen by any agency.

Clinical Management

In oral exposure, emesis is not indicated due to the irritant nature of charcoal. Dilution is recommended with 120–240 ml of water or milk, not exceeding 120 ml in children. In inhalation exposure, move patient to fresh air and monitor for respiratory distress. If cough or difficulty in breathing develops, the patient should be evaluated for respiratory tract irritation, bronchitis, or pneumonitis. Assist ventilation and administer oxygen as required. Bronchospasm can be treated with inhaled beta2 agonists and oral or parenteral corticosteroids. In eye exposure, wash exposed eyes with copious amounts of room-temperature water for at least 15 min and if pain, irritation, swelling, lacrimation, or photophobia persists, the patient should be seen in a health care facility.

Ecotoxicology

Charcoal in its original state is not harmful to the environment. No specific information is available on the effect of charcoal on animals or plants in the environment. No specific information is available on the effect of charcoal on aquatic life.

Exposure Standards and Guidelines

Drug products containing charcoal are offered over the counter for certain uses for instance in GI tract. Charcoal (activated) is included in antidiarrheal and digestive aid drug products.

US Consumer Product Safety Commission regulations require that two highly visible warning labels are included at the top of every bag of charcoal briquettes that identify the hazard of carbon monoxide poisoning.

US Occupational Safety and Health Administration: Hazardous by definition of Hazard Communication Standard (29 CFR 1910.1200). This product is on the European Inventory of Existing Commercial Chemical Substances. This product is not classified according to the EU regulations. Not applicable.

See also: Toxicity, Acute; Toxicity, Subchronic and Chronic; Gastrointestinal System; Carbon Monoxide.

Further Reading

Brown, J.A., Buckley, N.A., February 4, 2013. Carbon monoxide-induced death and toxicity from charcoal briquettes: comment. Med. J. Aust. 198 (2), 86.

Charcoal: powdered, compressed, willow and vine. Muse Art and Design. Muse Art and Design 7. http://museartanddesign.com/2011/09/charcoal-powdered-compressed-willow-and-vine/. Retrieved 27 May 2012.

Chyka, P.A., Seger, D., Krenzelok, E.P., Vale, J.A., 2005. American Academy of Clinical Toxicology; European Association of Poisons Centres and Clinical Toxicologists. Clin. Toxicol. (Phila) 43 (2), 61–87. Review.

Cunha, J.P., DO, FACOEP, "Activated Charcoal: Overview", eMedicineHealth, WebMD, Inc. http://www.emedicinehealth.com/activated_charcoal/article_em.htm. Retrieved 27 May 2012.

"Grilling Smackdown: Lump Charcoal vs. Briquettes". Serious Eats. SAY: Food. http://www.seriouseats.com/2008/05/grilling-smackdown-lump-charcoal-vs-briquette.html. Retrieved 27 May 2012.

Ojima, J., 2011. Generation rate of carbon monoxide from burning charcoal. Ind. Health 49 (3), 393–395.

Olson, K.R., June 2010. Activated charcoal for acute poisoning: one toxicologist's journey. J. Med. Toxicol. 6 (2), 190–198. http://dx.doi.org/10.1007/213181-010-0046-1.

Seger, D., March 2008. Single dose activated charcoal. J. Med. Toxicol. 4 (1), 65.

Using charcoal efficiently. http://www.fao.org/docrep/X5328E/x5328e0b.htm. Retrieved 2010-02-01.

Winder, C., September 17, 2012. Carbon monoxide-induced death and toxicity from charcoal briquettes. Med. J. Aust. 197 (6), 349–350.

Relevant Websites

http://www.inchem.org – International Program on Chemical Safety.

http://toxnet.nlm.nih.gov – Toxicology Data Network, US National Library of Medicine.

http://chem.sis.nlm.nih.gov/chemidplus – US National Library of Medicine: ChemIDplus Advanced: Search for: Charcoal.

http://www.cpsc.gov/en/Newsroom/News-Releases/1985/Burning-Charcoal-Causes-Deaths-From-Carbon-Monoxide/ – Consumer Product Safety Commission.

Chemicals Alternatives Assessments

MH Whittaker, ToxServices LLC, Washington, DC, USA

Introduction

Chemical alternatives assessment (CAA) is a process for identifying and comparing potential chemical and nonchemical alternatives to replace chemicals or technologies of concern on the basis of hazard, performance, and economic viability. CAAs are used to evaluate and manage hazards and subsequent health risks through the informed choice of safer chemicals. The CAA process is integral to the advancement of green chemistry, which can be defined as the design of chemical products and processes that reduce or eliminate the use and generation of hazardous substances. Historically, materials or chemicals have been selected during the design process based on the assessment and subsequent reduction of human health or environmental risks, as opposed to avoiding hazards or promoting continuous improvement in a chemical, material, product, system, production process, or function. CAA began its development in the late 1990s in the United States as a framework on which to avoid such hazards and promote safer alternatives. Prior to the inception of CAA, life cycle assessment (LCA) and risk assessment were the two primary tools used to select safer alternatives. Ideally, a CAA provides a science-based solution that identifies and characterizes chemical hazards, promotes the selection of less hazardous chemical ingredients, and avoids unintended consequences of switching to a poorly characterized and more hazardous chemical substitute or technology.

A number of regulatory initiatives at the state level in the United States (notably, in California, Washington, and Maine), voluntary hazard reduction initiatives such as the US Environmental Protection Agency's (EPA) Design for the Environment (DfE) Program, and EU and European-country funded initiatives such as SUBSPORT have contributed to the growth of CAA. CAA can be used as a process for identifying alternatives to a hazardous chemical, screening out alternatives of equal or greater hazard, and selecting a less hazardous alternative that is technically and economically viable.

Overview of CAA Frameworks

There are three primary CAA paradigms currently in use: The Lowell Center for Sustainable Production's Alternatives Assessment Framework (**Figure 1**), BizNGO's Chemical Alternatives Assessment Protocol (**Figure 2**), and DfE's Alternatives Assessment Criteria for Hazard Evaluation (**Figure 3**). More recently, the Interstate Chemicals Clearinghouse (IC2), an association of state, local, and tribal governments in the United States, has drafted Guidance for Alternatives Assessment and Risk Reduction. Internationally, the Austrian Environment Agency has proposed a draft methodology for the identification and assessment of substances that should be considered for restriction under the European Directive on the Restriction of the Use of Certain Hazardous Substances in Electrical and Electronic Equipment.

These CAA paradigms share many of the same attributes by placing initial emphasis on the assessment of hazards, with LCA and risk-related metrics such as exposure assessment, occurring later in the process. Core elements of a CAA comprise chemical hazard assessment (CHA), life cycle thinking, exposure assessment, technical/functional assessment, economic assessment, and social impact assessment.

Examples of CAAs published to date include the following:

- The University of Massachusetts at Lowell Toxics Use Reduction Institute's *Five Chemicals Alternatives Assessment Study* (2006)
  - This set of CAAs assessed the availability of technically and economically feasible safer alternatives for five hazardous chemicals (i.e., lead, formaldehyde, perchloroethylene, hexavalent chromium, and di(2-ethylhexyl)phthalate)
- DfE's Alternatives Assessment Project on Alternatives to Decabromodiphenyl ether (decaBDE) (2012)
  - This project assessed the toxicity and environmental fate of flame retardant chemicals that are potential alternatives to decaBDE when used in materials and products where decaBDE currently is, or previously was, used as a flame retardant.

Overview of CHA Frameworks

CHAs evaluate and manage human health and environmental hazards through the informed choice of safer chemicals. CHAs are based on primary data, data on chemical surrogates, and/or predictive modeling. Each CHA comprises literature search, identification of critical health and environmental effects, identification of data gaps, chemical analog selection and/or use of predictive modeling, including the use of QSAR software (when needed), and assignment of endpoint-specific hazard classifications (usually following the United Nation's Globally Harmonized System of Classification and Labeling of Chemicals (GHS)). All of these factors are applied to a broad set of toxicological and environmental hazard endpoints. The overall goal of a CHA is to determine whether a proposed chemical alternative is less hazardous to human health and the surrounding environment.

Two primary CHA paradigms in use today are the US EPA's DfE Alternatives Assessment (AA) protocol and Clean Production Action's GreenScreen™. Both CHA methods assess a broad range of health effects and environmental endpoints. As an example, the EPA's DfE AA paradigm estimates hazards for 17 individual health effects and environmental fate and toxicity endpoints, while GreenScreen assigns hazard classifications to 18 human health, environmental toxicity and fate, and physical characteristics of a chemical.

GreenScreen has grown in favor among those who perform CHA because it assigns a quantitative GreenScreen benchmark

 http://dx.doi.org/10.1016/B978-0-12-386454-3.01239-2

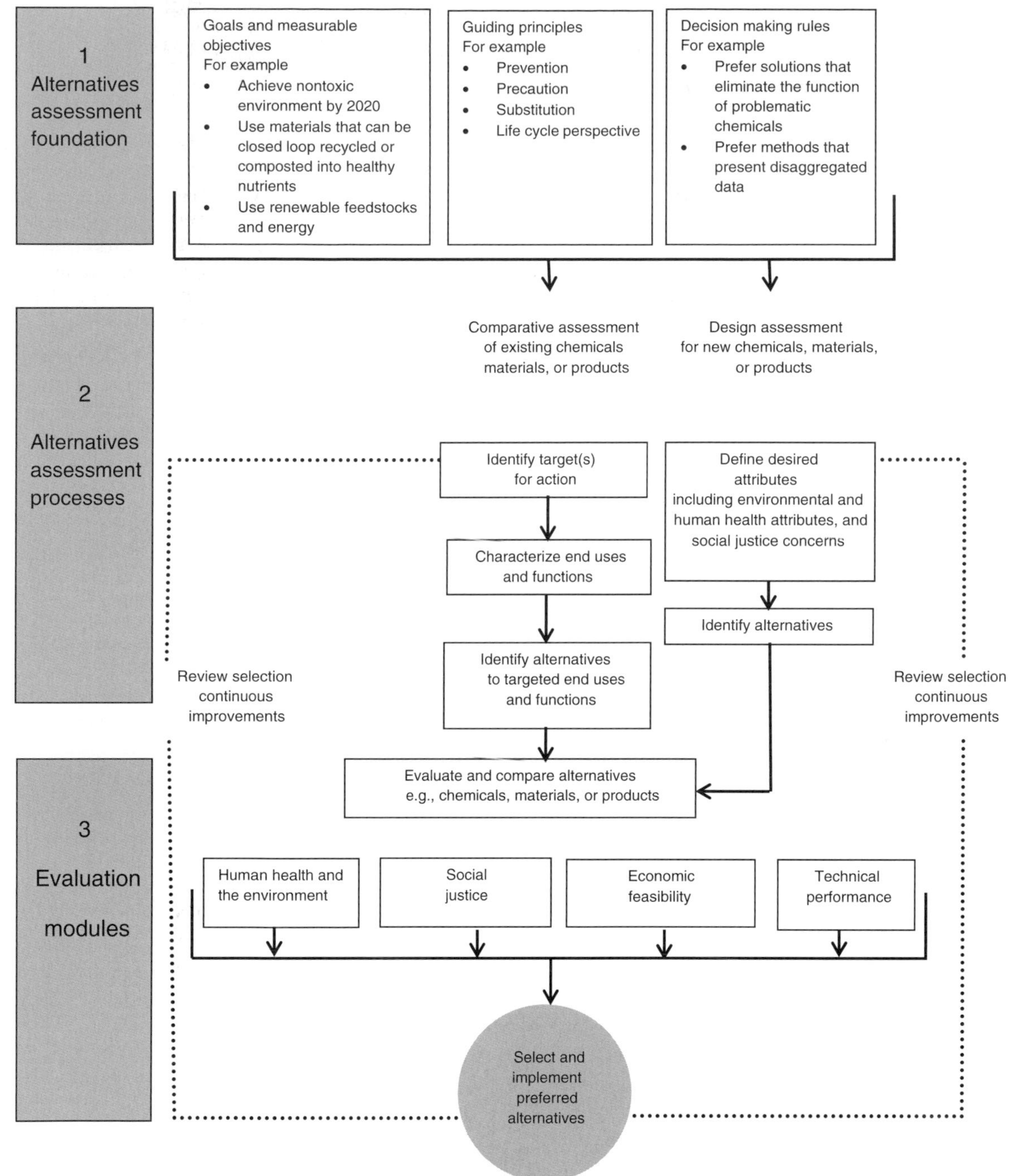

Figure 1 Lowell Center for Sustainable Production's alternatives assessment framework. Reproduced with permission from Rossi, M., Tickner, J., Geiser, K., 2006. Alternatives Assessment Framework of the Lowell Center for Sustainable Production. http://www.chemicalspolicy.org/downloads/FinalAltsAssess06.pdf.

score ranging from 1 to 4 according to specific combinations of hazard classifications, as shown in **Figure 4**:

- A GreenScreen score of 1 corresponds to 'Avoid. Chemical of High Concern'
- A GreenScreen score of 2 corresponds to 'Use But Search for Safer Substitutes'
- A GreenScreen score of 3 corresponds to 'Use But Still Opportunity for Improvement'
- A GreenScreen score of 4 corresponds to 'Prefer. Safer Chemical'

GreenScreen scores can be compared for individual chemicals or materials, assisting in the selection of less hazardous chemicals or materials during the design process. As an example, acetic acid received a GreenScreen benchmark score of 2 based on very high (vH) hazard scores for Group II and II* human toxicity endpoints, comprising system toxicity/organ

1. Identify chemical(s) of concern

2. Characterize end uses and function

3. Identify alternatives: are there potential alternatives including chemicals, material, products, or new designs?

No

3a. Implement best practices to reduce worker and community exposure

3b. Continue to research alternatives

Yes

4. Assess chemical hazards
Evaluate human and environmental health impacts of chemicals and deselect options of greatest concern

5. Evaluate technical and economic performance

6. Apply life cycle thinking
Is there potential for significant life cycle or exposure concerns?

Yes

6a. Life cycle concerns?

Yes

Life cycle evaluation

Depending on resources and needs complete partial or fill evaluation of life cycle impacts

6b. Exposure concerns?

Yes

Risk assessment (RA)

Depending on resources and needs complete partial or full RA to assess risks

No

7. Select and implement safer alternatives

Figure 2 BizNGO Chemical Alternatives Assessment Protocol (v.1.1) screening logic for selecting safer alternatives to chemicals of concern to human health or the environment*. Reproduced with permission from BizNGO, 2011. BizNGO Chemical Alternatives Assessment Protocol (v.1.1). November 2011. http://www.bizngo.org/safer.php.

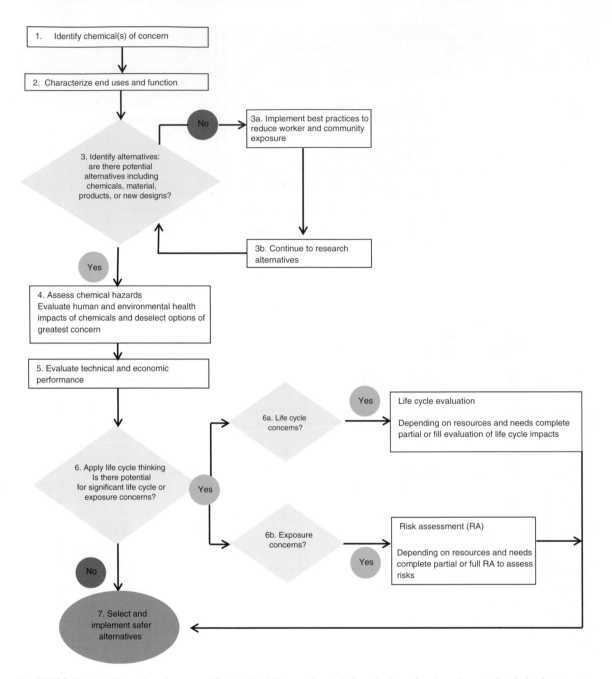

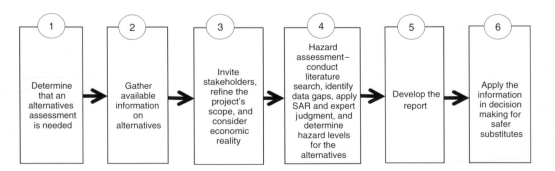

Figure 3 US EPA's DfE alternatives assessment criteria for hazard evaluation.

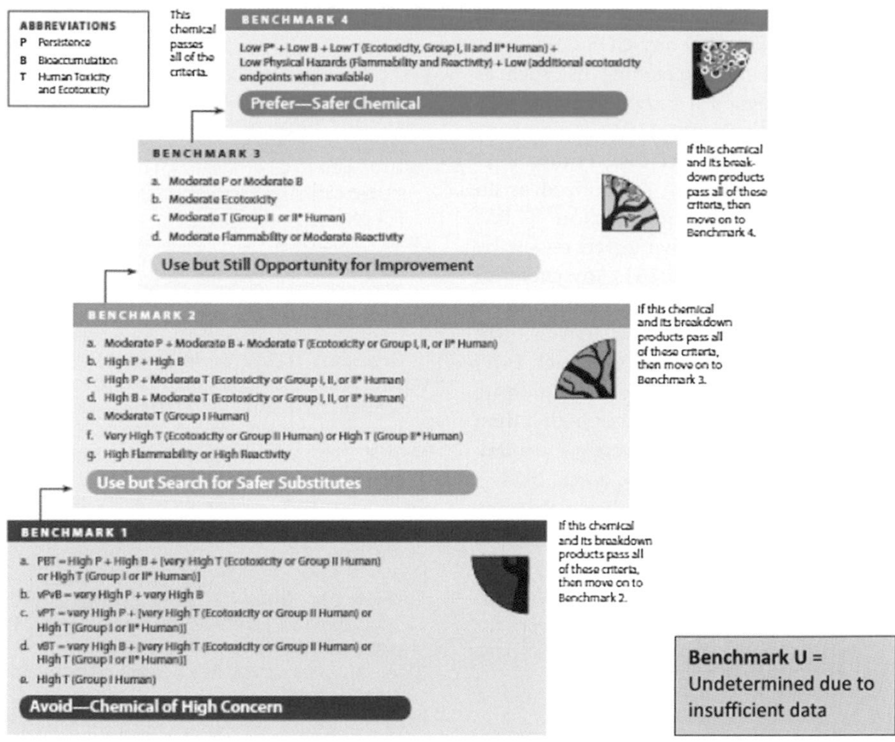

Figure 4 GreenScreen™ benchmarks. Reproduced with permission from Clean Production Action (CPA), 2011. GreenScreenTM Benchmarks. http://www.cleanproduction.org/library/greenScreenv1-2/GreenScreen_v1-2_Benchmarks_REV.pdf.

effects, skin and eye irritation, neurotoxicity, and skin and respiratory sensitization. Acetic acid's GreenScreen hazard rating table is illustrated in **Table 1**. Additional GreenScreen assessments can be viewed through Clean Production Action's GreenScreen website.

Acetic acid received a GreenScreen benchmark score of 2 based on hazard scores of very high (vH) for the following endpoints: systemic toxicity (single dose) (ST), skin irritation/corrosivity (IrS), eye irritation/corrosivity (IrE). This corresponds to benchmark classification 2f (very high for any ecotoxicity or Group II and II* human health endpoint) on the GreenScreen benchmarking scheme as shown in **Figure 4**.

Acetic acid is classified as a GHS Category 1 specific target organ toxicity chemical based on an inhalation effect level of 1.1 mg l^{-1} following a single dose, 4 h inhalation exposure in an acute inhalation study in rats. In addition, acetic acid is present on the GHS-Japan screening list as a Category 1 substance (blood) for single exposure systemic toxicity. According to GHS criteria, a specific target organ toxicant following single exposure is categorized as a Category 1 substance ('have the potential to produce significant toxicity in humans') in instances where significant toxicity is seen in humans or from studies in experimental. Specifically, the GHS guidance concentration value for a substance to be categorized as a Category 1 single dose inhalation toxicant (vapor form) is

Table 1 GreenScreen™ hazard ratings for acetic acid (2013)

Group I human					*Group II and II* human*									*Ecotox*		*Fate*		*Physical*	
						ST		*N*											
C	*M*	*R*	*D*	*E*	*AT*	*Single*	*Repeated**	*Single*	*Repeated**	*SnS**	*SnR**	*IrS*	*IrE*	*AA*	*CA*	*P*	*B*	*Rx*	*F*
L	***L***	*DG*	***L***	L	***M***	***vH***	***L***	***L***	L	*DG*	***M***	***vH***	***vH***	***M***	***L***	***vL***	**vL**	M	***M***

(AA) acute aquatic toxicity
(AT) acute mammalian toxicity
(B) bioaccumulation
(C) carcinogenicity
(CA) chronic aquatic toxicity
(E) endocrine activity
(F) flammability
(P) persistence
(N) neurotoxicity
(Rx) reactivity
(IrE) eye Irritation/corrosivity
(IrS) skin irritation/corrosivity
(M) mutagenicity and genotoxicity
(R) reproductive toxicity
(SnS) sensitization – skin
(SnR) sensitization – respiratory
(ST) systemic/organ toxicity
(Cr) corrosion/irritation (skin/eye)
(D) developmental toxicity
(DG) data gap

Note: Hazard levels – Very High (vH), High (H), Moderate (M), Low (L), Very Low (vL) in *italics* reflect estimated values and lower confidence. Hazard levels in **BOLD** font reflect values based on test data (See Guidance). Group II Human Health endpoints differ from Group II* Human Health endpoints in that they have four hazard scores (i.e., vH, H, M, and L) instead of three (i.e., H, M, and L), and are based on single exposures instead of repeated exposures.

equal to or less than 10 mg l^{-1} following a 4 h period of exposure. GreenScreen criteria states that any GHS Category 1 substance, or one that is listed on a screening list such as GHS-Japan, is automatically assigned a hazard score of very high (vH) for systemic toxicity (single dose).

Acetic acid is associated with the EU Risk Phrase R:35 ('Causes severe burns'). Risk phrases are categorized as an authoritative list that Clean Production Action (CPA) considers to be based on a comprehensive expert review by a recognized authoritative body (CPA, 2013). Any chemical assigned the EU R-phrase 34 or 35, which correspond to 'causes burns' and 'causes severe burns,' respectively, will automatically be assigned a hazard score of very high (vH) for IrS. Finally, data from human and animal studies indicate that acetic acid at concentrations equivalent to or higher than 3% in an aqueous solution is likely to be a severe eye irritant. In addition, the ocular damage induced by acetic acid is irreversible. GHS criteria for eye irritation indicate that any substance shown to produce irreversible ocular damage is classified as a Category 1 eye irritant (UN, 2009). CPA criteria state that any GHS Category 1 substance will automatically be assigned a hazard score of very high (vH) for IrE. Acetic acid was assigned a score of moderate (M) for acute aquatic toxicity.

CAA Tools

Another set of tools that industry can use to drive sustainability are online databases, such as Pharos, CleanGredients, and SUBSPORT, which promote safer chemical selection and hazardous chemical elimination. The Pharos Building Product Library evaluates more than 1000 products used in buildings, and scores materials and products on endpoints, including volatile organic compound content, toxic content, manufacturing toxics, renewable materials, and renewable energy. The Pharos Chemical and Material Library profiles health and environmental hazards of chemicals throughout various life cycle phases. CleanGredients is an online database that identifies less hazardous chemicals divided by functional use categories, such a less hazardous chelants, solvents, surfactants, among other functional classes. SUBSPORT is an EU, Germany, and Austrian-funded website designed to provide information about, and tools relating to, the substitution of hazardous chemicals. SUBSPORT developed a substitution steps paradigm companies can follow to phase out hazardous chemicals, and it also features an overview and electronic links to substitution/alternative assessment models and tools available around the world, such as the German GHS Column Model, Clean Production Action's GreenScreen, the Swedish Chemicals Inspectorate's PRIO database and tool, among others.

See also: Sustainability; Green Chemistry; Hazard Ranking; The Globally Harmonized System for Classification and Labeling of the GHS; Chemicals in Consumer Products.

Further Reading

BizNGO, November 2011. BizNGO Chemical Alternatives Assessment Protocol (v.1.1). http://www.bizngo.org/safer.php.

BizNGO, 2012. BizNGO Guide to Safer Chemicals. Version 1.0. http://www.bizngo.org/pdf/GuideToSaferChemicals-v1_2.pdf.

Clean Production Action (CPA), 2011. GreenScreen™ Benchmarks. http://www.cleanproduction.org/library/greenScreenv1-2/GreenScreen_v1-2_Benchmarks_REV.pdf.

Clean Production Action (CPA), 2013. The GreenScreen™ for Safer Chemicals Hazard Assessment Procedure. Version 1.2 Guidance. Dated: August 31, 2013. Available: http://www.cleanproduction.org/Greenscreen.php.

Clean Production Action (CPA), 2012a. GreenScreen™ Version 1.2 (2e) Hazard Criteria. Dated: November 2012 http://www.cleanproduction.org/library/GreenScreen_v1_2-2e_CriteriaDetailed_2012_10_10w_all_Lists_vf.pdf.

Clean Production Action (CPA), 2012b. GreenScreen™ for Safer Chemicals. Version 1.2 Specified Lists. February 2012 http://www.cleanproduction.org/library/greenscreen-translator-benchmark1-possible%20benchmark1.pdf.

Geiser, K., 2001. Materials Matter: Toward a Sustainable Materials Policy (Urban and Industrial Environments). MIT Press.

Interstate Chemicals Clearinghouse (IC2), March 2013. Draft Guidance for Alternatives Assessment and Risk Reduction. http://www.newmoa.org/prevention/ic2/aaguidance.cfm.

Lavoie, E.T., Heine, L.G., Holder, H., Rossi, M.S., Lee, R.E., Connor, E.A., Vrabel, M.E., DiFiore, D.M., Davies, C.L., 2010. Chemical alternatives assessment: enabling substitution to safer chemicals. Environ. Sci. Technol. 44 (24), 9244–9249. http://pubs.acs.org/doi/abs/10.1021/es1015789.

O'Brien, M., 2000. Making Better Environmental Decisions. An Alternative to Risk Assessment. MIT Press.

Rossi, M., Tickner, J., Geiser, K., 2006. Alternatives Assessment Framework of the Lowell Center for Sustainable Production. http://www.chemicalspolicy.org/downloads/FinalAltsAssess06.pdf.

United Nations, 2011. The Globally Harmonized System of Classification and Labelling of Chemicals (GHS), fourth revised ed. http://www.unece.org/trans/danger/publi/ghs/ghs_rev04/04files_e.html.

United States Environmental Protection Agency (U.S. EPA), August 2011. Design for the Environment Program Alternatives Assessment Criteria for Hazard Evaluation. Version 2.0. http://www.epa.gov/dfe/alternatives_assessment_criteria_for_hazard_eval.pdf.

Whittaker, M.H., Heine, L., 2013. Chemicals alternatives assessment (CAA): tools for selecting less hazardous chemicals. In: Chemicals Alternatives Assessments (Issues in Environmental Science and Technology). RSC Publishing, London.

Relevant Websites

http://www.cleanproduction.org/Greenscreen.php – Clean Production Action (CPA). 2013. GreenScreen™ for Safer Chemicals version 1.2 website.

http://www.epa.gov/dfe/alternative_assessments.html – Design for the Environment (DfE). 2013. Alternatives Assessments.

www.subsport.eu – European SUBSPORT. 2013. European Substitution Portal (SUBSPORT).

http://www.cleangredients.org/home – GreenBlue. 2013. CleanGredients database.

http://www.ecy.wa.gov/programs/hwtr/ChemAlternatives/index.html – State of Washington. 2013. Assessing the Safety of Chemical Alternatives. Department of Ecology.

http://www.turi.org/Our_Work/Research/Alternatives_Assessment – Toxics Use Reduction Institute (TURI). Alternatives Assessment. University of Massachusetts Lowell.

Chemical Hazard Communication and Safety Data Sheets

MJ Ramos-Peralonso, Green Planet Environmental Consulting, Madrid, Spain

This article is a revision of the previous edition article by Michele R. Sullivan & Patricia M. Nance, volume 1, pp 505–515, © 2005, Elsevier Inc.

Introduction

The use of chemical products is a widespread practice worldwide and it is clear that chemical products have enhanced and improved our life. However, alongside the benefits of these products, many chemicals have also the potential to cause adverse effects on human health and the environment. Some chemicals have intrinsic properties which create particular concerns. These properties include some physical properties, such as flammability or corrosion, as well as health concerns related to its toxicity to humans or animals or environmental concerns related to its ecotoxicity for environmental organisms. The identification of the specific hazards of each chemical substance is essential for their safe management, including manufacturing, transport, use, and disposal. The identification of the relevant hazards of each chemical product is also essential for their risk and safety assessment and should be communicated through the supply change to ensure that all users, including consumers, are aware of these potential hazards and take the appropriate protective measures.

The hazard communication strategy must consider the needs of the different target audiences. Chemicals are used worldwide in the workplace and by consumers; in addition, there are specific communication needs during their transport and in the case of emergencies.

Employers and workers manufacturing and using the chemicals need to know the specific hazards of the chemicals they are or may be exposed to in the workplace, the protective measures required to avoid the adverse effects that might be caused by those hazards, the proper storage conditions, and the mitigation measures to be adopted in case of emergencies. Labeling is the primary source of information but it is combined with other elements such as the safety data sheet (SDS), and training in hazard identification and prevention can be easily implemented.

In principle, consumers have similar needs but the label is, in most cases, the sole source of information; in addition, specific training is much more difficult to implement. There are two different approaches in the hazard communication to consumers, one focus on effectiveness and is based on the likelihood of injury, the other focuses on the 'right to know and to take educated decisions' and is based on the communication of hazards independently of the likelihood for those hazards to result in adverse effects.

The transport of dangerous chemical products requires communication on safe practices to different types of dedicated workers, from drivers to those handling directly the products. The main elements are the conditions for proper handling, e.g., during storage, loading, and unloading, as well as in the case of accident. Similarly, emergency responders have specific hazard communication needs in order to facilitate immediate and adequate responses. The needs for firefighters, those involved in the contention, cleaning, and risk assessment, or the medical personnel treating the victims are very different and should be considered.

The chemical hazard communication is mostly based on the classification and labeling system, which supports additional downstream implementation tools. The chemicals with dangerous properties are classified as hazardous and must be labeled when distributed to users and marketed. The classification system not only identifies that the chemical is a hazardous one, but it also identify which particular hazards are relevant for each chemical substance as well as its potency. During the twentieth century, different countries and regions developed their own classification and labeling systems, creating confusion and reclassification, and relabeling obligations when hazardous chemicals were transported among countries/regions.

The harmonization of the classification and labeling systems of chemicals started in fact in relation to the need for safe transport of dangerous goods. The United Nations Economic and Social Council's Committee of Experts on the Transport of Dangerous Goods (UNCEDTG) worked to harmonize physical hazards and acute toxicity in the transport sector. However, transport requirements in countries were often not harmonized with those of other sectors in that country and particularly in relation with the workplace or consumer sectors.

Chapter 19 of Agenda 21, adopted at the United Nations Conference on Environment and Development (UNCED, 1992), provided the international mandate to develop a single, globally harmonized system (GHS) to address classification of chemicals, labels, and SDSs. The work was coordinated and managed under the auspices of the Interorganization Programme for the Sound Management of Chemicals (IOMC) Coordinating Group for the Harmonization of Chemical Classification Systems (CG/HCCS). It required a long-term commitment from the three technical focal points:

- the International Labour Organization (ILO) for the hazard communication;
- the Organization for Economic Cooperation and Development (OECD) for the classification of health and environmental hazards; and
- the United Nations Sub-Committee of Experts on the Transport of Dangerous Goods (UNSCETDG) and ILO for the physical hazards.

The examination of existing systems at that moment clarified that although many countries had some requirements; four 'major' existing systems need to be considered:

1. Requirements of systems in the United States for the workplace, consumers, and pesticides.
2. Requirements of Canada for the workplace, consumers, and pesticides.
3. European Union directives for classification and labeling of substances and preparations.

 http://dx.doi.org/10.1016/B978-0-12-386454-3.00460-7

4. The UN recommendations on the transport of dangerous goods.

These systems were the basis for developing the GHS of classification and labeling of chemicals.

The GHS of Classification and Labeling of Chemicals

The first version of the GHS was adopted in December 2002 by the Sub-Committee on the GHS (SCEGHS), and endorsed by the Committee on the Transport of Dangerous Goods and the GHS of Classification and Labelling of Chemicals. The first version of the GHS was published in 2003. The system has been amended biannually.

The first revised edition of the GHS (GHS Rev. 1, published in 2005) included various revised provisions concerning classification and labeling, new provisions for aspiration hazards, and new guidance on the use of precautionary statements and pictograms and on the preparation of SDSs.

The second revised edition of the GHS (GHS Rev. 2, published in 2007) included new and revised provisions concerning the classification and labeling of explosives, respiratory and skin sensitizers, toxic by inhalation gases and gas mixtures, additional guidance on the interpretation of the building block approach and on the evaluation of the carcinogenic potential of chemicals, and the codification of hazard and precautionary statements.

The third revised edition of the GHS (GHS Rev. 3, published in 2009) included new provisions for the allocation of hazard statements and for the labeling of small packaging, two new subcategories for respiratory and skin sensitization, the revision of the classification criteria for long-term hazards (chronic toxicity) to the aquatic environment, and a new hazard class for substances and mixtures hazardous to the ozone layer.

The fourth revised edition of the GHS (GHS Rev. 4, published in 2011) included new hazard categories for chemically unstable gases and nonflammable aerosols, further rationalization of precautionary statements, and further clarification of some of the criteria to avoid differences in their interpretation. This revised version contains four parts and 10 annexes:

- Part 1: Introduction
- Part 2: Physical hazards
- Part 3: Health hazards
- Part 4: Environmental hazards
- Annex 1: Allocation of label elements
- Annex 2: Classification and labeling summary tables
- Annex 3: Codification of hazard statements, codification and use of precautionary statements and examples of precautionary pictograms
- Annex 4: Guidance on the preparation of SDSs
- Annex 5: Consumer product labeling based on the likelihood of injury
- Annex 6: Comprehensibility testing methodology
- Annex 7: Examples of arrangements of the GHS label elements
- Annex 8: An example of classification in the GHSs
- Annex 9: Guidance on hazards to the aquatic environment
- Annex 10: Guidance on transformation/dissolution of metals and metal compounds

The GHS describes the classification criteria and the hazard communication elements by type of hazard and covers the classification and labeling of chemical substances in its own and of mixtures. It covers 16 physical hazard classes, 10 health hazard classes, and 2 environmental hazard classes. It also includes details on the labeling and guidance on other hazard communication elements such as the SDS.

Classification of Chemical Substances and Mixtures

Classification is the process for identifying the physical, health, and environmental hazards of a substance or a mixture and it is done by comparing their intrinsic properties, measured through standardized assays or coming from other information sources, with defined criteria in order to arrive at a classification of the substance or mixture. It follows three consecutive steps: (1) the identification and examination of relevant data regarding the potential hazards of the substance or mixture; (2) the comparison of the data with the classification criteria; and (3) the decision on whether the substance or mixture shall be classified as hazardous in relation to each of the hazard classes, and the degree of hazard, where appropriate.

The classification system is based on a set of hazard classes which describe the nature of the physical, health, or environmental hazard, and a set of categories, within each class, which describe the severity of the harm. These categories may represent the potency with quantitative criteria for the allocation of the chemical within the category, e.g., in the case of acute toxicity or aquatic toxicity, or the extend/type of evidence, e.g., for carcinogens or chemicals toxic to reproduction.

For example, acute toxicity is based on the adverse effects occurring after the administration of a single dose (or multiple doses within 24 h for oral and dermal routes and 4 h for inhalation) and is mostly based on the oral/dermal LD_{50} and inhalation LC_{50} observed in animals under experimental standardized conditions. This hazard class contains five categories (Category 1–5) for each exposure route defined by fixed ranges in the oral/dermal LD_{50} and inhalation LC_{50}. Consequently, chemicals with similar acute toxicity potencies are classified within the same category.

Regarding carcinogenicity, the criteria are based on the strength and type of the evidence and distinguish three different types: chemicals known to have carcinogenic potential for humans, chemicals presumed to have carcinogenic potential for humans (mostly based on evidence on animals), and suspected human carcinogens. The potency or dose at which the effects have been observed is not part of the criteria and the classification does not provide information on the level of expected human cancer risk associated to a particular level of exposure.

Mixtures can be classified similarly to substances, e.g., by comparing directly their intrinsic properties measured through standardized methods with the classification criteria or by considering the properties and hazards of their components.

The classification in a particular hazard class and category implies the need to communicate this information through the labeling and other hazard communication elements such as the SDS.

Labeling of Hazardous Chemical Substances and Mixtures

As described above, each hazard class and category has a set of associated labeling requirements. The GHS labeling approach is based on four complementary label elements: the symbol, the signal word, the hazard statements, and the precautionary statements.

The nine GHS hazard symbols are basically similar to those used in the UN transport system, except one specific for certain health hazards but are presented in a specific graphic composition (shape, border, background pattern, and color), the pictogram, which is GHS specific: a square set at a point with a black symbol on a white background with a red frame (Figure 1).

The signal words are words used to indicate the relative level of severity of the hazard and to alert the reader to a potential hazard on the label. The word 'danger' is used for the more severe hazard categories and the word 'warning' is used for intermediate categories, while no signal word is allocated to the less severe categories.

The hazard statements are phrases assigned to each hazard class and category describing the nature of the hazards and its degree when appropriate. Each hazard statement is associated to a code, which starts with the letter 'H,' the number 2, 3, or 4 for physical, health, and environmental hazards, respectively, and two additional digits with sequential numbering.

The precautionary statements are phrases (and/or pictograms) that describe the measures recommended to minimize or prevent adverse effects resulting from the exposure to a hazardous product or its improper storage or handling. Each precautionary statement is associated to a code which starts with the letter 'P,' the number 1, 2, 3, 4, or 5 for general, prevention, response, storage, and disposal statements, respectively, and two additional digits with sequential numbering.

The label should also include a product identifier and information on the supplier.

Safety Data Sheets

SDSs, previously named as material SDSs in the United States and other jurisdictions, are the complementary hazard communication tool in the workplace. The SDS provides employers and workers, including those involved in transport and emergency personnel, with procedures for handling and storing the substance or mixture in a safe manner, advice on safety precautions, and to react properly in the case of accidental spills, mishandling, or emergencies.

The SDS is in fact the main tool for transferring detailed information on hazardous substances, as such or in mixtures, to workers and professional users through the supply chain. It is product specific and according to the GHS should be provided

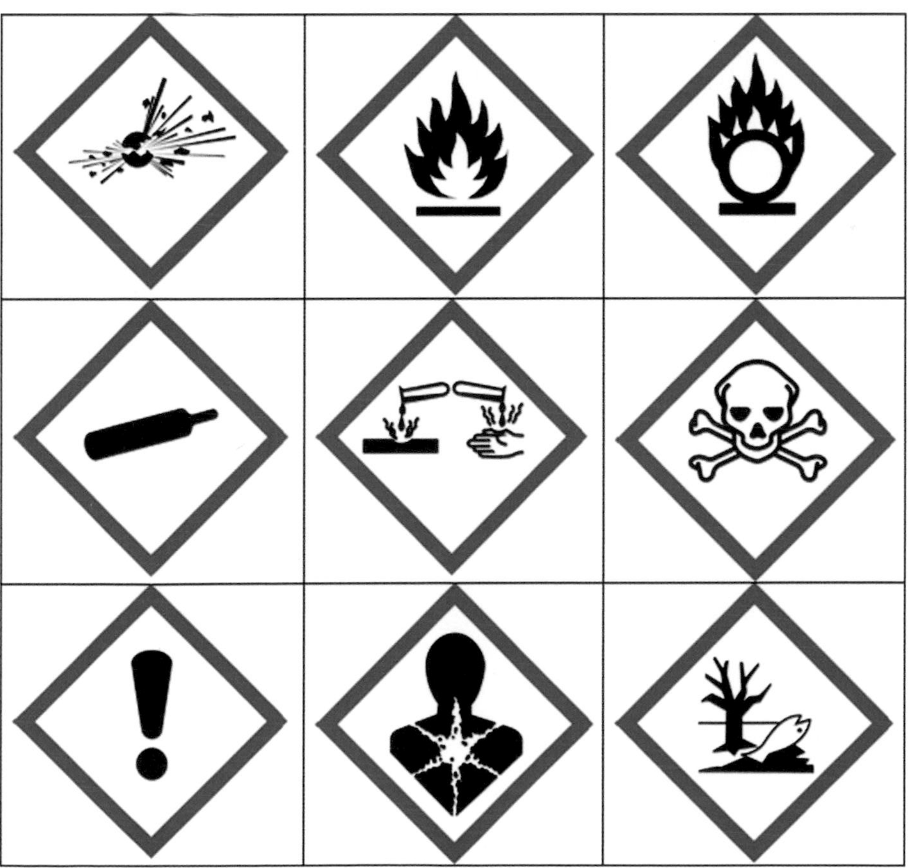

Figure 1 GHS pictograms.

at least for all substances and mixtures that meet one or more of the classification criteria, as well as for mixtures which contain ingredients that meet the criteria for carcinogenic, toxic to reproduction or specific target organ toxicity in concentrations exceeding the selected cutoff criteria. The competent authorities may also choose to require SDSs for mixtures not meeting the criteria for classification as hazardous but which contain hazardous substances in certain concentrations.

The information in the SDS has been also harmonized and should be presented using 16 specific headings:

1. Identification
   - GHS product identifier.
   - Other means of identification.
   - Recommended use of the chemical and restrictions on use.
   - Supplier's details (including name, address, phone number, etc.).
   - Emergency phone number.
2. Hazard(s) identification
   - GHS classification of the substance/mixture and any national or regional information.
   - GHS label elements, including precautionary statements. (Hazard symbols may be provided as a graphical reproduction of the symbols in black and white or the name of the symbol, e.g., flame, skull, and crossbones.)
   - Other hazards which do not result in classification (e.g., dust explosion hazard) or are not covered by the GHS.
3. Composition/information on ingredients (Note: For information on ingredients, the competent authority rules for CBI take priority over the rules for product identification)
   - For substances
     a. Chemical identity.
     b. Common name, synonyms, etc.
     c. CAS number, EC number, etc.
     d. Impurities and stabilizing additives which are themselves classified and which contribute to the classification of the substance.
   - For mixtures
     a. The chemical identity and concentration or concentration ranges of all ingredients which are hazardous within the meaning of the GHS and are present above their cutoff levels.
4. First aid measures
   - Description of necessary measures, subdivided according to the different routes of exposure, i.e., inhalation, skin and eye contact, and ingestion.
   - Most important symptoms/effects, acute, and delayed.
   - Indication of immediate medical attention and special treatment needed, if necessary.
5. Firefighting measures
   - Suitable (and unsuitable) extinguishing media.
   - Specific hazards arising from the chemical (e.g., nature of any hazardous combustion products).
   - Special protective equipment and precautions for firefighters.
6. Accidental release measures
   - Personal precautions, protective equipment, and emergency procedures.
   - Environmental precautions.
   - Methods and materials for containment and cleaning up.
7. Handling and storage
   - Precautions for safe handling.
   - Conditions for safe storage, including any incompatibilities.
8. Exposure controls/personal protection
   - Control parameters, e.g., occupational exposure limit values or biological limit values.
   - Appropriate engineering controls.
   - Individual protection measures, such as personal protective equipment.
9. Physical and chemical properties
   - Appearance (physical state, color, etc.).
   - Odor.
   - Odor threshold.
   - pH.
   - Melting point/freezing point.
   - Initial boiling point and boiling range.
   - Flash point.
   - Evaporation rate.
   - Flammability (solid and gas).
   - Upper/lower flammability or explosive limits.
   - Vapor pressure.
   - Vapor density.
   - Relative density.
   - Solubility(ies).
   - Partition coefficient: *n*-octanol/water.
   - Autoignition temperature.
   - Decomposition temperature.
   - Viscosity.
10. Stability and reactivity
    - Reactivity.
    - Chemical stability.
    - Possibility of hazardous reactions.
    - Conditions to avoid (e.g., static discharge, shock, or vibration).
    - Incompatible materials.
    - Hazardous decomposition products.
11. Toxicological information: Concise but complete and comprehensible description of the various toxicological (health) effects and the available data used to identify those effects, including:
    - information on the likely routes of exposure (inhalation, ingestion, and skin and eye contact);
    - symptoms related to the physical, chemical, and toxicological characteristics;
    - delayed and immediate effects and also chronic effects from short- and long-term exposure; and
    - numerical measures of toxicity (such as acute toxicity estimates).
12. Ecological information
    - Ecotoxicity (aquatic and terrestrial, where available).
    - Persistence and degradability.
    - Bioaccumulative potential.
    - Mobility in soil.
    - Other adverse effects.
13. Disposal considerations: Description of waste residues and information on their safe handling and methods of disposal, including the disposal of any contaminated packaging.

14. Transport information
    - UN number.
    - UN proper shipping name.
    - Transport hazard class(es).
    - Packing group, if applicable.
    - Environmental hazards (e.g., marine pollutant (yes/no)).
    - Special precautions which a user needs to be aware of or needs to comply with in connection with transport or conveyance either within or outside their premises.
15. Regulatory information: Safety, health, and environmental regulations specific for the product in question.
16. Other information

The GHS Implementation

New Zealand was the first country in implementing the GHS. Since then, the GHS has been already implemented, at least partially, in different countries and jurisdictions and is in the implementing stage in many others worldwide.

Examples of these implementations are the Model Work Health and Safety (WHS) legislation in Australia, the Standard ABNT NRB 14725:2009 in Brazil, the standards GB T 16483–2008: SDS for chemical products content and order of sections, GB 13690–2009: General rules for preparation of precautionary labels for chemicals, and GB 15258–2009: General rules for classification and hazard communication of chemicals in China, the National Technical Standard NTE INEN 2-266:2000 in Ecuador, the National Standard JIS in Japan, the national standard NMX-R-019-SCFI-2011 in Mexico, the Industrial Safety and Health Act (ISHA) and the Toxic Chemicals Control Act (TCCA) in the Republic of Korea, seven GOST national standards in Russia, the revised ordinances SR 813.11 and SR 813.12 in Switzerland, the revised Hazard Communication Standard (HCS) in the United States, the Decrees 307/009 of 3 July 2009 and 346/011 of 28 September 2011 in Uruguay, and the Regulation (EC) No. 1272/2008 of the European Parliament and of the Council of 16 December 2008, the CLP Regulation, in the European Union (EU) and European Economic Area (EEA).

Through these implementation procedures some authorities, e.g., in New Zealand and Japan, have created public inventories informing on the classification of dangerous substances. The largest and most extensive inventory has been created in the EU as part of the requirements of the CLP Regulation. The inventory includes the self-classification by manufacturers and importers of all substances marketed, as such or in mixtures, in the EU and contains ca.900 000 entries.

The EU Extended SDSs with Exposure Scenarios

The SDS information acts as a reference source for the management of hazardous chemicals in the workplace. The SDS is product related and, usually, is not able to provide specific information that is relevant for any given workplace where the product may finally be used. Instead, the information is designed to enable employers to develop active programs for worker protection measures specific to individual workplaces and to consider any measures, which may be necessary to protect the environment.

However, the new EU chemicals legislation implemented through the REACH and CLP Regulations has gone a step further, considering that the SDS should also provide specific information relevant to the assessment of each use. The UE legislation requires extended SDS indicating the uses that are covered by the provider of the substance (and the uses advised against and the reasons for this advice); in addition, the exposure scenarios for each relevant use should be attached. These exposure scenarios present clear indications regarding the operational conditions for proper handling of the substance, the risk reduction measures that should be applied to reduce the exposure and risk and the resulting exposure level, covering the workplace, the environment, and consumers when relevant, if possible in quantitative terms.

This EU approach combines the standard approach of SDS as a hazard (not risk) communication tool, with additional information on use patterns and expected exposure. Consequently, it offers new opportunities for the employers, facilitating their obligation to ensure a safe use of hazardous chemicals in the workplace, including environmental emissions. European downstream users are expected to implement the operational conditions and risk management measures indicated in the extended SDS for each described use pattern, as part of their obligations to ensure a safe handling and use of hazardous products. If a downstream user is unable to implement these conditions, must conduct its own safety assessment, which in certain cases should be notified to ECHA.

The use pattern and the associated exposure assessment are based on a use descriptor system, based on five separate descriptor lists which in combination with each other form a brief description of use. The five descriptors are the following:

1. The sector of use category (SU) describes in which sector of the economy the substance is used. This includes mixing or repacking of substances at formulator's level as well as industrial, professional, and consumer end-uses.
2. The chemical product category (PC) describes in which types of chemical products (=substances as such or in mixtures) the substance is finally contained when it is supplied to end-uses (by industrial, professional, or consumer users).
3. The process category (PROC) describes the application techniques or process types defined from the occupational perspective.
4. The environmental release category (ERC) describes the broad conditions of use from the environmental perspective.
5. The article category (AC) describes the type of article into which the substance has eventually been processed. This also includes mixtures in their dried or cured form (e.g., dried printing ink in newspapers; dried coatings on various surfaces).

In addition to their description function, these use descriptors define the name of the exposure scenario and support the identification of the suitable exposure estimation. In fact, some descriptors are directly associated to one of the available Tier 1 exposure estimation tools developed for the implementation of REACH, allowing an initial release/exposure estimation based on default values, which can be used for demonstrating safe use or as the starting point for the exposure refinement if needed.

As a complement, the EU REACH Regulation has extended the need to provide SDS to other chemicals not covered by the GHS criteria. These include the PBT and vPvB substances. In addition, an SDS should be provided for mixtures that contains at least one substance on the candidate list of substances of very high concern (SVHC) and the individual concentration of this substance in the mixture is $\geq$0.1% (w/w) for nongaseous mixtures if the substance is persistent, bioaccumulative, and toxic (PBT) or very persistent and very bioaccumulative (vPvB).

Chemical Hazard Communication for Substances in Articles

The communication of the hazards related to substances in articles has received less attention. The classification and labeling approach is restricted to 'chemical products': substances in its own or as mixtures. The hazards, of chemical or other nature in articles intended for industrial, professional, or consumer use, are communicated as elements in the label or just as indications in the instruction pamphlets that are distributed with the articles. With few exceptions, these obligations have not been harmonized and defined labeling requirements for covering specifically chemical risks in articles have not been developed yet. A typical exception is the classification of explosive articles in the EU, as the CLP Regulation applies the GHS principles to explosive articles.

Nevertheless, the need to communicate the chemical hazards of articles to users, including consumers, is receiving significant attention. In the European Union, the REACH Regulation has created new hazard communication obligations for those substances identified as of very high concern and included in the 'candidate list' of SVHC. EU or EEA suppliers of articles which contain substances on the candidate list in a concentration above 0.1% (w/w) have to provide sufficient information to allow safe use of the article to their customers. However, no specific indications on how to provide this information have been developed yet.

The obligation is also applied to consumers' articles if requested by the consumer. This information must contain as a minimum the name of the substance, and as a complement, ECHA has published in the web page the notifications received from producers and importers of articles regarding the presence of SVHC in their articles. However, additional efforts are still needed in order to fully implement the societal concerns for access to the information and the 'right to know' in a way that could really allow educated decisions by each consumer regarding personal assessments of the risk and benefits related to the presence of hazardous chemicals in consumer articles.

See also: Candidate List of Substances of Very High Concern (SVHC), Reach; The European Classification and Labeling (C&L) Inventory; Import/Export of Hazardous Chemicals; Chemical Safety Assessment; Risk Management.

Further Reading

ECHA, 2010. Guidance on Information Requirements and Chemical Safety Assessment. (Chapter R.12). Use descriptor system. ECHA-2010-G-05-EN. Available at: http://echa.europa.eu/documents/10162/13632/information_requirements_r12_en.pdf.

ECHA, 2011. Guidance on the Compilation of Safety Data Sheets. ECHA-2011-G-08.1-EN. Available at: http://echa.europa.eu/documents/10162/13643/sds_en.pdf.

ECHA, 2011. Guidance on Labelling and Packaging in Accordance with Regulation (EC) No 1272/2008 ECHA-11-G-04-EN. Available at:. http://echa.europa.eu/documents/10162/13562/clp_labelling_en.pdf.

UNCED, 1992. Agenda 21. Report of the United Nations Conference on Environment and Development (UNCED). UNEP.

UNECE, 2011. Globally Harmonized System of Classification and Labelling of Chemicals (GHS). Available at: fourth revised ed. http://www.unece.org/trans/danger/publi/ghs/ghs_rev04/04files_e.html.

Relevant Websites

http://echa.europa.eu – ECHA, European Chemicals Agency.

http://www.schc.org/ – Society for Chemical Hazard Communication.

http://www.unece.org/trans/danger/publi/ghs/ghs_welcome_e.html – United Nations Economic Commission for Europe: Globally Harmonized System of Classification and Labelling of Chemicals (GHS).

http://www.unece.org/trans/danger/publi/ghs/implementation_e.html – United Nations Economic Commission for Europe: GHS implementation.

http://www.osha.gov/dsg/hazcom/index.html – US Occupational Safety and Health Administration Hazard Communication web site.

Chemical Interactions

C Pope, Oklahoma State University, Stillwater, OK, USA

In reality, people are never exposed to individual chemicals in isolation. For example, multitudes of chemicals comprise the food we eat (both in the food itself and as contaminants on or in food), and there are many contaminating chemicals in air and drinking water, around the home, and in the workplace. Thus, there is a continual possibility of interactions among chemicals within our bodies. There are four basic types of interactions between chemicals that can modulate toxic outcome: additivity, antagonism, synergism, and potentiation. These interactions are based on additions of effect, which simply combines the measurable effect, or of dose, which considers the chemicals to be additive as if they were dilutions of each other.

Antagonism refers to the ability of one chemical to impair or limit the toxicity of another, or the joint interference with the toxic action of two or more chemicals. To illustrate these examples, let us consider two chemicals referred to as A and B, using an effect-addition approach. In measuring functional toxicity, a graded scale has been devised for recording the severity of response from 0 (i.e., no signs of toxicity) to 6 (lethality). If chemical A alone elicits an average response of 4 on the toxicity scale while chemical B elicits no toxicity on its own (i.e., an average response of 0), but both chemicals given together yield an average toxicity score of only 2, then it can be concluded that chemical B antagonized the toxic action of chemical A.

Treatment	*Toxicity score*
Chemical A	4
Chemical B	0
Both A and B	2

If on the other hand, chemical A and chemical B both elicited some degree of toxicity using this same scale, for example, chemical A caused an average response of 3 and B also elicited an average response of 3, but when given together a response of only 1 was noted, it is concluded that both chemicals antagonized the toxic actions of each other.

Treatment	*Toxicity score*
Chemical A	3
Chemical B	3
Both A and B	1

A simple mathematical description of antagonism is:

$T_{\text{Both}} < T_A + T_B$ (effect addition)

where T_{Both} is the degree of toxic response when both chemicals are given together, whereas T_A and T_B represent the degree of toxic response when either chemical A or chemical B is given alone. Antagonism is a relatively common phenomenon, and antidotal strategies are often based on this type of interaction. Chemical antagonism is a simple interaction between two chemicals in which the formed complex is less toxic. Functional antagonism occurs when two chemicals have opposing actions on physiology, their combined effects counteract each other. Kinetic or dispositional antagonism occurs when the absorption, distribution, elimination, or biotransformation of a chemical is altered by another such that less toxicant reaches its target site. Finally, receptor antagonism occurs when two chemicals bind to a specific receptor in the body, and competition between the two leads to lesser toxicity.

Synergism refers to a greater toxic response with exposure to two chemicals than would be expected under a specific definition of additivity, based on the toxic response elicited by either of the chemicals alone. Potentiation is similar to synergism in that greater toxicity is seen with exposure to two chemicals than expected based on the responses elicited by those chemicals alone, but in this case one of the chemicals has no overt capacity to elicit the toxic response on its own. With the mock toxicity grading scale used in the preceding, examples of synergism and potentiation in effect addition can be considered.

Treatment	*Toxicity score*
Synergism	
Chemical A	1
Chemical B	1
Both A and B	5
Potentiation	
Chemical A	2
Chemical B	0
Both A and B	6

A simple mathematical description of synergism or potentiation is:

$T_{\text{Both}} > T_A + T_B$ (effect addition)

where T_{Both} is the degree of toxic response when both chemicals are given together, whereas T_A and T_B represent the degree of toxic response when either chemical A or chemical B is given alone.

Under dose-addition theory, the combined effect of chemicals is described as the observed effect at the sum of doses A plus B, where the dose of A can be expressed in relation to a dose of B. Another way to consider dose-additivity is that, given a specified effect such as ED_{50}:

$dA/ED50_A + dB/ED50_B = 1$

 http://dx.doi.org/10.1016/B978-0-12-386454-3.00110-X

where dA and dB are the doses of A and B in the mixture, respectively, and $ED50_A$ and $ED50_B$ are the point estimates for each. When the sum = 1, the mixture is considered dose additive; by extension, sums less or greater than 1 represent antagonism or synergism, respectively. Dose-additivity is often a default assumption with chemicals that act through a common mode of action.

It is possible that two or more chemicals can elicit a toxic response that is additive in nature. Understanding how multiple toxicants that act through a common mechanism or pathway interact to yield cumulative toxicity is an important endeavor in risk assessment. Under default assumptions, multiple chemicals that elicit toxicity by a common mechanism are considered to exhibit dose-additivity; that is, the total dose is equal to the sum of the individual chemical doses, scaled according to their potency relative to an index chemical. A number of studies using various toxicological endpoints have observed apparent dose-additivity with multiple chemical interactions. It should be noted, however, that these studies necessarily use exposure levels much higher than would typically occur in humans. Chemical interactions and their cumulative effects as well as effects of multiple chemicals working through different mechanisms will continue to be an active area of research and important in understanding real-world risks.

As noted, people are exposed to many chemicals at any given time through various environmental media. Although interactions between two chemicals are relatively straightforward and easy to understand, with more than two chemicals the analysis becomes exceedingly complicated. However, study of the interactive effects of chemicals can often provide specific information on their mechanisms of action.

See also: Common Mechanism of Toxicity in Pesticides; Mixtures, Toxicology, and Risk Assessment; Dose–Response Relationship.

Further Reading

Eaton, D.L., Klaassen, C.D., 2001. Principles of toxicology. In: Klaassen, C.D. (Ed.), Casarett and Doull's Toxicology, sixth ed. McGraw-Hill, New York, pp. 11–34.

Moser, V.C., MacPhail, R.C., Gennings, C., 2003. Neurobehavioral evaluations of mixtures of trichloroethylene, heptachlor, and di(2-ethylhexyl)phthlate in a full-factorial design. Toxicology 188 (2–3), 125–137.

Murphy, S.D., 1980. Assessment of the potential for toxic interactions among environmental pollutants. In: Galli, G.L., Murphy, S.D., Paolletti, R. (Eds.), The Principles and Methods in Modern Toxicology. Elsevier, Amsterdam, pp. 277–288.

Pope, C.N., Padilla, S., 1990. Potentiation of organophosphorus-induced delayed neurotoxicity by phenylmethylsulfonyl fluoride. J. Toxicol. Environ. Health 31, 261–273.

Walker, N.J., Crockett, P.W., Nyska, A., Brix, A.E., Jokinen, M.P., Sells, D.M., Hailey, J.R., Easterling, M., Haseman, J.K., Yin, M., Wyde, M.E., Bucher, J.R., Portier, C.J., 2005. Dose-additive carcinogenicity of a defined mixture of "dioxin-like compounds". Environ. Health Perspect. 113, 43–48.

Wolansky, M.J., Gennings, C., DeVito, M.J., Crofton, K.M., 2009. Evidence for dose-additive effects of pyrethroids on motor activity in rats. Environ. Health Perspect. 117: 1563–1570.

Relevant Website

http://ec.europa.eu/environment/chemicals/pdf/report_Mixture%20toxicity.pdf.

Chemical Mixtures, Toxicology and Risk Assessment *see* Mixtures, Toxicology and Risk Assessment

Chemical Safety Assessment

European Chemicals Agency, Annankatu, FI Helsinki, Finland

Background

In 2006, the European Union (EU) adopted a new regulation on chemicals and their safe use called REACH. It deals with the registration, evaluation, authorization, and restriction of chemical substances. According to the regulation, companies submitting a registration dossier to the European Chemicals Agency (ECHA) have to perform a chemical safety assessment (CSA) for their chemical substance if it is manufactured or imported at volumes above 10 t year^{-1}. The assessment needs to be recorded in a chemical safety report.

The Assessment

CSA is the process used to identify and explain the conditions under which the manufacturing and use of a substance can be considered as safe. It can be divided into three steps:

1. Hazard assessment for human health, physicochemical properties, and the environment and a persistent, bioaccumulative, and toxic (PBT), and very persistent and very bioaccumulative (vPvB) substances assessment
2. Exposure assessment
3. Risk characterization

The first step, hazard assessment, involves the collection and evaluation of all relevant available information on a substance to decide if it classified as 'dangerous' and to set the derived no effect levels (DNELs) for human health effects and the predicted no effect concentrations (PNECs) for environmental effects. It should include information on substance properties, manufacture, use, and related emissions and exposures. If the existing information is insufficient under the requirements of the REACH Regulation, the registrant needs to generate further information. If the outcome of the hazard assessment is that the substance does not meet the criteria for 'classification' as hazardous and does not have PBT or vPvB properties, the CSA is finished, otherwise steps 2 and 3 are also required to complete the process.

The second step is the exposure assessment for the manufacture and all the uses of the substance. This step develops exposure scenarios to estimate the exposure to humans and the relevant environmental compartments. Exposure scenarios describe the different uses and manufacture in terms of the operating conditions and risk management measures. From these estimates of release, exposures can be made using standard models or better estimates using adapted models or actual measurements. The exposure scenarios cover all the identified uses and life stages of a substance.

The third step is risk characterization, which compares the levels of exposure with the threshold levels that are considered safe for humans (as described by DNELs) and the environment (as described by PNECs). Where it is not possible to determine a threshold level for one effect (the DNEL or PNEC is not applicable), a qualitative or semiquantitative approach is used. For risk characterization of physicochemical properties, the likelihood and severity of an adverse event occurring are assessed.

Under the REACH Regulation, risks are regarded as controlled when the exposure levels to the substance are below the threshold levels, both for humans and for the environment. For risks to be considered as under control for effects with no threshold levels, the users of the substance need to ensure that the emissions and exposures are minimized or avoided.

If risks are under control, the CSA ends here. If risks are not under control, the assessment has to be refined, either by obtaining more data on the properties of the substance, exposure, and emission or by changing the conditions for its manufacture or use. The CSA process is iterative and will continue until the risks are shown to be under control. Manufacturers and importers communicate these conditions to their customers in exposure scenarios.

Chesar

To help registrants deal with exposure and risk assessments, the ECHA has developed Chesar, a software tool that supports the harmonization of the CSA and report. The main features of the tool are to:

- allow the use of data in the IUCLID format (International Uniform Chemical Information Database), i.e., use the data from the registration dossiers;
- allow exposure estimation and risk characterization;
- support building and recording of exposure scenarios;
- support in documenting the measures recommended for controlling the risks of the substance during its use.

Chesar helps registrants to generate consistent and transparent chemical safety reports and exposure scenarios. For the communication of the conditions of safe use, the exposure scenarios are attached to safety data sheets, which in turn are generated on the basis of the chemical safety reports. Chesar also facilitates the reuse of assessments that the registrants or their industry associations have already conducted for REACH or other purposes.

 http://dx.doi.org/10.1016/B978-0-12-386454-3.00575-3

Acknowledgment

With thanks to the consulted experts at ECHA for their collaboration on this work.

See also: The European Chemicals Agency; REACH; REACH-IT.

Further Reading

European Chemicals Agency, 2011. Guidance on Information Requirements and Chemical Safety Assessment Part A – Introduction to the Guidance Document. pp. 1–45.

European Chemicals Agency, 2010. Chesar Manual – Introduction. pp. 1–35.

European Chemicals Agency, 2010. Chesar Manual – Parts 1–6.

Relevant Websites

http://chesar.echa.europa.eu/ – the Chesar website provides up-to-date information on the software tool which helps companies carry out their chemical safety assessments and prepare their chemical safety reports.

http://iuclid.echa.europa.eu the IUCLID website provides up-to-date information and download of the software tool which companies have to use to store data on chemicals and prepare for their REACH registration dossiers to the Agency.

http://echa.europa.eu – the website of the European Chemicals Agency is a one-stop-shop for information about the legislation it manages.

http://echa.cdt.europa.eu – ECHA-term is a multilingual terminology database with more than 900 key REACH and CLP terms and their definitions in 22 EU languages

Chemical Safety Assessment and Reporting Tool (Chesar), REACH

MJ Ramos-Peralonso, Green Planet Environmental Consulting, Madrid, Spain

Introduction

The CHEmical Safety Assessment and Reporting tool (Chesar) is an application developed by the European Chemicals Agency (ECHA) to help companies carry out their chemical safety assessments (CSAs) under the European REACH Regulation and to prepare their chemical safety reports (CSRs) that must be included in the REACH registration dossiers and the exposure scenarios (ES) that also should be added to the extended safety data sheets (SDSs) for communication in the supply chain.

The CSR is a regulatory requisite that must be included in the registration dossiers for chemicals registered under the REACH Regulation and manufactured or imported above 10 tons per year. Basically, Chesar has implemented as an IT tool the principles related to the CSA as described in the ECHA "Guidance on Information Requirements and Chemical Safety Assessment." Chesar is directly connected to IUCLID, the electronic database system for storing and presenting the information on the substance identity, its uses, and the hazard information (physical–chemical properties, ecotoxicology, and toxicology end-points). Chesar has been developed as a 'plug-in' for IUCLID5.

Chesar provides a structured workflow for carrying out a standard safety assessment for the different uses of a substance, but provides enough flexibility to accommodate specific situations. The tool also helps to structure the information needed for the exposure assessment and risk characterization, facilitating the generation of a transparent CSR.

Chesar allows both quantitative and qualitative risk assessments. The quantitative assessments are based on predicted no-effect levels for human health and for the environment. Under REACH, the predicted no-effect levels for human health assessment are named DNELs, Derived No-Effect Levels, and those for environmental protection, PNECs, Predicted No-Effect Concentrations. Regarding the quantitative exposure assessment, Chesar has combined three complementary generic exposure assessment models, the ECETOC TRA models for workers and for consumers and the EUSES 2.1 fate model for predicting the environmental concentrations. Chesar can also be used in assessments based on other exposure estimation tools or measured data; however, no automated calculation of exposure estimates can be performed in these cases, and the exposure data should be introduced manually.

Qualitative risk characterization approaches are used when hazards are identified for a substance but the information does not permit setting predicted no-effect levels. In these cases Chesar supports ES building with qualitative risk characterization.

The main aim of Chesar is to increase the efficiency when conducting CSAs under REACH and to provide consistency between CSAs and the information communicated to downstream users, with the automated generation of CSRs and ESs.

Chesar facilitates the reuse (or update) of assessment elements generated in Chesar or imported from external sources, and has considered developments by industry, such as generic exposure scenarios (GESs) or specific environmental release categories (SpERCs). It also enables the use of the phrase catalog and the information exchange format for ESs that have been developed under Cefic's ESCom project.

Chesar Workflows

Chesar is divided into seven major groups of functionalities called Boxes. All Boxes are connected and contribute to the generation of the CSR and/or the ES for the extended SDS:

- **Box 1: Manage substance.** It is used for importing the hazard information from the IUCLIC dossier. This includes the conclusions from the hazard assessment, directly determining the scope of exposure assessment and the type of required risk characterization (qualitative or quantitative). Chesar is used once the hazard assessment according to Annex I of REACH has been finalized, and consequently all the information related to those substances' intrinsic properties (single end-point summaries and overall toxicological and ecotoxicological summaries) needed for the exposure assessment and risk characterization is available in IUCLID. This information is imported into Chesar with the Box 1 functionalities, which also allow import and export of full CSAs, e.g., for exchange with other assessors.
- **Box 2: Use management.** Here the uses of the substance are described in a structured way to ensure consistency between use description, the exposure assessments, and the exposure scenario building. The information is presented using Chesar's life-cycle tree structure, reporting the relevant uses of the substance, considering human health and environmental aspects as well as the tonnage breakdown to the different uses. For each use one environmental contributing scenario is automatically created. Other contributing scenarios for human health and for the environment can be created in addition. The labels (names), the appropriate set of use descriptors according to REACH, and further specifications are included here to be used later on for setting a default conservative exposure assessment. This Chesar element also allows import or export of CSA building blocks (life-cycle tree or parts of it with corresponding exposure assessment).
- **Box 3: Assessment management.** One or more quantitative exposure assessments for each contributing scenario are conducted here. Chesar allows the selection of different exposure assessment methods, while the route/types of effects (for humans) and environmental compartments to be covered have been determined when importing the hazard conclusions from IUCLID in Box 1. Depending on the substance properties and the uses, the plugged in exposure estimation tools could be sufficient or not to demonstrate that the expected exposure is lower than the no-effect thresholds (the DNELs for human effects and the

 http://dx.doi.org/10.1016/B978-0-12-386454-3.00548-0

PNECs in the case of environmental assessments). Additional assessment methods may be needed in some cases, for example when the uses or the specific use conditions are not covered by the plugged-in tools included in Chesar, or when even after considering all refinement options, Chesar predicts an unacceptable level of risk (exposure exceeding the derived no-effect levels). In such situations other exposure assessment methods or measured data should be included manually to demonstrate a safe use. Alternatively, additional risk management options or significant changes in the operational conditions may be considered. Chesar supports the systematic and transparent manual reporting of such assessments.

- **Box 4: CSR management.** In this part the final exposure scenarios are built by consolidating the assessments carried for the contributing scenarios conducted in Box 3. At this stage hazards without DNELs or PNECs are also taken into account, and appropriate conditions of use are added, if needed to reach a sufficient level of exposure minimization for these hazards. Chesar offers quantitative and qualitative approaches as appropriate for completing the risk characterization. The justifications and final assessment can be clarified by entering explanations on single exposure scenarios or on the overall assessment approach. These explanations will be transferred automatically to the Chemical Safety Report. In Box 4 it is also possible to report risk management measures that are applicable to all uses, and do not result from the exposure assessment carried out for each specific use.
- **Box 5: SDS ES management.** It covers the establishment of the exposure scenarios for communicating the information to downstream users. These scenarios are meant to transport selected parts of the information documented in the Chemical Safety Report to the users. The exposure scenarios are expected to be use-specific and to describe how the substance can be safely used. This includes operational conditions and risk management measures. The scenarios are identified by a short title, which should enable the user of the substance to identify whether the exposure scenario contains information relevant to him. The short titles of the exposure scenarios for a substance shall be consistent with the brief general description of uses in IUCLID. The information should allow downstream users to establish whether or not they work within the conditions for which a safe use has been demonstrated by the registrant in the CSA. (Note that Box 5 is currently not available in Chesar 2.0.)
- **Box 6: Library management.** Box 6 includes the functionalities of the Chesar library. The library enables creation, storage, import, and export of objects that the assessor may need in his Chemical Safety Assessment work process. Chesar 2.0 can manage two library objects: Determinant Types and SpERCs. In the context of Chesar, a 'Determinant' is a condition or measure driving the exposure of a substance to man or the environment, for example, the amount of substance used per day at a site, or local exhaust ventilation (LEV) installed at a workplace. A 'Determinant Type' is a set of information systematically characterizing a determinant (including metadata) and defining the values it could take. SpERCs are used for environmental assessments. They correspond to sets of information describing specific conditions of use and the corresponding release estimates (to water, air, soil and waste). These library objects are meant to be used across various assessments, contributing to the harmonization and efficiency of the assessments conducted under REACH.
- **Box 7: User management.** Box 7 covers those aspects related to the user and role management. For example users can use this section for assigning a legal entity to objects created in the library, identifying the author (and therefore the source) of the object.

Exposure Assessments in Chesar

The exposure assessment under REACH is required for hazardous substances (those classified according to the CLP/GHS criteria) and for PBT/vPvB substances. The exposure assessment should present a quantitative or qualitative estimate of the dose/concentration of the substance to which humans and the environment are or may be exposed. The exposure assessment is expected to be an interactive process, but the reporting process for REACH registration is limited to the last step, once the use is considered safe by the registrant, and should include the description of use conditions proposed for ensuring a safe use. Chesar implements these fundamental principles, but may be also used for exchanging preliminary results among registrants and within the supply change.

Exposure assessment under REACH includes two elements. The first element is the characterization/definition of the operational conditions and risk management measures for the identified uses; based on this first step, the exposure to humans and to the environment occurring under these conditions should be predicted as a second element of the exposure assessment. The exposure assessment results are used later on during the risk characterization process.

Quantitative risk assessments require quantitative exposure estimates, and those are generated in Chesar Box 3. The identification of operational conditions and risk management measures driving this exposure estimation is an essential element for these quantitative exposure assessments.

Based on Box 3 results, the final exposure scenarios are built in Box 4, considering also the integration of conditions and measures needed to control risks from hazards for which a qualitative exposure assessment is considered.

Human Exposure Assessment

The human exposure assessment estimates the expected exposure for workers and consumers and the indirect exposure via the environment of the general population.

For workers, two exposure assessment methods are available, the ECETOC TRA workers v3 method and the exposure assessment based on measured data. In addition, Chesar allows the use of external exposure estimation tools, which results are later manually incorporated to be reported in the CSA.

The ECETOC Targeted Risk Assessment (TRA) tool consists of three separate models for estimating exposures to workers, consumers, and the environment that arise during a series of events (ESs). Version 3 of the workers model has been incorporated in Chesar and includes a number of enhancements for increasing the overall accuracy and utility of the ECETOC tool, while still ensuring that the information and skill requirements necessary to develop the associated exposure predictions remain compatible with Tier 1 expectations.

The ECETOC TRA workers plugged-in tool covers three routes of exposure: inhalation acute exposure, inhalation long-term exposure, and dermal long-term exposure. In all three cases, local and/or systemic effects can be assessed.

In order to run the ECETOC TRA tool, information on the substance properties (e.g., molecular weight, physical state of the substance, vapor pressure if liquid) is needed for estimating the exposure concentrations. The assumptions are defined by the use conditions (e.g., the assigned Product Category (PROC)) and a PROC has to be assigned to the selected contributing scenario.

The default exposure assessment with ECETOC TRA workers is based on the conditions of use representing worst case assumptions.

Additional information on the ECETOC TRA approach is available in the ECETOC Technical Reports and in the user guidance document.

The exposure estimation based on measured data requires the manual introduction for each route of all exposure estimation data (exposure value, units, and explanations on the source and representativity of those values). In addition, the conditions of use associated to the measured data set should be introduced. If the exposure estimates based on measured data will be used as key information for the risk characterization (not just as supportive information), determinant types for the use conditions should be created in the library under Box 6; to ensure that the related conditions of use are part of the ES.

Chesar allows the incorporation of exposure estimates obtained using external exposure estimation tools. Commonly used tools (e.g., Stoffenmanager for workers) can be directly selected from a pop-up window, but other tools can be used with a proper explanation. All exposure estimations data (exposure values, units, and explanations on the exposure value if relevant) have to be manually entered for each route. In addition, relevant determinants reporting the conditions of use should be added and transferred to the ES. Standard sets of determinants corresponding to the input parameters of the tool can be used. Chesar allows exposure estimation tool owners to provide sets of determinants in the appropriate Chesar format.

Similar exposure assessment methods are considered for consumers estimations, although the ECETOC TRA for consumer is not available in Chesar 2.0 and will be made available in Chesar 2.1.

Regarding the indirect human exposure via the environment, these calculations are part of the environmental exposure assessment described as follows.

Environmental Exposure Assessment

The environmental protection targets considered in Chesar are aquatic and sediment dwelling organisms (freshwater and marine), predators in the aquatic food chain (freshwater and marine), sewage treatment plant functioning, agricultural soil organisms, predators in the terrestrial food chain, and air. In addition, exposure estimates are generated for intakes by humans via the environment, estimating the concentration of substance in air, drinking water, and different food items (e.g., root crops, dairy products, meat, and fish).

Chesar allows two complementary assessment types: the 'Measured Data Assessment' when there is good quality information on the environmental exposure levels for one or more environmental protection targets, and the 'EUSES Assessments' where the exposure is estimated on the basis of selected scenarios.

In the EUSES Assessments, exposure concentrations in the different environmental compartments are estimated by combining the expected or measured release rates to water, air, and soil with the EUSES 2.1 fate model.

Chesar offers four possibilities for setting the release rates to each environmental compartment:

- Default release estimations based on the **Environmental Release Categories (ERC-based release estimations)** for any of the release route: water, air, and soil. This is the release method selected by default and corresponds to a worst case estimate of release under the assumption that no specific risk management measures have been put in place.
- Targeted estimations based on Specific Environmental Release Category **(SpERC-based release estimations)** describing the expected release under specific conditions of use and the corresponding release estimates to water, air, soil, and waste, covering all release routes.
- Ad hoc **release factors** for water, air, and/or soil (reported as the percentage of the daily tonnage released to each compartment). An explanation and justification giving details on the source and quality of these release factors must be provided.
- **Measured release** for water and air for the local release rate (kg/day) for each release route. In addition to the release rate, an explanation and justification giving details on the source for these measured release values should be provided.

Based on the outcome of these release estimations, Chesar estimates the exposure for the relevant compartments according to the EUSES 2.1 fate model. The EUSES 2.1 fate model uses a set of default parameters and assumptions, which can be modified and adapted to more realistic conditions.

The exposure assessment for uses at industrial sites and wide dispersal uses differ from each other, and these conditions are systematically differentiated in Chesar.

Uses at industrial sites are assessed for one generic representative site per use. It is assumed that a certain tonnage is used at this one single generic site and that a certain fraction of the use tonnage at this site is released (depending on the conditions of use). As explained above, the release factor depends on the operational conditions and risk management assumed for the generic site. As there may be very large and very small industrial sites for one use, two contributing scenarios (or even the definition of two different uses) may be needed to reflect the difference in conditions and tonnage. By default it is assumed that the discharge from the site is treated in a municipal sewage treatment plant (STP) and the STP sludge is applied to agricultural soil. In addition, it is assumed that the tonnage released from the site is diluted in the sewage system and further by an additional dilution factor when the sewage is discharged into the receiving river water. The Chesar plug-in tool has incorporated the default values and assumptions used in the EUSES fate model, these assumptions can be changed in Chesar if needed.

For wide dispersal uses it is assumed that the market tonnage is evenly distributed in space and time. The assessment is carried out for a standard town with 10 000 inhabitants and a corresponding use tonnage (fraction of the market tonnage). Thus wide dispersal uses are those uses that correspond to consumer activities, services in a municipality or housing. Depending on the conditions of use, a certain fraction of this tonnage is assumed to be released to the sewage system. It is also assumed that the tonnage released from the 10 000 inhabitants is diluted within the 2000 m^3 of wastewater generated by this population (average of 200 l of wastewater per person and day) and then by a generic additional factor of 10 in the receiving river water. By default it is assumed that the STP-sludge is applied to agricultural soil. Usually, the assessor will define one contributing scenario per use and will not overwrite the default assumptions on the local conditions for a substance marketed across Europe. The releases from all uses into the municipal sewage system are aggregated to derive an exposure estimate.

The Predicted Environmental Concentrations (PECs) for the generic site or generic town are estimated taking into account the so-called 'local concentrations' (Clocal) and 'regional concentrations.' The regional concentration results from all the uses of a substance and is calculated by EUSES in the background. The regional concentration is added to the local concentration for deriving the local PEC, in order to take into account that a single site or a single town do not discharge into a virgin environment but just add to emissions released by other site or towns. Measured regional concentrations for one or several compartments can also be reported in Chesar. When measured concentrations are reported they are automatically used as regional concentrations (overwriting the EUSES estimates), and thus also impact on the local PECs for each contributing scenario. Consequently, only very reliable regional concentrations should be reported.

For substances considered to be PBT or vPvB, only local concentrations for water are provided. This is due to the large uncertainties of the regional estimations that should predict the fate, distribution, and long-term effects of such substances in the environment, in particular regarding accumulation in the food chain.

Detailed explanations of environmental exposure assessment are available in the Guidance on Information Requirements and Chemical Safety Assessment Chapter R16: Environmental Exposure estimation and in the EUSES user manual and supplementary information.

See also: Society for Chemical Hazard Communication (SCHC); Derived Minimal Effect Level (DMEL); Derived No-Effect Level (DNEL); IUCLID (International Uniform Chemical Information Database); Predicted No Effect Concentration (PNEC); REACH; Chemical Safety Assessment; Risk Management Measures (RMM).

Further Reading

ECETOC, 2004. Technical Report No 93: Targeted Risk Assessment. Available at: http://www.ecetoc.org/tra.

ECETOC, 2009. Technical Report No 107: Addendum to TR 93(2009). Available at: http://www.ecetoc.org/tra.

ECETOC, 2012. Technical Report No 114: ECETOC TRAv3: Background and Rationale for the Improvements. Available at: http://www.ecetoc.org/tra.

ECHA, 2008. Guidance on Information Requirements and Chemical Safety Assessment. Available at: http://guidance.echa.europa.eu/guidance_en.htm.

ECHA, 2012. Chesar User Manuals. Available at: http://chesar.echa.europa.eu/web/chesar/support/manuals-tutorials.

EC-JRC, 2012. EUSES User Manual. Available at: http://ihcp.jrc.ec.europa.eu/our_activities/public-health/risk_assessment_of_Biocides/euses/EUSES_2.1/EUSES_2.1_documentation/EUSES_2.1_User_Manual.pdf.

Relevant Websites

http://chesar.echa.europa.eu/ – Chesar, home page.

http://www.ecetoc.org/tra – European Centre for Ecotoxicology and Toxicology of Chemicals Target Risk Assessment consumer tool.

http://www.ecetoc.org/tra – European Centre for Ecotoxicology and Toxicology of Chemicals Target Risk Assessment worker tool.

http://echa.europa.eu – ECHA, European Chemicals Agency.

http://ihcp.jrc.ec.europa.eu/our_activities/public-health/risk_assessment_of_Biocides/euses – European Union System for the Evaluation of Substances, home page.

Chemicals in Consumer Products

L Molander, Stockholm University, Stockholm, Sweden

Chemicals in Consumer Products – A Global Concern

Production of Chemicals and Consumer Products is Increasing

During the second half of the twentieth century, the global chemical production increased from around 7 million tons to over 400 million tons per year, and it is expected to continue to grow. In 2001, the Organisation for Economic Co-operation and Development (OECD) calculated that global chemical production would show an 85% increase between 1995 and 2020. It is estimated that over 100 000 chemical substances are commercially available on the global market. Chemical production has to a large extent shifted from the OECD countries to low-income countries and economies in transitions, mainly to Brazil, Russia, India, and China, over the last decade.

One important explanation for the increasing production of chemicals is the rapidly increasing production of consumer products, such as textiles, toys, and electrical and electronic equipment. The international trade with products has tripled since the 1970s.

Chemicals are present in products for different reasons. They can, for example, be used as constituents for the manufacturing of materials, such as plastics, or added to the material for it to achieve certain functions or properties. Examples of such chemicals are perfluorinated compounds (PFCs), which are water and grease repelling, and phthalates, which are used as plasticizers. Other applications include the treatment of products with biocides and finishing with paints and lacquers. Traces of chemical substances used in the manufacturing process may unintentionally remain in the finished product where they no longer serve any purpose.

The increasing production of consumer products is closely related to our lifestyles. As our way of living and consuming has changed much during the last 50 years, chemical exposure has also changed. There has been a shift from exposure to a limited number of substances, mainly in the occupational setting, to exposure to numerous chemicals at the same time, where indoor environments and food have become important sources.

The Life Cycle Perspective

Chemicals can be released from consumer products during all steps of the life cycle – manufacturing, use, waste handling and disposal, and recycling – thereby posing a potential risk to human health and the environment.

During the use phase, chemicals can be released from products through leakage of additive substances, washing and wearing, or via the formation of small particles. Humans and nontarget organisms in the environment may subsequently be exposed via several different routes. Humans can be orally exposed via food and drink, for example, to chemicals that have migrated from food contact materials. Chemicals that come into contact with the skin may result in dermal absorption. Human exposure also occurs via inhalation of particles in air and dust. Organic chemicals, such as brominated flame retardants (BFRs) which can be released from electronic devices and textile products, have been found to accumulate in indoor dust. Children who spend much time close to the floor are especially exposed to chemicals in dust.

Even if the chemical emission from a single type of product may be insignificant, the total emission of one chemical from several sources or the combined emissions of several chemicals may be important sources to human exposure and environmental pollution. Emissions from consumer products incorporated or treated with hazardous chemicals may result in long-term exposure to humans and the environment. However, knowledge about the mechanisms involved in the diffuse emissions of substances from products and consequent exposures of humans and the ambient environment is currently insufficient.

The fast turnover of consumer products leads to increased resource consumption, generates massive amounts of wastes, and prompts the need for safe and efficient recycling. Hazardous substances in waste may be released and pose risks via incineration or landfills as well as in the recycling process. Risks to human health and the environment are difficult to assess due to the lack of information about the presence of hazardous substances in consumer products. The information that is available is often not disseminated from producers and importers to the waste stage. Thus, hazardous chemicals may be reintroduced to the market via reused and recycled products and materials.

Manufacturing of many materials and consumer products that are sold and consumed on the EU or US markets takes place in countries having less restrictive and comprehensive chemical rules for protecting human health and the environment. The manufacturing of consumer products may therefore result in high occupational exposures and environmental releases of dangerous chemicals. Another stage of the life cycle chain closely associated with health and environmental problems in low-income countries is the waste stage. A recognized problem is that waste electrical and electronic equipment is being exported to countries where there are few risk management measures in place for minimizing negative impacts of its chemical content on human health or the environment.

Association with Adverse Outcomes

Humans of all ages, including children, unborn babies, and other sensitive subpopulations, are continuously exposed to multiple chemicals at the same time, many of which are commonly used in consumer products.

Biomonitoring studies of human chemical exposure have found that numerous chemicals representing different chemical classes are present in the human body at various levels.

 http://dx.doi.org/10.1016/B978-0-12-386454-3.00452-8

These include chemicals commonly incorporated in, and known to be released from, consumer products, such as BFRs, PFCs, bisphenol A, and phthalates as well as banned but still widespread persistent environmental contaminants, for example, polychlorinated biphenyls. Analyses conducted on blood samples from three generations in 13 EU member states showed, for example, that BFRs are detected in higher levels and more frequently in the blood of younger generations than in older generations. Research on male reproductive health conducted in Denmark and Finland has indicated a relationship between levels of a group of BFRs, polybrominated diphenyl ethers, in mothers' breast milk and cryptorchidism in their sons, that is, the testes have not descended in the scrotum by the time of birth.

Significant adverse effects of a number of chemicals used in consumer products are reported from both *in vitro* and *in vivo* toxicity and ecotoxicity experimental studies, but many relationships remain to be supported by epidemiological studies. However, it is very difficult to link health impacts to exposure to a specific substance, or a mixture of substances, in epidemiological studies due to statistical constraints and the many confounding factors. As the assessment of health and environmental impacts of chemicals involves many complex parameters and uncertainties, assessments are sometimes subject to both scientific and policy debates. Current such topics include the reliability and relevance of so-called low-dose effects (different definitions of *low-dose* exist, but often it refers to doses below the no observed adverse effect level or to doses in the range of typical human or environmental exposures) of endocrine-disrupting chemicals (EDCs) reported in experimental studies for human health risk assessment, mixture toxicity and risks of nanomaterials.

Risk Reduction Strategies

Both regulatory and voluntary strategies are used for managing health and environmental risks posed by hazardous chemicals emitted from consumer products. These may include bans or restrictions on certain substances, mixtures, or uses, requirements such as to disseminate information, and economic incentives for promoting substitution of hazardous chemicals to safer alternatives.

Regulatory Instruments

While some chemical sectors are relatively well regulated, regulations of industrial chemicals, and in particular the use of chemicals in consumer products, have been criticized for not being protective enough with regard to human health and the environment.

In the last decade, the EU chemicals legislation has essentially been completely renewed. When the industrial chemicals legislation REACH (Registration, Evaluation, Authorisation, and restriction of CHemicals) went into force on 1 June 2007, it replaced about 40 pieces of chemicals legislation. Important reasons behind the development of REACH were that data on chemical properties should be required for all industrial chemicals, despite the date of their entry to the market, as well as shifting the responsibility for assessing the safety of the chemicals from authorities to the chemical producers and importers.

The trade with consumer products is global and thus chemicals control within the EU affects and is affected by international conditions. The US national chemicals legislation, the Toxic Substances Control Act (TSCA), is also currently under debate concerning its renewal. The Safe Chemicals Act of 2011 is being proposed as a law for addressing problems identified with TSCA. It aims, for example, to improve the safety of chemicals used in consumer products and to increase public access to information on chemical safety.

Increasingly more of the production of consumer products is located in areas with fast economic growth, such as parts of Asia and Latin America, where chemicals control is less restrictive than in the EU. China is an important producer and supplier of consumer products to the northwestern part of the world. As a response to the regulatory gap created by the introduction of REACH, Chinese chemicals regulations were revised in 2010 and 2011 in order to improve human health and environmental protection and to overcome trade barriers. In the case of electrical and electronic equipment, the EU directive on Restriction of the use of certain Hazardous Substances (RoHS) has led to the implementation of similar legislations in other parts of the world. The EU RoHS Directive has thereby contributed to a more protective standard on hazardous substances in electronics on a global level.

A central problem in chemicals control is that data on toxicological and ecotoxicological properties are lacking or are too insufficiently required for many chemicals for enabling a robust health or environmental risk assessment. In the EU, what data are required by REACH to be submitted to the European Chemicals Agency (ECHA) is volume dependent; the higher the production volume of the substance, the more information about the substance is required. For chemical substances produced or imported in less than 1 ton per year no data are required, and for substances in the tonnage band between 1 and 10 tons the data requirements are very limited. This has the implication that a great number of chemicals cannot be adequately risk assessed or classified according to the hazard criteria as set out in the European regulation on classification, labeling, and packaging of substances and mixtures (CLP). The CLP hazard classifications are central in EU chemicals policy as they are often used as a basis for priority of substances for restrictions and requirements.

Another problematic issue for risk assessment and risk management is that information about the chemical content of consumer products is rarely available to regulators, professional buyers, or consumers. The assessment of health and environmental risks associated with the use of chemicals in consumer products is thus often hampered by the lack of important information.

The candidate list under REACH is the basis for the authorization process and a tool for increasing and disseminating information on the presence of substances of very high concern (SVHCs) in products, particularly in the supply chain, but also to consumers upon request. Since many supply chains are global, the information requirements connected to the SVHCs will have impacts also outside the EU. As the candidate list is regularly updated, it has been identified to promote chemical companies to work proactively with substitution and to find out the chemical content of their products. However, considering the large number of chemicals in commercial use, the authorization and information requirements currently apply only to a very small share of the chemicals on the EU market; approximately 0.1% has been identified as an SVHC. Decisions on what risk management measures to take, for example, what substances to select for authorization, is not solely based on health or environmental risk assessment conclusions, but also takes into account political, social, economic, and technological implications, including the availability of feasible and less toxic substitute substances.

Voluntary Approaches

To accelerate the work towards achieving a safe and sustainable use of chemicals in consumer products, voluntary approaches can be used to complement regulatory restrictions and bans. Such approaches include, for example, different kinds of information efforts.

Common voluntary information instruments are targeted information campaigns or positive labeling. These may increase the receivers' knowledge and perception of hazards and risks, and potentially lead to changes in attitudes and behavior. Consumers who are provided with information about content of hazardous chemicals in products in a user-friendly format may thus change their consumption patterns. Increased knowledge will enable consumers and purchasers, for example, in procurement, to make more informed choices, take precautionary actions, and ask for alternatives. This will put pressure on producers and suppliers of consumer products and may ultimately lead to the phase-out of chemicals with unwanted properties.

Along with the increasingly global trade of consumer products, the need for international cooperation increases with regard to the management of associated chemicals risks. The United Nation's Strategic Approach to International Chemicals Management (SAICM) is an international policy framework, which has identified chemicals in products as an 'emerging policy issue.' The overall aim of SAICM is to achieve the goal agreed upon in Johannesburg in 2002 at the World Summit on Sustainable Development that by 2020 chemicals should be "used and produced in ways that lead to minimization of significant adverse effects of human health and the environment." An important step toward this goal is that all actors, including consumers, have increased access to information on chemicals in products throughout the products' entire life cycle, including the waste stage.

Economic instruments have proven to sometimes constitute effective incentives for reaching environmental goals. The use of economic incentives such as taxes and fees has, however, been practiced only to a limited extent for minimizing the use of hazardous or untested chemicals. Internationally, existing chemicals control through economic incentives mainly concerns waste, packaging, and single substances. The use of economic instruments for managing risks associated with the use of chemicals in different consumer products is also possible, although it is more complicated than for single substances. The challenge is due to the limited knowledge of which products contain hazardous chemicals and in what concentrations.

Urgent Problems and Challenges

Emerging issues with regard to chemicals in consumer products include the need to increase the requirements on the generation of effect and exposure data, information on the chemical content of products, and information dissemination in the supply chain. This will facilitate substitution of hazardous chemicals to safer alternatives and enable supply chain actors and other stakeholders to improve the management of risks.

Furthermore, the life cycle perspective in chemicals control needs to be extended. To obtain improved resource efficiency and a sustainable development, it is necessary to minimize the input of hazardous chemicals into products. The majority of the commercially available chemicals are not restricted for use in consumer products, including substances that are considered especially hazardous, such as carcinogens, mutagens, and reprotoxicants; EDCs; persistent, bioaccumulative, and toxic substances; and strongly sensitizing chemicals. Lack of protective legislations can cause problems in all life cycle stages of a product. It has therefore been urged that hazardous chemicals should be avoided already at the stage of production. The EU environmental policy states that environmental damage should be rectified at source and that preventive and precautionary actions should be taken. Translated into the context of chemicals in consumer products, those principles could arguably hold that the input of hazardous chemicals into products should be avoided or minimized in order to prevent problems from arising at the end of pipe, such as difficulties in achieving environmental and health goals.

See also: Bisphenol A; Polybrominated Diphenyl Ethers; Surfactants, Perfluorinated; Mixtures, Toxicology, and Risk Assessment; Toy Safety and Hazards; Hazardous Waste; Import/Export of Hazardous Chemicals; Risk Management; Candidate List of Substances of Very High Concern (SVHC), REACH; Environmental Risk Assessment, Cosmetic and Consumer Products; The European Classification and Labeling (C&L) Inventory; Electronic Waste; Risk Assessment, Uncertainty; REACH; Chemical Safety Assessment; Environmental Life Cycle Assessment; PBT (Persistent, Bioaccumulative, and Toxic) Chemicals; Strategic Approach to International Chemicals Management (SAICM); Phthalates; Toxic Substances Control Act; Green Chemistry.

Further Reading

Articles

Beronius, A., Rudén, C., Håkansson, H., Hanberg, A., 2010. Risk to all or none? A comparative analysis of controversies in the health risk assessment of bisphenol A. Reprod. Toxicol. 29, 132–146.

Hansson, S.O., Molander, L., Rudén, C., 2011. The substitution principle. Regul. Toxicol. Pharmacol. 59, 454–460.

Molander, L., Rudén, C., 2012. Narrow-and-sharp or broad-and-blunt – regulations of hazardous chemicals in consumer products in the European Union. Regul. Toxicol. Pharmacol. 62, 523–531.

Molander, L., Breitholtz, M., Andersson, P.L., Rybacka, A., Rudén, C., 2012. Are chemicals in articles an obstacle for reaching environmental goals? – Missing links in EU chemical management. Sci. Total Environ. 435–436, 280–289.

Ruden, C., Hansson, S.O., 2010. Registration, Evaluation, and Authorization of Chemicals (REACH) is but a first step – how far will it take us? Six further steps to improve the European chemicals legislation. Environ. Health Perspect. 118 (1), 6–10.

Tsydenova, O., Bengtsson, M., 2011. Chemical hazards associated with treatment of waste electrical and electronic equipment. Waste Manag. 31, 45–58.

Reports

Centers for Disease Control and Prevention (CDC), 2009. Fourth National Report on Human Exposure to Environmental Chemicals. Available at: http://www.cdc.gov/exposurereport (accessed 17.06.2013).

Massey, R.I., Hutchins, J.G., Becker, M., Tickner, J., 2008. Toxic Substances in Articles: The Need for Information. The Nordic Council of Ministers, Copenhagen. TemaNord, p. 596.

WHO/UNEP, 2013. The State-of-the-Science of Endocrine Disrupting Chemicals – 2012 (Bergman, Å., Heindel, J.J., Jobling, S., Kidd, K.A., Zoeller, R.T., eds). ISBN: 978 92 4 150503 1.

Relevant Websites

http://www.saicm.org – Strategic Approach to International Chemicals Management (SAICM), 2012. Introducing SAICM (accessed 17.06.2013).

http://echa.europa.eu/web/guest/regulations/reach – European Chemicals Agency (ECHA), 2013. REACH (accessed 17.06.2013).

Chemicals of Environmental Concern

MM Schultz, The College of Wooster, Wooster, OH, USA

This article is a revision of the previous edition article by Steve J. D'Surney and Mike D. Smith, volume 1, pp 526–530, © 2005, Elsevier Inc.

Introduction

Chemicals of environmental concern are any physical, chemical, biological, or radiological substance or matter that has an adverse effect on air, water, soil, or living organisms. A reasonable definition of a pollutant is a substance present in greater than normal concentration as a result of human activity and having a detrimental effect on its environment or on something of value in that environment. Contaminants, which are not classified as pollutants unless they have some detrimental effect, cause deviations from the normal composition of an environment. Pollutants can enter through direct dumping, piped outflow, and channeled waste streams as localized point sources, or as diffuse nonpoint sources they can enter rivers, lakes, streams, and groundwater through runoff and soil percolation. Nonpoint sources are considered to be major contributors to air, water, and soil pollution that include runoff from paved streets and parking lots, agricultural lots, soil erosion from logging, and atmospheric deposition of acidic or toxic air pollutants. The source is particularly important, because it is the logical place to eliminate pollution. Common sources of contaminants to the environment include mining and mineral processing, fossil fuel combustion, agricultural and forestry, industrial production, and consumerism (**Table 1**). After a pollutant is released from a source, it may act on a receptor. The receptor is anything, both biotic and abiotic, that is affected by the pollutant. Humans whose eyes water from atmospheric oxidants are receptors. Juvenile trouts that die after exposure to pesticides in water are also receptors. Eventually, if the pollutant is long lived, it may be deposited in a long-term sink such as aquatic sediments and soils.

Table 1 Common sources of contaminants to the environment

Sources	*Contaminants*
Mining and mineral processing	Heavy metals, chemicals via cyanide and acids, hydrocarbon products resulting from spills and coal mining, and metallic salts
Fossil fuel combustion	Sulfur dioxide, carbon dioxide, nitric oxide, ozone, acids, polycyclic aromatic hydrocarbons, and volatile organic compounds
Agriculture and forestry	Pesticides, nitrates, phosphates, greenhouse gases, and mineral salts
Industrial production	Numerous synthetic organic and inorganic compounds, organochlorines, dioxins, heavy metals, hydrocarbons, chlorinated phenols, sulfates, sulfides, surfactants, solvents, acids, bases, salts, pharmaceuticals, plastics, resins, explosives, and natural organics
Consumerism	Residential and commercial chemicals, pesticides, fertilizers, hydrocarbons, solvents, surfactants, paints, sealants, pharmaceuticals and personal care products, volatile organic compounds, resins, plastics, metals, salts, acids, and bases

Mineral and Energy Exploration

The largest quantitative source of contamination derives from mining and energy extraction. Mining and mineral processing use a variety of chemicals for extraction, ore processing, water treatment, and many other supporting activities such as overburden removal. Mining and energy extraction generate large volumes of waste and have the potential to cause a number of environmental problems if improperly managed. Water and soil degradation can result from salinization, acidification, and chemical contamination. Streams and rivers can also experience severe siltation. Coarse tailings and rock blasting produce large amounts of dust and mobilize heavy metal contaminants, such as lead, copper, aluminum, and zinc, which can leach into the surface and subsurface waters. Cyanide and mercury are used to extract gold from soil and pulverized rock. Mineral processing generates a great deal of particulate matter released from bauxite and coal processing. Acid leaching into soil, groundwater, and riparian environments from mine wastes is common. Acid drainage from mine tailings, ore, and waste dumps contains sulfur and sulfides such as iron sulfide, which can be converted to acids through bacterial oxidation in the presence of moisture and oxygen.

Metal contaminants may become mobilized under acidic conditions to cause potential health and environmental problems resulting from leaching into soil, water, and sediment. Acid mine drainage and slag leachate can contain high concentrations of heavy metals and acids. Sulfuric acid can be formed via oxidation of sulfides. As a great deal of attention is paid to the containment and remediation of acid mine drainage, the neutralization of acid pH usually results in the precipitation of many contaminants, usually as metallic salts. These salts would then become soluble and may enter surface and groundwater. Oil spills and coal mining command considerable attention from the media because they are often large scale and visually very dramatic. Nothing seems worse than a mass of toxic crude oil and tarry hydrocarbons smeared over the natural habitats of some foreshore or the sight of strip mining operations. As a result, there is a massive public response and a frenzy of activity by agencies, community groups, and politicians. There are demands for 'the environment to be saved.' Often, as in the case of large spills such as Exxon Valdez or Deepwater Horizon, very large sums of money change hands in order to mobilize whatever resources can be found to clean up the mess. For many spills, however, the ecological issues are different from those being touted in public discussion. There is, in fact, plenty of evidence that chronic, low-level contamination of habitats by complex exogenous agents may be more compromising in terms of environmental outcomes. In addition, coupled with the destruction, deterioration, and fragmentation of natural habitats, there exists considerably greater threats to long-term sustainability of coastal biodiversity. Attempts to disperse oil spills with surfactants may be potentially hazardous.

 http://dx.doi.org/10.1016/B978-0-12-386454-3.01004-6

Hydraulic fracturing, or more commonly known as fracking, has been used commercially since the 1940s to extract petroleum and natural gas from fractures in the Earth's rock layer that result from the injection of pressurized fracturing fluids. Proponents of hydraulic fracturing argue that this extraction process allows access to fossil fuels that are otherwise inaccessible. However, hydraulic fracturing has raised environmental and regulatory concerns. These concerns have included groundwater contamination and risks to air quality resulting from methane leaks originating from wells. Other toxic hydrocarbons, including benzene, xylene, and naphthalene, have also been detected in air and water near hydraulic fracturing sites. Additional environmental concerns with hydraulic fracturing include water consumption (especially in arid regions); migration of gases and hydraulic fracturing chemicals to the surface and subsequent contamination of surface waters and soil; waste disposal of flowback, which may include brines, heavy metals, radionuclides, and organic chemicals; and the health effects due to exposure of all these chemicals.

Fossil Fuel Combustion

Humanity's major sources of energy are derived from fossil fuels, principally oil, gas, coal, and wood. The major combustion by-products of fossil fuel burning include sulfur dioxide (SO_2), carbon dioxide (CO_2), and nitric oxide (NO_2), and partially oxidized hydrocarbons. The process of burning fossil fuels in thermal power plants, factories, homes, and motor vehicles emits enormous amounts of the aforementioned pollutants. The most important environmental concerns resulting from fossil fuel use are global climate change, acid rain, surface ozone, and particulate- and aerosol-bound toxins.

Over 97% of climate scientists agree in anthropogenic sources for climate change. A component of the climate warming observed since the 1880s is likely attributed to increases in the concentration of the 'greenhouse gases' such as the fossil fuel combustion product CO_2 in the atmosphere. Another side effect of fossil fuel burning is acid rain. In the process of burning organic fuels, some gases, in particular SO_2 and NO_2, combine with atmospheric water vapor to form sulfuric and nitric acids. Acidified rainwater can attain pH values below 3. Acid rain can cause damage to plant life, in some cases seriously affecting the growth of forests and lakes due to acid-stimulated metal leaching from soils and rock.

Besides gaseous fossil fuel emissions that contribute to global climate change and acid rain, emissions of particulate matter from incomplete burning also contribute to poor air quality. Coal burning and diesel engines are a major source of particulate organic particles. Additionally, fuel combustion and evaporative emissions from motor vehicles are also major sources of anthropogenic volatile organic compounds (VOCs). Motor vehicles account for a considerable fraction of the total emissions of nitrogen oxides, particulate hydrocarbons, and VOCs in developed countries. Of particular concern is the production of polycyclic aromatic hydrocarbons (PAHs) resulting from incomplete combustion of fossil fuels. These compounds, especially diesel soot emissions, contain some of the most potent mutagens and carcinogens known to humankind.

Compared with solid fossil fuels, natural gas and oil are less polluting. Natural gas is the least polluting fossil fuel. The main environmental problems resulting from the production and transportation of primary energy are related to mining of solid fuels (mainly coal) and oil transportation. Coal mining operations produce large amounts of slag wastes and result in acid water drainage. The continuous acid discharges from mines seriously affect aquatic ecosystems, since acid waters containing heavy concentrations of dissolved heavy metals will support only limited water flora, and will not sustain fish and many invertebrates. The major impacts from oil are associated with accidental spillages during transportation both at sea and on land. The resultant damage to coastal areas and marine life can be dramatic in the short term and may also have long-term consequences. Solid wastes and ash disposal (spoil tips) from coal mines lead to the contamination of water percolating through slag heaps that cause groundwater and soil pollution. The combustion of liquefied petroleum gas causes the problems of liquid residual disposal.

Agriculture and Forestry

The global concentration of greenhouse gases has increased measurably over the past 250 years, partly due to land use activities such as agriculture and forestry. According to the fourth assessment report of the Intergovernmental Panel on Climate Change, carbon dioxide, methane, and nitrous oxide emissions have increased by ~41, 149, and 16%, respectively, since 1750. Agriculture and forestry practices have contributed to trends in emissions of these greenhouse gases through fuel consumption, land use conversions, cultivation and fertilization of soil, production of ruminant livestock, and management of livestock manure. Additionally, the irrigation of formerly arid lands leaches minerals from soils at accelerated rates resulting in toxic concentrations of agricultural pollutants, which include nutrients (nitrogen and phosphorus), pesticides, pathogens, selenium, and salts. While farmers do not intend for these materials to move from the field or enterprise, they often do, carried by rainfall, snowmelt, or irrigation water. After passage of the Reclamation Act of 1902, the US government began building and subsidizing irrigation projects to foster settlement and development of the arid and semiarid areas of the western United States. A wide variety of pesticides are applied to agricultural crops to control insect pests (insecticides), weeds (herbicides), fungi (fungicides), and rodents (rodenticide). Pesticide residues reaching surface water systems may harm freshwater and marine organisms, damaging recreational and commercial fisheries. Pesticides in drinking water supplies may also pose risks to human health. Long-lived pesticides such as dichlorodiphenyltrichloroethane (DDT), aldrin, dieldrin, and mercuric and arsenic compounds still persist in the environment. Shorter lived pesticides such as chlorpyrifos, methyl parathion, 2,4-D herbicides, and numerous new compounds are a global concern. Atrazine, a commonly used, relatively short-lived herbicide (half-life in soil ranges from 13 to 261 days) in the United States, is at the center of a regulatory battle in the United States. It has been used in the United States for over 50 years and is primarily applied to corn and sorghum fields to increase their crop yields. Atrazine is banned in the European Union due to persistent groundwater contamination and because research has suggested that atrazine is an endocrine-disrupting chemical that induces the production of aromatase, an enzyme that converts androgens (male sex hormones) to estrogens (female sex hormones). Atrazine exposure has also been linked to birth defects, low birth weights, cancer, and fertility problems.

Industrial Production

The global expansion of industrial and consumer-oriented societies is linked to large-scale industrial production and consumerism that use a vast array of numerous chemical compounds. The listings of such chemicals are too vast to present here but some examples are discussed here. Environmental contaminants in nature typically involve complex mixtures, partitioning factors, chemical transformations, and abiotic and biotic interactions. The biological and environmental effects are complex and may be additive, synergistic, and even antagonistic in nature. Pulp and paper mill sludge is a complex and changeable mixture of dozens or even hundreds of compounds. Some are well known, like natural wood extractives, organochlorines, organosulfides, and dioxins. Priority pollutants and chemicals of concern that must be analyzed in pulp mill residues include heavy metals, chlorinated hydrocarbons, chlorobenzenes, PAHs, chlorinated phenols, chlorinated catechols, chlorinated guaiacols, phthalates, resin acids, alkylphenols and alkylphenol ethoxylates, and plant sterols.

In 1775, PAHs were the first group of compounds known to cause cancer in humans. Nowadays, many of these compounds are well-known carcinogens in humans and animals. PAHs are produced in the environment as the result of heating organic matter to high temperatures like tobacco smoke, soot, coal tar, creosote production, wood burning, smoked foods, roasted coffee, charbroiled meat, and fossil fuel combustion exhaust. However, the major environmental source comes from asphalt, tar, used motor oil, diesel exhaust, and coal burning. Dioxins, a by-product of herbicide and pulp and paper production, are highly toxic members of a class of organochlorine chemicals including polychlorinated dibenzo-*p*-dioxins (PCDDs), polydibenzofurans (PCDFs), polychlorinated biphenyls (PCBs), polybrominated dibenzo-*p*-dioxins (PBDDs), polybrominated dibenzofurans (PBDFs), and polychlorinated pesticides. Dioxins and its related compounds are cytotoxic and genotoxic, and have hormonal effects that may disrupt the endocrine system and cellular signaling pathways in wildlife and humans. Dioxins have both estrogenic and antiestrogenic effects, depending on the organ or tissue affected. Exposure to relatively low levels of these chemicals has had catastrophic effects on populations of Beluga whales, alligators, turtles, mink, otters, bald eagles, osprey, cormorants, terns, herring gulls, migratory birds, chickens, lake trout, chinook and coho salmon, etc throughout the United States and Canada.

PCDFs are formed as inadvertent by-products in the production and use of PCBs, formerly used as an insulator in electrical transformers and, in combination with PCDDs, in the production of chlorophenols and have been detected as contaminants in these products. PCDFs and PCDDs also may be produced in thermal processes such as incineration and metal processing and in the bleaching of paper pulp with free chlorine. PCDFs are also found in residual waste from the production of vinyl chloride and the chloralkali process for chlorine production. The relative amounts of PCDF and PCDD congeners produced depend on the production or incineration process and vary widely.

Like PCDDs, PCDFs are ubiquitous in soil, sediments, and air. Excluding occupational or accidental exposures, most background human exposure to PCDFs occurs as a result of eating meat, milk, eggs, fish, and related products, as PCDFs are persistent in the environment and accumulate in animal fat. High exposures have occurred in relation to incidents in Japan (*yusho*) and Taiwan (*yucheng*) involving contamination of rice oil and in accidents involving electrical equipment containing PCBs. Occupational exposures also may occur in metal production and recycling, and in the production and use of chlorophenols and PCBs. Chemical wood preservatives account for the single largest pesticide use in the United States and one of the greatest pesticide threats to public health and the environment. Wood preservatives protect wood products from fungus and insect decay. The three principal wood preservatives include chromated copper arsenate (CCA), pentachlorophenol (penta), and creosote. The US Environmental Protection Agency (EPA) has classified many chemicals and even certain heavy metal contaminants as known or probable carcinogens, teratogens, cellular toxins, endocrine disrupters, and reproductive toxins. The arsenic in CCA, certain PAHs, and dioxins are known human carcinogens and are linked to disorders and birth defects.

Consumerism

Everything we put down the drain or flush down the drain ends up in our watersheds via wastewater treatment, which can affect the health of terrestrial and aquatic wildlife, plants, the atmosphere, and the water quality in our area. Large amounts of pharmaceuticals and personal care products (PPCPs) are released into the environmental every day through wastewater treatment by way of domestic waste from human excretion, direct disposal of unused or expired drugs in toilets, or rinsing of personal care products down the drain. Additional sources of consumer environmental contaminants include cleaning agents, surfactants, pesticides, fertilizers, lawn and garden treatments, paints, and sealants. It is imperative that those seeking a healthy lifestyle and reduction in pollutant exposure choose with care the products they use to clean and maintain their homes, yards, and pets. When one purchases a hazardous product for the home, it creates a market for these toxic chemicals. Once we use the hazardous substance, the vapors released or the water contaminated pose a risk to ecosystems and human populations alike.

Early examples of consumer-based environmental contaminants include the invention of chlorofluorocarbons (CFCs) in the late 1920s and early 1930s. CFCs were developed in response to the need for safer alternatives to the sulfur dioxide and ammonia refrigerants used at the time.

Chlorofluorocarbons were chosen for their safety and for their advantageous chemical properties. These compounds are low in toxicity, nonflammable, noncorrosive, and nonreactive with other chemical species, and have desirable thermal conductivity and boiling point characteristics. These features led to increased demand as more applications arose for CFC use. However, CFCs are human-made substances that release chlorine atoms which destroy ozone in the atmosphere, specifically in the stratosphere, which causes an increase in UV radiation at the ground level. The amount of CFCs produced (and therefore likely released into the atmosphere) steadily increased over several decades until an international agreement called the Montreal Protocol was signed in September 1987. In this agreement, the world's nations agreed to phase out CFC production. As a result, most stratospheric CFC concentrations have leveled off or are decreasing. To date, the Montreal Protocol is considered the most successful international environmental agreement.

In 1962, Rachel Carson's novel, *Silent Spring*, implicated pesticides such as DDT for the decline of some wildlife populations. Continued research in the late 1960s and 1970s discovered elevated use of manufactured organic chemicals in industrial and domestic applications. Chemicals of concern included PCBs, 2,3,7,8-tetrachloro-dibenzo-*p*-dioxin (TCDD), and related dioxin and furan congeners, PAHs, and various organic solvents. Regulatory efforts by the EPA and international efforts (e.g., Stockholm Convention of Persistent Organic Pollutants) resulted in a decreased production of these xenobiotics.

Consumerism and Chemicals of Emerging Environmental Concern

An active area of environmental research is in the area of 'emerging contaminants.' What is an emerging contaminant? Emerging contaminants are not only chemicals that have recently been released into the environment, but are broadly defined "as any synthetic or naturally occurring chemical or any microorganism that is not commonly monitored in the environment but has the potential to enter the environment and cause known or suspected adverse ecological and (or) human health effects." The majority of emerging contaminants differ from 'conventional' or 'historical' environmental chemicals of concern (e.g., pesticides, metals, PAHs, PCBs, dioxins) because many emerging contaminants are present in consumer products and are routinely used in households. Emerging contaminants encompass a wide variety of chemicals, including many pharmaceuticals and PPCPs. Examples of personal care products are fragrances, antimicrobial agents, sunscreens, and fluorescent whitening agents. As already mentioned, a primary route into the environment for PPCPs is via wastewater treatment, because many of these chemicals are flushed or rinsed down the drain and are not removed by conventional wastewater treatment. Since many of these PPCPs are biologically active, they may pose a risk to ecosystems and human populations alike. Since wastewater effluent often discharges to drinking water sources, there is the potential for drinking water to contain PPCPs. Recent studies provide evidence that PPCPs may contaminate drinking water, although it is currently unclear if the concentrations are significant enough to pose any risk to human health.

Many chemicals of emerging environmental concern are also potential endocrine-disrupting chemicals. An endocrine-disrupting chemical can be a natural or synthetic chemical that interferes with the hormonal system. Many of the previously discussed chemicals of concern are also classified as endocrine-disrupting chemicals, including DDT, PCBs, dioxins, and pesticides (e.g., dieldrin, atrazine, methoxychlor). Developing organisms are particularly vulnerable to the effects of the endocrine-disrupting chemicals. Exposure early in life (often during a critical or sensitive developmental period) to an endocrine-disrupting chemical can induce permanent, nonreversible effects. These effects often do present themselves until adolescence or adulthood as in the (unfortunate) case of diethylstilbestrol, more commonly known as DES. DES, a synthetic nonsteroidal estrogen, was prescribed to women during the 1940s–70s to prevent miscarriage. Although there have been few documented adverse effects in the mothers who took DES during their pregnancies, many of their daughters and sons who were exposed to DES *in utero* developed problems associated with their reproductive organs. Many daughters are sterile and a small percentage have developed a rare form of vaginal or cervical cancer. The prenatally exposed sons have an increased incidence of abnormalities in their sexual organs, decreased sperm counts, and a higher incidence of testicular cancer.

Suspected endocrine-disrupting chemicals are found in a wide variety of products, including insecticides, herbicides, fumigants, and fungicides that are used in agriculture as well as in the home. Other endocrine disruptors are found in industrial and consumer chemicals such as detergents, resins, plasticizers, organometals, halogenated aromatic hydrocarbons, monomers in many plastics, and PPCPs. Exposure to these chemicals occurs through direct contact in the workplace or at home, or through ingestion of contaminated water, food, or air. Substances that are considered both chemicals of emerging environmental concern and endocrine disruptors that are of regulatory concern to the EPA include polybrominated diphenyl ethers (PBDEs), long-chain perfluorinated chemicals (PFCs), short-chained chlorinated paraffins (SCCPs), phthalates, bisphenol-A (BPA), and triclosan. PBDEs are flame retardants that are used extensively in consumer products ranging from textiles to electronics. PFCs have widespread applications as liquid repellants for paper, packaging, textile, leather, and carpets, as well as in industrial solvents, additives, coatings, and fire-fighting foams. SCCPs, phthalates, and bisphenol-A are all used as plasticizers to increase the flexibility of the plastic material and are present in countless consumer products, including many children's toys. Triclosan is an antimicrobial additive in many personal care products that not only include antibacterial soaps, toothpaste, and mouthwash, but increasing use in household items including garden hoses, toys, cutting boards, and furniture.

Conclusions

The twentieth century has brought with it tremendous gains in science and technology as well as gains in the quality of human life and longevity. However, these gains have been accompanied by certain hazards, many associated with the 100 000 chemicals that are now commonly in use. As stated earlier, environmental contaminants are materials that can pollute our surroundings and adversely impact living organisms. Often these pollutants are chemical compounds produced by human endeavors, although environmental contamination can also come from nonhuman sources such as naturally occurring metals, animal waste, oil seeps, and algal blooms. Environmental contaminants may pollute soil, surface water, or aquatic sediments. Many compounds also leach through soils into groundwater, potentially impacting drinking water supplies. Numerous pollutants are discharged directly into the atmosphere by human industry, where winds may transport them to Earth's most remote corners. It is important, however, to note that industry is not the sole source of contaminants; individuals also contribute to this problem through the use of household pesticides and fertilizers, improper disposal of hazardous materials (e.g., used motor oil, paints, cleaning products), and by using many consumer products. Consequently, sites with one predominant contaminant are a rarity; complex mixtures and subsequent exposures define the real world.

See also: Atrazine; Bisphenol A; Carbon Dioxide; DDT (Dichlorodiphenyltrichloroethane); Estrogens IV: Estrogen-Like Pharmaceuticals; Perfluorooctanoic Acid; Persistent Organic Pollutants; Pesticides; Pharmaceuticals Effects in the Environment; Pollution Prevention Act, United States; Pollution, Air in Encyclopedia of Toxicology; Indoor Air Pollution; Pollution, Soil; Pollution, Water; Polybrominated Diphenyl Ethers; Polychlorinated Biphenyls (PCBs); Polycyclic Aromatic Hydrocarbons (PAHs); TCDD (2,3,7,8-Tetrachlorodibenzo-*p*-dioxin); Toxic Substances Control Act; Volatile Organic Compounds.

Further Reading

Daughton, C.G., Ternes, T.A., 1999. Pharmaceuticals and personal care products in the environment: agents of subtle change? Environ. Health Perspect. 107, 907–938.

Grossman, E., 2009. Chasing Molecules. Island Press, Washington.

Hites, R.A., 2011. Dioxins: an overview and history. Environ. Sci. Technol. 45, 16–20.

Kolpin, D.W., Furlong, E.T., Meyer, M.T., et al., 2002. Pharmaceuticals, hormones, and other organic wastewater contaminants in U.S. Streams, 1999–2000: a national reconnaissance. Environ. Sci. Technol. 36, 1202–1211.

Richardson, S.D., Ternes, T.A., 2011. Water analysis: emerging contaminants and current issues. Anal. Chem. 83, 4614–4648.

Snyder, S.A., Westerhoff, P., Yoon, Y., Sedlak, D.L., 2003. Pharmaceuticals, personal care products, and endocrine disruptors in water: implications for the water industry. Environ. Eng. Sci. 20, 449–469.

Steingraber, S., 2010. Living Downstream: An Ecologist's Personal Investigation of Cancer and the Environment, second ed. Da Capo Press, Philadelphia.

Relevant Websites

http://www.actio.net/default/index.cfm/actio-blog/list-of-lists-of-chemicals-of-concern-in-us-states/ – ACTIO: List: state by state chemicals of concern.

http://www.dtsc.ca.gov/AssessingRisk/EmergingContaminants.cfm – California Department of Toxic Substances Control: Emerging Chemicals of Concern.

http://www.ecy.wa.gov/programs/eap/toxics/chemicals_of_concern.html – Department of Ecology State of Washington: Chemicals of Concern.

Chemical-Specific Adjustment Factor (CSAF)

MA Rezvanfar, Tehran University of Medical Sciences, Tehran, Iran

This article is a revision of the previous edition article by Bette Meek, volume 1, pp 530–533 © 2005, Elsevier Inc.

Introduction

Uncertainty is a very important component of risk assessment because it influences the probability (risk) that an adverse effect will occur. Uncertainty occurs because of a lack of knowledge; therefore, it can often be reduced by collecting more and better data. The level of uncertainty associated with the conclusions of a risk assessment is conditional on available data and the models used to estimate exposure concentrations, assumptions in estimating exposure, and the methods used to develop toxicity factors. Uncertainties in the risk assessment process could result in an underestimation or overestimation of risk. However, it is standard in risk assessment practice (per US Environmental Protection Agency (EPA) guidance) to use health protective assumptions when uncertainty in quantifying risks exists, so as not to underestimate potential risk. The reference concentration (RfC) and reference dose (RfD) values used to evaluate noncancer risk and the inhalation unit risk (IUR) values used to quantify cancer are often derived from limited toxicity databases. This can result in substantial qualitative and quantitative uncertainty. To account for this uncertainty, the US EPA derives RfCs, RfDs, and IURs in a way that is intentionally conservative (protective of human health). In the development of reference or tolerable concentrations or doses, where kinetic and/or dynamic data are adequate, human health risk assessment has begun to depart from the traditional methods by replacement of the commonly adopted default values for interspecies differences and human variability with more certain, reasonable, data-driven, so-called chemical-specific adjustment factors (CSAFs) based on chemical-specific data. CSAFs represent part of a broader continuum of approaches to incorporate increasing amounts of data to reduce uncertainty, ranging from default (presumed protective) to more biologically based predictive approaches. Guidance for the adequacy of data to serve as the basis for development of CSAFs is available. For example, the CSAF concept and the International Programme on Chemical Safety (IPCS) guidelines have been used in the assessment of risk from chronic exposure to ethylene glycol and intraspecies variability of acetone toxicokinetics in the general and occupationally exposed populations.

Framework for Development of CSAFs

In the health risk assessment of chemicals, the determination of a no observed adverse effect level (NOAEL) is often based on data only from animal experiments. A safety or uncertainty factor of 100 is used to convert an NOAEL from an animal toxicity study to an acceptable daily intake (ADI) value for human intake, ADI = NOAEL/100. Historically, the assessment factor of 100 intended to cover interspecies (animal to human) and interindividual (human to human) variations has often been used as a default value.

In 2001, the IPCS, a cooperative program of the World Health Organization (WHO), International Labor Organization (ILO), and the United Nations (UN), published the Guidance Document for the Use of Data in the Development of Chemical Specific Adjustment Factors (CSAFs) for Interspecies Differences and Human Variability in Dose/Concentration Response Assessment to provide guidance to health risk assessors on the use of quantitative toxicokinetics and toxicodynamic data to address interspecies and interindividual differences in dose/concentration–response assessment. WHO's IPCS guidance for deriving CSAFs was finalized in 2005. The principal objectives of this document were to: (1) increase common understanding and to encourage the incorporation of relevant quantitative data on interspecies differences or human variability in toxicokinetics and toxicodynamics into dose/concentration–response assessment and (2) to more fully delineate appropriate avenues of research to enable more predictive estimates of risk. The latter objective includes the use of ethically derived human data to inform the selection of appropriate adjustment factors for interspecies and human variability.

A framework was proposed to address kinetics and dynamics separately in considering uncertainty related to interspecies differences and interindividual variability in the development of reference or tolerable concentrations/doses. Quantitation of this subdivision is supported by data on kinetic parameters and pharmacokinetic–pharmacodynamic (PKPD) modeling for a range of pharmacological and therapeutic responses to pharmaceutical agents. This framework allows the incorporation of quantitative chemical-specific data, relating to either toxicokinetics or toxicodynamics, to replace part of the usual 100-fold default uncertainty factor for interspecies differences or interindividual variability but reverts to the usual 100-fold default in the absence of appropriate information (**Figure 1**). Owing to the nature of the data on which the subdivision is based, in the context of the framework, toxicokinetics relates to the movement of the chemical around the body (i.e., absorption, distribution, metabolism, and excretion). Toxicodynamics refers to the actions and interactions of the toxicant within the organism and describes processes at organ, tissue, cellular, and molecular levels.

Important distinctions between IPCS (2005) and the present US EPA guidance are: IPCS restricts toxicokinetic evaluations to the central compartment, disallowing local tissue metabolism to be quantified as part of the toxicokinetic processes; uneven division of the animal to human extrapolation, attributing a greater fraction of default uncertainty to toxicokinetics than to toxicodynamics; and the general level of depth. The US EPA's approach to calculating extrapolation values based on data uses data-derived extrapolation factors (DDEFs). DDEFs are similar in concept to IPCS/WHO's CSAFs

 http://dx.doi.org/10.1016/B978-0-12-386454-3.00594-7

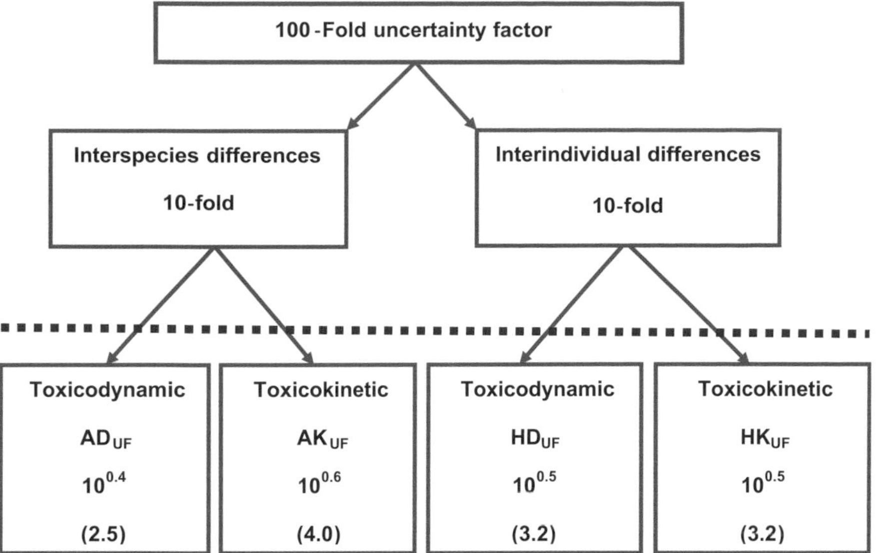

Figure 1 Subdivision of the 100-fold uncertainty factor to allow chemical-specific data to replace part of the default factor. ADUF, animal to human dynamic uncertainty factor; AKUF, animal to human kinetic uncertainty factor; HDUF, human variability dynamic uncertainty factor; HKUF, human variability kinetic uncertainty factor. Chemical-specific data can be used to replace a default uncertainty factor (UF) with an adjustment factor (AF).

in that the standard extrapolation factors are separated into toxicokinetic and toxicodynamic components, and kinetic and mechanistic data are used to derive refined interspecies or intraspecies extrapolation factor(s). Conceptually, CSAFs and DDEFs may not be limited to a specific chemical but may also apply to chemicals with common structural characteristics, common mode of action (MOA), or common toxicokinetic characteristics or determinants.

Basic Questions

The important question before comparison of toxicokinetic and/or toxicodynamic data is whether it is the parent compound or a metabolite that causes the critical effect(s) and whether there is enough information on the mechanism of action for the toxic effect(s). Another important aspect is whether the effect is related to a maximal concentration of the compound/metabolite in the target organ or to the overall dose. The relevance of the human study group, the route of exposure, the levels of exposure, and the number of subjects and samples (statistics) are other important issues.

Chemical-Specific Toxicokinetic Adjustment Factors (AK_{AF}, HK_{AF})

In order to obtain quantitative toxicokinetic data for comparisons between individuals or between animals and humans, human data are needed. These can be derived from *in vivo* experimentation in human volunteers using parameters such as area under the plasma or tissue concentration–time curve (AUC), the maximum measured concentration in blood (C_{max}), or clearance (Cl).

For interspecies differences, this is generally determined on the basis of comparison of the results of *in vivo* kinetic studies with the active compound in animals and a representative sample of the healthy human population. The IPCS mentions that the doses for animal experiments should preferably be close to the NOAEL and doses given in human studies should be similar to the estimated or potential human exposure. For humans, relevant data on AUC, C_{max}, or Cl are generally derived from *in vivo* experimentation in volunteers given very low doses of the relevant chemical. Alternatively, relevant information on such parameters may be derived from *in vitro* enzyme studies combined with suitable scaling to determine *in vivo* activity.

For interindividual variability, most often, factors responsible for clearance mechanisms are identified (e.g., renal clearance, CYP-specific metabolism, etc.) and a CSAF is derived based on measured or physiologically based pharmacokinetically (PBPK) modeled human variability in the relevant physiological and biochemical parameters. The population distribution for the relevant metric (e.g., AUC, C_{max}, Cl) for the active entity is analyzed and the CSAF (HK_{AF}) calculated as the difference between the central values for the main group and the given percentiles (such as 95th, 97.5th, and 99th) for the whole population (**Figure 2**). These differences are analyzed separately for any potentially susceptible subgroup (**Figure 2**).

Chemical-Specific Toxicodynamic Adjustment Factors

The CSAFs for toxicodynamic components are simply ratios of the doses that induce the critical toxic effect or a measurable related response *in vitro* in relevant tissues of animals and a representative sample of the healthy human population (interspecies differences) or in average versus sensitive humans

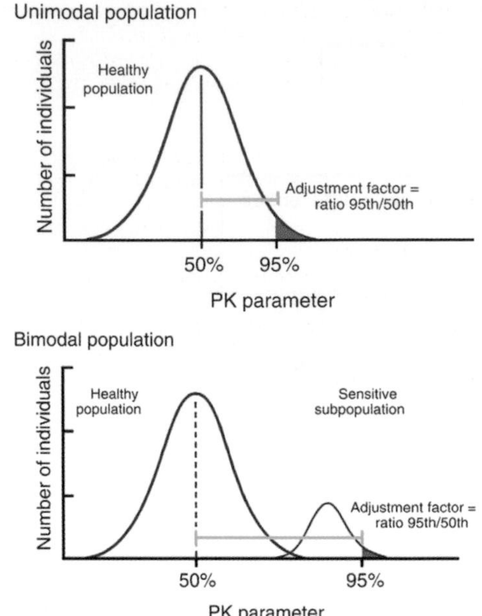

Figure 2 Development of CSAFs for interindividual variability.

(interindividual variability). At its simplest, then, a replacement for the dynamic component of the default factor for interspecies differences is the ratio of the effective concentrations in critical tissues of animals versus humans (e.g., $EC_{10\ animal}/EC_{10\ human}$) for interspecies differences and in healthy human and susceptible subpopulations for interindividual variability (e.g., the $EC_{10\ average}/EC_{10\ sensitive}$). *In vitro* studies are generally inadequate for the assessment of human variability. In practice, there is a lack of human *in vivo* data, and comparisons between animal and human toxicodynamics have to be based on parallel *in vitro* dose–response studies with animal and human tissue samples. It is crucial that the *in vitro* system is representative of what happens *in vivo*, and that the end point measured is either the critical toxic effect or closely linked to the critical effect.

Guidance for Development of CSAF

The IPCS provides guidance on several aspects of the development of CSAF, which are only briefly outlined here. For example, data for application in the four components of the framework must relate to the active form of the chemical. For the components of the framework addressing toxicokinetics (AK_{AF} and HK_{AF}), the choice of the appropriate metric is also an essential first step.

The choice of the appropriate end point is critical for the components addressing toxicodynamics (AD_{AF} and HD_{AF}). The selected measured end point must either be the critical effect itself or intimately linked thereto (with similar concentration–response and temporal relationships) based on an understanding of the mode of action.

In addition, the metric for toxicokinetics or the measure of effects for toxicodynamics as a basis for CSAF needs careful consideration in relation to the delivery of the chemical to the target organ. Measures of various end points *in vivo* may represent purely toxicokinetics, or toxicokinetics and part or all of the toxicodynamic processes, as defined based on the subdivision of defaults. This necessitates consideration of the impact of specific data to replace the toxicokinetic and potentially a proportion or all of the toxicodynamic components of the default uncertainty factors.

For data that serve as the basis for all components, the relevance of the population, the route of exposure, the dose/concentration, and adequacy of numbers of subjects/samples must also be considered and the potential impact on the validity of the calculated ratio addressed. For example, for *in vitro* studies that inform primarily dynamic components (AD_{AF}) and (HD_{AF}), the quality of the samples should be considered, and evidence provided that they are representative of the target population, for example, viability, specific content, or activity of marker enzymes. The most critical questions are whether the study population is relevant and representative, the number of subjects/samples is adequate, and the dose–response data are adequate. The relevance of route and dose is, of course, also important. If *in vitro* data are used, there must be a clear link to the mechanism of toxicity.

Example

To replace default toxicokinetic and toxicodynamic uncertainty factors for interspecies differences and human variability, a CSAF or a physiologically based toxicokinetic model has been proposed when compound-specific data are available as recommended by the WHO. This approach has recently been explored for the risk assessment of cadmium in food for which a physiologically based pharmacokinetic model was developed from human data and a human benchmark dose (BMD)/benchmark dose lower confidence limit (BMDL) was derived from a meta-analysis of the published studies relating urinary cadmium and biomarkers of renal effects (2-β microglobulin). In this case, the provisional tolerable weekly intake (PTWI) for cadmium was derived without the need to extrapolate from animals to humans and the use of the 100-fold uncertainty factor was replaced by the physiologically based pharmacokinetic model together with the use of a CSAF for cadmium variability in toxicodynamics.

Conclusions

The chemical-specific approach is attractive because it attempts to use scientific data. Advantages of the application of CSAFs include reduction of uncertainty through reliance on considerably more of the available chemical-specific data and the capacity to more meaningfully protect susceptible subgroups. Ultimately, use of CSAFs based on the development of relevant data strives to ensure scarce resources are appropriately directed to the highest priorities. In considering these approaches, however, it is important to note that acceptance of adjustment factors varies with the regulatory situation across different sectors of the chemicals industry. For example, the use of chemical-specific data to derive adjustment factors that are smaller than the default is rare in the case of pesticides. Also, the chemical-specific approach requires human studies, which may be difficult or impossible to accomplish for ethical reasons.

See also: Acceptable Daily Intake (ADI); Benchmark Dose; Margin of Exposure (MOE); Margins of safety; NOAEL; Oral/Dermal Reference Dose (RfD)/Inhalation Reference Concentration (RfC); Reference Dose (RfD); Risk assessment; Tolerable Daily Intakes (TDIs); Toxicodynamics; Pharmacokinetics; Uncertainty Factors.

Further Reading

Creton, S., Billington, R., Davies, W., Dent, M.P., Hawksworth, G.M., Parry, S., Travis, K.Z., 2009. Application of toxicokinetics to improve chemical risk assessment: implications for the use of animals. Regul. Toxicol. Pharmacol. 55, 291–299.

Dorne, J.L., 2010. Metabolism, variability and risk assessment. Toxicology 9, 156–164.

EFSA (European Food Safety Authority) Scientific Report, 2009. Technical report of EFSA prepared by assessment methodology unit on meta-analysis of dose–effect relationship of cadmium for Benchmark dose evaluation. EFSA Scientific Report 254, 1–62. Available at: http://www.efsa.europa.eu/en/efsajournal/doc/254r.pdf.

Falk-Filipsson, A., Hanberg, A., Victorin, K., Warholm, M., Wallén, M., 2007. Assessment factors—applications in health risk assessment of chemicals. Environ. Res. 104 (1), 108–127.

IPCS, 2005. Chemical-Specific Adjustment Factors (CSAFs) for Interspecies Differences and Human Variability: Guidance Document for the Use of Data in Dose/Concentration-Response Assessment. WHO/IPCS/01.4, 1–96. International Panel on Chemical Safety, World Health Organization, Geneva, Switzerland.

Meek, M.E., 2001. Categorical default uncertainty factors – interspecies variation and adequacy of database. Hum. Ecol. Risk Assess. 7, 157–163.

Meek, M.E., Ohanian, E., Renwick, A., et al., 1999. Guidelines for Application of Data-Derived Uncertainty Factors in Risk Assessment. Report of a Meeting by Toxicology Excellence for Risk Assessment for US EPA/Health Canada, Washington. March 25–26.

Mörk, A.K., Johanson, G., 2010. Chemical-specific adjustment factors for intraspecies variability of acetone toxicokinetics using a probabilistic approach. Toxicol. Sci. 116, 336–348.

Palmer, R.B., Brent, J., 2005. Derivation of a chemical-specific adjustment factor (CSAF) for use in the assessment of risk from chronic exposure to ethylene glycol: application of international programme for chemical safety guidelines. Toxicol. Appl. Pharmacol. 207, 576–584.

Renwick, A.G., 1993. Data-derived safety (uncertainty) factors for the evaluation of food additives and environmental contaminants. Food Addit. Contam. 10 (3), 275–305.

Renwick, A.G., Lazarus, N.R., 1998. Human variability and noncancer risk assessment – an analysis of the default uncertainty factor. Regul. Toxicol. Pharmacol. 27 (1 Pt 2), 3–20.

Renwick, A.G., Dorne, J.-L.C.M., Walton, K., 2001. Pathway-related factors: the potential for human data to improve the scientific basis of risk assessment. Hum. Ecol. Risk Assess. 7 (2), 165–180.

Relevant Websites

http://www.who.int/ipcs/methods/harmonization/areas/uncertainty/en/index.html: IPCS, 2005. Chemical-specific Adjustment Factors for Interspecies Differences and Human Variability: Guidance Document for Use of Data in Dose/Concentration–Response Assessment. World Health Organization, Geneva, Available at:

http://www.ipcsharmonize.org: International Programme on Chemical Safety (IPCS) (2001) Guidance Document for the Use of Data in Development of Chemical-Specific Adjustment Factors (CSAFs) for Interspecies differences and Human Variability in Dose/Concentration–Response Assessment. Geneva: World Health Organization, International Programme on Chemical Safety.

Chemical Warfare

SA Burr, Plymouth University Peninsula Schools of Medicine and Dentistry, Plymouth, UK

Prohibition

There have been several international agreements attempting to limit and ultimately abolish chemical warfare. The Brussels Declaration in 1874 (unratified) forbade parties 'to employ poison or poisoned arms.' The Hague Conference signed in 1899 (entered into force in 1900 and updated in 1907) forbade the "use of projectiles the object of which is the diffusion of asphyxiating or deleterious gases." The Geneva Protocol signed in 1925 (entered into force in 1928) forbade "the use in war of asphyxiating, poisonous or other gases, and of all analogous liquids, materials or devices." Most recently the Convention on the Prohibition of the Development, Production, Stockpiling and Use of Chemical Weapons and their Destruction of 1993 (entered into force in 1997) is administered by the Organisation for the Prohibition of Chemical Weapons (OPCW). This Chemical Weapons Convention has been ratified by all member states of the United Nations with the following exceptions: Israel and Myanmar have signed but not ratified; and Angola, Egypt, North Korea and South Sudan have neither signed nor acceded (as of October 2013). For Schedule 1 chemicals with no known general purpose use other than as a weapon (e.g., tabun, sarin, soman, cyclosarin, VX, lewisite, nitrogen mustard, sulfur mustard, ricin, saxitoxin, and the precursors chlorosarin, and chlorosoman), no more than 100 g^{-1} year can be produced for use in research. For Schedule 2 chemicals with established small-scale alternative applications (e.g., the lewisite precursor arsenic trichloride, which is also used in ceramic manufacture, the mustard gas precursor thiodiglycol, which is also used as a solvent for inks, and the sarin precursor dimethyl-methyl-phosphonate, which is also used as a flame retardant), facilities producing more than 1 kg, 100 kg, or 1 ton per year (depending on the specific chemical) must be declared and inspected. For Schedule 3 chemicals (e.g., phosgene and hydrogen cyanide) with established large-scale alternative applications, facilities producing more than 30 tons per year must be declared and inspected.

Many consider chemical weapons emotive, while others consider that the injuries inflicted are no more immoral than those inflicted by explosive agents. Furthermore, chemical weapons could be considered less environmentally destructive and hence preferable to nuclear weapons. Indeed, prohibition of chemical weapons means that the only remaining proportional response to an attack with a weapon of mass destruction would be to counterattack using nuclear weapons.

Historical Use of Chemical Agents

The use of poison-coated arrowheads and spearheads are referred to in some of the earliest historical records of warfare, which themselves are predated by references in mythological accounts. The poisoning of water supplies during sieges was first reported in the sixth century BC (when the Assyrians used ergot and Greeks used hellebore). The first recorded device for delivery is possibly the poisonous (probably arsenic and croton) smoke bomb used by the Chinese Sung dynasty in 1161 AD. Many more devices were developed over the centuries culminating in the modern delivery systems detailed in the previous section. It is estimated that 125 000 tons of chemical weapons (in descending order of quantity employed: chlorine, phosgene, diphosgene, chloropicrin, sulfur mustard, and cyanides) were used on the battlefield by both sides during WWI (from 1915 to 1918), causing more than 1 million casualties. As Germany sought to increase food production in the face of shortages following the Treaty of Versailles, research into organophosphates for new pesticides led to the discovery of the G-series nerve agents. More agents have been developed since then and been actively used on a comparatively small scale by several nations.

Exposure and Toxic Effects

Exposure is normally intended to be through breathing or skin contact, but can be through ingesting water or food, or via wounds. The predominant adverse effect of an agent is usually on the nervous system (increasing secretions and causing paralysis), skin (causing irritation, blisters, and burns) or lungs (causing edema; see **Table 1**). Onset of effects is generally quicker following inhalation than percutaneous exposure. However, having effective respiratory and dermal absorption dictates that both breathing and skin countermeasures are required for protection. Protective countermeasures may be circumvented by a combination of agents to compromise the integrity of protective equipment (e.g., addition of an emetic such as diphenyl chloroarsine (DA) to act as a 'mask breaker,' forcing the removal of breathing apparatus in order to vomit, or a corrosive agent such as phosgene oxime (CX) to penetrate barriers), or by achieving surprise and rapidly causing debilitating effects (e.g., hydrogen cyanide). thus preventing the effective use of countermeasures. High potency reduces the quantity needed to be delivered for coverage of any given target area, but is often offset by the higher expense of a more complex manufacturing process (e.g., VX).

Personal Protective Equipment

Major incident planning (for public health protection and counterterrorism) by local government emergency services includes provision for personal protective equipment. Emergency civilian personnel (i.e., police, fire and ambulance services) wear hazardous materials ('hazmat') suits for first response recovery and decontamination tasks (e.g., following spillages). Different degrees of protection for breathing and skin are available based on knowledge of the type of agent, concentration, and associated risk. Suit levels in the United States are designated A–D: Level A provides most protection, B provides more respiration protection than C, and D provides

 http://dx.doi.org/10.1016/B978-0-12-386454-3.01003-4

Table 1 Comparison of the effects of scheduled chemical warfare agents

OPCW schedule	Name	Code	Primary effect(s)	Onset	Potency: Inhalation LCt_{50} mg min^{-1} m^{-3}	Potency: Dermal LD_{50} mg kg^{-1}
1	Tabun = *O*-ethyl *N,N*-dimethyl phosphoramidocyanidate	GA	Paralysis (nerve)	Seconds (fatal 1–10 m after inhaling, 1–2 h after dermal)	100–200	14–57
	Sarin = *O*-isopropyl methylphosphonofluoridate	GB			70–100	28
	Soman = *O*-pinacolyl methylphosphonofluoridate	GD			70	5
	O-ethyl *S*-2-diisopropylaminoethyl methyl phosphonothiolate.	VX			39–70	0.142
	Sulfur mustards: bis(2-chloroethyl) sulfide	H (HD when distilled)	Blister (vesicant)	4–24 h	300–1500	20–100
	2-Chloroethylchloromethylsulphide					
	Bis(2-chloroethylthio)methane	HK				
	Sesquimustard = 1,2-bis (2-chloroethylthio)ethane	Q				
	1,3-Bis(2-chloroethylthio)-*n*-propane					
	1,4-Bis(2-chloroethylthio)-*n*-butane					
	1,5-Bis(2-chloroethylthio)-*n*-pentane					
	Bis(2-chloroethylthiomethyl)ether					
	O-mustard = bis(2-chloroethylthioethyl)ether	T				
	Lewisite 1 = 2-chlorovinyldichloroarsine	L1		10–20 s	1500	37
	Lewisite 2 = bis(2-chlorovinyl)chloroarsine	L2				
	Lewisite 3 = tris(2-chlorovinyl)arsine	L3				
	Nitrogen mustard 1 = bis(2-chloroethyl) ethylamine	HN1		1–12 h		
	Nitrogen mustard 2 = bis(2-chloroethyl) methylamine	HN2				
	Nitrogen mustard 3 = tris(2-chloroethyl)amine	HN3				
	Saxitoxin	TZ	Paralysis (nerve)	Minutes (fatal afte r 15 m)	5	Via flechettes, iv = 0.57 μg kg^{-1}
	Ricin	W	Gut lining (cytotoxic)	3–24 h	40	Via flechettes, iv = 5 μg kg^{-1}
2	1,1,3,3,3-Pentafluoro-2-(trifluoromethyl)-1-propene	PFIB	Choking (pulmonary)	5 m–4 h	320	Irritant, poorly absorbed
	3-Quinuclidinyl benzilate	BZ	Mental confusion (incapacitating), but effects are unpredictable	0.5–20 h	3800–200 000 (ICt_{50} = 110–112)	Poorly absorbed
3	Phosgene = carbonyl dichloride	CG	Choking (pulmonary)	20 m–24 h	120–3200	Potent irritant, poorly absorbed
	Cyanogen chloride	CK	Asphyxiation (metabolic)	15 s (fatal after 30 s–30 m)	11 000	100
	Hydrogen cyanide	AC	Asphyxiation (metabolic)		1000–5000, (NB. detoxified at 17 μg kg^{-1} min^{-1})	100
	Chloropicrin = trichloronitromethane	PS	Choking (pulmonary)	3–30 s	2000	Potent irritant, poorly absorbed

Where: s = seconds, m = minutes, and h = hours. NB. VG (Amiton = *O,O*-diethyl *S*-[2-(diethylamino)ethyl] phosphorothiolate) has similar properties to VX although with one-tenth the potency and hence is classified as schedule 2.

the least protection of all (inversely proportional to impingement of dexterity and comfort). Suit types in Europe are designated 1–6: Type 1 is gas tight (equivalent to A in the United States), 2 protects against gases and liquids but is not gas tight (B in the United States), 3 protects against liquids rather than gases and is liquid tight, 4 is spray tight (C in the United States), 5 protects most of the body against liquids (D in the United States), and 6 protects parts of the body against liquids. Individuals may use a self-contained breathing apparatus, air-purifying respirator, air-purifying escape respirator, self-contained escape respirator, or powered air-purifying respirator. It is also possible to provide collective protection using shelters that can be fixed, mobile, or improvised. Military personnel wear equivalent nuclear biological chemical/chemical biological radiological nuclear suits that are designed for uses extending to several days, and protection may be augmented by the use of prophylactic medication.

Decontamination

Dissipation of non-persistent gases (e.g., chlorine, phosgene, sarin) may be facilitated by exhaust fans in enclosed areas. Neutralization of persistent liquids can be achieved chemically using liquid sodium dichlorocyanate (Fischor), or by absorption using powdered aluminum silicate (Fullers' earth). Contaminated items need to be collected and contained for disposal, and protective equipment and people should be washed with hot water and soap (or 10% sodium carbonate or 5% household bleach) by blotting (rather than wiping) and rinsing. Pulmonary resuscitation and emetics are not normally recommended due to the increased risk of contaminating additional people. Subsequent to decontamination, individuals should not be confined in small spaces with poor ventilation, or wrapped so as to contain any residual agent next to the body. Medical treatment will depend on the specific agent and development of systemic signs and symptoms.

See also: Arsenical Vomiting Agents; Blister Agents/vesicants; 3-Quinuclidinyl Benzilate (BZ): Psychotomimetic Agent; Chemical Warfare Delivery Systems; Cyclosarin (GF); G-Series Nerve Agents; Lewisite; Nerve Agents; Nitrogen Mustards; Sarin (GB); Soman; Tabun; V-Series Nerve Agents: Other than VX; VX.

Further Reading

Everley, P.A., Dillman 3rd, J.F., October 20, 2010. Genomics and proteomics in chemical warfare agent research: recent studies and future applications. Toxicol. Lett. 198 (3), 297–303.

Kim, K., Tsay, O.G., Atwood, D.A., Churchill, D.G., September 14, 2011. Destruction and detection of chemical warfare agents. Chem. Rev. 111 (9), 5345–5403.

Kuca, K., Pohanka, M., 2010. Chemical warfare agents. EXS 100, 543–558.

Marrs, T.C., Maynard, R.L., Sidell, F.R., 2007. Chemical Warfare Agents: Toxicology and Treatment. John Wiley & Sons, Ltd, Chichester, UK.

Moshiri, M., Darchini-Maragheh, E., Balali-Mood, M., November 28, 2012. Advances in toxicology and medical treatment of chemical warfare nerve agents. Daru 20 (1), 81.

Rodgers, Jr, G.C., Condurache, C.T., September 2010. Antidotes and treatments for chemical warfare/terrorism agents: an evidence-based review. Clin. Pharmacol. Ther. 88 (3), 318–327.

Smirnov, I., Belogurov, A., Friboulet, A., Masson, P., Gabibov, A., Renard, P.-Y., 2013. Strategies for the selection of catalytic antibodies against organophosphorus nerve agents. Chem. Biol. Interact. 203, 196–201.

Relevant Websites

http://www.opcw.org – Organisation for the Prohibition of Chemical Weapons, Search for Convention.

http://toxnet.nlm.nih.gov – TOXNET, Toxicology Data Network, National Library of Medicine, Search for Chemical Weapon.

Chemical Warfare Agents *see* Anthrax; Arsenical Vomiting Agents; Bio Warfare and Terrorism: Toxins and Other Mid-Spectrum Agents; Blister Agents/Vesicants; Botulinum Toxin; 3-Quinuclidinyl Benzilate (BZ): Psychotomimetic Agent; Chlorine

Chemical Warfare Delivery Systems

SA Burr, Plymouth University Peninsula Schools of Medicine and Dentistry, Plymouth, UK

Chemical Agent Properties and Targeted Dispersion

The suitability of a chemical agent for delivery as a weapon depends on the effect required. To cause personnel casualties, the agent needs the appropriate volatility and density for adequate dispersal in the target environment (e.g., hydrogen cyanide is lighter than air and quickly lost unless used in an enclosed space). Non-persistent gases such as chlorine are useful for areas that require rapid occupation. Persistent liquids such as VX need to be nonvolatile and oily, with a larger droplet size to contaminate surfaces, and thickened (e.g., with an acryloid copolymer) to make them gelatinous and sticky to present a contact hazard. Accurate topographical maps and weather forecasting increase the success of agent laydown on target. Vegetation can absorb agents. Atmospheric pressure, temperature, humidity, and wind can affect vaporization. Wind speed, direction and consistency, and terrain can all divert delivery. Recognition of color, odor, and early onset warning signs and symptoms may enable protective countermeasures to be employed (e.g., the smell of phosgene is not unusual nor unpleasant and rapidly fades, while the onset of adverse effects may be delayed for several hours after exposure, by which time it is too late to avoid or use protection). Explosive detonation of a central 'burster' charge can be used to spread a small volume of agent. Explosive delivery methods are noticeable, but exposure is near instantaneous. However, it is difficult to optimize the size of droplets produced explosively. Some agent may be lost due to projection into surfaces and incineration, whereas flammable agents such as VX may ignite and be lost due to flashing. In contrast, nonflammable agents such as BZ may depend on thermal aerosolization. All agents need to be sufficiently stable to deliver predictable concentrations after storage, transportation, and delivery. Corrosive properties complicate the design of delivery systems (e.g., sarin is slightly corrosive to steel, and phosgene is highly corrosive in the presence of moisture). Unstable agents with short shelf-lives may require the addition of stabilizers (e.g., tributylamine to prevent hydrolysis of sarin, or diisopropylcarbodiimide when containing sarin in aluminum). Rapid environmental degradation enables takeover of the affected area (e.g., saxitoxin or ricin) via flechettes, whereas slow degradation requires personal protection or environmental decontamination to overcome exclusion areas (e.g., later, nitrogen mustards were developed for volatility, potency, and longer persistence). Persistence can be affected by many factors such as atmospheric transport, sedimentary binding, and microorganism biodegradation, in addition to reactions with water and photochemically produced hydroxyl radicals (see **Table 1**).

Manual Delivery

Manual delivery systems have the most efficient chemical agent fill to delivery system weight ratio. However, such systems also pose the greatest risk to friendly personnel due to close proximity during release and were largely replaced by projectile- and air-delivery systems after World War I.

Cylinders

Fritz Haber personally directed the first chlorine gas attack in 1915, releasing 180 000 kg from 5730 cylinders, which then successfully drifted over entrenched French and Algerian troops at Ypres. Cylinder release is highly dependent on wind, which can reverse and return gas to the attacker.

Hand Bombs

The 2.7 kg (British 6 lb) ground bomb had a 2 min delay fuse with an ejection charge to blow out the end of the bomb and release 1.6 kg of mustard gas.

Landmines

The 15 kg KhF-1/KhF-2 (Russian) bounding gas mine (345 × 150 mm) was electronically triggered by remote operator or tripwire to fire the mine vertically out of its container into the air and after a delay of 1.5 s to fragment at a height of 4–8 m and release 4.5 l of agent to cover a 10 m diameter area. The 4.9 kg M1 landmine (204 × 75 mm) consisted of a fuel can that released 4.5 kg of mustard gas after detonation of an external bursting charge. The 10 kg M23 landmine (330 mm diameter by 127 deep) was activated by a pressure-plate triggering a fuse to detonate an internal burster charge that ruptured the mine and heated 4.7 kg of VX for dispersal as an aerosol mist.

Projectile Delivery

Mortars

The 190 mm Livens Projector combined the gas volume of a cylinder with the range of artillery, firing a 14 kg, 550 mm

 http://dx.doi.org/10.1016/B978-0-12-386454-3.01002-2

Table 1 Comparison of factors affecting agent dispersion, detection, and persistence

Name	Code	Boiling point/state at 20 (°C)	Vapor density (relative to air)	Color	Odor/threshold (mg m^{-3})	Environmental $T_{1/2}$ at 20 °C & pH 7 photolysis/hydrolysis	Persistence	
							At 4–16 °C	At 21–32 °C
Tabun = *O*-ethyl *N,N*-dimethyl phosphoramidocyanidate	GA	240/Liquid	5.6	Pale amber	None (mild fruity almond if impure)	8 h/8.5 h	1–2 d	2–4 d
Sarin = *O*-isopropyl methylphosphonofluoridate	GB	147/Liquid	4.86	None	None-mild fruity/1.5	9.6 h/75 h	0.5–24 h	24–36 h
Soman = *O*-pinacolyl methylphosphonofluoridate	GD	167/Liquid	6.3		Camphor/3.3	8 h/82 h	1–2 d	2–4 d
O-ethyl *S*-2-diisopropylaminoethyl methyl phosphonothiolate	VX	298/Liquid	9.2	Amber	None/3.9	2.5 h/57 h	10–30 d	30–90 d
Sulfur mustards: bis(2-chloroethyl) sulfide	H (HD when distilled)	215–7/Oily liquid	5.4	Pale yellow	Garlic/0.015 – desensitizes within 3–8 m	50 h/4–16 m	1–2 d	2–4 d
2-Chloroethylchloromethylsulphide								
Bis(2-chloroethylthio)methane (HK)	HK							
Sesquimustard = 1,2-bis (2-chloroethylthio)ethane	Q							
1,3-Bis(2-chloroethylthio)-*n*-propane								
1,4-Bis(2-chloroethylthio)-*n*-butane								
1,5-Bis(2-chloroethylthio)-*n*-pentane								
Bis(2-chloroethylthiomethyl)ether								
O-mustard = bis (2-chloroethylthioethyl)ether	T							
Lewisite 1 = 2-chlorovinyldichloroarsine	L1	190/Oily liquid	7.1		Mild geramiums/0.14	1.3 m/1.2 m	18–36 h	2–3 d
Lewisite 2 = bis(2-chlorovinyl)chloroarsine	L2							
Lewisite 3 = tris(2-chlorovinyl)arsine	L3							
Nitrogen mustard 1 = bis (2-chloroethyl)ethylamine	HN1	194/Liquid	7.1	Dark-pale yellow	Fishy-soapy/0.6	24–36 h/9 d	1–3 d	2–6 d
Nitrogen mustard 2 = bis (2-chloroethyl)methylamine	HN2							
Nitrogen mustard 3 = tris(2-chloroethyl)amine	HN3							
Saxitoxin	TZ	Water soluble solid (melts at 236)	NA	White	NA	9–28 d in water	Aerosol decays 17% m^{-1}, 12 w for particulates	
Ricin	W	Water soluble solid (melts at 230)				14 h on wet metal, >14 d on dry concrete	7–14 d	12–19 d
1,1,3,3,3-Pentafluoro-2-(trifluoromethyl)-1-propene	PFIB	7/Gas	6.9	None	None (metallic taste)	5.7 d/rapid	Highly stable in the absence of water	
3-Quinuclidinyl benzilate	BZ	Water soluble solid (melts at 164)	NA	White	NA	3–4 w in moist air	10–20 d	30–60 d
Phosgene = carbonyl dichloride	CG	8.2/Gas	3.4	Pale yellow	Hay/1.5 – desensitizes rapidly	44 y/0.026 s	30 m	60 m
Cyanogen chloride	CK	13/Gas	1.98	None	Acrid/2–2.5	Not susceptible/5.25 h to AC unless alkaline	15–30 m	30–60 m
Hydrogen cyanide	AC	25.6/Liquid-gas	0.94	Very pale blue-white	Almond/0.9	14–22 w/slow		
Chloropicrin = trichloronitromethane	PS	112/Oily liquid	5.7	Very pale yellow	Flypaper/7.96	3–18 w/11 y	1 d–10 w	

Where: m = minutes, h = hours, d = days, w = weeks, and y = years.

long cylinder (Livens drum) up to 1.5 km. It was inaccurate but simple and inexpensive, enabling use en masse (the use of 1000s delivering saturation coverage of high gas concentrations) in an electrically triggered simultaneous barrage of projectiles that burst on impact to disperse the agent (most commonly phosgene or chloropicrin were employed by the British between 1916 and 1918). The 107 mm diameter (11.3 kg) 60 mm M2 mortar (range 4 km) was capable of delivering a M2A1 2.7 kg distilled mustard, 60% mustard to 40% *o*-mustard mix (i.e., HT for higher volatility), phosgene, or white phosphorous ammunition round.

Artillery Shells

The 155 mm (44 kg, 68 cm long) shell (range 14–30 km) had several variants, adapted to deliver various chemicals: M104 for 5.3 kg of mustard or distilled mustard, M110 for 7 kg of mustard, distilled mustard, or white phosphorus, and M121A1 for 2.9 kg of sarin or 2.7 kg of VX. The 105 mm (17.6 kg, 53 cm long) M60 shell (range 11–17 km) contained 1.4 kg of distilled mustard, and was adapted as the (14.5 kg, 50 cm long) M360 containing 725 g of sarin. The 203 mm (90 kg, 89 cm long) M426 shell (range 17–34 km) contained 7.2 kg of sarin or 6.4 kg of VX. Shells usually comprise a hollow one-piece steel shell that is press-fitted with a burster casing. Detonation depends on the fuse type selected. Fuse functioning detonates an explosive charge, which ruptures the projectile and heats and disperses the agent as an aerosol. The 155 mm (60 cm long) M687 shell (range 14–30 km) contained GB2: two canisters separated by a rupture disk (breached by acceleration when fired, with the spinning of the shell causing mixing, and sarin being produced in flight), one canister contained methylphosphonyl difluoride (DF in M20 canister) and the other contained isopropyl alcohol and isopropyl amine (OPA in M21 canister). Shells are typically more robust and safer to handle, store, and transport than other chemical munitions Conventional artillery equipment can be used without specialist adaptation and can maintain a sustained rate of fire. Range and trajectory can be used to calculate the fuse time delay needed to cause detonation at the desired altitude.

Self-Propelled Projectiles

The 115 mm (25 kg, 2 m long) M55 rocket contained 4.8 kg of sarin or 4.5 kg of VX, delivered up to a range of 6.5 km M55 rockets could be fired individually or via an M91 trailer-mounted multiple-rocket launcher, simultaneously firing 45 M55s (arranged 5 × 9). M55s were dangerous in long-term storage as the degradation of the propellant stabilizer could lead to autoignition and degraded sarin corroded the casing, causing leaks. The tactical ballistic missiles (0.88 × 11.35 m) R-300 Elbrus/R-17 Elbrus (employed by the USSR during the Cold War) and Hwasong-5 (a copy, reverse-engineered by Korea) were assigned by NATO as SS-1c Scud-B, with SS-1d Scud-C and SS-1e Scud-D variants having improved guidance control mechanisms. Following a 1 h launch sequence these 'Scuds' could deliver 555 kg VX warheads up to 500 km range. Missiles deliver the equivalent to an artillery barrage in a single strike and without the need for closer positioning and repeated firing of multiple artillery units. The reduced warning minimizes the likelihood of a target implementing effective protective countermeasures.

Air delivery

Unitary Bomb

A fuse detonates an internal burster charge, which ruptures the bomb and heats the agent for dispersal as an aerosol mist. The M47 required anticorrosion linings to carry chemical agents and was developed by the United States as the M47A1 for white phosphorus or M47A2 for 161 kg of mustard. The 329 kg MC-1 (41 × 127 cm) was a dumb bomb developed to deliver 100 kg of sarin, whereas the 200 kg Mark-94 (28 × 152 cm) could deliver 49 kg of sarin. The 238 kg Mark-116 Weteye (36 × 216 cm) was developed to deliver 157 kg of liquid sarin and was originally intended as a guided bomb.

Cluster Bombs

The 453 kg M34 (36 × 218 cm) contained 76 (arranged 4 × 19) 4.5 kg cylindrical 92 mm M125 E54R6 bomblets each containing 1.2 kg of sarin, delivering a total payload of 91 kg. Three hundred and fifty-six spherical 115 mm M134 E130R1 bomblets were developed for use in the 2640 kg (8.3 m long) MGR-1 M190 Honest John rocket, to deliver a total payload of 210 kg sarin up to 32 km. Later, 52 spherical M139 E130R2 bomblets were developed for use in the (4.4 m long) MGR-3 M206 Little John rocket, to deliver a total payload of 31 kg sarin up to 24 km. Finally, 330 M139s could be carried by the 4590 kg M212 MGM-29 Sergeant rocket, to deliver a total payload of 195 kg sarin up to 140 km. The M139 bomblet contained 590 g of sarin in two compartments around a central burster charge, with a 22° glide angle; en masse the bomblets could saturate a 1 km diameter area. The 340 kg M43 cluster bomb (41 × 228 cm) contained 57 (3 banks of 19) 72 mm diameter 4.5 kg M138 bomblets each containing 180 g of BZ mixed with an equal quantity of incendiary agent (as pyromix), which was ignited by a fuse following impact, to thermally aerosolize 10.3 kg of BZ, covering an area of 0.1–0.9 ha. The 79 kg M44 general cluster bomb (38 × 152 cm) contained 3 M16 generators, each of which in turn contained 42 M6 canisters (arranged 3 × 14), and a total of 126 M6s each containing 142 g of BZ (for a total M44 payload of 17.8 kg BZ). Such devices were developed for use against intelligence targets or when friendly and enemy forces co-occupied areas (e.g., hostage rescue situations). However, BZ has a very slow onset and is visible as a white cloud, enabling avoidance measures and consequently decreasing the effectiveness of the agent.

Aircraft Spray Tanks

Spraying overcomes the drawbacks of detonation. However, spraying is affected by speed and direction of both wind and aircraft, with delivery usually needing to occur within the boundary layer (i.e., below an altitude of 300 feet) to ensure the target is reached. Knowledge of fluid dynamics and aerodynamics is needed to facilitate production of optimal droplet size and dispersal as a mist. Polymeric thickening may be required so that the liquid forms large enough droplets so as to not evaporate before it reaches the ground. The 878 kg (4.7 m long) TMU-28 was developed to deliver 615 kg of VX.

Binary Glide Bomb

The contents of two compartments would mix after bomb release to produce an agent that is then sprayed during descent. Such devices were technically challenging due to pressure build-up and variable delivery associated with changing altitude. The 270 kg (2.28 m long) VX2 BLU-80 Bigeye was developed to combine NE (elemental sulfur) with QL (isopropyl aminoethylmethyl phosphonite) during flight and deliver 82 kg of VX.

Improvised Weapons

Any nation with an active military development program has the capability to convert conventional munitions to carry chemical agents. Terrorist groups with sufficient financial backing who are also able to persuade both a chemist to synthesize a suitable agent and an engineer to manufacture a delivery device could also produce a sophisticated chemical weapon. However, the simplest device could just be a sealed container (e.g., plastic bag) that is opened (e.g., punctured by a sharp object) via a timer-triggered mechanism on location. Such a weapon is likely to be manually placed in a densely populated area or to disrupt an essential service. Alternative methods of delivery include aerial release (e.g., from radio-controlled drones, balloons, or private light/microlight aircraft), or a shuttle vehicle that transfers painted or powdered agent by contact (e.g., contamination of currency, post, public transport, food or water sources). Unconventional chemical agents could include misappropriated pharmaceuticals (e.g., psychiatric or anesthetic drugs), industrial waste (e.g., carcinogenic or endocrine-disrupting chemicals), or biologically produced toxins (e.g., botulinum).

Storage, Transport, and Safe Handling

Ton containers were used for the bulk storage and transport of chemical agents. Ton containers were made of steel (2.1 m long, 725 kg when empty) and had fittings to permit the closed-system transfer of chemical agents. Delivery systems under development can be tested using chemical agent simulants (e.g., methylacetoacetate or di(2-ethylhexyl)phthalate replacing sarin). Binary systems facilitate easier handling and transport by having two safer agents that when combined produce the final agent, given the designation '-2' (e.g., GB2 for binary sarin). The Chemical Agent Transfer System (CHATS) is a protective, airtight glove box for manually draining agent from a ton storage container by attaching a pump followed by triple rinsing the container interior using spray nozzles. When dry, the container interior could be checked using a borescope before removal from the CHATS for reuse or disposal.

Detection

Active release or leakage can be detected by use of remote air sampling, optical detection (e.g., using a Raman spectrometer), and identification of biomarkers (e.g., degradation or metabolic sequelae). Passive evaluation of indeterminate munitions can be achieved by portable digital radiography and computed tomography, using X-rays to scan a suspected chemical munition placed vertically on a rotating platform. The resulting digital image can be reviewed to determine whether the contents are a liquid chemical agent. In addition, portable isotopic neutron spectroscopy enables the identification of chemical agents within closed munitions by using gamma rays. Detection of characteristic gamma-ray peaks reveals the presence and concentration of specific chemical agents.

Decommissioning, Neutralization, and Incineration

Tens of thousands of tons of chemical munitions were disposed of by dumping at sea (from 1946 to 1970), until chemical neutralization and incineration took over. Single Chemical Agent Identification Set (CAIS) Access and Neutralization System (SCANS) is a hand-held 3.8 l container designed to access and treat CAIS items containing up to 100 g of mustard or lewisite. The Explosive Destruction System (EDS) uses cutting charges to explosively access chemical munitions, eliminating their explosive capacity before the chemical agent is neutralized. A sealed steel vessel contains the blast, vapor, and fragments. The EDS is transportable for on-site treatment of chemical munitions. Larger scale destruction of chemical munitions by incineration requires three furnaces and pollution abatement. The Liquid Incinerator Chamber destroys liquid chemical agent and contaminated liquids after their removal from munitions or following decontamination processes. The liquid is pumped from a tank and sprayed into the incinerator through injection nozzles, for burning in a primary chamber at 2700 °F followed by a secondary chamber at 2000 °F. The Deactivation Furnace System is a rotary kiln for incineration of chopped rockets, propellants, explosives, and residual chemical agents. The Metal Parts Furnace decontaminates the metal from emptied munitions and other containers at 1500 °F (with a 2000 °F afterburner) before recycling or disposal. The Pollution Abatement System is a two tower wet scrubber system to cool gases and remove pollutants from gases following incineration. First, the quench tower uses water to lower gas temperatures from 2000 to 150 °F. The scrubber tower then uses sodium hydroxide to neutralize acids. Two Venturi filters remove large particles (before and after the scrubber tower), then a mist eliminator removes fine particles, and finally a carbon filter removes any trace amounts of metal and organic material.

See also: Arsenical Vomiting Agents; Blister Agents/vesicants; 3-Quinuclidinyl Benzilate (BZ): Psychotomimetic Agent; Chemical Warfare; Cyclosarin (GF); G-Series Nerve Agents; Lewisite; Nerve Agents; Nitrogen Mustards; Sarin (GB); Soman; Tabun; V-Series Nerve Agents: Other than VX; VX.

Further Reading

Marrs, T.C., Maynard, R.L., Sidell, F.R., 2007. Chemical Warfare Agents: Toxicology and Treatment. John Wiley & Sons, Ltd, Chichester, UK.

Relevant Websites

http://www.fas.org/nuke/guide/usa/cbw/cw.htm and http://www.fas.org/programs/bio/chemweapons/index.html – Federation of American Scientists.

http://toxnet.nlm.nih.gov – TOXNET, Toxicology Data Network, National Library of Medicine, Search for Chemical Weapon.

http://www.cma.army.mil – US Army Chemical Materials Agency, Search for Fact File.

Chemotherapeutic Agents *see* Cancer Chemotherapeutic Agents

Chernobyl

RK Chesser and BE Rodgers, Texas Tech University, Lubbock, TX, USA

This article is a revision of the previous edition article by Amy Bickham Baird and Ronald K. Chesser, volume 1, pp 533–534, © 2005, Elsevier Inc.

Background

Chernobyl's nuclear reactor number four was a graphite-moderated, 3140-megawatt (MW) thermal (1000-MW electric) power facility located 180 km north-north west of Kiev, Ukraine. The reactor was commissioned for operation by the Soviet Union in December 1983. The reactor had 1659 fuel rods containing 172 550 kg of uranium enriched to 2.1% ^{235}U. A significant power surge occurred during an experiment conducted in April 1986, which resulted in a loss of reactor control and inadequate flow of coolant water. Generation of hydrogen gas caused a series of explosions at 1.24 a.m. on 26 April 1986 that breached containment and spewed radioactive particles into the surrounding environment (**Figure 1**). The meltdown, explosion, and 10-day graphite fire at the Chernobyl nuclear power plant reactor four was the worst nuclear disaster in history. The initial hydrogen explosion destroyed the reactor containment vessel and ejected over 6000 kg of nuclear fuel particles and graphite into the environment along a narrow, westerly path of intense radiation. Fuel elements remaining in the core were resuspended into the atmosphere on the second day by drops of sand from multiple helicopter sorties. After the first day, the heat buildup in the exposed reactor core was sufficient to propel aerosols and oxidized volatile elements such as ^{134,137}Cesium, ^{131}Iodine, and ^{135}Xenon high into the stratosphere. These volatile nuclides were dispersed over a very broad geographic area, primarily affecting Ukraine, Belarus, Russia, and Scandinavia (**Figure 2**). The total radioactivity released by the accident was $3.7–5.5 \times 10^{18}$ Becquerels (Bq), or 100–150 million Curies (Ci). Thirty-one deaths were officially attributed to the explosion and radiation exposure to the personnel working in or near the facility. In 2008, the United Nations' Scientific Council on Effects of Atomic Radiation (UNSCEAR) updated the mortality estimates to a total of 64 deaths of persons diagnosed with acute radiation syndrome from Ukraine and Belarus.

The impact of the Chernobyl accident was exacerbated by the lack of a secondary containment structure in the RBMK-1000 reactor facility. The hydrogen explosion dislodged the 5000 metric ton biological shield and exposed the nuclear fuel to the environment. Fuel rods nearing the end of their fuel cycle, such as at Chernobyl, have accumulated over 100 different radionuclides as a product of 3 years of fission and neutron activation. Expulsion of nuclear fuel into the environment at Chernobyl was the main reason that this accident contributed significantly greater number of radioactive nuclides and higher radiation levels than at Fukushima, Japan, in 2011. At Fukushima, the nuclear fuel was damaged by partial meltdown, but primary and secondary containment structures prevented dispersion by explosive fragmentation. Venting of hydrogen gas at Fukushima did create explosions that damaged the superstructure of the facilities, but prevented rupture of the containment safety measures. Escaping gas and coolant water nevertheless contained considerable quantities of radioactive cesium, iodine, and xenon that had aerosolized from the damaged fuel. Although estimates of total releases are technically difficult, it appears that the total radiation release at Fukushima was 100–150 times less than that at Chernobyl. The accident at Japan's Fukushima Daiichi facility is estimated to have released about 40×10^{15} Bq contributed principally by the volatile elements (cesium, iodine, and xenon). The release of radiocesium at Fukushima, however, was more comparable, reaching 20–40% of that released at Chernobyl. Design inadequacies associated with the RBMK-type reactors led to the closure of the Chernobyl nuclear power plant in 2000. The aftermath of the Chernobyl accident helped shape safety measures in nuclear power plants and advance our understanding of the consequences of exposure to radiation.

Social, Health, and Environmental Impacts: Dose Estimates

Evacuation of the 45 000 citizens of the city of Pripyat, Ukraine, located only 2.9 km from Chernobyl's reactor four, commenced at 2.30 p.m. on 27 April, using buses sequestered from surrounding cities (**Figures 3 and 4**). Prior to that time, plumes of radiation had already been deposited and heavy contamination enveloped the city. Although citizens of Pripyat accumulated an average external radiation dose of only 0.0115 Sieverts (Sv) over their 37 h of exposure, their doses would have been much greater had the initial plume moved directly through the city. All 90 000 inhabitants within a 30-km radius around the reactor (exclusion zone) were evacuated from 3 to 5 May. After 1986, about 220 000 additional persons were relocated, and relocation continued until 1992. In all, over 350 000 persons were resettled. It was estimated that the later (non-Pripyat) exclusion zone evacuees received average and maximum external doses of 0.00182 and 0.383 Sv, respectively, before they left the exclusion zone. Efforts were made to limit doses to Chernobyl liquidators, those who

 http://dx.doi.org/10.1016/B978-0-12-386454-3.00080-4

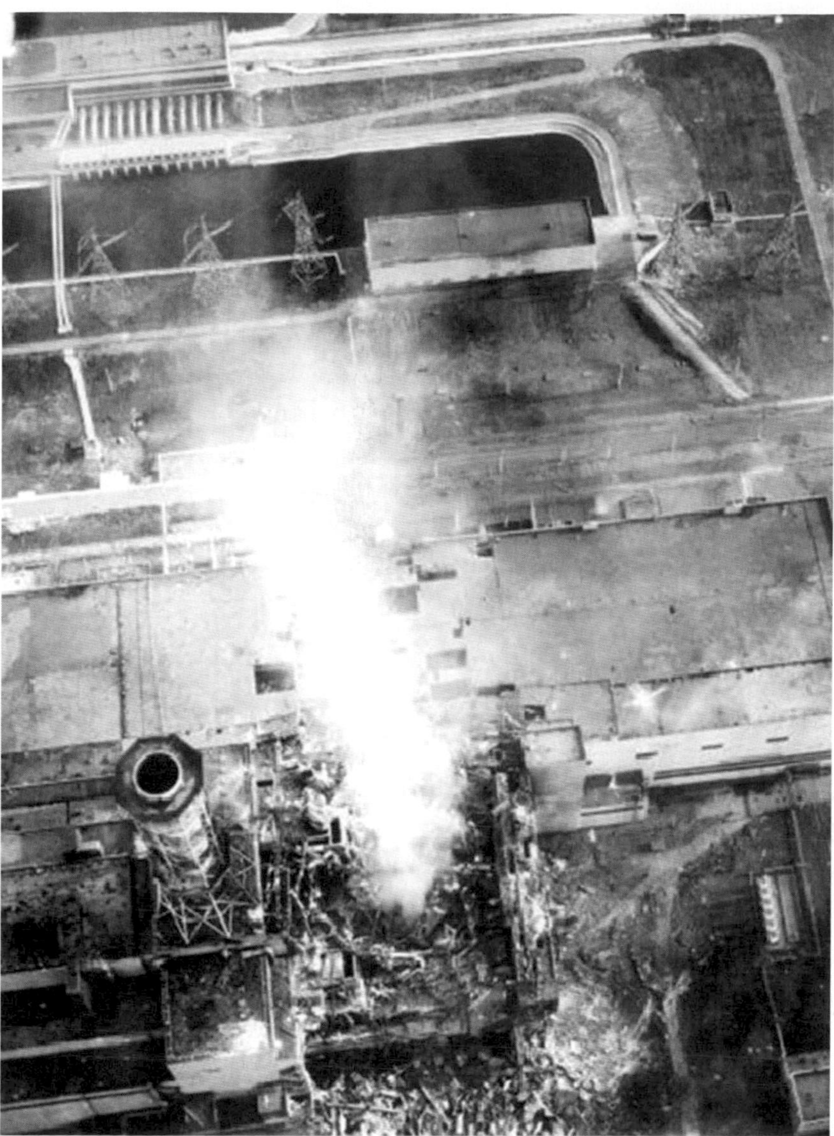

Figure 1 Aerial photograph of Chernobyl reactor four on 3 May 1986.

assisted with the cleanup of the Chernobyl power plant, to a total of 0.25 Sv. However, many were exposed to much higher doses as a consequence of their increased proximity to the reactor as well as possible ingestion or inhalation of contamination. Radiation doses to firemen and reactor personnel exposed shortly after the explosion reached as high as 15 Sv, leading to the deaths of 29 persons (two died as a direct result of the explosion) within 4 months. An additional 25 persons were later diagnosed with radiation doses exceeding 4 Sv, which led to their deaths months after the accident. There were 72 confirmed cases and 96 suspected cases of nonfatal acute radiation sickness in persons exposed to Chernobyl fallout.

The World Health Organization estimated 4000 excess cancer deaths can be expected for persons affected by radiation released from Chernobyl. Estimates made by UNSCEAR were higher, yielding 9335 excess cancer deaths as a result of Chernobyl. Of this total, UNSCEAR estimated 2350 excess cancer deaths in emergency workers, 165 in exclusion zone evacuees, 1660 in zones with ^{137}Cs deposits greater than 555 kBq m^{-2}, and 5160 in residents of other contaminated areas. Predictions were that about 12% of these cases would result in leukemia; the remainder would result in solid tumors. Despite these predictions, however, there has been no confirmed increase in leukemia in children, in the emergency workers, or in the general population exposed to radioactivity linked to the Chernobyl accident. Exposure of adolescents to ^{131}I in Chernobyl fallout has likely contributed to an increased number of cases of thyroid cancers in northern Ukraine and southern Belarus. About 1800 cases of thyroid cancer, predominantly in adolescents, were reported in Belarus, the Russian Federation, and Ukraine during the period 1990–1998. Factors other than ionizing radiation, such as closer scrutiny of this cohort, are believed to have contributed to the reported increase in thyroid cancer risks. Thyroid cancers are usually treatable and have not led to substantial increases in deaths attributable to Chernobyl.

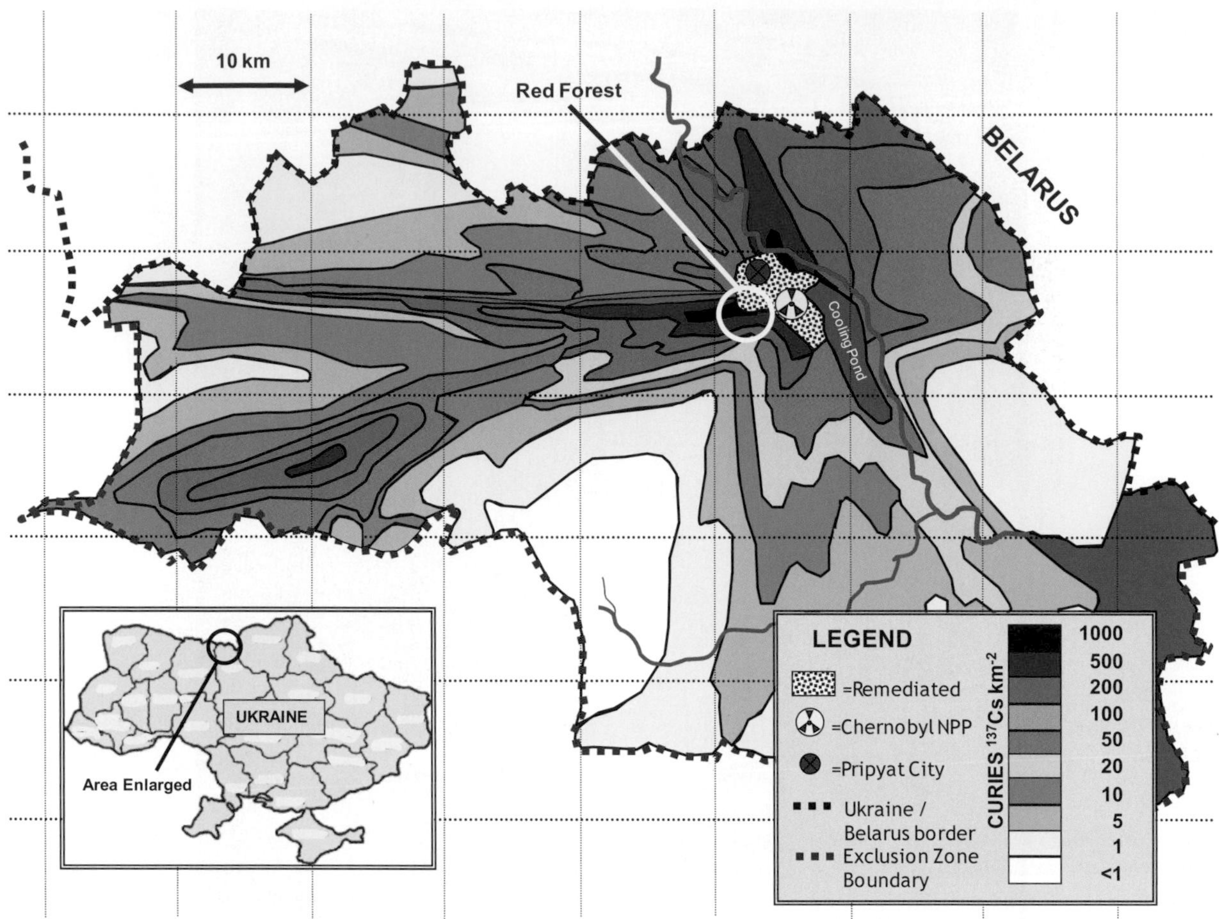

Figure 2 Map of cesium-137 fallout patterns in northern Ukraine and southern Belarus. *From Chesser, R.K., Baker, R.J., 2006. Growing up with Chernobyl.* American Scientist *94: 542–549.*

Environmental and Genetic Impacts: Empirical Evidence

Dose rates in the habitats surrounding reactor four were highly variable due to distinct plumes of radioactive fallout released subsequent to the explosion. The first plume, designated the Western Trace, yielded doses in excess of 6 Sv h^{-1} in some areas, resulting in the death of over 400 ha of Scotch pine (*Pinus sylvestris*) forest (**Figure 5**). Although this plume flow did not affect any metropolitan areas, it undoubtedly caused the extirpation of most resident species of birds, mammals, and reptiles in a narrow path about 2 km wide and extending to about 8–10 km from the reactor. After 2 years, the physical decay of short-lived radionuclides would have reduced dose rates sufficiently to permit gradual recolonization and reproduction in the affected habitats. By 2010, the most affected forests (Red Forest) west of the reactor have not yet recovered the loss of pine trees, except in areas where soil remediation and replanting of vegetation took place.

Ninety-eight percent of the isotopes released at Chernobyl have now dissipated. Dose rates rapidly declined subsequent to the Chernobyl accident and ensuing fire (**Figure 6**). Most of the isotopes released had short half-lives, so their energy caused rapid accumulation of radiation doses. The predominant radionuclides remaining are ^{137}Cs and ^{90}Sr, each with a half-life of ~30 years. These isotopes have high biological affinities and are readily incorporated into living tissues. Because of this affinity, the animals living in the Red Forest are the most radioactive organisms living in otherwise natural environments. Some rodents, for example, are receiving up to 0.1 Sv day^{-1} from ^{137}Cs in their muscles and ^{90}Sr in bone. Small mammals in these habitats are now completing all portions of their normal life cycles. Documenting the doses received at Chernobyl is an important step in performing empirical studies for observing and noting the responses to exposure to the radiation (**Figure 7**).

There have been no documented instances of radiation-induced genetic variations that have transcended generations in Chernobyl wildlife. While damage to genetic material (DNA strand breakage, micronuclei, chromosomal aberrations) has been shown to be significantly elevated in some species in radioactive environments, the impacts are ephemeral and apparently do not persist in affected lineages. Efforts to document adaptation of individuals to the radioactive environment have also shown no significant results; however, some anecdotal conclusions to the contrary have been reported. The vast

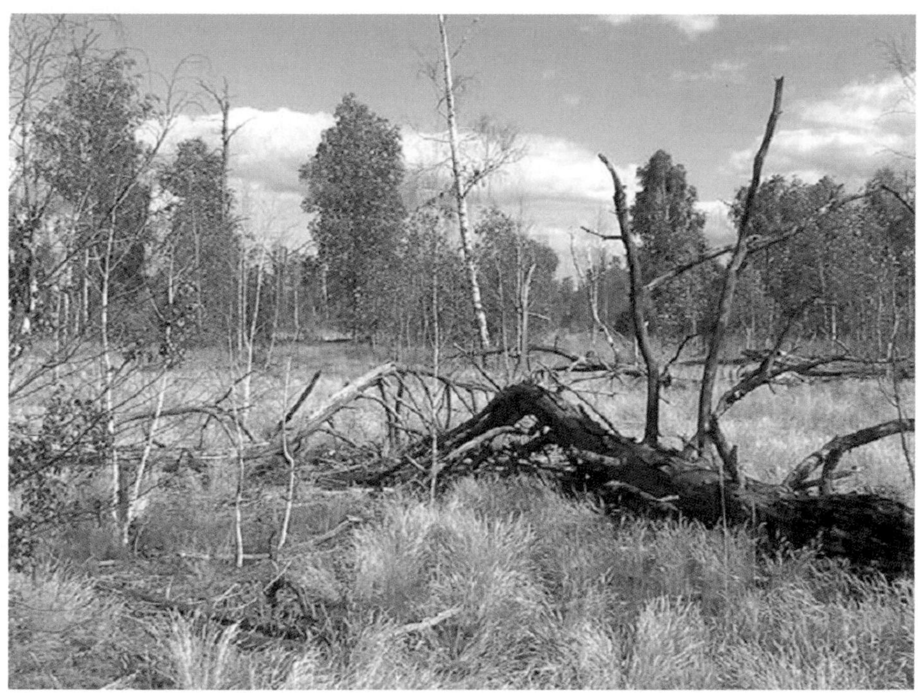

Figure 3 The Red Forest showing dead pine trees and surviving birch trees. This area is where the first plume of radiation was deposited. *Photograph by R.K. Chesser.*

literature on wildlife exposed to radiation at Chernobyl contains conclusions ranging from significant individual and population impacts to no measurable effects. Conclusions drawn from the results of field studies should be considered carefully. Readers should consider whether the authors documented absorbed radiation dose and how the dose was calculated and confirmed. Experimental design is extremely important in such studies and although controls may be difficult, researchers should address the confounding factors of naturally occurring geographic and temporal variation in their

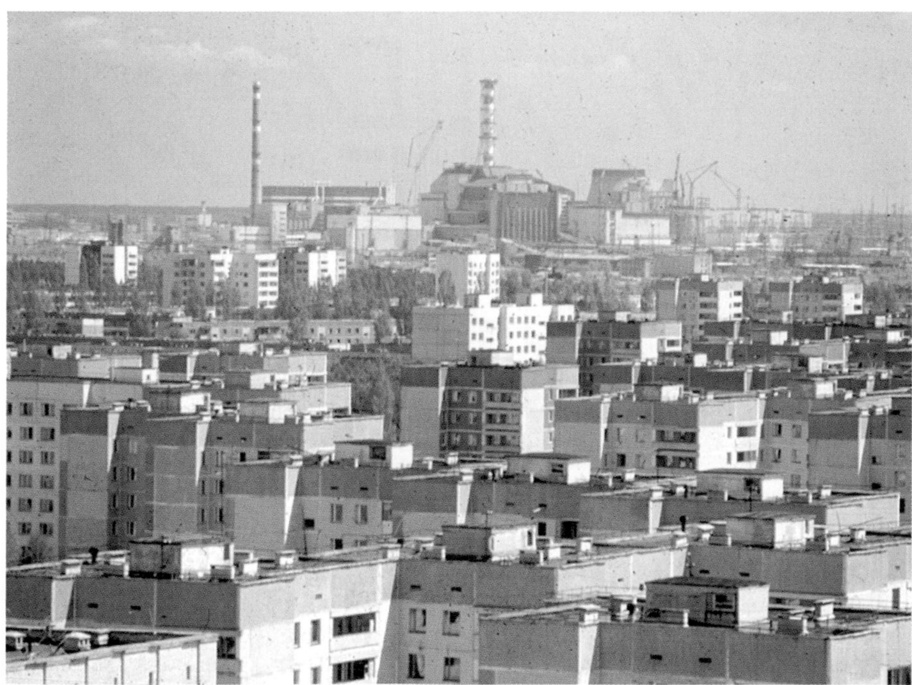

Figure 4 The abandoned city of Pripyat, Ukraine. The Chernobyl reactor four is shown in the background. *Photograph by R.K. Chesser.*

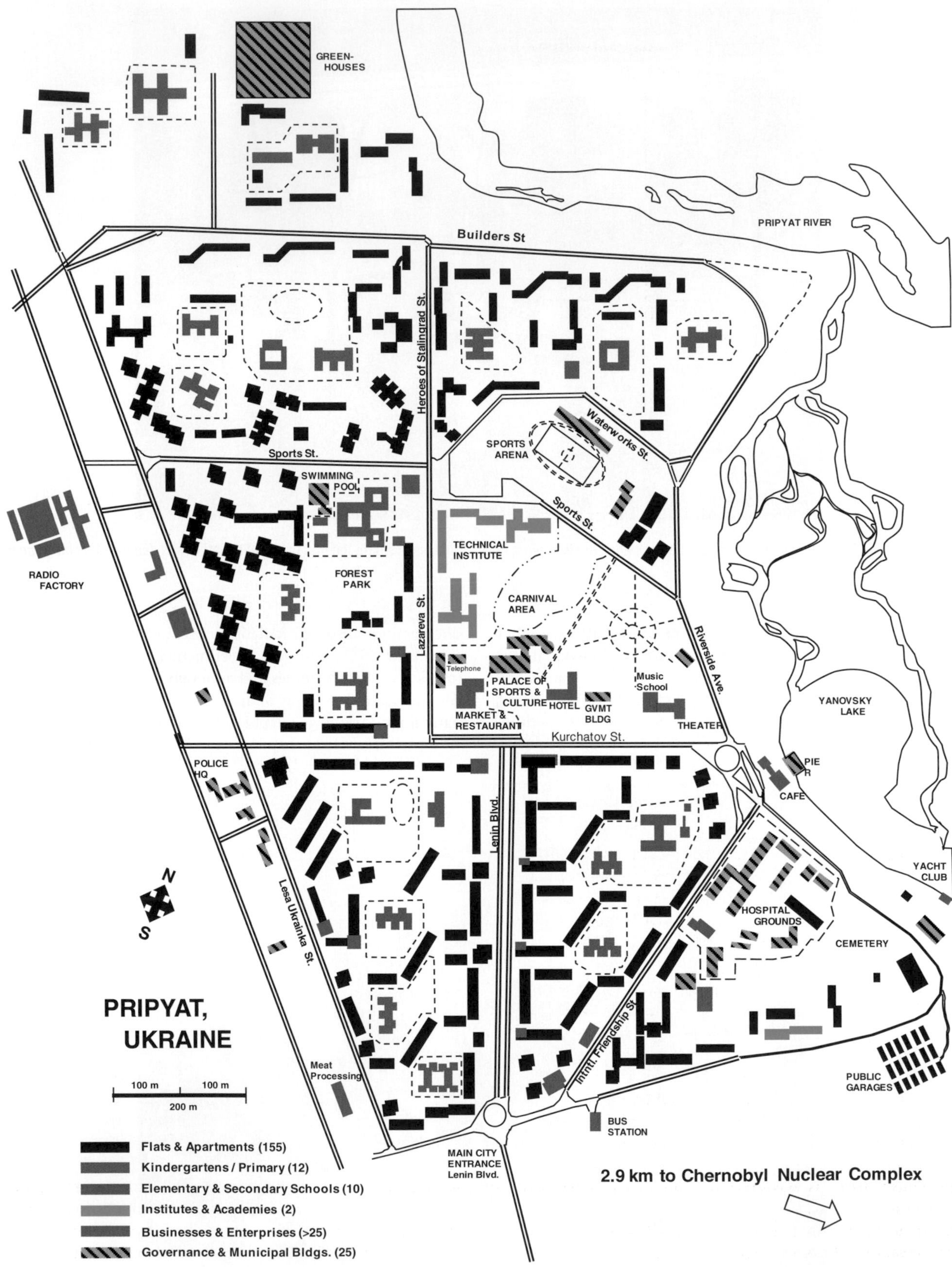

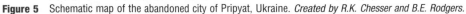

Figure 5 Schematic map of the abandoned city of Pripyat, Ukraine. *Created by R.K. Chesser and B.E. Rodgers.*

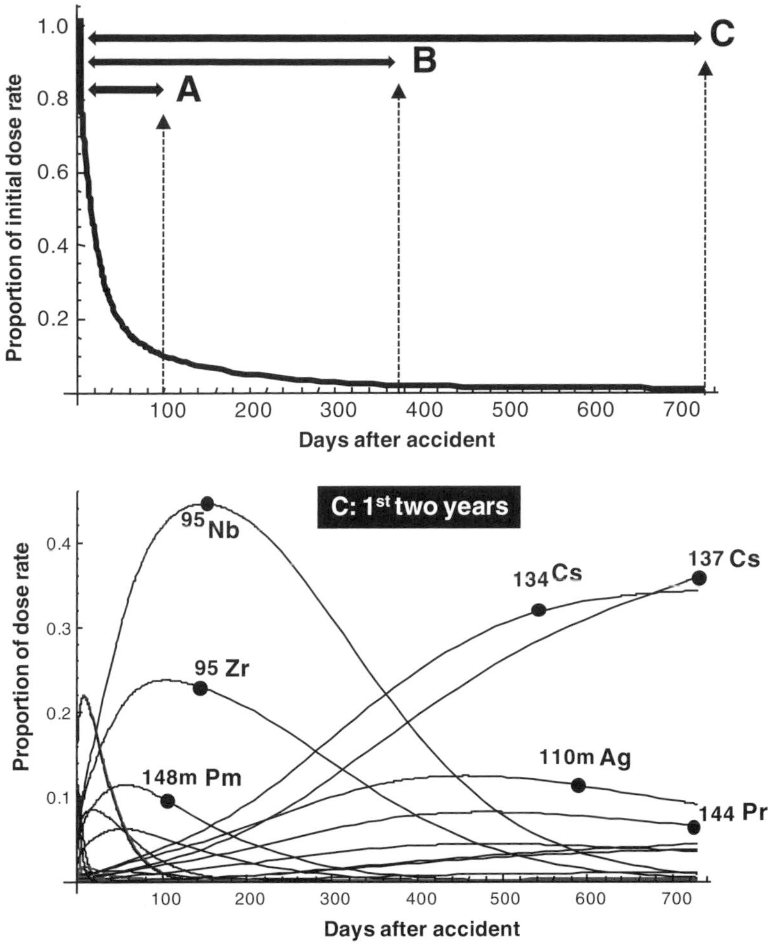

Figure 6 Graphic (upper) showing the rapid decrease in radiation doses after the accident (A = 100 days, B = 1 year, C = 2 years). The lower graph shows the changes in the nuclides responsible for radiation doses over the 2-year period. *Data from R.K. Chesser.*

reporting. There is little doubt that radiation doses immediately following the accident induced measurable genetic damage in exposed wildlife. However, it appears that the biological impact on wildlife species near Chernobyl has been subtle and difficult to document at either the individual or the population level.

Although present-day radiation doses experienced by wildlife species in limited areas near Chernobyl are unprecedented, they are nevertheless well below those documented to cause substantial genetic damage and are not sufficient to limit population growth. Lifetime doses in all but a very narrow tract of the Western Trace are below 0.1 Sv and are thereby classified as low-dose radiation. In fact, population recovery has likely been hastened by the evacuation of 135 000 people from the exclusion zone. Ecological recovery of habitats previously used as pasturelands and orchards has led to a rebound of many species to levels higher than before the accident. The Chernobyl exclusion zone is now being used in conservation efforts to recover the endangered Prezwalski's horse and European bison. Populations of these species have been released into the zone and are free from interference from excessive human activity.

Lessons from the Chernobyl Accident

In the aftermath of the Chernobyl accident there have been many valuable refinements to the design and operation of nuclear reactors. Refinements of operating power, the number and design of control elements, inclusion of automated emergency procedures, and enhanced training of operators have improved the safety of nuclear reactors. The RBMK-type reactor, although still in operation in some areas of the Russian Federation and Eastern Europe, is considered to be unstable due to its inability to withstand loss of cooling water and general lack of sufficient containment structures.

It was clear after Chernobyl that there was insufficient planning for a nuclear emergency involving substantial releases of radiation that could affect human populations. The 45 000 citizens of the city of Pripyat, Ukraine, were spared massive doses of radiation only by the fortuitous directions of the wind during the 37 h prior to evacuation. Because radioactive particles and aerosols of volatile elements may flow for very long distances from the source, it is imperative that communications of releases be accurately and immediately transmitted across political borders to permit protective

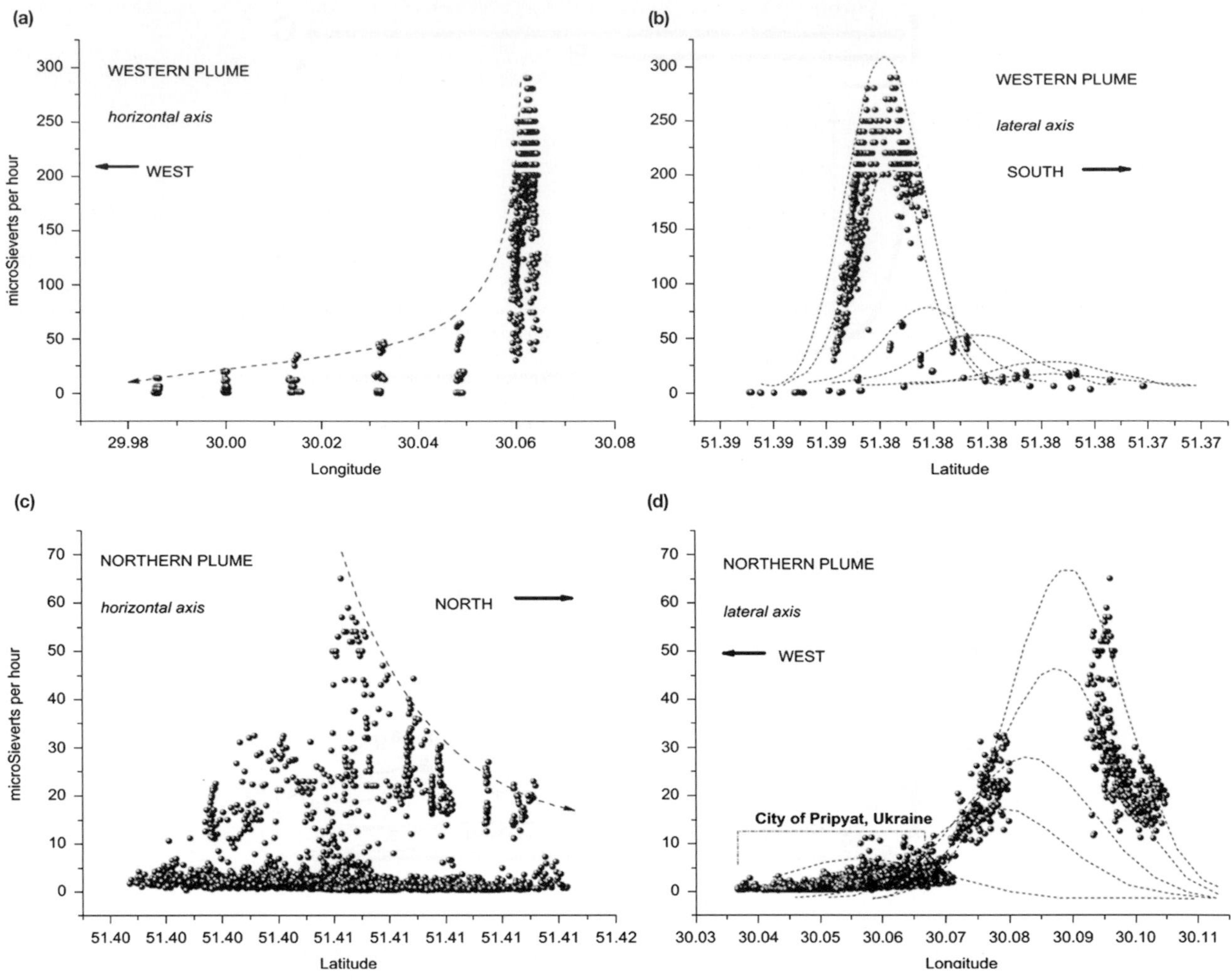

Figure 7 Graphics showing the radiation dose rates (in 2005) in the Western Plume (A and B) and in the Northern Plume (C and D). *From Chesser, R.K., Rodgers, B.E., 2008. Near-field particle dynamics and empirical fallout patterns in Chernobyl's Western and Northern Plumes.* Atmospheric Environment *42: 5124–5139.*

actions to be put into place. Prophylaxes, such as potassium iodide and cesium chloride tablets, should be immediately available to potentially affected communities. The studies at Chernobyl show that human and environmental health is affected predominantly during the first few days/weeks after a major radiation release by a reactor breach. Rapid decay of short-lived radionuclides, while producing large radiation doses over a short time period, will decay rapidly enough to sufficiently reduce exposure risks in the long term. At Chernobyl, even the most contaminated habitats began to recover most of their ecological diversity within a few years after the accident.

See also: Aerosols; Apoptosis; Carcinogenesis; Cesium; Chromosome Aberrations; Ecotoxicology; Emergency Response and Preparedness; Genetic Toxicology; Hormesis; Iodine; LD_{50}/LC_{50} (Lethal Dosage 50/Lethal Concentration 50); Plutonium; Radiation Toxicology, Ionizing and Nonionizing; Risk Characterization; Strontium; Three Mile Island; Uranium.

Further Reading

Cardis, E., 2003. Reconstruction of doses for Chernobyl liquidators. OECD Papers 3 (1) OECD, 2003.

Chesser, R.K., Rodgers, B.E., Wickliffe, J.K., et al., 2001. Accumulation of ^{137}cesium and ^{90}strontium from abiotic and biotic sources in rodents at Chornobyl, Ukraine. Environ. Toxicol. Chem. 20, 1927–1935.

Chesser, R.K., Sugg, D.W., DeWoody, A.J., et al., 2000. Concentrations and dose rate estimates of ^{134,137}cesium and ^{90}strontium in small mammals at Chornobyl, Ukraine. Environ. Toxicol. Chem. 19, 305–312.

Chesser, R.K., Baker, R.J., 2006. Growing up with Chernobyl. Am. Sci. 94, 542–549.

Chesser, R.K., Rodgers, B.E., 2008. Near-field particle dynamics and empirical fallout patterns in Chernobyl's western and northern plumes. Atmos. Environ. 42, 5124–5139.

Chumak, V.V., Likhtarjov, I.A., Riepin, V.S., 1996. Irradiation doses of evacuated population. In: Baryakhtar, V.G. (Ed.), Chornobyl Catastrophe, 1997. National Academy of Sciences of Ukraine, Kyiv Editorial House, Kiev, Ukraine, pp. 422–424.

Howell, E.K., Gaschak, S.P., Griffith, K.D.W., Rodgers, B.E., 2011. The effects of environmental low-dose irradiation on tolerance to chemotherapeutic agents. Environ. Toxicol. Chem. 30 (3), 640–649.

Imanaka, T., Koide, H., 2000. Assessment of external dose to inhabitants evacuated from the 30-km zone soon after the Chernobyl accident. Radiatsionnaya biologiya. Radioecologiya 20 (5).

Kashparov, V.A., Lundin, S.M., Zvarych, S.I., Yoshchenko, V.I., Levchuk, S.E., Khomutinin, Y.V., Maloshtan, I.M., Protsak, V.P., 2003. Territory contamination with the radionuclides representing the fuel component of Chernobyl fallout. Sci. Total Environ. 317 (1–3), 105–119.

Likhtarev, I.A., Chumack, V.V., Repin, V.S., 1994. Retrospective reconstruction of individual and collective external gamma doses of population evacuated after the Chernobyl accident. Health Phys. 66, 643–652.

Rodgers, B.E., Holmes, K.M., 2008. Radio-adaptive response to environmental exposures at Chernobyl. Dose Response 6 (2), 209–221.

Rodgers, B.E., Baker, R.J., et al., 2000. Frequencies of micronuclei in bank voles from zones of high radiation at Chornobyl, Ukraine. Environ. Toxicol. Chem. 19, 1644–1649.

Saenko, V., Ivanov, V., Tsyb, A., Bogdanova, T., Tronko, M., Demidchik, Y., Yamashita, S., 2011. The Chernobyl accident and its consequences. Clin. Oncol. 23 (4), 234–243.

Talerko, N., 2005. Reconstruction of (131) I radioactive contamination in Ukraine caused by the Chernobyl accident using atmospheric transport modelling. J. Environ. Radioact. 84 (3), 343–362.

UNDP and UNICEF, 2002. The Human Consequences of the Chernobyl Nuclear Accident.

UNSCEAR 2008 Report. Volume II. Effects of Ionizing Radiation. United Nations, Vienna, Austria.

Wickliffe, J.K., Bickham, A.M., Rodgers, B.E., et al., 2003. Exposure to chronic, low-dose rate gamma-radiation at Chernobyl does not induce point mutations in big blue mice. Environ. Mol. Mutagen. 42, 11–18.

Relevant Websites

http://lowdose.energy.gov – US Dept. of Energy: Low Dose Radiation Research Program.

http://www.bellona.org/articles/articles_2011/norwegian_estimates – Bellona: New Norwegian report says Fukushima radiation releases twice initial estimates.

http://www.iaea.org/Publications/Booklets/Chernobyl/chernobyl.pdf – International Atomic Energy Agency.

http://www.unscear.org/unscear/en/publications/2008_2.html – United Nations Scientific Committee on the Effects of Atomic Radiation.

http://www.un.org/ha/chernobyl/docs/report.pdf – United Nations.

http://www.who.int/ionizing_radiation/chernobyl/en/ – World Health Organization.

Children's Environmental Health

PJE Quintana, San Diego State University, San Diego, CA, USA

Introduction

Children are among the populations most vulnerable to environmental pollutants. The World Health Organization refers to the following categories of youth: 'newborns' (1–28 days), 'infants' (28 days–12 months), 'children' (1–10 years), and 'adolescents' (10–19 years). The term 'children' in this article refers to persons aged 1–19 years, unless otherwise specified. There are several reasons for children's increased vulnerability to toxic agents relative to adults. These include increased susceptibility due to physiological reasons, such as the fact that children are rapidly growing and developing, and that they often metabolize chemicals differently from adults. Children's behaviors also differ from adults and these can increase exposures through certain pathways, for example, hand-to-mouth behavior puts children at risk from toxicants in house dust. Children are also often more active, such as when on a playground, and when playing the increase in breathing rate and blood flow can increase absorption of air pollutants. Children are also powerless and are in close association with adults, which can, for example, lead them to be highly exposed to indoor air pollution from secondhand tobacco smoke and cooking smoke. Children have some unique exposures, for example, to toxicants in breast milk and infant formula. Children also are exposed early in life, and have a longer life expectancy and a longer period to develop adverse effects such as cancer. The following paragraphs will address each of these issues and provide examples of toxicants that greatly affect children's health, such as lead, and will finish by giving some approaches to protect children's health in the environment, such as ongoing research initiatives including the National Children's Study.

Children's Physiological Susceptibility to Environmental Toxicants

Children drink more water, breathe more air, and eat more food, pound for pound than does an adult. This increases their dose per kg of body weight, which can increase the likelihood of toxic responses. Children also absorb nutrients and also toxicants in a different way than adults. Soluble lead salts are more easily absorbed by children (>40% of ingested dose absorbed) than by adults (<15% absorbed). If children are deficient in nutrients they can also absorb more toxicants. Deficiencies of iron in the diet leading to anemia and also low calcium intake can further increase lead uptake in children. Children's growth rate is rapid and they are fashioning organs and systems that will last through their lifetimes. Growth occurs not only in young children, but also continues through late adolescence.

Protective mechanisms operating to reduce adult exposure to toxicants may be deficient or absent in children. For infants, the blood–brain barrier (a tight-knit cellular junction that prevents chemicals and drugs from crossing into the brain) has not fully developed, permitting toxicants such as mercury to cross from the blood to the brain. Also, metabolic enzymes that detoxify dangerous toxicants may not be functioning at adult levels. For example, an enzyme that detoxifies certain organophosphate pesticides is called paraoxonase, from the gene called PON1, and studies in farmworker children in the Salinas Valley have documented that this enzyme is present in very low levels in newborns as compared to adults. Therefore, a newborn exposed to certain pesticide residues may have a much higher risk of a toxic response as compared to an adult. An analysis of drugs metabolized by group of enzymes called the P450 enzymes found much slower elimination in newborns and infants. This group of enzymes catalyzes many reactions that eliminate environmental toxicants from the body.

Children's Behaviors and Environments That Increase Susceptibility to Environmental Toxicants

Children have special behaviors that put them at risk for environmental exposures. One is their hand-to-mouth behavior, which results in their ingesting much more soil and house dust per kg than do adults. The hand-to-mouth behavior results in a much higher risk to children from contaminated house dust and soils. In addition, activity level results in an increased resuspension of house dusts and soil in air near the ground or floor, which can then be inhaled due to their small stature. Chemicals such as household pesticides that have applied near the floor have also been shown to have a higher vapor concentration at children's breathing zone height as compared to an adult's level. Dermal exposure and absorption can also be increased due to touching behavior and thin skin. The United States Environmental Protection Agency (US EPA) has published an exposure factors handbook for children, which details differences in uptake in children due to physiological and behavioral factors. Children also are very active, which can increase their exposure to indoor airborne toxicants and to outdoor air pollutants such as ozone. Children's susceptibility due to their activity level at polluted locations is illustrated by a study conducted by the University of Southern California, which found that a major risk factor for children developing asthma was playing sports outdoors in the afternoon in areas with high ozone levels. Ozone is a major component of 'smog' air pollution that is found mainly outdoors and peaks in the late afternoon.

Children are also powerless to escape their environment and also spend much of the day in close proximity to adults, and this proximity may result in increased exposure. For example, a major factor in children's exposure to secondhand smoke is if one or more parents smoke. Even in California, a state that has some of the most strict antismoking laws in the United States, almost a million children were estimated to live

 http://dx.doi.org/10.1016/B978-0-12-386454-3.00801-0

with one or more smokers in 2011, and African American children, rural children, and low-income children were the most likely to be exposed. Globally, exposure to children to smoke from biomass burning, such as the use of wood or cow dung for heating or cooking, is a major cause of morbidity and mortality, often from pneumonia. Since women do the majority of the cooking and children stay close to the women, children are often directly exposed to high levels of particulates that equal or surpass levels from secondhand smoke.

Special and unique exposures for children include exposure to contaminants in breast milk and infant formula. Breast milk can contain many fat-soluble toxicants such as persistent organic pollutants. In areas such as the former East Germany, levels have been shown to be very high in mothers, and these levels are related to a high maternal body burden. However, the great and immediate health benefits of breast feeding outweigh the long-term risk from ingesting these toxicants, and breast milk is monitored as an indicator of population exposure rather than a toxic exposure. Contaminated formula and water presents risks to infants. The well-publicized intentional contamination of Chinese infant formula with melamine that resulted in kidney damage and deaths illustrates the vulnerability of infants to formula. Melamine is a plastic that was intentionally added to formula to make it appear that the protein content was sufficient. Formula made with contaminated water may also present a risk. Nitrates are pollutants associated with agricultural runoff and other sources and they have been shown to contaminate well water in the United States and worldwide. Blue baby syndrome is a condition where the infant's gut activates ingested nitrates to nitrites, which is a reaction that occurs more efficiently in infants than older children. The nitrites oxidize the iron in hemoglobin to make a form called methemoglobin that interacts with oxygen in a different way and does not release oxygen to tissues in sufficient amounts. The lack of oxygen makes the baby appear blue, especially at the lips and other thin-skinned areas, and can cause adverse effects on growth and development.

Selected Toxicants of Concern

Arsenic

Arsenic can be in inorganic (not combined with carbon) or organic forms. Children can be exposed through drinking water, as many sources of water worldwide are contaminated with arsenic. Highly exposed populations can be found in Taiwan, Chile, Bangladesh, and India, among others. Children can also be exposed through play structures made from preserved wood products treated with arsenic compounds, being near a smelter, and food. A number of recent studies have documented potential high exposures through consumption of rice, especially brown rice. Inorganic arsenic is classified as a known human carcinogen by the International Agency for Research on Cancer, and exposure has been associated with cancers of the skin, bladder, and lung in adults, though little information is available for children. It also causes skin lesions and has been reported to be associated with lowered IQ in children exposed to contaminated groundwater.

Lead

A main source of lead exposure to children in the United States is through ingestion of lead from leaded paint in homes, which can occur via ingestion of house dust or paint chips, or inhalation of air during refinishing operations involving lead paint. Children may also be exposed to lead through drinking water, contaminated toys, and cultural exposures such as Mexican candies or pottery containing lead. Internationally, children are still exposed to lead through the sale of leaded gasoline in some countries, although there is a worldwide movement to ban lead in gasoline. One of the single greatest interventions that has significantly improved children's environmental health was the ban on lead in gasoline and paint in the United States in the 1970s. The ban of lead in gasoline was followed by a precipitous drop of lead in blood samples taken from children of the United States, from almost 90% with a blood concentration over 10 $\mu g\ dl^{-1}$ in 1976 to <1% in 2008. Lead in paint is another target for global children's health. Leaded paint is still sold in many countries. Significant exposures also occur through artisanal gold mining, which can even lead to children dying of acute lead poisoning, as occurred in Nigeria in recent years. The health effects of lead exposure are covered in more detail elsewhere in the Encyclopedia, but are especially significant for children including lowered IQ, attention disorders, and other neurological findings. Childhood exposure might also affect risk for adult hypertension. The Centers for Disease Control and Prevention (CDC) has recently lowered the level of concern for children's blood lead from 10 $\mu g\ dl^{-1}$ to 5 $\mu g\ dl^{-1}$ based on the findings of adverse health effects at levels lower than 10 $\mu g\ dl^{-1}$.

Pesticides

Pesticides pose a hazard to children through acute poisonings, in addition to concerns about chronic exposures. Along the United States–Mexico border, studies have found that households often store pesticides in unmarked containers or in soda bottles or other food packaging. Children have died or been injured due to improper application of pesticides during pest control. In 2010, the US EPA restricted residential use of the pesticide Fumitoxin (active ingredient aluminum phosphide) after the death of two young Utah children when it was used near their home. The potential sensitivity of young children to certain pesticides due to lack of metabolic enzymes to detoxify the pesticide was discussed above. Concern about potential risks from pesticide residues in foodstuffs commonly consumed by children such as applesauce led to a reform of pesticide regulations and risk assessments by the US EPA with the Food Quality Protection Act of 1996. This act required the Agency to consider risks to children when assessing allowable amounts of pesticide residues in food.

Air Pollution

Air pollution exposures can be a significant risk to children both indoors and outdoors. Outdoor pollutants associated with adverse lung function and asthma risk include ozone and particulate matter, especially fine particulate matter ($PM_{2.5}$, less than an aerodynamic diameter of 2.5 μm) which are particles small enough to penetrate into the deep lung and even bloodstream. Many urban areas in the United States are in violation of air standards for these pollutants and globally, levels can be very high in urban areas such as Mexico City, Teheran, Bangkok, Beijing, and many other places where many children live and play. Indoors, major sources of $PM_{2.5}$ that lead to high indoor levels include tobacco smoke and cooking smoke. Recently, focus has turned to the health effects of near-traffic exposures with the realization that very high levels of pollutants can be found near roadways and that strong spatial gradients exist for toxic gases such as carbon monoxide, nitrogen dioxide, toxic vapors such as benzene, diesel exhaust particles measured as black carbon, and very small particles known as ultra fine particulate matter ($PM_{0.1}$). Children exposed to traffic pollutants near roadways have documented increased asthma and other respiratory issues, reduced lung growth and development, a potentially increased risk of leukemia, and a potential increased risk of autism in recent studies. The Children's Health Study at the University of Southern California has one of the most long-running studies on this issue and has an excellent web site on the health effects of traffic exposure.

Protecting Children from Environmental Hazards

The first step in protecting children is to document what hazards exist and what levels are harmful. For many health outcomes of concern, such as autism, the condition is relatively rare and therefore difficult to study. A large sample size is needed to find associations. The key to linking exposures and health effects is also to have accurate markers of exposure. Recent scientific studies to examine the effect of the environment and children's health include large cohort studies such as the National Children's Study. This is a large prospective study that is planned to have 105 000 children throughout the United States enrolled from before birth to 21 years, with extensive measures of their environment and health. In other efforts, the CDC monitors levels of pollutants in children in samples collected as part of the CDC's National Health and Nutrition Examination Survey. These are detailed by pollutant in the National Report on Human Exposure to Environmental Chemicals and provide an important reference for baseline levels and change over time. These samples document the drop in serum cotinine levels in children as a result of reductions in secondhand smoke exposure. Cotinine is a metabolite of nicotine and used as a marker for tobacco smoke exposure. Another focus area is the increased emphasis on environmental justice. The concept of environmental justice arose from the realization that poor and minority populations and children often bear the brunt of environmental exposures. President Clinton signed Executive Order 12898 "Federal Actions to Address Environmental Justice in Minority Populations and Low-Income Populations" in 1994, which directed federal agencies to consider disproportionately high adverse health effects of their actions on minority and low-income populations. The US EPA and other agencies now actively consider environmental justice in studying environmental exposures to children.

See also: Arsenic; Biomonitoring; Lead; Pesticides; Air Pollution; p450 Metabolism; Tobacco Smoke; Lead.

Further Reading

Ginsberg, G., Hattis, D., Sonawane, B., Russ, A., Banati, P., Kozlak, M., Smolenski, S., Goble, R., Apr 2002. Evaluation of child/adult pharmacokinetic differences from a database derived from the therapeutic drug literature. Toxicol. Sci. 66 (2), 185–200.

Gordon, B., Mackay, R., Rehfuess, E., 2004. Inheriting the World: The Atlas of Children's Health and the Environment. Retrieved from:. A WHO publication http://www.who.int/ceh/publications/atlas/en/.

Holland, N., Furlong, C., Bastaki, M., Richter, R., Bradman, A., Huen, K., Beckman, K., Eskenazi, B., Jul 2006. Paraoxonase polymorphisms, haplotypes, and enzyme activity in Latino mothers and newborns. Environ. Health Perspect. 114 (7), 985–991.

Landrigan, P.J., Goldman, L.R., 2011. Children's vulnerability to toxic chemicals: a challenge and opportunity to strengthen health and environmental policy. Health Aff. (Millwood) 30 (5), 842–850. http://dx.doi.org/10.1377/hlthaff.2011.0151.

Roberts, J.W., Dickey, P., 1995. Exposure of children to pollutants in house dust and indoor air. Rev. Environ. Contam. Toxicol. 143, 59–78.

U.S. EPA, 2008. Child-Specific Exposure Factors Handbook (Final Report). U.S. Environmental Protection Agency, Washington, DC. EPA/600/R-06/096F http://cfpub.epa.gov/ncea/cfm/recordisplay.cfm?deid=199243.

Relevant Websites

http://www.epa.gov/environmentaljustice/ – Environmental Justice. US EPA.

http://www.who.int/ceh/en/ – Global Plan of Action for Children's Health and the Environment. World Health Organization.

http://www.who.int/heli/risks/indoorair/indoorair/en/index.html – Indoor air pollution and household energy. Health and Environment Linkages Initiative – HELI. WHO/UNEP.

http://www.cdc.gov/nceh/lead/ – Lead. Centers for Disease Control and Prevention.

http://www.cdc.gov/exposurereport/ – National Report on Human Exposure to Environmental Chemicals. CDC.

http://www.nationalchildrensstudy.gov – The National Children's Study.

http://www.epa.gov/teach/ – Toxicity and Exposure Assessment for Children's Health (TEACH). US EPA.

http://hydra.usc.edu/cehc/research_findings.html – University of Southern California Children's Environmental Health Center. Key Research Findings.

Chloral Hydrate

M Troendle and BK Wills, Richmond, VA, USA

This article is a revision of the previous edition article by Michael Wahl, volume 1, pp 535–536, © 2005, Elsevier Inc.

- Name: Chloral Hydrate
- Chemical Abstracts Service Registry Number: 302-17-0
- Synonyms: Mickey Finn, Knockout drops, Noctec, Hydrated chloral, Chloralex
- Molecular Formula: $CCl_3CH(OH)_2$
- Chemical Structure:

Cl OH
Cl
Cl OH

Background

Chloral hydrate was first synthesized in 1832 by Justus von Liebig and was the first synthetic central nervous system (CNS) depressant. It was used to treat delirium tremens, insomnia, and anxiety, although it is considered an unapproved drug by the US Food and Drug Administration. Initially considered to be a safer alternative to opium, it was noted to produce rapid unconsciousness when combined with ethanol. Physical dependence can occur with chronic use.

Uses

Chloral hydrate is used as a sedative hypnotic, more commonly in pediatrics. With the advent of newer sedative hypnotics, its use has significantly decreased. It is also a drug of abuse, particularly in combination with ethanol to produce an amnestic effect in an individual who ingests it unknowingly.

Environmental Fate and Behavior

Chloral hydrate has been detected at 5 $\mu g\,l^{-1}$ in the US drinking water supply. Although chloral hydrate does not exist naturally, it can be produced as a by-product of chlorination of water at water treatment facilities, specifically in exposed water with high amounts of humic and fulvic substances.

Exposure and Exposure Monitoring

Most exposures are through ingestion. It is available as tablets, capsules, oral solution, and rectal suppositories. Toxicity may occur in patients as a result of unknowingly ingesting chloral hydrate. Cases are often with a coingestion of ethanol and/or other sedatives.

Toxicokinetics

Chloral hydrate is rapidly and well absorbed in the gastrointestinal (GI) tract. It is lipid soluble with an onset of action of approximately 30 min and half-life of only a few minutes. Chloral hydrate has a volume of distribution of 0.6–0.75 $l\,kg^{-1}$, and is rapidly metabolized by hepatic alcohol dehydrogenase to trichloroethanol. This active metabolite is responsible for the hypnotic effects and has a plasma half-life of 4–12 h. Trichloroethanol includes three elimination pathways. It can be conjugated with glucuronic acid to urochloralic acid, which is then renally excreted. Trichloroethanol can also be oxidized by aldehyde dehydrogenase to trichloroacetic acid, an inactive metabolite. Less than 10% of trichloroethanol is excreted unchanged by the kidneys.

Mechanism of Toxicity

Chloral hydrate is a CNS depressant, but its mechanism of action is not well known. Coingestion with ethanol produces enhanced effects by several mechanisms. First, ethanol competes for alcohol and aldehyde dehydrogenase, which then prolongs the half-life of ethanol. The metabolism of ethanol generates the reduced form of NADH, which is a cofactor for the metabolism of chloral hydrate to its active metabolite trichloroethanol. Finally, ethanol inhibits the conjugation of trichloroethanol to its inactive form urochloralic acid. This results in enhanced CNS depression.

Acute and Short-Term Toxicity

Animal

Chloral hydrate is used in veterinary medicine as a sedative hypnotic, and toxic effects are similar in humans and animals.

Human

Chloral hydrate is irritating to the GI tract, resulting in nausea, vomiting, and hemorrhagic gastritis. It may also rarely cause gastric and intestinal necrosis, which could lead to perforation and stricture formation. The major cause of death is believed to be secondary to cardiac dysrhythmias. Chloral hydrate and its metabolites can decrease myocardial contractility, shorten the refractory period, and increase sensitivity to catecholamines. Serious dysrhythmias can include ventricular fibrillation, ventricular tachycardia, and torsades de pointes. Respiratory failure can develop as a result of therapeutic use. As expected, patients can develop significant CNS depressions. Interestingly, case reports of seizure activity and a paradoxical central stimulant reaction has been reported.

Chronic Toxicity

Human

Chronic use may result in renal damage, skin eruptions, and gastritis. Physical dependence can also occur and withdrawal symptoms can be severe, including seizures and delirium.

Reproductive Toxicity

Chloral hydrate is listed as a category C agent.

Genotoxicity

Chloral hydrate has been shown to cause aneuploidy and stop mitosis.

Carcinogenicity

Chloral hydrate has not been identified as a carcinogen. Studies in rats given high doses during the lifetime did not produce carcinogenic concerns. However, chloral hydrate is structurally similar to known carcinogens.

Clinical Management

Activated charcoal can be used if the patient has a normal level of consciousness. There is no specific antidote and supportive care is the mainstay of treatment. Intubation should be performed if the patient is obtunded with loss of protective airway reflexes. Few hospital-based laboratories have the ability to rapidly detect chloral hydrate or its metabolites. Hypotension should be managed with intravenous crystalloids and dopamine. There is no role for forced diuresis. Hemodialysis and hemoperfusion could theoretically be useful in severe cases, although rarely employed.

Exposure Standards and Guidelines

The World Health Organization recommends concentrations limited to 10 $\mu g\ l^{-1}$. The US Environmental Protection Agency limits drinking water concentrations to 60 $\mu g\ l^{-1}$.

See also: Anxiolytics; Ethanol; Drugs of Abuse; Benzodiazepines.

Further Reading

Han, P., Song, H., Yang, P., Xie, H., Kang, Y.J., June 2011. Cardiac arrhythmias induced by chloral hydrate in rhesus monkeys. Cardiovasc. Toxicol. 11 (2), 128–133.

Pershad, J., Palmisano, P., Nichols, M., 1999. Chloral hydrate: the good and the bad. Pediatr. Emerg. Care. 6, 432–435.

Salmon, A.G., Kizer, K.W., Zeise, L., Jackson, R.J., Smith, M.T., 1995. Potential carcinogenicity of chloral hydrate–a review. J. Toxicol. Clin. Toxicol. 33 (2), 115–121. Review.

Sing, K., Erickson, T., Amitai, Y., Hryhorczuk, D., 1996. Chloral hydrate toxicity from oral and intravenous administration. J. Toxicol. Clin. Toxicol. 1, 101–106.

Chlorambucil

N Gupta, Phoenix VA Health Care System, Phoenix, AZ, USA
JR Salvatore, University of Arizona, Phoenix, AZ, USA

This article is a revision of the previous edition article by Larry J. Dziuk, volume 1, pp 536–538, © 2005, Elsevier Inc.

- Name: Chlorambucil
- Chemical Abstracts Service Registry Number: 305-03-3
- Synonyms: CB-1348, Chlorambucilum, Chlorambucyl, Chloraminophene, Chlorbutinum, Clorambucilo, Klórambucil, Klorambucil, Klorambusiili, Klorambusil, NSC-3088, WR-139013
- Molecular Formula: $C_{14}H_{19}Cl_2NO_2$
- Chemical Structure:

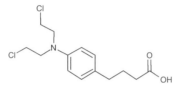

Background

Chlorambucil, approved by the Food and Drug Administration (FDA) in 1957, is an antineoplastic/alkylating agent with a broad spectrum of antitumor activity used to treat chronic lymphocytic leukemia (CLL), Hodgkin's and non-Hodgkin's lymphomas.

Uses

Chlorambucil is FDA indicated for the treatment of CLL, Hodgkin's and non-Hodgkin's lymphomas, and mycosis fungoides. It has also been known to treat other conditions such as polycythemia vera, uveitis, hairy cell leukemia, ovarian carcinoma, and Waldenstrom's magroglobulinemia.

Environmental Fate and Behavior

The chemical is of a white to pale slight odorous powder, insoluble in water. It is very slightly dispersible in diethyl ether and acetone. It has a melting point of 69 °C, boiling point of 424 °C, and 5.75 pK_a. The partition coefficient is 4.07 and has a molecular weight of 304.22 g mol^{-1}.

Exposure and Exposure Monitoring

The primary targets in overdose are the hematopoietic, gastrointestinal (GI), and neurological systems. Consistently reported findings are vomiting, ataxia, seizures, coma, and pancytopenia. The most common route of exposure is oral, through tablet or suspension. The tablets have been reformulated requiring refrigeration, or can be stored at room temperature (up to 86 °F) for up to 1 week. Maintenance doses for chlorambucil may be as low as 0.03 mg kg^{-1} per day but not to exceed 0.1 mg kg^{-1} per day. Pulse dosing is sometimes done up to 0.4 mg kg^{-1}. The usual dose for CLL is 4–10 mg per day for the average adult patient. For those adults with severe renal impairment, consider dose reduction by 25% with creatinine clearance (CrCL) from 10 to 50 ml min^{-1}, and by 50% if CrCL is less than 10 ml min^{-1}.

Possible human exposure includes inhalation, incidental ingestion, and dermal contact. Splash goggles, lab coat, dust respirator should be used for personal protection.

No information on environmental levels is available, however, due to its extensive metabolism in the treated patients environmental emissions are considered of low concern.

Toxicokinetics

Chlorambucil is rapidly and completely absorbed in the GI tract, food reduces its bioavailability by 10–20%. It is extensively metabolized in the liver to phenylacetic acid mustard, and its metabolites are extensively bound to plasma and tissue proteins. After a single dose, about 15–60% of chlorambucil appears in the urine after 24 h. However, less than 1% is actually intact drug and overall has low urinary excretion.

Mechanism of Toxicity

The mechanism of action of chlorambucil is thought to be an alkylating agent and an aromatic nitrogen mustard derivative; it interferes with DNA replication and RNA transcription by alkylation and cross-linking the strands of DNA.

Acute and Short-Term Toxicity

Neurologic toxicity such as seizures has been observed, myoclonus and abnormal vision in addition to psychiatric effects such as hallucinations and agitation were also observed. Hematologic toxicity such as anemia, leukopenia, neutropenia, and a black box warning for myelosuppression can occur. Dermatologic toxicity, GI upset, respiratory effects such as pulmonary fibrosis, renal and hepatotoxicity, and immunologic effects are also potential adverse effects.

Chronic Toxicity

Chlorambucil is known to cause severe bone marrow suppression. It is known to be leukemogenic, and can lead to

 http://dx.doi.org/10.1016/B978-0-12-386454-3.00478-4

slow and progressive lymphopenia during or following treatment. Neutropenia can also occur.

Immunotoxicity

Immune hypersensitivity reaction and drug fever have been shown. Administration of live vaccines to immunocompromised persons should be avoided.

Carcinogenicity

Chlorambucil has been reevaluated by International Agency for Research on Cancer (IARC) in 2012. It is considered as a direct-acting alkylating agent that is carcinogenic via a genotoxic mechanism. According to IARC, there is sufficient evidence in humans and experimental animals regarding the carcinogenicity of chlorambucil, and therefore it is concluded that chlorambucil is carcinogenic to humans (Group 1).

Reproductive Toxicity

Black-boxed warning for human fertility effects is a probable mutagenic and teratogenic agent. Reproductive effects including infertility, sexual dysfunction, and disorder of menstruation have been reported. Chlorambucil crosses the placenta, and case reports showed unilateral agenesis for those exposed in the first trimester. Reversible and permanent infertility has been seen in females and males, and mutagenicity with chromosome damage.

Clinical Management

There is no specific antidote for chlorambucil, and it is not dialyzable. For oral/parenteral exposure, induced emesis with ipecac is not recommended due to chance of seizures. However, activated charcoal or gastric lavage can be performed. Seizures toxicity may be managed with IV benzodiazepine. Pancytopenia should be monitored for up to 3 weeks, and fluid/electrolyte replacement in persistent vomiting.

Exposure Standards and Guidelines

The FDA regulates chlorambucil prescription drug labeling and other requirements. The Institute for Safe Medication Practices includes chlorambucil as a drug with heightened risk of causing significant harm to patients when used in error.

See also: Semustine.

Further Reading

IARC Monographs on the Evaluation of Carcinogenic Risks to Humans. Pharmaceuticals, Chlorambucil, vol. 100A, 2012, pp 47–55 http://monographs.iarc.fr/ENG/Monographs/vol100A/mono100A-7.pdf.

Rai, K.R., Peterson, B.L., Appelbaum, F.R., Kolitz, J., Elias, L., Shepherd, L., Hines, J., Threatte, G.A., Larson, R.A., Cheson, B.D., Schiffer, C.A., 2000. Fludarabine compared with chlorambucil as primary therapy for chronic lymphocytic leukemia. N. Engl. J. Med. 343 (24), 1750–1757. http://dx.doi.org/10.1056/NEJM200012143432402.

Takimoto, C.H., Calvo, E., 2008. Principles of oncologic pharmacotherapy. In: Pazdur, R., Wagman, L.D., Camphausen, K.A., Hoskins, W.J. (Eds.), Cancer Management: A Multidisciplinary Approach, eleventh ed.

Relevant Websites

http://www.sciencelab.com – Sciencelab.com (Chemical & Laboratory Equipment): Search for Chlorambucil).

http://www.micromedex.com – Truven Health Analytics: Micromedex 2.0.

http://www.accessdata.fda.gov/drugsatfda_docs/label/2011/010669s032lbl.pdf – US FDA: Prescribing information for Leukeran® (chlorambucil) tablets.

http://ntp.niehs.nih.gov/ntp/roc/twelfth/profiles/Chlorambucil.pdf – US National Institutes of Health: Report on Carcinogens - Chlorambucil.

Chloramphenicol

M Abdollahi and S Mostafalou, Tehran University of Medical Sciences, Tehran, Iran

This article is a revision of the previous edition article by Greene Shepherd, volume 1, pp 538–539, © 2005, Elsevier Inc.

- Name: Chloramphenicol
- Chemical Abstracts Service Registry Number: CAS 56-75-7
- Mixture Name: Chloromyxin; Elase-Chloromycetin; Ophthocort
- Synonyms: Amphicol, Amseclor, Aquamycetin, Biocetin, Biophenicol, Chlomycol, Chloramex, Chloramficin, Chloramsaar, Chlorocaps, Chlorocid, Chlorocol, Chloromax, Chloromycetin, Chloronitrin, Chloramex, Chloroptic, Chlornitromycin, Cloramfenicol, Cloramficin, Cloramicol, Cloromisan, Cylphenicol, Detreomycin, Enteromycetin, Farmicetina, Fenicol, Globenicol, Ismicetina, Kemicetine, Klorocid S, Leukomyan, Leukomycin, Levomicetina, Micloretin, Novomycetin, Ophthochlor, Paraxin, Quemicetina, Romphenil, Septicol, Sintomicetina, Tevcocin, Tifomycine, Unimycetin
- Dictionary: Jarisch–Herxheimer reaction: Is a reaction to endotoxins released by the death of harmful organisms. It resembles bacterial sepsis and can occur after the start of antibacterials such as chloramphenicol.
- Chemical Class: Antibiotic with both bacteriocidal and bacteriostatic properties
- Molecular Formula: $C_{11}H_{12}Cl_2N_2O_5$
- Chemical Structure:

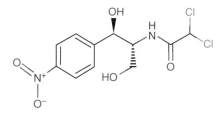

Background (Significance/History)

Chloramphenicol was first isolated from cultures of *Streptomyces venezuelae* in 1947 but now is produced synthetically. As the first discovered broad-spectrum antibiotic, it acts by interfering with bacterial protein synthesis.

Uses

Chloramphenicol as an antibiotic is active against gram-positive and gram-negative bacteria and anaerobic microorganisms. It was originally introduced as a treatment for typhoid but now it is rarely used for this purpose because of the prevalence of multiple drug-resistant *Salmonella typhi*. As it has an excellent blood–brain barrier penetration, chloramphenicol is the antibiotic of choice for brain abscesses caused by staphylococci and mixed or unknown microorganisms. Chloramphenicol is used in the treatment of meningitis when there is allergy to penicillin or cephalosporin. It may also be effective against vancomycin-resistant enterococci.

Environmental Fate and Behavior

Routes and Pathways Relevant Physicochemicals Properties

Chloramphenicol is a white to greyish-white or yellowish-white fine crystalline powder or fine crystals, needles, or elongated plates and it is bitter to taste. Chloramphenicol has a solubility of 25 000 mg l^{-1} (25 mg ml^{-1}) in water at 25 °C and it is very soluble in methanol, ethanol, butanol, ethyl acetate, acetone, and chloroform. Waste streams of drug industries producing chloramphenicol can be the source of its release to the environment. If released to the air, an estimated vapor pressure of 1.7×10^{-12} mm Hg at 25 °C indicates that chloramphenicol will exist solely in the particulate phase, which can be removed from the atmosphere by wet and dry deposition. This vapor pressure indicates chloramphenicol is not expected to be volatile from dry soil surface. Based on the estimated Henry's Law constant of 2.3×10^{-18} atm-cu m mol^{-1} for chloramphenicol, volatilization from water and moist soil surface is not plausible.

Partition Behavior in Water, Sediment, and Soil

In the aquatic system, chloramphenicol is not expected to adsorb to suspended solids and sediments given by the K_{oc} (Soil Organic Carbon–Water Partitioning Coefficient) value of 99.

Environmental Persistency (Degradation/Speciation)

Chloramphenicol solutions are susceptible to direct photolysis by sunlight or high temperatures and decompose to form hydrochloric and dichloric acid. Hydrolysis of chloramphenicol is not anticipated under environmental conditions because it lacks a functional group to hydrolyze. Chloramphenicol has been reported to degrade 86.2% with a biodegradation rate of 3.3 mg COD per gram per hour using adapted activated sludge as the inoculums. It can also be degraded by intestinal bacteria via amidolysis to 18 observed metabolites.

Long Range Transport

In terrestrial systems, the K_{oc} value of 99 suggests that chloramphenicol has high mobility in the soil.

Bioaccumulation and Biomagnifications

An estimated bioconcentration factor <1 for chloramphenicol indicates that the potential of bioconcentration in aquatic organisms is low.

 http://dx.doi.org/10.1016/B978-0-12-386454-3.00709-0

Exposure and Exposure Monitoring

Routes and Pathways (Including Environmental Release)

Manufacturing of chloramphenicol with subsequent waste streams and usage as an antibiotic can result in its release to the environment.

Human Exposure

People who work in the field of producing, manufacturing, or in administering chloramphenicol can be exposed to chloramphenicol through inhalation and dermal contact with this compound. For general population, exposure to chloramphenicol is likely to happen via use of pharmaceutical products containing this compound. Its use in food like certified shrimp aquaculture operations is banned worldwide.

Environmental Exposure (Monitoring Data in Air, Water, Sediment, Soil, and Biota)

Chloramphenicol has been reported in the low micrograms per liter range in the surface and sewage water as studied in Germany.

Toxicokinetics

Chloramphenicol is prepared as capsules, tablet, ear drop, eye drop, and ointment. It is also formulated as the palmitate in suspension for oral administration and as the succinate in vials for injection. When ingested, chloramphenicol is rapidly absorbed and achieves its maximum serum concentration of 10–13 mg ml^{-1} within 2–3 h. Water-soluble form of chloramphenicol for parenteral use is an inactive prodrug sodium succinate, which is hydrolyzed by esterases. Serum concentrations of intravenous and intramuscular administration of chloramphenicol are only 70% of those achieved when given orally. Having the volume of distribution of 0.2–3.1 l kg^{-1}, about 50% of the chloramphenicol is bound to plasma proteins (primarily albumin) and is widely distributed in body fluids particularly cerebrospinal fluid, where values range from 45 to 99% of those in plasma in the presence and absence of meningitis. It also diffuses into breast milk and placental fluid resulting in a fetal blood level of 30–80% of maternal serum concentrations. Chloramphenicol is mostly inactivated by conjugation with glucuronide in the liver and excretion of this metabolite and itself in the urine is the predominant route of elimination. Over a 24 h period, 75–90% of an orally administered dose is excreted. An elimination half-life of 1.6–4.6 h has been established for chloramphenicol, which correlates with plasma bilirubin concentrations and is considerably longer in neonates because their ability to conjugate drugs is not yet developed significantly. Accordingly, dosage adjustment are required in neonates and in patients with impaired hepatic function or cirrhosis but not necessary in cases of renal insufficiency or hemodialysis.

Mechanism of Toxicity

As an antibiotic, chloramphenicol enters the target cells by facilitated diffusion and binds reversibly to the 50S ribosomal subunit. This prevents the interaction between peptidyl transferase and its amino acid substrate, which results in the inhibition of peptide bond formation. Indeed, it is an inhibitor of protein synthesis in the bacteria and to a lesser extent, in eukaryotic cells. Chloramphenicol can also inhibit mitochondrial protein synthesis in mammalian cells particularly erythropoietic cells, which are sensitive to the drug.

Acute and Short-Term Toxicity (to Include Irritation and Corrosivity)

Animal

Chloramphenicol, as a common veterinary antibiotic, has a low level of animal toxicity. The acute LD_{50} of chloramphenicol in mice has been estimated 200 and 1320 mg kg^{-1} after IV and IP administration, respectively. Chloramphenicol has an LD_{50} in rats after IV administration of 170 mg kg^{-1}.

Human

Chloramphenicol toxicity in humans can cause nausea and vomiting, dysgeusia or unpleasant taste, diarrhea, perineal irritation, hypotension, and hypothermia. Blurring of vision, digital paresthesias, neurotoxic reactions, and peripheral neuritis are more uncommon toxic effects of this drug. Tissues with high rates of oxygen consumption are particularly susceptible to chloramphenicol with encephalopathy and cardiomyopathy resulting from chloramphenicol toxicity to the myocardium and central nervous system. Hypersensitivity to chloramphenicol is relatively uncommon although rarely macular or vesicular skin rashes, fever, angioedema, and Jarisch–Herxheimer reactions have been reported. Gray baby syndrome may occur in neonates exposed to excessive doses of chloramphenicol. It is a state of cardiovascular collapse and usually begins 2–9 days after start of treatment. The primary symptoms include vomiting, refusal to suck, irregular and rapid respiration, abdominal distention, periods of cyanosis, and passage of loose and green stools. After 24 h, the children become flaccid, hypothermic, and severely ill while turning an ashen-gray color. Death occurs in about 40% of patients within 2 days of initial symptoms. The developmental deficiency of glucuronyl transferase and inadequate renal excretion of unconjugated drug in neonates are two responsible mechanisms for the development of Gray baby syndrome. Topical application of chloramphenicol ophthalmic solution to the eye may cause transient burning or stinging. Hypersensitivity or inflammatory reactions including contact conjunctivitis, itching or burning, angioneurotic edema, urticaria, and vesicular and/or maculopapular dermatitis rarely occur following topical application of chloramphenicol in patients who are sensitive to the drug or to other ingredients in the formulation.

Chronic Toxicity

Animal

Intraperitoneal injections of chloramphenicol at 20, 40, or 100 mg kg^{-1} for 3 months in mice have been reported to cause splenomegaly, hepatomegaly, lymphadenopathy, and hypertrophy of the thymus. Elevated incidence of lymphomas has been reported in mice administered chloramphenicol for 2 years.

Human

Bone marrow suppression is a common and reversible side effect of chloramphenicol treatment due to its inhibitory action on mitochondrial protein synthesis in erythroid precursors and subsequent impairment of iron incorporation into heme. It primarily manifests as a fall in hemoglobin levels and occurs when chloramphenicol reaches a plasma concentration of 25 μg ml^{-1} or higher. Thrombocytopenia and leucopenia may also occur. Chloramphenicol can also produce severe, idiosyncratic bone marrow toxicity resulting in aplastic anemia, which is the most serious side effect. It is not dose-dependent and may occur more commonly in patients who undergo prolonged therapy. The incidence of aplastic anemia is low (1 in approximately 30 000) but it has a high rate of fatality. The incidence of acute leukemia in those who recover is high. There is a link between chloramphenicol exposure and acute leukemia, just as the risk increases with the length of treatment.

Immunotoxicity

There is no evidence on immunotoxicity of chloramphenicol in animals or human.

Reproductive Toxicity

Chloramphenicol diffuses easily into placental fluid and breast milk and is classified as FDA pregnancy category C, which requires caution in pregnancy. Maternal exposure to chloramphenicol in rats has been reported to cause malformations including hydrocephaly, cleft palate, umbilical hernia, and also impairment of avoidance learning in offspring. Higher incidence of embryonic and fetal death and fetal growth retardation were shown in rats, mice, and rabbits given high doses of chloramphenicol. Defects of neural tube development have been reported in chick embryos. Increased seizure threshold and decreased learning ability and performance in an open-field test were reported in offspring of mice administered with chloramphenicol during pregnancy.

Genotoxicity

According to acceptable data, the genotoxic hazard of chloramphenicol is considered low. The result of drosophila test as the genotoxicity assay *in vivo* for chloramphenicol was negative. Based on studies *in vitro*, chloramphenicol has been reported to cause some genetic damages like mutations in mouse lymphoma cells and sister chromatid exchange in Chinese hamster ovary (CHO) cells.

Carcinogenicity

Based on the findings from animal studies, chloramphenicol use has been associated with increased risk of certain malignancies such as lymphomas. Chloramphenicol also induces aplastic anemia, which is related to the occurrence of leukemia. Chloramphenicol is listed as reasonably anticipated to be a human carcinogen.

Clinical Management

In case of intoxication, standard emergency supportive cares should be instituted. As it causes hypothermia and hypotension, the patient should be slowly warmed using blankets, warm IV fluids, or warm mist inhalation. Administration of activated charcoal is the preferable measure of decontamination. Vitamins B6 and B12 have been recommended for neuritis, while L-phenylalanine can be used for bone marrow effects.

Ecotoxicology

Chloramphenicol has been reported to cause severe ultrastructural changes in leukocytes of toads. These changes were similar to those induced by chemical carcinogen 7, 12-dimethylbenz(α)anthracene and also similar to those in leukocytes reported in humans with leukemia.

Other Hazards

Chloramphenicol is an inhibitor of hepatic cytochrome P450 isozymes (CYPs) which can prolong the half-life of drugs metabolized by this system, including warfarin, dicumarol, phenytoin, chlorpropamide, antiretroviral protease inhibitors, rifabutin, and tolbutamide so that severe toxicity and death have been reported because of failure to recognize such effects. Conversely, drugs inducing CYPs like phenobarbital or rifampin can shorten the half-life of chloramphenicol, which may result in subtherapeutic drug concentrations.

Exposure Standards and Guidelines

Workplace environmental exposure level: 8 h time-weighted average is 0.5 mg m^{-3}. Because of the dose-independent character of chloramphenicol-induced aplastic anemia, an allowed daily intake could not be set for this drug.

Miscellaneous

In addition to safety concerns, resistance is a new reason for chloramphenicol not to be a first line antimicrobial agent anymore. Three mechanisms of resistance to chloramphenicol are reduced membrane permeability, elaboration of chloramphenicol acetyltransferase, and mutation of the 50S ribosomal subunit. Nonetheless, the global problem of ongoing bacterial resistance to newer antibiotics has led to the renewed interest in its use for some infections.

See also: Carboxylesterases; Cardiovascular System; Molecular Toxicology: Recombinant DNA Technology.

Further Reading

Berendsen, B., Stolker, L., de Jong, J., Nielen, M., Tserendorj, E., Sodnomdarjaa, R., Cannavan, A., Elliott, C., 2010. Evidence of natural occurrence of the banned antibiotic chloramphenicol in herbs and grass. Anal. Bioanal. Chem. 397 (5), 1955–1963.

National Toxicology Program, 2011. Chloramphenicol. In: Report on Carcinogens, vol. 12, pp. 92–94.

Wiest, D.B., Cochran, J.B., Tecklenburg, F.W., April 2012. Chloramphenicol toxicity revisited: a 12-year-old patient with a brain abscess. J. Pediatr. Pharmacol. Ther. 17 (2), 182–188.

Relevant Websites

http://www.inchem.org – IPCS International Program on Chemical Safety.
http://www.nlm.nih.gov/medlineplus – MedlinePlus: Search for Chloramphenicol.
http://health.nytimes.com/health/guides/disease/gray-syndrome/overview.html – The New York Times - Gray Syndrome.
http://toxnet.nlm.nih.gov – Toxicology Data Network, US National Library of Medicine.

Chlordane

SE Koshlukova and NR Reed, California Environmental Protection Agency, Sacramento, CA, USA

This article is a revision of the previous edition article by Benny L. Blaylock, volume 1, pp 540–542, © 2005, Elsevier Inc.

Background

Chlordane is a chlorinated cyclodiene manufactured for use as an insecticide. Technical chlordane is a mixture of *cis*- and *trans*-chlordane, lesser amounts of heptachlor, nonachlor and chlordenes, and other related compounds. Chlordane represents the oldest generation of the chloride channel blocker insecticides with marked mammalian toxicity.

Chlordane was first registered in the United States in 1948, and was extensively used to control agricultural and structural pests. In the late 1970s, concerns regarding carcinogenicity potential, toxicity to developing nervous and immune systems, environmental persistence, and bioaccumulation in the food chain led to its ban in many countries by 1998.

More than two decades after its ban, chlordane is still present in certain foods, water, air, and soils. Chlordane and oxychlordane are found in over 170 of the 1684 National Priorities List (NPL) sites (the most hazardous waste sites in the United States). Both chemicals are on the 2011 Comprehensive Environmental Response, Compensation, and Liability Act priority list for substances with the highest frequency, toxicity, and potential for human exposure at the NPL sites. Chlordane is on the United Nations Environment Program list of persistent organic pollutants, for which international action is required to reduce risks to humans and the environment.

Chemical Profile

- Technical Chlordane: Mixture of over 140 related compounds. Sixty percent to 95% of technical chlordane consists of stereoisomers *cis*- and *trans*-chlordane with a ratio of about 3:1. Both *cis*- and *trans*-isomers have insecticidal activity.
- Chemical Abstracts Service Registry Number: CAS 57-74-9 (analytical grade), CAS 12789-03-6 (technical grade), CAS 5103-71-9 (*cis*- or α-chlordane), CAS 5103-74-2 (*trans*- or γ-chlordane)
- Chemical Name: 1,2,4,5,6,7,8,8-octachloro-2,3,3a,4,7,7a-hexahydro-4,7-methanoindene
- Synonyms: Chlordane (technical), 1,2,4,5,6, 7,8,8-octa-chloro-2,3,3a,4,7, 7a-hexahydro-4,7 -methano-1H-indene; Chlorindan; Chlor; Corodan; Kypchlor; Niran; Octachlor; Topichlor; Toxichlor; Velsicol-1068
- Chemical Class: Chlorinated cyclodiene; insecticide
- Chemical Structure: (from Pubchem) http://pubchem.ncbi.nlm.nih.gov/image/structurefly.cgi?cid=24860539&width=400&height=400

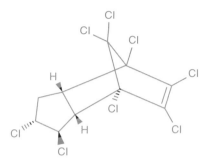

- Molecular Formula: $C_{10}H_6C_8$
- Molecular Weight: 409.779 g mol^{-1}
- Density: 1.59–1.63 g cm^{-3}
- Vapor Pressure: 0.0005–0.00001 mm Hg at 25 °C
- Boiling Point: 175 °C (technical grade)
- Melting Point: 107 °C (*cis*-isomer), 104 °C (*trans*-isomer)
- Flash Point: 107.2 °C
- Conversion Factor: 1 ppm = 16.75 mg m^{-3} at 25 °C
- Appearance: Amber-colored viscous liquid (technical chlordane)
- Odor: Pungent, chlorine like
- Odor Threshold: 0.0084–0.0419 mg m^{-3}

Uses

From 1948 to 1978, chlordane was extensively used to control termites in homes by underground applications around the foundation. It was widely applied as an insecticide on agricultural crops (e.g., corn and citrus); on lawns and gardens; as a wood preservative to control borers, termites, and dry rot; for protective treatment of underground cables; and as a fumigating agent. Prior to the severe worldwide restricted use in 1980s, the estimated annual production was 9500 tons in the United States and 70 000 tons globally. In 1978, the US Environmental Protection Agency (EPA) canceled its use on food crops and phased out the remaining uses. All uses and sale in the United States were prohibited in 1988, and production for export ceased in 1998. Chlordane was banned in the European Union in 1981, Canada in 1995, Australia in 1997, and Mexico in 1998. Despite these major actions to eliminate the use of chlordane, production facilities exist in China, Singapore, India, and Argentina; its insecticidal use continues in the developing countries.

Environmental Fate and Behavior

Chlordane is soluble in organic solvents (e.g., cyclohexanone, benzene) but practically insoluble in water (0.056 mg l^{-1}

solubility at 25 °C). The Henry's law constant of 0.00005 atm m^3 mol^{-1} indicates significant volatilization from surface water. In air, chlordane reacts with photochemically generated hydroxyl radicals with an estimated half-life of 5.2–51.7 h.

Chlordane does not undergo significant biotic and abiotic degradation in soil and water. Chlordane may persist for >20 years in soil. The degradation rate under field conditions is 4–28% per year. In river water under sunlight, 85% of chlordane persisted to the end of the 8-week experiment. Abiotic degradation (hydrolysis, oxidation, dechlorination, or direct photolysis) is also not an important environmental fate process. The estimated Log K_{oc} of 3.5–4.6 predicts strong soil adsorption and resistance to leaching to groundwater.

Chlordane in soil and sediment can be taken up by organisms and plants. Due to its stability, it can travel long distances and contaminate areas remote from its use. The measured Log K_{ow} of 5.4 indicates extensive bioaccumulation in food chains.

Exposure and Exposure Monitoring

Before its ban, human exposure to chlordane happened directly from its insecticidal use. Today, exposure to chlordane continues due to its persistence in the environment and bioaccumulation. The main exposure route is through ingestion of contaminated water and foods (particularly fish and meat). Enforceable levels are established in water and foods (chlordane, oxychlordane, nonachlor, and chlordene). Action levels were established in 1990 for the unavoidable environmental contamination.

Inhalation of vapors from contaminated soil and water or direct dermal contact with residual chlordane from past pesticide applications is also possible. Chronic indoor air exposure is possible in homes previously treated for termite control. Chlordane has been detected in indoor air 15 years after treatment, and an estimated over 50 million people have been exposed to chlordane in their homes in the United States. Occupational exposure remains in countries where chlordane is produced and used. The exposure is likely higher for the general public living near hazardous waste sites where chlordane has been detected. At a given exposure concentration, children generally have higher body burden due to their higher intake (inhalation volume, amount of food intake) or contact on a per-body-weight basis.

Toxicokinetics

The estimated oral absorption of chlordane is 80% in rats and above 50% in rabbits. Human oral, dermal, and inhalation absorptions are evident by the presence of chlordane compounds in blood and tissues, and in the observed systemic toxicity. Peak blood level of chlordane and its metabolites occurs 2–4 h after dosing in rats and after 8 h in mice.

Chlordane is extensively metabolized by the liver cytochrome P450 enzymes (CYP) in animals and humans. Hydroxylation followed by dehydration results in the more toxic oxychlordane. Dehydrochlorination produces heptachlor with subsequent formation of heptachlor epoxide. Dechlorination and replacement of chlorine atoms by hydroxyl group forms mono-, di-, and trihydroxy-metabolites. Chlordane residues are highest in fat and lower in liver, kidneys, brain, and muscles. The main metabolite in humans, monkeys, rats, and mice is the epoxide oxychlordane, which is very slowly metabolized and persists in fat. Chlordane is found in cow and human milk. Transplacental transport is evident through chlordane in maternal placenta, umbilical cord, and blood of newborns. Other persistent residues in human tissues include *trans*-nonachlor and pentachlorocyclopentene, as components of technical chlordane.

The feces are the major route of elimination in rats and mice, where 65–90% of a single oral dose is recovered within 7 days after dosing, while 2–8% is excreted in urine. Enterohepatic circulation is significant. Breast milk is another significant excretion route. Rabbits excreted a higher percentage (28–47%) of the dose in urine, possibly due to increased formation of soluble conjugates of chlordane metabolites. The elimination half-lives for chlordane are several weeks to several months in rats and humans.

Mechanism of Toxicity

The primary target for chlordane toxicity is the central nervous system. Like other cyclodiene insecticides, chlordane acts as a noncompetitive antagonist of the chloride ion channel of the $GABA_A$-receptor. When activated by GABA, the $GABA_A$-receptor increases Cl^- conductance into the neurons and prevents excessive nerve stimulation. Chlordane binds to the Cl^- channel of the receptor and thereby blocks the actions of GABA. Seizures, vomiting, and convulsions are typical symptoms associated with antagonism of GABA. The action of chlordane in the brain is very complex due to its biotransformation to more toxic metabolites and the presence of toxic components. Molecular modeling and binding studies indicate that the metabolites oxychlordane and heptachlor epoxide also block the brain GABA-gated Cl^- channels. The structurally similar component nonachlor causes toxicity symptoms typically associated with antagonism of GABA receptors.

Liver is another target of chlordane toxicity (hypertrophy, necrosis, and tumors). However, the mechanism is unknown. Chlordane induces hepatic cytochrome CYP enzymes. In mouse brain and liver, chlordane initiated signal transduction processes characteristic for known mitogens, that is, alter cellular Ca^{2+} levels and induce protein kinase C. Other potential targets include adenosine triphosphatase functions, nervous system development, inflammatory cytokines, macromolecule synthesis, DNA methylation, steroid metabolism, testosterone and neurotransmitter receptors, and lipid peroxidation.

Acute and Short-Term Toxicity

Animal

Chlordane is classified by the US EPA as a moderate oral toxicant (Category II). The acute oral LD_{50} for rats, mice, rabbits, and hamsters ranges from 83 to 1720 mg kg^{-1}. In rats, the oral LD_{50} is 20 mg kg^{-1} for oxychlordane and 39 mg kg^{-1} for heptachlor epoxide, indicating a greater toxicity than chlordane. The oral LD_{50} for *trans*-nonachlor in rats is 500 mg kg^{-1}. Chlordane dermal LD_{50} in rats is 530–840 mg kg^{-1} day^{-1} and the 4-h inhalation LC_{50} in rats is >200 mg l^{-1}. No reliable dermal or eye irritation studies are available.

The targets of chlordane toxicity after short-term inhalation and oral exposures are the liver, nervous and immune systems, and the developing offspring. Clinical signs of neurotoxicity include salivation, abnormal respiratory movements, hyperexcitability, convulsions, and paralysis.

Human

Deaths from accidental dermal exposure or intentional ingestion of chlordane are reported. The estimated acute oral lethal dose is 25–50 mg kg^{-1}. Initial signs involve confusion and convulsions.

Nonlethal acute signs of poisoning are headaches, tremors, seizures, numbness, nausea, fatigue, gastrointestinal symptoms, skin and eye irritation, and unconsciousness. The exposure level or duration is generally unknown. Incoordination, excitability, hyporeflexia, and convulsions occur at about 0.15 mg kg^{-1}.

Chronic Toxicity

Animal

Mortality occurred in rats after 50–163 days at 6–32 mg kg^{-1} day^{-1} and in mice within 42 days to18 months at 4–21 mg kg^{-1} day^{-1}. Rapid weight loss and convulsions were reported in rats prior to death.

Liver is the most common nonlethal target in 28 days to 2 years oral and inhalation studies in rats and mice. Increased liver weights, changes in serum liver enzyme activities and triglycerides, hypertrophy, necrosis, fat in the hepatocytes, and fatty degeneration occurred at the lowest observed effect levels (LOELs) of 0.06–8 mg kg^{-1} day^{-1} and 1–28 mg m^{-3}. These changes are often referred to as the chlorinated hydrocarbon insecticide rodent liver type. Similar effects were reported for oxychlordane and heptachlor epoxide. The LOELs for other tissue toxicity included 6 mg kg^{-1} day^{-1} for decreased thymus weight of rats, 16–50 mg kg^{-1} day^{-1} for reduced body weight in rats, and 1.7–50 mg kg^{-1} day^{-1} for neurological disturbance (e.g., hyperexcitability, hypersensitivity to touch, tremors, seizures, and convulsions) in rats and mice. Liver tumors occurred in mice at 1.2–8.3 mg kg^{-1} day^{-1}.

Human

Adverse health outcomes are described in humans who had increased blood and fat levels of oxychlordane, heptachlor, and *trans*-nonachlor. Neurological effects in apartment occupants exposed for up to 7 years to airborne chlordane at about 0.0005 mg m^{-3} included slowing of reaction time, balance dysfunction, reduction in cognitive function, and deficit of immediate and delayed recall. Exposure to oxychlordane is associated with an increased waist circumference and an increased prevalence of diabetes, possibly through adipocyte dysfunction.

Immunotoxicity

Animal

Oral studies in mice showed altered immune systems from chlordane exposure during gestation days (GDs) 1–18 and throughout lactation period. The LOEL for suppression of cell-mediated immunity (depressed delayed-type hypersensitivity reaction), granulocyte-macrophage, and spleen-forming stem cells in the bone marrow was 4–8 mg kg^{-1} day^{-1}. Reduced thymus weight and increased leukocyte counts occurred in rats exposed to 1–28 mg m^{-3} chlordane in air for 28–90 days. Altered levels of serum immunoglobulin M, G1, and G2 were reported in rats that received 25 mg kg^{-1} day^{-1} chlordane orally for 28 days. In the same study, the component nonachlor at 2.5–25 mg kg^{-1} day^{-1} decreased the ability to combat bacterial infections. *In vitro*, chlordane impaired the lymphocyte functions in monkeys.

Human

Chlordane (oxychlordane and *cis*- and *trans*-nonachlor) in umbilical cord blood from 300 newborns was associated with lower levels of the proinflammatory cytokine IL-1β.

Studies using *trans*-nonachlor and chlordane in fat biopsies as markers of chlordane exposure at home or at work revealed an association with immunological disregulation (distribution of lymphocytes and decreased response to foreign antigens). The exposure was 3 days to 15 months, but the immunological test was followed for 4 months to 10 years, indicating lasting impact on immune functions.

Reproductive and Developmental Toxicity

Reduced size of seminiferous tubules, degeneration of spermatogenic epithelium, and increased androgen receptor sites in ventral prostate were reported in mice treated orally with 100–300 mg kg^{-1} day^{-1} and in rats treated with 20 mg kg^{-1} day^{-1} for 30 days.

Decreased pup survival (up to 55%) was observed when pregnant rats received 21–28 mg kg^{-1} day^{-1} chlordane orally on GD 6–19 and pregnant mice at 8 mg kg^{-1} day^{-1} throughout gestation (GD 1–18). Plasma corticosterone in the surviving offspring was drastically elevated at the 0.16 mg kg^{-1} day^{-1} dose level, possibly due to diminished liver metabolic activity. Mice fed chlordane during late gestation (GD 12–19) exhibited normal pregnancy, offspring, and lactation; however, pups at 38 days of age showed depressed acquisition of avoidance response, increased seizure threshold, and exploratory activity at the LOEL of 1 mg kg^{-1} day^{-1}.

Genotoxicity

Chlordane is tested negative in several gene mutation systems, including in *Salmonella typhimurium* and *Escherichia coli*, and in rat hepatocytes hypoxanthine-guanine phosphoribosyl transferase. Chlordane is negative for dominant lethality in mice and recessive lethality in *Drosophila melanogaster*. It is also tested negative for DNA damage/repair in *S. typhimurium* and *E. coli*;

in rat, mouse, and hamster hepatocytes; and in human SV-40 transformed fibroblasts (with metabolic activation). The relatively fewer positive reports include mitotic gene conversion in *Saccharomyces cerevisiae* (with metabolic activation), prophage induction in *E. coli*, forward mutation in mouse lymphoma L5178Y cells (without metabolic activation), ouabain-resistant mutation in Chinese hamster V79 cells, and sister chromatid exchange in human lymphoid cells.

Carcinogenicity

Rodent dietary inclusion bioassays with chlordane and mixtures with heptachlor and heptachlor epoxide showed increased liver neoplasm in multiple strains of mice (adenoma, carcinoma, and hemangioma) and rats (adenoma), and thyroid follicular–cell adenomas and carcinomas in rats. Promotion of mouse liver neoplastic lesions initiated by *N*-nitrosodiethylamine was also reported.

Several investigations of different sample sizes and methods (e.g., self-reporting, employment records, and biomarkers) pertaining to occupational (manufacturing and pesticide applicators) and nonoccupational exposures were inadequate for carcinogenicity evidence in humans. Increased non-Hodgkin's lymphoma was reported among farmers. Possible associations to brain and lymphohematopoietic cancers in children were reported in a small study. No notable increase was found for breast, endometrial, or pancreatic cancers, leukemia, soft-tissue sarcoma, or multiple myeloma. Concomitant exposure to other chemicals (e.g., organochlorines and pesticides) was a common confounder in these studies.

Taking into consideration the carcinogenicity profiles of the common impurities heptachlor and heptachlor epoxide, the International Agency for Research on Cancer in 2001 classified chlordane and heptachlor as possibly carcinogenic to humans (Group 2B). The US EPA classified chlordane as a probable human carcinogen (Group B2) with an upper bound lifetime cancer potency of 0.35 per (mg kg^{-1} day^{-1}). The corresponding unit risk (risk per unit concentration) is 1×10^{-5} per (mg l^{-1}) in drinking water.

Clinical Management

Currently, there is no specific antagonist to the effects of chlordane. However, benzodiazepines and barbiturates are used to control chlordane-induced seizures. Cholestyramine is recommended for increased elimination of chlordane. Gastric lavage is performed for exposures to potentially life-threatening doses of chlordane.

Ecotoxicology

Chlordane is highly toxic to aquatic life. The 96 h LC_{50} for freshwater invertebrates and fish ranged widely. The mean values from all data for each of the following species are 0.058 mg l^{-1} in *Daphnia magna*, 0.0063 mg l^{-1} in freshwater shrimp, 0.037 mg l^{-1} in fathead minnow, 0.003 mg l^{-1} in carp, 0.025 mg l^{-1} for rainbow trout, 0.056 mg l^{-1} in salmon, 0.059 mg l^{-1} in bluegill, and 0.19 mg l^{-1} in guppy. The LC_{50} for saltwater species also ranged widely: 0.0004 mg l^{-1} in pink shrimp, 0.006 mg l^{-1} in eastern oyster, 0.012 mg l^{-1} in striped bass, 0.018 mg l^{-1} in sheepshead minnow, and 0.12 mg l^{-1} in threespine stickleback.

Chronic toxicity data are sparse. Sheepshead minnow did not survive after 10 days at 7.1 μg l^{-1}. The lowest observed effect concentration (LOEC) from a life-cycle test is 0.32 μg l^{-1} for brook trout, 1.22 μg l^{-1} for bluegill, and 1.7 μg l^{-1} for midges.

The 8-day dietary LD_{50} of chlordane is 331 mg kg^{-1} in bobwhite quail, 430 mg kg^{-1} in pheasant, and 858 mg kg^{-1} in mallard ducks. Chlordane is highly toxic to bees and earthworms.

Other Hazards

Concomitant exposure to other chlorinated cyclodiens with similar mechanism of action may result in cumulative toxicity. Chlordane acute toxicity is increased by liver metabolic enzyme inducers (e.g., aldrin, dieldrin, dichlorodiphenyltrichloroethane (DDT), or phenobarbital) through increased conversion to oxychlordane and heptachlor epoxide. Chlordane toxicity may also be modified by chemicals (e.g., lindane, organophosphate, and carbamate insecticides) that share same biotransformation pathways. Rats fed low-protein diets had approximately twofold lower acute LD_{50}. Age is a modifying factor for the acute toxicity of chlordane. Fetal exposures may lead to lasting changes in the immune system function. Individuals with chronic liver disease or impaired liver function may have greater sensitivity to chlordane. Individuals with idiosyncratic responses to chlordane may be prone to development of blood dyscrasia (i.e., aplastic anemia and leukemia).

Exposure Standards and Guidelines

- American Conference of Governmental Industrial Hygienists threshold limit value: 0.5 mg m^{-3} (30 ppb) Time Weighted Average (TWA); skin: A3 – confirmed animal carcinogen with unknown relevance to humans
- National Institute for Occupational Safety and Health (NIOSH) recommended exposure level: 0.5 mg m^{-3} (30 ppb) (up to 10-h workday during a 40-h workweek TWA; skin; a potential occupational carcinogen)
- NIOSH immediately dangerous to life or health concentration: 100 mg m^{-3} (6 ppm; a potential occupational carcinogen)
- Occupational Safety and Health Administration permissible exposure limit: 0.5 mg m^{-3} (30 ppb) (8-h TWA; skin – potential for dermal absorption)
- US EPA) drinking water maximum contaminant level: 0.002 mg l^{-1} (20 ppb)
- World Health Organization acceptable daily intake: 0.5 μg kg^{-1}

See also: Behavioral Toxicology; Developmental Toxicology; Chlordane; Cyclodienes; Neurotoxicity; Organochlorine Insecticides; Pesticides; National Institute for Occupational Safety and Health; Carcinogen Classification Schemes;

Carcinogenesis; Federal Insecticide, Fungicide, and Rodenticide Act, US; Genetic Toxicology; Immune System; International Agency for Research on Cancer; Regulation, Toxicology and; Risk Assessment, Human Health; Occupational Exposure Limits; Ecotoxicology; ACGIH® (American Conference of Governmental Industrial Hygienists); Children's Environmental Health; CERCLA; Revised as the Superfund Amendments Reauthorization Act (SARA); Safe Drinking Water Act; Bioaccumulation; Environmental Fate and Behavior.

Further Reading

Agency for Toxic Substances and Disease Registry (ATSDR), 1994. Toxicological Profile for Chlordane. Public Health Service, U.S. Department Of Health And Human Services. http://www.atsdr.cdc.gov/ToxProfiles/tp31.pdf.

American Conference of Governmental Industrial Hygienists (ACGIH), 2001. Chlordane: TLV® Chemical Substances 7th Edition Documentation. Publication #7DOC-297.

European Food Safety Authority (EFSA), 2007. Chlordane as undesirable substance in animal feed1. Scientific panel on contaminants in the food chain. EFSA J. 582, 1–53. http://www.efsa.europa.eu/en/efsajournal/doc/CONTAM_op_ej582_chlordane_en,3.pdf.

National Institute for Occupational Safety and Health (NIOSH), September 2007. Pocket Guide to Chemical Hazards. DHHS (NIOSH) Publication No. 2005-149. Department Of Health And Human Services, Centers for Disease Control and Prevention. http://www.cdc.gov/niosh/docs/2005-149/pdfs/2005-149.pdf.

USEPA, 1997. Toxicological Review of Chlordane (Technical). United States Environmental Protection Agency. http://www.epa.gov/iris/toxreviews/0142tr.pdf.

World Health Organization (WHO), 2006. Chlordane. Poisons Information Monograph 574. International Programme on Chemical Safety (IPCS), WHO. http://www.inchem.org/documents/pims/chemical/pim574.htm.

Relevant Websites

http://www.atsdr.cdc.gov/toxprofiles/index.asp – Agency for Toxic Substances and Disease Registry.

http://toxnet.nlm.nih.gov – Hazardous Substance Data Bank.

http://npic.orst.edu/ – National Pesticide Information Center.

http://www.epa.gov – United States Environmental Protection Agency.

Chlordecone

S Biswas, Birla Institute of Technology and Sciences-Pilani, Hyderabad, India
B Ghosh, Center for Human Genetic Research, Center for System Biology, Harvard Medical School, Harvard University, Boston, MA, USA

This article is a revision of the previous edition article by Harihara M. Mehendale and Zhengwei Cai, volume 1, pp 542–544, © 2005, Elsevier Inc.

- Name: Chlordecone
- Chemical Abstracts Service Registry Number: CAS 143-50-0
- Synonyms: 1,3,4-Methano-2H-cyclobuta-(cd)pentaten-2-one; 1,1α,3,3α,4,5,5,5α,5β,6-Decachloroctahydro; Kepone; GC1189; Ciba8514; ENT16,391; NCI-C00191; Decachloroketone; Decachlorotetracyclodecanone; Decachlorotetrahydro-4,7-methanoindeneone
- Chemical/Pharmaceutical/Other Class: Polycyclic chlorinated hydrocarbons
- Molecular Formula: $C_{10}Cl_{10}O$
- Chemical Structure:

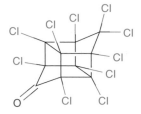

Uses

Chlordecone had wide application as insecticide and fungicide.

Background Information

Chlordecone, commonly known as kepone, is a tan to white crystalline odorless solid that was used primarily as insecticide. Specific application included control of the rust mites in non-fruit-bearing citrus trees, control of wireworms in tobacco fields, grass mole crickets, slugs, snails, and fire ants. Chlordecone was first produced in the United States in the early 1950s and introduced commercially in 1958. A huge quantity of this compound (3.6 million pounds) was produced in the United States between 1951 and 1975. Production of chlordecone stopped in 1975 after the incidence of intoxication of workers from severe industrial exposure from only chlordecone manufacturing plants. During 1974–75, Life Science Products associated with Allied Chemical Corporation, who was the sole producer of kepone in the United States, experienced kepone-related intoxication in over half of their 133 employees. Kepone illegally discharged in the nearby James river by the factory also resulted in extensive contamination in the water and marine life throughout the tidewater region in Virginia. The production plant was officially shut down in 1975. Typical symptoms of chlordecone intoxication include nervousness, headache, and tremor.

Exposure Routes and Pathways

Ingestion is the most common route of exposure. However, inhalation via the respiratory tract to the lung and dermal routes are also common. Chlordecone is very well absorbed following oral exposure. After its passage through the gastrointestinal tract (GI), it is mainly concentrated in the liver. Main metabolites include chlordecone alcohol, glucuronide conjugates of chlordecone, and chlordecone alcohol.

Toxicokinetics

Chlordecone absorption in humans via ingestion, inhalation, and dermal contacts has been investigated by the measurement of chlordecone concentration in blood, subcutaneous fat, and other body fluids and tissues. Workers were divided into subjective and objective depending on their neurological symptoms such as nervousness, tremulousness, and ataxia. The blood concentration of chlordecone was 0.009 and 11.8 ppm, respectively, for subjective and objective workers. Chlordecone blood concentrations for workers without neurological symptoms were between 0.003 and 4.1 ppm. Neurological symptoms were also detected in the blood of community residents living near the chlordecone plant, with concentrations ranging from 0.005 to 0.0325 ppm. The routes of exposure were inhalation of chlordecone associated with fine particulate matter and ingestion of contaminated soil and drinking water.

Chlordecone was readily absorbed from the GI tract in animals and establishes equilibrium of distribution among most tissues within 24–48 h. In one experiment, male Sprague-Dawley rats received a single dose of 40 mg kg^{-1} [^{14}C]-labeled chlordecone orally in corn oil solution. Approximately 10% of the total radioactivity was excreted on the first day, indicating approximately 90% of the dose was absorbed in the body. Chlordecone has limited absorption through the skin. A complete biodistribution study done in 32 workers exposed to chlordecone for a period of 3–16 months indicated that high concentrations of chlordecone were present in blood, liver, and subcutaneous fat tissues whereas a modest amount of chlordecone was found in muscle, gallbladder, bile, and stool. In addition, trace amount were detected in aqueous body fluids such as urine, saliva, gastric juice, cerebrospinal fluids, etc. It has also been found that, compared to other chlorinated organic pesticides, chlordecone has a strong affinity for fat tissues, resulting in a high ratio of concentration of fat to blood (7:1). In addition, it has been reported that 75% of chlordecone in blood binds with albumin and high-density lipoproteins. The main deposition organ for chlordecone is liver. Preferential uptake and slow elimination from liver were observed in laboratory animals. While studying the

 http://dx.doi.org/10.1016/B978-0-12-386454-3.00275-X

distribution of chlordecone in rats receiving a single oral dose of 40 mg kg^{-1} [^{14}C]-labeled chlordecone in corn oil, initial distribution, i.e. high level of radioactivity, was observed in adrenal gland followed by liver, lung, and fat tissues. However, 3 days after the treatment, the highest concentration of chlordecone was found in liver and eliminated at the slowest rate from liver as compared to other tissues (the concentration ratio in liver: blood increased from 28:1 on day 1 to 126:1 on day 84). The reason for the preferential retention of chlordecone by the liver is due to its binding to plasma proteins and lipoproteins: 75% of chlordecone in blood is bound with albumin and high-density lipoproteins. Chlordecone is mainly stored in liver tissues, followed by adipose tissues in both humans and animals.

Metabolism of chlordecone to chlordecone hydrate and then to the more stable metabolite chlordecone alcohol begins with the hydration of a ketone group by aldo-keto reductase enzyme. Activity of reductase enzyme was detected in liver cytosol of humans, rabbits, and gerbils, but was absent in laboratory animals, including rats, mice, hamsters, and guinea pigs. There was a 38% increase in chlordecone reductase activity in gerbils pretreated with a single oral dose of chlordecone. Metabolism of chlordecone to chlordecone alcohol was also found in pigs. Induction of chlordecone reductase activity in pigs was suggested when an increase in the ratio of chlordecone alcohol to chlordecone was observed in the gallbladder bile. Chlordecone induces cytochrome P450 mixed function oxidase enzyme systems in rats. In humans, the hydrate and alcohol form of chlordecone undergo glucuronide conjugation by α-D-glucuronic acid. Metabolites of chlordecone do not impart significant toxicity. It is not subjected to metabolism in laboratory animals. Fecal excretion is the main route of elimination. Only minimal amounts are eliminated through kidney. Study showed that by 84 days, 65% of the dose is excreted through feces whereas only 1.6% through urine.

Mechanism of Toxicity

A cardinal feature of chlordecone intoxication in humans is tremor, which occurs due to the alteration in neurotransmitter activity in dopaminergic, serotonergic, and α-noradrenergic systems. At the cellular levels, changes in ATPase activity and calcium homeostasis in the nervous system were observed. Calcium uptake in animals decreased and calcium concentration in total protein-bound myelin and synaptosomal calcium following daily oral doses of 25 mg kg^{-1} in mice was observed. *In vitro* study results suggested alteration of calcium regulation as a main reason for neurological disorder. Chlordecone-induced inhibition of brain mitochondrial and synaptosomal membrane-bound Na^+, K^+, ATPase, and oligomycin-sensitive Mg^{2+}-ATPase activity was observed, which may result in blocked cellular uptake and storage of neurotransmitters such as catecholamines and γ-aminobutyric acid, leading to neurotoxicity. Significant decrease in the level of dopamine in whole brain and striatum was seen in animals exhibiting tremor.

Chlordecone-induced hepatic biliary dysfunction could be due to the inhibition of Mg^{2+}-ATPase, resulting in decreased hepatic mitochondrial energy production. Chlordecone at high doses induces the hepatic microsomal drug-metabolizing system. It decreases the tolerance of carbon tetrachloride, and 67-fold increase in the toxicity of a nonlethal dose of carbon tetrachloride in laboratory rats was observed. The hepatotoxicity could be due to decreased energy owing to the disrupted intracellular calcium hemostasis.

Acute and Short-Term Toxicity (or Exposure)

Animal

Tremor and hyperexcitability are the main neurological symptoms observed in chlordecone-treated mice. The animals also experienced loss of body weight owing to decreased water and food consumption. Reversal of the condition in surviving animals was observed upon withdrawal of chlordecone administration. A high degree of mortality was observed in animals treated with chlordecone and the rate of mortality was dose dependent. Mortality in mice dosed with 50 mg kg^{-1} day^{-1} started at day 4 and reached 100% at day 6, whereas mortality at a dose of 25 mg kg^{-1} day^{-1} started at day 6 and reached 100% at day 11, and mortality at a dose of 10 mg kg^{-1} day^{-1} started at day 12 and reached 90% at day 24. Orally administered chlordecone (in corn oil) demonstrated LD_{50} values as 71, 126, 250, and 480 for rabbits, rats, dogs, and chickens, respectively. Dermally administered chlordecone demonstrated an LD_{50} value of 434 mg kg^{-1}.

Human

All information about the adverse side effects of chlordecone administration in human came from the studies of occupational workers (group of 133 men) exposed to chlordecone in a chlordecone manufacturing plant in Hopewell, Virginia. Even though there are many effects found upon long-term exposure; however, no death in humans exposed to chlordecone was reported. The main affected target organs for chlordecone toxicity in humans are the nervous system, skin, liver, and reproductive system.

Chronic Toxicity (or Exposure)

Animal

In one chronic animal study, rats were administered a low dose of chlordecone (1 ppm) for 21 months. There was no difference in survival and weight gain in treated and control rats. However, histopathological findings indicated increased incidence of lesions in the liver and thyroid among the chlordecone-treated group. In another study by the National Cancer Institute (NCI), to assess carcinogenicity, rats were administered chlordecone in the diet for 80 weeks at doses of 0, 15, 30, or 60 ppm for male rats and 0, 30, and 60 ppm for female rats. The incidence of tremor and other clinical signs such as rough hairs, dermatitis, and anemia was low to moderate during the first year, but gradually increased during the second year of the study. High-dose female and male rats developed dose-dependent hepatocellular carcinomas, which were described as large, poorly circumscribed masses that were well differentiated without vascular invasion and metastases. Tumors in other organs and the endocrine and reproductive systems were observed. However, incidence rates for all tumor types were not statistically increased as compared to control, and no dose–response trend was observed. A similar experiment conducted in mice by NCI demonstrated a similar result. In another study, growth retardation of fetus was observed in pregnant rats given 2 mg kg^{-1} day of chlordecone, in mice fed 40 ppm, in laying hen fed 75 ppm, and in quail fed 300 ppm. Liver toxicity was observed in rats, quail, mice, and dogs chronically treated with chlordecone.

Human

Health effects of occupational workers (133 men) who were working only in a chlordecone manufacturing plant were extensively studied. Out of 133 men, 76 experienced neurological symptoms such as nervousness, headache, and tremors that persisted for 9–10 months, even after cessation of exposure. Other neurological symptoms included irritability, poor recent memory, muscle weakness, gait ataxia, incoordination, and slurred speech. Another side-effect registered was oligospermia. Sperm count and motility had returned to normal 5–7 years following cessation of chlordecone exposure and treatment with cholestyramine. Liver enlargement was noticed in 20 out of 32 workers with high blood levels ($>0.6\ \mu g\ ml^{-1}$) of chlordecone. However, no evidence of significant liver toxicity, such as liver neoplasia, fibrosis, cholestasis, and hepatocellular necrosis, was observed. Reversal of chlordecone toxicity was observed upon removal of the drug and cessation of exposure.

Clinical Management

Cessation of exposure by removing the individual from the source would be the first step. In case of ingestion, emesis could be induced followed by administration of activated charcoal and cathartics. Oil-based cathartics are avoided. To prevent the reabsorption of chlordecone in the GI tract, cholestyramine was used for chlordecone intoxication. It binds with chlordecone and increases the fecal excretion. Cholestyramine is an anion-exchange resin that binds chlordecone, and the complex does not get absorbed in the GI tract. Cholestyramine treatment reduces the average $t_{1/2}$ of chlordecone in the blood from 165 to 80 days.

Ecotoxicology

Chlordecone does not get degraded in the environment. Chlordecone does not undergo hydrolysis or photolysis. Microorganisms can degrade chlordecone slowly. It gets absorbed to soil and sticks to suspended particulate matter in water. Chlordecone accumulates significantly in fish and other aquatic organisms.

See also: Developmental Toxicology; Occupational Toxicology; Neurotoxicity; Organochlorine Insecticides.

Further Reading

Guzelian, P.S., 1982. Comparative toxicology of chlordecone (kepone) in humans and experimental animals. Annu. Rev. Pharmacol. Toxicol. 22, 89–113.

Plaa, G.L., 2010. Chlorinated methanes and liver injury: highlights of the past 50 years. Annu. Rev. Pharmacol. Toxicol. 40, 42–65.

Toxicological Review of Chlordecone (Kepone), 2009. US Environmental Protection Agency, Washington, DC. EPA/635/R-07/004F. http://www.epa.gov/iris/toxreviews/1017tr.pdf.

Tsai, W.T., 2010. Current status and regulatory aspects of pesticides considered to be persistent organic pollutants (POPs) in Taiwan. Int. J. Environ. Res. Public Health 7 (10), 3615–3627.

Chlordimeform

LG Costa, University of Washington, Seattle, WA, USA

This article is a revision of the previous edition article by Paul R. Harp, volume 1, pp 544–546, © 2005, Elsevier Inc.

- Chemical Abstract Service Registry Numbers: CAS 6164-98-3 (base); CAS 19750-95-9 (hydrochloride salt)
- Synonyms: Chlorphenamidine; ENT 27335 (base); ENT 27567 (salt); Chlorphenamide; Galecron™
- Molecular Formula: $C_{10}H_{13}ClN_2$
- Chemical Name: *N*′-(4-Chloro-2-methylphenyl)-*N*,*N*-dimethylformamidine
- Chemical Structure:

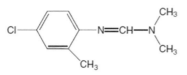

Background

Chlordimeform is a member of the formamidine family of insecticides/acaricides, now represented by Amitraz [*N*′-2,4-(dimethylphenyl)-*N*-((2,4-dimethylphenyl)imino)methyl-*N*-methanimidamide], as chlordimeform was withdrawn from the market in 1992 because of potential carcinogenicity. Formamidines are a unique class of insecticides as they target the adrenergic nervous system. In insects they activate the octopamine receptors, whereas in mammals a primary target is represented by the alpha$_2$-adrenergic receptors.

Uses

Chlordimeform was used as a broad spectrum acaricide and insecticide. It is particularly effective against mites and ticks, and some *Lepidoptera* insects. It was extensively used in agriculture, particularly in fruits such as apples, cherries, and strawberries, as well as in rice and cotton. It was also used in veterinary medicine as an acaricide. In 1976 its use was suspended because of suspected carcinogenicity, but it was re-introduced in most countries in 1978 for insect control in cotton. In the late 1980s to early 1990s, production and use ceased worldwide because of carcinogenicity of one of its major metabolites.

Environmental Fate and Behavior

Chlordimeform has a relatively high volatility, and low water solubility, although the salt is highly water soluble. Chlordimeform undergoes rapid microbial degradation in soil, and is rapidly degraded in plants. There is no evidence of bioaccumulation of chlordimeform in the food chain.

Exposure and Exposure Monitoring

Exposure to chlordimeform occurred in occupational settings (manufacture, formulation, use) and was primarily caused by dermal exposure with minor contribution from inhalation. Some exposure may have occurred in the general population on aerial spraying in cotton fields. Exposure also occurred because of residues present in raw and processed foods. Cases of accidental or intentional oral exposure to chlordimeform have also been reported, particularly in China.

Toxicokinetics

Chlordimeform is well absorbed from all routes of exposure. The base is better absorbed dermally than the hydrochloride salt. Chlordimeform undergoes significant metabolism and is rapidly excreted, primarily through the urine. Chlordimeform's metabolism plays a most relevant role in its toxicity, as the two demethylated metabolites demethylchlordimeform and didemethylchlordimeform have higher acute toxicity than the parent compound. Two other metabolites of chlordimeform, 4-chloro-o-toluidine and *N*-formyl-4-chloro-*o*-toluidine, are believed to be responsible for the carcinogenic effects of chlordimeform. Neither chlordimeform nor any of the metabolites accumulate in tissues. However, despite its discontinued use since 1993, low levels of chlordimeform have been found in human adipose tissue in residents of Southeast China as late as 2008.

Mechanism of Toxicity

Earlier studies indicated that a primary mechanism of chlordimeform's toxicity was inhibition of monoamine oxidase; however, subsequent findings suggested that this biochemical effect does not play a significant role in its acute toxicity. Other reported effects of chlordimeform include inhibition of oxidative phosphorylation and inhibition of calcium channels. The chemical structure of chlordimeform is similar to that of norepinephrine and other sympathetic amines. In insects, chlordimeform exerts its toxicity by activating octopamine receptors. The equivalents of the latter in mammals are the alpha$_2$-adrenergic receptors. Chlordimeform acts as an agonist at alpha$_2$-adrenoceptors, and its demethylated metabolite, which is more acutely toxic, is also 400-fold more potent toward alpha$_2$-adrenoceptors. Signs and symptoms of chlordimeform's acute exposure can be explained by activation of alpha$_2$-adrenergic receptors.

Acute and Short-Term Toxicity

Animal

Chlordimeform has a moderate acute toxicity in rodents (oral LD_{50} = 200–300 mg kg^{-1} bw). Main signs of acute exposure are hypotension, hypothermia, hyperglycemia, and bradycardia. Anemia, and kidney and liver damage have also been reported in short-term animal studies.

 http://dx.doi.org/10.1016/B978-0-12-386454-3.00112-3

Human

Effects of chlordimeform in humans include severe hypotension, cardiac toxicity, nausea, and vomiting; central nervous system depression, and blurred vision are common. In some cases, impairments of kidney and liver functions have also been reported.

Chronic Toxicity

Animals

The main adverse effect of chlordimeform is carcinogenicity.

Humans

Cases of hematuria were reported in workers in a chlordimeform packaging plant. Various studies in individuals exposed to chlordimeform indicate an increased risk of bladder cancer, primarily when exposure to 4-chloro-*o*-toluidine also occurred. Chlordimeform is classified by IARC and EPA as a probable human carcinogen (Group 2A and B2, respectively), based on the findings in mice and on limited information in humans.

Immunotoxicity

There no evidence that chlordimeform induces significant immunotoxic effects.

Reproductive Toxicity

No significant treatment-related effects were found in multigenerational reproductive studies in rodents. Chlordimeform does not appear to be a teratogen.

Genotoxicity

Chlordimeform is negative in most *in vitro* tests for mutagenicity and genotoxicity in both bacterial and mammalian systems. In contrast, 4-chloro-*o*-toluidine tested positive in various *in vitro* tests for DNA damage and cell transformation.

Carcinogenicity

The main adverse effect of chlordimeform on chronic exposure is carcinogenicity, and two metabolites, 4-chloro-*o*-toluidine and *N*-formyl-4-chloro-*o*-toluidine, appear to be responsible for this effect. 4-Chloro-*o*-touidine in particular is a more potent carcinogen than chlordimeform, and is believed to be responsible for the tumors observed in rodents and humans. The exact mechanism of carcinogenicity by 4-chloro-*o*-toluidine is unclear, but may involve genotoxic mechanisms.

In mice, a dose-dependent incidence of hemangioendotheliomas, particularly in liver, kidney, and spleen, has been found in two studies. Hemangiomas and hemangiosarcomas were also found in mice on chronic dietary exposure to the chlordimeform metabolite 4-chloro-*o*-toluidine. No treatment related increase tumor incidence was reported in rats.

Clinical Management

Treatment for chlordimeform intoxication is supportive and symptomatic. Adequate ventilation should be supported. Diazepam may be used for seizures, and atropine for bradycardia. Hypotension may respond to the use on an inotrope. Gastric lavage may be considered shortly after ingestion, and oral activated charcoal would be appropriate later. Antagonists of alpha$_2$-adrenergic receptors, such as yohimbine, have been shown to reverse acute toxicity in animals, but their efficacy has not been assessed in humans.

Ecotoxicology

Limited studies indicate that chlordimeform has moderate to low toxicity toward fish and avian species.

Exposure Standards and Guidelines

The last available temporary ADI (Acceptable Daily Intake) for chlordimeform was 0.0001 mg kg^{-1} day^{-1}, established in 1978. The temporary ADI was withdrawn in 1987.

See also: Amitraz; Pesticides.

Further Readings

Costa, L.G., Olibet, G., Murphy, S.D., 1988. Alpha$_2$-adrenoceptors as a target for formamidine pesticides: in vitro and in vivo studies in mice. Toxicol. Appl. Pharmacol. 93, 319–328.

Popp, W., Schmieding, W., Speck, M., Vahrenholz, C., Norpoth, K., 1992. Incidence of bladder cancer in a cohort of workers exposed to 4-chloro-*o*-toluidine while synthesizing chlordimeform. Br. J. Ind. Med. 49, 529–531.

Relevant Website

http://www.inchem.org – Chlordimeform (Environmental Health Criteria 199); International Programme on Chemical Safety.

Chlorfenvinphos

SE Koshlukova and NR Reed, California Environmental Protection Agency, Sacramento, CA, USA

Background

Chlorfenvinphos is a chlorinated organophosphorus ester manufactured as an insecticide and acaricide. Like other organophosphorus pesticides (OPs), its most prominent toxicity is associated with binding and thereby inhibiting the enzyme acetylcholinesterase (AChE) in insects and mammals. Chlorfenvinphos represents the oldest generation of OPs that exhibit marked mammalian toxicity. It is a direct-acting cholinesterase (ChE) inhibitor and does not require metabolic activation to yield anti-ChE activity.

Chlorfenvinphos was registered in the United States in 1963 and extensively used to control insect pests on domestic animals, in households, and animal buildings. Concerns regarding high acute toxicity and developmental and reproductive effects led to the cancelation of all its uses in 1991. Chlorfenvinphos was banned in Canada in 1999 and in the European Union (EU) in 2006. It continues to be used in the developing countries, and in Australia and New Zealand as an important veterinary medicine for ectoparasites in livestock.

Chlorfenvinphos has been detected in at least one of the 1684 National Priorities List sites (the most hazardous waste site) in the United States. It is regulated under "The Emergency Planning and Community Right-to-Know Act of 1986," which requires manufacturers or users to report annual release to any environmental media. Chlorfenvinphos is also one of the 38 high-priority hazardous chemicals and chemical warfare agents for which the US Environmental Protection Agency is developing advisory levels for exposure in case of large-scale disasters or environmental contamination.

Chemical Profile

- Technical Chlorfenvinphos: mixture of E and Z isomers of the phosphate with a Z:E ratio of 8.6:1. Both E and Z isomers have insecticidal activity
- Chemical Abstracts Service Registry Number: CAS 470-90-6 (EZ), CAS 18708-86-6 (E), CAS 18708-87-7 (Z)
- Chemical Name: ((EZ)-2-chloro-1-(2,4-dichlorophenyl) ethenyl) diethyl phosphate
- Synonyms: Chlorfenvinphos, Clofenvinfos, 2-Chloro-1-(2,4-dichlorophenyl)vinyl diethyl phosphate, Chlorfenvinphos solution, Clorfenvinfos, Clofenvinfos (INN), Supona (TN), AC1NTBS1, AC1Q3MCM, 2-Chloro-1-(2,4-dichlorophenyl)ethenyl diethyl phosphate
- Chemical Class: Organophosphate; Insecticide, Acaricide
- Chemical Structure: (from Pubchem): http://pubchem.ncbi.nlm.nih.gov/image/structurefly.cgi?cid=5377791&width=400&height=400

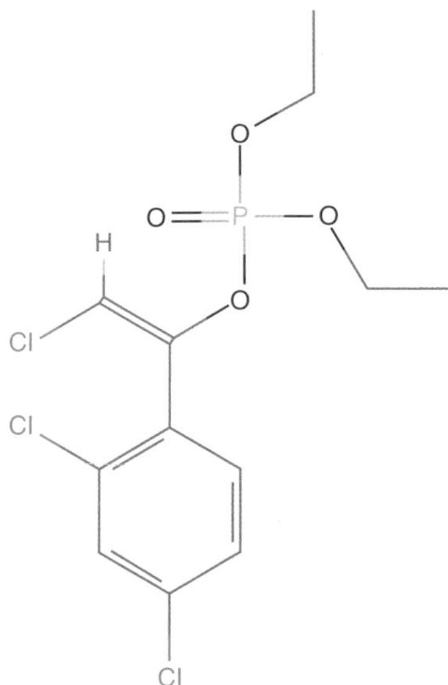

- Molecular Formula: $C_{12}H_{14}Cl_3O_4P$
- Molecular Weight: 359.57 g mol^{-1}
- Density: 1.53 g cm^{-3} at 25 °C
- Vapor Pressure: 0.000008 mm Hg at 25 °C
- Boiling Point: 120 °C
- Melting Point: −23 to −19 °C
- Flash Point: No data
- Conversion Factor: 1 ppm = 14.7 mg m^{-3} at 25 °C
- Appearance: Colorless to amber liquid
- Odor: Mild odor

Uses

From 1963 until the early 1990s, chlorfenvinphos was extensively used in veterinary products (dip, dust, and collars) for flea and tick control on pets and domestic animals, and in dairy barns, milk rooms, poultry houses, and other animal buildings. Agriculturally, it was used on potatoes, rice, and maize, and for control of soil insects and nematodes. All uses were canceled in the United States in 1991 and phased out in EU in 2006. Chlorfenvinphos continues to be used in Australia and New Zealand in veterinary products for combating ectoparasites on cattle and sheep.

Environmental Fate and Behavior

Chlorfenvinphos is soluble in organic solvents (e.g., ethanol, acetone) and has moderate solubility in water (145 mg l^{-1} solubility at 23 °C). The calculated Henry's law constant of 0.00000002 atm m^3 mol^{-1} indicates that surface water

 http://dx.doi.org/10.1016/B978-0-12-386454-3.01110-6

volatilization is unlikely an important fate process. The estimated half-life for reacting with photochemically generated hydroxyl radicals in the air is 7–92 h. Photolysis of chlorfenvinphos produces dechlorinated products or isomerization of the Z to the E isomer.

Chlorfenvinphos undergoes abiotic hydrolysis, photodegradation, and biotic degradation in soil and water. Depending on the soil type and climate, its soil persistence varies from 14 days to over 210 days. Half-lives in river waters range from 13 to 51 days. The rate of hydrolysis depends on the acidity of the environment. Chlorofenvinphos hydrolyzes slowly in neutral and acidic solutions with a half-life of 388–483 days. The main degradates are 2,4-dichloro-1-(1 hydroxyethyl)benzene, 2,4-dichloro-chloromethyl ketone, 2,4-dichlorobenzoic acid, and 2-hydroxy-4-chlorobenzoic acid. The estimated $\log K_{oc}$ of 2.45 indicates moderate soil adsorption and the potential for groundwater leaching.

Chlorfenvinphos in soil and sediment can be taken up by organisms and plants. Based on the measured $\log K_{ow}$ of 3.81–4.22, chlorfenvinphos is not expected to bioaccumulate in food chains. Australian studies reported a half-life of 57 days in greasy wool of merino sheep with over 29% of the applied pesticide recovered in the grease to be processed into lanolin products.

Exposure and Exposure Monitoring

Human exposure to chlorfenvinphos happens directly from its insecticidal use. Dermal and inhalation pathways are likely to dominate workers' exposures from handling treated cattle, sheep and wool wax, or reentering treated fields.

In countries like the United States where chlorfenvinphos is banned, exposures may continue from runoff and leaching from hazardous waste disposal sites. Exposure to the general public may occur by ingesting imported foods and lanolin-containing pharmaceutical products. Occupational exposure remains possible for workers at contaminated waste sites or in legal production for export. The exposure is likely higher for the general public living near hazardous waste sites, where chlorfenvinphos has been detected in surface and ground waters and soil samples. At a given exposure concentration, children generally have higher body burden due to their higher intake (inhalation volume, amount of food intake) or contact on a per bodyweight basis.

Toxicokinetics

The estimated oral absorption of chlorfenvinphos is 86–94% in rats, dogs, and humans. In rats, peak blood level of chlorfenvinphos and its metabolites occurs between 25 min and 1 h after dosing. The dermal and inhalation absorptions in humans are evident in the detection of the parent compound and metabolites in tissues and organs, and by the inhibition of ChE activities.

In rats, dogs, and humans, chlorfenvinphos is extensively metabolized through oxidative dealkylation by the liver cytochrome P450 (CYP) enzymes and produces 2-chloro-1-(2,4-dichlorophenyl)vinyl ethyl hydrogen phosphate, 2,4-dichloromandelic acid, and acetaldehyde possibly through epoxide intermediates. In humans, chlorfenvinphos and its metabolites are found in serum, cervical mucus, follicular and sperm fluids, and milk. It also binds to plasma proteins, e.g., albumin. Chlorfenvinphos is detected in omental fat of sheep 3 days after applications in a dip or spray race. Chlorfenvinphos metabolism in liver slices is more rapid in dogs, rabbits, and mice than in rats.

Urine is the main route of elimination where 86–89% of a single oral dose is found over 4 days in rats and dogs, and 94% is excreted within 26 h in humans. About 2–16% is excreted in the feces. Chlorfenvinphos was detected in cow milk. The major metabolites in excreta are 2-chloro-1-(2,4-dichlorophenyl)vinyl ethyl hydrogen phosphate, 1-(2,4-dichlorophenyl)ethanol, 1-(2,4-dichlorophenyl)ethanediol, 2,4-dichloromandelic acid, 2,4-dichlorobenzoyl glycine, and glucuronide conjugates. An elimination half-life ($t_{1/2}$) of 24 h is reported in rabbits.

Mechanism of Toxicity

The mechanism of toxicity of chlorfenvinphos is related to its binding and inhibition of the serine hydrolase AChE. In the nervous system, AChE hydrolyzes the neurotransmitter acetylcholine, thereby terminating its synaptic action. AChE inhibition increases the availability of acetylcholine at the neural synapse, leading to cholinergic overstimulation, autonomic and neuromuscular dysfunction, and at higher levels, resulting in coma and death. Major metabolites of chlorfenvinphos do not inhibit ChE. Chlorfenvinphos inhibits butyrylcholinesterase which may function as a molecular scavenger for anti-ChE compounds in the blood or substitute for AChE where it is low.

The stress responses to acute exposure of chlorfenvinphos are evidenced in rats by rapidly increased plasma corticosterone concentrations and a prolonged reduced sensitivity to psychostimulants such as amphetamine. These effects were attributed to the hyperactivity of the cholinergic system from ChE inhibition, leading to persistent alterations of the brain cholinergic–dopaminergic balance.

Other potentially more sensitive non-ChE targets that may influence the overall toxicity of chlorfenvinphos include lipid metabolism, oxidative stress, aromatic amino acid transferases, and cytotoxicity. Chlorfenvinphos may act via central noradrenergic mechanisms to induce hypotension by accelerating the noradrenaline turnover in the brain. Chlorfenvinphos induces hepatic CYPs.

Acute and Short-Term Toxicity

Animal

Marked difference between species exists in the acute oral LD_{50} values of chlorfenvinphos. These are 9.7–39 mg kg^{-1} for rats, 117–250 mg kg^{-1} for mice and guinea pigs, 300 mg kg^{-1} for rabbits, and >5000 mg kg^{-1} for dogs. The species sensitivity may reflect the rate of metabolic detoxification of chlorfenvinphos to 2-chloro-1-(2,4-dichlorophenyl) vinyl ethyl hydrogen phosphate. *In vitro*, rats had much lower conversion rate than mouse, rabbit, and dog. Rats were shown to be protected from acute toxicity of chlorfenvinphos by CYP inducers (e.g., dieldrin), possibly through enhanced detoxification. The rat dermal LD_{50} is $30\,mg\,kg^{-1}\,day^{-1}$ and the inhalational LC_{50} is $0.133\,mg\,l^{-1}$. Chlorfenvinphos is not irritating to the eye and is a weak skin sensitizer. Based on its acute toxicity, the WHO classified in 1992 chlorfenvinphos as extremely hazardous.

The main target of chlorfenvinphos toxicity after short-term oral exposure is the nervous system. Muscarinic and nicotinic cholinergic syndromes include hypersalivation, respiratory distress, miosis, muscular twitches, tremors, ataxia, diarrhea, and vomiting. Other nonlethal effects are metabolic and liver enzyme changes, elevation of plasma corticosteroids, hypotension, and alteration in noradrenaline levels and aromatic aminotransferase activity in the brain and sleep disturbance. Chlorfenvinphos has not been tested for delayed neuropathy in hens.

Human

Human deaths occurred due to intentional ingestion of chlorfenvinphos. Pulmonary congestion and edema were reported in one case at about $830\,mg\,kg^{-1}$. Postmortem, chlorfenvinphos was detected in the stomach, liver, blood, and urine. Nonlethal effects involve central nervous system, cardiovascular system, and respiratory system.

Common cholinergic signs are lacrimation, salivation, tremors, nausea, miosis, and muscle incoordination. Unconsciousness, absence of tendon reflexes, severely inhibited blood and red blood cell (RBC) ChE, respiratory failure, and hypersecretion occurred after a single oral dose of about $360\,mg\,kg^{-1}$. In clinical studies with adults, the lowest observed effect level (LOEL) for plasma and RBC ChE inhibition is $1\,mg\,kg^{-1}$ orally and $5\,mg\,kg^{-1}$ dermally.

Over 200 records of nonoccupational poisonings are available during 1995–2010 from the Spanish Poison Control Center Database. The majority were accidental oral exposure from chlorfenvinphos veterinary products.

Chronic Toxicity

Animal

Reproductive two- and three-generation studies in rats (see Reproductive and Developmental Toxicity Section) showed decreased pup survival at $10\,mg\,kg^{-1}\,day^{-1}$. Nonlethal LOELs reported in 30 days to 2 years oral studies with chlorfenvinphos included $0.8\,mg\,kg^{-1}$ for gastrointestinal effects in rats, $1.5–7\,mg\,kg^{-1}\,day^{-1}$ for increased liver weight and decreased thymus and kidney weight in rats and mice, $93\,mg\,kg^{-1}\,day^{-1}$ for hypertrophy and hyperplasia of adrenal cortex in mice, $1.9–10\,mg\,kg^{-1}\,day^{-1}$ for neuromuscular effects and decreases in bodyweight, bodyweight gains, and food consumption in rats, $0.5–0.7\,mg\,kg^{-1}\,day^{-1}$ for 17–48% plasma, RBC, and brain ChE inhibition in rats and dogs after 1 week–2 years of oral exposures.

Human

Adverse health outcomes are described in humans occupationally exposed to chlorfenvinphos for up to 15 years. Workers involved in production of chlorfenvinphos showed impaired immune system, respiratory muscle and liver function, inhibition of plasma ChE, and changes in electromyographic voltage measured in the ulnar nerve region. Most of these studies involved exposures to other pesticides and cannot be ascribed to chlorfenvinphos alone.

Immunotoxicity

Chlorfenvinphos administered to mice, rats, and rabbits for 84–90 days at $1.5–10\,mg\,kg^{-1}\,day^{-1}$ produced various immunological/lymphoreticular changes. The LOEL for reduction of thymus weight, involution of the thymus, and stimulation of spleen colonies was $1.5\,mg\,kg^{-1}\,day^{-1}$ in mice. This is the basis for the Agency for Toxic Substances and Disease Registry (ATSDR) to establish the minimal risk level (MRL) for intermediate-duration oral exposure to chlorfenvinphos, in addition to setting the acute and chronic MRLs based on ChE inhibition. Decreased number of hemolysin-producing cells and E-rosette-forming cells, increased interleukin-1 activity, and delayed hypersensitivity reaction occurred at higher doses. In rats and rabbits, reduced spleen weight, spleen cytomorphological changes, elevated serum hemagglutinin and hemolysin activity, and increased number of nucleated lymphoid cells producing hemolytic antibody to sheep erythrocytes occurred at $3–10\,mg\,kg^{-1}\,day^{-1}$.

Reproductive Toxicity

The available data suggest that chlorfenvinphos adversely affects reproduction and pre- and postnatal development. In prenatal developmental studies, pregnant rats received chlorfenvinphos up to $3\,mg\,kg^{-1}\,day^{-1}$ orally on gestation days (GDs) 6–15 or pregnant rabbits received up to $100\,mg\,kg^{-1}\,day^{-1}$ on GDs 6–18. Preimplantation losses were reported in rabbits at the LOEL of $25\,mg\,kg^{-1}\,day^{-1}$. Chlorfenvinphos at $50\,mg\,kg^{-1}\,day^{-1}$ increased the incidence of open eyes and edema in hamster dams and decreased the weight and length of hamster fetuses.

In two- and three-generation studies, rats fed with $0.05–30\,mg\,kg^{-1}\,day^{-1}$ of chlorfenvinphos mated normally and exhibited normal pregnancy. However, pup viability and lactation index were severely impacted at $5–10\,mg\,kg^{-1}\,day^{-1}$. Marked decreases in fertility (50–84%) and birth index, reduction in maternal and pup bodyweight gain, and inhibition of plasma and brain ChE had the lowest LOEL of $0.5\,mg\,kg^{-1}\,day^{-1}$.

No developmental neurotoxicity data on chlorfenvinphos are available in laboratory animals or in humans.

Genotoxicity

Chlorfenvinphos shows mostly negative results in genotoxicity tests. It was negative for mutation in *Escherichia coli* (WP2 hcr), *Bacillus subtilis* (H17 Rec+ and M45 Rec−), and in multiple studies in multiple strains of *Salmonella typhimurium*. The only positive report was in TA100 strain with decreased potency in the presence of metabolic activation. A pesticide mixture containing 0.3% chlorfenvinphos was tested negative in male rat bone marrow micronucleus assay from oral exposures and for chromosomal aberration in human lymphocytes *in vitro*.

Clinical Management

The muscarinic signs of chlorfenvinphos poisoning are antagonized by atropine, which blocks acetylcholine but only at muscarinic receptors. Oximes are used to treat the nicotinic effects (e.g., muscle paralysis) by reversing the AChE phosphorylation before the onset of its aging. CYP inducers such as antipsychotics (triflupromazine) and analgesics (aspirin, morphine) are used to accelerate the detoxification of chlorfenvinphos. Gastric lavage is performed for exposures to potentially life-threatening doses of chlorfenvinphos.

Ecotoxicology

Chlorfenvinphos is highly toxic to freshwater *Daphnia*, with reported acute LC_{50} at <0.1–$10\ mg\ l^{-1}$ and a 21-day reproductive toxicity lowest observed effect concentration (LOEC) at $0.0003\ mg\ l^{-1}$. In fish, the acute LC_{50} is $<0.1\ mg\ l^{-1}$ for tilapia and carp, 0.1–$1\ mg\ l^{-1}$ for rainbow trout, and 1–$10\ mg\ l^{-1}$ for guppy. The LOEC is $0.1\ mg\ l^{-1}$ for a 7-day brain AChE inhibition in rainbow trout and $0.003\ mg\ l^{-1}$ for an 84-day reproduction in striped catfish. Toxicity to avian species varied, with acute oral LD_{50} ranged from $<10\ mg\ kg^{-1}$ in starlings to 50–$500\ mg\ kg^{-1}$ to mallards, chickens, pheasants, and quail. The 28-day No Observed Effect Level for brain AChE inhibition is $3\ mg\ kg^{-1}$ in adult starlings. The LD_{50} of chlorfenvinphos to bees ranged widely, with a mid value of 0.004 mg per bee.

Other Hazards

Concomitant exposure to other OPs and carbamates with similar mechanism of action may result in cumulative toxicity. Among those having greater sensitivity to the acute toxicity of chlorfenvinphos are the young who have lower CYP level for detoxification and those with low plasma ChE, which acts to reduce the availability of chlorfenvinphos to the neuromuscular tissue. Data in animals showed that chlorfenvinphos toxicity is decreased by CYP inducers, and is increased by agents that inhibit liver metabolic enzymes (ethyl isocyanide and halogenated alkanes and alkenes).

Exposure Standards and Guidelines

USA ATSDR MRL for oral exposure: $0.002\ mg\ kg^{-1}\ day^{-1}$ for acute and intermediate durations; $0.0007\ mg\ kg^{-1}\ day^{-1}$ for chronic duration.

Joint FAO/WHO Meeting on Pesticide Residues Chronic Oral Acceptable Daily Intake: $0.0005\ mg\ kg^{-1}\ day^{-1}$.

See also: Behavioral Toxicology; Developmental Toxicology; Toxicity Testing, Developmental; Cholinesterase Inhibition; Common Mechanism of Toxicity in Pesticides; Neurotoxicity; Organophosphorus Compounds; Pesticides; Cytochrome P450; Federal Insecticide, Fungicide, and Rodenticide Act, US; Genetic Toxicology; Immune System; Regulation, Toxicology and; Toxicity Testing, Reproductive; Risk Assessment, Human Health; Ecotoxicology; Children's Environmental Health; Epidemiology; Environmental Fate and Behavior.

Further Reading

Agency for Toxic Substances and Disease Registry (ATSDR), 1997. Toxicological Profile for Chlorfenvinphos. Public Health Service, U.S. Department of Health and Human Services. http://www.atsdr.cdc.gov/toxprofiles/tp.asp?id=932&tid=193.

Australian Pesticides and Veterinary Medicine Authority (APVMA), 2011. Chlorfenvinphos Review. Australian Government, Canberra, Australia. http://www.atsdr.cdc.gov/toxprofiles/tp.asp?id=932&tid=193.

Martinez, M.A., Ballesteros, S., 2012. Two suicidal fatalities due to the ingestion of chlorfenvinphos formulations: simultaneous determination of the pesticide and the petroleum distillates in tissues by gas chromatography-flame-ionization detection and gas chromatography-mass spectrometry. J. Anal. Toxicol. 36, 44–51.

World Health Organization (WHO), 1994. Chlorfenvinphos. Pesticide Residues in Food. Part II Toxicology. International Programme on Chemical Safety (IPCS), WHO. http://www.inchem.org/documents/jmpr/jmpmono/v94pr03.htm.

Relevant Websites

http://www.atsdr.cdc.gov – Agency for Toxic Substances and Disease Registry.
http://www.apvma.gov.au – Australian Pesticides and Veterinary Medicine Authority.
http://npic.orst.edu – National Pesticide Information Center.
http://www.epa.gov – United States Environmental Protection Agency.
http://toxnet.nlm.nih.gov – Hazardous Substance Data Bank.

Chlorination Byproducts

SS Anand, DuPont Haskell Global Centers for Health and Environmental Sciences, Newark, DE, USA
BK Philip, Drug Safety Evaluation, Bristol-Myers Squibb, Vernon, IN, USA
HM Mehendale, University of Louisiana at Monroe, Monroe, LA, USA

This article is a revision of the previous edition article by S. Satheesh Anand and Harihara M. Mehendale, volume 1, pp 546–553, © 2005, Elsevier Inc.

Introduction

Drinking water disinfection is a worldwide practice to eliminate the microbial contaminants and is considered to be one of the greatest public health advances in this century. Ever since the use of disinfectants, there is a significant decrease in waterborne infectious diseases such as typhoid, cholera, hepatitis, and polio, which for decades posed threat to public health. The most widely used disinfectants are chlorine, ozone, chlorine dioxide, and chloramines. Among these, chlorine is the most effective and efficient in inactivating most microbes. The noteworthy biocidal effects of chlorine have been somewhat offset by the formation of potential toxic and carcinogenic chlorination byproducts (CBPs). Additionally, several adverse birth outcomes are implicated to CBP exposure. Hence, in order to balance between microbial and chemical risks, it is essential to better understand the chemistry, toxicology, and epidemiology of CBPs.

Formation of CBPs

Chlorine is applied as chlorine gas, powdered calcium hypochlorite ($Ca(OCl)_2$), or liquid sodium hypochlorite (NaOCl; bleach). Chlorine reacts with the organic (natural organic matter (NOM)) or inorganic (bromide ion (Br^-)) precursors in the water to form chlorine disinfection byproducts (DBPs), including trihalomethanes (THMs), haloacetic acids (HAAs), haloacetonitriles (HANs), haloketones, chloral hydrate, and chloropicrin. Humic and fulvic acids are the predominant NOMs. When bromine exists, the chlorine oxidizes it to hypobromous acid/hypobromite ion ($HOBr/OBr^-$) to form bromo THMs (bromodichloromethane (BDCM) and dibromochloromethane (DBCM)), HAAs, and HANs. The formation of CBPs is influenced by pH, temperature, ammonia, carbonate alkalinity, chlorine dose, contact time, removal of NOM (is higher in the surface water compared to groundwater) before chlorine application, etc. Moreover, the composition of these mixtures may change seasonally resulting in higher CBPs during warm season compared to cold season. The formation of THMs increases at high pH levels and decreases at low pH levels, whereas the opposite is true of HAAs. Generally, chlorinated THM, HAA, and HAN species dominate over brominated species, although the opposite may be true in high bromide waters. More than 600 DBPs have been identified in drinking water; despite intense efforts, a significant percentage of the total organic halogens still remain unaccounted for.

Toxicology of CBPs

Drinking water ingestion is a predominant pathway of CBP exposure. However, exposure via inhalation, dermal contact, and also exposure during showering, bathing, and swimming can occur. The toxicity of the CBPs is highly dependent on the species and strain of the rodents. The dominance of chlorine DBP groups generally decreases in the order of THMs, HAAs, and HANs. Among the THMs, chloroform ($CHCl_3$) and BDCM are the first and second most dominant species. Among HAAs, dichloroacetic acid (DCA) and trichloroacetic acid (TCA) are the first and second most dominant species. A brief review of findings relevant to the toxicity of important CBPs follows.

Trihalomethanes

The THMs are volatile liquids at room temperature and a variety of toxic effects have been associated with short-term and long-term exposures of experimental animals at high doses. Each of the four most common THMs – $CHCl_3$, BDCM, DBCM, and bromoform – has been shown to be carcinogenic to rodents in high-dose chronic studies. $CHCl_3$ is generally the predominant and the most extensively studied chemical of this class. THMs administered by corn oil gavage cause significantly more toxicity than equivalent doses administered in an aqueous emulsion. However, administration via drinking water did not show any signs of toxicity. Nonetheless, bulk of the studies has been conducted using oil vehicle. The maximum annual average of THMs detected in local water supplies cannot exceed 80 ppb as per EPA regulations.

Chloroform

Toxicokinetics

$CHCl_3$ absorption is rapid and extensive after oral, dermal, and inhalation routes. $CHCl_3$ appears to distribute widely throughout the body, with high levels in liver and fat and lower levels in blood, brain, muscle, lung, and kidney. However, high levels were found in the kidney of male mice. $CHCl_3$ is rapidly metabolized and it undergoes both oxidative and reductive biotransformations through cytochrome P450. While the oxidative metabolism produces phosgene, causing toxic effects, the reductive biotransformation forms dichloromethyl radical, which may react with the phospholipids to form adducts. However, oxidative metabolism is predominant. $CHCl_3$ metabolism is species and strain specific. It is metabolized primarily by CYP2E1, whereas at high levels CYP2B1/2 is also involved in the metabolism. $CHCl_3$ biotransformation occurs mainly in the liver and kidney (only in male mice). In humans, about 80 and 90% of the $CHCl_3$ is absorbed under inhalation and oral exposures, respectively. Absorption of dermal exposure was approximately equivalent to inhalation exposure. Human CYP2E1 catalyzes the oxidation of $CHCl_3$.

Toxicity

The LD_{50}s ranging from 36 to 3245 mg kg^{-1} have been reported in rats and mice depending upon strain, vehicle, and route of exposure. Acute and short-term exposures to $CHCl_3$ affect the liver, kidney, central nervous system (CNS), and immune system. Cell proliferation preceding liver and kidney toxicity, higher lipid peroxidation, and glutathione (GSH) depletion were noted in rodents following $CHCl_3$ administration. The extent of $CHCl_3$-induced damage via drinking water is significantly lower than other modes of administration. $CHCl_3$ is teratogenic. Signs of maternal toxicity (decreased body weight and changes in organ weight) were reported in rats, rabbits, and/or mice. Reproductive effects were reported in a three-generation study in mice. $CHCl_3$ produces liver tumors in male and female mice, kidney tumors in male mice and rats, and liver tumors in female rats. The tissue-, species-, strain-, and sex-specific metabolism and toxicity of $CHCl_3$ correlate well with tumor formation. There is only weak evidence for genotoxicity of chloroform in *in vivo* experiments and in mammalian cells *in vitro*. Nausea, lassitude, dry mouth, flatulence, depression, scalding urination, and higher frequency of hepatitis were observed in workers exposed to $CHCl_3$ in occupational settings. $CHCl_3$ anesthesia may result in death in humans due to respiratory and cardiac arrhythmias and cardiac failure. Because of the relatively high frequency of 'late $CHCl_3$ poisoning' (liver toxicity), its use as anesthetic has been abandoned. International Agency for Research on Cancer (IARC) concluded that there is inadequate evidence for the carcinogenicity of chlorinated drinking water in humans and classified $CHCl_3$ as possible carcinogen (group 2B).

Mode of Action

There is, however, compelling evidence that $CHCl_3$ produces cancer in rodents through a nongenotoxic/cytotoxic mode of action, with carcinogenesis resulting from events secondary to $CHCl_3$-induced cytotoxicity and regenerative cell proliferation.

Bromodichloromethane

Bromine substitution generally decreases volatility and enhances lipid solubility (uptake into tissues), which increases biotransformation. Among the four THMs commonly found in drinking water, BDCM appears to be the more potent rodent toxicant and carcinogen. A recent study has shown that showering, bathing, and other water uses involving dermal contact will lead to much greater systemic BDCM doses than ingestion of water. However, studies concerning BDCM toxicities are limited.

Toxicokinetics

Absorption of BDCM appeared to be rapid, but fairly complete and eliminated rapidly. The highest levels were found in the liver, stomach, and kidney. With aqueous vehicle the absorption and elimination were rapid as compared with oil vehicle. Like $CHCl_3$, BDCM also undergoes P450-mediated oxidative and reductive metabolisms and produces phosgene and dichloromethyl radical, respectively. Cytochrome P450, CYP2E1, and CYP2B1/2, as well as a theta-class GST, have been implicated in the metabolism of BDCM in animals. CYP2E1 is responsible for BDCM metabolism in humans.

Toxicity

The oral LD_{50}s ranging from 450 to 969 mg kg^{-1} were reported in mice and rats. Following acute and short-term exposures, pathological changes in liver, kidney, adrenals, lung, and brain and clinical observations including ataxia, sedation, and anesthesia were noted. Males appear to be slightly more susceptible than females. Increased incidence of sternebral anomalies in fetus in rats was observed at maternally toxic dose. Chronic exposure to BDCM caused nonneoplastic lesions in liver and kidney and tumors in liver, kidney, and large intestine. Animal studies provide convincing evidence that BDCM is carcinogenic. BDCM has shown some genotoxic activity (chromosome aberrations) in mammalian cells *in vitro* and has caused sister chromatid exchange (SCE) in bone marrow in mice *in vivo*. The GSH conjugate of BDCM (but not that of chloroform) is much more mutagenic in bacteria than the parent compound and such a conjugation activity takes place also in mammalian cells. Epidemiological studies have suggested a correlation between BDCM exposure and spontaneous abortions, stillbirths, and neural tube defects. IARC concluded that there is sufficient evidence for its carcinogenicity in experimental animals and inadequate evidence for its carcinogenicity in humans and assigned to 2B class.

Mode of Action

BDCM is a relatively weak mutagen, and its conjugation with GSH may lead to genotoxicity. It is proposed that BDCM induces cancer through cytotoxicity leading to regenerative hyperplasia and direct mutation of metabolites. The extent to which each of these processes contributed to the induction of tumors is at present unclear.

Dibromochloromethane

Compared to $CHCl_3$ and BDCM, the toxic potency of DBCM is lower.

Toxicokinetics

The pattern of distribution and elimination of DBCM was very similar to that observed with BDCM, but it is the least studied THM. Presumably, metabolism proceeds via the same routes of biotransformation as described for BDCM. Oxidative metabolism of DBCM would be expected to yield a bromochlorocarbonyl rather than phosgene, and reductive dehalogenation would produce a bromochloromethyl radical.

Toxicity

Acute oral LD_{50}s ranging from 800 to 1200 mg kg^{-1} and clinical signs such as ataxia, sedation, and anesthesia were noted in rodents. Acute or repeated administration of DBCM caused decreased response rates and reduced aggressive behavior in mice and hamsters. Hepatotoxicity, nephrotoxicity, cardiotoxicity, necrosis in salivary glands, and depression in immune function were noted in the repeat dose studies. DBCM did not cause developmental toxicity, but reduced fertility in a two-generation study. DBCM was not carcinogenic in rats. However, according to National Toxicology Program (NTP), there is equivocal evidence of DBCM carcinogenicity since hepatocellular adenomas and carcinomas were significantly increased in females and marginally increased in the male mice at the high dose in the NTP 2-year carcinogenicity study. Due to the inadequate evidence for its carcinogenicity in humans and limited evidence for its carcinogenicity in experimental animals this compound was assigned to group 3 (not classifiable as to carcinogenicity to humans) by IARC.

Mode of Action

The greater propensity for the metabolism of this compound and bromoform as compared with BDCM is difficult to reconcile with its lower carcinogenicity. A possible explanation is less bioavailability resulting from the greater lipophilicity of this compound and the use of corn oil as the vehicle of administration. However, *in vitro* studies showed that DBCM is more potent mutagenic than other THMs.

Bromoform

Toxicokinetics

The distribution and elimination of bromoform resembled those of $CHCl_3$. Bromoform (and organic metabolite) elimination via exhaled breath was greater than that for all other THMs in the rat, but less than that for all other THMs in the mouse. While both oxidative and reductive pathways were involved in bromoform metabolism, oxidative metabolism seems predominant. Bromoform, like DBCM, has a much greater potential than BDCM to be conjugated by GSH to form a mutagenic intermediate.

Toxicity

The acute oral LD_{50}s ranging from 1147 to 1550 mg kg^{-1} in mice and rats were noted. Lethargy, shallow breathing, and ataxia were observed in rats following drinking water administration of bromoform. Acute and repeated exposures (gavage and inhalation) caused liver and kidney toxicity, but the magnitude of liver and kidney effects was less than that observed with the other THMs. Fetotoxic response was observed after gavage administration of bromoform. No reproductive effects were observed. Bromoform showed positive for *in vitro* mutagenicity tests. Slight liver and kidney damages occurred after chronic exposure to high dose of bromoform. While chronic exposure caused dose-related increase in squamous metaplasia of the prostate gland and higher incidences of adenomatous polyps or adenocarcinomas in rats, no neoplastic effects were associated with the exposure of mice to bromoform. There was some evidence of genotoxicity (SCEs) of bromoform in mammalian cells *in vitro* and *in vivo*. Studies are not available to evaluate the chronic human toxicity of bromoform except the deaths reported following overdose of bromoform-containing sedative. The principal causes for death were severe CNS depression and respiratory failure. IARC classified bromoform as group 3.

Mode of Action

Although bromoform seems to have a greater propensity for metabolism and is a more potent mutagen than BDCM, it appears to be a less potent toxicant and carcinogen. As with DBCM, a possible explanation is less bioavailability resulting from the greater lipophilicity of this compound and the use of corn oil as the vehicle of administration.

Halo Acids

Halo acids are the second most frequently found CBPs after THMs. To date, the chlorinated acetic acids have been more thoroughly characterized toxicologically than their brominated analogs. HAAs, unlike THMs, are nonvolatile and they have low dermal absorption (at low concentrations). The DCAs and TCAs occur in significantly higher concentrations than the monohaloacetates. TCA and DCA are metabolites and ultimate carcinogenic forms of rodent carcinogens, trichloroethylene (TCE) and perchloroethylene (PERC). The maximum annual average of HAAs permitted by EPA regulations is 60 ppb.

Dichloroacetic Acid

This compound exists in drinking water as salt; however, most of the experiments employed the free acid. Therefore, the applicability of the results of such studies to estimating human risks will be uncertain because of the large pH artifacts that can be expected when administering a strong acid.

Toxicokinetics

Absorption of DCA is rapid from the intestinal tract into the bloodstream. Once in the bloodstream, DCA is distributed to the liver and muscles, and then in smaller quantities to the fat, kidney, and other tissues such as the brain and testes. The systemic clearance of DCA is significantly higher. The metabolism of DCA is mediated by a novel GST, GST-zeta, found in cytosolic fraction that catalyzes the conversion of DCA to glyoxylate. This enzyme appears to be subjected to autoinhibition by DCA.

Toxicity

DCA is not very toxic when administered acutely to rodents. The LD_{50}s of 4.5 and 5.5 g kg^{-1} in rats and mice, respectively, have been reported for sodium salt of DCA. Following short-term exposure, dogs were more sensitive than rats to DCA. The most overt toxicity in rats was hind limb paralysis at the highest dose and relative liver weights were significantly increased at all doses. Histopathological changes were observed in the brain and testes of both species. At high repeated doses, DCA caused kidney damage. The effects such as reduced weights of accessory organs (epididymis, cauda epididymis, and preputial gland) changes in sperm motion, delayed spermiation and formation, and distorted sperm heads have been observed when administered in drinking water. DCA induces soft tissue abnormalities in fetal rats. DCA produces a severe hepatomegaly and liver tumors in rats following chronic exposure.

DCA was used as a potential orally effective hypoglycemic agent. Although there is no conclusive evidence, DCA is proposed to cause neurotoxic effects in humans. Therefore, DCA was not fully developed as a hypoglycemic agent. IARC classified DCA as a group 3 compound for its carcinogenicity.

Mode of Action

A number of potential modes of DCA-induced hepatocarcinogenicity have been proposed, including direct genotoxicity, tumor promotion, inhibition of apoptosis, etc. However, available data are not adequate to indicate the exact mode(s) of action responsible for the hepatic carcinogenicity in rats and mice to DCA exposure. Peroxisome proliferation likely contributes to tumor development in the liver at high doses but the histopathological and other analyses suggest that other mechanisms may be more important at low doses. Most data now suggest that it is the parent compound that is responsible for the effects related to carcinogenicity by interfering with the cellular signaling mechanisms.

Trichloroacetic Acid

Like DCA, TCA exists almost exclusively in salt form at pH found in drinking water.

Toxicokinetics

TCA is readily absorbed from the gastrointestinal tract in experimental animals and humans and its clearance from blood is relatively slow relative to other HAAs. Approximately half of the administered dose was eliminated unchanged. There are substantial differences in this clearance by different species. Clearance is much faster in mice than in rats and human clearance is very slow. TCA produces same metabolites as DCA with or without being converted to DCA.

Toxicity

The oral LD_{50} of TCA (neutralized to pH 6–7) is found to be $3.32\,g\,kg^{-1}$ in rats and $4.97\,g\,kg^{-1}$ in mice when administered in aqueous solution. The most obvious target organ for TCA is the liver. Repeated administration of TCA in drinking water only produced minimal evidence of liver toxicity. TCA administration resulted in body weight reductions, soft tissue malformations, and interventricular septal defect. TCA (neutralized) induces hepatic tumors in male and female mice, but not in rats when administered via drinking water. After short-term exposures, TCA induces basophilic liver foci in mice, similar to those caused by several peroxisome proliferators.

TCA is a strong acid. It is widely recognized that skin contact of TCA has the potential to produce acid burns, and ingestion of TCA has the potential to damage tissues of the gastrointestinal tract or produce systemic acidosis, even though specific studies of these effects do not appear in the literature. TCA is frequently utilized for chemical peeling by physicians practicing dermatologic surgery. TCA is a major metabolite of commonly used solvents such as TCE and PERC and occupational exposures to these solvents have been quite high in the past, but few, if any, effects of the solvents in humans have been attributed to TCA. So it is reasonable to presume that TCA is relatively nontoxic to humans under circumstances of low exposures such as those encountered in chlorinated drinking water. In addition, the mode of tumor induction – peroxisomal proliferation – in animals is not relevant for humans. IARC has classified TCA as a group 3 compound for its carcinogenicity.

Mode of Action

TCA causes carcinogenicity mainly by peroxisomal proliferation mechanism. Additional mechanisms suggested are increased oncogene expression via DNA hypomethylation and promotion of spontaneous liver tumors.

Other Chlorination Byproducts

Brominated HAAs are formed in waters that contain bromide. There are very limited data available on the toxicity of these chemicals.

Toxicological data in experimental animals and humans for the haloketones and haloacetaldehydes are extremely limited. Slight liver and CNS effects were observed. Hepatocellular carcinomas in mice were reported, probably due to mutagenic effect.

Members of this class have been identified as key metabolites of chemicals such as TCE, vinyl chloride, and dibromochloropropane. Trichloroacetaldehyde and chloral hydrate are important compounds of this group. Chloral hydrate is primarily known for its depressant effects on the CNS and doses of 500–2000 mg produce CNS depression in humans. It is also known to cause liver damage.

Epidemiological Studies

Numerous epidemiological studies have attempted to assess the association between cancer and the long-term consumption of disinfected drinking water. A wide range of cancer sites such as gall bladder, esophagus, kidney, breast, liver, pancreas, prostate, stomach, bladder, colon, and rectum were found to be associated with the use of chlorinated surface water in humans. Additionally, published epidemiological data suggest the possibility that increased spontaneous abortion rates may be related to DBPs in drinking water. The epidemiological evidence is inconclusive and equivocal for an association between cancer and noncancer effect exposure to CBPs in drinking water. The quality of information about water disinfection exposures and potential confounding characteristics differs dramatically between these studies. The confounding factors such as smoking, drinking, and exposure to other chemicals make the matter more complicated. In addition, occurrence of cancer incidence at one place and nonoccurrence at other places further complicate the interpretation.

It is noteworthy that there is little support in the animal data for certain target organs that are prominently associated with chlorinated drinking water in epidemiological studies (e.g., bladder cancer). Therefore, the possibility has to be left open that the carcinogenic effect of CBPs may be dependent on genetically determined characteristics of a target organ (or tissue) that make it more susceptible than the same organ in test animals. It also suggests that toxicology evaluation of whole CBPs including unidentified byproducts is needed. To address this problem, US EPA initiated 'Integrated Disinfection Byproducts Mixtures Research: Toxicological and Chemical Evaluation of Alternative Disinfection Treat Treatment Scenarios', also known as the 'Four Lab Study', with the collaboration of four national Laboratories. This ongoing study evaluated toxicological effects of complex CBP mixtures, with an emphasis on reproductive and developmental effects and recommended a new procedure for producing chlorinated drinking water concentrate for animal toxicology. The next phase of this work is a larger battery of toxicological endpoints and focused on chlorinated drinking water.

Conclusions

Chlorination has been the major disinfection process of drinking water in many countries for many years despite the availability of alternative disinfectants. There is a widespread concern about cancer, noncancer, and reproductive effects of CBPs based on animal and epidemiological studies. However, most of these studies were conducted with a single chemical, at high doses and using corn oil vehicle, a potentially confounding factor in toxicological evaluations of drinking water contaminants. These conditions are irrelevant to human exposure. Importantly, carcinogenic effects of individual CBPs may not represent the risk posed by the mixtures, as disinfected drinking water is a very complex mixture of chemicals. Although some epidemiological studies linked CBPs to the incidence of cancer and adverse reproductive effects in humans, there is no scientific basis for the proposed association and none of the CBPs studied individually to date is a potent carcinogen at concentrations normally found in drinking water. In addition, the toxic effects of many CBPs remain largely unknown and many of them remain unidentified. Hence, it is not possible to make sound scientific judgment. It is important to evaluate all CBPs individually or as mixtures in a systematic manner to provide comparative toxicity and to better understand the exposure concentrations in the drinking water based on daily ingestion, inhalation, swimming, bathing, etc. in the risk assessment paradigm. A complicating factor when assessing risk from CBPs is that they occur in complex mixtures that vary by location, disinfection process, distance from the treatment plant, changing conditions of the source water, and even weather conditions. Moreover, the effects may be altered by factors such as coexposure to other compounds age and lifestyle. Nonetheless, safe drinking water is a substantive health concern and a balance should be achieved between reducing exposure to CBPs and maintaining control of waterborne diseases.

See also: Bromoform; Chloroform, Bromoform, Chloroacetic Acid, Trihalomethanes; Chlorine; Chlorine Dioxide; Chloroform; Trihalomethanes; International Agency for Research on Cancer; Pharmacokinetics; Drinking-Water Criteria (Safety, Quality, and Perception); Clean Water Act (CWA), US; Environmental Protection Agency, US.

Further Reading

Diduch, M., Polkowska, Z., Namieśnik, J., 2011. Chemical quality of bottled waters: a review. J. Food Sci. 76 (9), R178–R196.

Doria Mde, F., Pidgeon, N., Hunter, P.R., 2009. Perceptions of drinking water quality and risk and its effect on behaviour: a cross-national study. Sci. Total Environ. 407 (21), 5455–5464.

Hrudey, S.E., Hrudey, E.J., 2007. A nose for trouble – the role of off-flavours in assuring safe drinking water. Water Sci. Technol. 55 (5), 239–247.

Loo, S.L., Fane, A.G., Krantz, W.B., Lim, T.T., 2012. Emergency water supply: a review of potential technologies and selection criteria. Water Res. 46 (10), 3125–3151.

Ngwenya, N., Ncube, E.J., Parsons, J., 2013. Recent advances in drinking water disinfection: successes and challenges. Rev. Environ. Contam. Toxicol. 222, 111–170.

Sun, F., Chen, J., Tong, Q., Zeng, S., 2007. Integrated risk assessment and screening analysis of drinking water safety of a conventional water supply system. Water Sci. Technol. 56 (6), 47–56.

Yang, H., Bain, R.E., Bartram, J., et al., 2012 Dec 31. Water safety and inequality in access to drinking-water between rich and poor households. Environ. Sci. Technol. [Epub ahead of print].

World Health Organization (WHO). Guidelines for drinking-water quality, fourth ed. World Health Organization, Geneva. 2011.

Relevant Websites

http://www.cdc.gov/safewater/chlorination-byproducts.html – Centers for Disease Control and Prevention.

http://water.epa.gov/drink/contaminants/index.cfm – United States Environmental Protection Agency (USEPA). National primary drinking water standards.

Chlorine

A Suryanarayanan, Manchester University College of Pharmacy, Fort Wayne, IN, USA

This article is a revision of the previous edition article by Sanjay Chanda and Harihara M. Mehendale, volume 1, pp 553–555, © 2005, Elsevier Inc.

- Name: Chlorine
- Chemical Abstracts Service Registry Number: CAS # 7782-50-5
- Synonyms: Bertholite, Chloor, Chlor, Chlore, Molecular chlorine, Cloro, RTECS FO2100000, UN1017
- Molecular Formula: Cl_2
- Chemical Structure:

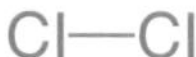

Background Information

Chlorine is a greenish-yellow, noncombustible gas at room temperature and atmospheric pressure. It can also be generated when bleach is mixed with other cleaning products. For more than 100 years now, industry has exploited this highly reactive chemical produced from one of nature's inexhaustible minerals – common salt. Today, chlorine is used in a vast range of processes to create many products that serve our everyday needs at work, home, and play. Some properties of chlorine are listed:

Property	*Information*
Molecular weight	70.91
Density at 0 °C and 760 mm Hg	3.21 g l^{-1}
Melting point at 760 mm Hg	−101 °C
Boiling point at 760 mm Hg	−34.6 °C
Water solubility at 0 °C and 760 mm Hg	14.6 g l^{-1}
Vapor pressure at 0 °C and 760 mm Hg	3.61

Uses

1. A bacteriostat, disinfectant, odor control, and demulsifier in the treatment of drinking water, swimming pools, and sewage
2. Use in the paper and pulp and textile industries for bleaching cellulose for artificial fibers
3. Manufacture of chlorinated lime; chemical warfare
4. To control biofouling in cooling systems
5. Chlorinating and oxidizing agent in organic and inorganic synthesis
6. Manufacture of pharmaceuticals, cosmetics, lubricants, flameproofing, adhesives, in special batteries containing lithium or zinc, and in hydraulic fluids
7. Processing of meat, fish, vegetables, and fruit
8. Manufacture of synthetic rubber, plastics, resins, elastomers, pesticides, automotive antifreeze, refrigerants, antiknock compounds, chlorinated hydrocarbons, polyvinyl chloride, and chlorinated lime
9. Detinning and dezincing iron, and to shrink-proof wool
10. Disinfectant in laundries, dishwashers, cleaning powders, cleaning dairy equipment
11. In metallurgy, chlorine is used as a fluxing, purification, and extraction agent.

Exposure Routes and Pathways

Dermal or ocular contact and inhalation are the most common exposure pathways. Chlorine can be absorbed into the body by all routes. The extent of the injury depends on the concentration of the gas. This can range from mild mucous membrane irritation (after 1 h) to toxic lung disease and water-logged lungs or death within a few minutes. After inhalation, chlorine causes irritation of the eyes, nose, and throat, followed by coughing and wheezing, shortage of breath, nausea, vomiting, sputum production, and chest pain. Heightening of anxiety is seen in those prone to neurosis. Larger exposures may lead to heart and lung failure. Severe exposure can also lead to severe tracheobronchitis, pulmonary edema, and acute hypoxemic respiratory failure; short-term, high-level exposures can also aggravate preexisting heart diseases, producing electrocardiographic changes and congestive heart failure; and at sufficiently high doses (i.e., wartime conditions) chlorine can cause shock, coma, respiratory arrest, and death. Those surviving exposure may have persistent cough for up to 14 days or even several months. Symptoms may include chest pains, vomiting, and coughing. After skin contact, chlorine causes irritation, pain, redness, blister, and burns. Liquid chlorine may cause burns on contact. After eye contact, symptoms are conjunctival irritation, watering of eyes, and inflammation.

In human poisoning incidents involving accidental ingestion of household bleach, chlorine caused a burning sensation in the mouth and throat, irritation to the digestive tract and stomach, and vomiting. Exposure to chlorine gas causes effects ranging from bronchitis, asthma, and swelling of the lungs, to headaches, heart disease, and meningitis. Swimmers have reported a bleaching effect of chlorine on their hair; some have developed 'green hair' and chemical conjunctivitis. There have also been occasional reports of asthma precipitated by exposure to chlorinated water.

Probable Routes of Human Exposure

The National Institute for Occupational Safety and Health (NIOSH) (National Occupational Exposure Survey (NOES), 1981–83) has statistically estimated that 182 873 workers (22 083 of these are female) are potentially exposed to chlorine in the United States. Individuals may be exposed to chlorine when mixing a cleaning product that contains an acid with a solution containing sodium hypochlorite (bleach). The misuse of swimming pool chemicals may also potentially expose the general population to chlorine.

 http://dx.doi.org/10.1016/B978-0-12-386454-3.00277-3

Exposures most commonly result from either storage or transportation accidents involving the pressurized liquid form. Other poisonings occur in industrial accidents, school chemistry experiments, accidental release of chlorine from swimming pool operations, and mixing of cleaning agents (adding acidic cleaning agents to hypochlorite bleach releases chlorine gases).

Toxicokinetics

Chlorine persists as an element only at a very low pH (<2), and at the higher pH found in living tissue it is rapidly converted into hypochlorous acid. In this form, it can penetrate the cell and form *N*-chloro-derivatives that can damage cellular integrity. The intermediate water solubility of chlorine accounts for its effect on the upper airway and the lower respiratory tract. In addition, the density of the gas is greater than that of air, causing it to remain near ground level and increasing exposure time. The odor threshold for chlorine is approximately 0.3–0.5 parts per million (ppm).

Chlorine is eliminated primarily in urine and feces, mainly (81% of ingested label) as the chloride ion.

Mechanism of Toxicity

Chlorine reacts with body moisture to form acids. The acids form acid proteinates. Under physiological conditions (pH 7.4, 37 °C), chlorine reacts with water to produce hypochlorous acid. Evidence suggests that chlorine produces oxygen radicals. Elemental chlorine, hypochlorous acid, hydrogen chloride, and oxygen are all thought to contribute to the biological activity. Apparently, hypochlorous acid can penetrate the cell wall, disrupting its integrity and permeability, and by reacting with sulfhydryl groups in cysteine, can inhibit various enzymes.

Acute and Short-Term Toxicity (or Exposure)

Animal

A single exposure of several hours to a chlorine concentration of 29–87 mg m^{-3} (10–30 ppm) induced definite adverse effects, including high mortality rates, in rodent species tested. Repeated exposure to chlorine concentrations of 2.9–26 mg m^{-3} (1–9 ppm), for a period of several weeks to months, induced dose-related pulmonary and other adverse effects. A level of 2 mg m^{-3} (0.7 ppm) was reported to be a no observed adverse effect level, for rabbits and guinea pigs, repeatedly exposed to chlorine through inhalation.

Exposure of cats to a concentration of 900 mg m^{-1} (300 ppm) for 1 h may cause death after a period during which the conjunctiva is inflamed; coughing and dyspnea are also present. Dogs rarely die following a 30 min exposure to 650 ppm and never die following a 30 min exposure to less than 280 ppm. The pulse rate of dogs is retarded during exposure to concentrations of 200 ppm or greater.

In studies designed to evaluate the effects of chlorine exposure on resistance to disease, repeated exposure to 261 mg m^{-3} (90 ppm) for 3 h day^{-1}, during a 20 day period, had a greater effect on rats with spontaneous pulmonary disease (SPD) than on those that were specific pathogen free. A higher mortality rate and a greater incidence of pulmonary tract abnormalities were noted among the SPD rats. At lower levels, guinea pigs, exposed to chlorine at 5.0 mg m^{-3} (1.7 ppm) for 5 h day^{-1}, over 47 days, before or after injection with a virulent strain of human tuberculosis, showed decreased average survival rates compared with unexposed, injected animals.

Acute exposure/lethal time for 50% mortality/(LT_{50}) values for male mice that had undergone a single exposure to a chlorine concentration of 841 or 493 mg m^{-3} (290 or 170 ppm) were 11 and 55 min, respectively. This study confirmed the importance of delayed death in chlorine toxicity studies, with some deaths occurring up to 30 days after exposure. Exposure of mice to chlorine at 841 mg m^{-3} (290 ppm) for 25 ± 6 min (mean ±SD) resulted in about 100% mortality over 30 days. About 80% mortality was recorded in mice exposed to 841 mg m^{-3} (290 ppm) for 15 ± 2 min. Whereas exposure to 841 mg m^{-3} (290 ppm) for 9 ± 1 min caused almost 40% mortality, limiting the exposure to 6 min allowed all the mice to survive. Exposure of mice to a chlorine concentration of 493 mg m^{-3} (170 ppm) for 120 ± 40 or 52 ± 13 min caused almost 80 and 50% mortality, respectively. When exposure at 493 mg m^{-3} (170 ppm) was limited to 28 ± 8 min, there were no immediate deaths, but about 10% delayed mortality occurred over the 30 day observation period.

Human

Liquid chlorine causes burns to skin and eyes and frostbite. It may cause lung injury if inhaled. Chlorine causes smarting of the skin and first-degree burns on short exposure; it may cause secondary burns in long exposures. Inhalation of low concentrations causes mild mucous membrane irritation and upper respiratory tract irritation. Inhalation of high concentrations of the gas causes necrosis of the tracheal and bronchial epithelium as well as pulmonary edema, atelectasis, emphysema, and damage to the pulmonary blood vessels. Acute exposure may also cause anxiety and vomiting. Exposure to 500 ppm can be lethal over 30 min, while a 1000 ppm exposure can be lethal within a few minutes.

A meta-analysis study of epidemiological studies in humans concluded that long-term consumption of chlorinated water is associated with bladder cancer, particularly in men. The pool chlorine hypothesis postulates that the rise in childhood asthma in the developed world could result at least partly from the increasing exposure of children to toxic gases and aerosols contaminating the air of indoor chlorinated pools. A study involving schoolchildren attending a public pool concluded that pool use by young children is strongly linked to development of childhood asthma.

Skin, Eye, and Respiratory Irritations

Chlorine is irritating to nose and throat at 5 ppm or above and highly irritating, especially to the mucous membranes of the eyes and respiratory tract. Potential symptoms of overexposure are burning of eyes, nose, and mouth; lacrimation, rhinorrhea; coughing, choking, and substernal pain; nausea, vomiting;

headache, dizziness; syncope; pulmonary edema; pneumonia; hypoxemia; dermatitis; and eye and skin burns.

Populations at Special Risk

Individuals with pulmonary disease, breathing/problems/, bronchitis, or chronic lung conditions.

Chronic Toxicity (or Exposure)

Animal

Chlorine gas was not carcinogenic in mice and rats exposed to varying concentrations. Chlorine administered in drinking water produced lymphomas and/or leukemia in rats, but was not carcinogenic in a third study.

Human

A4; Not classifiable as a human carcinogen.

In a series of 75 tests on three subjects, a chlorine concentration of 0.52 ppm elicited heightened light sensitivity, but exposure to a concentration of 0.28 ppm did not induce any effects. Changes in sensitivity to light became evident only at, or above the odor perception threshold level.

Twenty-nine students were exposed to 0, 0.5, 1.0, or 2.0 ppm chlorine for 4–8 h. Sensations of itching or burning of the nose and eyes and general discomfort were reported, primarily during exposures to 1.0 or 2.0 ppm. Few subjects reported experiencing feelings of nausea, headache, dizziness, or fatigue at these concentrations, although several reported experiencing shortness of breath for several hours after the 8 h exposure to 1 ppm. No subjects reported any sensory perception related to exposure the morning after the exposure. Statistically significant reductions in pulmonary function were found following the 8 h exposure to 1 ppm, but not 0.5 ppm.

Chronic exposure causes permanent, although moderate, reduction in pulmonary function and corrosion of teeth.

In vitro Toxicity Data

In a series of *in vitro* experiments on a human lymphocyte culture system, it was reported that chlorine induced chromatid and chromosome breaks, translocations, dicentric chromosomes, and gaps.

Immunotoxicity

Epidemiologic surveys show a higher prevalence of nasal symptoms among subjects with seasonal allergic rhinitis than nonrhinitic subjects after provocation with chlorine in the air.

Reproductive and Developmental Toxicity

No adverse effects were observed in pregnant rabbits or their offspring following exposure of the rabbits, through inhalation, to chlorine concentrations of 1.7–4.4 mg m^{-3} (0.6–1.5 ppm). Furthermore, adverse effects were not seen in seven generations of rats given highly chlorinated water (100 mg l^{-1} daily) throughout the entire life span.

Genotoxicity

In a series of *in vitro* experiments on a human lymphocyte culture system, it was reported that chlorine concentration 2–20 times those normally found in drinking water induced chromatid and chromosome breaks, translocations, dicentric chromosomes, and gaps. Mutations have been detected in *Salmonella typhimurium*, and chromosome aberrations have been detected in human lymphocytes.

Carcinogenicity

In humans, lymphoma has been observed in relation to water treatment with chlorine. Associations with increased renal, bladder, and gastric cancers have also been found, but firm conclusions cannot be drawn because of mixed exposures with caustic acids.

Clinical Management

Exposure should be terminated as soon as possible by removal of the patient to fresh air. The skin, eyes, and mouth should be washed with copious amounts of water. A 15–20 min wash may be necessary. Contaminated clothing and jewelry should be removed and isolated. Contact lenses should be removed from the eye to avoid prolonged contact of the chemical with the area. Affected areas should not be rubbed. If breathing has stopped, artificial respiration should be given. If breathing is difficult, oxygen should be given.

Treatment Overview

1. Inhalation exposure
   a. Management of mild toxicity: Provide supplemental oxygen to maintain PaO2 of 60 mm Hg or greater. Bronchodilators (inhaled albuterol or other beta-agonists, and anticholinergics) have been used frequently for the management of respiratory symptoms. A 1% lidocaine solution added to nebulized albuterol results in analgesic and cough-suppressant actions. Nebulized sodium bicarbonate (3.75%) has been used. Perform an ophthalmologic exam in any patient with persistent eye irritation.
   b. Management of severe toxicity: Aggressive use of inhaled beta-agonists, lidocaine, and nebulized sodium bicarbonate for bronchospasm. Corticosteroids may also be useful for severe bronchospasm. Early intubation for laryngospasm or severe respiratory distress. Treat respiratory failure with positive-pressure ventilation. Positive end-expiratory pressure (8–10 mm Hg) and inverse ratio ventilation may be beneficial in acute lung injury.
   c. Decontamination

i. Prehospital: Remove the individual from the toxic environment. Administer humidified oxygen if respiratory irritation develops. Remove contaminated clothing.
ii. Hospital: Irrigate exposed eyes with copious amounts of normal saline. Remove contaminated clothing and wash exposed skin with water.

d. Airway management: Perform endotracheal intubation if indicated (e.g., persistent hypoxemia, severe bronchospasm, stridor, severe respiratory distress, or laryngeal edema).

Medical Surveillance

Medical histories should include sufficient detail to document the occurrence of bronchitis, tuberculosis, or pulmonary abscesses. A complete history and physical examination, an eye examination, cardiac status, and teeth should be stressed. The skin should be examined for evidence of chronic disorders. Simple tests of olfactory ability should be carried out, along with respiratory function tests.

Environmental Fate

The stability of free chlorine in natural water is very low because it is a strong oxidizing agent and rapidly oxidizes inorganic compounds. It also oxidizes organic compounds, but more slowly than inorganic compounds.

Ecotoxicology

Chlorine is highly toxic to all forms of aquatic life; there is no potential for bioaccumulation or bioconcentration. In a study designed to test chlorine toxicity to early life stages of freshwater mussels (Bivalvia: Unionidae), Valenti et al. conducted tests with glochidia from several species and 21 day bioassays with 3-month-old *Epioblasma capsaeformis* and 3-, 6-, and 12-month-old *Villosa iris* juveniles. The authors observed significant declines in growth and survival in the 21 day test with *E. capsaeformis* at 20 μg total residual chlorine (TRC) per liter. Lowest observed adverse effect concentrations in bioassays with juvenile *V. iris* were higher (30–60 μg TRC per liter) but showed a significant trend of declining toxicity with increased age. The authors concluded that although endpoints were above water quality criteria set by the US Environmental Protection Agency, the long life spans of unionids and potential implications of chronic exposure to endangered juvenile mussels warrant concern.

In another study by Grizzle et al., chlorination was implicated as a factor contributing to the induction of papilloma development in caged bullhead catfish exposed to effluent of a wastewater treatment plant.

Exposure Standards and Guidelines

The current Occupational Safety and Health Administration permissible exposure limit for chlorine is 1 ppm (3 mg m^{-3}) as a ceiling limit. A worker's exposure to chlorine shall at no time exceed this ceiling level.

NIOSH has established a recommended exposure limit for chlorine of 0.5 ppm (1.5 mg m^{-3}) as a time-weighted average (TWA) for up to a 10 h workday and a 40-h workweek and a short-term exposure limit (STEL) of 1 ppm (3 mg m^{-3}). The NIOSH limits are based on the risk of severe eye, mucous membrane, and skin irritation.

The American Conference of Governmental Industrial Hygienists (ACGIH) has assigned chlorine a threshold limit value of 0.5 ppm (1.5 mg m^{-3}) as a TWA for a normal 8 h workday and a 40 h workweek and a STEL of 1.0 ppm (2.9 mg m^{-3}) for periods not to exceed 15 min. Exposures at the STEL concentration should not be repeated more than four times a day and should be separated by intervals of at least 60 min. The ACGIH limits are based on the risk of eye and mucous membrane irritation.

Reported Fatal Dose

A reported fatal dose was 430 ppm, lethal after 30 min, and 1000 ppm, fatal within a few minutes.

See also: Detergent; Pollution, Air in Encyclopedia of Toxicology; Pollution, Soil; Surfactants, Anionic and Nonionic.

Further Reading

Abdel-Rahman, M.S., Suh, D.H., Bull, R.J., 1984. Pharmacodynamics and toxicity of chlorine in drinking water in the rat. J. Appl. Toxicol. 4, 82–86.
Florentin, A., Hautemanière, A., Hartemann, P., 2011. Health effects of disinfection by-products in chlorinated swimming pools. Int. J. Hyg. Environ. Health 214 (6), 461–469.
Jonasson, S., Koch, B., Bucht, A., January 2013. Inhalation of chlorine causes long-standing lung inflammation and airway hyperresponsiveness in a murine model of chemical-induced lung injury. Toxicology 7 (303), 34–42.
Krasovskii, G.N., Egorova, N.A., 2003. Chlorination of water as a high hazard to human health. Gig. Sanit. 1, 17–21.
Samal, A., Honovar, J., White, C.R., Patel, R.P., 2010. Potential for chlorine gas-induced injury in the extrapulmonary vasculature. Proc. Am. Thorac. Soc. 7 (4), 290–293.
Vetrano, K.M., 2001. Molecular chlorine: health and environmental effects. Rev. Environ. Contam. Toxicol. 170, 75–140.
Winder, C., 2001. The toxicology of chlorine. Environ. Res. 85, 105–114.

Chlorine Dioxide

VM Gómez-López, CEBAS-CSIC, Espinardo, Spain

This article is a revision of the previous edition article by Zhengwei Cai, volume 1, pp 555–556, © 2005, Elsevier Inc.

- Name of Chemical: Chlorine dioxide
- Chemical Abstracts Registry Service Number: 10049-04-4
- Synonyms: Chlorine peroxide, Chloroperoxyl, Chloryl radical, Chlorine(IV) oxide, Anthium dioxcide.
- Chemical Class: Chlorine dioxide and its byproducts are collectively called oxychlorines
- Molecular Formula: ClO_2
- Chemical Structure: O=Cl=O

O
\\
Cl—O ·

Background (Significance/History)

Chlorine dioxide is an oxidant used as an industrial bleaching agent and water disinfectant. The British chemist and inventor Sir Humphrey created chlorine dioxide in 1814. It was first used to disinfect water at a spa in Ostend, Belgium. Chlorine dioxide gas was used for anthrax spore decontamination of the Hart Senate Office Building in 2001 and other American buildings in 2002 and 2004. It has been studied as a substitute of chlorine because it produces almost no chlorinated disinfection byproducts.

Uses

Chlorine dioxide is a strong oxidizing agent, bactericide, fungicide, algicide, and antiseptic. It can be applied as gas or in solution. It is used in bleaching cellulose, paper pulp, leather, flour, fats and oils, textiles, and beeswax, and in deodorizing and purifying water. It is currently considered an alternative to chlorine as a disinfectant for public water supplies in the United States, and it is used for drinking water disinfection in several European countries, in swimming pools, and in commercial water cooling systems. The US Food and Drug Administration (FDA) allows the use of chlorine dioxide as an antimicrobial agent in water used in poultry processing, and in water used to wash fruits and vegetables. Gaseous chlorine dioxide has been used as fumigant against spores of the causative agent of anthrax. It is also used in the manufacture of many chlorite salts.

Environmental Fate and Behavior

Chlorine dioxide is not expected to persist in the environment because it is unstable and also quickly reacts with organic matter. It decomposes to chlorine gas and oxygen after release to air. When added to raw water, chlorine dioxide is rapidly reduced to chlorite, a persistent byproduct of health concern. It persists up to minutes in air and up to hours in water and soil. Chlorine dioxide is easily photolyzed.

Exposure and Exposure Monitoring

Routes and Pathways

Consumption of drinking water is the most probable route of exposure to chlorine dioxide and its byproducts for the general public. Workers in factories that produce or use it are the most exposed populations. Inhalation and contact with eyes and skin are exposure routes for these workers. Patients undergoing hemodialysis may be directly exposed to chlorine dioxide through dialysis water disinfected with chlorine dioxide. Poultry, fruits, and vegetables washed with chlorine dioxide solutions could be a potential entry route to the human body of this substance and its byproducts; however, the US FDA states that an additional process step such as rinsing must be used for fruits and vegetables after chlorine dioxide washings. Environmental release may occur to the air and in wastewater streams from chlorine dioxide–related factories.

Environmental Exposure (Monitoring Data in Air)

The OSHA procedure for monitoring chlorine dioxide in air uses a midget fritted glass bubbler containing buffered potassium iodide. STEL samples are collected until a volume of 7.5 l and TWA until 120 l. Samples are analyzed later by ion chromatography, although other methods can opt for a simpler iodometric titration with sodium thiosulfate.

Toxicokinetics

Chlorine dioxide can be rapidly absorbed through the gastrointestinal tract. Peak blood concentration levels can be reached within 1 h after a single dose administered orally. It can also be slowly absorbed through shaved skin with a half absorption time of 22 h. It seems unlikely that intact chlorine dioxide is absorbed by inhalation giving its highly reactive nature; it is more likely that its derivatives can be absorbed. Chlorine dioxide is metabolized to chlorite, chlorate, and mostly chloride. Most administered chlorine dioxide and its metabolites remain in plasma followed by kidneys, lungs, stomach, intestine, liver, and spleen. About 43% of orally administered chlorine dioxide is eliminated in the urine and feces within 72 h. It is not excreted via the lungs.

 http://dx.doi.org/10.1016/B978-0-12-386454-3.00278-5

Mechanism of Toxicity

The toxicity of chlorine dioxide is attributed to the oxidative stress caused by this compound and its byproducts or metabolites. Animal studies and *in vitro* experiments with human red blood cells indicate that chlorine dioxide and its byproducts, especially chlorite, oxidize hemoglobin to methemoglobin by inhibiting methemoglobin reductase, decreasing erythrocyte glutathione levels, stimulating erythrocyte hydrogen peroxide production, and causing hemolytic anemia.

Acute and Short-Term Toxicity

Animal

Delayed death occurred in animals after exposure to 150–200 ppm of gas for less than 1 h. Rats repeatedly exposed to 10 ppm of gas died after 10–13 days of exposure. The oral LD_{50} in rats is 292 mg kg^{-1}. 'Chlorine' derived from aqueous chlorine dioxide is absorbed by the oral route, with a wide distribution and rapid and extensive elimination. In one study, groups of four rats received a single oral dose of approximately 1.5 or 4.5 mg $^{36}ClO_2$ kg^{-1} body weight. Blood samples were collected for up to 48 h postadministration, and at 72 h, upon sacrifice. Kidneys, lungs, small intestine, liver, spleen, thymus, bone marrow, and testes were collected to detect levels of ^{36}Cl. It was found in all tissues except testes, skin, and the remaining carcass, although levels in these tissues each were found to be less than 1% of the administered dose. Approximately 40% of a single dose of ^{36}Cl was recovered in urine, expired air, and feces, although the urine accounted for most (about 30%). The rapid appearance of ^{36}Cl in plasma following oral administration of chlorine dioxide ($^{36}ClO_2$) or chlorite ($^{36}ClO_2^-$) has been shown in laboratory animals.

Human

Chlorine dioxide gas is highly irritating to the skin and mucous membranes of the respiratory tract. Symptoms of exposure by inhalation include eye and throat irritation, headache, nausea, nasal discharge, coughing, wheezing, bronchitis, and delayed onset of pulmonary edema. It is explosive in the form of concentrated vapor or solution (10 vol% in the air). When involved in a fire, chlorine dioxide is a source of oxygen. Daily ingestion of 1 l of water containing 0.7 mg of chlorine dioxide has been reported to cause nausea. Exposure of a worker to 19 ppm for an unspecified time was reported to be fatal. Ingestion of 250 ml of a 40 mg l^{-1} solution of chlorine dioxide causes symptoms within 5 min of ingestion that disappear 5 min later.

Chronic Toxicity

Animal

Chronic exposure of rats and rabbits to chlorine dioxide gas has revealed lung damage, including lesions to the alveoli and blood abnormalities.

Human

Human exposure to chlorine dioxide, both in controlled prospective studies and in actual use situations in community water supplies, has failed to reveal adverse health effects. However, glucose-6-phosphate dehydrogenase-deficient individuals and infants are groups thought to be at higher risk to chlorine dioxide toxicity due to their susceptibility to oxidant-induced methemoglobinemia. The chronic toxicity signs are mainly dyspnea and asthmatic bronchitis, and in certain cases irritation of the gastrointestinal tract. Chronic exposure of workers to airborne chlorine dioxide has caused symptoms of ocular and respiratory irritation.

Immunotoxicity

There is no concern about possible immunotoxicity of chlorine dioxide.

Reproductive Toxicity

Studies performed in rats with orally administrated chlorine dioxide solutions have not shown evidence of effects on reproduction.

Genotoxicity

Positive and negative results have been reported for chlorine dioxide genotoxicity in animals, and no reports were found for humans. Surface water used for human consumption treated with chlorine dioxide can produce formation of genotoxic halogenated disinfection byproducts.

Carcinogenicity

According to the US Environmental Protection Agency (EPA), chlorine dioxide is not classifiable as to human carcinogenicity because of inadequate data.

Ecotoxicology

Chlorine dioxide can be highly toxic to aquatic organisms, although is very unstable and it is will not persist in the environment. It has been classified as a moderate toxicant to fish. According to studies performed on rainbow trout, it is more toxic than chlorite but it persists less.

Exposure Standards and Guidelines

The maximum residual chlorine dioxide level allowed by the US EPA in drinking water is 0.8 mg l^{-1}. The exposure limits have been set for concentration in air. OSHA PEL: 0.1 ppm (0.3 mg m^{-3}) TWA. ACGIH TLV: 0.1 ppm (0.28 mg m^{-3}) TWA, 0.3 ppm (0.83 mg m^{-3}) STEL. NIOSH REL: 0.1 ppm TWA,

0.3 ppm (0.9 mg m^{-3}) STEL, and IDLH 5 ppm. HSE WEL: 0.1 ppm (0.28 mg m^{-3}) long-term exposure, 0.3 ppm (0.84 mg m^{-3}) STEL.

See also: Anthrax; Oxidative Stress; Recommended Exposure Limits; LD_{50}/LC_{50} (Lethal Dosage 50/Lethal Concentration 50)

Further Reading

Akamatsu, A., Lee, C., Morino, H., Miura, T., Ogata, N., Shibata, T., 2012 Feb 21. Six-month low level chlorine dioxide gas inhalation toxicity study with two-week recovery period in rats. J. Occup. Med. Toxicol. 7 (2). http://dx.doi.org/10.1186/1745-6673-7-2.

Environmental Toxicants: Human Exposures and Their Health Effects, third ed. Oxford: Wiley.

Filby, A.L., Shears, J.A., Drage, B.E., et al., 2010. Effects of advanced treatments of wastewater effluents on estrogenic and reproductive health impacts in fish. Environ. Sci. Technol. 44 (11), 4348–4354.

Maffei, F., Carbone, F., Forti, G.C., et al., 2009. Drinking water quality: an *in vitro* approach for the assessment of cytotoxic and genotoxic load in water sampled along distribution system. Environ. Int. 35 (7), 1053–1061.

Nishikiori, R., Nomura, Y., Sawajiri, M., Masuki, K., Hirata, I., Okazaki, M., 2008. Influence of chlorine dioxide on cell death and cell cycle of human gingival fibroblasts. J. Dentistry 36 (12), 993–998.

Qingdong, X., Guangming, Z., Li, W., 2006. Study on subchronic toxicity of chlorine dioxide and by-products in water. J. Environ. Sci. Health A Tox. Hazard Subst. Environ. Eng. 41 (7), 1347–1353.

White, C.W., Martin, J.G., 2010. Chlorine gas inhalation: human clinical evidence of toxicity and experience in animal models. Proc. Am. Thor. Soc. 7 (4), 257–263.

Relevant Websites

http://pubchem.ncbi.nlm.nih.gov – Pubchem: Search for Chlorine Dioxide.
http://www.cdc.gov/niosh/ – Centers for Disease Control.
http://www.epa.gov/iris/ – Environmental Protection Agency.

Chloroacetic Acid

M Abdollahi and S Karami-Mohajeri, Tehran University of Medical Sciences, Tehran, Iran

- Names: Chloroacetic acid and Monochloroacetic acid
- Chemical Abstracts Service Registry Number: 79-11-8
- Synonyms: Acide chloroacetique, Acide monochloracetique, Acide monochloracetique, Acidomonocloroacetico, BRN, Caswell No. 179B, Chloracetic acid, Chloroacetic acid, Chloroethanoic acid, Kyselina chloroctova, Monochloorazijnzuur, Monochloracetic acid
- Molecular Formula: $C_2H_3ClO_2$
- Structure:

Cl O OH

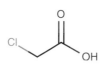

Background

Chloroacetic acid (CAA) is a monohalogenated acetic acid (m-HAA) that is used as a photosensitizing agent and in industrial synthesis of certain organic chemicals such as indigoid dyes. The m-HAAs are a major class of drinking water disinfection by-products during chlorination of drinking water.

Uses

CAA is one of these agents used in the topical treatment of warts in most European countries and also as an herbicidal agent and a bleaching agent for silkworm cocoons. It can be found in wines and beers using static headspace extraction coupled with gas chromatography–mass spectrometry. CCA is the main toxic metabolite of vinyl chloride. CAA and volatile organochlorines are suspected to contribute to forest dieback and stratospheric ozone destruction.

Environmental Fate and Behavior

CCA's Henry's law constant of 9.42×10^{-9} atm-m^3 mol^{-1}, vapor pressure of 0.065 mmHg at 25 °C, and water solubility of $8.58 \times 10^{+5}$ mg l^{-1} at 25 °C indicate that volatilization from moist soil and water surfaces is expected to be an important fate process and also it can be volatilized from dry soil surfaces and exist as a vapor in the atmosphere. *Burkholderia* strains are capable of degrading CAA.

Exposure and Exposure Monitoring

Occupational exposure to CAA can occur through inhalation and dermal contact with this compound at workplaces where it is produced or used. The general population can be exposed to CAA via ingestion of chlorinated or chloraminated drinking water.

The atmospheric photochemical oxidation of some volatile organochlorine compounds is one source of CAAs in the environment. CAA can be generated during water disinfection processes and during metabolic detoxification of industrial solvents such as trichloroethylene.

Toxicokinetics

In rat at the subtoxic oral dose, concentration of CAA peaked at 0.1% of dose by 2 h. Most of the dermal dose rapidly penetrated into the skin. In oral poisoning, peak plasma concentration was reached within 0.25 h. The plasma half-life was 2 h for oral and 4 h for dermal administration. The pattern of distribution of CAA shows an initial fast distribution into lipid-poor tissue and then uptake into lipid-rich tissues such as the brain. The absorbed dose was metabolized by liver and eliminated through bile. Fecal elimination is negligible. Urinary excretion is 64–72% of the dose. Metabolites of CCA are eliminated through bile.

Mechanism of Toxicity

CCA by inhibition of the pyruvate-dehydrogenase, aconitase, and α-ketoglutarate dehydrogenase that contribute in tricarboxylic acid cycle and also inhibition of glyceraldehyde-3-phosphate dehydrogenase can impair production of cellular energy and conversion to anaerobic glycolysis, resulting in increasing acidosis with accumulation of glycolic acid, oxalate, and lactate production. CCA can also affect cellular components via sulfhydryl groups. Both of these effects may contribute to central nervous system (CNS), cardiovascular, renal, and hepatic effects. The metabolites glycolic acid and oxalate may contribute to CNS and renal toxicity (myoglobin and oxalate precipitation in the tubuli). Binding of calcium to oxalates probably causes the hypocalcemia, but hypocalcemia can be secondary to rhabdomyolysis. CAA by reduction of cellular glutathione can cause oxidative stress. Inhibition of mitochondrial aconitase causes hypoglycemia.

Acute and Short-Term Toxicity

CAA is a strong organic acid that is irritating and corrosive to the skin and mucous membranes of the mouth, throat, lung, and esophagus, with immediate pain and dysphagia. A typical skin lesion is hyperemia with a central white zone. Early signs of systemic poisoning are vomiting, diarrhea, and CNS excitability with disorientation, delirium, convulsions, and cerebral edema. CAA induces metabolic acidosis, rhabdomyolysis, and renal failure. There is a report of hemolytic uremic syndrome after intentional suicidal ingestion of it with vomiting, hematochezia,

 http://dx.doi.org/10.1016/B978-0-12-386454-3.01111-8

oliguanuria, severe renal failure, metabolic acidosis, anemia, and thrombocytopenia with evidence of intravascular hemolysis. Vapors from CAA have apparently caused corneal epithelial injury. Atmospheric concentration in air of 5.7 mg m^{-3} was said to be the irritation threshold of respiratory mucous membrane. In rat, hypoglycemia is caused by the acute cutaneous CCA exposure.

Subacute and Chronic Toxicity

Chronic exposure may result in hepatoxicity (hepatocellular cytoplasmic vacuolization) and teratogenic effects. Exposure to 20.8 mg m^{-3} of CAA for 4 months reduced body weight, inflamed the lungs, reduced blood hemoglobin levels, lowered rectal temperature, and decreased oxygen uptake. Cholinesterase levels were significantly decreased in female mice receiving 150 or 200 mg kg^{-1} over 13 weeks. The decreased levels may have been a reflection of hepatic toxicity. A significant dose-related induction in blood urea nitrogen, alanine aminotransferase, and aspartate aminotransferase occurred in male and female rats receiving 90–150 mg kg^{-1} and 60–150 mg kg^{-1} over 3 weeks, respectively.

Reproductive Toxicity

It can cause pregnancy loss and eye malformations (anophthalmia, microphthalmia).

Genotoxicity

Most of the altered mRNA expressions were associated with genes responding to DNA damage and those regulating cell cycle. CAA did not induce DNA strand breaks in human lymphoblastic leukemia cells. There are several reports of chronic cytotoxicities in cell lines. CAA has mutagenic potential in *Rattus norvegicus* by chromosomal aberrations (breaks, gaps, exchanges, rings, and multiple aberrations) and micronuclei induction.

Carcinogenicity

Not classifiable as a human carcinogen.

Clinical Management

Liver and kidney function tests and examination of the nervous system should be performed. Prolonged exposure of the skin results in corrosion (severe burns), but if the skin is quickly washed well, only rubefaction of the skin occurs.

Ecotoxicology

CAA has a very low log octanol/water partition coefficient, 0.22, and therefore would not be expected to bioconcentrate in fish. At 560 mg l^{-1}, the following effects were observed in zebrafish: difficulty at hatching and spinal deformations.

Exposure Standards and Guidelines

Workplace standards are 0.3 ppm for 8-h work periods and 1 ppm for 15-min work periods. Acceptable daily intake (ADI) is unknown.

See also: Mitochondrial Toxicity; Kidney; Oxidative Stress; Environmental Exposure Assessment; Environmental Fate and Behavior; Bioaccumulation; Environmental Protection Agency, US; Toxicity Testing, Mutagenicity; Toxicity Testing, Carcinogenesis; Toxicity Testing, Inhalation; Mechanisms of Toxicity; Toxicity, Acute; Toxicity, Subchronic and Chronic; Toxicity Testing, Dermal.

Further Reading

Attene-Ramos, M.S., Wagner, E.D., Plewa, M.J., 2010. Comparative human cell toxicogenomic analysis of monohaloacetic acid drinking water disinfection byproducts. Environ. Sci. Technol. 44, 7206–7212.

Baser, N.T., Yalaz, B., Yilmaz, A.C., Tuncali, D., Aslan, G., 2008. An unusual and serious complication of topical wart treatment with monochloroacetic acid. Int. J. Dermatol. 47, 1295–1297.

Cardador, M.J., Gallego, M., 2012. Development of a method for the quantitation of chloro-, bromo-, and iodoacetic acids in alcoholic beverages. J. Agric. Food Chem. 60, 725–730.

Faisal Siddiqui, M., Ahmad, R., Ahmad, W., Hasnain, A.U., 2006. Micronuclei induction and chromosomal aberrations in *Rattus norvegicus* by chloroacetic acid and chlorobenzene. Ecotoxicol. Environ. Saf. 65, 159–164.

Horisaki, T., Yoshida, E., Sumiya, K., et al., 2011. Isolation and characterization of monochloroacetic acid-degrading bacteria. J. Gen. Appl. Microbiol. 57, 277–284.

Kato, J., Dote, T., Shimizu, H., et al., 2006. Lethal acute lung injury and hypoglycemia after subcutaneous administration of monochloroacetic acid. Toxicol. Ind. Health 22, 203–209.

Komaki, Y., Pals, J., Wagner, E.D., Marinas, B.J., Plewa, M.J., 2009. Mammalian cell DNA damage and repair kinetics of monohaloacetic acid drinking water disinfection by-products. Environ. Sci. Technol. 43, 8437–8442.

Laturnus, F., Fahimi, I., Gryndler, M., et al., 2005. Natural formation and degradation of chloroacetic acids and volatile organochlorines in forest soil–challenges to understanding. Environ. Sci. Pollut. Res. Int. 12, 233–244.

Liviac, D., Creus, A., Marcos, R., 2010. Genotoxicity testing of three monohaloacetic acids in TK6 cells using the cytokinesis-block micronucleus assay. Mutagenesis 25, 505–509.

Narotsky, M.G., Best, D.S., McDonald, A., et al., 2011. Pregnancy loss and eye malformations in offspring of F344 rats following gestational exposure to mixtures of regulated trihalomethanes and haloacetic acids. Reprod. Toxicol. 31, 59–65.

Nayak, S.G., Satish, R., 2007. An unusual toxic cause of hemolytic-uremic syndrome. J. Toxicol. Sci. 32, 197–199.

Pals, J.A., Ang, J.K., Wagner, E.D., Plewa, M.J., 2011. Biological mechanism for the toxicity of haloacetic acid drinking water disinfection byproducts. Environ. Sci. Technol. 45, 5791–5797.

Plewa, M.J., Simmons, J.E., Richardson, S.D., Wagner, E.D., 2010. Mammalian cell cytotoxicity and genotoxicity of the haloacetic acids, a major class of drinking water disinfection by-products. Environ. Mol. Mutagen. 51, 871–878.

Saghir, S.A., Rozman, K.K., 2003. Kinetics of monochloroacetic acid at subtoxic and toxic doses in rats after single oral and dermal administrations. Toxicol. Sci. 76, 51–64.

Sakai, A., Shimizu, H., Kono, K., Furuya, E., 2005. Monochloroacetic acid inhibits liver gluconeogenesis by inactivating glyceraldehyde-3-phosphate dehydrogenase. Chem. Res. Toxicol. 18, 277–282.

Schmidt, M.M., Rohwedder, A., Dringen, R., 2011. Effects of chlorinated acetates on the glutathione metabolism and on glycolysis of cultured astrocytes. Neurotoxicity Res. 19, 628–637.

Zhang, S.H., Miao, D.Y., Liu, A.L., et al., 2010. Assessment of the cytotoxicity and genotoxicity of haloacetic acids using microplate-based cytotoxicity test and CHO/HGPRT gene mutation assay. Mutat. Res. 703, 174–179.

Relevant Websites

http://www.iarc.fr – International Agency for Research on Cancer.

http://www.inchem.org – International Programme on Chemical Safety: INCHEM: Chloroacetic Acid.

http://toxnet.nlm.nih.gov – Toxnet (Toxicology Data Network): search under Toxline for Chloroacetic Acid.

http://chem.sis.nlm.nih.gov/chemidplus – US National Library of Medicine: ChemIDplus Advanced: Search for Chloroacetic Acid.

Chlorobenzene

SD Pravasi, Bristol Myers Squibb (PPD), Hopewell, NJ, USA

This article is a revision of the previous edition article by Linda A. Malley, volume 1, pp 556–559, © 2005, Elsevier Inc.

- Name: Chlorobenzene
- Chemical Abstracts Service Registry Number: 108-90-7
- Synonyms: Benzene chloride, Chlorobenzol, Monochlorobenzene, Phenyl chloride, Tetrosin SP
- Molecular Formula: C_6H_5Cl
- Chemical Structure:

Background

Chlorobenzene production has been declining since its peak in 1969, and is likely to continue declining due to the substitution of more environmentally friendly chemicals. Chlorobenzene is produced by chlorination of benzene in the presence of a catalyst, and is produced as an end product in the reductive chlorination of di- and trichlorobenzenes. This compound is extensively used in the manufacture of phenol, aniline, and DDT; as a solvent for paints; and as a heat transfer medium. It is also occasionally used in the dry cleaning industry.

Chlorobenzene's production and use as a chemical intermediate, solvent, and heat transfer medium may result in its release to the environment through various waste streams. If released to air, chlorobenzene will exist solely as a vapor in the atmosphere. Photochemically produced hydroxyl radicals will ultimately degrade vapor-phase chlorobenzene in less than 24 h. Exposure of chlorobenzene to direct sunlight (absorbs at >290 nm) will cause photolysis. Occupational exposure to chlorobenzene may occur through inhalation and dermal contact with this compound at workplaces where chlorobenzene is produced or used. Monitoring data indicate that the general population may be exposed to chlorobenzene via inhalation of ambient air, ingestion of food and drinking water, and dermal contact with this compound.

Uses

Historically, chlorobenzene was used to make phenol and DDT. Chlorobenzene is used as a solvent for pesticide formulations, and in auto parts degreasing. It is a chemical intermediate in the production of diphenyl oxide, diisocyanates, and nitrochlorobenzene. It has also been used as a fiber-swelling agent and as a dye carrier in textile processing.

Environmental Fate and Behavior

In the ambient atmosphere, chlorobenzene will exist as a vapor, and will be degraded by reaction with photochemically produced hydroxyl radicals, with an estimated half-life of 21 days. It can be removed from the air by rain. Photolysis half-lives of 4–18 h were measured in aqueous media. If released to soil, chlorobenzene is expected to have very high to moderate mobility based on a K_{oc} range of 4.8–313. Moist soil surfaces will favor volatilization based upon Henry's Law constant of 3.11×10^{-3} atm-cu m mol^{-1}. Chlorobenzene may volatilize from dry soil surfaces as well. If released into water, chlorobenzene may adsorb to suspended solids and sediment based on the K_{oc} values. Volatilization from water surfaces is expected to be an important fate process based on this compound's Henry's Law constant. Estimated volatilization half-lives for a model river and model lake are 3.4 h and 4.3 days, respectively. Reported bioconcentration in aquatic organisms is low to high, provided the compound is not metabolized by the organism. Hydrolysis is not expected to be an important environmental fate process since this compound lacks functional groups that hydrolyze under environmental conditions. Biodegradation results are variable based on soil type and microbial diversity. In river water, the biodegradation half-life was reported to be 150 and 75 days in the sediment.

Chlorobenzene has a boiling point of 131.7 °C, melting point of −45.2 °C, density/specific gravity of 1.1058 g cm^{-3} at 20 °C, octanol/water partition coefficient of $\log K_{ow} = 2.84$, solubility in water of 498 mg l^{-1} at 25 °C, Henry's Law constant of 3.11×10^{-3} atm-cu m mol^{-1} at 25 °C, and vapor density of 3.88.

Exposure and Exposure Monitoring

Probable routes of human exposure are inhalation, ingestion, and eye and skin contact. Chlorobenzene's production and use as a chemical intermediate, solvent, and heat transfer medium may result in its release to the environment through various waste streams.

Toxicokinetics

Data in rabbits indicate that the toxicity from a single dermal application is minimal, with only slight reddening of the skin observed. Continuous skin contact with chlorobenzene for 1 week resulted in moderate erythema and slight superficial necrosis. Absorption in amounts sufficient to cause toxicity can also occur as a result of ingestion or inhalation. Because chlorobenzene is highly lipophilic and hydrophobic, it is thought to be distributed throughout the total body water, with body lipids being a major deposition site.

The kinetics of metabolism and excretion was investigated in rabbits administered a single oral dose of 0.5 mg kg^{-1} or doses of 0.5 g twice daily for 4 days. In the single-dose study, 27% of the administered dose was excreted unchanged in the expired air. The majority of the remainder was excreted in the urine as a glucuronide (25%), ethereal sulfate (27%), and mercapturic acid (20%). Similarly, rabbits administered

 http://dx.doi.org/10.1016/B978-0-12-386454-3.00279-7

repeated doses of chlorobenzene excreted the majority of the dose in the urine, and only small amounts were detected in the tissues and feces. Rats administered a single intraperitoneal dose of chlorobenzene also excreted metabolites in the urine, which were identified as 4-chlorocatechol, 2-chlorophenol, 4-chlorophenol, and 3-chlorophenol. In addition, chlorobenzene was covalently bound to DNA, RNA, and proteins in the liver, kidney, and lung 22 h following a single intraperitoneal injection. Chlorobenzene is first oxidized to 3,4-epoxide, which then can follow one of several pathways. One leads to the formation of the l-mercapturic acid conjugate following glutathione conjugation. A second pathway results in the formation of 4-chlorocatechol, and the third pathway ends with the formation of 4-chlorophenol and its conjugates. Data collected from exposed workers and volunteers indicate that for humans, the primary pathways are formation of the *p*-mercapturic acid conjugate and 4-chlorocatechol.

Mechanism of Toxicity

Similar to other volatile organic chemicals, chlorobenzene is a central nervous system (CNS) depressant. In addition, lesions of the liver and kidneys have also been observed following toxic doses. Exposure to chlorobenzene induces the release of monocyte chemoattractant protein 1 (MCP-1) by lung epithelial cells, a chemokine involved in inflammatory reactions. To characterize the underlying mechanisms, the influence of chlorobenzene on the activation of two intracellular signaling pathways, the nuclear factor-kappa B (NF-κβ) and the p38 mitogen-activated protein kinase (MAPK) pathways, were investigated. Exposure of lung epithelial cells to chlorobenzene resulted in an activation of NF-κβ and p38 MAPK and a release of the chemokine MCP-1. In the presence of IKK-NBD, a specific NF-κβ inhibitor, or the inhibitors of the p38 MAPK, the chlorobenzene-related MCP-1 release was suppressed, suggesting an involvement of both pathways in the chlorobenzene-induced expression of MCP-1.

Acute and Short-Term Toxicity

Animal

The oral LD_{50} values for rats, mice, and rabbits were 2290, 2300, and 2830 mg kg^{-1}, respectively. The approximate inhalation LD_{50} (2 h) is 4300 ppm for mice. Application of chlorobenzene to the skin of rabbits caused slight reddening; prolonged skin contact was irritating. Ocular contact in rabbits caused a transient conjunctival irritation that resolved within 48 h. Tremors, CNS depression, and death were observed in cats administered a single inhalation exposure of 3700 ppm and above.

Several repeated-exposure oral studies have been conducted in various species. Although the doses at which effects were observed are variable between species, the primary effects of chlorobenzene were observed in the liver and kidneys. Rats and mice were administered daily doses of 60–750 mg kg^{-1}, 5 days per week, for 13 weeks. Survival was lower in rats at 500 mg kg^{-1} and above and in mice at 250 mg kg^{-1} and above. Pathological changes in the liver and kidneys and changes in the hematopoietic system (spleen, bone marrow, and thymus) were observed in both species at 250 mg kg^{-1} and above. In another study, rats were administered doses ranging from 14.4 to 376 mg kg^{-1} per day, 5 days per week, over a period of 192 days. Doses of 144 mg kg^{-1} per day and above caused changes in liver and kidney weights and liver morphology. Doses of 18.8 mg kg^{-1} per day and below did not cause any adverse effects. Dogs were administered oral doses ranging from 27.2 to 272.5 mg kg^{-1} per day, 5 days per week, for 93 days. There were no effects at 54.5 mg kg^{-1} per day and below. At 272.5 mg kg^{-1} per day, changes in clinical chemistry parameters were observed, four of eight dogs died, and pathological changes were observed in the liver, kidney, gastroenteric mucosa, and hematopoietic tissue. Repeated-exposure inhalation studies have been conducted in several species. Rats, rabbits, and guinea pigs were exposed to airborne concentrations ranging from 200 to 1000 ppm for 7 h per day, 5 days per week, for a total of 32 exposures. At 475 ppm and above, organ weight changes and histopathological changes were observed. There were no effects detected at 200 ppm. In another study, changes in hematology parameters and pathological changes in the adrenal cortex, kidney, and liver were observed in rats and rabbits exposed to airborne concentrations of 75 or 250 ppm chlorobenzene vapors for 7 h per day, 5 days per week for 24 weeks.

Human

The human literature primarily consists of case reports. In the industrial environment, symptoms including headache, numbness, skin irritation and redness, eye irritation and redness, irritation and redness of the upper respiratory tract, bronchitis, dizziness, somnolence, loss of consciousness, hematopoietic effects, gastritis, hepatitis, and neuromuscular changes have been reported. Accidental ingestion of 5–10 ml of a cleaning agent containing chlorobenzene caused loss of consciousness, vascular paralysis, and heart failure in a child (~2 years old).

Chronic Toxicity

Lesions of the liver and kidneys have been observed following absorption of toxic doses. The histological changes may progress as exposure becomes more severe or as the period of exposure is lengthened. Liver injury may progress to necrosis and parenchymous degeneration.

Carcinogenicity

Animal

In a study determining the carcinogenic potential of chlorobenzene, rats were administered daily doses of 0, 60, or 120 mg kg^{-1} per day, 5 days per week, for 103 weeks, and mice were similarly administered 30 or 60 mg kg^{-1} per day. No increased tumor incidences were observed in female rats or in male or female mice. Male rats administered 120 mg kg^{-1} per day had an increased incidence of hepatic neoplastic nodules (8% for untreated control, 4% for vehicle control, 8% for 60 mg kg^{-1}, and 16% for 120 mg kg^{-1}). Based on these results, the US Environmental Protection Agency (EPA) classified chlorobenzene as 'D' (not classifiable as to carcinogenicity in humans).

Human

There were no epidemiology studies in humans regarding long-term exposure to chlorobenzene.

However, based on the results of a chronic toxicity study in rats, the US EPA classified chlorobenzene as D (not classifiable as to carcinogenicity in humans).

In addition, the American Conference of Governmental Industrial Hygienists (ACGIH) classified chlorobenzene as A3 (confirmed animal carcinogen with unknown relevance to humans).

Immunotoxicity

Mice exposed to chlorobenzene at >250 mg kg^{-1} per day by gavage for 13 weeks showed thymic necrosis and lymphoid or myeloid depletion of bone marrow, spleen, or thymus. while histopathologic evidence suggests that chlorobenzene is immunotoxic.

Reproductive Toxicity

Chlorobenzene has no reproductive toxicity to rats and no developmental toxicity including embryotoxicity and teratogenicity to rats and rabbits.

Genotoxicity

Chlorobenzene showed positive results in some *in vitro* and *in vivo* genotoxicity studies. It showed negative results in the majority of the studies on *in vitro* gene mutation, chromosomal aberration, DNA damage and unscheduled DNA synthesis (UDS), and *in vivo* sister chromatid exchange (SCE) experiments. From overall evaluation of these results, chlorobenzene is considered not to be genotoxic.

Clinical Management

Treatment is symptomatic and supportive. For ocular contact, the eyes should be irrigated immediately with abundant running water. If the material contacts the skin, the affected areas should be washed with soap and water promptly. If inhalation exposure occurs, the exposed person should be moved to fresh air immediately and should be provided with respiratory support (oxygen or artificial respiration) if necessary. Bronchospasm can be treated with inhaled beta2 agonist and oral or parenteral corticosteroids.

If the material has been ingested, vomiting should not be induced. For ingestion, gastric lavage (followed by saline catharsis) should be performed or activated charcoal should be administered. The trachea should be protected from aspiration. Renal and hepatic function should be monitored and supported if necessary. Hepatic injury caused by chlorobenzene can be treated with *N*-acetylcysteine and alprostadil. Hypotension should be treated with dopamine or norepinephrine.

Ecotoxicology

In acute toxicity of chlorobenzene to algae, a 96 h EC_{50} (growth inhibition) for freshwater alga was 12.5 mg l^{-1}. The acute toxicity of chlorobenzene to invertebrates is reported in freshwater and seawater crustaceans. A 48 h EC_{50} (immobilization) for the freshwater water flea was 0.59 mg l^{-1}.

The acute toxicity of chlorobenzene to fish is reported in rainbow trout, bluegill, and fathead minnow, and the 96 h LC_{50} values were 4.7 mg l^{-1} for the rainbow trout, 7.4 mg l^{-1}, for the bluegill, and 7.7 mg l^{-1} for the fathead minnow. The long-term toxicity to fish in the early life stage has been reported in rainbow trout, goldfish, and largemouth bass, and the reliable lowest LC_{50} was the 7.5 day LC_{50} of 0.05 mg l^{-1} for 4 day posthatch of the largemouth.

Other Hazards

Chlorobenzene is highly flammable, and the vapors are heavier than air. They will spread along the ground and collect in low or confined areas. The lower flammable limit is 1.8%, the upper flammable limit is 9.6%, and the flash point is 851 °F (29.21 °C closed cup). The explosive limit value ranges from 7.1 to 1.3% at 150 °C.

Combustion of chlorobenzene can form phosgene and hydrogen chloride gases. Chlorobenzene reacts with strong oxidizing materials, powdered sodium, and phosphorus trichloride and sodium.

Exposure Standards and Guidelines

Based on the results of a chronic toxicity study in rats, the US EPA classified chlorobenzene as group D (not classifiable as to carcinogenicity in humans). In addition, the American Conference of Governmental Industrial Hygienists classified chlorobenzene as A3 (confirmed animal carcinogen with unknown relevance to humans). The current exposure standards and guidelines are summarized in **Table 1**.

Table 1 Summary of exposure criteria for chlorobenzene

Agency	*Criteria*	*Averaging time*
ACGIH	TLV-TWA, 10 ppm	8 h day, 40 h week
National Institute for Occupational Safety and Health	IDLH, 1000 ppm	NA
Occupational Safety and Health Administration	PEL (TWA), 75 ppm (350 mg cu m^{-1})	8 h day, 40 h week

IDLH, immediately dangerous to life or health; PEL, permissible exposure limit; TLV, threshold limit value; TWA, time-weighted average.

See also: Dichlorobenzene; Hexachlorobenzene; Bromobenzene; Benzene.

Further Reading

Chang, E.E., Wei-Chi, W., Li-Xuan, Z., Hung-Lung, C., 2010. Health risk assessment of exposure to selected volatile organic compounds emitted from an integrated iron and steel plant. Inhal. Toxicol. 22 (Suppl. 2), 117–125.

Chin, J.Y., Godwin, C., Jia, C., et al., 2013. Concentrations and risks of *p*-dichlorobenzene in indoor and outdoor air. Indoor Air 23 (1), 40–49.

Faisal Siddiqui, M., Ahmad, R., Ahmad, W., Hasnain, A.U., 2006. Micronuclei induction and chromosomal aberrations in *Rattus norvegicus* by chloroacetic acid and chlorobenzene. Ecotoxicol. Environ. Saf. 65 (2), 159–164.

Feltens, R., Mögel, I., Röder-Stolinski, C., et al., 2010. Chlorobenzene induces oxidative stress in human lung epithelial cells *in vitro*. Toxicol. Appl. Pharmacol. 242 (1), 100–108.

Guerrero, P.A., Corsi, R.L., 2012. Emissions of *p*-dichlorobenzene and naphthalene from consumer products. J. Air Waste Manag. Assoc. 62 (9), 1075–1084.

Hu, H., Guo, Y., Sun, X., et al., May 3, 2013. Determination of chlorobenzenes in water samples by solid-phase disk extraction and gashromatography-electron capture detection. J. Chromatogr. Sci. (Epub ahead of print).

Lehmann, I., Röder-Stolinski, C., Nieber, K., Fischäder, G., June 2008. *In vitro* models for the assessment of inflammatory and immuno-modulatory effects of the volatile organic compound chlorobenzene. Exp. Toxicol. Pathol. 60 (2–3), 185–193.

Leslie, H.A., Hermens, J.L., Kraak, M.H., 2004. Baseline toxicity of a chlorobenzene mixture and total body residues measured and estimated with solid-phase microextraction. Environ. Toxicol. Chem. 23 (8), 2017–2021.

Logue, J.M., McKone, T.E., Sherman, M.H., Singer, B.C., 2011. Hazard assessment of chemical air contaminants measured in residences. Indoor Air 21 (2), 92–109.

Nagyeri, G., Valkusz, Z., Radacs, M., et al., 2012. Behavioral and endocrine effects of chronic exposure to low doses of chlorobenzenes in wistar rats. Neurotoxicol. Teratol. 34 (1), 9–19.

Röder-Stolinski, C., Fischäder, G., Oostingh, G.J., et al., 2008. Chlorobenzene induces the NF-kappa B and p38 MAP kinase pathways in lung epithelial cells. Inhal. Toxicol. 20 (9), 813–820.

Ryan, R.P., Terry, C.E., Leffingwell, S.S., Toxicology Desk Reference, fifth ed. vol. 1. Taylor & Francis, NY, pp. 313–316.

Satoh, K., Nonaka, R., Ohyama, K., et al., 2008. Endocrine disruptive effects of chemicals eluted from nitrile-butadiene rubber gloves using reporter gene assay systems. Biol. Pharm. Bull. 31 (3), 375–379.

Wang, C., Xi, J.Y., Hu, H.Y., 2008. Chemical identification and acute biotoxicity assessment of gaseous chlorobenzene photodegradation products. Chemosphere 73 (8), 1167–1171.

Wang, C., Xi, J.Y., Hu, H.Y., 2009. Reduction of toxic products and bioaerosol emission of a combined ultraviolet-biofilter process for chlorobenzene treatment. J. Air Waste Manag. Assoc. 59 (4), 405–410.

Zhang, L., Anderson, W.A., 2013. Effect of ozone and sulfur dioxide on the photolytic degradation of chlorobenzene in air. Ind. Eng. Chem. Res. 52 (9), 3315–3319.

Zhang, T., Li, X., Min, X., et al., 2012. Acute toxicity of chlorobenzenes in tetrahymena: estimated by microcalorimetry and mechanis. Environ. Toxicol. Pharmacol. 33 (3), 377–385.

Relevant Websites

www.clean.cise.columbia.edu – CEPSR Clean Room at Columbia University.

http://ijerst.com/ijerstadmin/upload/ijerst_509d32db95e16.pdf – International Journal of Engineering Research and Science & Technology.

www.toxnet.nlm.nih.gov – National Institutes of Health-National Library of Medicine.

http://toxnet.nlm.nih.gov/cgi-bin/sis/search/r?dbs+hsdb:@term+@rn+@rel+108-90-7 – National Library of Medicine-Hazardous Substances Data Bank.

http://www.epa.gov/ttnatw01/hlthef/chlorobe.html – US Environmental Protection Agency.

Chlorobenzilate

DM Janz, Toxicology Centre, University of Saskatchewan, Saskatoon, SK, Canada

- Name: Chlorobenzilate
- Chemical Abstracts Service Registry Number: 510-15-6
- Synonyms: Ethyl-4,4-dichlorobenzilate; Ethyl-4,4-dichlorophenylglycollate; Ethyl 2,2-bis(4-chlorophenyl)-2-hydroxyacetate; Chlorobenzylate
- Molecular Formula: $C_{16}H_{14}Cl_2O_3$
- Chemical Structure:

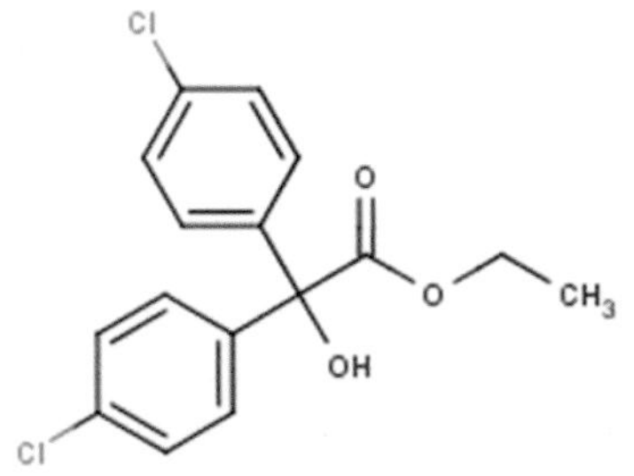

Background

Chlorobenzilate is an organochlorine pesticide belonging to the same class as dichlorodiphenyltrichloroethane (DDT). It was originally developed by Ciba–Geigy and introduced in 1952.

Uses

The primary use of chlorobenzilate is as an acaricide for mite control on citrus crops and in beehives. It has a narrow insecticidal action, killing only mites and ticks. Historically, chlorobenzilate was used as a synergist for DDT. Although now banned for use in the United States and Europe, it is believed to be used on crops other than citrus in other countries.

Environmental Fate and Behavior

The historical use of chlorobenzilate resulted in its release into the environment. It has low water solubility ($\log K_{ow} = 4.74$) and adsorbs strongly to sediment and suspended particulate matter in aquatic environments. Chlorobenzilate has low soil mobility due to an estimated K_{oc} of 1500 and thus is not expected to leach into groundwater. Decomposition via photolysis or hydrolysis is not considered significant. The half-life of chlorobenzilate in fine sandy soils was estimated to be 10–35 days, with degradation being primarily microbial. In silty clay loam and clay soils, the half-life of chlorobenzilate was estimated to be 10.8–15.1 and 29.5–169.1 days, respectively. Volatilization from water or soil is not appreciable due to an estimated Henry's law constant of 7.2 atm m^3 mol^{-1}. If released into air, chlorobenzilate will exist in both vapor and particulate phases. The half-life of vapor-phase chlorobenzilate in ambient air was estimated to be 3.2 days. Chlorobenzilate in the particulate phase is expected to be removed from the atmosphere by wet or dry deposition. There is no evidence for long-range transport of chlorobenzilate. Bioaccumulation in aquatic organisms is moderate to high due to a reported bioconcentration factor range of 224–709 in fish.

Exposure and Exposure Monitoring

Occupational exposure to chlorobenzilate may occur through inhalation or dermal contact during its production and use as an acaricide. Exposure to the general population may occur via contaminated food and drinking water. Although these exposure routes are likely low or nonexistent in Europe and the United States due to ceased use, potential current use of chlorobenzilate in other areas of the world is not known.

Toxicokinetics

Due to its high lipid solubility, chlorobenzilate is readily absorbed from the gastrointestinal tract following oral exposure. Dermal absorption also occurs following exposure to commercial (oil-based) formulations. No significant storage of chlorobenzilate in adipose tissue of dogs was reported following daily oral administration of 12.8 mg kg^{-1} for 35 weeks. Dichlorobenzilic acid, dichlorobenzhydrol, chlorobenzoic acid, and dichlorobenzophenone were the major metabolites produced when chlorobenzilate was incubated in the presence of rat liver homogenates. Urinary excretion of these metabolites in addition to significant excretion of unchanged chlorobenzilate in the feces was reported in dogs and rats after oral administration. Although structurally similar to DDT, chlorobenzilate appears to be much more rapidly excreted following absorption in mammals.

Mechanism of Toxicity

Similar to other organochlorine pesticides in this structural class, chlorobenzilate causes disruption of normal flow of Na^+ and K^+ across axonal membranes in the central nervous system (CNS) and peripheral nervous system and may also antagonize gamma-aminobenzoic acid-mediated inhibition in the CNS. The net result is a hyperexcitable state of neurotransmission.

Acute and Short-Term Toxicity (Animal/Human)

The oral LD_{50} for chlorobenzilate in rats, mice, and hamsters ranges from 700 to 729 mg kg^{-1}. The dermal LD_{50} is greater than 10 000 mg kg^{-1} in rats and rabbits. In humans, symptoms

 http://dx.doi.org/10.1016/B978-0-12-386454-3.00113-5

of acute poisoning are similar following ingestion, inhalation, or dermal absorption of chlorobenzilate and include nausea, dizziness, vomiting, incoordination, confusion, and muscle weakness or pain. Death may result from respiratory collapse or arrhythmias.

Chronic Toxicity (Animal/Human)

Chronic exposure to chlorobenzilate may cause similar symptoms as those observed following acute exposure. Abnormal electrical activity in the CNS has been observed following chronic occupational exposure in humans. Chronic dietary exposure studies in male and female rats showed significant decreases in body weight but no effect on survival. Chlorobenzilate is an eye irritant and causes conjunctivitis following chronic exposure. Chronic skin exposure may cause skin inflammation (dermatitis).

Reproductive Toxicity

Chlorobenzilate has been shown to cause testicular atrophy in mice and rats following chronic dietary exposure. In a three-generation reproduction study in rats, chlorobenzilate had no effect on litter size, weaning survival, or the number of uterine implants. No significant changes in body weight or teratogenicity of progeny were observed in this study.

Genotoxicity

Chlorobenzilate produced negative results when tested for mutagenicity using the standardized Ames assay with five strains of *Salmonella* in the presence or absence of hepatic microsomes.

Carcinogenicity

Chronic dietary chlorobenzilate exposure in male and female mice resulted in a significantly increased incidence of hepatocellular carcinoma. Carcinogenicity bioassays in rats have produced equivocal results. No carcinogenicity data are available in humans. Thus, chlorobenzilate is considered a probable human carcinogen. The study in mice resulted in the banning of chlorobenzilate for agricultural use in the United States and Europe.

Clinical Management

Only symptomatic treatment is available. An airway should be established and if necessary assisted ventilation provided. The cardiac rhythm should be monitored and treatment for arrhythmia should be given if required. For eye exposure, eyes must be flushed immediately with water or saline and irrigation maintained during transport. For ingestion, oral administration of activated charcoal is indicated. For skin contamination, the exposed area should be washed with soap and water.

Ecotoxicology

Ecotoxicological data are limited but suggest that chlorobenzilate has very low acute toxicity to aquatic and terrestrial animals. Acute lethality (48- and 96-h LC_{50} values) in aquatic invertebrates and fish ranges from 0.55 to 1.0 $mg\,l^{-1}$. Acute lethality (7- to 8-day LD_{50} values) following dietary exposure in mallard ducks and bobwhite quail ranges from 3375 to 5620 $mg\,kg^{-1}$. Chlorobenzilate is practically nontoxic to bees. There are no chronic toxicity data available in aquatic or terrestrial vertebrates.

Other Hazards

No other hazards have been noted.

Exposure Standards and Guidelines

The acceptable daily intake and reference dose for chlorobenzilate is 0.02 $mg\,kg^{-1}\,day^{-1}$.

See also: DDT (Dichlorodiphenyltrichloroethane); Organochlorine Insecticides.

Further Reading

Smith, A.G., 2001. DDT and its analogs. In: Krieger, R. (Ed.), Handbook of Pesticide Toxicology, second ed. Academic Press, San Diego, pp. 3–56.

Relevant Website

http://toxnet.nlm.nih.gov/cgi-bin/sis/htmlgen?HSDB – Hazardous Substances Data Bank.

Chlorodibenzofurans (CDFs)

RD Kimbrough, Washington, DC, USA

- Name: Chlorinated dibenzofurans
- Chemical Abstracts Service Registry Number: 136677-10-6
- Molecular Weight: 203.6472
- Chemical Structure:

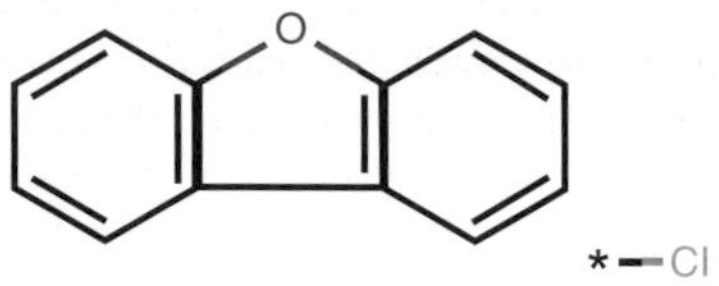

Background

Polychlorinated dibenzofurans (PCDFs) are a group of 135 aromatic congeners with the basic structure shown here. From one to eight chlorine atoms may be substituted on the phenyl rings.* The degree of toxicity of the individual congeners is determined by the position of the chlorines on the rings. The most toxic members of this group are the planar, coplanar, or nearly planar compounds where at least three or four lateral positions are occupied by chlorines,* such as the 2,3,7,8-tetrachlorodibenzofuran.

Their chemical inertness tends to increase with chlorination. PCDFs are usually present in the environment and in tissues together with polychlorinated dibenzo-*p*-dioxins (PCDDs) and other chlorinated aromatic compounds. When their presence is determined in the environment, the results are often reported as toxic equivalencies (TEQs) based on toxic equivalency factors (TEFs). Toxicity values are assigned to the congeners of PCDD/Fs relative to the toxicity of 2,3,7,8-tetrachlorodibenzo-*p*-dioxin (TCDD). When a TEF is multiplied by the concentration of a congener in a matrix, TEQ is obtained. The sum of all congener TEQs in a specimen (total TEQ) can be used to compare dioxinlike activity among specimens. TCDD is the most toxic chemical among the PCDD/Fs congeners. The toxicity values are based on their structure–activity relationship for binding and activation of the aryl hydrocarbon receptor (AHR), an initial but insufficient step in the development of TCDD-type toxicity. The variation in the effect on the AHR among congeners with dioxinlike activity is 10 000 fold. Most of the research on structure–activity relationship has been done with TCDD. The substantial species variation is not considered in this approach.

PCDFs may be formed in small amounts as impurities during the industrial production of some chlorinated aromatic chemicals. PCDFs are lipid and only very slightly water soluble. Since PCDFs are usually present in trace amounts in the environment and in tissues, their measurement is difficult, particularly the measurement of individual isomers.

The presence of PCDD/Fs in the environment before the industrial age has also been determined. In 1980, it was first reported that PCDDs are the product of fire. Similarly, PCDFs are formed by combustion. They have been formed as long as fire has existed. How much wildfires and volcanoes add to the global mass balance of PCDDs/Fs is poorly understood. It has been estimated that total global deposition of PCDD/Fs from the atmosphere to land is about 12 500 kg year^{-1} and 610 kg year^{-1} to the oceans. The total annual emissions from human activities, namely municipal waste incineration, biomass combustion, steel, copper mill, cement kiln, and automobile emissions, have been estimated to be 3000 kg. Since the global deposition is about four times greater, many sources of PCDDs/Fs are not well characterized.

Uses

PCDFs have no commercial use and are not deliberately produced by industry. Small amounts of a few congeners have been synthesized in the laboratory for research purposes.

Environmental Behavior, Fate, Routes, and Pathways

No recent information was available on PCDD/Fs concentrations in ambient air. The key sources of PCDD/Fs are from fire and other combustion processes. Emissions have been detected in flue gas and fly ash from municipal and industrial incinerators and oil-fired power plants, and in vehicular exhaust and cigarette smoke. The relative contributions of these and other unidentified sources to the presence of PCDD/Fs in the atmosphere are not known. When PCDD/Fs were measured in atmospheric samples of cities in New York, levels of up to 8.8 pg m^{-3} of total PCDD/Fs were found. Atmospheric concentrations of PCDD/Fs in rural and remote areas of the United States were in the low fg m^{-3} range.

PCDFs are lipid soluble and present in water in extremely low concentrations. They may contaminate surface water and groundwater in areas with point sources. They usually adhere to soil or sediment particles. Their presence has not been reported in municipal drinking water.

PCDD/Fs were determined in samples of archived surface soils collected in the early 1880s, in contemporary surface soils, and in archived subsurface soils collected in 1870/1880 and stored in Rothamsted experimental station in Lancaster, UK PCDFs were detected in most samples. The homolog compositions of PCDFs in earlier soils were similar to patterns in more recent soils, suggesting that similar sources of atmospheric emissions of PCDFs are operating currently as in the past in Europe. The homolog pattern, in samples from Thailand and Australia were different.

$P_{4\text{-}8}$CDD/Fs in archival soils ranged from 6 to 520 ng kg^{-1} (ppt) of dry weight. PCDD/Fs in contemporary samples ranged

 http://dx.doi.org/10.1016/B978-0-12-386454-3.01113-1

from 200 to 2000 ng kg^{-1} (ppt) of dry weight. Samples from Cyprus and arctic Norway were close to the limit of detection of 15 ng kg^{-1} of dry weight.

PCDD/Fs have also been found in clay. The average TEFs for raw and processed samples were 1513 and 966 (ng kg^{-1}) ppt of dry weight, respectively. Levels of PCDFs with 2,3,7,8 substitution were 2–3 orders of magnitude lower than the PCDDs or PCDFs were not detected. The presence of these chemicals in prehistoric clay samples was attributed to natural geological processes.

The natural formation of chlorinated phenols and PCDD/Fs in the humic layer of a Douglas fir forest is assumed to have resulted from processes involving microorganisms. Thus, PCDD/Fs are formed naturally in the environment.

Dated sediment core studies have shown that PCDF concentrations started to increase from around 1930 until about 1970, when they began to decline. The increase in emissions and in dated sediment samples matched the time when a variety of industrial activities were increasing. The subsequent decreases in core sediment levels can be attributed to the decrease of open burning, particulate control on combustors, phase-out of leaded gasoline, bans on the manufacture and use of polychlorinated biphenyls (PCBs), 2,4,5-trichlorophenoxy acid (2,4,5 T), and hexachlorophene, and restrictions on the use of pentachlorophenol. This decline is also reflected in the decrease of human body burdens.

Food

The inadvertent intake of PCDD/Fs in the United States and in Western Europe has decreased over the past 25 years. For the US population, the primary source of exposure to PCDD/Fs is food, mostly meat, dairy products, and local fresh water fish. Based on the US Food and Drug Administration's total diet study and on the US Department of Agriculture most recent food consumption estimates, the mean PCDD/F intake for the US. Population is 0.38 pg TEQ kg^{-1} of body weight (bw) per day and 1.21 pg kg^{-1} of bw per day at the 95th percentile. The mean intake for children ranges from 0.93 to 1.20 pg TEQ kg^{-1} of bw per day.

Human Exposure and Exposure Monitoring

Human lipid serum levels of PCDFs have decreased and are frequently below the limit of detection of the analytical method in younger age groups. Subpopulations live in areas with above-background levels of PCDFs in soil and sediment in their immediate environment. However, this environmental contamination makes only a negligible contribution to their overall exposure. The ingestion of contaminated fish or occupational exposure is usually identified as the source of elevated blood or adipose tissue levels.

The concentration of PCDFs in human blood of the general population is lower than that of PCDDs. Particularly the octa-CDF may be as much as 100 times less than octa-CDD. In the US National Health and Nutrition Examination Survey subsample study of 2002–03, many measurements were below the limit of detection. Only the following congeners in lipid adjusted sera had demonstrable 90th percentile levels: 1,2,3,4,6,7,8-heptachlorodibenzofuran, 1,2,3,4,7,8-hexachlorodibenzofuran, 1,2,3,6,7,8-hexachlorodibenzofuran. Geometric means could only be calculated for 2,3,4,7,8-pentachlorodibenzofuran.

Toxicokinetics

PCDFs are lipid soluble, concentrating in adipose tissue. They are absorbed from the gastrointestinal tract by passive diffusion. At equilibrium, in adipose tissue concentrations are similar to concentrations in serum and human milk on a lipid basis. However, at toxic levels, concentrations primarily in the liver may be higher than in adipose tissue. The less halogenated PCDFs and those with unsubstituted vicinal carbon atoms are metabolized and more rapidly excreted. The highly halogenated congeners are not easily absorbed but are more persistent and bioaccumulate at a greater rate. Half-lives vary among species. In humans, half-lives of PCDFs are positively associated with body mass and age and are excreted much faster in infants and children than in adults, particularly older adults. They are excreted by first order kinetics primarily in the feces as unchanged PCDFs or as hydroxylated or sulfur containing metabolites. More polar metabolites are also excreted in urine. Degree of metabolism, half-lives of different congeners are dose-dependent and range from days in hamsters to many months to years in humans.

Mechanism of Action

It is assumed that the mechanism of action of PCDFs is similar to that of PCDDs. The effects of PCDFs are generally attributed to their initial interaction with the AHR. The function of the AHR is transcriptional regulation. It is a ligand-activated transcription factor with a basic region/helix-loop-helix (bHLH) motif. While the interaction with the receptor appears to be necessary for many PCDF effects, by itself it is insufficient. It requires the product of a second locus that encodes a protein product referred to as the Ah receptor nuclear translocator (ARNT). However, ARNT is not required for nuclear translocation per se. Binding to the AHR mediates induction of enzymes such as the P450 cytochromes, which are expressed in more than 17 isoforms. In different strains of mice, AHR ligand-binding affinity varies. The polymorphism responsible for reduced ligand-binding affinity of the human AHR is characteristic of that of nonresponsive mouse strains. The toxicity of PCDD/Fs results from their ability to dysregulate or down regulate genes that are under the control of the AHR. Pronounced differences in the AHR gene structure in laboratory animals result in a variation of responses to their toxicity. Humans have relatively few polymorphisms that result in only a modest variation of downstream effects. The amino acid sequence of the human AHR and murine receptors of resistant mice responsible for the reduced ligand-binding affinity of the AHR receptor is the same in both species. This may explain why humans are relatively resistant to the adverse effects of PCDD/F.

Aryl hydrocarbon hydroxylase (AHH) inductive properties have been correlated with toxic effects. The order by which PCDFs induce enzymes in AHH-responsive mouse strains is as follows: 2,3,7,8-TCDF, >1,2,3,7,8-penta-CDF, >2,3,4,7,8-penta-CDF, >1,2,3,7,8-penta-CDF, >2,3,4,7,8-penta-CDF, >2,3,4,6,7-penta-DCF, 1,2,3,4,7,8-hexa-CDF, >2,3,6,7-tetra-CDF. The 2,4,6,8-TCDF and 1,3,6,8-TCDF are poor *in vitro* inducers of AHH and ethoxyresorufin-*o*-diethylase (EROD) activities but have high binding capacity to the cytosolic receptor protein. Their administration together with 2,3,7,8-TCDD served as an antagonist for AHH and EROD induction. In general, mixtures of compounds that compete for the same receptor may partially or completely antagonize each other. Thus, there are exceptions to the assumed additive effect of the toxicity of mixtures of these chemicals. It is not clear how prevalent this is since for the most part the less toxic congeners, which may have pronounced binding affinity, are usually not measured in mixtures. There is some information that the PCDFs similarly to 2,3,7,8-TCDD may alter the total binding capacity of cellular receptors such as the epidermal growth factor and estrogen and glucocorticoid receptors. Even though additivity is assumed with the TEQ scheme, few to no data are available for mixtures of several PCDFs to substantiate this assumption.

Toxicity

Toxicity data on the 135 PCDF congeners is spotty, with few of the congeners having been studied. When PCDFs or mixtures of PCDFs with other chemicals were studied, additivity, agonism, and antagonism may be observed because of their competitive binding to the AHR. The TEQ approach may therefore not necessarily reflect the actual toxicity of mixtures of these chemicals.

Animal Toxicity

The acute and organ-specific toxicity varies among species. For mammals, the guinea pig is the most sensitive species followed by the monkey, rabbit, rat, and mouse. In small species, death is delayed by a few weeks, while death may be delayed longer in larger animals such as horses and cows. Toxicity among strains of rats and mice differs as well. Hamsters are very resistant to these compounds. The oral LD_{50} in guinea pigs is between 5 and 10 μg kg^{-1} of bw for 2,3,7,8-TCDF, for 2,3,4,7,8-penta-CDF it is <10 μg kg^{-1} of bw, and for 2,3,4,6,7,8-hexa-CDF it is 120 μg per kg of bw. Doses as high as 6 mg kg^{-1} of bw of 2,3,7,8-TCDF did not result in lethality in C57 Bl/6fh (J67) 6-week-old male mice. The bull frog (>1000 μg kg^{-1} of bw) and the hamster (>1154–5000 μg kg^{-1} of bw) can tolerate similar high doses exemplified by 2,3,7,8-TCDD, the most toxic congener among this group of chemicals. In small animals, weight loss occurs in a few days as one of the first signs of toxicity while in larger animals such as cows, horses, dogs, and nonhuman primates it is not observed as quickly. This 'wasting syndrome' is only partially explained by reduced food intake. In birds, particularly chickens, weight loss and edema referred to as chick edema are very prevalent.

Doses of 2,3,4,7,8-penta-CDF between 6 and 200 ng kg^{-1} of bw per day given to Harlan Sprague–Dawley rats for 30 weeks caused dose-dependent lipid peroxidation, production of superoxide anions, and single-strand DNA breaks in liver and brain tissue.

Dietary levels of 5 and 50 μg kg^{-1} of bw of 2,3,7,8-TCDF for 6 and 2 months, respectively, caused sickness and some deaths in two groups of three rhesus macaques each. The principal pathological findings were atrophy (metaplasia) of the sebaceous glands, involution of the thymus, and hypoplasia of the bone marrow. Among survivors, recovery was complete after 3 months of a diet without 2,3,7,8-TCDF. Hyperplasia of the epithelium of the intestinal tract and the biliary tract may also occur in monkeys. Retention cysts of the Meibomian glands of the eyelids and hyperkeratosis of the pilar pores of the skin, facial edema, and loss of facial hair, including eyelashes, have been reported in monkeys following exposure to PCDFs. In rats and mice, the liver and thymus are primary target organs.

Among chicks fed 2,3,7,8-TCDF of 1 and 5 μg kg^{-1} of bw per day for 21 days, mortality was 16 and 100%, respectively. At 5 μg kg^{-1} of bw per day the liver was affected, and thymic atrophy and edema were observed. Porphyria may also occur in chickens and has been reported in rats dosed with technical pentachlorophenol contaminated with PCDDs and PCDFs. However, it was not determined whether the pentachlorophenol also contained hexachlorobenzene a known porphorinogenic substance.

Immunotoxicity

Toxic doses of 2,3,7,8-tetra-CDF and 2,3,4,7,8-penta-CDF cause severe thymic atrophy in the guinea pig, mouse, and rat. Humoral antibody production is also inhibited. However, 2,3,7,8-TCDF is 30 times less effective than 2,3,7,8-TCDD. The degree of PCDF-induced immunotoxicity is influenced by the genetic background of different laboratory animal species. Reductions in thymus weight and the number of spleen cells were seen in C57B1/6J mice after a single dose of 100 μg kg^{-1} of bw of 2,3,7,8-tetra-CDF. Humeral immunity was also affected. The LD_{50} for 2,3,7,8-tetra-CDF in these mice is >6000 μg kg^{-1} of bw. Adult guinea pigs were dosed once weekly with 2,3,7,8-tetra-CDF for 6 weeks. Thymus weight was reduced at 1.0 and 0.5 μg kg^{-1} of bw and the body weight gain was reduced. Leukocyte counts were depressed. A marked depression of antibody responses was observed.

Reproductive and Developmental Toxicity

Single doses of 2,3,7,8-TCDF of 100–1000 μg kg^{-1} of bw on days 10–13 of pregnancy produced cleft palate and hydronephrosis in mice. The teratogenic ED_{50}s for 2,3,4,7,8-penta-CDF, 1,2,3,7,8-penta-CDF, and 1,2,3,4,7,8-hexa-CDF were 40, 100, and 400 μg kg^{-1} of bw, respectively. Similar ED_{50} values have been reported in other studies. In rats, fetal deaths and suggestive fetal cleft palates have been observed.

Genotoxicity

Mutagenicity was studied in several Salmonella strains and cell fractions obtained from rats. The 2,3,7,8-, 2,8-, 3,6-, and octa-PCF were all nonmutagenic.

Carcinogenicity

Cholangiocarcinomas and hepatomas were observed in Harlan Sprague–Dawley rats given daily doses of 44, 92, and 200 ng kg^{-1} of bw 2,3,4,7,8-penta-CDF. Dosing was by gavage 5 days $week^{-1}$ for up to 2 years.

Human Toxicity

No information is available for PCDFs per se. However, two poisoning outbreaks occurred, in 1968 in Japan and in 1979 in Taiwan. PCBs were used as a heat transfer agents during the production of rice bran oil. In Japan and in Taiwan, the heat-degraded PCBs accidentally contaminated the oil because of holes in the PCB-filled coils. Analysis of the heat transfer fluid and the contaminated oil eventually revealed the presence of PCBs, PCDFs, PCDDs, and polychlorinated quaterphenyls (PCQs). Later, polychlorinated quaterphenyl ethers (PCQEs) and polychlorinated terphenyls (PCTs) were also identified. It is assumed that the PCDFs were the primary cause of illness. The total number of registered Yusho patients in Japan was 1860, and over 2000 people were affected in Taiwan. In the late 1970s and mid-1980s, the estimated average intake during the intoxication period for Yusho was 633, 3.4, and 596 mg and for Yucheng 973, 3.8, and 586 mg for PCBs, PCDFs, and PCQs, respectively. However, these estimates do not include the PCDDs, which were found later in additional analyses. In 1989, with improved analytical methods, 0.826 mg kg^{-1} PCDDs, 11.6 mg kg^{-1} PCDFs, and 380 mg kg^{-1} PCBs were found in two rice oil samples. It is unclear how representative these oil samples were. Since the contamination was accidental, it was not uniform. It appears that the most highly contaminated oil had been consumed by the time the outbreaks were investigated.

In adult Yusho and Yucheng patients, the primary signs were chloracne, hyperpigmentation of the skin and mucous membranes, eye discharge, liver toxicity, and paresthesias. In neonates, dark brown pigmentation of the skin and mucous membranes, edematous faces, and prematurely erupted teeth were noted. Abnormal laboratory tests such as elevated triglycerides were also found. In many individuals, these signs regressed over time. The brownish pigmentation of the babies disappeared in 2–3 months. In adults, signs and symptoms also diminished over time. Half of the Yusho patients complained of respiratory stress, and infections of the respiratory tract were prevalent. Some immunoglobulins were decreased. The physical and mental development of the Yusho babies was normal, while the Yucheng children at ages 6–7 had poorer cognitive development than matched controls. They scored approximately five points lower (0.40 SD) on the Wechsler Intelligence Scale Revised. It is unclear whether these children were breastfed, since formula feeding also affects these tests. Results of follow-up studies in this population suggest that there is no difference in relative survival if compared to the general population. However, a mortality study with 40-year follow-up suggests that the standardized mortality ratios (SMR) for all cancers (SMR 1.37; CI 1.11–1.66), cancer of the liver (SMR 1.82; CI 1.06–2.91), and lung cancer (SMR 1.75; CI 1.14–2.57) among males were statistically significantly elevated but tended to decrease over time, suggesting potential confounding.

Ecotoxicology

No definitive information for CDFs was available. Studies in mink suggest that they tolerate higher doses of PCDFs than implied by the most recent TEFs. Wood ducks seem to be more sensitive to these types of compounds than other bird species.

Exposure Standards and Guidelines

No specific guidelines or standards have been set for PCDFs. Some environmental guidelines such as clean-up levels in contaminated areas exist only for the combination of PCDDs and PCDFs and sometimes also included PCBs. These guidelines are based on the TEF approach and vary in different locales.

See also: Glyphosate; Hexachlorobenzene; Chlorination Byproducts; Chloromethyl Ether, Bis-; Chlorophenols; Dibenzofuran; Jet Fuels; Interactive Toxicity; *S*-(1,2-Dichlorovinyl)-L-Cysteine; Polychlorinated Biphenyls (pcbs); Ethanol; Dioxins; Strontium; TCDD (2,3,7,8-Tetrachlorodibenzo-*p*-dioxin).

Further Reading

Brzuzy, L.P., Hites, R.A., 1996. Global mass balance for polychlorinated dibenzo-*p*-dioxins and dibenzofurans. Environ. Sci. Technol. 30, 1797–1804.

Centers for Disease Control and Prevention (CDC), 2005. Third National Report on Human Exposure to Environmental Chemicals. Georgia, Atlanta.

Charnley, G., Kimbrough, R.D., 2006. Overview of exposure, toxicity and risk to children from current levels of 2,3,7,8-tetrachlorodibenzo-*p*-dioxin and related compounds in the USA. Food. Chem. Toxicol. 44, 601–615.

Green, N.J.L., Jones, J.L., Johnston, A.E., Jones, K.C., 2001. Further evidence for the existence of PCDD/Fs in the environment prior to 1900. Environ. Sci. Technol. 35, 1974–1981.

Green, N.J.L., Hassanin, A., Johnston, A.E., Jones, K.C., 2004. Observations on historical, contemporary and natural PCDD/Fs. Environ. Sci. Technol. 38, 715–723.

Kimbrough, R.D., Jensen, A.A., 1989. Halogenated biphenyls, terphenyls, naphthalenes, dibenzodioxins and related products. Top. Environ. Health 4. Elsevier Science Publishers B.V., Amsterdam, The Netherlands.

Okey, A.B., 2007. An aryl hydrocarbon receptor odyssey to the shores of toxicology: the Deichmann Lecture, International Congress of Toxicology-XI (2007). Toxicol. Sci. 98, 5–38.

Report on a WHO Working Group, Abano Terme/Padua, 16–19 February 1987. In: Grandjean, P., Tarkowski, S., Kimbrough, R., Yrjänheikki, E., Rantanen, J.H. (Eds.), Assessment of Health Risks in Infants Associated with Exposure to PCBs, PCDDs and PCDFs in Breast Milk. Environmental Health, vol. 29. World Health Organization Regional Office for Europe, Copenhagen.

Schmidt, V.J., Bradfield, C.A., 1996. AH receptor signaling pathways. Annu. Rev. Cell Dev. Biol. 12, 55–89.

Van den Berg, M., De Jongh, J., Poiger, H., Olson, J.R., 1994. The toxicokinetics and metabolism of polychlorinated dibenzo-*p*-dioxins (PCDDs) and dibenzofurans (PCDFs) and their relevance for toxicity. Crit. Rev. Toxicol. 24, 1–74.

Van den Berg, M., Birnbaum, L.S., Denison, M., De Vito, M., Farland, W., Feeley, M., et al., 2006. The 2005 World Health Organization reevaluation of human and mammalian toxic equivalency factors for dioxins and dioxin-like compounds. Toxicol. Sci. 93, 223–241.

Walker, N.J., Crockett, P.W., Nyska, A., Brix, A.E., Jokinen, M.P., Sells, D.M., et al., 2005. Dose additive carcinogenicity of a defined mixture of dioxin-like compounds. Environ. Health Perspect. 113, 43–48.

Chloroethane

S Milanez, Oak Ridge National Laboratory, Oak Ridge, TN, USA

- Name: Chloroethane
- Synonyms: Ethyl chloride; Monochloroethane
- Molecular Formula: C_2H_5Cl
- Chemical Structure:

$$H_3C\!-\!CH_2\!-\!Cl$$

Background

Chloroethane is a flammable, colorless, gas or liquid (below 54 °F), with a pungent, etherlike odor. It is not found naturally, but is produced by the hydrochlorination of ethylene, and as a by-product of polyvinyl chloride synthesis. It is a lipophilic compound that is moderately soluble in water, but readily soluble in organic solvents.

Uses

Chloroethane is used in the manufacture of tetraethyl lead, ethyl cellulose, agrichemicals, butyl rubber, dyes, perfumes, and medicinal drugs. It is applied as a topical spray skin analgesic for the temporary relief of pain. Its former predominant uses to make the gasoline additive tetraethyl lead and as a general anesthetic and refrigerant have been curtailed.

Environmental Fate and Behavior

Chloroethane's production and uses may result in its release to the environment, primarily to air. In ambient air, chloroethane will exist as a gas, which is degraded by reaction with photochemically produced hydroxyl radicals with a half-life of >23 days. Chloroethane can be removed from air by wet or dry deposition, since it is only moderately water soluble. It is expected to have very high mobility in soil and could leach into groundwater, and can volatilize from moist and dry soil surfaces. In water, chloroethane is not expected to adsorb to suspended solids and sediment, or to hydrolyze appreciably, and is expected to volatilize from the water surface. Bioconcentration in aquatic organisms is low. The primary routes for human chloroethane exposure are inhalation and dermal contact.

Exposure and Exposure Monitoring

Potential routes of human exposure include inhalation, ingestion, and eye and skin contact. Workers may be exposed by inhalation and dermal contact where chloroethane is used or synthesized, and the general population may be exposed by inhaling ambient air, drinking contaminated water, from dermal contact with consumer products (solvents, paints, and refrigerants), and from its use as a topical numbing agent. Chloroethane can be released to the environment by emissions from its production and use as a chemical intermediate, by fumes from plastics and refuse combustion, by wastewater effluent treatment facilities, and by leaching from landfills.

Toxicokinetics

Humans and animals rapidly absorbed inhaled chloroethane, and ingested chloroethane was largely absorbed from the gastrointestinal (GI) tract in rodents. Skin absorption has not been determined, but is expected to be minor based on chloroethane's physical properties. *In vitro* tissue/air partition studies showed that chloroethane has a greater affinity for fat than for muscle, liver, or blood. High concentrations of chloroethane were found *in vivo* in the brain and medulla oblongata.

Inhalation studies with rats and mice showed that only a fraction of absorbed chloroethane is metabolized, and the majority is exhaled unchanged. One major metabolic pathway is oxidation via liver microsomal cytochrome P450IIE1 to form acetaldehyde, which is quickly metabolized to acetic acid by aldehyde dehydrogenase. The second major pathway is conjugation with glutathione to form S-ethyl-glutathione, catalyzed by glutathione-S-transferase, with subsequent metabolism to more hydrophilic forms that are excreted in the urine. Mice had a greater capacity than rats to metabolize chloroethane by both the P450 and glutathione conjugation pathways. Dechlorination was not a significant metabolic pathway for chloroethane.

Chloroethane is quickly eliminated from the body, primarily through the lung as the unchanged compound, with the rest excreted in the urine, feces, and sweat.

Mechanisms of Toxicity

The mechanism of chloroethane toxicity, which primarily affects the central nervous system (CNS), heart, liver, and kidneys, has not been defined. Chloroethane is a small lipophilic compound that can cross membranes by simple diffusion. The anesthetic effect in humans and animals caused by inhalation of high concentrations may be due to chloroethane interaction with the lipid layer of the cellular membrane, or with hydrophobic areas of specific membrane-bound cellular proteins. *In vitro* studies have shown that chloroethane interferes with calcium-mediated excitation–contraction coupling, leading to a reduction in ATP use, possibly due to disruption of the lipid structure of the transverse tubule walls. Inhalation of high concentrations of chloroethane sensitizes the heart to the effects of catecholamines. This, together with ethyl

 http://dx.doi.org/10.1016/B978-0-12-386454-3.01114-3

chloride-induced euphoria, excitement, asphyxia, and hypoxia can result in arrhythmias and death. It has been proposed that chloroethane may depress atrioventricular nodal conduction, causing atrioventricular block.

Acute and Short-Term Toxicity

Animal

The minimum lethal concentration of chloroethane in a 2-h exposure study was ~55 000 ppm in rats and mice. Guinea pigs died from a 9-h exposure to 40 000 ppm, and had pathological changes in the lung, heart, liver, spleen, and kidneys, and signs of CNS toxicity (dizziness, ataxia). Dogs exposed to anesthetic concentrations of chloroethane exhibited muscle twitching and tremors, and had cardiac depression due to vagal nerve stimulation. This led to ventricular tachycardia, asystole, and death.

Mice exposed to ~5000 ppm continuously for 11 days had increased relative liver weight and slightly increased hepatocellular vacuolation, but no other significant toxicity in numerous examined organs. The most notable effects in rats, mice, and dogs exposed discontinuously for 2 or 3 weeks to 10 000–19 000 ppm, and in rats and mice exposed for 13 weeks to 19 000 ppm, were slight CNS depression, lethargy, and slightly increased liver weight in rats.

Human

Chloroethane vapor is irritating to eyes, nose, and throat, and the liquid is irritating to the skin and eyes. Exposure to 13 000 ppm for 12 min caused subjective intoxication and decreased reaction times. A few breaths of 20 000–40 000 ppm resulted in eye irritation, mild abdominal cramps, nausea, vomiting, and dizziness, whereas exposure for ~10 min caused intoxication, incoordination, and unconsciousness. Anesthetic concentrations of chloroethane have caused cardiac depression due to vagus nerve stimulation, which has in some cases led to arrhythmia and resulted in the death. Symptoms of frostbite can result from prolonged dermal exposure to chloroethane.

Chronic Toxicity

Animal

A chronic toxicity and carcinogenicity study with rats and mice showed no histopathological changes in the respiratory tract, cardiovascular system, GI tract, or liver after exposure for 6 h per day, 5 days per week to up to 15 000 ppm chloroethane for 2 years. Mild nephrotoxicity was seen in mice exposed to 15 000 ppm, and consisted of tubular regeneration and minimal glomerulosclerosis in females, and slight enlargement of renal tubular cell nuclei in males.

Human

Case reports of long-term inhalation abuse of high concentrations of chloroethane showed the greatest adverse effects on the nervous system. Symptoms included jerking eye movements, an inability to control voluntary movements, difficulty in speaking clearly, sluggish lower limb reflexes, seizures, disorientation, short-term memory loss, and hallucinations. Nerve damage, an enlarged liver, and mild transient disturbance of liver function were also seen following exposure to high concentrations.

Repeated dermal exposure to chloroethane has resulted in contact sensitivity, as shown by positive patch tests.

Immunotoxicity

Contact dermatitis has been reported following dermal application of chloroethane. In animals, no treatment-related effects were seen on organs or tissues of the immune system of mice after continuous inhalation exposure of 4800 ppm for 11 days, or in mice and rats treated intermittently with up to 15 000 ppm for 2 weeks to 2 years. Anemic or congested spleens were noted in guinea pigs exposed for 90 min to ~40 000 ppm chloroethane.

Reproductive Toxicity

Pathological changes were not seen in reproductive organs of animals exposed to chloroethane by inhalation for up to 2 years. No maternal toxicity or adverse effects on reproductive or fetal parameters were seen in mice exposed to chloroethane during gestation days 6–15, except for a small but statistically significant increase in the incidence of unossified bones of the skull at the high dose (5000 ppm). Dogs anesthetized with chloroethane had decreased uterine motility and muscle tone. Rats and mice exposed to chloroethane had decreased glutathione levels in a number of organs, the greatest decrease being in the uterus. Mice exposed to high concentrations of chloroethane had decreased uterine weight and slightly longer estrous cycle duration.

Genotoxicity

Chloroethane yielded mixed results in standard genotoxicity assays. It caused cytotoxicity in two independent BALB/c-3T3 cell transformation assays, but elicited morphological transformation in only one of the tests. It was mutagenic in the Ames test in *Salmonella typhimurium* strains TA1535 and TA100, but not in strains TA98 or TA1537. Chloroethane did not induce unscheduled DNA synthesis in mouse hepatocyte primary culture or micronuclei in bone-marrow cells from mice exposed by inhalation, but was mutagenic at the *hprt* locus in Chinese hamster ovary cells.

Carcinogenicity

No epidemiological studies were available that examined the carcinogenic potential of chloroethane. The National Toxicology Program (NTP) conducted 2-year toxicology and carcinogenesis studies of chloroethane with both sexes of rats and mice. The evidence of carcinogenic activity was equivocal for male rats (benign and malignant skin neoplasms), female rats (malignant brain astrocytomas), and male mice (alveolar/bronchiolar neoplasms). The female mice had a clear increase in uterine carcinomas, which parallels the finding in other studies that glutathione depletion was greater in the uteri of female mice than in other organs of mice or in rats. PBPK models of chloroethane disposition in mice and humans have been recently developed, and for rats have been expanded. The models allow for comparison of predicted internal dose metrics between the three species, and help determine the mechanism of uterine carcinogenicity.

Clinical Management

Chloroethane vapors can be irritating to the eyes, skin, and mucous membranes, and cause symptoms that include headache, blurred vision, dizziness, ataxia, stupor, CNS depression, vomiting, abdominal cramps, and liver or kidney toxicity. Chloroethane increases myocardial sensitivity to catecholamines, and can cause cardiac arrhythmias. Eczema and allergic contact dermatitis have been reported.

Persons exposed by inhalation should be moved to fresh air and monitored for respiratory effects. Bronchospasm should be treated with inhaled beta2-agonist and oral or parenteral corticosteroids, and seizures with benzodiazepine. The electrocardiogram (ECG) should be monitored in cases of heavy exposure. If the eyes have been exposed, they should be irrigated at least 15 minutes with room-temperature water. For dermal exposure, contaminated clothing should be removed and the affected area should be washed thoroughly with soap and water. Dermal hypersensitivity reactions can be treated with systemic or topical corticosteroids, or antihistamines.

Ecotoxicity

Scant information was available regarding the ecotoxicity of chloroethane. EC_{50} values of $58\,\mathrm{mg\,l^{-1}}$ and $39\,\mathrm{mg\,l^{-1}}$ were obtained for *Daphnia magna* and the algae *Scenedesmus subspicatus*, respectively. An EC_{10} of $>140\,\mathrm{mg\,l^{-1}}$ was determined for the soil bacterium *Pseudomonas putida*.

Exposure Standards and Guidelines

The U.S. Occupational Safety and Health Administration (OSHA) established a permissible exposure limit (PEL) of 1000 ppm as a time-weighted average (TWA) inhalation concentration for chloroethane, with a skin designation. The American Conference of Governmental Industrial Hygienists (ACGIH) determined an 8-h TWA threshold limit value (TLV-TWA) of 100 ppm, with a skin designation and defined excursion levels.

The California Environmental Protection Agency (EPA) (2001) derived a no significant risk level (NSRL) of 0.15 mg per day as the daily intake level posing a 10^{-5} lifetime risk of cancer, based on the female mouse uterine carcinoma data in an NTP study (NTP, 1989). Based on delayed fetal ossification in CF-1 mice in a developmental toxicity inhalation study, the California EPA derived a chronic reference exposure level of $30\,\mathrm{mg\,m^{-3}}$, the U.S. EPA Integrated Risk Information System (IRIS) program developed a reference concentration (RfC) of $10\,\mathrm{mg\,m^{-3}}$, and the Agency for Toxic Substances Disease Registry (ATSDR) developed an acute inhalation minimal risk level (MRL) of 15 ppm. IRIS did not develop a reference dose for chronic oral exposure (RfD).

The International Agency for Research on Cancer (IARC) has concluded that chloroethane is not classifiable as to its carcinogenicity to humans, and the ACGIH has classified it as a confirmed animal carcinogen with unknown relevance to humans. The National Institute for Occupational Safety and Health (NIOSH) considers chloroethane to be a potential occupational carcinogen, because of its structural similarity to other animal carcinogens. The IRIS does not currently present a carcinogenicity assessment for lifetime exposure to chloroethane.

See also: Anesthetics; Developmental Toxicology; Neurotoxicity; Kidney; Cardiovascular System.

Further Reading

ATSDR (Agency for Toxic Substances and Disease Registry), 1998. Toxicological Profile for Chloroethane (Update). U.S. Department of Health and Human Services, Public Health Service, Atlanta, GA. Available online at: http://www.atsdr.cdc.gov/ToxProfiles/tp105.pdf.

California Environmental Protection Agency, 2001. No significant risk level (NSRL) for the proposition 65 carcinogen, chloroethane. Office of Environmental Health Hazard Assessment (OEHHA). Available online at: http://www.oehha.org/prop65/law/pdf_zip/chloroethaneNSRL.pdf – No Significant Risk Level (NSRL) for the proposition 65 carcinogen Chloroethane.

Gargas, M.L., Sweeney, L.M., Himmelstein, M.W., et al., 2008. Physiologically based pharmacokinetic modeling of chloroethane disposition in mice, rats, and women. Toxicol. Sci. 104, 54–66.

HSDB (Hazardous Substances Data Bank), 2012. Ethyl chloride. National Library of Medicine TOXNET database, National Institutes of Health, USA. Available online at: http://toxnet.nlm.nih.gov.

IARC (International Agency for Research on Cancer), 1999. IARC monographs on the evaluation of carcinogenic risks to humans. Geneva: World Health Organization. Available online at:http://monographs.iarc.fr/index.php.

IUCLID (International Uniform Chemical Information Database), 2000. Dataset for-chloroethane (75-00-3). Created by the European Commission – European Chemicals Bureau on 19-Feb-2000. Available online at: http://esis.jrc.ec.europa.eu/doc/IUCLID/data_sheets/75003.pdf.

Landry, T.D., Ayres, J.A., Johnson, K.A., Wall, J.M., 1982. Ethyl chloride: a two-week inhalation toxicity study and effects on liver non-protein sulfhydryl concentrations. Fundam. Appl. Toxicol. 2, 230–234.

Landry, T.D., Johnson, K.A., Phillips, J.E., Weiss, S.K., 1989. Ethyl chloride: 11-day continuous exposure inhalation toxicity study in B6C3F1 mice. Fundam. Appl. Toxicol. 13, 516–522.

National Toxicology Program (NTP), 1989. Toxicology and Carcinogenesis Studies of Chloroethane (CAS No. 75-00-3) in F344/N Rats and B6C3F1 Mice Inhalation Studies. Technical Report Series No. 346. NIH Publication No. 90-2801. U.S. Department of Health and Human Services, Public Health Service, National Institutes of Health.

NIOSH (National Institute for Occupational Safety and Health), 2007. Ethyl chloride. NIOSH Pocket Guide to Chemical Hazards. Department of Health and Human Services, Centers for Disease Control and Prevention. DHHS (NIOSH) Publication No. 2005-149, p. 135. Available online at: http://www.cdc.gov/niosh/docs/2005-149/pdfs/2005-149.pdf, and at http://www.cdc.gov/niosh/npg/npgd0267.html.

Scortichini, B.H., Johnson, K.A., Momany-Pfruender, J.J., Hanley, T.R., 1986. Ethyl Chloride: Inhalation Teratology Study in CF-1 Mice. Dow Chemical Company. EPA Document #86–870002248.

US EPA (Environmental Protection Agency), 1988. Summary Review of Health Effects Associated with Monochloroethane: Health Issue Assessment. Office of Research and Development, Office of Health and Environmental Assessment, Environmental Criteria and Assessment Office, Research Triangle Park, NC. Report no. EPA/600/8–88/080.

U.S. EPA (Environmental Protection Agency), 1991. Ethyl chloride. Integrated Risk Information System (IRIS). National Center for Environmental Assessment, Washington, DC. Assessment last revised 04/01/1991. Available online at: http://www.epa.gov/iris/subst/0523.htm. (accessed 8/2012).

Chlorofluorocarbons

WT Tsai, National Pingtung University of Science and Technology, Pingtung, Taiwan

Background

It is recognized that nontoxic and nonflammable refrigerants (Freon or chlorofluorocarbon (CFC)) were commercialized in the manufacture of chlorofluoro- derivatives of methane and ethane until the 1930s. Since that time, studies on the synthesis of CFCs and their applications have progressed in many directions, such as aerosol, blowing agent for foam manufacture, fire extinguisher, cleaning solvent, and refrigerant. Due to the potential environmental and health effects of ozone depletion and greenhouse effect, the use of Freons has been reduced by international agreements since the end of the 1980s. Under a treaty known as the Montreal Protocol on Substances that Deplete the Ozone Layer, which was first established in 1987, several interim replacements for CFCs were thus developed in the 1990s, i.e., partially or fully fluorinated or partially chlorofluorinated alkanes, including hydrochlorofluorocarbons (HCFCs), hydrofluorocarbons (HFCs) and perfluorocarbons (PFCs). **Table 1** lists the chemical identities and the information on ozone depletion potential (ODP), global warming potential (GWP), and partition property of common CFCs, including trichlorofluoromethane (CFC-11), dichlorodifluoromethane (CFC-12), 1,1,2-trichloro-1,2,2-trifluoroethane (CFC-113), 1,2-dichlorotetrafluoroethane (CFC-114), and chloropentafluoroethane (CFC-115).

Obviously, these CFCs contain only the elements chlorine, fluorine, and carbon. Thus, they are usually colorless gases or liquids that evaporate easily at room temperatures. They are generally unreactive and stable, nontoxic, and nonflammable. It means that the atmosphere is the most likely fate for their accumulations of emissions. CFCs are also a part of the group of chemicals known as the volatile organic compounds. On the other hand, it can be seen in **Table 1** that the values of log K_{ow} for CFCs are below 3.5, showing that these fluorocarbons have very low potential bioaccumulation in the environment. Herein, some CFCs, including chlorotrifluoromethane (CFC-13), 1,1,1,2-tetrachloro-2,2-difluoroethane (CFC-112a), and 1,1,2,2-tetrachloro-1,2-difluoroethane (CFC-112), are not discussed.

Mode of Action

CFCs are characterized by high chemical and thermal stabilities, nonflammability, and low toxicity. Although CFCs are physiologically inert, they can cause cardiac sensitization (i.e., sensitization of the heart to the body's adrenalin) at high concentrations (e.g., above 10% in air). This can lead to cardiac arrhythmia, resulting in irregular heartbeat and sometimes cardiac arrest.

Major Uses

The chemical inertness, thermal stability, low toxicity, and nonflammability of these CFCs coupled with their unique physical properties are used in many application fields, including refrigerant for air conditioning, aerosol (propellant), blowing agent for foam manufacture, fire extinguisher, cleaning agent, dielectric fluid, and ion implantation of semiconductor device. However, it should be noted that the timetable of phase-out of these compounds was regulated by the Montreal protocol (i.e., the production of CFCs ended by 1 January 1996 and their applications banned).

Environmental Hazards

GWP expresses the relative increase in earthward IR radiation flux due to the emission of organic compounds. Notably, all CFCs have high GWP values relative to the reference compound, carbon dioxide (seen in **Table 1**). Furthermore, these saturated halocarbons are considered not easily biodegradable based on the data of octanol/water partition coefficients also listed in **Table 1**. With respect to ecotoxicity, it was also revealed to be not very toxic to aquatic organisms (i.e., algae, water fleas, and fish) and terrestrial plants. For example, CFC-113, which was one of the most used solvents, shows a very low toxicity toward aquatic species such as Daphnia and fish. As described, the most significant environmental hazard for CFCs should be the ozone depletion, which is caused by chlorine molecules in these so-called ozone-depleting substances that migrate to the stratosphere and then react catalytically with ozone, thus destroying it. In addition, from the view of the effect on air quality, CFCs have been listed as having 'negligible photochemical reactivity' and do not contribute to smog formation and ground-level ozone. Therefore, they are exempt from volatile organic compound regulations according to the US Clean Air Act Amendments of 1990.

Table 1 Environmental properties of common chlorofluorocarbons (CFCs)

CFCs (abbrev.)	*CAS no.*	*Molecular formula*	*Mol. wt. (g mol^{-1})*	*Lifetime (years)*	*ODP*[a]	*GWP*[b]	*Log K_{ow}*
Trichlorofluoromethane (CFC-11)	75-69-4	CCl_3F	137.38	45	1.0	4750	2.53
Dichlorodifluoromethane (CFC-12)	75-71-8	CCl_2F_2	120.91	100	1.0	10 900	2.16
1,1,2-Trichloro-1,2,2-trifluoroethane (CFC-113)	76-13-1	CCl_2FCClF_2	187.40	85	0.8	6130	3.16
1,2-Dichlorotetrafluoroethane (CFC-114)	76-14-2	$CClF_2CClF_2$	170.93	300	1.0	10 000	2.82
Chloropentafluoroethane (CFC-115)	76-15-3	$CClF_2CF_3$	154.47	1700	0.6	7370	2.30

[a]Ozone depletion potential (relative to the ODP of CFC-11 = 0) in Montreal Protocol.
[b]Global warming potential with 100-year time horizon (relative to GWP of CO_2 = 1).

Table 2 Toxicity data and exposure limits of common chlorofluorocarbons (CFCs)

CFCs	*LC_{50}[a] (ppm)*	*LOEL[b] (ppm)*	*OSHA-PEL[c] (ppm)*	*ACGIH-TLV[d] (ppm)*	*TLV-basis*
CFC-11	26 200	5000	1000	1000	Cardiac sensitization
CFC-12	760 000	50 000	1000	1000	Cardiac sensitization
CFC-113	52 000	5000	1000	1000	Central nervous system impairment
CFC-114	600 000	25 000	1000	1000	Pulmonary function
CFC-115	> 800 000	150 000	1000	1000	Cardiac sensitization

[a]LC_{50}: Lethal concentration for 50% of test animals (rat).
[b]LOEL: Lowest observed effect level at which sensitization occurs in dog with epinephrine challenge.
[c]OSHA-PEL: US Occupational Safety and Health Administration permissible exposure limit based on 8-h time-weighted average.
[d]ACGIH-TLV: American Conference of Governmental Industrial Hygienists-Threshold Limit Value based on 8-h time-weighted average.

Exposure Routes and Pathways

Inhalation (pulmonary route) is the main source of exposure to CFCs. Skin absorption or contact (dermal exposure) and eye contact may also occur. Because they are no longer used as refrigerants and blowing agents, human exposure to CFCs may occur via inhalation from accidental leaks or spills from a refrigeration system of recycling system for electronic appliances where they are still used.

Acute (Short-Term) Health Effects

Due to the physiochemical properties of CFCs, there is only a low potential for human toxicity based on the results of mammalian (i.e., rat) tests, and no significant acute health risk is expected. Briefly, the biotransformation of CFCs has been shown to undergo cytochrome P450-catalyzed oxidation or reduction reactions. The formed acyl halides are further hydrolyzed to give excretable haloacetic acid (e.g., trifluoroacetic acid) in urine. Although CFCs are physiologically inert, exposure to pressurized CFCs like liquid nitrogen, such as may occur with a refrigerant leak, can cause frostbite as well as to the upper airway if inhaled, possibly resulting in asphyxiation and cardiac sensitization (i.e., sensitization of the heart to the body's adrenalin) at high concentrations. The data on lowest observed effect level and lethal concentration for 50% of specimens (LC_{50}) for common CFCs are also listed in **Table 2**. It should be noted that repair of air-conditioning systems could involve welding operations and possibly cause the occupational exposure to decomposition toxic products, including hydrogen fluoride (HF), hydrogen chloride (HCl), carbon monoxide (CO), phosgene ($COCl_2$), and carbonyl fluoride (COF_2).

Chronic (Long-Term) Health Effects

In general, occupational workers exposed to CFCs at the exposure standards/limits (described below) showed no adverse health effects. In experimental animals exposed to CFCs for long-term tests, no significant effects were seen. Regarding the carcinogenic, reproductive, and developmental effects of CFCs, their potential for chronic effects is low.

Exposure Standards/Limits

Basically, CFCs have only a low potential for toxicity, and are considered not readily biodegradable, with very low ecotoxicity. Thus, the exposure limits for these chemicals, based on the permissible exposure limit by the US Occupational Safety and Health Administration and the threshold limit value (TLV) by the American Conference of Governmental Industrial Hygienists, are mostly set at 1000 ppm, as shown in **Table 2**. However, there are some exceptions as in the cases of CFC-112a and CFC-112. They will cause liver and kidney damage to experimental animals subjected to repeated exposure at high concentration; therefore, TLV-time-weighted average values of 100 ppm and 50 ppm are set for CFC-112a and CFC-112, respectively.

See also: Aerosols; Ozone; Global Climate Change and Environmental Toxicology.

Further Reading

American Conference of Governmental Industrial Hygienists, 2009. Documentation of the Threshold Limit Values and Biological Exposure Indices. ACGIH, Cincinnati, Ohio, USA.

Dekant, W., 1996. Toxicology of chlorofluorocarbon replacements. Environ. Health Perspect. 104 (Suppl. 1), 75–83.

Mackay, D., Shiu, W.Y., Ma, K.C., Lee, S.C., 2006. Handbook of Physical-chemical Properties and Environmental Fate for Organic Chemicals, second ed. CRC Press, Boca Raton, FL, USA.

National Institute for Occupational Safety and Health, 2004. NIOSH Pocket Guide to Chemical Hazards. NIOSH, Atlanta, GA, USA.

Sekiya, A., Yamabe, M., Tokuhashi, K., Hibino, Y., Imasu, R., Okamoto, H., 2006. Evaluation and selection of CFC alternatives. In: Tressaud, A. (Ed.), Fluorine and the Environment: Atmospheric Chemistry, Emissions, & Lithosphere. Elsevier, Amsterdam, pp. 33–87.

United Nations Environment Programme, 2011. Scientific Assessment of Ozone Depletion: 2010. UNEP, Geneva.

Relevant Websites

http://www.inchem.org/ – Fully Halogenated Chlorofluorocarbons (Environmental Health Criteria 113).

http://toxnet.nlm.nih.gov/ – National Library of Medicine's Toxicology Data Network (TOXNET).

http://www.des.nh.gov/ – New Hampshire Department of Environmental Services, Chlorofluorocarbons (CFCs): Health Information Summary (ARD-EHP-34).

Chloroform

J Estévez and E Vilanova, Universidad Miguel Hernández de Elche, Elche, Spain

This article is a revision of the previous edition article by Anna M. Fan, volume 1, pp 561–565, © 2005, Elsevier Inc.

- Name: Chloroform
- Chemical Abstracts Service Registry Number: 67-66-3
- European Inventory of Existing Commercial Chemical Substances Number: 200-663-8
- Synonyms: Methane trichloride, Trichloromethane, Methenyl trichloride, Methyl trichloride, Trichloroform
- Molecular Formula: $CHCl_3$
- Chemical Structure:

Cl
Cl
Cl

Background

Chloroform was discovered in 1831 independently by Liebig J., Soubeiran E., and Guthrie S. Chloroform was used in surgery by Ives E., but Simpson J.Y. first used chloroform in midwifery (1847). The anesthetic properties had been described by Flourens M.J.P. In 1906, Brown used a warmed mixture of nitrous oxide and oxygen, followed by ether and chloroform.

Very soon sudden deaths were reported and a specific effect on the heart was suspected. In 1911, Levy A.G. proved in experiments with animals that chloroform could cause cardiac fibrillation. Between 1865 and 1920, chloroform was used in 80–95% of all narcosis performed in UK and German-speaking countries. The discovery of hexobarbital in 1932 was the beginning to the gradual decline of chloroform narcosis. The clinical use of chloroform ended in 1976. Classification of the chloroform hazard according to the Globally Harmonized System (GHS) is shown in **Table 1**. It is classified as carcinogen category 2 (suspected of causing cancer) and also for oral acute toxicity, skin irritation, and for long-term effect.

Uses

Chloroform is mainly used as a raw material in the production of hydrochlorofluorocarbon-22 (HCFC 22), as a production and extraction solvent especially in the pharmaceutical industry (e.g., in the extraction of penicillin and other antibiotics), and it is also used as a solvent, degreasing agent, or chemical intermediate in industries like adhesives, pesticides, fats, oils, etc. Chloroform is a by-product in the manufacture of vinyl chloride/polyvinyl chloride (VC/PVC, IUPAC name: Polychloroethene) products and other chlorinated bulk chemicals. Similarly, chloroform is an important building block for fluorinated polymers and copolymers.

Chloroform has been used in the United States as an insecticidal fumigant on stored grains and as mildew fungicide for tobacco seedlings, but these applications are not registered in the European Union (EU). Elsewhere, unintended emissions of chloroform are observed in water chlorination processes or chlorination for paper bleaching.

Environmental Fate and Behavior

Routes and Pathways

Chloroform in soil or surface water volatilizes readily; at equilibrium, greater than 99% is expected to partition to the atmosphere. Some wet deposition of atmospheric chloroform may occur, but subsequent revolatilization is likely to be extensive. Chloroform is not expected to partition significantly to soils or sediments, because its affinity for organic carbon and lipids is low. Compartmental partitioning has been reported to be 99.1, 0.9, 0.01, and 0.01% in air, water, soil, and sediment, respectively. The preferred target compartment in the environment at equilibrium is the air compartment.

Physical and Chemical Properties

Chloroform is a volatile, heavy, colorless liquid. It is nonflammable and possesses a characteristic sweet odor. The physical and chemical properties of chloroform are summarized in **Table 2**.

Partition Behavior in Water, Sediment, and Soil

Chloroform is considered as nonbiodegradable in water. Hydrolysis is an unimportant fate process at a neutral pH value

Table 1 Chloroform classification according to the Globally Harmonized System of Classification and Labeling of Chemicals

Hazard class and category code(s)	*Hazard statement code(s) and meaning*	*Pictogram signal word code(s)*
Acute tox. 4	H302 harmful if swallowed	GHS08
Carc. 2	H351 suspected of causing cancer	GHS07
STOT RE 2	H372 may cause damage to organs through prolonged or repeated exposure	Wng
Skin irrit. 2	H315 causes skin irritation	

Source: Annex VI. Table 3.1 of European Regulation 1272/2008.

 http://dx.doi.org/10.1016/B978-0-12-386454-3.00479-6

Table 2 Physical and chemical properties of the substance

Property	*Value*
Molecular weight	119.5 g mol^{-1}
Relative density	1480 kg m^{-3}
Melting point	63.5 °C
Boiling point	61.3 °C
Vapor pressure	209 hPa at 20 °C
Relative density	1.4 at 20 °C
Surface tension	0.0271 N m^{-1} at 20 °C
Partition coefficient	Log K_{ow} 1.97
Henry's law	Constant $H = 367$ Pa m^3 mol^{-1} at 25 °C
Water solubility	8700 mg l^{-1} at 23 °C
Partition coefficient octanol/water	1.97
Flash point	None
Flammability	No

Source: European Union Risk Assessment Report of chloroform.

and direct photolysis in water is not expected too. In surface water, the principal removal process is volatilization with estimated half-lives of 1.5 days and 9–10 days in a river and a lake, respectively. Most studies have indicated little biodegradation up to 25 weeks in aquatic systems under aerobic conditions. The principal fate of chloroform at the soil surface is temperature-dependent volatilization due to its volatile nature and low soil adsorption.

Environmental Persistency

In air, a half-life value of 105 days is estimated. Chloroform emitted to air reacts primarily with photochemically generated hydroxyl radicals in the troposphere. The reaction products include phosgene, dichloromethane, formyl chloride, carbon monoxide, carbon dioxide, and hydrogen chloride.

The chemical degradation in sediments and soil is not rapid, except under anaerobic methanogenic conditions. Chloroform biodegradation is observed in anaerobic sediment and a half-life in sediment is estimated at 15 days. The major degradation products under anaerobic conditions are carbon dioxide, methane, and hydrogen chloride, with smaller amounts of dichloromethane. A K_{oc} value of 185 l kg^{-1} has been estimated.

Bioaccumulation and Biomagnification

The octanol/water partition coefficient and the bioconcentration factor measured for fish (see **Table 3**) indicate that chloroform is unlikely to bioaccumulate to any significant extent in aquatic biota.

Exposure and Exposure Monitoring

Routes and Pathways

The environmental exposure of chloroform is based on the expected releases of the substance during the life cycle stages of the production of this substance, the use as an intermediate (HCFC 22 production, dyes, pesticides production, and other), the use as a solvent (chemical and pharmaceutical industry), the unintended formation (by-product during chemical and VC/PVC products manufacturing), the water chlorination (drinking water, municipal wastewater, swimming pools, cooling water), the pulp and paper bleaching, atmospheric reaction of high tonnage chlorinated solvents, vehicle emissions, landfills, incineration processes, and natural sources. The major global sources for tropospheric chloroform would be direct emissions from the surface ocean, soils, and fungi, although biological processes are not well defined. Estimated emissions from anthropogenic sources account for 10% of the total emitted and the amounts emitted from fires represented only 0.4%. Chlorination of soil organic matter is one possible source of chloroform.

Human Exposure

Environmental Exposure

Based on concentrations determined in Canadian air (national surveys), food in Canada and the United States, and drinking water, the average estimated intake from food, drinking water, and air varied from 0.6 to 10 μg kg^{-1} body weight per day. Upper-bounding estimates were ranged from 40 to 95 μg kg^{-1}

Table 3 Results from bioaccumulation experiments in different species of fish studied in flow through

Species	*Exposure (d)*	*Water conc. (μg l^{-1})*	*Depuration*	*BCF (bioaccumulation factor)*
Cyprinus carpio	42	1000	–	1.4–4.7
Cyprinus carpio	42	100	–	4.1–13
Oncorhynchus mykiss	1	1000	Total depuration within 24 h	3.4–10.4
Lepomis macrochirus	1	1000	Total depuration within 24 h	1.6–2.5
Micropterus salmoides	1	1000	Total depuration within 24 h	2.1–2.2
Ictalurus punctatus[a]	1	1000	91% depuration within 26 h	3–3.4

[a]Equilibrium has not been reached.
Source: European Union Risk Assessment Report of chloroform.

body weight per day. The estimated total daily dose was 54.8 μg kg^{-1} body weight per day in the EU Risk Assessment Report on chloroform.

Occupational Exposure

Mean time-weighted average (TWA) exposures of 13, 2, and 1 mg m^{-3} for production operators, drummers/bottle fillers, and maintenance/utility personnel at one pesticide plant with levels of 10–1000 mg m^{-3} in a Polish pharmaceutical plant, an 8-h TWA of 77.4 mg m^{-3} (range 13–227 mg m^{-3}) in a police forensic laboratory, and (during 1968–72) levels of 34–830 mg m^{-3} (mean 230 mg m^{-3}, 79 samples) in a film manufacturing plant using a solvent containing 22% chloroform, have been reported.

Toxicokinetics

Chloroform is well absorbed, metabolized, and eliminated by mammals after oral, inhalation, or dermal exposure and widely distributed in the entire organism, via blood circulation and preferentially in fatty tissues and in the brain due to its liposolubility. The half-life in humans was 7.9 h following inhalation exposure. An oral-exposure study found most of the chloroform dose being eliminated within 8-h postexposure.

Chloroform is mainly metabolized in liver; the major metabolite is carbon dioxide. The oxidative pathway *in vivo* generates also reactive metabolites including phosgene, whereas the reductive pathway generates the dichloromethylcarbene free radical. Both pathways proceed through a cytochrome P450-dependent enzymatic activation step and their balance depends on species, tissue, dose, and oxygen tension. Phosgene is produced by oxidative dechlorination of chloroform to trichloromethanol, which spontaneously dehydrochlorinates.

The chloroform toxicity is due to its metabolites. Transplacental transfer of chloroform has been reported in mice and in the fetal blood in rats and it is expected to appear in human colostrum and is excreted in mature breast milk.

Inhalation, dermal, and oral absorptions are considered to be 80, 10, and 100%, respectively, in animals and humans.

Mechanism of Toxicity

The chloroform elicits the same symptoms of toxicity in humans as in laboratory animals. Oral administration to rats and mice resulted in central nervous system depression and nasal lesions in rats and liver damage in both species and in mice by gavage, and in dogs. Rats exposed by inhalation for 4–6 months showed liver damage (necrosis) and increased kidney weight. Cell proliferation was seen in the nasal tissues of rats and mice inhaling chloroform for 13 weeks.

Chloroform-induced kidney tumors in male mice exposed by inhalation or by ingestion in a toothpaste vehicle, but not when given in corn oil. Mice and female rats were not susceptible to chloroform-induced kidney cancer. Chronic inhalation caused ossification, necrosis, hyperplasia, and metaplasia in the nasal tissues of rats and mice, but not nasal tumors.

The molecular mechanism by which chloroform metabolism results in cellular toxicity is not certain. Oxidative metabolism of chloroform also produces hydrochloric acid, which may contribute to the toxic effect.

Acute and Short-Term Toxicity

Acute toxicity varies depending upon the strain, sex, and vehicle. **Table** 4 shows LC_{50} and LD_{50} for different species.

Extensive necrosis of the skin and degenerative changes in the kidney tubules after chloroform exposure under occlusive conditions have been reported in rabbits exposed by dermal route. An oral no observed adverse effect level (NOAEL) of 30 mg kg^{-1} has been reported in rats for serum enzyme changes indicative of liver.

The mean lethal oral dose for an adult is estimated to be about 45 g in humans but with large interindividual differences.

Some studies on clinical use and accidental human exposure have also been reported with inhalation lowest observable adverse effect concentration (LOAEC) $\leq$249 mg m^{-3} and the oral lowest observed adverse effect level (LOAEL) $<$107 mg kg^{-1}.

Studies in rabbits demonstrated that chloroform is an irritant substance for skin, eye, and upper airways and caused chemical dermatitis in humans. The LOAEC reported in rats was 50 mg m^{-3} by inhalation.

Chronic Toxicity

Laboratory animal studies identify the liver, kidneys, and the nasal cavity as the key target organs for chloroform's toxic potential. Different LOAEL, LOAEC, and effects in mice and rats are summarized in **Table 5**. Gastrointestinal symptoms, toxic hepatitis, and other effects including jaundice, nausea, and vomiting, without fever were manifested in workers exposed to different concentrations of 2–400 ppm. In humans, limited data on repeated dose toxicity suggest that the liver and kidneys are the likely target organs.

Table 4 Acute toxicity properties of chloroform

	Oral LD_{50} mg kg^{-1}	*LC_{50} (6-h inhalation exposure) g m^{-3}*
Mice	36–1366	6.2
Rats	450–2000	9.2

Source: European Union Risk Assessment Report of chloroform.

Table 5 Subchronic and chronic toxicity properties of chloroform

Study	*Species*	*LOAEL (oral) mg kg^{-1} per day*	*NOAEC (inhalation) mg m^{-3}*	*Effect*
Chronic	Dog (liver)	15		Hepatic effect (fatty cysts and elevated ALAT levels)
90-day study	Mice	50		Hepatic effect
14-day study	Mice	37		Renal effect
90-day study	Mice (male)		25	Renal effect
90-day study	Mice (male)		25	Hepatic effect
104 weeks	Mice		25	Increased renal cytoplasmic basophilia (males and females). Increased atypical tubule hyperplasia and nuclear enlargement in the kidneys (males).
Subchronic inhalation exposure	Rat		9.8	Cellular degeneration and regenerative hyperplasia in nasal passage tissues.
Subchronic oral exposure	Rats	34		Lesions and cell proliferation in the olfactory epithelium and changes in the nasal passages were observed.

Source: European Union Risk Assessment Report of chloroform.

Reproductive Toxicity

Exposure of animals to chloroform during pregnancy results in reproductive or developmental toxicity at the same or higher doses as those, which cause effects on the dam. The enzyme responsible for chloroform metabolism (CYP2E1) is low or absent in the fetus. No association was clearly established between exposure to chloroform and reduced fetal weight, stillbirth, and cleft defects. By inhalation, the effects of chloroform include effects on pregnancy rate, resorption rate, litter size and live fetuses, at concentrations causing a decrease of maternal weight and food consumption, fetal weight and CRL decrease, and skeletal and gross abnormalities.

Regarding fertility, an increased mice abnormal sperm following exposure to an air concentration of 400 or 800 ppm chloroform, epididymal lesions or increased right epididymis weight (oral no observed adverse effect concentration (NOAEC) 15.9 mg kg^{-1}) has been observed.

One occupational case study reported asthenospermia in association to chloroform exposure.

Genotoxicity

The reviews of several organizations concluded that chloroform is not a strong mutagen but a weak genotoxic effect was not excluded. Negative *in vivo* results are reported. Chloroform could induce micronuclei and chromosomal aberrations. Positive results are observed in the target organ (kidney) or in bone marrow cells, which might be consistent with a mechanism of oxidative damage due to glutathione depletion. Besides, it should be noted that micronucleus and chromosomal aberration tests performed in rats were all positive whereas mixed results were observed in mice. These studies suggested that chloroform is a slightly genotoxic compound *in vivo*.

Carcinogenicity

In animals, chloroform causes increased incidence of liver and kidney tumors in several species by several exposure routes. This carcinogenic response occurs only at high dose levels that result in cytotoxicity, and the carcinogenic responses observed in animals are associated with regenerative hyperplasia. Phosgene and other metabolites formed via the oxidative route of metabolism are responsible for the cytotoxic effects and subsequent cell proliferation and development of tumors in the kidney following exposures to chloroform.

Although some studies in humans have found increased risks of bladder cancer associated with long-term ingestion of chlorinated drinking water and cumulative exposure to trihalomethanes, results were inconsistent between men and women and between smokers and nonsmokers.

The current human data are insufficient to establish a causal relationship between exposure to chloroform in drinking water and increased risk of cancer.

The NOAEC via inhalation for the kidney adenoma/carcinoma was identified at 5 ppm in mice, for nasal lesions an LOAEC of 5 ppm was determined. Oral treatment with chloroform was associated with increased incidence of moderate to severe kidney lesions in CBA and CF/1 mice (NOAEL = 17 mg kg^{-1}).

Clinical Management

Human exposure to chloroform may occur by inhalation, ingestion, or dermal contact. In cases of ingestion, ipecac-induced emesis is not recommended and activated charcoal slurry with or without saline cathartic or sorbitol can be given. If exposed, skin should be decontaminated by repeated washing with soap, and eyes should be irrigated with copious amounts of water at room temperature for at least 15 min.

Management comprises early decontamination, supportive and symptomatic treatment with respiratory and cardiac monitoring (respiratory assistance, defibrillation, possible fluid replacement), and treatment of liver and/or kidney failure (renal dialysis) if they occur. Catecholamine drugs have to be avoided. No specific antidote is known.

Ecotoxicology

Freshwater/Sediment Organisms Toxicity

Chloroform has a moderated to low acute toxicity to aquatic organisms; acute fish LC_{50} range from 18 mg l^{-1} for *Oncorhynchus mykiss* to 171 mg l^{-1} for *Pimephales promelas* and values within this range have also reported for aquatic invertebrates. The chronic no observed effect concentration (NOEC) values are higher than 1 mg l^{-1}, suggesting also low chronic toxicity on aquatic species. The acute toxicity data in different species are summarized in **Table 6**.

The chronic toxicity results are summarized in **Table 7**.

In the methanogenesis study in a sediment/water suspension, EC_{10} (11 d) was 5.5 mg kg-dw^{-1} and EC_{50} (11 d) was 6.9 mg kg-dw^{-1}. Long-term studies on *Chironomus riparius* and *Lumbriculus variegatus* have been reported (**Table 8**).

Marine Organisms Toxicity

In *Penaeus duorarum*, 72-h LC_{50} and NOEC values of 81.5 and 32 mg l^{-1}, respectively, were reported. A 24-h EC_{50} of 30 mg l^{-1} for immobilization was recorded in 30-h posthatch larvae of a marine shrimp. The 48-h LC_{50} was 1 mg l^{-1} from a graph in larvae of *Crassostrea virginica*. A lowest observed effect concentration (LOEC) of 50.4 mg l^{-1} and an NOEC of 80.4 mg l^{-1} were estimated in oyster embryos.

Terrestrial Organisms Toxicity (Soil Microorganisms, Plants, Terrestrial Invertebrates, and Terrestrial Vertebrates)

There is little information on the toxicity of chloroform to terrestrial microorganisms. Single application of chloroform at 1000 mg kg^{-1} to a silty loam soil caused microbial respiration to increase for several days before returning to control levels 6 days after treatment. In sandy soils, it caused an initial depression in microbial respiration followed by a stimulation period and a return to control levels 6 days after treatment. Fumigation treatments with chloroform apparently did not eliminate microbial populations.

The data are also limited in terrestrial invertebrates. A study with *Eisenia fetida* classified chloroform as moderately toxic in comparison with the other chemicals. Other study demonstrated that the fumigation with chloroform eliminated protozoans from the soil but nematodes were not affected. The potential harm of chloroform in soil cannot be estimated with current data.

Table 6 Toxicity properties in different species of fish

Species	*Endpoint (duration)*
Limanda limanda	LC_{50} (96 h) = 28 mg l^{-1}
Lepomis macrochirus	LC_{50} (96 h) = 18 mg l^{-1} (mean LC_{50} of five tests)
Poecilia reticulata	LC_{50} (96 h) = 300 mg l^{-1}
Leuciscus idus	LC_0 (48 h) = 51 mg l^{-1}
	LC_{50} (48 h) = 92 mg l^{-1}
	LC_{100} (48 h) = 151 mg l^{-1}
Oncorhynchus mykiss	LC_{50} (48 h) = 20 mg l^{-1}
	LC_{50} (96 h) = 18 mg l^{-1} (mean LC_{50} of five tests)
Brachydanio rerio	LC_{50} (48 h) = 100 mg l^{-1}
	LC_{50} (96 h) = 121 mg l^{-1}
Oryzias latipes	LC_{50} (48 h) = 117 mg·l^{-1}
Cyprinus carpio	LC_{50} (3–5 days) = 97 mg l^{-1}(toxicity to carp embryos)
Ictalurus punctatus (Juvenile catfish)	LC_{50} (96 h) = 75 mg l^{-1}
Pimephales promelas	LC_{50} (96 h) = 71 mg l^{-1}
Micropterus salmoides	LC_{50} (96 h) = 51 mg l^{-1} (mean LC_{50} of three tests)
Poecilia reticulata	Experimental: LC_{50} (14 days) = 102 mg l^{-1}
	Calculated: LC_{50} (14 days) = 154 mg l^{-1}

Source: European Union Risk Assessment Report of chloroform.

Table 7 Results of the studies in freshwater organisms

	24-h EC_{50} mg l^{-1}	*48-h LC_{50} mg l^{-1}*	*NOEC mg l^{-1}*	*NOEC (9 days) mg l^{-1}*	*NOEC (16 days) mg l^{-1}*	*NOEC (21 days) mg l^{-1}*
Daphnia magna		29–90		3.4	15	6.3
Artemia salina	31–37					
Chlamydomonas reinhardtii			3.61			

Source: European Union Risk Assessment Report of chloroform.

Table 8 Results of the studies in sediment organisms

	Emergence (proportion of larvae emerged) ratio EC_{50} value mg kg^{-1}	*NOEC mg kg^{-1}*	*LOEC mg kg^{-1}*	*Development rate NOEC mg kg^{-1}*	*Development rate LOEC mg kg^{-1}*
Chironomus riparius	20.1	10	20.4	10 (females) 4.5 (males)	20.4 (pooled male and female) 10 (males)
Lumbriculus variegatus	12.9	36.9			

Source: European Union Risk Assessment Report of chloroform.

Other Hazards

The toxic effects of chloroform exposure include cytotoxicity in liver, kidney, and nasal epithelium, with neurological effects. The concurrent exposure to chemicals, which induce liver cytochrome P450 increases the risk to effects of chloroform. Persons with underlying liver, kidney, or neurological diseases are in higher risk to effects of chloroform.

Exposure Standards and Guidelines

The EU Directive 2000/39 proposed the indicative limit value for time weight average of 10 mg m^{-3} on the basis of 8-h work, 40 h per week. The Occupational Safety and Health Administration has set a maximum allowable concentration of chloroform of 50 ppm in workroom air during an 8-h workday in a 40-h workweek.

The European Commission and US Environmental Protection Agency have set a drinking water standard of 100 mg l^{-1} for total trihalomethanes (including chloroform).

The European regulation for Registration, Evaluation, Authorization and Restriction of Chemicals restricts the use and place of chloroform and mixtures containing concentrations equal to or greater than 0.1% chloroform by weight on the market for the general public. The use is restricted in industrial installations only.

See also: Carbon Dioxide; Volatile Organic Compounds; The Globally Harmonized System for Classification and Labeling of the GHS; Hydrochloric Acid; Phosgene; Solvents.

Further Reading

Baskerville, C., 1911. The chemistry of anesthetics. Science 34 (867), 161–176.
Elmer, S.P., Park, S., Pande, V.S., 15 Sept 2005. Foldamer dynamics expressed via Markov state models. I. Explicit solvent molecular-dynamics simulations in acetonitrile, chloroform, methanol, and water. J. Chem. Phys. 123 (11), 114902.
European Union Risk Assessment Report. Chloroform, 2008. ESIS database.
Flanagan, R.J., Pounder, D.J., 15 Apr 2010. A chloroform-related death: analytical and forensic aspects. Forensic Sci. Int. 197 (1–3), 89–96. Epub 13 Jan 2010.
Lionte, C., Jul 2010. Lethal complications after poisoning with chloroform–case report and literature review. Hum. Exp. Toxicol. 29 (7), 615–622. Epub 5 Jan 2010.
U.S. Environmental Protection Agency (EPA), 2001. Toxicological Review of Chloroform. Washington, DC.
Wawersik, J., 1997. History of chloroform anesthesia. Anaesthesiol. Reanim. 22 (6), 144–152.
Wexler, P., 2005. Encyclopedia of Toxicology, second ed. Elsevier.
World Health Organization (WHO), 2004. Chloroform, Concise International Chemical Assessment Document 58. Geneva.

Relevant Websites

http://echa.europa.eu/web/guest/information-on-chemicals/registered-substances – European Chemicals Agency (ECHA): Registered Substances.
http://esis.jrc.ec.europa.eu/ – European Chemical Substances Information System (ESIS).
http://toxnet.nlm.nih.gov/cgi-bin/sis/htmlgen?HSDB – Hazardous Substances Data Bank (HSDB).
http://www.who.int – World Health Organization (WHO).

Chloromethane

S Milanez, Oak Ridge National Laboratory, Oak Ridge, TN, USA

- Name: Chloromethane
- Synonyms: Methyl chloride; Monochloromethane
- Molecular Formula: CH_3Cl
- Chemical Structure:

$$H_3C - Cl$$

Background

Chloromethane is a ubiquitous colorless gas with a slight, sweet tasting, ethereal odor. It is formed naturally in the ocean, and by microbial fermentation and biomass fires, which accounts for the vast majority of chloromethane in the atmosphere. Chloromethane is primarily synthesized from methanol and hydrogen chloride, and also by the chlorination of methane.

Uses

The primary use of chloromethane is in the manufacture of silicones. Less common uses are in the production of methylcellulose, agrichemicals, butyl rubber, and quaternary amines. It was formerly used as a refrigerant and an anesthetic.

Environmental Fate and Behavior

Under ambient conditions, chloromethane exists as a gas in the air due to its high vapor pressure (4.3×10^3 mm Hg at 25 °C). Chloromethane discharged into the air is subjected to transport and diffusion into the stratosphere. Chloromethane gas is degraded in the atmosphere by reaction with photochemically produced hydroxyl radicals, with a half-life of $\sim$1 year. In water, it can degrade by hydrolysis or by biodegradation, but its main fate is volatilization, with a calculated half-life of 2.5 h for surface water, and 18 days for lake water. In groundwater, however, hydrolysis may be more significant, with an estimated half-life of 2.1 years at 20 °C under neutral conditions. Chloromethane has a low soil adsorption coefficient and is expected to have high mobility in soil. Any present near the soil surface is expected to volatilize, and any present in lower layers is expected to leach to lower horizons or to diffuse to the surface and volatilize. Chloromethane has a low potential for bioconcentration in aquatic organisms. It may be biodegraded in groundwater and soil.

Exposure and Exposure Monitoring

Chloromethane may be released into waste streams as a result of its production and use as a chemical intermediate. Workers may be exposed to chloromethane by inhalation and dermal contact where chloromethane is used or synthesized. The general population may be exposed to chloromethane by inhaling ambient air or drinking water containing chloromethane.

Toxicokinetics

Inhalation is the primary route of human exposure to chloromethane. The lungs quickly absorb the gas, blood levels reaching a steady-state concentration. Chloromethane has mixed uptake kinetics in rats, dogs, and humans, composed of a slow first-order process and a rapid, saturable, process that drives the overall uptake rate. Chloromethane is distributed to most organs and tissues, and there is limited evidence that it can be distributed transplacentally. The vast majority (>90%) of absorbed chloromethane is metabolized, approximately half of which is exhaled as CO_2.

The primary chloromethane metabolite is formaldehyde, which is formed by a glutathione (GSH)-mediated pathway. Formaldehyde is oxidized to formate by the GSH-dependent enzyme formaldehyde dehydrogenase. Formate enters the one-carbon pool, and can be incorporated into macromolecules (proteins, DNA, RNA) or converted to CO_2 via folate-dependent single-carbon pathways. The primary urinary metabolite in humans is S-methylcysteine. The urinary levels of S-methylcysteine in humans who inhale chloromethane fall into two groups, due to polymorphisms in the glutathione-S-transferase (GST) isozyme GSTT1-1. The isozyme has been found in human erythrocytes, liver, and kidneys. Examination of the GST activity toward chloromethane in erythrocyte preparations from a group of 45 volunteers showed that 60% had variable GST activity ('conjugators' or 'rapid metabolizers'), and the rest had no detectable activity ('non-conjugators' or 'slow metabolizers'). Results were not gender dependent. It is unknown if GST genotype affects the toxicological risk from chloromethane.

Mechanisms of Toxicity

The most marked effect of exposure to chloromethane in humans is central nervous system (CNS) toxicity, characterized by headache, nausea, vision disturbance, ataxia, muscle spasms, convulsions, and respiratory depression. Degenerative changes occur in the brain and spinal cord, and lesions are also seen in the liver, kidneys, lung, heart, and gastrointestinal (GI) tract. Similar toxic effects occurred in animal studies, including decrements in neurofunctional tests, weakness, cerebellar and testicular degeneration, and lesions in the liver, kidneys, and spleen.

The mode by which chloromethane causes toxicity in the CNS and other organs has not been elucidated. It has been

 http://dx.doi.org/10.1016/B978-0-12-386454-3.01115-5

proposed that chloromethane may be metabolized to methanethiol, which causes neurotoxic effects similar to those of chloromethane. The acute toxicity of chloromethane in the liver, kidneys, and brain of rats and mice was shown to be dependent on the presence of GSH, as pretreatment with inhibitors of GSH synthesis prevented the toxic effects. Chloromethane inhalation was shown to deplete the nonprotein sulfhydryl content and/or GSH levels in the liver, kidneys, and lungs in rats. The chloromethane-induced GSH depletion was associated with lipid peroxidation paralleling hepatocellular toxicity. The GSH depletion also inhibited the GSH-dependent enzyme formaldehyde dehydrogenase, which was postulated to lead to the accumulation of formaldehyde in tissues. Co-treatment with the anti-inflammatory agent BW755C reduced brain, liver, and kidney toxicity caused by chloromethane, suggesting that chloromethane may disturb prostaglandin or leukotriene metabolism.

Acute and Short-Term Toxicity

Animal

One study was located in which chloromethane was administered orally, in which rabbits were gavaged with chloromethane in olive oil for 60 doses over 83 or 85 days. The only treatment-related effect was toxicity of the spleen, characterized by congestion, phagocytosis, and hemosiderosis. In acute inhalation studies, cerebellar degeneration was the primary adverse effect in mice, rats, guinea pigs, dogs, and cats. Other effects included weakness and decrements in psychomotor performance. Lesions were seen in the testes and/or liver in some studies.

Human

No studies of human exposure to chloromethane by the oral or dermal route were located. Volunteers exposed to 20–150 ppm chloromethane for up to 7.5 h per day over 2–5 consecutive days had no detrimental effects on physiological, clinical, neurological, or cognitive parameters. Volunteers exposed for 3 h to 200 ppm had marginally decreased performance in several psychomotor tasks. Acute inhalation exposure to unspecified concentrations of chloromethane resulted in multiple symptoms of CNS depression, including headache, nausea, dizziness, disturbed vision, slurred speech, incoordination, muscle spasms, convulsions, respiratory depression, unconsciousness, and coma, and possibly elevated mortality from cardiovascular disease. Death resulted from acute exposure to $\geq$30 000 ppm in a number of case reports. Severe CNS toxicity was accompanied by degeneration of the brain and spinal cord, and also caused toxic changes in the liver, kidneys, lung, heart, and GI tract.

Chronic Toxicity

Animal

Chronic exposure led to cerebellar degenerative lesions, testicular lesions, renal toxicity, splenic atrophy, and hepatocellular lesions in rats and/or mice. In some cases, the effects occurred at concentrations that were lethal. The female C57BL/6 mouse appeared to be more susceptible to cerebellar lesions than the male, and both sexes of $B6C3F_1$ mice.

Human

No studies of human exposure to chloromethane by the oral or dermal route were located. Long-term inhalation of low levels of chloromethane ($<$50 ppm) was associated with CNS toxicity including fatigue, nausea, headache, disequilibrium, blurred vision, ataxia, confusion, personality changes, and short-term memory loss. Most of the effects were considered reversible.

Reproductive Toxicity

Rats exposed to $\geq$1000 ppm chloromethane had pathological changes in the testes and epididymis, low sperm count and quality, and dominant lethal effects were seen upon mating with unexposed females. Male rats exposed to 1500 ppm were infertile.

Heart malformations occurred in $B6C3F_1$ mouse fetuses exposed during gestation to 500–1500 ppm, more frequently in females than males. No embryotoxicity was seen in rats exposed to up to 1500 ppm during gestation.

Genotoxicity

Chloromethane is generally considered a weak mutagen. It had mutagenic or clastogenic activity in several test systems, albeit at high concentrations that were in some cases cytotoxic: exposure to $\geq$1000 ppm by inhalation *in vivo,* or to 0.5–30% v/v *in vitro.* Chloromethane was weakly mutagenic in several *Salmonella* strains, induced unscheduled DNA synthesis and sister chromatid exchanges, and enhanced viral transformation *in vitro.* Inhalation of chloromethane resulted in DNA–protein cross-links and DNA single-strand breaks in kidney tissue of male mice, sex-linked recessive lethal mutations in *Drosophila,* and dominant lethal effects in Sprague–Dawley rats, although the last was likely due to cytotoxic effects on the testes and epididymides.

Carcinogenicity

Several epidemiological studies found no association between occupational exposure to chloromethane and cancer at any site, or all cancers. In a 2-year inhalation study with rats and mice of both sexes, an increase in tumors was seen in only male mouse kidneys, and the relevance of this finding to humans was questionable. Due to the lack of adequate evidence in humans and experimental animals, the International Agency for Research on Cancer (IARC) concluded that chloromethane is not classifiable as to its carcinogenicity to humans (Group 3), and the U.S. EPA places it in carcinogenicity weight-of-evidence Group D – not classifiable as to its human carcinogenicity.

Clinical Management

Symptoms of severe chloromethane inhalation poisoning appear in humans after a latency period of 3–48 h, and include CNS effects (dizziness, visual changes, confusion, ataxia, drowsiness, delirium, convulsions, coma), respiratory effects (bronchospasm, respiratory failure, cyanosis), GI effects (nausea, vomiting, abdominal pain), anemia, hepatic and renal damage, and death. Chronic exposure symptoms include confusion, irritability, incoordination, vision disturbance, slurred speech, depression, and insomnia. Individuals exposed by inhalation should be moved to fresh air. Respiratory difficulty can be treated with oxygen and assist ventilation, and bronchospasm with inhaled beta2-agonists and oral or parenteral corticosteroids. Seizures can be treated with diazepam or lorazepam. Exposed persons should be monitored for hypotension, dysrhythmias, respiratory depression, urinary albumin and cells, fluid and electrolyte balance, liver enzymes, and blood counts. Recovery can occur within 5–6 h, but may take 30 days or more with very high exposure.

Direct skin contact with the liquefied gas or concentrated vapor can result in frostbite, anesthesia, erythema, and vesiculation. Persons exposed dermally should remove any contaminated clothing and wash the exposed area with soap and water. Eye exposure to chloromethane can result in irritation, pain, swelling, lacrimation, and photophobia. Exposed eyes should be irrigated 15 or more minutes with room temperature water unless frost injury has occurred. Persistent symptoms following dermal or eye exposure should be evaluated at a health care facility.

Ecotoxicity

Chloromethane has relatively low toxicity to aquatic organisms. The 96-h acute toxicity values for the freshwater fish bluegill sunfish (*Lepomis macrochirus*) and largemouth bass (*Micropterus salmoides*), and for the saltwater fish tidewater silverside (*Menidia beryllina*) ranged from 270 to 1500 mg l^{-1}. Toxicity threshold values in the 7-day cell multiplication inhibition test were 550 mg l^{-1} for the cyanobacteria *Microcystis aeruginosa*, 1450 mg l^{-1} for the green algae *Scenedesmus quadricauda*, and >8000 mg l^{-1} for the protozoa *Entosiphon sulcatum*. The 48-h EC_{50} value for *Daphnia magna* exposed in a closed system was 200 mg l^{-1}.

Gas production was inhibited in methanogenic bacteria at chloromethane concentrations of 50 mg l^{-1} and in *Nitrobacter* at >2 g ml^{-1}, and cell multiplication was inhibited at 500 mg l^{-1}. Exposure to $\geq$5000 mg m^{-3} chloromethane was toxic to a number of plant species, including wheat, soy beans, sugar beets, tomatoes, and sunflowers.

Exposure Standards and Guidelines

The U.S. Occupational Safety and Health Administration established a permissible exposure limit of 100 ppm as a time-weighted average (TWA) inhalation concentration for chloromethane, and a 200 ppm ceiling with a 5-min maximum peak of 300 ppm in any 3-h period. The American Conference of Government Industrial Hygienists determined a TWA threshold limit value (TLV-TWA) of 50 ppm and a short-term exposure limit of 100 ppm for occupational inhalation exposure.

The U.S. EPA Integrated Risk Information System (IRIS) program developed a reference concentration for chronic inhalation exposure of 9×10^{-2} mg m^{-3}, which was based on cerebellar lesions seen in female C57BL/6 mice exposed by inhalation continuously (22–22.5 h per day) for 11 days. IRIS did not develop a reference dose for chronic oral exposure.

The 2012 edition of the U.S. EPA Drinking Water Standards and Health Advisories lists 1- and 10-day health advisories of 9 mg l^{-1} and 0.4 mg l^{-1}, respectively, for a 10-kg child.

The Agency for Toxic Substances Disease Registry (ATSDR) developed an acute inhalation Minimal Risk Level (MRL) of 0.5 ppm based on impaired motor coordination and cerebellar lesions in female mice exposed by inhalation continuously for 11 days. The ATSDR based the intermediate inhalation MRL of 0.2 ppm on increased activities of liver enzymes in male mice after 6 months of intermittent chloromethane inhalation, and a chronic inhalation MRL of 0.05 ppm on axonal swelling seen after 2 years in male mice in the same study.

See also: Anesthetics; Neurotoxicity.

Further Reading

ATSDR (Agency for Toxic Substances and Disease Registry), December 1998. Toxicological Profile for Chloromethane (Update). Atlanta, GA.

ATSDR, June 24, 2009. Addendum to the Toxicological Profile for Chloromethane. Atlanta, GA.

CIIT (Chemical Industry Institute of Toxicology), 1981. Final Report on a Chronic Inhalation Toxicology Study in Rats and Mice Exposed to Methyl Chloride. Report Prepared by Battelle Columbus Laboratories for the Chemical Industry Institute of Toxicology. EPA/OTS Doc #878212061, NTIS/OTS0205952.

Dodd, D.E., Bus, J.S., Barrow, C.S., 1982. Nonprotein sulfhydryl alterations in F-344 rats following acute methyl chloride inhalation. Toxicol. Appl. Pharmacol. 62, 228–236.

HSDB (Hazardous Substances Data Bank), 2012. Methyl chloride. National Library of Medicine TOXNET database, National Institutes of Health, USA. Online at: http://toxnet.nlm.nih.gov – Toxnet (Toxicology Data Network): search under Toxline for Chloromethane.

SIDS (Screening Information Data Set for High Production Volume Chemicals), 2004. SIDS for methyl chloride. Online at: http://www.inchem.org/documents/sids/sids/CLMETHANE.pdf.

U.S. EPA (Environmental Protection Agency), 1986. Health and Environmental Effects Profile for Methyl Chloride. Document no. EPA/600/X-86/156. U.S. EPA Environmental Criteria and Assessment Office, Office of Health and Environmental Assessment, Office of Research and Development, Cincinnati, OH.

U.S. EPA, 1987. Health Effects Assessment for Chloromethane. Document no. EPA/600/8–88/024. U.S. EPA Environmental Criteria and Assessment Office, Office of Health and Environmental Assessment, Office of Research and Development, Cincinnati, OH.

U.S. EPA (Environmental Protection Agency), 2001a. Methyl chloride. Integrated Risk Information System (IRIS). Assessment last revised 7/17/2001. Online at: http://www.epa.gov/iris/subst/1003.htm. (accessed 8/2012).

U.S. EPA, 2001b. Toxicological review of methyl chloride in support of summary information on the Integrated Risk Information System (IRIS). National Center for Environmental Assessment, Washington, DC. Available online at: http://www.epa.gov/iris/toxreviews/1003tr.pdf#page=69.

U.S. EPA (Environmental Protection Agency), 2012. The 2012 edition of the drinking water standards and health advisories. Office of Water, U.S. Environmental Protection Agency Washington, DC. EPA 822-S-12-001. Spring 2012. Date of update: April, 2012. Online at: http://water.epa.gov/action/advisories/drinking/upload/dwstandards2012.pdf.

Chloromethyl Ether, Bis-

CV Rao,

- Name: Bis(choromethyl) ether
- Chemical Abstracts Service Registry Number: 542-88-1
- Synonyms: BCME, *sym*-Dichloromethyl ether, Dichloromethyl ether, Dichloromethyl ether
- Chemical/Pharmaceutical/Other Class: Alkyl organic synthetic compound with a strong unpleasant odor
- Molecular Formula: $C_2H_4OCl_2$
- Chemical Structure: $ClCH_2$–O–CH_2Cl

Uses

Bis(choromethyl) ether (BCME) is primarily used in the synthesis of polymers, ion exchange resins, and plastics. It is used as a chemical intermediate for the synthesis of other complex organic alkyl compounds as well as chloromethylating (cross-linking) reaction mixture in anion exchange resins. It is used as a dental restorative material.

In textile industry, it is used in laminating and as adhesive in the flocking of fabrics and in the finishing product of the fabrics as a mixture with formaldehyde containing reactants and resins. Nonwoven textile industry uses it as binder and thermosetting of acrylic emulsion.

Exposure Routes and Pathways

Primary routes of human exposure to BCME are inhalation and dermal contact, which might occur in chemical plants that make or use BCME. Also, some BCME may exist in chemical waste sites, which may be inhaled by breathing the air containing BCME vapors. The risk of potential occupational exposure to BCME is greatest for chemical plant workers, ion exchange resin makers, laboratory workers, and polymer makers. BCME is highly unstable in water, quickly breaking down into formaldehyde and hydrochloric acid. Therefore, exposure through water pollution is limited.

Toxicokinetics

BCME is rapidly absorbed through skin and lung surface. On contact with body fluids, it is quickly broken down to formaldehyde and hydrochloric acid and interacts with cells and tissues at various levels. Absorption by the body depends on the proximity to the source of production at the industry and at the waste dump site. BCME is mainly metabolized in the liver but to some extent it is also metabolized in the lung tissue. On metabolism, BCME is converted into an epoxide, which is a reactive species of free radical capable of reacting with any organic substance. Metabolites of BCME cause alkylation of DNA leading to mutagenesis and carcinogenesis. Glutathione *S*-transferase, sulfotransferase, and glucuronidation help in removal of toxic metabolites.

Mechanism of Toxicity

In humans, acute exposure to BCME may cause skin, mucous membrane, and respiratory tract irritation. Lung irritation, congestion, edema, and hemorrhage have been observed in rats and hamsters following acute inhalation exposure. BCME is irritating to the skin of mice and rabbits. Corneal opacity has been observed in rabbits. Acute animal tests in rats, mice, hamsters, and rabbits have demonstrated BCME to have extreme acute toxicity via inhalation and high acute toxicity via oral and dermal exposure. Chronic bronchitis, chronic cough, and impaired respiratory function have been observed in humans following chronic inhalation exposure. However, exposure to BCME usually occurs concurrently with exposure to chloromethyl methyl ether, which itself is a lung irritant. Chronic inhalation exposure of mice to BCME has been reported to cause respiratory distress.

Chronic Toxicity (or Exposure)

Animal

The International Agency for Research on Cancer (IARC) (1974, 1979, 1982, 1987) reported that there is sufficient evidence of carcinogenicity of BCME. When BCME is administered through subcutaneous route to mice of both sexes, it induced pulmonary tumors, papillomas, and fibrosarcomas; local sarcomas in female mice; and fibromas and fibrosarcomas in female rats. BCME is also an initiator of skin tumors in mice. It produced low incidence of tumors of respiratory tract in rats and hamsters after exposure by inhalation. When administered by inhalation, BCME induced lung tumors in mice and squamous cell carcinoma of the lung and esthesioneuroepitheliomas of the nasal cavity in rats. When applied topically, BCME induced papillomas, most of which developed into squamous cell carcinoma in female mice.

Human

BCME is known to be a human carcinogen based on sufficient evidence of carcinogenicity in humans. Numerous epidemiological studies and case reports from around the world have documented that workers exposed to BCME have an increased risk of lung cancer. Two studies of workers exposed to BCME showed an increased risk of lung cancer, mainly small cell carcinoma. Two subsequent studies have shown a positive association between atypical cells in bronchial excretion on exposure to BCME. Among heavily exposed workers, the relative risk of cancer is 10-fold or greater. Risks increase with duration and cumulative exposure. Maximal relative risks appear to occur 15–20 years after first exposure, and latency is shortened among workers with heavier exposure. Excess respiratory cancer mortality was most markedly increased in workers less than 55 years of age.

 http://dx.doi.org/10.1016/B978-0-12-386454-3.00280-3

The American Conference of Governmental Industrial Hygienists time-weighted average threshold limit value is 0.001 ppm (0.0047 mg m^{-3}) with the notation that material is a confirmed human carcinogen.

Clinical Management

There is no antidote recommended for poisoning by BCME. Administration of free radical scavengers should alleviate the toxicity.

Environmental Fate

No information is available on the transport and partitioning of BCME in the environment. Due to the relatively short half-life in both air and water, it is unlikely that significant partitioning between media or transport occurs. Primary process for BCME degradation in air is believed to be reaction with photochemically generated hydroxyl radicals to yield chloromethyl formate ClCHO, formaldehyde, and HCl. Atmospheric half-life due to reaction with hydroxyl radicals is estimated to be 1.36 h. Hydrolysis in the vapor phase is found to be slower with an estimated half-life of 25 h.

BCME is rapidly hydrolyzed in water to yield formaldehyde and HCl, and the hydrolysis rate constant is estimated to be 0.018 s^{-1} at 20 °C, which is equal to a half-life of ~35 s.

No information is available on the fate of BCME in soil. It is probable that BCME would rapidly degrade upon contact with moisture in soil. Due to its high volatile nature, it is not expected that BCME would persist in soil for significant periods.

Exposure Standards and Guidelines

The US Environmental Protection Agency (EPA) recommends that levels in lakes and streams should be limited to 0.0000038 ppb parts of water to prevent possible health effects from drinking water or eating fish contaminated with BCME. Any release to the environment greater than 10 lbs of BCME must be reported to the EPA.

The EPA calculated an inhalation unit risk estimate of 0.062 $\mu g^{-1} m^3$. The EPA estimates that, if an individual were to continuously breathe air containing BCME at an average of 0.000016 $\mu g\, m^{-3}$ (1.6×10^{-8} mg m^{-3}) over his or her entire lifetime, that person would theoretically have no more than a 1 in 10^6 increased chance of developing cancer as a direct result of breathing air containing this chemical. Similarly, the EPA estimates that breathing air containing 0.00016 $\mu g\, m^{-3}$ (1.6×10^{-7} mg m^{-3}) would result in not greater than a 1 in 10^5 increased chance of developing cancer, and air containing 0.0016 $\mu g\, m^{-3}$ (1.6×10^{-6} mg m^{-3}) would result in not greater than a 1 in 10^4 increased chance of developing cancer.

The EPA has calculated an oral cancer slope factor of 220 mg^{-1} kg day. The Occupational Safety and Health Administration has set a limit of 1 ppb as the highest acceptable level in workplace air, and strict controls have been established to minimize exposure to this chemical.

The Agency for Toxic Substances and Disease Registry has established an intermediate inhalation minimal risk level (MRL) of 0.0014 mg m^{-3} (0.0003 ppm) based on respiratory effects in rats. The MRL is an estimate of the daily human exposure to a hazardous substance that is likely to be without appreciable risk of adverse noncancer health effects over a specified duration of exposure. It is not a direct estimator of risk but rather a reference point to gauge the potential effects. At exposures increasingly greater than the MRL, the potential for adverse health effects increases.

See also: Polymers; Chemicals in Consumer Products.

Further Reading

American Conference of Governmental Industrial Hygienists (ACGIH), 1999. 1999 TLVs and BEIs. Threshold Limit Values for Chemical Substances and Physical Agents. Biological Exposure Indices. ACGIH, Cincinnati, OH.

Budavari, S. (Ed.), 1989. The Merck Index. An Encyclopedia of Chemicals, Drugs, and Biologicals, eleventh ed. Merck and Co. Inc., Rahway, NJ.

International Agency for Research on Cancer (IARC), 1974. IARC Monographs on the Evaluation of the Carcinogenic Risk of Chemicals to Man: Some Aromatic Amines, Hydrazine and Related Substances, *N*-Nitroso Compounds and Miscellaneous Alkylating Agents, Vol. 4. World Health Organization, Lyon, France.

International Agency for Research on Cancer (IARC) Monographs (1974, 1979, 1982, 1987).

Chlorophenols

M Badanthadka, Torrent Research Centre, Gujarat, India
HM Mehendale, University of Louisiana at Monroe, Monroe, LA, USA

- Representative Compound: Pentachlorophenol (PCP)
- Name: Pentachlorophenol
- Chemical Abstracts Service Registry Number: 87-86-5
- Synonym: 1-Hydroxy-2,3,4,5,6-pentachlorobenzene
- Molecular Formula: C_6HCl_5O
- Chemical Structure:

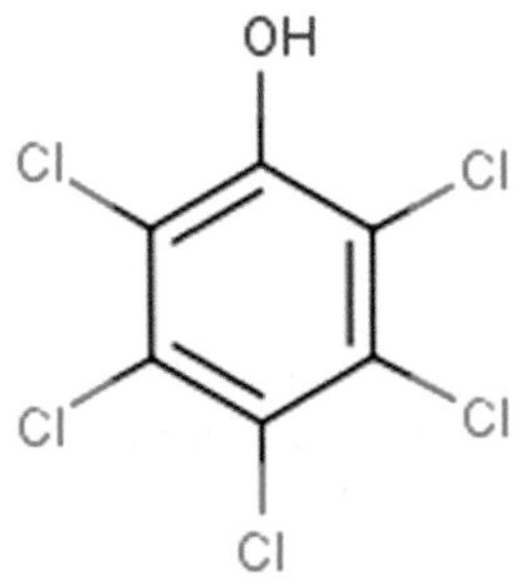

Background

Pentachlorophenol (PCP) is a synthetic substance made from other chemicals and does not occur naturally in the environment. At one time, it was one of the most widely used biocides in the United States. Since 1984, the purchase and use of PCP have been restricted to certified applications. It is no longer available to the general public. Before use restrictions, PCP was widely used as a wood preservative. It is now used industrially as a wood preservative for power line poles, cross arms, and fence posts.

PCP can be found in two forms: PCP and the sodium salt of PCP. The sodium salt dissolves easily in water but PCP does not. The physical properties of these two forms are different but their toxic effects are expected to be similar.

Humans are generally exposed to technical-grade PCP, which usually contains toxic impurities such as polychlorinated dibenzo-*p*-dioxins and dibenzofurans. In addition to workplace exposure, humans can be exposed to very low levels of PCP in indoor and outdoor air, food, soil, and drinking water. Exposure may also result from dermal contact with wood treated with preservatives that contain PCP.

Uses

Chlorophenols are used in the synthesis of dyes, fungicides, herbicides, wood preservatives, and as ingredients in alcohol denaturants.

Environmental Fate and Behavior

Production of PCP may result in its release to the environment through various waste streams; its use as a wood preservative and surface disinfectant can result in its direct release to the environment. Vapor-phase PCP is degraded into hydroxyl radicals by photochemical reaction. The half-life for this reaction in air is estimated to be 29 days.

If released into soil, PCP is expected to have low to no mobility based on measured values for the organic carbon partition coefficient (K_{oc}) ranging from 1250 for the dissociated form to 25 000 for the undissociated form. The dissociation constant (pK_a) of PCP is 4.70, indicating that this compound exists almost entirely in the anion form in the environment and anions generally do not adsorb more strongly to soils. Volatilization from moist soil is not expected because the acid exists as an anion and anions do not volatilize. PCP may not volatilize from dry soil surfaces based on its vapor pressure.

If released into water, PCP is expected to adsorb to suspended solids and sediment based on its measured K_{oc} values. Bioconcentration factor (BCF) values from approximately 5 to 5000 indicate that the bioconcentration of PCP in aquatic organisms is low to high; the value is greatly influenced by environmental pH. PCP is not expected to undergo hydrolysis in the environment due to the lack of functional groups that hydrolyze under environmental conditions.

The environmental impact of PCP increases when its many degradation products are taken into consideration. Biodegradation has been extensively studied in *Sphingobium chlorophenolicum* [ATCC 39723]. In water and under ambient conditions of temperature and pressure, it is completely destroyed at catalyst/substrate ratio of 1:715 within minutes.

Exposure and Exposure Monitoring

Exposure to chlorophenols may occur through ingestion, inhalation, or dermal contact at workplaces where it is used or produced. The major occupational exposure is to workers in the wood products industry. Air and urine samples taken at 25 factories using PCP as a wood preservative showed that the average worker's exposure in air was 0.013 mg m^{-3}. Elevated levels were found in the urine and serum of workers.

Toxicokinetics

Absorption of PCP is rapid through oral, dermal, or inhalation exposure. The major tissue deposits vary somewhat between species. In humans, the liver, kidneys, brain, spleen, and fatty tissue are the major deposition sites. In the mouse, the gall bladder is a principal storage site. In the rat, it is the kidneys. The primary route of elimination is through the kidneys in

 http://dx.doi.org/10.1016/B978-0-12-386454-3.00281-5

unchanged form. Labeled PCP given to rats by injection or oral route yielded 41–43% unchanged PCP in the urine. One metabolite, tetrachlorohydroquinone (5–24%), was identified. The elimination half-life for PCP may be up to 20 days in chronically exposed individuals.

In one study, a single dose of PCP (15 mg kg^{-1}) was administered intravenously and orally to B6C3F1 mice. After intravenous administration, the clearance values and volume of distribution were 0.057 ± 0.007 l h^{-1} kg^{-1} and 0.43 ± 0.06 l h^{-1} kg^{-1}, respectively. The elimination half-life was 5.2 ± 0.6 h. After oral administration, the peak plasma concentration (28 ± 7 μg ml^{-1}) occurred at 1.5 ± 0.5 h and bioavailability (1.06 ± 0.09) was complete. The elimination half-life was 5.8 ± 0.6 h. Only 8% of the PCP dose was excreted unchanged in the urine. PCP was primarily recovered in urine as glucuronide and sulfate conjugate metabolites. A portion of the dose was recovered in urine as tetrachlorohydroquinone (5%) and its conjugates (15%). For both PCP and tetrachlorohydroquinone, sulfates accounted for 90% or more of the total conjugates.

There are marked gender differences in the biological half-life in non-human primates. The biological half-life for excretion in Rhesus monkeys was 41 and 92 h in males and females, respectively.

Mechanism of Toxicity

Chlorophenols block ATP production without blocking the electron transport chain. They inhibit mitochondrial oxidative phosphorylation, thereby causing accelerated aerobic metabolism. This increases the basal metabolic rate and body temperature, which leads to clinical hyperthermia. As body temperature rises, heat-dissipating mechanisms are overcome and metabolism is accelerated. ADP and other substrates accumulate and stimulate the electron transport chain further. This process demands more oxygen in a futile effort to produce ATP. This oxygen demand quickly surpasses the oxygen supply, and energy reserves of the body become depleted.

Acute and Short-Term Toxicity

Animal

The lethal dose 50% (LD_{50}) for PCP in laboratory animals ranges from 30 to 100 mg kg^{-1}.

Human

The most prevalent signs and symptoms after ingestion of 30–250 ml of chlorophenols are corrosion of tissue, profuse sweating, intense thirst, nausea, vomiting, diarrhea, convulsions, pulmonary edema, cyanosis, and coma. If death from respiratory failure is not immediate, jaundice and oliguria or anuria may occur.

Chronic Toxicity (or Exposure)

Human Toxicity

Repeated exposure may cause symptoms of acute poisoning. Skin sensitivity reactions occur occasionally. Prolonged skin contact with chlorophenols may cause bladder tumors, hemolytic anemia, and lens opacities.

Pathologic findings after death due to chlorophenols include necrosis of mucous membranes, cerebral edema, and degenerative changes in the liver and kidneys.

Immunogenicity

The immunogenic effects of PCP were evaluated by checking the frequency of lymphocyte phenotypes, functional responses, serum immunoglobulin levels, and autoantibodies in 38 individuals who were exposed to PCP in manufacturer-treated log houses. A comparison of subjects with controls revealed that the exposed individuals had activated T cells, autoimmunity, functional immunosuppression, and B-cell dysregulation. Autoimmunity was shown by elevation of TA1 phenotype frequencies and a 21% incidence of anti-smooth muscle antibody. Functional immunosuppression was shown by the significantly reduced responses to all mitogens tested and to allogeneic lymphocytes in the mixed lymphocyte culture test. There was a significant elevation of CD10, and an 18% increase or decrease in serum immunoglobulins was noted. A striking anomaly was the enhanced natural killer activity found in exposed females but not in males.

An *in vitro* experimental study showed a significant decrease in the tumor-killing (lytic) function of human natural killer cells indicating signs of immune alteration.

Reproductive Toxicity

Overexposure may cause reproductive disorder(s) based on tests with laboratory animals.

PCP was administered to dams and their offspring via drinking water (6.6 mg l^{-1}) during gestation and the lactation period. Tissue samples were obtained from dams, 3-week-old weanling pups, and 12-week-old pups. The results show that PCP exposure during development causes thyroid function vulnerability, testicular hypertrophy in adults, and aberrations in brain gene expression.

Embryo–fetal toxicity and the teratogenic potential of PCP were studied following oral gavage to presumed pregnant female Sprague–Dawley rats. Doses of 0 (corn oil), 10, 30, and 80 mg kg^{-1} day^{-1} were administered to the rats at concentrations of 0, 2, 6, and 16 mg ml^{-1}, respectively, from day 6 to day 15 of presumed gestation. The dose volume was 5 ml kg^{-1}. Rats were sacrificed on day 20 of presumed gestation and necropsied. The no observed adverse effect level (NOAEL) for maternal toxicity and developmental NOAEL in rats were also found to be 30 mg kg^{-1} day^{-1}. The lowest observed adverse effect level (LOAEL) for PCP developmental toxicity (80 mg kg^{-1} day^{-1}) was associated with increased resorption, reduced live litter size, and fetal body weight, and caused increased malformations and variations.

The potential of PCP to induce general and reproductive/developmental toxicity was evaluated in Crl Sprague–Dawley rats, using a two-generation reproduction toxicity study. PCP was administered by gavage at doses of 0, 10, 30, and

60 mg kg^{-1} day^{-1}. It was concluded that 30 mg kg^{-1} day^{-1} is the LOAEL and 10 mg kg^{-1} day^{-1} is the NOAEL for both reproductive and general toxicity. In addition, the results did not indicate bioaccumulation and thereby PCP did not selectively affect reproduction or development of the offspring of rats at a dose of 10 mg kg^{-1} day^{-1}, a dose that is much higher than human exposure.

Genotoxicity

PCP seems to be a weak inducer of DNA damage and has gentotoxic potential. It does not produce DNA strand breaks or clear differential toxicity to bacteria in the rec-assay in the absence of metabolic activation. Also in the sister–chromatid exchange induction assay, no increase can be observed *in vivo*, but PCP was found to be marginally active in *in vitro* experiments.

An *in vivo* study on the genotoxic effects of PCP was carried out using freshwater fish (*Channa punctatus*). The fish were exposed to three sublethal doses of PCP (0.2, 0.4, and 0.6 ppm) by medium treatment. The results confirmed the genotoxicity of PCP in this organism.

Chromosome analyses were carried out on peripheral lymphocytes from 22 male workers employed at a factory producing PCP. A small but significant increase in the frequency of dicentrics and acentrics was observed, suggesting that PCP has a genotoxic effect.

Carcinogenicity

There is limited evidence of carcinogenicity of PCP in humans. The evidence is based on assays that utilized less than pure PCP. Contaminants of PCP include tri- or tetrachlorophenol, hexachlorobenzene, polychlorinated dibenzo-*p*-dioxins, or polychlorinated dibenzofurans. Indications are that the positive evidence for carcinogenicity is from the contaminant(s) and not the PCP. This product is, or contains, a component that has been reported to be possibly carcinogenic based on its International Agency for Research on Cancer (IARC), American Conference of Governmental Industrial Hygienists (ACGIH), National Toxicology Program (NTP), or Environmental Protection Agency (EPA) classification. Additionally, there is sufficient evidence in experimental animals for the carcinogenicity of PCP. Therefore, PCP is a probable human carcinogenic agent based on inadequate human data and sufficient evidence of carcinogenicity in animals.

Clinical Management

After exposure by ingestion, if corrosive injury is absent, decontamination to prevent further absorption may be achieved using activated charcoal. Emesis by syrup of ipecac may be considered, but is not preferred. Next, milk should be given to drink. Gastric lavage and emesis are contraindicated in the presence of esophageal injury. In the case of dermal exposure, the poison should be removed by washing the affected skin or mucous membrane with copious amounts of water for at least 15 min.

Ecotoxicology

Classification and K_{oc} values indicate that PCP is expected to adsorb to suspended solids and sediment in water. pK_a values indicate that PCP exists almost entirely in the anion form at pH 5–9 and, therefore, volatilization from water surfaces is not expected to be an important fate process. BCF values suggest that the bioconcentration in aquatic organisms is low to very high; this value is greatly influenced by the environmental pH. PCP rapidly photodegrades in surface water when exposed to direct sunlight; the half-life for photolysis in solution has been reported to be 0.86 h.

Effect of PCP on Aquatic Organisms

Organism	*Effect*
Golden orfe	LC_{50} 0.60 mg l^{-1} (96 h)
Rainbow trout	LC_{50} 0.12–0.26 mg l^{-1} (96 h)
Water flea	LC_{50} 0.33–0.41 mg l^{-1} (96 h)
Bacteria (div.)	NOEC 12.3 mg l^{-1} (30 min), growth
Algae	EC_{50} 10–7000 μg l^{-1} (96 h), growth

EC_{50}, half maximal effective dose; LC_{50}, lethal concentration 50%; NOEC, no observed effect concentration.

Toxicity to Marine Organisms

Reported lethal (effect) concentration 50% [L(E)C_{50}] data ranging from 0.6 to 19.5, 2.55 to 29.7, and 5 to 7 mg l^{-1} for algae, crustaceans, and fish, respectively, indicate moderate to high acute toxicity.

The toxicity of chlorophenols to aquatic organisms increases with an increase in the degree of chlorination and substitution away from the *ortho* position. The higher toxicity of the more highly chlorinated congeners can be ascribed to an increase in lipophilicity, which leads to a greater potential for uptake into the organism. *Ortho*-substituted congeners are generally of lower toxicity than the *meta*- and *para*-substituted compounds, as the close proximity of the *ortho*-substituted chlorine to the OH group on the molecule appears to shield the OH, which apparently interacts with the active site in aquatic organisms, causing the observed toxic effects. Toxicity also depends on the extent to which the chlorophenol molecules are dissociated in the exposure medium.

No data could be located for sediment-dwelling organisms.

Exposure Standards and Guidelines

The Occupational Safety and Health Administration permissible exposure limit is 0.5 mg m^{-3} for the 8-h time-weighted average (TWA). The threshold limit value is 0.5 mg m^{-3} for the 8-h TWA. The National Institute of Occupational Safety and Health recommended exposure limit is 0.5 mg m^{-3} for the 10-h TWA.

See also: Chlorophenoxy Herbicides; Drugs of Abuse; Dyes and Colorants.

Further Reading

Aoyama, H., Hojo, H., Takahashi, K.L., et al., 2005. A two-generation reproductive toxicity study of 2,4-dichlorophenol in rats. J. Toxicol. Sci. 30, 59–78.

Bernard, B.K., Hoberman, A.M., 2001. A study of the developmental toxicity potential of PCP in the rat. Int. J. Toxicol. 20, 353–362.

Bernard, B.K., Hoberman, A.M., Brown, W.R., Ranpuria, A.K., Christian, M.S., 2002. Oral (gavage) two-generation (one litter per generation) reproduction study of pentachlorophenol (penta) in rats. Int. J. Toxicol. 21, 301–318.

Farah, M.A., Ateeq, B., Ali, M.N., Ahmad, W., 2003. Evaluation of genotoxicity of PCP and 2,4-D by micronucleus test in freshwater fish Channa punctatus. Ecotoxicol. Environ. Safety 54, 25–29.

Gupta, S.S., Stadler, M., Noser, C.A., et al., 2002. Rapid total destruction of chlorophenols by activated hydrogen peroxide. Science 296, 326–328.

Huang, Y., Xun, R., Chen, G., Xun, L., 2008. Maintenance role of a glutathionyl-hydroquinone lyase (PcpF) in pentachlorophenol degradation by Sphingobium chlorophenolicum ATCC 39723. J. Bacteriol. 190, 7595–7600.

Jensen, J., 1996. Chlorophenols in the terrestrial environment. Rev. Environ. Contam. Toxicol. 146, 25–51.

Kawaguchi, M., Morohoshi, K., Saita, E., et al., 2008. Developmental exposure to pentachlorophenol affects the expression of thyroid hormone receptor beta1 and synapsin I in brain, resulting in thyroid function vulnerability in rats. Endocrine 33, 277–284.

McLellan, I., Carvalho, M., Silva Pereira, C., et al., 2007. The environmental behaviour of polychlorinated phenols and its relevance to cork forest ecosystems: a review. J. Environ. Monitor. 9, 1055–1063.

Nnodu, U., Whalen, M.M., 2008. Pentachlorophenol decreases ATP levels in human natural killer cells. J. Appl. Toxicol. 28, 1016–1020.

Triebig, G., Csuzda, I., Krekeler, H.J., Schaller, K.H., 1987. Pentachlorophenol and the peripheral nervous system: a longitudinal study in exposed workers. Br. J. Indus. Med. 44, 638–641.

Relevant Websites

http://toxnet.nlm.nih.gov – TOXNET, Specialized information Service, National Library of Medicine, Search for Chlorophenols.

http://www.atsdr.cdc.gov – Agency for Toxic Substances and Disease Registry. Toxicological Profile for chlorophenols.

http://www.inchem.org – IPCS – International Programme on Chemical Safety, search for pentachlorophenol.

http://www.epa.gov – Advanced search for chlorophenols

Chlorophenoxy Herbicides

S Karanth, Charles River Laboratories, Reno, NV, USA

- Name: Chlorophenoxy herbicides
- Chemical Structure: 2,4-D

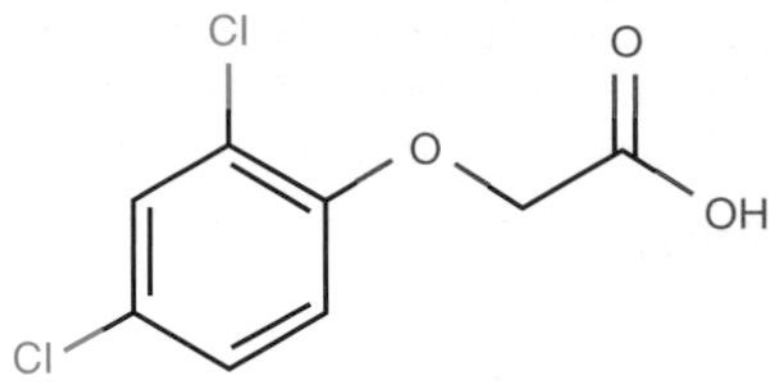

Background

A mixture of the chlorophenoxy herbicides 2,4-dichlorophenoxy acetic acid (2,4-D) and 2,4,5-trichlorophenoxy acetic acid (2,4,5-T), known as Agent Orange, was extensively used by the US military during Vietnam War in order to destroy forest and other vegetation from the premises of US bases. About 19 million gallons of Agent Orange was used on approximately 3.6 million acres of land in Vietnam and Laos during the period from 1962 to 1971. Some lots of 2,4,5-T were contaminated with dioxins formed during manufacturing. Because dioxins resist degradation and remain in the environment for years, they are considered persistent organic pollutants. The main dioxin present in Agent Orange, 2,3,7,8-tetrachlorodibenzo-*p*-dioxin, or TCDD, is one of the most acutely toxic synthetic chemicals known. TCDD levels were found to be higher among veterans serving in Vietnam compared to those serving elsewhere at the same time. Concerns that these and other health problems may have been associated with exposure to Agent Orange stimulated a series of scientific studies, health care programs, and compensation programs directed in support of veterans.

Uses

Chlorophenoxy herbicides are commonly used for controlling broadleaf weeds in agriculture. They are extensively used for the control of vegetation along highways, maintenance of parks, golf courses, home lawns, and gardens.

Environmental Fate

Chlorophenoxy herbicides are generally not persistent in the environment. Common herbicides such as 2,4-D, 2-(4-chloro2-methylphenoxy)propionic acid, and dicamba are readily biodegraded by soil and aquatic microorganisms. 2,4-D and dicamba are commonly found in public drinking water systems. Typical half-life in water ranges from 10 to 15 days and biodegradation is the primary route of elimination.

Exposure and Exposure Monitoring

Chlorophenoxy herbicides can be absorbed into the body by inhalation of its aerosol, through the skin, and by ingestion. The most common exposure pathway is accidental or intentional ingestion. The monitoring data indicate that 2,4-D is detected in groundwater and surface water.

Toxicokinetics

Chlorophenoxy herbicides are readily absorbed through the gastrointestinal tract and distributed throughout the body. They are excreted unchanged mainly in the urine and are generally not stored in the body. Studies in laboratory rats given 1, 5, or 10 mg kg^{-1} of ^{14}C 2,4-D have shown that 94–99% is eliminated from the body unchanged within 72 h. Biological half-life ranged from 10 to 33 h.

Mechanism of Toxicity

The mechanism of action of chlorophenoxy herbicides in mammals is not clearly known. They are believed to elicit toxicity by cell membrane damage, uncoupling of oxidative phosphorylation, or disruption of acetylcoenzyme A metabolism. Myotonia (stiffness and incoordination of hind extremities) is commonly observed following overdose of 2,4-D. In addition, high doses can cause significant metabolic acidosis and renal failure in humans. Formulations of chlorophenoxy herbicides were often contaminated by complex chlorinated hydrocarbons; for example, dibenzodioxins. TCDD, which is highly toxic to mammals, was one of the common dioxin pollutants in Agent Orange.

Acute and Short-Term Toxicity

Animal

Chlorophenoxy herbicides exhibit low mammalian toxicity. The acute oral LD_{50} for 2,4-D in rats is 4300 mg kg^{-1}. Dogs are more susceptible to 2,4-D poisoning with an oral LD_{50} of 100 mg kg^{-1}.

Human

Ingestion of high doses of chlorophenoxy herbicides can lead to burning of the mouth, vomiting, abdominal pain, and gastrointestinal hemorrhage. Acute exposure may also cause severe metabolic acidosis, myotonia, and muscle weakness, which can persist for a long period of time.

 http://dx.doi.org/10.1016/B978-0-12-386454-3.00114-7

Chronic Toxicity

Animal

Long-term feeding studies in rats have revealed that exposure to a daily dosage of 300 mg kg^{-1} day^{-1} does not cause any adverse effects while exposure to higher doses can result in body weight loss.

Human

Chronic exposure to some common chlorophenoxy herbicides such as 2,4-D through drinking water can potentially cause damage to the nervous system, kidneys, and liver. Chronic exposure to 2,4-D has also been linked to immune system suppression and endocrine disruption. 2,4-D and 4-chloro-2methyl-phenoxy acetic acid, which are commonly used in wheat production, have been linked to birth defects. While carcinogenic potential of these herbicides is not clear, case-control studies conducted in Sweden showed a statistically significant association between exposure to chlorophenoxy herbicides and the occurrence of soft-tissue sarcomas.

Immunotoxicity

A study evaluating the overall immunologic spectrum of the Vietnam War Korean veterans exposed to Agent Orange contaminated with TCDD suggested an overall association between Agent Orange exposure and immune homeostasis resulting in dysregulation of B- and T-cell activities.

Reproductive Toxicity

Reproductive toxicity, characterized as an increase in gestation length, was observed following exposure to 2,4-D at a dose level above the threshold of saturation of renal clearance. Developmental toxicity, characterized mainly as an increased incidence of skeletal abnormalities in the rat, was observed following exposure to 2,4-D and its amine salts and esters at dose levels that were at or above the threshold of saturation of renal clearance. Similarly, developmental toxicity was observed in a rabbit study following exposure to 2,4-D (abortions) and diethanolamine salt of 2,4-D (DEA) (increased number of litters with fetuses having seventh cervical ribs) at or above the threshold of renal clearance. Reduced fetal viability was observed in hamsters following maternal dosing at 40 mg kg^{-1} day^{-1} during pregnancy, although these effects did not follow a dose–response relationship.

Genotoxicity

2,4-D is not genotoxic. There is considerable evidence that TCDD does not damage DNA directly through the formation of DNA adducts; however, TCDD may be indirectly genotoxic.

Carcinogenicity

The Institute of Medicine studies concluded that there was sufficient evidence of an association between Agent Orange and soft-tissue sarcomas, non-Hodgkin's lymphoma (NHL), Hodgkin disease, and chronic lymphocytic leukemia. Regulatory agencies have relatively similar conclusions regarding carcinogenicity of chlorophenoxy herbicides and TCDD. The US National Toxicology Program does not list chlorophenoxy herbicides (including Agent Orange) as carcinogens, but lists 2,3,7,8-TCDD as 'known to be a human carcinogen.' The International Agency for Research on Cancer has not rated Agent Orange itself, but the chlorophenoxy herbicides including 2,4-D and 2,4,5-T are categorized as 'possibly carcinogenic to humans' while 2,3,7,8-TCDD is categorized as 'known to be carcinogenic to humans.' In contrast, the US Environmental Protection Agency has not classified either chlorophenoxy herbicides or TCDD as to carcinogenicity.

Clinical Management

Chlorophenoxy compounds are moderately irritating to skin. In case of dermal or eye exposure, the contaminated area should be bathed or flushed with copious amounts of water for at least 15 min, and if irritation persists a physician should be contacted. Ingestion of substantial amounts of these chemicals results in spontaneous emesis. If the patient is fully alert and there are no apparent signs of emesis, emesis should be induced with syrup of ipecac (adults, 30 ml; children <12 years, 15 ml), followed by one to two glasses of water. In order to limit the absorption of the herbicide in the gut, 30–50 g of activated charcoal can be administered in approximately 6–8 ounces of water. Severe intoxication with chlorophenoxy compounds may result in renal failure. To avoid toxicant buildup in the kidney and to accelerate excretion, intravenous fluids (saline or dextrose) can be administered and serum electrolytes should be monitored. Early initiation of forced alkaline diuresis with sodium bicarbonate may be useful in the management of acute poisoning.

Ecotoxicology

Some of the commercial products containing chlorophenoxy herbicides are highly toxic to aquatic invertebrates and other beneficial nontarget plants.

Exposure Standards and Guidelines

Acceptable daily intake for 2,4-D = 0.01 mg kg^{-1} body weight.

Chronic reference dose for 2,4-D = 0.005 mg kg^{-1} day^{-1}.

See also: Ecotoxicology; Pesticides.

Further Reading

Boers, D., Portengen, L., Turner, W.E., Bueno-de-Mesquita, H.B., Heederik, D., Vermeulen, R., 2012. Plasma dioxin levels and cause-specific mortality in an occupational cohort of workers exposed to chlorophenoxy herbicides, chlorophenols and contaminants. Occup. Environ. Med. 69, 113–118.

Kim, H.A., Kim, E.M., Park, Y.C., Yu, J.Y., Hong, S.K., Jeon, S.H., Park, K.L., Hur, S.J., Heo, Y., 2003. Immunotoxicological effects of Agent Orange exposure to the Vietnam War Korean veterans. Ind. Health 41, 158–166.

Ünal, F., Yüzbaşõoğlu, D., Yilmaz, S., Akinci, N., Aksoy, H., October 2011. Genotoxic effects of chlorophenoxy herbicide diclofop-methyl in mice in vivo and in human lymphocytes in vitro. Drug Chem. Toxicol. 34 (4), 390–395.

Von Stackelberg, K., 2013. A systematic review carcinogenic outcomes and potential mechanisms from exposure to 2,4-D and MCPA in the environment. J. Toxicol. 2013, 53. http://dx.doi.org/10.1155/2013/371610. Article ID 371610.

Relevant Websites

http://www.cancer.org – American Cancer Society.

http://edis.ifas.ufl.edu/pdffiles/PI/PI12000.pdf – University of Florida: Pesticide Toxicity Profile: Chlorophenoxy Herbicides.

http://extoxnet.orst.edu – Extension Toxicology Network, Oregon State University.

http://infoventures.com – US Department of Agriculture, Forest Service.

http://www.epa.gov/teach/chem_summ/24D_summary.pdf – Environmental Protection Agency.

http://www.inchem.org/documents/iarc/suppl7/chlorophenoxyherbicides.html – International Programme on Chemical Safety, INCHEM.

Chloropicrin

P Raman, Northeast Ohio Medical University, Rootstown, OH, USA

- Name: Chloropicrin
- Chemical Abstracts Service Registry Number: 76-06-2
- Synonyms: Trichloronitromethane; Nitrochloroform; Nitrotrichloromethane; Acquinite; Larvicide
- Molecular Formula: CCl_3NO_2
- Chemical Structure:

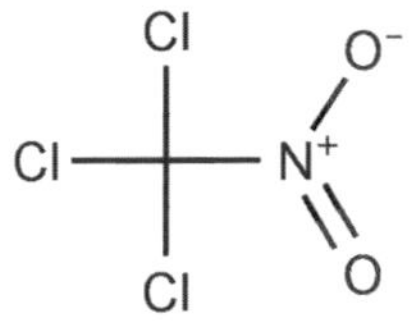

Background

Chloropicrin is a colorless to faint-yellow oily liquid with an intensely irritating and sharp odor with characteristics of tear gas. Some common trade names of products containing chloropicrin include Dolochlor, Aquinite, Nemax, Pic-Chlor, Timberfume, Profume A, Tri-Clor, and Microlysin. It has a molecular weight of 164.38, water solubility of 2000 mg l^{-1} at 25 °C, and melting and boiling points of −64 and 112 °C, respectively. Chloropicrin is nonflammable and has a vapor density of 5.7 compared to the vapor density of one assigned to air. Heating above 234 °F results in explosive decomposition of chloropicrin, leading to the release of toxic gases, including nitrogen oxides, phosgene, nitrosyl chloride, chlorine, and carbon monoxide. Chloropicrin is a widely used fungicide that is primarily used for preplant soil fumigation. Chloropicrin is used to fumigate stored grain and to treat soil against fungi, insects, and nematodes either as a stand-alone treatment or in combination with other fumigants like methyl bromide and sulfuryl fluoride for enhanced potency. Chloropicrin is also used to prevent internal decay of wood poles and timber caused by fungi and insects.

Chloropicrin was first synthesized in 1848 by a Scottish chemist named John Stenhouse by interaction of a chlorinating agent with picric acid. It was patented as an insecticide in 1908 and has been extensively used since then as a soil fumigant at high application rates of 18 lb $acre^{-1}$. Chloropicrin was extensively used as a chemical warfare and riot control agent during World War I; however, it is not authorized for military use any longer. It is manufactured by reacting nitromethane with sodium hypochlorite. It is extremely toxic (Category: 5), and estimated probable oral lethal dose for humans ranges from 5 to 50 mg kg^{-1}; between seven drops and one teaspoonful for a 70 kg person (150 lb). Additional reports suggest that exposure to chloropicrin at 2.00 mg l^{-1} (300 ppm) for 10 min or 0.80 mg l^{-1} (120 ppm) for 30 min was lethal.

The most recent large-scale exposure occurred in Kern County, California, in 2003. One hundred sixty-five people developed symptoms as a result of off-site drift of chloropicrin from a nearby agricultural site. Peak concentrations of chloropicrin were estimated to exceed one part per million. Nearly all (99%) of those exposed experienced eye pain, burning, or lacrimation. Fifty-one percent experienced respiratory symptoms, including cough, dyspnea, or upper respiratory irritation. Nearly half (47%) complained of gastrointestinal complaints such as nausea, vomiting, abdominal pain, or diarrhea, and 25% complained of headache.

Uses

Chloropicrin is classified as a Toxicity Category I pesticide by the US Environmental Protection Agency (EPA) for acute oral, dermal, and inhalation toxicity. The EPA classified all products containing more than 2% chloropicrin as restricted use pesticides to be used only under the supervision of certified applicators, owing to its acute inhalation toxicity. Chloropicrin-containing products are registered as preplant fumigants for crops such as asparagus, broccoli, carrots, cauliflower, celery, eggplant, lettuce, and onions and fruit crops such as melons, grapes, pineapples, raspberries, strawberries, as well as floral and nut crops.

Environmental Fate and Behavior

The half-life of chloropicrin in sandy loam soil was 8–24 h and 4.5 days, with carbon dioxide being the terminal breakdown product. Chloropicrin can be produced during chlorination of drinking water in the presence of nitrated organic contaminants. If released to air, a vapor pressure of 23.8 mm Hg at 25 °C indicates chloropicrin will exist solely as a vapor in the atmosphere. Vapor-phase chloropicrin will be degraded in the atmosphere by reaction with photochemically-produced hydroxyl radicals; the half-life for this reaction in air is estimated to be 123 days. Chloropicrin absorbs UV light in the 280–390 nm range and therefore may be susceptible to direct photolysis. The photolysis products of chloropicrin are phosgene, nitric oxide, chlorine, nitrogen dioxide, and dinitrogen tetroxide. Chloropicrin dissipates from soil primarily via volatilization followed by chemical degradation and microbial decomposition. Under reducing conditions, chloropicrin is capable of undergoing reductive dechlorination. The calculated Henry's Law constant is 2.51×10^{-3} atm-m^3 mol^{-1} at 25 °C. Chloropicrin does not move rapidly in aquatic environment, since it is only slightly water soluble. Field volatility data suggest that substantial portions of applied chloropicrin are emitted from soil. Chloropicrin is susceptible to rapid degradation in soil both under aerobic and anaerobic conditions.

Exposure Routes and Pathways

Chloropicrin has strong lacrimatory properties and is a potent skin irritant. Thus, dermal and eye exposures are the most common routes of chloropicrin toxicity. It is also an inducer of

 http://dx.doi.org/10.1016/B978-0-12-386454-3.00282-7

vomiting, bronchitis, and pulmonary edema in humans. As a fumigant, the respiratory tract is the principal target of chloropicrin toxicity. The primary lesion following ingestion of chloropicrin is manifested by corrosive effects on the forestomach tissue. The intraperitoneal LD_{50} in mice is 25 mg kg^{-1}. Human exposure to chloropicrin also occurs from trace levels in drinking water disinfected by chlorination.

Toxicokinetics

The toxic effects of chloropicrin occur very rapidly. The liver is the primary site of metabolism of this compound. Reductive dechlorination of chloropicrin serves as the basis for its multiple types of toxic action. Following an intraperitoneal or oral administration of chloropicrin, urine is the major route for excretion of its metabolites, mostly (43–47%) within the first 24 h. The urinary metabolites at 24 h are polar and nonvolatile.

Mechanism of Toxicity

Recent studies identify a new metabolic pathway for chloropicrin involving a rapid dechlorination to $CHCl_2NO_2$ and conversion of glutathione (GSH) to glutathione disulfide (GSSG) plus possible adduct formation with thiol proteins. In this newly discovered pathway, chloropicrin is metabolized to thiophosgene, characterized as the cyclic cysteine adduct (raphanusamic acid) in mice urine. The initially formed $GSCCl_2NO_2$ metabolite is proposed to either react further with GSH or is cleaved by cysteine-β-lyase, ultimately leading to raphanusamic acid, which is excreted. Chloropicrin is an SN_2 alkylating agent with an activated halogen group and reacts with sulfhydryl groups, 'fixing' enzymes. Oxidation of protein thiols with chloropicrin is accompanied with the formation of internal and cross-linked disulfide bonds, leading to the suggestion that inhibition of pyruvate dehydrogenase (PDH) and succinate dehydrogenase (SDH) with critical SH groups in their active sites is involved in acute mammalian toxicity. Both PDH and SDH complexes are inhibited *in vitro* by chloropicrin with moderate potency ($IC_{50} = 4$–13 μmol l^{-1}). Chloropicrin also has the additional toxic effect of interfering with oxygen transport by its reaction with SH–groups in hemoglobin. Thus, chloropicrin toxicity in mice is linked to the accumulation of oxyhemoglobin in tissues, particularly the liver. Chloropicrin may also undergo a photochemical transformation to phosgene.

Acute and Short-Term Toxicity (or Exposure)

Animal

Chloropicrin is 10 times more potent than its dehalogenated metabolites. It has been reported to inhibit porcine heart pyruvate and mouse liver succinate dehydrogenase complexes with IC_{50} values of 4 and 13 μmol l^{-1}, respectively. Mice treated intraperitoneally with chloropicrin at 50 mg kg^{-1} showed a dose-dependent increase in liver oxyhemoglobin, hemoprotein, and total hemoglobin levels. Acute toxicity of chloropicrin in mice is due to the parent compound or metabolites other than $CHCl_2NO_2$ or CH_2ClNO_2. In rats, the respiratory tract is the primary target on inhalation exposure. Chloropicrin is intensely irritating with an intraperitoneal LD_{50} of 25 mg kg^{-1} in mice. Rabbits exposed to an intravenous injection of chloropicrin at a dosage of 15 mg kg^{-1} died within 15–240 min; clinical and autopsy findings were typical of acute pulmonary edema. Chloropicrin induces lesions in the lower respiratory tract with an RD_{50} (concentration that elicits a respiratory rate decrease of 50%) values of 8 ppm. The no observed adverse effect level (NOAEL) for systemic toxicity following chloropicrin exposure is reported to be 1.0 ppm and greater than 1.5 ppm for developmental toxicity and reproductive parameters. The NOAEL for maternal toxicity has been established to be 0.4 ppm, and the NOAEL for fetal toxicity is 1.2 ppm suggesting that the developing fetus is not a target tissue for chloropicrin toxicity.

Human

Exposure to chloropicrin causes eye and respiratory tract irritation accompanied by vomiting and diarrhea. The primary signs and symptoms following inhalation exposure to chloropicrin include coughing, nasal and pharyngeal mucosal edema, and erythema, lacrimation, and rhinorrhea. Fatal pulmonary edema has been reported with an onset of 3 h postexposure. Chloropicrin is a strong eye irritant, producing ocular burning, eye pain, and lacrimation following eye exposure. These effects may last up to 30 min or longer. Redness and edema may be noted 1 or 2 days following exposure. Dermal exposure to chloropicrin produces severe skin irritation.

Chronic Toxicity (or Exposure)

Animal

Following an oral gavage for 90 days, the no-effect dose is 8 mg kg^{-1} per day, with severe forestomach tissue lesions characterized by inflammation, necrosis, acantholysis, hyperkeratosis, and epithelial hyperplasia. Mice exposed to 8 ppm chloropicrin vapor for 6 h day^{-1} for 5 days developed moderate to severe degeneration of the respiratory and olfactory epithelium as well as fibrosing peribronchitis and peribronchiolitis of the lung.

Human

Following exposure to chloropicrin vapor in an agricultural chemicals facility, persistent chest wall pain as well as an increase in creatine phosphokinase levels has been reported. Severity of symptoms and degree of biochemical abnormalities were reported to occur in a dose-dependent pattern. Inhalation exposure to very high levels of chloropicrin can lead to pulmonary edema, unconsciousness, and even death. Chloropicrin has not been reported to cause significant reproductive or teratogenic effects. *In vitro* genetic toxicity studies failed to reveal a potential for chloropicrin to produce significant mutagenic effects. Chloropicrin has not been reported to produce any carcinogenic effects in any species tested by the three routes of exposure.

In Vitro Toxicity Data

Chloropicrin is a bacterial mutagen and induces sister chromatid exchanges in cultured human lymphocytes, but is not considered as carcinogenic. Mutagenicity assays establish chloropicrin to be toxic but not mutagenic at 500 nmol per plate.

Carcinogenicity

Chloropicrin is a strong electrophile due to its chlorine and nitro groups. Therefore, it is capable of covalently binding to nucleophiles, such as DNA. Chloropicrin tested positive in a number of tests for genotoxicity. Carcinogenicity studies were carried out using both mice and rats (oral, one inhalation). One oral chronic toxicity study was conducted in dogs. Many of these studies met Federal Insecticide, Fungicide, and Rodenticide Act (FIFRA) guidelines. The effects observed with oral exposure included reduced survival, ptyalism, emesis, diarrhea, hunched posture, squinted or reddened eyes, reddened ears, urogenital stains, reduced body weights, hematological and clinical chemistry changes, nonneoplastic lesions in the forestomach/nonglandular stomach and liver, and neoplastic lesions in the mammary gland and stomach. The lowest no observed effect level (NOEL) with oral exposure was 0.1 mg kg^{-1} per day based on reduced body weights and periportal hepatocyte vacuolation in rats. The effects seen with inhalation exposure included reduced survival, reduced body weights and food consumption, increased lung weights, and nonneoplastic and neoplastic lesions in the respiratory tract. The lowest NOEL with inhalation exposure was 0.1 ppm (0.67 mg m^{-3}) in both rats (hamster embryo cells (HEC) = 0.029 ppm) and mice (HEC = 0.054 ppm).

Mutagenicity

Chloropicrin tested positive in eight reverse mutation assays with *Salmonella typhimurium* strains with and without activation; however, only one of these studies met FIFRA guidelines. One study found that the addition of GSH alone also converted chloropicrin to a mutagenic metabolite either through reductive dechlorination or through the formation of a reactive intermediate GSH conjugate, such as $GSCCl_2NO_2$ or $GSCHClNO_2$. In addition, chloropicrin tested positive in a reverse mutation assay with Escherichia coli WP2 *hcr*. Chloropicrin was negative in a mouse lymphoma assay that met FIFRA guidelines. Results from chromosomal aberrations assays were mixed. One study, which met FIFRA guidelines, reported that chloropicrin induced chromosomal aberrations in Chinese hamster ovary cells without S-9. In a published report, no increase in chromosomal aberrations was seen in human lymphocytes with or without S-9; however, an increase in sister chromatid exchanges was observed with and without S-9. No increase in micronuclei was seen *in vitro* with TK6 cells and human lymphocytes and *in vivo* with newt larvae or mice. Only the *in vivo* assay with mice met FIFRA guidelines. There was no increase in unscheduled DNA synthesis either *in vitro* with rat primary hepatocytes or *in vivo* with rats. Both of these studies met FIFRA guidelines. Increased DNA damage was seen in three published, nonguideline studies, a SOS chromotest with *Escherichia coli*, a Comet assay with TK6 cells, and a single-cell gel electrophoresis assay with CHO cells. Repair kinetics in the Comet assay indicated this damage was readily repaired. Chromosomal aberrations in the absence of a metabolic activation system were observed. No increase in forward mutation frequency was seen using the mouse lymphoma mutagenicity assay with L5178Y mouse lymphoma cells. Some investigators found no increase in unscheduled DNA synthesis in rat primary hepatocytes.

Clinical Management

Following an eye exposure to chloropicrin, the affected eyes should be irrigated with copious amounts of tepid water for at least 15 min. If irritation persists following decontamination, ophthalmic corticosteroids or local anesthetic ointments may be used. In case of an inhalation exposure, the patient should be monitored for respiratory distress. Emergency airway support and 100% humidified supplemental oxygen with assisted ventilation may be needed. Following dermal exposure to chloropicrin, the exposed area must be washed thoroughly with soap and water. If dermatitis persists, topical treatment with wet dressings of Burow's solution 1:40, followed by corticosteroid creams or calamine lotion may be given. Burn injuries to the skin are treated with standard burn management techniques, including use of medicated bandages. Secondary infection may necessitate antibiotic therapy. Oral antihistamines may be useful for pruritus.

In case of respiratory distress, medications that are used to treat asthma (such as bronchodilators and steroids) may also be used to assist breathing. Albuterol and aminophylline may be beneficial in cases involving signs of bronchoconstriction. Use supplemental humidified oxygen in cases of respiratory compromise. In severe respiratory compromise, ventilatory support is mandatory. No specific drug therapy or antidote is available for chloropicrin toxicity. For methemoglobinemia greater than 10–20%, consider the use of methylene blue. Signs of pulmonary edema may not be evident early after exposure. Observation for 24–48 h for progression or worsening of symptoms is recommended.

Ecotoxicology

Chloropicrin is highly toxic to fish, the 96 h LC_{50} for trout and bluegill being 0.0165 and 0.105 mg l^{-1}, respectively. However, little information is available about the effects of chloropicrin on birds. If released to soil, chloropicrin is expected to have high mobility based on a K_{oc} of 81. Volatilization from moist soil surfaces is expected to be an important fate process based on a Henry's Law constant of 2.05×10^{-3} atm-m^3 mol^{-1}. Chloropicrin may volatilize from dry soil surfaces based on its vapor pressure. Half-lives in soil ranging from 0.2 to 4.5 days at 20 °C suggest that biodegradation is an important environmental fate process in soil. If released into water, chloropicrin is not expected to adsorb to suspended solids and sediment based on the K_{oc}. A half-life of 0.5 days in activated sludge suggests that biodegradation may be an important environmental fate process in water. Volatilization from water surfaces is expected to be an important fate process based on this compound's estimated Henry's Law constant. An estimated BCF of eight suggests the potential for bioconcentration in aquatic organisms is low. Chloropicrin is stable to hydrolysis in neutral aqueous solution. Monitoring data indicate that the general population may be exposed to chloropicrin via inhalation of ambient air following adjacent agricultural applications and ingestion of drinking water.

Exposure Standards and Guidelines

Chloropicrin is a class I toxicity, restricted use pesticide, labeled with the signal word 'Danger.' The only exposure guidelines available for chloropicrin are those of permissible exposure level (PEL) and threshold limit value (TLV), both having a value of 0.1 ppm. It has an inhalation reference exposure level of 0.4 μg m^{-3}.

Occupational Safety and Health Administration: The PEL for chloropicrin is reported to be 0.7 ng m^{-3} for both general and construction industry.

American Conference of Governmental Industrial Hygienists: The TLV is 0.1 ppm, 0.67 ng m^{-3} time-weighted average (TWA) (not classifiable as a human carcinogen).

National Institute for Occupational Safety and Health: The recommended exposure limit is 0.1 ppm TWA.

See also: Pesticides.

Further Reading

Barry, T., Oriel, M., Verder-Carlos, M., et al., 2010. Community exposure following a drip-application of chloropicrin. J. Agromedicine 15 (1), 24–37.

Condie, L.W., Daniel, F.B., Olson, G.R., Robinson, M., 1994. Ten and ninety-day toxicity studies of chloropicrin in Sprague-Dawley rats. Drug Chem. Toxicol. 17 (2), 125–137.

Oriel, M., Edmiston, S., Beauvais, S., Barry, T., O'Malley, M., 2009. Illnesses associated with chloropicrin use in California agriculture, 1992–2003. Rev. Environ. Contam. Toxicol. 200, 1–31.

Pesonen, M., Vähäkangas, K., Halme, M., et al., 2010. Capsaicinoids, chloropicrin and sulfur mustard: possibilities for exposure biomarkers. Front. Pharmacol. 1, 140.

Pesonen, M., Pasanen, M., Loikkanen, J., et al., 2012. Chloropicrin induces endoplasmic reticulum stress in human retinal pigment epithelial cells. Toxicol. Lett. 211 (3), 239–245.

Schneider, M., Quistad, G.B., Casida, J.E. Glutathione activation of chloropicrin in the Salmonella mutagenicity test. Mutat. Res. 439 (2), 233–238.

Sparks, S.E., Quistad, G.B., Li, W., Casida, J.E., 2000. Chloropicrin dechlorination in relation to toxic action. J. Biochem. Mol. Toxicol. 14 (1), 26–32.

TeSlaa, G., Kaiser, M., Biederman, L., Stowe, C.M., 1986. Chloropicrin toxicity involving animal and human exposure. Vet. Hum. Toxicol. 28 (4), 323–324.

Xuan, R., Yates, S.R., Ashworth, D.J., Luo, L., 2012. Mitigating 1,3-dichloropropene, chloropicrin, and methyl iodide emissions from fumigated soil with reactive film. Environ. Sci. Technol. 46 (11), 6143–6149.

Relevant Websites

http://www.cdc.gov/niosh/ershdb/EmergencyResponseCard_29750034.html – Centers for Disease Control and Prevention.

http://pmep.cce.cornell.edu/profiles/extoxnet/carbaryl-dicrotophos/chloropicrin-ext.html – Cornell University Extension Toxicology Network.

http://emedicine.medscape.com/article/832637-overview – eMedicine.

http://toxnet.nlm.nih.gov – Toxnet (Toxicology Data Network): search under HSDB for Chloropicrin.

http://www.epa.gov/opptintr/aegl/pubs/chloropicrin_interim.pdf – US Environmental Protection Agency.

http://www.cdpr.ca.gov/docs/emon/pubs/tac/part_b_0210.pdf – USA: California-Environmental Protection Agency.

Chloroprene

HE Hurst, University of Louisville, School of Medicine, Louisville, KY, USA

- Name: Chloroprene
- Chemical Abstracts Service Registry Number: 126-99-8
- Synonyms: Beta-chloroprene CD; 2-chloro-1,3-butadiene; Chlorobutadiene; Cloroprene
- Molecular Formula: C_4H_5Cl
- Chemical Structure:

Background

Chloroprene, 2-chloro-1,3-butadiene, is a colorless, volatile synthetic liquid that has a pungent ether-like odor. Synthesis of chloroprene was first reported by chemists of the E. I. du Pont de Nemours Company in 1931 following studies of acetylene polymerization with the objective of producing synthetic rubber. The chloroprene monomer differs from isoprene, the fundamental monomer of natural rubber, only by substitution of chlorine for the methyl group of isoprene. Chloroprene was observed to polymerize much more quickly than did isoprene. In industrial processes prior to 1960, chloroprene was produced in relatively high yields by reacting vinyl acetylene with hydrogen chloride. Today, chloroprene is produced more efficiently by chlorination of 1,3-butadiene.

When compared with natural rubber the chloroprene synthetic polymer, polychloroprene, was noted to be much denser, more resistant to water and hydrocarbon solvents, less permeable to many gases, and was more resistant to degradation by oxygen, ozone, hydrogen chloride, hydrogen fluoride, and other chemicals. Due to desirable physical and chemical properties, polychloroprene and its latex polymers are produced in quantities exceeding 200 000 metric tons at a limited number of facilities around the world. Chloroprene production is closely tied to demand for polychloroprene.

Uses

More than 90% of chloroprene produced annually is used to make polychloroprene, which constitutes the widely known DuPont product Neoprene. This solvent-resistant elastomer, made by free radical initiated polymerization of chloroprene, is used to make many automotive rubber products, such as tires, hoses, and belts. Polychloroprene is formulated into adhesives and latex emulsions for dip coated goods. Other products made from polychloroprene are rubber personal protection garments including gloves, shoes, and wetsuits. Polychloroprene is used in conveyor and transmission belts, sealing materials, and electrical insulating materials.

Environmental Fate and Behavior

Physical and chemical properties of chloroprene are listed in Table 1.

Chloroprene is not generally available from chemical supply firms. Concentrated chloroprene is extremely reactive unless stored cold, under inert gas, and in presence of oxidation inhibitors and free radical scavengers. With pure chloroprene multiple undesirable reactions can occur, including spontaneous dimerization, polymerization, oxidation, epoxide formation, and nitration. Due to its reactivity, handling and transportation of chloroprene are carefully regulated; shipment of uninhibited chloroprene is forbidden by statute.

Chloroprene is not known to occur naturally. It is not widely distributed in the environment due its reactivity and its use at a limited number of facilities worldwide. Industrial production of chloroprene is accomplished in sealed reactor systems with very limited fugitive emissions. Polymerization processes are designed to be sealed, but must be opened to remove and manipulate formed polymer. Such opening causes most environmental release of chloroprene, the majority of which enters the atmosphere. From National Library of Medicine Toxics Release Inventory 2010 data, more than 270 000 pounds of chloroprene was released into the environment. Of that amount more than 97% was released into air at one site in Louisiana, USA.

Chloroprene is not considered a persistent environmental pollutant due its reactivity, nor is it known to undergo bioaccumulation or biomagnification because it is readily metabolized. Given its significant vapor pressure, most released chloroprene will be gaseous and will react with photochemically

Table 1 Physical properties of chloroprene

Atmospheric OH reaction rate constant	2.21×10^{-11} cm^3 $molecule^{-1}s^{-1}$
Boiling point	59.4 °C
Conversion factor, 1 ppm to mg $(m^3)^{-1}$	3.62 mg $(m^3)^{-1}$ ppm^{-1}
Conversion factor, 1 mg $(m^3)^{-1}$ to ppm	0.276 ppm $(mg\ (m^3)^{-1})^{-1}$
Henry constant	56 l-atm mol^{-1}
Melting point	−130 °C
Molecular weight	88.54 g mol^{-1}
Octanol–water partition coefficient (log P)	2.53
Specific gravity	0.96 at 20 °C
Vapor pressure	216 mm Hg at 25 °C
Water solubility	875 mg l^{-1}

Sources: U.S. National Library of Medicine Specialized Information Services Chemical Information, reference "chloroprene," "Physical Properties," http://chem.sis.nlm.nih.gov/chemidplus/; Hurst, H.E., 2007. Toxicology of 1,3-butadiene, chloroprene, and isoprene. Rev. Environ. Contam. Toxicol. 189, 131–179.

 http://dx.doi.org/10.1016/B978-0-12-386454-3.01116-7

produced hydroxyl radicals and ozone molecules. Half-lives of these reactions have been estimated to be 18 h and 10 days, respectively. Chloroprene would be expected to evaporate from soil and water toward the same fate. It has been detected in industrial wastewaters of the People's Republic of China and in Russia.

Exposure and Monitoring

Excluding serious industrial accidents, industrial exposure to chloroprene occurs primarily to polymer workers manufacturing polychloroprene rather than those involved in the closed processes of chloroprene manufacturing and storage. Important means of human exposures include respiratory and dermal routes, for which limiting values have been developed.

Human exposure data taken from personnel monitoring records during the period of 1976–96 indicate that US polymer workers have been exposed to ambient levels of the order of 1–8 ppm, while monomer production worker exposures were in the range of 1–2 ppm or less during that period. More recent environmental air monitoring in neighborhoods around a now-closed chloroprene polymerization facility in Louisville, Kentucky, noted air concentrations in the low ppb range. Dry solid polychloroprene is reported not to yield detectable chloroprene at a limit of detection of 0.5 ppm.

Toxicokinetics

Chloroprene is readily absorbed through the respiratory tract, as determined by animal inhalation studies. It is distributed into fatty tissues due to large partition coefficients for fatty tissues. Upon mammalian exposure chloroprene is metabolized similarly among species, although the quantities of specific metabolites differ, by cytochrome P450 enzymes (CYP 2E1). This system forms several metabolites through addition of oxygen, including reactive epoxides, aldehydes, and α,β-unsaturated ketones.

The stable but reactive, genotoxic epoxide ((1-chloroethenyl)oxirane, CEO) is produced as oxidation occurs at the vinyl group not substituted with chlorine. Estimates of the extent of CEO formation in rodent studies have been 2–5% of dose. Given the asymmetry produced in the structure by the chlorine atom, this epoxide metabolite exists as *R*-CEO and *S*-CEO enantiomers. As these epoxide enantiomers are reactive electrophiles, they bind covalently at nucleophilic biochemical sites, including nucleic acids, amino acids, and thiols. These CEO enantiomers are detoxified by hydrolysis via epoxide hydrolase and through glutathione conjugation facilitated by glutathione *S*-transferase. Species differ in CEO enantiomer formation and detoxification rates by epoxide hydrolase. Research has indicated that the *S*-CEO enantiomer is more rapidly detoxified by glutathione-dependent mechanisms in mouse red cells than is the *R*-CEO enantiomer.

No stable epoxide of the chlorinated vinyl group has been detected and confirmed in biological systems. However, oxidation to 2-chloro-2-ethenyloxirane can be inferred through detection of glutathione conjugates of likely rearrangement products, which include reactive aldehydes and α,β-unsaturated ketones.

Mechanism of Toxicity

The mechanisms of chloroprene toxicity differ depending on the extent and duration of exposure. An acute exposure to large concentration causes central nervous system depression typical of exposure to hydrocarbons. Organ and cellular toxicities due to reactions of chloroprene or metabolites with cellular constituents are evident. Detailed mechanisms of acute toxicities such as formation of edema and hemorrhage in tissues following large exposures are not yet known. Chronic toxicity is related to the mutagenic potential of oxidative metabolites of chloroprene, as these react with specific nucleoside sites in DNA.

Acute and Short-Term Toxicity

An early industrial report of human exposures from chloroprene rubber facilities noted symptoms of nervous system depression, lung, liver and kidney injuries, and irritation of mucous membranes and the skin, along with respiratory complications. Dermatitis and hair loss have been reported with dermal exposure to chloroprene.

Acute lethal human exposure to chloroprene is associated with nervous system intoxication, pulmonary edema, narcosis, and respiratory arrest. Chloroprene is acutely lethal to rats exposed to 2300 ppm for 4 h, with gross toxic effects including pulmonary hemorrhage and edema, as well as hepatic necrosis. A threshold exposure for chloroprene-induced acute hepatotoxicity in rats was noted to be between 106 and 180 ppm during 4-h exposures. Experimental exposures of rats at concentrations of greater that 161 ppm for 2–4 weeks caused deaths with olfactory epithelial degeneration, decreased red blood cell counts, and centrilobular hepatic necrosis. Subchronic 90-day inhalation studies in rats at 80 ppm produced similar effects of olfactory epithelium metaplasia and loss of nonprotein sulfhydryl content of lungs and liver. A similar 90-day inhalation study in mice noted deaths at 200 ppm with hyperplasia of the forestomach epithelium.

Chronic Toxicity

Chronic toxicity from exposures to lower concentrations is a concern because of potential genotoxicity, mutagenicity, and carcinogenicity due to formation of electrophilic metabolites.

Immunotoxicity

Limited detailed information is available regarding effects of chloroprene on immune function. A few reports published in Chinese and Russian literature suggest that chloroprene has inhibitory effects on cellular primary and humoral immune function. Depression of complement activity was noted in serum of workers manufacturing chloroprene rubber. Mice treated subchronically by inhalation of chloroprene concentrations of 25–110 ppm exhibited decreases in peripheral T lymphocytes and NK cell activity. These effects were related to toxic effects on the thymus and bone marrow.

Reproductive Toxicity

No human data indicate reproductive or developmental effects to date. Early studies exposing pregnant rats by inhalation noted embryotoxic effects at concentrations higher than 0.035 ppm, and by oral dosage of 0.5 mg kg^{-1} body weight during gestation. Later studies have noted increases in fetal resorption and decreased fetal body weights following inhalation exposures of female rats to 10 ppm 4 h day^{-1} during gestation. Reproductive capability of male rats appeared unaffected. National Toxicology Program (NTP) studies of reproductive toxicity of chloroprene noted slight but significant reduction of sperm motility, but estrus cycle length was unchanged in mice and rats.

Genotoxicity

Although direct genotoxicity of chloroprene per se has not been demonstrated unambiguously, its metabolites exhibit genotoxic potential. Tests for genotoxicity by studies using the Ames *Salmonella* reverse mutation tests have been mixed, apparently depending on experimental conditions. Most reverse mutation tests using freshly distilled chloroprene alone were not positive. Others indicated direct mutagenic effects from compound that had been stored for one or more days at $-20\,^{\circ}C$. Increasing mutagenicity correlated with formed chloroprene decomposition products, particularly cyclic dimers of chloroprene. These studies suggest that genotoxicity is caused by products of chloroprene reaction or degradation rather than chloroprene.

Additional reverse mutation studies that included liver homogenate to enable metabolic activation of chloroprene have indicated genotoxicity. Studies using the metabolite chloroprene epoxide (CEO) indicated mutagenic potential of CEO comparable to that of the butadiene metabolite epoxybutene. However, chloroprene exhibits lower potential metabolic genotoxicity than butadiene, as chloroprene does not readily form a stable diepoxide metabolite. This difference may be due to potential of the butadiene metabolite diepoxybutadiene to form interstrand DNA cross-links as it is a bifunctional electrophile. Although weaker than that of diepoxybutadiene, chloroprene epoxide may exhibit cross-linking activity similar to that of epichlorohydrin. A mechanism has been proposed involving rearrangement and reactive dechlorination after initial reaction of CEO with nucleophilic sites in DNA.

Studies of chloroprene epoxide in reactions with nucleosides *in vitro* have indicated a variety of DNA alkylation products. Similar reactions of CEO with double-stranded calf thymus DNA gave predominant adducts *N*7-(3-chloro-2-hydroxy-3-buten-1-yl)-guanine, formed by electrophilic attack with epoxide ring opening of CEO at the nucleophilic *N*7 nitrogen atom of 2′-deoxyguanosine, and *N*3-(3-chloro-2-hydroxy-3-buten-1-yl)-uridine, formed by attack of CEO at the N3 position with deamination of 2′-dexoycytidine. As these adducts are difficult to repair, they are genotoxic and believed to be involved in mutagenic actions of the CEO metabolite of chloroprene.

The impact of these reactions from active metabolites of chloroprene has been observed in chronic cancer bioassays in rodents. Formation of lung tumors in the 2-year NTP bioassay using $B6C3F_1$ mice noted a high proportion of the chloroprene-induced lung tumors exhibited mutations in the K-*ras* tumor suppressor gene. Such mutations often correlate with MAP-kinase activation of cell mitosis and play a significant role in mouse lung carcinogenesis.

Carcinogenicity

In animal studies to date, strain and species differences appear to have yielded negative as well as positive carcinogenicity indications. Chronic tests for carcinogenicity by the National Cancer Institute National NTP noted dose-related cancers in many tissues. These included increased bronchiolar/alveolar adenomas and carcinomas in lungs of male and female $B6C3F_1$ mice. Hemangiosarcoma, Harderian gland adenomas or carcinoma, forestomach squamous cell papillomas, and renal tubule adenomas were observed. Additionally, hepatocellular carcinomas and carcinomas of Zymbal's gland were noted in female mice. Similar chronic tests for cancers in NTP studies using male and female F344 rats noted squamous cell papillomas or carcinomas of the oral cavity, follicular cell adenoma or carcinomas, mammary fibroid adenomas in females, and renal tubule adenomas or carcinomas.

One clarifying toxic dose metric has been offered for differences among strains and species, as percentages of animals with tumors were related to the total amounts of chloroprene metabolized per weight of lung tissue per day. This finding is consistent with the hypothesis that carcinogenic potential arises from active metabolite(s) of chloroprene.

Given the weight of evidence from toxicological studies, chloroprene is characterized in the US Integrated Risk Information System (IRIS) as likely to be carcinogenic to humans. This determination was based on statistically significant dose response data demonstrating development of multiple tumors in multiple animal species, evidence of liver cancer risk associated with occupational exposure, suggestive evidence of association between occupational exposure and lung cancer risk, the proposed mutagenic action, and similarities of chloroprene with butadiene and vinyl chloride, which are known human carcinogens.

The International Agency for Research on Cancer in its 1999 chloroprene monograph classifies it in Group 2B, as possibly carcinogenic to humans. The latter designation is used when there is limited or inadequate evidence of carcinogenicity in humans, but there is evidence of carcinogenicity in experimental animals.

Clinical Management

As reports of acutely poisoned humans are very rare, successful treatment and clinical management have not been described in recent times. Presumably such would involve supportive care, as there is no antidote for exposure.

Insight to human intoxication is available in a recent report of chloroprene-induced fatality that notes its concentrations in lipid tissues, particularly brain, following human poisoning. This intoxication was caused by unprotected entry into a nominally empty chloroprene industrial vessel, 1.6-m diameter and 3-m depth, via a manway hatch. A worker wearing no upper torso garments but a respiratory mask without external air supply was found unconscious at the tank bottom about 20 min following his last sighting. He presented with cardiac arrest, pupils dilated and rigid. Reanimation efforts were unsuccessful. Beginning edema of the brain was indicated by computer tomography.

Postmortem examination indicated nonspecific macromorphological findings, but the corpse and internal organs gave off an intense chemical odor that interfered with progress of the autopsy. Lungs were heavy and edematous, the brain indicated severely increased intracranial pressure, and all internal organs were congested with blood. Headspace gas chromatographic analysis indicated tissue concentrations in brain ($120\,\mu g\,g^{-1}$), kidney ($25\,\mu g\,g^{-1}$), liver ($16\,\mu g\,g^{-1}$), myocardial tissue ($13\,\mu g\,g^{-1}$), heart blood ($3.8\,\mu g\,ml^{-1}$), and femoral blood ($1.1\,\mu g\,ml^{-1}$). Cause of death was believed due to asphyxia and chloroprene intoxication due to inhalation and probable dermal absorption.

Ecotoxicology

Little information has been published concerning ecotoxicology of chloroprene. One report has addressed ecotoxicological issues of chloroprene through mathematical modeling. This study involved fuzzy logic clustering of chloroprene among 90 chemicals using 10 chemical parameters. These included oil–water partition coefficient; Henry constant; biodegradability score; degradation in water and air; toxicities to microbes, aquatic invertebrates, and vertebrates, and mammals; and carcinogenicity, mutagenicity, or teratogenicity. Chloroprene was clustered within a group that had slightly increased aquatic toxicity with no other significant parameters.

Other Hazards

Chloroprene is known to be flammable.

Exposure Standards and Guidelines

ACGIH TLV: 8-h time weighted average (TWA): 10 ppm, skin. OSHA PEL: 8-h TWA, 25 ppm or 90 mg $(m^3)^{-1}$.

See also: Epichlorohydrin; Butadiene, 1,3-; Carcinogen Classification Schemes; Carcinogenesis; International Agency for Research on Cancer; Isoprene; ACGIH® (American Conference of Governmental Industrial Hygienists); Ames Test; Polymers; Toxicity Testing, Carcinogenesis; Toxicity Testing, Mutagenicity; Vinyl Chloride; Environmental Protection Agency, US; The National Toxicology Program.

Further Reading

Carothers, W.H., 1931. Acetylene polymers and their derivatives. II. A new synthetic rubber: chloroprene and its polymers. J. Am. Chem. Soc. 53, 4203–4225.

Cottrell, L., Golding, B.T., Munter, T., Watson, W.P., 2001. In vitro metabolism of chloroprene: species differences, epoxide stereochemistry and a de-chlorination pathway. Chem. Res. Toxicol. 14, 1552–1562.

Himmelstein, M.W., Carpenter, S.C., Hinderliter, P.M., 2004. Kinetic modeling of β-chloroprene metabolism: I. *in vitro* rates in liver and lung tissue fractions from mice, rats, hamsters, and humans. Toxicol. Sci. 79, 18–27.

Himmelstein, M.W., Carpenter, S.C., Evans, M.V., Hinderliter, P.M., Kenyon, E.M., 2004. Kinetic modeling of β-chloroprene metabolism: II. The application of physiologically based modeling for cancer dose response analysis. Toxicol. Sci. 79, 28–37.

Hurst, H.E., 2007. Toxicology of 1,3-butadiene, chloroprene, and isoprene. Rev. Environ. Contam. Toxicol. 189, 131–179.

Hurst, H.E., Ali, M.Y., 2007. Analyses of (1-chloroethenyl)oxirane headspace and hemoglobin N-valine adducts in erythrocytes indicate selective detoxification of (1-chloroethenyl)oxirane enantiomers. Chem. Biol. Interact. 166, 332–340.

Lynch, M., 2001. Manufacture and use of chloroprene monomer. Chem. Biol. Interact. 135–136, 155–167.

Melnick, R.L., Sills, R.C., Portier, C.J., et al., 1999. Multiple organ carcinogenicity of inhaled chloroprene (2-chloro-1,3-butadiene) in F344/N rats and B6C3F$_1$ mice and comparison of dose-response with 1,3-butadiene in mice. Carcinogenesis 20, 867–878.

Munter, T., Cottrell, L., Watson, W.P., Hill, S., Kronberg, L., Golding, B.T., 2002. Identification of adducts derived from reactions of (1-chloroethenyl)oxirane with nucleosides and calf thymus DNA. Chem. Res. Toxicol. 15, 1549–1560.

Munter, T., Cottrell, L., Golding, B.T., Watson, W.P., 2003. Detoxication pathways involving glutathione and epoxide hydrolase in the *in vitro* metabolism of chloroprene. Chem. Res. Toxicol. 16, 1287–1297.

Munter, T., Cottrell, L., Ghai, R., Golding, B.T., Watson, W.P., 2007. The metabolism and molecular toxicology of chloroprene. Chem. Biol. Interact. 166, 323–331.

Rickert, A., Hartung, B., Kardel, B., Teloh, J., Daldrug, T., 2012. A fatal intoxication by chloroprene. Forensic Sci. Int. 215, 110–113.

Valentine, R., Himmelstein, M.W., 2001. Overview of the acute, subchronic, reproductive, developmental and genetic toxicology of beta-chloroprene. Chem. Biol. Interact. 135–136, 81–100.

Wadugu, B.A., Ng, C., Bartley, L.B., Rowe, R.J., Millard, J.T., 2012. DNA interstrand cross-linking activity of (1-chloroethenyl)oxirane, and metabolite of β-chloroprene. Chem. Res. Toxicol. 23, 235–239.

Relevant Websites

http://www.inchem.org/documents/icsc/icsc/eics0133.htm – International Programme on Chemical Safety information on chloroprene

http://monographs.iarc.fr/ENG/Monographs/vol71/mono71-9.pdf – IARC Monograph on chloroprene

http://chem.sis.nlm.nih.gov – National Library of Medicine Chemical Information Services substance search

http://www.cdc.gov/niosh/npg/npgd0133.html – NIOSH Pocket Guide to Chemical Hazards - chloroprene

Chloropropionitrile, 2-

M Abdollahi and S Karami-Mohajeri, Faculty of Pharmacy and Pharmaceutical Sciences Research Center, Tehran University of Medical Sciences, Tehran, Iran

- Name: 2-Chloropropionitrile
- Chemical Abstracts Service Registry Number: 1617-17-0
- Synonyms: 1-Chloro-2-Cyanoethane, 3-Chloropropanenitrile, Beta-Chloropropionitrile, 3-Chloropropionitrile, Propanenitrile
- Molecular Formula: C_3H_4ClN
- Structure:

H_3C N Cl

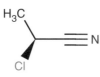

Background

2-Chloropropionitrile (2-CPN) is a colorless flammable liquid with a characteristic acrid odor.

Uses

Major uses of this chemical are in pharmaceutics and polymer synthesis.

Environmental Fate and Behavior

According to Henry's law constant of 1.43×10^{-5} atm-$m^3\ mol^{-1}$, vapor pressure of 2.770 mm Hg and water solubility of $45\ g\ ml^{-1}$ at 25 °C are expected to indicate that volatilization from moist soil and water surfaces is expected to be an important fate process and also it can be volatilized from dry soil surfaces and exist as a vapor in the atmosphere.

When heated to decomposition, it emits very toxic fumes of chlorine-containing compounds: nitrogen oxides, hydrogen cyanide, and hydrogen chloride.

Exposure and Exposure Monitoring

Pharmaceutical, industrial residues, and wastewater can be major routes of its environmental release. Occupational exposure via inhalation and dermal contact may occur in industries.

Toxicokinetics

2-CPN readily penetrates the skin to produce systemic cyanide poisoning.

Mechanism of Toxicity

Most of the toxicity of propionitrile results from release of cyanide. Cause of death is due to lack of oxygen to the body's cells, especially to the brain and heart cells.

Acute and Short-Term Toxicity

This chemical is toxic by the inhalation, dermal, and oral exposure routes. It is a lachrymatory agent. Massive doses may produce loss of consciousness, metabolic acidosis, and death from respiratory arrest. Upon ingestion, bitter and burning taste is followed by feeling of constriction or numbness in throat. Lacrimation, excessive salivation, nausea, and vomiting may also occur.

Chronic Toxicity

Duodenal ulcers with perforation of the liver and pancreas were seen in rats chronically fed the related compound propionitrile.

Immunotoxicity

No immunotoxicity was reported for 2-CPN.

Reproductive Toxicity

No reproductive studies were found but related nitrile compounds have been teratogenic in experimental animals.

Clinical Management

Evaluation of vital signs including pulse and respiratory rate, mechanical respiration (if not breathing), administering 100% oxygen to all victims, gastric lavage after ingestion of a large amount of poison without induction of emesis, and administration of activated charcoal, dopamine, or norepinephrine for treatment of hypotension can be useful.

Exposure Standards and Guidelines

Minimum lethal human exposure is unknown and exposure standards are not listed in safety agencies.

See also: Acrylonitrile; Polymers; Cyanide; Environmental Fate and Behavior; Environmental Protection Agency, US; Toxicity Testing, Mutagenicity; Toxicity Testing, Carcinogenesis; Toxicity Testing, Inhalation.

Further Reading

Bismuth, C., Baud, F.J., Djeghout, H., Astier, A., Aubriot, D., 1987. Cyanide poisoning from propionitrile exposure. J. Emerg. Med. 5, 191–195.

Mumtaz, M.M., Farooqui, M.Y., Cannon-Cooke, E.P., Ahmed, A.E., 1997. Propionitrile: whole body autoradiography, conventional toxicokinetic and metabolism studies in rats. Toxicol. Ind. Health 13, 27–41.

Wiberg, K.B., Wang, Y.G., Wilson, S.M., Vaccaro, P.H., Cheeseman, J.R., 2005. Chiroptical properties of 2-chloropropionitrile. J. Phys. Chem. A. 109, 3448–3453.

Relevant Websites

http://toxnet.nlm.nih.gov – Toxnet (Toxicology Data Network): search under Toxline for 2-Chloropropionitrile.

http://www.inchem.org – International Programme on Chemical Safety: INCHEM: 2-Chloropropionitrile.

http://chem.sis.nlm.nih.gov/chemidplus – US National Library of Medicine: ChemIDplus Advanced: 2-Chloropropionitrile.

http://www.iarc.fr – International Agency for Research on Cancer.

Chloroquine/Hydroxychloroquine

M Qozi and FL Cantrell, California Poison Control System San Diego, CA, USA

This article is a revision of the previous edition article by F. Lee Cantrell, volume 1, pp 573–574, © 2005, Elsevier Inc.

- Name: Chloroquine and hydroxychloroquine
- Chemical Abstracts Service Registry Number: 54-05-7
- Synonyms: SN 7618, Sanoquin, Tresochin, Silbesan, Artichin, Bipiquin, Avlocluor, Tanakan, Resochin, Resoquine, Aralen
- Chemical/Pharmaceutical/Other Class: Aminoquinoline antimalarial/antirheumatic
- Molecular Formula: $C_{18}H_{26}ClN_3$
- Chemical Structures:

Chloroquine

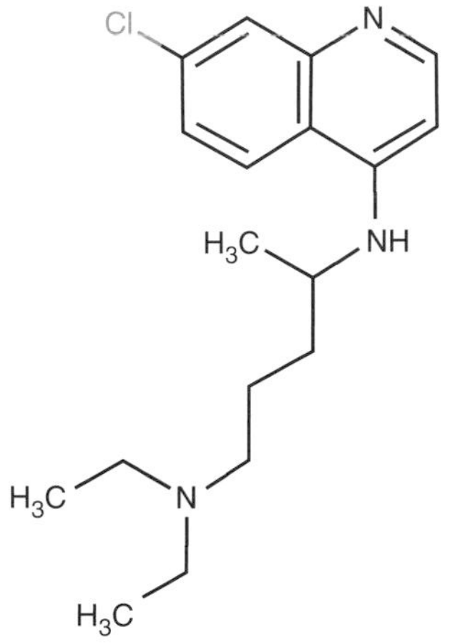

Hydroxychloroquine

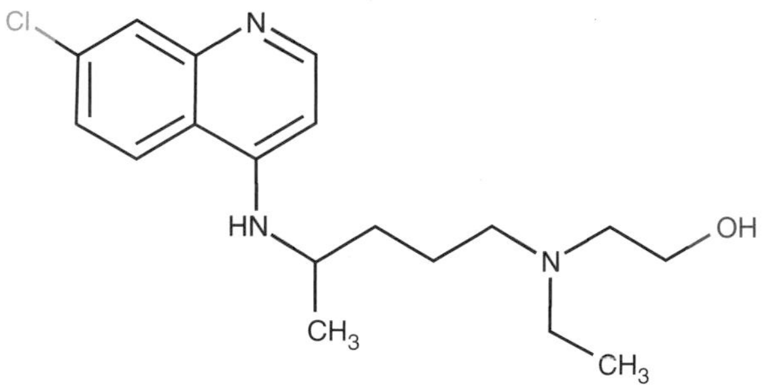

Background

Chloroquine (CQ) and hydroxychloroquine (HCQ) are synthetic 4-aminoquinolines. CQ has been used as an antimalarial drug since World War II. Later, CQ's use expanded to include management of systemic lupus erythematosus (SLE) and rheumatoid arthritis (RA). It has mild adverse effects when used short term, however, chronic use for autoimmune indications can cause irreversible ocular toxicity. HCQ was synthesized by adding a β-hydroxyl group to one of the *N*-ethyl groups on the CQ molecule in hopes of reducing its toxicity. HCQ was first approved by the Food and Drug Administration in 1955 for malaria. It is not as effective for treatment of malaria when compared to CQ but is considered to be a safer option for SLE and RA given its lower risk of ocular toxicity.

Uses

CQ and HCQ are both used as anti-inflammatory and antimalarial drugs.

Environmental Fate and Behavior

Physicochemical Properties

CQ is a white or slightly white odorless crystalline powder. It has a melting point from 87 to 92 °C. CQ is slightly soluble in water, and also in chloroform, ether, and dilute acids. Solutions of chloroquine phosphate and hydroxychloroquine sulfate have a pH of 4.5.

Exposure Routes and Pathways

CQ is available in oral and intravenous forms. HCQ is only available orally.

Toxicokinetics

CQ and HCQ have similar pharmacokinetics. Both drugs are absorbed rapidly and almost completely from the gut; peak serum concentrations of both drugs are attained within 1 or 2 h. CQ plasma protein binding is ~55, and 30–40% for HCQ given the variability in specific enantiomer protein binding. The two drugs exhibit very large volumes of distribution; 116–285 l kg^{-1} for CQ and 596–614 l kg^{-1} for HCQ. CQ may be found in 500 times greater concentration within the liver, spleen, kidneys, lungs, and leukocytes (compared with plasma).

The primary route of metabolism for CQ is deethylation, producing desethylchloroquine. HCQ undergoes *N*-dealkylation of the tertiary amine along with oxidative deamination of the primary amines leading to carboxylic acid derivatives, desethylhydroxychloroquine and desethylchloroquine. Elimination is significantly reduced in the presence of hepatic disease. Nearly 50% of CQ and 25% of HCQ are recovered in urine as unchanged drugs. The metabolites are cleared renally as well. The terminal half-life of CQ varies from 12 to 60 days. The half-life of HCQ varies from 32 to 50 days in healthy volunteers to 15.5–31 h in overdose.

Both drugs cross the placenta readily. A very small amount of both drugs is transmitted into breast milk as well.

 http://dx.doi.org/10.1016/B978-0-12-386454-3.00710-7

Mechanism of Toxicity

The exact mechanism of action of CQ and HCQ is not completely understood but involves inhibition of DNA and RNA polymerase. They are also direct myocardial depressants that impair cardiac conduction through membrane stabilization. It is unclear how they work in autoimmune diseases.

Acute and Short-Term Toxicity (or Exposure)

Animal

CQ and HCQ are not commonly used therapeutically in domestic animals. HCQ was used safely at a maximum dose of 10 mg kg^{-1} for 9 months in dogs with exfoliative cutaneous lupus erythematosis.

Human

There are few published cases of acute HCQ toxicity, however, it appears that it mimics CQ in overdose. Symptoms of overdose occur within 1–2 h and include nausea, vomiting, transient visual or auditory deficits, drowsiness, and seizures followed by severe cardiac arrhythmias, shock, or cardiorespiratory arrest. Hypotension may be severe and intractable, producing metabolic acidosis and end organ failure. Hypokalemia occurs due to intracellular potassium shift and the degree of hypokalemia correlates with the severity of overdose. Cardiac conduction disturbances include complete atrioventricular dissociation, QRS and QT prolongation, severe bradycardia, and ventricular fibrillation. Acute ingestions of 30–50 mg kg^{-1} of CQ in adults and as little as 300 mg in children are potentially fatal. Unlike CQ, there is no established lethal dose for HCQ given the limited reported cases of overdose in the literature. From what is reported so far, it appears that ingestion of 4 g can lead to significant toxicity and symptoms can occur as early as 30 min from the time of ingestion.

Chronic Toxicity (or Exposure)

Animal

Rats chronically administered CQ in food for up to 2 years demonstrated dose related inhibition of growth compared with controls. High-dose (from 100 to 1000 mg kg^{-1} diet over 2 years) studies in rats showed myocardial and other muscle damage, centrilobular liver necrosis, and testicular damage. Both drugs caused acute cardiotoxicity when given in high repeated doses to dogs.

Human

Chronic use of CQ may produce cinchonism, a syndrome characterized by headache, visual changes, and gastrointestinal disturbances. Visual disturbances are associated with retinal artery spasm. Ototoxicity may also occur. Dermatologic reactions, particularly a lichenoid skin eruption, may result from chronic CQ use. Long-term therapeutic use of HCQ appears to be less retinotoxic than CQ based on the number of reported cases in the literature.

In Vitro Toxicity Data

Studies in cultured chick brains demonstrated inhibition of retinal pigment epithelium viability at concentrations similar to those seen *in vivo* for patients experiencing CQ-induced retinopathy.

Carcinogenicity

There is no evidence to suggest that CQ or HCQ are carcinogenic.

Reproductive Toxicity

4-Aminoquinolines have been shown to accumulate selectively in melanin structures of fetal eyes. No teratogenic effects have been reported with therapeutic doses of CQ. CQ in doses used for malaria prophylaxis appears to be safe for use during pregnancy. CQ can, however, cross the placenta and bilateral cochlea-vestibular disturbances have been reported in children of mothers who have been treated with high doses of CQ throughout their pregnancy. CQ is not contraindicated during pregnancy but high doses or prolonged administration can cause toxicity and should be avoided. CQ is found in the breast milk in only insignificant amounts when taken by lactating mothers.

Clinical Management

Management for both drugs is the same. Basic and advanced life-support measures should be implemented as necessary. In patients presenting within 1 h of ingestion, activated charcoal should be administered. In the event of depressed consciousness or seizures, airway protection should first be secured. Sodium bicarbonate, epinephrine, and high-dose diazepam should be used to treat cardiotoxicity. Potassium repletion should be handled with extreme care given the intracellular potassium shift. Diazepam is recommended for the treatment of seizures. Methods of extracorporeal drug removal such as hemodialysis are ineffective given the drugs' large volume of distribution and protein binding. Extracorporeal treatments, however, may facilitate supportive cares. Sodium bicarbonate should be administered in bolus doses for signs of membrane-depressant toxicity such as QRS widening on the electrocardiogram.

See also: Poisoning Emergencies in Humans; The QT Interval of the Electrocardiogram; Quinidine; Quinine.

Further Reading

Childhood chloroquine poisoning – Wisconsin and Washington. Morb. Mortal. Wkly. Rep. 37, 1988, 437–439.

Furst, D.E., 1996. Pharmacokinetics of hydroxychloroquine and chloroquine during treatment of rheumatic diseases. Lupus 5, S11–S15.

Gunja, N., Roberts, D., McCoubrie, D., Lamberth, P., Jan, A., Simes, D.C., Hackett, P., Buckley, N.A., 2009. Survival after massive hydroxychloroquine overdose. Anaesth. Intensive Care 37 (1), 130–133.

Iron dextran. In: AHFS Drug Information, 2008. American Society of Health Systems Pharmacists, Bethesda, MD, pp. 854–861.

Jordan, P., Brookes, J.G., Nicolic, G., Couteur, D.G., 1999. Hydroxychloroquine overdose: toxicokinetics and management. Clin. Toxicol. 37, 861–864.

Marquardt, K., Albertson, T.E., 2001. Treatment of hydroxychloroquine overdose. Am. J. Emerg. Med. 19, 420–424.

Maudlin, E.A., Morris, D.O., Brown, D.C., Casal, M.L., 2010. Exfoliative cutaneous lupus erythematosus in German shorthaired pointer dogs: disease development, progression of the three immunomodulatory drugs (cyclosporine, hydroxychloroquine, and adalimumab) in a controlled environment. Vet. Dermatol. 21, 373–382.

Nelson, L.S., Lewin, N.A., Howland, M.A., et al., 2011. Goldfrank's Toxicologic Emergencies, ninth ed. McGraw-Hill Companies, Inc, New York.

Olson, K.R., 2012. Poisoning & Drug Overdose, sixth ed. McGraw Hill, San Francisco.

Piette, J.C., Guillevin, L., Chapelon, C., 1987. Chloroquine cardiotoxicity. N. Engl. J. Med. 317, 710–711.

Rynes, R.I., 1997. Antimalarial drugs in the treatment of rheumatologic diseases. Br. J. Rheumatol. 36, 799–805.

Williams, D.A., Lemke, T.L., 2002. Foye's Principles of Medicinal Chemistry, fifth ed. Lippincott Williams & Wilkins, Baltimore.

Yanturali, S., Aksay, E., Demir, O.F., Atilla, R., 2004. Massive hydroxychloroquine overdose. Acta Anaesthesiol. Scand. 48, 379–381.

Yaylali, S.A., Sadigov, F., Erbil, H., Ekinci, A., Akcakaya, A.A., March 2, 2013. Chloroquine and hydroxychloroquine retinopathy-related risk factors in a Turkish cohort. Int. Opththalmol. (Epub ahead of print).

Relevant Websites

http://www.cdc.gov/malaria/about/history/ – Centers for Disease Control and Prevention: The History of Malaria, an Ancient Disease.

http://emedicine.medscape.com/article/1229016-overview – Chloroquine and Hydroxychloroquine Toxicity – eMedicine at Medscape online.

http://webeye.ophth.uiowa.edu/eyeforum/cases/139-plaquenil-toxicity.htm – Eye Institute at the University of Iowa Health Center online resource – hydroxychloroquine (Plaquenil) ocular toxicity and recommendations for screening.

http://www.inchem.org/documents/pims/pharm/chloroqu.htm – Inchem online resource for chloroquine toxicity – from toxicokinetics, mechanism of toxicity as well as human and animal data to treatment recommendations.

http://archopht.jamanetwork.com/article.aspx?articleid=1106671 – Journal of the American Medical Association online resource – article describing chloroquine and hydroxychloroquine toxicity.

Silicon Tetrachloride

S López and J Bergueiro, Universidad de Santiago de Compostela, Santiago de Compostela, A Coruña, Spain
J Fidalgo, IES Rosalía de Castro Rúa de San Clemente, Santiago de Compostela, A Coruña, Spain

- Name: Silicon Tetrachloride
- Chemical Abstracts Service Registry Number: 10026-04-7
- Synonymus: Silicon chloride, Tetrachlorosilane, Tetrachlorosilicon
- Molecular Formula: $SiCl_4$

Background

Chlorosilanes (general formula $R_nH_mSiCl_{4-n-m}$, where R is an alkyl, aryl, or olefin group) are compounds in which silicon is bound to between one and four chlorine atoms, bonds with hydrogen and/or organic groups making its total number of bonds up to four. Chlorosilanes react with water, moist air, and steam, producing heat and toxic, corrosive hydrogen chloride fumes. Contact between gaseous hydrogen chloride and metals may release gaseous hydrogen, which is inflammable and explosive. Chlorosilanes react vigorously with oxidizing agents, alcohols, strong acids, strong bases, ketones, and aldehydes.

Uses

Chlorosilanes are chemical intermediates used in the production of silicon and silicon-containing materials, and in the semiconductor industry; they are also protecting agents for intermediates in pharmaceutical syntheses. The most important industrially utilized silicon halides are trichlorosilane and silicon tetrachloride.

Silicon tetrachloride ($SiCl_4$) can be manufactured by chlorination of silicon compounds such as ferrosilicon or silicon carbide, or by heating silicon dioxide and carbon in a stream of chlorine. It can also be obtained as a by-product in the production of zirconium tetrachloride, and in the past substantial quantities were produced by this route, which in recent decades has lost importance owing to the reduced demand for zirconium in nuclear facilities. Nowadays, industrial silicon tetrachloride is produced either by direct reaction of hydrogen chloride with silicon – this product mainly being employed as an intermediate in fumed silica production – or as the by-product of the production of silane for the microelectronics industry by disproportionation of trichlorosilane.

Silicon tetrachloride is used as an intermediate in the manufacture of high-purity silicon because its boiling point is convenient for purification by repeated fractional distillation. Once purified, it can be reduced to silicon by gaseous hydrogen for use in the semiconductor industry; hydrolyzed to high-purity fused silica; or oxidized to pure silica in the presence of oxygen in the manufacture of optical fibers by processes such as modified chemical vapor deposition, a widely used method for the fabrication of high quality optical fiber preforms, that require it to be free of hydrogen-containing impurities such as trichlorosilane. Silicon tetrachloride is also used as a 'blocking agent' in organic synthesis, and to produce military smoke screens.

Environmental Fate and Behavior

Silicon tetrachloride is a colorless, noninflammable, volatile liquid with a pungent, suffocating odor. It fumes in air and is corrosive to metals and tissues in the presence of moisture. In experiments at Argonne National Laboratory in which it was mixed with water and stirred under room conditions, about 35% of the theoretical yield of HCl evolved as a gas in the first minute. It also reacts very rapidly with alcohols, primary and secondary amines, ammonia, and other compounds containing active hydrogen atoms. Thermal decomposition or burning may produce dense white clouds of silicon oxide particles and hydrogen chloride.

Silicon tetrachloride is a by-product in the production of polysilicon, the key component of sunlight-capturing wafers in solar energy panels, and for each ton of polysilicon produced, at least four tons of silicon tetrachloride liquid waste are generated. Pollution by silicon tetrachloride has been reported in China, associated with the increased demand for photovoltaic cells that has been stimulated by subsidy programs.

Exposure and Exposure Monitoring

The main exposure route for humans is through inhalation, ingestion, and skin and/or eye contact.

Acute and Short-Term Toxicity

Mechanism of Toxicity

Studies of rats subjected to acute inhalation of 10 structurally similar chlorosilanes, including tetrachlorosilane, suggest that the acute toxicity of chlorosilanes is largely due to the hydrogen chloride hydrolysis product. The observed effects were similar to those of HCl inhalation both qualitatively (clinical signs) and quantitatively (molar equivalents of hydrogen chloride at the atmospheric LC_{50}).

Animal Data

Rats

Although toxicity data are available for few individual chlorosilanes, and for those few are limited, well-conducted inhalation toxicity studies have been performed on rats for a series of chlorosilanes including tetrachlorosilane. In each case, groups of five male and five female Fischer 344 rats were exposed to varying concentrations of a chlorosilane for 1 h and were observed for up 14 days. Nominal chlorosilane concentrations were used to calculate LC_{50} values. In general, the LC_{50} values of monochlorosilanes were approximately twice those of dichlorosilanes and three times those of trichlorosilanes. Tetrachlorosilane had an LC_{50} of 1312 ppm, similar to those of the trichlorosilanes. The clinical signs exhibited by the

 http://dx.doi.org/10.1016/B978-0-12-386454-3.01236-7

experimental animals were consistent with hydrogen chloride exposure and indicative of severe irritation/corrosion. They included lacrimation, salivation, dry material around or on the eyes and/or nose, green staining around the nose and mouth, and perineal urine staining. Labored breathing, rales, hypoactivity, closed or partially closed eyes, prostration, corneal opacity or opaqueness, and swollen and/or necrotic paws were also observed. Hemorrhage, congestion and/or consolidation of the lungs, ectasia of the lungs, gaseous distension of the gastrointestinal tract, absence of body fat, nostrils that were obstructed, alopecia around the eyes, and discoloration of hair were observed at necropsy.

Rabbits

The application of $SiCl_4$ to shaved rabbit skin produced complete denaturation and tissue sloughing within 10 min of exposure, with the appearance of blanched patches and blisters. When instilled into the eye, even a dose as low as 0.05 ml caused severe burns on the cornea and lids. Gastrointestinal tissue corrosion has been observed in animals given a single oral dose.

Human Data

The only human exposure data located concerned an accidental release of silicon tetrachloride at a chemical plant in a South San Francisco industrial park in 1984. Several thousand people were evacuated and 28 sought medical attention. Most of the affected individuals suffered transient eye and upper airway irritation that cleared within 24 h. Six employees involved in clean-up operations (all male smokers, aged 25–56 years) developed transient symptoms, including lacrimation, rhinorrhea, burning in the mouth and throat, headaches, coughing, and wheezing. The results of pulmonary function studies were normal except that four patients exhibited mild obstructive airway disease that may have been due either to the silicon tetrachloride exposure or to smoking. Two patients also complained of pedal dysesthesias after the accident. Although the temporal relationship between the exposure and onset of these symptoms is striking, no definite etiological relationship could be established. No values for silicon tetrachloride or hydrogen chloride air concentrations during the incident were reported.

Assuming the toxicity of silicon tetrachloride to be due to hydrogen chloride, and given the known effects of the latter, the effects of $SiCl_4$ exposure may be expected to be as follows. Inhalation may cause severe irritation of the upper respiratory tract, resulting in coughing, choking, and a feeling of suffocation; continued inhalation may produce ulceration of the nose, throat, and larynx, and deep inhalation edema of the lungs. Vapor severely irritates the eyes, causing pain, excess lachrymation (tears), closure of the eyelids, marked excess redness, and swelling of the conjunctiva. High concentrations of hydrogen chloride vapor, if formed, could injure the cornea. Splash contamination may cause severe conjunctivitis, seen as marked excess redness and swelling of the conjunctiva, discharge, iritis, and severe corneal injury that, if untreated, could result in permanent blindness. Skin contact with liquid $SiCl_4$ may cause full-thickness burns; repeated contact with dilute solutions or exposure to concentrated vapors may cause dermatitis. Ingestion causes severe internal injuries in the mouth, throat, esophagus, and stomach, intense thirst, difficulty in swallowing, nausea, vomiting, and diarrhea; in severe cases, collapse and unconsciousness may result. Silicon tetrachloride may affect the nervous system.

Chronic Toxicity

Prolonged or repeated exposure to hydrogen chloride vapor may cause corrosion (discoloration and erosion) of the teeth, ulceration of the nasal mucosa, and bleeding of nose and gums.

Genotoxicity

Tetrachlorosilane was not mutagenic in studies of *Salmonella typhimurium* strains TA98, TA100, TA1535, TA1537, and TA1538; *Saccharomyces cerevisiae* strain D-4; and *Escherichia coli* strains W3110/polA^+ and P3478/polA^- with and without metabolic activation. It also tested negative in an L5178Y mouse lymphoma assay.

Carcinogenicity

Inorganic chlorosilanes are not listed by the National Toxicology Program, the US Occupational Safety and Health Administration (OSHA), or the International Agency for Research on Cancer. Silicon tetrachloride has not been tested for its ability to cause cancer in animals.

Ecological Effects

The ultimate fate of chlorosilanes in the troposphere is probably determined by hydrolysis of the silicon–chlorine bonds in water droplets. In arid regions, some transport to the stratosphere might occur. In the stratosphere, photolysis by short-wavelength light is expected. Chlorosilanes do not generate any ozone-depleting chemicals.

The instant hydrolysis of silicon tetrachloride upon contact with water generates hydrogen chloride and silicic acid gel, and shifts pH into the acidic range. Chlorosilanes are not listed as marine pollutants by the US Department of Transportation (DOT).

In the light of its bioaccumulation-relevant properties (fast hydrolysis, formation of nonpersistent inorganic substances) and toxicity assessment (it is not classified as having long-term human health effects or aquatic toxicity), silicon tetrachloride does not meet the criteria for consideration as a very persistent, and very accumulative substance or a persistent, bioaccumulative, and toxic substance. Its susceptibility to hydrolysis means that adsorption on soil, volatilization, biodegradation, and bioaccumulation are not expected to be important fate processes.

Other Hazards

Inhalation may aggravate asthma and inflammatory or fibrotic pulmonary disease. Skin irritation may aggravate an existing dermatitis.

Exposure Standards and Guidelines

Silicon tetrachloride is on the Right-to-Know Hazardous Substance List of a number of US states because it is listed by DOT and the National Fire Protection Association. More specifically, it is on the Special Health Hazard sublist.

Inorganic chlorosilanes are considered hazardous by the OSHA Hazard Communications Standard.

The following exposure limits are for gaseous hydrogen chloride, which is produced when silicon tetrachloride reacts with water or moisture in the air. In no case should the concentration of hydrogen chloride in air exceed the limit at any time.

OSHA permissible exposure limit: 5 ppm

National Institute for Occupational Safety and Health recommended airborne exposure limit: 5 ppm

American Conference of Governmental Industrial Hygienists threshold limit value : 2 ppm

See also: Silane.

Further Reading

Jean, P.A., Gallavan, R.H., Kolesar, G.B., Siddiqui, W.H., Oxley, J.A., Meeks, R.G., 2006. Chlorosilane acute inhalation toxicity and development of an LC_{50} prediction model. Inhal. Toxicol. 18, 515–522.

Kizer, K.W., Garb, L.G., Hine, C.H., 1984. Health effects of silicon tetrachloride-report of an urban accident. J. Occup. Med. 26, 33–36.

National Research Council, 2011. "Selected Chlorosilanes". Nineteenth Interim Report of the Committee on Acute Exposure Guideline Levels: Part A; Committee on Acute Exposure Guideline Levels; Committee on Toxicology. The National Academies Press, Washington D.C.

Relevant Website

http://www.washingtonpost.com/wp-dyn/content/article/2008/03/08/AR2008030802595_pf.html. – The Washinton Post: Solar Energy Firms Leave Waste Behind in China.

Chlorothalonil

P Raman, Northeast Ohio Medical University, Rootstown, OH, USA

- Name: Chlorothalonil
- Chemical Abstracts Service Registry Number: 1897-45-6
- Synonyms: 2,4,5,6-Tetrachlorobenzenedicarbonitrile; Tetrachloroisophthalonitrile; Bravo; Daconil; Forturf
- Molecular Formula: $C_8Cl_4N_2$
- Chemical Structure:

Cl
N N
Cl Cl
Cl

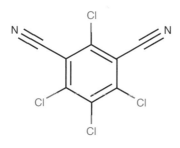

Background

Chlorothalonil is an aromatic halogen compound that appears as a grayish to colorless crystalline solid that is odorless or has a slightly pungent odor. It has a molecular weight of 265.92, water solubility of 0.6 mg l^{-1} at room temperature, a melting point of 250–251 °C, and a boiling point of 350 °C. Chlorothalonil is only slightly soluble in acetone, dimethyl sulfoxide, cyclohexane, and xylene. It is noncorrosive and stable in moderately alkaline or acidic aqueous solutions. At high temperatures, chlorothalonil decomposes to emit hydrochloric acid. Some popular trade names for chlorothalonil include Bravo, Daconil 2787, Echo, Exotherm Termil, Nopcocide, Repulse, and Tuffcide. This compound can be found in formulations with many other pesticide compounds. Chlorothalonil is an important broad-spectrum, nonsystemic, organochlorine fungicide that has been widely used for more than 30 years as an effective disease management tool for potatoes, peanuts, turf, and vegetable and fruit crops. It is also used to control fruit rots in cranberry bogs and is used in paints. Chlorothalonil is classified as a general use pesticide by the US Environmental Protection Agency (EPA). Typical chlorothalonil application rates are 1 kg ha^{-1} with four to nine applications per growing season. Chlorothalonil can enter surface waters through rainfall runoff, spray drift, or atmospheric deposition, subsequently having an impact on the aquatic biota. Most common routes of exposure to chlorothalonil are via the skin and eyes; it may also be ingested or inhaled.

Uses

Chlorothalonil is an extensively used pesticide in agriculture, silviculture, and urban settings. It is also used as a fungicide, bactericide, and nematocide. It is used as a wood preservative in some countries and is used as a mildew-preventing agent in paints.

Environmental Fate and Behavior

Chlorothalonil's production and use as a broad-spectrum, nonsystemic, protectant pesticide results in its direct release to the environment. Its uses as a wood protectant, antimold and antimildew agent, bactericide, microbiocide, algaecide, insecticide, and acaricide are additional routes of release. If released to air, chlorothalonil will exist in both the vapor and particulate phases in the ambient atmosphere. Vapor-phase chlorothalonil will be degraded slowly in the atmosphere by reaction with photochemically produced hydroxyl radicals (reaction half-life ~7 years). Direct photolysis may also occur. Chlorothalonil is removed from the atmosphere by wet and dry deposition. If released to soil, chlorothalonil is expected to have low mobility or be immobile, based on K_{oc} values in the range of 900–7000 measured in four soils. Volatilization from moist or dry soil surfaces is not expected to be important based on a Henry's Law constant of 2.5×10^{-7} atm-cu m mol^{-1}. Aerobic biodegradation half-lives of chlorothalonil in four different soils ranged from 10 to 40 days. If released into water, chlorothalonil is expected to adsorb to suspended solids and sediment in the water column.

Biodegradation is expected to be an important fate process given aerobic aquatic degradation half-lives of 8.1 and 8.8 days measured in marine water, and anaerobic degradation half-lives ranging from 5 to 15 days measured in flooded soils. Hydrolysis does not occur under acidic conditions or at pH 7; however, a hydrolysis half-life of 38.1 days was observed for chlorothalonil at pH 9. An aqueous photolysis half-life of 65 days was measured for chlorothalonil, suggesting photolysis in sunlit surface waters is possible. Bioconcentration factor values of 9.4–264 measured in different species of fish suggest bioconcentration in aquatic organisms can be low to high. The principal breakdown product of chlorothalonil in the soil is 4-hydroxy-2,5,6-trichloroisophthalonitrile, which is slightly toxic to aquatic organisms and moderately toxic to birds and mammals. Soil moisture and temperature both promote degradation of chlorothalonil. It has a high degree of binding and low mobility in silty loam and silty clay loam soils, while having a relatively low binding and moderate mobility in sand. Residues of chlorothalonil remain on above-ground crops at harvest but are prone to dissipate overtime. It is a relatively persistent fungicide on plants, based on its rate of application. Chlorothalonil is almost insoluble in water and does not evaporate easily.

Exposure Routes and Pathways

Dermal and eye exposures are the most common routes of accidental exposure to chlorothalonil. It may also be ingested or inhaled.

 http://dx.doi.org/10.1016/B978-0-12-386454-3.00283-9

Toxicokinetics

Chlorothalonil is rapidly absorbed both orally and via inhalation. However, the amount of material absorbed is limited and dose related. Thus, while ~30% of an administered dose of up to 50 mg kg^{-1} is absorbed, absorption at high doses decreases relatively. There is also a marked species-dependent variation in chlorothalonil absorption. Chlorothalonil is only poorly absorbed by the dermal route of exposure. Absorbed chlorothalonil undergoes rapid distribution among body tissues in rats, tissue concentration being in the order of kidney > liver > whole blood. Conjugation with glutathione constitutes the primary route of metabolism of chlorothalonil. Liver represents the major site for chlorothalonil conjugation. In the enzymatic reaction, 4-(glutathione-*S*-yl)-2,5,6-trichloroisophthalonitril is formed initially. This is also a substrate for glutathione-*S* transferases (GSTs), resulting in the substitution of a second chlorine atom to give 4,6-bis(glutathione-*S*-yl)-2,5-dichloroisophthalonitril. Hydrolysis studies indicated that the metabolism of chlorothalonil is pH dependent. Thus, 4-hydroxy-2,5,6-trichloroisophthalonitrile and 3-cyano-2,4,5,6-tetrachlorobenzamide are formed at pH 9 but not at pH 7. The metabolism of chlorothalonil was recently investigated in liver and gill cytosolic and microsomal fractions from channel catfish using high performance liquid chromatography. The reports indicate that chlorothalonil is detoxified *in vitro* by GST-catalyzed glutathione conjugation. However, no human data are currently available for the biotransformation of chlorothalonil. Chlorothalonil is primarily eliminated via the kidneys. Following administration of 1 mg kg^{-1} chlorothalonil endotracheally, orally, or dermally to rats, less than 6% was recovered in blood or urine within 48 h. The major route of elimination following oral administration to rats is in the feces (>80%), with 5.4–11.5% being excreted in the urine as the dose increases from 5 to 200 mg kg^{-1}. Marked species differences exist in the pharmacokinetic behavior of chlorothalonil. Thus, following oral administration of 50 mg kg^{-1} chlorothalonil, dogs and rhesus monkeys excrete up to 98 and 92% of the dose, respectively, in the feces compared with ~82% in rats.

Mechanism of Toxicity

Glutathione conjugation represents a bioactivation reaction for chlorothalonil resulting in the formation of *S*-conjugates toxic to the kidney. Chlorothalonil acts as an alkylating agent and reacts with cellular sulfhydryl compounds. Alkylation of biological molecules results in effects on cellular function and viability. Chronic damage to the proximal tubular epithelium may be involved in the mechanism of chlorothalonil tumorigenicity to the kidneys.

Animal Toxicity

Forestomach and the renal proximal tubule are the primary target tissues of chlorothalonil toxicity in Sprague–Dawley rats. Toxicity is characterized by hypertrophy, hyperplasia, vacuolization, and degeneration of renal tubular epithelium and acanthosis, hyperkeratosis, and hyperplasia of the squamous epithelium of the forestomach. Chlorothalonil is a well-known skin and eye irritant. Sustained contact with the squamous epithelium of the forestomach can lead to an inflammatory response. The earliest observation following chlorothalonil administration at 175 mg kg^{-1} day^{-1} to rats for varying periods of time for up to 91 days has been characterized by multifocal ulceration and erosion of the mucosa, subsequently progressing to hyperplasia and hyperkeratosis. These lesions have been observed in subchronic and chronic studies in rats and mice (no observed effect level (NOEL) ~2 mg kg^{-1} day^{-1}) and in chronic studies appear to be closely related with incidence of neoplasia (NOEL ~4–21 mg kg^{-1} day^{-1}). Undiluted chlorothalonil is a strong irritant and produces irreversible corneal, iridal, and conjunctival effects in rabbits. Weakness and sedation precede death in animals given acute toxic doses intraperitoneally. Chronic oral administration to rats results in ataxia. Hematuria, vaginal bleeding, and epistaxis are seen in rats following chronic oral exposure. In chronic dermal exposures to chlorothalonil dissolved in acetone, the no-effect level for irritation is 0.001%. The 0.01% concentration is a mild irritant and 0.1% a moderate irritant. Prolonged exposure of rodents to chlorothalonil results in nephrotoxicity and renal tubular hyperplasia, and these effects, if sustained, can lead to a tumorigenic response. Chlorothalonil produced a dose-related increased incidence of renal tubular adenomas and adenocarcinomas in rats. The oral LD_{50} in rats is greater than 10 g kg^{-1}. Chlorothalonil is predicted to be a rodent carcinogen via a nongenotoxic mechanism.

Some of the LD_{50} values for a variety of experimental animals are as follows:

1. Mouse model: i.p. – 2500 mg kg^{-1}; oral – 3700 mg kg^{-1}
2. Rat model: i.p. – 2500 mg°kg^{-1}; dermal – 10 000 mg kg^{-1}
3. Rabbit: percutaneous – >5000 mg kg^{-1}

Human Toxicity

Facial dermatitis has been reported in occupational exposures and can occur in the absence of direct skin contact, presumably due to the high volatility of chlorothalonil. Chlorothalonil is a strong primary skin irritant and may also cause allergic contact urticaria and anaphylaxis. Patch testing with concentrations greater than 0.01% may produce primary irritant reactions. Hypersensitivity reactions characterized by facial erythema, periorbital erythema and edema, eczema, and pruritus have been observed following chlorothalonil exposure. Photosensitivity reactions were seen in some individuals. High concentrations of chlorothalonil produce delayed irritant reactions. Delayed dermal irritant effects have also been noted 48–72 h after cessation of exposure. Immediate respiratory reactions such as tightness of chest and throat may occur following inhalation exposure to chlorothalonil. A recent review of the potential cancer risks of chlorothalonil to operators and consumers conducted in the United Kingdom for the Pesticide Advisory Committee (UK, 1994) provided evidence that chlorothalonil is not genotoxic. The primary potential for human exposure to chlorothalonil is to forest service applicators applying the fungicide. Chlorothalonil does not have any adverse reproductive or teratogenic effects at expected exposure levels. Data suggesting carcinogenic potential of chlorothalonil remain inconclusive at the present time.

Reproductive Effects

Long-term administration of chlorothalonil at high doses to both males and female rats did not affect reproduction or the litters that were produced. However, weight gains in both sexes decreased generation after generation. Administration of high doses of chlorothalonil to pregnant rabbits through the stomach during the sensitive period of gestation resulted in abortion. These studies suggest that chlorothalonil will not affect human reproduction except at very high doses. In second- and third-generation reproductive toxicity studies, rats showed decreased food consumption, lower body weights, kidney lesions, and forestomach lesions after exposure to chlorothalonil in the diet. The only effect in the pups was a reduction in body weight exposed to chlorothalonil or SDS-3701 *in utero*.

Developmental Toxicity

Chlorothalonil did not cause developmental toxicity in rats or rabbits.

However, dams treated with chlorothalonil showed increased mortality, clinical signs (excess lacrimation, vaginal and nose discharges, and anogenital stains), decreased food consumption, and reduced body weight.

Teratogenic Effects

Female rats given high doses of chlorothalonil through the stomach during the sensitive period of gestation had normal fetuses, even though that dose was toxic to the mothers. Limited study disclosed rabbits had no effects. Based on these observations, chlorothalonil is expected to produce no birth defects in humans.

Mutagenic Effects

Mutagenicity studies on various animals, bacteria, and plants indicate that chlorothalonil does not cause any chromosomal changes. The compound is therefore not expected to pose mutagenic risks to humans. Chlorothalonil (>97% pure; up to 10 μg plate^{-1}) was not mutagenic in Ames assays with strains TA98, TA100, TA1537, or TA1538 with and without rat liver S-9 homogenate pretreated with Aroclor 1254. Chlorothalonil (up to 50 μg plate^{-1}) was also not mutagenic in the above strains with and without rat kidney S-9 homogenate. Chlorothalonil (97.3% pure) was not mutagenic when tested at 0.3 μg ml^{-1} in Chinese hamster lung fibroblasts (V79) cells, at 0.3 μg ml^{-1} with activation (rat liver S-9 homogenate pretreated with Aroclor 1254) in mouse BALB/3T3 fibroblasts, and at 0.03 μg ml^{-1} without activation in BALB/3T3 cells. However, chlorothalonil was positive in some chromosomal aberration assays and a DNA damage study. An epigenetic mechanism has been suggested for chlorothalonil-induced DNA damage in isolated human lymphocytes.

Carcinogenic Effects

There is sufficient evidence in experimental animals for the carcinogenicity of chlorothalonil. Chlorothalonil is a potential human carcinogen, known to affect the kidney, ureter, and bladder in experimental animals. Both sexes of rats fed chlorothalonil daily over a lifetime developed carcinogenic and benign kidney tumors at the higher doses. In an unsettled study, mouse fed daily high doses of chlorothalonil for 2 years developed tumors in the forestomach area in females and carcinogenic and benign kidney tumors in males. A long-term National Toxicology Program study concluded that under the conditions of this bioassay, chlorothalonil is carcinogenic to Osborne–Mendel rats, but not to B6C3F1 mice.

Clinical Management

One of the primary forms of treatment is to support respiratory and cardiovascular function. Dilution and dermal or eye decontamination are primary considerations. Following oral exposure, immediate dilution with 4–8 ounces of milk or water is recommended. Vomiting must be induced if victim is conscious. If inhaled, victim must be immediately moved to fresh air. And if not breathing, artificial respiration should be provided. In case of dermal exposure to chlorothalonil, the exposed area should be thoroughly washed with soap and water. Allergic contact dermatitis may be treated with antihistamines, topical steroids, or systemic steroids. Following an eye exposure, the affected eyes should be irrigated with copious amounts of tepid water for at least 15 min. Immediate medical attention for the eyes is also recommended. Exposure may cause temporary allergic side effects. Symptoms include redness of the eyes, mild bronchial irritation, and redness or rash on exposed skin. Temporary allergic reactions can be treated with antihistamines or steroid creams and/or systemic steroids upon consultation with the physician.

Ecotoxicology

Chlorothalonil and its metabolites are highly toxic to fish, aquatic invertebrates, and marine organisms. Chlorothalonil levels of less than 1 ppm have been reported to produce noticeable toxicity in fish such as the rainbow trout (LC_{50} of 0.25 mg l^{-1}), bluegills (LC_{50} of 0.3 mg l^{-1}), and channel catfish (LC_{50} of 0.43 mg l^{-1}). However, it is relatively nontoxic to birds, mammals, and bees.

Exposure Standards and Guidelines

Owing to its potential for causing eye irritation, chlorothalonil is also classified as a toxicity class II, moderately toxic chemical. Based on the increased incidence of renal tumor in female rats, EPA currently lists chlorothalonil as a Group B2 (probable human) carcinogen, the Q* value being 0.007 66 mg kg^{-1} day^{-1}. Chlorothalonil has an acceptable daily intake and a reference dose value of 0.03 and 0.015 mg kg^{-1} day^{-1}, respectively.

American Conference of Governmental Industrial Hygienists threshold limit value: none.

National Institute for Occupational Safety and Health recommended exposure limit: none.

See also: Nematicides; Pesticides.

Further Reading

Andre, V., Lebailly, P., Pottier, D., et al., 2003. Urine mutagenicity of farmers occupationally during a 1-day use of chlorothalonil and insecticides. Int. Arch. Occup. Environ. Health 76 (1), 55–62.

Bellas, J., 2008. Prediction and assessment of mixture toxicity of compounds in antifouling paints using the sea-urchin embryo-larval bioassay. Aquat. Toxicol. 88 (4), 308–315.

Budai, P., Szabó, R., Lehel, J., et al., 2012. Toxicity of chlorothalonil containing formulation and Cu-sulphate to chicken. Commun. Agric. Appl. Biol. Sci. 77 (4), 449–454.

de Castro, V.L., Chiorato, S.H., Pinto, N.F., 2000. Biological monitoring of embrio-fetal exposure to methamidophos or chlorothalonil on rat development. Vet. Hum. Toxicol. 42 (6), 361–365.

DeLorenzo, M.E., Fulton, M.H., July 2012. Comparative risk assessment of permethrin, chlorothalonil, and diuron to coastal aquatic species. Mar. Pollut. Bull. 64 (7), 1291–1299.

Farag, A.T., Karkour, T.A., El Okazy, A., 2006. Embryotoxicity of oral administered chlorothalonil in mice. Birth Defects Res. B Dev. Reprod. Toxicol. 77 (2), 104–109.

Garron, C., Knopper, L.D., Ernst, W.R., Mineau, P., 2012. Assessing the genotoxic potential of chlorothalonil drift from potato fields in Prince Edward Island, Canada. Arch. Environ. Contam. Toxicol. 62 (2), 222–232.

Godard, T., Fessard, V., Huet, S., et al., 1999. Comparative in vitro and in vivo assessment of genotoxic effects of etoposide and chlorothalonil by the comet assay. Mutat. Res. 444 (1), 103–116.

Hernández-Hernández, C.N., Valle-Mora, J., Santiesteban-Hernández, A., Bello-Mendoza, R., 2007. Comparative ecological risks of pesticides used in plantation production of papaya: application of the SYNOPS indicator. Sci. Total Environ. 381 (1–3), 112–125.

King, K.W., Balogh, J.C., 2013. Event based analysis of chlorothalonil concentrations following application to managed turf. Environ. Toxicol. Chem. 32 (3), 684–691.

McMahon, T.A., Halstead, N.T., Johnson, S., et al., 2011. The fungicide chlorothalonil is nonlinearly associated with corticosterone levels, immunity, and mortality in amphibians. Environ. Health Perspect. 119 (8), 1098–1103.

Mozzachio, A.M., Rusiecki, J.A., Hoppin, J.A., et al., 2008. Chlorothalonil exposure and cancer incidence among pesticide applicator participants in the agricultural health study. Environ. Res. 108 (3), 400–403.

Phyu, Y.L., Palmer, C.G., Warne, M.S., et al., 2013. Assessing the chronic toxicity of atrazine, permethrin, and chlorothalonil to the cladoceran *Ceriodaphnia cf. dubia* in laboratory and natural river water. Arch. Environ. Contam. Toxicol. 64 (3), 419–426.

Sherrard, R.M., Murray-Gulde, C.L., Rodgers Jr., J.H., Shah, Y.T., 2003. Comparative toxicity of chlorothalonil: *Ceriodaphnia dubia* and *Pimephales promelas.* Ecotoxicol. Environ. Saf. 56 (3), 327–333.

Suzuki, T., Nojiri, H., Isono, H., Ochi, T., 2004. Oxidative damages in isolated rat hepatocytes treated with the organochlorine fungicides captan, dichlofluanid and chlorothalonil. Toxicology 204 (2–3), 97–107.

Wu, X., Cheng, L., Cao, Z., Yu, Y., 2012. Accumulation of chlorothalonil successively applied to soil and its effect on microbial activity in soil. Ecotoxicol. Environ. Saf. 81, 65–69.

Yu, S., Wages, M.R., Cobb, G.P., Maul, J.D., July 15, 2013. Effects of chlorothalonil on development and growth of amphibian embryos and larvae. Environ. Pollut. http://dx.doi.org/10.1016/j.envpol.2013.06.017 pii: S0269-7491(13)00334-5. (Epub ahead of print).

Relevant Websites

http://www.cdpr.ca.gov/docs/emon/surfwtr/presentations/syngenta_presentation_2012.pdf – California Environmental Protection Agency.

http://www.cdpr.ca.gov/docs/risk/rcd/chlorothalonil.pdf – California. Gov.

http://pmep.cce.cornell.edu/profiles/extoxnet/carbaryl-dicrotophos/chlorothalonil-ext.html – Cornel University, Extension Toxicology Network.

http://toxnet.nlm.nih.gov/cgi-bin/sis/search/r?dbs+hsdb:@term+@rn+@rel+1897-45-6 – National Library of Medicine-Hazardous Substances Data Bank.

http://nj.gov/health/eoh/rtkweb/documents/fs/0415.pdf – New Jersey. Gov.

http://www.state.nj.us/dep/enforcement/pcp/bpc/wps/chlorothalonil.pdf – New Jersey Department of Environmental Protection.

http://www.pesticideinfo.org/Detail_Chemical.jsp?Rec_Id=PC34550 – Pesticide Action Network.

Chlorpheniramine

EJ Hall, Coastal Valley Veterinary Services, LLC, Old Lyme, CT, USA
GJ Hall, United States Coast Guard Academy, New London, CT, USA

This article is a revision of the previous edition article by Brenda Swanson-Biearman, volume 1, pp 577–578, © 2005, Elsevier Inc.

- Name: Chlorpheniramine
- Chemical Abstracts Service Registry Number: 132-22-9
- Synonyms: 3-(4-chlorophenyl)-*N*,*N*-dimethyl-3-pyridin-2-yl-propan-1-amine (IUPAC); Chlor-Trimeton®
- Chemical Formula: $C_{16}H_{19}ClN_2$
- Chemical Structure:

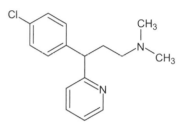

Uses

Chlorpheniramine is a drug in the class of first-generation antihistamines, used to help alleviate symptoms of allergic reactions potentiated by histamine release. Though it is included in many multisymptom over-the-counter cold relief medications, the Food and Drug Administration (FDA) issued a safety alert in March 2011 detailing some risks associated with these medications. The safety alert also indicated that increased enforcement of FDA laws governing the marketing of these drugs would occur, as many of the products had not been approved in their current formulations for safety, effectiveness, and quality.

Since the mechanism of bronchial asthma and systemic anaphylactic reactions involves many other mechanisms than just histamine release, histamine antagonists are used only as adjunctive therapy to epinephrine after the acute reactions have been controlled. Antihistamines may also be used to help ameliorate allergic reactions during blood or plasma transfusions.

Chlorpheniramine is commonly used in small-animal veterinary medicine for its antihistaminic/antipruritic effects, especially for the treatment of pruritus in cats, and occasionally as a mild sedative.

Exposure Routes and Pathways

Chlorpheniramine is available in oral and injectable formulations; thus, ingestion and injection are routes of intentional and unintentional exposure.

Pharmacokinetics

Chlorpheniramine is well absorbed after oral administration and has a serum half-life of approximately 20 h in adults. It undergoes a relatively high degree of first-pass metabolism in the gastrointestinal (GI) mucosa and liver; therefore, only about 25–60% of the drug is available systemically. The drug and its metabolites (desmethylchlorpheniramine and didesmethylchlorpheniramine) are excreted almost exclusively through the kidneys. The elimination half-life is more rapid in children, 9.5–13 h vs 14–24 h in adults.

Mechanisms of Toxicity

Toxicity of antihistamines is usually related to their anticholinergic effects and may include loss of appetite, nausea, vomiting, diarrhea or constipation, and other GI effects, as well as dizziness, tinnitus, lassitude, incoordination, fatigue, blurred vision, diplopia, euphoria, nervousness, insomnia, and tremors. Acetylcholine is competitively blocked at muscarinic receptors, resulting in symptoms of anticholinergic poisoning. Concurrent use of alcohol, tricyclic antidepressants, monoamine oxidase inhibitors, or other central nervous system (CNS) depressants along with antihistamines may exaggerate and extend the anticholinergic and CNS depressant effects of antihistamines; concurrent use is not recommended.

Products that were marketed prior to the FDA safety alert but not approved by the FDA included multisymptom cold medications comprised of drug combinations of chlorpheniramine with decongestants, antitussives, and analgesics. Risks associated with the use of these products included improper use in children and infants, potentially risky combination of ingredients, and patients receiving too much or too little medication because of problems with the way some 'extended-release' products were made. Newborn and premature infants are even more prone to anticholinergic side effects and an increased susceptibility toward convulsions; thus, this drug is not recommended at all in this age group. Geriatric patients are also more prone to anticholinergic effects, and a paradoxical reaction characterized by hyperexcitability may occur in some children taking antihistamines. Overdosage may also produce central excitation resulting in convulsions.

Acute and Short-Term Toxicity or Exposure

Animal

CNS stimulation (excitement to seizures) or depression (lethargy to coma) may follow overdosage, as well as previously mentioned anticholinergic effects, respiratory depression, or death. Normal dosage range for veterinary use in small animals is 0.2–0.8 mg kg^{-1}; one report of a puppy ingesting 25 mg kg^{-1} described signs of ataxia, tremors, bradycardia, coma, and cardiac arrest, eventually resulting in death within 11 h of ingestion. Treatment includes emesis if the patient is alert and CNS status is stable, followed by saline cathartic and/or

 http://dx.doi.org/10.1016/B978-0-12-386454-3.00711-9

activated charcoal. Supportive and symptomatic care should be used to treat other clinical signs.

Human

CNS stimulation is more common in children than adults following overdosage. Overdosage in adults usually causes CNS depression (lethargy to coma) followed by excitement, seizures, and postictal depression, as well as previously mentioned anticholinergic effects. Cardiovascular effects may include tachycardia with prolonged QTc and QRS intervals and nonspecific ST and T-wave changes, hypo- or hypertension, dysrhythmias, and cardiac arrest; extreme overdose may result in cerebral edema, coma, cardiovascular or respiratory arrest, or death. Symptoms may appear 30 min to 2 h after exposure, and death may occur several days after onset of initial symptoms.

Chronic Toxicity or Exposure

Animal

Animal feeding models designed to test for carcinogenicity and mutagenicity following chronic exposure have so far proved negative. The FDA categorizes this drug as category B for use during pregnancy (animal studies have not yet demonstrated risk to the fetus, but there are no adequate studies in pregnant women; or animal studies have shown an adverse effect, but adequate studies in pregnant women have not demonstrated a risk to the fetus in the first trimester of pregnancy, and there is no evidence of risk in later trimesters).

Human

Studies of chronic dosing in adults and children have shown expected side effects of drowsiness and sedation in therapeutic doses.

Genotoxicity

Ames Salmonella and mouse lymphoma tests for mutagenicity have been negative.

Clinical Management

Symptomatic and supportive care including advanced life-support measures should be implemented as necessary. Induction of emesis and gastric lavage are indicated if the time of ingestion was recent and the patient is conscious with stable CNS signs. Agitated patients with tachycardia may benefit from sedation with benzodiazepines. Patients who have taken large overdoses should have electrocardiogram monitoring performed, though the use of antidysrhythmics associated with prolongation of the QT interval should be avoided (class Ia agents such as quinidine, disopyramide, procainamide, and aprindine and most class III agents such as *N*-acetylprocainamide and sotalol). Intravenous benzodiazepines and phenytoin have been used to treat seizures cased by antihistamine toxicity in humans; barbiturates and diazepam are not recommended. Physostigmine administration may be indicated in cases where severe anticholinergic symptoms are refractory to conventional treatment.

See also: Diphenhydramine; Benzodiazepines.

Further Reading

Gilman, A.G., Rall, T.W., Nies, A.S., Taylor, P. (Eds.), 1990. Goodman and Gilman's the Pharmacological Basis of Therapeutics, eighth ed. Pergamon Press, New York, NY, p. 586.
Monte, A.A., Chuang, R., Bodmer, M., December 2010. Dextromethorphan, chlorphenamine and serotonin toxicity: case report and systematic literature review. Br. J. Clin. Pharmacol. 70 (6), 794–798.
Murphy, L., October 2001. Antihistamine toxicosis. Vet. Med., 752–765.
USP Convention, 1995. USPDI – Drug Information for the Health Care Professional, fifteenth ed., vol. 1. United States Pharmacopeial Convention, Inc., Rockville, MD (Plus Updates), p. 306.
Wogoman, H., Steinberg, M., Jenkins, A.J., 1999. Acute intoxication with guaifenesin, diphenhydramine, and chlorpheniramine. Am. J. Forensic Med. Pathol. 20, 199–202.
Wyngaarden, J.B., Seevers, M.H., 1951. The toxic effects of antihistaminic drugs. J. Am. Med. Assoc. 145, 277–282.

Relevant Website

http://www.nlm.nih.gov/medlineplus/druginfo/meds/a682543.html – MedlinePlus.

Chlorpromazine

RD Beckett, Manchester University College of Pharmacy, Fort Wayne, IN, USA

This article is a revision of the previous edition article by Linda A. Malley, volume 1, pp 578–582, © 2005, Elsevier Inc.

- Name: Chlorpromazine
- Chemical Abstracts Service Registry Number: 50-53-3
- Synonyms: 2-Chloro-10-[3-(dimethylamino)propyl]phenothiazine; Chlorpromazine hydrochloride; CPZ; Thorazine
- Molecular Formula: $C_{17}H_{19}ClN_2S$
- Chemical Structure:

CH3 N H3C N Cl S

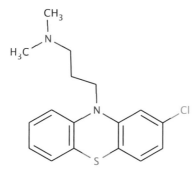

Background

Chlorpromazine is a first-generation ('typical') antipsychotic approved by the US Food and Drug Administration (FDA) in 1957. First-generation antipsychotics were the most commonly used class of medications for the treatment of schizophrenia until the 1990s, when second-generation ('atypical') antipsychotics (e.g., olanzapine, quetiapine, risperidone) gained popularity due to their decreased risk for extrapyramidal adverse reactions. Structurally, chlorpromazine is classified as a phenothiazine, along with fluphenazine, prochlorperazine, promethazine, and thioridazine. Toxicity due to chlorpromazine presents similarly to, but less severely than, that due to tricyclic antidepressants (TCA).

Uses

Chlorpromazine is approved by FDA for use in humans for the management of psychotic disorders (i.e., control of mania, treatment of schizophrenia); control of nausea and vomiting; relief of apprehension before surgery; acute intermittent porphyria; adjunctive treatment of tetanus; intractable hiccups; combativeness or explosive hyperexcitable behavior in children aged 1–12 years; and short-term treatment of hyperactivity in children with symptoms of impulsivity, difficulty sustaining attention, aggressiveness, mood lability, and poor frustration tolerance. Chlorpromazine is commonly used off-label for treatment of behavioral symptoms associated with dementia in the elderly and psychosis and agitation related to Alzheimer's dementia; however, it carries a boxed warning regarding increased risk of death in patients with dementia-related psychosis. Chlorpromazine is also used off-label for managing agitation in terminal cancer patients, autonomic dysreflexia, cancer pain, adjunctive treatment of cholera, migraine headaches, opioid withdrawal, ocular pain, paralytic ileus, and phantom limb syndrome.

In veterinary medicine, the use of chlorpromazine has been largely replaced by the phenothiazine acepromazine due to its more favorable pharmacokinetic profile. Chlorpromazine may be used as an antiemetic for small animals or for preoperative sedation. Chlorpromazine may also be used for management of hypertension in dogs and cats.

Environmental Fate and Behavior

Chlorpromazine occurs as a white, crystalline solid that is nearly water insoluble but freely soluble in alcohol. The melting point of chlorpromazine is approximately 60 °C. Chlorpromazine is commercially available as a hydrochloride salt, a white, crystalline powder that is soluble in water ($1\ g\ ml^{-1}$) and alcohol ($667\ mg\ ml^{-1}$) at 25 °C. The commercially available product has a pH of 3–5 and may contain inactive ingredients benzyl alcohol and sulfites, as well as others. Chlorpromazine is photosensitive; it should be protected from light, moisture, and temperatures outside of 20–25 °C. Chlorpromazine significantly adsorbs to plastic; such tubing should be avoided clinically.

Chlorpromazine exists as both a vapor and particulate at ambient atmospheric conditions. Chlorpromazine vapor is degraded by photochemically produced hydroxyl radicals with an estimated half-life of 1.6 h. Chlorpromazine particulate is removed by wet or dry deposition. Chlorpromazine is likely to be immobile in soil (K_{oc} 9900, pK_a 9.3) and to adsorb to sediment if released into water. It is not expected to volatilize from soil or water. There is high potential for bioconcentration.

Exposure and Exposure Monitoring

Chlorpromazine is administered orally, by deep intramuscular (IM) injection, intravenous (IV) injection, or IV infusion. Chlorpromazine is not administered subcutaneously due to the risk for dermal irritation. Pharmacists, physicians, and nurses dispensing or administering chlorpromazine could be exposed through dermal or inhalational contact. Personnel involved in chlorpromazine production may also be exposed.

Therapeutic drug concentrations can be monitored; however, this is not commonly done clinically. There is wide variation in the plasma level at which clinical response occurs among patients with schizophrenia.

Toxicokinetics

- Absorption: Chlorpromazine is rapidly absorbed orally and from parenteral sites of injection with peak plasma levels occurring at 2–4 h following oral administration and 15–30 min following IM injection. Due to significant first-pass hepatic metabolism and intestinal wall metabolism that vary among individual patients, interindividual oral absorption is erratic. Drug information references cite 20–32% bioavailability; absorption following IM administration is expected to be 10-fold higher. Following administration, oral tablets are expected to elicit pharmacological action within 30–60 min; IM injection has an onset time of 15 min.
- Distribution: Chlorpromazine distributes to most fluids and body tissues with a volume of distribution ranging from 8 to 160 $l\,kg^{-1}$; concentrations in the central nervous system (CNS) are five times higher than in plasma as chlorpromazine efficiently crosses the blood–brain barrier. Chlorpromazine is highly protein-bound, particularly to albumin, with a plasma protein binding rate of 90–99%; protein binding in the CNS ranges from 19 to 72%. Chlorpromazine and its metabolites have been found to distribute to fetal plasma, amniotic fluid, and neonatal urine following intramuscular doses given to pregnant women prior to delivery. Rapid placental transfer, with fetal levels approaching 50% of maternal values within 10 min, has also been observed in animal studies. Chlorpromazine distributes to breast milk.
- Metabolism: Chlorpromazine undergoes extensive hepatic metabolism to 10–12 metabolites, both active and inactive. The *N*-dimethylaminopropyl side chain of chlorpromazine is demethylated and metabolized to an *N*-oxide while positions 3 and 7 of the phenothiazine nucleus undergo hydroxylation. The quantitatively important metabolites of chlorpromazine are nor2-chlorpromazine, chlorphenothiazine, methoxy and hydroxyl products, and glucuronide conjugates of hydroxylated compounds. Several of these metabolites are active, including nor2-chlorpromazine, nor2-chlorpromazine sulfoxide, and 3-hydroxy chlorpromazine.
- Elimination: Less than 1% of a chlorpromazine dose is excreted in the urine as unchanged drug; most elimination of a single 120 $mg\,m^{-2}$ dose occurred within 6 h. Chlorpromazine and its metabolites may be detected up to 6–18 months following treatment. Twenty-three to 37% of a chlorpromazine dose is excreted as unchanged drug or metabolites. The two major metabolites of chlorpromazine found in the urine are *N*-dedimethylchlorpromazine and 7-hydroxychlorpromazine. Elimination occurs faster in children than in adults. Twenty percent of the chlorpromazine dose excreted in the urine consists of unconjugated unchanged drug, demonomethylchlorpromazine, dedimethylchlorpromazine, sulfoxide metabolites, and chlorpromazine-*N*-oxide. Eighty percent of the chlorpromazine dose excreted in the urine consists of conjugated *O*-glucuronides, ethereal sulfates of mono- and dihydroxy-chlorpromazine derivatives. The half-life of chlorpromazine is cited as 6 h; however, values ranging from 2 to 119 h have been reported. Chlorpromazine is also eliminated in the feces. Chlorpromazine is not dialyzable.

Mechanism of Toxicity

Acute and chronic toxicity due to chlorpromazine generally manifests as an extension of normal pharmacological activity. The precise mechanism of action of chlorpromazine, and other phenothiazines, is unknown; however, it is thought to primarily involve antagonism of dopaminergic (D2) neurotransmission at synaptic sites and blockade of postsynaptic dopamine receptor sites at the subcortical levels of the reticular formation, limbic system, and hypothalamus. This activity contributes to chlorpromazine's extrapyramidal reactions. Chlorpromazine also has strong central and peripheral activity directed against adrenergic receptors and weak activity against serotonergic, histaminic (H1), and muscarinic receptors. Chlorpromazine has slight ganglionic blocking action. Chlorpromazine is known to depress vasomotor reflexes medicated by the hypothalamus and/or brain stem; inhibit release of growth hormone; antagonize secretion of prolactin release-inhibiting hormone; and reduce secretion of corticotropin-regulatory hormone.

Chlorpromazine also has direct effects on cardiac myocytes; it can induce early after-depolarizations, block depolarizing sodium channels, and cause significant prolongation of the QTc interval.

Chlorpromazine may be irritating to eyes, mucous membranes, and skin. Contact and inhalation should be avoided.

Acute and Short-Term Toxicity

Animal

The oral 50% lethal dose (LD_{50}) for rats is 142–225 $mg\,kg^{-1}$. Single and repeated exposures to oral chlorpromazine have been conducted in several species, including cats, dogs, horses, and rats at doses ranging from 2 to 30 $mg\,kg^{-1}\,day^{-1}$. The primary effects of chlorpromazine were cardiac arrhythmia, decreased activity, stimulation of hepatic microsomal enzyme activity, hormonal changes, hypotension, impaired motor activity, ocular lesions, photosensitization, tachycardia, and reduced bile flow, and reduced red blood cell count and hemoglobin.

The IV LD_{50} for rats is 23 $mg\,kg^{-1}$. When administered parenterally at doses ranging from 1.5 to 100 $mg\,kg^{-1}$ in dogs, mice, and rats, chlorpromazine was associated with ataxia, CNS depression, decreased hemoglobin, hypotension, and stimulation of hepatic microsomal enzyme activity.

When administered to pregnant rats, chlorpromazine was administered at IV doses ranging from 5 to 45 $mg\,kg^{-1}\,day^{-1}$ and associated with delays in bone ossification, decreased body weight, increased fetal and maternal mortality, and skeletal malformations at higher doses.

Human

Acute toxicity and/or overdosage of phenothiazines, such as chlorpromazine, is expected to present as an extension of normal adverse effects observed at therapeutic doses; the most commonly reported manifestations of acute toxicity are severe extrapyramidal reactions, hypotension, and sedation. Patients with early or mild intoxication may present with confusion, disorientation, drowsiness, excitement, or restlessness. Patients in the late stage may present with CNS stimulation and convulsions followed by respiratory and/or CNS depression. Other signs of intoxication include cardiovascular shock, cardiovascular conduction abnormalities, dysrhythmias, agitation, anticholinergic effects, changes in body temperature, vomiting, difficulty breathing, and pulmonary edema.

Severity of toxic effects is dose-related. For phenothiazines, doses at least 10 times the defined daily dose are considered to be potentially lethal; for chlorpromazine, this value is approximately 3000 mg day^{-1}. Due to the varied, dose-related nature of chlorpromazine toxicity, typical therapeutic blood concentrations (i.e., 0.02–3.0 mg l^{-1}) overlap with reported lethal blood concentrations (i.e., 1–44 mg l^{-1}). Fatalities have been reported at doses as low as 350 mg in infants and at therapeutic doses in adults. Conversely, adult survival has been reported following doses as high as 10 and 17 g.

Chronic Toxicity

Human

In general, patients with a history of long-term treatment of any antipsychotic should be periodically reevaluated to determine whether continued therapy is warranted due to the potential for adverse reactions associated with long-term therapy. The following additional syndromes may occur at normal or toxic doses of chlorpromazine. Up to 60% of patients receiving antipsychotics, including chlorpromazine, experience extrapyramidal reactions, including dystonic reactions, feelings of motor restlessness, and parkinsonian manifestations (i.e., hypersalivation, tremors, shuffling gait, slowed speech, dysphagia, akinesia, or bradykinesia). Patients may also experience tardive dyskinesia, presenting as potentially irreversible, involuntary, dyskinetic movements. Tardive dyskinesia may remit partially or completely if the causative agent is removed; however, there is no established, reliable treatment. Toxicity due to chlorpromazine may also present as neuroleptic malignant syndrome (NMS), manifesting as hyperpyrexia, muscle rigidity, altered mental status, and autonomic instability (i.e., cardiac dysrhythmias, diaphoresis, irregular heart rate or blood pressure, tachycardia). Patients receiving antipsychotics may experience an encephalopathic syndrome consisting of confusion, extrapyramidal symptoms, fever, and lethargy.

Additional potential adverse reactions associated with chlorpromazine include anticholinergic adverse effects, cardiac arrest, cerebral edema, convulsive seizures, drowsiness, fever following large IM doses, jaundice, hematological disorders including agranulocytosis, lactation, peripheral edema, postural hypotension, psychotic symptoms, systemic lupus erythematosus-like syndrome, and tachycardia. The following adverse reactions are particularly related to long-term therapy: skin hyperpigmentation in patients receiving the drug for at least 3 years, deposition of particulate matter in the lens and cornea and development of opacities following treatment for at least 2 years, and development of multifocal tics and vocalizations following 6 years of treatment. See the FDA-approved prescribing information for a complete list of adverse drug effects and reactions.

Immunotoxicology

Chlorpromazine is contraindicated for use for patients with hypersensitivity to any phenothiazine due to the potential for crossover allergic reactions. Additionally, the parenteral product may cause anaphylaxis, life-threatening asthmatic episodes, or less severe asthmatic episodes in susceptible patients due to sulfites present in the formulation. Asthmatics are at heightened risk for this effect. Chlorpromazine hydrochloride injection may cause contact dermatitis; direct contact to skin should be avoided. In rare reported cases, this can progress to a persistent photosensitivity.

Reproductive Toxicity

Chlorpromazine is considered to be pregnancy category C. Rigorous animal studies have not been performed to evaluate the safety of chlorpromazine during pregnancy or breastfeeding. Two observational studies found no evidence of a relationship between chlorpromazine and perinatal mortality, defects, or malformations, while a second found a higher rate of malformations with phenothiazines compared with placebo (3.5% vs. 1.6%). Reported malformations attributed to chlorpromazine include syndactyly, microcephaly, clubfoot/hand, muscular abdominal aplasia, endocardial fibroelastosis, and brachymesophalangy. Microcephaly due to phenothiazines has been reported elsewhere.

Exposure to any phenothiazine during the third trimester of pregnancy is associated with increased neonatal risk for extrapyramidal reactions and/or withdrawal symptoms. Symptoms include agitation, feeding disorder, hypertonia, hypotonia, respiratory distress, somnolence, tardive dyskinetic-like symptoms, and tremor. It is important to note that in many reported cases of neonatal phenothiazine withdrawal, the mother was receiving multiple medications; however, some cases suggested risk with chlorpromazine alone.

Overall, chlorpromazine is not considered to be teratogenic. In one animal study, oral chlorpromazine was associated with ovarian toxicity and reduced fertility at doses of at least 10 mg kg^{-1}. Despite distributing to breast milk, no adverse events in breastfed babies have been reported.

Genotoxicity

In animal studies, certain phenothiazines have been associated with chromosomal aberrations in spermatocytes and abnormal sperm.

Carcinogenicity

Animal studies have shown increased risk for development of mammary neoplasms following long-term administration of prolactin-stimulating antipsychotics. Phenothiazines, including chlorpromazine, should be used with caution in patients with a history of breast cancer due to this theoretical risk. Current evidence is inconclusive as to the absolute risk associated with this issue.

Clinical Management

Patients suspected of overdose should be immediately transferred to a health care facility, a careful patient history should be taken to characterize present and previous exposures to chlorpromazine and other neuroleptics. Concurrent ingestion of TCAs should be ruled out. Chlorpromazine should be discontinued. Electrocardiogram (ECG), electrolytes, and arterial blood gases should be measured on admission. The recommended treatment for chlorpromazine overdose, and overdose of phenothiazines in general, is normal supportive and symptomatic care; no antidote is available at the time of writing. Continuous or repeat ECG is often necessary to continue to rule out development of dysrhythmia. If an ECG is abnormal, monitoring should continue for at least 24 h. Regular measurement of electrolytes, particularly potassium and magnesium, is intended to identify additional dysrhythmia risk. Arterial blood gases help rule out development of respiratory acidosis, which itself can increase dysrhythmia risk. Plasma chlorpromazine concentrations are recommended as helpful in clinical management of suspected overdose. Abnormalities in electrolytes and acid-base balance should be corrected.

Gastrointestinal decontamination with activated charcoal may be used for patients who present within 1 h of ingesting a potentially lethal dose. Repeat use of activated charcoal may enhance elimination; however, continued use increases risk for ileus. Additionally, gastric lavage may be used. Since phenothiazines can decrease gastrointestinal motility, gastric lavage may be effective up to several hours following ingestion. Forced emesis, cathartics, and whole bowel irrigation are not recommended due to lack of benefit and increased risk for decreased consciousness, aspiration, seizures, dystonia, and paralytic ileus.

If a patient develops extrapyramidal reactions as part of an overdosage, anticholinergic antiparkinsonian drugs may be used. The preferred agent for acute treatment is benztropine 1–2 mg IV or IM; for persistent dystonias, benztropine 2–8 mg day^{-1} in oral, divided doses or trihexyphenidyl 5–15 mg day^{-1} in divided doses can be used.

Little data are available regarding preferred treatment for chlorpromazine- or phenothiazine-induced dysrhythmias; however, sodium bicarbonate has been suggested due to its effectiveness in similar cardiac conduction defects in TCA toxicity. If a patient develops ventricular or supraventricular dysrhythmia, heart block, or a QRS interval wider than 120 ms, sodium bicarbonate may be given at doses of 1–3 mEq kg^{-1} IV bolus administered at 3- to 5-min intervals to a maximum blood pH of 7.55; lidocaine, phenytoin, isoproterenol, ventricular pacing, and defibrillation may also be warranted for second-line treatment depending on the clinical scenario. If sodium bicarbonate is ineffective in reducing a case of torsades de pointes, magnesium sulfate may be used. Medications that prolong the QTc interval (e.g., procainamide, quinidine) should be avoided due to risk of dysrhythmia development during concomitant use with chlorpromazine.

If patients develop hypotension, IV fluids and pressors should be used to maintain perfusion. Norepinephrine or phenylephrine are preferred pressors, as chlorpromazine reverses the effects of epinephrine and dopamine. Stimulants (i.e., amphetamine, destroamphetamine, caffeine with sodium benzoate) that do not increase seizure threshold may be used for patients with severe CNS depression. Benzodiazepines (e.g., diazepam 5–20 mg IV) are preferred for treatment of seizures; barbiturates should be relegated to second-line treatment due to their potential to induce respiratory depression.

Development of NMS will require management in an intensive care setting with similar supportive care as described. Additionally, bromocriptine 2.5–10 mg orally three to four times daily or dantrolene 1–3 mg kg^{-1} day^{-1} IV in four divided doses is recommended for treatment of severe cases and consideration for nonsevere cases. Concomitant development of acute renal failure should be addressed per normal guidelines. Chlorpromazine can be restarted under supervision at low doses after several weeks.

Ecotoxicology

Chlorpromazine may be released into the environment through its production and clinical use; its theoretical risk for bioconcentration in fish is high assuming that the organism does not metabolize the drug.

Other Hazards

When heated to decomposition, fumes of hydrogen chloride, nitroxides, and sulfoxides are emitted.

Exposure Standards and Guidelines

Clinically, doses should be titrated to patient response using the lowest dose possible. For most adult psychotic patients, oral doses of 500 mg day^{-1} are sufficient for chronic treatment; however, the maximum recommended total daily IM dose during acute psychosis is 2400 mg.

For psychotic pediatrics at least 6 months of age, the maximum recommended oral dose for chronic treatment is 0.55 mg kg^{-1} every 4 h. During acute episodes, IM doses up to 0.55 mg kg^{-1} every 6 h may be used. Maximum dose for patients younger than 5 years of age or less than 22.7 kg is 40 mg IM day^{-1}; maximum dose for patients aged 5–12 years and weighing 22.7–45.5 kg is 75 mg IM day^{-1}.

There are no occupational exposure standards for chlorpromazine.

See also: Anticholinergics; Phenothiazines; Tricyclic Antidepressants.

Further Reading

Buckley, N.A., 2004. Antipsychotic drugs (neuroleptics). In: Dart, R.C. (Ed.), Medical Toxicology, third ed. Lippincott Williams & Wilkins, New York, pp. 861–870.
Chlorpromazine [Prescribing Information], 2011. Sandoz Inc., Princeton, NJ.

Kelly, D.L., Weiner, E., Wehring, H.J., 2010. Schizophrenia. In: Chisholm-Burns, M.A., Schwinghammer, T.L., Wells, B.G., Malone, P.M., Kolesar, J.M., DiPiro, J.T. (Eds.), Pharmacotherapy: Principles & Practices, second ed. McGraw Hill Medical, Chicago, IL, pp. 631–652.

McEvoy, G.K. (Ed.), 2012. AHFS Drug Information. American Society of Health-Systems Pharmacists, Bethesda, MD.

Relevant Websites

Thomson Micromedex. DrugDex: Chlorpromazine. Available at: http://thomsonhc.com.

National Library of Medicine. Hazardous Substances Data Bank: Chlorpromazine. Available at: http://toxnet.nlm.nih.gov/cgi-bin/sis/search/f?./temp/~k36qkp:1.

Chlorpyrifos

SE Koshlukova and NR Reed, Environmental Protection Agency, Sacramento, CA, USA

This article is a revision of the previous edition article by Anuradha Nallapaneni and Carey N. Pope, volume 1, pp 583–585, © 2005, Elsevier Inc.

Chemical Profile

- Chemical Abstracts Service Registry Number: CAS 2921-88-2
- Chemical Name: *O,O*-Diethyl *O*-3,5,6-trichloropyridin-2-yl phosphorothioate
- Synonyms: Brodan, Detmol UA, Dowco 179, Dursban, Empire, Eradex, Lorsban, Paqeant, Piridane, Scout, Stipend
- Chemical Class: Organophosphate, Insecticide, Acaricide, Nematocide
- Chemical Structure: (from Pubchem) http://pubchem.ncbi.nlm.nih.gov/image/structurefly.cgi?cid=2730&width=400&height=400
- Molecular Formula: $C_9H_{11}Cl_3NO_3PS$
- Molecular Weight: 350.59 g mol^{-1}
- Density: 1.51 g cm^{-3} at 21 °C
- Vapor Pressure: 0.00002 mm Hg (0.003 Pa) at 25 °C
- Boiling Point: >320 °C
- Melting Point: 41–42 °C
- Flash Point: >200 °F
- Conversion Factor: 1 ppm = 14.31 mg m^{-3} at 25 °C
- Appearance: Colorless to white, crystalline solid
- Odor: Mild mercaptan

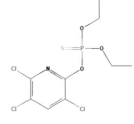

Background

Chlorpyrifos is a chlorinated organophosphorus (OP) ester manufactured as an insecticide, acaricide, and miticide. Like the other OP insecticides, the most prominent toxicity of chlorpyrifos is associated with binding and inhibition of the enzyme acetylcholinesterase (AChE) in insects and mammals. Chlorpyrifos requires metabolic activation to chlorpyrifos oxon to yield anticholinesterase activity.

First sold in 1965, chlorpyrifos is used globally to control agricultural and structural pests and mosquitos. In the 1990s, chlorpyrifos ranked as one of the top selling pesticides in the world, for the most part, replacing the persistent organochlorine insecticides. Over the last decade, concerns regarding toxicity to the developing nervous system have limited its use. By 2001, residential uses and uses in schools and parks were prohibited, and many agricultural uses were restricted and the US Residential use limitations were also imposed in Canada, Australia, and the European Union (EU). It continues to be used in large quantities to control crop damage worldwide. In the developing countries, excessive agricultural application and lack of protective devices result in hundreds of thousands of deaths yearly.

Uses

Chlorpyrifos is one of the most widely used OPs insecticides worldwide. During 1987–98, over 20 million pounds were used in the United States. Although registered for many fruits, vegetables, and grain crops, over 60% of chlorpyrifos is applied to four crops: corn, tree nuts, tree fruits, and soybeans. Once among the most widely applied pesticides in the US homes to control termites, cockroaches, and fleas, such uses were banned in 2001. Roach bait is the only residential use exempted from cancelation, because it is not expected to result in a significant exposure. Today, nonagricultural uses in the United States are limited to mosquito control for public health purposes and insect control on golf courses. In 2006, the major manufacturers of chlorpyrifos in the United States and the EU began a global phase out of nonagricultural uses of chlorpyrifos. However, other manufactures may continue to support residential uses outside the United States and EU.

Environmental Fate and Behavior

Chlorpyrifos is soluble in organic solvents (e.g., isooctane, methanol), but has low solubility in water (<2 mg l^{-1} solubility at 25 °C). The calculated Henry's law constant of 0.00001 atm m^3 mol^{-1} indicates possibility of volatilization from surface water. The odor threshold of chlorpyrifos is 0.14 mg m^{-3} (10 ppb). The estimated half-life for reacting with photochemically generated hydroxyl radicals in the air is 6.3 h. Photolysis of chlorpyrifos produces dechlorinated products.

Chlorpyrifos undergoes abiotic hydrolysis, photodegradation, and biotic degradation in soil and water. Depending on the soil type and climate, its soil persistence varies from 2 weeks to over 1 year. Microbial degradation is indicated by the shorter half-lives in natural soils than sterile soils. Chemical hydrolysis produces *O*-ethyl-*O*-3,5,6-trichloro-2-pyridyl phosphorothioate or 3,5,6-trichloro-2-pyridinol (TCP) and phosphorthioic acid at alkaline conditions. Half-lives in river and well waters vary from 4.8 to 38 days, with the rate of hydrolysis increasing with temperature and alkalinity. The estimated Log K_{oc} of 3.73 predicts strong adsorption to soil and resist leaching to groundwater. Chlorpyrifos can persist indoors for several months.

Oxidation of chlorpyrifos to its more toxic metabolite chlorpyrifos oxon could occur through photolysis, aerobic metabolism, and chlorination. Water chlorination is the major route of chlorpyrifos oxon formation. It is subsequently rapidly

 http://dx.doi.org/10.1016/B978-0-12-386454-3.00115-9

hydrolyzed to TCP. TCP and its glucuronide conjugates have been detected in fish tissues. The measured K_{ow} of 4.8 indicates a potential for bioaccumulation in aquatic and terrestrial food chains.

Exposure and Exposure Monitoring

Exposure to chlorpyrifos may occur through ingestion of residues in the diet, inhalation of vapors, and dermal absorption following skin contact. Prior to 2001, residential exposure to chlorpyrifos was widespread. Today, exposure to the general public occurs principally via the diet. Residential exposure is still possible from the remaining registered uses for mosquito control and on golf course turf. Indoor air and house dust exposures may add to the total in-home exposures in heavily agricultural areas. Dermal and inhalation exposure pathways are likely to dominate workers' exposures from handling chlorpyrifos or reentering treated fields.

Enforceable maximum residue levels of chlorpyrifos (or 'tolerances' in the United States) are established for more than 100 food commodities. These are the highest levels allowable in or on these commodities. At a given exposure concentration, children generally have higher body burden due to their higher intake (inhalation volume, amount of food intake) or contact on a per body weight basis.

Toxicokinetics

The estimated oral absorption of chlorpyrifos is 70–99% in rats and humans. In rats, peak blood level of chlorpyrifos and its metabolites occurs between 3 and 6 h after dosing. The estimated dermal absorption is 3–10% based on the urinary recovery of metabolites. The inhalation absorption is mostly indicated by the inhibition of ChE activities.

In animals and humans, chlorpyrifos is extensively metabolized by the liver cytochrome P-450 enzymes (CYP). Oxidative desulfuration results in the potent ChE inhibitor chlorpyrifos oxon. Dearylation of chlorpyrifos and chlorpyrifos oxon by CYP produces TCP and diethyl thiophosphate (DETP). Hydrolyses of chlorpyrifos oxon by A-esterases (paraoxonases, PON1) forms TCP and diethylphosphate (DEP). Extrahepatic metabolism may occur in tissues such as brain and intestine. In animals, the highest levels of chlorpyrifos are found in the fat. It also binds to plasma proteins, such as albumin. Chlorpyrifos is detected in rat and human milk. In rats, transplacental transfer to the fetus is evidenced by the ChE inhibition in fetal plasma and brain and by the presence of chlorpyrifos in the fetal liver, brain, placenta, umbilical cord, and amniotic fluid.

The urine is the main route of elimination for chlorpyrifos, where 84% of a single oral dose in rats is found within 72 h. About 5% is excreted in the bile/feces. The major urinary metabolites are TCP, DEP, DETP, glucuronide, and sulfate conjugates. In humans, 70% is excreted in urine as conjugated TCP within 5 days of a single oral exposure. Levels of urinary TCP are commonly used in human biomonitoring studies. The elimination half-life for chlorpyrifos in rats and humans is 10–27 h.

Mechanism of Toxicity

The classical mechanism of toxicity of chlorpyrifos is related to the ability of its oxon metabolite to bind and inhibit the serine hydrolase AChE. The nervous system is the primary target because AChE hydrolyzes the neurotransmitter acetylcholine thereby terminating its synaptic action. Inhibition of AChE increases the availability of acetylcholine at the neural synapse leading to excessive stimulation of the cholinergic pathways in the central and peripheral nervous systems. Significant inactivation of AChE causes acute cholinergic effects, morbidity, or death.

Chlorpyrifos oxon interacts with other esterases such as butyrylcholinesterase, neuropathy target esterase (NTE), carboxylesterase, and PON1. Carboxylesterases and PON1 are key enzymes involved in detoxification of chlorpyrifos. Carboxylesterases act as alternative targets to AChE for chlorpyrifos oxon thereby decreasing its concentration in blood. Gender and age differences are observed in the carboxylesterase activity in animals. PON1 is a polymorphic enzyme with allozymes differing in their ability for hydrolytic detoxification of chlorpyrifos oxon. The PON1 status is an important determinant in modulating the acute toxicity of chlorpyrifos. Butyrylcholinesterase may function as a molecular scavenger for chlorpyrifos in the blood or substitute for AChE where it is low. NTE may be involved in the OP-induced delayed neurotoxicity syndrome.

Chlorpyrifos itself is a week ChE inhibitor. In risk assessment, the co-occurrence of chlorpyrifos and chlorpyrifos oxon is addressed by applying a toxicity equivalence factor or relative potency factor of 10 to chlorpyrifos oxon.

Concerns were raised regarding regulatory standards of chlorpyrifos established based on its inhibitory effects on ChE activity that may overlook potentially more sensitive non-cholinergic mechanisms. Besides AChE, potential targets include neurogenesis, nervous system development, cytotoxicity, macromolecule synthesis, neurotransmitter receptors, oxidative stress, cell signaling, nuclear transcription factors, and neuronal-glial cell interactions.

Acute and Short-Term Toxicity

Animal

Chlorpyrifos is classified by US Environmental Protection Agency (USEPA) as a moderate oral toxicant (Category II). The acute oral LD_{50} is 32 mg kg^{-1} for hens and 82–504 mg kg^{-1} for rats, mice, and guinea pigs. The oral LD_{50} for chlorpyrifos oxon is >100 mg kg^{-1} in male rats and 300 mg kg^{-1} in female rats. The oral toxicity of chlorpyrifos oxon may be attenuated by extensive hepatic metabolism before entering systemic circulation. Chlorpyrifos dermal LD_{50} in rats is 202 mg kg^{-1} day^{-1}. The 4-h inhalation LC_{50} in rats is >2 mg l^{-1}. Chlorpyrifos is a Category IV skin and eye irritant (slight conjunctival and dermal irritation).

The main targets of chlorpyrifos toxicity after short-term oral exposure are the nervous system and the developing offspring. Cholinergic syndromes from overstimulation of the muscarinic and nicotinic-type acetylcholine receptors include hypersalivation, respiratory distress, miosis, muscular twitches, tremors, ataxia, diarrhea, and vomiting. Other nonlethal effects are hematological and liver enzyme changes, chromodacryorrhea, tachycardia, renal effects, hypothermia, and body weight decreases. No delayed neuropathy was observed in hens receiving a single or 20 repeated oral doses of chlorpyrifos.

Young animals are three- to fourfold more sensitive to ChE inhibition than adults. Applying the Benchmark Dose (BMD) analysis, USEPA established a lower bound of BMD (BMDL) at 0.36 mg kg^{-1} day^{-1} based on 10% red blood cell (RBC) ChE inhibition in postnatal day (PND) 11 pups after a single oral exposure. For acute chlorpyrifos oxon exposure, the similarly determined BMDL is 0.08 mg kg^{-1} day^{-1}.

Pregnant animals are 2- to12-fold more sensitive than nonpregnant adults to ChE inhibition, which may reflect the capacity of key detoxification enzymes such as paraoxonase and P450 isozymes.

Human

Human deaths are reported due to accidental exposure or intentional ingestion of chlorpyrifos. The exposure level or duration is generally unknown. Death is caused by respiratory and cardiovascular failure.

Nonlethal acute poisoning affects the central nervous system and cardiovascular and respiratory systems. Common clinical signs of cholinergic toxicity in humans are numbness, dizziness, tremor, abdominal cramps, sweating, lacrimation, salivation, and blurred vision. High doses (>300 mg kg^{-1}) lead to unconsciousness, convulsions, cyanosis, and uncontrolled urination. In some acute poisoning cases, sequelae (intermediate syndrome) characterized by muscle paralysis were reported 1–4 weeks after exposure. In clinical studies of male adults, the lowest observed effect level (LOEL) for inhibition of plasma ChE is 0.5 mg kg^{-1}.

Chronic Toxicity

Animal

Mortality occurred in pregnant rats at 5 mg kg^{-1} day^{-1} and pregnant mice at 25 mg kg^{-1} day^{-1}. Nonlethal LOELs for nonpregnant adults included 2–15 mg kg^{-1} day^{-1} for increased adrenal gland, brain, and heart weight in rats, 3–45 mg kg^{-1} day^{-1} for increased liver weight and hepatocyte vacuolation in dogs and mice, 15 mg kg^{-1} day^{-1} for changes in hematologic parameters in rats, 1.2–25 mg kg^{-1} day^{-1} for decreases in body weight, bodyweight gains, and food consumption in mice and rats, and 45 mg kg^{-1} $day^{-1}$for ocular opacity and hair loss in mice. USEPA established a BMDL of 0.09 mg kg^{-1} day^{-1} based on 10% RBC ChE inhibition in PND 11 male rats after 11 days of oral exposures.

Human

Effects reported in workers chronically exposed to chlorpyrifos included impaired memory, disorientation, speech difficulties, nausea, and weakness. In clinical studies, the LOEL for inhibition of plasma ChE for repeated 28-day oral exposures is 0.01 mg kg^{-1} day^{-1}, 50-fold lower than for a single oral exposure.

Both population-based multiyear biomonitoring (e.g., National Health and Nutrition Examination Survey (NHANES)) and longitudinal farming-related monitoring provide data that facilitate recent efforts to relate the exposure to OP toxicity in human population. Epidemiological studies using chlorpyrifos specific markers are discussed under Developmental Neurotoxicity.

Immunotoxicity

Studies in rodents, cats, and dogs conducted over the past four decades indicate that at doses causing significant ChE inhibition, chlorpyrifos does not alter the immune system function.

Reproductive and Developmental Toxicity

Animal

In prenatal developmental studies, pregnant rats and mice received chlorpyrifos up to 15–25 mg kg^{-1} day^{-1} orally on gestation days (GD) 6–15 or pregnant rabbits received 140 mg kg^{-1} day^{-1} on GD 7–19. Fetal growth retardation and malformations were observed in the presence of maternal toxicity.

In two- and three-generation studies, rats fed 0.3–5 mg kg^{-1} day^{-1} chlorpyrifos mated normally and exhibited normal pregnancy, offspring, and lactation, although maternal and fetal body weights were impacted at 5 mg kg^{-1} day^{-1}. Available data suggest that chlorpyrifos is not teratognic and does not adversely affect reproduction. Inhibition of RBC ChE activity had the lowest LOEL of 0.1–0.3 mg kg^{-1} day^{-1}.

Human

Collective results from three major prospective cohort studies indicated association of indoor and outdoor exposure to chlorpyrifos during pregnancy to decreased birth size, decreased gestational age at birth, and decreased head circumference, especially at low maternal PON1 levels. These studies evaluated pre- and postnatal pesticide exposure in mother–infant pairs and birth and developmental outcomes in neonates, infants, and young children. The Columbia University in New York City study focused on chlorpyrifos levels in the umbilical cord and maternal plasma as a direct biomarker for chlorpyrifos *in utero* fetal exposure. The other two studies from Mount Sinai Hospital in New York City and from the University of California at Berkeley measured TCP (a metabolite of chlorpyrifos and chlorpyrifos methyl) and nonspecific OP metabolites in maternal urine.

Studies in men using urinary TCP as an indicator for chlorpyrifos exposure revealed an association with decreased testosterone or alterations in the homeostasis of thyroid and sex steroid hormones. Their TCP levels fall within the range of the NHANES data for the general US population.

Developmental Neurotoxicity

Chlorpyrifos causes developmental neurotoxicity at doses not altering pregnancy and general health of the offspring, and in the absence of fetal brain ChE inhibition. At a subtoxic dose (i.e., 1 mg kg^{-1} day^{-1}), gestational and early postnatal exposure in rats and mice produced long-lasting impairment of locomotor activity (exploration and rearing), deficit in the cognitive function (spatial learning and memory), and social interaction (aggression and maternal behavior in adulthood). A number of noncholinergic mechanisms have been suggested for the neurodevelopmental perturbations; however, evidence for alternative targets is not conclusive.

The developmental neurotoxicity reported in rats and mice provides implications for humans with documented developmental exposure, such as the participants in the epidemiologic studies previously described who had measured chlorpyrifos levels in maternal and umbilical cord blood. At 3 years of age, children from higher chlorpyrifos levels in the umbilical cord plasma showed delays in cognitive and motor functions and problems with attention.

Genotoxicity

Several limited assays showed that chlorpyrifos is negative for gene mutation (*Salmonella*, *Escherichia coli*, Chinese hamster ovary cell hypoxanthine-guanine phosphoribosyl transferase forward mutation) and chromosomal aberration (rat lymphocytes, mouse bone marrow micronucleus). DNA damage assays were negative in mammalian cells (unscheduled DNA synthesis in WI-38 human embryonic lung fibroblast cell line and rat hepatocytes) but positive in yeast, *E. coli*, and *Bacillus subtilis*.

Carcinogenicity

No evidence of carcinogenicity through dietary exposures was found in F344 rats and CD-1 mice.

Ecotoxicology

The acute LC_{50} for estuarine algae is 140–300 ppb. The 96-h LC_{50} for aquatic invertebrates varies with species, e.g., 0.04 ppb for mysid shrimp, 0.38 ppb for stonefly, and 6.0 for crayfish. The 48-h LC_{50} for *Daphnia magna* is 0.6 ppb. The acute LC_{50} for fish also showed wide species variations, e.g., 0.6 ppb for striped bass and 130–163 ppb for fathead minnow. The toxicity increases with increasing temperature, e.g., for rainbow trout, LC_{50} is 51, 15, and 7.0 ppb at 1.6, 7.2, and 12.7 °C, respectively. The chronic no observed adverse effect concentration (NOAEC) for reproduction is <0.0046 ppb for mysid shrimp, 0.04 ppb for *D. magna*, 0.28 ppb for Atlantic silverside, and 0.57 ppb for fathead minnow.

The acute avian species LD_{50} is $10\ mg\ kg^{-1}$ for house sparrow and 136 ppm in the diet for mallard duck. The chronic dietary no observed adverse effect level for reproduction is 25 ppm for mallard duck. Toxicities to mammals are presented in the acute and chronic toxicity sections.

Based on estimates of risk quotients in 2006, USEPA concluded high risk of chlorpyrifos to aquatic invertebrate species, fish, birds, and small mammals from a single outdoor application and prolonged risk from multiple applications. Aquatic birds and mammals are additionally at risk from chlorpyrifos bioconcentrating in water bodies.

Other Hazards

Simultaneous exposure to other OPs that are detoxified by carboxylesterase (e.g., malathion, diazinon, azinphos methyl, parathion) results in more extensive toxicity in terms of lethality, clinical signs, and ChE inhibition than with chlorpyrifos alone. Inhibition of carboxylesterase activity may be the cause of these toxicological interactions.

Chlorpyrifos is a potent inhibitor of the human metabolism of environmental chemicals (carbaryl, fipronil, N,N-diethyl-3-methylbenzamide, and the jet fuel components nonane and naphthalene) that are substrates of common CYPs (CYP3A4, CYP2B6) and share biotransformation pathways. Metabolic interactions are reported with endogenous substrates (testosterone and estradiol) and with the antidepressant drug imipramine possibly through competition for CYP3A4 and CYP1A2. All of the CYP inhibitions, also known as 'suicidal or mechanism-based inhibition,' are irreversible and result from the formation of reactive sulfur during chlorpyrifos desulfuration. In rats, chlorpyrifos alters the serotonin systems during neurodevelopment.

Exposure Standards and Guidelines

American Conference of Governmental Industrial Hygienists Threshold Limit Value: $0.1\ mg\ m^{-3}$ Time-weighted average (TWA); Inhalable fraction and vapor (skin) (A4 – Not Classifiable as a Human Carcinogen)

National Institute for Occupational Safety and Health Recommended Exposure Limit: $0.2\ mg\ m^{-3}$ TWA; $0.6\ mg\ m^{-3}$ Short-term exposure limit; (Skin)

USEPA population-adjusted dose (oral): $0.0036\ mg\ kg^{-1}\ day^{-1}$ (acute); $0.0003\ mg\ kg^{-1}\ day^{-1}$ (chronic)

See also: Behavioral Toxicology; Developmental Toxicology; Toxicity Testing, Developmental; A-esterase; Fermentation (Industrial): Media for Industrial Fermentations; Carboxylesterases; Cholinesterase Inhibition; Common Mechanism of Toxicity in Pesticides; Neurotoxicity; Organophosphorus Compounds; Pesticides; Cytochrome P450; National Institute for Occupational Safety and Health; Carcinogen Classification Schemes; Federal Insecticide, Fungicide, and Rodenticide Act, US; Genetic Toxicology; International Agency for Research on Cancer; Regulation, Toxicology and; Toxicity Testing, Reproductive; Risk Assessment, Human Health; Ecotoxicology; ACGIH® (American Conference of Governmental Industrial Hygienists); Food Quality Protection Act; Children's Environmental Health; Epidemiology; Environmental Fate and Behavior.

Further Reading

Agency for Toxic Substances and Disease Registry (ATSDR), 1997. Toxicological Profile for Chlorpyrifos. Public Health Service, U.S. Department of Health and Human Services. http://www.atsdr.cdc.gov/toxprofiles/tp84.pdf.

American Conference of Governmental Industrial Hygienists (ACGIH), 2003. Chlorpyrifos: TLV® Chemical Substances, seventh ed. Documentation. Publication #7DOC-134.

Eaton, D.L., et al., 2008. Review of the toxicology of chlorpyrifos with an emphasis on human exposure and neurodevelopment. Crit. Rev. Toxicol. 38 (2), 1–125. www.sciencepartners.com/html/pdf/Chlorpyrifos.pdf.

National Institute for Occupational Safety and Health (NIOSH), 2007. Pocket Guide to Chemical Hazards. Department of Health and Human Services, Centers for Disease Control and Prevention. DHHS (NIOSH) Publication No. 2005-149. September 2007. http://www.cdc.gov/niosh/docs/2005-149/pdfs/2005-149.pdf.

Testai, E., Buratti, F.M., Di Consiglio, E., 2010. Chlorpyrifos. In: Kreiger, R. (Ed.), Hayes' Handbook of Pesticide Toxicology, third ed. Academic Press, San Diego, USA, pp. 1505–1519.

USEPA, 2011. Chlorpyrifos: Preliminary Human Health Risk Assessment for Registration Review. United States Environmental Protection Agency. EPA-HQ-OPP-2008-0850-0025. http://www.regulations.gov/#!documentDetail;D=EPA-HQ-OPP-2008-0850-0025.

Relevant Websites

http://www.atsdr.cdc.gov – Agency for Toxic Substances and Disease Registry.
http://toxnet.nlm.nih.gov – Hazardous Substance Data Bank.
http://npic.orst.edu – National Pesticide Information Center.
http://www.epa.gov – United States Environmental Protection Agency.
http://www.osha.gov – United States Occupational Safety and Health Administration.

Chlorsulfuron

M Battalora, MD McCoole, and CM Hirata, DuPont Crop Protection, Stine-Haskell Research Center, Newark, DE, USA

- Name: Chlorsulfuron
- Chemical Abstracts Service Registry Number: 64902-72-3
- Synonyms: Glean®, Telar®
- Molecular Formula: $C_{12}H_{12}ClN_5O_4S$
- Chemical Structure:

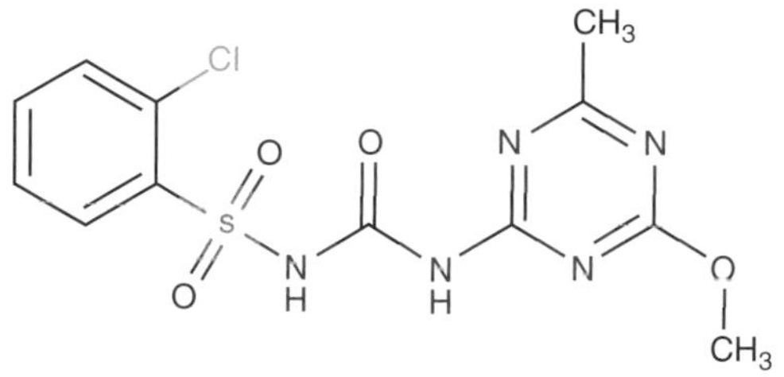

Background

Chlorsulfuron is one of the first sulfonylurea herbicides developed and commercialized by DuPont. Dr George Levitt and his team at DuPont first synthesized chlorsulfuron in 1976, and it was commercialized for use as a herbicide in 1981. It is currently registered by DuPont in the United States, Canada, the European Union, Russia, the Ukraine, Australia, New Zealand, South Africa, Saudi Arabia, and in several countries of South America.

Compared with many other herbicides that are applied at levels of pounds per acre (or kilograms per acre), sulfonylureas are highly effective at use rates of less than an ounce per acre (approximately 6 g per acre for chlorsulfuron).

Uses

Chlorsulfuron is used as a postemergence herbicide for the control of dicotyledonous weeds, with excellent safety for wheat and other cereals crops. While chlorsulfuron is primarily used to control weeds in cereals, it can also be used in range and pasture applications. It is currently only used to a minor extent for nonfood industrial applications and right-of-way purposes.

Environmental Behavior, Fate, Routes, and Pathways

Chlorsulfuron has a moderate to short-lived fate in the environment. It does not bioaccumulate and is not volatile. In the environment, chlorsulfuron degrades via a combination of biotic and abiotic processes. Chlorsulfuron degrades in acidic solutions and soil by cleavage of the sulfonylurea bridge, *O*-demethylation, and hydroxylation. Chlorsulfuron is metabolized by soil microbes to numerous minor degradation products, is mineralized to CO_2, and sequestered as nonextractable residues. Photodegradation is not a significant pathway of dissipation for chlorsulfuron in the environment. Hydrolytic processes are not expected to be a major contributing factor in the environmental degradation of chlorsulfuron, and would only be significant at acidic pH. While the hydrolysis of chlorsulfuron is significant at pH 5, with a first-order half-life of ~23 days at 25 °C, it is essentially stable at pH 7 and 9.

Exposure

Since the use rates are very low, there is expected to be very little exposure to the pesticide applicator. Additionally, very little exposure due to residues in commodities is expected.

Toxicokinetics

Following oral exposure, chlorsulfuron was extensively absorbed at both low and high doses in rats. It was rapidly excreted mostly in the unmetabolized form. Urine was the predominant route of elimination, with lesser excretion in the feces. Cleavage of the sulfonylurea bridge by hydrolysis occurred to a minor extent. Tissue clearance was rapid, with less than 1% remaining in the tissues at 120 h.

Mechanisms of Action

Chlorsulfuron, as a sulfonylurea, functions as a herbicide by inhibiting amino acid synthesis. It operates specifically as an acetolactate synthase inhibitor, which catalyzes the first step in branched-chain amino acid synthesis. Inhibition of this enzyme essentially starves plant cells by blocking the biosynthesis of essential amino acids such as valine and isoleucine needed for new growth. This enzyme is not present in animals.

In regard to animal toxicity, few specific effects have been observed. The main findings in toxicity studies are related to body weight decreases. There have been some transient observations of decreased red cell parameters observed in repeated dose studies at high doses.

Acute and Short-Term Toxicity

Results of acute toxicity studies in rats indicate that chlorsulfuron has no significant acute toxicity via the oral, dermal, or inhalation route of exposure. In animal studies, chlorsulfuron was not a skin or eye irritant in rabbits. It did not cause skin sensitization in guinea pigs.

The acute oral LD_{50} value in rats is $>5000\ mg\ kg^{-1}$ body weight. The acute dermal LD_{50} value in rabbits is $>3400\ mg\ kg^{-1}$

body weight (highest dose tested). Finally, the acute inhalation LC_{50} value in rats is >5 mg l^{-1} (4-h exposure).

In shorter-term repeated dose studies by oral feeding (90-day rat and mouse studies, 6-month to 1-year studies in dogs), the effects of chlorsulfuron were characterized primarily by reductions in body weight parameters and/or nutritional status. A few effects on clinical pathology parameters, including reductions in red blood cell mass, were observed in the 90-day mouse study and the 1-year dog study. These clinical pathology changes were not observed consistently across species and, when observed, did not occur in both sexes. The hematology effects observed in the subchronic mouse study were considered to be nonadverse. The effects in female dogs were considered to be adverse or potentially adverse but reversible. When considering these three species, the dog was the most sensitive species, based on reductions in indicators of circulating erythrocyte mass and slight body weight changes in the 1-year feeding study. The no observed adverse effect level in this study was approximately 60 mg kg^{-1} body weight per day^{-1}.

Neurotoxicity studies have not been performed with chlorsulfuron; however, there is no indication of a neurotoxic effect in the toxicity studies performed with chlorsulfuron. Furthermore, this compound is a herbicide and its mode of action differs from the mode(s) of action of insecticides that have neurotoxic effects. In addition, several sulfonylureas have been tested in acute and subchronic neurotoxicity studies, but no findings that suggest a clear neurotoxicological effect have been reported.

Chronic Toxicity

The main findings in the long-term studies in rats and mice were based on body weight and/or nutritional decrements. In rats, effects were observed mainly during the first year of the study, although male rats had lower body weight and food efficiency throughout the study. Likewise, in mice the main effects were body weight and nutritional decrements.

Immunotoxicity

No specific immunotoxicity studies have been performed with chlorsulfuron. However, in the regulatory toxicology studies, organs of the immune system have not been observed to be a target. Furthermore, several sulfonylureas have been tested in immunotoxicity studies, and none have produced an effect supportive of immunotoxicity.

Reproductive and Developmental Toxicity

Developmental and reproductive toxicity studies with chlorsulfuron that were conducted in the early 1980s suggested a possible impact in this area. Specifically, effects in the rabbit developmental toxicity study suggested a possible test substance-related increase in resorptions. Likewise, the reproduction study in rats suggested a possible test substance-related decrease in the fertility index. Subsequently, guideline-compliant studies were conducted using higher doses. In the guideline study in rabbits there were no increases in resorptions observed. The modern multigeneration reproduction study in rats did not indicate any decrease in fertility. Hence, the original findings were merely spurious in the case of the rabbit developmental toxicity study, and due to a lack of consideration of the historical control data in the case of the reproduction study. No specific effects on offspring were observed in the study with rats at doses that were not maternally toxic.

Genotoxicity

A full battery of *in vitro* studies with chlorsulfuron was conducted in bacteria and in mammalian cells. Additionally, *in vivo* genetic toxicity studies in rats and mice were also performed. Results from all studies were negative. There was no indication of a genotoxic effect.

Carcinogenicity

Two-year dietary feeding studies were conducted in rats and mice with chlorsulfuron. There was no indication of a carcinogenic effect in mice. There was a slight increase in unilateral interstitial cell tumors but no increase in bilateral tumors in male rats at the highest dose tested. The number of tumors was within the historical control range. Since survival was increased in the high-dose group, the marginal increase in these tumors is likely a result of the increased longevity observed at this dose. The United States Environmental Protection Agency (US EPA) assessed these data and reported in 2005 that chlorsulfuron showed no evidence of carcinogenicity.

Ecotoxicology

Regulatory testing has shown that chlorsulfuron exhibited no toxicity to mammals, birds, fish, aquatic invertebrates, bees and other insects, or soil organisms. Chlorsulfuron has been shown not to bioaccumulate in the environment, further reducing the likelihood of adverse effects from exposure. Chlorsulfuron is highly active on some terrestrial and aquatic plants and has been shown to have effects on nontarget plant species. This sensitivity of nontarget plants to chlorsulfuron has been shown to be the result of differential metabolism. Because of its high efficacy at low concentrations, effects on nontarget plant species need to be considered. However, potential exposure to the environment and nontarget organisms is reduced through low use rates of chlorsulfuron.

Exposure Standards and Guidelines

The European Union set an acceptable daily intake level for dietary risk assessment at 0.02 mg kg^{-1} body weight per day^{-1}, based on the 2-year rat study (European Union, 2010). The US EPA also set a chronic reference dose of 0.02 mg kg^{-1}

body weight per day^{-1} based on the same study in 2002 (US EPA, 2002).

The European Union has set maximum residue limits for various commodities (0.1 mg kg^{-1} for cereals, 0.05 mg kg^{-1} for most other plant commodities, and 0.01 mg kg^{-1} for animal commodities) (European Union, 2008). The US EPA has set a range of tolerances for various commodities (0.1 ppm for wheat, barley, and oat grains, 0.5 ppm for their straws, and 20 ppm for oat and wheat forage, 0.1 ppm for milk, 0.3 ppm for other animal tissues, 11 ppm grass forage, and 19 ppm grass hay) (US EPA, 2002).

References

European Union, 2008. Commission Regulation (EC) No 149/2008, amending Regulation (EC) No 396/2005 of the European Parliament and of the Council by establishing, Annexes II, III and IV setting maximum residue levels for products covered by Annex I thereto.

European Union, 2010. *Chlorsulfuron, SANCO/198/08 – final. Review report for the active substance Chlorsulfuron*, Finalised in the Standing Committee on the Food Chain and Animal Health at its meeting on, 26 February 2009, in view of the inclusion of Chlorsulfuron in Annex I of Directive 91/414/EEC.

US EPA, Wednesday, August 14, 2002. Federal Register, vol. 67, No. 157, *Chlorsulfuron; Pesticide Tolerance*. pp. 52866–52873.

Chlorzoxazone

KN Thakore, California Department of Public Health, Richmond, CA, USA
HM Mehendale, University of Louisiana at Monroe, Monroe, LA, USA

- Name: Chlorzoxazone
- Chemical Abstracts Service Registry Number: 95-25-0
- Synonyms: 5-Chloro-3(*H*)-2-benzoxazolone, 5-Chloro-2-benzoxazolol, Paraflex, Biomioran, Solaxin
- Molecular Formula: $C_7H_4ClNO_2$
- Chemical Structure:

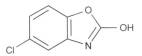

Chlorzoxazone (CAS RN 95-25-0)

Background

Chlorzoxazone is a muscle relaxant. It acts by blocking nerve impulses or pain sensations that are sent to brain. Typically, it is used together with rest and physical therapy to treat skeletal muscle conditions such as pain or injury. Chlorzoxazone, 5-chloro-2-benzoxazolione, is synthesized by a heterocyclization reaction of 2-amino-4-chlorophenol with phosgene. Skeletal muscle relaxants have conventionally been classified into one group; however, they are actually a heterogeneous group of medications commonly used to treat two different types of underlying conditions – spasticity from upper motor neuron syndromes and muscular pain or spasms from peripheral musculoskeletal conditions. Medications classified as skeletal muscle relaxants are baclofen, carisoprodol, chlorzoxazone, cyclobenzaprine, dantrolene, metaxalone, methocarbamol, orphenadrine, and tizanidine. These drugs may impair mental and/or physical abilities required for driving vehicles. As a class, skeletal muscle relaxants have central nervous system (CNS)-related side effects: drowsiness, dizziness, decreased alertness, blurred vision, and ataxia. Their use has been associated with a twofold increase in the risk for motor vehicle crashes. Muscle relaxants are included in the 'Beers List' of potentially inappropriate medications in older adults. Most muscle relaxants are poorly tolerated by elderly patients because they cause anticholinergic adverse effects, sedation, and weakness. Although extremely uncommon, this compound may yield to idiosyncratic and unpredictable type of liver toxicity. The concomitant use of alcohol or other CNS depressants may have an additive effect. Individuals on chlorzoxazone containing drugs should be monitored for abnormal liver enzymes (e.g., aspartate transaminase (AST), alanine transaminase (ALT), alkaline phosphatase, bilirubin, etc.).

Uses

Chlorzoxazone is used as a centrally acting skeletal muscle relaxant and as an analgesic. It is also a strong oxidizing agent.

Environmental Fate and Behavior

It is a white to off-white solid. It is soluble in organic solvents such as ethanol, methanol, and dimethyl sulfoxide (DMSO).

Exposure and Exposure Monitoring

When heated to decompose, chlorzoxazone emits acrid smoke and irritating fumes.

Toxicokinetics

Chlorzoxazone is rapidly absorbed and eliminated by oral route. The half-life for an oral dose is about 1 h. The decay of its plasma concentration is also rapid after intravenous administration. The concentration of chlorzoxazone in fat is twice the plasma level. Chlorzoxazone is rapidly metabolized in the liver by CYP1A2 and CYP2E1 to 6-hydroxychlorzoxazone which conjugates with glucuronide. This glucuronide conjugate is then eliminated in urine.

Mechanism of Toxicity

Chlorzoxazone is metabolized by the CYP1A2 and CYP2E1 microsomal enzymes to a toxic metabolite 6-hydroxychlorzoxazone.

Acute and Short-Term Toxicity

Animal

In rat, the oral and intraperitoneal LD_{50} values are 763 and 150 mg kg^{-1} bw, respectively. In mouse, the oral, intraperitoneal, and subcutaneous LD_{50} values are 440, 50, and 170 mg kg^{-1} bw, respectively. In the hamster, the oral and intraperitoneal LD_{50} values are 662 and 166 mg kg^{-1} bw, respectively.

Human

Exposure to chlorzoxazone is harmful through inhalation, dermal, and oral routes. It causes drowsiness; CNS effects such as headache, dizziness, and blurred vision; nausea and vomiting; and eye, skin, and mucous membrane irritation. The liver, nerves, and skeletal muscles are the target organs. Multiple exposures to chlorzoxazone by ingestion can cause increase in morbidity and mortality.

Clinical Management

In case of contact, the eyes and skin should be flushed immediately with water for at least 15 min. If the victim is not

 http://dx.doi.org/10.1016/B978-0-12-386454-3.00285-2

breathing, artificial respiration should be administered; if breathing with difficulty, oxygen should be given. If the patient is in cardiac arrest, cardiopulmonary resuscitation should be provided. If swallowed, the mouth should be washed out with water provided the person is conscious. Life-support measures should be continued until medical assistance has arrived. An unconscious or convulsing person should not be given liquids or induced to vomit.

Exposure Standards and Guidelines

Engineering controls, standard work practices, and personal protective equipment, including respirators are employed to prevent worker exposure to chlorzoxazone. After use, the clothing and equipment should be placed in an impervious container for decontamination or disposal.

See also: Musculoskeletal System; Neurotoxicity; Oxidative Stress.

Further Reading

Ahn, C.Y., Bae, S.K., Jung, Y.S., et al., 2008. Pharmacokinetic parameters of chlorzoxazone and its main metabolite, 6-hydroxychlorzoxazone, after intravenous and oral administration of chlorzoxazone to liver cirrhotic rats with diabetes mellitus. Drug Metab. Dispos. 36 (7), 1233–1241.

Ahn, C.Y., Kim, E.J., Lee, I., et al., 2003. Effects of glucose on the pharmacokinetics of intravenous chlorzoxazone in rats with acute renal failure induced by uranyl nitrate. J. Pharm. Sci. 92 (8), 1604–1613.

Anon., 1996. Chlorzoxazone hepatotoxicity. Med. Lett. Drugs Ther. 38 (974), 46.

Gao, N., Zou, D., Qiao, H.L., 2013. Concentration-dependent inhibitory effect of Baicalin on the plasma protein binding and metabolism of chlorzoxazone, a CYP2E1 probe substrate, in rats in vitro and in vivo. PLoS One 8 (1), e53038. http://dx.doi.org/10.1371/journal.pone.0053038.

Kim, R.B., O'Shea, D., 1995. Interindividual variability of chlorzoxazone 6-hydroxylation in men and women and its relationship to CYP2E1 genetic polymorphisms. Clin. Pharmacol. Ther. 57 (6), 645–655.

Lenga, R.E., 1988. Chlorzoxazone. In: Lenga, R.E. (Ed.), The Sigma Aldrich Library of Chemical Safety Data, second ed., vol. 1. Sigma Aldrich Co, USA, p. 871.

Lewis, R.J., 2012. Chlorzoxazone. In: Lewis, R.J. (Ed.), Sax's Dangerous Properties of Industrial Materials, twelth ed., vol. 2. John Wiley & Sons, Inc, New York, pp. 932–933.

Li, L., Porter, T.D., 2009. Chlorzoxazone hydroxylation in microsomes and hepatocytes from cytochrome P450 oxidoreductase-null mice. J. Biochem. Mol. Toxicol. 23 (5), 357–363.

Powers, B.J., Cattau Jr., E.L., Zimmerman, H.J., 1986. Chlorzoxazone hepatotoxic reactions: an analysis of 21 identified or presumed cases. Arch. Intern. Med. 146 (6), 1183–1186.

Richards, B.L., Whittle, S.L., Buchbinder, R., 2012. Muscle relaxants for pain management in rheumatoid arthritis. Cochrane Database Syst. Rev. 1, Art No. CD008922. http://dx.doi.org/10.1002/14651858.CD008922.pub2.

Rossoff, I.S., 2002. Chlorzoxazone. In: Rossoff, I.S. (Ed.), Encyclopedia of Clinical Toxicology. The Parthenon Publishing Group, New York, p. 254.

Relevant Websites

http://toxnet.nlm.nih.gov – Chlorzoxazone: 'HSDB database.'

http://www.rxlist.com/parafon-forte-drug/patient-avoid-while-taking.htm – RxDrug List.

Choline

VJ Drake and G Angelo, Oregon State University, Corvallis, OR, USA

This article is a revision of the previous print edition article by Brad Hirakawa, volume 1, pp 587–588, © 2005, Elsevier Inc.

- Name: Choline
- Chemical Abstracts Service Registry Numbers: CAS 62-49-7; CAS 123-41-1 (choline hydroxide)
- Synonyms: Bursine; Ethanaminium; Fagine; Gossypine; Luridine; Sincaline; Sinkalin; Sinkaline; Vidine; (2-Hydroxyethyl)trimethylammonium hydroxide
- Molecular Formula: $C_5H_{15}NO_2$
- Chemical Structure:

OH⁻ H_3C N^+ OH H_3C CH_3

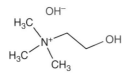

Background

Choline was first discovered in 1864 by Adolph Strecker and was first chemically synthesized a few years later, in 1866. Choline is considered an essential nutrient as it plays a role in acetylcholine release from neurons and consequentially brain function. It is most similar to B vitamins.

Uses

Choline is used as a direct cholinergic agonist in therapeutics and as a research tool.

Although humans can synthesize small amounts of choline, it is considered an essential nutrient that must also be obtained from dietary sources. Choline is used to make phospholipids, the neurotransmitter acetylcholine, and the methyl donor betaine.

Environmental Fate and Behavior

Dermal and oral contacts are the most common exposure pathways.

Exposure and Exposure Monitoring

Little is known about environmental release or environmental exposures.

Toxicokinetics

Choline is metabolized to trimethylamine, which is excreted in skin, lungs, and kidney.

Mechanism of Toxicity

Choline is a cholinergic agonist, choline acetyltransferase substrate; therefore, it exerts toxicity by directly hyperstimulating the postganglionic cholinergic receptors. This may lead to stimulation of gastrointestinal, urinary, uterine, bronchial, cardiac, and vascular receptors.

Acute and Short-Term Toxicity

Animal

Acute choline overexposure results in hyperstimulation of the cholinergic nervous system.

Human

The estimated oral lethal dose for humans is 200–400 g. Vital signs may include bradycardia (decreased heart rate), hypotension, hypothermia, miosis (small pupils), salivation and lacrimation (tearing), ocular pain, blurred vision, bronchospasm, muscle cramps, fasciculation (muscle twitching), weakness, nausea, vomiting, diarrhea, and involuntary urination.

High oral doses of choline (≥ 8 g day^{-1}) have been associated with fishy body odor, vomiting, salivation, sweating, and hypotension. Based on reports of hypotension and fishy body odor in several small human trials, a dose of 7.5 g day^{-1} has been defined as the lowest observed adverse effect level.

Chronic Toxicity

Little is known about the chronic toxicity of choline in laboratory animals or humans.

Clinical Management

Atropine sulfate is the drug of choice. Epinephrine may assist in overcoming severe cardiovascular or bronchoconstriction. Diazepam, phenytoin, and phenobarbital may be given in cases of seizures. Induction of emesis is not necessary due to spontaneous vomiting. Activated charcoal slurry with or without saline cathartic may be used. Sorbitol should not be used because it may contribute to the nausea and diarrhea. Skin decontamination should be accomplished by repeated washing with soap. Exposed eyes should be irrigated with copious amounts of room-temperature water for at least 15 min.

Other Hazards

Choline base solutions are corrosive and are extremely destructive to tissue of the mucous membranes and upper respiratory tract, eyes, and skin.

 http://dx.doi.org/10.1016/B978-0-12-386454-3.00986-6

See also: Anticholinergics; Cholinesterase Inhibition; Neurotoxicity.

Further Reading

Rajaie, S., Esmaillzadeh, A., 2011. Dietary choline and betaine intakes and risk of cardiovascular diseases: review of epidemiological evidence. ARYA Atheroscler. 7, 78–86.

Spencer, M.D., Hamp, T.J., Reid, R.W., et al., 2011. Association between composition of the human gastrointestinal microbiome and development of fatty liver with choline deficiency. Gastroenterology 140, 976–986.

Zeisel, S.H., 2011. Nutritional genomics: defining the dietary requirement and effects of choline. J. Nutr. 141, 531–534.

Relevant Websites

http://www.cdc.gov/niosh – The U.S. National Institute for Occupational Safety and Health (NIOSH) website.

http://www.nap.edu/openbook.php?record_id=6015&page=390 – U.S. Institute of Medicine website.

Cholinesterase Inhibition

BW Wilson, University of California, Davis, CA, USA

Introduction and History

Cholinesterases (ChEs) are a ubiquitous group of enzymes that hydrolyze esters of choline. A well-known example is acetylcholinesterase (AChE, acetylcholine hydrolase, EC 3.1.1.7), the enzyme responsible for hydrolyzing the important neurotransmitter acetylcholine (ACh). Another ChE is butyrylcholinesterase (BuChE, acylcholine acylhydrolase, EC 3.1.1.8), also known as nonspecific cholinesterase. The preferred substrate for AChEs is ACh; BuChEs prefer to hydrolyze esters such as butyrylcholine and propionylcholine. Both AChE and BuChE are inhibited by some organophosphate (OP) and carbamate (CB) esters and also by other chemicals.

Many ChE inhibitors act at the catalytic site of the enzyme, forming enzyme–inhibitor complexes that are slow to hydrolyze. The use of ChE inhibitors as insecticides and chemical warfare agents, their toxicity to humans, and their impact on wildlife have made them important to toxicology researchers, and public health and environmental health officials.

This article focuses on ChE inhibitions by OPs and CBs. Other chemicals, such as tacrine, cocaine, and succinylcholine, are also briefly discussed.

One of the first ChE inhibitors to be studied was a CB, physostigmine (eserine), an alkaloid from the Calabar bean (*Physostigma venenosum*) used in a 'trial by ordeal' in West Africa. The accused were forced to eat the poisonous beans; survivors were proclaimed innocent. The drug has been used as a treatment for glaucoma since 1877. In 1931, Englehart and Loewi showed it blocked ChE activity. Soon after, neostigmine, an analog, was shown to be effective in the symptomatic treatment of myasthenia gravis.

OPs with high toxicity were synthesized as chemical warfare agents in the late 1930s and early 1940s. During this period, Schrader discovered the insecticidal properties of OPs, resulting in the synthesis of tetraethyl pyrophosphate in 1941 and parathion in 1944. Synthetic CBs developed as pesticides have been in commercial use since the 1950s. Some OPs and CBs exhibit toxicities in addition to their direct inhibitions of ChEs. These include long- and short-term damage to nerves and muscles, mutagenicity, and effects on reproduction.

Acetylcholinesterase, Butyrylcholinesterase, and Other Esterases

AChEs and BuChEs are specialized carboxylic ester hydrolases that preferentially hydrolyze choline esters. They are classed among the B-esterases, enzymes that are inhibited by OPs. Another B-esterase is neuropathy target esterase (NTE), an enzyme associated with organophosphate-induced delayed neuropathy (OPIDN). Enzymes that actively hydrolyze OPs are known as A-esterases. They provide an important route of detoxification. Examples are paraoxonase and DFPase (**Table 1**). The tertiary structure and amino acid sequences of several AChEs and BuChEs have been elucidated.

ChEs are widely distributed in the body. AChEs regulate excitation at cholinergic synapses by destroying the neurotransmitter ACh. These enzymes are some of the most active known, cycling within a few milliseconds. AChEs are found in excitable tissues at synapses, neuromuscular junctions, myotendinous junctions, central nervous system (CNS) neuron cell bodies, axons, and muscles (**Table 2**). AChEs are also found in the erythrocytes (red blood cells [RBCs]) of mammals, the serum of some birds and mammals, and the blood platelets of rodents (rats and mice) and ruminants (sheep). For example, the serum ChE activity of the American kestrel, a small falcon, consists almost entirely of AChE, and the serum ChE of the laboratory rat is high in both AChE and BuChE activities. The AChE activity of human blood is localized to its RBCs. AChE activity occurs in the serum of developing mammals and birds and precursors of formed blood elements in some species; it decreases to adult levels after birth.

BuChEs are also widely distributed. They are found at synapses, motor endplates, and muscle fibers together with AChE. BuChE activity in blood is restricted to serum.

Substrate preferences of AChE and BuChE enzymes vary with species. For example, although both mammal and bird AChEs rapidly hydrolyze ACh and its thiocholine analog acetylthiocholine, avian AChEs also readily hydrolyze acetyl β-methylcholine and acetyl β-methylthiocholine, whereas mammalian AChEs do not. AChEs and BuChEs respond differently to increasing substrate concentration. AChEs are inhibited by excess substrate (often >2 mM); BuChEs are less sensitive to substrate inhibition.

AChEs and BuChEs have multiple molecular forms and complicated life histories (**Figures 1 and 2**). Some of the forms move from site to site within cells, others are secreted into body fluids. AChEs consist of asymmetric and globular

Table 1 Esterase classes

A-esterases
Hydrolyze OPs to inactive products
Found in liver and HDL in plasma
High activity in mammals
Lower activity in birds
Examples: paraoxonase and DFPase
B-esterases
Widely distributed in cells and tissues
Inhibited by OPs and CBs
Slow hydrolysis of OP–enzyme complex
Relatively rapid hydrolysis of CB–enzyme complex
Examples: AChE, BuChE, CaE, and NTE

OP, organophosphate ester; HDL, high-density lipoprotein; CB, carbamate; AChE, acetylcholinesterase; BuChE, butyrylcholinesterase; CaE, carboxylesterase; NTE, neuropathy target esterase.

 http://dx.doi.org/10.1016/B978-0-12-386454-3.00116-0

Table 2 Cholinesterase properties

All
Hydrolyze ACh and other choline esters
AChE
Prefers ACh, is inhibited by excess substrates
Found at neural junctions and in mammal RBCs and plasma and platelets of some vertebrates
BuChE
Prefers butyrylcholine, propionylcholine
Widely distributed in vertebrate tissues and plasma

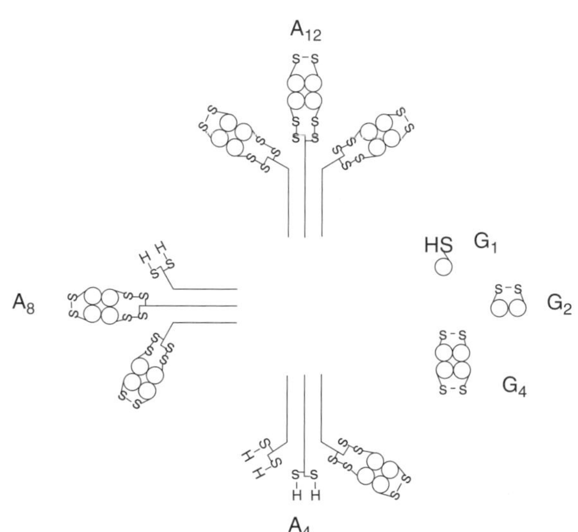

Figure 1 Subunit structure of the multiple molecular forms of ChEs. G, globular forms; A, asymmetric forms with collagen-like tails. Each circle is a catalytic subunit; disulfide bridges indicated by S–S, as found in the electric organ of the electric eel. Modified from Brimijoin, W.S., 1992. US EPA Workshop on Cholinesterase Methodologies.

forms. The asymmetric forms tend to be localized at synapses and motor endplates; they have glycosylated heads joined together by sulfhydryl groups containing the active sites, and collagen tails that attach the enzymes to cell surfaces. The globular forms lack collagen tails; they are made up of the catalytic subunits.

AChE and BuChE subunits are synthesized within cells (e.g., nerve, muscle, liver, and some megakaryocytes), glycosylated within the Golgi apparatus, and secreted. Collagen-tailed forms become attached to the cell surface at specific binding sites. Globular forms are released into body fluids or bind to cell surfaces by ionic bonds. Antibodies have been prepared to several purified AChEs and BuChEs, and protein and nucleic acid sequences have been determined.

The three-dimensional structure of AChE from the electric organ of *Torpedo californica* has been established. One interesting feature is that the active site is embedded in a 'gorge' of ~20 Å that reaches halfway into the protein. The postulated 'anionic site,' theoretically invoked to bind the quaternary ammonium ion of ACh, appears to be represented by aromatic

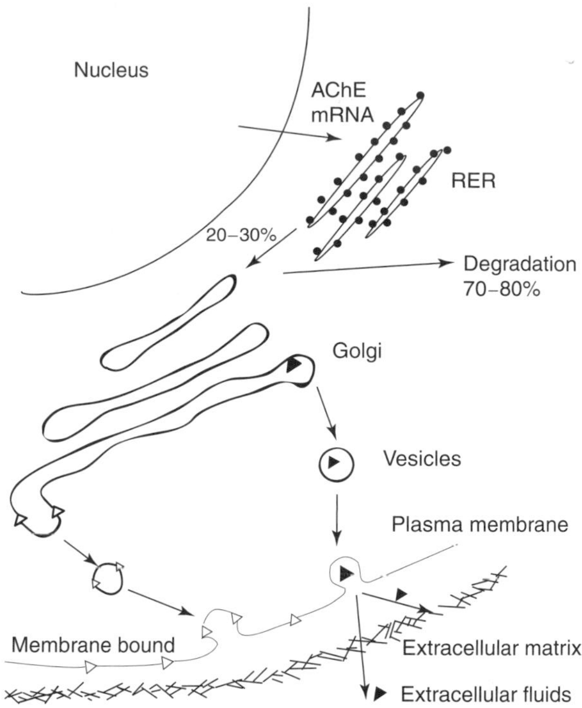

Figure 2 Life cycle of ChEs. AChE is synthesized as a monomer globular form (G_1). Up to 80% is degraded by intracellular processes. Secretory forms are separated from membrane-bound forms, collagen tails are added to asymmetric forms, and the enzyme is glycosylated and becomes enzymatically active. After secretion, globular forms may escape into the body fluids, whereas asymmetric forms are bound to the synaptic basal lamina. Modified from Brimijoin, W.S., 1992. US EPA Workshop on Cholinesterase Methodologies.

amino acids in the gorge itself; these and charges in the active center are believed to stabilize the choline group. In addition, some inhibitions, such as that caused by excess substrate, are believed to result from a 'peripheral site.' Elucidation of the structure of ChE molecules may open the way to a new generation of 'designer' anti-ChE agents with improved specificities of action.

Functions of Cholinesterases

$$E + AX \underset{k_{-1}}{\overset{k_{+1}}{\longleftrightarrow}} EAX \overset{k_2}{\longleftrightarrow} EA \overset{k_3}{\longleftrightarrow} E + A$$

where E is the enzyme, AX is the substrate (ACh) or inhibitor, EAX is the reversible enzyme complex, and *k*s are reaction rate constants.

A century of research has established that a major function of AChE is to hydrolyze the ACh released by cholinergic neurons, regulating the course of neural transmission at synapses, motor endplates, and other effector sites. The reaction is multistep involving formation of a reversible enzyme–substrate complex (EAX), the acetylation of the catalytic site of the enzyme (EA), the hydrolysis of the enzyme–substrate complex to yield acetic acid, choline, and the regenerated enzyme (E + A). One generally accepted mechanism has (1) an electrostatic attraction between the positive charge on the quaternary nitrogen atom of ACh and the negative charge of an 'anionic site' on the enzyme to form the enzyme–substrate complex, (2) the acetylation of a serine hydroxyl, followed by (3) a rapid deacetylation restoring the enzyme and cleaving acetylcholine into acetate and choline. A similar reaction scheme is believed to apply to BuChEs. The new information on the conformation of these molecules should result in a greater understanding of the biophysical mechanisms underlying their catalytic actions.

In contrast with the functional information available for the roles of ACh and AChE, the function of nonspecific ChEs is less established. One idea is that they protect the body from natural anti-ChE agents (e.g., physostigmine) encountered during the evolution of the species. Another idea is that they have specific but still unknown roles in tissues. For example, there are reports that inhibition of BuChE activity blocks adhesion of neurites from nerve cells in culture, and that AChE promotes outgrowth of neurites as if the enzymes had roles in cell adhesion and differentiation.

Toxicities

The toxicities of OPs and CBs often roughly parallel their effectiveness as inhibitors of brain AChE. For example, **Figure 3** shows the relationship between the toxicity *in vivo* of directly acting OPs and their inhibition of AChE *in vitro*, plotting intraperitoneal LD_{50} versus the PI_{50} in mice. The LD_{50} is the dose resulting in 50% mortality; the PI_{50} is the negative logarithm of the concentration of toxicant resulting in 50% inhibition of the enzyme. Only two of the chemicals tested did not 'fit' the curve.

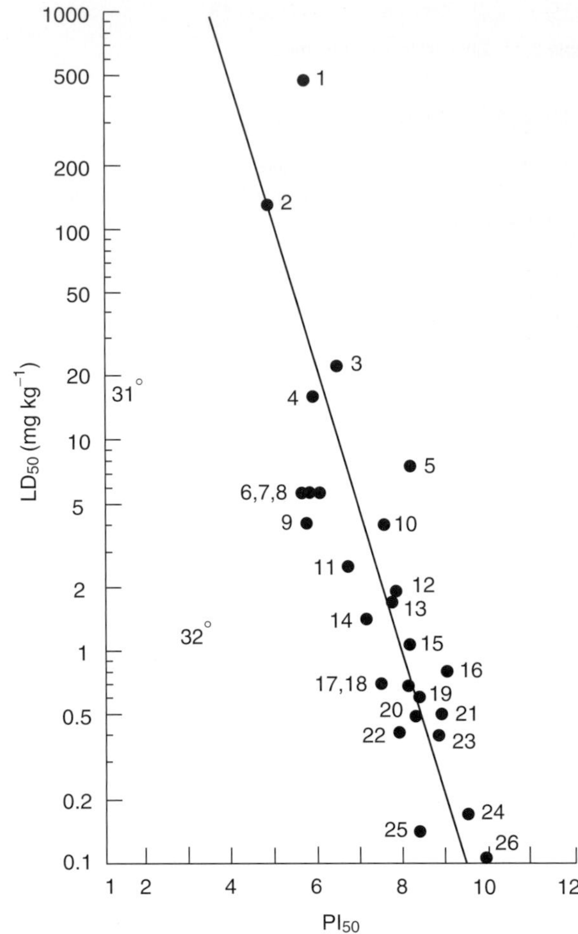

Figure 3 Relationship of the toxicity *in vivo* (LD_{50}) of directly acting OPs to AChE inhibition *in vivo* (PI_{50}). 1, dipterex; 2, *O,O*-diethyl-4-chlorophenylphosphate; 3, *O,O*-diethyl-bis-dimethylpyrophosphoramide (*sym*); 4, TIPP; 5, *O,O*-diethylphosphostigmine; 6, isodemeton sulfoxide; 7, isodemeton; 8, isodemeton sulfone; 9, DFP; 10, diethylamidoethoxyphosphoryl cyanide; 11, *O,O*-dimethyl-*O,O*-diisopropyl pyrophosphate (asym); 12, diethylamidomethoxyphosphoryl cyanide; 13, tetramethyl pyrophosphate; 14, *O,O*-diethylo phosphorocyanidate; 15, *O,O*-dimethyl-*O,O*-diethyl pyrophosphate (asym); 16, soman; 17, TEPP; 18, *O*-isopropylethylphosphonofluoridate; 19, tabun; 20, amiton; 21, diethylamido ispropoxyphosphoryl cyanide; 22, *O,O*-diethyl-*S*-(2-diethylaminoethyl) phosphorothioate; 23, sarin; 24, *O,O*-diethyl-*S*-(2-triethylammoniumethyl) thiophosphate iodide; 25, echothiophate; 26, methylfluorophosphorylcholine iodide; 31, schradan; 32, dimefox. Adapted from Gallo, L. 1991. Organophosphorus insecticides. In: Hayes, W.J., Jr. Laws, E.R., Jr. (Eds.), Handbook of Pesticide Toxicology, vol. 2, p. 932. Academic Press, San Diego, CA.

In general, many of the physiological effects of anti-ChEs are attributable to excess ACh at junctions in the nervous system. The precise symptoms and the time course of ChE inhibition depend on the chemicals and localization of the receptors affected. The properties of some cholinergic receptors are listed in **Table 3**. Cholinergic junctions are classified into several categories based on their pharmacological sensitivities to nicotine, muscarine, atropine, and curare. Early symptoms of cholinergic poisoning represent stimulation of neuroeffectors of the parasympathetic system. These effects are termed muscarinic – stimulated by muscarine and blocked by atropine. Such effects include slowing of the heart (bradycardia), constriction of the pupil of the eye (miosis), diarrhea, urination, lacrimation, and salivation. Actions at skeletal neuromuscular junctions (motor endplates) are termed nicotinic – stimulated by nicotine, blocked by curare, but not by atropine. Overstimulation results in muscle fasciculation (disorganized twitching) and, at higher doses, muscle paralysis. A third site of action of anti-ChEs is the cholinergic junctions of the sympathetic and parasympathetic autonomic ganglia. These junctions are also nicotinic – stimulated by nicotine but not affected by muscarine, atropine, or curare, except at high concentrations. Their actions affect the eye, bladder, heart, and salivary glands, with one set often antagonizing the actions of another. Finally, there are the junctions of the CNS: Some are stimulated by nicotine, and some are affected by atropine. They are not responsive to muscarine or curare. CNS symptoms include hypothermia, tremors, headache, anxiety, convulsions, and coma. Death generally occurs when the agents extensively affect the respiratory centers in the brain. Whether or not there are consistent behavioral effects at low dose levels of OPs and CBs, such as deficits in learning and memory, is a matter of current research.

The excess ACh produced at motor endplates brings about a transient myopathy in experimental animals. Experiments *in vivo* and *in vitro* of Dettbarn, Wecker, Salpeter, and others using cholinergic drugs and ACh receptor blockers indicate that

Table 3 Properties of cholinergic receptors

Muscarinic PNS
Parasympathetic nervous system
Muscarine stimulates
Atropine blocks
Nicotinic PNS
Skeletal muscle motor endplates
Nicotine stimulates
Curare blocks
Atropine has no effect
Nicotinic CNS
Autonomic NS antagonist
Sympathetic and parasympathetic NS
Nicotine stimulates respiratory center

PNS, peripheral nervous system; CNS, central nervous system.

excess ACh leads to an influx of Ca^{2+} ions and other cations into the postsynaptic cell, resulting in regions of necrosis in the muscle fibers around the motor endplates. From 10 to 30% of the fibers may be damaged and recovery may take several weeks or more. A disorder known as intermediate syndrome in humans involves prolonged muscle weakness and some muscle damage lasting several weeks or longer after exposure to high levels of some OPs, including methyl parathion, fenthion, and dimethoate.

Although most of the effects of OPs and CBs are considered to be caused by AChE inhibition, there is evidence that anti-ChEs directly affect ACh receptors in the CNS and PNS and that some anti-AChE pesticides depress the immune system in experimental animals.

A few OPs, such as tri-ortho cresyl phosphate (TOCP), leptophos, mipafox, methamidophos, isofenphos, and chlorpyrifos, cause OPIDN, a neuropathy that results in the death of some motor and sensory neurons in humans and experimental animals. Some, such as chlorpyrifos and isofenphos, require very high dose levels to be neuropathic – higher levels than could occur if the chemicals were used as directed. TOCP, an industrial chemical, has been responsible for the paralysis of thousands of people since the turn of the century. Inhibition of ~70% or more of the carboxylesterase NTE is often associated with the disorder. It is known as a 'delayed' neuropathy because onset of the disorder is usually 10 days to several weeks after exposure. Discussion of this neuropathy is beyond the scope of this article, except to note that neuropathic chemicals that are the most dangerous often are those that are better NTE inhibitors than AChE inhibitors, permitting a higher dose of the chemical to be reached before cholinergic symptoms or death occurs. Agricultural chemicals are routinely screened for OPIDN using hens because chickens are sensitive to the disorder.

The action of many toxicants, including anticholinergic compounds, often involves specific sites on molecules and cells. Such finely tuned molecular events suggest the possibility of discovering 'genocopies,' genetic abnormalities that mimic chemically induced disorders. For example, patients have been reported with smaller than normal motor endplates, defective in AChE and suffering from muscle weakness. There are no reported human AChE-less mutants; it is likely that such a genetic disaster would be lethal. There are humans with inherited differences in their serum BuChEs with decreased activity of the enzyme in their blood. Possessors of these genotypes usually are symptomless, unless they are given succinylcholine (or a similar drug) during surgery to bring about muscle relaxation. Lack of sufficient blood BuChE to speedily destroy the drug intensifies and prolongs the activity of succinylcholine, sometimes with fatal consequences. BuChEs may also play a detoxifying role in cocaine intoxication by hydrolyzing the drug. Several studies on experimental animals indicate that depressing ChEs with anti-ChEs intensifies the toxic effect of cocaine. A 'knock-out' genetically manipulated mouse lacking AChE studied by Oksana Lockridge and colleagues seems to use BuChEs as a substitute to destroy excess ACh.

Organophosphorus Cholinesterase Inhibitors

OP inhibitors are substituted phosphoric acids of the form

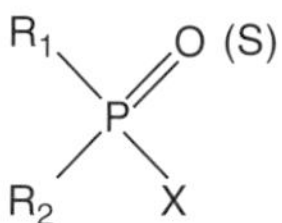

where R_1 and R_2 are usually alkyl or aryl groups linked either directly or via O or S groups to the P atom. According to one classification, X, termed the leaving group, may be (1) a quaternary nitrogen; (2) a fluoride; (3) a CN, OCN, SCN, or a halogen other than F; or (4) other groups. See **Figure 4** for representative organophosphorus cholinesterase inhibitors.

- OPs containing quaternary nitrogen (phosphorylcholines) are strong inhibitors of ChEs and directly acting cholinergics. One, echothiophate iodide, is used in the treatment of glaucoma.
- Fluorophosphates are also highly toxic and relatively volatile. Sarin and soman are chemical warfare agents. Diisopropyl fluorophosphate (DFP) is often used by biochemists to study serine-active enzymes. Mipafox and DFP cause OPIDN in humans and experimental animals.
- An example of a CN-containing nerve gas is Tabun.
- Most OP pesticides are in the fourth and largest category. Many are dimethoxy or diethoxy compounds. OPs used in agriculture tend to be manufactured in the relatively stable P=S form. They are less toxic than OPs with the P=O (oxon) group.

Three important chemical reactions that underlie ChE inhibitions are hydrolysis, desulfuration, and alkylation.

- Hydrolysis: The rate of hydrolysis is a function of the acid and alcohol groups, pH, and temperature. It usually increases with increasing pH, temperature, and UV light.
- Desulfuration: An important oxidation is the conversion of the P=S group of phosphorothionates to P=O, the oxon form, increasing the intensity of ChE inhibition.
- Alkylation: Alkyl substituents, especially methoxy groups, may act as alkylating agents. They are capable of altering nucleic acids, leading some to be concerned about OPs as mutagens.

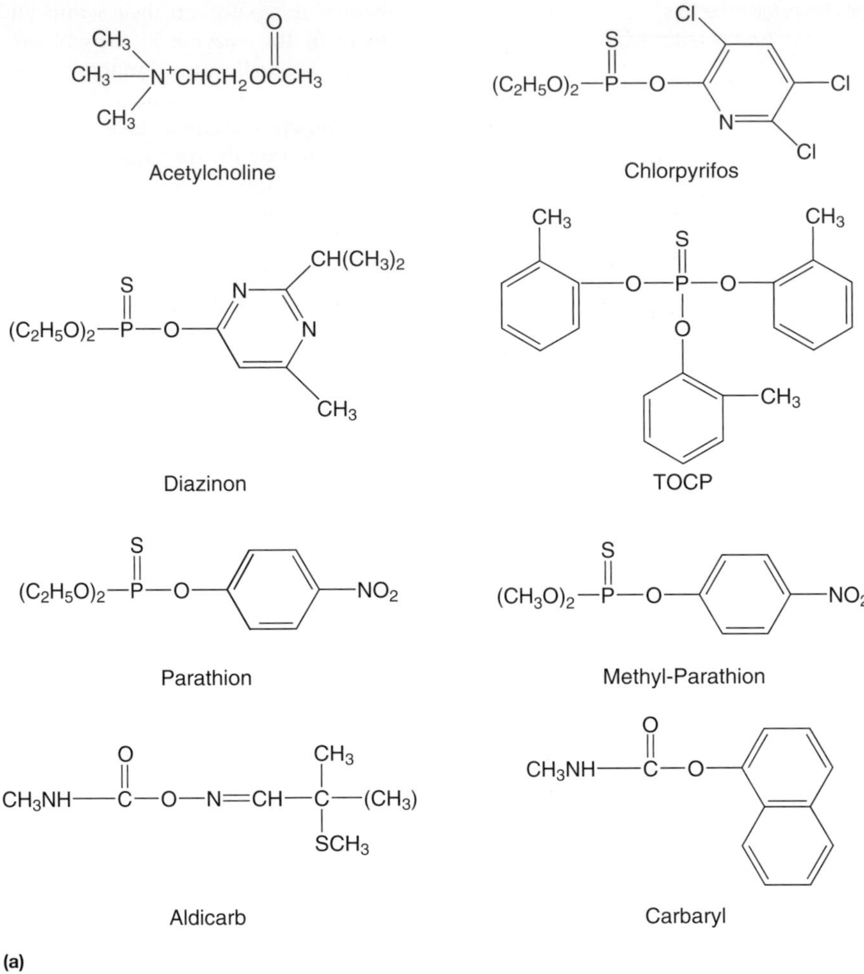

Figure 4 Representative organophosphorus (a) and organocarbamate cholinesterase (b) inhibitors.

Carbamate Cholinesterase Inhibitors

The CBs used as pesticides are N-substituted esters of carbamic acid. CBs developed in the 1950s as insect repellents were found to have insecticidal activity, leading to the development of the naphthyl CBs with high anti-ChE activity and selective toxicity against insects. One example is carbaryl; it is widely used because of its low toxicity to mammals and its degradability. Aldicarb, a plant systemic, is more toxic than carbaryl. Aldicarb was associated with a July 4th holiday incident in which residents on the west coast of the United States complained of anticholinergic symptoms after eating aldicarb-contaminated watermelons.

Most *N*-methyl and *N,N*-dimethyl carbamates are better AChE inhibitors than BuChE inhibitors. However, *N*-carbamylated AChE spontaneously reactivates faster than *N*-carbamylated BuChE. AChE activity may recover as rapidly as 30 min following exposure – much faster than after exposure to OPs.

Although phosphorylation of AChE by OPs is heavily influenced by the electron-withdrawing power of the leaving group, carbamylation by methyl carbamates is also greatly dependent on molecular complementarity with the conformation of the enzyme as well as reactivity of the molecule. In general, phenolic and oxime moieties are more reactive than benzyl alcohol groups.

N-methyl carbamates do not need activation to inhibit ChEs. However, at least in the case of aldicarb, inhibition increases with metabolism. Aldicarb is rapidly oxidized to the relatively stable aldicarb sulfoxide, which in turn is more slowly metabolized to aldicarb sulfone, a stronger AChE inhibitor. These products are then detoxified by conversion to oximes and nitriles, which in turn are degraded to aldehydes, acids, and alcohols. Procarbamate derivatives were developed to reduce the toxicity of CBs to mammals. The hydrogen atom on the carbamate nitrogen is replaced by a wide variety of nucleophiles – many with a sulfur atom – causing reduction in anti-ChE activity. The bond is rapidly broken in insects, restoring the activity and toxicity of the parent compound.

The rapid spontaneous reactivation of carbamates can be a problem in determining ChE activity. For example, some testing routines require that animals be put on a control diet for 24 h before sampling. With CBs, the inhibitions may have disappeared by the time the assays are performed. In addition, the dilutions specified in some assays may reduce the inhibition and high concentrations of substrate may compete with the carbamate to further reactivate the enzyme.

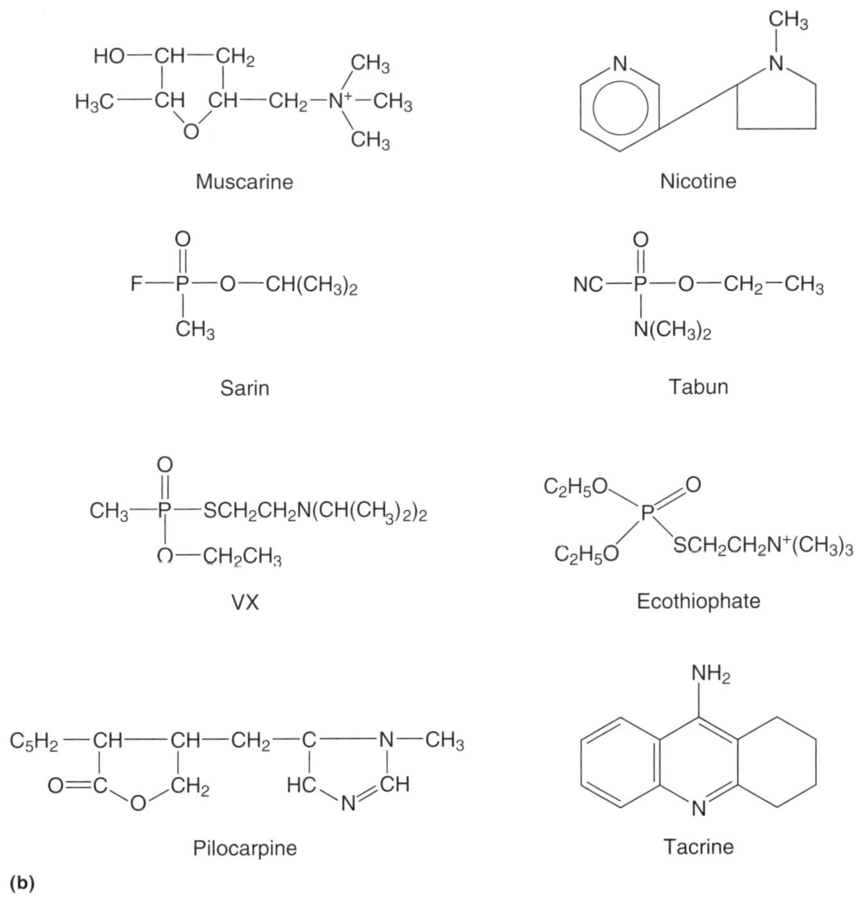

Muscarine

Nicotine

Sarin

Tabun

VX

Ecothiophate

Pilocarpine

Tacrine

(b)

Figure 4 (*continued*).

Chemical Warfare Anticholinesterase Agents

Anticholinesterase chemical warfare agents have been stockpiled since their development immediately before and during World War II. Several countries have active programs researching their toxicity and control. P=O groups confer potent anti-ChE inhibition properties and, in addition, the toxicity of agents such as soman and VX may be caused in part by their actions on receptors, perhaps as well as other proteins. The toxicity of the nerve agents is greater than that of agricultural chemicals. For example, the dermal LD_{50} of agent VX is estimated to be 0.04–0.14 mg kg^{-1} for humans, which is at least an order of magnitude more toxic than most pesticides. LD_{50}s for representative agricultural OPs and CBs are shown in **Table 4**.

Assay Techniques

An early assay for ChE activity was a manometric method in which the change in pH caused by ACh hydrolysis released CO_2 from a reaction buffer. A common technique (that of Michel) directly determines ACh hydrolysis by changes in pH. Another assay, that of Hestrin, utilizes the reaction of ACh with hydroxylamine and ferric chloride, producing a reddish–purple complex. A test developed by Okabe and coworkers oxidizes the choline released from ACh hydrolysis and determines the H_2O_2 produced. Several assays use radioactive ACh; one method counts the acetate produced by the reaction by separating it into an organic phase, leaving the unhydrolyzed ACh behind in an aqueous phase. Another common approach utilizes thioanalogs of ACh and other esters. In the assay developed by Ellman and coworkers, hydrolysis of thiocholines such as acetylthiocholine is measured at 410 nm with the color reagent dithionitrobenzoate. Although assays that rely on pH or radioactivity of ACh have the advantage of using a natural substrate, assays utilizing thiocholine esters are inexpensive, readily automated, and do not require expensive disposal of radioactive wastes. Negative features are the possibility of interference of hemoglobin in RBC samples and a nonlinear reaction of the reduced glutathione in some RBCs with the color reagent. Some of the methods have been adapted for field use. Whatever the assay, it is important that its conditions be validated for the species, tissues, and chemicals under study. Unfortunately, there are no national or international standards for ChE assays, making it difficult to compare results from one clinical laboratory with another. The state of California specified a version of the Ellman assay as its clinical standard, and required all laboratories monitoring blood ChEs to comply or harmonize with this standard methodology.

Table 4 Representative acute LD_{50}s of selected organophosphates and carbamates

Compound	*LD_{50} (mg kg^{-1})*	
	Oral	*Dermal*
Organophosphates		
Dimethoxy compounds		
Azinphosmethyl (*O,O*-dimethyl-*S*-[(4-oxo-1,2,3-benzotriazin-3(4*H*)-yl)methyl]phosphorodithioate)	13	220
Malathion (*O,O*-dimethyl-*S*-(1,2-dicarbethoxyethyl) phosphorodithioate)	1375	>4000
Methyl parathion (*O,O*-dimethyl-*O*-(*p*-nitrophenyl) phosphorothioate)	14	67
Diethoxy compounds		
Parathion (*O,O*-diethyl-*O*-(4-nitorphenyl) phosphorothioate)	13	21
Diazinon (*O,O*-diethyl-*O*-(2-isopropyl-6-methyl-4-pyrimidnyl)phosphorothioate)	108	200
Carbamates		
Aldicarb (2-methyl-2-(methylthio)propylideneamino-*N*-methylcarbamate)	0.8	3.0
Carbaryl (1-naphthyl-*N*-methylcarbamate)	850	>4000

Adapted from Gaines, T.B., 1969. Acute toxicity of pesticides. Toxicol. Appl. Pharmacol. 14, 515–534.

Biochemistry of Cholinesterase Inhibition

The inhibition of the activity of ChEs by OPs and CBs proceeds in a manner similar to the action of the enzymes on ACh. However, instead of forming a rapidly hydrolyzed acetyl–enzyme complex, the OPs and CBs, respectively, phosphorylate and carbamylate the catalytic sites of the enzymes. The major biochemical features of the inhibition of ChEs by OPs and CBs involve (1) activation of the inhibitors, (2) detoxification, (3) reaction of the inhibitor with the serine-active site of the enzyme and loss of a 'leaving group', (4) hydrolysis of the complex and spontaneous reactivation of the enzyme, (5) loss of a second group, known as aging, and (6) recovery by synthesis of new enzyme.

One way to visualize the biochemical mechanisms underlying the toxicity of OPs and CBs is to trace the fate of an OP such as parathion from its entry into the body. Mixed function oxidases (MFO) in the liver (or other tissues) convert parathion, a thionophosphate, to its oxygen analog, paraoxon, increasing its anti-ChE potential by orders of magnitude. The paraoxon may exert its toxic action by inhibiting AChE or be inactivated by conjugation with glutathione, reaction with glutathione transferases, further oxidation by MFO, or hydrolysis by A-esterases, in this case paraoxonase. Such reactions may lead to a loss in toxicity of either parathion or paraoxon. Paraoxon may also be inactivated by binding and reacting with B-esterases other than AChE, such as BuChE and carboxylesterases.

The reaction of an OP with AChE, BuChE, or other B-esterases is similar to the reaction of AChE with ACh, except that the hydrolysis step is much slower or, in some cases, may not occur at all. Its basis is a phosphorylation of the enzyme via a nucleophilic attack. The electronegative serine hydroxyl at the catalytic site reacts with the electropositive phosphorus atom of the inhibitor to form an OP–ChE complex and loss of a side group on the phosphorus atom, known as the leaving group (X). In time, the phosphorylated enzyme may reactivate by rehydrolysis. A similar set of reactions leads to carbamylation, except that the spontaneous reactivation tends to be more rapid than that for an OP. Spontaneous reactivation of an OP may take hours to days, whereas CBs may reactivate as soon as 30 min. In addition, OPs undergo a further reaction known as 'aging,' in which a second group (often an alkyl group) is lost from the phosphate, stabilizing the OP–ChE complex.

Structure/Activity

Some general rules for OPs based on their structures include the following:

- The P=O group is more toxic than the P=S group because it is more reactive. It is more reactive because of its higher electronegativity, which causes a more electropositive P atom, facilitating its reaction with the serine hydroxyl at the active site.
- The electron-withdrawing ability of the leaving group X is predicted by the strength of its acid. For example, fluoride is a more powerful leaving group than nitrophenol because HF is a strong acid.
- Reactivity of the R groups is in the order methoxy > ethoxy > propoxy > isopropoxy > amino groups. The more difficult a compound is to hydrolyze, the weaker is likely to be its ChE inhibition.
- Steric effects are also important. The longer and more branched a compound, the more reduced is its rate of inhibition, probably because of the conformation of the proteins around the catalytic site.

The terms 'reversible' and 'irreversible' are often misused in describing ChE inhibitions. For example, statements such as "OPs are irreversible inhibitors and CBs are reversible inhibitors" are useful insofar as they refer to the stability of the aged OP–enzyme and the more rapid hydrolysis of the CB–enzyme compared with that of the un-aged OP–enzyme. Technically, one could argue that the term 'reversible' should be reserved for cases in which there is an equilibrium between the substrate and the enzyme–substrate complex.

Spontaneous Reactivation of Organophosphates

Table 5 lists the half-lives of recovery for some OP-inhibited AChEs. In general, OP–AChE complexes from dimethoxy-substituted OPs (e.g., malathion) spontaneously dephosphorylate faster than diethoxy (e.g., parathion) or diisopropoxy (e.g., DFP) complexes. Eto pointed out in 1974 that the stability of a phosphorylated AChE may be predicted from the stability of the specific OP inhibitor itself. One possibility is that methyl groups have less steric hindrance and greater electronegativity than ethyl or isopropyl groups.

Chemical Reactivation of Organophosphates

It has been more than 50 years since Irwin Wilson observed that nucleophiles, oximes such as hydroxamic acid, reactivated OP-inhibited AChE above and beyond that occurring from

Table 5 Half-lives of spontaneous reactivation and aging of selected organophosphates

Compound	*Tissue*	$t_{1/2}$ *Reactivation (h)*	$t_{1/2}$ *Aging (h)*
Malathion	Human RBC	0.85	3.9
Methamidophos	Bovine RBC	0.13	0.54
Chlorpyrifos	Bovine RBC/mouse brain	58	36
Diazinon	Human RBC	58	41
Parathion	Rat brain/bovine RBC	103	58
Tabun	Human RBC	ND	13
Sarin	Human RBC	ND	3.0
DFP	Human RBC	ND	4.6
Soman	Human RBC	ND	0.02

Adapted from Wilson et al. (1992) In: Chambers, J.E., Levi, P.E. (Eds.), Organophosphates: Chemistry, Fate, Effects. Academic Press, New York.

spontaneous reactivation, opening the way to a treatment for OP poisoning. The oxime registered for use in the United States as Protopam is 2-pralidoxime chloride (2-PAM); its methanesulfonate salt (P2S) is used in Europe. Oxime therapy should be recommended with caution for carbamate poisonings. Although beneficial in the case of aldicarb, there is evidence that 2-PAM treatment increases the toxicity of carbaryl.

The mechanism of action of oxime reactivation involves transfer of the substituted phosphate or phosphonate residue from the catalytic site of the enzyme to the oxime. In addition, 2-PAM may react directly with the free OP molecule itself. Other oximes such as TMB-4, obidoxime, and HI-6 are reported to be superior to 2-PAM as reactivators and antidotes to chemical warfare agents. Oxime therapy should not be used in the absence of ChE inhibition because 2-PAM itself is a weak ChE inhibitor. In addition to the reactions discussed previously, direct effects of these compounds on muscle contraction and nicotinic receptors led Albuquerque and colleagues to propose that oximes also act directly on cholinergic receptors.

Aging

Research on oximes revealed an important phenomenon: the extent of reactivation of an OP–AChE complex decreases with time and depends on the OP used. This 'aging' prevents both spontaneous and chemical reactivation. Evidence indicates that aging is caused by the loss of a second group from the phosphorus atom. In 1966, Harris and colleagues demonstrated the percentage of loss of an alkyl group from a soman–AChE complex correlated with the percentage of enzyme resistant to oxime activation. In general, OP–ChE complexes that spontaneously reactivate slowly tend to age rapidly. Exceptions are dimethoxy-phosphorylated AChEs, which both rapidly age and spontaneously reactivate. In general, agricultural chemicals (e.g., malathion, parathion, and diazinon) have half-lives of aging of hours and longer, while chemical warfare agents age rapidly (e.g., <2 min for soman).

Treatment for Anticholinesterase Poisoning

The information included here is educational; it should not be construed as specific recommendations for treatment of patients.

Table 6 Treatments for anticholinesterase poisoning

Atropine
2 mg intravenously, at 15- to 30-min intervals as needed to suppress symptoms
2-Pralidoxime
1 g either intramuscularly or intravenously two or three times per day or to suppress symptoms
Diazepam
10 mg subcutaneously or intravenously, repeated as required

Adapted from WHO, 1986. Environmental Health Criteria 63.

Inhibition of AChE by OPs or CBs is one of the few types of toxicity for which there are antidotes. The usual treatment for OP poisoning is atropine and 2-PAM (**Table 6**). The presence of atropine reduces the effectiveness of the ACh receptors, counterbalancing the excess ACh present. The recommended doses for humans are 1 g 2-PAM (intramuscular or intravenous) two or three times a day and 2 mg atropine (intravenous) at 15- to 30-min intervals as needed. Higher doses may be used depending on the extent of the OP intoxication. Environmental Health Criteria No. 63 describes the case of a patient who drank a large amount of dicrotophos while inebriated. Treatments were progressively increased up to 6 mg atropine intravenously every 15 min with continuous infusion of 2-PAM at 0.5 g h^{-1}. All told, 92 g of 2-PAM and 3912 mg of atropine were given to the patient, who was discharged after 33 days.

Much of the research on treatments of ChE inhibitions has concerned chemical warfare agents, providing little direct information for the treatment of agricultural chemicals.

Considerable attention has been given to treatments to protect military units and civilian populations in the event of either accidental or deliberate release of nerve gas agents. One kit contains a combination of atropine, 2-PAM, and the tranquilizer, diazepam. Diazepam is included to lessen CNS symptoms. Another contains pyridostigmine, a carbamate, which is given prophylactically. The use of pyridostigmine is based on the idea that a readily rehydrolyzable carbamate will compete for AChE catalytic sites with the high-affinity binding nerve gas agents, reducing the percentage of AChE that becomes 'irreversibly' inhibited. Using these agents is not without risk because they are themselves toxic. Issuance of atropine kits to the general population in Israel during the Persian Gulf crisis led to the accidental injection of more than 200 children; some had systemic effects but fortunately there were no fatal consequences.

The discovery of methods to isolate relatively large amounts of ChE enzymes in essentially pure form has led to an alternate method of treating OP intoxication – that of adding purified ChEs to the blood. Several experiments indicate enough of the OPs bind to the ChEs to reduce their toxicity in experimental animals.

Treatments with Anticholinesterase Agents

Several anticholinesterase agents have been used to treat human disorders.

Alzheimer's Disease

The finding that senile dementia of the Alzheimer's type was accompanied by a loss of AChE activity (as well as other neurochemical markers for cholinergic neurons) in parts of the brain has stimulated study of cholinergic nerve activity, learning and memory, and the use of anti-ChE compounds in the treatment of Alzheimer's disease. The strategy is to increase the effective level of ACh by reducing the activity of the AChE present. Tacrine (tetrahydroaminoacridine) was the first drug to be evaluated for this purpose. Tacrine is a weakly binding anti-ChE agent approved for treatment by the US FDA. The dose of Tacrine recommended (100 mg day^{-1}) was chosen on the basis of the side effects the drug has on liver function rather than on an unequivocal demonstration of its effectiveness. A subsequent cholinesterase inhibitor approved for use was donepezil (E 2020; Aricept). This drug appears less capable of eliciting adverse side effects. Other cholinesterase inhibitors evaluated for use in Alzheimer's disease include physostigmine and trichlorfon.

Glaucoma

Glaucoma is a disorder of vision accompanied by an increase in ocular pressure. Although mostly replaced by other drugs (e.g., beta blockers and pilocarpine), anti-ChE drugs such as echothiophate are still used in the treatment of these common disorders.

Myasthenia Gravis

Myasthenia gravis is a progressive disorder characterized by muscle weakness; eye muscles are often the first affected. Research has shown it to be an autoimmune disease in which the victim forms antibodies to his or her nicotinic acetylcholine receptors at motor endplates. It is characterized by fatigability and weakness of the skeletal muscles, especially those of the eyes. Approximately 90% of the patients have droopy eyelids and double vision. Treatments include corticosteroids and thymectomy to reduce the actions of the immune system and anti-ChE agents such as pyridostigmine to improve the effectiveness of the receptors that remain.

Wildlife and Domestic Animal Exposures

The recognition that chlorinated hydrocarbons are a persistent danger to wildlife led to a decrease in their use as agricultural chemicals and to an increase in the use of OPs and CBs. In general, OPs and CBs do not bioaccumulate as do chlorinated hydrocarbons and they are relatively biodegradable. However, they are more acutely toxic than chlorinated hydrocarbons to humans and wildlife. A thorough discussion of the comparative toxicology of OPs and CBs is outside the scope of this entry. ChE inhibitions are generally the same, regardless of the animal; differences between species are often in the overall pharmacokinetics and metabolism. For example, although birds have higher brain AChE activities than mammals, they also have less hepatic MFOs to activate OPs and less A-esterases to hydrolyze them. Much research has been done on the toxicology of OPs to wild birds from sparrows to hawks and eagles. For example, Hill et al. of the US Fish and Wildlife Service studied the toxicity of 19 OPs and 8 CBs to 35 species of birds. In general, such studies showed that more than 50% of OPs and 90% of CBs have LD_{50}s of <40 mg kg^{-1} for most birds.

Route of exposure may have much to do with the recovery from OPs. When pigeons were treated orally with an OP, inhibition of blood ChE was rapid, and recovery of activity occurred within a few days. However, when the treatment was conducted dermally, putting the OP on the feet, recovery of enzyme activity took several weeks, implying the presence of a depot for OPs and the possibility that birds can accumulate OPs by flying from site to site. The possibility of bioaccumulation of OPs in a food chain (usually considered to be a characteristic of chlorinated hydrocarbons) was demonstrated by the report of an eagle poisoned by an OP (Warbex) in magpies that, in turn, had obtained the OP by ingesting hair from a steer that had been treated with it for parasites.

Beef cattle, horses (more than sheep), goats, and swine are treated several times each year with OPs to control parasites, and some are fed tetrachlorvinphos to prevent fly larvae hatching in their feces. Carbaryl is commonly used for flea and tick control. Oehme states that insecticides are a common cause of poisoning of domestic animals and that "the majority of insecticide problems in domestic animals result from ignorance or mismanagement." Indeed, there is some epidemiological evidence that animal technicians in pet grooming and veterinary hospitals are exposed to the OP and CB chemicals used to control fleas and ticks while washing the animals. Sheep 'dipping' methods have been changed to minimize exposure to the worker.

Exposures in the Workplace

Worldwide, estimates of the number of humans requiring treatment because of anti-ChE chemicals run into many thousands annually. Concern for those who manufacture and use agricultural chemicals has resulted in studies of pesticide residues, protective clothing, urinary metabolites, and blood ChE levels of farm workers, greenhouse workers, and spray applicators. In general, the rule has been to consider decreases of blood cholinesterases of 20–30% or more as meaningful, signifying the worker should be removed from contact with the agent. In the United States, California requires workers to be monitored; however, until recently there was no single standard method to determine ChE activities even there.

Chemical Warfare and Terrorism

The use of chemical weapons, nerve gases, mustard gases, and blistering agents is banned by international treaty. Nerve agents were inadvertently released from storage sites during the 1991 Persian Gulf conflict. The role that nerve agents played, whether alone or in company with other chemicals, in a baffling set of symptoms known as the Gulf War syndrome is still unclear.

Millions of pounds of chemical warfare agents are stockpiled throughout the world. Their destruction by incineration at high temperatures, up to 2500 °F (1480 °C) is planned or underway in several countries. These include eight sites in the United States, such as the Tooele Army Depot in Utah and the Johnston Atoll in the Pacific, which is 750 miles from Hawaii. Some of the ordinance has been stored since World Wars I and II. Complaints have been lodged by citizens' groups concerned about possible risks to residents during the destruction of the chemicals.

Sadly, chemical warfare weapons are also dangerous instruments of terror. Two episodes in which sarin was used by terrorists in Japan cast a cloud over attempts to control the use of these weapons. Sarin was released in a residential area of the city of Matsumoto, on 27 June 1994, and in a crowded Tokyo subway less than a year later, on 20 March 1995. In Matsumoto, about 600 residents and rescuers were affected and 7 died. More than 5500 people were poisoned and 12 died in the Tokyo incident. Many more might have perished if it were not for the quick action and bravery of firemen, police, and others, as well as the availability of antidotes in Japanese hospitals. (Two subway attendants died removing containers of sarin from subway cars.)

Significance of Blood Cholinesterase Levels

There has been a continuing discussion of the significance of monitoring blood ChEs of humans and wildlife. The setting of no-observed-adverse-effect levels (NOAELs) is an example. (NOAELs are the highest dose levels at which no important effect of a toxicant is observed.) Determining NOAELS is an important step in assigning risks and safe levels for the use of a toxic chemical. Some propose that batteries of behavioral tests performed under controlled laboratory conditions provide the best data for setting safe levels of exposure. Under field conditions, others propose that measurements of residues on skin and clothing, urinary metabolites of agricultural workers, and fecal metabolites of wild animals provide evidence of exposure to chemicals without invasive procedures. Proponents of the use of ChE levels point out that they represent standardized, relatively inexpensive measurements that directly demonstrate a biochemical effect of an exposure to a toxic chemical rather than merely providing evidence of the exposure itself. Recent technology permits determinations of enzyme activities on 100 µl or less of blood, obtainable by a finger prick.

Regardless, as long as millions of pounds of OPs and CBs are used annually, ChE measurements will be an important tool in the protection of humans, domestic animals, and wildlife from overexposure to these toxic agents.

Acknowledgments

Barry Wilson would like to acknowledge the assistance of J.D. Henderson who did a major job of proofing this article.

See also: A-esterase; Anticholinergics; Carbamate Pesticides; Carboxylesterases; Neurotoxicity; Nerve Agents; Organophosphorus Compounds; Pesticides; Veterinary Toxicology.

Further Reading

Ballantyne, B., Marrs, T.C., 1992. Clinical and Experimental Toxicology of Organophosphates and Carbamates. Butterworth-Heinemann, Stoneham, MA.

Chambers, J.E., Levi, P.E. (Eds.), 1992. Organophosphates: Chemistry, Fate, Effects. Academic Press, New York.

Hoffman, W.E., Kramer, J., Main, A.R., Torres, J.L. Clinical enzymology, Loeb, W.F., Quimby, F.W., (Eds.), 1989. The Clinical Chemistry of Laboratory Animals. Taylor & Francis, Philadelphia, PA, pp. 237–278.

Krieger, R.I. (Ed.), 2001. Handbook of Pesticide Toxicology, third ed. Academic Press, San Diego, CA.

Reiner, E., Massoulie, J., Rosenberry, T., et al., (guest eds.), 2010. Special issue: 10th international meeting on cholinesterase. Chem. Biol. Interact. 187 (1–3), 1–446. London: Elsevier.

Taylor, P., 2011. Chapter 10. Anticholinesterase agents. In: Brunton, L.L., Chabner, B.A., Knollman, B.C. (Eds.), Goodman & Gilman's The Pharmacological Basis of Therapeutics, twelfth ed. McGraw-Hill, New York.

US EPA, 1992. Workshop on Cholinesterase Methodologies, Office of Pesticide Programs. US EPA, Washington, DC.

World Health Organization, 1986. Carbamate Pesticides: A General Introduction. Environmental Health Criteria No. 64. World Health Organization, Geneva.

Cholinesterases *see* Cholinesterase Inhibition

Chromium

SC Gad, Gad Consulting Services, Cary, NC, USA

This article is a revision of the previous edition article by Abbi Heilig, volume 1, pp 600–602, © 2005, Elsevier Inc.

- Name: Chromium
- Chemical Abstracts Service Registry Number: 7440-47-3
- Synonyms: Chrome, Chromium(II) compounds, Chromium(III) compounds, Chromium, elemental
- Molecular Formula: Cr, Cr^{3+}, Cr^{5+}, Cr^{6+}

Background

Chromium as a metallic element was first discovered over 200 years ago, in 1797. But the history of chromium really began several decades before this. In 1761, in the Beresof Mines of the Ural Mountains, Johann Gottlob Lehmann obtained samples of an orange-red mineral, which he called 'Siberian red lead.' He analyzed this mineral in 1766 and discovered that it contained lead "mineralized with a selenitic spar and iron particles." The mineral he found was crocoite, a lead chromate ($PbCrO_4$).

In 1770, Peter Simon Pallas also visited the Beresof Mines and observed the same type of mineral. He described it as "a very remarkable red lead mineral which has never been found in any other mine. When pulverized, it gives a handsome yellow guhr which could be used in miniature painting…." Chromium from the Beresof Mines and Siberia was used as a paint pigment. Due to its rarity, this later became a collector's item and increased in popularity in the paint industry. A bright yellow made from crocoite fast became the fashionable color for the carriages of the nobility in both France and England.

In 1797, chromium received its name from a professor of chemistry and assaying at the School of Mines in Paris, Nicolas-Louis Vauquelin. He received some samples of crocoite ore, and his subsequent analysis revealed a new metallic element, which he called chromium after the Greek word 'khroˆma,' meaning color. After further research, he detected trace elements of chromium in precious gems – giving the characteristic red color of rubies and the distinctive green of emeralds, serpentine, and chrome mica.

In 1798, Lowitz and Klaproth independently discovered chromium in a sample of a heavy black rock found farther north of the Beresof Mines, and in 1799 Tassaert identified chromium in the same mineral from a small deposit in the Var region of southeastern France. The chromite ore deposits discovered in the Ural Mountains greatly increased the supplies of chromium to the growing paint industry and even resulted in a chromium chemicals factory being set up in Manchester, England around 1808. In 1827, Isaac Tyson identified deposits of chromite ore on the Maryland-Pennsylvania border, and the United States became the monopoly supplier for a number of years.

But high-grade chromite deposits were found near Bursa in Turkey in 1848, and with the exhaustion of the Maryland deposits around 1860, Turkey then became the main source of supply. This continued for many years until the mining of chromium ore started in India and Southern Africa around 1906. And although paint pigments remained the main application for many years, chromium was finding other uses: Kochlin introduced the use of potassium dichromate as a mordant in the dyeing industry in 1820. The use of chromium salts in leather tanning was adopted commercially in 1884. While chromite was first used as a refractory in France in 1879, its real use started in Britain in 1886.

The first patent for the use of chromium in steel was granted in 1865, but the large-scale use of chromium had to wait until chromium metal could be produced by the alumino-thermic route, developed in the early 1900s, when the electric arc furnace could smelt chromite into the master alloy, ferrochromium.

Uses

Chromium is a transitional element with many industrial uses. It is mainly used in imparting a shiny appearance to metal surfaces. In the early 1800s, the mineral, now known as chromite, was widely used in the production of paint as well as in the production of chromium compounds. These compounds can be used in a variety of applications. For example, potassium dichromate is used in the dyeing industry and chromium salts are used in leather tanning and wood preservation. Today, perhaps its most important use is in the production, in combination with iron, of stainless steel, as well as applying shiny finishes.

Environmental Fate and Behavior

Chromium enters the air, water, and soil mostly in the chromium(III) and chromium(VI) forms. In air, chromium compounds are present mostly as fine dust particles, which eventually settle over land and water. Chromium can strongly attach to sediment and soil, and only a small amount is expected to dissolve in water and leach though the soil to groundwater. Fish do not accumulate much chromium in their bodies.

 http://dx.doi.org/10.1016/B978-0-12-386454-3.00828-9

Most chromium exposure in the general population is through ingestion of the chemical in food containing chromium(II), although exposure is also possible as a result of drinking contaminated well water, or living near uncontrolled hazardous waste sites containing chromium or industries that use chromium. Inhalation of chromium dust and skin contact during use in the workplace are the main routes of occupational exposure.

Studies have shown that inhalation and oral and dermal exposures can result in chromium deposits in liver, kidney, heart, and lungs. Chromium in the breast milk of mothers can be passed down to infants, and fetuses can be exposed to chromium that passes through the placenta.

Exposure and Exposure Monitoring

Routes and Pathways

Inhalation, ingestion, and dermal absorption.

Human Exposure

Human exposure in three different routes: through the airways, through gastrointestinal (GI) tract, or through the skin.

Environmental Exposure

Chromium is ubiquitous in nature, and chromium in air comes from erosion of shales, clay, and other kind of soil. There is only limited information on chromium concentrations in the environmental atmosphere.

Toxicokinetics

The toxicokinetics of a given chromium compound depend on the valence state of the chromium atom and the nature of its ligands. In contrast to chromium(III), which is bound to plasma proteins such as transferrins, chromium(VI) entering the blood stream is taken up selectively by erythrocytes, reduced, and bound predominantly to hemoglobin.

The absorption of chromium(VI) into the blood system through the skin has been reported but not investigated extensively, mainly because the reported health effects are rare. Once absorbed into the blood system, there are various antioxidants that act as reducing agents, such as glutathione and ascorbate, which rapidly reduce chromium(VI) to chromium(III). Chromium absorbed through the lungs into the blood system is excreted by the kidneys and the liver. The kidney appears to absorb chromium from the blood through the renal cortex and releases it into the urine. Thus, sampling of urine for chromium can be used for biological monitoring of certain types of welding fumes that contain water-soluble chromium(VI).

Mechanism of Toxicity

Chromium may cause adverse health effects following inhalation, ingestion, or dermal exposure. The toxicity of chromium is mainly caused by hexavalent compounds as a result of a higher cellular uptake of chromium(VI) compounds than chromium(III). This is explained by the fact that the chromate anion $(CrO_4)^{2-}$ can enter the cells via facilitated diffusion through nonspecific anion channels (similar to phosphate and sulfate anions). Absorption of chromium(III) compounds is via passive diffusion and phagocytosis.

Hexavalent chromium is unstable in the body and is reduced intracellularly (by many substances, including ascorbate and glutathione), providing very reactive pentavalent chromium and trivalent chromium. Both of these intermediates can alter DNA.

Acute and Short-Term Toxicity (or Exposure)

Animal

Chromium can cause irritation in both the eyes and skin. Hexavalent chromium is corrosive to the skin and eyes.

Human

Ingesting large amounts of chromium(VI) can cause stomach upsets and ulcers, convulsions, kidney and liver damage, and even death. Skin contact with certain chromium(VI) compounds can cause skin ulcers. Some people are extremely sensitive to chromium(VI) or chromium(III). Allergic reactions consisting of severe redness and swelling of the skin have been noted.

Chronic Toxicity (or Exposure)

Animal

The hexavalent form of chromium is a potent teratogen, primarily affecting bone formation. However, trivalent chromium was not found to be teratogenic. Animal studies also show an increase in the risk of cancer after exposure to chromium(VI) compounds.

Human

Chromium(III) is an essential nutrient that helps the body use sugar, protein, and fat. Chronic liver and kidney damage due to long-term exposure of chromium(VI) has been reported. However, chronic low-level exposure to chromium does not appear to produce measurable renal damage. Dermal exposure to chromium compounds can cause irritant dermatitis and skin ulcerations (chrome holes). Breathing high levels of chromium(VI) can cause irritation to the nose, such as runny nose, nosebleeds, and ulcers and holes in the nasal septum. Inhalation of chromium(VI) compounds is also associated with lung cancer, and these compounds are classified as human carcinogens.

Immunotoxicity

There are insufficient data on the immunotoxic effects of chromium.

Reproductive Toxicity

Long-term (12 weeks) ingestion of Cr(VI) of $1000\,mg\,l^{-1}$ in drinking water is shown to reduce the number of females impregnated by males, and both the number of viable fetuses and the number of implantations were reduced. Also, similar results were found when adding Cr(III) compounds ($5000\,mg\,l^{-1}$) to drinking water. Exposure Cr(VI) (1000 ppm) and Cr(III) (1000 ppm) in drinking water seemed to reduce the sexual activity of male rats.

Genotoxicity

A strong clastogen, Cr(VI) produces chromosome aberrations and sister chromatid exchanges, as well as DNA strand breaks, oxidized base damage, and DNA–DNA and DNA–protein crosslinks. Hexavalent chromium is also a mutagen.

Several studies of chromosomal aberrations and sister chromatid exchange were conducted, some reported positive and some reported negative results. Thus, these studies are limited by factors such as lack of exposure data, coexposure to other potentially genotoxic agents, and too few workers for meaningful statistical analysis.

Carcinogenicity

Some evidence on animal studies show that Cr(VI) compounds can cause cancer in various tissues due to the low water insolubility. Cr(VI) compounds are more potent cancer inducers in humans than in animals. Other studies reported on different applications of Cr(VI) and Cr(III) compounds such as intramuscularly, by implantation, and intratracheally. Some studies have caused tumors at the injection side, and chromates administered by intramuscular and intraperitoneal routes in animals studies have led to significant excesses of malignant tumors. Inhaled hexavalent chromium is a potent nasal carcinogen.

Clinical Management

There are no specific antidotes for chromium poisoning. Prompt administration of ascorbic acid after acute exposure to chromium(VI) can prevent or limit nephrotoxicity. Since most human overexposure is by ingestion, gastric lavage is appropriate in some cases. However, emesis should not be induced. Maintaining the proper fluid balance is critical due to the impact on the kidney's ability to reabsorb fluid. It is necessary to establish that there is no impairment with breathing due to fluid accumulation in the lungs. Another important step is to decrease the intake of dietary supplements that contain chromium.

Ecotoxicology

While chromium(III) is insoluble, hexavalent chromium is readily soluble and therefore leaks and leaches into surface waters and into the water table. Predominantly produced as a result of industrial activity, dumping sites near industries that produce hexavalent chromium can cause high toxicities in the surrounding marine/aquatic life. Known to be highly toxic to fish, particularly freshwater, this can generate high risk for any wildlife exposed to hexavalent chromium.

Exposure Standards and Guidelines

The Occupational Safety and Health Administration permissible exposure limit time-weighted averages (TWAs) for chromium compounds are chromium(0) and salts: $1.0\,mg\,m^{-3}$, and for chromium(II) and chromium(III): $0.5\,mg\,m^{-3}$. The American Conference of Governmental Industrial Hygienists' threshold limit value – TWA for chromium(VI) is $0.01\,mg\,m^{-3}$. The US Environmental Protection Agency maximum contaminant level in drinking water is $0.1\,mg\,l^{-1}$. Both the International Agency for Research on Cancer and the National Toxicology Program classify certain chromium compounds as carcinogens.

See also: Cardiovascular System; Metals; Respiratory Tract Toxicology.

Further Reading

Basketter, D.A., Angelini, G., Ingber, A., Kern, P.S., Menne, T., 2003. Nickel, chromium and cobalt in consumer products: revisiting safe levels in the new millennium. Contact Derm. 49 (1), 1–7.

Dayan, A.D., Paine, A.J., 2001. Mechanisms of chromium toxicity, carcinogenicity and allergenicity: review of the literature from 1985 to 2000. Hum. Exp. Toxicol. 20 (9), 439–451.

Langard, S., Costa, M., 2007. Chromium. In: Nordberg, G.F., Fowler, B.A., Nordberg, M., Friberg, L.T. (Eds.), Handbook on the Toxicology of Metals. Academic Press, San Diego, CA, pp. 487–510.

Nickens, K.P., Patierno, S.R., Ceryak, S., 2010 Nov. Chromium genotoxicity: a double-edged sword. Chem.-Biol. Interact. 188 (2), 276–288.

Shrivastava, R., Upreti, R.K., Seth, P.K., Chaturvedi, U.C., 2002. Effects of chromium on the immune system. FEMS Immunol. Med. Microbiol. 34 (1), 1–7.

Velma, V., Vutukuru, S.S., Tchounwou, P.B., 2009 Apr–Jun. Ecotoxicology of hexavalent chromium in freshwater fish: a critical review. Rev. Environ. Health 24 (2), 129–145.

Wise, J.P., Wise, S.S., Kraus, S., Shaffey, F., Grau, M., Chen, T.L., Perkins, C., Thompson, W.D., Zheng, T., Zhang, Y., Romano, T., O'Hara, T., 2008 Jan. Hexavalent chromium is cytotoxic and genotoxic to the North Atlantic Right Whale (*Eubalaena glacialis*) lung and testes fibroblasts. Mutat. Res. 650 (1), 30–38.

Yao, H., Guo, L., Jiang, B.H., Luo, J., Shi, X., 2008. Oxidative stress and chromium (VI) carcinogenesis. J. Environ. Pathol. Toxicol. Oncol. 27 (2), 77–88.

Relevant Websites

http://www.atsdr.cdc.gov – Agency for Toxic Substances and Disease Registry. Toxicological Profile for Chromium.

http://toxnet.nlm.nih.gov/ – Toxnet homepage, search for chromium.

Chromosome Aberrations

RJ Preston, National Health and Environmental Effects Research Laboratory, US, Environmental Protection Agency, NC, USA

This article is a revision of the previous edition article by Antone L. Brooks, volume 1, pp 606–607, © 2005, Elsevier Inc.

A cell consists of two major sections, the nucleus and the cytoplasm, that are separated by the nuclear membrane. The nucleus consists of a great extent of the cell's DNA, which is the carrier of the genetic information that defines a particular cell's characteristics. DNA has the extremely important capability of being able to self-replicate, such that the genetic information can be transmitted from parent cell to daughter cell and, for whole organisms, from one generation to the next. The several meters of DNA in a human cell is specifically folded and segregated into a number of separate units called chromosomes. Following DNA duplication, each chromosome consists of two identical subunits called chromatids. In a normal (euploid) human cell, for example, there are 46 chromosomes (22 pairs of autosomes plus two sex chromosomes; for mammals XX in females and XY in males) and in a mouse cell, there are 40 chromosomes. These chromosomes can be distinguished microscopically to some extent by their overall size; they contain different amounts of DNA. The chromosome complement of a cell is known as its karyotype. Each chromosome has several landmarks. The ends are capped by short DNA sequence repeats that form a hairpin structure with associated proteins is called the telomere. There is also a region of specific DNA to which is bound a set of proteins forming the centromere, which is involved in the separation of chromosomes at the time of cell division. The centromere is the site of attachment of the spindle fibers that aid in chromosome segregation and help to ensure that each daughter cell contains the correct euploid chromosome complement. The position of the centromere along a chromosome varies from chromosome pair to chromosome pair, allowing for further differentiation among the chromosomes of a cell. In addition to DNA, a chromosome also contains a number of proteins, most notably histones that are structural and functional components. The integrity of the chromosomes, both in overall structure and in organization, is essential for the normal functioning of cells. If this integrity is compromised, then cellular alterations can ensue and these can, for example, eventually lead to cancer or to birth defects in the offspring.

The karyotype of a cell can be altered in several ways: the number of chromosomes in a cell can be increased (hyperploidy) or decreased (hypoploidy); the structure of chromosomes can be altered when regions of chromosomes are exchanged, inverted, deleted, or duplicated. The general term used to describe all these classes of change is chromosome aberrations. These aberrations can be produced by errors of normal cellular processes such as DNA replication, DNA repair, transcription, and cell division. The frequency of these errors can increase with age and so the frequency of chromosome aberrations generally increases with increasing age. They can also be induced by exposures from environmental stressors such as ionizing (e.g., X-rays) and nonionizing (ultraviolet light) radiation, and natural and manufactured chemicals (e.g., polyaromatic hydrocarbons, cigarette smoking). At the structural level, aberrations can involve both chromatids at identical sites giving rise to chromosome-type aberrations or involve only one of the two chromatids resulting in chromatid-type aberrations.

The classic method for studying chromosome aberrations is to histologically stain the DNA with a specific dye (e.g., Giemsa) and view chromosomes during cell division, at metaphase, when they are somewhat contracted and clearly visible under a microscope at about a 1200× magnification. Note is made of numerical alterations from the normal karyotype or structural alterations when these are discernible. The types of alterations that are most reliably quantifiable by this method are chromosome deletions and a class of interchange called a dicentric. A dicentric is formed when two chromosomes are broken and the pieces rejoin such that the two pieces containing the centromere join together to form the dicentric and the two noncentromeric pieces join to a form an acentric fragment. Dicentrics are typically cell lethal events because of the loss of the acentric fragment and its associated, quite extensive, genetic information at the time of cell division. Similarly, chromosome deletions are cell lethal events. Thus, these types of readily observable alterations can be used as indicators of a response and estimators of a level of exposure but not as predictors of longer-term responses such as cancer. The identification of specific chromosomes can be conducted using one of several different types of banding techniques. The general aim is to use a pretreatment of chromosomes to partially denature the DNA and then stain with Giemsa giving the result of a specific banded pattern to the chromosomes (G-banding) (**Figure 1**). Chromosome aberrations can be identified as alterations in the banding pattern from that for the normal karyotype. The method is quite technically challenging and the analysis is very time consuming. More recently, a number of sophisticated methods based on molecular biology principles and methods have been developed that allow for fluorescent painting of specific chromosomes or chromosomal regions through the use of DNA sequence or chromosome specific labeled probes. The method is broadly referred to as fluorescence in situ hybridization (FISH) (**Figure 2**). Using these probes with fluorescence microscopy allows for all types of chromosome aberrations to be observed, especially those that are frequently not cell lethal, such as chromosomal inversions and reciprocal translocations, and thus, can have longer-term consequences (**Figures 3 and 4**). These specific classes of aberrations are very difficult or impossible to detect by classic methods. In addition, fluorescent analysis of chromosomal aberrations can be conducted on nondividing cells, which allows for observation on a much broader set of cellular models both *in vitro* and *in vivo*.

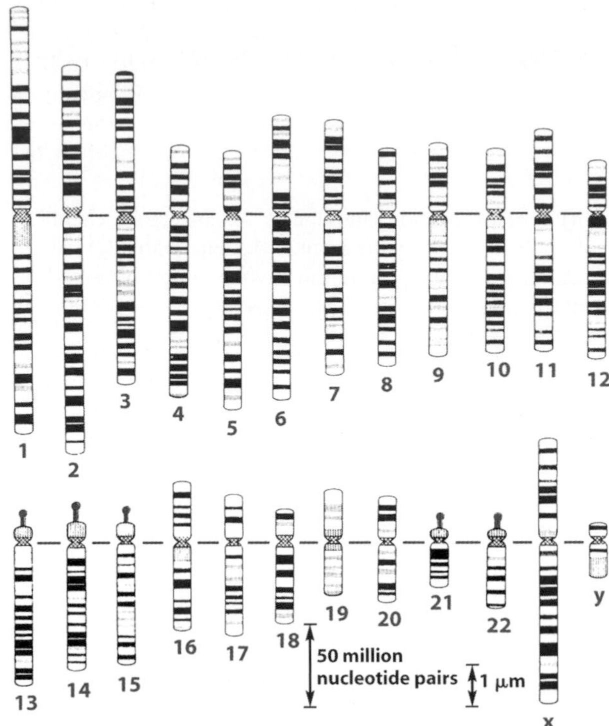

Figure 1 Schematic karyotype of a human cell showing the G-banding pattern. The Biology of Cancer, ed. By Robert A. Weinberg, 2006 by Garland Science.

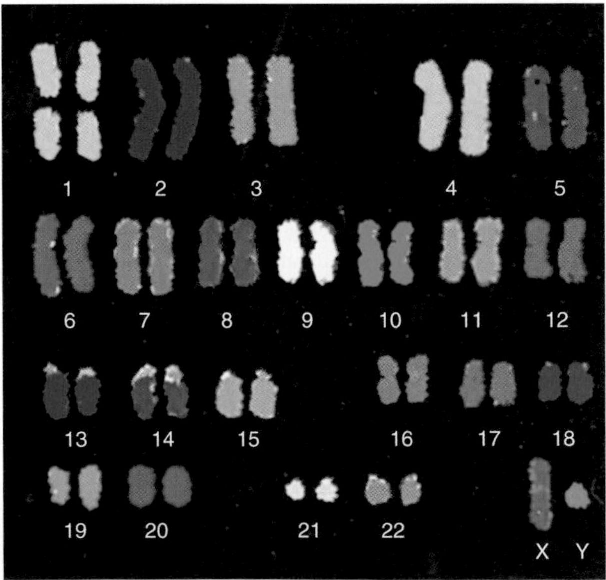

Figure 2 Karyotype of a human cell using FISH; appropriate chromosome probe sets allow for each chromosome pair to be computer colorized so that it has a specific color for analysis. The Biology of Cancer, ed. By Robert A. Weinberg, 2006 by Garland Science.

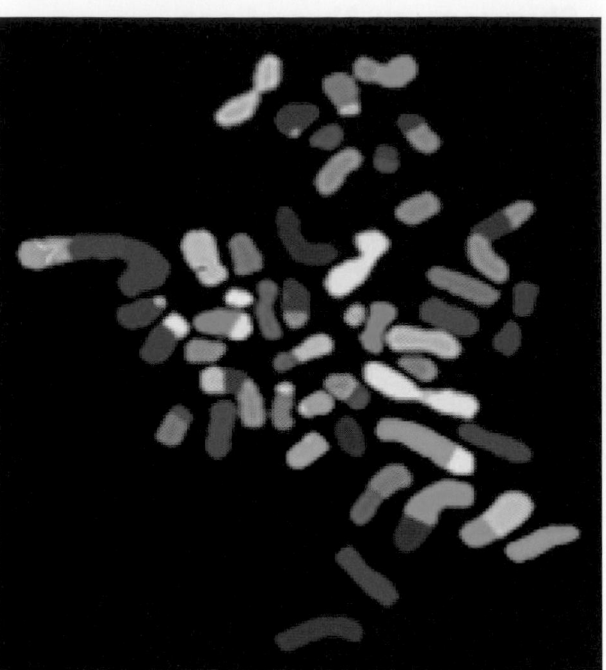

Figure 3 Human breast cancer cell showing aneuploidy for some chromosomes and translocations. The Biology of Cancer, ed. By Robert A. Weinberg, 2006 by Garland Science.

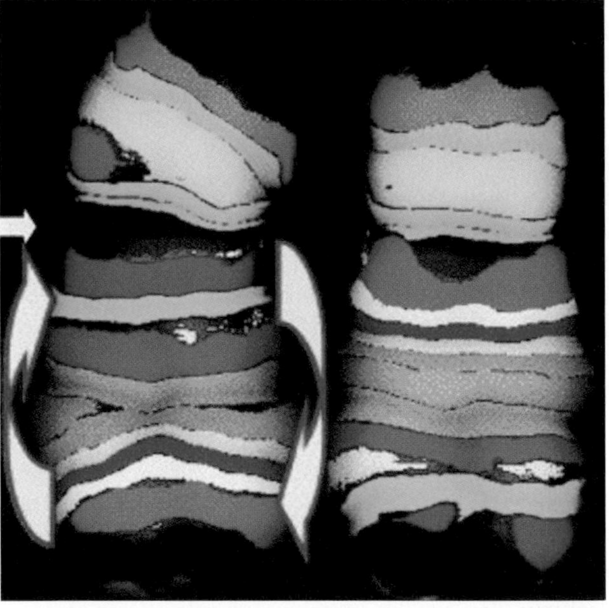

Figure 4 Region of human chromosome 5 stained by M-FISH; the left-hand segment has been inverted as can be seen when compared with the right-hand normal segment. The Biology of Cancer, ed. By Robert A. Weinberg, 2006 by Garland Science.

The analysis of chromosome aberrations, qualitatively and quantitatively, has both a practical benefit in terms of identifying potential exposures and predicting subsequent adverse outcomes, and a scientific benefit in assisting with the understanding of mechanisms and etiology of disease. Chromosome aberrations can serve as biomarkers of exposure and effect (i.e., as surrogates for an adverse outcome); specific chromosome aberrations, for example, can be considered as key events along a pathway from a normal cell to a transformed one and as such are predictors of cancer itself. Thus, they can be considered to be bioindicators of the apical end point – cancer in this case. It is possible to use such bioindicators as part of the risk characterization step of a risk assessment.

There is a long history of studies that have shown the role of chromosome aberrations in the production of adverse health outcomes, particularly for reproductive effects, developmental abnormalities, and cancer. A summary is provided in the following paragraphs.

Based on a number of quite extensive studies, it has been shown that approximately 50% of products of spontaneous abortions have abnormal karyotypes, particularly three copies of one or more chromosomes, instead of the normal 2. Balanced and unbalanced translocations are present in about 5%, with other chromosomal abnormalities also being found, but at lower frequencies. The great majority of trisomies are embryo lethal, although individuals with trisomy for chromosome 21 (Down syndrome), chromosome 18 (Edwards syndrome) or chromosome 13 (Patau syndrome) are viable as live births. Overall, the approximate frequencies of these trisomies are Down 1 in 800 live births; Edwards 1 in 3000 live births; and Patau 1 in 15 000 live births. It is readily possible to assess the karyotype of a fetus, when this is indicated or recommended, using either amniocentesis (sampling the amniotic fluid) or, more recently, by analyzing fetal cells in a maternal blood sample. The analysis can be conducted using regularly stained metaphase preparations or FISH with interphase cells.

Since 2006, tremendous progress has been made in identifying specific genetic alterations that are associated with tumor formation for several different tumor types. Tumors in general are characterized by their high degree of genomic instability, including both gene and chromosomal alterations. It has been highly informative to classify these alterations as being drivers or passengers, where drivers are essential to the cancer process and passengers are consequences of the cell transformation genotype. An additional important observation from tumor cytogenetic analysis is that, in a number of cases, specific chromosome aberrations can be identified. The most clear-cut cases involve the hematopoietic tumors (leukemias and lymphomas). For example, some 80% of chronic myeloid leukemia cases in humans involve a very specific translocation between chromosome 22 and chromosome 9 (known as the 9/22 translocation); part of chromosome 9 becomes attached to chromosome 22 and vice versa. The consequence is that a chimeric protein is produced from the region at the chromosomal breakpoint on chromosome 22 and this protein has a specific new cellular activity that results in enhanced cell division. This leads eventually to the leukemia. In fact, this chimeric protein has been used as a target for chemotherapy for chronic myeloid leukemia. Similar types of translocation involving other chromosome pairs have been identified in other leukemias and lymphomas. Less precise chromosomal alterations have been identified for a wide range of tumor types. In fact, all tumors have an unstable karyotype, although the specific chromosomal aberration drivers have not been identified at this time. The use of sophisticated molecular cytogenetic methods will allow for rapid progress in this area.

An understanding of the mechanism of formation of chromosome aberrations can provide some insights into the potential etiology of disease and aid in the identification of susceptible subgroups. In general terms, structural chromosome aberrations arise from errors of repair of induced DNA damage or from errors of replication on an altered or damaged DNA template. There are some errors that result from the processes of repair and replication themselves, but estimates suggest that the frequencies of these types of error are low. DNA damage consists of several general classes including single- and double-strand DNA breaks (induced by ionizing radiation and radiomimetic chemicals); base damage (induced by oxidative processes produced by ionizing radiation and DNA-reactive chemicals); clustered DNA damage (ionizing radiation); DNA adducts (DNA-reactive chemicals); DNA–DNA crosslinks. During replication at or repair of these damaged sites, there can either be (1) a failure to repair leading to a chromosome deletion or (2) DNA from adjacent chromatids or chromosomes coincidentally undergoing replication or repair can interact to produce interchromosome exchanges (dicentrics or translocations) or intrachromosome exchanges (inversions or duplications). Because chromosomes tend to occupy specific domains within the nucleus, it is likely that chromosome aberrations involving specific pairs of chromosomes will be produced at greater frequencies than predicted from random events. Such nonrandom events can have ramifications for disease likelihood where specific chromosome aberrations are involved in their production. For example, individuals with genotypes that lead to increases in errors of DNA repair and/or replication will therefore be at an enhanced risk of converting DNA damage into chromosome aberrations, and have the potential to be susceptible to adverse outcomes such as cancer or birth defects.

Thus, the analysis of chromosome aberrations is an essential component of a risk assessment toolbox: specific aberrations can be key events in an adverse outcome pathway for disease development; aberrations in general can be harbingers of an adverse outcome without being predictive. More sophisticated molecular methods for identification and characterization will enhance these capabilities and increase the predictive value of chromosome aberrations.

See also: Aneuploidy; Radiation Toxicology, Ionizing and Nonionizing; Sister Chromatid Exchanges; Carcinogenesis; Genetic Toxicology; Risk Assessment, Human Health; Carcinogen–DNA Adduct Formation and DNA Repair; Toxicity Testing, Mutagenicity; Environmental Biomarkers; Biomonitoring.

Further Reading

Brenner, J.C., Chinnaiyan, A.M., 2009. Translocations in epithelial cancers. Biochim. Biophys. Acta 1796, 201–215.

Faas, B.H., Cirigliano, V., Bui, T.H., 2011. Rapid methods for targeted prenatal diagnosis of common chromosome aneuploidies. Semin. Fetal Neonatal Med. 16, 81–87.

Folle, G.A., 2008. Nuclear architecture, chromosome domains and genetic damage. Mutat. Res. 658, 172–183.

Hada, M., Wu, H., Cucinotta, F.A., 2011. mBAND analysis for high- and low-LET radiation-induced chromosome aberrations: A review. Mutat. Res. 711, 187–192.

Igbokwe, A., Lopez-Terrada, 2011. Molecular testing of solid tumors. Arch. Pathol. Lab. Med. 135, 67–82.

Natarajan, A.T., Palitti, F., 2008. DNA repair and chromosomal alterations. Mutat. Res. 657, 3–7.

Preston, R.J., 1999. Chromosomal changes. In: McGregor, D.B., Rice, J.M., Venitt, S. (Eds.), Short/Medium Term Carcinogenicity Tests and Genetic and Related Effects. IARC Monograph No. 146. International Agency for Research on Cancer, Lyon, pp. 395–408.

Preston, R.J., Hoffmann, G.R., 2008. Genetic toxicology. In: Klaassen, C.D. (Ed.), Casarett and Doull's Toxicology, seventh ed. McGraw-Hill, York, PA, pp. 381–414.

Sakata, K., Someya, M., Matsumoto, Y., Hareyama, M., 2007. Ability to repair DNA double-strand breaks related to cancer susceptibility and radiosensitivity. Radiat. Med. 25, 433–438.

Savage, J.R., 1976. Classification and relationships of induced chromosomal structural changes. J. Med. Genet. 13, 103–122.

Stratton, M.R., Campbell, P.J., Futreal, P.A., 2009. The cancer genome. Nature 458, 719–724.

Tucker, J.D., 2007. Low-dose ionizing radiation and chromosome translocations; a review of the major considerations for human biological dosimetry. Mutat. Res. 659, 211–220.

Chronic Toxicity *see* Toxicity, Chronic and Subchronic

Chrysene

S Biswas, Birla Institute of Technology and Sciences-Pilani, Hyderabad, India
B Ghosh, Harvard University, Boston, MA, USA

This article is a revision of the previous edition article by Linda A. Malley, volume 1, pp 607–610, © 2005, Elsevier Inc.

- Name: Chrysene
- Chemical Abstracts Service Registry Number: CAS-218-01-9
- Synonyms: 1,2,5,6-Dibenzonaphthalene; 1,2-Benzophenanthrene; Benz(*a*)- phenanthrene; Benzo(*a*) phenanthrene
- Molecular Formula: $C_{18}H_{12}$
- Chemical Structure:

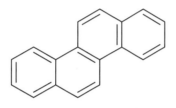

Background Information

Chrysene is a polycyclic aromatic hydrocarbon (PAH) with the molecular formula $C_{18}H_{12}$. It is one of the natural constituents in coal tar, from which it was first isolated and characterized. It is produced as a gas during combustion of coal, gasoline, garbage, animal, and plant materials and usually found in smoke and soot. Chrysene usually combines with dust particles in the air and is carried into water and soil and onto crops. Creosote, a chemical used to preserve wood contains chrysene. High concentration of chrysene in the air is typically found during open burning and home heating with wood and coal. People are exposed to chrysene from a variety of environmental sources such as air, water, and soil and from cigarette smoke and cooked food. General population is usually exposed to chrysene along with a mixture of similar chemicals. Chrysene is a by-product of many industrial processes and thereby released in the atmosphere. Chrysene is lipophilic, insoluble in water, slightly soluble in other polar solvents such as alcohol, ether and moderately soluble in benzene and toluene. However, it readily dissolves in benzene and toluene at an elevated temperature. The name 'Chrysene' originates from the Greek word *chrysos*, meaning 'gold,' and is due to the golden yellow color of the slightly impure crystals. However, in pure state, chrysene is a colorless, crystalline solid. It has characteristic red–blue fluorescence under UV light. Some important properties of chrysene are summarized below. **Table 1** summarizes some of the important properties of chrysene.

Chrysene has very low volatility as indicated by very low vapor pressure of the compound. High K_{ow} indicates its lipophilicity and poor water solubility. In the environment, it has been detected in automobile exhaust, cigarette smoke, wood smoke, and soot from premixed acetylene–oxygen flames. It has also been found in petroleum products including clarified oils, waxes, petroleum, tar oil, coal tar, creosote, cracked petroleum residues, etc. Depending on the orientation of the phenyl ring in the molecule, chrysene has many structural isomers such as naphthacene, triphenylene, benzo(*c*)phenanthrene, and benzo(*a*)anthracene.

Uses

Used strictly for research purposes.

Environmental Fate and Behavior

Generally, disposal of PAH from the industrial plants, accidental release from the containers, smoke from plant, combustion, or automobile exhaust causes chrysene and other PAHs to enter the environment. Because of the poor water solubility and low vapor pressure, chrysene has limited chance to get washed away or evaporate in the environment. Therefore, it remains immobile in soils. If exposed to water, it gets absorbed on the particulate matters and either float or sediment on the riverbed. The rate of biodegradation in soil ranges from 77 to 387 days depending on the soil type. Chrysene does not undergo hydrolysis due to the lack of hydrolyzable functional groups. However, it undergoes photochemical oxidations when exposed to the environment. Dihydrodiol is the common degradation product of chrysene. Half-life of

Table 1 Important properties of chrysene

Molecular weight (g mol^{-1})	228.3
Melting point (°C)	255–256
Boiling point (°C)	448 (760 mm Hg)
Octanol/Water partition coefficient (K_{ow})	8.138×10^5
Log K_{ow}	5.910
Aqueous solubility (mass%)	0.000 000 19
Henry's law constant (K_h)	4.32×10^{-7}
Vapor pressure (mm Hg)	6.38×10^{-9}

degradation of chrysene, absorbed to soot particles and exposed to sunlight in air containing 10 ppm nitrogen oxides is 26 days. The National Research Council (NRC 1983) noted that the PAHs adsorbed to soot particles are more resistant to photochemical reactions than pure compounds.

Exposure Routes and Pathways

Release of chrysene to the environment is widespread since it is the product of incomplete combustion. Of all the estimated environmental releases of chrysene, 93% are found in the air and in the remaining 7%, equal amounts are present in water and land.

It is associated in high proportion with particulate matter, soils, and sediments. Human exposure occurs from inhalation of contaminated air from the populated area, from automobile exhaust, and consumption of contaminated food and water. Moreover, high exposure occurs through the cigarette smoking and ingestion of smoked or charcoal broiled meats and fish. Workers who handle or are involved in the manufacture of PAH-containing materials or in the coal tar production plants have found greatest exposure.

If disposed on the ground, it gets absorbed to the soil and does not leach appreciably in the groundwater because of its low water solubility. If released in surface water through discharges from industrial plants and wastewater treatment plants, chrysene gets strongly associated with sediments and particulate matters. If released to air, it undergoes rapid photoactivated free radical reactions with hydroxyl radicals. The estimated half-life of the gas phase chrysene in the atmosphere is 1.25 h due to photolysis. Absorption to various materials may affect the rate of photolysis. The half-life of chrysene on near surface of solid particles, upon direct photolysis from exposure to sunlight (midday in midsummer at latitude 40 °N) is 4.4 h. Chrysene may be biodegraded in the water system.

Toxicokinetics

High lipophilicity of chrysene causes its partition in lipids and adipose tissues and has rapid systemic absorption by dermal, oral, and inhalation route of exposure. Following oral administration in rats, peak concentration of chrysene in blood and liver has been obtained in 1 h. The majority of administered dose gets eliminated in the feces within 2 days. Major metabolites of chrysene found in rat liver homogenates are 1,2-, 3,4-, and 5,6-dihydrodiols and some mono hydroxy derivatives including 1- and 3-phenols. Microsomal oxidation in rat liver is responsible for the conversion of chrysene to dihydrodiol metabolites. The dihydrodiol derivatives undergo further transformation to form 1,2-diol-3,4-epoxide and 3,4-diol-1,2-epoxide. Chrysene *trans*-3,4-dihydrodiol is the major metabolite of the parent compound.

Mechanism of Toxicity

Compounds under the class of PAH are potent carcinogens. Carcinogenicity of chrysene is due to the mutagenic activity of its metabolites, 1,2-dihydrodiol and 1,2-diol-3,4-epoxide. Compounds containing the bay-region (sterically hindered cup-shaped area between carbon 10 and 11 of benzo[*a*]pyrene or 1 and 12 of benzo[*a*]anthracene) in their structure are considered to be the potent carcinogen because of their reactivity to enzymes. Chrysene has a bay-region in its structure, which is metabolized by mixed function oxidases to reactive 'bay-region' diol epoxides. These diol epoxides get converted to carbocations, which are mutagens and initiators of carcinogenesis. This compound together with other PAHs may be more toxic or carcinogenic than a single compound. It has been reported that the heavier PAHs (4,5 and 6-rings) such as chrysene tend to be greater carcinogenic than lighter PAHs. Within the aromatic series, acute toxicity increases with increasing alkyl substitution on the aromatic nucleus. The metabolites of chrysene, 1,2-dihydrodiol and 1,2-diol-3,4-epoxide are mutagenic in *in vitro* mammalian and bacterial cell cultures and have induced pulmonary adenomas in newborn mice. In addition, the 1,2-dihydrodiol was a tumor-initiating agent in mouse skin. All PAHs act as carcinogens through biotransformation to chemically relevant intermediates that covalently bind to cellular macromolecules such as DNA, which leads to mutation and tumor initiation. They also induce P450 isoenzyme, important for the metabolism of PAHs.

Acute and Short-Term Toxicity (or Exposure)

Animal

Chrysene caused increased incidence of liver tumors in male and female mice, upon intraperitoneal injections of chrysene in dimethyl sulfoxide (DMSO). The dose used for this study was 0, 160, and 640 μg per mouse and the days of administration were days 1, 8, and 15 of age. A statistically significant increase in the incidence of liver adenomas occurs in low dose, whereas the majority of tumors were carcinomas in high dose treated mice. The LD_{50} of chrysene in mice upon intraperitoneal injection is 320 mg kg^{-1}.

Human

Chrysene is still considered a probable human carcinogen. However, there are no human data that specifically prove the exposure of chrysene to human cancers. Chrysene is a component of the mixture of PAH found in coal tar, soot, coke oven emissions, and cigarette smoke that has been directly associated with human cancer. However, in general, PAH have low acute toxicity.

Chronic Toxicity (or Exposure)

Animal

There is sufficient evidence of carcinogenicity in animals treated with chrysene. Intraperitoneal chrysene injections in male mice demonstrated an increased incidence of liver tumors, malignant lymphomas, and lung tumors. Chrysene caused skin carcinomas in mice following dermal exposure. Long-term toxicity included chromosomal abnormalities in Chinese hamsters, hamster spermatogonia, and mouse oocytes after gavage exposure of 450 or 900 mg kg^{-1}. Chrysene showed positive result in bacterial gene mutation assays and transformed mammalian cells exposed in culture. Chrysene was shown to be a potent carcinogen when tested in carcinogenic and cancer initiating activity in mouse skin painting assays. Chrysene demonstrated positive result for initiating activity and produced skin papillomas and carcinomas when combined with various promoting agents such as decahydronaphthalene, croton oil, etc. in several mouse strains (C3H, ICR/Ha Swiss, Ha/ICR/Mil Swiss, CD-1, Sencar). Therefore, most of the treatment protocols resulted in an increased incidence of tumors at the site of injection.

Human

According to the American Conference of Governmental Industrial Hygienists (ACGIH), chrysene is classified as A2, which indicates it as a suspected human carcinogen. Environment Protection Agency (EPA) Integrated Risk Management System has classified chrysene as B2 (probable human carcinogen). There are no specific reports of toxicity or carcinogenicity in humans resulting from exposure to chrysene is available. However, chrysene is one of the components of PAH, which caused increased incidences of skin, bladder, lung tumors, and tumors of the GI tract among exposed workers. The Department of Health and Human Services has determined that among the components of PAH, benz[*a*]anthracene, benzo[*b*]fluoranthene, benzo[*k*]fluoranthene, benzo[*a*] pyrene, dibenz[*a,h*]anthracene, and indeno[1,2,3-*c,d*]pyrene are well known carcinogens to human whereas Benzo[*b*]fluoranthene, benzo[*j*]fluoranthene, benzo[*k*]fluoranthene, and indeno[1,2,3-*c,d*]pyrene are possibly carcinogenic to human. Few other PAHs such as anthracene, benzo[*g,h,i*]perylene, benzo[*e*]pyrene, chrysene, fluoranthene, fluorene, phenanthrene, and pyrene are not classifiable as carcinogen to humans. Several epidemiologic studies have shown increased incidence of lung cancer in humans exposed to coke oven emissions, roofing-tar emissions, and cigarette smoke. Each of these mixtures contains chrysene as one of the PAHs. It is impossible to evaluate the contribution of individual PAH to the total carcinogenicity. However, chrysene along with benzo [*a*]pyrene, benz[*a*]anthracene, benzo[*b*]fluoranthene, and dibenz[*a,h*]anthracene causes human cancer.

In Vitro Toxicity Data

Mutagenic effect of chrysene was determined in bacterial, fungal, and mammalian cell culture systems *in vitro*. In bacteria, chrysene produced negative results in *Escherichia coli* and *Saccharomyces*, the mutagenic effect was found in *Salmonella typhimurium* in TA100. Chrysene produced positive result in Syrian hamster embryo cells *in vitro*. Chrysene induced aryl hydrocarbon hydroxylase in cultured human lymphocytes.

Immunotoxicity

The immunotoxicity of PAHs is thought to be related to their carcinogenic potency. It has been suggested that immunosuppression by chrysene is not related to its metabolites. Current thought centers around the correlation between PAH carcinogenicity and immunotoxicity and the role of the AhR and bioactivated metabolites in PAH-induced immunosuppression.

Reproductive Toxicity

Administration of chrysene as 0.1% solution in petroleum hydrocarbon mixture (known to have low embryotoxicity) to the eggshell of Mallard duck embryos resulted in embryotoxic and teratogenic effects in the ducklings. A single oral dose of chrysene to the pregnant rats on 19th day of gestation induced hepatic P450 enzymes in the fetal rat liver. Chrysene also induced activity of benzo(*a*)pyrene hydroxylase in the placenta.

Genotoxicity

Studies suggest that metabolites of chrysene are possibly genotoxic.

Carcinogenicity

Chrysene belongs to PAH, which are potent carcinogens. Its carcinogenicity is due to the mutagenic effects of its metabolites.

Chrysene causes increased incidence of liver tumors, malignant lymphomas, skin sarcomas, and lung tumors in mice.

The EPA Integrated Risk Management System classifies chrysene as B2 (a probable human carcinogen), and the ACGIH classifies it as A2 (a suspected human carcinogen). However there are no specific reports of carcinogenicity in humans resulting from exposure to chrysene available, as it is impossible to evaluate the contributions of individual components of PAH to the total carcinogenicity of PAH.

Clinical Management

Generally, chronic exposure of PAHs leads to toxicities such as carcinogenicity. The evidence of carcinogenicity in humans are primarily from occupational studies of workers exposed to PAHs from the areas of coke production, roofing, oil refining, coal gasifications, etc. Human cancers from PAH are predominantly lungs and skin from inhalation and dermal exposure respectively. Studies on animals demonstrate that PAHs tend to affect proliferating tissues such as bone marrow, gonads, lymphoid organs, and intestinal epithelium. No minimum risk levels for PAHs have been derived, as there are no adequate human or animal dose-response data available that identify the safe level that does not produce carcinogenicity. Generally, a common practice to reduce the absorption following acute exposure to PAHs include removing the individual from the source of exposure, remove contaminated clothing, and decontaminating the exposed areas of the body by proper washing with detergents. Administration of charcoal following ingestion of PAH is recommended for PAH absorption, however, it has not been proved to reduce absorption of PAHs in the gastrointestinal system. Use of emetics as gastrointestinal decontaminant of PAHs is not recommended, as there is a risk of causing pneumonitis. In case of inhalation exposure, if difficulty in breathing develops, oxygen is administered and assisted ventilation is provided. Symptoms of bronchospasm can be treated with inhaled beta-2-agonist and/or oral or parenteral corticosteroids or inhaled sympathomimetic agents. For eye exposure, thorough washing followed by eye evaluation would be made. For dermal exposure, after thorough washing, if hypersensitivity develops, topical or systemic corticosteroids or antihistamines could be applied. The follow-up evaluations to check complete blood count, liver, and renal functions are recommended to rule out possible systemic toxicity. In case of abnormal data from any of the evaluations, supportive treatment for particular organ should be undertaken.

Ecotoxicology

The LC_{50} in fish for 96 h was greater than 1 mg l^{-1}. The 24 h LC_{50} in amphibians was greater than 6.7 mg l^{-1}. The LC_{50} for 24 h in insects was 1.7 mg l^{-1}. The LC_{50} in 2 h in *Daphnia magma* was 1.9 mg l^{-1}.

Other Hazards

Emission of smoke and fumes following heating of chrysene at elevated temperature is observed.

Exposure Standards and Guidelines

No specific reports of toxicity or carcinogenicity in humans resulting from exposure to chrysene alone have been registered. However, a mixture of PAHs including chrysene as one of the components cause occupational health hazards in workers subjected to long-term exposure. Increased incidences of skin, bladder, and lung tumors and tumors of the GI tract among workers are reported.

See also: Coal Tar; Polycyclic Aromatic Hydrocarbons (PAHs); Toxicity, Subchronic and Chronic; Developmental Toxicology; Carcinogenesis.

Further Reading

Chang, R.L., Wood, A.W., Huang, M.T., et al., 2013. Mutagenicity and tumorigenicity of the four enantiopure bay-region 3,4-diol-1,2-epoxide isomers of dibenz[*a,h*] anthracene. Carcinogenesis 34, 2184–2191.

Fisnera, M., Taniguchic, S., Moreira, F., et al., 2013. Polycyclic aromatic hydrocarbons (PAHs) in plastic pellets: variability in the concentration and composition at different sediment depths in a sandy beach. Mar. Pollut. Bull. 70 (1–2), 219–226.

Jennings, A.A., 2012. Worldwide regulatory guidance values for surface soil exposure to carcinogenic or mutagenic polycyclic aromatic hydrocarbons. J. Environ. Manage. 110, 82–102.

Kemble, N.E., Hardesty, D.K., Christopher, G., et al., 2013. Contaminants in stream sediments from seven United States metropolitan areas: part II – sediment toxicity to the amphipod *Hyalella azteca* and the midge Chironomus dilutes. Arch. Environ. Contam. Toxicol. 64, 52–64.

Landrum, P.F., Chapman, P.M., Neff, J., Page, D.S., 2013. Influence of exposure and toxicokinetics on measures of aquatic toxicity for organic contaminants: a case study review. Integr. Environ. Assess. Manage. 9, 196–210.

Lauer, F.T., Walker, M.K., Burchiel, S.W., 2013. Dibenzo[def,p]chrysene (DBC) suppresses antibody formation in spleen cells following oral exposures of mice. J. Toxicol. Environ. Health A 76 (1), 16–24.

National Toxicology Program, 2011a . Polycyclic aromatic hydrocarbons: 15 listings – benz[*a*]anthracene, benzo[*b*]fluoranthene, benzo[*j*]fluoranthene, benzo[*k*]fluoranthene, benzo[*a*]pyrene, dibenz[*a,h*]acridine, dibenz[*a,j*]acridine, dibenz[*a,h*] anthracene, 7H-dibenzo[*c,g*]carbazole, dibenzo[*a,e*]pyrene, dibenzo[*a,h*]pyrene, dibenzo[*a,i*]pyrene, dibenzo[*a,l*]pyrene, indeno[1,2,3-cd]pyrene, 5-methylchrysene. Reprod. Carcinogen. 12, 353–361.

National Toxicology Program, 2011b . Nitroarenes (selected): 6-nitrochrysene. Reprod. Carcinogen. 12, 290–291.

Selbig, W.R., Bannerman, R., Corsi, S.R., 2013. From streets to streams: assessing the toxicity potential of urban sediment by particle size. Sci. Total Environ. 444, 381–391.

Shorey, L.E., Castro, D.J., Baird, W.M., et al., 2012. Transplacental carcinogenesis with dibenzo[def,p]chrysene (DBC): timing of maternal exposures determines target tissue response in offspring. Cancer Lett. 317 (1), 49–55.

Shorey, L.E., Madeen, E.P., Atwell, L.L., et al., 2013. Differential modulation of dibenzo [def, p]chrysene transplacental carcinogenesis: maternal diets rich in indole-3-carbinol versus sulforaphane. Toxicol. Appl. Pharmacol. 270 (1), 60–69.

Siddens, L.K., Larkin, A., Krueger, S.K., et al., 2012. Polycyclic aromatic hydrocarbons as skin carcinogens: comparison of benzo[*a*]pyrene, dibenzo[def,p]chrysene and three environmental mixtures in the FVB/N mouse. Toxicol. Appl. Pharmacol. 264 (3), 377–386.

Williams, D.E., 2012. The rainbow trout liver cancer model: response to environmental chemicals and studies on promotion and chemoprevention. Comp. Biochem. Physiol. C Toxicol. Pharmacol. 155 (1), 121–127.

Yan, Z., Yuan, J., Zhu, G., et al., 2013. A new strategy based on cholesterol-functionalized iron oxide magnetic nanoparticles for determination of polycyclic aromatic hydrocarbons by high-performance liquid chromatography with cholesterol column. Anal. Chim. Acta 780, 28–35.

Relevant Websites

http://www.nature.nps.gov/hazardssafety/toxic/chrysene.pdf – Environmental Contaminants Encyclopedia. Chrysene Entry. National Park Service. July 1, 1997.

http://nj.gov/health/eoh/rtkweb/documents/fs/0441.pdf – NJ Department of Health.

http://toxnet.nlm.nih.gov/cgi-bin/sis/search/a?dbs+hsdb:@term+@DOCNO+2810 – NLM's Toxnet.

Ciguatoxin

MA Darracq, University of California, San Diego, CA, USA

This article is a revision of the previous edition article by David Eldridge and Christopher P. Holstege, volume 1, pp 610–611, © 2005, Elsevier Inc.

Chemical Profile

- Synonyms: CTX 1, P-CTX 1, Pacific ciguatoxin 1
- Molecular Formula: $C_{60}H_{86}O_{19}$
- Chemical Structure:

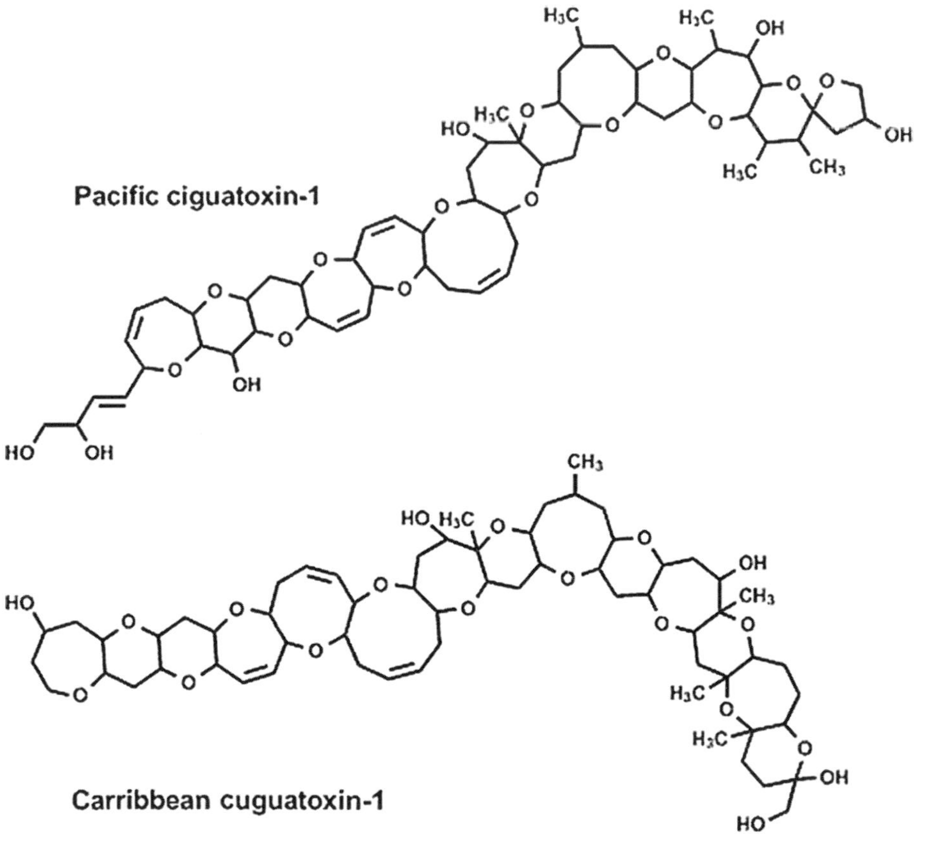

Pacific ciguatoxin-1

Carribbean cuguatoxin-1

Parrot fish, Red snapper, Reef cord, Sea bass, Swordfish, and Yankee whiting.

Ciguatera poisoning may occur after consumption of these fish. Ciguatera poisoning is also known as ciguatera fish poisoning or ichthyosarcotoxism. Unfortunately, ciguatoxin-containing fish look, smell, and taste normal, thereby preventing easy identification of contaminated fish. Laboratory-based detection methods (gas and liquid chromatography/ mass spectroscopy) for the presence of ciguatoxins in fish are available; however, they remain labor and time intensive. To date, there are no laboratory tests commercially available for the detection of ciguatoxins in human blood and diagnosis remains based on the characteristic signs and symptoms and on the history of fish consumption. Expanding trade from ciguatoxin endemic areas has contributed to a wider distribution and increasing frequency of reported disease in nonendemic areas where poisoning may be underrecognized or under appreciated. Ciguatera is responsible for the highest reported incidence of food-borne illness attributable to finfish in the United States

Background

The ciguatoxins are a group of heat-stable, colorless, odorless, and lipid-soluble compounds with a polyether ring structure. They bind avidly to and open voltage-gated sodium channels with symptoms of characteristic neuroexcitability that may last for days to months. There are 12 known ciguatoxins found in Caribbean and tropical Atlantic waters and 29 reported ciguatoxins in Pacific waters. Ciguatoxins may be found in the flesh and viscera of predatory coral-reef fish from waters predominantly between 35° south and 35° north latitude. Implicated species of fish are predatory reef fish, including Amberjack, Barracuda, Cinnamon, Coral trout, Dolphin, Eel, Emperor, Spanish mackerel, Surgeon fish, Grouper, Kingfish, Paddletail, and worldwide with 50 000 cases reported annually; however, underreporting is likely in endemic areas. Most exposures are reported following the exposure to fish caught in Pacific, Indian, or Caribbean waters.

Exposure Routes and Pathways

Ciguatera occurs after the consumption of ciguatoxic fish listed above, including Grouper, Red snapper, Barracuda, and Amberjack. These large carnivorous and predatory reef fish accumulate toxin after consumption of smaller reef fish, which have fed on toxic dinoflagellates such as *Gambierdiscus toxicus* and related species. Bottom-dwelling dinoflagellates synthesize ciguatoxins for unclear purposes. Ciguatoxins become concentrated up the food chain, with humans at the top. Contaminated fish accumulate ciguatoxins in the flesh, muscle, skin, and viscera. In Pacific waters, as ciguatoxin moves up the food chain, biotransformation occurs resulting in a more oxidized form of ciguatoxin with increased toxicity. Ciguatoxin is one of the most potent natural toxins known. One pacific ciguatoxin (P-CTX-1) poses a health risk at concentrations as low as 0.08–0.1 $\mu g\,kg^{-1}$ in man. Most fish do not concentrate sufficient ciguatoxin to be lethal to humans. Neither cooking nor freezing can inactivate the toxin. Fishermen in endemic areas may rub fish organ tissue across their gums to determine safety with the sensation of tingling denoting an unsafe fish.

Toxicokinetics

Signs and symptoms of toxicity occur 30 min to 30 h (average 6 h) after consumption of the contaminated fish. To date, no study has evaluated the toxicokinetics of ciguatoxin in humans. A rat model using one of the Pacific ciguatoxins (P-CTX-1) demonstrated a peak blood concentration at 1.97 h after oral exposure. Ciguatoxin elimination from the blood was slow with a terminal half-life of 82 h. Ciguatoxin activity was measured in rat liver, muscle, and brain 96 h after exposure. Small amounts of ciguatoxin appeared in the urine; however, the main route of excretion was in the feces.

Mechanism of Toxicity

Ciguatoxins have been demonstrated to bind to and modulate the activity of cell membrane voltage-gated sodium channels. Ciguatoxins bind at site 5 on the alpha subunit, resulting in the opening of the channels at resting membrane potential. Sodium influx causes membrane depolarization and spontaneous or repetitive firing of action potentials. *In vitro* studies using mammalian dorsal root ganglia demonstrated an increased recovery of sodium channels from the inactivated state with resultant neuroexcitability. The influx of sodium into the neuronal tissue results in cellular swelling with decreased conduction velocity and neurotransmission. This excess neuroexcitation is thought to be the etiology of the neurological symptoms often described by patients. Recovery from ciguatoxin binding and modulation may take months to years as new receptors are synthesized.

Acute and Short-Term Toxicity (or Exposure)

Human

Gastrointestinal and neurological symptoms are most commonly described following ciguatoxin exposure; however, the pattern is highly geographically variable and likely reflects differences in the effects and relative potencies of different types of ciguatoxins. In the Caribbean, gastrointestinal symptoms such as nausea, vomiting, diarrhea, and abdominal pain are reported to occur prior to the development of neurological symptoms. In Pacific and Indian waters, neurological symptoms predominate with minimal gastrointestinal effects. Nausea, vomiting, diarrhea, and abdominal pain may occur within 6–24 h of consumption of fish with spontaneous resolution in 1–4 days. Early in the disease course, cardiovascular toxicity manifested by hypotension and bradycardia may occur and requires prompt resuscitative medical care. Neurological symptoms present within a few days of exposure and are quite variable between patients. Parasthesias (numbness and tingling) of the oral region and extremities, generalized itching, myalgias, hot/cold temperature sensation reversal, and dysthesias have been reported. Hot/cold reversal is considered characteristic of ciguatera; however, not all patients describe this sensation. Neurotoxic shellfish poisoning caused by the neurotoxin brevitoxin may also produce a hot/cold dysthesia. Dental pain has also been described following ciguatoxin exposure. Neuropsychiatric symptoms such as anxiety, subjective memory loss, depression, and difficulty in concentrating may occur. More marked disturbances such as hallucinations, giddiness, ataxia or incoordination, and coma have been reported following exposure to Pacific ciguatoxins. Ciguatera fish poisoning is rarely fatal; however, death may occur from complications related to bradycardia, hypotension, or respiratory muscle paralysis if not appropriately treated.

Chronic Toxicity (or Exposure)

Human

After the initial period of gastrointestinal symptoms has abated, patients may continue to experience chronic neurological and neuropsychiatric symptoms. Feelings of subjective weakness, extremity parasthesias, malaise, headaches, and fatigue may persist for weeks to months. In one study of 12 ciguatera patients, there was no difference between exposed patients and healthy controls on measures of neuroexcitation and neuropsychiatric complaints at 6-month postexposure. Rarely, symptoms lasting for years have been reported; however, these case reports suffer from potential confounding due to other medical or psychiatric illnesses. Regional differences in ciguatoxins may mediate some symptom chronicity; however, symptoms lasting longer than 1 year should prompt evaluation for other etiologies.

Reproductive and Developmental Toxicity

The effects of ciguatoxins on pregnancy are not well known or described. Spontaneous abortion, premature labor, and neurological deficits in the newborn have been described in epidemiological surveys in endemic areas and small case series of pregnant patients diagnosed with ciguatera. It is also speculated that ciguatoxins may be passed through breast milk and the placenta. However, additional case reports suggest normal pregnancy and no adverse effects to the developing fetus following ciguatera poisoning. Further studies and research are needed.

In Vitro Toxicity Data

All ciguatoxins bind specifically and with high affinity for voltage-dependent sodium channels in the rat brain. Relatively small chemical differences between ciguatoxin molecules result in significant differences in the affinity for the sodium channel. Ciguatoxins have also demonstrated direct cytotoxic effects on mouse neuroblastoma cells. Toxicity is likely secondary to modulation of voltage-gated sodium channels but may involve other cellular effects. Other *in vitro* animal studies suggest blockade of potassium channels in cultured rat cerebellar cells.

Clinical Management

Treatment for ciguatoxin poisoning is predominantly supportive in nature and symptomatic. Analgesics may be necessary for muscle cramping and pain, antihistamines for pruritis, and antiemetics for nausea and vomiting. Advanced interventions including cardiovascular support and vasopressors may be necessary for those patients who experience bradycardia, hypotension, or cardiovascular collapse. Mannitol (20%, 5–10 ml kg^{-1} over 1 h) is often recommended to potentially ameliorate or reverse neurological dysfunction. Previous case reports and uncontrolled trials have demonstrated a benefit in 60% of cases when given within the first 24 h of the symptoms. Other studies suggest a benefit up to 2 months. Mannitol remains controversial, however, as a clear mechanism of action has not been elucidated and controlled studies have demonstrated no benefit in reversing or reducing neurological symptoms. Proposed mechanisms for mannitol include reduction of neuronal swelling, prevention of sodium channel opening, prevention of binding of ciguatoxin to receptors, or neutralization of circulating ciguatoxin. The ideal treatment, however, for ciguatera fish poisoning remains unclear.

Patients who have experienced ciguatera in the past are extremely sensitive to reexposure with more severe symptoms often described. Alcohol, mushrooms, nuts, caffeine, any type of fish, shellfish, pork, chicken, and chocolate may also exacerbate symptoms and should be avoided. Any type of physical exertion has similarly been reported to exacerbate symptoms.

Ecotoxicology

It remains unclear both why ciguatoxins are produced by dinoflagellates and if there are any significant adverse clinical effects of ciguatoxins on fish. Several studies suggest that ciguatoxins may alter the color of scales in barracuda; however, whether this effect occurs in other species of fish or is functionally relevant is unknown. Further studies are necessary to determine the effects of ciguatoxins on fish as it is bioconcentrated along the food chain.

See also: Food Safety and Toxicology; Marine Venoms and Toxins; Neurotoxicity; Scombroid; Shellfish Poisoning, Paralytic.

Further Reading

Bottein, M.Y., Wang, Z., Ramsdell, J.S., 2011. Toxicokinetics of the ciguatoxin P-CTX-1 in rats after intraperitoneal or oral administration. Toxicology 284 (1–3), 1–6.

Dickey, R.W., Plakas, S.M., 2010. Ciguatera: a public health perspective. Toxicon 56 (2), 123–136.

Dickey, R., Bottein, M.Y., Backer, L., Ayyar, R., Weisman, R., Watkins, S., Granade, R., Reich, A., 2008. Ciguatera fish poisoning: treatment, prevention and management. Mar. Drugs 6 (3), 456–479.

Bagnis, R.A., Legrand, A.-M., 1987. Clinical features on 12 890 cases of ciguatera (fish poisoning) in French Polynesia. In: Gopalakrishnakone, P., Tan, C.K. (Eds.), Progress in Venom and Toxin Research. National University of Singapore, Singapore, pp. 372–384.

Pearn, J.H., Harvey, P., De Ambrosis, W., Lewis, R., McKay, R., 1982. Ciguatera and pregnancy. Med. J. Aust. 1, 57–58.

Rivera-Alsina, M.E., Payne, C., Pou, A., Payne, S., 1991. Ciguatera poisoning in pregnancy. Am. J. Obstet. Gynecol. 164 (1 Pt 2), 397.

Senecal, P.E., Osterloh, J.D., 1991. Normal fetal outcome after maternal ciguateric toxin exposure in the second trimester. J. Toxicol. Clin. Toxicol. 29 (4), 473–478.

Relevant Websites

http://www.fda.gov/Food/FoodSafety/FoodborneIllness/FoodborneIllnessFoodbornePathogensNaturalToxins/BadBugBook/ucm070772.htm – US Food and Drug Administration (FDA) Bad Bug Book

Accessed May 1, 2012

http://www.cdc.gov/nceh/ciguatera/ – US Centers for Disease Control and Prevention (CDC) Harmful Algal Blooms

Accessed May 1, 2012

Ciprofloxacin

T Dodd-Butera, California State University, San Bernardino, CA, USA
M Broderick, California Poison Control System, San Diego, CA, USA

- Chemical Abstracts Service Registry Number: 85721-33-1
- Synonyms: Cyclopropyl-6-fluoro-1,4-dihydro-4-oxo-7-(1-piperazinyl)-3-quinolinecarboxylic acid; 1-Cyclopropyl-6-fluoro-4-oxo-7-(1-piperazinyl)-1,4-dihydro-3-quinolinecarboxylic acid; Cipro; Cipro XR; Proquin XR; Cipro IV
- Molecular Formula: $C_{17}H_{18}FN_3O_3$
- Chemical Structure:

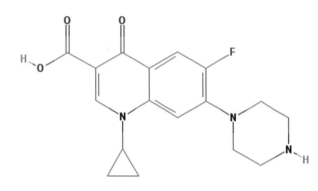

Background

Ciprofloxacin hydrochloride (Chemical Abstracts Service Registry Number 85721-33-1) is a fluoroquinolone antimicrobial agent. It is a yellow crystalline substance and the monohydrochloride monohydrate salt of cyclopropyl-6-fluoro-1,4-dihydro-4-oxo-7-(1-piperazinyl)-3-quinolinecarboxylic acid. The drug has antibacteriocidal properties and is a nucleic acid synthesis inhibitor. Bayer AG first patented the drug in 1983, and it was given approval in 1987 by the US Food and Drug Administration (FDA). Since the approval by the FDA, ciprofloxacin has been utilized as both a treatment and prophylactic regimen against serious infections. Clinical indicators for postexposure anthrax prophylaxis with ciprofloxacin were obtained during the anthrax bioterrorism events of October 2001 in the United States.

Uses

Ciprofloxacin is used in the treatment of infections from a wide range of aerobic gram-positive and aerobic gram-negative microorganisms (**Table 1**). It has been shown to be effective against inhalational anthrax and reduce the incidence or progression of disease following exposure to aerosolized *Bacillus anthracis*. It is also used in select respiratory infections, urinary tract infections, typhoid fever, some sexually transmitted diseases, and septicemia. Infectious diarrhea may be caused by organisms found in food or water and transferred by person-to-person contact. This may have a devastating effect, globally, especially in immunocompromised individuals. Ciprofloxacin is effective against those organisms that may contribute to infectious diarrhea, such as *Escherichia coli* (enterotoxigenic strains), *Campylobacter jejuni*, and select strains of *Shigella*; and is utilized when antibacterial therapy is medically indicated. Ciprofloxacin has also been utilized as a secondary agent in the treatment of tuberculosis.

Exposure and Exposure Monitoring

Exposure to ciprofloxacin in therapeutic settings may be via tablets or oral suspension, intravenous, ophthalmic, or otic drops. Monitoring ciprofloxacin blood serum concentrations has been used as representative of indication for therapeutic

Table 1 Selected organisms and infections for ciprofloxacin use

Organisms	*Urinary tract infections*	*Typhoid fever (Enteric fever)*	*Skin and skin structure infections*	*Lower respiratory tract infections*
Escherichia coli	x		x	x
Klebsiella pneumoniae	x		x	x
Enterobacter cloacae	x		x	x
Serratia marcescens	x			
Proteus mirabilis	x		x	x
Providencia rettgeri	x			
Morganella morganii	x		x	
Citrobacter diversus	x			
Citrobacter freundii	x		x	
Pseudomonas aeruginosa	x		x	x
Methicillin-susceptible *Staphylococcus*	x			
Salmonella typhi	x	x		
Stretococcus p pneumonia				x
Haemophilus influenzae			x	x

 http://dx.doi.org/10.1016/B978-0-12-386454-3.00011-7

benefit against inhalational anthrax. Occupational exposure may occur by inhalation of particles or dermal exposure.

Mechanism of Action

The antimicrobial action of the drug is due to inhibition of the enzymes required for bacterial DNA function. Topoisomerase II (DNA gyrase) and topoisomerase IV are necessary for bacterial DNA replication, transcription, strand repair, and recombination. Thus, ciprofloxacin cytotoxicity may be caused by the loss of mtDNA encoded functions.

Toxicokinetics

Ciprofloxacin hydrochloride is absorbed from the gastrointestinal tract following oral administration. The oral bioavailability of the drug is 50–85% in healthy, fasting adults, with peak serum concentrations attained in 0.5–2 h. The serum elimination half-life of ciprofloxacin in adults with normal renal function is approximately 3–5 h. Following intravenous and oral exposure, the drug is widely distributed into body tissues and fluids. The drug is eliminated by renal excretion, and the biliary system of the liver, to a lesser degree. Ciprofloxacin inhibits the CYP3A4 and CYP1A2 enzyme systems, and thus has the potential for adverse drug interactions. Concurrent use of ciprofloxacin and other drugs, such as the methylxanthines, primarily metabolized by CYP1A2, can increase plasma concentrations of drugs, such as theophylline, to potentially toxic levels. Multiple drugs are reported to potentially interact with ciprofloxacin, so concurrent use of any substance should be reported to a health care provider.

Acute and Short-Term Toxicity

Animal

Single oral doses, in general, were tolerated in mice, rats, and dogs. However, crystalluria without nephropathy was noted in rhesus monkeys with single oral doses. A dose–response relationship to adverse gastrointestinal symptoms did occur in some studies with dogs. In rabbits, doses greater than 2500 mg kg^{-1} were lethal, although response was delayed to periods of weeks following administration. In studies on mice, rats, rabbits, and dogs, neurotoxicity was noted, including seizure activity with intravenous exposure. Concomitant administration of nonsteroidal anti-inflammatory drugs in mice enhanced an excitatory response the central nervous system. In dogs and rhesus monkeys, intravenous administration produced hypotension, although the results were more consistent in dogs.

Human

Case reports of acute overdose indicate neurotoxicity, and acute renal failure may occur. The renal failure was characterized by acute tubular necrosis and distal nephron apoptosis, in some instances. Severe hypersensitivity reactions have also been reported in one-time therapeutic doses.

Chronic and Long-Term Toxicity

Animal

Reports of arthropathy in various animal species have been noted in investigations of immature animals. Joint damage was also noted in juvenile dogs and rats. Crystalluria occurred in laboratory animals, although alkaline conditions of the urine may decrease the ciprofloxacin solubility.

Acute topical administration was investigated in ocular exposure in rabbits, and inflammation was found to increase penetration into aqueous and vitreous humor with repeated use.

Human

Adverse incidents from therapeutic exposures may occur with ciprofloxacin usage, although the drug is generally well tolerated and offers benefit for select bacterial infections. Mild to moderate severity of response may be mitigated with discontinuation of the drug. Inflammation and joint pain, swelling or tearing of a tendon, especially in the Achilles' tendon of the heel may occur; noted with concomitant use of steroids. Age may contribute to the risk of tendon rupture. Ciprofloxacin-induced cholestatic liver injury and associated renal failure have been reported. Cardiovascular effects, such as arrhythmias, hypertension, pulmonary edema, and cardiopulmonary arrest have also occurred in patients taking ciprofloxacin. In addition, neurotoxicity, altered mental status, hematologic effects, bleeding disorders, altered kidney function, crystalluria, increases in liver enzymes, and fatal hepatic failure have been reported with use. More commonly, gastrointestinal effects, such as nausea and abdominal discomfort, may be experienced.

Immunotoxicity

Immunologic reactions, such as hypersensitivity, vasculitis, rashes, and anaphylaxis, have occurred with acute and chronic exposures.

Reproductive and Developmental Toxicity

Ciprofloxacin is an FDA pregnancy category C drug, indicating it is unknown whether or not this substance will harm an unborn baby. A review from the Teratogen Information System indicated that teratogenic risk was low from therapeutic doses, but that insufficient data existed to conclude the absence of risk. Studies examining spontaneous abortions, prematurity, and low birth weight did not indicate an increase in adverse conditions of pregnancy with ciprofloxacin use. However, maternal toxicity in some animal studies resulted in increased incidence of abortion. There were no clinically significant musculoskeletal anomalies or dysfunction noted, despite evidence in animal species that ciprofloxacin causes arthropathy and histological changes in weight-bearing joints of juvenile animals resulting in lameness. Ciprofloxacin crosses the placenta, however, and is distributed in the amniotic fluid in humans. Thus, use in pregnancy should be discussed with a health care provider to determine if benefit outweighs risk. More extensive studies are required to ascertain the full measure of safety or risk of in utero exposures to ciprofloxacin.

Regarding use in nursing mothers, the American Academy of Pediatrics has determined that therapeutic use of ciprofloxacin is compatible with breast-feeding. However, the drug is also distributed into human milk; and pseudomembranous colitis has been reported in a nursing infant with maternal use of ciprofloxacin. The arthropathies and cartilage erosion in immature animals indicate the need for evaluation of use in nursing mothers by a health care provider, considering the toxicity to developing joints in animal studies.

Genotoxicity

Mutagenicity test results have been varied for chromosomal aberration. Positive results for *in vitro* studies with mammalian cells may be secondary to inhibition of topoisomerase II. *In vivo* genotoxicity tests were negative for clastogenicity and DNA damage in comprehensive and comparative studies using the micronucleus test in bone marrow of mice, cytogenetic chromosome analysis in Chinese hamster, dominant lethal assay in male mice, and unscheduled DNA synthesis tests in primary rat and mouse hepatocytes.

Carcinogenicity

In studies with mice, possible skin carcinogenicity was noted with exposure to ciprofloxacin and irradiation with ultraviolet A (UVA) over a protracted period of time. Future studies are needed to ascertain the full risk of carcinogenicity.

Ecotoxicology

Ciprofloxacin has been detected in wastewater streams from effluents in municipal treatment plants and from hospital disposables. The drug is not readily biodegradable and if released into water, it is expected to adsorb to soil and sediment. Aqueous solutions may photolyze in sunlight. If released into air, ciprofloxacin is expected to remain in the particulate phase in the atmosphere.

Clinical Management

Overdosing

In the event of an acute overdose, (reversible) renal toxicity, which may require dialysis, is a potential risk. Avoid alkalinizing the urine, due to risk of crystalluria. Supportive care and emergency treatment are indicated, as determined necessary by a health care provider.

Therapeutic Dosing

Indicating conditions of tendon problems, myasthenia gravis, seizure disorders, neurological conditions, asthma, liver dysfunction, previous drug allergies, QT prolongation on an electrocardiogram, renal dysfunction, joint problems, diabetes, psychiatric disorders, or administration of prescription or over-the-counter substances is important information to share with a health care provider, in order to establish safety measures while on ciprofloxacin. There are many potential drug interactions that range from mild to severely toxic, so caution must be exercised with concomitant use of other substances. Photosensitivity is increased with ciprofloxacin use, so limited sun and UVA exposure is recommended. As with other antibiotics, pseudomembranous colitis is a potential risk, and symptoms must be reported immediately, if they occur. Emerging resistance of organisms to ciprofloxacin is a potential public health concern, so judicious use of this and other antibiotics is indicated, in consultation with a health care provider.

See also: Kidney; Immune System.

Further Reading

Fisher, L.M., Lawrence, J.M., Josty, I.C., Hopewell, R., Margerrison, E.E., Cullen, M.E., 1989 Nov 30. Ciprofloxacin and the fluoroquinolones. New concepts on the mechanism of action and resistance. Am. J. Med. 87 (5A), 2S–8S.

Goodman, Gilman's, 1996. The Pharmacological Basis of Therapeutics, ninth ed. McGraw-Hill, New York.

Herbold, H.A., Brendler-Schwaab, S.Y., Jurgen Ahr, H., 2001. Ciprofloxacin: in vivo genotoxicity studies. Mutat. Res. 498, 193–205.

Mäkinen, M., Forbes, P.D., Stenbäck, F., 1997 Feb. Quinolone antibacterials: a new class of photochemical carcinogens. J. Photochem. Photobiol. B 37 (3), 182–187.

Relevant Website

http://www.ncbi.nlm.nih.gov/sites/entrez?db=pccompound&term=ciprofloxacin – NCBI PubChem Compound.

Circadian Clock Effects/Chronotoxicology

CB Spainhour, Spainhour Consulting Services, South Abington Township, PA, USA

The study of the kinetics, pharmacodynamics, toxicological responses, and side effects of drugs, toxins, chemicals, xenobiotics, etc., relative to the temporal rhythms of living organisms is referred to as chronotoxicology. These temporal rhythms are driven by circadian (24 h time period) or solar time cycles, which are in turn based on periodic photostimuli received from sunlight and potentially further influenced by other local time signals.

The biological rhythm of living organisms has been well known for several decades as a result of numerous and various reports in the published literature of cell biology, physiology, and pharmacology. Temporal variations can and do simply explain why the same xenobiotics, etc., regardless of origin, do not induce the same efficacy or other effects in a living organism, if administered at different times of the day or at different seasons of the year. Rhythmic or circadian changes in the sensitivity or susceptibility to xenobiotics were actually first reported as far back as 1958 in experiments with mice. A few years later it was demonstrated that German cockroaches (*Blatella germanica*) exhibited a rhythmic susceptibility over a 24 h period of time to a standard dose of potassium cyanide, when organisms were exposed to the toxin at different times within the day.

The mammalian circadian system is organized in a prioritized manner with a highly important, centrally located pacemaker within the suprachiasmatic nucleus (SCN) of the hypothalamic region of the brain. This structure is located proximal to the optic chiasm and receives transmitted light within the wavelength range of 460–480 nm. The reception of this light is via nonvisual photosensitive retinal ganglion cells, which contain the substance melanopsin and are located within the retinohypothalamic tract of the brain. This center controls and synchronizes the circadian receivers or oscillators in millions of peripherally located cells all over the body. These cells themselves are not responsive to light, but do respond to neural and humoral signals from the SCN. Major timing signals in the synchronization of many of these peripheral clocks include sleep and activity periods and feeding and fasting cycles. This has suggested to researchers in the field that the temporal coordination of metabolism and proliferation is a major effort of the mammalian timing, circadian, or circannual system. Taken together, the complete chronosystem directs and controls precisely timed events that sustain life by regulating physiological function of the cardiovascular, hemodynamic, metabolic, nervous, digestive, immune, reproductive, and endocrine systems. Rhythmic fluctuations in absorption, distribution, metabolism, and excretion regulate the detoxification of toxic substances, drug toxicity, and drug efficacy. This watch-like control of xenobiotic catabolism and detoxification provides the molecular and biochemical basis for the dosing time dependence of both drug toxicities and drug efficacy. The inactivation of noxious food components by intestinal, hepatic, and renal detoxification systems is among the processes regulated in a circadian fashion. Many of these chronologic processes are further regulated at the genetic level by actual clock genes, which establish basic transcriptional–translational feedback oscillation loops under the control of such entities as *Per* 1–3, *Cry* 1,2, Rev-erbα, Rev-erbβ, Rorα, Rorβ, and cAMP response element-binding protein along with the circadian locomotor output cycles kaput/brain and muscle ARNT-like protein 1 (CLOCK/BMAL 1) heterodimers. Knowledge and understanding of these clock-based processes continues to grow and expand and can be used for improving or designing therapeutic treatment regimens.

It has not been an uncommon finding that some studies in the area of chronotoxicology are also susceptible to seasonal variability. Reports have shown that some circadian peak times of susceptibility found during one season may be totally different from that observed in a different season. The exposure of mice via intraperitoneal injection to mercuric chloride at four different times a day over 6 months of the year revealed that the same dose of mercury (5 mg kg^{-1}) induced different mortality rates when administered in January, June, or September. Let us consider the subacute toxicity of amikacin. Urinary enzyme activity in animals in autumn is enhanced by a factor of about 5 when amikacin is administered at 20.00 h and by a factor only a little more than 1 when administration occurs at 14.00 h. Alternatively, in the spring of the year, this increase in enzymatic activity is very weak at 20.00 h and significantly elevated by about 4–7 times when administration occurs at 14.00. Seasonal variation has been observed in the degree of acute toxicity of X-rays, cyclophosphamide, and arabinosylcytosine in rodents. The toxicity of phenobarbital has been studied in mice. It has been reported that a dose of 190 mg kg^{-1} administered at 16.00 h killed no animals in July but killed 90% of the mice in January. A dose of 270 mg kg^{-1} of phenobarbital administered at 04.00 h killed all animals in October and only 40% of the mice in July. Rat tolerance of cisplatin is twice as high in the winter as it is in the summer. Murine tolerance to doxorubicin and donomycin was optimal in autumn and poorest in the spring and summer. These studies clearly indicate that not only the time of the day is important, but also the month of the year. It has become obvious that the wavelike high or low phases of susceptibility or tolerance in an organism can totally reverse themselves according to the season. It is important to keep in mind that the severity of potential damage to organs exposed to the administration of metals, antibiotics, anticancer agents, etc. is dependent not only on the circadian time but also on the season of the year. These annual cycles or rhythms of tolerance and susceptibility may indeed be controlled at least in part by the levels of hormones (testosterone, estrogen, luteinizing hormone, thyroxin, oxytocin, etc.), which can possibly affect organ or tissue defense mechanisms. Research continues in this area.

The examples that will be provided of alterations in the acute, subchronic, or chronic toxicities or side effects of drugs, chemicals, etc., as a result of the temporality of administration do raise the question as to what exactly the mechanism or mechanisms are that drive or control these differences of tolerance or susceptibility. Original attempts have led to

 http://dx.doi.org/10.1016/B978-0-12-386454-3.00964-7

investigations of biotransformation and pharmacokinetics. It is known that the liver and kidneys do undergo a circadian-dependent synthesis of their enzymes and changes in membrane structure and function and nuclear components. A complete understanding of the chronophysiology of the liver and kidneys does make it possible to explain the chronopharmacological variations in hepatic and/or renal elimination and the metabolism of drugs. Time studies of the activities of glycogen phosphorylase and glycogen synthetase copy exactly the activities of hexobarbital oxidase and barbiturate-induced sleep duration. Similarly, the circadian changes in the hemodynamics of the kidneys are well correlated with cortical accumulation and elimination. This all brings us to the introduction of another new term, chronesthesy. This is defined as the rhythmic changes of any biological system with regard to its susceptibility or tolerance. The biological system can be a living organism, cell, tissue, or organ.

The immune system, not surprisingly exhibits a clocklike regulation. When mice were administered *Bacillus Calmette-Guerrin* in the middle of the day, 75% of the exposed animals survived. However, when the mice were injected in the latter portion of the night period, only 50% were found to survive.

Studies involving the assessment of gastric chronotoxicology using gastric mucosal integrity have revealed that there is indeed a time-related damage component caused by the well-characterized aspirin and nonsteroidal anti-inflammatory agents. Although still somewhat controversial, it appears that night-time administration of these types of agents are better tolerated than the day-time administration of the same. In humans, using endoscopic visualization, it was determined that the administration of 1300 mg of aspirin at 08.00 versus 20.00 h resulted in the development of almost 40% fewer gastric mucosal lesions if the medicine was administered in the evening. In a study utilizing osteoarthritic patients, it was discovered that the administration of a sustained-release formulation of indomethacin at 08.00 h resulted in a significantly greater number of undesirable effects than if the medication was administered at 20.00 h.

Hearing has been evaluated in rats exposed to kanamycin. Kanamycin was administered to female Sprague-Dawley rats four times a day via a subcutaneous route at 02.00, 08.00, 14.00, and 20.00 h of each day under light-synchronized conditions for a study duration of 6 weeks. Observations at 2 weeks postdosing revealed that the 8.00 h dose group showed significant hearing loss, while there were minimal changes recorded in the other animals and dose groups. However, it was discovered that after 6 weeks of exposure, the 8.00 and 14.00 h groups both demonstrated similar dramatic hearing loss, with other animals revealing minimal changes. The conclusion of the study stated that it appeared that kanamycin-induced auditory damage is more dramatic during the day (rest period) than during the night (activity period). The improved night-time tolerance was discovered also to be correlated with the peak of body temperature – another possible rhythm marker in aminoglycoside-induced toxicity.

Unfortunately, damage to the kidneys is very common as a result of exposure to drugs or toxins. This is no surprise because approximately a quarter of cardiac output flows through the kidneys, which are a major route of elimination of many substances. Moieties are filtered through the glomerular barrier and enter the tubular lumen in the tubular fluid. The structure and function of membrane structures in the kidney can be significantly altered as a result of exposure to aminoglycoside antibiotics, impairing the elimination processes. Xenobiotics may indeed reach very high levels of intracellular concentrations and therefore produce renal cell injury by one of three different metabolic pathways. Substances, even if extrarenal and if stable enough and whether metabolized or not, may inflict direct toxicity to the kidney. Second, a substance may enter renal tubular cells and interfere directly with cellular functions. Third, materials may be metabolized within renal cells to highly reactive metabolites that may bind covalently to structural or functional proteins or even initiate lipid peroxidation.

The kidneys are a prime target for heavy metals, because these substances are chiefly concentrated in the renal cortex. This accumulation leads to the development of well-characterized pathological changes in the proximal tubules. The initial response of rat kidneys to the administration of a single dose of a heavy metal is the development of a focal necrosis in the midthird of the proximal tubule (*pars recta*). If mercury is used as an example, within 3 h after exposure, tubular cell brush borders become fragmented and by 6 h postexposure the epithelial cells of the *pars recta* begin to swell and protrude into the tubular lumen, creating tubular blockage. The prevalence of intracellular vacuoles in the cytoplasm substantially increases. At 12 h postexposure, a significantly increased number of lysosomal structures are appearing within the cells and the mitochondria are swelling. Eventually, cell necrosis results with the release of whole cells and cell parts into the tubular lumen. Over the years, cadmium, platinum, and mercury have been popular heavy metal renal toxins for studies that populate the literature. It is now accepted that the lethality of heavy metals is highly dependent on the timing of exposure. The exposure of rodents to cisplatin was monitored via histopathological evaluation and the determination of blood levels of serum urea and *N*-acetyl-glucosamidase (NAG). Using these methods of evaluation, it was determined that rats exposed to cisplatin in the middle of the night demonstrated trivial changes from control kidneys and renal damage was minimal. However, a fourfold increase in NAG as well as a significant increase in serum urea was correlated with exposure to cisplatin during the day time hours. Mercuric chloride's renal toxicity is well known and highly characterized. Single, sublethal doses of mercuric chloride administered via the subcutaneous route to rats at four different time points during a 24 h period were evaluated for toxicity by measuring the levels of various tubular nephrotoxicity biomarker enzymes. It was discovered that if the mercuric chloride was administered in the middle of the day or light period, urinary levels of the biomarkers approached increases of almost 2000%, but if the administration was performed in the middle of the dark period (high activity period of rats), the elevations of these biomarkers were only approximately 1000%. When one looks at the location of mercury or cisplatin in the kidney after exposure to cisplatin or mercuric chloride, if the exposure was performed at the end of the light period, mercury or cisplatin concentrations were found to be highest in the renal tissue and lowest in the urine. Simply put, these chemicals were excreted in larger amounts when animals were exposed during their active period as opposed to exposure during their rest phase (day). Similar results have been found in mice. Indeed, it has also been found that mice better tolerate the administration of adriamycin if exposure was during the latter half of the animal's rest period (day) and that cisplatin was best tolerated when administered in the latter half of the animal's activity period (night). Shifting now to the clinical arena, when patients were exposed to adriamycin in the morning and cisplatin in the evening or adriamycin in the evening and cisplatin in the morning, complications and side effects were significantly worse for patients receiving adriamycin in the evening and cisplatin in the morning. Similar results have been found in studies using human subjects exposed to 5-fluorouracil, cisplatin, or vindesine. If administrations of antineoplastics for advanced-stage colon and rectal cancers were modulated over time rather than just constantly administered over time, a significantly greater degree of effectiveness was observed. Similar effects or expressions of toxicity are observed with the administration of a variety of antibiotics cleared through the kidneys and many antineoplastic agents that are also cleared through the kidneys.

Over the years, a variety of agents have been reported in the literature as being hepatotoxic, and the solvent carbon tetrachloride has been a popular agent studied. After a single dose exposure of carbon tetrachloride, centrilobular necrosis and lipidoses occur in the livers of all animals. Mitochondrial damage can be observed by 5–6 h after exposure. Other lesions develop by 12 h postexposure, and severe hepatic necrosis has developed by 24 h postexposure. Studies have demonstrated that the circadian susceptibility of animals to hepatotoxicity has been found to be at least in part dependent on the timing of toxin uptake and metabolism. Similar correlations with chronotoxicity have been found in studies with the agents chloroform, trichloroethylene, and 1,1-dichloroethylene and the drug acetaminophen. Rats have been found to be most susceptible to chloroform exposure when the administration is performed within a 2 h period after the initiation of their active period (night) (21.00 h). The lowest level of susceptibility was observed when exposure was at 09.00 h (day). Even though rats exposed to chloroform at both 21.00 and 09.00 h revealed depressed levels of glutathione, hepatic levels of glutathione were found to be more significantly depressed at 21.00 h than at 09.00 h. If the serum activities of glutamic-pyruvic-transaminase, isocitrate dehydrogenase, ornithine-carbamyl-transferase, and sorbitol dehydrogenase were measured in rats after exposures to carbon tetrachloride at eight different time points within a day, it was revealed that significant increases (in some cases approaching 400%) were observed with the administration of carbon tetrachloride at 18.00 or 20.00 h, but remained unchanged if exposure was at 10.00 h.

Although trichloroethylene is a well-known and highly characterized hepatotoxin, it is also a potent neurotoxin. For example, if trichloroethylene is administered to rats via the intraperitoneal route at four different time points within a day and toxicity assessed by evaluating muscle tone, it was determined that the time of the most significant neurotoxic effect of trichloroethylene was early in the active phase (21.00 h). Interestingly, the plasma concentrations of trichloroethylene and two of its major metabolites are found to be at minimal levels at 21.00 h. Accordingly, it appears that neurotoxicity of trichloroethylene is accentuated when hepatic elimination is at its lowest level of activity.

It is important to know and realize that it is not just chemical agents that can be associated with time-dependent toxicological effects. These same patterns of timing have also been associated with exposures to viruses, fungi, venoms, toxins, and bacteria. The toxins released by these agents as part of their 'infective' or invasive activities can effect mortality and/or cell damage, the severity of which can be strongly related to the time of exposure. Scorpion (*Heterometrus fulvipes*) venom has demonstrated a circadian-dependent toxicity in tropical mice (*Mus booduga*) as evaluated with the measurement of the blood levels of acetylcholine and acetylcholinesterase. Mice exposed to *Brucella* endotoxin exposed at night time lived for approximately 75 h, but those exposed during the day time survived only 37 h. Circadian-dependent changes in locomotor activity in hamsters has been observed with exposure to the protein synthesis inhibitor anisomycin. The locomotor phase change is delayed if the anisomycin is administered at midnight, but accelerated if administered at midday. Mice injected with *Escherichia coli* endotoxin at 0.00 and 16.00 h showed survival rates of 85% and 20%, respectively. Tetrodotoxin (*Spheroides rubripes*) exposure results in significant changes in vasopressin release from the SCN in the rat. However, if tetrodotoxin is perfused into the rat at night (12 h period), no alterations of vasopressin release were observed, but when tetrodotoxin was perfused into rats during the day (12 h), the levels of vasopressin were almost suppressed. Interestingly, the induction of seizures by the presence of white noise (100 dB for 60 s) in mice has been shown to be circadian dependent, and X-ray irradiation has been similarly demonstrated to be circadian dependent as measured by the mortalities observed in both *Drosophila* and mice. With regard to the irradiation, a dose of 555 R administered at night resulted in 100% mortality, but if done during the day the exposure was not lethal at all.

All of the studies mentioned for the most part have been performed in rodents or humans as part of clinical trials or other evaluations. A big reason for this is the fact that the maintenance of synchronized and strictly defined conditions can be most cost-effectively managed with rodents, which also then permit the use of sufficient numbers of animals for statistical power. However, studies in the area of chronotoxicology have also been performed and reported in other species, including both fish and insects. Circadian rhythms have been observed in rainbow trout. In the case of rainbow trout, a seasonality to the lethality of cyanide exposure was discovered. The study of chronobiology in insects could lead to the more efficient and efficacious use of pesticides and improved ecological outcomes. For example, if one looks at houseflies and yellow fever mosquito (*Aedes aegypti*) larvae and their exposure to malathion and/or dursban, investigations have shown that differing potencies of lethality are observed to the same concentration of pesticide depending on the timing of exposure. Ninety percent of insect larvae can be killed if they are exposed during the latter half of the night and only 20% if exposed at the end of the day period.

Toxicologists have many times taken issue with some results reported in the literature and the discrepancies that were found to exist. The data from this relatively new area of research mandate that it is necessary to critically evaluate and reevaluate toxicity, especially if mortality is involved with respect to exposures and the time of the day and even the time of the year. The examples provided demonstrate that both circadian and circannual patterns do indeed exist and can significantly alter the susceptibility ad response levels of living organisms. It is now fundamental for toxicology reports and studies to state not only the lighting schedule for animals on a given study but also the exact hour of the day and the month of the year to be able to fairly and accurately compare toxicity results. The lack of adequate consideration of this timing parameter can result in significantly altered efficacy profiles, toxicity profiles, therapeutic indices, safety factors, and tolerance.

See also: Cyclosporine; Radiation Toxicology, Ionizing and Nonionizing; Toxicity, Acute; Toxicity, Subchronic and Chronic; Cancer Chemotherapeutic Agents; Chemical Interactions; Malathion; Neurotoxicity; Organochlorine Insecticides; Pesticides; Acetaminophen; Cell Cycle; Cell Proliferation; Cisplatin; Cyanide; Kidney; Lipid Peroxidation; Mechanisms of Toxicity; Mercuric Chloride ($HgCl_2$); Distribution; Endocrine System; Excretion; Resistance to Toxicants; Toxicology; Trichloroethylene; Veterinary Toxicology; How Toxicology Impacts Other Sciences; *Bacillus Thuringiensis*; Ecotoxicology; Aquatic Ecotoxicology; Avian Ecotoxicology; Genetic Ecotoxicology; Ecotoxicology, Aquatic Invertebrates; Ecotoxicology Terrestrial; Ecotoxicology; Wildlife; Species Sensitivity Distributions; Safety Testing, Clinical Studies; The History of Toxicology; Angiotensin Converting Enzyme (ACE) Inhibitors; Acetylsalicylic Acid; Barbiturates; Ibuprofen; Sedatives; Scorpions; Snakes; Spiders; Tetrodotoxin; Modifying Factors of Toxicity; Translational Toxicology; Animal Models; LD_{50}/LC_{50} (Lethal Dosage 50/Lethal Concentration 50); Mercury; Metallothionein; Metals; SSRIs (Selective Serotonin Reuptake Inhibitors); Toxicity Testing, Alternatives; Toxicity Testing, Behavioral; Toxicity Testing, Carcinogenesis; Toxicity Testing, Dermal; Toxicity Testing, Inhalation; Toxicity Testing, Mutagenicity; Toxicity Testing, Sensitization; Natural Products; Animals, Poisonous and Venomous; *Escherichia coli* (Escherichia Coli).

Further Reading

Batalla, A., Malmary, M.F., Cambar, J., Labat, C., Oustrin, J., 1994. Dosing-time dependent nephrotoxicity of cyclosporin A during 21 days administration to Wistar rats. Chronobiol. Int. 11 (3), 195.

Bélanger, P.M., 1987. Chronobiological variation in the hepatic elimination of drugs and toxic chemical agents. Annu. Rev. Chronopharmacol. 4, 1–46.

Bruckner, J.V., Luthra, R., Lakatua, D., Sackett-Lunden, L., 1984. Influence of time of exposure to carbon tetrachloride on toxic liver injury. Annu. Rev. Chronopharmacol. 1, 373–376.

Cal, J.C., Dorian, C., Cambar, J., 1985. Circadian and circannual changes in nephrotoxic effects of heavy metals and antibiotics. Annu. Rev. Chronopharmacol. 2, 143–176.

Cambar, J., L'Azou, B., Cal, J.C., 1992. Chronotoxicology. In: Touitou, Y., Haus, E. (Eds.), Biologic Rhythms in Clinical and Laboratory Medicine. Springer, Berlin, Heidelberg, New York, pp. 138–150.

Cambar, J., Pons, M., 2010. New trends in chronotoxicology. In: Redfern, P.H., Lemmer, B. (Eds.), Physiology and Pharmacology of Biological Rhythms, Handbook of Experimental Pharmacology, vol. 125. Springer-Verlag, Berlin, Heidelberg, Germany, pp. 557–588.

Dorian, C., Catroux, P., Cambar, J., 1988. Chronobiological approach to aminoglycosides. Arch. Toxicol. 12, 151–157.

Earnest, D.J., Digiogio, S.M., Sladek, C.D., 1991. Effects of tetrodotoxin on the circadian pacemaker mechanism in suprachiasmatic explants *in vitro*. Brain Res. Bull. 26, 677–682.

Fisch, J., Yonovitz, A., Smolensky, M., 1984. Effects of circadian rhythm on kanamycin-induced hearing loss. Annu. Rev. Chronopharmacol. 1, 385–388.

Hayes, D.K., Morgan, N.O., 1988. Insects as animal models for chronopharmacological research. Annu. Rev. Chronopharmacol. 5, 243–246.

Lévi, F., Schibler, U., 2007. Circadian rhythms: mechanisms and therapeutic implications. Annu. Rev. Pharmacol. Toxicol. 47, 593–628.

Lévi, F., Boughattas, N.A., Blazsek, I., 1988. Comparative murine chronotoxicity of anticancer agents and related mechanisms. Annu. Rev. Chronopharmacol. 4, 283–331.

Motahashi, Y., Miyazaki, Y., 1990. Temporal variations in acute neurotoxicity of trichloroethylene in the rat. Annu. Rev. Chronopharmacol. 7, 177–180.

Prat, M., Bruguerolle, B., 1988. Chronotoxicity and chronokinetics of two local anaesthetic agents, bupivacaine and mepivacaine, in mice. Annu. Rev. Chronopharmacol. 5, 263.

Walker, C.A., Soliman, M.R., Soliman, K.F., 1983. Chronopharmacology and chronotoxicology of CNS drugs: interrelationships with neuromodulators. Int. J. Toxicol. 2 (6), 359–370.

Relevant Websites

http://www.circadian.com – Circadian Rhythms.
http://www.circadian.org/links.html – Circadian Rhythms.
http://www.nigms.nih.gov – Circadian Rhythms.

Cisplatin

TG Towne and A Murray, Manchester University College of Pharmacy, Fort Wayne, IN, USA

This article is a revision of the previous edition article by Linda A. Malley, volume 1, pp 614–616, © 2005, Elsevier Inc.

- Name: Cisplatin
- Chemical Abstracts Service Registry Number: CAS 15663-27-1
- Synonyms (National Health Services HAZ-MAP): [1]CDDP *cis*-Platin; *cis*-Platinum(II); Peyrone's chloride
- Molecular Formula: $Cl_2H_6N_2Pt$
- Chemical Structure:

```
            Cl⁻
   H         |        H
    \        |       /
H —  N ——— Pt2+ ——— N — H
    /        |       \
   H         |        H
            Cl⁻
```

Background Information

Cisplatin was the first compound of the platinum-antineoplastic medications approved for use in humans in 1978. However, this compound was originally known as 'Peyrone's chloride,' as it was first prepared in 1845 by an Italian chemist, Michele Peyrone. A Swiss chemist, Alfred Werner played a central role in the characterization of the compound, winning a Nobel Prize in 1913 for his work. Cisplatin was later found to be an anticancer drug by Barnett Rosenberg during the 1960s. Rosenberg had originally tested the effects of an electric field on the bacteria *Escherichia coli* and found that the bacteria ceased to divide when placed in this environment. The inhibition of bacterial division was found to occur due to the platinum electrode rather than the electrical field. Because of this discovery, platinum-containing compounds were investigated for their effects in anticancer treatments. Cisplatin is an important compound in treating cancer and is widely used today in various malignancies. Its discovery has also led to the development of other platinum-antineoplastic medications and advancement in treating malignancies.

Uses

Cisplatin has many therapeutic uses in treating various oncologic malignancies. FDA-approved indications for this compound include metastatic malignant tumor of the testis in combination with other chemotherapy agents, metastatic ovarian tumors, and advanced transitional cell carcinoma of the bladder. There are many other malignancies cisplatin is used for; however, these are non-FDA labeled indications. Research in the field of oncology continues to play an important role in determining other uses for antineoplastic medications such as cisplatin. Although not listed as an FDA-approved indication, cisplatin is also used as first line therapy in combination with other chemotherapy agents for treatment of small cell and nonsmall cell lung cancer. It is also frequently used in combination with radiation for treatment of head and neck cancer. In the future, cisplatin may be found to be useful in various other malignancies.

Environmental Fate and Behavior

The production of *cis*-diaminedichloroplatinum may result in its release, potentially into soil. Conversion to ionic species by abiotic or biotic processes can further enhance its adsorption to soil. In water *cis*-diaminedichloroplatinum will slowly convert to *trans* diaminedichloroplatinum. In this form, *trans*-diaminedichloroplatinum will remain dissolved until it is adsorbed to suspended particles or it precipitates into sediment.

Exposure and Exposure Monitoring

Cisplatin is a parenteral agent used for intravenous injection. It is available as either a solution or as a dry, lyophilized powder for reconstitution. Both the solution and the powder when reconstituted have a standardized concentration of 1 mg cisplatin/1 ml solution. During production and preparation of cisplatin formulations it is possible for dermal, oral, or inhalation exposure to occur. In addition, dermal exposure may occur during the administration of cisplatin to either the administrator of the agent or its recipient.

Toxicokinetics

The distribution of cisplatin following intravenous administration has been investigated in both humans and animals. Following administration and exposure to physiologic pH, the chloride atom of cisplatin may be displaced by a nucleophile such as water or a sulfhydryl group. The result of this chemical reaction is two primary molecular species, cisplatin (the parent compound) and monohydroxymonochloro *cis*-diammine platinum(II) (the platinum component). When a normal therapeutic dose of cisplatin is administered, concentrations of platinum are highest in the liver, kidneys, and prostate. Other organs with uptake of platinum include bladder, testes, muscle, spleen, pancreas and to a much lesser degree the bowel, adrenal, heart, lung, cerebrum, and cerebellum. Within the actual tumor, concentrations of platinum are generally lower than the organ where the tumor is located.

The excretion of cisplatin in the urine is highly dependent on the method of administration. When given as a single bolus dose 10–40% of platinum is excreted in the urine over a 24-h period. With repeated dosing on five consecutive days, the mean total elimination of platinum was 35–51%. The majority of platinum is eliminated rapidly from the body within the first 4 h due to the extensive protein binding of the compound.

While the use of cisplatin is typically limited to intravenous administration, intraperitoneal delivery may provide some benefit for solid tumors of intraperitoneal cavity. Due to the direct administration, the intraperitoneal cavity is exposed to 10–20 times more platinum than if the drug was administered by standard intravenous infusion. Much of the drug (~86%) will rapidly pass through the plasma-peritoneal barrier, reaching the systemic circulation and distributing to the extent that was described in the preceding paragraphs.

Mechanism of Toxicity

Cisplatin reacts covalently with several of amino acids leading to a variety of platinum-DNA adducts. The effects on cross-linking with DNA appear to differ among cell type; however, these may involve signal-transduction pathways such as cell-cycle arrest, programmed cell death, and impaired recognition and repair of cisplatin-induced DNA damage. In addition to its effects on DNA, cisplatin inhibits a number of enzymes containing a catalytically active sulfhydryl group.

Acute and Short-Term Toxicity (or Exposure)

Animal

When cisplatin was tested in rats, the oral LD_{50} was 25.8 mg kg^{-1}, the intravenous LD_{50} was 8 mg kg^{-1}, the intraperitoneal LD_{50} was 6.4 mg kg^{-1}, and the intramuscular LD_{50} was 9.2 mg kg^{-1}. The toxic effects observed in rats included leukopenia, decreased numbers of circulating platelets, lymphoid depletion, intestinal epithelial injury, bone marrow depression, and sloughing of the renal tubular epithelium.

In mice, the oral LD_{50} was 32.7 mg kg^{-1}, the intravenous LD_{50} was 11 mg kg^{-1}, the intraperitoneal LD_{50} was 6.6 mg kg^{-1}, and the intramuscular LD_{50} was 17.9 mg kg^{-1}.

The minimum lethal dose for dogs was single intravenous injection of 2.5 mg kg^{-1} or five consecutive daily injections of 0.75 mg kg^{-1}. In rhesus monkeys, the minimum lethal dose was five daily doses of 2.5 mg kg^{-1}. Toxic symptoms such as severe hemorrhagic enterocolitis and severe damage to the bone marrow and lymphoid tissue were observed in both species. Renal necrosis and renal nephrosis were observed in dogs and monkeys, respectively. Occasionally, pancreatitis was also observed in dogs and myocarditis in monkeys.

Human

Cisplatin is corrosive to the skin, and dusts cause eye and respiratory irritation. Renal dysfunction is the major, dose-limiting toxic effect of this drug. It can occur as a result of a single dose; however, usually manifests with multiple-course therapy. It reduces the single-nephron glomerular filtration rate and causes a back leak of inulin across the renal tubule. Additional toxic effects that are commonly observed in the acute setting include ototoxicity, myelosuppression, and nausea/vomiting/diarrhea. Other toxicities such as peripheral neuropathy (paresthesias), central extrapyramidal disorders, loss of deep tendon reflexes, metabolic acidosis, headaches, taste disturbance, retrobulbar neuritis, seizures, thirst, metallic taste, leukopenia, allergic reactions, azotemia, hypokalemia, hypophosphatemia, hypocalcemia, and hypomagnesemia may also occur following treatment with cisplatin. Some patients have also experienced anaphylactic reactions to treatment with platinum-containing compounds.

Chronic Toxicity (or Exposure)

Animal

Studies in animals indicate that cisplatin increases the occurrence of tumors. Cisplatin was administered once weekly by intraperitoneal injection to mice for 10 weeks for a total dose of 108 mol kg^{-1}. Cisplatin treated mice had a significantly higher incidence (100%) of pulmonary adenomas compared to similarly treated control mice (26%). In another study, mice received weekly intraperitoneal injections of cisplatin 1.62 mg kg^{-1} in 5 ml saline for 16 weeks, followed by dermal application of croton oil, dermal application of croton oil alone (control), or saline alone (control). Mice treated with croton oil and cisplatin had a higher incidence of skin papillomas compared to cisplatin alone or the control groups.

Female rats were administered twice weekly intraperitoneal injections of cisplatin for a cumulative dose of 15 or 34 mg kg^{-1}. Following the last dose, sensory and motor nerve conduction velocities were determined. Both doses of cisplatin significantly decreased sensory nerve conduction velocity. In addition, the level of cisplatin DNA binding in dorsal root spinal ganglion satellite cells equaled that in liver cells; however, the level of cisplatin DNA binding in spinal cord and brain was very low.

Human

Within 2 months of the initiation of treatment, the use of cisplatin usually causes azoospermia. Following the cessation of treatment, sperm counts recover in 1–2 years in most patients.

Immunotoxicity

Myelosuppression is a known and relatively frequent adverse effect associated with the use of cisplatin. The severity of the suppression of leukocytes is dose dependent and usually resolves within 1–2 months. Additionally, acute leukemia has been noted in patients receiving cisplatin in addition to other agents to treat malignancy.

Reproductive Toxicity

Intraperitoneal administration to rats and mice demonstrated high levels of embryo toxicity at levels far below the therapeutic dose used in human adults. For rats, the embryonic LD_{50} values were 2.88, 1.28, and 1 mg kg^{-1} for day 6, 8, and 11 postgestation, respectively. The embryonic LD_{50} in mice was 5.24 mg.

Surviving fetuses exhibited mitochondrial and skeletal abnormalities, DNA adduct formation, and a higher incidence of tumor formation throughout the body.

Cisplatin will cause azoospermia in men; however, this is usually reversible several years after cessation of therapy. Teratogenicity has been noted with the use of cisplatin during all trimesters of pregnancy. The US Food and Drug Administration classifies cisplatin as a pregnancy category D agent, meaning its use is likely to cause fetal harm, but its use may be justified for life-threatening maternal diseases. It is known to cross the placental barrier; however, its safety in breastfeeding is not well defined.

Genotoxicity

Cisplatin was mutagenic in *Salmonella typhimurium* strains G46/pkM101, TA100, and TA98, without metabolic activation. Cisplatin also induced increased mutations in Chinese hamster ovary cells and V79 Chinese hamster cells. Postreplication repair was induced in V79 cells and in HeLa cells; and sister chromatid exchanges were induced in V79 cells. Chromosomal damage and sister chromatid exchanges were also induced by cisplatin in human lymphocyte cultures. Similar to the *in vitro* data, intraperitoneal injection of mice with 13.85 $mg\,kg^{-1}$ cisplatin induced a significant increase in sister chromatid exchanges and in chromosome aberrations.

Carcinogenicity

Cisplatin administered in combination with etoposide is carcinogenic in humans.

Clinical Management

Risk of nephrotoxicity may be minimized by intravenous hydration and mannitol over a 6–8 h period, surrounding the infusion of cisplatin. The extent of nephrotoxicity will also impact electrolyte concentrations which will need to be monitored and supplemented as necessary. Nausea and vomiting may be managed with antiemetics. Management of an anaphylactic reaction would include the administration of epinephrine and corticosteroids with or without antihistamines. If accidental exposure to the eyes or skin occurs, the affected skin should be washed thoroughly with soap and water, and the eyes should be flushed with copious amounts of tepid water for at least 15 min.

Ecotoxicity

No aquatic organism toxicity to cisplatin was reported.

Other Hazards

Contact with aluminum causes the degradation of cisplatin. Therefore during the production, distribution, and administration of this agent all contact with aluminum and aluminum-containing products should be avoided. For those solutions having a low chloride concentration, cisplatin is not compatible. Upon heating and decomposition of cisplatin, toxic fumes such as hydrogen chloride and nitrogen oxide are emitted. Caution and protective measures should be in place to avoid exposure.

Exposure Standards and Guidelines

An 8-h time weighted average (TWA) of 0.002 $mg^{-3}m^{3}$ is the recommended threshold limit value (TLV) by the American Conference of Governmental Industrial Hygienists. Furthermore, workers having exposure to cisplatin may exceed an exposure of three times the TLV–TWA for a maximum of 30 min per working day, never exceeding five times the TLV–TWA.

See also: Cancer Chemotherapeutic Agents; Carcinogen–DNA Adduct Formation and DNA Repair; Cyclophosphamide; Melphalan; Dacarbazine;

Further Reading

Barnes, K.R., Lippard, S.J., 2004. Cisplatin and related anticancer drugs: recent advances and insights. Met. Ions Biol. Syst. 42, 142–177.

Bischin, C., Lupan, A., Taciuc, V., Silaghi-Dumitrescu, R., 2011. Interactions between proteins and platinum-containing anti-cancer drugs. Mini Rev. Med. Chem. 11 (3), 214–224 (Review).

Feldman, D.R., Schaffer, W.L., Steingart, R.M., 2012. Late cardiovascular toxicity following chemotherapy for germ cell tumors. J. Natl. Compr. Canc. Netw. 10 (4), 537–544.

Hoff, P.M., Saad, E.D., Costa, F., et al., 2012. Literature review and practical aspects on the management of oxaliplatin-associated toxicity. Clin. Colorectal Caner 11 (2), 93–100.

Jaggi, A.S., Singh, N., 2012. Mechanisms in cancer-chemotherapeutic drugs-induced peripheral neuropathy. Toxicology 291 (1–3), 1–9.

Rossi, A., Di Maio, M., Chiodini, P., et al., 2012. Carboplatin- or cisplatin-based chemotherapy in first-line treatment of small-cell lung cancer: the COCIS meta-analysis of individual patient data. J. Clin. Oncol. 30 (14), 1692–1698.

US Department of Health & Human Services/National Toxicology Program, Tenth Report on Carcinogens. Cis-Diaminedichloroplatinum (15663-27-1).

van As, J.W., van den Berg, H., van Dalen, E.C., 2012. Medical interventions for the prevention of platinum-induced hearing loss in children with cancer. Cochrane Database Syst. Rev. 5 CD009219.

Yorgason, J.G., Luxford, W., Kalinec, F., 2011. In vitro and in vivo models of drug ototoxicity: studying the mechanisms of a clinical problem. Expert Opin. Drug Metab. Toxicol. 7 (12), 1521–1534.

Clean Air Act (CAA), US

RW Kapp, Jr., BioTox, Monroe Township, NJ, USA

Title: CAA
Agency: US Environmental Protection Agency (EPA)
Year Enacted: 1963, amended 1967, Clean Air Act Extension of 1970, amended 1977 and 1990

Background

There were a number of air pollution events that have brought pressure to bear on governments to be proactive in controlling air contaminants. Three events were instrumental in bringing air pollution to national attention in the United States:

1. The St Louis, MO smog incident began on 28 November 1939 with a temperature inversion which trapped coal burning emissions close to the ground and lasted for 9 days. While there were no reports of any health problems, the city council passed a smoke ordinance requiring cleaner coal supplies, more efficient furnaces, and public education campaign to improve air quality in the city.
2. The Donora, PA smog incident began on 27 October 1948 with a temperature inversion that trapped sulfur dioxide, nitrogen dioxide, and fluorine emissions from US Steel's Donora Zinc Works and the American Steel and Wire Plant and lasted until 31 October 1948. This event resulted in 20 human and 800 animal deaths. Some claim that about one-third of the town's 14 000 residents were taken ill by the exposure.
3. The London Great Smog incident began with a period of cold weather combined with an anticyclone and windless conditions causing a temperature inversion that trapped pollutants from burning coal on 5 December 1952 and lasted through 9 December 1952. It is estimated that this incident resulted in over 4500 excess deaths that week and over 13 500 excess deaths by March 1953.

These and many other factors resulted in the first US federal legislation dealing with controlling air pollution at its source was Public Law 84–159, the Air Pollution Control Act of 1955. The legislation granted $5 million annually for 5 years for research by the Public Health Service. While the act did not prevent any air pollution, it did provide research and technical assistance to air pollution control efforts. In 1960, the Act was amended to extend research for four additional years. In 1962, the Act was further amended to add research by the US Surgeon General to determine the health effects of various motor vehicle exhaust substances.

The Clean Air Act (CAA) of 1963 (Public Law 88–206) was passed to improve, strengthen, and accelerate programs for the prevention and abatement of air pollution. This legislation granted $95 million over a 3-year period to state and local governments and air pollution control agencies to conduct research and create control programs. This Act encouraged the development of emissions standards for motor vehicles and from stationary sources which led to research on the removal of sulfur from high sulfur coal and oil fuels. The Act was amended in 1965 to establish standards for automobile emissions. It was further amended in 1966 and 1967 to expand local air pollutions control programs. The 1967 Amendment established national emissions standards for stationary sources and created Air Quality Control Regions as a means of monitoring ambient air. The states were given fixed timetables in which to implement State Implementation Plans to meet emission standards.

Overview of CAA

The CAA is the federal law designed to assure that the air is safe to breathe. While public health is the primary goal, the Act also seeks to prevent environmental damage caused by air pollution. The fundamentals of the CAA were set up in the CAA of 1970 under President Richard Nixon and have been amended several times since then. The basic framework of the Act and the objective of public health have remained intact.

The CAA of 1970 (Public Law 81–604) essentially rewrote the original CAA of 1963, by making it a more effective program to improve the quality of the ambient air. The legislation set ambitious National Ambient Air Quality Standards (NAAQS) to protect the public health with six 'criteria' pollutants, which are listed below:

1. Carbon monoxide
2. Nitrogen dioxide
3. Ozone
4. Sulfur dioxide
5. Lead
6. Particulate matter (PM) with aerodynamic size less than or equal to 10 mm (PM_{10})

The CAA also set New Source Performance Standards that strictly regulated emissions of any new sources of air pollution entering an area. It also established two categories of air-quality standards: Primary Standards set limits to protect public health, and Secondary Standards set limits to protect against public welfare effects, such as damage to farm crops and vegetation. The CAA further required leaded gasoline be phased out by the mid-1980s.

The CAA also established the National Emissions Standards for Hazardous Air Pollutants which are emissions standards for 189 hazardous air pollutants not covered by NAAQS that may cause an increase in fatalities or in serious illness. The standards require a maximum degree of emission reduction as determined by Environmental Protection Agency (EPA) known as the maximum achievable control technology (MACT) for which the EPA must establish emissions standards for sources that emit any listed pollutant. There was considerable debate concerning the costs of emissions control, which came to

 http://dx.doi.org/10.1016/B978-0-12-386454-3.00829-0

a head in 1986 when CAA issued a standard for vinyl chloride. This standard was set aside by the courts; however, the court case (*Natural Resources Defense Council, Inc.* v. *United States Environmental Protection Agency*, 1987) set a precedent by recognizing that the EPA could, in fact, consider costs in deciding if any additional margin of safety (MOS) was necessary. In addition, the Act allowed citizens the right to take legal action against anyone or any organization, including government itself, who was in violation of the emissions standards. Eight years after the technology-based MACT standards are issued for a source category, EPA is required to review those standards to determine whether any residual risk exists for that source category and, if necessary, revise the standards to address such risk.

In 1977, this Act was amended to extend the deadline of meeting the motor vehicle emissions standards. These amendments also made a first attempt to control stratospheric ozone and created the New Source Review, which required older 'grandfathered' facilities to install pollution control technologies as they modernized.

In 1990, the CAA was again amended and rewritten (Public Law 101–549). These amendments extended the prohibition of leaded gasoline to 1995. However, additional changes drastically strengthened the measures for attaining air quality standards provided in the CAA, which include the following:

- Provisions relating to mobile pollution sources
- Expanding the regulation of hazardous air pollutants as set forth in Section 112
- Requiring substantial reductions in power plant emissions for control of acid rain (SO_2 and NO_x abatement). Utilities had the choice of using any of the following ways to meet the standard annual emissions allowance limit:
  - Using cleaner fuel or choosing lower sulfur coal or fuel blending
  - Obtaining additional allowances
  - Installing flue gas desulfurization equipment (scrubbers)
  - Using previously implemented controls
  - Retiring units
  - Boiler repowering
  - Establish operating permits for all major sources of air pollution
  - Establish provisions for stratospheric ozone protection
  - Expand enforcement powers and penalties

The 1990 amendments replaced the health-based standard with a two-tiered system of regulation. Under the newly revised Section 112, EPA must first issue standards that are technology based, designed to require the MACT available. If the MACT values are insufficient to protect human health with an 'ample margin of safety,' EPA must issue residual risk standards as well. These amendments define a sufficient MOS for carcinogens by requiring EPA to establish residual risk standards for any pollutant that poses a lifetime excess cancer risk of greater than 1:1 000 000.

In 1997, the Act was again amended to tighten the permissible ozone levels from 0.12 ppm per 1 h to 0.08 ppm per 8 h. In addition, the amendment revised the 24-h PM up to 10 mm in diameter (PM_{10}) to simplify data handling requirements. Finally, new PM up to 2.5 mm ($PM_{2.5}$) standards with an annual limit of 15 mg m^{-3} was also added to the Act.

Milestones in US Air Regulations

- July 1955 – Air Pollution Control Act.
- December 1963 – CAA of 1963.
- December 1973 – EPA requires reduction of leaded gasoline to 1.1 g per gallon by 1982.
- April 1975 – Federal Government will not award contracts, grants, or loans to organizations that are air polluters.
- September 1978 – EPA announced it final atmospheric air quality standard for airborne lead.
- December 1979 – EPA 'Bubble' policy added to assist industry plants to clean up air pollution. With this policy, an imaginary bubble is drawn around the whole plant and the company can find the most efficient way of controlling the plant's emissions as a whole.
- March 1985 – EPA sets limit of 0.1 g of lead per gallon by January 1986.
- September 1987 – Montréal Protocol signed joining international partners in efforts to protect the ozone layer.
- November 1990 – Acid Rain Controls reducing sulfur dioxide emissions and controls to phase out ozone-depleting substances enacted through the CAA Amendments. Hazard Substance regulated under the revised Section 112.
- November 1993 – EPA schedules end of manufacture of chlorofluorocarbons by 1996.
- 28 July 1995 – EPA announces a rule to reduce pollution at 192 petroleum refineries and any future sites.
- December 1995 – EPA has also issued final rules to control emissions of certain air toxics from solid waste combustion facilities.
- January 1996 – Leaded gasoline is completely phased out.
- August 1998 – EPA launches air pollution information by ZIP code.
- July 1999 – The Regional Haze Rule calls for state and federal agencies to work together to improve visibility in 156 national parks and wilderness areas.
- December 1999 – EPA announces tailpipe emissions standards for cars, sport utility vehicles, minivans, and trucks must be 77–95% cleaner.
- April 2003 – Virginia Electric Power agrees to spend $1200 million to reduce emission in largest CAA settlement to date.
- January 2004 – Clean School Bus Program implemented to reduce diesel particulate exposure.
- May 2004 – The Clean Air Nonroad Diesel Rule implemented to cut emission levels from construction, agricultural, and industrial diesel-powered equipment by 90%.
- June 2006 – National Clean Diesel Campaign – refiners required to produce diesel fuel with 97% less sulfur.
- September 2006 – EPA issues the strongest national air quality standards for particle pollution in our country's history.
- October 2007 – BP pays the largest criminal fine $62 million criminal fine, plus $400 million on safety upgrades to date.

- March 2008 – New tough emissions standards to be implemented by 2015 to cut pollution from locomotive and marine diesel engines by up to 90%.
- October 2008 – Stronger lead standards implemented to 0.15 $\mu g\, m^{-3}$ of air.
- March 2009 – Initiative to monitor levels of toxic air pollutants near schools.
- April 2009 – EPA sets greenhouse gas emissions standards for cars.
- December 2009 – EPA determines that greenhouse gases that lead to climate change can be regulated under the CAA.
- January 2010 – EPA implements stricter smog health standards.
- October 2010 – EPA implements greenhouse gas fuel economy standards for trucks and cars.
- November 2010 – Greenhouse gas reporting implemented with significant carbon dioxide emitters.
- July 2011 – The Cross-State Air Pollution Rule requiring states to significantly improve air quality by reducing power plant smokestack emissions that contribute to ozone and/or fine particle pollution in other states.
- August 2011 – Fuel efficiency and greenhouse gas pollution standards announced for heavy-duty vehicles built in 2014 through 2018.
- December 2011 – EPA proposed changes in the CAA emissions standards for large and small boilers and incinerators that burn solid waste.
- December 2011 – EPA proposes national standards for mercury pollution from power plants to be implemented in 4 years.

See also: Environmental Protection Agency, US; Environmental Toxicology; Pollution, Air in Encyclopedia of Toxicology; Donora: Air Pollution Episode.

Further Reading

EPA, 2012. History of the Clean Air Act. http://epa.gov/oar/caa/caa_history.html.

Jacobson, M.Z., 2002. Atmospheric Pollution: History, Science, and Regulation. Cambridge University Press, Cambridge, UK.

Kenney, R., Gastman, A., 2012. Clean Air Act, United States. The Encyclopedia of Earth. http://www.eoearth.org/article/Clean_Air_Act.

Relevant Website

http://www.epa.gov/; http://www.law.cornell.edu/lii/get_the_law

Clean Water Act (CWA), US

RW Kapp, Jr., BioTox, Monroe Township, NJ, USA

Title: CWA
Agency: US EPA
Years enacted: 1948, amended and reauthorized 1972; major amendments in, 1977 and 1987

Background

Water pollution is not a recent phenomenon. For instance, the Cuyahoga River in Cleveland, Ohio, has presented several instances of fire hazards due to pollution such as debris and oil slicks as early as 1868. While there are other instances of river pollution, the Cuyahoga is the most well known. Federal legislation on water began when Congress enacted the River and Harbor Act of 1886 that was recodified in the Rivers and Harbors Act of 1899. The Federal Water Pollution Control Act is a comprehensive statute aimed at restoring and maintaining the chemical, physical, and biological integrity of the nation's water. It was originally enacted in 1948. Again in 1952, the oil slick and debris polluting the Cuyahoga River caught fire causing over $1 million in damage. The Water Pollution Control Act Amendments of 1956 were subsequently passed strengthening enforcement by no longer requiring the federal government to receive consent from the States. The Water Quality Act of 1965 (Public Law 89–234) provided for the setting of enforceable water quality standards and the basis for interstate water quality standards. The Clean Water Restoration Act of 1966 (Public Law 89–753) imposed fines ($100 per day) on polluters who failed to submit a required report. Then on 29 June 1969, the Cuyahoga River debris caught fire. This event became a significant national news event when *Time Magazine* ran a story describing the river as not only a fire hazard but also "having no visible life, not even low forms such as leeches and sludge worms that usually thrive on wastes" and that "oozes rather than flows" because of the severe pollution.

There is no agreement among historians that the legislation was a direct result of the events on the Cuyahoga River; however, the US Environmental Protection Agency (EPA) website indicates that "By bringing national attention to water pollution issues, the Cuyahoga River fire was one of the events that led to the creation of the federal Environmental Protection Agency (in 1970)." The Water Quality Improvement Act of 1970 (Public Law 91–224) further expanded federal authority to certify water quality. These various amendments created cumbersome legislation that was, at best, difficult to implement. Growing public concern for controlling water pollution in the environment led the enactment of the Federal Water Pollution Control Act Amendments of 1972 (Public Law 92–500). Subsequently, this law was amended in 1977 and became known as the Clean Water Act (CWA).

Overview of CWA

In a step toward resolving numerous administrative and implementation problems with the previous water pollution legislation, the 1972 amendments to the Federal Water Pollution Control Act restructured water pollution control under the authority of the Administrator of the EPA. The objective of the 1972 reauthorization was to restore and maintain the chemical, physical, and biological integrity of the nation's surface waters. This original legislation did not deal directly with ground water or with water quality issues. Initially, there were two critical goals:

1. The elimination of the discharge of all pollutants into the navigable waters by 1985.
2. The creation of an interim level of water quality to provide for the protection of fish, shellfish, and wildlife and recreation by 1 July 1983.

The 1972 legislation also required federal effluent limitations and state water quality standards, required permits for the discharge of pollutants into navigable water, provided enforcement mechanisms, and authorized funding for wastewater treatment works construction grants to states and tribes for their water quality programs. The 1972 legislation basically changed the enforcement from regulating the quality of existing water to regulating the amount of effluents being discharged from particular point sources. (Point source defined as "any discernible, confined, and discrete conveyance from which pollutants are or may be discharged.")

The EPA Administrator originally published guidelines for 63 chemicals and a host of other materials – sewage, garbage, dirt, discarded equipment, even heat – that could not be indiscriminately dumped in the water. The Act was amended in 1977 (Public Law 95–217) to include 126 materials, which EPA had identified as toxic under newly developed health-based 'water quality criteria.' The Act also addressed previously unrecognized but widespread sources of water pollution such as municipal storm water, and new sources, such as land application of manure from Confined Animal Feeding Operations. To meet this challenge, the most recent water act, the 1998 National Pollutant Discharge Elimination System (NPDES), focused not just on waterways but on watersheds. The Act authorized numerous research programs to study the prevention, reduction, and elimination of water pollution. The act authorized the development of plans for the control of pollution within all or any part of the watersheds of the Great Lakes. In 1992, it authorized EPA to conduct a comprehensive survey of data on aquatic sediment quality and report the findings to Congress. The Act prohibited the discharge of pollutants except those in compliance with the effluent limitations with the best practicable control technology.

The Act provided for construction grants and loans to publicly owned treatment works (POTWs) to implement improved water pollution control measures. Another significant feature of the Act was the creation of a national pollutant NPDES. The NPDES basically required POTWs as well as industrial sources to acquire a permit that mandated certain effluent limitations had to be met before any discharges could

 http://dx.doi.org/10.1016/B978-0-12-386454-3.00830-7

occur in navigable waters. Other water pollution issues covered by the Act included the Clean Lakes Program, thermal discharges, nonpoint source pollution, estuaries, marine sanitation devices, oil and hazardous substance liability, and sewage sludge.

The pollutants regulated under the CWA include biochemical oxygen demand, fecal coliform, total suspended solids, oil and grease, and pH ('conventional pollutants'). Also included in the CWA are 'priority pollutants,' that is, toxic pollutants as well as 'nonconventional pollutants' not identified as either conventional or priority.

The critical requirements of the CWA include the following:

1. Direct discharges from 'point source' limitations. Point sources include sewers, pipes, drainage ditches, etc. Any facility that intends to discharge into a lake or stream or river must obtain a permit prior to initiating the discharge. The discharge must meet conditions and effluent limitations set by the state and/or EPA.
2. Pretreatment requirements for indirect discharges into POTWs must meet pretreatment requirements as set forth in 40 CFR403.6 National Pretreatment Standards: Categorical Standards. Effluent guidelines for direct discharges and pretreatment standards for specific chemical industry manufacturers and users are listed in the Code of Federal Regulations as follows:
   40 CFR 414 Organic Chemicals, Plastics, and Synthetic Fibers,
   40 CFR 415 Inorganic Chemicals Manufacturing,
   40 CFR 417 Soap and Detergent Manufacturing,
   40 CFR 418 Fertilizer Manufacturing,
   40 CFR 422 Phosphate Manufacturing,
   40 CFR 428 Rubber Manufacturing,
   40 CFR 446 Paint Formulation,
   40 CFR 447 Ink Formulation,
   40 CFR 454 Gum and Wood Chemicals Manufacturing,
   40 CFR 455 Pesticide Chemicals,
   40 CFR 457 Explosives Manufacturing,
   40 CFR 458 Carbon Black Manufacturing.

1. Storm water runoffs were addressed in the 1987 CWA Amendments. These regulations required that manufacturers with any sort of storm sewer connected with any aspect of the chemical process apply for a permit under these conditions: (1) a discharge is associated with industrial activity, (2) a discharge from a large or medium municipal storm sewer system, or (3) a discharge, which has been determined to contribute to a violation of any, water standard or is a significant contributor of pollutants to waters of the nation. These specific regulations are located in 40 CFR 122.26.
2. Oil and hazardous substance spill prevention and responses are generally incorporated into the Comprehensive Environmental Response, Compensation, and Liability Act (CERCLA) and the Emergency Planning and Community Right-to-Know Act regulations. However, the Spill Prevention, Control, and Countermeasure plan applies to any facility that has oil or hazardous materials that has the potential to reach the nation's waters. These regulations are located in 40 CFR 112.
3. Wetlands modifications and/or the placement of dredge and fill materials into surface waters is covered by a permit program administered by the US Army Corps of Engineers. The CWA defines surface waters to include wetlands; hence, activities that involve any modification of wetlands are covered by the US Army Corps of Engineers. The regulations governing this permit program are located in 40CFR 404.

Milestones in US Water Regulations at the EPA

- December 1970 – EPA is officially established to protect human health by safeguarding the nation's air, water, and land.
- April 1972 – Great Lakes Water Quality Agreement in which the United States and Canada agree to clean up the Great Lakes.
- October 1972 – Federal Water Pollution Control Amendments enacted expanding the Federal Water Pollution Control Amendments of 1948.
- October 1972 – CWA is enacted to eliminate additional water pollution by 1985 and ensure surface waters would meet standards by 1983.
- October 1972 – Ocean Dumping Act enacted to reduce ocean pollution.
- March 1973 – First wastewater permits are issued permitting licensees authority to discharge treated wastewater into navigable waters in Indiana.
- December 1974 – Safe Drinking Water Act was enacted authorizing the EPA to regulate the quality of public drinking water.
- April 1975 – Federal government legislation to discontinue awarding contracts, grants, or loans to organizations that are water polluters.
- October 1976 – Resource Conservation and Recovery Act enacted primarily to permit control of solid and hazardous waste and also established monitoring groundwater regulations.
- June 1977 – Safer Drinking Water Act was enacted which put into place drinking water standards.
- July 1979 – EPA Ocean Survey Vessel named The Antelope is launched to study waste disposal sites.
- December 1980 – CERCLA or the 'Superfund' was enacted which was extensive regulatory legislation that covered numerous environmental hazards and also permitted the EPA to regulate groundwater.
- December 1983 – Chesapeake Bay Pollution Cleanup initiated joint clean up of the Chesapeake Bay between federal, state, and local authorities.
- June 1986 – Safe Drinking Water Act Amendments enacted expanding EPA authority to regulate over 100 contaminants by 1991.
- October 1986 – EPA announces the creation of the Office of Wetlands Protection to protect estuaries which includes swamps, marshes, bogs, and similar areas.
- December 1987 – Water Quality Act of 1987 was passed amending the 1972 Act encouraging new water treatment methods for toxic pollutant controls.

- November 1988 – Sewage Ocean-Dumping Ban is enacted banning ocean dumping of sewage sludge and industrial waste.
- June 1992 – New York City ceases dumping sewage into the ocean under the Ocean Dumping Ban Act of 1988.
- August 1996 – Amendments to the Safe Drinking Water Act implemented to improve protections for safe drinking water.
- April 1997 – Great Lakes Cleanup Plan enacted in conjunction with Canada to remove toxic substances from the Great Lakes by 2006.
- August 1998 – EPA launches water pollution information by ZIP code.
- February 2002 – EPA officially moves to cleanup polychlorinated biphenyl contamination in the Hudson River.
- July 2006 – EPA creates the WaterSense program which seeks to protect the nation's water supply through less use.
- October 2006 – EPA issues Ground Water Rule to reduce risk of contaminations in public water systems.
- December 2008 – Tennessee Value Authority Kingston Fossil Plant releases 1100 million gallons of coal fly ash on land and into the waterways resulting in an EPA review of coal ash sites nationally.
- May 2009 – Chesapeake Bay Executive Order signed by President Obama calling on a renewed effort by the federal government to restore and protect the Chesapeake and its watershed.
- October 2010 – Gulf Coast Ecosystem Restoration Task Force Executive Order signed by President Obama to implement restoration programs and projects in the gulf coast region.
- December 2010 – EPA establishes the Chesapeake Bay Total Maximum Daily Load identifying necessary reductions of nitrogen, phosphorus, and sediment from local jurisdictions to be in place by 2025.

See also: CERCLA; Revised as the Superfund Amendments Reauthorization Act (SARA); Drinking-Water Criteria (Safety, Quality, and Perception); Effluent Biomonitoring; Environmental Toxicology; National Environmental Policy Act, USA; Pollution Prevention Act, United States; Pollution, Water; Resource Conservation and Recovery Act (USA); Safe Drinking Water Act; Toxicity Testing, Aquatic.

Further Reading

Adler, R.W., Landman, J.C., Cameron, D.M., 1993. The Clean Water Act 20 Years Later. Island Press, Washington, DC.

Adler, J.H., Connolly, K.D., Gardner, R.C., Johnson, S.M., Latham, M., 2007. The Supreme Court and the Clean Water Act: Five Essays. Vermont Law School, South Royalton, VT. http://www.vermontlaw.edu.

USEPA, 2004. Office of Inspector General. Evaluation Report: Effectiveness of Effluent Guidelines Program for Reducing Pollutant Discharges Uncertain Report No. 2004-P-00025, 24 August 2004.

Relevant Website

http://www.epa.gov/; http://www.law.cornell.edu/lii/get_the_law

Clinical Chemistry

SC Gad, Gad Consulting Services, Cary, NC, USA

The function of clinical chemistry in toxicology (as well as in human and veterinary medicine) is to provide, via laboratory analysis, evaluations of the qualitative and quantitative characteristics of specific endogenous chemical components present in samples of blood, urine, feces, spinal fluid, and tissues. The purpose is to help identify abnormal or pathological changes in organ system functions. The most common specimens used in clinical chemistry are blood and urine, and many different tests exist to test for almost any type of chemical component in blood or urine, for example, blood glucose, electrolytes, enzymes, hormones, lipids (fats), other metabolic substances, and proteins. The tests used were all initially applied to human clinical medicine, and may not possess the same utility when performed as part of nonclinical toxicity studies in a wide variety of other species.

Clinical chemistry evaluations are commonly recommended in animal toxicology studies. Regulatory agencies such as the US Food and Drug Administration and the US Environmental Protection Agency have set guidelines for clinical pathology testing in nonclinical toxicity and safety studies. Measurement of chemical components of biological fluids allows the toxicologist to do serial sampling, detect metabolic injury or organ-specific effects, and perhaps gain additional information helpful in establishing the no-effect level and determining the mechanism of toxicity. When using serum enzymes as markers of tissue or organ damage, the enzyme of interest must reasonably reflect pathological change in a specific tissue, organ, or group of organs and must be easily measured.

The tests that are traditionally and routinely performed provide information concerning hepatocellular and biliary integrity and function, renal function, carbohydrate, protein, and lipid metabolism, and mineral and electrolyte balance. Modern analytical techniques require only small sample volumes to make accurate determinations, allowing

Table 1 Association of changes in biochemical parameters with actions at particular target organs

Parameters	*Blood*	*Heart*	*Lung*	*Kidney*	*Liver*	*Bone*	*Intestine*	*Pancreas*	*Notes*
Albumin				↓	↓				Produced by the liver. Very significant reductions indicate extensive liver damage
ALP					↑	↑	↑		Elevations associated with wholestasis. Bone alkaline phosphatase tends to be higher in young animals
Bilirubin (total)	↑				↑				Usually elevated due to cholestasis, either due to obstruction or hepatopathy
BUN				↑	↓				Estimates blood-filtering capacity of the kidneys. Does not become significantly elevated until the kidney function is reduced by 60–75%
Calcium				↑					Can be life threatening and result in acute death
Cholinesterase				↑	↓				Found in plasma, brain, and RBC
CPK		↑							Most often elevated due to skeletal muscle damage but can also be produced by cardiac muscle damage. Can be more sensitive than histopathology
Creatinine				↑					Also estimates blood-filtering capacity of kidney as BUN does
Glucose								↑	Alterations other than those associated with stress are uncommon and reflect an effect on the pancreatic islets or anorexia
GGT					↑				Elevated in cholestasis. This is a microsomal enzyme and levels often increase in response to microsomal enzyme induction
HBDH		↑			↑				
LDH		↑	↑	↑	↑				Increase usually due to skeletal muscle, cardiac muscle, or liver damage. Not very specific
Protein (total)				↓	↓				Absolute alterations are usually associated with decreased production (liver) or increased loss (kidney). Can see increase in case of muscle 'wasting' (catabolism)
AST				↑	↑			↑	Present in skeletal muscle and heart and most commonly associated with damage to these
ALT					↑				Elevations usually associated with hepatic damage or disease
SDH					↑↓				Liver enzyme that can be quite sensitive but is fairly unstable. Samples should be processed as soon as possible

↑, increase in chemistry values; ↓, decrease in chemistry values.

ALP, alkaline phosphatase; BUN, blood urea nitrogen; CPK, creatinine phosphokinase; GGT, gamma glutaryl transferase; HBDH, hydroxybutyric dehydrogenase; LDH, lactic dehydrogenase; RBC, red blood cells; SDH, sorbitol dehydrogenase; AST, aspartate amino transferase (also known as SGOT, serum glutamic oxaloacetic transaminase); and ALT, alanine amino transferase (also known as SGPT, serum glutamic pyruvic transaminase).

 http://dx.doi.org/10.1016/B978-0-12-386454-3.00831-9

in-life evaluations of effects in rats and larger species at multiple times during the course of a study without compromising animal health. More recently, Food and Drug Administration and European Medicines Agency have accepted a new specific biomarker set for kidney toxicity in nonclinical studies. This panel includes Kim-1, albumin, total protein, β2 microglobulin, crystatin C, clusterin, and trefoil factor-3.

Table 1 summarizes the routinely measured end points and the probable causes behind findings.

See also: Toxicity, Subchronic and Chronic.

Further Reading

Burtis, C.A., Ashwood, E.R., Bruns, D.E. (Eds.), 2006. Tietz Textbook of Clinical Chemistry, fourth ed. Saunders, Philadelphia, PA.

Evans, G.O., 2009. Animal Clinical Chemistry, second ed. CRC Press, Boca Raton, FL.

Kurtz, D.M., Prescott, J.S., Travlos, G.S., 2011. Loeb and Quimby's Clinical Chemistry of Laboratory Animals, third ed. CRC Press, Boca Raton, FL.

Relevant Websites

http://www.aacc.org – American Association for Clinical Chemistry (AACC) website. Also considering accessing the AACC Listservs http://www.clinchem.org – Clinical Chemistry: International and Journal of Molecular Diagonistics and Laboratory Medicine.

http://www.e-c4.org – European Communities Confederation of Clinical Chemistry and Laboratory Medicine.

Clofibrate

S Betharia, Manchester University College of Pharmacy, Fort Wayne, IN, USA

This article is a revision of the previous edition article by Sanjay Chanda and Harihara M. Mehendale, volume 1, pp 622–623, © 2005, Elsevier Inc.

- Name: Clofibrate
- Chemical Abstracts Service Registry Number: 637-07-0
- Synonyms: 2-(*p*-Chlorophenoxy)-2-methylpropionic acid ethyl ester, α-*p*-Chlorophenoxyisobutyryl ethyl ester, Amotril, Angiokapsul, Anparton, Antilipid, Ateculon, Ateriosan, Atheropront, Atromid, Atromidin, Hyclorate, Lipavin, Liponorm, Liporil, Lipofaction, Neo-atromid, Normet, Regelan, Serotinex
- Molecular Formula: $C_{12}H_{15}O_3Cl$
- Molecular Weight: 242.7 g mol^{-1}
- Chemical Structure:

Cl O H_3C O CH_3 O CH_3

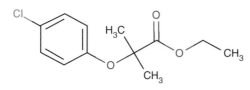

Background

Researchers in France observed in 1953 that structures derived from dehydrocholic acid, phenylethyl acetic acid, and certain other disubstituted acetic acids exhibited hypocholesterolemic properties in rats and humans. Several years later, Thorp and Waring discovered clofibrate as an effective compound for lowering lipids in animal models, with minimal toxicity. Its mode of action was initially attributed to seasonal variations in adrenal and thyroid function, and the administration of androsterone was found to potentiate the hypocholesterolemic effect of this compound. Subsequently, several clinical trials were performed which showed that clofibrate decreases lipid levels in hypercholesterolemic patients, mainly as the result of a reduction in the very-low-density lipoprotein (VLDL), and less in the low-density lipoprotein (LDL) fraction, and that the coadministration of androsterone was not necessary for its hypolipidemic effect. Despite reported hepatomegaly in rats following long-term treatment with clofibrate, this drug was approved in the United States in 1967 for the treatment of hyperlipidemias.

Clofibrate can be chemically synthesized by the condensation of phenol with ethyl 2-chloro-2-methylpropionate in the presence of a dehydrochlorinating agent, followed by chlorination and purification. It can also be synthesized by the condensation of *p*-chlorophenol with acetone and chloroform followed by esterifying the resultant acid to give clofibrate.

Uses

Clofibrate is a lipid-lowering agent (antilipidemic) used for controlling high cholesterol (anticholesteremic) and triacylglyceride levels in the blood. It increases lipoprotein lipase activity to promote the conversion of VLDL to LDL, thereby reducing VLDL levels. It is indicated only in subjects with increased concentrations of VLDL and intermediate-density lipoproteins (IDL) who have failed to respond adequately to gemfibrozil or nicotinic acid. Clofibrate is of limited utility for patients with either familial hypercholesterolemia or polygenic hypercholesterolemia, as comparatively more effective drugs are available for lowering the concentration of LDL in these patients.

Clofibrate has no effect on hyperchylomicronemia, nor does it affect concentrations of high-density lipoproteins (HDL). Thus, clofibrate appears to have specific efficacy only in patients with familial type-III hyperlipoproteinemia. There is no substantial evidence proving efficacy of clofibrate in preventing deaths from coronary artery disease. Clofibrate has been used to prevent or control polydipsia, polyuria, and dehydration in a limited number of patients with mild to moderate neurohypophyseal diabetes insipidus. A 5-year multicenter study reported failure of clofibrate in reducing or preventing mortality in cardiovascular disorders, which has provided a setback for the prophylactic use of this drug.

Environmental Fate and Behavior

Clofibrate is a clear, colorless liquid with a density of 1.14 g ml^{-1} (at 25 °C). The boiling point of clofibrate is 148–150 °C at 25 mm Hg. This drug is a stable, colorless to pale-yellow liquid with a faint odor and characteristic taste. Its melting point is below 25 °C, it is soluble in common solvents but not in water, and its solubility or log *P* (octanol/water) is 3.620.

Exposure and Exposure Monitoring

Exposure to clofibrate is primarily intentional and for medical reasons; however, accidental overdose or ingestion can occur. Response to clofibrate can be variable, and therefore serum cholesterol and triglyceride concentration should be determined prior to and regularly during clofibrate therapy. It is recommended that liver function tests, blood cell counts, and the LDL, VLDL, and HDL fractions should also be determined and the LDL fraction rechecked during the first few months of clofibrate therapy.

Toxicokinetics

Clofibrate is rapidly and completely absorbed from intestine after oral administration and is hydrolyzed to clofibric acid during absorption and passage through the liver. The peak plasma concentration of 49–53 μg ml^{-1} occurs within 4–6 h after oral administration of a single 500 mg dose in a healthy individual. Concomitant administration of cholestyramine

 http://dx.doi.org/10.1016/B978-0-12-386454-3.00289-X

with clofibrate has been shown to decrease the rate of absorption of clofibrate. Clofibrate can transfer across the placenta and into the milk, as reported in a study with newborn rats whose mothers were fed clofibrate. A major fraction of clofibric acid is bound to plasma albumin. Plasma concentration of unbound clofibric acid is increased in patients with renal failure and low serum albumin concentrations. Elimination of this metabolite proceeds in two kinetic phases, with a slower exponential phase having a mean half-life of nearly 15 h. Sixty percent of it is excreted as glucuronide conjugate in the urine. Some is secreted into the bile and is reabsorbed. The plasma elimination half-life is between 12 and 25 h in healthy individuals, and between 29 and 88 h in patients with renal failure.

Clofibrate is known to interact with various other nutrients in the body. It has been found to impair absorption of vitamin B_{12}, vitamin E, iron, carotene, glucose, and medium-chain triglycerides. Other drug interactions also reported include those with statins, niacin, insulin, blood thinners, oral antidiabetic medications, and probenecid. While statins and fibrates have synergistic effects on plasma lipid levels, coadministration can lead to side effects such as rhabdomyolysis and acute renal necrosis.

Mechanism of Action

Clofibrate characteristically reduces plasma triglycerides by lowering the concentration of VLDL within 2–5 days after initiation of therapy. In a majority of patients, total cholesterol and LDL concentrations in plasma fall slightly. However, some patients who exhibit a large fall in VLDL may show a paradoxical rise in LDL, resulting in minimal net effect on total cholesterol levels.

The drug has several proposed antilipidemic actions, including increased triglyceride and VLDL clearance, mobilization of cholesterol from tissues, increased fecal excretion of neutral sterols, decreased hepatic lipoprotein synthesis and/or secretion, decreased free fatty acid release, and decreased triglyceride synthesis. The precise mechanisms by which clofibrate lowers serum concentrations of triglycerides and cholesterol are not known.

Acute and Short-Term Toxicity

Rats given food containing 1% clofibrate or subcutaneous injections of 0.3–0.9 g kg^{-1} daily for 2 days showed spontaneous electromyographic responses in hind limbs. In newborn rats, clofibrate has been shown to induce relative enlargement of the liver in proportion to the body as well as an abnormal fetal thrombosis syndrome. The latter consisted of an extension of the normal thrombosis in the umbilical arteries, which caused necrosis of the tail or parts of the hind limbs.

The oral LD_{50} for clofibrate has been established as 940 mg kg^{-1} (rat), 1220 mg kg^{-1} (mouse), and 2400 mg kg^{-1} (hamster). The intraperitoneal LD_{50} values established are 910 mg kg^{-1} (rat), 540 mg kg^{-1} (mouse), and 1260 mg kg^{-1} (hamster). For mammals, the oral LD_{50} value has been set at 3000 mg kg^{-1}.

In humans, initiation of clofibrate therapy may result in side effects such as stomach upset, nausea, loose stools, bloating, gas, dizziness, drowsiness, or headache. Mouth sores, dry or itchy skin, brittle hair, decreased sexual function, or muscle aches have also been reported. A characteristic flu-like syndrome, associated with severe muscle cramps and tenderness, stiffness, and weakness, is now associated with this drug, and recurs whenever the drug is taken. Accident application to the eye can lead to significant damage. Contact with abraded skin should be avoided, as skin contact can produce a reaction known as nonallergic contact dermatitis. Patients on therapy are advised to consult their doctor if they suffer from chest pain, an irregular heartbeat, severe stomach pains, vomiting, skin rash, breathing trouble, decreased urine output, blood in the urine, swelling of the feet or ankles, fever, chills, weight gain, or muscle aches/pain/weakness. It has thus been recommended that clofibrate be used only in patients with significant hyperlipidemia and high risk of arterial disease, and only in treatment of primary hyperlipidemias when other dietary means are ineffective. Clofibrate therapy is contraindicated in patients with peptic ulcers, hepatic or renal dysfunction, primary biliary cirrhosis, or known hypersensitivity to the drug. Administration of clofibrate also increases the lithogenicity of bile and is associated with a high incidence of cholelithiasis and cholecystitis.

Chronic Toxicity

Clofibrate causes hepatic tumors in rodents. Male Fischer rats fed clofibrate at a dietary concentration of about 250 mg kg^{-1} body weight per day for up to 28 months showed development of one or more hepatocellular carcinomas in a significant number of animals. In addition, pancreatic exocrine acinar carcinomas, dermatofibrosarcoma, and leiomyoma of the intestine were also reported in a small percentage of rats, while no such tumors were observed in controls.

In humans, long-term use of this medication has been found to increase the risk of developing gallstones twofold. The World Health Organization cooperative trial on primary prevention of ischemic heart disease using clofibrate to lower serum cholesterol reported an excess mortality in the clofibrate-treated group despite successful cholesterol lowering. A prolonged use of this drug can result in persistent fever, which after being resolved with drug discontinuation, can develop again upon rechallenge. Because of the possibility of undesirable side effects, clofibrate should be used only in certain patients after other treatments have failed to lower the levels of cholesterol.

Reproductive Toxicity

Reproduction studies in both dogs and monkeys using clofibrate dosages approximately 4–6 times the usual human dosage have demonstrated arrest of spermatogenesis. Adverse genitourinary effects of clofibrate include decreased libido in men and impotence. It is stated by the manufacturer of this drug that clofibrate must not be used during pregnancy, and that women of child-bearing age must use reliable birth control methods while using this medication. Further, if a pregnancy is planned, clofibrate should be stopped several months before becoming pregnant. Clofibrate can build up dangerously in unborn babies, who do not yet have the ability to successfully metabolize and excrete this drug. This medication passes into breast milk and must not be used while breast-feeding.

Developmental Toxicity

With doses of 200 mg kg^{-1} body weight per day given to both male and female rats, both before and during gestation, a significant decrease in litter size has been reported. With doses of 500 mg kg^{-1} body weight, the number of pregnancies was reported to be decreased from 7/8 to 0/8.

Genotoxicity

Clofibrate was not mutagenic to *Salmonella typhimurium* strains, with or without metabolic activation by rat liver microsomes. Although clofibrate suppressed the incorporation of ^{3}H-thymidine into replicating DNA in primary cultures of stimulated mouse splenic lymphocytes, the effect was reversible upon removal of the drug. This is in contrast to the action of several DNA-binding carcinogens, and therefore it was concluded that clofibrate does not cause DNA damage.

Carcinogenicity

In a large, randomized clinical trial conducted to determine the potential of clofibrate to lower the incidence of ischemic heart disease in men, the incidence of nonfatal myocardial infarction was reduced in clofibrate-treated group. However, there were significantly more deaths in this group, many of which were due to malignant neoplasms. Presently, there is inadequate evidence in humans and limited evidence in animals for the carcinogenicity of clofibrate. Therefore, clofibrate is not classifiable as a carcinogen in humans.

Clinical Management

Exposure should be terminated as soon as possible. If toxic amount in overdose is unknown, then gastric decontamination is required, but should be considered only if the amount ingested is several times the daily therapeutic dose. Activated charcoal as a slurry (30 g charcoal in 240 ml water) should be given at a dose of 1 g kg^{-1} (infants less than 1 year), 25–50 g (children 1–12 years), and 25–100 g (adults/adolescents).

Exposure Standards and Guidelines

Manufacturers, packers, and distributors of drug and drug products for human use are responsible for complying with the labeling, certification, and usage requirements as prescribed by the Federal Food, Drug, and Cosmetic Act.

See also: Carcinogenesis; Gastrointestinal System; Lipid Metabolism Modifying (Statins, Cholesterol); Toxicity Testing, Dermal.

Further Reading

Clofibrate. IARC Monographs on the Evaluation of Carcinogenic Risks to Humans, vol. 66, 391–426.

Cohen, A.J., Grasso, P., 1981. Review of the hepatic response to hypolipidemic drugs in rodents and assessment of its toxicological significance to man. Food. Cosmet. Toxicol. 19, 585–605.

Oliver, M.F. Retrospective commentary: the clofibrate saga. Br. J. Clin. Pharmacol., in press.

Penna, F., Bonelli, G., Baccino, F.M., Costelli, P., 2010. Cytotoxic properties of clofibrate and other peroxisome proliferators: relevance to cancer progression. Curr. Med. Chem. 17 (4), 309–320.

Rao, M.S., Reddy, J.K., 1996. Hepatocarcinogenesis of peroxisome proliferators. Ann. N. Y. Acad. Sci. 804, 573–587.

Strauss, V., Mellert, W., Wiemer, J., et al., 2012. Increased toxicity when fibrates and statins are administered in combination – a metabolic approach with rats. Toxicol. Lett. 211, 187–200.

Takahashi, K., Kamijo, Y., Hora, K., Hashimoto, K., Higuchi, M., Nakajima, T., Ehara, T., Shigematsu, H., Gonzalez, F.J., Aoyama, T., 2010. Pretreatment by low-dose fibrates protects against acute free fatty acid-induced renal tubule toxicity by counteracting PPARα deterioration. Toxicol. Appl. Pharmacol. 252 (3), 237–249.

Yamana, D., Shimizu, T., Fan, Y., Miura, T., Nanashima, N., Yamada, T., Hakamada, K., Tsuchida, S., 2011. Decrease of hepatic stellate cells in rats with enhanced sensitivity to clofibrate-induced hepatocarcinogenesis. Cancer Sci. 102 (4), 735–741.

Clostridium perfringens

BA McClane, University of Pittsburgh School of Medicine, Pittsburgh, PA, USA

This article is a revision of the previous edition article by Lee R. Shugart, volume 1, p 625, © 2005, Elsevier Inc.

Description

Clostridium perfringens is a gram-positive, spore-forming rod. This bacterium requires anaerobic conditions for growth, but is more tolerant of air (aerotolerant) than most other anaerobes. *C. perfringens* is widely distributed throughout the environment and frequently occurs in low numbers in the intestines of humans and domestic animals. Vegetative cells and, particularly, spores of the organism persist in soil, sediments, and areas subject to human or animal fecal pollution. Any raw food, but particularly meats, poultry, and seafood, may contain vegetative cells or spores of this bacterium.

Mechanism of Toxicity

The pathogenesis of all clostridial diseases is attributable to potent exotoxins released by the organism. *C. perfringens* exemplifies this pathogenic strategy, being capable of producing over 17 different toxins. These toxins include epsilon toxin, which is a Centers of Disease Control (CDC) class B select toxin and the third most potent clostridial toxin, ranking behind only tetanus toxin and the botulinum toxins.

When *C. perfringens* toxins contact host cells, they usually bind and then act in various ways. Alpha toxin has both phospholipase C and sphingomyelinase activities, which can damage the plasma membrane. In addition, hydrolysis of phosphatidylcholine by alpha toxin produces diacyl glycerol, a second messenger that activates host cell signaling pathways. Iota toxin is internalized into host cells, where the A component of this toxin then produces ADP-ribosylates actin, causing cytoskeletal changes. Several other important *C. perfringens* toxins (perfringolysin O, enterotoxin (CPE), epsilon toxin, and beta toxin) bind to cells by receptors and then oligomerize into toxin complexes. These toxin complexes then insert into the membranes to form pores that lead to cell death.

Patterns of toxin production vary considerably amongst different *C. perfringens* strains. In large part, these strain-to-strain differences in toxin production reflect the presence of many toxin genes on plasmids, whose presence varies between individual strains. For classification purposes, *C. perfringens* strains are commonly divided into five types (A–E) based on their production of four typing toxins (alpha, beta, epsilon, and iota). All strains produce alpha toxin, but type C strains also produce beta toxin, type D strains also produce epsilon toxin, type E strains also produce iota toxin, and type B strains also produce both epsilon and beta toxins. In addition to producing one or more typing toxins, strains may express additional toxins (e.g., about 5% of strains produce *C. perfringens* enterotoxin (CPE)).

Nature of Disease

The diversity in toxin production amongst *C. perfringens* strains allows this bacterium to cause a broad spectrum of diseases in both humans and livestock. For example, *C. perfringens* is considered the most important clostridial species causing histotoxic tissue infections in humans. Among those histotoxic infections, *C. perfringens* is the most common cause of traumatic clostridial myonecrosis (death of muscle tissue), also known as gas gangrene. In clostridial myonecrosis, *C. perfringens* grows in muscles using fermentation, which results in the presence of gas in muscle tissue and explains why the disease is often referred to as gas gangrene. During this *in vivo* growth, the bacterium also produces toxins, particularly alpha toxin, that produce necrotic tissue, which, due to its low oxidation–reduction potential, allows progressive spread of the infection by this anaerobic bacterium. In addition, the toxins can enter the circulation and cause effects on distant organs. Clostridial myonecrosis is typically rapidly fatal without prompt initiation of therapy, which is described later.

Besides causing histotoxic infections, *C. perfringens* is also responsible for numerous infections that originate in the gastrointestinal tract of humans or livestock. The most common of these infections for humans is *C. perfringens* type A food poisoning. This illness currently ranks as the second most common bacterial food-borne infection in the United States, where nearly a million cases occur annually. In most instances, poor temperature control during cooking or holding foods is the cause of this food poisoning, especially when large quantities of food such as meats, meat products, gravy, and poultry are prepared several hours before serving. The *C. perfringens* strains causing food poisoning are typically type A strains that produce *C. perfringens* enterotoxin (CPE, discussion below). In addition, spores (and to a lesser extent, vegetative cells) of these food poisoning strains are often highly resistant to food stresses such as heating, storage at low temperature (refrigerators or freezers), and preservatives such as nitrites. This resistance phenotype likely facilitates bacterial survival in foods and is attributable, in large part, to the ability of these food poisoning strains to produce spores containing a variant of a small acid-soluble protein named SASP-4. This variant SASP-4 protein binds tightly to spore DNA, thus offering exceptional protection from the food stresses described above.

After the highly resistant *C. perfringens* spores contaminate foods, they can later germinate back to actively growing vegetative cells when stresses such as high temperature are removed. Those *C. perfringens* vegetative cells then rapidly multiply in foods due to the short doubling time of this bacterium, which can be as little as 10 min at 43 °C. After ingestion of a contaminated food containing large numbers of vegetative cells, the organism starts to sporulate in the small intestinal lumen. It is during this *in vivo* sporulation that CPE is produced, so this food poisoning is typically an infection rather than an intoxication.

CPE accumulates in the cytoplasm of the sporulating cell until that cell lyses at the completion of sporulation to release the mature endospore. This lysis also releases CPE into the small intestine, where the toxin binds to receptors present on enterocytes. These receptors include certain members of the

 http://dx.doi.org/10.1016/B978-0-12-386454-3.00081-6

claudin family of mammalian tight junction proteins. Once bound to these claudin receptors, the enterotoxin oligomerizes into a hexamer, which then inserts into host cell plasma membranes. As briefly mentioned earlier, insertion of this CPE hexamer results in pore formation, which causes a calcium influx into enterocytes that activates calpain and results in cell death from either apoptosis (caused by low CPE doses) or oncosis (caused by high CPE doses). Death of enterocytes produces tissue damage (including epithelial desquamation, epithelial necrosis, and villus blunting/shortening) in the small intestine. This histologic damage apparently induces fluid secretion that manifests clinically as diarrhea.

C. perfringens type A food poisoning is characterized by intense abdominal cramps, as well as diarrhea, that begin 8–22 h after consumption of tainted food. The illness is usually over within 24 h; however, it can be fatal in the elderly or in patients receiving medication that produces significant constipation. Due to food preparation issues (i.e., holding large volumes of prepared foods for long periods before serving), this food poisoning often occurs in institutional settings.

CPE-producing type A strains of *C. perfringens* also cause 3–15% of all cases of human non-food-borne gastrointestinal diseases, which include sporadic diarrhea and antibiotic-associated diarrhea. Interestingly, the symptoms of these non-food-borne diarrheic illnesses can persist for much longer (up to several weeks) than those of the food poisoning. Also, relative to food poisoning strains, spores of the *C. perfringens* type A strains causing sporadic or antibiotic diarrhea are much less resistant to heat and other stresses. In addition, they carry their enterotoxin gene on a plasmid, in contrast to the chromosomal location of the enterotoxin gene in ~75% of food poisoning strains.

Non-type A *C. perfringens* strains are also responsible for human and veterinary diseases that originate in the intestines. For example, type C isolates cause enteritis necroticans in humans, which occurs sporadically in malnourished people throughout the developing world and, occasionally, in diabetics in developed countries. However, enteritis necroticans is historically most closely associated with the Papua New Guinea highlands, where it is known as pigbel. During the 1970s, pigbel was the leading cause of death in young children in the Papua New Guinea highlands.

Enteritis necroticans develops in people with low intestinal trypsin activity, which can result from a diet rich in trypsin inhibitor and/or from low intestinal trypsin levels due to a protein-poor diet or disease. The importance of low trypsin levels for developing enteritis necroticans reflects the importance of trypsin as a host defense against toxins (particularly beta toxin) produced in the intestines by type C isolates. In individuals with low intestinal trypsin activity, beta toxin persists to cause hemorrhagic necrotizing enteritis. This pore-forming toxin can also be absorbed into the circulation to damage other internal organs, resulting in a condition referred to as enterotoxemia. Besides human disease, type C isolates also cause similar, often fatal, necrotizing enteritis and enterotoxemia in several livestock species. Young animals are particularly affected, probably due to the anti-trypsin activity present in colostrum.

Type B and D strains of *C. perfringens* also rank as important veterinary pathogens, causing potentially fatal enteritis or enterotoxemias in numerous livestock species. For type D strains, the pore-forming epsilon toxin is considered of particular pathogenic importance, while it appears likely that both epsilon toxin and beta toxin contribute to the virulence of type B strains. Type E strains producing iota toxin occasionally cause enteritis in calves and perhaps other livestock.

Control

In most instances, poor temperature control of prepared food is the cause of acute *C. perfringens* type A food poisoning. Therefore, to reduce the occurrence of this food poisoning, it is important to keep hot foods above 60 °C and cold foods at or below 5 °C before serving. Since this food poisoning is usually a mild, self-limiting disease, symptomatic and supportive therapy, including fluid and electrolyte replacement, is normally adequate intervention. The disease symptoms are produced by the enterotoxin, so antibiotics play no role in its management.

For preventing enteritis and enterotoxemias caused by *C. perfringens* type B–D isolates, crude vaccines have been developed using inactivated culture supernatants. A type C vaccine was introduced in 1980 and proved very efficacious in reducing the frequency of pigbel amongst young children in Papua New Guinea. Once pigbel occurs, the major therapeutic intervention requires surgical removal of affected bowel tissue; however, this procedure must be performed early in the disease before extensive intestinal necrosis or enterotoxemia develops. Similarly, crude vaccines against type B, C, and D strains are often used to prevent enteritis and enterotoxemia in livestock.

Currently, vaccines are not used to prevent or treat *C. perfringens* histotoxic infections, including gas gangrene. Instead the major therapeutic approach involves surgical debridement of infected tissues, along with antibiotic therapy. Surgical debridement to treat clostridial myonecrosis must be initiated early during infection, before the infection has spread too far and too many toxins have entered the circulation. Hyperbaric oxygen conditions are sometimes also used as supportive therapy for gas gangrene, with the aim of increasing the oxidation–reduction potential of tissue in the patient and thus inhibiting bacterial growth.

See also: Gastrointestinal System.

Further Reading

McClane, B.A., 2007. *Clostridium perfringens.* In: Doyle, M.P., Beuchat, L.R. (Eds.), Food Microbiology: Fundamentals and Frontiers, third ed. ASM Press, Washington, DC, pp. 423–444.

Stevens, D.L., Rood, J.I., 2006. Histotoxic clostridia. In: Fischetti, V.A., Novick, R.P., Ferretti, J.J., Portnoy, D.A., Rood, J.I. (Eds.), Gram-positive Pathogens, second ed. ASM Press, Washington, DC, pp. 715–725,.

McClane, B.A., Uzal, F.A., Miyakawa, M.F., Lyerly, D., Wilkins, T., 2006. The enterotoxic clostridia. In: Dworkin, M., Falkow, S., Rosenburg, E., Schleifer, H., Stackebrandt, E. (Eds.), The Procaryotes, third ed. Springer-Verlag, New York, pp. 688–752.

CN Gas

H Salem, Edgewood Chemical Biological Center, Aberdeen, MD, USA
SA Katz, Rutgers University, Camden, NJ, USA
M Feasel, Edgewood Chemical Biological Center, Aberdeen, MD, USA
B Ballantyne[†]**,** Consultant, Charleston, WV, USA

This article is a revision of the previous edition article by Harry Salem, Bryan Ballantyne, and Sidney A. Katz, volume 1, pp. 626–628, © 2005, Elsevier Inc.

- Name: 2-Chloroacetophenone
- Chemical Abstracts Service Registry Number: 532-27-4
- Synonyms: Tear gas, Less-than-lethal, Nonlethal, Lacrimator, Harassing agent, Incapacitant, 2-Chloro-L-phenylethanone, 2-Chloroacetophenone, Chloroacetophenone, Phenacyl chloride, Chloromethyl phenyl ketone
- Molecular Formula: C_8H_7ClO
- Structure:

O H
|| |
—C—C—Cl
|
H

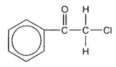

Background (Significance/History)

Chloroacetophenone was first synthesized in 1870 by the Germans. It is used as a riot control agent (RCA) due to its potency as a lachrymatory agent. It got its fame after World War I when it was given the trade name Mace®, the first American manufacturer of CN devices and sold for personal and commercial protection. Generically, it is known as tear gas. It was used in US military systems until its replacement by CS (o-chlorobenzylidene malononitrile) in 1959. However, CN is still sold commercially in the United States and is used by militaries and police all over the world.

Uses

CN is used as a nonlethal or less-than-lethal chemical in riot control situations to distract, deter, incapacitate, disorient, or disable disorderly people; to clear facilities or areas; to deny areas; or for hostage rescue. It can also be used in peacekeeping operations. It is also used in military training as a confidence builder for the protective mask.

Environmental Fate and Behavior

In Soil

CN has a half-life under aerobic conditions of 672 h and can be biodegraded in most moist, nutrient-rich soil.

In Water

Biodegradation in water is similar to degradation in soil. Howard et al. (1991) reports the same 672 h half-life for CN in aerobic surface water. This half-life is extended up to 2688 h for anaerobic aqueous degradation.

Volatile losses of CN from surface waters can be another significant process for CN disappearance in water. For instance, Olajos and Stopford (2004) calculated that CN contamination in a river would have a half-life of approximately 14 days, while CN contamination in a lake would have a half-life of approximately 110 days.

In the Atmosphere

CN reacts with hydroxyl radicals in the atmosphere. A half-life of 8 days has been estimated (Toxnet).

Decontamination

Contaminated clothing should be removed and sealed in a plastic bag. Disposable rubber gloves should be used when handling contaminated clothes. The eyes should be irrigated copiously with saline for 15–20 min. Contaminated skin should be washed thoroughly with copious amounts of water, alkaline soap and water, a mildly alkaline solution (sodium bicarbonate or sodium carbonate), or mild liquid soap and water. Sodium hypochlorite solution will exacerbate the skin lesions and should not be employed: Only a saline irrigation should be used over vesiculated skin.

Table 1 describes tear agent breakdown in water/alkaline solutions. CS shows to be the easiest to decontaminate as it readily hydrolyzes in water, and does so even more rapidly in alkaline solutions. CR and CN show low vulnerability to hydrolysis, rendering them mild environmental risks.

Exposure and Exposure Monitoring

Exposure Routes and Pathways

CN is a white solid with low vapor pressure that can be dispensed as a fine powder or as a jet or stream of solution from small or large spray tanks, as well as aerosols or smokes by pyrotechnic generation. Its solubility in water is limited, but it is soluble in organic and chlorinated organics. Exposure of eyes, nose, mouth, skin, and respiratory tract produces irritation and pain. If swallowed, CN may produce vomiting.

† Deceased.

Table 1 Decontamination of riot control agents

Compound	*($t_{1/2}$) Hydrolysis in water*	*($t_{1/2}$) Water + alkaline*
CS	(15 min) Rapid	(1 min) Rapid
CR	Little–none	Little–none
CN	Very slow	Very slow

Includes half-life of CS in water/alkaline solution.

Human Toxicology

The incapacitating effects of CN in human volunteers during exposure included lacrimation, some blurring of vision, and conjunctivitis. On the nose and throat, CN causes a tingling sensation, irritation, pain, and some increase in secretions; on the respiratory tract it causes irritation, burning, and pain. CN on the skin causes burning in the periorbital area and other areas of tender skin, especially where sweating is present. Occasionally, nausea and gagging occur during and soon after exposure. Most of these effects disappear within 20 min after exposure, but conjunctivitis and blepharospasm usually disappear after a few days leaving no after-effect. Incapacitating dosages (ICt_{50}) of CN have ranged from 20 to 50 mg min m^{-3}. The estimates of human LCt_{50} values, extrapolated from animals exposed to CN dispersed from a solvent, is 7000 mg min m^{-3}, and 14 000 mg min m^{-3} when dispersed from commercially available grenades. Other estimates range from 8500 to 25 000 mg min m^{-3}. The maximum safe inhalation dosage of CN for humans is estimated to be 500 mg min m^{-3}. Acute injuries to the eyes, primarily from effects of blast and missiles, may occur from tear-gas weapons such as pen guns. The immediate effects of these injuries include swelling and edema of the lids with penetration of skin, conjunctivitis, cornea, sclera, or globe by gunpowder and CN. Conjunctival ischemia and chemosis, corneal edema, erosion, inflammation or ulceration, and focal hemorrhage have been reported. A few hand injuries resulting from accidental discharges of tear gas guns at close range have been reported. Surgery was required in all to relieve pain and to remove the foreign material. All of these few victims suffered continuing pain and some loss of sensation, apparently from the toxic action of CN on nerves.

Toxicokinetics

Evaporation of organic solvent may concentrate CN in the eyes and intensify damage. Hydrolysis of CN is very slow in water and is difficult to decompose. Environmental contamination may be persistent and difficult to remove.

Mechanism of Toxicity

CN is considered less than lethal or nonlethal because it has a large safety ratio. That is, its effective dose or concentration ECt_{50} is low compared to its lethal dose or concentration (LCt_{50}). In the body, CN is converted to an electrophilic metabolite. It is an SN2 alkylating agent that reacts with SH groups and other nucleophilic sites of biomolecules. Alkylation of SH-containing enzymes leads to enzyme inhibition with disruption of cellular processes. CN was found to inhibit human plasma cholinesterase via a non-SH interaction, and some of the toxic effects may be due to alkylation of SH-containing enzymes.

CN as well as CS is an SN2-alkylating agent with activated halogen groups that react readily at nucleophilic sites. The prime targets include sulfhydryl-containing enzymes such as lactic dehydrogenase. Alkylation of $^{-}$SH-containing enzymes leads to enzyme inhibition with disruption of cellular processes. It has been suggested that tissue injury may be related to inactivation of certain of these enzyme systems. The initial response to the inhalation of CN or other sensory irritants is consistent with the Kratschmer reflex and the Sherrington pseudoaffective response. These aerosols stimulate the pulmonary irritant receptors to produce bronchoconstriction and increased pulmonary blood volume by augmenting sympathetic tone. The chlorine atoms released from CN on contact with skin and mucous membranes are reduced to hydrochloride acid, which can cause local irritation and burns. CN was also found to inhibit human plasma cholinesterase via a non-SH interaction.

CS, CR, and CN are all potent agonists to the transient receptor potential A1, or TrpA1, cation-selective channel. This receptor is part of the same family of receptors as TrpV1, the receptor through which oleoresin capsicum (OC), or pepper spray, works. TrpA1 differs structurally from the other Trp receptors, mainly by having amino terminal ankyrin repeat domains and an 1125 amino acid carboxy-terminal chain, both intracellularly. The receptor has been shown to generate action potentials based on pain and inflammatory stimuli experienced at these sites. This includes agonism by the tear agents CN, CS, and CR. These agents possess an electrophilic carbon that binds covalently to cysteine thiol residues in the TrpA1 receptor. This covalent bond is reversible, however, accounting for the temporary effects of these agents. In this study by Brone, in fact, the researchers were merely looking for TrpA1 receptor agonists and when synthesizing some of these noticed a pungent irritation of the eyes and nose. They then realized they were synthesizing compounds structurally similar to CR. From there, they reviewed the biological activity of the riot control agents and decided to test *their* affinity and efficacy for the TrpA1 receptor instead of synthesizing new compounds.

Upon agonism by these riot control agents, the TrpA1 receptor opens and selectively allows for the flux of sodium (Na^{+}) and calcium (Ca^{2+}) ions into the cell. This depolarizes the sensory neuron and sends an afferent signal to the CNS that is interpreted as pain. CN allows for the least calcium influx in the longest amount of time into the cell, establishing it as the least potent tear agent of the three. CR is the most potent followed by CS with respect to the amplitude and time to peak of calcium influx. This study, therefore establishes that CS, CR, and CN do in fact work through the TrpA1 receptor. Studies went on further to test for cross-reactivity with other Trp receptors, and the tear agents were deemed TrpA1 selective, with no agonism found within this family of receptors.

The sensory effects seen with tear gas exposures are due to the afferents formed by trigeminal neurons that express high concentrations of TrpA1 receptors. For example, stimulation of the tearing reflex transduces a signal through the trigeminal

Table 2 Tear gas potencies

Compound	TC_{50} (mg m^{-3})	IC_{t50} (mg min m^{-3})
CR	0.004	0.7
CN	0.3	20–50
CS	0.004	3.6
OC	0.0003–0.003	NA

TC_{50}, Threshold concentration; IC_{50}, Incapacitating concentration.
OC Included for comparison and is not a TrpA1 agonist.
Reproduced from Blain, P.G., 2003. Tear gases and irritant incapacitants. Toxicol. Rev. 22 (2), 103–110.

nerve and registers as pain. That being said, antagonists for the TrpA1 receptor could be potential therapeutic targets for tear gas overexposure treatments. With regard to TrpA1 activation, the potencies of the tear agents are described in **Table 2**.

Acute and Short-Term Toxicity (Animal/Human) (To Include Irritation and Corrosivity)

Acute and sublethal effects following aerosol exposure from commercially available thermal grenades or from acetone solutions in experimental animals were lacrimation, conjunctivitis, copious nasal secretions, salivation, hyperactivity, lethargy, and dyspnea, which occurred in all animals. Effects on the skin of exposed animals were primarily erythema. The estimated LCt_{50} values calculated for CN in the various animal species were 8878 mg min m^{-3} in the rat, 7984 mg min m^{-3} in the guinea pig, and 7033 mg min m^{-3} in the dog. The pathological findings in the animals that died from inhalation of CN consisted of congestion of the alveolar capillaries, alveolar hemorrhage, and excessive secretions in the bronchi and 628 Coal Tar bronchioles, as well as areas of acute inflammatory cell infiltration of the trachea, bronchi, and bronchioles. The early deaths exhibited lesions of the upper respiratory tract, with marked pseudomembrane formation, excessive salivation, and nasal secretion. The animals that died later exhibited edema, and hemorrhage of the lungs.

At high concentrations, CN may result in chemical injury to the eye with corneal and conjunctival edema, erosion or ulceration, chemosis, and focal hemorrhages. CN-induced ocular effects on the rabbit eye following exposure to various formulations included lacrimation, chemosis, iritis, blepharitis, and keratitis, with severity dependent on the formulation.

CN is also a potent skin irritant that may cause serious injury to the skin that includes severe generalized itching, diffuse and intense erythema, severe edema, and vesication. CN is considered a potent skin irritant and sensitizer.

Chronic Toxicity (Animal/Human)

In repeated exposures for 10 consecutive days in guinea pigs, dogs, and monkeys, the toxicity of CN was found to be considerably less when administered in divided doses. Overall, studies demonstrated a lack of cumulative toxicity. Changes in biochemical endpoints measured following multiple exposures of CN in mice were a decrease in hepatic glutathione and increased lipid peroxidation. Hepatic acid phosphatase increased after the 5-day exposure to CN, and the glutathione levels decreased after 10-day CN exposures. CN-induced elevation in acid phosphatase levels reflected the release of lysosomal enzymes from the liver, indicative of tissue injury. Additionally, hyperglycemia was observed after exposure to CN. Stress-mediated release of epinephrine is known to elevate glucose levels and thus may be responsible for the hyperglycemia. Significant decreases in body weight gain were also noted on exposure to CN. Histopathologic changes following CN exposures included hemorrhage, perivascular edema, congestion of the alveolar capillaries, occluded bronchioles, and alveolitis. Renal histopathology demonstrated congestion and coagulative necrosis in the cortical renal tubules in CN-exposed mice. Hepatic histopathology consisted of cloudy swelling and lobular and centrolobular necrosis of hepatocytes following CN exposures.

More recently, in a 2-year study with 60 male and 60 female rats exposed to 0, 2, or 4 mg m^{-3} CN 6 h per day, 5 days per week, death rates were unaffected by exposure.

Immunotoxicity

There have been very few studies of the immunotoxicity of CN. Kumar et al. (1993) found that CN suppressed pulmonary macrophages. More specifically, this study demonstrated that inhalation of CN decreases the phagocytic capacity of pulmonary macrophages.

Reproductive Toxicity

No modern mammalian studies have been conducted to assess the reproductive toxicity of CN. However, past studies have found that millimolar concentrations of CN in alcohol solutions have affected embryonic development in chicken embryos.

Carcinogenicity

In 2-year carcinogenicity inhalation bioassays in rats and mice, there were no indications of carcinogenicity in male rats, while equivocal evidence was found in female rats. These findings were evidenced by increased fibroadenomas of the mammary gland. In these 2-year inhalation studies in mice, there was no evidence of carcinogenic activity in males or females.

Clinical Management

Effects of exposure in open air are generally self-limiting and require no specific therapy. Most effects disappear in 15–30 min following exposure, although erythema may persist for an hour or longer.

CN can produce intense blepharospasm, pain, lacrimation, conjunctival erythema, periorbital edema, and a rise in intraocular pressure. These generally diminish within 30-min post-exposure. CN also produces rhinorrhoea, nasal irritation and congestion, bronchorrhoea, sore throat, cough, sneezing, and unpleasant taste and burning of the mouth immediately after exposure. These effects rapidly resolve within minutes postexposure. Symptomatic treatment of ocular irritation consists of use of a topical solution to relieve the irritation with topical antibiotics. The eyes should be examined for corneal abrasions. Treatment with oral analgesics, topical antibiotics, and mydriatics should be considered. Since CN is a solid, it is possible for a particle or clump to become embedded in the cornea or conjunctiva and cause tissue damage. Medical care for eye pain after exposure should include thorough decontamination of the eyes and a thorough ophthalmological examination. The injured eye should be carefully irrigated with isotonic saline and the remaining powder removed with a cotton swab. Any remaining stromal particles should be removed with a needle tip under slit lamp illumination. Airway problems may occur in individuals with lung disease, especially if exposed to higher than average field use concentrations. If these occur, the immediate priority is removal from the exposure and to ensure a patent airway.

Severe and prolonged erythema or severe dermatitis may occur several hours after exposure followed by vesiculation. These are generally second-degree burns and should be treated as such.

If the release of irritant incapacitants is in a confined, unventilated space, exposure may be to very high concentrations. Some individuals may be more susceptible to high concentrations, possibly because of an existing medical condition such as asthma, and will require intensive supportive medical treatment postexposure.

Ecotoxicology

Little ecotoxicology data exist for CN. However, Summerfelt and Lewis (1967) did determine that CN in concentrations from 0.5 to 2.0 mg l^{-1} repel the green sunfish. At levels as low as 0.05 mg l^{-1}, an avoidance response was detected in the same animal model. Despite the insolubility of CN in water, CN is an effective repellent even without a solvent. It should be noted that this study found that concentrations equal to or greater than 2.0 mg l^{-1} of CN in water produced 100% mortality in the green sunfish study.

Exposure Standards and Guidelines

- TLV (ACGIH): 0.05 ppm
- PEL (OSHA): 0.05 ppm
- IDLH (NIOSH): 2 ppm

See also: Arsenical Vomiting Agents; Blister Agents/vesicants; 3-Quinuclidinyl Benzilate (BZ): Psychotomimetic Agent; CS; Nerve Agents; Nonlethal Weapons; Riot Control Agents.

Further Reading

Blain, P.G., 2003. Tear gases and irritant incapacitants. Toxicol. Rev. 22 (2), 103–110.

Brone, B., Peeters, P., Marrannes, R., Mercken, M., Nuydens, R., Meert, T., Gijsen, H., 2008. Tear gasses CN, CR and CS are potent activators of the human TrpA1 receptor. Tox. Appl. Pharm. 231, 150–156.

Dray, A., Perkins, M., Mar 1993. Bradykinin and inflammatory pain. Trends Neurosci. 16 (3), 99–104.

Giksen, H., Berthelot, D., Zaja, M., Brone, B., Geuens, I., Mercken, M., 2010. Analogues of morphanthridine and the tear gas dibenz[b, f][1,4]oxazepine (CR) as extremely potent activators of the human transient receptor potential ankyrin 1 (TrpA1) channel. J. Med. Chem. 53, 7011–7020.

Howard, P.H., Boethling, R.S., Jarvis, W.F., Meylan, W.M., Michalenko, E.M., 1991. Handbook of Environmental Degradation Rates. Lewis Publishers, Printup, H.T., Chelsea, MI.

Kumar, P., Zacharaiah, K., Vijayaraghavan, R., 1993. Effects of w-chloro-acetophenone (CN) vapor inhalation on pulmonary immune system of mice. Bull. Environ. Contam. Toxicol. 50, 69–76.

Lakahai, M.S., 1962. The effect of chloroacetophenone on chick embryos cultured *in vitro*. J. Embryol. Exp. Morphol. 10, 373–382.

Moran, M., McAlexander, M., Biro, T., Szallasi, A., Aug 2011. Transient receptor potential channels as therapeutic targets. Nat. Rev. 10, 601–620.

Olajos, E.J., Stopford, W., 2004. Riot Control Agents: Issues in Toxicology, Safety, and Health. CRC Press, Boca Raton, FL.

Romano Jr., J.A., Lukely, B.J., Salem, H. (Eds.), 2008. Chemical Warfare Agents: Chemistry, Pharmacology, Toxicology, and Therapeutics, second ed. CRC Press, Taylor & Francis Group, Boca Raton, FL.

Summerfelt, R.C., Lewis, W.M., 1967. Repulsion of green sunfish by certain chemicals. J. Water Pollut. Control Fed. 39 (12), 2030–2038.

Thornburn, K.M., 1982. Injuries after use of the lacrimatory agent chloroacetophenone in a confine space. Arch. Environ. Health 37 (3), 182–186.

Relevant Websites

http://www.bt.cdc.gov – US Centers for Disease Control and Prevention, Agency for Toxic Substances and Disease Registry, Chemical Agents.

http://sis.nlm.nih.gov – US National Library of Medicine, Specialized Information Services, Chemical Warfare Agents.

Coal Tar

L Roberts, Chevron Energy Technology Company, San Ramon, CA, USA

This article is a revision of the previous edition article by Richard D. Phillips, volume 2, pp 628–631, © 2005, Elsevier Inc.

- Name: Coal Tar
- Chemical Abstracts Service Registry Number: 8007-45-2
- Synonyms: Coke oven emissions; Crude coal tar; Coal tar distillates
- Molecular Formula: Unspecified
- Chemical Structure: UVCB (Unknown or Variable composition, Complex reaction products or Biological materials)

Background (Significance/History)

Coal tar is a complex hydrocarbon mixture produced by thermal destruction (pyrolysis) of coal, typically a dark viscous liquid or semisolid with a smoky or naphthenic odor. The composition of coal tar will be influenced by the process used for pyrolytic distillation as well as by the original composition of the coal; however all coal tars will be comprised of a variable mixture of organic compounds including benzene, toluene, xylenes, cumenes, coumarone, indene, benzofuran, naphthalene, acenaphthene, methylnaphthalenes, fluorine, phenol, cresols, pyridine, picolines, phenanthracene, carbazole, quinolines, fluoranthene, and pyrene. The number of specific chemical constituents is in the thousands. Coal tar creosotes and coal tar distillates, oily liquids generally lighter in color and of lower viscosity than coal tar, are fractions produced by additional distillation of crude coal tar. Coal tar pitch is a highly viscous dark semisolid byproduct of coal pyrolysis. Coal tar volatiles are the vapors produced from heated coal tar or coal tar pitch, containing lower molecular weight (smaller ring number) polycyclic aromatic hydrocarbons (PAHs).

Coal tar is noteworthy as one of the first – if not the first – chemical substances documented to cause cancer through occupational exposures. In the eighteenth century, Sir Percival Pott, a British surgeon, noticed a higher incidence of cancers in chimney sweeps chronically exposed to soot and coal tar. He then demonstrated excess cancers occurring in laboratory animals when coal tar is applied to the ears and skin. In the early twentieth century, polycyclic aromatic compounds isolated from coal tar were identified as chemical carcinogens.

Uses

Coal tar is primarily used as a raw material in the manufacture of plastics, solvents, dyes, and in the manufacturing of other chemicals. Most coal tar undergoes further distillation. Industries that use coal tar include road paving, roofing, smelting, and coking. Coal tar creosote is used as a wood preservative. Coal tar products are also ingredients in medicine (Coal Tar United States Pharmacopeia) used to treat skin diseases such as psoriasis or eczema.

Environmental Fate and Behavior

Environmental partitioning will vary dependent upon the chemical characteristic of various constituents of coal tar. Photochemical degradation may occur in the atmosphere. If entered into aquatic systems, light hydrocarbon constituents such as benzene will volatilize in the air. Biodegradation in aquatic ecosystems will occur at various rates for different constituents. Large molecules such as PAHs are likely to adsorb to soil and sediment, undergoing slow degradation. Other hydrocarbons, such as phenols, may be readily degraded under aerobic conditions.

Exposure and Exposure Monitoring

Many of the constituents in coal tar are expected to be absorbed via skin contact or inhalation of vapors. Exposure and systemic absorption can be confirmed by analysis of urinary samples for 1-hydroxypyrene, pyrene, or total PAHs. Another noninvasive assay for exposure to coal tar or materials containing PAHs is measurement of arylhydrocarbon hydroxylase (AHH) in hair follicles; AHH activity is induced by coal tar and PAHs.

Toxicokinetics

The wide range of chemicals in coal tar are expected to differ in their rates of absorption and metabolism. Coal tar constituents can be absorbed via oral, dermal, or inhalation exposures. Regional differences in dermal absorption have been measured, with the shoulder demonstrating the highest rate of absorption and the ankle and palm the lowest.

PAHs found in coal tar are metabolized by cytochrome P450 isozymes found in many cell types, including liver and skin. Oxidative biotransformation produces reactive epoxides that can form DNA adducts. Metabolites of coal tar constituents include phenols, dihydrodiols, quinones, with potential conjugation prior to elimination.

Mechanisms of Toxicity

Due to the variability in composition, it is not possible to describe all potential mechanisms of toxicity for coal tar. The reader is recommended to review additional references for individual constituents found in the Table of Contents. It is likely that acidity of some constituents, such as phenols, and the defatting potential of some hydrocarbons, contribute to the irritancy of coal tar. Phototoxicity of PAHs is likely to be a main cause of contact irritation.

The carcinogenicity of PAH constituents is believed to lie in their potential for their reactive metabolites to be bound to macromolecules such as DNA. The mechanism of therapeutic value as a topical agent in the treatment of skin diseases is unknown but is thought to involve decreased epidermal proliferation.

Acute and Short-Term Toxicity (Animal and Human)

Coal tar is irritating to skin and eyes; vapors can irritate the respiratory tract. Symptoms may include coughing and swollen nasal passages. Phototoxicity can be produced by the combination of UVA radiation (340–430 nm wavelength) and coal tar and coal pyrolysis materials such as coal pitch and creosote; symptoms include delayed erythema, hyperpigmentation, and skin pain (tar smarts). Eye irritation testing in rabbits found that irritation produced in the presence of ultraviolet radiation was much more severe than without UV light. In the eyes, this can produce persistent conjunctivitis. Overexposure to coal tar vapors may produce symptoms of central nervous system depression and dizziness.

Repeated exposure testing in laboratory studies for 3 months identified the thymus and bone marrow as target organs for coal tar. Rats exposed by inhalation at 690 mg m^{-3} displayed thymic atrophy and hypocellular bone marrows with decreased red and white blood cell counts.

Chronic Toxicity

Chronic exposure to coal tar or coal tar volatiles can be harmful to human health. Various forms of skin lesions in humans may be similar to acne, appear as a rash with or without desquamation, and/or may be characterized by hyperkeratosis or hyperpigmentation. Benign skin growths, papillomas, may also occur. Workers with long-term inhalation of dust from coke tar distillation were found to have an increased risk of chronic respiratory diseases.

Immunotoxicity

Repeated exposure to coal tar produces thymic atrophy in laboratory studies (rodents). In humans exposed to coal tar products for treatment of psoriasis, significantly decreased levels of immunoglobulins IgG and IgM were measured in serum.

Reproductive Toxicity

No conclusive reproductive toxicity studies were found; subchronic testing with coal tar produced a significant reduction in relative ovary weights with decreased amount of ovarian luteal tissue noted microscopically. Coal tar and coal tar distillates produced developmental toxicity (increased resorptions, reduced prenatal growth, cleft palate) concurrently with maternal toxicity in rats and mice. Maternal thymus weights were significantly reduced while spleen weights were significantly increased. PAHs produce a similar developmental toxicity profile in laboratory studies.

Genetic Toxicity

Coal tar produces evidence of genetic toxicity in mutation, DNA repair, and chromosomal aberration assays. Significant increases in chromosomal abnormalities and sister chromatid exchanges were detected in the peripheral blood lymphocytes of workers with occupational exposure to coal tar. Coal tar and a polycyclic aromatic constituent, benzo[a]pyrene, form DNA adducts. Various PAHs in coal tar have been shown to differ in genetic toxicity potency, with the 5-ring benzo[a]pyrene demonstrating greater potency than the 4-ring benz[a] anthracene.

Carcinogenicity

Coal tar is classified as a human carcinogen, with multiple types of cancer reported at increased risk (respiratory tract, kidney, prostate). Elevated mortality rates from cancers of the respiratory tract, genitourinary tract, and skin have been reported. Both inhalation and dermal routes of exposure are considered hazardous. For dermal contact, long-term exposure to PAHs such as dimethylbenzanthracene and benzo[a]pyrene can produce 'tar warts,' keratotic papillomas that may progress to squamous cell carcinoma. Exposure to coal tar and simultaneous UV radiation from sunlight increases the likelihood of lesion development. Workers exposed chronically to coal tar volatiles have been found to have an increased risk of lung cancer.

Chronic inhalation studies in rodents with coal tar or coal tar pitch produced a dose-responsive increase in lung tumors. Other tumor types, such as liver, kidney, and spleen, were also induced, as were cancers of the digestive tract following dietary exposure. Chronic skin painting studies with coal extracts or coal tar extracts produce tar warts, papillomas, and malignant tumors. Adducts of benzo[a]pyrene were detected in forestomach tumors.

Clinical Management

If coal tar contacts the eye, flush eyes with water to thoroughly remove the material. If ingested, the mouth should be rinsed to remove any material in the oral cavity; if the individual is conscious, drinking water can dilute the ingested amount. Vomiting should not be induced. Coal tar on skin should be removed thoroughly. Remove to fresh air if vapors are above the occupational exposure limit.

Ecotoxicity

Aquatic toxicity to ecosystems is likely to be a factor of smaller aromatic constituents such as phenols.

Exposure Standards and Guidelines

Occupational Safety and Health Administration, American Conference of Governmental Industrial Hygienists: Coal tar pitch volatiles (CAS 65996-93-2) TWA = 0.2 mg m^{-3} (confirmed human carcinogen).

See also: Anthracene; Benz[a]anthracene; Benzene; Benzo(a) pyrene; Chrysene; Creosote (Coal Tar Creosote and Wood Creosote); Naphthalene; Phenanthrene; Phenol; Polycyclic Aromatic Hydrocarbons (PAHs); Pyrene; Pyridine.

Further Reading

ATSDR, 2002. Toxicological Profile for Wood Creosote, Coal Tar Creosote, Coal Tar, Coal Tar Pitch, and Coal Tar Pitch Volatiles. U.S. Department of Health and Human Services.

ATSDR, 2009. Addendum to the toxicological profile for creosote. http://www.atsdr.cdc.gov/toxprofiles/creosote_addendum.pdf

HSDB, 2007. Coal Tar. http://toxnet.nlm.nih.gov/cgi-bin/sis/search/a?dbs+hsdb:@term+@DOCNO+5050

Miller, J.A., 1970. Carcinogenesis by chemicals: an overview – G.H.A. Clowes memorial lecture. Cancer Res. 30, 559–576.

U.S. EPA (1989, updated version 2002) Integrated Risk Information System: Coke oven emissions.

Waldron, H.A., 1983. A brief history of scrotal cancer. Br. J. Indust. Med. 40, 390–401.

Relevant Websites

http://www.atsdr.cdc.gov/toxprofiles/tp85.pdf – Agency for Toxic Substances and Disease Registry, 2002. Toxicological profile for wood creosote, coal tar creosote, coal tar, coal tar pitch, and coal tar pitch volatiles.

http://www.atsdr.cdc.gov/toxprofiles/creosote_addendum.pdf – ATDSR - Addendum to the toxicological profile for Creosote.

http://toxnet.nlm.nih.gov/cgi-bin/sis/search/a?dbs+hsdb:@term+@DOCNO+5050 – Hazardous Substances Data Bank, 2007. Coal Tar.

Cobalt

SC Gad, Gad Consulting Services, Cary, NC, USA

- Chemical Abstracts Service Registry Number: 7440-48-4
- Synonyms: Kobalt, Aquacat, Cobalt-59, Super cobalt, C.I. 77320
- Molecular Formula: Co^{2+}
- Valence States: 0, +1, +2, +3, +4, +5

Background

Cobalt was discovered by George Brandt in 1737. Cobalt exists in valence states from 0 to 5, with the most stable (+2 and +3) being the most common. Although there is only one stable isotope of cobalt, there are a number of unstable isotopes. Two of these, cobalt-60 and cobalt-57, are in use commercially. Cobalt-60 is used for cancer treatment and food irradiation. Cobalt-57 has research applications.

Uses

Cobalt is a relatively rare metal produced primarily as a by-product of the mining of other metals, chiefly copper. It is the essential trace element found in cyanocobalamin (vitamin B_{12}). This vitamin protects against pernicious anemia and is required in the production of red blood cells. Medicinally, cobalt salts have been used to stimulate the formation of red blood cells in individuals suffering from anemia.

Commercially, cobalt is used primarily in high temperature alloys, tungsten carbide tools, and (with iron and nickel) permanent magnets. Cobalt salts are used in pigments and paint dryers and as catalysts in the petroleum industry.

Environmental Fate and Behavior

The sources of cobalt in the environment are both natural and synthetic (anthropogenic). Natural sources include soil, seawater spray, volcanic eruptions, and forest fires. Anthropogenic sources include combustion of fossil fuels, metal smelting, sewage sludge, and processing of cobalt alloys. Cobalt is found in the atmosphere in particulate form and returns to the Earth's surface through dry deposition and with rain or snow. Once in surface water, cobalt generally moves into sediment. Cobalt does not appear to biomagnify significantly in the aquatic food chain. The cobalt that does accumulate in fish is largely found in the nonedible parts of the fish. Seventy-nine percent of the cobalt is transported by rivers globally and precipitates in estuaries.

Under normal environmental conditions, cobalt is expected to bind strongly to soil; thus, migration through soil is very limited. Cobalt in soil can be taken up by plant roots and root vegetables, but does not translocate to the aboveground parts of plants.

Exposure and Exposure Monitoring

For the general population, ingestion is the primary exposure pathway for cobalt. For persons working in industrial settings, inhalation is a significant pathway (e.g., carbide industry emissions and airborne particulate from grinding processes), as is dermal exposure. There can also be an internal exposure from implanted medical devices.

Toxicokinetics

Oral ingestion of cobalt salts results in ready absorption, probably in the jejunum. Although cobalt is readily absorbed, increased levels do not tend to cause significant accumulation. The majority (80%) of cobalt is excreted in the feces of rats and cattle. In contrast, in humans, ~80% of absorbed cobalt is excreted via the urine and 15% is excreted in the feces by an enterohepatic pathway. Breast milk and sweat are secondary routes of excretion. The total body burden for the average person is estimated at 1.1 mg. Muscle generally contains the greatest mass of cobalt, but the highest concentrations are found in fat. Cobalt present in the blood is associated with the red blood cells.

Mechanism of Toxicity

Cobalt most often depresses the activity of enzymes, including catalase, amino levulinic acid synthetase, and P-450, enzymes involved in cellular respiration. The Krebs citric acid cycle can be blocked by cobalt resulting in the inhibition of cellular energy production. Cobalt can replace zinc in a number of zinc-required enzymes such as alcohol dehydrogenase. Cobalt can also enhance the kinetics of some enzymes, such as heme oxidase in the liver. Cobalt interferes with and depresses iodine metabolism, resulting in reduced thyroid activity. Reduced thyroid activity can lead to goiter.

Acute and Short-Term Toxicity (or Exposure)

Human

Ingestion of cobalt may result in the production of an unusually high number of red blood cells (similar to a cancer of red blood cells [polycythemia vera]). Ingestion of cobalt salts (once added to beer as a defoaming agent) has resulted in cardiomyopathy. The signs and symptoms of cardiomyopathy caused by beer consumption are similar to those of congestive heart failure. Autopsy results indicated a 10-fold increase in cobalt

 http://dx.doi.org/10.1016/B978-0-12-386454-3.00832-0

concentrations in heart tissue. The alcohol may have potentiated cobalt absorption or toxic effects.

Chronic Toxicity (or Exposure)

Animal

When implanted intramuscularly or subcutaneously in rats, cobalt metal produced fibrosarcomas at the site, but no other routes of exposure have elicited a carcinogenic response. This is considered a rodent-specific solid state tumor (SST) phenomenon.

Human

Cobalt is an essential nutrient at low levels ($\sim$40 mg day^{-1}). In industrial settings, inhalation of high concentrations of cobalt compounds has led to hard-metal pneumoconiosis, which may result in interstitial fibrosis. Workers with this condition typically develop hypersensitivity to cobalt compounds (symptoms include coughing and wheezing). A few workers have developed skin hypersensitivity after dermal contact with cobalt and its compounds. Cobalt can cause cardiomyopathy and (if inhaled as a dust) interstitial lung disease.

Immunotoxicity

Cobalt is a common dermal allergen and its salts are also irritants.

Reproductive Toxicity

No studies were located regarding reproductive effects in humans after inhalation exposure to cobalt.

Both rats exposed to cobalt (as cobalt chloride) at 13.3–58.9 mg kg^{-1} body weight per day for 2–3 months in drinking water or diet and mice exposed to cobalt (cobalt chloride) at 43.3 mg kg^{-1} body weight per day for 13 weeks in drinking water exhibited testicular degeneration and atrophy.

Long-term exposure of cobalt-containing aerosols resulted in effects on reproductive end points. Testicular atrophy was reported in rats, but not in mice, exposure to 10 mg cobalt per m^3 as cobalt sulfate over 16 days. Following exposure of mice to cobalt for 13 weeks, a decrease in sperm motility was found at 1.14 mg cobalt per m^3, and testicular atrophy was found at 11.4 mg cobalt per m^3.

Carcinogenicity

In experimental animals, studies found in local tumors at injection sites and lung tumors after intratracheal instillation with cobalt oxides. Other studies conducted with cobalt metal alone or alloyed with chromium and molybdenum did not provide evidence of carcinogenicity except local site tumors induced after injection. Cobalt sulfate has been recommended to be listed as "reasonably anticipated by the National Toxicology Program to be a human carcinogenicity on the basis of sufficient evidence in animals," is classified as a category 2 carcinogen (labeled R49; 'can cause cancer by inhalation') by the European Union, and IARC has concluded that there was sufficient evidence in experimental animals for the carcinogenicity of cobalt sulfate.

Clinical Management

The oil-soluble BAL (British anti-Lewisite; 2,3-dimercaptopropanol) appears to be the antidote of choice for cobalt poisoning.

Animal studies have tested various chelating agents in models of cobalt toxicity. Animal experiments suggested that *N*-acetylcysteine may be helpful, but there are no human studies to corroborate these findings. Chelation therapy with calcium disodium ethylenediaminetetraacetic acid or dimercaprol may be useful; however, definitive clinical studies are lacking.

Ecotoxicology

It does not bioaccumulate and is not known to be toxic to marine or freshwater organisms.

Other Hazards

In the 1960s, heart failure in high-volume beer drinkers, known as 'beer drinkers' cardiomyopathy was characterized by pericardial effusion, elevated hemoglobin concentrations, and biventricular congestive heart failure. Mortality approached 50%.

Exposure Standards and Guidelines

The American Conference of Governmental Industrial Hygienists (ACGIH) threshold limit value time-weighted average for cobalt (elemental and inorganic compounds) is 0.02 mg m^{-3}. ACGIH classifies cobalt as an animal carcinogen.

See also: Metals; Vitamins.

Further Reading

Basketter, D.A., Angelini, G., Ingber, A., Kern, P.S., Menne, T., 2003. Nickel, chromium and cobalt in consumer products: revisiting safe levels in the new millennium. Contact Derm. 49 (1), 1–7.

De Boeck, M., Kirsch-Volders, M., Lison, D., 2003. Cobalt and antimony: genotoxicity and carcinogenicity. Mutat. Res. 533 (1–2), 135–152 (Erratum in Mutation Research 2004; 548(1–2):127–128).

Goyer, R.A., Klaassen, C.D., Waalkes, M.P., 1995. Metal Toxicology. Academic Press, San Diego, CA.

Henretig, F., Joffe, M., Baffa, G., et al., 1998. Elemental cobalt toxicity and effects of chelation therapy. Vet. Hum. Toxicol. 30, 372–378.

Lison, D., De Boeck, M., Verougstraete, V., Kirsch-Volders, M., 2001. Update on the genotoxicity and carcinogenicity of cobalt compounds. Occup. Environ. Med. 58 (10), 619–625.

Nordberg, G.F., Fowler, B.A., Nordberg, M., Friberg, L.T., 2007. Handbook on the Toxicology of Metals, third ed. Associated Press, London.

Relevant Website

http://www.atsdr.cdc.gov – Agency for Toxic Substances and Disease Registry. Toxicological Profile for Cobalt.

Cocaine

M Siegrist, Huther Doyle, Rochester, NY, USA
TJ Wiegand, Strong Memorial Hospital, University of Rochester Medical Center (URMC), Rochester, NY, USA

This article is a revision of the previous edition article by Michael Wahl, volume 1, pp 632–634, © 2005, Elsevier Inc.

- Name: Cocaine
- Chemical Abstracts Service Registry Number: 50-36-2
- Molecular Formula: $C_{17}H_{21}NO_4$
- Cocaine (50-36-2) is a central nervous system stimulant, vasoconstrictor, and drug of abuse.
- Synonyms: Chemical: Ecgonine methyl ester benzoate, Benzoylmethylecgonine; [1R-(exo–exo)]-3-(benzoyloxy)-8-methyl-8-azabicyclo[3,21]octane-2-carboxylic acid methyl ester, Ecgonine methyl ester benzoate; Slang: Blow, C, Caine, Charlie, Coke, Crack, Dama blanca (White Lady in Spanish), Perico (slang 'Little Perrot'), Snow, Toot, Uptown, White Lady, White
- Chemical Structure:

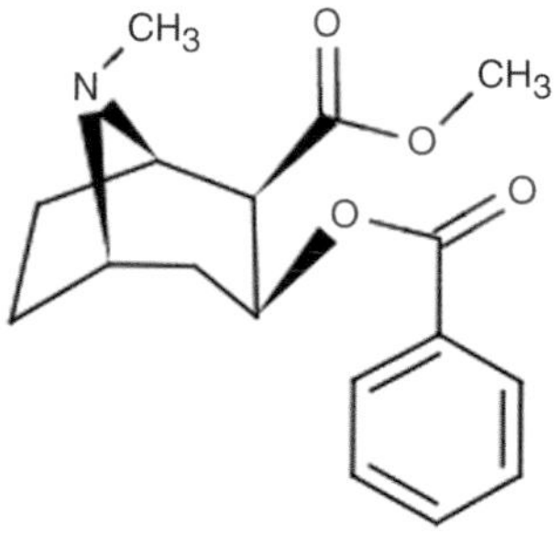

Background

For thousands of years, indigenous people of South America and other areas around the globe have chewed coca leaves as a mild stimulant. The leaves also provided nutritional benefit when eaten. When the Spanish arrived in South America, they taxed the leaves and used them as currency of sort. In 1855, cocaine was isolated from the coca leaf by the German chemist Friedrich Gaedcke. He named the alkaloid, 'erythroxyline' and published his findings in the journal *Archiv der Pharmazie*. An improvement on Gaedke's extraction was done by another German chemist, Albert Niemann, and described in his PhD dissertation, 'On a New Organic Base in the Coca Leaves,' which was published in 1860. Niemann named the alkaloid 'cocaine' from the Quechua word from 'cuca.' The ending 'caine' was added as this suffix was used to form names of synthetic local anesthetic, and cocaine had local anesthetic properties. Cocaine prohibition began in 1914 when the Harrison Act required that it be dispensed only with a doctor's order. At the turn of the century, in 1900, cocaine was popular with laborers, the underclass, and marginalized segments of society, including prostitutes. The current US cocaine market is worth nearly 100 million dollars annually. Cocaine powder remains popular, with use increasing in the late 1990s and early 2000s, and the development and popularization of the freebase form of cocaine, 'crack,' introduced cocaine to lower socioeconomic groups. Use of 'crack' cocaine has remained widespread since first becoming popular in the early 1980s.

Uses

Medicinal

Cocaine is used medically as the hydrochloride salt. A topical solution is available for local anesthesia of mucous membranes and it can be injected locally for both local anesthetic and vasoconstrictive effects. It is also used in otolaryngology to control bleeding during nasal and head and neck surgeries. Current medicinal use of cocaine is primarily confined to intraoperative surgical use for nasal and dermal lacerations.

Illicit

Cocaine is used illicitly in various forms and through multiple routes. As cocaine hydrochloride (powdered cocaine), the primary route of use is intranasal (insufflation). It can also be taken orally or rectally or dissolved in water and injected. As a freebase form (or as crack), cocaine can be volatilized and thus inhaled or 'smoked.' Freebase cocaine can also be dissolved in acidic solutions (i.e., vinegar, citrate, or other acidic solutions). The subsequent salt is also soluble in water. In areas where freebase or crack cocaine is more widely available, injection drug users will solubilize the freebase form and inject it in this manner.

Environmental Fate and Behavior

Physicochemical Properties

Cocaine hydrochloride is a nearly odorless, bitter-tasting chemical that appears as white crystals. It is soluble in water at a rate of 200 g per 100 ml. In alcohol, 25 g is soluble in 100 ml. Cocaine hydrochloride is insoluble in ether. The melting point of cocaine hydrochloride is 197 °C, and a 1% solution is of neutral (7) pH.

Cocaine freebase is volatile, anhydrous, and bitter tasting and appears as white or slightly yellow crystals. It is minimally soluble in water (0.17 g per 100 ml), somewhat soluble in alcohol (15.4 g per 100 ml), and soluble in ether (28.6 g per 100 ml). The melting point of cocaine freebase is 98 °C and the boiling point is 187–188 °C.

Street cocaine is often cut with various diluents and toxicity, and effect is often affected by the products used to cut cocaine (i.e., levamisole).

Exposure Routes and Pathways

- *Smoking* the base alkaloid (as crack or freebase) remains the most common route of exposure.
- *Nasal insufflation* of the hydrochloride salt.
- *Intravenous injection* of the water-soluble forms.
- *Application of the hydrochloride salt to mucous membranes* is a therapeutic as well as a method of abuse.

Toxicity and clinical effects often depend on not only the amount ingested but also the manner in which cocaine is used, including the route of exposure. Smoking the freebase form of cocaine (volatilizing) leads to the most rapid rise in concentrations and greatest rates of increase of dopamine in the reward circuitry in the brain (thus 'smoking' is the most 'addictive' route of use). Insufflation is done through the use of hydrochloride salt. Intravenous injection can occur with water-soluble forms, including the hydrochloride (standard powdered cocaine), or with other 'salts,' including the citrate and acetate forms of cocaine.

Toxicokinetics

Cocaine toxicokinetics depends on the route of use. Smoked cocaine is rapidly absorbed from the lungs and peak plasma concentrations occur within minutes. In a study involving 20 and 40 mg doses, the peak plasma concentrations of smoked cocaine occurred at 2 min after the 20 and 40 mg doses. When cocaine is absorbed across mucous membranes, an initial rapid rise in plasma concentrations occurs, which slows as the vasoconstrictive effects of cocaine influence the rate of absorption. Peak plasma concentrations occur within 1 h after oral ingestion and nasal application. By oral or intranasal routes, about 60–80% of a cocaine dose is absorbed. In acidic environments, such as the stomach, cocaine is ionized and uptake into cells is limited. In alkaline environments, there is less ionization and the absorption is increased. Bioavailability is decreased when cocaine is ingested orally as hydrolysis occurs in the gastrointestinal tract.

There are three primary routes of metabolism for cocaine: hydrolysis within the liver and peripherally by hepatic and plasma cholinesterases. This route leads to the formation of ecgonine methyl ester through loss of the benzoyl group. The secondary route is spontaneous hydrolysis, which is most likely nonenzymatic and leads to benzoylecgonine demethylation. The final metabolism leads to ecgonine from both benzoylecgonine and ecgonine methyl ester through demethylation. Norcocaine is formed as a minor metabolite through *N*-demethylation processes. Cocaine metabolism is dose dependent and at high doses, in particular during binge use episodes, metabolism may be significantly prolonged. Cocaine is widely distributed in the body and has an apparent volume of distribution (Vd) of 1.2–1.9 $l\ kg^{-1}$. Cocaine rapidly appears in the central nervous system (CNS), where it inhibits the dopamine transporters within 4–5 s of intravenous injection. This effect peaks at 30 s following intravenous use. In a comparison of inhalation (smoked) and intravenous use of cocaine, the time to peak subjective effects occurred significantly faster for smoked (1.4 ± 0.5 min) than for intravenous cocaine (3.1 ± 0.9 min). Peak effects for intranasal cocaine use occurred much slower (14.6 ± 8 min). Cocaine crosses the placenta. The elimination half-life of cocaine is approximately 1 h at doses of less than 2 mg kg^{-1}. Cocaine can be measured at low concentrations, however, in chronic users, due to prolongation of metabolism and half-life of elimination. Cocaine is concentrated in adipose tissue and in the CNS after large and repeated doses. Low doses of cocaine are excreted primarily in the urine as metabolites, with less than 10% of the dose found as unchanged cocaine in the urine.

Mechanism of Toxicity

Cocaine primary organs of effect are the central nervous system and the cardiovascular system. Effects depend on the dose, the route of exposure, adulterants, impurities, and other substances ingested as well as individual differences in susceptibility to toxicity from cocaine. Cocaine acts as a reuptake inhibitor for the neurotransmitters serotonin, norepinephrine, and dopamine. In the periphery norepinephrine causes alpha-1 agonism, leading to vasoconstrictive effects and tachycardia. Cocaine also has nonspecific sodium channel antagonism, leading to local anesthetic effects. In overdose, cocaine can cause slowing of myocardial sodium channels similar to the quinidine-like effect seen in other sodium channel antagonists such as tricyclic antidepressants, lamotrigine, and even diphenhydramine (at high doses). This can lead to QRS widening and decreases in contractility. In addition to direct toxicity from cocaine, specific adulterants of illicit cocaine can be particularly toxic. In recent years, levamisole has emerged as a common adulterant, with nearly 80% of the world's cocaine supply found to have significant concentrations of levamisole (up to 20% by weight). Levamisole can cause immunosuppression and vasculitis. Deaths from levamisole-mediated toxicity including infections (neutropenia-associated infections) and vasculitis have occurred. When cocaine is ingested in the presence of ethanol, cocaethylene is synthesized. Cocaethylene has similar actions to cocaine; however, it has a longer duration of action. Cocaine also can cause increases in platelet aggregation through its serotonergic effects and has direct end-organ toxicity primarily through vasoconstrictive effects.

Adulterants

Cocaine in nonmedical use form may contain adulterants that occur during the manufacture, conversion for shipping, additions used to disguise the cocaine from detection, dilution for distribution and sale, and substances used to enhance the euphoria. These adulterants may be a major cause of toxicity. It has also been proposed that some adulterants are added to track shipments by the cocaine producers and distributors.

One such agent is levamisole, which causes cutaneous vasculitis or agranulocytosis associated in levamisole-adulterated cocaine. Levamisole is found in more than 80% of illicit cocaine seized within US borders.

Combinations

Cocaine is sometimes used in combination or within other drugs of abuse, complicating the elucidation of its toxicity. A common example combination is its use in a 'speed ball' where it is used after it is combined with heroin. In the presence of ethanol, cocaine is also metabolized to cocaethylene, which may alter the toxidromes picture.

Acute and Short-Term Toxicity (or Exposure)

Animal

Animal models have demonstrated acute toxicity similar to that present in humans. Dogs develop toxicity at lower doses than rats, and death appears to be associated with the development of hyperthermia. The functional status of organ enervation and the presence of anesthetics may alter cocaine toxicity in animal models.

Human

Cocaine toxicity can present after a wide range of doses, with reports of toxicity at doses of less than 1 mg kg^{-1} in adults. In nonmedical use, acute toxicity may be due to the adulterants further complicating treatment of cocaine-related toxicity. Toxicity occurs in most organ systems and cocaine use increases the risk of trauma as well as infections. Acute tolerance to the many CNS and cardiovascular effects of cocaine may develop. Kindling and lowering of seizure threshold with repeated subtoxic doses can also occur. The CNS toxicity of cocaine includes in a dose-dependent fashion with simple stimulation at lower doses followed by euphoria, anxiety/agitation, seizures, intracranial hemorrhage, and excited delirium. Chest pain is the most common post-use side effect leading to emergency room visits. Acute ischemic stroke, intracranial hemorrhage, and subarachnoid hemorrhage have been shown to result from acute cocaine use. Mesenteric ischemia and perforated gastric and duodenal ulcers can occur from vasoconstrictive and other effects of cocaine. Cardiovascular toxicity can include tachycardia, hypertension, coronary artery spasm, myocardial ischemia, infarction, and myocarditis. Bradycardia, hypotension, cardiovascular collapse, dysrhythmias, and sudden death occur as cocaine toxicity progresses. Pulmonary toxicity after smoking the alkaloid form of cocaine includes hemorrhage, barotrauma including pneumomediastinum, pulmonary edema and 'crack lung,' a hypersensitivity reaction that includes fever, productive sputum, pulmonary infiltrates, and bronchospasm. Other toxicities seen with acute cocaine use include hyperpyrexia (fever), rhabdomyolysis, and metabolic acidosis. The lethal dose of cocaine in humans is estimated at 0.5–1.3 g per day by mouth, 0.05–5 g per day intranasal, and 0.02 g via parenteral route (there is a wide margin of variation in toxic effects depending on individual susceptibility to toxic effects of cocaine).

Chronic Toxicity (or Exposure)

Animal

Animal models of chronic, self-administered cocaine use show regular patterns of use and abstinence. Administration of cocaine during a period of self-induced abstinence from cocaine restarts this cycle. Animals with free access to 24 h per day cocaine showed weight loss, self-mutilation, and death within 2 weeks.

Human

Toxicity associated with chronic use is not as well described as acute toxicity and may be a function of dose and route/type of administration as well as impurities and adulterants in street cocaine. Addiction and dependence can occur in certain individuals with access to cocaine over a period of time. Organ toxicity including increased rates of cardiovascular disease is seen in chronic and heavy cocaine users, in particular crack cocaine users, as atherosclerosis is increased and the risk of myocardial infarction substantially increased. Toxicity from cocaine is difficult to separate from other drugs often used by individuals who chronically use cocaine (i.e., tobacco, alcohol, and other illicit substances).

Immunotoxicity

Cocaine has been demonstrated to covalently modify proteins *in vitro*. This finding has been seen in animals and humans chronically exposed to cocaine. Modified proteins are immunogenic and may explain why some people develop autoimmune effects after chronic cocaine exposure. 'Crack lung' is thought to be a hypersensitivity reaction that includes fever, productive sputum, pulmonary infiltrates, and bronchospasm.

Genotoxicity

Cocaine is not known to be mutagenic.

Reproductive Toxicity

Cocaine use during pregnancy can result in an increased risk of abruption placentae, spontaneous abortion, and low-birth-weight infants with congenital malformations and potentially neurobehavioral impairment. Freebase cocaine crosses the placenta and norcocaine persists for 4–5 days in amniotic fluid, even when it is no longer detectable in maternal blood. A meta-analysis in humans showed an increased rate in congenital malformations in the offspring of cocaine users, including limb, urogenital, cardiovascular, and digestive abnormalities.

Carcinogenicity

Cocaine has not been shown to be carcinogenic in humans.

Clinical Management

The initial management of acute cocaine intoxication should include an assessment and management of the patient's airway, breathing, and circulation. Supplemental oxygen and a benzodiazepine are frequently indicated when agitation or general CNS stimulation occurs. Hyperpyrexia, seizures, and rhabdomyolysis should be managed using the basic treatment approaches for the complication (sedation, hydration, and treatment with GABAergic agents such as benzodiazepines). Concurrent use of alcohol and other drugs is frequent and should be considered during the initial assessment. Beta-blockers are contraindicated in tachycardia or chest pain and myocardial infarction due to the potential for unopposed alpha-agonism and worsening of hypertension and vasoconstriction, in particular in the coronary arteries. If a beta-blocker is used, a short-acting agent is preferred (i.e., esmolol). Nitrates, opiates, thrombolytics, and cardiac catheterization may be used when appropriate clinical and laboratory findings occur in the setting of potential myocardial infarction. When sodium channel antagonism occurs (i.e., QRS widening), in particular in the setting of acidosis, intravenous sodium bicarbonate should be administered as bolus at 1–2 Meq kg^{-1}. In severe intoxications, paralysis may facilitate aggressive cooling strategies and hasten clinical improvement. Cocaine 'body packers' and 'body stuffers' are unique populations associated with significant risk of toxicity. A 'stuffer' is someone who ingests hastily wrapped drugs in an attempt to hide evidence or evade police detection. Absorption of significant amounts of cocaine can occur in this setting. Monitoring and symptomatic care are the cornerstones of the treatment. Asymptomatic patients (stuffers) should be monitored for a period of time and gastrointestinal decontamination should be considered in these patients (i.e., activated charcoal and even whole bowel irrigation); however, data do not support aggressive treatment in all supposed body stuffers for cocaine. In body packers (i.e., drug mules) transporting large amounts of usually more fastidiously wrapped cocaine, the potential for severe or catastrophic toxicity from packet rupture exists. These patients require packet removal. Consultation with a toxicologist and poison specialist should be done in cases of body packer or stuffer ingestion of cocaine.

See also: Drugs of Abuse; Marijuana; Poisoning Emergencies in Humans.

Further Reading

Baselt, R.C., Cravey, R.H., 1989. Disposition of Toxic Drugs and Chemicals in Man, third ed. Yearbook Medical Publishers, Chicago. 208–213.

Brownlow, H.A., Pappachan, J., 2002. Pathophysiology of cocaine abuse. Eur. J. Anaesthesiol. 19 (6), 395–414.

Chiriboga, C.A., Bateman, D.A., Brust, J.C.M., 1993. Neurologic findings in neonates with intrauterine cocaine exposure. Pediatr. Neurol. 9, 115–119.

De Giorgi, A., Fabbian, F., Pala, M., Bonetti, F., Babini, I., Bagnaresi, I., Manfredini, F., Portaluppi, F., Mikhailidis, D.P., Manfredini, R., June 2012. Cocaine and acute vascular diseases. Curr. Drug Abuse Rev. 5 (2), 129–134.

Goldfrank, L.I., Hoffman, K.S., 1991. The cardiovascular effects of cocaine. Ann. Emerg. Med. 20, 165–175.

Harvey, J.A., 2004. Cocaine effects on the developing brain: current status. Neurosci. Biobehav. Rev. 27 (8), 751–764.

Heard, K., Palmer, R., Zahniser, N.R., 2008. Mechanisms of acute cocaine toxicity. Open Pharmacol. J. 2 (9), 70–78. http://dx.doi.org/10.2174/1874143600802010070.

Hollander, J.E., Shih, R.D., Hoffman, R.S., 1997. Predictors of coronary artery disease in patients with cocaine-associated myocardial infarction. Am. J. Med. 102, 158–163.

Jenkins, A.J., Keenan, R.M., Henningfield, J.E., Cone, E.J., October 2002. Correlation between pharmacological effects and plasma cocaine concentrations after smoked administration. J. Anal. Toxicol. 26 (7), 382–392.

Karch, S.B., Mari, F., Bartolini, V., Bertol, E., July 26, 2012. Aminorex poisoning in cocaine abusers. Int. J. Cardiol. 158 (3), 344–346 (Epub July 20, 2011).

Knuepfer, M.M., 2003. Cardiovascular disorders associated with cocaine use: myths and truths. Pharmacol. Ther. 97 (3), 181–222.

Larocque, A., Hoffman, R.S., April 2012. Levamisole in cocaine: unexpected news from an old acquaintance. Clin. Toxicol. (Phila.) 50 (4), 231–241.

Leikin, J.B., Krantz, A.J., Zell-Kanter, M., Barkin, R.L., Hryhorczuk, D.O., 1989. Clinical features and management of intoxication due to hallucinogenic drugs. Med. Toxicol. Adverse Drug Exp. 4, 324–350.

McKinney, C.D., Postiglione, K.F., Herotid, D.A., 1992. Benzocaine-adulterated street cocaine in association with methemoglobinemia. Clin. Chem. 38 (4), 596–597.

Miranda, C.H., Pazin-Filho, A., 2013. Crack cocaine-induced cardiac conduction abnormalities are reversed by sodium bicarbonate infusion. Case Rep. Med. 2013, 396401. http://dx.doi.org/10.1155/2013/396401 (Epub May 23, 2013).

MMWR Morb. Mortal. Wkly. Rep. 58 (49), December 18, 2009, 1381–1385.

MMWR, July 2010. Poison Issues Unintentional Drug Poisoning in the United State.

Odeleye, O.E., Watson, R.R., Eskelson, C.D., 1993. Enhancement of cocaine-induced hepatotoxicity by ethanol. Drug and Alcohol Depend. 31, 253–263.

Roncero, C., Daigre, C., Grau-Lopez, L., Rodriguez-Cintas, L., Barral, C., Perez-Pazos, J., Gonzalvo, B., Corominas, M., Casas, M., 2013. Cocaine-induced psychosis and impulsivity in cocaine-dependent patients. J. Addict. Dis. 32 (3), 263–273.

Sullivan, D., Pinsonneault, J.K., Papp, A.C., Zhu, H., Lemeshow, S., Mash, D.C., Sadee, W., January 2013. Dopamine transporter DAT and receptor DRD2 variants affect risk of lethal cocaine abuse: a gene-gene-environment interaction. Transl. Psychiatry 22 (3), e222.

Sanchez, E.J., Hayes, R.P., Barr, J.T., Lewis, K.M., Webb, B.N., Subramanian, A.K., Nissen, M.S., Jones, J.P., Shelden, E.A., Sorg, B.A., Fill, M., Schenk, J.O., Kang, C., July 19, 2013. Potential role of cardiac calsequestrin in the lethal arrhythmic effects of cocaine. Drug Alcohol Depend. pii: S0376-8716(13) 00231-7.

Treadwell, S.D., Robinson, T.G., 2007. Cocaine use and stroke. Postgrad. Med. J. 83 (980), 389–394.

Volkow, N.D., Wang, G.J., Fischman, M.W., Foltin, R., Fowler, J.S., Franceschi, D., Franceschi, M., Logan, J., Gatley, S.J., Wong, C., Ding, Y.S., Hitzemann, R., Pappas, N., August 11, 2000. Effects of route of administration on cocaine induced dopamine transporter blockade in the human brain. Life Sci. 67 (12), 1507–1515.

Yachoui, R., Kolasinski, S.L., Eid, H., 2012. Limited cutaneous vasculitis associated with levamisole. J. Clin. Med. Res. 4 (5), 358–359 (Epub Septenber 12, 2012).

Yorgason, J.T., Jones, S.R., España, R.A., 2011. Low and high affinity dopamine transporter inhibitors block dopamine uptake within 5 seconds of intravenous injection. Neuroscience.

Relevant Websites

http://www.inchem.org/documents/pims/pharm/pim139e.htm – Cocaine at inChem an online resource for chemistry, properties, pharmacology and toxicology related to cocaine.

http://emedicine.medscape.com/article/813959-overview – Cocaine toxicity – *eMedicine* website on overview, clinical presentation, treatment and other discussion on cocaine intoxication.

http://emedicine.medscape.com/article/813959-overview – Cocaine Toxicity in Emergency Medicine.

http://www.emedicinehealth.com/cocaine_abuse/article_em.htm – *eMedicine* website (Medscape) on cocaine abuse including overview, diagnosis, symptoms and treatment.

http://www.drugabuse.gov/publications/drugfacts/cocaine – National Institute on Drug Abuse website on cocaine (DrugFacts).

http://oas.samhsa.gov/cocaine.htm – SAMHSA Office of Applied Studies on cocaine.

http://store.samhsa.gov/term/Cocaine – Substance Abuse Mental Health Services Administration (SAMHSA) website on cocaine resources and publications (ordering).

http://www.asam.org/ – The American Society of Addiction Medicine online resource.

www.erowid.org/chemicals/cocaine/cocaine.shtml – Vault of erowid cocaine information.

Coke Oven Emissions

FF Farris, Manchester University, Fort Wayne, IN, USA

This article is a revision of the previous edition article by Shashi K. Ramaiah and Harihara M. Mehendale, volume 1, pp 635–637, © 2005, Elsevier Inc.

- Name: Coke oven emissions
- Chemical Abstracts Service Registry Number: No individual number has been assigned
- Synonyms: Primary synonym is coal tar pitch volatiles such as benzene soluble organics. However, synonyms vary depending on the specific constituents in the emissions; RTECS No. GH0346000
- Molecular Formula: Coke oven emissions are a complex mixture of substances and have no single molecular formula
- Chemical Structure: Coke oven emissions are a complex mixture of substances and have no single structure

Background

Coke is a fuel of high carbon content (typically about 90%) that produces a clean, intense heat when burned. It is an important fuel in the smelting of iron and other metallic ores in the production of metals in blast furnaces. Smelting of iron and most other ores commonly requires three primary ingredients, coke being one of them. The remaining two ingredients are flux materials such as limestone and the ore itself. The flux serves as a purifying or cleaning agent that helps remove the gangue of the ore as slag. Coke actually serves two purposes in the smelting process. First, it serves as fuel for the furnace. As a fuel, coke (28 000–31 000 kJ kg^{-1}) contains approximately 50% more energy per unit weight than bituminous coal (17 000–23 000 kJ kg^{-1}) and about the same as anthracite (32 500–34 000 kJ kg^{-1}). Second, carbon in the coke serves as a reducing agent, removing oxygen from the ore and leaving behind the purified metal.

Coke is the solid residue that remains after extensive baking of carbonaceous materials at high temperatures in the absence of air. Coke is produced in coke ovens that typically operate at temperatures ranging between 1800 and 3600 °F (1000–2000 °C). At these temperatures, in the absence of air, volatile constituents are driven off. The fused residue that remains (coke) is primarily carbon with small amounts of impurities such as ash and sulfur.

Coke is usually made from low-ash, low-sulfur bituminous coal. These cokes are gray, hard, and porous. Bituminous coal must meet certain criteria for use as coking coal. These criteria include moisture, ash, sulfur, and tar content and are necessary in order to produce coke that will have characteristics appropriate for use in blast furnaces.

Coke oven emissions are defined as the benzene-soluble fraction of the particulate matter produced during coke production. The chemical and physical properties of coke oven emissions vary depending on the constituents of the coal. The greater the noncarbonaceous content of the coal, the greater the amount of volatile by-products that are produced during coke production. Volatile products released during the production of coke include primarily water, coal gas, and coal tar. Coal gas is a mixture of various volatile compounds, including hydrogen, carbon monoxide, carbon dioxide, sulfur dioxide, nitric oxides, methane, benzene, and other volatile hydrocarbons. Coal tar is a high viscosity black liquid mixture of phenols, aromatic compounds, polycyclic aromatic hydrocarbons (PAHs), heterocyclic compounds, and metals including arsenic, cadmium, and mercury. More than 60 organic compounds, including more than 40 PAHs, have been identified in air samples collected at coke plants.

The significance of coke oven emissions as a public health, as well as an occupational health, issue has diminished considerably in the United States during the last half century. In 1970, there were 64 coking plants in the United States operating more than 13 000 coke ovens, with an estimated 10 000 coke oven workers. By 1998, it had declined to 23 coking plants operating about 3800 ovens. Increased efforts to minimize and monitor exposures to workers have also been instituted.

Uses

The primary use of coke is as a fuel reductant, a component in the smelting of iron ore and the production of iron in blast furnaces. Chemicals recovered from coke oven emissions are used for the production of various products including plastics, solvents, dyes, paints, roads coverings, roofing, insulation, and sealants. Coal gas is used as a fuel. Coal tar can be used in medicated shampoo, soap, and ointment, as a treatment for dandruff and psoriasis. It may also be used in the extemporaneous preparation of topical medications in the clinical treatment of skin disorders such as eczema, dermatitis, and psoriasis.

Environmental Fate and Behavior

Coke oven emissions represent a complex mixture of individual chemicals, so a discussion of the environmental fate and behavior of these emissions would require an extensive discussion. Approximately 80% of coal tar is composed of mixed carbon chains (C_{18}–C_{22}). Coal tar volatiles include benzene, toluene, and xylene. Among the most toxicologically important emissions are metals and PAHs, including benzo(*a*) pyrene (BaP), benzanthracene, chrysene, and phenanthrene. PAHs are a concern because they can be relatively persistent in the environment and have many toxic effects. Individual PAHs vary in behavior. Some can be easily volatilized and inhaled. Although PAHs are not particularly soluble in water, low levels may still be found in water systems.

Exposure and Exposure Monitoring

The primary routes of potential human exposure to coke oven emissions are inhalation and dermal contact. Occupational exposure to coke oven emissions may occur for those workers in the aluminum, steel, graphite, electrical, and construction industries. Workers at coking plants and coal tar production plants, as well as people who live near these plants, have a high risk of possible exposure to coke oven emissions. Studies have indicated that exposure of employees to coke oven emissions depends on the individual's working proximity to the oven during the coking process.

The Occupational Safety and Health Administration (OSHA) has established a Permissible Exposure Limit (PEL) to coke oven emissions at 150 $\mu g\ m^{-3}$ of air determined as an average over an 8 h period. Respirators must be worn by workers that may be exposed to levels that exceed this limit. Workers must wear appropriate, clean, protective clothing and equipment to protect them from repeated skin contact with coke oven emissions and from the heat generated during the coking process. Any individual working in a regulated area for at least 30 days per year must be provided with a medical examination every year. The initial examination includes a posterior–anterior chest X-ray reading, pulmonary function tests, weight, urinalysis, skin examination, and a urinary cytologic examination, for detection of urinary cancer. These tests serve as the baseline for comparing the employee's future test results.

Toxicokinetics

Since coke oven emissions are complex mixtures of coal and coke particles, specific information is not available. In general, coke oven emissions are well absorbed from the respiratory tract, skin, and the conjunctiva. Disposition of absorbed chemicals will vary with the individual compound but is expected to follow kinetic behavior typical of that compound.

Mechanism of Toxicity

Complex chemical mixtures in coke oven emissions are known to result in DNA adduct formation. Free oxygen radicals and CYP450 are implicated in the pathogenesis. PAHs, which are primary compounds in coke oven emissions generated by the coking process, cause cancer and mutagenesis by a multitude of mechanisms including DNA adduct formation and metabolism.

Acute and Short-Term Toxicity

Animal

Animal studies have reported weakness, depression, dyspnea, general edema, and effects on the liver from acute oral exposure to coke oven emissions.

Human

Acute exposure to coke oven emissions produces irritation of the eyes, respiratory symptoms like cough, dyspnea, and wheezing.

Chronic Toxicity

Animal

Chronic oral dosing of coke oven emissions has been reported to cause liver toxicity in experimental animals. Chronic exposure to emissions from coke ovens has also been associated with the development of various types of cancers.

Human

Chronic exposure to coke oven emissions in humans results in conjunctivitis, severe dermatitis, and lesions of the respiratory system and digestive tract. Chronic exposure to emissions from coke ovens has also been associated with the development of various types of cancers.

Immunotoxicity

PAHs have been reported to suppress immune reactions in rodents. The precise mechanism responsible for this effect has not been identified.

Reproductive Toxicity

No specific information is available on the reproductive or developmental effects of coke oven emissions in animals or humans but several of the individual components have been studied in animals.

Studies on the embryotoxicity of the PAH BaP after oral administration of 120 $mg\ kg^{-1}$ bw day^{-1} to pregnant mice (during days 2–10 of gestation) indicated that it is embryotoxic in certain strains but not others, dependent primarily on their aryl hydrocarbon receptor status and the inducibility of cytochrome P450 enzymes. Fetal malformations were seen in some strains but not others. This dose of BaP was also reported to cause maternal toxicity.

In another study, CD1 mice were given 10, 40, or 160 $mg\ kg^{-1}$ bw day^{-1} of BaP by gavage on days 7–16 of pregnancy. Reduced survival of the pups was observed at the two highest doses and body weight was reduced at all dose levels. The fertility of the male offspring was markedly affected; pups exposed to the two highest doses were sterile, and there was a 20% decrease in fertility at the lowest dose. Exposure to PAHs from coke oven emissions could contribute to increased levels of bulky DNA adducts in sperm.

A number of metals (e.g., arsenic, cadmium and mercury) found in coke oven emissions have well-known reproductive and developmental toxicities.

Genotoxicity

Again, because coke oven emissions are a mixture of numerous chemicals, genotoxicity must reflect the genotoxicity of the individual components. PAHs have been demonstrated to be genotoxic *in vivo* in rodents and *in vitro* using mammalian cell lines. Many of the parent PAH molecules are not genotoxic themselves but must be activated by metabolism. For example BaP undergoes a series of metabolic steps to reach the ultimate mutagen, the diol epoxide, which reacts with DNA.

Carcinogenicity

In animals, extracts and condensates of coke oven emissions were found to be carcinogenic in both inhalation studies and skin painting bioassays. The mutagenicity of whole extracts and condensates, as well as their individual components, provides supportive evidence for carcinogenicity. In addition, several inhalation exposure studies in laboratory animals have provided evidence of the carcinogenic effect of aerosols of coal tar and its fractions. The extract was found to produce papillomas and skin carcinomas in the mice and acted as an initiating agent, although the extent to which this extract is representative of coke oven emissions is uncertain since the sample was contaminated with particulate matter from ambient air. Numerous carcinogenicity studies have shown that coal tar samples applied topically to the skin of laboratory animals produce local tumors.

Coke oven emissions are classified by the Environmental Protection Agency as a Group A, known human carcinogen. The cancer sites include the skin, respiratory system, kidneys, and urinary bladder. Studies of coke oven workers have shown increased risk of mortality from cancer of the lung, trachea, and bronchus; cancer of the kidneys; cancer of the prostrate; and cancer at all sites combined. Depending on the segment of the population considered, the respiratory cancer risk for coke oven workers was as high as four and a half times the risk for non-oven workers. To evaluate a biologically effective exposure dose in human biomonitoring studies, DNA carcinogen adduct analysis is frequently used. OSHA has not identified thresholds for carcinogens that will protect 100% of the population. It usually recommends that occupational exposures to carcinogens be limited to the lowest detectable concentration. To ensure maximum protection from carcinogens through the use of respiratory protection, only the most reliable and protective respirators are recommended. The OSHA PEL for benzene-soluble fraction of coke oven emissions is 0.150 mg m^{-3}.

Clinical Management

The exposed person should be moved to fresh air at once. If breathing has stopped, mouth-to-mouth resuscitation should be performed. The affected person should be kept warm and at rest. Exposed eyes should be washed immediately with large amounts of water; the lower and upper lids should be lifted occasionally. Medical attention should be obtained immediately.

Ecotoxicology

Once released into the environment, the individual components that make up coke oven emissions will act differently. PAHs often absorb to dust particles in the air and can be widely dispersed, ultimately settling to the land or water. If exposed to direct sunlight they may undergo photooxidation and be degraded in a period of days to weeks. Even so, PAHs are moderately persistent in the environment. PAHs are insoluble in water but enter aquatic systems by absorption to particulates that precipitate as sediments, or by dissolving in oily materials that contaminate water.

The acute toxicity of PAHs to aquatic life and birds is moderate and mammals can absorb these compounds through dermal contact, inhalation, or ingestion. Bioaccumulation and biomagnification of PAHs can be significant in fish and shellfish. Bioaccumulation has also been shown in terrestrial invertebrates but metabolism of PAHs is sufficient to prevent biomagnification.

Metals are also emitted as particulates during coke production. They can be dispersed into the atmosphere or deposited in soil or water. Either way, they will enter the normal biogeochemical cycle characteristic of that metal.

Exposure Standards and Guidelines

The OSHA standard for coke oven emissions is a PEL of 0.15 mg m^{-3} as an 8 h time-weighted average (TWA). Under this standard, specific engineering and work practice control requirements became effective. OSHA has also promulgated a PEL of <0.2 mg m^{-3} as an 8 h TWA for coal tar pitch volatiles. National Institute for Occupational Safety and Health and OSHA have recommended work practices to minimize the harmful effects of exposure to coke oven emissions.

All OSHA standards are listed and described in the Code of Federal Regulations (2011), Title 29 (Labor), Part 1910 (Occupational Safety and Health), Subpart Z (Toxic and Hazardous Substances), Section 1910.1029 (Coke Oven Emissions).

Miscellaneous

Coke production in the United States steadily increased between 1880s and 1950s, peaking at 72 million tons in 1951. In 1976, the United States ranked number in the world with 52.9 million tons of coke or 14.4% of the world production. By 1998 the number had declined to 23 coking plants operating about 3800 ovens. Although, the by-product process is designed to collect the volatile materials given off during the coke process, emissions escape because of structural defects around the doors or changing lids, improper use of engineering controls, improper work practices, and insufficient engineering controls.

See also: Coal Tar; Occupational Toxicology; Benz[a]anthracene; Benzo(a)pyrene; Chrysene; Creosote (Coal Tar Creosote and Wood Creosote); Arsenic; Cadmium; Mercury; Phenanthrene.

Further Reading

Chao, M.R., Wang, C.J., Wu, M.T., et al., 2008. Repeated measurements of urinary methylated/oxidative DNA lesions, acute toxicity, and mutagenicity in coke oven workers. Cancer Epidemiol. Biomarkers Prev. 17 (12), 3381–3389.

Chen, M.L., Mao, I.F., Wu, M.T., et al., 1999. Assessment of coke oven emissions exposure among coking workers. Am. Ind. Hyg. Assoc. J. 60, 105–110.

Code of Federal Regulations (CFR) 29,1926.1129. U.S. Government Printing Office, Supt. of Documents, Washington, DC 20402.
Costantino, J.P., Redmond, C.K., Bearden, A., 1995. Occupationally related cancer risk among coke oven workers 30 years of follow up. J. Occup. Environ. Med. 37, 597–604.
Hu, Y., Chen, B., Qian, J., et al., 2010. Occupational coke oven emissions exposure and risk of abnormal liver function: modifications of body mass index and hepatitis virus infection. Occup. Environ. Med. 67 (3), 159–165.
Jeng, H.A., Pan, C.H., Lin, W.Y., et al., 2013. Biomonitoring of polycyclic aromatic hydrocarbons from coke oven emissions and reproductive toxicity in nonsmoking workers. J. Hazard. Mater. 244–245, 436–443.
Keimig, D.G., Slymen, D.J., White Jr, O., 1986. Occupational exposure to coke oven emissions from 1979–1983. Arch. Environ. Health 41, 363–367.
Khare, P., Baruah, B.P., 2011. Estimation of emissions of SO2, PM2.5, and metals released from coke ovens using high sulfur coals. Environ. Prog. Sustain. Energy 30, 123–129.
National Toxicology Program, 2011. Coke-oven emissions. In: Report on Carcinogens, vol. 12, pp. 120–122.
Report on Carcinogens, 2011. Coke Oven Emissions, twelfth ed. National Toxicology Program, Department of Health and Human Services. p. 120.
Toxicological Profile for Polycyclic Aromatic Hydrocarbons, 1995. U.S. Department of Health and Human Services, Public Health Service, Agency for Toxic Substances and Disease Registry.
U.S. Department of Health and Human Services, 1993. Hazardous Substances Data Bank (HSDB, Online Database). National Toxicology Information Program, National Library of Medicine, Bethesda, MD.
U.S. Environmental Protection Agency, 1999. Integrated Risk Information System (IRIS) on Coke Oven Emissions. National Center for Environmental Assessment, Office of Research and Development, Washington, DC.
Zhai, Q., Duan, H., Wang, Y., et al., 2012. Genetic damage induced by organic extract of coke oven emissions on human bronchial epithelial cells. Toxicol. *In Vitro* 26 (5), 752–758.

Relevant Websites

http://www.osha.gov/dts/chemicalsampling/data/CH_229200.html – US Dept. of Labor.
http://www.cdc.gov/niosh/npg/npgd0149.html – Centers for Disease Control and Prevention: NIOSH Pocket Guide to Chemical Standards: Coke oven emissions.
http://www.cdc.gov/niosh-rtecs/GH54790.html – National Institute for Occupational Safety and Health: Coke oven emissions.
http://www.epa.gov/ttnatw01/hlthef/cokeoven.html – US Environmental Protection Agency - Technology Transfer Network - Air Toxics Web Site: Coke oven emissions.
http://www.epa.gov/iris/subst/0395.htm – US Environmental Protection Agency - Integrated Risk Information System: Coke oven emissions.
http://ntp.niehs.nih.gov/ntp/roc/twelfth/profiles/CokeOvenEmissions.pdf – Report on Carcinogens, Twelfth Edition (2011): Coke-Oven Emissions.
https://www.osha.gov/pls/oshaweb/owadisp.show_document?p_table=STANDARDS&p_id=10049 - US Department of Labor - Occupational Safety & Health Administration: Coke oven emissions substance information sheet.

Colchicine

HA Spiller, Central Ohio Poison Center, Columbus, OH, USA

- Name: Colchicine
- Chemical Abstracts Service Registry Number: 64-86-8
- Description: Colchicine is obtained from the autumn crocus, *Colchicum autumnale*, or the glory lily, *Gloriosa superba*
- Pharmaceutical Class: Naturally occurring alkaloid
- Molecular Formula: $C_{22}H_{25}NO_6$
- Chemical Structure:

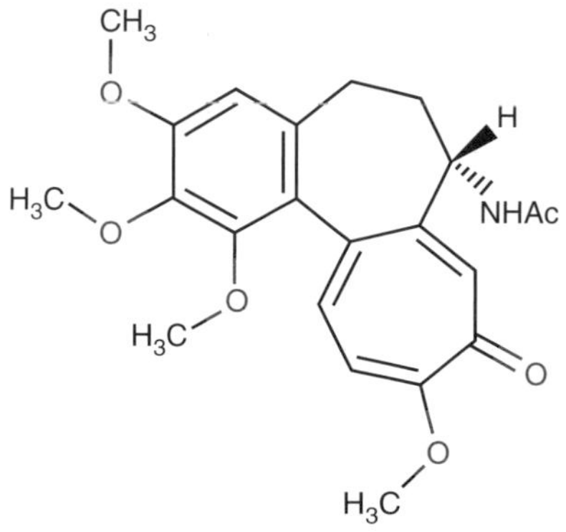

Uses

Colchicine is used in the treatment of acute gouty arthritis. Unlabeled uses include treatment of familial Mediterranean fever, neoplasms of the skin, Behcet's disease, scleroderma, sarcoidosis, and cirrhosis of the liver. Colchicine has been recently gaining acceptance as a treatment for acute and recurrent pericarditis. It is also available as a pesticide for moles and gofers.

Background Information

Descriptions regarding use of *Colchicum autumnale* (meadow saffron) for swelling and types of inflammatory arthritis date back to the first century AD. Use of the extract was described in the Ebers Papyrus (an Egyptian papyrus). *Colchicum* plants were introduced to the Americas by Benjamin Franklin who suffered from gout and used an extract to treat his condition. Colchicine was first isolated from *C. autumnale* in 1820 by the French chemists Pelletier and Caventou.

Environmental Fate

Physicochemical Properties

Colchicine is a phenanthrene derivative and a pale yellow chemical that darkens upon exposure to light. It is odorless and has a melting point of 153–157 °C. The pH of a 0.5% solution is acidic at 5.9. Colchicine is soluble in water at 45 g l^{-1} at 20 °C. It is also soluble in ethanol and chloroform.

No information is currently available on breakdown in soil, groundwater, or surface water. Colchicine alkaloids withstand storage, drying, and boiling.

Exposure Pathways

Ingestion is the most common route of both accidental and intentional exposure to colchicine. It is available as an oral tablet and solution for injection.

Toxicokinetics

Colchicine is readily absorbed from the gastrointestinal tract. In therapeutic dosing, peak serum levels occur in 30–120 min. Colchicine undergoes deacetylation and hydrolysis in the liver. It has a rapid initial distribution phase, with a plasma half-life of 19 or 20 min, suggesting swift uptake by the tissues. The volume of distribution is 2.2 l kg^{-1}. Up to 40% of colchicine is excreted in the urine, with 20–30% of this as unchanged drug. The majority of the drug undergoes enterohepatic recirculation and is excreted via bile and feces. The average elimination half-life is 20 h.

Mechanism of Toxicity

Colchicine binds to tubulin and prevents its polymerization into microtubules, subsequently disrupting microtubule function. Consequently, it alters nuclear structure, intracellular transport, and cytoplasmic motility, ultimately causing cell death. Colchicine is a potent inhibitor of cellular mitosis.

Acute Toxicity

Human Toxicity

Colchicine toxicity has been divided into three stages. The first stage, from 2 to 24 h, is the gastrointestinal phase, notable for abdominal pain, vomiting, diarrhea, and a prominent leukocytosis. The gastrointestinal symptoms may be relieved by atropine, but this does not prevent or alter the onset of the second stage. The second stage is marked by multisystem failure. Most life-threatening symptoms occur 24–72 h postexposure. Confusion, delirium, coma, seizures, and cerebral edema may occur. Progressive respiratory distress and pulmonary edema can occur. After an initial leukocytosis, bone marrow depression is seen with a nadir between the fourth and the seventh day. Bone marrow depression, coupled with potential gastrointestinal hemorrhages and a hemolytic anemia, may produce profound anemia. Consumptive coagulopathy may also be seen. Renal function may be affected by direct organ damage as well as by decreased perfusion from profound and persistent hypotension. Cardiovascular instability along with metabolic

 http://dx.doi.org/10.1016/B978-0-12-386454-3.00717-X

acidosis may develop due to volume depletion, cardiac failure, and arrhythmias. Most deaths result from shock in the 24- to 72-h period. Stage three is the recovery phase. If patients survive to this convalescent phase, the main complication is sepsis.

Animal Toxicity

Animal toxicity is primarily related to ingestion of the plant *C. autumnale*. Colchicine is available as a pesticide for burrowing animals. The estimated toxic dose for cows is 10 g kg^{-1} with fresh leaves or 2 or 3 g kg^{-1} with dried leaves. Symptoms may include gait disorders, hypersalivation, bloody vomitus, and diarrhea. Death within 72 h has occurred secondary to shock. It is only slightly toxic to cold-blooded and hibernating animals.

Chronic Toxicity

Chronic toxicity seen with colchicines is similar to that seen during acute exposure for both humans and animals.

Immunotoxicity

Colchicine can inhibit the production of neutrophils and lymphocytes and also cause bone marrow inhibition at high doses. Hypersensitivity reactions have been reported.

Genotoxicity

Colchicine is genotoxic. It causes gene mutations, DNA damage, and chromosomal damage in *in vitro* and *in vivo* assays.

Reproductive Toxicity

Animal studies have indicated that colchicine may be teratogenic. Teratogenic effects were observed in mice and hamsters given 0.5 and 10 mg kg^{-1} colchicines, respectively. In a case of an 18-year-old pregnant patient exposed to 40 mg of colchicine, the fetus was aborted on day 7 after poisoning and the patient developed acute respiratory distress syndrome although survived. In women treated with colchicines for familial Mediterranean fever, 7 out of 28 pregnancies ended in miscarriage. All the 16 infants born in this group were healthy. Azospermia, that is reversible, has been reported in males taking colchicines and two cases of Down syndrome have been reported in babies born to mothers taking colchicines. Some authors recommend that amniocentesis for karyotyping and reassurance be recommended in mothers taking colchicines during pregnancy. Colchicine is eliminated in the breast milk and should be avoided during breast-feeding.

Carcinogenicity

Since colchicine is a known mutagen it is thought to be potentially carcinogenic.

Clinical Management

Basic and advanced life-support measures should be utilized as necessary. Treatment of colchicine toxicity is largely supportive. Activated charcoal effectively adsorbs colchicine and should be administered. Aggressive early gastrointestinal decontamination may be lifesaving. However, activated charcoal may be of use up to 24 h postingestion. Severe anemia may require packed red blood cell replacement. Coagulopathies may respond to vitamin K and fresh frozen plasma. Hypotension may be unresponsive to fluid replacement and pressor support. Due to rapid tissue distribution and the large volume of distribution, hemoperfusion and hemodialysis are ineffective. Colchicine Fab fragments have effectively reversed hypotension and increased survival in animals and humans in the research setting but are not commercially available.

Ecotoxicity

Colchicine is extremely dangerous for water. It is water danger class III (German Regulation) and should not reach groundwater, sewage, or water treatment system.

See also: Atropine; Charcoal; Omics and Related Recent Technologies; Pesticides; Poisoning Emergencies in Humans.

Further Reading

Baud, F.J., Sabouraud, A., Vicaut, E., Taboulet, P., Lang, J., Bismuth, C., Rouzious, J.M., Scherrmann, J.M., 1995. Brief report: treatment of severe colchicine overdose with colchicines-specific fab fragments. N. Engl. J. Med. 332 (10), 642–645.

Imazio, M., Brucato, A., Cemin, R., Ferrua, S., Maggiolini, S., Begaraj, F., Demarie, D., Forno, D., Ferro, S., Maestroni, S., Belli, R., Trinchero, R., Spodick, D.H., Adler, Y., August 2013. A randomized trial of colchicines for acute pericarditis. N. Engl. J. Med. (Epub ahead of print).

Lauer, E., Widmer, C., Versace, F., Staub, C., Mangin, P., Sabatasso, S., Augsburger, M., Deglon, J., May 16, 2013. Body fluid and tissue analysis using filter paper sampling support prior to LC-MS/MS: application to fatal overdose with colchicines. Drug Test. Anal. http://dx.doi.org/10.1002/dta.1496 (Epub ahead of print).

Lilly, L.S., 2013. Treatment for acute and recurrent idiopathic pericarditis. Circulation 127 (16), 1723–1726.

Little, A., Tung, D., Truong, C., Lapinsky, S., Burry, L., 2013. Colchicine overdose with coingestion of nonsteroidal anti-inflammatory drugs. CJEM 15 (0), 1–5.

Maxwell, M.J., Muthu, P., Pritty, P.E., 2002. Accidental colchicine overdose. A case report literature review. Emerg. Med. J. 19, 265–266.

Montiel, V., Huberlant, V., Vincent, M.F., Bonbled, F., Hantson, P., 2010. Multiple organ failure after an overdose of less than 0.4 mg/kg of colchicine: role of coingestants and drugs during intensive care management. Clin. Toxicol. 48, 845–848.

Sapra, S., Bhalla, Y., Nandani, Sharma, S., Singh, G., Nepali, K., Budhiraja, A., Dhar, K.L., 2013. Colchicine and its various physicochemical and biological aspects. Med. Chem. Res. 22 (2), 531–537.

Relevant Websites

http://www.inchem.org/documents/pims/pharm/colchic.htm – Inchem – website for toxicology information regarding colchicines.

http://livertox.nih.gov/Colchicine.htm – National Library of Medicine – Liver Tox database and description of colchicines and mechanism of hepatotoxicity.

Combustion Toxicology

SC Gad, Gad Consulting Services, Cary, NC, USA

This article is a revision of the previous edition article by Barbara C. Levin, Erica D. Kuligowski, volume 1, pp 639–652, © 2005, Elsevier Inc.

Combustion toxicity research is the study of the adverse health effects caused by exposure to fire atmospheres. A fire atmosphere is defined as all of the effluents generated by the thermal decomposition of materials or products regardless of whether that effluent is produced under smoldering, nonflaming, or flaming conditions. The objectives of combustion toxicity research are to identify potentially harmful products from the thermal degradation of materials, to distinguish those materials that produce unusual or greater quantities of toxic combustion products, to determine the best measurement methods for the identification of the toxic products as well as the degree of toxicity, to determine the effect of different fire exposures on the composition of the toxic combustion products, and to establish the physiological effects of such products on living organisms. The ultimate goals of this field of research are to reduce human fire fatalities due to smoke inhalation, to determine effective treatments for survivors, and to prevent unnecessary suffering of fire casualties caused by smoke inhalation.

Fire Death Statistics

The latest statistics from the US National Fire Protection Association (NFPA) report that the fire death rate in the United States was 1.3 times higher (2.1 times more if the New York City deaths from the 11 September 2001 terrorist attacks are included) than in the United Kingdom, 1.16 times more than in Sweden, 1.3 times less than for Japan (or 1.3 times more if the deaths from the 11 September 2001 terrorist attacks are included), and about the same as that in Canada. Although the reasons are still being debated, the number of fire deaths per capita since 1977 have been higher in the United States and Canada than in most of the other industrialized nations outside of the former Union of Soviet Socialist Republics.

Fire statistics collected by NFPA indicated that 1 687 500 fires were reported in the United States in 2002, the latest year for which complete statistics are available at the time of this writing. Calculated another way, these statistics translate into a reported fire occurring in the United States every 19 s, in an outside property every 38 s, in a structure every 61 s, in a residence every 67 s, and in a motor vehicle every 96 s. These fires caused ~3380 civilian deaths and 18 425 reported injuries in 2002. Excluding New York City's World Trade Center deaths from the 11 September 2001 terrorist attacks, in which 2326 civilian deaths occurred, the number of deaths in 2002 decreased by almost 10% from the previous year. However, there was still one civilian fire death every 156 min and one fire injury every 28 min. The number for injuries is believed to be less than the actual number, since many injuries are not reported.

In 2002, residential fires accounted for only 24% of the total fires, but were responsible for 79% of all the fire deaths and 76% of the reported injuries. Although in the years 1977–2002 the number of civilian fire fatalities in homes dropped from 5865 to 2670, fires in homes still cause the greatest concern to the fire community. Statistics show that children under 5 and adults over 65 years of age are the most frequent casualties of residential fires. This is attributed to their inherent difficulties in trying to escape. Statistics also show that males are more likely to die in fires than females. More fires and higher fire death rates occur in the South than any of the other geographical areas of the United States; the geographical region with the next highest fire death rate and number of fires is the Northeast.

One must distinguish between the causes of fires and the causes of fire deaths. The primary causes of residential fires have been shown to be heating and cooking. Lack of central heat and the incorrect use of portable space heaters are two of the reasons given for the high fire and death rate in the South. Heating fires result in the highest property losses, primarily because cooking fires are usually noticed and extinguished before getting out of control. Fire deaths, however, usually result from fires ignited by cigarettes. The most common fire scenario leading to fire deaths is one in which a person (usually intoxicated) falls asleep in an upholstered chair while smoking. The cigarette falls into a crevice and starts the upholstered chair smoldering. The individual awakes and goes to bed. The chair can smolder for an extended period of time (in laboratory tests, an hour was not unusual) before bursting into flames. It is after the flaming starts that the smoke fills the room and escapes to other rooms. It is common to find people who have died from smoke inhalation (not burns) in or near their beds, indicating that the little or no effort to escape was probably due to lack of awareness of the danger. Smoke detectors in this type of scenario would save many lives. Statistics have shown that working smoke detectors double one's probability of escaping alive. Recent statistics have also shown that many homes have nonfunctioning smoke detectors due to being disconnected after a false alarm (usually from smoke from cooking or a wood stove) or when the beeping indicating the need for a new battery became annoying.

Since most of the deaths from fires occur in residences, the NFPA proposes the following safety initiatives to improve fire safety:

1. Increase fire safety education on fire prevention and what to do if a fire occurs.
2. Install smoke detectors in all homes and check them periodically to ensure they are working properly.
3. Practice escape plans with the entire family.
4. Install residential home sprinklers to prevent fires from spreading once they start.
5. Develop products for the home that are more fire safe and produce fewer and lower masses of toxic combustion products (the latter is proposed by the authors).
6. Study the needs of the populations most at risk (the young, the elderly, and the poor) and implement preventative measures.

 http://dx.doi.org/10.1016/B978-0-12-386454-3.00596-0

The US Fire Administration has issued the following Home Fire Safety Checklist:

- Smoke detectors, are they:
  - Placed near bedrooms.
  - On every floor.
  - Places away from air vents.
  - Checked regularly for working batteries.
- Electrical wiring, is it:
  - Replaced if frayed or cracked
  - Not placed under rugs, over nails, or in high traffic areas
  - Are the outlets:
    - Not overloaded
    - Cool to the touch, not hot
    - Covered with cover plates
- Electrical space heaters, are they:
  - Plugged directly into a wall socket with no extension cords.
  - Unplugged when not in use.
- Kerosene heaters, are they:
  - Used only in permitted geographical areas.
  - Filed only with K-1 kerosene, never gasoline or camp stove fuel.
  - Only refueled outdoors and when cool.
- Woodstoves and fireplaces, are they:
  - Used only with seasoned wood, never used with green wood, Wolmanized chromate copper arsenate (CCA)-treated wood, pressure-treated wood, artificial logs, or trash.

After 30 December 2003, Wolmanized CCA-treated wood (also called Wolmanized pressure-treated wood) was no longer be produced for nonindustrial applications. This wood had been preserved by pressure treatment with a US-registered pesticide containing CCA to protect it from termite attack and decay. Wood treated with CCA should be used only where such protection is important. Exposure to CCA or its combustion products presents certain hazards. Therefore, the following precautions should be taken both when handling the treated wood and in determining where to use and how to dispose of the treated wood. Treated wood should not be burned in open fires or in stoves, fireplaces or residential boilers because toxic chemicals are produced as part of the smoke and ashes (see section 'Relevant Websites'). The Journal of the American Medical Association (in 1984) reported that a Wisconsin family who had burned CCA-containing wood scraps in their home furnace for heating purposes experienced their hair falling out, rashes, severe reoccurring nosebleeds, extreme fatigue, and debilitating headaches. The parents spoke of black-out periods that would last for several hours with long periods of extreme disorientation following them. The two children also reported experiencing frequent seizures. Since arsenic affects not just humans but any pets and wildlife, the family noticed their houseplants and fish had died as well. Later, all the serious health effects were attributed to the family breathing in minute amounts of arsenic dust that had accumulated in the ashes.

  - Protected by screens
  - Cleaned regularly along with flues, interiors, hearths, and chimneys.
- All alternate heaters, are they:
  - Used only in well-ventilated rooms
  - Stable such that they cannot be easily knocked over
  - Never used to dry clothing or other items
  - Kept at a safe distance from curtains or furniture
- Home escape plan
  - Is it practiced every 6 months
  - Are the emergency numbers, a whistle, and a flashlight kept near the telephone
  - Is the outside meeting place identified

Generation of Toxic Gases in Fires: Adverse Effects of Particulates

Eighty percent of the residential fire deaths are attributed to smoke inhalation, not to burns. Smoke is defined by ASTM International (ASTM, formerly the American Society for Testing and Materials) as "the airborne solid and liquid particulates and gases evolved when a material undergoes pyrolysis or combustion." The adverse effects from smoke inhalation are believed to be due mainly to the exposure to toxic gases, although the role of particulates alone and in combination with fire gases needs further investigation. The importance, therefore, of determining the identities and concentrations of toxic gases produced from materials thermally decomposed under various fire conditions is evident. In addition, the increased variety of plastics in buildings and homes has raised the issue of whether synthetic materials may produce unusually or extremely toxic combustion products. In 1975, the journal Science documented a case in which an experimental rigid polyurethane foam containing a fire retardant produced a very unusual toxic combustion product identified as 4-ethyl-1-phospha-2,6,7-trioxabicyclo[2.2.2]octane-1-oxide (commonly referred to as a bicyclic phosphate ester). Bicyclic phosphate compounds have been shown to cause seizures at very low concentrations. Based on these test results, this product never became commercially available. To a large extent, however, it was this case that generated the burgeoning interest in the field of 'combustion toxicology' and the widespread concern about the potential formation of 'supertoxicants.' Although research since the 1970s has shown that this concern is largely unfounded, the bicyclophosphate ester case and at least one other product that generated extremely toxic combustion products have indicated the need to test new formulations or materials containing new combinations of compounds to ensure that extremely or unusually toxic products are not generated.

The gas composition of smoke depends on the chemical composition, the molecular structure, and polymer formulation of the burning material, which may include a variety of additives, plasticizers, stabilizers, flame retardants, cross-linking agents, fillers, and blowing agents. In addition, the conditions of thermal degradation, for example, temperature, oxygen availability, and ventilation, will affect the nature of the combustion atmosphere. In a series of reviews of the combustion products and toxicity of seven plastics (acrylonitrile-butadiene-styrenes (ABS), nylons, polyesters, polyethylenes, polystyrenes, poly(vinyl chlorides) (PVC), and rigid polyurethane foams) commonly found in residences, and decomposed under various thermal and atmospheric conditions, over 400 different decomposition products were noted. Many of these products were common to more than one plastic. In addition, there are probably many other combustion products that were not detected. The toxicity of most of these individual compounds is currently unknown, and little has been done to tackle the enormous problem of determining the toxicity of combinations of these compounds. It is important to note that lack of detection of a specific combustion product from a material may only mean that the particular analytical techniques used were not suitable to detect that compound or that the investigator did not specifically analyze for that combustion product. Toxicity testing, for example, on animals, becomes important to ensure that an unsuspected and therefore undetected toxic by-product has not been formed.

Since the number of compounds one can reasonably analyze in any one test is limited, knowledge of the chemical composition, molecular structure, and formulation of the polymer can be used to provide some indication of the main gaseous products that may or may not be generated under specified experimental conditions. However, one needs to be cautious when predicting the combustion products from generic materials of unknown formulations. For example, one would expect nitrogen-containing materials (e.g., ABS, nylons, rigid and flexible polyurethanes) to produce hydrogen cyanide (HCN) and would not expect HCN from a material like PVC. However, a PVC-containing zinc ferrocyanide (an additive designed to suppress smoke) as well as a vinyl chloride-vinylidene chloride copolymer was found to generate HCN. In a similar fashion, based on the chemical composition, PVC is the only one of the seven plastics mentioned that would be expected to generate chlorinated combustion products. However, widespread usage of halogenated fire retardants in plastic formulations makes predicting which materials will products halogenated products extremely difficult.

Temperature also plays an important role in influencing the production of decomposition products. In general, as the temperature and thus the rate of decomposition increase, the quantity of the more complex compounds and heavier hydrocarbons decreases and the concentrations of carbon monoxide (CO), carbon dioxide (CO_2), and nitrogen dioxide (NO_2) increase. The generation of HCN has also been shown to increase as a function of temperature. Another example is hydrogen chloride (HCl), the detection of which begins when stabilized PVC is heated to $\sim$200 °C; rapid dehydrochlorination then occurs at $\sim$300 °C. On the contrary, more acrolein was generated from polyethylene under lower temperature, nonflaming conditions than under higher temperature, flaming conditions.

As mentioned earlier, more work is needed to examine the adverse effects of the particulate matter produced when these materials are thermally decomposed. Examination of the smoke particulate and condensable matter is important for a number of reasons. First, many of the thermal degradation products may condense or be adsorbed by the soot particles and be transported along with the smoke into the body. Hydrogen chloride is one example of a compound that may be transported in such a fashion and can form a corrosive acid mist in moist air, such as that found in the lung. One study of the particulate matter that formed during the smoldering decomposition of rigid polyurethane foam showed that many of the compounds detected in the soot fraction were not found in the volatile fraction. Free radicals, which form in fires and are of toxicological concern due to their high reactivity, are usually considered to have very short life spans; however, if adsorbed onto soot particles, their lifetimes can be considerably longer and, if the soot particles are the correct size, they can be inhaled into the individual's deep lungs. In addition, the particulate matter may interfere with the escape and rescue of individuals by causing the obscuration of vision, eye irritation (the eyes clamp shut and the victim is unable to see), and upper respiratory distress. An extreme case indicating the adverse effect of particulates was noted in experiments conducted at the US National Institute of Standards and Technology (NIST). Rats exposed for 30 min to the smoke from polystyrene died during the exposures, and the level of CO in the blood, even in combination with CO_2, was too low to be fatally toxic. Pathological examination of these rats showed that their respiratory passages were completely blocked by soot and that suffocation was the likely cause of death.

Toxic Potency versus Fire Hazard versus Fire Risk

Death in a fire may be caused by:

1. Carbon monoxide (CO)
2. Toxic gases in addition to CO
3. Oxygen (O_2) at levels too low to sustain life
4. Incapacitation – either physical (inability to escape) or mental (incorrect decision-making)
5. Bodily burns from flame contact
6. Very high air temperatures
7. Smoke density or irritants in smoke that affect vision and interfere with ability to escape
8. Psychological effects (e.g., fear, shock, and panic)
9. Physical insults (e.g., building or ceiling collapses, broken bones from jumping from upper floors)

Research in the field of combustion toxicology is primarily concerned with items 1–4, all of which are related to the toxic potency of the fire gas effluent. Toxic potency is defined by ASTM as "a quantitative expression relating concentration (of smoke or combustion gases) and exposure time to a particular degree of adverse physiological response, for example, death on exposure of humans or animals." This definition is followed by a discussion, which states, "The toxic potency of smoke from any material or product or assembly is related to the composition of that smoke which, in turn, is dependent upon the conditions under which the smoke is generated." One should add that the LC_{50} is a common end point used in laboratories to assess toxic potency. In the comparison of the toxic potencies of different compounds or materials, the lower the LC_{50} (i.e., the smaller the amount of material necessary to reach the toxic end point), the more toxic the material.

It is important to note that a toxicity assessment based on lethality due to toxic gases is only part of the total fire hazard that needs to be evaluated, especially when one is making choices as to the best material for a specific end use. ASTM defines 'fire hazard' as the potential for harm associated with fire. The discussion that follows this definition states, "A fire may pose one or more types of hazards to people, animals, or property. These hazards are associated with the environment and with a number of fire-test-response characteristics of materials, products, or assemblies including but not limited to ease of ignition, flame spread, rate of heat release, smoke generation and obscuration, toxicity of combustion products and ease of extinguishment." Other factors that need to be evaluated when considering a material for use in a given situation include the quantity of material needed, its configuration, the proximity of other combustibles, the volume of the compartments to which the combustion products may spread, the ventilation conditions, the ignition and combustion properties of the material and other materials present, the presence of ignition sources, the presence of fire protection systems, the number and type of occupants, and the time necessary to escape.

'Fire risk' is defined by ASTM as "an estimation of expected fire loss that combines the potential for harm in various fire scenarios that can occur with the probabilities of occurrence of those scenarios." The discussion following the definition of fire risk states, "Risk may be defined as the probability of having a certain type of fire, where the type of fire may be defined in whole or in part by the degree of potential harm associated with it, or as potential for harm weighted by associated probabilities. Risk scales do not imply a single value of acceptable risk. Different individuals presented with the same risk situation may have different opinions on its acceptability." A simple way to explain the difference between fire risk is to compare the fire to skydiving, a very hazardous sport; however, if one never goes skydiving, no risk is incurred.

Toxicity Assessment: Animal Exposures

In most combustion toxicology experiments, the biological end point has been lethality or incapacitation of experimental animals, usually rats or mice. Incapacitation in a fire can be as perilous as lethality if an individual becomes incapable of correct decision-making or physically unable to move. Under these circumstances, the ability to escape will be lost and death will occur unless the individual is rescued. Therefore, many fire scientists are concerned with the levels of combustion products or amounts of materials that when combusted will cause incapacitation. However, an incapacitation model for use in laboratory testing has been especially difficult to develop. Most of the tests for incapacitation that have been designed are based on the physical–motor capability of an experimental animal to perform some task (e.g., running in a motorized wheel, jumping onto a pole or lifting a paw to escape a shock, running in a maze, or pushing the correct lever to open a door to escape from an irritating atmosphere). The concentration of toxic combustion products that cause the loss of these types of physical–motor capabilities is usually close to the concentration that is lethal and does not usually add much additional information. More recently, however, there have been attempts at examining neurological end points such as measuring the increased number of errors by humans doing mathematical problems while exposed to low levels of CO or exposing rats and pigeons to a complete neurobehavioral battery of 15 tests following nonlethal toxic exposures.

Whether one needs to examine incapacitation or lethality depends on the problem one is trying to solve. To determine the best material for a particular end-use application, the lethality end point has proved to be more definitive and will flag the materials that produce extremely toxic combustion products better than at incapacitation end point. There are at least two reasons for this: (1) Incapacitation is only measured during the exposure, which is usually 30 min or less, but lethality can also occur during the postexposure observation period, which can be 2 weeks or longer. A material that causes only delayed effects during the postexposure period (e.g., a material that generates HCl) can thus have an LC_{50} value that is lower than the incapacitation EC_{50} value. The amount needed to kill can be less than the amount needed to incapacitate because the amount of thermally decomposed material necessary to cause postexposure deaths can be less than the amount needed to cause incapacitation during the exposure. (2) In many cases in which the combustion products contain high concentrations of irritant gases, the animals would only appear to be incapacitated (i.e., they would stop responding to the test indicator due to the high irritant quality of the smoke), but when removed from the combustion atmosphere, would immediately start responding normally.

Other delayed effects from exposures to combustion atmospheres, such as tissue or organ injury, mutagenicity, carcinogenicity, and teratogenicity also need to be studied since they may ultimately lead to permanent disability and death. The current advances in the field of genetics provide investigators with new opportunities to examine the effects of combustion products at the molecular level. One objective could be to determine whether these toxic products cause DNA damage or mutations or both. Specific problems of interest include the following: Does the damage occur in nuclear DNA and/or mitochondrial DNA? Are certain areas of the DNA more prone to these mutations (i.e., are there hot spots?)? Can we categorize the types of mutations (e.g., transitions, transversions, deletions, insertions)? How efficient are the repair mechanisms? Are there mutagens also known to be carcinogens?

Toxicity Assessment: Predictive Models

In the 1970s, there were essentially two experimental strategies to examine the issues raised by the field of combustion toxicology: (1) an analytical chemical method and (2) an animal exposure approach. In the analytical chemical method, investigators thermally decomposed materials under different experimental conditions and tried to determine every combustion product that was generated. This approach generated long lists of compounds. The toxicity of most of these individual compounds was unknown and the concept of examining the toxicity of all the various combinations of compounds was and still is considered a formidable task. An additional problem with the analytical approach was that, as mentioned earlier, the detection and identification of the toxic combustion products depended on the analytical method used. Therefore, one could not be certain that every toxic product was detected and identified. This approach enabled one to identify many of the multiple products that were generated, without knowing the toxic potency of all the identified compounds, either singly or combined.

In the animal exposure approach, the animals (usually rats or mice) serve as indicators of the degree of toxicity of the combustion atmospheres. The materials of concern are thermally decomposed under different combustion conditions and the animals are exposed to the combined particulate and gaseous effluent. Multiple animal experiments (each with multiple animals) with different concentrations of material are conducted to determine an EC_{50} (incapacitation) or an LC_{50} (lethality) for a specific set of combustion conditions. Each material would then have a particular EC_{50} or LC_{50} value that can be used to compare the toxicities of different materials decomposed under the same conditions. The lower the EC_{50} or LC_{50} value, the more toxic the combustion products from that material are considered to be. In this approach, one knows the relative toxicity of a material as compared to another material, but does not know which of the toxic gases are responsible for the adverse effects.

In the 1980s, investigators at NIST began examining the possibility of combining the analytical chemical method with the animal exposure approach to develop empirical mathematical models to predict the toxicity. These predictions were based on actual experiments with animals and their response to each of the main toxic combustions gases; CO, CO_2, low O_2, HCN, NO_2, HCl, HBr, and various combinations of these gases. The advantages of these predictive approaches are that (1) the number of necessary test animals can be reduced by first predicting the toxic potency from a limited chemical analysis of the smoke; (2) smoke may be produced under conditions that simulate any fire scenario of concern; (3) fewer tests are needed, thereby reducing the overall cost of the testing; and (4) information is obtained on both the toxic potency of the smoke (based on the mass of material burned) and the responsible gases (based on the primary toxic gases in the mixture). The prediction is checked with one or two animal tests to ensure that an unexpected gas or toxic combination has not been generated. The results of using these empirical mathematical models indicated that, in most cases, one could predict the toxic potency of a combination atmosphere based on the concentrations of the main toxic gases and did not need to worry about the effects of minor or more obscure gases.

Primary Toxic Combustion Gases

Complete combustion of a polymer containing carbon, hydrogen, and oxygen in an atmosphere with sufficient O_2 yields CO_2 and water. It is during incomplete combustion under various atmospheric conditions in either flaming or nonflaming modes that compounds of greater toxicological concern are generated. When oxygen is limited, the primary gases formed during the combustion of most organic materials are CO, CO_2, and water. If the materials contain nitrogen, HCN and NO_2, the two principal thermo-oxidative products of toxicological concern, are also likely to be generated. Halogenated or flame-retardant materials generally produce HCl or HBr. Other commonly found fire gases include nitrogen oxides, ammonia, hydrogen sulfide, sulfur dioxide, and fluorine compounds. One also needs to consider that in fire situations, oxygen levels drop and exposure to low oxygen atmospheres will have additional adverse physiological effects. Some of these toxic combustion gases produce immediate asphyxiant symptoms, while others (e.g., HCl, HBr, NO_2) fall into an irritant category and produce symptoms following the exposures.

The N-Gas Models

The N-gas models for predicting smoke toxicity were founded on the hypothesis that a small number (N) of gases in the smoke will account for a large percentage of the observed toxic potency. These predictive models were based on an extensive series of experiments conducted at NIST on the toxicological interactions of the primary gases found in fires. Both the individual gases and complex mixtures of these gases were examined. To use these models, materials are thermally decomposed using a bench-scale method that stimulates realistic fire conditions, the concentrations of the primary gases are measured, and the toxicity of the smoke using the appropriate N-gas model is predicted. The predicted toxic potency is checked with a small number of animal (Fischer 344 male rate) tests to ensure that an unanticipated toxic gas was not generated or an unexpected toxicological effect (e.g., synergism or antagonism) did not occur. The results indicate whether the smoke from a material or product is extremely toxic (based on mass consumed at the predicted toxic level) or unusually toxic (the toxicity cannot be explained by the combined measured gases). These models have been shown to correctly predict the toxicity in both bench-scale laboratory tests and full-scale room burns of a variety of materials of widely differing characteristics chosen to challenge the system. The six-gas model (without NO_2) is now included in two national toxicity test method standards (ASTM E1678), approved by ASTM, and NFPA 269, approved by the NFPA. It is also included in an international standard (ISO 13344) that was approved by 16 member countries of the ISO technical committee 92 (TC92). All three of these standards were published in 1996.

The objectives for developing the N-gas models were:

- To establish the extent to which the toxicity of a material's combustion products could be explained and predicted by the interaction of the major toxic gases generated from that material in the laboratory or whether minor and more obscure gases needed to be considered.
- To develop a bioanalytical screening test and a mathematical model that would predict whether a material would produce extremely toxic or unusually toxic combustion products.
- To predict the occupant response from the concentrations of primary toxic gases present in the environment and the time of exposure.
- To provide data for use in computer models designed to predict the hazard that people will experience under various fire scenarios.

The Six-Gas N-Gas Model

The six-gas model was based on studies at NIST on the toxicological interactions of six gases: CO, CO_2, HCN, low O_2, HCl, and HBr. First, individual gases in air were tested for LC_{50} both during and including postexposure observation periods of 14 days. The studies on HCl and HBr were conducted at Southwest Research Institute (SwRI) under a grant from NIST. Similar measurements for various combinations of these gases indicated whether the toxicity of the mixtures of gases was additive, synergistic, or antagonistic.

Based on these empirical results, the following six-gas model was developed:

$$\frac{m[CO]}{[CO_2]-b}+\frac{[HCN]}{LC_{50}HCN}+\frac{21-[O_2]}{21-LC_{50}O_2}+\frac{[HCl]}{LC_{50}HCl}+\frac{[HBr]}{LC_{50}HBr}=N-\text{gas value} \quad [1]$$

where the terms in brackets indicate the time-integrated average atmospheric concentrations during a 30 min exposure period (ppm × min) per min or for O_2 (% × min) per min. The other terms are described in the following paragraphs.

Under the experimental conditions used at NIST and with Fischer 344 male rate, the 30 min LC_{50} value of CO_2 is 47% (470 000 ppm) with 95% confidence limits of 43–51%. No deaths occurred in rats exposed to 26% CO_2 min. In a real fire, the highest theoretically possible concentration of CO_2 is 21%, a concentration that could occur only if all the atmospheric O_2 were converted to CO_2, a highly improbably event. Therefore, CO_2 concentrations generated in fires are not lethal. However, CO_2 is a respiratory stimulant, causing an increase in both respiratory rate and tidal volume. It also increases the acidosis of the blood. When combined with any of the other tested gases, CO_2 has a synergistic toxicological effect. Empirically, however, it was found that the effect of CO_2 can only be added into the six-gas N-gas equation once. Therefore, the CO_2 effect was included with the CO factor since there were more data on the effect of different concentrations of CO_2 on the toxicity of CO and CO is the toxicant most likely to be present in all fires. The results on the synergistic effect of CO_2 on CO indicated that as the concentration of CO_2 increases (up to 5%), the toxicity of CO increases. Above 5% CO_2, the toxicity of CO starts to revert back toward the toxicity of the CO by itself. The terms m and b in the equation define this synergistic interaction and equal -18 and 122 000, respectively, if the CO_2 concentrations are 5% or less. For studies in which the CO_2 concentrations are above 5%, m and b equal 23 and -38 600, respectively.

In rats, the 30 min LC_{50} for CO is 6600 ppm, and with 5% CO_2, this value drops to 3900 ppm. Exposure to CO in air produced deaths only during the actual exposures and not during the postexposure observation period; however, exposures to CO and CO_2 also caused deaths in the postexposure period. Carbon monoxide is a colorless, odorless, tasteless, and non-irritating poisonous gas. The toxicity of CO comes from its binding to the hemoglobin in red blood cells and the formation of carboxyhemoglobin (COHb). The presence of CO on the hemoglobin molecule prevents the binding of O_2 to hemoglobin (O_2Hb) and results in hypoxia in the exposed individual. Since the binding affinity of hemoglobin for CO_2 is 210 times greater than that for O_2, only 0.1% CO (1000 ppm) is needed to compete equally with O_2, which is normally present at 20.9% in the air (20.9%/210 ≈ 0.1%). Thus, only 1000 ppm of CO in the atmosphere is enough to generate 50% COHb, a value commonly quoted (but not necessarily proved) as the concentration that is lethal to humans. The time to get to 50% COHb at 1000 ppm CO would be longer than 30 min.

The LC_{50} value of HCN is 200 ppm for 30 min exposures or 150 ppm for 30 min exposure plus the postexposure observation period. HCN caused deaths both during and following the exposures.

The 30 min LC_{50} of O_2 is 5.4%, a value that is included in the model by subtracting the combustion atmospheric O_2 concentration from the normal concentration of O_2 in the air, that is, 21%. The LC_{50} values of HCl and HBr for 30 min exposures plus postexposure times are 3700 and 3000 ppm, respectively. HCl and HBr at levels found in fires cause only postexposure effects.

The pure and mixed gas studies showed that if the value of the six-gas N-gas equation is 1.1 ± 0.2, then some fraction of the test animals would die. Below 0.9, no deaths would be expected, and above 1.3, all the animals would be expected to die. Since the concentration–response curves for animal lethalities from smoke are very steep, it is assumed that if some percentage (not 0 or 100%) of the animals die, the experimental leading is close to the predicted LC_{50} value. Results using this method show good agreement (deaths of some of the animals when the N-gas values were above 0.9) and the good predictability of this approach.

This model can be used to predict deaths that will occur only during the fire exposure or deaths during and following the fire. To predict the deaths that would occur both during and following the exposures, the six-gas N-gas equation is used as presented. To predict deaths that would occur only during the exposures, HCl and HBr, which have only postexposure effects, should not be included in the equation. In small-scale laboratory tests and full-scale room burns, the equation was used successfully to predict combustion products from numerous materials. In the case of PVC, the model correctly predicted the results as long as the HCl concentration was greater than 1000 ppm; therefore, it is possible that HCl concentrations under 1000 ppm may not have any observable effect on the model even in the postexposure period. More experiments are necessary to show whether a true toxic threshold for HCl does exist.

Although most of the work at NIST concentrated on deaths during or following 30 min exposures, the LC_{50} values of many of these gases, both singly and mixed, were determined at other times ranging from 1 to 60 min, and in all the cases examined, the predictive capability of the equation holds if the LC_{50} values for the other times are substituted into the equation.

The Seven-Gas Model; Addition of NO_2 to the N-Gas Model

Nitrogen dioxide is an irritant gas that will cause lachrymation, coughing, respiratory distress, increases in methemoglobin (MetHb) levels, and lung edema. Single brief exposures to less than lethal concentrations can cause lung damage, emphysema, or intestinal fibrosis. Low levels have been alleged to increase one's susceptibility to respiratory infections and aggravate one's reactions to allergens. Impairment of dark adaptation has also been noted. Delayed serious effects can be observed as late as 2–3 weeks following exposures. In the lungs,

NO_2 forms both nitric (HNO_3) and nitrous (HNO_2) acids, which are most likely responsible for the observed damage to the lung cells and connective tissue.

In fires, NO_2 may arise from atmospheric nitrogen fixation, a reaction that is material independent, or from the oxidation of nitrogen from nitrogen-containing materials. To examine the generation of NO_2 from nitrogen fixation, a small study was undertaken at NIST. In two small-scale fires of rooms in which the main source of fuel was polystyrene-covered walls, only low levels of NO_x (10 and 25 ppm) were found, indicating little nitrogen fixation under these conditions. A real example of burning nitrogen-containing materials was the 1929 Cleveland Clinic (Ohio, USA) fire in which 50 000 nitrocellulose X-ray films were consumed. The deaths of 97 people in this fire were attributed mainly to NO_x. An additional 26 people died between 2 h and 1 month following the fire, and 92 people were treated for nonfatal injuries. In laboratory tests of nitrogen-containing materials under controlled conditions, 1–1000 ppm of NO_x were measured. In military tests of armored vehicles penetrated by high-temperature ammunition, NO_2 levels above 2000 ppm were found.

Individual and Binary Mixtures

In small-scale laboratory tests of NO_2 in air, deaths of Fischer 344 male rats occurred only in the postexposure period and the LC_{50} value following a 30 min exposure is 200 ppm. Carbon dioxide plus NO_2 shows synergistic toxicological effects. The LC_{50} for NO_2 following a 30 min exposure to NO_2 plus 5% CO_2 is 90 ppm (postexposure deaths) (i.e., the toxicity of NO_2 doubled) (**Table 1**).

As mentioned, CO produces only within-exposure deaths, and its 30 min LC_{50} is 6600 ppm. In the presence of 200 ppm of NO_2, the within-exposure toxicity of CO doubled (i.e., its 30 min LC_{50} became 3300 ppm). An exposure of ~3400 ppm CO plus various concentrations of NO_2 showed that the presence of CO would also increase the postexposure toxicity of NO_2. The 30 min LC_{50} value of NO_2 went from 200 to 150 ppm in the presence of 3400 ppm of CO. A concentration of 3400 ppm of CO was used as that concentration would not be lethal during the exposure and any postexposure effects of NO_2 would become evident; the LC_{50} of CO would have caused deaths of the animals during the 30 min exposure.

The 30 min LC_{50} of O_2 is 5.4%, and the deaths occurred primarily during the exposures. In the presence of 200 ppm of NO_2, the within-exposure LC_{50} of O_2 and its toxicity increased to 6.7%. In the case of O_2, increased toxicity is indicated by an increase in the value of the LC_{50} since it is more toxic to be adversely affected by a concentration of O_2 ordinarily capable of sustaining life. Exposure of the animals to 6.7% O_2 plus various concentrations of NO_2 showed that the NO_2 toxicity doubled (i.e., its LC_{50} value decreased from 200 to 90 ppm).

Table 1 Synergistic effects of CO_2

Gas	LC_{50} values	
	Single gas	With 5% CO_2
CO_2	470 000 ppm[a]	N/A
CO	6600 ppm[a]	3900 ppm[b]
NO_2	200 ppm[a]	90 ppm[c]
O_2	5.4%[a]	6.4%[b]

All gases were mixed in air; 30 min exposures of Fischer 344 rats.
[a]Deaths occurred during the exposure.
[b]Deaths occurred during and following the exposures.
[c]Deaths occurred during the postexposure period.

One of the most interesting findings was the antagonistic toxicological effect noted during the experiments on the combinations of HCN and NO_2. As mentioned, the 30 min LC_{50} for NO_2 alone is 200 ppm (postexposure) and the 30 min within-exposure LC_{50} for HCN alone is also 200 ppm. This concentration of either gas alone is sufficient to cause death of the animals (i.e., 200 ppm HCN or 200 ppm NO_2 would cause 50% of the animals to die either during the 30 min exposure or following the 30 min exposure, respectively). However, in the presence of 200 ppm of NO_2, the within-exposure HCN LC_{50} concentration increases to 480 ppm or, stated in other words, the toxicity of HCN decreases by a factor of 2.4.

The mechanism for this antagonistic effect is believed to be as follows. In the presence of water, NO_2 forms nitric acid (HNO_3) and nitrous acid (HNO_2). These two acids are the most likely suspects responsible for the lung damage, leading to the massive pulmonary edema and subsequent deaths noted following exposure to high concentrations of NO_2. Nitrite ion (NO_2^-) formation occurs in the blood when the nitrous acid dissociates. The nitrite ion oxidizes the ferrous ion in oxyhemoglobin to ferric ion to produce MetHb (eqn [2]). MetHb is a well-known antidote for CN^- poisoning. MEtHb binds to cyanide, forming cyanmethemoglobin, which keeps the cyanide in the blood and prevents it from entering the cells. In the absence of MetHb, free cyanide will enter the cells, react with the cytochrome oxidase, prevent the utilization of O_2, and cause cytotoxic hypoxia. If, on the other hand, cyanide is bound to MetHb in the blood, it will not be exerting its cytotoxic effect. Therefore, the mechanism of the antagonistic effect of NO_2 on the toxicity of cyanide is believed to be due to the conversion of oxyhemoglobin [$O_2Hb(Fe^{2+})$] to methemoglobin [$MetHb(Fe^{3+})$] in the presence of nitrite (eqn [2]).

$$\begin{aligned} & 2H^+ + 3NO_2^- + 2O_2Hb\left(Fe^{2+}\right) \\ & = 2MetHb\left(Fe^{3+}\right) + 3NO_3^- + H_2O \end{aligned} \qquad [2]$$

Tertiary Mixtures of NO_2, CO_2, and HCN

Earlier work indicated that the presence of 5% CO_2 with either HCN or NO_2 produced a more toxic environment than would occur with either gas alone. The antagonistic effects of NO_2 on HCN indicate that the presence of one LC_{50} concentration of NO_2 (~200 ppm) will protect the animals from the more toxic effects of HCN during the 30 min exposures, but not from the postexposure effects of the combined HCN and NO_2. Thus, it was of interest to examine combinations of NO_2, CO_2, and HCN. In this series of experiments, the concentrations of HCN were varied from almost 2–2.7 times its LC_{50} value (200 ppm). The concentrations of NO_2 were approximately equal to one LC_{50} value (200 ppm) if the animals were exposed to NO_2 alone and approximately half the LC_{50} (90 ppm) if the animals were exposed to NO_2 plus CO_2; the concentrations of CO_2 were maintained at ~5%, and the O_2 levels were kept above 18.9%. The results indicated that CO_2 does not make the situation worse, but rather provided additional protection even during the postexposure period. In each of the six experiments, some or all of the animals lived through the test even though they were exposed to greater than lethal levels of HCN plus lethal levels of NO_2. In addition, in four tests, some of the animals lived through the postexposure period even though the animals were exposed to combined levels of HCN, NO_2, and CO_2 that would be equivalent to 4.7–5.5 times the lethal concentrations of those gases. One possible reason that CO_2 seems to provide an additional degree of protection is that NO_2 in the presence of 5% CO_2 produces four times more MetHb than does NO_2 alone.

Mixtures of CO, CO_2, NO_2, O_2, and HCN

The initial design of these experiments was to look for additivity of the CO/CO_2, HCN, and NO_2 factors, keeping each at about one-third of its toxic level while keeping the O_2 concentration above 19%. When these initial experiments produced no deaths, we started to increase the concentrations of CO up to one-third of the LC_{50} of CO alone (6600 ppm), HCN was increased to 1.3 or 1.75 times its LC_{50} depending on whether the within-exposure LC_{50} (200 ppm) or the within- and postexposure LC_{50} (150 ppm) is being considered, and NO_2 was increased up to a full LC_{50} value (200 ppm). The results indicated that just adding an NO_2 factor (e.g., $[NO_2]/LC_{50}\ NO_2$) to eqn [1] would not predict the effect on the animals. A new mathematical model was developed and is shown as eqn [3]. In this model, the differences between the within-exposure and postexposure predictability are as follows: (1) the LC_{50} value used for HCN is 200 ppm for within-exposure or 150 ppm for within-exposure and postexposure lethality, and (2) the HCl and HBr factors are not used to predict the within-exposure lethality, only the within-exposure and postexposure lethality. According to eqn [3], animal deaths will start to occur when the N-gas value is above 0.8, and 100% of the animals will die when the value is above 1.3. The results indicated that in those few cases where above 0.8 and no deaths occurred, the animals were severely incapacitated (close to death) as demonstrated by no righting reflex or eye reflex.

$$\begin{aligned} \text{N}-\text{gas value} = {} & \frac{m[\text{CO}]}{\text{CO}_2 - b} + \frac{21-[\text{O}_2]}{21-\text{LC}_{50}(\text{O}_2)} + \left(\frac{[\text{HCN}]}{\text{LC}_{50}(\text{HCN})} \right. \\ & \left. \times \frac{0.4[\text{NO}_2]}{\text{LC}_{50}(\text{NO}_2)}\right) + 0.4\left(\frac{[\text{NO}_2]}{\text{LC}_{50}(\text{NO}_2)}\right) \\ & + \frac{[\text{HCl}]}{\text{LC}_{50}(\text{HCl})} + \frac{[\text{HBr}]}{\text{LC}_{50}(\text{HBr})} \end{aligned} \quad [3]$$

The N-Gas Model Including NO_2

For an explanation of these terms, see the paragraphs following eqn [1]. Equation [3] should be used to predict the within-exposure plus postexposure lethal toxicity of mixtures of CO, CO_2, HCN, reduced O_2, NO_2, HCl, and HBr. The LC_{50} values will be the same as those given for eqn [1] using 150 ppm for HCN and 200 ppm for NO_2. If one wishes to predict the deaths that will occur only during the exposure, the LC_{50} value used for HCN should be 200 ppm and the HCl and HBr factors should not be included. To predict the lethal toxicity of atmospheres that do not include NO_2, eqn [1] is to be used.

Combustions Toxicity Test Methods

The toxicity of the combustion products from any new material formulation or product containing additives or new combinations of additives needs to be examined. Material and polymer chemists are currently trying to develop new 'fire safe' materials. The terms 'fire safe' or 'fire resistant' are not the same as noncombustible. Unless these new materials are noncombustible, some thermal decomposition will occur when the materials are exposed to fire conditions. The toxic gases and the irritants that are present in all smoke need to be considered potential dangers. The toxic products can cause both acute and delayed toxicological effects. It is the acute and extremely short-term effects that prevent escape from burning buildings by causing faulty judgment, incapacitation, and death. The irritants in the smoke can also interfere with the ability to escape by causing severe coughing and choking and by preventing those exposed from keeping their eyes open long enough to find the exits. In addition, the delayed effects, such as tissue or organ injury, mutagenicity, carcinogenicity, and teratogenicity, need to be studied since they may ultimately lead to permanent disability and post-exposure deaths.

Toxicity screening tests for both the acute and delayed effects are, therefore, needed to evaluate the combustion products, including any irritants that may be present in newly proposed materials and products. It is imperative that the materials and products be tested under experimental conditions that simulate realistic fire scenarios of concern (e.g., flashover conditions emanating from first, smoldering and then, flaming of upholstered furniture in homes, or smoldering fires in concealed spaces in aircraft). The ideal tests should be simple, rapid, inexpensive, use the least amount of sample possible (since, in many cases, only limited amounts of new experimental materials may be available), use a minimum number of test animals, and have a definitive toxicological end point for comparison of the multiple candidates. While faulty judgment and incapacitation are significant causes of worry since they can prevent escape and cause death, they are extremely difficult and complex end points to define and measure in non-human test subjects. Death of experimental animals (e.g., rats), on the other hand, is a more definitive and easily determined end point and can be used to compare the relative toxicities of alternate materials deemed suitable for the same purpose. The assumption made here is that if the combustion products of material X are significantly more lethal than those of material Y, the combustion products of X would probably cause more incapacitation and more impairment of judgment than Y as well. The number of experimental animals can be significantly reduced by utilizing one of the predictive mathematical models developed for combustion toxicology such as the N-gas models previously discussed in this article. The six-gas N-gas model is currently indicated in two national standards (ASTM E1678 and NFPA 269) and one international standard (ISO 13344).

Many test methods for the determination of the acute toxicity of combustion products from materials and products have been developed over the last two decades and continue to be developed and/or improved. In 1983, 13 of the methods published up to that time were evaluated by Arthur D. Little, Inc. to assess the feasibility of incorporating combustion toxicity requirements for building materials and finishes into the building codes of New York State. On the basis of seven different criteria, only two methods were found acceptable. These two methods were the flow-through smoke toxicity method developed at the University of Pittsburgh and the closed-system cup furnace smoke toxicity method developed at NIST (known at that time as the National Bureau of Standards (NBS)). Standard Reference Materials and protocols (SRM 1048 and SRM 1049) were developed at NIST and are available to the users of these methods to provide assurance that they are performing the methods correctly (see 'Relevant Websites' section). Based on the results of the Arthur D., Little report, the State of New York under Article 15, Part 1120 of the New York State Fire Prevention and Building Code decided to require that building materials and finished be examined by the method developed at the University of Pittsburgh and that the results be filed with the state. It is important to note, however, that although the results are filed, New York does not regulate any materials or products based on the results of this or any other toxicity test. Although not regulated, the process of testing by the developer should prevent any unduly toxic products from appearing in the marketplace.

New methods that have been developed since 1983 to examine acute combustion toxicity include the University of Pittsburgh II radiant furnace method, a radiant furnace smoke toxicity protocol developed by NIST and SwRI, and the National Institute of Building Sciences (NIBS) toxic hazard test method. All three use radiant heat to decompose materials.

The NIST radiant test and the NIBS toxic hazard test use the same apparatus, consisting of three components: a radiant furnace, a chemical analysis system, and an animal exposure chamber. The chemical analysis system and animal exposure system are identical to that developed for the NBS cup furnace smoke toxicity method. Although the apparatus of both the methods is essentially the same, the methods have different toxicological end points. In the NIST method, an approximate LC_{50}, based on the mass of material needed to cause lethality in 50% of the test animals during a 30 min exposure or a 14 day postexposure period or both, is the determinant of toxicity. The number of animals needed to run the test is substantially reduced by first estimating the LC_{50} by the six-gas N-gas model. This estimate is then verified with one or two animal tests to ensure that no unforeseen gas was generated. The toxicological end point of the NIBS toxic hazard test is the IT_{50}, the irradiation time (the time that the material is exposed to the radiant heat) that is required to kill 50% of the animals during a 30 min exposure or 14 days postexposure time. The actual results of the NIBS test with 20 materials indicated that the test animals died in very short periods of time (personal communication) and the test was unable to discriminate very well between materials. These results substantiate the thesis that mass (the smaller the mass necessary for an LC_{50}, the more toxic the material) is a better indicator of acute toxicity than time.

Both the NIST and NIBS test procedures are designed to simulate a post-flashover scenario. The premise for simulating a post-flashover fire is that most people who die from inhalation of toxic gases in residential fires are affected in areas away from the room of fire origin. Smoke and toxic gases are more likely to reach these distant areas following flashover. This scenario may not be relevant in certain circumstances (e.g., aircraft interior fires, where a smoldering fire in a concealed space may cause significant problems if the plane is over a large body of water and unable to land for a considerable period of time, or fire in the Station Nightclub in the early 2000s in West Warwick (Rhode Island, USA) that killed 100 and injured over 200 people and resulted from a combination of the use of pyrotechnics inside the nightclub, the use of a highly flammable foam on the walls, no sprinkler system, and outdated fire codes).

The NIST radiant test has been accepted by ASTM as a US national standard designated ASTM E1678 and entitled 'Test Method for Measuring Smoke Toxicity for Use in Fire Hazard Analysis.' In 1995, the ISO Technical committee 92, Subcommittee 3 (ISO/TC92SC3) on Toxic Hazards in Fire published an international standard for combustion toxicity that was approved by 16 countries. This standard – ISO/IS 13344 entitled 'Determination of the Lethal Toxic Potency of Fire Effluents' – describes the mathematical models (including the six-gas N-gas model) available for predicting the toxic potency of fire atmospheres based on the toxicological interactions of the main combustion gases present. In the international standard, investigators have the flexibility of designing or choosing a system that will simulate conditions relevant to their fire scenario rather than having to accept a designated combustion system.

Toxicant Suppressants

Fire scientists are very familiar with fire-retardant chemicals, which are defined by ASTM as "chemical[s] which, when added to a combustible material, delay ignition and combustion of the resulting material when exposed to fire." The discussion adds "a fire-retardant chemical can be a part of the molecular structure, an admixture or an impregnant." The term 'toxicant suppressant,' however, is a new term arising from research at NIST that demonstrated that the addition of copper compounds to flexible polyurethane foam (FPU) significantly reduced the generation of HCN as well as the toxicity of the combustion products when the foam was thermally decomposed. These experiments were designed to simulate the nonflaming and then flaming stages of a chair ignited by a cigarette (a two-phase heating system which simulated the fire scenario that results in the most fire deaths in the United States). The term toxicant suppressant may be defined as a chemical that, when added to a combustible material, significantly reduces or prevents one or more toxic gases from being generated when that material undergoes thermal decomposition. The resultant gas effluent should be less toxic than that from the untreated material; that is, the toxic gas, whose concentration is being reduced, should not be converted to an equally or more toxic product.

The results of these studies at NIST indicated that:

1. Hydrogen cyanide concentrations in the thermal decomposition products from a flexible polyurethane foam were reduced ~85% when the foam was treated with 0.1 or 1.0% Cu_2O by weight and thermally decomposed via a two-phase heating system in the NIST Cup Furnace Smoke Toxicity Apparatus.
2. The copper or copper compounds could be added to the foams during or after the foams were formulated and still reduce the HCN yield and toxicity of the combustion products. (NIST added the copper after formulation; the BASF Corporation added the Cu_2O during formulation.) The addition of the copper or copper compounds during formulation did not affect the foaming process or the physical appearance of the foams except for a slight change of color.
3. Low levels of the copper compounds were effective. In particular, when cupric oxide (CuO) was used, the concentration of copper needed was only 0.08% by weight, and when cuprous oxide (Cu_2O) was used, only 0.07% by weight was needed to significantly reduce the generation of HCN.
4. Full-scale room burns indicated that the presence of Cu_2O in the flexible polyurethane foam reduced the HCN generation by ~50–70% when the experimental plan was designed to simulate a realistic scenario (the foams contained 1.0% Cu_2O by weight, were covered with a cotton upholstery fabric, and were arranged to simulate a chair; smoldering was initiated with cigarettes and flaming occurred spontaneously).
5. Under small-scale conditions, less than 3 ppm of NO_x was generated from the untreated foams, whereas a range of 3–33 ppm of NO_x was measured from 0.1 to 1.0% by weight of Cu_2O-treated foams. About 6% of the HCN appeared converted to NO_x. In the full-scale room tests, ~23% of the HCN appeared to be converted to NO_x. Since we have shown at NIST that NO_2 acts as an antagonist to HCN, this amount of NO_x may also act to counteract the immediate toxic effects of any residual HCN.
6. Since atmospheric O_2 concentrations can reach very low levels in real fires, it was important to know whether the reduction of HCN by copper would occur under low O_2 conditions. Small-scale tests with the ambient O_2 concentrations as low as 6% indicated that the HCN levels were reduced by as much as 82% when the flexible polyurethane foam was treated with 0.1% Cu_2O by weight.
7. The toxicity of the gas effluent was also reduced (an indication that HCN was not being converted into some compound that was even more toxic). Fewer animal (Fischer 344 rats) deaths occurred during the 30 min exposures to the flexible polyurethane foam treated with the copper and copper compounds compared to the untreated flexible polyurethane foam. Toxicity based on LC_{50} values was reduced 40–70% in the small-scale tests with 0.1% Cu_2O-treated foams. The blood cyanide levels in the animals exposed to the combustion products from the CuO-treated foams for 30 min were one-half to one-quarter of those measured in the animals exposed to the smoke from the same amount of untreated foam.
8. Postexposure deaths were also reduced in the animals exposed to the combustion products from the Cu- and Cu_2O-treated FPU foams in the small-scale tests. These delayed postexposure deaths have not been observed in animals exposed to combustion products from flexible polyurethane foams decomposed in large-scale room fire tests. The specific cause of these postexposure deaths is not known.
9. No differences in flammability characteristics between the 0.1% Cu_2O-treated and untreated flexible polyurethane foam were observed. These characteristics were examined to ensure that the positive effect on the toxicity was not contradicted by negative effects on the flammability properties. The flammability characteristics examined were (1) ignitability in three systems (the NIST cup furnace smoke toxicity method, the cone calorimeter, and the lateral ignition and flame spread test (LIFT)); (2) heat release rates under small-scale (cone calorimeter) and medium-scale (furniture calorimeter) conditions; (3) heats of combustion under small-scale (cone calorimeter) and medium-scale (furniture calorimeter) conditions, CO/CO_2 ratios under small-scale (cone calorimeter) and medium-scale (furniture calorimeter) conditions, (5) smoke obscuration (cone calorimeter); and (6) rate of flame spread (LIFT).
10. Research conducted at the BASF Corporation indicated that the physical properties of the 1.0% Cu_2O-treated flexible polyurethane foam were not significantly different from the comparable untreated flexible polyurethane foam. The physical properties examined were tensile strength, elongation, tear strength, resilience, indentation force deflection, support factor, compression sets, and airflow.
11. One of the additives being used in combustion-modified flexible polyurethane foams is melamine. Small-scale tests conducted at NIST indicated that a melamine-treated flexible polyurethane foam generated six times more HCN than an equal amount of foam that did not contain melamine. The presence of Cu_2O reduced the HCN generated from the melamine foam by 90%. Melamine-treated flexible polyurethane foam is one of two flexible polyurethane foams currently allowed in Great Britain.

In the late 1970s, research by Jellinek et al. at Clarkson College of Technology also showed that the concentrations of HCN generated from the thermal decomposition of a polyurethane at 300 and 400 °C decreased when flowed through copper compounds. In their studies, the polyurethane films were usually 15 μm thick (50 mg). In some experiments, the metal powder was mixed with the polymer and, in others, copper metal films of 400–1000 Å were deposited on top of the polymer films. In most cases, the percentage of copper was 10% or greater. The lowest concentrations that they tested was a 2.6% copper film, which inhibited the evolution of HCN by 66%. Their experiments indicated that copper probably acts as an oxidative catalyst that decomposes gaseous HCN into N_2, CO_2, H_2O, and small amounts of nitrogen oxides. Further research is needed to determine whether this is the actual molecular mechanism that allows copper to act as an HCN toxicant suppressant.

Research by Levin et al. (1992) at NIST differed from that of Jellinek in that much larger samples of flexible polyurethane foam (including full-scale room burns of cushions and simulated chairs), and much smaller concentrations of copper were used. The toxicity of the combustion products from the copper-treated flexible polyurethane foam was also examined.

Unpublished data of Levin et al. (1992) also indicated that a wool fabric treated with copper would generate 50% less HCN than the untreated fabric. These results demonstrate a more universal effect, namely that treating nitrogen-containing materials with copper compounds will probably reduce the HCN generated when that material is exposed to fire conditions. Taking these results one step further, one could develop other toxicant suppressants that, when added to materials and products, would now prevent or significantly reduce the toxic effluents generated when they are thermally decomposed. Since 80% of fire deaths are the result of smoke inhalation, a less toxic smoke could significantly increase the time available for escape and reduce the number of injuries and deaths from fires.

Not well recognized is that the fine particulates generated in fires adhere reactive toxic species to their surfaces, and that these are effectively point sources of toxicity and therefore of a very different and extremely toxic compound.

Most recent concerns in the area of combustion toxicology have centered on its occurrence in closed environments (e.g., aircraft, spacecraft, submarines).

See also: Carbon Dioxide; Carbon Monoxide; CCA-Treated Wood; LD_{50}/LC_{50} (Lethal Dosage 50/Lethal Concentration 50).

Further Reading

Baxter, C.S., 2013. Smoke and combustion products. In: Bingham, E., Cohrssen, B. (Eds.), Patty's Toxicology, sixth ed., vol. 6. Wiley, Hoboken NJ, pp. 399–417.

Chaturvedi, A.K., 2010. Aviation combustion toxicology. J. Anal. Toxicol. 34, 1–16.

Hardman, J.G., Limbird, L.E., Molinoff, P.B., Ruddon, R.W., Gilman, A.G. (Eds.), 1996. Goodman and Gilman's the Pharmacologic Basis of Therapeutics, ninth ed. McGraw-Hill, New York.

Kaplan, H.L., Grand, A.F., Hartzell, G.E., 1983. Combustion Toxicology, Principles and Test Methods. Technomic Publishing Co, Lancaster, PA.

Karter Jr., M.J., 2003. 2002 US fire loss. NFPA J. 97, 59–63.

Levin, B.C., 2001. Smoke and combustion products. In: Bingham, E., Cohrssen, B., Powell, C.H. (Eds.), Patty's Toxicology, Chapter 108, fifth ed. Col VIII. Wiley, New York, pp. 648–668.

Levin, B.C., Braun, E., Paabo, M., Harris, R.H., Navarro, M., 1992. Reduction of Hydrogen Cyanide Concentrations and Acute Inhalation Toxicity from Flexible Polyurethane Foam Combustion Products be the Addition of Copper Compounds. Part IV. Effects of Combustion Conditions and Scaling on the Generation of Hydrogen Cyanide and Toxicity from Flexible Polyurethane Foam with and without Copper Compounds. NISTIR 4989. National Institutes of Standards and Technology, Gaithersburg, MD.

National Research Council, National Materials Advisory Board, 1995. Fire- and Smoke-Resistant Interior Materials for Commercial Transport Aircraft. Publication Number NMAB-477-1. National Academy Press, Washington, DC.

Nelson, G.L. (Ed.), 1995. Fire and Polymers II; Materials and Tests for Hazard Prevention. ACS Symposium Series 599. American Chemical Society, Washington, DC.

Relevant Websites

http://www.wolmanizedwood.com – Information on Wolmanized pressure-treated wood.

http://ts.nist.gov – NIST website providing information of standard reference materials and protocols developed.

Comet Assay

Solange Costa and João Paulo Teixeira, Portuguese National Institute of Health, Porto, Portugal

Introduction

Comet Assay or single cell gel electrophoresis (SCGE) is a versatile, simple, and adaptable method to measure DNA damage and repair at individual cell level.

It is based on the capacity of negatively charged loops/fragments of DNA to be pulled through an agarose gel in response to an electric field, appearing like a 'comet.'

In the last two decades the Comet Assay became very popular and today is probably one of the most used assays for the assessment of DNA damage and repair. It combines the simplicity of biochemical techniques for detecting DNA single-strand breaks (strand breaks and incomplete excision repair sites), alkali-labile sites (ALS), and cross-linking, with the single cell approach typical of cytogenetic assays.

The main advantages of the Comet Assay include: (1) sensitivity for detecting low levels of damage, (2) use of any monodispersed cell population, proliferating as well as non-proliferating, (3) single cell data collection, allowing more robust statistical analyses, (4) requirement for a small number of cells per sample, (5) low cost, rapid, and ease of application, and (6) flexibility to use fresh or frozen samples.

The popularity of the assay is largely due to the fact that any eukaryote cell that can be obtained as a single cell suspension like cells isolated from blood, cells from tissue biopsies that can be homogenized, buccal cells, whole blood, and cultured cells can be used. Nonetheless for some cell types, such as plant cells and sperm cells, a few modifications to the classical protocol are required. Overall, for most purposes, well-characterized cell lines or primary cells (e.g., peripheral blood mononuclear cells) used in classical genetic toxicology testing assays are preferred.

The assay as also a few limitations, it is not able to detect aneugenic effects and epigenetic mechanisms (indirect) of DNA (effects on cell-cycle checkpoints). In addition, since Comet Assay is not able to detect the DNA fragments that result from apoptosis or necrosis processes, cytotoxicity can potentially lead to false positive/negative results.

Although initially developed to measure variation in DNA damage and repair capacity within a population of mammalian cells, Comet Assay applications now range from human and ecological biomonitoring (e.g., DNA damage in mussels living in polluted estuarine sites) to measurement of DNA damage in specific genomic sequences.

Versions

Comet Assay principles were first introduced in 1984 by Ostling and Johanson.

The assay was based on previous work published in the late 1970s by Cook and colleagues, who developed a method to investigate nuclear structure of eukaryotic cells based on high salt lysis with nonionic detergents. The proposed model was a supercoiled DNA arranged as a series of loops attached at intervals to the nuclear matrix. By adding an intercalating agent, the supercoiled DNA was relaxed and loops expanded out from the nuclear structure, called a nucleoid, to form a 'halo.' After irradiating with γ-rays the size of the halo was approximately proportional to the irradiation dose.

The SCGE approach by Ostling and Johanson produced a 'tail.' described as being a halo of relaxed loops pulled to one side (toward the anode) by the electrophoretic field. As described in the original, protocol lysis and electrophoresis were done under neutral conditions.

The Ostling and Johanson SCGE procedure was later adapted under alkaline conditions by Singh et al. (1988) ($pH > 13$), which led to a more sensitive version of the assay that could assess double- and single-strand DNA breaks as well as ALS (apurinic/apyrimidic sites), crosslinks, and incomplete DNA repair sites.

In a parallel but independent work, Olive et al. also optimized the original technique of Ostling and Johanson so that the Comet Assay after alkali treatment was followed by electrophoresis at either neutral or mild alkaline (pH 12.3) conditions to detect single-strand DNA breaks. Both methods are identical in principle and similar in practice, but Singh method, depending on the agent, was found to be more responsive.

Since its development, the SCGE technique has been modified at various steps (lysis/unwinding and/or electrophoresis) to improve reproducibility and sensitivity, and to provide suitable ways to assess various kinds of damage in different cells. Employing neutral pH (8–10) condition mainly facilitates the detection of strand breaks; a pH 12 enables the detection of double- and single-strand breaks and incomplete excision repair sites; while a $pH \geq 13$ expresses ALS in addition to all types of lesions appointed above.

Alkaline Comet Assay

Several versions of the Comet Assay are currently in use the most popular being the alkaline version first introduced by Singh et al.

In short, cells embedded in agarose are placed on a microscope slide and lysed with detergent at high salt concentration.

During lysis, cellular membranes, cytoplasmic and nucleosplasmic constituents, and histones are removed. After lysis, what remains is the nucleoid, containing RNA, proteins, and negatively supercoiled DNA attached to the nuclear matrix. The immobilized nucleoid is then denaturated in an alkali buffer and electrophoresed in same buffer.

Electrophoresis results in structures resembling comets, with a distinct head, comprising intact DNA and a tail of extended DNA loops and DNA fragments (**Figure 1**).

 http://dx.doi.org/10.1016/B978-0-12-386454-3.01072-1

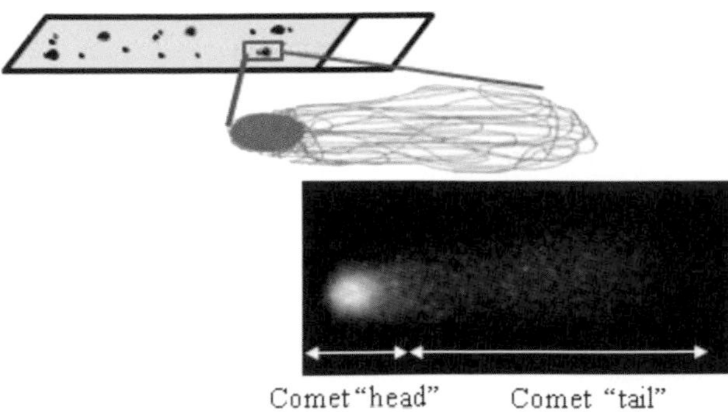

Figure 1 Schematic picture representing a comet of a damaged cell and a comet image of a damaged cell.

The 'comet' can be visualized with a fluorescence microscope after staining with a DNA staining dye (e.g., ethidium bromide, acridine orange). The size and shape of the comet and the distribution of DNA within the comet correlate with the extent of DNA damage present in the individual cell (**Figure 2**).

Some technical sources of variability were detected in the assay that can have an impact on the results, namely, the agarose gel density, the temperature and the duration of alkaline unwinding treatment, electrophoresis time, voltage across the gel, and temperature of lysis. Several guidelines have been published for the Comet Assay; however, a standardized protocol is still lacking.

Although the assay enables the assessment of low levels of DNA damage, the type of lesions detected such as single-strand breaks is short-lived and is generally repaired. Also measuring DNA migration gives limited information about the class of lesion that is being detected, as it is an estimate of different types of DNA lesions.

Enzyme-Comet Assay

In order to improve Comet Assay's sensitivity and selectivity, Collins et al. (1996) introduced an extra step after lysis: incubation with lesion-specific enzymes that are used to convert damaged bases to DNA breaks. Enzymes that have been used include: formamidopyrimidine glycosylase that detects oxidized purines (e.g., 8-oxoguanine) as well as other lesions; hOGG1 identifies 8-oxoguanine; endonuclease III (EndoIII) reveals oxidized pyrimidines; T4 endonuclease V exposes UV induced cyclobutane pyrimidine dimmers and uracil glycosylase that recognize uracil bases in the DNA sequence.

Scoring "Comets"

Comets can be analyzed by visual scoring, by computerized image analysis, or by recently developed fully automatic computerized image analysis. There is a range of different software available to analyze comets.

In visual scoring the comets are divided into five categories ranging from class 0, undamaged cells, to classes 1–4 representing increasing relative tail intensities, and therefore increasing damaged cells.

Computerized scoring is reported using a range of different parameters. The most frequently used endpoints are %DNA in tail, tail moment, and tail length. The different ways of scoring cells have different advantages and limitations. Nonetheless Azqueta et al. recently compared visual scoring, computerized scoring, and automatic computerized scoring and concluded that all three scoring methods are reliable, and results from the three methods are, to a certain extent, comparable.

Applications

Broadly used to measure cellular responses to DNA damage, Comet Assay has been applied in genotoxicity testing, ecological studies, and in human biomonitoring and clinical studies. The assay has been used under a variety of exposures, including *in vitro*, *in vivo*, and *in situ*. Despite the general consensus of the usefulness of Comet Assay there is still no OECD guideline for its design, presently it is under international validation process.

Genotoxicity Test

Currently the Comet Assay is being used as a genotoxicity test to assess the safety of new drug candidates. It is a valuable tool for early and reliable genotoxicity screening of novel chemicals or pharmaceuticals. The protocol used is the alkaline Comet Assay for measuring DNA migration.

Ecological Monitoring

Environmental anthropogenic-mediated toxicants can have a deleterious influence in genetic diversity both at the individual and ecosystem levels and may also affect the genetic structure of populations. The Comet Assay in combination with suitable organisms can be used as sentinels for measuring toxicants (metals and organics) often present in the environment.

The SCGE method demonstrated to have broad applicability for both aquatic and terrestrial animals in terms of organisms, tissues, and cell types.

DNA damage, measured by Comet Assay, in aquatic animals collected from contaminated sites was associated with effects on growth, reproduction, and population dynamics (e.g., mussels from marine and estuarine systems

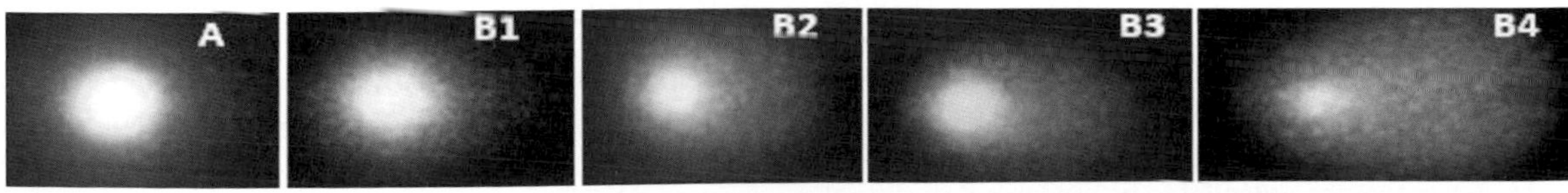

Figure 2 Comet Assay images. (a) Untreated cell exhibiting intact DNA, without a tail. (b) Cells exhibiting increased DNA migration after treatment with a DNA-damaging agent; images B1–B4 represent different classes of DNA damage.

contaminated by oil spillage). This assay was also used to assess immunotoxicity in dolphins, with increased DNA damage correlating with a decreased ability of the T cells to proliferate, which relates to the ability of the animals to respond to infection.

Moreover, tadpoles from two frog species (*Rana clamitans* and *Rana pipiens*) collected from areas with heavy agriculture and industrial activity, respectively, showed significantly higher damage compared to tadpoles from nonagricultural and nonindustrial areas.

DNA damage in earthworms from toxic waste sites proved to be a valuable tool for monitoring and detection of genotoxic compounds in polluted soils. Rodents (*Ctenomys torquatus*) from an area close to a coal mine had significantly higher damage in lymphocytes compared with animals from a region where no coal mines were found.

Human Studies

During the last decade the Comet Assay was introduced as a useful biomarker for risk assessment in human biomonitoring studies. In recent years, several comprehensive reviews have come into view in relation to Comet Assay methodology and application areas and its response as an indicator of carcinogen exposure. It has been shown to be a valuable tool for acquiring knowledge about current levels of internal exposure to toxicants agents, and for identifying hot spots or trends in exposure risks of human populations. Applications include monitoring occupational exposure to genotoxic chemicals or radiation, environmental exposure (air pollutants, living close to mining sites), assessment of oxidative stress associated with various human diseases, and detection of DNA damage associated with smoking.

While biomonitoring studies employing cytogenetic techniques are limited to circulating lymphocytes and involve proliferating cell populations, the SCGE technique can be applied to proliferating and nonproliferating cells, and cells of those tissues which are the first sites of contact with mutagenic carcinogenic substances (e.g., oral and nasal mucosa cells).

Another reason for the increased use of the Comet Assay as a biomarker for risk assessment is the similarity of results between this assay and validated biomarkers extensively used in human studies. Nevertheless, the usefulness of this assay depends on the toxicants involved, their molecular mechanisms of action, as well as the experimental design (e.g., use of control groups, timing of sample collection).

Recently the Comet Assay has been used to investigate DNA damage and repair efficiency in a wide range of tumor cells in response to a variety of DNA-damaging agents. These studies include both investigations on human tumor cell lines and on tumor cells extracted from cancer patients. Many of these studies show that the data produced by the Comet Assay provide important information about the particular characteristics of the cancer, which could be used by oncologists to decide the best possible course of intervention. In addition, the Comet Assay has also the potential to be used to aid in clinical diagnosis (e.g., xeroderma pigmentosum and Nijmegen breakage syndrome).

Emerging Applications

Fluorescence *in situ* Hybridization

Fluorescence *in situ* hybridization (FISH) is a method used to locate specific DNA sequences within interphase chromatin and metaphase chromosomes and to identify both structural and numerical chromosome changes. FISH coupled with Comet Assay can provide unique knowledge about the DNA damage and repair in specific genes and DNA sequences. By hybridizing fluorescently labeled probes to DNA after electrophoresis, DNA damage in particular genes and DNA sequences can be measured by the Comet Assay. If the DNA of the gene is found in the comet tail, this indicates that a DNA break had occurred in the proximity of the gene. In addition, Comet-FISH can be applied as a first look of the three-dimensional organization of genomic loci and elucidation of mechanisms of comet formation and DNA organization in comets.

Chromosome

This recent application is based on the chromosome isolation protocols used for whole chromosome mounting in electron microscopy, in combination with Comet Assay, to visualize putative DNA damage in subnuclear structures. The results show that migrant DNA fragments can be visualized in whole nuclei and isolated chromosomes and that they exhibit patterns of DNA migration that depend on the level of DNA damage produced.

DNA Repair

In addition to evaluate DNA damage, the Comet Assay can be used in different ways to measure the DNA repair capacity at cellular level.

One simple approach is to treat cells with a DNA-damaging agent, incubate them in a culture medium (37 °C, CO_2 chamber), and monitor the speed with which they remove the lesions. At intervals, samples are taken for analysis with Comet Assay. The rate at which the damage is removed indicates the efficiency of repair.

Alternatively the repair capacity of cells extract can be assessed in an *in vitro* assay and applied in population studies.

DNA repair is a major factor in individual susceptibility to cancer. However, little is known about the degree of variation of intra- and interindividual capacity for DNA repair, which can be explained by the limitations of the available methods. One option is to measure the expression of DNA repair genes, but results often do not correlate with the enzymatic repair activity.

Modified versions of the Comet Assay are able to measure enzyme repair activity and hence be used in human biomonitoring studies.

DNA repair capacity is evaluated by extracting DNA repair enzymes from cells and measure the extract's ability to repair DNA lesions in a substrate. The substrate is composed of cells previously treated with a DNA-damaging agent, appropriate for the type of repair being measured. After lysis the cells with induced DNA damage are incubated with the extract containing DNA repair enzymes. The extract's incision activity (the first step in the repair process) on DNA damage is measured by the

Comet Assay. Thus the efficiency of both base excision repair and nucleotide excision repair pathways can be assessed.

Validation

The growing popularity of Comet Assay among researchers along with the increasing awareness of its versatility and potential use across virtually all areas in biomonitoring studies arises the need to validate this assay as a valuable tool in cancer risk assessment.

One important aspect of the validation process is international multilaboratory validation studies, which can demonstrate the Comet Assay's inter- and intralaboratory reproducibility and reliability, and therefore expose potential sources of variability in results.

At this time no standardized protocol exists for Comet Assay, although several guidelines for the procedure have been published. Hence there are still some considerable differences between the protocols used by different research groups, which impair the interlaboratory comparison of results.

In this sense several collaboration efforts are being made by international agencies namely JaCVAM, ICCVAM, and ECVAM to evaluate the validity of the assay. As a consequence a number of international workgroups and networks were established to address this important issue, within the current OECD regulatory strategy for genotoxicity testing.

The main objectives are to thoroughly evaluate the reliability and accuracy of the assay and to produce a standardized protocol with maximum acceptability by international regulatory agencies.

An important point is to evaluate the ability of the *in vivo* rodent alkaline Comet Assay to identify genotoxic carcinogens, as a potential replacement for the *in vivo* rodent hepatocyte unscheduled DNA synthesis assay.

See also: Biomarkers, Human Health; Environmental Toxicology; Genetic Toxicology; Health Assessments; Occupational Toxicology; Oxidative Stress; Regulation, Toxicology and; Risk Assessment, Ecological; Risk Assessment, Human Health; Toxicity Testing, Aquatic.

Further Reading

Azqueta, A., Meier, S., Priestley, C., et al., 2011. The influence of scoring method on variability in results obtained with the comet assay. Mutagenesis 26, 393–399.

Collins, A.R., Dušinská, M., Gedik, C.M., Stetina, R., 1996. Oxidative damage to DNA: do we have a reliable biomarker? Environ. Health Perspect. 104, 465–469.

Collins, A.R., Oscoz, A.A., Brunborg, G., et al., 2008. The comet assay: topical issues. Mutagenesis 23, 143–151.

Cook, P.R., Brazell, I.A., 1975. Supercoils in human DNA. J. Cell Sci. 19, 261–279.

Cook, P.R., Brazell, I.A., Jost, E., 1976. Characterization of nuclear structures containing superhelical DNA. J. Cell Sci. 22, 303–324.

Cotelle, S., Férard, J.F., 1999. Comet assay in genetic ecotoxicology: a review. Environ. Mol. Mutagen. 34, 246–255.

Dušinská, M., Collins, A.R., 2008. The comet assay in human biomonitoring: Gene environment interactions. Mutagenesis 23, 191–205.

Möller, L., Godschalk, R.W., Langie, S.A., et al., 2009. Variation in the measurement of DNA damage by comet assay measured by the ECVAG inter-laboratory validation trial. Mutagenesis 25, 113–123.

Olive, P.L., 2002. The comet assay. An overview of techniques. Methods Mol. Biol. 203, 179–194.

Ostling, O., Johanson, K.J., 1984. Microelectrophoretic study of radiation-induced DNA damages in individual mammalian cells. Biochem. Biophys. Res. Commun. 123, 291–298.

Shaposhnikov, S., Frengen, E., Collins, A.R., 2009. Increasing the resolution of the comet assay using fluorescent *in situ* hybridization—a review. Mutagenesis 24, 383–389.

Singh, N.P., McCoy, M.T., Tice, R.R., Schneider, E.L., 1988. A simple technique for quantitation of low levels of DNA damage in individual cells. Exp. Cell Res. 75, 184–191.

Relevant Websites

http://cometassay.com/ – Comet Assay Interest Group

http://www.comnetproject.org/ – ComNet Project

http://www.ecnis.org/ – Environmental Cancer Risk, Nutrition and Individual Susceptibility

http://ecvam.jrc.it/ – European Centre for the Validation of Alternative Methods

http://www.nationalacademies.org/nrc/ – National Research Council

http://www.newgeneris.org/ – NewGeneris

http://www.oecd.org/home/ – Organization for Economic Cooperation and Development

http://iccvam.niehs.nih.gov/ and http://iccvam.niehs.nih.gov/methods/milestones.htm – US Interagency Coordinating Committee on the Validation of Alternative Methods

Common Mechanism of Toxicity in Pesticides

BE Mileson, Technology Sciences Group Inc., Washington, DC, USA

Background

Common mechanism of toxicity is a phrase used to characterize the toxicological actions of two or more agents that act by the same cellular and molecular mechanisms leading to a common adverse effect on the structure or function of a living organism. An understanding of all steps that comprise a common mechanism of toxicity for given toxicants is rarely achieved, but identification of the crucial events following chemical interaction with an organism can be sufficient to describe a common mechanism of toxicity.

The concept of common mechanism of toxicity in pesticides gained prominence in the United States after Congress passed the Food Quality Protection Act of 1996 (FQPA), which requires the US Environmental Protection Agency (USEPA) to consider the effects of human exposure to all pesticides and other chemicals that act by a common mechanism of toxicity when they derive tolerances (acceptable levels) for pesticide use on crops. As a result of the FQPA, the term common mechanism of toxicity has a regulatory connotation in addition to a toxicological definition. The USEPA Office of Pesticide Programs (OPP) makes an official determination to identify specific pesticides that act by a common mechanism of toxicity. After the common mechanism group is identified, USEPA OPP conducts a cumulative risk assessment of exposure to all the pesticides in the common mechanism group when establishing, modifying, leaving in effect, or revoking a tolerance for a pesticide chemical residue, as specified in the FQPA.

Common Mechanism Groups

The USEPA OPP has issued guidance to identify pesticides and other chemicals that act by a common mechanism of toxicity. The first step in this guidance is to determine whether a group of pesticides should be considered a 'preliminary grouping' of compounds that may act by a common mechanism of toxicity. Characteristics suggested by USEPA OPP, which may be an indication that substances act by a common mechanism of toxicity include (1) compounds share a structural similarity, (2) pesticides have a similar mechanism of insecticidal action, (3) compounds act by the same general mechanism of mammalian toxicity, and/or (4) compounds cause a particular toxic effect.

The USEPA OPP refines the evaluation of a preliminary common mechanism group by considering the biochemical and toxicological actions of each toxicant to determine if they all act by a common mechanism of toxicity, or if they should be separated into more than one common mechanism group for cumulative risk assessment. To determine if a preliminary group of compounds all act by a common mechanism of toxicity, the actions of these chemicals are evaluated based on whether they cause the same critical effect, act on the same molecular target at the same target tissue, act by the same biochemical mechanism, and/or share a common toxic intermediate. To evaluate mechanisms of toxicity, the USEPA OPP relies on data from studies submitted in support of pesticide registration, data from the public literature, and data from government reports.

The Pest Management Regulatory Agency (PMRA) of Health Canada proposed to harmonize with the USEPA policy on common mechanism of toxicity. PMRA issued guidance for identifying pesticides that have a common mechanism of toxicity that was adapted from the USEPA guidance document.

Examples of Pesticides That Act by a Common Mechanism of Toxicity

An example of a group of toxicants that act by a common mechanism of toxicity is the organophosphorus (OP) pesticides. OP pesticides are an otherwise structurally diverse group of chemicals that all contain phosphate atoms that are pentavalent and tetracoordinate. The primary molecular mechanism of action of most of the OP pesticides is the inhibition of acetylcholinesterase (AChE), a serine esterase that occurs throughout the central and peripheral nervous systems of vertebrates. The normal physiological action of AChE is to hydrolyze the neurotransmitter acetylcholine (ACh) so that activation of cholinergic receptors is transient. Inhibition of AChE results in accumulation of ACh at the synapses, overstimulation of cholinergic neurons, and resultant signs of cholinergic toxicity. Clinical signs of cholinergic toxicity include increased lacrimation and salivation, bronchoconstriction, bronchosecretion, miosis, gastrointestinal cramps, diarrhea, urination, bradycardia, tachycardia, hypertension, muscle fasciculations, tremors, and muscle weakness, among other signs. OP pesticides have been determined to act by a common mechanism of toxicity if they inhibit AChE by phosphorylation and elicit any spectrum of cholinergic effects in exposed animals or humans. AChE enzymes inhibited by an OP pesticide may be reactivated, but this is a slow process that can take anywhere from several hours to days depending on the specific OP structure and the resulting stability of the phosphorylated enzyme.

The N-methyl carbamate (NMC) pesticides comprise another common mechanism group identified by the USEPA OPP. The common mechanism shared by the NMC pesticides is inhibition of AChE by carbamylation of the serine hydroxyl group in the active site of the enzyme. This mechanism of toxicity is similar to that of the OP pesticides in that both groups inhibit AChE. The NMC mechanism of toxicity is distinct from the OP mechanism in that the NMC carbamylation of AChE is transient and readily reversible, such that signs of toxicity generally resolve within a few hours.

Triazine pesticides are considered a common mechanism group by the USEPA OPP. The common mechanism shared by the triazines, atrazine, simazine, propazine, and a few degradants, is disruption of the hypothalamic–pituitary–gonadal (HPG) axis. The triazines in this group test positive for

 http://dx.doi.org/10.1016/B978-0-12-386454-3.00117-2

mammary gland tumors in female Sprague Dawley rats. The alterations in the HPG axis as demonstrated in the rat model are initiated with a decrease in the release of gonadotropin-releasing hormone by the hypothalamus and consequent attenuation of the daily surge in luteinizing hormone during the estrous cycle. This prolongs the estrous cycle, resulting in increased estrogen exposure that stimulates prolactin secretion from the pituitary. The combination of hormonal alterations produces conditions that are conducive to the development of mammary gland tumors in the rat. There are a number of pesticides that contain a triazine ring structure that do not share this mechanism of toxicity according to USEPA OPP, including ametryn, prometon, metsulfuron methyl, trisulfuron, chlorsulfuron, and melamine. These compounds do not cause the carcinogenic profile identified for atrazine, simazine, and propazine, and there is no known common mechanism of toxicity that would unite these in a single group.

A fourth group of pesticides evaluated by the USEPA OPP and identified as a common mechanism group is the chloroacetanilide pesticides. This pesticide group is known to produce tumors of the nasal olfactory epithelium in rats. The chloroacetanilide pesticides, alachlor, acetochlor, and butachlor, cause nasal turbinate tumors *via* the generation of a common tissue reactive metabolite (a quinoneimine) that leads to sustained cytotoxicity and regenerative proliferation of the nasal epithelium resulting in neoplasia.

Examples of Pesticides That Do Not Act by a Common Mechanism of Toxicity

Two preliminary groups of pesticides identified by the USEPA OPP as potential common mechanism groups ultimately were not combined in common mechanism groups for cumulative risk assessment. Thiocarbamate pesticides initially were believed to induce a common effect of neuropathy of the sciatic nerve, but on closer examination, there was insufficient evidence to support a common mechanism of toxicity for these pesticides. Similarly, dithiocarbamate pesticides were a preliminary common mechanism group, but the available evidence did not support grouping the dithiocarbamates based on a common mechanism for neuropathology.

Conclusion

Many classes of pesticides are composed of structurally similar compounds that act by a common mechanism of toxicity. The fact that groups of pesticides act by a common mechanism of toxicity is predictable since these chemicals were designed to resemble one another structurally and elicit similar pesticidal effects.

See also: Carbamate Pesticides; Cholinesterase Inhibition; Dithiocarbamates; Organophosphorus Compounds; Cumulative (Combined Exposures) Risk Assessment

Further Reading

Breckenridge, C.B., Holden, L., Sturgess, N., Weiner, M., Sheets, L., Sargent, D., Soderlund, D.M., Choi, J.S., Symington, S., Clark, J.M., Burr, S., Ray, D., 2009. Evidence for a separate mechanism of toxicity for the Type I and the Type II pyrethroid insecticides. Neurotoxicology 30 (Suppl. 1), S17–S31.

Mileson, B.E., Chambers, J.E., Chen, W.L., Dettbarn, W., Ehrich, M., Eldefrawi, A.T., Gaylor, D.W., Hamernik, K., Hodgson, E., Karczmar, A.G., Padilla, S., Pope, C.N., Richardson, R.J., Saunders, D.R., Sheets, L.P., Sultatos, L.G., Wallace, K.B., 1998. Common mechanism of toxicity: a case study of organophosphorus pesticides. Toxicol. Sci. 41, 8–20.

Relevant Websites

http://www.epa.gov/oppsrrd1/cumulative/methods_tools.htm – US Environmental Protection Agency's Office of Pesticide Programs: Cumulative Risk Assessment Methods and Tools.

Coniine

M Badanthadka, Torrent Research Centre, Gandhinagar, Gujarat, India
HM Mehendale, University of Louisiana at Monroe, Monroe, LA, USA

- Name: Coniine
- Chemical Abstract Service Registry Numbers: 458-88-8 and 3238-60-6
- Synonyms: CASRN – 458-88-8: (+)-Coniine; (*S*)-(+)-Coniine; (*S*)-2-Propylpiperidine; (*S*)-Beta-propylpiperidine; (*S*)-Coniine; Cicutin; Cicutine; Conicine; Coniin; Coniine; D-Conicine; Koniin; Piperidine, 2-propyl-, (*S*)-; CASRN – 3238-60-6: (±)-Coniine
- Molecular Formula: $C_8H_{17}N$
- Chemical Structure:

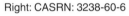

Left: CASRN: 458-88-8

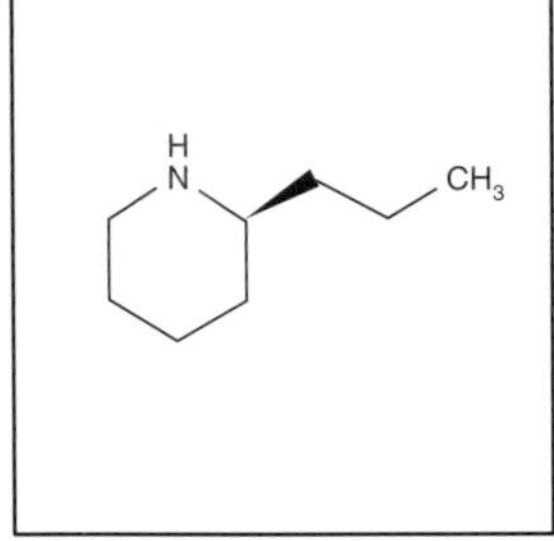

MW: 127.2293

Right: CASRN: 3238-60-6

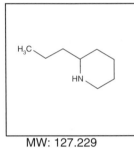

H3C
HN

MW: 127.229

Background

Coniine is a neurotoxin and toxic to humans and all classes of livestock. Dose less than 200 mg is fatal to humans, with death caused by respiratory paralysis. Historically, Socrates was put to death by this poison in 399 BC. Coniine has two stereoisomers: (*S*)-(+)-coniine, and (*R*)-(−)-coniine. Coniine was first synthesized by Albert Ladenburg in 1886.

Uses

Poison hemlock has been used as a sedative, antispasmodic, and antiarthritic drug. It has a narrow therapeutic index.

Environmental Fate and Behavior

It is an extremely poisonous alkaloid present to the extent of 2% in the leaves and unripe fruits. The concentrations of alkaloids vary with the age of the plant. Plants up to ~1-year-old have very low alkaloid content in roots, ~0.15% in stems, and 0.3–0.6% in leaves. Plants in their second year have an alkaloid content of ~1% in all their parts. Geographic latitude and drying will also affect the coniine content of the plant.

Exposure and Exposure Monitoring

The most common route of coniine exposure is by ingestion, although there are reports of dermal and eye irritation upon direct contact. The general signs of poisoning are similar in all species and include dilation of the pupils, weakness, and a staggering gait; the pulse, at first slow and becomes rapid; respiration becomes slow, labored, and irregular and is arrested before the heart ceases to beat. Consciousness is not usually lost. However, at higher doses death occurs rapidly (less than 3 h) with the most prominent signs and symptoms referable to peripheral paralysis and loss of sensation. Symptoms include drowsiness, paresthesias, weakness, ataxia, nausea, profuse salivation, and bradycardia followed by tachycardia. Death is due to respiratory arrest from paralysis of respiratory muscles. Central depression may play a role after very large doses.

Toxicokinetics

Coniine is rapidly absorbed from the gastrointestinal tract. Coniine is eliminated from the body through the lungs and kidneys and the peculiar mousy odor of the urine and exhaled air is diagnostic.

Mechanism of Toxicity

Coniine acts on the autonomic ganglia and produce initial stimulation of skeletal muscle followed by neuromuscular blockade. The actions of coniine are similar to those of nicotine that produce paralysis of greater numbers of central nervous system (CNS) and skeletal muscle nerve endings leading to respiratory paralysis. As a consequence, oxygen availability to the brain and heart is progressively decreased, ultimately leading to death.

Acute or Short-Term Toxicity

Animal

Certain small birds (skylarks, chaffinches, and robins) are not susceptible to coniine poisoning. Coniine toxicity has been reported in cows, goats, horses, pigs, sheep, ewes, rabbits, and chickens. The general signs of poisoning are similar in all species and include dilation of the pupils, weakness, and a staggering gait. Initially the pulse is slow and becomes rapid and respiration becomes slow, labored, and irregular and is arrested before the heart ceases to beat. Consciousness is not usually lost. The oral LD_{50} of coniine in the mouse is ~100 mg kg^{-1}. There are limited data in cattle, goats, and sheep suggesting developmental abnormalities to the musculoskeletal system of offspring when pregnant mothers are

 http://dx.doi.org/10.1016/B978-0-12-386454-3.00292-X

exposed orally to coniine (70 mg kg^{-1} for cattle and 484 mg kg^{-1} for goats and sheep). Coniine poisoned cattle developed signs of bloating, increased salivation and lacrimation, depression, respiratory distress, ataxia, and death after ingestion of hay that contained large amounts of poison hemlock. In another study, coniine caused arthrogryposis and spinal curvature in calves whose mothers were gavaged with the plant, *Conium maculatum* between 50 and 75 days of gestation.

Human

Toxic doses of the plant extract are difficult to determine due to differing concentrations of eight piperidinic alkaloids in the plant. Ingestion of poison hemlock in a 2-year-old boy had the onset of abdominal pain and weakness after 2 h of ingestion. He had a rapidly progressive muscular weakness and was intubated for respiratory failure. A toxic dose of coniine is estimated to be 60 mg and a lethal dose is estimated to be 100–300 mg for an adult. Death occurs rapidly (within 3 h) with the most prominent signs and symptoms of peripheral paralysis and loss of sensation. The principal manifestations of coniine poisoning are nausea and vomiting, salivation, fever, and gradually increasing muscular weakness followed by paralysis with respiratory failure leading to death.

Reproductive Toxicity

Congenital defects were reported in calves born to cows gavaged with the fresh green plant during 50–75 days of gestation. Both arthrogryposis and spinal curvature were reported with coniine. The arthrogrypotic manifestations of the condition markedly increased in severity as the animals aged. Animals gavaged dry plant had either normal or equivocally deformed offspring. No congenital defects in offspring from maternal inhalation of coniine.

Carcinogenicity

In a different study, cows, ewes, and mares varied considerably in susceptibility to toxic effects after the oral administration of coniine. Cows were most and ewes were least susceptible. Only calves had teratogenic effects from maternal administration of coniine during gestation; lambs and foals were apparently resistant. Results suggest that the marked differences between cattle and sheep are probably not due to variation in gut absorption or rumen metabolism.

Clinical Management

No antidote exists for coniine poisoning. Treatment is directed at removing ingested toxin and providing supportive care. Gastric lavage may be used to remove the ingested plant or plant extract. However, this method may not effectively remove large pieces of plant material. Intragastric administration of activated charcoal is recommended to reduce absorption in the gastrointestinal tract. Due to the rapid onset of CNS depression and seizures, emesis is generally not recommended. Difficulty to breath is treated by artificial respiration with oxygen. Convulsions are controlled with diazepam. A poisoned person may recover if artificial ventilation is maintained until the toxin is removed from the receptor.

See also: Hemlock; Poison; Plants, Poisonous (Humans); Poison Management; First Aid.

Further Reading

Arihan, O., Boz, M., Iskit, A.B., Ilhan, M., 2009. Antinociceptive activity of coniine in mice. J. Ethnopharmacol. 125 (2), 274–278.

Forsyth, C.S., Frank, A.A., 1993. Evaluation of developmental toxicity of coniine to rats and rabbits. Teratology 48, 59–64.

Forsyth, C.S., Speth, R.C., Wecker, L., Galey, F.D., Frank, A.A., 1996. Comparison of nicotinic receptor binding and biotransformation of coniine in the rat and chick. Toxicol. Lett. 89 (3), 175–183.

Frank, A.A., Reed, W.M., 1990. Comparative toxicity of coniine, an alkaloid of *Conium maculatum* (poison hemlock), in chickens, quails, and turkeys. Avian Dis. 34, 433–437.

Galey, F.D., Holstege, D.M., Fisher, E.G., 1992. Toxicosis in dairy cattle exposed to poison hemlock (*Conium maculatum*) in hay: isolation of *Conium* alkaloids in plants, hay, and urine. J. Vet. Diagn. Invest. 4, 60–64.

Lee, S.T., Green, B.T., Welch, K.D., Pfister, J.A., Panter, K.E., 2008. Stereoselective potencies and relative toxicities of coniine enantiomers. Chem. Res. Toxicol. 21 (10), 2061–2064.

López, T.A., Cid, M.S., Bianchini, M.L., 1999. Biochemistry of hemlock (*Conium maculatum* L.) alkaloids and their acute and chronic toxicity in livestock. A review. Toxicon 37 (6), 841–865.

Panter, K.E., James, L.F., Gardner, D.R., 1999. Lupines, poison-hemlock and *Nicotiana* spp: toxicity and teratogenicity in livestock. J. Nat. Toxin. 8 (1), 117–134.

Radulović, N., Đorđević, N., Denić, M., et al., 2012. A novel toxic alkaloid from poison hemlock (*Conium maculatum* L., Apiaceae): identification, synthesis and antinociceptive activity. Food Chem. Toxicol. 50 (2), 274–279.

Reynolds, T., 2005. Hemlock alkaloids from socrates to poison aloes. Phytochemistry 66 (12), 1399–1406.

Vetter, J., 2004. Poison hemlock (*Conium maculatum* L.). Food Chem. Toxicol. 42, 1373–1382.

West, P.L., Horowitz, B.Z., Montanaro, M.T., Lindsay, J.N., 2009. Poison hemlock-induced respiratory failure in a toddler. Pediatr. Emerg. Care 25 (11), 761–763.

Relevant Websites

http://chem.sis.nlm.nih.gov/chemidplus/ – National Library of Medicine, Search for Coniine.

http://toxnet.nlm.nih.gov/ – TOXNET, Specialized Information Service, National Library of Medicine, Search for Coniine.

Consumer Product Safety Commission

MA Babich, Directorate for Health Sciences, U.S. Consumer Product Safety Commission, Bethesda, MD, USA

- Relevant Chemicals and Chemical Abstracts Service Registry Numbers: asbestos (1332-21-4), butyl benzyl phthalate (85-68-7), dibutyl phthalate (84-74-2), di(2-ethylhexyl) phthalate (117-81-7), di-*n*-octyl phthalate (117-84-0), diisononyl phthalate (28553-12-0, 68515-48-0), diisodecyl phthalate (26761-40-0, 68515-49-1), lead (7439-92-1), and methylene chloride (dichloromethane) (75-09-2)

Consumer Product Safety Commission

The U.S. Consumer Product Safety Commission (CPSC) is an independent federal regulatory agency created by Congress in 1972. The agency's mission is to protect the public against unreasonable risks of injury from consumer products through education, safety standards activities, regulation, and enforcement. The CPSC has jurisdiction over thousands of types of products used in and around the home, in schools, and in recreation. Products under the jurisdiction of the CPSC include clothing, children's articles, household appliances, home furnishings, cleaners, and consumer fireworks. The CPSC does not have jurisdiction over foods, drugs, cosmetics, pesticides, certain radioactive materials, products that emit radiation, and automobiles, which are regulated by other federal agencies. Although the CPSC does not regulate drugs or cosmetics, it can require special packaging (i.e., child-resistant) for drugs, cosmetics, and household chemicals and can regulate medical devices in certain limited circumstances under the Federal Hazardous Substances Act (FHSA). The CPSC is directed by five commissioners, each of whom is appointed by the President of the United States, with one of the commissioners nominated by the President to the position of Chairman. (This information has been prepared by CPSC staff, has not been reviewed or approved by, and may not reflect the views of, the commissioners. Because this material was prepared by CPSC staff in their official positions, it is in the public domain and may be freely copied or reprinted.)

Statutes Administered by CPSC

To carry out its mission, the CPSC administers several statutes including Children's Gasoline Burn Prevention Act, Consumer Product Safety Act (CPSA) as amended by the Consumer Product Safety Improvement Act (CPSIA) of 2008, FHSA, Flammable Fabrics Act (FFA), Poison Prevention Packaging Act (PPPA), Refrigerator Safety Act, and the Virginia Graeme Baker Pool and Spa Safety Act. Toxicological issues arise most frequently under the CPSA, FHSA, and PPPA. CPSC regulations implementing these statutes may be found at Title 16 of the Code of Federal Regulations (CFR) and are available on the Commission's website at www.cpsc.gov.

The CPSIA amended the CPSA. (Public Law 110-314. The CPSIA was amended in 2011 by Public Law 112-28, which had further clarifications regarding bans related to lead and phthalates in certain children's products among other things.) Several sections specifically address toxicological issues. Section 101 of the CPSIA limits the concentration of lead in most children's products to 100 ppm, except for inaccessible component parts and certain electronic devices. Section 108 permanently prohibits the sale of any 'children's toy' or 'child care article' individually containing concentrations of more than 0.1% of dibutyl phthalate, butyl benzyl phthalate, or di(2-ethylhexyl) phthalate (DEHP). Section 108 prohibits, on an interim basis, the sale of 'any children's toy' that can be placed in a 'child's mouth' or 'child care article' containing concentrations of more than 0.1% of di-*n*-octyl phthalate, diisononyl phthalate, or diisodecyl phthalate. The interim prohibitions will be reevaluated in 2012, following review by a Chronic Hazard Advisory Panel (CHAP) on phthalates. Section 102 of the CPSIA requires manufacturers of certain children's products to certify that their products have been tested by a third party laboratory and are certified to comply with all applicable standards, including limits on lead and phthalates.

CPSA regulations include a ban of certain products that contain respirable, free-form asbestos. 16 CFR part 1304. In 1998, the Commission issued guidance requesting manufacturers to eliminate the use of hazardous liquid chemicals (e.g., methanol, methylene chloride, and petroleum distillates) from children's products, such as 'rolling balls, bubble watches, necklaces, pens, paperweights, key chains, liquid timers, and mazes.' 16 CFR § 1500.231.

In 1992, the Commission issued guidelines for assessing chronic hazards under the FHSA, including carcinogenicity, neurotoxicity, reproductive/developmental toxicity, exposure, bioavailability, risk assessment, and acceptable risk. 57 FR 46626–46674. The chronic hazard guidelines are intended to assist manufacturers in complying with the FHSA. A summary of the chronic hazard guidelines appears in the CPSC's regulations at 16 CFR § 1500.135 and is available on the Commission's website at www.cpsc.gov.

The CPSC is required to convene a CHAP before issuing certain mandatory requirements for substances that are associated with cancer, birth defects, or gene mutations. A CHAP is composed of seven independent scientists nominated by the National Academy of Sciences. CHAP members may not be employed by the federal government, except for the National Institutes of Health, National Toxicology Program, or the National Center for Toxicological Research, and they may not be employed by manufacturers, distributors, or retailers of consumer products.

The Labeling of Hazardous Art Materials Act (LHAMA) amended the FHSA to provide additional requirements for arts and crafts materials. Under regulations implementing LHAMA, each producer or repackager of an art material must describe, in

 http://dx.doi.org/10.1016/B978-0-12-386454-3.00597-2

writing, and submit to the Commission, the criteria used to determine whether an art material has the potential for producing chronic adverse health effects. 16 CFR § 1500.14 (b)(8). The producer or repackager must also submit a list of art materials requiring chronic hazard labeling. 16 CFR § 1500.14 (b)(8)(ii)(C). In addition, the CPSC regulations require art materials to have a statement of conformance and bear an emergency management telephone number. 16 CFR § 1500.14 (b)(8)(ii)(C).

Under the PPPA, to require child-resistant packaging for household substances, the Commission must find that special packaging is needed to protect children from serious personal injury or illness from handling, using, or ingesting a substance and that special packaging can be developed and mass produced that will protect the integrity of the product. Chemicals are regulated under the PPPA on a case-by-case basis.

Regulatory Options

If Commission action is needed to address a particular hazard, a range of regulatory options is available. Commission actions may include staff participation in the development of voluntary standards, mandatory labeling, mandatory performance standards, recalls, bans, and information and education. In general, for the Commission to issue standards or bans under the CPSA, FHSA, or FFA, findings must be made concerning costs and benefits, regulatory alternatives, issues raised by the public comments, and the adequacy of any relevant voluntary standards. Certain provisions of the CPSIA provide a different regulatory framework for toys, durable infant or toddler products, and children's products containing phthalates.

CPSC Programs

CPSC activities are organized into two major programs: Compliance and Hazard Identification and Reduction (HIR). Both programs are organized by the type of hazard: chemical, children's, combustion, electrical, fire and burn, and mechanical. The Compliance program encompasses activities related to ensuring compliance with or enforcement of existing regulations. In recent years, the CPSC has increased its focus on the safety of imported products and has added staff at major US ports to monitor such imports. Imported products are identified with the assistance of U.S. Customs and Border Protection staff. The HIR program identifies and assesses hazards to consumers and develops risk-reduction approaches, such as voluntary standards and mandatory regulations. Scientific and technical analyses of product hazards are carried out by HIR staff. For example, the HIR laboratory staff routinely tests thousands of products for compliance with regulations.

An essential tool of the HIR program is the National Electronic Injury Surveillance System (NEISS). NEISS is a stratified sample of approximately 100 emergency departments that report injuries associated with consumer products. Information such as the type and seriousness of the injury and identification of the product is entered into a database that provides estimates of consumer product-related injuries for the United States. NEISS is used to identify emerging hazards and to assess risk. Researchers and consumers can search NEISS online.

CPSC Staff

HIR activities are performed by staff in five technical directorates: Economic Analysis, Epidemiology, Engineering Sciences, Health Sciences, and Laboratory Sciences. The Directorate for Health Sciences employs scientists with advanced degrees in several disciplines, including toxicology, pharmacology, physiology, and chemistry at the CPSC's offices in the Washington, DC area. Health scientists generally work in multidisciplinary teams whose members also include engineers, statisticians, economists, attorneys, and experts in psychology, child development, and industrial and systems engineering who specialize in the field of Human Factors. The CPSC also maintains engineering and chemistry laboratories, with special expertise in combustion emissions, indoor air quality, and exposure assessment. Employment opportunities are listed on the CPSC's website and USAjobs.gov.

Contacting CPSC

Consumers may contact the CPSC to report an unsafe product or product-related injury; find out whether a product has been recalled; request injury data; or obtain CPSC publications, including press releases, staff reports, and regulations. Consumers can report a dangerous product or a product-related injury to the CPSC, as well as sign up to receive recall notifications and other announcements at www.saferproducts.gov. Consumers can contact the CPSC's hotline by phone at (800) 638-2772 or by e-mail at info@cpsc.gov. A teletypewriter for the deaf is available at (301) 595-7054.

See also: Asbestos; Chemicals in Consumer Products; Children's Environmental Health; Environmental Protection Agency, US; Food and Drug Administration, US; Lead; Nanotoxicology; The National Toxicology Program; Phthalates; Proposition 65, California; Recalls, Drugs and Consumer Products; Regulation, Toxicology and; Risk Assessment, Human Health; Toy Safety and Hazards; Toxic Substances Control Act.

Further Reading

Code of Federal Regulations. Consumer Products, vol. 16. http://www.gpo.gov/fdsys/pkg/CFR-2012-title16-vol1/content-detail.html (Chapter II) January 2012.

The National Electronic Injury Surveillance System, March 2000. A Tool for Researchers. U.S. Consumer Product Safety Commission. http://www.cpsc.gov/neiss/2000d015.pdf.

U.S. Consumer Product Safety Commission (CPSC), 1992. Labeling requirements for art materials presenting chronic hazards; guidelines for determining chronic toxicity of products subject to the FHSA; supplementary definition of "toxic" under the Federal Hazardous Substances Act; final rules. 57 Fed. Reg. 46626–46674. http://www.cpsc.gov/BUSINFO/chronic.pdf.

Relevant Websites

Consumer Product Safety Commission www.cpsc.gov

CPSC regulations. Code of Federal Regulations. Volume 16, Chapter II. Consumer Products. http://www.access.gpo.gov/nara/cfr/waisidx_03/16cfrv2_03.html

National Electronic Injury Surveillance System (NEISS) http://www.cpsc.gov/library/neiss.html

To report an injury or dangerous product www.saferproducts.gov

Product ingredients http://hpd.nlm.nih.gov/

Environmental Protection Agency www.epa.gov

Food and Drug Administration www.fda.gov

Contract Research Organizations

CB Spainhour, Spainhour Consulting, PA, USA

Contract research organizations, otherwise known by the acronym CROs, are service organizations located all over the world that provide services to a wide variety of businesses in a broad spectrum of industries. However, for the purposes of this work, the scope will be restricted to the pharmaceutical and biotechnology industries. CROs are alternatively known as contract service organizations and pharmaceutical development organizations. CROs range in size from small niche service providers to the large full ('we do it all') service CROs. CROs provide services that exist within the domains of good laboratory practice (GLP), good manufacturing practice, and good clinical practice as well as outside the boundaries of such areas. Some providers incorporate service offerings that include more than one of these areas. Specific areas of expertise can include biology, chemistry, clinical science, pharmaceutics, and regulatory expertise. Within the biology niche, offerings can include both the *in vitro* and the *in vivo* screening of test articles for lead identification and lead optimization as well as efficacy modeling, genetic toxicology, animal toxicology, immunotoxicology, pharmacokinetics, and metabolism. For chemistry services, one would expect to find synthesis and the scale-up synthesis of test articles, active pharmaceutical ingredient (API) manufacture, radiosynthesis, and analytical and bioanalytical method development and validation. Clinical services would include the availability of actual Phase 0 and Phase I Centers, data and site management services along with the services of statisticians, and clinical research associates along with report writing services. These latter services are also typically available for studies conducted at Phase II/III sites. Services within the discipline of pharmaceutics would include formulation development and drug product manufacture. Finally, organizations that specialize in the area of regulatory services in addition to the provision of regulatory advice also offer compilation and writing for an Investigational New Drug Application (IND), New Drug Application (NDA), Investigational Device Exemption, 510(k), Premarket Approval, Common Technical Document, Drug Master File, and Annual Updates.

Contract Research organizations have been around for a long time. The oldest in the United States was Food and Drug Research Laboratories, which opened for business in the 1930s in suburban New Jersey and closed for business in the 1980s. Starting around 1975, a number of different toxicology laboratories came into existence and after varying periods of time, went out of business. Some, but not all of these laboratories were Bioassay Systems, Tegaris, Bushy Run, Utah Biomedical Biotesting Laboratory, HTI, and Oread. Over the years, especially recent years, in addition to closures, there have been a number of acquisitions and mergers of different laboratories. Hazleton has evolved into Covance and Charles River has accumulated a number of smaller organizations all ultimately assembled under the 'Charles River Laboratories' name. All these activities are ultimately driven by the drive for the generation of top line revenue and the maximization of profit. Various economic pressures have also forced some of these changes (mergers and closures) in the pharmaceutical contract research industry.

Starting in the mid-1990s, a business strategy emerged with CROs in which the attitude was to 'touch' clients as much and as long as possible during the course of the drug development process, starting from actual discovery through the introduction of the product into the marketplace. Hence, the giant or behemoth CRO emerged. The concept was to keep the client as long as possible by just handing-off the client from one division to another division as the client progressed down the drug development path and their needs changed. Theoretically, this kept a persistent revenue stream from any given client. The problem with this is that no one company can realistically be expected to provide the same high-quality level of services in all the different disciplines that are required to develop a pharmacological entity or device for market. Alternatively, the smaller to mid-size CROs made conscious business decisions to not offer everything from 'soup to nuts' and focus on doing just a few things well. When it comes to the utilization of CROs, some individuals prefer to work with one large organization as a matter of convenience and pseudosecurity. Yet others prefer to work with a series of smaller to mid-size CROs despite any perceived enhanced monitoring and management effort in order to take advantage of each given organization's expertise.

A discussion of business philosophy is not inappropriate at this time. It is a well-known and recognized fact in business that to succeed a business must focus on three areas: operations, technology, and service. To really distinguish oneself, an organization must pick one area from these three and be better than their competitors in that chosen area and be at least as good as their competitors in the remaining two areas. So let's look more closely at these individual areas.

For CROs that elect to excel in technology, one can expect to see a catalog listing that includes each and every new technology that has arisen and is available. It does not matter whether or not there is regulatory support for such studies and the data generated from them. These data can be useful early in the drug development process, in the discovery stage, but is of questionable value when regulated studies are the main focus. The client needs to be wary of purchasing more than they need and generating too much data from assays and procedures that are not well recognized or accepted (at least wholly) by regulators and are possibly not properly validated, are imprecise, have poor predictive values, or translate poorly to prognostications of human safety. The data from such ancillary efforts can in turn rather than provide answers to questions and generate a lot more questions to be asked by regulators with concomitant delays in the attainment of milestones. However, to be fair, sometimes these tests are appropriate to run depending upon the timing, available time, and the questions that need to be answered.

Some CROs elect to pursue the service strategy. While everyone claims to provide excellent service, in actuality not all

 http://dx.doi.org/10.1016/B978-0-12-386454-3.00965-9

organizations do. The prospective client needs to look at references and ascertain whether the claims of outstanding service are indeed warranted. Specific areas of concern should be effectiveness of communication, timeliness of communication, flexibility of services, personalization or customization of services, responsiveness, on-time-delivery rate, total quality management procedures, and methods of resolution of mistakes and conflict.

Finally, for those CROs choosing to focus on operations, typically a giant lumbering machine is constructed. This machine can provide comfort to the prospective client in the fact that it is huge and very possibly the biggest or near the largest – so that if something goes wrong, the client can then tell his or her superior that "... I went with the biggest and everybody has heard of them ...," a statement carrying the inherent message that "nobody else would have gotten it right either." Not uncommonly these giants are rigid, inflexible, slowly responsive, and not very service oriented. So in the end, a potential Sponsor looking to outsource work needs to look at not only the type of work that needs to be done but also the business strategy and business philosophy of the organization where the work is to be placed to make sure that it is compliant with the attitude of the Sponsor himself or herself.

To place studies at a CRO, one must first identify a CRO with which to work. A variety of lists and advertisements exist in trade journals, professional journals, and books that can be extremely helpful. CROs usually attend scientific meetings, and so a great volume of information can be obtained by visitation and personal interaction at these functions. Professional colleagues are also a good source of information; however, be careful of potential bias, either positive or negative in these discussions. Follow through with your own investigation and make your own decisions. If one is looking to place highly specialized work, such as inhalation studies, then the options may indeed be few. From all these, an initial listing of laboratories can be constructed. For ease of management, the list should not exceed six to nine laboratories.

Once a list of laboratories has been identified, then the selection process begins. A good place to start is to visit the Food and Drug Administration (FDA) website and look for copies of laboratory inspection reports that have been conducted by federal agencies and are available for free under the Freedom of Information Act. While some specific information may and probably will have been purged from the reports, they are still of great value with regard to laboratory operations and systems. Since the inspection procedures used by the government are very consistent, these reports facilitate the comparison of different laboratories when evaluating the form and function of different systems. Keep in mind that effort must be made to put findings and citations in the proper perspective. All points mentioned on an audit report are not necessarily of equal importance and severity, and indeed some may even be considered to be trivial in nature. When it comes to visits to the various laboratories, one may wish to perform actual visits or interviews themselves of the various CROs under consideration or work through an intermediary, such as a suitably qualified toxicology or safety assessment consultant. Regardless, the critical areas of consideration in the selection of a laboratory should be (1) dependability, (2) actual prior experience with the activity or specific study (do not be scared by being the first program of its type, but rather look to see if the proper systems and resources are in place to do the project properly), (3) training of personnel, (4) status and type of equipment required to perform the project, (5) cost of the project, (6) state of facilities, (7) regulatory history, (8) state of IT systems, (9) financial soundness, (10) physical location and accessability, (11) references and reputation, (12) procedures in place to protect client confidentiality, (13) acceptability of study scheduling, (14) special considerations, (15) the wording and terms of the Master Services Agreement, (16) the format and detail of a study protocol, (17) company position on authorship, (18) the on-time report delivery record, and (19) openness to inspections by the Sponsor.

Historically, CROs that provided services in support of the development of pharmacologic moieties and medical devices were located in just a few places, such as the United States, Great Britain, Canada, Japan, Western Europe, and Israel. This is no longer the case. Driven in part by the desire and possibility to get into human trials outside of the United States and accelerate the drug development process, both China and India have led the way in the burgeoning of new CROs. Brazil, Korea, Singapore, Australia, and Eastern and Central European countries are now also represented. There are over 1100 CROs (30% nonclinical and 70% clinical) located all over the world, but the vast majority of capacity still exists in the original group of countries first listed above. Indeed, CROs are now and have been appearing all over the world. These organizations operate in almost all of the areas supporting drug development listed previously, but with varying degrees of success. The founding and development of these new CROs are a result of improved technology and capabilities in the various countries housing these new CROs, a desire of these various countries to enter the health care and R&D business sector and a perceived economic opportunity to sate the appetite for cheaper study costs and larger pools of available patients. The key factors attracting both US and European companies to CROs in these new countries include significantly cheaper pricing, fewer animal rights issues and concerns, a strategy to capture work from the large, growing economies in the new CRO host countries, and access to larger and new groups of subjects for clinical trials. This is, however, offset by the realities of the far too frequently observed: lack of quality, poor regulatory compliance, inadequate documentation of work and data, poor protection of intellectual property, poor security, communication problems, significant cultural differences affecting work performance, and lack of clear adherence to patient protection procedures.

So what should be the approach with regard to the use of CROs in these new countries? First, perform extensive and thorough qualification audits. Second, spend the time to develop proper, detailed, specific, and effective standard operating procedures and protocols. Third, maximize on-site monitoring of critical phases of studies conducted at such facilities. Fourth, place work and conduct business with laboratories that have some documented track record of performing regulated studies and submitting reports to the FDA and European Medicines Agency (EMEA).

But, let's take a closer look at the main two new players, India and China. Most Indian toxicology laboratories follow OECD protocol. There is one good Indian laboratory dealing primarily with agrochemicals, which has claimed to have performed over 80 studies for foreign sponsors and even to have passed GLP inspections from some European agrochemical and environmental regulatory authorities. While this is all good, this laboratory still lacks significant experience in dealing with toxicities observed with potential medicines and medical devices. Indian CROs have a lack of trained and suitably experienced veterinary histopathologists to detect early signs of drug-induced cardiotoxicity, hepatotoxicity, neurotoxicity, nephrotoxicity, and immunotoxicity. The growth and development of clinical pathology laboratories in India approved by the US-based College of Pathologists is limited, but growing. The costs of some Indian laboratories are relatively high for rodent studies, when compared to Chinese laboratories and while the work may be considered to be of GLP quality in India, are truly not of GLP quality. The modernization of facilities for the housing of animals and the implementation of proper procedures for feeding and animal management will require significant long-term investment, persistent training of personnel, and the establishment and enforcement of the highest standards of animal care and cleanliness. There is also a tendency of Indian laboratories to issue overly clean toxicology reports for purposes of local registration, by excluding diseased, dead, and out of range animals in reports, leading to an overestimation of safety and an underestimation of toxicity. Guidelines and rules set by the Committee for the Purpose of Control and Supervision of Experiments on Animals (CPCSEA) were revised in 2000 to require a central approval by the CPCSEA for all experiments on large animals (canines, nonhuman primates, and swine). Indian laboratories still need to implement in their operations, a comprehensive veterinary health program that includes adequate bacteriological, viral, parasitological, immunological, and pathological testing to monitor and establish the health integrity of animals used for studies. Toxicology laboratories in India need to better understand the techniques and procedures required for the development and validation of bioanalytical methods for the detection of test article in biological fluids and tissues. There have been reports that samples from the same animal have been repeated in order to save on the costs of the purchase of solid phase extraction cartridges. This repeated use of items intended for single use persists commonly in India. The level of training and experience of personnel performing bioanalytical work for toxicology laboratories in India, as a general rule, may not pass the scrutiny of an international analytical audit. There is a significant and essential need in India for a system, which implements consistent, strict, regular (annual) auditing procedures and clearly identifies certification procedures and standards for all toxicology, pharmacology, drug metabolism, and animal pharmacokinetic laboratories using animals for research. Interestingly, up to only a few years ago, it was illegal for any Indian toxicology laboratory to test a New Chemical Entity/New Molecular Entity (NCE/NME) discovered outside of India. However, toxicology studies have been and are still being performed in India for foreign clients.

Historically, Chinese CROs have focused on services in such areas as biology and chemistry. They have performed quite well in identifying moieties and combinations with the potential for use as therapeutic agents. They also have developed a reasonable reputation with regard to the manufacture of API for generic drugs. China currently has about 138 CROs, no animal rights activist problems, and an abundant supply of nonhuman primates. Accordingly, China has evolved into an attractive destination for animal testing. Worth noting is the fact that in order to sell drugs to China, pharmaceutical companies are required to conduct additional testing in China to obtain local approvals. Still, the biggest concern about placing toxicology work in China is the single fear that the FDA or EMEA will reject a Chinese GLP quality study, because it does not meet global regulatory expectations. Such an event would cause the loss of time and money in repeat of the work and theoretically loss of market opportunity. While this view is reasonable, there is in actuality no evidence that such a view is justified. Indeed, the facts are that the use of a high-quality Chinese CRO to perform a GLP toxicology study puts a program at no more significant risk than the use of a Western-based CRO.

GLP toxicology data from Chinese CROs have been used to support at least 30 (US) INDs and several NDAs since 2006. The China Preclinical Management Service has monitored over 20 GLP studies at Chinese CROs and data from these studies have been used to support three (US) INDs. Each of these INDs has been opened with no questions regarding the quality or the validity of the GLP studies involved. The US FDA recently opened permanent offices in China and has audited all of the CROs that have submitted GLP toxicology studies conducted in support of the filings of various INDs and NDAs. No studies evaluated in any of these audits were disqualified for any reason. Chinese animal technicians at the major top-tier Chinese CROs are perceived to be of very high-quality, well-educated, highly trained, and very committed to their jobs.

Regardless of where work is placed, if proper procedures as outlined here are followed for the identification and selection of CRO, success should be attainable with adequate management and supervision of the work.

Despite the best intentions and plans, there will always be unforeseen problems that develop during the course of the execution of a project. The best strategy in dealing with these is to educate oneself ahead of time so as to be prepared to deal with the challenges as they arise. To this end, seeking the advice of colleagues who have had to work through similar if not identical challenges can be very useful. Some common examples of areas in which problems might arise are (1) changes in key study or organizational personnel; (2) lack of clarity in lines of authority and signatory responsibilities; (3) lack of adherence to and slippage in attainment of timed milestones; (4) lack of regulatory compliance; (5) failures in quality control procedures and/or quality assurance procedures; (6) poor or inappropriate selection of proper technology to generate data; (7) actual closure of the testing facility (a more common concern these days); (8) acts of nature; (9) miscommunication, ineffective communication, or stretching the truth; (10) the use of silent or stealth subcontractors; (11) the existence of potential conflict of interest alliances; (12) overpromising and under-delivering, or in other words overly committing to too much work for the available resources at hand; and (13) simple extraneous events associated with the perpetration of errors.

Geographically, work can be placed at any number of CROs all over the world and despite every effort and extensive planning, unfortunate events can still happen. But proper research and planning are essential and in the end the essence that it all distills to is the integrity of the people and the organization working together.

See also: Behavioral Toxicology; High Throughput Screening; American College of Toxicology; The Hamner Institutes for Health Sciences; EUROTOX; Food and Drug Administration, US; Good Clinical Practice (GCP); National Center for Environmental Health-ATSDR; National Center for Toxicological Research, US; National Institute for Occupational Safety and Health; The National Institute of Environmental Health Sciences; National Institutes of Health; Occupational Safety and Health Administration; Genetic Toxicology; International Union of Toxicology; Occupational Safety and Health Act, US; Regulation, Toxicology and; Toxicity Testing, Reproductive; Toxicology; Veterinary Toxicology; Risk Assessment, Human Health; Toxicity Testing, Aquatic; Ecotoxicology; Aquatic Ecotoxicology; Avian Ecotoxicology; Genetic Ecotoxicology; Ecotoxicology, Aquatic Invertebrates; Ecotoxicology Terrestrial; Ecotoxicology; Wildlife; European Centre for Ecotoxicology and Toxicology of Chemicals; Ecological Quality Standards (EQS) Global; REACH; European Union and Its European Commission; The History of Toxicology; Information Resources in Toxicology; Animal Models; Biocompatibility; Food, Drug, and Cosmetic Act, US; Good Laboratory Practices; *In Vitro* Tests; *In Vivo* Tests; The International Conference on Harmonisation; Investigative New Drug Application; The QT Interval of the Electrocardiogram; Toxic Substances Control Act; Toxicity Testing, Alternatives; Toxicity Testing, Behavioral; Toxicity Testing, Carcinogenesis; Toxicity Testing, Dermal; Toxicity Testing, Inhalation; Toxicity Testing, Mutagenicity; Toxicity Testing, Sensitization; Cosmetics and Personal Care Products; Environmental Protection Agency, US; Environmental Toxicology; Toxicology Forum.

Further Reading

Gad, S.C., 2009. Drug Safety Evaluation, second ed. John Wiley & Sons, Inc, Hoboken, NJ.

Gad, S.C., 2011. Safety Evaluation of Pharmaceuticals and Medical Devises. International Regulatory Guidelines. Springer, New York.

Gad, S.C., McCord, M.G., 2008. Safety Evaluation in the Development of Medical Devices and Combination Products, third ed. Informa Healthcare USA, Inc., New York.

Gad, S.C., Spainhour, C.B., 2011. Contract Research and Development Organization Their Role in Global Product Developments. Springer, New York.

Gad, S.C., Taulbee, S.M., 1996. Handbook of Data Recording, Maintenance, and Management for the Biomedical Sciences. CRC Press, Boca Raton, FL.

Gralla, E.J., 1981. Scientific Considerations in Monitoring and Evaluating Toxicological Research. Hemisphere Publishing Corporation, Washington, DC.

Guarino, R.A., 1987. New Drug Approval Process. Marcel Dekker, New York.

Mathieu, M., 2000. New Drug Development: A Regulatory Overview. Parexel, Waltham, MA.

Matoren, G.M., 1984. The Clinical Research Process in the Pharmaceutical Industry. Marcel Dekker, New York.

Parikh, D., 2001. Formulation development. Contract Pharma October 60–64.

Silverman, J., Suckow, M.A., Murthy, S. (Eds.), 2007. The IACUC Handbook, second ed. CRC Press, Boca Raton, Fl.

Smith, C.G., 1992. The Process of New Drug Discovery and Development. CRC Press, Boca Raton, FL.

Sneader, W., 1986. Drug Development: From Laboratory to Clinic. John Wiley & Sons, Inc, New York.

Snyder, S., 2009. Working with study directors. Contract Pharma July/August 28–30.

Swarbrick, J., Boylan, J.C., 2002. Encyclopedia of Pharmaceutical Technology, second ed. Marcel Dekker, New York.

Relevant Websites

Chemistry Consultants www.chemconsultants.com
CRO Registry www.technomark.com
CRO Registry www.inpharm.com
Freedom of Information Documents
www.fda.gov/RegulatoryInformation/foi/default.htm
Inspected Nonclinical Laboratories
www.fda.gov/org/compliance ref/bimo/GLP/default.htm
Inspection of Quality Systems
www.fda.gov/ora/inspect_ref/igs/qsit/QSITGUIDE.PDF
Outsourcing www.bioportfolio.com
Outsourced Project Management www.arachnova.com
Toxicology Consultants www.toxconsultants.com
Web-based CRO Selection System www.dataedge.com

Copper

SC Gad, Gad Consulting Services, Cary, NC, USA

- Chemical Abstracts Service Registry Number: 7440-50-8
- Chemical/Pharmaceutical/Other Class: Metals
- Molecular Formula: Cu^{2+}
- Valence States: +1, +2, +3, +4

Background

Copper has long been used by humans for a variety of reasons. The name copper derives from the Latin for the metal, *cuprum*, which is named for the Roman source, the island of Cyprus. Copper has been used in a variety of alloys; of particular importance among copper alloys is bronze, which comprised most of the tools and weapons of the age that bears its name. Brass, a copper–zinc alloy, is also highly used, for example, in brass musical instruments. Copper has also long been used as a building material, and owing to the metal's malleability, as well as high thermal and electric conductivity, continues to find new uses. Copper and its compounds are naturally present in the earth's crust. Natural discharges to air and water may be significant. Therefore, it is important to consider the background levels that are commonly found and distinguish these from high levels that may be found as a result of anthropogenic activity. Copper is emitted into the air naturally from windblown dust, volcanoes, and anthropogenic sources, the largest of which are being primary copper smelters and ore processing facilities. It is associated with particulate matter. The mean concentration of copper in the atmosphere is 5–200 ng m^{-3}.

Uses

Copper is an essential trace element. Adequate daily requirements are 2–3 mg day^{-1}. It is widely distributed in nature and extensively used in industry. It is used as an electrical conductor, as a component in a variety of alloys (including gold and silver alloys), and as a constituent in paints and ceramic glazes. Because it corrodes at a very slow rate, it is used extensively for water pipes. In addition, copper sulfate mixed with lime is used as a fungicide.

Medicinally, copper sulfate is used as an emetic. It has also been used as an antihelminthic (antiparasitic agent) based on its astringent and caustic actions.

Environmental Fate and Behavior

Copper is slightly soluble in dilute acid, and slowly soluble in ammonia water. Some copper compounds are water soluble, such as copper sulfate and copper chloride.

The largest release of copper by far is to land, and the major sources of release are mining and milling operations, agriculture, solid waste, and sludge from publicly owned treatment works. Sediment is an important sink and reservoir for copper. In relatively clean sediment, the copper concentration is <50 ppm; polluted sediment may contain several thousand ppm of copper.

Copper is released to water as a result of natural weathering of soil and discharges from industries and sewage treatment plants. Copper compounds may also be intentionally applied to water to kill algae. Of special concern is copper that gets into drinking water from the water distribution system.

The major species of soluble copper found in freshwater, seawater, and a combination of the two over a range of pHs is Cu^{2+}, $Cu(HCO_3)^+$, and $Cu(OH)_2$. At the pH values and carbonate concentrations characteristic of natural waters, most dissolved Cu(II) exists as carbonate complexes rather than as free (hydrated) cupric ions.

The transport of copper is largely dependent on source characteristics as well as particle size; however, it can bind to many inorganic ligands. Some copper compounds are water soluble, and this can increase transport distance, as well as likelihood the metal will be taken up by organisms or adsorb to organic residues.

The bioconcentration factor (BCF) of copper in fish obtained in field studies is 10–100, indicating a low potential for bioconcentration. The BCF is higher in mollusks (i.e., oysters), where it may reach 30 000, possibly because they are filter feeders. There is a good deal of evidence that there is no biomagnification of copper in the food chain.

Exposure and Exposure Monitoring

The primary exposure pathway for copper is ingestion (e.g., food and water). Many foods contain copper, especially legumes, organ meats, and oysters. Water carried through copper pipes is also a source of this element. Inhalation is only a significant exposure pathway in industrial settings (e.g., near copper refineries).

Many workers are exposed to copper in agriculture, industries connected with copper production, metal plating, and other industries. Little information is available concerning the forms of copper to which workers are exposed. Copper has been identified at many National Priorities List hazardous waste sites in the United States.

Toxicokinetics

Approximately 50% of ingested copper is absorbed from the stomach. Although copper can be absorbed from the gastrointestinal tract, a modifying biological mechanism regulates total copper absorbed. Copper is transformed in the blood by first binding to albumin and then to a copper-specific protein (ceruloplasmin). Copper also binds to metallothionein more firmly than zinc or even cadmium. Copper is stored in the liver and bone marrow as the metallothionein.

 http://dx.doi.org/10.1016/B978-0-12-386454-3.00834-4

Copper-dependent enzymes include tyrosinase (which is involved in melanin pigment formation) and the various oxidases (i.e., cytochrome oxidase, superoxide dismutase, amine oxidase, and uricase). Copper plays a major role in the incorporation of iron into the heme of hemoglobin. Copper deficiency is characterized by hypochromic, microcytic anemia resulting from defective hemoglobin synthesis.

Copper levels in the human body vary with age. Copper levels in the brain increase with age, whereas in some tissues (e.g., liver, lungs, and spleen), copper levels are higher in newborns than in adults. Tissue levels gradually decline up to age 10 and remain relatively constant thereafter. Copper is normally excreted in bile, which plays a primary role in copper homeostasis.

Mechanism of Toxicity

Copper reduces glutathione, which is necessary for normal cell viability. The amino acid transferases are inhibited in the presence of excess copper; lipid peroxidation also occurs. Copper combines with thiol groups, which reduces the oxidation state II to I in copper and oxidizes the thiol groups to disulfides, especially in the cell membrane.

Acute and Short-Term Toxicity (or Exposure)

Animal

Copper produces lung damage by inhalation. Intratracheal administration of copper has produced lung damage in rodents; macrophages increased with degenerative membrane structure and hemoglobin values decreased. In larger animals, excess copper intake resulted in iron-deficient anemia and gastric ulcers.

Human

Although copper is an essential element, it is much more toxic to cells than such nonessential elements as nickel and cadmium. Acute poisoning from ingestion of excessive amounts of copper salts, most frequently copper sulfate, results in nonspecific toxic symptoms, a metallic taste, nausea, and vomiting (with vomitus possibly a blue-green color). The gastrointestinal tract can be damaged by ulceration.

Chronic Toxicity (or Exposure)

Animal

No statistically significant increases in tumor formation were noted in mice fed copper for ~1 year. Subcutaneous and intramuscular injection of copper compounds showed a low incidence of sarcomas. The current data are adequate to assess the carcinogenicity of copper.

Human

Severe symptoms include hypotension, coma, jaundice, and death. Liver necrosis has also been observed. In some cases, copper toxicity can result in an inability to urinate. Treatment with copper compounds can induce hemolytic anemia.

It is believed that the increased susceptibility to copper toxicity seen in infants and children is owing to the normally high hepatic copper levels in early life and the fact that homeostatic mechanisms are not fully developed at birth.

Copper is associated with two genetic inborn errors of metabolism. The first, Menke's disease or Menke's kinky-hair syndrome is associated with severe copper deficiency, owing to a defect in an ATPase gene resulting in the inability of the gastrointestinal tract to absorb copper. It is a sex-linked trait characterized by peculiar hair, failure to thrive, severe neurological degradation in the brain, and death before 3 years of age. The cerebral cortex and white matter degenerates; mental retardation ensues before death. The second disease, Wilson's disease or hepatolenticular degeneration, is associated with severe copper excess, owing to a defect in another ATPase gene resulting in the inability of the liver to excrete copper in the bile. It is characterized by an unusual concentration of copper in the brain, kidneys, cornea, and especially in the liver (which may become abnormally large). Mental retardation is not associated with this disease. This disease is usually treated with a chelating agent such as penicillamine or triethylene tetramine.

Immunotoxicity

Of copper compounds, only copper sulfate has been tested as to its immunotoxicity. Hamsters exposed to inhaled copper sulfate experiences reduced pulmonary macrophage activity. In mice a number of immunotoxic effects have been observed, such as a decrease in the lymphoproliferative response, among other immunodepressant activities.

Genotoxicity

Mutagenesis results are dependent on the bacterial strain and copper compound evaluated. Mammalian cell tests indicate a positive mutagenic response.

Reproductive Toxicity

Insufficient data exist to truly classify copper and its compounds as to their reproductive toxicity; however, studies have revealed no link between abortion and placental copper, but a positive birth weight correlation with increasing copper concentrations.

Carcinogenicity

There are not enough animal data and no human data to classify copper as a human carcinogen, it has therefore been classified as class D, not classifiable as to human carcinogenicity. Some data do exist suggesting a connection, but there is not enough specificity and an overabundance of confounding factors in these studies.

Clinical Management

For acute toxicity, emesis is recommended. Treatment is symptomatic. A combination of BAL (British anti-Lewisite; 2,3-dimercaptopropanol) and calcium ethylene diamine tetraacetic acid has been used successfully in a poisoned infant. Penicillamine has also been used. Recently, oral administration of 2,3-dimercapto1-propane sulfonate was found to be effective in experimental rodents. Electrolyte balance must be maintained when gastric lavage is indicated. Potassium ferrocyanide should be added to precipitate the copper.

Ecotoxicology

Nearly all organisms require copper for proper functioning, and many are able to regulate internal levels. Mollusks accumulate more copper than other organisms; however, it appears to not have negative effects until at extraordinarily high levels. Plants require trace amounts of copper to aid in photosynthesis; however, if on contaminated soil, even moderate levels can have severe deleterious effects on plants.

Exposure Standards and Guidelines

The American Conference of Governmental Industrial Hygienists threshold limit value time-weighted average is 0.2 mg m^{-3} for copper fume and 1 mg m^{-3} for copper dusts and mists.

The Environmental Protection Agency drinking water limit is 1.3 ppm. The median concentration of copper in natural water is 4–10 ppb.

Daily intakes of copper and other essential minerals are estimated and can be found as part of the Food and Drug Administration's Total Diet Study.

Miscellaneous

Copper used in construction settings can often be seen in its oxidized state, which changes its appearance from a lustrous red-orange to a matte light green.

See also: Metallothionein; Metals; Pollution, Water.

Further Reading

Brewer, G.J., 2008 Nov. The risks of free copper in the body and the development of useful anticopper drugs. Curr. Opin. Clin. Nutr. Metab. Care 11 (6), 727–732.

Brewer, G.J., 2010 Feb. Risks of copper and iron toxicity during aging in humans. Chem. Res. Toxicol. 23 (2), 319–326.

Gaetke, L.M., Chow, C.K., 2003. Copper toxicity, oxidative stress, and antioxidant nutrients. Toxicology 189 (1–2), 147–163.

Georgopoulos, P.G., Roy, A., Yonone-Lioy, M.J., Opiekun, R.E., Lioy, P.J., 2001. Environmental copper: its dynamics and human exposure issues. J. Toxicol. Environ. Health B Crit. Rev. 4 (4), 341–394.

Goyer, R.A., Klaassen, C.D., Waalkes, M.P., 1995. Metal Toxicology. Academic Press, San Diego, CA.

Grass, G., Rensing, C., Solioz, M., 2011. Metallic copper as an antimicrobial surface. Appl. Environ. Microbiol. 77 (5), 1541–1547.

Hostynek, J.J., Maibach, H.I., 2003. Copper hypersensitivity: dermatologic aspects – an overview. Rev. Environ. Health 18 (3), 153–183.

Nordberg, G.F., Fowler, B.A., Nordberg, M., Friberg, L.T., 2007. Handbook on the Toxicology of Metals, third ed. Associated Press, London.

Relevant Websites

http://www.atsdr.cdc.gov – Agency for Toxic Substances and Disease Registry. Toxicological Profile for Copper.

http://www.inchem.org/documents/ehc/ehc/ehc200.htm – International Program on Chemical Safety, Environmental Health Criteria.

Coprine *see* Mushrooms, Coprine

Corrosives

MM Purcell and JM Marraffa, Upstate Medical University, Syracuse, NY, USA

This article is a revision of the previous edition article by Greene Shepherd, volume 1, p 668, © 2005, Elsevier Inc.

Background

Corrosive materials are present in almost every workplace, and injuries following exposure are often more severe than other exposures because industrial products are more concentrated than those found in the home. Caustics (which include acids or alkalis) and other chemicals may be corrosive; however, acids and bases are most often responsible for corrosive exposures. Common corrosive acids include hydrochloric acid, sulfuric acid, nitric acid, chromic acid, acetic acid, and hydrofluoric acid. Common corrosive bases are ammonium hydroxide, potassium hydroxide (caustic potash), and sodium hydroxide (caustic soda).

Uses

Corrosive materials are present in almost every workplace. Household cleaning substances (for example, toilet bowl or drain cleaners) can contain potentially corrosive substances. Corrosives have also been used as disinfectant and sterilizing agents in medical and dental settings as well as other uses.

Acute and Short-Term Toxicity (or Exposure)

Corrosives can burn and destroy body tissues on contact. Stronger or more concentrated corrosives, or longer contact with the skin or mucosal tissues, result in more serious injuries.

Corrosives are harmful if they come in contact with the skin or eyes, inhaled, or swallowed. Direct contact with the skin can severely irritate or even badly burn and blister the skin. Severe corrosive burns over a large part of the body can cause death. Corrosive materials can severely irritate, or in some cases, burn the eyes. This could result in scars or permanent blindness. The stronger or more concentrated the corrosive material is and the longer it contacts with the eyes, the worse the injury will be. Breathing in corrosive vapors or particles irritates and burns the inner lining of the nose, throat, windpipe, and lungs. In serious cases, this results in pulmonary edema, a buildup of fluid in the lungs that can be fatal. Swallowing corrosives burns the lining of the mouth, throat, esophagus, and stomach. In nonfatal cases, severe scarring of the throat may occur and could result in losing the ability to swallow due to stricture formation.

Clinical Management

For oral exposure, perform endoscopy to assess burns and evaluate for stricture formation. For inhalation exposure, endotracheal intubation and airway management may be needed for patients with upper airway edema or respiratory distress. Copious irrigation and removal of contaminated clothing are needed after dermal exposure. For ocular exposure, copious irrigation is needed until pH is neutral.

Exposure Standards and Guidelines

The Occupational Safety and Health Administration divides corrosives into three subcategories based on observations of corrosive damage to the skin of laboratory animals. All subcategories of skin corrosives are regulated as Category 1, which is the most severe toxicity category.

Other Issues

Many acid and base corrosives attack and corrode metals. Under these circumstances, flammable and explosive hydrogen gas can be formed.

See also: Hydrochloric Acid; Sulfuric Acid; Nitric Acid; Chromic Acid; Acetic Acid and Hydrofluoric Acid; Ammonium Hydroxide; Potassium Hydroxide; Sodium Hydroxide.

Further Reading

Edlich, R.F. Treatment and Prevention of Chemical Injuries (updated September 18, 2013). Available at: http://emedicine.medscape.com.

Naik, R.R.R., Vadivelan, M., 2012. Corrosive poisoning. Indian J. Clin. Pract. 23 (3), 131–134.

Relevant Website

http://www.ccohs.ca/ – Corrosive Materials – Hazards.

Corticosteroids

B Spoelhof and SD Ray, Manchester University College of Pharmacy, Fort Wayne, IN, USA

This article is a revision of the previous edition article by Prathibha S. Rao, volume 1, pp 669–670, © 2005, Elsevier Inc.

- Name: Corticosteroids
- Chemical Abstracts Service Registry Number: 8001-02-3
- Synonyms: Cortisone; Prednisone (Deltasone®, Orasone®); Dexamethasone (Decadron®); Hydrocotisone (Cortef®, Westcort®); Aldosterone; Fludrocotrisone (Florinef®)
- Molecular Formula: Varies depending on agent
- Chemical Structure:

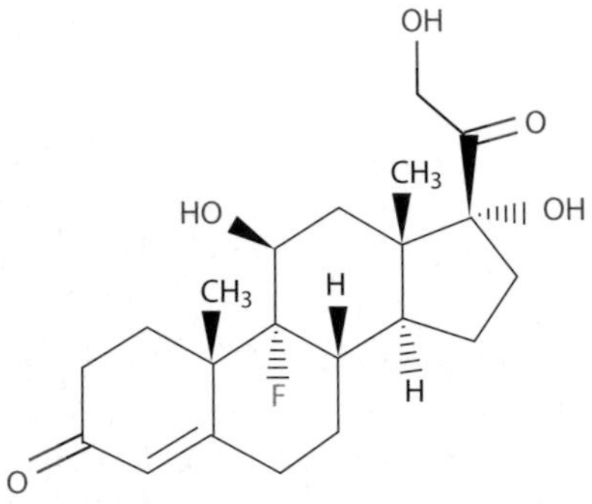

Fludrocortisone

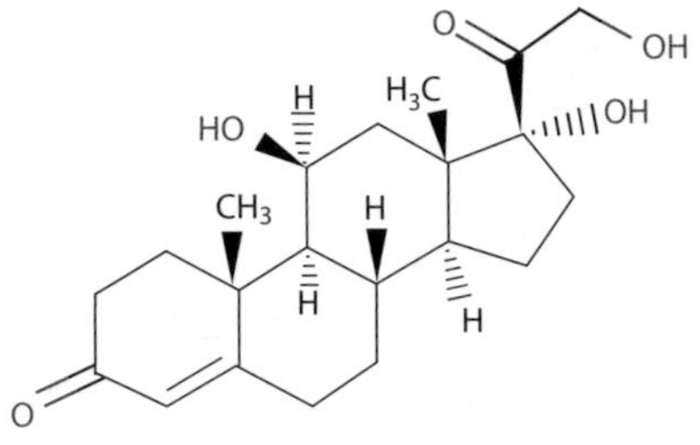

Cortisol/Hydrocortisone

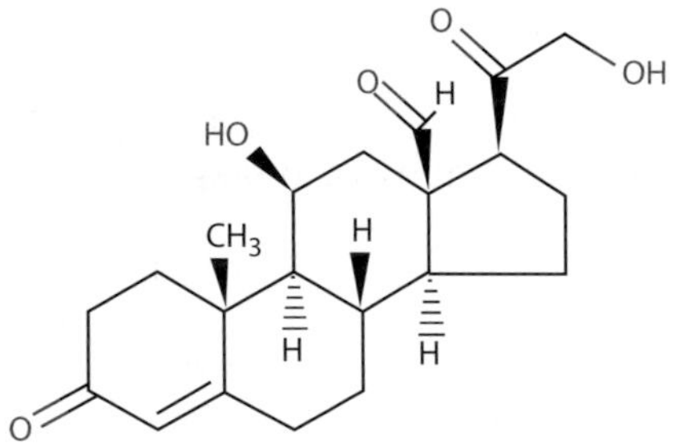

Aldosterone

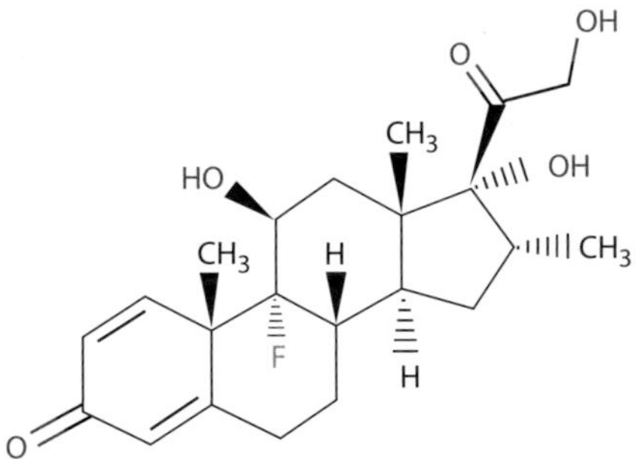

Dexamethasone

effects. There are two classes of corticosteroids, glucocorticoids and mineralocorticoids that have predominant effects on metabolic and electrolyte processes, respectively. Beyond the carbohydrate, protein, and lipid metabolism; water and electrolyte management; corticosteroids also exert effects by regulating normal function of the cardiovascular, immune, kidney, skeletal, endocrine, and nervous systems. Furthermore, in part due to the physiological responses during times of survival and noxious stimuli, corticosteroids have been termed the *stress hormones*.

Background

Addison first described in the mid-nineteenth century that destruction of the adrenal glands led to fatal outcomes. Further studies identified the adrenal cortex as a chief regulator of metabolic, water, and electrolyte homeostasis, and by the 1930s, the structure of several compounds important in glucose metabolism had been described. Nearly a century later, research by Kendall and colleagues led to the discovery of cortisone as an effective antiinflammatory agent for patients with rheumatoid arthritis.

Corticosteroids are a broad class of both endogenous and exogenous compounds that exert a wide range of physiological

Mechanisms of Action

General Mechanism of Action

Corticosteroids exert their physiological effects via activation of either glucocorticoid receptor (GR) or the mineralocorticoid receptor (MR) in target tissues to alter the expression of corticosteroid-responsive genes. For example, the GR in the cell cytoplasm binds with steroid ligands to form hormone–receptor complexes that eventually translocate to the cell nucleus. These complexes bind to specific DNA sequences and alter their expression. The complexes may induce the transcription of mRNA leading to synthesis of new proteins. Though less studied than glucocorticoids, mineralocorticoids have a similar mechanism of action in gene regulation.

Antiinflammatory Mechanism of Action

Lipocortin, a protein known to inhibit PLA2a is one such protein that is upregulated and thereby blocks the synthesis of prostaglandins, leukotrienes, and platelet activating factor (PAF). Glucocorticoids also inhibit the production of other mediators including amino acids metabolites such as cyclooxygenase, cytokines, the interleukins, adhesion molecules, and enzymes such as collagenase.

Metabolic Mechanism of Action

In order to provide a mode of preservation for highly energy-dependent organ systems such as heart and brain tissues, glucocorticoids lead to increased serum glucose levels. Though poorly understood peripheral uptake of glucose is inhibited, it leads to decreased glucose utilization. Furthermore, gluconeogenesis is stimulated by inducing the transcription of enzymes such as phosphoenolpyruvate carboxykinase, fructose-1,6-biphosphatase, and glucose-6-phosphatase.

Electrolyte Homeostasis Mechanism of Action

Aldosterone is the prototypical mineralocorticoid. MRs located on the distal tubule and collecting duct upregulate sodium potassium pumps to increase reabsorption of sodium within the nephron. As a result, potassium and hydrogen ions are excreted and water is retained.

Available Agents and Routes of Administration

Corticosteroids are available as a variety of dosage forms. Oral administration can be facilitated via tablet, capsules, or liquid preparations. Furthermore, several commercially available devices exist for administration of dry powder, nebulized, and aerosolized drug. Corticosteroids can be topically applied as solutions, foams, shampoos, creams, ointments, and suspensions to the skin, eyes, or ears. Suppositories for rectal administrations and parenteral preparations for intramuscular or intravenous administration also exist. These preparations are available as either over-the-counter or prescription only. In addition, they may also be supplied in combination with other therapeutic agents (ciprofloxacin, nystatin).

Uses

Synthetic pharmaceutical drugs with corticosteroid-like effect are used in a variety of conditions, ranging from brain tumors to skin diseases. Dexamethasone and its derivatives are almost pure glucocorticoids, while prednisone and its derivatives have some mineralocorticoid action in addition to the glucocorticoid effect. Fludrocortisone (Florinef) is a synthetic mineralocorticoid. Hydrocortisone (cortisol) is available for replacement therapy, e.g., in adrenal insufficiency and congenital adrenal hyperplasia. See **Table 1** for relative dosing and antiinflammatory/mineralocorticoid activity.

The most common use for corticosteroids today is for their antiinflammatory effects. Both oral and topical agents are used as treatment options for patients with conditions such as contact dermatitis. Autoimmune disorders or other inflammatory diseases such as ulcerative colitis, Crohn's disease, temporal arteritis, systemic lupus erythematosus, or multiple sclerosis can all be treated with oral or intravenous therapy. National treatment guidelines recommend the use of inhaled corticosteroids as maintenance therapy for patients with mild persistent asthma and a short course of oral therapy for moderate or severe persistent asthma.

Corticosteroids have been widely used in treating people with traumatic brain injury. A systematic review identified 20 randomized controlled trials and included 12 303 participants, compared patients who received corticosteroids with patients who received no treatment. The authors recommended people with traumatic brain injury should not be routinely treated

Table 1 Relative dosing and potency of select corticosteroids

	Approximate equivalent dose (mg)	*Relative antiinflammatory potency*	*Relative mineralocorticoid potency*	*Half-life plasma (min)*
Short-acting				
Cortisone	25	0.8	0.8	30
Hydrocortisone	20	1	1	90
Intermediate-acting				
Methylprednisolone	4	5	0	180
Prednisolone	5	4	0.8	200
Prednisone	5	4	0.8	60
Triamcinolone	4	5	0	300
Long-acting				
Betamethasone	0.75	25	0	100–300
Dexamethasone	0.75	25–30	0	100–300
Mineralocorticoids				
Fludrocortisone	–	10	125	200

Asare, K., 2007. Diagnosis and treatment of adrenal insufficiency in the critically ill patient. Pharmacotherapy 27 (11), 1512–1528.

with corticosteroids, as it may lead to increased mortality. Furthermore, a Cochrane review found limited evidence for the use of methylprednisolone in spinal cord injury patients. If used, it must be given within 8 h of initial injury and continued for 24–48 h.

Corticosteroids can also be given during moments of adrenal insufficiency. Addison's disease is a disorder in which endogenous production of corticosteroids is either limited or completely ceased. This can occur for many reasons such as Hypothalamic–pituitary–adrenal axis (HPAA) suppression, moments of overt and high stress such as septic shock, or genetic abnormalities.

Side Effects and Adverse Reactions

The potent effect of corticosteroids can result in serious side effects, which mimic Cushing's disease, a malfunction of the adrenal glands resulting in an overproduction of cortisol. The list of potential side effects is long and includes: increased appetite and weight gain; deposits of fat in chest, face, upper back, and stomach; water and salt retention leading to swelling and edema; high blood pressure; diabetes; black and blue marks; slowed healing of wounds; osteoporosis; cataracts; acne; muscle weakness; thinning of the skin; increased susceptibility to infection; stomach ulcers; increased sweating; mood swings; psychological problems such as depression; and adrenal suppression and crisis.

Side effects can be minimized by following doctor's orders and keeping to the lowest dose possible. It is also important to avoid self-regulation of the dosage, either by adding more or stopping the medication without a schedule.

Acute and Short-Term Toxicity

Human

Acute exposure of methylprednisolone has been associated with seizure activity and cardiac dysrhythmias such as atrial fibrillation, myocardial infarction, asystole, and sudden death.

Patients may develop hypertension, electrolyte abnormalities, and increased glucose following acute exposure.

Chronic Toxicity (or Exposure) Animal

Animal

Chronic exposure to high serum levels of corticosterone induced a significant impairment of inhibitory avoidance learning in rats. In another study, corticosterone elevated over a period of 21 days impaired the formation of a longer-term form of memory, most likely reference memory. Impairments in spatial working memory were seen only after longer durations of corticosterone administration.

Human

Chronic administration leads to hypothalamic–pituitary–adrenal axis suppression. Chronic exogenous administration of corticosteroids provides a negative feedback to decrease corticotropin-releasing hormone (CRH) and adrenocorticotropic hormone (ACTH) release by the hypothalamus and the pituitary, respectively. When the exogenous steroids are removed, an Addisonian state is induced and patients may develop an Addison's crisis characterized by hypoglycemia, low blood pressure, and several electrolyte derangements.

Fluid and electrolyte disturbances, hypertension, hyperglycemia, and glycosuria of acute toxicity may also occur. It also increases the susceptibility to infections including tuberculosis; causes peptic ulcers, osteoporosis, behavioral disturbances, posterior subcapsular cataracts, growth arrest, Cushing's habitus, 'buffalo hump,' enlargement of supraclavicular fat pads, 'central obesity,' striae, ecchymoses, acne, and hirsutism.

Genotoxicity

Very few studies with the natural or synthetic corticosteroids have been published. Data on cortisol and corticosterone are not available. Data on hydrocortisone are minimal. There is weak evidence that dexamethasone could have clastogenic and sister-chromatid exchange (SCE)-inducing potential.

Toxicokinetics

Generally, the biological half-lives of corticosteroids can be classified as short (8–12 h), intermediate (12–36 h), or long (36–72 h). See **Table 1** for relative half-lives of various corticosteroids. Cortisone and cortisol are examples of short-lived corticosteroids. Prednisone, prednisolone, and triamcinolone are of the intermediate class. Dexamethasone and β-methasone are associated with the longer-lived class.

The adrenocortical steroids and their synthetic congeners require a double bond in the 4,5 position and a ketone group at C3 for biological activity. The reduction of the 4,5 double bond, resulting in an inactive compound, occurs by both hepatic and extrahepatic metabolisms. Glucocorticoids are absorbed systemically from sites of local administration in amounts that may be sufficient to suppress the HPAA. Following absorption, ~90% of cortisol (or its synthetic analogs) is reversibly bound to plasma proteins, primarily corticosteroid binding globulin, and albumin. Only the unbound portion is available to exert physiological and pharmacological effects. At very high steroid concentrations, protein-binding capacity may be exceeded. Most of the ring A-reduced metabolites can be conjugated at the 3-hydroxyl position with sulfate or glucuronic acid forming water-soluble metabolites enhancing excretion by the kidney.

Agents That Affect Corticosteroids

There are several agents that affect corticosteroids throughout the body. Ketoconazole, for example, is an antifungal but at high doses inhibits the cholesterol side chain cleavage preventing steroids synthesis. Similar agents that block steroids production have been identified such as aminoglutethimide,

Table 2 Representative toxins that are known to deregulate corticosteroid homeostasis *in vivo*

Name of the compound	*Model system*	*Reference*
Aflatoxin B_1	Rat liver	Pratt, R.M., 1985. Environ. Health Perspect. 61, 35–40.
Chlordane	Rat	Cassidy, R.A., Toxicol. Appl. Pharmacol. 126 (2), 326–337.
Cadmium	Rat	Singh, P.K., et al., 2012. Drug Chem. Toxicol. 35 (2), 167–177.
Ethanol	DBA/2J (D2) mice	Ford, M.M., et al., 2013. Psychoneuroendocrinology S0306-4530(13) 00228-X.
MPTP	Mice	Ben-Shaul, Y., et al., 2006. Eur. J. Neurosci. 23 (11), 2915–2922.
TCDD	C57BL/6N mice	Kensler, T.W., et al., 1976. Biochim. Biophys. Acta 437 (1), 200–210.

metyrapone, trilostane, and abiraterone. Mifepristone at high doses blocks the GRs.

There are also two commercially available agents, spironolactone and eplerenone, that are used as mild diuretics in hypertension and heart failure. They act by antagonizing mineralocorticoid activity.

Table 2 describes several other agents that act upon the homeostasis of corticosteroids in the body.

Clinical Management

Acute overdose probably would not result in toxicity. Should oral overdosage occur, standard emergency and supportive care procedures should be followed. If anaphylaxis should occur, epinephrine may be given as 0.3–0.5 ml (0.3–0.5 mg) subcutaneously of a 1:1000 solution for adults and children should receive 0.01 mg kg^{-1}.

Administrations of benzodiazepines for seizures are recommended.

If chronic toxicity should occur, it is important to reduce the dosage of corticosteroid to a minimal maintenance dose at the first sign of toxicity. Because of the risk that patients have developed HPAA suppression, it is important to taper corticosteroids and not abruptly discontinuing them. Debate exists about the length and dosage required to develop HPAA suppression and proper tapering techniques. Tapering should be guided based on clinical symptoms of withdrawal.

Population at Risk

Glucocorticoids should be used with caution in patients with hypothyroidism or cirrhosis, because such patients often show exaggerated response to the drugs. Glucocorticoids should be used with caution in psychotic patients or patients with hypertension or congestive heart failure, patients with recent myocardial infarction, in patients with viral infections or bacterial infections not controlled by antiinfectives, in patients with active or latent peptic ulcer, diverticulitis, nonspecific ulcerative colitis (if there is a probability of impending perforation, abscess, or other pyogenic infection), and in those with recent intestinal anastomoses.

Glucocorticoids may cause fetal damage when administered to pregnant women. One retrospective study of 260 women who received pharmacological dosages of glucocorticoids during pregnancy revealed two instances of cleft palate, eight stillbirths, one spontaneous abortion, and 15 premature births. Another study reported two cases of cleft palate in 86 births. Occurrence of cleft palate in these studies is higher than in the general population but could have resulted from the underlying diseases as well as from the steroids. Other fetal abnormalities that have been reported following glucocorticoid administration in pregnant women include hydrocephalus and gastroschisis. Women should be instructed to inform their physicians if they become or wish to become pregnant while receiving glucocorticoids. If glucocorticoids must be used during pregnancy or if the patient becomes pregnant while taking one of these drugs, the potential risks should be carefully considered.

Routes of Exposure

The National Institute for Occupational Safety and Health statistically estimated that 30 657 workers (17 738 of these are females) are potentially exposed to dexamethasone in the United States. Occupational exposure to dexamethasone may occur through dermal contact with this compound at workplaces where dexamethasone is produced or used.

See also: Anabolic Steroids; Lipid Peroxidation.

Further Reading

Asare, K., 2007. Diagnosis and treatment of adrenal insufficiency in the critically ill patient. Pharmacotherapy 27 (11), 1512–1528.

Bracken, M.B., 2012. Steroids for acute spinal cord injury. Cochrane Database Syst. Rev. 1, CD001046.

Barshes, N.R., Goodpastor, S.E., Goss, J.A., 2004. Pharmacologic immunosuppression. Front. Biosci. 9, 411–420.

McEvoy, G.K. (Ed.), 2007. American Hospital Formulary Service. AHFS Drug Information. American Society of Health-System Pharmacists, Bethesda, MD, pp. 3034–3035.

Miller, L.W., 2002. Cardiovascular toxicities of immunosuppressive agents. Am. J. Transplant. 2, 807–818.

Nikkanen, H.E., Shannon, M.W., 2007. Endocrine toxicology. In: Shannon, M.W., Borron, S.W., Burns, M.J. (Eds.), Haddad and Winchester's Clinical Management of Poisoning and Drug Overdose, fourth ed. Saunders Elsevier, Philadelphia, PA (Chapter 16).

Takeda, Y., Tomino, Y., 2004. Immunosuppressive therapy for nephrotic syndrome and strategy for adverse side effects from that therapy. Nihon Rinsho 62, 1875–1879.

Ventura, M.T., Buquicchio, R., Cecere, R., et al., 2013. Anaphylactic reaction after the concomitant intravenous administration of corticosteroids and gastroprotective drugs: two case reports. J. Biol. Regul. Homeost. Agents 27 (2), 589–594.

Williams, J.S., Williams, G.H., 2003. 50th anniversary of aldosterone. J. Clin. Endocrinol. Metab. 88 (6), 2364–2372.

Weissman, D.E., Dufer, D., Vogel, V., Abeloff, M.D., 1987. Corticosteroid toxicity in neuro-oncology patients. J. Neurooncol. 5 (2), 125–128.

Relevant Websites

http://arthritis.about.com/cs/steroids/a/corticosteroids.htm – Arthritis & Joint Conditions at About.com: Facts about corticosteroids.

http://www.merckvetmanual.com – The Merck Veterinary Manual.

http://umm.edu/health/medical/ency/articles/corticosteroids-overdose – University of Maryland Medical Center.

Corticosterone *see* Corticosteroids

Cortisone *see* Corticosteroids

Cosmetics and Personal Care Products

A Manayi and S Saeidnia, Tehran University of Medical Sciences, Tehran, Iran

Introduction and History

The application of cosmetics dates back to 6000 years of human history worldwide. Documented uses in ancient cultures include castor oil (a protective balm in ancient Egypt), beeswax (as skin cream in several ancient cultures), olive oil, and rose water (in ancient Rome). Cosmetics were also used in ancient Persia, Greek, Japan, China, Europe, and Africa. The literature reveals that among the first to decorate their lips were Mesopotamian women, who resided in an ancient region of southwestern Asia, in the area now known as Iraq. There are indications that they might have prepared lipsticks by crushing gemstones and applying them to decorate the lips. It is documented that an Arab-Andalusian cosmetologist named Abu al-Qasim al-Zahrawi provided solid lipsticks, which were formed as sticks rolling and pressing in particular molds. Some of these historical products contained ingredients later discovered to be highly toxic. Two examples are the white lead pigment known as ceruse, used to make faces fashionably pale, and belladonna alkaloids (atropine from *Atropa belladonna*), used to dilate pupils in order to enhance the attractiveness of the eyes by Italian women around the late nineteenth century. As another example, ancient Egyptians extracted red dye from red seaweeds, 0.01% iodine, as well as some brominated mannite, which caused serious toxicity. In the United States (nineteenth century), lipsticks were provided by using carmine dye, which was extracted from cochineal (scale insects native to Central America) mixed with aluminum or calcium salts.

In modern times, the number and variety of cosmetic and personal care products and their individual ingredients are almost overwhelming. In this article, the authors will focus on some of the most common products and key ingredients under typical conditions of use from both a functional and toxicological perspective. While accidental ingestion of some of these products (e.g., by children) can lead in some cases to significant systemic toxicity, a discussion of these conditions is outside the scope of this article and the reader is referred to other articles in this work and other published literature.

Hair-Care Products

Hair-Coloring Products

The ingredients in hair-coloring products or hair dyes are among the most reactive chemicals used in the cosmetic industry. Hair-coloring products are divided into oxidative (permanent) dyes and direct (temporary or semipermanent) dyes. Oxidative hair dyes contain the oxidizer hydrogen peroxide and a dye intermediate such as paraphenylenediamine (PPD), resorcinol, and aminophenol. PPD is an aromatic compound, widely used in almost all hair-coloring formulations, because oxidation of this substance with couplers produces colored reaction products. Direct dyes include semipermanent and temporary dyes. Temporary hair dyes contain azo, triphenylmethane, anthraquinone, or indamine dyes while semipermanent hair dyes contain nitrophenylenediamines, nitro-aminophenols, and some azo dyes. Permanent hair dyes differ from semipermanent or temporary dyes in that permanent hair dyes consist of two components that are mixed before use and generate the dye on/in the hair by a chemical reaction.

Although there are advantages of using PPD in hair dyes and colors, studies show this ingredient is a common allergen in humans. Cases of contact sensitization induced by PPD have been reported. Some of these cases are attributed to hypersensitivity of its para group or to the formation of oxidized products subsequent to oxidation by air exposure of PPD. N-Substitution of PPD influences its sensitization potential. Also, the length of the chain of the alkyl substituent often has an effect on the sensitization potential. There are also other types of dyes such as metal salts and natural dyes. Metal salts are mainly used for coverage of graying hair and are generally based on lead acetate while natural dyes use 'henna' as its pure dye ingredient.

The genotoxicity of various components of permanent hair dyes has been studied by various groups, with overall mixed results and findings. For example, the genotoxicity of six important phenylenediamines (PDs) were evaluated for their potential to induce various genotoxic end points. No single PD was found to be positive or negative for all end points evaluated.

Reproductive toxicity of PPD and other PDs has also been studied in animals. No definitive link between exposure to these compounds and adverse effects on the reproductive system was established.

A number of epidemiological studies have pointed to a potential risk of cancer among occupational groups like hairdressers and beauticians due to high exposure to hair dyes, generally citing a weak association. However, a recent study by Hueber-Becker et al. showed no evidence of increased risk of neoplastic disease. Current thinking is that use of personal

 http://dx.doi.org/10.1016/B978-0-12-386454-3.00979-9

protective equipment (e.g., gloves) and other safety precautions in the handling of hair dyes can protect users (including professional users) from adverse health effects.

Hair-Waving and Hair-Straightening Products

To achieve their intended effects, these products contain ingredients that involve the breaking and/or reforming of chemical bonds in hair. Consequently, they are chemically quite aggressive and care must be taken to avoid damage to the hair itself and also to surrounding skin and body structures (e.g., the eyes).

In general, 'permanent' hair-waving products make use of a reducing solution or lotion to break the disulfide bonds in the hair, which is wrapped around styling rods. Some of the oxidizing agents commonly used include ammonium thioglycolate or other thioglycolate salts, glyceryl thioglycolate, and thiolactate salts. Ammonium thioglycolate has long been safely used in home permanents. Hairdressers may, however, occasionally become sensitized to it. Glycerol monothioglycolate has been shown to cause sensitization in hairdressers and occasionally in their clients. It is generally recommended that skin contact with these substances be avoided, particularly by hairdressers who are exposed more frequently in the occupational setting than individual consumers applying the products on a relatively infrequent basis. Care must be taken to avoid contact with the eyes.

Hair-waving products also make use of neutralizing solutions containing hydrogen peroxide, sodium bromate, or perborate to re-form disulfide bonds and re-form the hair to the shape of the styling rods. Some permanent wave fixatives consist of 2–8% (w/v) mercuric chloride. Again, care must be taken to avoid contact of the neutralizing solution/fixative with the eyes and use of gloves is recommended, particularly for hairdressers. Accidental ingestion of any of the components of a permanent wave product can lead to severe gastrointestinal and central nervous system effects, along with damage to other organ systems (e.g., renal).

The majority of 'permanent' hair-straightening products fall into one of two classes: alkali based or alkaline thioglycolate based (or sulfite based). In the alkali-based products, the base cleaves the hair's disulfide bonds, which is quickly followed by the formation of new, monosulfide cross-links. Both classes of products make use of a neutralizing solution in a second step, but the function accomplished during the neutralizing step is quite different in the two classes. For the alkali-based products, the neutralizing solution simply removes the excess alkali from the hair by an acid-containing or acid-buffered shampoo. In the thioglycolate- or sulfite-based products, the neutralization step reforms disulfide bonds. For the alkali-based products, it is particularly important that the alkali component not be left on the hair for longer than directed to avoid significant and sometimes severe damage to the hair.

Depilatories

These are products employed to remove unwanted hair and generally contain sodium or calcium hydroxide (alkalis, which are quite toxic), barium sulfide, and thioglycollates. Because of the caustic nature of these products, care should be taken to minimize irritation to the surrounding skin and, particularly, mucous membranes. See also remarks above under hair-waving and hair-straightening products.

Hairstyling Products

These types of products contain synthetic film-forming polymers as the primary functional ingredients in water or water/alcohol solvent vehicles that also contain different additives to improve the properties of the film and other aspects of product application and function. The polymers, or resins, are typically acrylate-based copolymers, composed of vinyl acetate, acrylamide, and methyl vinyl ether. Aerosol hair sprays typically contain ethanol as the solvent and hydrocarbon, dimethyl ether, or carbon dioxide propellants. Common hydrocarbon propellant systems involve butane. Many of the ingredients or their residual monomers or impurities have the potential to cause respiratory problems if inhaled in sufficient amounts. Adequate ventilation is essential for their safe use.

Hair-Cleansing and Conditioning Products

Shampoos typically consist of an aqueous emulsion of several surfactants, at least one of which will have strong detergent properties, various additives to enhance cleansing performance or improve sensory attributes, one or more preservatives, and fragrance. Antidandruff shampoos can contain any one of a number of active ingredients, which function through very different mechanisms. An ingredient in some traditional shampoos in this category is coal tar, which is carcinogenic under certain conditions of exposure, but has been found safe for use under the conditions specified and customary for antidandruff shampoo.

Anionic surfactants tend to be the most effective cleansers, but at high concentration can be irritating to the scalp. Commonly used anionic surfactants with good cleansing and foaming properties include sodium lauryl sulfate, sodium laureth sulfate, and ammonium laureth sulfate; these can be irritating to the skin and are usually used in combination with nonionic surfactants, which tend to be milder. Baby shampoos are generally formulated with nonionic or amphoteric surfactants, which are even milder. Polyethoxylated surfactants are the largest group of nonionics; they may contain trace levels of ethylene oxide or 1,4-dioxane, both of which have been classified as probable carcinogens. A process known as 'vacuum stripping' is used during their manufacture to limit the levels of these incidental impurities. Diethanolamine and triethanolamine are two surfactants that have been identified as possible contributors to nitrosamine formation in formulations that contain other ingredients that produce nitrates on decomposition. Multiple authorities recommend that use levels be controlled and surfactant–preservative combinations that could lead to nitrosamine formation be avoided.

Because of the high water activity and use conditions of shampoos, they contain preservatives to inhibit microbial growth. Preservatives such as quaternium-15, imidiazolidinyl urea, and diazolidinyl urea function through the release of trace amounts of formaldehyde. Formaldehyde is a potential sensitizer and a known inhalation carcinogen. Various expert bodies recommend restrictions on the use levels of formaldehyde-releasing preservatives. Parabens, another class of preservatives used in shampoos and hair products, have shown some ability to weakly mimic estrogen and have been found in breast tumor tissue. No direct link between parabens and cancer has been established, however. The potential for various classes of chemicals used in a variety of consumer products to function as 'endocrine disruptors' in animals and/or humans is an active area of academic and government research and also examination by regulatory and public health agencies.

Hair conditioners, broadly speaking, are meant to restore those desirable components or qualities of hair that are removed or degraded by shampooing. The most commonly used types of products generally contain cationic surfactants, perfumes, and fatty acids and fatty alcohols in a water-based emulsion also containing a preservative system. The cationic surfactants function by adsorbing or absorbing to the hair shaft and modifying texture and appearance. They are mild and generally considered nontoxic. Preservative systems do not differ greatly from those used in shampoos and other water-based emulsion products of similar water content. Fragrance, as noted, is discussed further below.

Skin-Cleansing Products

Soap

Soap, in its most basic description, is an alkali salt of a long-chain fatty acid. Historically, they were produced by mixing animal fats with lye obtained from wood ashes. Today, bar soaps and cleansing bars are made from a wider variety of different fats and oils using more refined processes and include additives of different kinds such as additional surfactants, stabilizers and antioxidants, colorants, and fragrance. A limited treatment of toxicological issues related to surfactants was provided above; similar discussion for cosmetic colorants and fragrance components are provided in sections below.

Liquid Skin Cleansers

Commercial cleansers usually consist of alcohol and petroleum products to remove dirt and clean the skin, which also remove natural oils and cause skin dryness. The most commonly used nonionic surfactants used for their cleansing effect in these products are similar to those in shampoos, albeit often at lower levels. Different anionic and other modifying surfactants are used to achieve greater 'mildness,' particularly for use on facial skin, as well as other sensory properties important to consumers in use of face and body cleansers. The increasing popularity of cleansers making 'antibacterial' claims and containing preservative agents or other antibacterial substances at higher levels than for preservative function is deserving of mention. In addition to the potential toxicological issues of preservative agents that are connected with primary product use and fate, there is increasing concern over effects on human and animal health deriving from distribution of these substances or their breakdown products into the environment via the wastewater stream. Triclosan, which can ultimately degrade into dioxins, is an example of such a substance, where studies have shown effects on the immune system of aquatic organisms and the potential for endocrine disruption. A full discussion of environmental toxicity of cosmetic ingredients and breakdown products, and their ultimate cumulative effects on human health is, however, beyond the scope of this article and the reader is referred to other articles and the recommended readings cited therein.

Exfoliants and Scrubs

Scrubs contain exfoliating ingredients that remove dead skin. The vehicle for the exfoliating ingredients may be a liquid or paste that also provides some surfactant-based cleansing action. Many scrubs use 'microbeads' of polyethylene plastic as an exfoliating agent; others use natural substances such as ground nuts, seeds, or salt. Chemical exfoliants, in the form of alpha-hydroxy acids or beta-hydroxy acids, are used in certain of these products. As the intended effect is exfoliation, these substances are necessarily irritants. In addition, they can increase sensitivity of the skin to sun exposure. Consequently, in products intended for consumer use, levels are limited in order to prevent excessive irritation and burning and the use of sun protection is recommended.

Makeup Remover

Makeup removers are used to remove oily residues of decorative cosmetics such as eye makeup, foundation, etc. Typically, they are formulated as water-in-oil emulsions and their use is often followed with the use of the type of bar or liquid cleanser discussed above. They also generally contain preservatives (albeit generally at lower levels than in higher water content products), colorants, and fragrance.

Skin-Care Products

Lotions, Creams, and Other Moisturizers

These products are emulsions, whether oil in water (o/w, the most common), water in oil (w/o, cold cream is the classic example), aqueous gel, silicone in water, or combination emulsions of different types (which will not be discussed further). Various surfactants are used as emulsifying agents. The type of surfactant depends on both the emulsion type and end use/user of the product. Surfactants in these products, because they are not used for their detergency or cleansing power, are generally far milder than those used in cleansing products, and far less likely to be skin irritants. A variety of other chemicals are added to the basic emulsion mixture as moisturizing agents, thickeners, and preservatives. Mineral oil and petrolatum are common ingredients used to help skin retain moisture. They can contain small residual amounts of potentially carcinogenic polycyclic aromatic hydrocarbons. Proper sourcing and appropriate specifications for these raw materials effectively minimizes any human health risk. Propylene glycol, used as a moisture-carrying ingredient, is a known irritant, can cause contact dermatitis, as can lanolin, when not properly processed to remove allergenic impurities. Retinyl palmitate is included in many facial creams and lotions that claim to reduce wrinkles or otherwise function as 'antiaging' products. There is some mixed evidence that it may produce free radicals on exposure to ultraviolet (UV) light, damaging skin DNA, and possibly increasing the risk of skin cancer.

Shaving Creams

Conventional shaving creams are frequently based on water and contain foaming or lathering agents, binders and thickeners, fragrance, and other substances. For the aerosol types, consideration of potential inhalation exposure and toxicity is important. For example, isobutane, a common propellant ingredient, can contain residual amounts of butadiene, a carcinogen. It is important that incidental inhalation be minimized.

Toners and After Shave

Aftershaves are designed to soothe irritated skin, and are typically based on water and denatured alcohol. They are, however, heavily fragranced and serve as perfumes for men. Toxicological considerations related to fragrance components are discussed below.

Sun Protection

Sunscreens consist of chemical sunscreens, which absorb UV rays, and mineral sunscreens, which tend to physically block the sun's rays. Common UV absorbers (also referred to as UV filters) include para-aminobenzoic acid and its derivatives, cinnamates, salicylates, camphor derivatives, avobenzone, triazones, and benzophenones. Some countries regulate products providing sunscreen as drugs, others as cosmetics. Not all UV filters are permitted for use in all countries; where allowed, the permitted use levels can also vary. Some UV filters, e.g., avobenone and octyl methoxycinnamate, have been shown to cause adverse skin reactions, primarily irritation. Some contact and photocontact sensitivity to individual sunscreen active ingredients has been reported, but at relatively low levels in the context of their overall widespread use. The most common ingredients contained in mineral sunscreens are zinc oxide and titanium dioxide. These naturally occurring minerals function as sunblocks and are generally considered inert. However, the introduction and widespread use of nanoparticles of zinc oxide and titanium dioxide in sunscreens raises new concerns. It has been hypothesized that use of nanosized particles may allow these compounds to penetrate the skin more easily, leading to systemic exposure and possible toxicity. This is currently an area of active research. For aerosol spray sunscreens, the small particles created represent a possible inhalation hazard.

Deodorants and Antiperspirants

Deodorants contain aluminum and zinc salts, and fragrance to mask the smell of perspiration. Most conventional antiperspirants rely on aluminum compounds, like aluminum trichlorohydrex gly, which plug the sweat ducts, and stop sweat coming to the skin's surface. There is some evidence that many aluminum compounds are neurotoxic, cause skin irritation, and interfere with estrogen, which increases the incidence of breast cancer. Crystal deodorants are a popular alternative to conventional deodorants and antiperspirants. They typically contain either potassium alum or aluminum alum as active ingredients, which are believed to be less allergenic than other ingredients of similar function. Many products in this category contain substantial levels of fragrance. For aerosol products, toxicity of the propellant and its impurities is a consideration in formulation and in practical use. For example, isobutane, a propellant in aerosol sprays, can be contaminated with carcinogenic butadiene. Aerosol sprays create extremely small particles, which can be more deeply inhaled and this may increase their harmful effects.

Oral Care Products

Toothpastes, powders, and tooth liquids contain calcium phosphates, alumina, abrasives, and anionic surfactants. Mouthwashes usually contain alcohol, flavoring (essential oils), and sweeteners. Denture cleaners contain bicarbonates, borates, phosphates, and carbonates. While these products are not intended to be ingested, some incidental ingestion is to be expected and they must be formulated with this in mind. The reader is referred to other articles in this work for information regarding toxicity through ingestion exposure of key ingredients mentioned here.

Fragrance

Fragrances consist of a mixture of essential oils or other volatile aromatic compounds (often synthetic), solvents, and 'fixatives' (substance used to improve stability and reduce/slow evaporation). Typical solvents are ethanol or a mixture of ethanol and water. Essential oils are themselves complex mixtures of hydrocarbons, ethers, alcohols, esters, and ketones. Examples of essential oils are lemon, eucalyptus, peppermint, geranium, and rosewood. Several historical natural fragrance components such as ambergris and natural musk oil are no longer used, primarily for environmental reasons, but in some cases also because of safety concerns. Fragrance components are the most commonly implicated substances in cosmetic allergies. Specifically, contact allergy to fragrance ingredients may develop following skin contact with sufficient amount of these substances. Usually, this manifests as a localized contact dermatitis where perfume-type products, other heavily scented products, and antiperspirants or deodorants are applied and, of course on the hands. Upon reexposure to sufficient amounts of these fragrance components, eczema may develop (allergic contact dermatitis). Less frequently, irritation, contact urticarial, and photocontact dermatitis are encountered. In the European Union, 26 fragrance components with recognized potential to cause allergy are required to be identified on the label of cosmetic products in which they are present so that sensitive consumers may avoid them. Thirteen of the fragrance substances listed have been frequently reported as well-recognized contact allergens in consumers and are thus of most concern while others are less well documented (See **Table 1**.)

Decorative Cosmetics

This category is often referred to as 'color cosmetics.' The chief function of these products is to color or conceal and they contain among the highest levels of coloring substances of any cosmetic or personal care products. These coloring substances generally fall into two categories: synthetic organic or mineral pigments, although there are some other coloring substances

Table 1 List of 26 fragrance allergens designated by the European Union

Allergen	*CAS-No.*
Frequently reported	
Amyl cinnamal	122-40-7
Amylcinnamyl alcohol	101-85-9
Benzyl alcohol	100-51-6
Benzyl salicylate	118-58-1
Cinnamyl alcohol	104-54-1
Cinnamal	104-55-2
Citral	5392-40-5
Coumarin	91-64-5
Eugenol	97-53-0
Geraniol	106-24-1
Hydroxycitronellal	107-75-5
Hydroxymethylpentyl-cyclohexenecarboxaldehyde	31906-04-4
Isoeugenol	97-54-1
Less frequently reported	
Anisyl alcohol	105-13-5
Benzyl benzoate	120-51-4
Benzyl cinnamate	103-41-3
Citronellol	106-22-9
Farnesol	4602-84-0
Hexyl cinnamaldehyde	101-86-0
Lilial	80-54-6
D-Limonene	5989-27-5
Linalool	78-70-6
Methyl heptine carbonate	111-12-6
3-Methyl-4-(2,6,6-trimethyl-2-cyclohexen-1-yl)-3-buten-2-one	127-51-5
Oak moss	90028-68-5
Tree moss	90028-67-4

Reproduced from Scientific Committee on Consumer Safety (SCCS). Adopted 6/2012.

derived from natural sources. Most coloring substances contain residual amounts of impurities, typically reaction by-products and intermediates, heavy metals, and other co-occurring substances. The levels of these impurities are strictly limited and additional use restrictions applied by regulatory authorities in many countries. Coloring substance in products intended for use in the area of the eye or where there may be mucous membrane or secondary incidental ingestion exposure (e.g., the lips) are often subject to additional limits and restrictions because of the sensitivity of the body structures and/or the greater potential for systemic absorption. Some coloring substances can cause reactions in sensitive individuals and labels should be read carefully.

Face Makeup

This category includes foundation (sometimes referred to as 'formation' in some countries) and blusher, both of which may be in liquid, cream, or powder form, and other 'finishing' face powders. The liquid and cream products may be suspensions or emulsions (primarily o/w). Because these products are in prolonged contact with generally more sensitive facial skin, the emulsifying agents must be carefully chosen to minimize irritation. The oils used are generally those with low potential to block pores (comedogenicity) and result in black heads, white heads, and acne. Highly refined and purified mineral oil is often used because of its low comedogenicity and low potential for irritation. Lower grade mineral oils can be comedogenic and should be avoided. Both liquid and powdered foundations and blushers contain inorganic pigments (both for hiding and color), various polymers for enhancing application properties, silica, and fragrance. Blushers also contain organic colorants (e.g., D&C Red No. 7 calcium lake). While some of the powdered products are formulated without preservatives, the use of low levels is common and recommended to ensure microbiological safety. Suspension and emulsion products must contain preservatives to ensure safety (the most common preservatives are similar to those used in other cosmetic products and have been described in preceding sections).

Lip Makeup

Classical lipstick is a cosmetic product containing pigments, waxes, and oils and other emollients that lends color, texture, and protection to the lips and its use dates back to ancient times. Classical lipstick continues to be enormously popular, available in many shades and other surface appearance qualities. Modern products also include lip pencils, which use different combinations and specific ingredients from among the same basic ingredient groups as classical lipsticks and also include fillers and other additives needed to produce the physical form of the product.

Because there is some incidental ingestion exposure with this product, there has been great interest in determining and possibly limiting the levels of lead and other heavy metals in these products. Recent studies conducted in various parts of the globe (Saudi Arabia, European Union, and United States) have yielded a vast amount of data showing that for most lipsticks, lead levels are below those that would represent a public health concern but that there are some with levels in excess. This continues to be an active area of research and regulatory activity.

Eye Makeup

Products in this category include eye liner, eye shadow, and mascara. Modern eyeliners and mascara are liquid products. The majority of eye shadows are pressed powders, with liquid (cream) forms also marketed.

The most common types of eyeliners are composed of water, a gelling agent (gums, e.g., magnesium aluminum silicate), wetting agents (e.g., water soluble esters, such as Polysorbate 80), polyols (e.g., propylene glycol or butylene glycol), colorants, alcohol, preservative, and a polymeric film former. Mascaras are found as emulsions (both o/w and w/o) and anhydrous solvent-based suspensions. Ingredients classes used in all types include pigments, waxes, emulsifiers, polymers, and other film formers, and, importantly, preservatives. With respect to the polyols, some can be irritants (e.g., propylene glycol) and they are generally used at as low a level as possible, in part for this reason. With respect to certain of the polymers used in some products (e.g., polymethylmetharcrylate), residual monomers can function as irritants or potential sources of other toxicity. The levels of these residual substances are minimized through specific controls for ingredients.

Pressed powder eye shadows are formulated similarly to other pressed powder products, but the range of allowed colorants and pigments is narrower. Limitations on permitted particle size are also often in place, to minimize the potential for eye irritation and injury. The cream products contain solvents (often hydrocarbons or isoparaffins), waxes similar to some of those used in certain mascaras, emollients, gelling agents, fillers (e.g., talc, starches, and some polymers), and, of course, colorants and preservatives.

Regarding preservatives, it is critical that products used in the area of the eye be free of microbial pathogens and with numbers of any other microorganisms kept as low as possible to minimize the possibility of causing or exacerbating eye infections.

Nail Makeup

Nail polishes and lacquers are the most widely used nail makeup products. They are composed of a polymeric film former, modifying polymers or resins, plasticizing agents, and solvents. Nitrocellulose is the most commonly used film former, and the most commonly used modifying resin is para-toluene sulfonamide formaldehyde resin. Formaldehyde is a known sensitizer and this formaldehyde resin has been associated with allergic reactions in some users, prompting the development of some products that use other modifiers. A variety of plasticizers are used, most of which are considered relatively benign, with the exception of dibutyl phthalate, which has been shown to affect the immune system in animal studies. Concerns over these findings have resulted in reformulation of a great many products to reduce levels of this ingredient or eliminate it entirely. Nail lacquers also contain solvents at approximately 70% and for some of the solvents used in these products this has given rise to health concerns, particularly in the salon setting. In such settings, air levels can be much higher than in the home setting and inhalation exposure also much more prolonged for the salon professionals applying the products. Adverse effects that have been associated with high airborne levels of these substances include eye irritation and possible eye damage; nausea and vomiting with abdominal pain; chest pain and irregular heart beat; difficulty breathing and shortness of breath; balance problems; euphoria and hallucinations; and at very high exposure levels, seizures.

Regulations, Standards, and Testing

As noted previously, cosmetics and personal care products are defined and regulated differently across the globe. The authors will present examples of some of the key differences; for a fuller treatment, the reader is referred to the Additional Reading and Web Site References.

For example, according to the EU definition "cosmetics are any substance or preparation intended to be placed in contact with various external parts of the human body (epidermis, hair system, nails, lips, and external genitals) and with the teeth or mucous membranes of the oral cavity with a view exclusively or mainly cleaning them, perfuming them, changing their appearance and/or for protecting them or keeping them in a good condition." In the United States, cosmetics are defined a bit more narrowly as "articles to be rubbed, poured, sprinkled or otherwise applied to the human body or any part thereof for cleansing, beautifying, promoting attractiveness, or altering the appearance, and articles intended for use as a component of any such articles…" Certain products classified as cosmetics in the EU are regulated as over-the-counter (OTC) drugs in the United States, including (but not limited to) anticaries toothpaste, antiperspirants, antidandruff shampoos, sunscreen products, and more. In Japan, the definition of cosmetic categories more closely resembles that of the United States, but somewhat different, and in some cases more stringent requirements are applied. For example, many products that would be OTC drugs in the United States are termed 'quasi-drugs' in Japan and subject to a registration process that also requires submission of safety and efficacy information, unlike the process in the United States.

The manner in which ingredients are identified as safe/suitable for use in products differs significantly and is beyond the scope of this article. However, there is a core set of data and information that is pivotal to the safety assessment of most cosmetic ingredients: levels of use and physical/chemical data (including impurities), skin irritation and sensitization, dermal absorption/penetration data, and genetic toxicity data. In situations where oral intake is expected or if dermal absorption/penetration data indicate possibly significant systemic absorption, additional studies of different kinds may be needed. Photoinduced toxicity data are especially useful when a cosmetic ingredient/product is expected or intended to be used on sunlight-exposed skin. Human data are very useful and typically included in a comprehensive evaluation of a cosmetic product's safety. Changing perspectives on, and legal requirements governing the use of, animal testing in various parts of the globe are also changing perspectives and requirements regarding testing. The development of *in vitro* and so-called *in silico* alternatives to animal testing is an area of vigorous

Table 2 Common skin assays for testing cosmetic products/ingredients

Method	*End point*	*Test type*	*Endorsement/regulatory acceptance*
EpiSkin® human skin model	Skin corrosion	*In vitro*	ECVAM; ESAC; ICCVAM; OECD TG 431
EpiDerm™ human skin model	Skin corrosion	*In vitro*	ESAC; ICCVAM; OECD TG 431
Rat skin transcutaneous electrical resistance test	Skin corrosion	*Ex vivo*	ECVAM; ESAC; ICCVAM; OECD TG 430
SkinEthic™ human skin model	Skin corrosion	*In vitro*	ECVAM; ESAC; ICCVAM; OECD TG 431
Vitrolife-Skin™ human reconstructed epidermis assay	Skin corrosion	*In vitro*	JaCVAM; OECD TG 431
EpiSkin™ skin irritation test (with MethylThiazolyl Tetrazolium Assay (MTT) reduction)	Skin irritation	*In vitro*	ESAC; JaCVAM; OECD TG 431
EpiDerm™ skin irritation test (with MTT reduction)	Skin corrosion	*In vitro*	EU test method B.46 in COM regulation 440
EpiDerm™ SIT model (EPI-200) assay	Skin corrosion	*In vitro*	ECVAM; ESAC; JaCVAM; OECD TG 439
SkinEthic RHE model test	Skin corrosion	*In vitro*	ECVAM; ESAC; JaCVAM; OECD TG 439

ECVAM, European Center for the Validation of Alternative Methods; ESAC, ECVAM Scientific Advisory Committee; ICCVAM, Interagency Coordinating Committee on the Validation of Alternative Methods; OECD, Organization for Economic Cooperation and Development; and JaCVAM, Japanese Center for the Validation of Alternative Methods.

Table 3 Common skin sensitization assays for testing cosmetics ingredients/products

Method	*End point*	*Test type*	*Endorsement/regulatory acceptance*
Mouse local lymph node assay (LLNA)	Skin sensitization/immunotoxicity	*In vivo*	ICCVAM; ESAC; OECD TG 429;
Reduced LLNA: rLLNA	Skin sensitization/immunotoxicity	*In vivo*	ESAC; ICCVAM; JaCVAM; OECD TG 429
Nonradiolabeled LLNA	Skin sensitization/immunotoxicity	*In vivo*	ICCVAM; JaCVAM; OECD TG 442A
Nonradiolabeled LLNA: DA	Skin sensitization/immunotoxicity	*In vivo*	ICCVAM; JaCVAM; OECD TG 442B
LLNA for potency categorization of skin sensitizers	Skin sensitization/immunotoxicity	*In vivo*	ICCVAM; some US agencies
Human repeated insult patch tests	Skin sensitization/immunotoxicity	Human studies	ICCVAM
Human maximization test	Skin sensitization/immunotoxicity	Human studies	ICCVAM

ECVAM, European Center for the Validation of Alternative Methods; ESAC, ECVAM Scientific Advisory Committee; ICCVAM, Interagency Coordinating Committee on the Validation of Alternative Methods; OECD, Organization for Economic Cooperation and Development; and JaCVAM, Japanese Center for the Validation of Alternative Methods.

Table 4 Common eye (ocular) assays for testing cosmetic ingredients/products

Method	*End point/area of application (if applicable)*	*Test type*	*Endorsement/regulatory acceptance*
Bovine corneal opacity and permeability test	Eye corrosion (moderate to severe irritants)	*Ex vivo*	ICCVAM; ECVAM; JaCVAM; OECD TG 437
Cytosensor microphysiometer modified test	Eye corrosion/irritation	*In vitro*	ICCVAM; ECVAM; ESAC; Draft OECD TG 460
Hen's egg test – chorioallantoic membrane assay	Eye corrosion (severe irritants and mild/moderate for surfactants)	*In vitro*	–
Isolated chicken eye assay	Eye corrosion	*Ex vivo*	ICCVAM; ECVAM; JaCVAM; OECD TG 438
Isolated rabbit eye assay	Eye corrosion (severe irritants)	*Ex vivo*	–
EpiOcular	Eye irritation (moderate to mild irritants)	*In vitro*	ICCVAM
Human corneal epithelial cell assay (SkinEthic)	Eye irritation (differentiate between irritants vs nonirritants)	*In vitro*	ICCVAM
Rabbit low-volume eye test	Eye irritation (all irritants)	*In vitro*	ESAC; ICCVAM
Fluorescein leakage test method	Eye corrosion	*In vitro*	ECVAM; ESAC; Draft OECD TG

ECVAM, European Center for the Validation of Alternative Methods; ESAC, ECVAM Scientific Advisory Committee; ICCVAM, Interagency Coordinating Committee on the Validation of Alternative Methods; OECD, Organization for Economic Cooperation and Development; and JaCVAM, Japanese Center for the Validation of Alternative Methods; TG, testing guidance; –, no endorsement or regulatory acceptance.

Table 5 Common phototoxicity assays for testing cosmetic ingredients/products

Method	*End point*	*Test type*	*Endorsement/regulatory acceptance*
3T3 neutral reuptake photocytotoxicity	Photoirritation	*In vitro*	OECD
Guinea pig models	Photoallergy	*In vivo*	–

Note: There is no *in vitro* method currently accepted for photoallergy testing. OECD, Organization for Economic Cooperation and Development; –, no endorsement or regulatory acceptance.

research. A selection of assays for toxicological end points particularly important in assessing the safety of cosmetic products and ingredients is given in **Tables 2–5**.

Acknowledgments

The assistance of colleagues from the US Food and Drug Administration is gratefully acknowledged.

See also: Acetone; Acrylamide; Ammonia; Atropine; Belladonna Alkaloids; Boric Acid; Ethanol; Hydrogen Peroxide; Lead; Mercury; Phthalates; Turpentine; Xylene; Zinc.

Further Reading

Burlando, B., Verotta, L., Cornara, L., Bottini-Massa, E., 2010. Herbal Principles in Cosmetics. CRC Press, Taylor and Francis Group.

Nohynek, G.J., Antignac, E., Thomas, R., Toutain, H., 2010. Safety assessment of personal care products/cosmetics and their ingredients. Toxicol. Appl. Pharmacol 243, 239–259.

Paye, M., Barel, A., Maibach, H. (Eds.), 2006. Handbook of Cosmetic Science and Technology, second ed. CRC Press.

Schlossman, M. (Ed.), 2009. The Chemistry and Manufacture of Cosmetics, fourth ed. Allured Publishing Corporation.

Whitman, J.H. (Ed.), 1987. Cosmetic Safety – A Primer for Cosmetic Scientists. Marcel Dekker, Inc.

Wilhelm, K.-P., Zhai, H., Maibach, H. (Eds.), 2012. Dermatotoxicology, eighth ed. CRC Press.

Relevant Websites

http://ec.europa.eu/consumers/sectors/cosmetics/regulatory-framework/ – European Commission: Health and Consumers - Cosmetics Regulation.

http://www.fda.gov/Cosmetics/ – Food and Drug Administration.

http://www.hc-sc.gc.ca/cps-spc/cosmet-person/indust/require-exige/index-eng.php – Health Canada: Consumer Product Safety - General Requirements for Cosmetics.

http://www.mhlw.go.jp/english/ – Ministry of Health, Labour and Welfare.

Cotinine

JP Gray and GJ Hall, U.S. Coast Guard Academy, New London, CT, USA

This article is a revision of the previous edition article by Sanjay Chanda and Harihara M. Mehendale, volume 1, pp 673–674, © 2005, Elsevier Inc.

- Name: Cotinine
- Chemical Abstracts Service Registry Number: CAS 486-56-6
- Synonyms: (S)-1-methyl-5-(3-pyridyl)-2-pyrrolidinone; (S-)-1-methyl-5-(3-pyridyl)-2-pyrrolidone
- Molecular Formula: $C_{10}H_{12}N_2O$
- Chemical Structure:

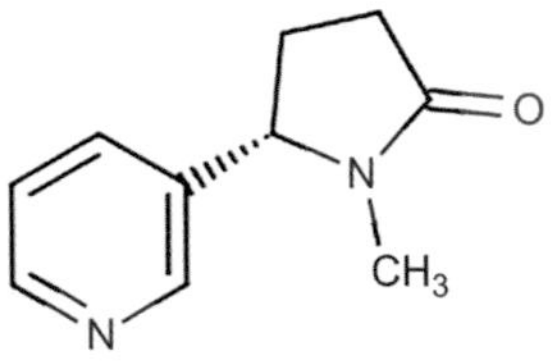

Background (Significance/History)

Cotinine is the major metabolite of nicotine. In the liver, nicotine is rapidly metabolized to cotinine (70–80%) by CYP2A6 and to nornicotine (5%) by CYP2A6 and CYP2B6. With a half-life about 10-fold longer than that of nicotine (15–19 h for cotinine versus 2–3 h for nicotine), cotinine induces plasma concentrations of 1–3 μM in smokers. After administration to rats, cotinine levels in the brain reach fourfold those of nicotine at 4 h following injection. Cotinine is not biotransformed in the brain, allowing accumulation of this substance to levels greater than that of nicotine.

Like nicotine, cotinine is able to induce dopamine release in smokers and in superfused rat striatal slices in a dose- and calcium-dependent manner via the nicotinic receptors, but only at concentrations higher than those normally seen in smokers. Indeed, administration of cotinine to smokers at levels 10-fold that is seen following smoking had no observable effect, suggesting that cotinine is not neuroactive at doses found in smokers. However, cotinine also acts as an inhibitor for nicotine binding in rat brain via desensitization of the nicotinic receptor.

At high doses in rats, cotinine reduces heart rate in a dose-dependent manner, reduces aldosterone levels, reduces blood pressure, and reduces heart rate. Although some studies report behavioral alterations in animals, these were performed using supraphysiological doses of cotinine and one report suggests contaminants playing a role in behavioral changes.

The presence of cotinine is sometimes used as an indicator for smoking: Active smokers typically have levels of cotinine that are higher (10–500 ng ml^{-1}) than those of nonsmokers (1–10 ng ml^{-1}). A different report gave mean serum levels of nicotine (0.12 μM) and cotinine (0.85 μM) in smokers.

Uses

Cotinine is primarily used in research. Cotinine is a biomarker for the consumption of tobacco and other nicotine-containing products.

Environmental Fate and Behavior

Cotinine has a vapor pressure of 3.8×10^{-4} mm Hg at 25 °C. Cotinine will be photochemically degraded with a half-life of 15 h. In sediment, cotinine is completely degraded to carbon dioxide within 72 h. It is not expected to bioaccumulate in aquatic organisms.

Exposure and Exposure Monitoring

Cotinine is a viscous liquid. Dermal or ocular contact is the most common exposure pathway. Because it is a predominant metabolite of nicotine, systemic exposure occurs after consumption of tobacco products. Exposure may also occur via second-hand smoke.

Toxicokinetics

The half-life of cotinine in human serum is approximately 15–19 h. Low levels of nicotine are also present in vegetables such as tomatoes and potatoes, presumably as a natural pesticide against insects.

Mechanism of Toxicity

Cotinine stimulates dopamine release in the nigrostriatal pathway by activating nicotinic acetylcholine receptors. However, its lower EC_{50} prevents significant activation of this pathway in smokers.

Acute and Short-Term Toxicity

Animal

The oral gavage LD_{50} for cotinine in mice is 1,604 mg kg^{-1}. The intraperitoneal LD_{50} in mice is 930 mg kg^{-1}. Cotinine induced excitement, somnolence, and dyspnea in mice.

Human

Most studies have found no correlation between cotinine treatment and changes in blood pressure or heart rate. Cotinine at a dose of 1800 mg day^{-1} exposure for 4–6 days in nonsmoking males did not elicit any adverse effects.

 http://dx.doi.org/10.1016/B978-0-12-386454-3.00294-3

Carcinogenecity

Cotinine is not recognized as carcinogenic by IARC, ACGIH, NTP, or OSHA. However, cotinine has been found to inhibit doxorubicin-induced cell death by suppression of caspase-mediated apoptosis through the PI3 kinase/Akt pathway. Individuals with reduced-function or null polymorphisms of CYP2A6 have less tobacco-related lung cancer. Because CYP2A6 is the primary enzyme responsible for the metabolism of nicotine to cotinine, these data suggest that cotinine enhances the risk of lung cancer.

Clinical Management

Artificial respiration is advised if the patient is not breathing. Monitor for shock, pulmonary edema, and seizures. Emetics are not advised.

See also: Nicotine; Tobacco.

Further Reading

Dwoskin, L.P., Teng, L., Buxton, S.T., Crooks, P.A., 1999. (S)-(-)-cotinine, the major brain metabolite of nicotine, stimulates nicotinic receptors to evoke [3H]dopamine release from rat striatal slices in a calcium-dependent manner. J. Pharmacol. Exp. Ther. 288, 905–911.

Hatsukami, D.K., Grillo, M., Pentel, P.R., Oncken, C., Bliss, R., 1997. Safety of cotinine in humans: physiologic, subjective, and cognitive effects. Pharmacol. Biochem. Behav. 57, 643–650.

Nakada, T., Kiyotani, K., Iwano, S., et al., 2012. Lung tumorigenesis promoted by anti-apoptotic effects of cotinine, a nicotine metabolite through activation of the PI3K/Akt pathway. J. Toxicol. Sci. 37, 555–563.

Relevant Websites

http://chem.sis.nlm.nih.gov/chemidplus/ProxyServlet?objectHandle=DBMaint&actionHandle=default&nextPage=jsp/chemidheavy/ResultScreen.jsp&ROW_NUM=0&TXTSUPERLISTID=0000486566

http://pubchem.ncbi.nlm.nih.gov/summary/summary.cgi?cid=408#x351

Coumarins

A Garrard, Upstate New York Poison Center, Syracuse, NY, USA

This article is a revision of the previous edition article by Betsy D. Carlton, volume 1, pp 674–676, © 2005, Elsevier Inc.

- Name: Coumarins
- Chemical Abstracts Service Registry Number: 91-64-5
- Synonyms: Coumarin; 2H-1-Benzopyran-2-one; 1,2-Benzopyrone; *cis-o*-Coumaric acid lactone; Coumarinic anhydride; 2-Oxo-1,2-benzopyran; Tonka bean camphor (note: Coumadin and warfarin are not synonyms for coumarin)
- Chemical/Pharmaceutical/Other Class: Benzopyrone
- Molecular Formula: $C_9H_6O_2$
- Chemical Structure:

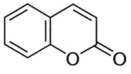

Background

Coumarin is a naturally occurring Benzopyrone compound. It is found in a large number of plants belonging to many different families including tonka beans, woodruff, lavender oil, cassia, melilot (sweet clover), and other plants. It is found in edible plants such as strawberries, cinnamon, peppermint, green tea, carrots, and celery, as well as in partially fermented tea, red wine, beer, and other foodstuffs. Concentrations range from 87 000 ppm in cassia and 40 000 ppm in cinnamon to 20 ppm in peppermint and 5 ppb in tangerines.

Uses

Coumarin is most often used as a fragrance ingredient, where it functions as a fragrance, as a fragrance enhancer, and as a stabilizer. Coumarin is widely used in perfumes, hand soaps, detergents, and lotions at concentrations from 0.01 to 2.4%. It is used to give pleasant aromas to household products or to mask unpleasant odors. The conservative estimate for systemic exposure of humans by using cosmetic products is 0.13 mg kg^{-1} day^{-1}, disregarding any corrections that should be made for absorption that is $<100\%$. Coumarin is used as a pharmaceutical for the treatment of high-protein lymphedema and for improved venous circulation, and has been tested in clinical trials as an antineoplastic. Although coumarin's use in foods is allowed via naturals such as cinnamon, at the present time, coumarin is not permitted for use as a direct food additive; however, it is used as a tobacco flavor. Coumarin is also used in the electroplating industry.

Environmental Fate

Coumarin is readily biodegradable. Coumarin is unlikely to bind to soil. Coumarin does not bioaccumulate; the bioconcentration factor has been determined to be <10–40. Various environmental fate studies have shown that coumarin in the environment would biodegrade and be lost to volatilization. Losses resulting from photolysis may also occur.

Exposure Routes and Pathways

Due to its common use in fragrances and fragrance-containing products, dermal exposure to coumarin is common. Coumarin is readily absorbed dermally, a fact that makes dermal dosing for lymphedema treatment a consideration. Human exposure to coumarin also occurs orally via natural foodstuffs, from pharmaceutical use, and from tobacco products. Coumarin is rapidly absorbed from the gut.

Toxicokinetics

The absorption, metabolism, and excretion of coumarin have been widely studied for many years. Advances in synthetic and analytical chemistry techniques in recent years have allowed a significant revision to our understanding of how coumarin is handled in the body, particularly in rodents and humans. While coumarin is readily available by both the oral and dermal routes in animals and humans, blood levels and toxicity profiles are influenced by the specific exposure mode. Plasma levels more than 20 times higher than those observed following exposure via the diet have been reported after a bolus oral dose at similar milligram coumarin per kilogram body weight levels. Dermal exposure bypasses the 'first-pass' effect of initial metabolism by the liver. Coumarin in the blood first passes through the lung, where significant amounts can be exhaled prior to being metabolized by the liver. Metabolic pathways are highly species specific and, sometimes, strain specific. DBA/2J mice have been reported to have a high level of coumarin hydroxylase activity, resulting in metabolism mainly to 7-hydroxycoumarin. CH3/HeJ mice, on the other hand, have been reported to have very little hydroxylase activity. In rats and many strains of mice other than the DBA/2J, oral coumarin exposure results in hepatic metabolism of coumarin, with the formation of the coumarin 3,4-epoxide (CE), which spontaneously rearranges extremely rapidly to the *o*-hydroxyacetaldehyde (*o*-HPA), the toxic metabolite. The *o*-HPA is then further metabolized to the nontoxic *o*-hydroxyacetic acid (*o*-HPAA) and *o*-hydroxyethanol (*o*-HPE). Rodents also metabolize coumarin by several lesser pathways, to the nontoxic 3-hydroxycoumarin and several other more minor metabolites. It is the balance between the formation of the toxic *o*-HPA and

 http://dx.doi.org/10.1016/B978-0-12-386454-3.00798-3

the nontoxic *o*-HPAA and *o*-HPE that is critical to the determination of hepatotoxicity at high exposure levels of coumarin. Mice form more *o*-HPA than do rats, but detoxify it much more rapidly and efficiently than do rats. The result is that hepatotoxicity at doses $\geq$150 mg coumarin per kilogram body weight is observed in rats, but not in mice. Similarly, when high doses of coumarin result in high plasma levels, mice demonstrate pulmonary toxicity, whereas rats do not. This is the result of the formation of higher levels of CE and *o*-HPA in the Clara cells in the lungs of mice, which is not observed in rats. In contrast to rodents, humans primarily metabolize coumarin not to the epoxide and *o*-HPA, but rather to the nontoxic metabolite, 7-hydroxycoumarin. Very high levels of coumarin are required to generate any *o*-HPA in human liver, and what is formed is rapidly detoxified. Humans have very few Clara cells in the lungs and do not generate CE and *o*-HPA in the lung, even at high coumarin doses. In a study using human hepatic microsomes with various CYP2A6 7-hydroxylation capacities, those samples that demonstrated a low capacity to utilize the 7-hydroxylatation pathway also showed a decreased capacity to form CE.

Mechanism of Toxicity

Coumarin toxicity is a function of blood and target tissue levels of coumarin relative to the metabolic capacity of the target organ. Cellular toxicity results when the formation of the toxic moieties exceeds the capacity of the cell to detoxify. This can have significant impact when comparing dosing by gavage to dietary exposure (see Toxicokinetics).

Acute and Short-Term Toxicity (or Exposure)

Animal

LD_{50} values ranging from 160 to 780 mg kg^{-1} body weight have been reported. The differences may relate to the species/strain of animal used and whether the animals were fasted at the time of dosing. Coumarin can be slightly irritating to the eye and skin. In rat studies, dietary exposure at levels $\geq$2500 ppm for 4 weeks or more may result in decreased food consumption, with resulting decreased body weight, and microscopic changes in the liver. Doses as high as 1–2% in the rodent's diet (10 000–20 000 ppm) have been given, usually resulting in a refusal of food and mortality. In rats exposed to doses that are sufficiently high to significantly affect food consumption, coumarin can decrease reproductive success. At lower dose levels, no adverse effects on reproduction or development have been reported.

Human

Coumarin exposure is common via cinnamon, green tea, sweet clover honey, and other foodstuffs. Bleeding has been reported from drinking herbal teas containing tonka beans, melilot, and sweet woodruff. When used as a pharmaceutical, doses have ranged from 70 to 7000 mg day^{-1}. The most common pharmaceutical dosage appears to be 200 mg once or twice per day. Infrequently, hepatotoxicity has been reported following pharmaceutical use. Hepatic enzyme changes have been reported to be reversible following cessation of administration, and occasionally are reversible despite continued use. The incidence rates reported have ranged from $<$0.1 to 6%, depending on the study population and, to a lesser extent, on the dose administered. Some deaths have been reported, but confounding factors such as preexisting medical conditions have precluded interpretation in most cases. Studies of CYP2A6 polymorphism in humans have not shown an association with coumarin-associated liver dysfunction. Coumarin has been tested for its ability to cause sensitization in several test systems including dermal application in guinea pigs, the mouse ear swelling test, and the local lymph node assay (LLNA). In all cases where pure coumarin was tested in animals, results were negative, including when tested at up to 50% in four recent LLNA studies. Also in LLNA studies, a chlorinated impurity (6-chlorocoumarin) and less-pure coumarin derived from *o*-cresol have been shown to be sensitizers, confirming reports of sensitization from various substituted derivatives of coumarin. In humans already sensitized to certain other substances such as balsam of Peru, coumarin has been reported to cross-react. While laboratory species are not likely to have been exposed to coumarin or cross-reacting substances before being tested, the human population is likely to have been previously exposed. This can make testing in humans more difficult to interpret. The furanocoumarins may cause photosensitivity in light-skinned humans. Some coumarins are similar to warfarin in their activity and may have an anticoagulant effect at large enough doses. Its anticoagulant activity is 1/50 000th of that of warfarin. Coumarin may also potentiate the effect of vitamin K antagonists as suggested by several case reports. This mechanism remains unknown. It is not teratogenic in humans (does not cause hemorrhagic syndrome) and has no reported adverse effects on human reproduction.

Chronic Toxicity (or Exposure)

Animal

Numerous long-term toxicity and/or carcinogenicity studies have been conducted. In general, the primary effects reported are decreased food consumption with resulting decreased body weight and liver toxicity (in rats). At doses that produce a significantly decreased body weight gain ($\geq$150 mg kg^{-1} body weight), liver toxicity and liver tumors are reported in rats. These tumors are nonmetastatic and nonlethal. Lung tumors have been reported in mice exposed by bolus (via stomach tube) administration at doses $\geq$150 mg kg^{-1} body weight, but not in mice exposed to comparable doses in the diet.

Human

In workers, dusts may be irritating to the respiratory system. Coumarin may be a weak dermal sensitizer in sensitive individuals. Purity of the material can play a significant role in this regard. No other long-term effects of coumarin have been reported in humans. The International Agency for Research on Cancer reviewed coumarin in 2000 and classified it into group 3, not classifiable as a carcinogen in humans.

In Vitro Toxicity Data

Coumarin is not mutagenic and does not bind to deoxyribonucleic acid. It is not clastogenic (i.e., it has no significant effect on chromosomes).

Reproductive Toxicity

In contrast to warfarin, coumarin is not teratogenic.

Genotoxicity

Coumarin has been shown to be void of any genotoxic effect and has even shown to be protective against doxorubicin-induced mutations.

Carcinogenicity

Coumarin has not been identified as a carcinogen and may even have antioxidant and antineoplastic effects.

Clinical Management

Due to the limited toxicity of coumarin, there is little data identified for clinical management of overdoses. Management could include gastric decontamination in large overdose via oral exposure. Furthermore, monitoring of international normalized ratio and liver function tests may be warranted.

Ecotoxicology

Coumarin is not very environmentally toxic, with 96-h LC_{50} values in fish of 56 mg l^{-1} and a 24-h EC_{50} in *Daphnia magna* of 55 mg l^{-1}. Algal respiration was depressed at laboratory test concentrations of 50 mmol l^{-1}. Coumarin in the environment will readily degrade.

See also: Cosmetics and Personal Care Products.

Further Reading

Blumenthal, M., Busse, W.R., Goldberg, A., et al., 1998. The Complete German Commission E Monographs: Therapeutic Guide to Herbal Medicines, first ed. American Botanical Council, Boston.

Born, S., Caudill, D., Smith, B.J., Lehman-McKeeman, L.D., 2000a. In vitro kinetics of coumarin 3,4-epoxidation: application to species differences in toxicity and carcinogenicity. Toxicol. Sci. 58, 23–31.

Born, S.L., Hu, J.K., Lehman-McKeeman, L.D., 2000b. *o*-Hydroxyphenylacetaldehyde is a toxic metabolite of coumarin. Drug Metab. Dispos. 28 (2), 218–223.

Born, S.L., Api, A.M., Ford, R.A., Lefever, F.R., Hawkins, D.R., 2003. Comparative metabolism and kinetics of coumarin in mice and rats. Food Chem. Toxicol. 41 (2), 247–258.

Bubols, G.B., Vianna Dda, R., Medina-Remon, A., von Poser, G., Lamuela-Raventos, R.M., Eifler-Lima, V.L., Garcia, S.C., March 2013. The antioxidant activity of coumarins and flavonoids. Mini Rev. Med. Chem. 13 (3), 318–334.

Burian, M., Freudenstein, J., Tegtmeier, M., et al., 2003. Single copy of variant CYP2A6 alleles does not confer susceptibility to liver dysfunction in patients treated with coumarin. Int. J. Clin. Pharmacol. Ther. 41 (1), 141–147.

Floc'h, F., Mauger, F., Desmurs, J.-R., et al., 2002. Coumarin in plants and fruits: implications in perfumery. Perfum. Flavor. 27, 32–36.

Ford, R.A., Hawkins, D.R., Mayo, B.C., Api, A.M., 2001. The in vivo dermal absorption and metabolism of [4-^{14}C] coumarin by rats and by human volunteers under simulated conditions of use in fragrances. Food Chem. Toxicol. 39, 153–162.

Hogan III, R.P., 1983. Hemorrhagic diathesis caused by drinking an herbal tea. J. Am. Med. Assoc. 49, 2679–2680.

IARC (International Agency for Research on Cancer), 2000. IARC Monographs on the Evaluation of Carcinogenic Risks to Humans. In: Some Industrial Chemicals, vol. 77, p. 193. Summaries & Evaluations. Coumarin (Group 3).

Lake, B., 1999. Coumarin metabolism, toxicity and carcinogenicity: relevance for human risk assessment. Food Chem. Toxicol. 37, 423–453.

Rezaee, R., Behravan, E., Behravan, J., Soltani, F., Naderi, Y., Emami, B., Iranshahi, M., 11 October 2013. Antigenotoxic activities of the natural dietary coumarins umbelliferone, herniarin and 7-isopentenyloxy coumarin on human lymphocytes exposed to oxidative stress. Drug Chem. Toxicol. (Epub ahead of print).

Crafts Materials *see* Arts, Crafts, Theater, and Entertainment

Creosote (Coal Tar Creosote and Wood Creosote)

JE Kester, NewFields, Wentzville, MO, USA

This article is a revision of the previous edition article by William S. Utley, volume 1, pp 677–678, © 2005, Elsevier Inc.

- Name: Coal tar creosote and wood creosote
- Chemical Abstracts Service Registry Numbers: 8021-39-4, 8001-58-9
- Molecular Formula: None
- Chemical Structure: None

Background

This article summarizes the physicochemical characteristics of wood creosote and coal tar creosote. Because there is relatively little toxicological information regarding wood creosote, and it is little used in the United States, attention is focused on the environmental fate, toxicokinetics, toxicology, and regulatory status of coal tar creosote.

Chemical Identity

The chemical identities of wood creosote and coal tar creosote are presented in **Table 1**.

Wood Creosote

Wood creosote (CASR# 8021-39-4) was first prepared in Germany in 1830. It is obtained from fractional distillation of beechwood or related plants, and consists mainly of phenols, cresols, guaiacols, and xylenols. It is a colorless or pale yellowish greasy liquid, with a smoky odor and burnt taste. Wood creosote has been used for medicinal purposes (as a disinfectant, laxative, and expectorant) since its discovery. Although it is not now a major pharmaceutical ingredient in the United States and other western countries, wood creosote is still listed in the Japanese and Korean pharmacopoeia for the treatment of diarrhea, and is used in these countries as a self-medication for gastrointestinal disorders, including diarrhea. Its use as a synthetic flavoring substance is permitted in the United States.

Because wood creosote is not widely used in the United States and has received relatively little toxicological evaluation, it is not further discussed in this article.

Coal Tar Creosote

Coal tar creosote (CASR# 8001-58-9) is a brownish-black/yellowish-dark green oily liquid with a characteristic sharp odor. Formed from distillation of coal tars (by-products of the carbonization of bituminous coal to produce coke and/or natural gas), it is a complex and variable mixture of hundreds to thousands of hydrocarbon compounds, with few contributing more than 1%.

Table 1 Chemical identity of coal tar and wood creosotes

	Coal tar creosote	*Wood creosote*
Synonym(s)	Creosote, creosote oil, dead oil, brick oil, coal tar oil, creosote P1, heavy oil, liquid pitch oil, wash oil, creosotum, cresylic creosote, naphthalene oil, tar oil, AWPA#1, Preserv-o-sote	Beechwood creosote, creosote, creasote
Identification numbers		
CAS registry	8001-58-9	8021-39-4
NIOSH RTECS	GF9615000	G05870000
EPA hazardous waste	U051	U051
UHM/TADS	No data	No data
DOT/UN/NA/IMCO shipping	UN 1136/1137; IMO 3.2/3.3	UN 2810; IMO 6.1
HSDB	6299	1979

CAS = Chemical Abstracts Services; DOT/UN/NA/IMCO = Department of Transportation/United Nations/North America/International Maritime Dangerous Goods Code; EPA = Environmental Protection Agency; HSDB = Hazardous Substance Data Bank; NIOSH = National Institute for Occupational Safety and Health; OHM/TADS = Oil and Hazardous Materials/Technical Assistance Data System; RTECS = Registry of Toxic Effects of Chemical Substances.
Information from Agency for Toxic Substances and Disease Registry (ATSDR), 2002. Toxicological Profile for Wood Creosote, Coal Tar Creosote, Coal Tar, Coal Tar Pitch, and Coal Tar Pitch Volatiles. U.S. Department of Health and Human Services, Public Health Service.

When used as a pesticide to preserve wood, coal tar creosote must conform to standards established by the American Wood Preservers Association, P1/P13 or P2. The chemical compositions of P1/P13 and P2 are listed in **Table 2**. There are six major classes of compounds in creosote: aromatic hydrocarbons (including polycyclic aromatic hydrocarbons (PAHs) and alkylated PAHs) with two, three, or four to five, which constitute up to 90% of creosote; phenolics; nitrogen-, sulfur-, and oxygen-containing heterocyclic compounds (including dibenzofurans); and aromatic amines. The PAHs may have two, three, four, or five fused aromatic rings. The principal PAHs in coal tar creosote are naphthalene, phenanthrene, fluoranthene, acenaphthene, fluorene, and pyrene, while the carcinogenic PAHs are minor constituents. Thus, the physical and chemical properties of the individual components of creosote vary widely.

Table 2 Mean fractional composition of P1/P13 and P2 coal tar creosote

Compound	*CAS#*	*P1/P13 fraction % (mean)*	*P2 fraction% (mean)*
Indole	120-72-9		0.20
Indene		NC	0.5
Benzo[*c*]thiophene		NC	0.40
Benzoquinoline-1 (7,8-benzoquinoline)	230-27-3		0.70
2-Methylphenanthrenes			0.60
Pyrene (benzo[def]phenanthrene	129-00-00		3.64
1,2-Benzofluorene (benzo[*a*]fluorene	–		0.73
Chrysene (benz[*a*]phenanthrene)	218-01-9		1.4
Benzo[ghi]perylene		<0.1	0.10
2-Phenylnaphthalene	–	0.20	0.47
Methylpyrene		0.20	0.30
3-Methyl biphenyl (3-phenyl toluene)	643-93-6	0.30	0.61
Benz[*e*]pyrene		0.3	0.50
Benz[*a*]anthracene	56-55-3	0.40	0.20
Benzo[*a*]pyrene		0.40	
1-Ethylnaphthalene		0.60	0.50
1,3-Dimethyl naphthalene	575-41-7	0.80	0.60
4-Methyldibenzofuran		0.80	0.40
Benz[*b*]fluoranthene	205-99-2	0.80	0.51
2,3-Benzofluorene	243-17-4	0.90	0.80
Quinoline	91-22-5	1.0	0.50
Dibenzothiophene	132-65-0	1.3	0.94
Chrysene		1.4	0.10
4H-cyclopenta [def]phenanthrene	203-64-5	1.5	1.74
Biphenyl	92-52-4	1.6	0.71
9H-carbazole	86-74-8	1.7	1.4
1-Methylnaphthalene	90-12-0	2.5	1.3
Anthracene	120-12-7	3.1	2.90
Dibenzofuran	132-64-9	4.3	2.3
Pyrene		4.7	4.0
Fluoranthene	206-44-0	5.5	4.60
2-Methylnaphthalene	91-57-6	5.6	2.80
Fluorene	86-73-7	6.0	4.03
9H-Fluorene		6.0	3.5
Naphthalene	91-20-3	6.2	17.3
Acenaphthene	83-32-9	7.7	4.40
Phenanthrene	85-01-8	12.8	9.60

Data from U.S. Environmental Protection Agency (EPA), 2008. Reregistration Eligibility Decision for Creosote (Case 0139). EPA 739-R-08–007. Prevention, Pesticides, and Toxic Substances.

Uses

Coal tar creosote is a fungicide, insecticide, and sporicide, primarily used as a wood preservative in the United States. Creosote formulations intended for wood treatment are restricted use pesticides. Wood treated with these preservatives is specified for commercial and industrial uses at outdoor sites. Approximately 70% of creosote wood preservatives are used to pressure-treat railroad ties and crossties, 15–20% is used for utility poles and cross arms, and the remainder for assorted lumber products (e.g., timbers, poles, posts, and groundline-support structures).

Environmental Transport and Distribution

The environmental transport and distribution of creosote constituents involve multiple complex processes. Differences in environmental behavior depend on the physicochemical characteristics of the individual compounds, which control their solubility, bioavailability, susceptibility to degradation, and capacity for depuration by organisms, as well as on their interactions with environmental matrices and environmental conditions. Volatile compounds (low–molecular weight PAHs, phenolics, and some heterocyclics) partition to air, polar compounds to water, and hydrophobic, higher molecular weight compounds may sorb to soil and sediment and/or accumulate in biota. As a result, creosote-contaminated soil and sediment usually contain relatively higher levels of hydrophobic PAHs than creosote itself. Creosote constituents can also enter the atmosphere as particulate matter. The predominant environmental sinks for creosote constituents are groundwater and soil and sediment, where they may persist for decades.

In the aquatic environment, coal tar creosote constituents can dissolve, volatilize, sorb to sediment, and/or enter biological tissues via bioconcentration and bioaccumulation. The bioavailability of individual constituents varies widely, and the majority of available data pertains to PAHs. Field monitoring studies at creosote-contaminated sites, relocation experiments, and laboratory and microcosm studies have demonstrated that aquatic invertebrates and fish can bioaccumulate certain PAHs from creosote. Although biomagnification of creosote PAHs in fish appears to be limited by their greater metabolic capacity, human exposure to lipophilic coal tar creosote constituents via consumption of contaminated seafood has been observed. PAHs derived from coal tar creosote in soil can also be taken up by terrestrial plants and animals, although to a lesser degree than in aquatic systems.

Environmental degradation of coal tar creosote constituents is likewise variable, dependent on structure and environmental conditions. Phenolic compounds and some heterocyclic compounds are quickly removed, whereas others are recalcitrant. Photochemical transformation seems to be the dominant mechanism of abiotic degradation of PAHs and heterocyclic and phenolic compounds in the atmosphere and, to a lesser extent, in water and soil. Aerobic biodegradation is generally more effective than anaerobic degradation. Degradability of PAHs appears to be inversely related to the number of aromatic rings. Thus, higher molecular weight compounds tend to be more persistent. However, PAHs sorbed to soil and sediment may undergo an aging process that results in reduced bioaccessibility and bioavailability over time.

Human Exposure Routes and Pathways

Coal tar creosote is not available for sale or use by homeowners, and must be applied in a controlled setting under closed process conditions, only by certified applicators or under direct supervision. Accordingly, the US Environmental Protection Agency (EPA) has determined that there is no potential for human exposure to creosote through food or drinking water. Wood treatment workers and workers involved in remediation of creosote-contaminated sites experience the greatest potential for exposure.

The primary route of occupational exposure to creosote constituents is dermal, through handling treated wood or contaminated media. Inhalation exposure is also possible, but less important. Members of the general public living near creosoting plants may be exposed to volatile components via air emissions. Creosote is not registered for residential use, and other pesticides are generally used for preservation of playground equipment. In its reregistration review in 2008, EPA determined that children's potential exposure to creosoted landscape ties was too brief and infrequent to be of concern. It should be noted that PAHs tend to be poorly absorbed from the gastrointestinal tract, particularly when associated with soil particles.

Toxicokinetics

Coal tar creosote constituents can be absorbed by passive diffusion across oral, dermal, and respiratory mucosae, at rates and in quantities dependent on the nature of exposure and their physicochemical characteristics. The EPA has estimated a dermal absorption fraction of 5% for humans. Although distribution studies with coal tar creosote have not been performed, it is reasonable to assume that studies on the individual constituents are reflective of their behavior in a mixture. Studies with both PAHs and phenolic compounds have found them to be rapidly and widely distributed in the tissues. Therefore, it is likely that absorption of coal tar creosote would result in a wide distribution of its constituents in the body.

Few studies on the metabolism of coal tar creosote are available, but many studies have examined PAH metabolism. PAHs are generally metabolized by microsomal oxidative enzyme systems, in particular the cytochrome P450 system, liver, lungs, skin, kidney, and other tissues. Certain PAHs can undergo hydroxylation, resulting in reactive epoxides that can bind to DNA and other macromolecules. The principal metabolic products identified are conjugates of phenols, dihydrodiols, quinones, and anhydrides. Phenolic compounds can undergo conjugation, hydroxylation, and oxidation.

Specific urinary metabolites detected after human occupational exposure to coal tar creosote include 1-naphthol, which is formed from naphthalene, and 1-pyrenol, which is formed from pyrene. Urinary concentrations of both 1- and 2-naphthol (also a naphthalene metabolite) were significantly higher in nonsmoking residents near a wood treatment plant in Canada than in controls, but similar to levels observed in smokers. In contrast, 1-pyrenol was not elevated in the residents.

Excretion of coal tar creosote constituents other than PAHs has been little studied. Regardless of the route of absorption, metabolized (and some unmetabolized) PAHs are excreted into bile and feces and, to a lesser extent, into urine. Reabsorption via hepatobiliary circulation may occur. Lipophilic PAHs can also be excreted into milk.

Toxicity

Acute and Subchronic Toxicity

Coal tar creosote formulations have a moderate degree of acute toxicity (Toxicity Category III) in experimental animals via the oral and dermal routes, and low toxicity (Toxicity Category IV) via inhalation (**Table 3**). However, they can cause moderate to substantial eye irritation, and are assumed to be dermal sensitizers.

Table 3 Acute mammalian toxicity data for creosote P1/P13 and P2 fractions

Test (species)	*P1/P13*	*Toxicity category*	*P2*	*Toxicity category*
Acute oral toxicity (rat) LD_{50}	2451 mg kg^{-1} (M) 1893 mg kg^{-1} (F)	III	2524 mg kg^{-1} (M) 1993 mg kg^{-1} (F)	III
Acute dermal toxicity (rabbit) LD_{50}	>2000 mg kg^{-1}	III	>2000 mg kg^{-1}	III
Acute inhalation toxicity (rat) LC_{50}	>5 mg l^{-1}	IV	>5.3 mg l^{-1}	IV
Primary eye irritation (rabbit)	Clear in 8–12 days	II	Clear in 7 days	III
Primary dermal irritation (rabbit)	Erythema to day 14	III	No irritation after 7 days	III

Human deaths have occurred within 14–36 h after ingestion of about 7 g of coal tar creosote by adults and 1–2 g by children. The primary cause of death appears to be cardiovascular collapse. Acute inhalation exposure in humans may result in irritation and burns of the skin and eyes and respiratory irritation. Similarly, oral exposure may cause irritation and damage to the gastrointestinal tract, with symptoms including salivation, vomiting, thready pulse, headache, and loss of pupillary reflexes. Reports of long-term self-medication have indicated symptoms of intoxication and visual disturbances.

Repeated-dose dermal studies conducted in rats indicated minimal toxic effects, with no observed adverse effect level (NOAEL) of 40–400 mg kg^{-1} day^{-1} depending on creosote type and animal sex. Subchronic (90 day) inhalation exposure to creosote produced a wider spectrum of effects, some of which were reversible following a 6-week recovery period. P1/P13 creosote caused myocardial pathology and altered hematological parameters in both sexes. The systemic NOAEL identified by the EPA for P1/P13 is 5.4 mg m^{-3}. P2 creosote also produced altered hematological parameters, and resulted in increased absolute and relative liver and thyroid weights, follicular cell hypertrophy, and lesions of the nasal cavity. The systemic NOAEL identified by the EPA for P2 is 4.7 mg m^{-3}.

Developmental Toxicity

There are no data regarding the developmental toxicity of creosote in humans. Animal studies provide little evidence of developmental toxicity, and treatment-related effects appear to be associated with maternal toxicity. In rats administered 25, 50, or 175 mg P1/P13 creosote per kg per day, both maternal toxicity and developmental toxicity (increased postimplantation loss, decreased body weights for male fetuses, and reduced numbers of live fetuses) were observed at the highest dose. Although the incidence of fetal malformations observed at 175 mg kg^{-1} day^{-1} dose level was low and plausibly due to maternal stress, EPA concluded that the teratogenic potential of P1/P13 creosote could not be ruled out. The EPA identified an NOAEL of 50 mg kg^{-1} day^{-1} for both maternal toxicity and developmental toxicity. In rabbits administered 1, 9, or 75 mg P1/P13 creosote per kg per day, maternal toxicity and reduced litter viability were noted at the highest dose level. EPA determined that the NOAEL for maternal toxicity was 9 mg kg^{-1} day^{-1}, and that for developmental toxicity was 75 mg kg^{-1} day^{-1}.

In rats, P2 creosote caused maternal toxicity at all doses (25, 75, and 225 mg kg^{-1} day^{-1}), but developmental toxicity (increased incidence of postimplantation loss, reduced numbers of viable fetuses, reduced fetal body weights, and crown rump length) was evident only at the highest dose. The EPA determined the NOAEL for maternal toxicity to be 75 mg kg^{-1} day^{-1}, although maternal toxicity at lower doses is suggested by the significantly decreased body weights at 25 mg kg^{-1} day^{-1}. The EPA determined the NOAEL for developmental toxicity to be 25 mg kg^{-1} day^{-1}, based on the observation of malformations that they deemed possibly treatment related at the middose level.

Reproductive Toxicity

A two-generation reproduction study was conducted in rats administered 25, 75, or 150 mg P1/P13 creosote per kg per day. A dose-related decrease in body weight was observed in parental animals. Decreased litter size and offspring viability were seen at the higher dose levels, perhaps resulting from decreased maternal body weight gain during gestation. Based on this study, EPA determined that parental systemic NOAEL is <25 mg kg^{-1} day^{-1}, the developmental NOAEL is <25 mg kg^{-1} day^{-1}, and the reproductive NOAEL is <25 mg kg^{-1} day^{-1}.

Endocrine Disruption

Little information regarding the endocrine-disrupting potential of creosote is available. A coal tar creosote mixture was examined for ability to bind and activate estrogen receptor and aryl hydrocarbon receptor in a battery of *in vitro* and *in vivo* assays. Creosote was found to bind to the mouse estrogen receptor and elicit partial agonist activity in reporter gene assays in transiently transfected MCF-7 cells. Based on the competitive binding assay, the estrogenic potency of creosote relative to estradiol is 0.000 165. Because cytotoxicity prevented determination of creosote's relative potency in the estrogen receptor-mediated reporter gene assay, relative inductive potency could not be determined. However, the maximal measured effect of creosote was three orders of magnitude lower than that of estradiol. Creosote effectively transformed the guinea pig aryl hydrocarbon receptor *in vitro*, and had a relative potency of 0.000 731 compared to TCDD in an aryl hydrocarbon receptor-mediated reporter gene assay. No aryl hydrocarbon receptor-mediated antiestrogenic activity of creosote was observed *in vitro*. *In vivo*, creosote significantly induced aryl hydrocarbon receptor-responsive liver enzyme activities, but did not cause estrogen receptor-mediated effects, possibly due to suppression of estrogenic responses by aryl hydrocarbon receptor-mediated antiestrogenic activity.

Genotoxicity

The mutagenic potential of coal tar creosote has been investigated both *in vitro* and *in vivo*. Positive results were obtained in several *in vitro* systems in the presence of S9. PAHs are thought to be primarily responsible for the mutagenicity of creosotes, but aromatic amines and azaarenes may also play a role. Interactions among the components of the complex mixture may be both synergistic and antagonistic. In contrast, results of *in vivo* mutagenicity tests have been both negative and positive. Neither P1/P13 nor P2 exhibited dominant lethal effects in a rat assay.

Chronic Toxicity and Carcinogenicity

Epidemiological studies of various designs have addressed the issue of chronic human health effects, including cancer, associated with creosote. Although older reports suggested a relationship between occupational creosote exposure and skin cancer, the overall weight of evidence indicates no serious chronic health conditions resulting from current levels of occupational creosote exposure. EPA has classified coal tar creosote as B1 (probable human carcinogen) based on "limited evidence of the association between occupational creosote contact and subsequent tumor formation, sufficient evidence of local and distant tumor formation after dermal application to mice, and some evidence of mutagenic activity, as well as the well-documented carcinogenicity of other coal tar products to humans." Similarly, the International Agency for Research on Cancer has classified it in Group 2A (probably carcinogenic to humans), based on limited data in humans and sufficient data in experimental animals.

Coal tar creosote is both an initiator and a promoter of skin cancer in animals when applied at high doses for prolonged periods of time. Both portal-of-entry and lung tumors were observed. However, none of the dermal studies in animals are appropriate for quantitative cancer risk assessment due to experimental design issues (lack of controls, poor characterization of exposure, intermittent exposures, coexposure to other initiators/promoters, less than lifetime exposures, small number of dose groups). Tumor responses in high-dose animal studies correlate with chronic irritation (with resulting cytotoxicity and hyperplasia). In the absence of appropriate data for creosote, EPA calculated cancer slope factors for use in health risk assessment based on data from studies of animals exposed to coal tar. Because coal tar contains a higher concentration of potentially carcinogenic compounds than creosote, this estimate is likely to overstate the potential human cancer risk of creosote.

Ecotoxicity

Leaching of coal tar creosote constituents from treated wood is the main source of exposure to both aquatic and terrestrial organisms. In its ecological risk assessment for coal tar creosote, EPA concluded that risk to birds and terrestrial mammals and plants is likely to be minimal, due to lack of exposure and the ability of these organisms to avoid creosote. A number of studies in aquatic microorganisms, plants, invertebrates, and fish have demonstrated the toxic (and/or phototoxic) potential of coal tar creosote constituents. Associations between heavy creosote contamination and increased incidence of neoplastic lesions in fish have been observed in field studies, and lower exposures can cause reproductive impairment and developmental effects.

EPA approached evaluation of potential risks to aquatic organisms by focusing on eight PAHs: acenaphthene, anthracene, chrysene, fluoranthene, fluorene, naphthalene, phenanthrene, and pyrene. These PAHs (1) comprise at least 2% of total PAHs in creosote; (2) are frequently detected in the water column and/or sediments in field and laboratory studies; (3) are EPA priority pollutants as identified under the Clean Water Act; and (4) are highly toxic to fish and aquatic invertebrates. Because the half-lives of these PAHs in aquatic organisms are only a few days, EPA concluded that biomagnification is not a concern. Acute and chronic toxicity data for salt- and freshwater fish and invertebrates are summarized in **Table 4**. Few data examining chronic toxicity are available. Anthracene, fluoranthene, and pyrene appear to be the most acutely toxic PAHs, and aquatic invertebrates and fish appear to be the most sensitive organisms.

Table 4 Acute and chronic toxicity of creosote PAHs to fish and invertebrates exposed in the water column

	Acute LC_{50}/EC_{50} ($\mu g\ l^{-1}$)		*Chronic NOEC ($\mu g\ l^{-1}$)*	
PAH	*Saltwater*	*Freshwater*	*Saltwater*	*Freshwater*
Acenapthene	160–2200	240–580	44.6–332	295–520
Anthracene	3.6	1.27–5.6		
Chrysene	<1000	1900		
Fluoranthene	0.58–0.8	0.97–6.8	11.1	10.4–10.6
Fluorene	1000	420–760		
Naphthalene	971–2400	890–1000		
Phenanthrene	17.7–108	96–234	5.5	5–57
Pyrene	0.89	4–25.6		

EC_{50} = effect concentration for 50% of test organisms; LC_{50} = lethal concentration for 50% of test organisms; NOEC = no observed effect concentration.
Data from U.S. Environmental Protection Agency (EPA), 2008. Reregistration Eligibility Decision for Creosote (Case 0139). EPA 739-R-08-007. Prevention, Pesticides, and Toxic Substances.

Regulation

Coal tar creosote is included in the EPA and Organisation for Economic Co-operation and Development high production volume programs. It is listed as a Resource Conservation and Recovery Act hazardous waste (U051), and has a reportable quantity of 1 pound under the Comprehensive Environmental Response, Compensation, and Liability Act. It is also an Emergency Planning and Community Right-to-Know Act Section 313 reportable substance.

The use of coal tar creosote is regulated by the EPA under the Federal Insecticide, Fungicide, and Rodenticide Act (FIFRA), and has been registered as a wood preservative active ingredient under FIFRA since 1948. In 1984, following an administrative review considering whether creosote uses should be canceled or modified, EPA determined that creosote would continue to meet FIFRA's statutory standard for registration if it was classified for restricted use (only by or under the supervision of certified applicators), and if certain protective clothing and other precautionary requirements for wood treatment workers were added to creosote labeling.

In 1986, EPA commenced a reregistration review of creosote as required under FIFRA for all pesticide active ingredients first registered prior to 1 November 1984. As a result of the voluntary cancellation of nonpressure treatment end-use registrations and removal of nonpressure treatment uses on other creosote products initiated by the creosote registrants in 2003, creosote is now a restricted use pesticide that can only be applied by pressure treatment. In 2008, EPA determined that creosote-containing products are eligible for reregistration, provided that risk mitigation measures are adopted and labels are amended accordingly.

See also: Coal Tar; Petroleum Distillates; Polycyclic Aromatic Hydrocarbons (PAHs).

Further Reading

Agency for Toxic Substances and Disease Registry (ATSDR), 2002. Toxicological Profile for Wood Creosote, Coal Tar Creosote, Coal Tar, Coal Tar Pitch, and Coal Tar Pitch Volatiles. U.S. Department of Health and Human Services, Public Health Service.

Bengtsson, G., Törneman, N., Yang, X., 2010. Spatial uncoupling of biodegradation, soil respiration, and PAH concentration in a creosote contaminated soil. Environ. Pollut. 158 (9), 2865–2871.

Borak, J., Sirianni, G., Cohen, H., Chemerynski, S., Jongeneelen, F., 2002. Biological versus ambient exposure monitoring of creosote facility workers. J. Occup. Environ. Med. 44, 310–319.

Bouchard, M., Pinsonneault, L., Tremblay, C., Weber, J.P., 2001. Biological monitoring of environmental exposure to polycyclic aromatic hydrocarbons in subjects living in the vicinity of a creosote impregnation plant. Int. Arch. Occup. Environ. Health 74, 505–513.

Elovaara, E., Heikkilä, P., Pyy, L., Mutanen, P., Riihimäki, V., 1995. Significance of dermal and respiratory uptake in creosote workers: exposure to polycyclic aromatic hydrocarbons and urinary excretion of 1-hydroxypyrene. Occup. Environ. Med. 52, 196–203.

Elovaara, E., Mikkola, J., Mäkelä, M., Paldanius, B., Priha, E., 2006. Assessment of soil remediation workers' exposure to polycyclic aromatic hydrocarbons (PAH): biomonitoring of naphthols, phenanthrols, and 1-hydroxypyrene in urine. Toxicol. Lett. 162, 158–163.

Fielden, M.R., Wu, Z.-F., Sinal, C.J., Jury, H.H., Bend, J.R., Hammond, G.L., Zacharewski, T.R., 2000. Estrogen receptor- and aryl hydrocarbon receptor-mediated activities of a coal-tar creosote. Environ. Toxicol. Chem. 19, 1262–1271.

Hiramoto, K., Yamate, Y., Kobayashi, H., Ishii, M., Miura, T., Sato, E.F., Inoue, M., 2012. Effect of the smell of Seirogan, a wood creosote, on dermal and intestinal mucosal immunity and allergic inflammation. J. Clin. Biochem. Nutr. 51 (2), 91–95.

Hultgren, J., Pizzul, L., Castillo Mdel, P., Granhall, U., 2010. Degradation of PAH in a creosote-contaminated soil. A comparison between the effects of willows (*Salix viminalis*), wheat straw and a nonionic surfactant. Int. J. Phytoremediation 12 (1), 54–66.

International Agency for Research on Cancer (IARC), 2010. IARC Monographs on the Evaluation of Carcinogenic Risks to Humans: Some Non-heterocyclic Polycyclic Aromatic Hydrocarbons and Some Related Exposures, vol. 92. World Health Organization.

Juhasz, A.L., Smith, E., Waller, N., Stewart, R., Weber, J., 2010. Bioavailability of residual polycyclic aromatic hydrocarbons following enhanced natural attenuation of creosote-contaminated soil. Environ. Pollut. 158 (2), 585–591.

Jung, D., Cho, Y., Collins, L.B., Swenberg, J.A., Di Giulio, R.T., 2009. Effects of benzo [a]pyrene on mitochondrial and nuclear DNA damage in Atlantic killifish (*Fundulus heteroclitus*) from a creosote-contaminated and reference site. Aquat. Toxicol. 95 (1), 44–51.

Kreitinger, J.P., Neuhauser, E.F., Doherty, F.G., Hawthorne, S.B., 2007. Greatly reduced bioavailability and toxicity of polycyclic aromatic hydrocarbons to *Hyalella azteca* in sediments from manufactured-gas plant sites. Environ. Toxicol. Chem. 26, 1146–1157.

Lee, K.-G., Lee, S.-E., Takeoka, G.R., Kim, J.-H., Park, B.-S., 2005. Antioxidant activity and characterization of volatile constituents of beechwood creosote. J. Sci. Food Agric. 52, 1580–1586.

Nyyssönen, M., Kapanen, A., Piskonen, R., Lukkari, T., Itävaara, M., 2009. Functional genes reveal the intrinsic PAH biodegradation potential in creosote-contaminated groundwater following in situ biostimulation. Appl. Microbiol. Biotechnol. 84 (1), 169–182.

Stout, S.A., Graan, T.P., 2010. Quantitative source apportionment of PAHs in sediments of Little Menomonee River, Wisconsin: weathered creosote versus urban background. Environ. Sci. Technol. 44 (8), 2932–2939.

Thierfelder, T., Sandström, E., 2008. The creosote content of used railway crossties as compared with European stipulations for hazardous waste. Sci. Total Environ. 402 (1), 106–112.

Thomson, N.R., Fraser, M.J., Lamarche, C., Barker, J.F., Forsey, S.P., 2008. Rebound of a coal tar creosote plume following partial source zone treatment with permanganate. J. Contam. Hydrol. 102 (1–2), 154–171.

U.S. Department of the Interior, 1987. Polycyclic aromatic hydrocarbon hazards to fish, wildlife, and invertebrates: a synoptic review. In: Biological Report 85(1,11). Contaminant Hazard Reviews Report no. 11. Fish and Wildlife Service.

U.S. Environmental Protection Agency (EPA), 2008. Reregistration Eligibility Decision for Creosote (Case 0139). EPA 739-R-08-007. Prevention, Pesticides, and Toxic Substances.

White, P.A., Claxton, L.D., 2004. Mutagens in contaminated soil: a review. Mutat. Res. 567 (2–3), 227–345.

World Health Organization (WHO), 1998. Selected non-heterocyclic polycyclic aromatic hydrocarbons. In: International Programme on Chemical Safety Environmental Health Criteria 202. WHO, Geneva.

World Health Organization, 2004. Coal tar creosote. In: Concise International Chemical Assessment Document 62. WHO, Geneva.

Relevant Websites

http://www.atsdr.cdc.gov – Agency for Toxic Substances and Disease Registry.

http://creosotecouncil.org/research-health.php – Toxicological Profile for Creosote.

http://www.epa.gov/iris/subst/0360.htm#carc – Integrated Risk Information System entry for Coal tar Creosote.

http://nj.gov/health/eoh/rtkweb/documents/fs/0517.pdf – NJ Dept of Health.

http://toxnet.nlm.nih.gov – TOXNET, Specialized Information Services, National Library of Medicine.

Cresols

M Badanthadka, Torrent Research Centre, Gujarat, India
HM Mehendale, University of Louisiana at Monroe, Monroe, LA, USA

- Name: Cresol (*o*-Cresol; *m*-Cresol; *p*-Cresol)
- Chemical Abstracts Service Registry Number: 1319-77-3 (*o*-Cresol: 95-48-7; *m*-Cresol: 108-39-4; *p*-Cresol-106-44-5)
- Synonyms: *o*-Cresol or 2-Methylphenol: 1-Hydroxy-2-methylbenzene 2-hydroxy toluene; *m*-Cresol or 3-Methylphenol: 1-Hydroxy-3-methylbenzene-3-hydroxy toluene; *p*-Cresol or 4-Methylphenoi: 1-Hydroxy-4-methylbenzene-4-hydroxy toluene
- Molecular Formula: C_7H_8O
- Chemical Structure:

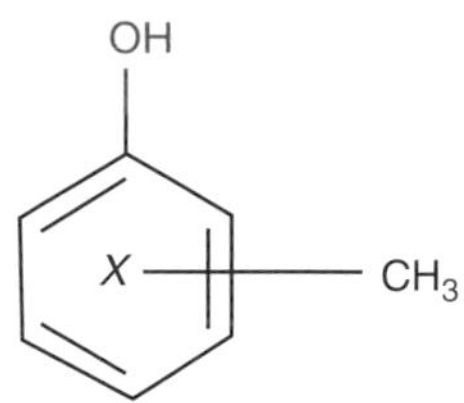

Background

Pure cresol is colorless, yellowish, brownish-yellow, or pinkish liquid, *o*-cresol, *m*-cresol, and *p*-cresol are the three structural isomers of cresol. Boiling point is 191.0 °C for *o*-cresol, 202 °C for *m*-cresol and 201.9 °C for *p*-cresol. Melting point for *o*-cresol is 29.8 °C, for *m*-cresol is 11.8 and 35.5 °C for *p*-cresol. The names of the three compounds indicate that hydrogen on the benzene ring of the molecule has been replaced. They are obtained from coal tar or petroleum. Because the boiling points of these three compounds are nearly the same, a separation of a mixture of the three into its pure components is impractical. The mixture of cresols obtained from coal tar is called cresylic acid, an important technical product used as a disinfectant and in the manufacture of resins and tricresyl phosphate. Cresols are useful as raw materials for various chemical products, disinfectants, and synthetic resins. The isomer *o*-cresol is a starting material for the herbicides 4,6-dinitro-*o*-cresol and 2-methyl-4-chlorophenoxyacetic acid. The isomers *m*-cresol and *p*-cresol are used in phenol–formaldehyde resins and are converted to tricresyl phosphate (a plasticizer and gasoline additive) and to di-*t*-butyl cresols (antioxidants called butylated hydroxytoluene).

Professions that involve dealing with the combustion of coal or wood may be exposed to higher levels of cresols than the general population. Environmental tobacco smoke is also a source of cresol exposure. Average cresol concentration may vary between the brand and type of cigarette in a 45-cubic meter chamber after six cigarettes had been smoked (ranged from 0.17 to 3.9 $\mu g\ m^{-3}$), although low levels of cresol can be detected in certain foods and tap water, and these do not constitute major sources of exposure for most population. Detectable levels of cresols have been reported in several consumer products including tealeaves, tomatoes, and ketchup as well as butter, oil, and various cheeses. Exposure to children occurs by the same routes that affect adults. Children are likely to be exposed to cresols through inhalation of contaminated air from automobile exhaust, waste incineration, and second-hand smoke.

Uses

Cresols (mixtures of the ortho-, meta-, and para-isomers) are synthesized by sulfonation or oxidation of toluene compounds or can be derived from coal tar and petroleum. Commercial grade crude cresol is generally a mixture of 20% *o*-cresol, 40% *m*-cresol, and 30% *p*-cresol. Phenol and xylenols are often found as minor contaminants. Manufacture of synthetic resins, tricresyl phosphate, salicylaldehyde, coumarin, and herbicides employ cresols. Degreasing compounds in textile scouring, paintbrush cleaners as well as fumigants in photographic developers, and explosives contains cresols. Cresols are also often used as antiseptics, disinfectants, and antiparasitic agents in veterinary medicine. Estimated breakdown of cresol and cresylic acid use is 20% phenolic resins, 20% wire enamel solvents, 10% agricultural chemicals, 5% phosphate esters, 5% disinfectants and cleaning compounds, 5% ore flotation, and 25% miscellaneous purposes. Overall, use of cresols as antimicrobial outweighs any other property.

Environmental Fate and Behavior

Cresol's production and use as a solvent, disinfectant, and chemical intermediate in the production of synthetic resins may result in its release to the environment through various waste streams. Cresols are also released to the environment through automobile exhaust and tobacco smoke. Cresols are a group of widely distributed natural compounds formed as metabolites of microbial activity and excreted in the urine of mammals. Cresols occur in various plant lipid and oil constituents. If released to air, an extrapolated vapor pressure range of 0.11–0.299 mm Hg at 25 °C for the various isomers indicates cresols will exist solely as a vapor in the ambient atmosphere. Vapor-phase cresols will be degraded in the atmosphere by photochemical reaction and produce hydroxyl radicals. The half-life for this reaction in air is estimated to be 6–9 h. If released to soil, cresols are expected to have high mobility based upon K_{oc} values of 22–49 measured in soil. Volatilization from moist soil surfaces is expected to occur slowly based upon Henry's Law constants. Cresols are not expected to volatilize from dry soil surfaces based upon the extrapolated vapor pressure range. Cresols biodegrade quickly in soils with half-lives of few days. If released into water, cresols do not adsorb to suspended solids and sediment in the water. Cresols biodegrade quickly in water with half-lives of several

 http://dx.doi.org/10.1016/B978-0-12-386454-3.00296-7

days to few weeks. Volatilization from water surfaces is expected to occur slowly based upon the range of Henry's Law constants for the various isomers. Estimated volatilization half-lives for a model river and model lake range from 21 to 29 and 235–327 days, respectively. Cresols are not expected to undergo hydrolysis since they lack functional groups that hydrolyze under environmental conditions. Direct photolysis in sunlit surface occurs and products occur at a much slower rate than biodegradation. Log bioconcentration factor values of 1.3 and 1.03 measured in ide and zebrafish respectively suggests that the potential for bioconcentration in aquatic organisms is low.

Exposure and Exposure Monitoring

Estimates indicate that nearly 1.2 million people are exposed to cresols each year via manufacturing, processing, and/or use activities. Cresols are released in to the atmosphere by auto and diesel exhaust, during coal tar and petroleum refining, wood pulping, and during its use in manufacturing, metal refining, etc. Wastewater from these industries as well as municipal wastewater treatment plants contain cresols. Occupational exposure is through inhalation and dermal contact either at workplace where the cresol isomers are produced or used. The general population may be exposed to cresols via inhalation of ambient air, use of tobacco products, and ingestion of food or contaminated drinking water, and dermal contact with this compound from consumer products containing cresol.

Toxicokinetics

Cresols are absorbed across the respiratory and gastrointestinal tracts, and through the skin. Gastrointestinal and dermal absorption are rapid and extensive. Cresols are distributed to all the major organs. The primary metabolic pathway for cresols is conjugation with glucuronic acid and inorganic sulfate. Minor metabolic pathways include hydroxylation of the benzene ring and side-chain oxidation. The major route for elimination is renal excretion in the form of conjugate metabolites.

Mechanisms of Toxicity

It acts by disruption of the cell membrane by denaturation of proteins and enzymes of the cell.

Acute or Short-Term Toxicity

Animal

Cresols are highly irritating to the skin and eyes of rabbits, rats, and mice. The mean lethal concentration of the cresol vapor or aerosol mixture is 178 mg m^{-3}. Clinical signs of toxicity-included irritation of mucous membranes and neuromuscular excitation that progressed from twitching of individual muscles to clonic convulsions. Hematuria was reported at very high concentrations. Microscopic examination revealed edematous changes in the lung and necrotic, and degenerative changes in the liver and kidneys. In another study, investigators reported that rats survived an 8 h exposure to substantially saturated cresol vapors at room temperature; the liquid penetrated the skin to a dangerous extent and caused severe skin and corneal injury.

Short-term oral exposure resulted in decreased body weight, organ weight, corrosion in the gastrointestinal tract and mouth of rats with similar effects as phenol. Kidney tubule damage, nodular pneumonia, and congestion of the liver with pallor and necrosis of the hepatic cells were also reported. More severe effects were reported in mice. At the highest concentrations, death resulted from exposure to *o*-, *m*-, and *p*-cresols but not from exposure to cresol itself.

Subchronic exposure in mice appeared to tolerate single, brief exposures of saturated vapors of cresol, but repeated exposures to saturated concentrations for 1 h day^{-1} for 10 days caused irritation of the nose and eyes and death of some mice.

Acute exposure for concentrated cresols instilled into the eyes of rabbits caused permanent opacification and vascularization. A drop of 33% solution of cresol applied to rabbit eyes and removed with saline irrigation within 60 s caused only moderate injury, which was reversible.

All three cresol isomers, either alone or in combination, are severely irritating to rabbit skin, producing visible and irreversible tissue destruction. Acute exposure can cause muscular weakness, GI disturbances, severe depression, collapse, and death.

Human

Cresols are highly irritating upon dermal contact, eye contact, and contact with any mucous membranes. Ingestion of cresols results in burning of the mouth and throat, abdominal pain, and vomiting. The target tissues/organs affected are the blood, kidneys, lungs, liver, heart, and CNS. In acute exposures, severe burns, anuria, coma, and death may result. Dermal exposure has been reported to cause severe skin burns, scarring, systemic toxicity, and death. Very few data are available regarding reproductive effects and there are no data on carcinogenicity in humans. At concentrations normally found in the environment, cresols do not pose any significant risk for the general population. However, under conditions of high exposure, people with renal insufficiency or enzyme deficiency will develop potential adverse health effects.

Chronic Toxicity

Animal

Exposure to vapors of *o*-, *m*-, and *p*-cresol resulted in weight loss, reduced locomotor activity, inflammation of nasal membranes and skin, and changes in the liver. Oral exposures to mice, rats, and hamsters for 13 weeks resulted in mortality, tremor, reduced body weights, hematological effects, increase in organ weight, hyperplasia of nasal, and stomach epithelium. Oral and inhalation exposure to cresol isomers results in lengthened estrus cycle, histopathological changes in the uterus and ovaries of rats as well as mice further support this finding. No adverse effects on spermatogenesis are observed. Mild fetotoxic effects have been reported upon exposure of pregnant mice. Some evidence of genotoxicity has been reported from *in vitro* experiment using sister-chromatid exchange (SCE) assay. However, cresol is not genotoxic after *in vivo* exposure.

Human

Prolonged or repeated absorption of low concentrations of cresol through the skin, mucous membranes, or respiratory tract may cause chronic systemic poisoning. Symptoms and signs of chronic poisoning include vomiting, difficulty in swallowing, salivation, diarrhea, loss of appetite, headache, fainting, dizziness, mental disturbances, and skin rash. Death may result if there has been severe damage to the liver and kidneys.

Immunotoxicity

Studies demonstrating the immunotoxicity of cresols by any exposure route in any species or gender are either scanty or not available.

Reproductive Toxicity

Ortho cresol causes mild effects on the body weight and pup weight in the second-generation mating trial. The relative reproductive toxicity of ortho cresol is absent at lower doses.

Mixture of *m*- and *p*-cresol was a reproductive toxicant in Swiss CD-1 mice, as evidenced by fewer F1 pups per litter, and reduced pup weight in both generations. There were also reductions in the weights of reproductive organs at necropsy at the high or middle and high dose levels. However, changes in pup growth and weights of somatic organs occurred at all dose levels. Thus, *m*- and *p*-cresols are not selective toxicants in Swiss CD-1 mice.

Genotoxicity

Studies on the induction of unscheduled DNA synthesis showed *p*-cresol to be positive in human lung fibroblast cells in the presence of hepatic homogenates, the mixture of the three isomers to be weakly positive in primary rat hepatocytes, and *o*-cresol to be negative in rat hepatocytes.

No isomer, when tested individually, induced SCEs *in vivo*, but the mixture of the three isomers induced SCEs in Chinese hamster ovary cells *in vitro*. Only *o*-cresol induced SCEs in human lung fibroblasts.

In a reverse mutation assay, a mixture of three cresol isomers at 0.005–50 μl per plate with or without S-9 from Aroclor-induced rats (activating system) was negative in *Salmonella typhimurium* strains at all doses.

In a forward mutation assay, a mixture of three cresol isomers at 0.488–750 nl ml^{-1}, with or without S-9 from Aroclor induced rats (activating system) produced dose related increase in mutation. In mouse lymphoma cell culture; without activation, results suggest weak mutagenic activity.

In an alternative *in vitro* test, in cell transformation assay using BALB/3T3 cells, a mixture of three cresol isomers was positive, and *o*-cresol was negative. Positive mutagenic responses were found at noncytotoxic doses.

Carcinogenicity

Based on increased incidence of skin papillomas in mice cresols are considered as possible human carcinogen. All the three cresol isomers produced positive results in genetic toxicity studies either alone or in combination.

Clinical Management

Oral exposure: Liquid intake should be avoided because dilution may enhance absorption. Immediate administration of activated charcoal is recommended to limit systemic toxicity. Ipecac-induced emesis is not recommended because of the potential for CNS depression and seizures. Gastric lavage is effective only within 1 h after ingestion. Patients should be treated symptomatically. Convulsions are controlled with diazepam.

Inhalation exposure: Victims should be removed to fresh air. Respiratory distress should be monitored and consult healthcare personnel.

Eye and dermal exposure: Decontamination with water is necessary. Copious dilution with room temperature water is appropriate after dermal and eye exposure. Consult a physician if required.

Ecotoxicology

A bioaccumulation factor for *m*-cresol is 20 in fish indicates no major bioaccumulation potential in higher trophic levels. A bioaccumulation factor of 4900 in algae indicates, however, a risk for bioaccumulation in lower organisms.

Aquatic toxicity of *m*-cresol

Species	*Duration*	*LC_{50} (mg l^{-1})*
Leuciscus idus (fish)	48	6
Brachydanio rerio (freshwater fish)	96	15.9
Salmo gairdneri (estuary, freshwater fish)	96	8.6
Daphnia magna (crustacea)	48	18.8
Daphnia magna (crustacea)	24	8.9

(Effect endpoint: immobilization).

Atmospheric Fate

Cresols are not expected to persist in the atmosphere because: (1) cresols have low estimated half-lives (less than 1 day); (2) they are sensitive to photolysis; and (3) the water solubility of cresols may cause transport of cresols from the atmosphere to the soil or aqueous environment. The photodegradation half-life of cresol isomers during the daytime is 8–10 h while at night it is approximately 2–4 min. Daytime half-lives would be reduced under smog conditions. Cresols are highly soluble compounds and gas scavenging will be an efficient removal process as is reflected by high concentrations in rain.

Terrestrial Fate

While there is substantial release of cresols to the soil, this route of environmental exposure is not expected to be a problem. Cresols are readily biodegraded by soil microflora and moves to lower layer of soil. Therefore, cresols will not persist in soils and will probably be leached, due to their water solubility, into the aquatic environment where they will be degraded by microorganisms. The degradation rates of cresols in soil may decrease at lower temperatures (−2 to 5 °C).

Aquatic Fate

Cresols do not contain any functional groups that are hydrolyzable. Therefore, hydrolysis of these compounds in aquatic media is unlikely. However, it will degrade primarily due to biodegradation in eutrophic waters, although photolysis may make a contribution in oligotrophic lakes based on modeling studies. Biodegradation generally occurs within 8 h after several days of acclimation, except in oligotrophic lakes, estuarine, and marine waters where degradation takes several days. Degradation is much slower under anaerobic conditions especially for the ortho isomer. *m*-Cresol biodegrades in water and its half-lives are in the range of 2–29 days (aerobic water) and 15–49 days (anaerobic water).

Two factors that may influence the biodegradation rate of cresols in natural aquatic media are the temperature and the quality of the water. In general, freshwater media have the maximum biotransformation rate for cresols. Rates for marine waters are much lower than freshwater. A decrease in temperature from 24 to 11 °C increased the biotransformation half-life by a factor of >20; however, the rate of biodegradation of cresols in marine water was so low that the lowering of water temperature would not change the biodegradation rate appreciably.

LC_{50} values for aquatic organisms

Gammarus fasciatus/(scud/immature stage)	7.0 mg l^{-1} 48 h^{-1a}
Asellus militaris/(aquatic sowbug/immature stage)	21.6 mg l^{-1} 48 h^{-1a}
Ophryotrocha diadema (polychaete worm)	33–100 mg l^{-1} 48 h^{-1}
Gammarus fasciatus/(scud/adult male)	24.9 mg l^{-1} 48 h^{-1}
– Do –, (adult female)	34.3 mg l^{-1} 48 h^{-1}
– Do –, oviparous female	33.9 mg l^{-1} 48 h^{-1a}
Asellus militaris/(aquatic sowbug/adult male)	65.4 mg l^{-1} 48 h^{-1}
– Do –, (adult female)	68.0 mg l^{-1} 48 h^{-1}
– Do –, oviparous females	61.9 mg l^{-1} 48 h^{-1a}
Pimephales promelas (fathead minnow, 29 days old, size 20.8 mm)	12.8 mg l^{-1} 96 h^{-1}
Gambusia affinis (mosquitofish, adult females)	22 mg l^{-1} 96 h^{-1a}
**Selenastrum capricornutum* (green alga, 14 day old culture; growth inhibition)	137 mg l^{-1} 14 $days^{-1a}$

*EC_{50} value, a, static.

Other Hazards

Fire-Fighting Measures

For small fires, use media such as alcohol foam, dry chemical, or carbon dioxide. For large fires apply water as far as possible. Use very large quantities (flooding) of water applied as a mist or spray; solid streams of water may be ineffective. Cool all affected containers with flooding quantities of water. Carbon oxides will generate from the substance or mixture. Wear self-contained breathing apparatus for fire fighting if necessary.

Accidental Release Measures

Wear respiratory protection. Avoid breathing vapors, mist, or gas. Ensure adequate ventilation. Remove all sources of ignition. Evacuate personnel to safe areas. Beware of vapors accumulating to form explosive concentrations and can accumulate in low areas. Prevent further leakage or spillage if safe to do so. Do not let product enter drains. Discharge into the environment must be avoided.

Spillage should be collected with a sponge or good absorbing material. Electrically operated vacuum cleaner should not be used. Keep disposals in suitable closed container to discard according to local regulations.

Precautions for Safe Handling and Storage

Skin and eye contacts should be avoided. Inhalation of vapor or mist should be avoided. Keep away from sources of ignition, no smoking near the product. Take measures to prevent the build-up of electrostatic charge. Store in cool place. Keep container tightly closed in a dry and well-ventilated place.

Exposure Standards and Guidelines

Occupational Safety and Health Administration permissible exposure limit is 5 ppm (22 mg m^{-3}) for 8 h time-weighted average (TWA). The threshold limit value for cresol and its isomers is 5 ppm for 8 h TWA. National Institute of Occupational Safety and health recommended exposure limit is 2.3 ppm (10 mg m^{-3}) for 10 h TWA for all isomers.

See also: Coal Tar; Pesticides.

Further Reading

Andersen, A., 2006. Final report on the safety assessment of sodium *p*-chloro-*m*-cresol, *p*-chloro-*m*-cresol, chlorothymol, mixed cresols, *m*-cresol, *o*-cresol, *p*-cresol, isopropyl cresols, thymol, *o*-cymen-5-ol, and carvacrol. Int. J. Toxicol. 25 (Suppl. 1), 29–127.

Aranha, M.M., Matos, A.R., Teresa Mendes, A., et al., 2007. Dinitro-*o*-cresol induces apoptosis-like cell death but not alternative oxidase expression in soybean cells. J. Plant Physiol. 164 (6), 675–684.

Chan, C.P., Yuan-Soon, H., Wang, Y.J., et al., 2005. Inhibition of cyclooxygenase activity, platelet aggregation and thromboxane B2 production by two environmental toxicants: *m*- and *o*-cresol. Toxicology 208 (1), 95–104.

Cuoghi, A., Caiazzo, M., Bellei, E., et al., 2012. Quantification of *p*-cresol sulphate in human plasma by selected reaction monitoring. Anal. Bioanal. Chem. 404 (6–7), 2097–2104.

Lesaffer, G., De Smet, R., D'Heuvaert, T., et al., 2003. Comparative kinetics of the uremic toxin *p*-cresol versus creatinine in rats with and without renal failure. Kidney Int. 64, 1365–1373.

Morinaga, Y., Fuke, C., Arao, T., Miyazaki, T., 2004. Quantitative analysis of cresol and its metabolites in biological materials and distribution in rats after oral administration. Leg. Med. (Tokyo) 6, 32–40.

Neirynck, N., Vanholder, R., Schepers, E., et al., 2013. An update on uremic toxins. Int. J. Urol. Nephrol. 45 (1), 139–150.

Onesios, K.M., Bouwer, E.J., 2012. Biological removal of pharmaceuticals and personal care products during laboratory soil aquifer treatment simulation with different primary substrate concentrations. Water Res. 46 (7), 2365–2375.

Peng, Y.S., Ding, H.C., Lin, Y.T., et al., 2012. Uremic toxin *p*-cresol induces disassembly of gap junctions of cardiomyocytes. Toxicology 302 (1), 11–17.

Suarez-Ojeda, M.E., Guisasola, A., Baeza, J.A., et al., 2007. Integrated catalytic wet air oxidation and aerobic biological treatment in a municipal WWTP of a high-strength *o*-cresol wastewater. Chemosphere 66 (11), 2096–2105.

Sun, C.Y., Chang, S.C., Wu, M.S., 2012. Uremic toxins induce kidney fibrosis by activating intrarenal renin-angiotensin-aldosterone system associated epithelial-to-mesenchymal transition. PLoS One 7 (3), e34026. http://dx.doi.org/10.1371/journal.pone.0034026. Epub March 30, 2012.

Sun, C.Y., Hsu, H.H., Wu, M.S., 2013. *p*-Cresol sulfate and indoxyl sulfate induce similar cellular inflammatory gene expressions in cultured proximal renal tubular cells. Nephrol. Dial. Transplant 28 (1), 70–78.

Watanabe, H., Miyamoto, Y., Honda, D., et al., 2013. *p*-Cresyl sulfate causes renal tubular cell damage by inducing oxidative stress by activation of NADPH oxidase. Kidney Int. 83 (4), 582–592.

Wu, M.L., Tsai, W.J., Yang, C.C., Deng, J.F., 1998. Concentrated cresol intoxication. Vet. Hum. Toxicol. 40 (6), 341–343.

Zhu, J.Z., Zhang, J., Yang, K., et al., 2012. *p*-cresol, but not *p*-cresylsulphate, disrupts endothelial progenitor cell function *in vitro*. Nephrol. Dial. Transplant. 27 (12), 4323–4330.

Relevant Websites

http://www.atsdr.cdc.gov/toxprofiles/tp34-c2.pdf – ATSDR-CDC.

http://www.seagrant.umn.edu/water/report/chemicalsofconcern/cresols/cresols.pdf – ATSDR database.

http://www.cdc.gov/niosh/idlh/cresol.html – CDC.

http://www.cdc.gov/niosh/docs/81-123/pdfs/0154.pdf – Occupational Safety and Health Guideline for Cresol, All Isomers, CDC, Atlanta, GA.

http://www.pesticideinfo.org/Detail_Chemical.jsp?Rec_Id=PC32877 – PAN Pesticide database.

http://webwiser.nlm.nih.gov/ – Substance List, Search for Cresol.

http://toxnet.nlm.nih.gov/ – TOXNET, Specialized Information Service, National Library of Medicine, Search for Cresols.

Criminal Enforcement of Environmental Laws

CM Perales, Uría Menéndez, Madrid, Spain

This article is a revision of the previous edition article by Grant R. Trigger, volume 1, pp 680–684, © 2005, Elsevier Inc.

In this section criminal environmental liability in the European Union is explained. We focus on the European Union Directive 2008/99/EC, of the European Parliament and of the Council, of 19 November 2008, on the protection of the environment through criminal law (hereinafter, the **Directive**), with a critical and practical approach. A brief reference to the situation in the United States is included at the end of the section.[1]

Environmental Criminal Liability in the European Union

1. The objective of Directive 2008/99 is to ensure a more effective protection of the environment, and it is with this aim that it establishes measures relating to criminal law in order to protect the environment more effectively (Article 1). Member States had to bring into force the laws, regulations, and administrative provisions necessary to comply with this Directive before 26 December 2010.

The justification for the enactment of the Directive was that the Community was concerned at the rise in environmental offenses, some of which may cause substantial damage to the air, including the stratosphere, and to soil, water, animals, or plants, including the conservation of species. In the opinion of the Directive, experience had shown that the then-existing systems of penalties had not been sufficient to achieve complete compliance with the laws for the protection of the environment. With the purpose of strengthening such compliance, the purpose of the Directive was to make available criminal penalties that demonstrate a social disapproval of a qualitatively different nature compared to administrative penalties or a compensation mechanism under civil law.

From a critical standpoint, it must be acknowledged that criminal liability may, and must, exist to protect the environment. However, it should not be considered as a solution to the deficiencies in the application of other liability regimes, namely tort and regulatory regimes. Consequently, and due to its very serious consequences (namely, prison for individuals) the scope of criminal liability should be restricted to the most serious negative effects on the environment. As it is explained in the following lines, this has not been the case of the Directive.

2. According to the Directive, the following conducts (including inciting, aiding, and abetting them[2]) constitute a criminal offense, when unlawful[3] and committed intentionally or with at least serious negligence (Article 3):

(a) The discharge, emission or introduction of a quantity of materials or ionizing radiation into air, soil, or water, which causes or is likely to cause death or serious injury to any person or substantial damage to the quality of air, the quality of soil or the quality of water, or to animals or plants.

This is what might be labeled as the 'typical' environmental crime, that is, the carrying out of harmful conducts consisting of emissions into the environment.

Two notes are worth highlighting, though: an environmental crime may exist even if no damage to the environment has been caused, since likelihood of causation of such damage suffices for considering that a crime has been committed; and not any damage (caused, or likely to be caused) is enough: it is necessary that it is a 'substantial' damage.

(b) The collection, transport, recovery, or disposal of waste, including the supervision of such operations and the aftercare of disposal sites, and including action taken as a dealer or a broker (waste management), which causes or is likely to cause death or serious injury to any person or substantial damage to the quality of air, the quality of soil, or the quality of water, or to animals or plants.

These are specific conducts that could have been included in the preceding paragraph (a). However, the Directive has put them separately, perhaps to avoid possible interpretations that would exclude them from the more general wording in (a). But the two notes referred to before remain: the crime exists even if no damage to the environment has been caused, since likelihood of causation is enough; and the damage (caused, or likely to be caused) to the environment must be substantial.

(c) The shipment of waste under Article 2.35 of Regulation 1013/2006 undertaken in a nonnegligible quantity, whether executed in a single shipment or in several shipments which appear to be linked.[4]

In this point the Directive is defective: there is utmost uncertainty as to what 'nonnegligible quantity' means. The

[1] This brief reference of the situation in the United States is a summary of the work prepared for the second edition of this Encyclopedia, by Grant R. Trigger; Honigman, Miller Schwartz and Cohn LLP, Detroit, MI, USA.

[2] Article 4 of the Directive.

[3] For the purposes of the Directive, 'unlawful' means infringing a variety of legislation (and decisions taken by a competent authority of a Member State) adopted pursuant to the EC Treaty as listed in Annex A of the Directive; this Annex refers to almost any element of the environment that deserves protection, from air pollution to waste, water, dangerous substances and preparations, natural habitats, wild fauna and flora, genetically modified organisms and micro-organisms, integrated pollution prevention and control. It also means infringing legislation with regard to activities covered by the Euratom Treaty, the legislation adopted pursuant to the Euratom Treaty and listed in Annex B.)

[4] Article 2.35 of Regulation 1013/2006 refers to the definition of illegal shipment of waste.

 http://dx.doi.org/10.1016/B978-0-12-386454-3.00481-4

Directive provides no clue in this respect. Bearing in mind that the Directive deals with criminal liability, on the basis of which prison could be imposed on individuals, this drafting is not acceptable. In addition, there is no need to cause a damage, nor that there is likelihood of the creation of any damage.

The same applies to another conduct included in the Directive, consisting of the production, importation, exportation, placing on the market, or use of ozone-depleting substances: it is irrelevant, for the purposes of the Directive, if the conduct refers to 1 g of substance or to 1 ton, or whether or not there is any damage.

A second criticism may be made to the conduct we are explaining: reference to the several shipments 'which appear to be linked' adds another element of uncertainty that should have been avoided.

These criticisms might be countered noting that Member States must implement the Directive by passing their own national rules, and it is in these rules where the uncertainties noted could be solved – namely, by adapting the penalties to the conduct so that, as per Articles 5 and 7, the conducts are punishable by effective, proportionate, and dissuasive criminal penalties. Therefore, the penalties will always exist, but their severity may be adapted to the actual nature or relevance of the conduct in question. It could be then argued that in the case of the conduct under this paragraph (c) penalties will vary depending of the amount of substance or risk involved.

This argument might be correct were it not for the fact that, in my view, there must be certain conducts below a certain threshold that do not deserve a criminal penalty. And this is not considered in the Directive.

(d) The Directive includes thereafter other conducts that pose no major problems of interpretation:
   - the operation of a plant in which a dangerous activity is carried out or in which dangerous substances or preparations are stored or used and which, outside the plant, causes or is likely to cause death or serious injury to any person or substantial damage to the quality of air, the quality of soil, or the quality of water, or to animals or plants;
   - the production, processing, handling, use, holding, storage, transport, import, export, or disposal of nuclear materials or other hazardous radioactive substances which causes or is likely to cause death or serious injury to any person or substantial damage to the quality of air, the quality of soil or the quality of water, or to animals or plants;
   - the killing, destruction, possession, or taking of specimens of protected wild fauna or flora species, except for cases where the conduct concerns a negligible quantity of such specimens and has a negligible impact on the conservation status of the species;
   - trading in specimens of protected wild fauna or flora species or parts or derivatives thereof, except for cases where the conduct concerns a negligible quantity of such specimens and has a negligible impact on the conservation status of the species; and
   - any conduct which causes the significant deterioration of a habitat within a protected site.

3. Three more ideas are worth highlighting in relation to the Directive:
   (i) As indicated, in all cases the conducts that may constitute an environmental crime must have been committed unlawfully (as defined) and intentionally (or with at least serious negligence); therefore, the Directive does not contemplate criminal strict liability.
   (ii) The Directive provides for minimum rules: Member States may adopt or maintain more stringent measures regarding the effective criminal law protection of the environment, provided that they are compatible with the treaty (re. whereas 12 of the Directive).
   (iii) Liability lies not only on natural persons who are the perpetrators, inciters, or accessories of the conduct in question, but also on legal persons when the crime has been committed for their benefit by any person who has a leading position within the legal person, acting either individually or as part of an organ thereof, based on a power of representation, an authority to take decisions on behalf of the legal person, or an authority to exercise control within it. Legal persons may also be held liable where the lack of supervision or control has made possible the commission of the person (Article 6)[5].

Environmental Criminal Liability in the United States

1. Initial environmental laws in the United States were focused on reducing the amount of contamination released to the environment. Over time, those who failed to comply with these requirements became the focus of enforcement officials, and the desire to encourage more widespread compliance resulted in pressuring individual corporate officials with the threat of personal liability to ensure greater compliance. These trends have eroded traditional principles of criminal law such that there may actually be greater jeopardy of being convicted of an environmental related crime than of a drug or robbery related offense. The 'shrinking' *mens rea* requirement of knowingly causing a violation of law is a potential issue for any environmental criminal litigation matter according to Marshall, Sims, and Castella (see Further Reading section). In other words, traditional criminal law punished the defendant for knowingly causing harm; however, the trend in environmental crimes is to convict due to the consequences rather than intent. For example, if a plant operator allows a discharge, he may be potentially criminally liable even if he did not know the content of the discharge was hazardous. For a contrary view, see the note authored by Escobar listed in the 'Further Reading' section.
2. Tampering with monitoring equipment and falsifying consumer certifications has been the basis of criminal convictions (*US v. Louisiana-Pacific Corp.*, No. 95-CR-215, D. Colo. 1998). In addition, inadequate resources devoted to environmental compliance can lead to criminal liability (*US v. United Technologies Corp.*, No. 2:91CR00028, D. Conn.

[5] The definition of 'legal person' in the Directive does not include States or public bodies exercising State authority, nor public international organizations.

1991). Moreover, liability exposure to individual officers or employees has expanded the scope of criminal liability and responsibility for not only the actions of individuals but also their respective corporate employers (*US v. Martin Envt'l Labs.*, No. 01-90040, E.D. Mich. 2 May 2002).

Expanding the 'reach' of the federal racketeering statute to environmental matters has broadened the basis for criminal environmental liability. On 10 August 2001, the US District Court for the Eastern District of Michigan, in the first successful case for convictions under the federal racketeering law for environmental crimes, sentenced the president/owner and operations manager of Hi-Po, Inc. to multiple-year prison terms. They were charged with dumping materials such as diesel fuel into streams and sewers so that their company would win contracts to clean up the polluted waters. The president and owner was sentenced to 33 months in prison, for violation of the Racketeer Influenced and Corrupt Organizations Act (RICO), followed by 3 years of supervised release. He was also ordered to pay $505 000 in restitution and to forfeit $500 000. The company's operations manager was sentenced to 27 months in prison, for violation of RICO, followed by 3 years of supervised release, and was ordered to pay $430 000 in restitution. The company itself was fined $50 000 for pleading guilty to two counts of violating the Clean Water Act (CWA) (*US v. Smith*, No. 00-80528, 10 August 2001).

In a case that further widened the scope of environmental criminal liability the court concluded that a defendant did not have to know that his conduct violated the law to be held criminally liable. The government prosecutors were only required to prove that the defendant had knowledge of the storage or disposal, that the material was waste, and that it was harmful to others or the environment (*US v. Kelley Technical Coatings, Inc.*, No. 96-6282, 157F.3d 432, 6th Cir. 1998).

However, in *US v. Ahmad*, 101 F.3d 386 (5th Cir. 1996), a federal appeals court held that the government must meet 'traditional' intent requirements of criminal law to obtain a conviction under the CWA. The court reversed and remanded the lower court's conviction and held that the law required the government to prove defendant's knowledge of each actual element of an offense and that the defendant had to know all the facts that made his actions illegal. The court also narrowed the 'public welfare doctrine' that allows the government to dispense with traditional intent requirements in prosecuting some environmental regulatory crimes and held that serious felonies should not fall within the public welfare exception absent a clear statement from Congress. Later decisions have distinguished themselves from *Ahmad* as being convictions based on 'mistakes in law' and not 'mistakes in fact.'

3. In the context of personal injury toxic tort liability, a defendant's apparent intentional disregard for the safety of his employees led to a criminal conviction.

For instance, on 26 June 1998, a five-count indictment was lodged against the owner of an Idaho fertilizer company who allegedly exposed workers to cyanide in 1996 without protective equipment, causing permanent brain damage to one employee. The owner was charged with endangering the safety and health of employees by ordering employees to clean out a 25 000 gal storage tank that contained cyanide. Count one was for knowing endangerment; and counts two through five were for illegal disposal of hazardous waste on three occasions and making a false statement by fabricating and backdating a safety plan on worker entry of the tank. The owner was sentenced to 17 years of imprisonment and ordered to pay $6 million in restitution to the family of one of his employees who suffered brain damage as a result of cleaning the tank without wearing appropriate protective gear (*US v. Allan Elias*, No. CR-98-070-BLW, D. Idaho 2 June 1998). On 23 October 2001, the US Court of Appeals for the Ninth Circuit upheld the conviction, but remanded the case to the district court to amend the sentence by deleting the restitution provision because the particular provision under which the owner was ordered to pay restitution (18 U.S.C. § 3663) did not allow the imposition of restitution (*US v. Elias*, No. 00-30145, 27 Fed. Appendix. 750, 9th Cir. 23 October 2001).

The potential liability for corporate officials has expanded even to those who are not in direct management control of environmental compliance activities. In *Doe Run Resources Corp. v. Neill* No. SC85451, 123 S.W. 3d 502 (Mo. S. Ct 10 February 2004), the Missouri Supreme Court concluded that a lead smelter's chief financial officer (CFO) likely would have had enough knowledge of the company's alleged polluting activities that he could have stopped or influenced those activities by his control over the company's finances and budget. As a result, the court held he could be sued personally under applicable Missouri law for harm caused by the company's breach of state and federal environmental laws. Although this case did not address criminal liability, it suggests that if a CFO can be held liable for environmental noncompliance of his company, then a criminal case based on little more may under case-specific circumstances lead to potential criminal liability.

4. As of the end of 2003, the US EPA had charged an average of about 330 criminal defendants per year (1998–2003), with no trends suggesting a decline in prosecutions. An average of over 183 years of sentences were issued and an average of over $84 million in fines were collected each year during this same time period. While these numbers do not reflect any assessment of tort claim recoveries, they do demonstrate the fact that criminal matters are not insignificant on a national scale and must be considered in reviewing any potential toxic tort matter.

See also: Chemicals of Environmental Concern; Clean Air Act (CAA), US; Clean Water Act (CWA), US; Resource Conservation and Recovery Act (USA).

Further Reading

Barker, D., 2002. Environmental crimes. Prosecutorial discretion, and the civil/criminal line. Va. Law Rev. 88, 1387.

Cardwell, P.J., French, D., Hall, M., Tackling environmental crime in the European Union: The case of the missing victim, http://inece.org/conference/9/papers/French%20D_Enviro%20Crime_FINAL%20v3.pdf.

Escobar, J., 2004. Holding corporate officers criminally responsible for environmental crimes. Collapsing the doctrine of piercing the corporate veil and the responsible corporate officer. N. Engl. J. Crim. Civ. Confin. 30, 305.

Glickman, R., Standifer, R., Stone, L., Sullivan, J., 2003. Environmental crimes. Am. Crim. Law Rev. 40, 413.

Marshall, R., Sims, R., Castella, J., 1999. When is a mistake a crime? The ever shrinking *Mens Rea* requirement for environmental crimes. Argent Environmental Liability, Enforcement & Penalties Reporter 10, 29.

Rice, P., 2003. Harmonization of criminal environmental liability throughout the EU. Environ. Claim. J. 15 (2), 281–286.

Relevant Websites

http://ec.europa.eu/environment/legal/crime/index.htm – Environmental Crime (page of the EU Commission).

http://ec.europa.eu/environment/legal/implementation_en.htm – Implementation of Community environmental legislation.

http://law.honigman.com – Nadeau S. Criminal enforcement of environmental laws. October 2002. Honigman Miller Schwartz and Cohn, 2290 First National Building, Detroit, MI 48226.

http://www.inece.org – The International Network for Environmental Compliance and Enforcement.

Cromolyn

FL Cantrell, California Poison Control System – San Diego Division, San Diego, CA, USA

- Name: Cromolyn
- Chemical Abstracts Service Registry Number: 16110-51-3
- Synonyms: Cromolyn sodium; Disodium cromoglycate; Disodium salt of cromolyn
- Chemical/Pharmaceutical/Other Class: Mast cell stabilizing antiallergic agent
- Chemical Formula: $C_{23}H_{14}Na_2O_{11}$
- Chemical Structure:

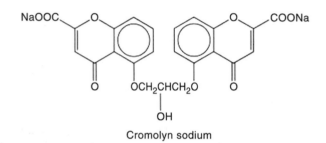

Cromolyn sodium

Background

Cromolyn is a synthetic analog of the plant extract khellin that was first developed in the late 1960s and introduced into clinical practice the following decade. It is continued to be used widely in the treatment of allergic rhinitis, asthma, mastocytosis, and conjunctivitis. It has an outstanding safety profile and can be readily obtained without prescription in many countries.

Uses

Cromolyn is used primarily for the prophylaxis of various types of asthma and in the treatment of allergic rhinitis, mastocytosis, and vernal conjunctivitis.

Environmental Fate and Behavior

Cromolyn is a mast cell stabilizer and typically marketed as the sodium salt in the United States. It is typically found in solution as a clear and colorless liquid. Cromolyn is soluble in water and the solution is completely soluble in water.

Physicochemical properties include the following:

Molar volume: 288.5 cm^3
Surface tension: 83.0 dyne cm^{-1}
Flash point: 263.9 ± 26.4 °C
Boiling point: 752.3 ± 60 °C at 760 mmHg
Polarizability: 43.3×10^{-24} cm^3
Density: 1.6 ± 0.1 g cm^{-3}
Vapor pressure: 0.0 ± 2.6 mmHg at 25 °C

Exposure Routes and Pathways

For use in asthma, cromolyn is administered by inhalation using solutions delivered by aerosol spray or nebulizer as well as a powdered drug mixed with lactose and delivered by a turbo inhaler. For use in mastocytosis, cromolyn is ingested in a liquid form. Cromolyn is available in ocular drop form for the treatment of vernal conjunctivitis.

Toxicokinetics

Oral absorption of cromolyn is less than 1%, although up to 10% of an inhaled dose of cromolyn can be absorbed systemically. After complete absorption, cromolyn is excreted unchanged in urine and bile in about equal proportions. Peak plasma concentrations occur 15 min after inhalation. The distribution of cromolyn in the lung and the extent of systemic absorption are enhanced by bronchodilation during drug delivery. The biological half-life following inhalation ranges from 45 to 100 min.

Mechanism of Toxicity

The major prophylactic effect of cromolyn is centered on inhibition of the degranulation of pulmonary mast cells causing a reduction in histamine release, reduced leukotriene production, and inhibition of release of inflammatory mediators from several cell types.

Acute and Short-term Toxicity (Animal/Human)

Animal

The acute toxicity of cromolyn, measured as the LD, has been determined in the rat (>2150 mg kg^{-1} orally and 6000 mg kg^{-1} subcutaneously) and the mouse (3300 mg kg^{-1} intravenously; 1000 mg kg^{-1} intraperitoneally; and 4400 mg kg^{-1} subcutaneously).

Chronic Toxicity (Animal/Human)

Animal

Studies of reproduction in mice, rats, and rabbits have not demonstrated fetal toxicity at doses up to 338 times the usual human dose.

Human

Because of its low toxicity, cromolyn is generally well tolerated. Adverse side effects, such as bronchospasm, cough, wheezing, laryngeal edema, joint swelling, joint pain, angioedema, headache, rash, and nausea, are rare (less than 1 in 10 000 patients). Documented instances of anaphylaxis have also been rare.

 http://dx.doi.org/10.1016/B978-0-12-386454-3.00719-3

Immunotoxicity

Anaphylactic reactions and severe asthma attacks have been rarely described following the therapeutic administration of cromolyn.

Reproductive Toxicity

Cromolyn is a pregnancy category B medication. It is not known whether cromolyn is distributed into breast milk.

Genotoxicity

Cromolyn is not believed to be genotoxic.

Carcinogenicity

Cromolyn is not believed to be carcinogenic.

Clinical Management

Toxicity is unlikely, but should adverse effects occur, general emergency management and supportive care procedures are indicated.

Ecotoxicology

Cromolyn solution, as the product administered to patients, presents a negligible impact on the environment.

Exposure Standards and Guidelines

Cromolyn solution is not classified as hazardous by Department of Transportation (DOT) regulations.

See also: Aerosols; Immune System; Respiratory Tract Toxicology.

Further Reading

Amin, K., Jan 2012. The role of mast cells in allergic inflammation. Respir. Med. 106 (1), 9–14.

Cockcroft, D.W., Mar 1999. Pharmacologic therapy for asthma: overview and historical perspective. J. Clin. Pharmacol. 39 (3), 216–222.

Dusinská, M., Jurák, B., Vlcková, A., Horáková, K., Feb 1998. Disodium cromoglycate is neither cytotoxic nor genotoxic in mammalian cells *in vitro*. Pharmacol. Toxicol. 82 (2), 103–107.

Glacy, J., Putnam, K., Godfrey, S., Falzon, L., Mauger, B., Samson, D., Aronson, N., July 2013. Treatments for Season Allergic Rhinitis (Internet). Agency for Healthcare Research and Quality (US), Rockville, MD.

Pacharn, P., Vichyanond, P., Oct 2013. Immunomodulators for conjunctivitis. Curr. Opin. Allergy Clin. Immunol. 13 (5), 550–557.

Settipane, G.A., Klein, D.E., Boyd, G.K., Sturam, J.H., Freye, H.B., Weltman, J.K., Feb 23 1979. Adverse reactions to cromolyn. JAMA 241 (8), 811–813.

Storms, W., Kaliner, M.A., Mar 2005. Cromolyn sodium: fitting an old friend into current asthma treatment. J. Asthma 42 (2), 79–89.

Relevant Websites

http://www.drugs.com/monograph/cromolyn-sodium.html – Drugs.com Monograph on Prescribing Cromolyn Including Pharmacokinetics, Toxicokinetics and Additional Information.

http://www.medicinenet.com/cromolyn/article.htm – MedicineNet.com Information on Cromolyn.

Crotonaldehyde

A Suryanarayanan, Manchester University College of Pharmacy, Fort Wayne, IN, USA

- Name: Crotonaldehyde
- Chemical Abstracts Service Registry Number: CAS 4170-30-3
- Synonyms: Beta-methylacrolein, Propylene aldehyde, Crotonic aldehyde, 2-Butenal, Topanel, Ethylene propionate, Trans-2-butenal, Crotonal, Topanel, Ethylene dipropionate
- Molecular Formula: C_4H_6O
- Chemical Structure:

Background

Crotonaldehyde is a clear, colorless to straw-colored liquid with a strong suffocating odor. It is highly flammable and produces toxic vapors at room temperature. Crotonaldehyde is found naturally in emissions of some vegetation and volcanoes; many foods contain crotonaldehyde in small amounts. Crotonaldehyde is an important environmental pollutant. It is formed during combustion of carbon-containing fuels and other materials. Lipari et al. calculated an emission of 140–2700 metric tons of crotonaldehyde per year in the United States due to burning of wood in fireplaces, based on the consumption of firewood. Concentrations of 0.02–17 mg m^{-3} were measured in automobile exhausts; however, surprisingly low concentrations of crotonaldehyde in the range of 1.1–2.1 μg m^{-3} were found near highways at a distance of 1 m. In addition, relatively high amounts of 72–228 μg of crotonaldehyde are formed from each smoked cigarette. Crotonaldehyde is evidently also formed during biological degradation of organic material such as plants. In exhausts of house garbage compost plants, amounts of 2.9 mg m^{-3} were measured. Strongly varying concentrations of crotonaldehyde are reported to occur in food, e.g., in fish (71–1000 μg kg^{-1}), in meat (10–270 μg kg^{-1}), and in fruits and vegetables (1–100 μg kg^{-1}). Crotonaldehyde was also found in alcoholic beverages like wine (0.3–1.24 mg l^{-1}) or whisky (30–210 μg l^{-1}). Crotonaldehyde is an important industrial chemical (e.g., for the synthesis of tocopherol (vitamin E), the food preservative sorbic acid, and the solvent 3-methylbutanol), but it is also a contaminant and by-product in various chemical processes.

Production

Crotonaldehyde is produced by the aldol condensation of acetaldehyde:

$$2CH_3CHO \rightarrow CH_3CH{=}CHCHO + H_2O$$

Uses

Crotonaldehyde is mainly used in the manufacture of sorbic acid, which is a yeast and mold inhibitor. Crotonaldehyde has been used as a warning agent in fuels, as alcohol denaturant, as stabilizer for tetraethyl lead, in the preparation of rubber accelerators, and in leather tanning.

Environmental Behavior, Fate, Routes, and Pathways

Chemical and physical properties of acetaldehyde:

1. Molecular weight: 70.09.
2. Boiling point (at 760 mm Hg): 104 °C (219.2 °F).
3. Specific gravity: 0.85 at 20 °C (68 °F).
4. Vapor density (air = 1): 2.41.
5. Melting point: −74 °C (−101.2 °F).
6. Vapor pressure at 20 °C (68 °F): 19 mm Hg.
7. Solubility: very soluble in water; soluble in alcohol, ether, acetone, and benzene.
8. Evaporation rate: data not available.

In food, (E)-crotonaldehyde has been found as a volatile component of raw beef, chickpea, mutton, chicken, and pork. (E)-Crotonaldehyde's production and use in the manufacture of butyraldehyde in locating breaks and leaks in pipes, in the manufacture of maleic acid, crotyl alcohol, butyl chloral hydrate, in rubber accelerators, in organic syntheses, as solvent in purification of mineral oils, in the manufacture of resins, rubber antioxidants, in chemical warfare, and as an intermediate for 2-ethylhexyl alcohol may result in its release to the environment through various waste streams.

Crotonaldehyde (steric form not reported) has been identified as a volatile emission product from the arboreous plant Chinese arborvitae. It has also been detected in gases emitted from volcanoes. (E)-Crotonaldehyde is emitted to the atmosphere from the combustion of wood and in exhaust from gasoline and diesel engines. It is also released to the environment from tobacco smoke, polymer combustion, and turbine exhaust.

(E)-Crotonaldehyde has been detected in drinking water and wastewater, and in human milk and expired air. If released to soil, (E)-crotonaldehyde will have very high mobility. Volatilization of (E)-crotonaldehyde may be important from moist and dry soil surfaces. Biodegradation studies suggest that (E)-crotonaldehyde may be biodegradable in soil and water, especially in anaerobic conditions. (E)-Crotonaldehyde readily polymerizes; therefore, if it is released to soil or water in a spill situation, a significant fraction may polymerize. If released to water, (E)-crotonaldehyde may not adsorb to suspended solids and sediment.

(E)-Crotonaldehyde may volatilize from water surfaces with estimated half-lives from a model river and a model lake of 1.7 and 15 days, respectively. An estimated bioconcentration factor value of 0.74 suggests that (E)-crotonaldehyde will not bioconcentrate in aquatic organisms. If released to the atmosphere, (E)-crotonaldehyde will exist in the vapor phase. Vapor-phase (E)-crotonaldehyde is degraded in the atmosphere by reaction

 http://dx.doi.org/10.1016/B978-0-12-386454-3.01212-4

with photochemically produced hydroxyl radicals with a half-life of about 11 h. Vapor-phase (E)-crotonaldehyde is also degraded in the atmosphere by reaction with ozone with a half-life of about 15.5 days. The general population can be exposed to (E)-crotonaldehyde through inhalation, ingestion, and dermal contact with food and other items containing (E)-crotonaldehyde.

Exposure and Exposure Monitoring

1. Crotonaldehyde is emitted from the combustion of gasoline, the burning of wood, and tobacco. Therefore, the general population may be exposed to crotonaldehyde through inhalation of tobacco smoke, gasoline and diesel engine exhausts, and smoke from wood burning.
2. Crotonaldehyde is a liquid chemical used to synthesize other chemicals. Therefore, workers employed in occupations where crotonaldehyde is used may inhale crotonaldehyde vapors or get the liquid on their skin. People living near uncontrolled hazardous waste sites may be exposed to higher than normal levels.

Crotonaldehyde in the air can irritate eyes, nose, throat, and lungs, causing cough, tightness of chest, and shortness of breath. High levels can cause fluid buildup in lungs, which can be fatal.

Some people may develop a reaction even to low levels of crotonaldehyde.

Upon oral ingestion, it can cause chemical burns of eyes, lips, mouth, throat, esophagus, and stomach.

Toxicokinetics

Predictive models have shown dermal fluxes of 0.627 and 0.326 $mg\,cm^{-2}\,h^{-1}$ for crotonaldehyde. Depending on the model applied, a 1-h exposure of both hands and forearms (surface area of about 2000 cm^2) would produce a total uptake of 1254 or 652 mg crotonaldehyde.

Mechanism of Action

Crotonaldehyde forms protein adducts and DNA–histone cross-links *in vitro*. After incubation with crotonaldehyde, cyclic 1,N_2-propanodeoxyguanosine adducts could be detected in isolated calf thymus DNA, cultured Chinese hamster ovary (CHO) cells, and human fibroblasts, and locally and systemically in various tissues of mice and rats treated *in vivo*. These adducts are to be considered as breakdown products from the reaction of the activated C–C double bond of crotonaldehyde with the exocyclic nitrogen of the deoxyguanosine remainder, analogous to a Michael reaction. Similar cyclic 1,N_2-propanodeoxyguanosine adducts are also formed endogenously *in vivo* in animals and humans.

It was shown in a study that crotonaldehyde induces cytotoxicity through induction of cellular oxidative stress with the depletion of intracellular glutathione and increase of reactive oxygen species in a human bronchial epithelial cell line. Crotonaldehyde caused both apoptosis and necrosis; necrosis was seen with increasing crotonaldehyde concentrations. Crotonaldehyde-induced apoptosis was mediated via cytochrome *c* release and caspases cascade. However, this study cannot rule out the possibility that apoptosis might be occurring through other caspase-independent pathways, such as apoptosis-inducing factor.

Acute and Short-Term Toxicity

Crotonaldehyde is very irritating to the eyes, skin, and mucous membranes. Corneal damage may occur from direct eye contact. Respiratory tract irritation and delayed noncardiogenic pulmonary edema are possible. Irritation of the nose and throat may occur. Gastrointestinal tract irritation may be predicted to occur following ingestion based on the other irritant properties of this substance. Allergic contact dermatitis may be seen. Seizures have been observed as a terminal event in exposed experimental rats. Damage to the thymus and adrenal glands has also been described in exposed animals.

Chronic Toxicity

Chronic oral administration of crotonaldehyde to rats has produced hepatic tumors. Chronically exposed Russian workers developed functional neuropsychiatric disorders.

Reproductive and Developmental Toxicity

Crotonaldehyde has been shown to cause sperm cell degeneration in mice. After intragastric administration of high doses of crotonaldehyde, DNA adducts were detected in liver, lung, and kidney of rats. These data support the systemic availability of crotonaldehyde. Degenerative changes in the nuclei in the various stages of spermatogenesis and significant increases in sperm head anomalies after intraperitoneal treatment indicate that crotonaldehyde reaches germ cells.

Chronically exposed Russian workers developed unspecified sexual disturbances, decreased androgynous function of the male endocrine glands, and menstrual disturbances.

Genotoxicity

Crotonaldehyde was found to be mutagenic in *Escherichia coli* and human fibroblasts transfected with plasmid pMY189 treated with 0–1.8 M crotonaldehyde. Human Cos-7 cells were transfected with plasmids pMS2 into which oligonucleotides for the α-*R*-methyl-γ-hydroxy-1,N_2-propanodeoxyguanosine and α-S-methyl-γ-hydroxy-1,N_2-propanodeoxyguanosine adducts had been inserted. Analysis of the mutations of the plasmid in DH10B *E. coli* cells yielded a rate of mutation of 5–6%, in which mainly transversions from G → T were found. In another study involving ^{32}P-postlabeling, crotonaldehyde was found to bind covalently to calf thymus DNA and dose dependently to the DNA of the CHO cells and the DNA of human fibroblasts. The DNA adducts have been identified as cyclic 1,N_2-propanodeoxyguanosine adducts.

In the comet assay with primary rat hepatocytes, crotonaldehyde concentrations of 2 and 5 mg ml^{-1} induced small, highly condensed areas within the round DNA spots in 89 and 94% of the images. In a comet assay with primary rat epithelial cells of the stomach and colon, the DNA damage increased dose dependently after a 30-min treatment with 0, 0.4, and 0.8 mM crotonaldehyde. Overall, the findings of chromosomal aberrations, micronuclei, and the micronuclei analysis by means of centromere-specific coloring unambiguously demonstrate a genotoxic effect of crotonaldehyde.

In vivo, after dermal application of 6.7 mg crotonaldehyde five times per week for 3 weeks, cyclic 1,N_2-propanodeoxyguanosine adducts were found in the epidermis of the *Sencar* mouse. Likewise, these adducts were investigated in liver, lung, kidney, and in the colon epithelium of Fischer 344 rats following a single treatment via gavage with 200 or 300 mg kg^{-1} body weight after 12 and 20 h. After doses of 200 and 300 mg kg^{-1} body weight, 29 and 34 adducts 10^{-9} nucleotides were found in the liver. No adducts were found in the liver of untreated rats. Twenty and nine adducts 10^{-9} nucleotides were detected in lung and kidney, respectively.

Genotoxicity of crotonaldehyde was studied in the bone marrow and germ cells of laboratory mice. A positive dose–response relationship between treatment and induction of chromosomal aberrations in the somatic and germ cells and dominant lethal mutation in the germ cells was found.

Carcinogenicity

Bittersohl carried out epidemiologic studies with workers. A majority of these workers were employed in an aldehyde factory for more than 20 years. The ambient air concentrations of crotonaldehyde (besides other aldehydes such as acetaldehyde) varied at the different workplaces between 1 and 7 mg m^{-3} air. Of the 150 workers, nine developed malignant tumors (two squamous cell carcinomas of the oral cavity, one adenocarcinoma of the stomach, one adenocarcinoma of the cecum, and five squamous cell carcinomas of the bronchi). Due to the tumor incidence observed, the author suggested that carcinogenic properties of acetaldol formed from acetaldehyde and a syncarcinogenic effect of the aliphatic aldehydes were responsible. There are no new studies available.

Environmental Protection Agency states that crotonaldehyde is a possible human carcinogen. Classification: C; possible human carcinogen. Basis for classification: based on no human data and an increased incidence of hepatocellular carcinomas and hepatic neoplastic nodules (combined) in male F344 rats. The possible carcinogenicity of crotonaldehyde is supported by genotoxic activity and the expected reactivity of croton oil and aldehyde. Crotonaldehyde is also a suspected metabolite of *N*-nitrosopyrrolidine, a probable human carcinogen.

Human carcinogenicity data: none.

International Agency for Research on Cancer states that it is not carcinogenic to humans, classification: Group 3. There is inadequate evidence in humans and experimental animals for the carcinogenicity of crotonaldehyde.

Overall evaluation: Crotonaldehyde is not classifiable as to its carcinogenicity to humans (Group 3).

Clinical Management

The following medical procedures should be made available to each employee who is exposed to crotonaldehyde at potentially hazardous levels:

1. Initial medical screening: Employees should be screened for history of certain medical conditions (listed below), which might place the employee at increased risk from crotonaldehyde exposure. Chronic respiratory disease: in persons with impaired pulmonary function, especially those with obstructive airway diseases, the breathing of crotonaldehyde has irritant properties. Skin disease: crotonaldehyde is a primary skin irritant. Persons with existing skin disorders may be more susceptible to the effects of this agent.
2. Periodic medical examinations: Any employee developing the above-listed conditions should be referred for further medical examination.

Baseline arterial blood gases and chest X-ray should be obtained for patients with significant respiratory exposure. Baseline liver and renal function tests and complete blood count with differential are suggested for patients with substantial exposure.

Treatment Overview

Oral Exposure

1. Because of the potential for gastrointestinal tract irritation and seizures, emesis should NOT be induced. Administer activated charcoal as slurry (240 ml water/30 g charcoal). Usual dose: 25–100 g in adults/adolescents, 25–50 g in children (1–12 years), and 1 g kg^{-1} in infants less than 1-year old. Significant esophageal or gastrointestinal tract irritation or burns may occur following ingestion. The possible benefit of early removal of some ingested material by cautious gastric lavage must be weighed against potential complications of bleeding or perforation. Consider gastric lavage only after ingestion of a potentially life-threatening amount of poison if it can be performed soon after ingestion (generally within 1 h). Protect airway by placement in the head down left lateral decubitus position or by endotracheal intubation. Control any seizures first. Gastric lavage is contraindicated if there is any loss of airway protective reflexes or decreased level of consciousness in unintubated patients; following ingestion of corrosives; hydrocarbons (high aspiration potential); patients at risk of hemorrhage or gastrointestinal perforation; and trivial or nontoxic ingestion.
2. Obtain baseline liver and renal function tests and complete blood count.
3. Observe patients with ingestion carefully for the possible development of esophageal or gastrointestinal tract irritation or burns. If signs or symptoms of esophageal irritation or burns are present, consider endoscopy to determine the extent of injury.

Inhalation Exposure

1. Move patient to fresh air: Monitor for respiratory distress. If cough or difficulty in breathing develops, evaluate for respiratory tract irritation, bronchitis, or pneumonitis.

Administer oxygen and assist ventilation as required. Treat bronchospasm with inhaled beta2-agonist and oral or parenteral corticosteroids.
2. Acute lung injury: Maintain ventilation and oxygenation and evaluate with frequent arterial blood gas or pulse oximetry monitoring. Early use of *positive end-expiratory pressure* and mechanical ventilation may be needed.

Eye Exposure

Decontamination: Irrigate exposed eyes with copious amounts of room temperature water for at least 15 min. If irritation, pain, swelling, lacrimation, or photophobia persists, the patient should be examined in a health care facility.

Dermal Exposure

1. Decontamination: Remove contaminated clothing and wash exposed area thoroughly with soap and water. A physician may need to examine the area if irritation or pain persists.
2. Treat dermal irritation or burns with standard topical therapy. Patients developing dermal hypersensitivity reactions may require treatment with systemic or topical corticosteroids or antihistamines.

Ecotoxicology

There are no studies on the bioaccumulation of crotonaldehyde. Bioaccumulation is not expected on the basis of the calculated log K_{OW} of 0.63. Crotonaldehyde was one of the 221 organic compounds measured in a roadway tunnel in Los Angeles, California, in 1993. In 1999, air samples were collected at the inlet and outlet of two highway tunnels near San Francisco, California, and Pennsylvania. Crotonaldehyde was one of the 10 most abundant carbonyls measured (0.23 $\mu g\, m^{-3}$ in California and 0.12 $\mu g\, m^{-3}$ in Pennsylvania). Crotonaldehyde was also detected in ambient air at the Oakland–San Francisco Bay Bridge tollbooth plaza in California during rush hour traffic, indicating that this compound is emitted by vehicles.

Exposure Standards and Guidelines

OSHA limits: 2 ppm crotonaldehyde of workroom air/8-h work shift, 40-h workweek.

Sources: ATSDR URL: http://www.atsdr.cdc.gov/toxfaqs/tf.asp?id=948&tid=197.

See also: Acetaldehyde; Carcinogen–DNA Adduct Formation and DNA Repair; Neurotoxicity.

Further Reading

Bittersohl, G., Epidemiologic investigations on cancer incidence in workers contacted by acetaldol and other aliphatic aldehyds. Arch Geschwulstforsch. 43 (2), 172–176.

Chen, H.J., Lin, W.P., 2009. Simultaneous quantification of 1, N_2-propano-2′-deoxyguanosine adducts derived from acrolein and crotonaldehyde in human placenta and leukocytes by isotope dilution nanoflow LC nanospray ionization tandem mass spectrometry. Anal. Chem. 81 (23), 9812–9818.

Kielhorn, J., Mangelsdorf, I., Ziegler-Skylakakis, K., 2008. World Health Organization, United Nations Environment Programme, International Labour Organisation, International Program on Chemical Safety (IPCS), Inter-Organization Programme for the Sound Management of Chemicals, Concise International Chemical Assessment Document 74.

Liu, X.Y., Yang, Z.H., Pan, X.J., Zhu, M.X., Xie, J.P., 2010. Crotonaldehyde induces oxidative stress and caspase-dependent apoptosis in human bronchial epithelial cells. Toxicol. Lett. 195 (1), 90–98.

Liu, X.Y., Yang, Z.H., Pan, X.J., Zhu, M.X., Xie, J.P., 2010. Gene expression profile and cytotoxicity of human bronchial epithelial cells exposed to crotonaldehyde. Toxicol. Lett. 197 (2), 113–122.

Stein, S., Lao, Y., Yang, I.Y., Hecht, S.S., Moriya, M., 2006. Genotoxicity of acetaldehyde- and crotonaldehyde-induced 1, N_2-propanodeoxyguanosine DNA adducts in human cells. Mutat. Res. 608 (1), 1–7.

Relevant Websites

https://www.osha.gov/dts/chemicalsampling/data/CH_230000.html – US Department of Labor - Occupational Safety & Health Administration: Crotonaldehyde.

http://www.inchem.org/documents/iarc/vol63/crotonaldehyde.html – IPCS Inchem: Crotonaldehyde.

Crude Oil *see* Oil, Crude

CS

H Salem*, Edgewood Chemical Biological Center, MD, USA
SA Katz, Rutgers University, Camden, NJ, USA
M Feasel*, Edgewood Chemical Biological Center, MD, USA
B Ballantyne[†], Consultant, Charleston, WV,USA

This article is a revision of the previous edition article by Harry Salem, Bryan Ballantyne, and Sidney A. Katz, volume 1, pp. 686–692, © 2005, Elsevier Inc.

- Name: Chlorobenzylidene malononitrile
- Chemical Abstracts Service Registry Number: 2698-41-1
- Synonym: Tear gas; Less-than-lethal; Nonlethal; Lacrimator, Harassing agent; Incapacitant; (2-Chlorophenyl) methylene; Propanedinitrile, (*o*-chlorobenzylidene) malononitrile; 2-Chlorobenzalmalononitrile
- Molecular Formula: $C_{10}H_5ClN_9$
- Structure:

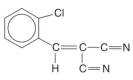

Background (Significance/History)

CS, or *o*-chlorobenzylidene malononitrile, is the current major riot control agent (RCA) used by U.S. military forces. It was originally synthesized in 1928 by Corson and Stoughton, and the U.S. Army designated the compound 'CS' for the authors' initials. CS replaced CN, chloroacetophenone, in 1959 as the U.S. Army's premier RCA due to its higher safety ratio over CN. CS is more effective as an RCA, that is to say, more potent and safer than its predecessor CN. CS can be disseminated pyrotechnically, or in the cases of CS_1 and CS_2, in powder formulations.

Uses

CS is used as a nonlethal or less-than-lethal chemical in riot control situations, to distract, deter, incapacitate, disorient, or disable disorderly people, to clear facilities, areas, deny areas, or for hostage rescue. It can also be used in peacekeeping operations. It is also used in military training as a confidence builder for the protective mask. In addition to the nonpersistent form of CS, two hydrophobic variations were created, CS_1 and CS_2. CS_1 is a micronized powder formulation containing 5% hydrophobic silica aerogel, which can persist for up to 2 weeks in normal weather conditions, and CS_2 is a siliconized microencapsulated form of CS_1 with a long shelf life, persistence, resistant to degradation, and ability to float on water, which could restrict or deny the use of water for military operations. CS is commonly used as an RCA and a simulant for training. Members of military organizations and law enforcement agencies are routinely exposed to heated CS during training. The heat vaporizes the CS for dispersion, which then condenses to form an aerosol.

Environmental Fate and Behavior

Decontamination

Contaminated clothing should be removed and sealed in a plastic bag. Disposable rubber gloves should be used when handling contaminated clothes. The eyes should be irrigated copiously with saline for 15–20 min. Contaminated skin should be washed thoroughly with copious amounts of water, alkaline soap and water, a mildly alkaline solution (sodium bicarbonate or sodium carbonate), or mild liquid soap and water. The use of sodium hypochlorite solution will exacerbate the skin lesions and should not be employed. Only a saline irrigation should be used over vesiculated skin.

Decontamination of material/clothing after contamination with CS can be done with sodium bicarbonate or carbonate 5–10% solution. If this means of decontamination cannot be accomplished (e.g., contaminated rooms and furniture), the only other means is by intensive air exchange – preferably with hot air.

Table 1 Decontamination of riot control agents

Compound	*($t_{1/2}$) Hydrolysis in water*	*($t_{1/2}$) Water + Alkaline*
CS	(15 min) Rapid	(1 min) Rapid
CR	Little–None	Little–None
CN	Very slow	Very slow

Includes half-life of CS in water/alkaline solution.

* The views of the authors do not purport to reflect the position of the US Department of Defense. The use of trade names does not constitute official endorsement or approval of the use of such commercial product.
† Deceased.

 http://dx.doi.org/10.1016/B978-0-12-386454-3.00598-4

If clothing is to be washed, cold water should be used because hot water will cause any residual CS to volatilize, leading to symptoms in attending staff.

Table 1 describes tear agent breakdown in water/alkaline solutions. CS is the easiest to decontaminate because it readily hydrolyzes in water, and does so even more rapidly in alkaline solutions. CR and CN have low vulnerability hydrolysis, rendering them mild environmental risks (**Table 1**).

Fate in Soil and Water

Tests conducted at Eglin Air Force Base near Ft. Walton Beach, Florida, concluded that CS in soil has a 'conservative' half-life of 3.9 days. Degradation of CS increases with soil and air moisture, and with light exposure as it undergoes a slow hydrolysis process. Olajos (2004) concluded that CS degrades to *o*-chlorobenzaldehyde and malononitrile, the former of which is ultimately converted to catechol under aerobic conditions. Nitriles such as the malononitrile degradation product of CS have a short half-life in soil and can be converted readily to organic acids. Anaerobically, microalgae have been reported to transform CS breakdown products into benzoate. The U.S. Army Edgewood Research Development and Engineering Center (USAERDEC) reports a solubility of 200 mg l^{-1}.

Fate in Air

CS concentrations attenuate in the atmosphere through three processes: reaction with hydroxyl radicals, hydrolysis reactions with atmospheric humidity, and deposition of particulate CS. It should be noted that vapor pressure increases with temperature, as should be expected. At 20 °C, CS vapor pressure is 3.5×10^{-5} mmHg, and at 60 °C, it is 5–7 mmHg.

Exposure and Exposure Monitoring

Routes and Pathways

CS at room temperature is a white solid, stable when heated, and with a low vapor pressure. The vapor is several times heavier than air. It can be dispersed as a fine powder, as a jet or stream of solution from small or large spray tanks, and as aerosols or smokes by pyrotechnic generation. Its solubility in water is limited, but it is soluble in organic and chlorinated organics. High-temperature dispersion may produce a number of organic thermal degradation products through rearrangements and loss of cyano and chlorine substituents on CS, possibly HCN and HCl. CS is rapidly hydrolyzed in water with a half-life of ~15 min at room temperature at pH 7. In alkaline solution (pH 9), the half-life is 1 min. Therefore, CS can be easily inactivated by a water/alkaline solution or by washing with soap and water.

Human Exposure

When CS was disseminated using spray nozzles from a 10% solution in acetone or in methylene or dichloride, or from a miniature M8 thermal grenade, the mass median diameter (MMD) of CS produced was 3.0 μm for the CS in acetone, 1.0 μm for the CS in methylene dichloride, and 0.51 μm for the miniature M18 CS thermal grenade. When properly fitted, protective masks fully protect against exposure to CS. In those who were unable to mask rapidly, panic was evident. Concentrations of 9–10 mg m^{-3} forced 50% of the subjects to leave the chamber within 30 s, 99% left when exposed to ~17 mg m^{-3}, and 100% left and were considered incapacitated at 40 mg m^{-3} or greater.

Spray devices in use by UK police are 5% CS in a methyl isobutyl ketone (MIK) propellant. MIK itself is a strong irritant, leading to much debate over the safety of CS sprayers. In addition, in pyrotechnic dissemination devices, it is possible to generate HCN and HCl at high temperatures (above 700 °C). These by-products are undesirable when attempting to avoid permanent health risks by using nonlethal devices.

Toxicokinetics

CS reacts covalently with plasma proteins to form compounds that may be antigenic. On contact with water, it hydrolyzes into *o*-chlorobenzaldehyde and malononitrile. The kidney excretes *o*-chlorobenzaldehyde as the metabolites *o*-chlorohippuric acid (major) and *o*-chlorobenzoic acid (minor). The malononitrile is metabolized to thiocyanate. The cyano groups of 2-chlorobenzylidene malononitrile are unlikely to cause systemic cyanide toxicity since no significant amounts of free cyanide appear in the plasma.

Mechanism of Toxicity

These agents are considered less than lethal and nonlethal because they have a very large safety ratio. That is, their effective dose or concentration ECt_{50} is very low compared to their lethal dose or concentration (LCt_{50}).

CS as well as CN is an SN2-alkylating agent with activated halogen groups that react readily at nucleophilic sites. The prime targets include sulfhydryl-containing enzymes such as lactic dehydrogenase. In particular, CS reacts rapidly with the disulfhydryl form of lipoic acid, a coenzyme in the pyruvate decarboxylase system. It has been suggested that tissue injury may be related to inactivation of certain of these enzyme systems. CS causes the release of bradykinin, which can cause pain without tissue injury. The initial response to the inhalation of CS or other sensory irritants is consistent with the Kratschmer reflex and the Sherrington pseudoaffective response. These aerosols stimulate the pulmonary irritant receptors to produce bronchoconstriction and increased pulmonary blood volume by augmenting sympathetic tone. The chlorine atoms released from CS on contact with skin and mucus membranes are reduced to hydrochloride acid, which can cause local irritation and burns.

Brone et al. in 2008 concluded that CS, CR, and CN all are potent agonists to the transient receptor potential A1, or TrpA1, cation-selective channel. This receptor is part of the same family of receptors as TrpV1, the receptor through which oleoresin capsicum (OC), or pepper spray, works. TrpA1 differs structurally from the other Trp receptors, mainly by having amino-terminal ankyrin repeat domains and an 1125

Table 2 Tear gas potencies (Blain, 2003)

Compound	*TC_{50} (mg m^{-3})*	*IC_{50} (mg min m^{-3})*
CR	0.004	0.7
CN	0.3	20–50
CS	0.004	3.6
OC	0.0003–0.003	NA

TC_{50} = Threshold concentration.
IC_{50} = Incapacitating concentration.
OC included for comparison and is not a TrpA1 agonist.

amino-acid carboxy-terminal chain, both intracellularly. The receptor has been shown to generate action potentials based on pain and inflammatory stimuli experienced at these sites. This includes agonism by CS. CS possesses an electrophilic carbon that binds covalently to cysteine thiol residues in the TrpA1 receptor. This covalent bond is reversible, however, accounting for the temporary effects of these agents. In this study by Brone, in fact, the researchers were merely looking for TrpA1 receptor agonists and when synthesizing some of these noticed a pungent irritation of the eyes and nose. They then realized they were synthesizing compounds structurally similar to CR. From there, they reviewed the biological activity of the riot control agents and decided to test *their* affinity and efficacy for the TrpA1 receptor instead of synthesizing new compounds.

Upon agonism by these RCAs, the TrpA1 receptor opens and selectively allows for the flux of sodium (Na^+) and calcium (Ca^{2+}) ions into the cell. This depolarizes the sensory neuron and sends an afferent signal to the central nervous system (CNS) that is interpreted as pain. CR allows for the most calcium influx in the shortest amount of time into the cell, establishing it as the most potent tear agent of the three. CS follows closely behind CR with respect to the amplitude and time to peak of calcium influx. CN trails the others in third place. This study, therefore establishes that CS, CR, and CN do in fact work through the TrpA1 receptor, but is that the only Trp receptor they antagonize? The study went on further to test for cross-reactivity with other Trp receptors, and the tear agents were deemed TrpA1 selective, as no agonism was found with the other receptors.

The sensory effects seen with tear gas exposures are due to the afferents formed by trigeminal neurons, which express high concentrations of TrpA1 receptors. For example, stimulation of the tearing reflex transduces a signal through the trigeminal nerve and registers as pain. That being said, antagonists for the TrpA1 receptor could be potential therapeutic targets for tear gas overexposure treatments. With regard to TrpA1 activation, the potencies of the tear agents are described in **Table 2**.

Acute and Short-Term Toxicity (To Include Irritation and Corrosivity)

Human

Persons who had been exposed previously to a high concentration developed a fear of the agent, and even though subsequently exposed to lower concentration, the time to incapacitation for trained men was shorter than expected. There were no significant differences noted in the time to incapacitation in subjects exposed to CS at 0–95 °F, although it was apparent that the subjects appeared unable to tolerate the agent as well as those exposed at ambient temperature. At 95 °F and a relative humidity of 35% or 97%, the skin-burning effects were much more prominent, possibly because of the excessive diaphoresis. Hypertensive subjects reacted similarly to and tolerated CS as well as normotensive individuals. However, their blood pressure elevation was greater and lasted longer than in normotensives, possibly because of the stress of exposure. The hypertensive subjects recovered as rapidly as normotensives.

One study has shown that emotional state has much to do with the response to CS exposure. Some of the first physiological signs and symptoms of CS exposure are hypertension and irregular breathing. However, in experiments that bypass the nose and upper airway by administering CS endotracheally, a *drop* in blood pressure occurs and *decreased* respiration is observed. This phenomenon is due to pain receptors in the nose and upper airway being bypassed and thus no emotional response due to pain is present to manifest the typical respiratory and circulatory effects of CS seen in the field.

Subjects with a history of peptic ulcer, jaundice, or hepatitis and those between the ages of 50 and 60 years reacted similarly to normal subjects. Persons with a history of drug allergy, hay fever, asthma, or drug sensitivity were able to tolerate CS exposure as well as the normal subjects; however, a higher percentage of this group had more severe chest symptoms than the normals. Although many of these lay prostrate on the ground for several minutes, no wheezing or ronchi were heard on auscultation, and recovery time was slightly prolonged, but only by 1–2 min. Although not significantly different, subjects exposed to CS disseminated from methylene dichloride appeared to tolerate the agent for a slightly longer period than those subjected to CS in acetone solution, nor were there many differences from CS disseminated from the miniature M18 CS smoke grenade. CS was effective within seconds. Although high concentrations for prolonged exposure in closed spaces can produce severe effects, no validated deaths in humans have been reported for CS. These effects were acute laryngotracheobronchitis in an infant, reactive airway dysfunction syndrome, hemoptysis and hypoxia, and erythroderma in adults, which were all treated successfully. Ingestion of CS may lead to abdominal cramping, pain, and diarrhea.

Animal

Various experimental animal species were exposed to aerosols of CS generated by various methods of exposure from 5 to 90 min. The toxic signs observed in mice, rats, guinea pigs, rabbits, dogs, and monkeys were immediate, and included hyperactivity, followed by copious lacrimation, and salivation within 30 s of exposure in all species except the rabbit. The initial level of heightened activity subsided, and within 5–15 min following initiation of the exposure, those exposed exhibited lethargy and pulmonary stress, which continued for about an hour following cessation of the exposure. All other signs disappeared within 5 min following removal from the

Table 3 Acute inhalation toxicity LCt_{50} (mg min m^{-3})

Animal	*CS smoke*	*CS aerosol*
Guinea pig	35 800	67 000
Rabbit	63 600	54 090
Rat	69 800	88 480
Mouse	70 000	50 110

exposure. When toxic signs were observed, they occurred following exposure by all of the dispersion methods.

Lethality estimates were expressed by calculation of LCt_{50} values. From acute exposures to CS dispersed from a 10% CS in methylene dichloride, the LCt_{50} values (in mg min m^{-3}) were as follows: mice, 627 000; rats, 1 004 000; and guinea pigs, 46 000. No deaths occurred in rabbits exposed to up to 47 000 mg min m^{-3}. CS at dosages up to 30 000 mg min m^{-3} did not cause any deaths in any of the monkeys with pulmonary tularemia. The combined LCt_{50} for mice, rats, guinea pigs, and rabbits was calculated to be 1 230 000 mg min m^{-3} for CS dispersed from methylene dichloride. Goats, pigs, and sheep did not exhibit hyperactivity on exposure to CS, and they were also resistant to its lethal effect. Therefore, no LCt_{50} values could be calculated for goats, pigs, or sheep. However, a combined LCt_{50} was calculated for all of the species tested, including mice, rats, guinea pigs, rabbits, dogs, monkeys, goats, pigs, and sheep, and was estimated to be 300 000 mg min m^{-3}. LCt_{50} values were also calculated for CS dispersed from M18 and M7A3 thermal grenades. These were (in mg min m^{-3}) 164 000 for rats and 36 000 for guinea pigs exposed to the M18 thermal grenade dissemination; for the M7A3 thermal grenade they were (in mg min m^{-3}) as follows: rats, 94 000; guinea pigs, 66 000; rabbits, 38 000; goats, 48 000; pigs, 17 000; dogs, 30 000; monkeys, 120 000.

All of the acute exposure results were combined and LCt_{50} values were calculated for all rodents to be 79 000 mg min m^{-3}, and for all nonrodent species tested to be 36 000 mg min m^{-3}, and for all the species it was 61 000 mg min m^{-3}. The LCt_{50} values for CS_2 were also calculated. CS_2 is 95% CS, 5% Cab-oSil R, and 1% hexamethyldisilazane, and the LCt_{50} values are rats, 68 000 mg min m^{-3}; guinea pigs, 49 000 mg min m^{-3}; dogs, 70 000 mg min m^{-3}; and monkeys, 74 000 mg min m^{-3}. The lethal effects in animals following inhalation exposures are caused by lung damage leading to asphyxia and circulatory failure, or bronchopneumonia secondary to respiratory tract injury. Pathology involving the liver and kidneys following inhalation of high dosages of CS is also secondary to respiratory and circulatory failure.

The acute inhalation toxicity of CS, generated in smoke and as an aerosol, was studied in several animal species, and the LCt_{50} data are presented in **Table 3**.

Chronic Toxicity

Animal

Repeated exposures of thermally dispersed CS were conducted in rats and dogs. They were exposed from 4 to 5 min per day, 5 days a week for 5 weeks. The 25-day cumulative dosage (Ct) to which the rats were exposed was 91 000 mg min m^{-3} (3640 mg min m^{-3} per day), while the dogs were exposed to a cumulative dosage of 17 000 mg min m^{-3} (680 mg min m^{-3} per day). No lethality occurred in the dogs, while the rats became hyperactive and aggressive, biting noses and tails of other rats, and scratching their own noses. No changes were found in blood values for sodium, potassium, protein, albumin, or creatinine throughout the tests. Five of the 30 rats exposed died, 2 following the cumulative dosage of 25 000 mg min m^{-3}, and 3 died after 68 000 mg min m^{-3}. Gross pathological examinations of the rats that died were negative, as were those of six other rats that were sacrificed after 5 weeks of exposure. The exposed rats lost 1% of body weight, while unexposed rats gained 20% during the 5 weeks. There were no significant differences in organ to body weight ratios for heart, kidneys, lungs, liver, or spleen following the 5-week exposures. It was concluded that repeated exposures did not make the animals more sensitive to the lethal effects of CS. The animals that died after exposure to CS showed increased numbers of goblet cells in the respiratory and gastrointestinal tracts and conjunctiva, as well as necrosis in the respiratory and gastrointestinal tracts, pulmonary edema, and occasionally hemorrhage in the adrenals. Death appeared to result from poor transfer of oxygen from the lungs to the blood stream, probably because of edema, hemorrhage in the lungs, and obstruction of the airways.

The effects of repeated exposures to CS in mice, rats, and guinea pigs to neat CS aerosols for 1 h per day, 5 days per week for 120 days demonstrated that high concentrations of CS were fatal to the animals after only a few exposures, while mortality in the low and medium concentrations did not differ significantly from the controls. It was concluded that CS concentrations below 30 mg m^{-3} were without deleterious effects.

Immunotoxicity

Studies conducted by Nagarkatti et al. (1981) concluded that CS has a direct effect on the immune system through their experimentation with mice. Mice were dosed with CS at two dose levels. The lower dose produced suppression of the humoral immune response to sheep red blood cell (SRBC) antigen. The higher dose produced elevated levels of corticosterone in the mice.

Reproductive Toxicity

The effects of CS inhalation were studied on embryonic development in rats and rabbits at concentrations consistent with those expected in riot control situations (10 mg m^{-3}). Although the concentrations were low and the duration of exposure (5 min) may not have been adequate to assess the fetotoxic and teratogenic potential of CS, no significant increases in the numbers of abnormal fetuses or resorptions were noted.

Genotoxicity

The mutagenic potential of CS and CS_2 was studied in microbial and mammalian bioassays. CS was negative in the Ames

Assay when tested in *Salmonella typhimurium* strains TA 98, TA 1535, and TA 1537 with and without metabolic activation. The mutagenic potential for CS and CS_2 in mammalian assays such as the Chinese hamster ovary test for the induction of sister chromatid exchange (SCE) and chromosomal aberration (CA), and the mouse lymphoma L5178Y assay for induction of trifluorothymidine (Tfi) resistance, indicated that CS_2 induced SCE, CAs, and Tfi resistance. The Committee on Toxicology of the (U.S.) National Research Council (1984) reported that, taken in their totality, the tests of CS for gene mutation and chromosomal damage provide no clear evidence of mutagenicity. Although most of the evidence is consistent with nonmutagenicity, in the committee's judgment, it is unlikely that CS poses a mutagenic hazard to humans.

Carcinogenicity

CS_2 was evaluated for carcinogenicity in the U.S. National Toxicity Program (NTP) 2-year rodent bioassay. Compound-related nonneoplastic lesions of the respiratory tract were observed. The pathologic changes observed in the exposed rats included squamous metaplasia of the olfactory epithelium, hyperplasia, and metaplasia of the respiratory epithelium. In mice, hyperplasia and squamous metaplasia of the respiratory epithelium were observed. Neoplastic effects were not observed in either rats or mice. It was concluded that the findings suggest that CS_2 is not carcinogenic to rats and mice. CS in methylene chloride was also tested in mice and rats for carcinogenicity in a 2-year study, and no tumorigenic effects were observed in the CS-exposed animals.

Clinical Management

Ocular exposure to CS produces intense blepharospasm, pain, lacrimation, conjunctival erythema, periorbital edema, and a rise in intraocular pressure. These effects generally diminish within 30 min postexposure. CS also produces rhinorrhea, nasal irritation and congestion, bronchorrhea, sore throat, cough, sneezing, unpleasant taste, and burning of the mouth immediately after exposure. These effects rapidly resolve within minutes postexposure. Symptomatic treatment of ocular irritation consists of the use of a topical solution to relieve the irritation with topical antibiotics. The eyes should be examined for corneal abrasions. Treatment with oral analgesics, topical antibiotics, and mydriatics should be considered. Since CS is a solid, it is possible for a particle or clump to become embedded in the cornea or conjunctiva and cause tissue damage. Medical care for eye pain after exposure should include thorough decontamination of the eyes and a thorough ophthalmologic examination. The eye with ocular injuries should be carefully irrigated with isotonic saline and the remaining powder removed with a cotton swab. Any remaining stromal particles should be removed with a needle tip under slit lamp illumination. Airway problems may occur in individuals with lung disease, especially if exposed to higher than average field use concentrations. If these occur, the immediate priority is the removal from the exposure and to ensure a patent, or open airway.

Severe and prolonged erythema or severe dermatitis may occur several hours after exposure that is then followed by vesiculation. These are generally second-degree burns and should be treated like second-degree chemical burns.

If the release of irritant incapacitants is in a confined, unventilated space, exposure may be to very high concentrations. Some individuals may be more susceptible to high concentrations, possibly because of an existing medical condition such as asthma, and will require intensive supportive medical treatment postexposure.

Ecotoxicology

Few studies have been done regarding the ecotoxicology of CS, but one study conducted by Morrison et al. (1974) concluded that it is highly toxic to woody terrestrial plants at concentrations from 60 to 120 $g\,m^{-3}$. Malononitrile, one of the hydrolysis products of CS, has shown to be toxic to duckweed, an aquatic plant, as well according to Worthley and Schott (1971) at levels above 5 $mg\,l^{-1}$.

Rainbow trout and the mumichog were both used as animal models to test the aquatic toxicity of CS in the 1970s and 1980s. Abram and Wilson report that malononitrile is less toxic than CS and *o*-chlorobenzaldehyde at the following molar concentrations: CS – 0.031 $mmol\,l^{-1}$, *o*-chlorobenzaldehyde – 0.032 $mmol\,l^{-1}$, and malononitrile – 0.17 $mmol\,l^{-1}$.

CS was found by Pearson (1975) to cause coughing and convulsions in the mumichog at levels at or above 6.3 $mg\,l^{-1}$, but no effect was seen when exposed to *o*-chlorobenzaldehyde at levels approaching 35.0 $mg\,l^{-1}$ in the same animal model. However, in a later study, Keller et al. (1986) found the lethal concentration threshold of CS in the mumichog to be 3.9 $mg\,l^{-1}$.

Pearson also studied the effects of CS on gold fish, *Carassius auratus*. Gold fish could tolerate 6 $mg\,l^{-1}$ of CS up to approximately 22 h, and 10 $mg\,l^{-1}$ for 2.7–5.3 h.

Exposure Standards and Guidelines

Ceiling (ACGIH): 0.05 ppm.

PEL (OSHA): 0.05 ppm.

"Human data: It has been reported that median incapacitating concentrations range from 12 to 20 $mg\,m^{-3}$ after about 20 s of exposure (U.S. Depts of Army and Air Force, 1963) and that a 2-min exposure to concentrations between 2 and 10 $mg\,m^{-3}$ was considered 'intolerable' by 6 of 15 persons (Army, 1961). In another study, 3 of 4 volunteers exposed to 1.5 $mg\,m^{-3}$ for 90 min developed headaches and 1 volunteer developed slight eye and nose irritation; human volunteers have found concentrations greater than 10 $mg\,m^{-3}$ to be extremely irritating and intolerable for more than 30 s because of burning and pain in the eyes and chest (Punte et al. 1963). Exposures above 14 $mg\,m^{-3}$ for 1 h produced extreme irritation, erythema, and vesication of the skin of volunteers (Weigand, 1969)." (Hazmap, 2012)

See also: Arsenical Vomiting Agents; Blister Agents/Vesicants; 3-Quinuclidinyl Benzilate (BZ): Psychotomimetic Agent; CN Gas; Nerve Agents; Nonlethal Weapons; Riot Control Agents.

Further Reading

Abram, F.S.H., Wilson, P., 1979. The acute toxicity of CS to rainbow trout. Water Res. 13, 631–635.

Army [1961]. U.S. Army, Chemical Corps Safety Directive No. 385-12. Safety guide for processing, filling, handling and decontamination of CS and CS1. Edgewood Arsenal, MD: CML C SD-385-12, p. 4.

Blain, P.G., 2003. Tear gases and irritant incapacitants. Toxicol. Rev. 22 (2), 103–110.

Brone, B., Peeters, P., Marrannes, R., Mercken, M., Nuydens, R., Meert, T., Gijsen, H., 2008. Tear gasses CN, CR and CS are potent activators of the human TrpA1 receptor. Tox. Appl. Pharm. 231, 150–156.

Chemical Warfare Agents, 2008. In: Romano Jr., J.A., Lukely, B.J., Salem, H. (Eds.), Chemistry, Pharmacology, Toxicology, and Therapeutics, second ed. CRC Press, Taylor & Francis Group (Print), Boca Raton, FL.

Dray, A., Perkins, M., Mar 1993. Bradykinin and inflammatory pain. Trends Neurosci. 16 (3), 99–104.

Giksen, H., Berthelot, D., Zaja, M., Brone, B., Geuens, I., Mercken, M., 2010. Analogues of morphanthridine and the tear gas Dibenz[b, f][1,4]oxazepine (CR) as extremely potent activators of the human transient receptor potential ankyrin 1 (TrpA1) Channel. J. Med. Chem. 53, 7011–7020.

Haz-Map: Information on Hazardous Chemicals and Occupational Diseases. Brown, Jay A., M.D., M.P.H. http://hazmap.nlm.nih.gov/category-details?id=355&table=copytblagents. Accessed November 2012.

Keller, William C., Elves, Robert G., Bonnin, John C. Assessment of CS Environmental Toxicity at Eglin AFB FL. USAFOEHL Report 86-058E00058HTB. Final Report. August 1986.

Moran, M., McAlexander, M., Biro, T., Szallasi, A., Aug 2011. Transient receptor potential channels as therapeutic targets. Nat. Rev. 10, 601–620.

Morrison, B., Dralle, D., Demaree, K., 1974. Effects of CS on Vegetation: ii. Field and Screening Studies, ECTR-74040, Edgewood Arsenal, Aberdeen Proving Ground, Maryland.

Nagarkatti, M., Nagarkatti, P.S., Raghuveeran, C.D., 1981. Short-term toxicity of *o*-chlorobenzylidene malononitrile on humoral immunity in mice. Toxicol. Lett. 8, 73–76.

National Academy of Sciences, 1984. Possible Long-Term Health Effects of Short-Term Exposure to Chemical Agents, Vol. 2. Cholinesterase Reactivators, Phychochemicals, and Irritants & Vesicants. National Academy Press, Washington, DC.

Olajos, E.J., Stopford, W., 2004. Riot Control Agents: Issues in Toxicology, Safety, and Health. CRC Press.

Pearson, J., and R. Renne. The Toxicity of the Riot Control Agent CS (o-chlorobenzylidene Malononitrile) and Its Hydrolysis Products to the Mummichog, Fundulus Heterolitus (Linnaeus). Edgewood Arsenal Technical Report EATR 74095. March 1975.

Punte, C.L., Owens, E.J., Gutentag, P.J., 1963. Exposures to ortho-chlorobenzylidene malononitrile: controlled human exposures. Arch Environ Health 6, 366–374.

Thornburn, K.M., 1982. Injuries after use of the lacrimatory agent chloroacetophenone in a confine space. Arch. Environ. Health 37 (3), 182–186.

U.S. Departments of the Army and Air Force [1963]. Military chemistry and chemical agents. Washington, DC: Army Technical Manual TM3-215; Air Force Manual AFM 355-7, December 1963.

Weigand DA [1969]. Cutaneous reaction to the riot control agent CS. Milit Med 134:437.

Worthley, E.G., Schott, C.D., 1971. The Comparative Effects of CS and Various Pollutants on Fresh Water Phytoplankton Colonies of Wolffia papulifer. Thompson Edgewood Arsenal Technical Report 4595. Department of Army, Edgewood Arsenal, Maryland.

Relevant Websites

http://www.bt.cdc.gov – Centers for Disease Control and Prevention: Emergency Preparedness and Response.

http://sis.nlm.nih.gov – US National Library of Medicine, Specialized Information Services, Chemical Warfare Agents.

Culture and Toxicology *see* Toxicology in the Arts, Culture, and Imagination

Cumene

S Nikfar, Tehran University of Medical Sciences, Tehran, Iran; Food and Drug Laboratory Research Center, Ministry of Health and Medical Education, Tehran, Iran
AF Behboudi, Chemical Engineering, Toronto, ON, Canada

This article is a revision of the previous edition article by Ralph Gingell, volume 1, pp 690–692 © 2005, Elsevier Inc.

- Chemical Abstracts Service Registry Number: 98-82-8.
- IUPAC Systematic Name: Benzene, (1-methylethyl)-
- Synonyms: (1-Methylethyl)benzene; 2-Fenilpropano; 2-Phenylpropane; Benzene, isopropyl; Cumol; Isopropilbenzene; Isopropyl-benzol; Isopropylbenzene; Propane, 2-phenyl
- Chemical Formula: C_9H_{12}
- Chemical Structure:

CH_3 CH CH_2

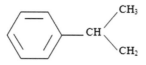

Background

Cumene is a common name for isopropylbenzene, an organic compound. Cumene is a volatile colorless liquid at room temperature with a characteristic sharp, penetrating, aromatic odor. It is insoluble in water but is soluble in alcohol and many other organic solvents. Cumene is structurally a member of the alkyl aromatic family of hydrocarbons, which also includes toluene (methylbenzene) and ethylbenzene. Cumene can be found in crude oil, refined fuels, and is a part of processed high-octane gasoline. Its chemical and physical properties are listed in **Table 1**.

Cumene is manufactured by reacting benzene with propylene at elevated temperature and pressure in the presence of a catalyst. It is considered an environmental pollutant because it is a natural component of petroleum and is present in tobacco smoke. Cumene vapor can be absorbed by the respiratory tract. Sufficiently high levels of exposure to cumene causes central nervous system (CNS) depression leading to death, internal bleeding of numerous organs, as well as irritation of the eyes and respiratory system, skin, and mucous membranes. Cumene is a high production volume chemical.

Table 1 Chemical and physical properties of pure cumene

Relative molecular mass	120.194
Description	Colorless liquid
Boiling point	152.4 °C
Melting point	−9.60*E*+01 °C
Log*P* (octanol–water)	3.66
Water solubility	61.3 mg l^{-1}
Vapor pressure	4.5 mm Hg at 25 °C
Henry's law constant	0.0115 atm m^3 mol^{-1} at 25 °C
Atmospheric OH rate constant	6.50E−12 cm^3 $molecule^{-1}$ s^{-1}

Data taken from ChemIDplus.

Uses

Around 98% of cumene is used in the production of phenol and its coproduct, acetone, using cumene hydroperoxide as chemical intermediate. However, the demand for cumene is largely dependent on the performance of phenol's derivatives, which have resulted in healthy growth rates in demand for cumene. It is also used as a starting material in the production of acetophenone, α-methylstyrene, diisopropylbenzene, and dicumylperoxide. Cumene is used as a thinner for paints, lacquers, and enamels. It is also used in the manufacture of acetophenone, methylstyrene, and other chemicals commonly found in home cleaning products. Minor uses of cumene include as a constituent of some petroleum-based solvents, such as naphtha; in gasoline blending diesel fuel and high-octane aviation fuel; and as a raw material for peroxides and oxidation catalysts such as polymerization catalysts for acrylic and polyester-type resins. It is also a good solvent for fats and resins and has been suggested as a replacement for benzene in many of its industrial applications.

Environmental Fate and Behavior

Cumene is released into the environment as a result of production and processing from petroleum refining and the evaporation and combustion of petroleum products. Cumene also occurs in a variety of natural substances including essential oils from plants and foodstuffs. When released to soil, cumene is expected to biodegrade and may volatilize from the soil surface. Cumene is expected to have low mobility based on its estimated adsorption coefficient (K_{oc}) of 820. Based on Henry's law constant of 0.0115 atm m^3 mol^{-1}, cumene volatilization from moist soil surfaces is expected to be an important environmental fate and it may volatilize from dry soil surfaces based on its vapor pressure. Cumene is expected to strongly adsorb to soils and is not expected to leach to groundwater.

 http://dx.doi.org/10.1016/B978-0-12-386454-3.00599-6

When released into water, cumene is expected to adsorb to sediment and suspended solids in water based on the estimated K_{OC}. The aerobic biodegradation rate of cumene in river water and sediment via mineralization was 0.02 per day, which equates to a half-life of 34.6 days. Cumene volatilization from the surface of water is expected with an estimated half-life of 4.4 days, which is an important environmental fate process based on Henry's law constant for this compound. Hydrolysis is not expected to occur due to the lack of hydrolysable functional groups. Cumene can be found as a natural component in plants and is widely detected in the atmosphere due to its presence in gasoline.

When released into the atmosphere, a vapor pressure of 4.5 mmHg at 25 °C indicates that cumene exists solely as a vapor in the ambient atmosphere. Cumene in the vapor phase reacts with photochemically generated hydroxyl radicals. The reaction of cumene in the vapor phase with ozone has an estimated half-life of 2.5 days. Cumene may also react with ozone radicals found in the atmosphere but not at an environmentally important rate.

Exposure and Exposure Monitoring

Cumene is a contaminant of air, sediments and surface, and drinking and groundwater, and a natural constituent of a variety of foods and vegetation. Cumene exposure may fall into two categories: environmental occurrence and natural occurrence. Primary sources of release of cumene into the environment include petrochemical refineries, spills of finished fuel products during transport or processing, and emissions from petrol stations and motor vehicles. Cigarettes and tobacco are also a source of cumene released during consumption. There are many other industries that release cumene during and after their production processes. These industries include operations involving vulcanization of rubber, building materials, jet engine exhaust, outboard motor operations, solvent uses, paint manufacture, pharmaceutical production, textile plants, leather tanning, iron and steel manufacturing, paving and roofing, paint and ink formulation, printing and publishing, ore mining, coal mining, organics and plastics manufacturing, pesticide manufacturing, electroplating, and pulp and paper production. Cumene release from all these sources was estimated to be about 9.5×10^6 kg annually.

Cumene occurs naturally in petroleum crudes and coal tar and also occurs in a variety of natural substances including essential oils from plants, marsh grasses, and a variety of foodstuffs such as papaya, sapodilla fruit, and Australian honey. Cumene has been also detected in fried chicken, tomatoes, Concord grapes, cooked rice, oat groats, baked potatoes, Beaufort cheese, fried bacon, dried legumes (beans, split peas, lentils), southern pea seeds, and Zinfandel wine.

Toxicokinetics

Cumene is a water-insoluble petrochemical used in the manufacture of several chemicals, including phenol and acetone. In humans and animals, cumene is metabolized primarily to the secondary alcohol 2-phenyl-2-propranol. This alcohol and its conjugates are major metabolites in both humans and animals. No data are available with which to quantify human exposure. Increases in organ weights, primarily the kidneys, are the most prominent effects observed in animals readily exposed to cumene by either the oral or inhalation route. Neither cumene nor its metabolites are likely to accumulate within the body.

Mechanism of Toxicity

CNS depression is the most commonly reported toxic effect and sensitive end point of exposure to cumene. It is characterized in animals by narcosis, decreased motor activity, incoordination, prostration, and impaired gait and reflexes to stimuli. The exact mechanism has not been discovered but it is believed to involve the similarity with which cumene is lipid-soluble and not water-soluble, for nerve tissue due to its high lipid content. Signs of CNS depression occurred in most of the available studies on acute and subchronic inhalation of cumene. Some of these studies showed that the CNS depressant effects occurred during exposure and shortly thereafter and the effects disappeared within 24 h. This is consistent with the rapid absorption and excretion of cumene shown in pharmacokinetic studies. Cumene also causes sensory irritation at neurotoxic concentrations. Some other studies on respiratory rate inhibition (RD_{50}) showed that the sensory irritation of cumene and related alkylbenzenes compounds is caused by a physical interaction with a receptor protein in a lipid layer, rather than by a chemical interaction.

Acute and Short-Term Toxicity

Cumene is not highly toxic to laboratory animals by inhalation, oral, or dermal routes of exposure. However, it is reported that cumene has a potent CNS depressant action characterized by a slow induction period and long duration of narcotic effects in animals. In mice, a lethal concentration 50% (LC_{50}) of 9800 mg cumene m^{-3} (2000 ppm) and for rats a 4-h inhalation LC_{50} of 39 200 mg m^{-3} (8000 ppm) were reported in several studies. More investigations reported that the acute oral lethal dose 50% (LD_{50}) values for rats range from 1400 to 2900 mg kg^{-1} body weight and intraperitoneal LD_{50} values for male mice were 2000 mg kg^{-1} body weight. Weakness, ocular discharge, collapse, and death were reported as acute clinical signs of oral toxicity in rats, and pathological findings in animals that died were hemorrhagic lungs, liver discoloration, and acute gastrointestinal inflammation.

Cumene is considered an ocular irritant. Ocular irritation includes immediate discomfort followed by redness of the conjunctiva and copious discharge. Ocular irritation was observed after instillation of undiluted cumene to rabbits; these effects were reversible within 120 h. Slight eye irritation was generated when cumene was applied to rabbit eyes. However, another study reported that cumene was harmless to rabbit eyes when applied undiluted. The concentration of cumene causing a 50% reduction in the respiratory (RD_{50}) rate in mice was determined to be 10 084 mg m^{-3} (2058 ppm) after 30 min of exposure. This concentration is quite high, and repeated exposure could cause death and morbidity in rats and rabbits.

No information was located regarding the toxicity of cumene in humans following acute exposure. The minimum lethal human exposure, dermal irritation, and sensitization to cumene have not been identified and reported in the literature. However, it is reported that acute inhalation exposure to cumene may cause CNS depression indicated by headaches, dizziness, drowsiness, slight incoordination, and unconsciousness in humans.

Chronic Toxicity

No information is available regarding the toxicity of cumene in humans following acute, subchronic, or chronic exposure. No epidemiology, case reports, or clinical studies of humans were located. There are no long-term *in vivo* bioassays addressing the issue of cancer. No data exist to support any quantitative cancer assessment.

Immunotoxicity

No studies were located that examined immunotoxicity in animals after exposure to cumene by any route. Cumene is known as a CNS depressant like many other solvents such as alcohol. The occurrence of neurological effects from inhalation exposure to cumene has been confirmed in several studies. These studies involve acute exposures that show neurotoxicological effects only at quite high concentrations. Neurotoxicological effects were not observed in the longer-term inhalation studies.

Reproductive Toxicity

No information is available on the reproductive or developmental effects of cumene in humans. Inhalation studies in rats and rabbits reported no significant adverse effects on reproduction or fetal development. No effects on sperm were observed in male rats exposed by inhalation. No multigeneration reproductive study exists for cumene by either the oral or inhalation route. There are no data concerning cumene exposure of females prior to mating, from conception to implantation, or during late gestation, parturition, or lactation.

Genotoxicity

The potential for genotoxicity of cumene is not possible to evaluate due to the lack of studies; however, most genotoxicity test data in animals with cumene are negative.

Carcinogenicity

Studies examining the carcinogenic activity of cumene in humans have not been published. Based on the US Environmental Protection Agency (EPA) Risk Assessment Guidelines, cumene is a class D carcinogen; not classifiable as to human carcinogenicity because no adequate data, such as well-conducted long-term animal studies or human epidemiological studies, are available for assessment that the substance does cause or does not cause cancer. Chronic toxicity or carcinogenicity studies in animals were not available in the literature.

Clinical Management

Handling petroleum hydrocarbon products is very critical, and clinical management in most cases is symptomatic. Attention must be paid to possible aspiration pneumonitis after ingestion of cumene; vomiting must not be induced. Cumene is flammable. Exposure could cause CNS effects and at high concentrations could result in unconsciousness. Oral or high concentration of exposure to vapor may cause CNS depression and the patient must be moved to fresh air.

Cumene is very hazardous in case of contact with skin, eye, ingestion, and inhalation. The potential effects of eye contact can be characterized by redness, watering, and itching. The effects of skin contact can be characterized by itching, scaling, reddening, and blistering. In case of contamination with material, clothing should be removed, and skin and eyes should be flushed with water.

Ecotoxicology

Cumene vapor can react chemically with sunlight and is quickly broken down when released into the atmosphere. In the atmosphere, cumene exists almost entirely in the vapor phase. Cumene does not absorb ultraviolet light at wavelengths greater than 290 nm, which suggests that cumene would not be subject to direct photolysis and oxidation by ozone in the atmosphere. Thus, reaction with ozone and direct photolysis are not expected to be important removal processes. Reaction with photochemically generated hydroxyl radicals appears to be the primary degradation pathway. Small amounts of cumene may be removed from the atmosphere during precipitation. Cumene has been assigned a photochemical ozone creation potential (POCP) value of 35 relative to ethylene at 100. POCP values represent the ability of a substance to form ground-level ozone as a result of its atmospheric degradation reactions.

When cumene is released to surface water, it volatilizes and biodegrades rapidly. In water, important fate and transport processes are expected to be volatilization and aerobic biodegradation. Chemical hydrolysis, oxidation, photolysis, and reaction with hydroxyl radicals are not expected to be important environmental fate processes.

When spilled on soil, cumene is expected to volatilize and biodegrade from the soil surface. Cumene strongly adsorbs to soils and is not expected to easily leak through the soils to the groundwater or underground drinking water.

Other Hazards

Cumene is flammable in the presence of open flames and sparks. The autoignition temperature is 424 °C. The flash point is 36 °C closed cup and 93.3 °C open cup. The flammable limit is between 0.9% and 6.5%. The flammable liquid is soluble or dispersed in water.

Exposure Standards and Guidelines

Cumene is not classified as a highly toxic chemical. The US EPA Office of Air Quality Planning and Standards for a hazard ranking under Section 112 (g) of the Clean Air Act Amendments evaluated cumene for chronic (long-term) toxicity and gave it a toxic score of 11. Scores range from 1 to 100, with 100 being the most toxic. The threshold limit value (time-weighted average) and odor threshold have been recorded as 50 ppm and 0.039 ppm, respectively, with skin notation based on the American Conference of Governmental Industrial Hygienists.

Miscellaneous

Vapors are heavier than air and may travel across the ground and reach remote ignition sources causing a flashback fire danger. Electrostatic charges may be generated during pumping and may cause fire. Exposure prevention includes proper eye, skin, and face protection, and a cartridge-type of self-contained breathing apparatus.

See also: Carcinogen Classification Schemes; Carcinogenesis; Chemical Hazard Communication and Safety Data Sheets; Chemical Safety Assessment and Reporting Tool (Chesar), REACH; Chemicals of Environmental Concern; Ecotoxicology; Environmental Toxicology; EU Risk Assessment Committees; Eye Irritancy Testing; Fuel Oils; High Production Volume (HPV) Chemicals; Petroleum Distillates; Petroleum Hydrocarbons; Risk Assessment, Ecological; Risk Assessment, Human Health; Standards and Guidelines for Toxicity Testing; Toxicity Testing, Carcinogenesis; Toxicity, Acute; Toxicity, Subchronic and Chronic.

Further Reading

Foureman, G.L., 1997. Toxicological Review of Cumene. U.S. Environmental Protection Agency, Washington, DC. Available at: http://www.epa gov/iris/toxreviews/0306tr.pdf.

Foureman, G., 1999. Concise International Chemical Assessment Document 18, Cumene. World Health Organization, Geneva.

National Advisory Committee, 2007. Acute Exposure Guideline Levels (AEGLs) for Cumene. NAC/AEGL Committee.

Relevant Website

Ohio Department of Health. (2009). *Cumene.* Retrieved from Bureau of Environmental Health: http://www.odh.ohio.gov

The Dow Chemical Company. (2011). *Cumene.* Retrieved from Dow Aromatics Products: http://www.dow.com/

U.S. Environmental Protection Agency (EPA). (2000). *Cumene.* Retrieved from Technology Transfer Network Ait Toxics Web Site: http://www.epa.gov

U.S. National Library of Medicine. (2011). *Cumene.* Retrieved from Hazardous Substances Data Bank (HSDB): http://toxnet.nlm.nih.gov/

Cumulative (Combined Exposures) Risk Assessment

A Emami, Food and Drug Administration (FDA), Center for Drug Evaluation and Research, Silver Spring, MD, USA
M Rajabi, Oak Ridge Institute for Science and Education, Oak Ridge, TN, USA
B Meek, University of Ottawa, Ottawa, ON, Canada

This article is a revision of the previous edition article by Jeffrey H. Driver, volume 1, pp 692–694, © 2005, Elsevier Inc.

In 2009, the National Research Council (NRC) recommended the need to include all the chemical, biological, physical, and social stressors in assessment of combined or cumulative exposures. The US Environmental Protection Agency (EPA) guidelines define cumulative risk assessment as analysis, characterization, and possible quantification of the combined risks to health or the environment from multiple elements. The EPA have also signified the need to include low income, depressed community property values, limited access to health care, psychosocial stress, and other stressors within the nonchemical category.

Recently, terminology for cumulative (combined exposures) risk assessment has been considered in an international initiative of the World Health Organization (WHO) International Programme on Chemical Safety (IPCS). Working definitions for key terms and concepts have been developed as a basis to increase understanding and better harmonize approaches among jurisdictions.

Exposure to the same substance from multiple sources and by multiple pathways and routes (referred to in some jurisdictions as aggregate exposure) was described as single chemical, all routes. Similarly, it was recommended that exposure to multiple chemicals by a single route be distinguished from exposure to multiple chemicals by multiple routes (referred to in some jurisdictions as cumulative exposure). Substances grouped together for evaluation of combined exposures were referred to as an assessment group.

Also relevant to combined exposures assessment is a common understanding of the mode of action, which has been defined previously by the IPCS. A postulated mode of action is a biologically plausible sequence of key events leading to an observed effect supported by robust experimental observations and mechanistic data. It describes key cytological and biochemical events; that is, those that are both measurable and necessary to the observed effect. It does not imply full understanding of the mechanism of action at the molecular level.

One of the objectives of assessment of combined exposures or cumulative risk assessment is to consider multichemical, multipathway risks in site-specific risk assessment that supports the regulation of specific chemicals or processes (e.g., pesticides, food additives, product safety). An example is the evaluation of aggregate (multimedia) exposures to pesticides with a common mechanism or mode of action.

The Food Quality Protection Act of 1996 (FQPA) required the US EPA to consider available information on the combined effects of such residues and other substances that have a common mechanism or mode of toxicity in establishing, modifying, leaving in effect, or revoking a tolerance for a pesticide chemical residue. The FQPA raised a number of scientific questions, such as what constitutes a common mechanism or mode of toxicity?

The US EPA describes a mechanism (mode) of toxicity as the major steps leading to an adverse health effect following interaction of a pesticide with biological targets. An understanding of all steps leading to an effect is not necessary, but identification of the crucial events following chemical interaction is required to describe a mechanism (mode) of toxicity.

The cumulative risk assessment process for pesticides includes the following steps:

1. **Identifying the common mechanism group (CMG)**: Identify a group of chemicals that possess a common toxic effect by a common mechanism (mode) of toxicity.
2. **Identifying the potential exposure source**: Evaluate the proposed and registered uses and use patterns to identify potential exposure pathways (i.e., food, drinking water, residential) and routes (oral, inhalation, dermal) for each CMG member.
3. **Characterization and selection of the common mechanism (mode)**: Evaluate common effects that arise from the common mechanism (mode) of toxicity across all exposure routes and durations of interest, determine the time frames of expression for the common toxicity, and assess the quality of the dose–response data for each CMG member. This can lead to recommending the end points/species/sex that can serve as a uniform basis for determining relative potency.
4. **Determining the need for cumulative (combined exposures) risk assessment**: Consider the number and types of possible exposure scenarios in conjunction with the associated residue values available. Assess the toxicological information on dose–response for the common effect. A screening-level assessment for the CMG may indicate that there is no risk concern for this group of chemicals and no further detailed assessment will be necessary. This evaluation may also suggest that a cumulative (combined exposures) assessment is simply not appropriate at this time.
5. **Determining the candidate risk assessment group (CAG)**: Select pesticides, pesticide uses, routes, and pathways from the CMG that have an exposure and hazard potential to result in cumulative effects for inclusion in the quantitative estimates of cumulative risk.
6. **Performing dose–response analyses and determining relative potencies and points of departure**: Select and apply an appropriate dose–response method to evaluate the common mechanism/mode of action effects and determine the relative toxic potencies of the CAG by each exposure route and duration of interest. Analyze the point(s) of departure for extrapolating the risk of the CAG.
7. **Sketching a detailed exposure scenario for all routes and duration**: Determine the role of all the uses remaining for

 http://dx.doi.org/10.1016/B978-0-12-386454-3.00600-X

each pesticide in the CAG to establish the magnitude of possible exposures. Decide the relative importance of the scenarios and the need for their inclusion in a quantitative assessment. Identify populations of interest and locations for evaluation in the assessment. Assess the co-occurrence of possible exposure scenarios.

8. **Establishing exposure input elements**: Determine the magnitude, frequency, and duration of all pertinent exposure pathway/route combinations. Identify appropriate sources of use/usage information, residues in all appropriate media, and any modifying factors necessary for inclusion in the assessment.
9. **Performing final cumulative (combined exposures) risk assessment**: Assign route/duration-specific risk metrics. Conduct a trial run and evaluate the output. Perform sensitivity analysis. Assess subpopulations of concern to determine group uncertainty and FQPA safety factors.
10. **Characterizing the cumulative (combined exposures) risk**: Describe the results and conclusions of the risk analysis, including the relative confidence in toxicity and exposure data sources and model inputs. Discuss major areas of uncertainty, the magnitude and direction of likely bias, and the impact on the final assessment. Evaluate the risk contributions from each pathway and route individually, as well as in combination. Identify risk contributors with regard to pesticide(s), pathway, source, time of year, and subpopulation affected (with particular attention to children). Conduct sensitivity analyses to determine those factors most likely to affect the risk. Determine need for uncertainty and safety factors.

Recently, an international framework that draws on experience in various countries including that on pesticides mentioned above has been developed to advance the risk assessment of combined exposure to multiple chemicals. The framework is designed to aid risk assessors in identifying priorities for risk management for a wide range of applications where co-exposures to multiple chemicals are expected. It is based on a hierarchical (phased) approach that involves integrated and iterative considerations of exposure and hazard at all phases, with each tier being more refined (i.e., less conservative and uncertain) than the previous one, but more labor and data intensive. It includes reference to predictive and probabilistic methodology in various tiers in addition to tiered consideration of uncertainty. Associated case studies, including application of the threshold of toxicological concern (TTC) for consideration of substances detected in drinking water, a screening assessment of polybrominated diphenyl ethers, and an in-depth assessment of a pesticide, have been developed to test and refine the framework.

In summary, combined exposures risk assessment can be described in three phases: (1) problem formulation/planning, (2) analysis, and (3) risk characterization. In the first phase, a team creates a conceptual model that establishes the stressors and the health or environmental effects to be evaluated. Next, the analysis plan lays out the available data, the approach to be taken, and the appropriate tier or level of analysis to meet specified assessment objectives. These result in a fit-for-purpose analysis of the risks associated with the multiple stressors to which the study population or populations are exposed. Finally, the risk characterization puts the risk estimates into perspective in terms of their significance, the reliability of the estimates, and the overall confidence in the assessment.

See also: Environmental Exposure Assessment; Environmental Risk Assessment, Pesticides and Biocides; Environmental Risk Assessment, Secondary Poisoning; Environmental Toxicology; Interactive Toxicity; Levels of Effect in Toxicology Assessment; Mechanisms of Toxicity; Mode of Action; Risk Assessment, Ecological; Risk Assessment, Human Health.

Further Reading

Framework for Cumulative Risk Assessment: http://www.epa.gov/raf/publications/framework-cra.htm

ILSI (International Life Sciences Institute), 1999. A Framework for Cumulative Assessment: An ILSI Risk Science Institute Workshop Report. ILSI Press, Washington, DC, ISBN 1-57881-055-8.

Lewis, A.R., Sax, A.S., Wason, S.C., Campleman, S.L., 2011. Non-chemical stressors and cumulative risk assessment: an overview of current initiatives and potential air pollutant interactions. Int. J. Environ. Res. Pub. Health 8, 2020–2073.

Meek, M.E., Boobis, A.R., Crofton, K.R., Heinemeyer, G., Van Raaij, C., Vickers, C., 2011. Risk assessment of combined exposures to multiple chemicals: a WHO/IPCS framework. Regul. Toxicol. Pharmacol. 60, S1–S14.

Mileson, B.E., Chambers, J.E., Chen, W.L., et al., 1998. Common mechanism of toxicity: a case study of organophosphorus pesticides. Toxicological Sciences 41, 8–20.

NRC, 1996. Understanding Risk: Informing Decisions in a Democratic Society. Committee on Risk Characterization, Commission on Behavioral and Social Sciences and Education. National Academy Press, Washington, DC. ISBN 0-309-05396-X.

Sonich-Mullin, C., Fielder, R., Wiltse, J., et al., 2001. IPCS conceptual framework for evaluating a mode of action for chemical carcinogenesis. Reg. Toxicol. Pharmacol. 34, 146–152.

US Department of Agriculture. Science and Technology Programs at AMS. http://www.ams.usda.gov/science/pdp

US Environmental Protection Agency (US EPA), 1999. Guidance for Conducting Health Risk Assessment of Chemical Mixtures. Risk Assessment Forum, Washington, DC.

US Environmental Protection Agency (US EPA), 1999. Guidance for Performing Aggregate Exposure and Risk Assessments. October 29. US EPA, Office of Pesticide Programs, Washington, DC.

US Environmental Protection Agency (US EPA), 2002. Guidance on Cumulative Risk Assessment of Pesticide Chemicals that Have a Common Mechanism of Toxicity. January 14. US EPA, Office of Pesticide Programs, Washington, DC. http://www.epa.gov/fedrgstr/EPA-PEST/1999/February/Day-05/6055.pdf.

US Environmental Protection Agency (US EPA), 2002. Organophosphate Pesticides: Revised OP Cumulative Risk Assessment. June 10. US EPA, Office of Pesticide Programs, Washington, DC.

US Food and Drug Administration. Center for Food Safety and Applied Nutrition: Pesticides, Metals, Chemical Contaminants & Natural Toxins. http://www.fda.gov/Food/FoodSafety/FoodContaminantsAdulteration/default.htm.

Curare (D-Tubocurarine)

SA Burr, Plymouth University Peninsula Schools of Medicine and Dentistry, Plymouth, UK
YL Leung, Musgrove Park Hospital, Taunton, UK

This article is a revision of the previous edition article by Susan M. Stejskal, volume 1, pp 694, © 2005, Elsevier Inc.

Chemical Profile

- Chemical Abstracts Service Registry Number: CAS 57-94-3
- Synonyms: Tubocurarine chloride; Intocostrin; Ourare; Ourari; Urare; Urari; Woorali; Wooralia; Woorara; Woorari; Wourali; Wouralia; Wourara; Wourari; CID 16051918
- Classification: Naturally occurring tetrahydroisoquinoline plant alkaloid
- Molecular Formula: $C_{37}H_{42}Cl_2N_2O_6$ (anhydrous), Molecular Weight = 681.645 18
- Chemical Structure:

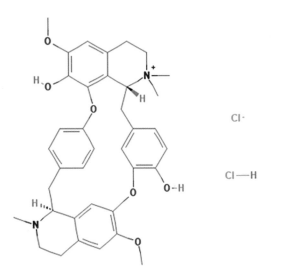

Background

The name curare is derived from the native Guyana Mukusi Indian word wurari. In 1596, Sir Walter Raleigh referred to curare in *The Discovery of the Large, Rich, and Beautiful Empire of Guiana*. In 1780, Abbe Felix Fontana identified the action of curare on voluntary muscles. In 1800, Alexander von Humboldt described the extraction of curare. In 1811, Sir Benjamin Collins Brodie determined that complete recovery from curare poisoning is possible provided artificial ventilation is maintained. In 1825, Charles Waterton brought curarep to Europe, and in 1835 Sir Robert Hermann Schomburgk classified and named the vine *Strychnos toxifera*. In 1850, George Harley demonstrated that curare could be used to treat tetanus and strychnine poisoning. By 1868, Claude Bernard and Alfred Vulpian had identified the site of action of curare as the motor end plate. From 1887, curare was marketed for medical use by Burroughs Welcome. In 1900, Jacob Pal recognized that physostigmine could be used to antagonize the effects of curare. In 1912, Arthur Lawen demonstrated the use of curare during surgery, but this potential was not realized as the finding was published in German. In 1914, Henry Hallett Dale described the action of acetylcholine. In 1935, Harold King isolated D-tubocurarine and described its structure, while in 1936 Dale revealed the role of acetylcholine in neuromuscular transmission and the mechanism of action for curare. In 1940, Abram Elting Bennett revealed that curare could be used to reduce trauma during metrazol-induced convulsive therapy for spastic disorders in children. In 1942, Harold Griffith and Enid Johnson used curare to augment general anesthesia when performing an appendectomy. Curare was used surgically until the development of safer synthetic neuromuscular blocking analogues such as Pancuronium (in 1964), Vecuronium (in 1979), Mivacurium (in 1993), and Rocuronium (in 1994).

Uses

Historically, curare was first used as a paralyzing arrow/dart poison by indigenous South Americans. Later, curare was used as a muscle relaxant during surgery. Previously, to enable deep surgery, increased relaxation could only be achieved by higher and hence riskier quantities of general anesthetic. Being able to control the degree of muscle relaxation independently of the depth of sedation greatly improves survival, although bringing an associated risk of awareness while anesthetized.

Exposure

Only effective if it enters the bloodstream directly.

Toxicokinetics

D-Tubocurarine contains one positively charged quaternary nitrogen atom and another which is usually protonated when in the body, which prevents it from being absorbed from the gastrointestinal tract (hence not orally toxic) or crossing the blood–brain barrier (hence retention of consciousness during paralysis).

Mechanism of Toxicity

D-Tubocurarine acts as a non-depolarizing competitive antagonist at nicotinic acetylcholine receptors on the motor end plate of the neuromuscular junction, causing the relaxation of skeletal muscle. D-Tubocurarine competes with at least an equal affinity to acetylcholine, and at the same position on nicotinic receptors. Hence curare does not affect cardiac muscle, smooth muscle, or glandular secretions. Flaccid paralysis begins within a minute and progressively prevents movement of the eyes, limbs, and finally trunk. Death due to respiratory paralysis can occur within 3–20 min.

 http://dx.doi.org/10.1016/B978-0-12-386454-3.00482-6

Acute and Short-Term Toxicity

Animal

LD_{50} values: dog = 1200 $\mu g\,kg^{-1}$ (intravenous), rabbit = 1300 $\mu g\,kg^{-1}$ (intravenous), and mouse = 140 $\mu g\,kg^{-1}$ (intravenous), 500 $\mu g\,kg^{-1}$ (subcutaneous), and 3200 $\mu g\,kg^{-1}$ (intraperitoneal).

Human

The lowest published lethal dose is 735 $\mu g\,kg^{-1}$ (route unreported).

Clinical Management

Artificial ventilation combined with an acetylcholinesterase (AChE) inhibitor (e.g., physostigmine) can be used to treat curare poisoning. AChE inhibitors block the degradation of acetylcholine, thus increasing the availability of acetylcholine for competitive binding at the neuromuscular junction nicotinic receptors.

See also: Neurotoxicity.

Further Reading

Bowman, W.C., 2006. Neuromuscular block. Br. J. Pharmacol. 147 (Suppl. 1), 277–286.

Relevant Website

http://toxnet.nlm.nih.gov – TOXNET, Toxicology Data Network, National Library of Medicine, Search for tubocurarine.

Cuyahoga River

NR Webber, Westerville, OH, USA
KL Mumy, Liberty Twp., OH, USA

This article is a revision of the previous edition article by Lee R. Shugart, volume 1, p 695, © 2005, Elsevier Inc.

The Cuyahoga River is a U-shaped river that spans 100 miles in northeastern Ohio (the United States) starting at Lake Erie and running through the cities of Cleveland and Akron. In the mid-1900s, the Cuyahoga River was so heavily polluted that it had caught fire at least nine times prior to the infamous fire that took place in 1969 and raised awareness toward the declining health of US waterways.

By 1968, the Cuyahoga River was considered to be in a state of disrepair. The lower portion of the river was used for waste disposal and was plagued with significant levels of debris, industrial wastes, oils, and sewage. Additionally, the river suffered from a severe lack of dissolved oxygen. Very few plant and animal species were able to survive under such poor conditions, and it was said that the lower portion of the river contained no visible life. Potential fires were a daily threat, such that fireboats routinely patrolled the Cuyahoga River to disperse oil slicks. Nevertheless, on Sunday, 22 June 1969, an oil slick and debris caught fire and burned for less than half an hour before it could be extinguished by firefighters. Flames from the fire reached a height of approximately five stories and caused $50 000 in damage to two key railroad tresses.

Interestingly, previous fires caused considerably more damage, including a large fire that took place in 1952 and caused over $1 million in damage to boats and an office building located along the riverfront. However, the 1969 fire was used to highlight the environmental crisis associated with pollution and improper disposal of industrial wastes and sewage. The event sparked national attention on the state of the waterways within the United States and provided support to clean and restore rivers. These efforts subsequently led to the passing of the Federal Clean Water Act of 1972 to establish a structure for regulating the discharge of pollutants into US waterways and maintaining quality standards for surface waters. The Great Lakes Water Quality Agreement was also signed in 1972 and serves to reaffirm the obligations of the United States and Canada to restore and maintain the integrity of the Great Lakes Basin Ecosystem. Furthermore, the attention toward such environmental issues and water pollution control activities helped to create the federal Environmental Protection Agency.

Legislative acts, including the Clean Water Act, and increased awareness have led to great strides in the restoration of the Cuyahoga River. The cities of Akron and Cleveland have improved their sewage treatment facilities to include tertiary treatment (i.e., processes to increase the quality of the effluent prior to its final release) and industrial waste discharge into the river has drastically been reduced. Aquatic life has returned to the Lower Cuyahoga River, including the presence of several fish species. While restoration is not yet complete, the river is now an area for 'full contact' recreation, and restaurants and entertainment have been rebuilt along the river. A large area between Akron and Cleveland was deemed The Cuyahoga National Recreation Area with a portion of the area becoming the Cuyahoga Valley National Park in 2000.

See also: Clean Water Act (CWA), US; Environmental Protection Agency, US; Pollution, Water.

Further Reading

Stradling, D., Stradling, R., 2008. Perceptions of the burning river: deindustrialization and Cleveland's Cuyahoga river. Environ. Hist. 13, 515–535.

Relevant Websites

http://www.epa.gov/glnpo/aoc/cuyahoga.html – Cuyahoga River Area of Concern.
http://www.epa.gov/glnpo/glwqa/1978/index.html – Great Lakes Water Quality Agreement.
http://www.epa.gov/lawsregs/laws/cwa.html – Summary of the Clean Water Act.
http://www.time.com/time/magazine/article/0,9171,901182,00.html – "The Cities: The Price of Optimism, 1969-08-01". Time (magazine). 1 August 1969.

 http://dx.doi.org/10.1016/B978-0-12-386454-3.01005-8

Cyanamide

P Kempegowda, Ealing Hospital NHS Trust, London UB1 3HW, UK

This article is a revision of the previous edition article by Leonard I. Sweet, volume 1, pp 695–698, © 2005, Elsevier Inc.

- Chemical Abstracts Service Registry Number: 420-04-2
- Synonyms: Amidocyanogen; Carbamonitrile; Carbimide; Cyanoamine; Carbodiamide; Carbodiimide; Cyanogenamide; Hydrogen cyanamide; Cyanogen nitride
- Chemical/Pharmaceutical/Other Class: Cyanamides
- Molecular Formula: CH_2N_2
- Chemical Structure:

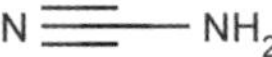

Background Characteristics and Uses

Cyanamide is a colorless, orthorhombic, hydrophilic, crystalline solid with a mild odor. It is similar to but not as toxic as cyanide. It is commonly used in liquid solution and is expected to be soluble in water, ether, benzene, acetone, phenols, amines, ketones, and alcohols. It is used mainly in agriculture as a rest-breaking agent and in pharmaceutical industries in the production of antihistamines, antihelminthics, and many other drugs.

Containing both nucleophilic and electrophilic sites on the same molecule, cyanamide exists as two tautomers – $NCNH_2$ and HNCNH. It is a highly reactive chemical and is a dangerous explosion hazard. It can release toxic fumes of cyanides and nitrogen oxides when heated to decomposition or contacted with acids, acid fumes, moisture, or 1,2-phenylenediamine salts. It is combustible when exposed to heat or flame. Cyanamide reacts with acids, strong oxidants, strong reducing agents, and water, causing explosion hazard.

Environmental Fate and Behavior

Adsorption–desorption studies in soil have estimated very low K_{oc} values (0–6.81 ml g^{-1}) indicating low adsorption and high mobility potential of cyanamide in soil; however, soil column leaching studies indicate that cyanamide is only slightly mobile. Volatilization is not expected to be an important fate and transport process based on the Henry's law constant and vapor pressure. When released into the air, vapor phase cyanamide is expected to have a half-life of less than 1 day. Aerobic biodegradation is expected to occur, with cyanamide serving as source of nitrogen and carbon. The estimated half-life of cyanamide from the water phase of the aquatic systems was 2.3 days for the river system and 4.3 days for the pond system, respectively. Bioconcentration and bioaccumulation potential is expected to be low, based on the estimated bioconcentration factor and experimental octanol–water partition coefficient.

Exposure and Exposure Monitoring

Exposure to cyanamide can occur through inhalation, ingestion, and eye or skin contact.

Toxicokinetics and Toxicodynamics

Cyanamide can gain entry through oral, inhalation, dermal, or eye contact with rapid absorption but variable bioavailability. The estimated half-life in humans after oral administration is expected to be less than 2 h. The oral, dermal, and intravenous LDs_{50} for rats are 125, 84, and 56 mg kg^{-1}, respectively. Similar values for humans are not known. The estimated fatal dose in humans ranges from 40 to 50 g cyanamide. The main mechanism of toxicity is due to inhibition of alcohol dehydrogenase resulting in disulfiram-like syndrome with concomitant alcohol use. The compound is mainly excreted in urine as *N*-acetylcyanamide with the remainder excreted in the feces or exhaled as carbon dioxide.

Effects of Acute Exposure

Acute toxicity has been historically reported to be accidental; however, recently acute toxicity with suicidal intent has been reported. Cyanamide is very toxic if taken orally and moderately toxic through dermal route. The toxic effects are due to overactivity of the parasympathetic nervous system and are similar both in animals and in humans. Contact with cyanamide in dust or liquid form can cause severe irritation of the eyes and ulceration of moist skin. Systemic exposure produces causing miosis, salivation, lacrimation, and twitching. Symptoms of severe poisoning include metabolic acidity and refractory shock.

Effects of Chronic Exposure

Chronic exposure to cyanamide is usually due to lack of training about handling the chemicals, inadequate personal protection equipments, and absence of engineering controls. Cyanamide causes inhibition of alcohol dehydrogenase resulting in accumulation of acetaldehyde in individuals concomitantly exposed to alcohol. The resulting disulfiram-like reaction is characterized by facial flushing, headache, nausea, vomiting, sweating, chest pain, hypotension, weakness, blurred vision, confusion, and difficulty in breathing.

Chronic overexposure may produce the following: pneumonitis and pulmonary edema on repeated inhalation; throat ulceration and esophageal irritation on oral ingestion; dermal ulceration, allergic dermatitis, and sensitization on skin exposure; and keratitis, conjunctivitis, or corneal ulceration on repeated contact with eyes.

Clinical Management

Acute Exposure

Individuals overexposed to cyanamide are removed from the source of exposure to prevent further toxicity. Contaminated clothing is removed and eyes are flushed with copious amounts of water. Skin contamination should be removed by washing with soap and water. Patients developing dermal hypersensitivity reactions may require treatment with topical or systemic corticosteroids or antihistamines. If ingested, vomiting should not be induced. If large doses have been ingested within an hour of exposure, gastrointestinal decontamination may be considered. If dosage was small or treatment is delayed, oral administration of activated charcoal and sorbitol may prove beneficial. Gastric lavage treatment may be given with caution and avoided if tracheal or esophageal ulceration is suspected. In cases of respiratory overexposure, the victim should be moved to fresh air immediately and treated according to severity of irritation.

As there is no known antidote for cyanamide toxicity, management of acute cyanamide toxicity is mainly symptomatic. The life-threatening complications due to acute cyanamide toxicity include acute lung injury resulting in respiratory depression, metabolic acidosis, and severe hypotension which need immediate management. For acute lung injury, ventilation and oxygenation should be maintained and evaluation should be done with frequent arterial blood gas or pulse oximetry monitoring. Arterial blood gas would also indicate the presence of metabolic acidosis. An early correction of acidosis is warranted to prevent serious complications such as cardiac arrhythmias. Hypotension should be treated by placing the patient in the Trendelenburg position, providing intravenous fluids, including plasma or blood if necessary, and vasopressor drugs.

Chronic Exposure

Effects of chronic exposure are mainly seen due to inhalation or dermal exposure. Management would include avoiding further exposure and educating regarding the toxic effects of exposure. Monitoring complete blood count, urinalysis, and liver and kidney functions test are suggested for patients with significant exposure. Chronic toxicity could be prevented by systematic program of medical surveillance of personnel who are under long-term exposure to cyanamide.

Ecotoxicology

Cyanamide is toxic to aquatic organisms, particularly invertebrates and daphnids, with acute $L(E)_{50}$ values around 1 $mg\,l^{-1}$, fish seems to be less sensitive with 96-h LC_{50} ranging between 40 and 90 $mg\,l^{-1}$. Low acute toxicity for earthworms has been observed; however, spray applications have shown that cyanamide may be hazardous for some arthropod species. The toxicity for birds has been studied on the Northern Bobwhite quail; the single oral dose LD_{50} was 350 mg a.i. per kg of bodyweight. In chronic studies, the 22 weeks no observed effect level was 152 mg a.i. per kg of diet.

Occupational Exposure Standards and Guidelines

The guidelines for cyanamide exposure limits vary across the world. Some of the established standards include the following:

- American Conference of Governmental Industrial Hygienists (2 $mg\,m^{-3}$ ppm time-weighted average (TWA));
- Australia (2 $mg\,m^{-3}$ TWA);
- Belgium (2 $mg\,m^{-3}$ TWA);
- Canada (2 $mg\,m^{-3}$ TWA);
- China (2 $mg\,m^{-3}$ TWA);
- Denmark (2 $mg\,m^{-3}$ TWA);
- France (2 $mg\,m^{-3}$ TWA);
- Germany (2 $mg\,m^{-3}$ TWA inhalable fraction);
- Mexico (2 $mg\,m^{-3}$ TWA);
- Sweden (4 $mg\,m^{-3}$ short-term exposure limit);
- United Kingdom (2 $mg\,m^{-3}$ TWA); and
- US Occupational Safety and Health Administration vacated permissible exposure limit (2 $mg\,m^{-3}$ TWA).

Further Reading

de Haro, L., 2009. Disulfiram-like syndrome after hydrogen cyanamide professional skin exposure. J. Agromed. 14, 382–384.

Schep, L., Wayne, T., Beasley, M., 2009. The adverse effects of hydrogen cyanamide on human health: an evaluation of inquiries to the New Zealand National Poisons Centre. Clin. Toxicol. 47, 58–60.

Sheshadri, S.H., Sudhir, U., Kumar, S., Kempegowda, P., 2011. DORMEX-hydrogen cyanamide poisoning. J. Emerg. Trauma Shock 4, 435–437.

Relevant Websites

http://toxnet.nlm.nih.gov – TOXNET, Specialized Information Services, National Library of Medicine. Search for Cyanamide.

http://www.inchem.org – International Chemical Safety Card from the International Programme on Chemical Safety. Cyanamide.

http://www.state.nj.us – Hazardous Substance Fact Sheet from the New Jersey Department of Health and Senior Services. Cyanamide.

http://echa.europa.eu/web/guest/information-on-chemicals/registered-substances?p_p_id=48_INSTANCE_Rfk8&_48_INSTANCE_Rfk8_iframe_q=420-04-2&_48_INSTANCE_Rfk8_iframe_legal=true. (ECHA registered substances)

Cyanide

SA Burr, Plymouth University Peninsula Schools of Medicine and Dentistry, Plymouth, UK
YL Leung, Musgrove Park Hospital, Taunton, Somerset, UK

This article is a revision of the previous edition article by Zhengwei Cai, volume 1, pp 698–701, © 2005, Elsevier Inc.

- Name: Cyanide
- Chemical Abstracts Service Registry Numbers: 57-12-5 (CN); 74-90-8 (Hydrogen cyanide); 143-33-9 (Sodium cyanide); 151-50-8 (Potassium cyanide); 75-05-8 (Methyl cyanide)
- Synonyms: Cyanide ion, Isocyanide, Cyanide anion, Nitrile anion, Cyanide anion, Cyanide ion, CID 5975
- Classification: A compound containing a monovalent CN group. Inorganic cyanides are salts of HCN. Organic cyanides are nitriles.
- Molecular Formula: CN−
- Molecular Weight: 26.0174
- Chemical Structure: HCN (hydrogen cyanide/hydrocyanic acid/prussic acid); NaCN (sodium cyanide); KCN (potassium cyanide); CH_3CN (methyl cyanide/acetonitrile)

$$^{-}C \equiv N$$

Background

Cyanide is found naturally as cyanogenic glycosides as a defense against consumption in the seeds of several plants. Amygdalin in bitter almonds forms hydrogen cyanide (HCN) when in contact with emulsion in saliva. The bitter taste usually prevents a dangerous dose (10–20 bitter almonds could be fatal if eaten raw). Similarly, fruit of the *Prunus* genus in the rose family, such as apples, apricots, cherries, peaches, and plums, contain prunasin. Taxiphyllin is found in immature bamboo shoots. Linamarin and lotaustralin are particularly concentrated in the skin of both cassava and lima beans, while sorghum roots are rich in dhurrin, as a defense against insects such as rootworm. Other exposures are through industrial manufacturing and use of HCN and its salts. Cyanide poisoning can be treated with several antidotes, with differing mechanisms of action and diverse toxicological, clinical, and risk–benefit profiles. Depending on the type of exposure, Cyanokit (hydroxocobalmin) or the Cyanide Antidote Kit (amyl nitrite pearls administered by inhalation; sodium nitrite and sodium thiosulfate administered by infusion) can be used.

Historically, Zyklon B (40% HCN dissolved onto calcium sulfate) was devised by Fritz Haber 20 years prior to World War II and was initially used for parasite control in buildings. Zyklon B was eventually used by the Nazis as their preferred method for the extermination of over 5 million people sent to concentration camps. Thus cyanide has been used to assassinate more people than any other single toxin. Cyanide was also the method of death for the largest mass suicide in modern history: Jim Jones' religious cult moved to Guyana and established the Peoples Temple of Jonestown. In 1978, 909 cult members (276 of whom were children) died on the same day by either swallowing or injecting a mixture of valium (anxiolytic), chloral hydrate (sedative), and cyanide.

Uses

Inorganic cyanide salts are used in large quantities for the extraction of precious metals from low-grade deposits of ground-up ore-bearing rock, as cyanide binds to gold (and silver). The refinement process also forms mercury–cyano complexes (further electrolytic processes release mercury as a vapor). Other uses include case hardening of iron and steel; electroplating and metal polishing; manufacture of dyes such as Prussian blue (which is used to produce photographic blueprints); and enclosed-space insecticide fumigation (especially of ships and warehouses). Lesser uses include NaCN solution used illegally to stun coral reef fish and catch them for the aquarium trade; and NaCN solid used in the US M44 trap to exterminate predators such as coyotes (when the bait is removed, a spring propels the salt into the animal's face). Cyanide salts can be moved in large quantities and relatively easily handled in solid form, but are highly dangerous when combined with acid. Organic nitrile compounds are used extensively in manufacturing: fibers such as nylon are derived from adiponitrile, and synthetic rubber and polyurethane plastics are derived from acrylonitrile (increasing the danger from smoke inhalation in enclosed fires burning such materials).

Environmental Fate

HCN is highly volatile, having a boiling point of 26 °C. It is less dense than air and readily disperses, leading to a low outdoor risk.

Exposure

Industrial workers may experience dermal exposure, contaminated food or water may be ingested, and inhalation may occur during fumigation of confined spaces. HCN is a colorless gas with an almond smell above 0.4–4.4 ppm, although 20–40% of people lack the genetic trait that enables detection of the odor.

Toxicokinetics

Cyanide is rapidly absorbed through the skin, mucosal, and respiratory membranes, becoming distributed throughout the blood within a few minutes. CH_3CN is metabolized by cytochrome P450 (CYP2E1) to cyanohydrin, which then undergoes peroxidation to HCN; metabolism results in a latent period of 3–12 h after ingestion before toxic effects occur. KCN and NaCN produce HCN on contact with water or acid; ingestion of

 http://dx.doi.org/10.1016/B978-0-12-386454-3.00297-9

cyanide salt may delay toxic effects by up to an hour. Cyanide has a high affinity for sulfur, with which it binds to form thiocyanate during metabolism in the presence of mercaptopyruvate sulfur transferase and/or the mitochondrial enzyme rhodanese. Some cyanide will bind to methemoglobin. Some binds to vitamin B_{12} and becomes incorporated into cysteine and hence proteins. With sublethal doses, 80–90% is metabolized to thiocyanate within 3 h, which is then excreted in urine.

Mechanism of Toxicity

Cyanide reversibly binds to the ferric (Fe^{3+}) ions of cytochrome *c* oxidase (a-a_3 complex), inhibiting electron transport and the production of ATP using oxygen. Thus cyanide is a metabolic poison to all cells, blocking the final step of mitochondrial oxidative phosphorylation, leading to anaerobic metabolism and lactic acidosis.

Acute and Short-Term Toxicity

Animal

LD_{50} values: KCN in mouse = 6.7–7.9 mg kg^{-1} (intravenous bolus); KCN in dog = 2.4 mg kg^{-1} (0.1 mg kg^{-1} min^{-1} intravenous infusion); NaCN in rat = 4.6–15 mg kg^{-1} (intravenous bolus); HCN mouse = 117 ppm (inhalation) with death in 29 min (17 min for 266 ppm, and 40 s for 873 ppm).

Human

The lethal dose for HCN is 100 mg kg^{-1} (dermal) and 0.5–1.0 mg kg^{-1} (oral). For KCN or NaCN it is 3–7 mg kg^{-1} (oral). Exposure to 20 ppm HCN causes symptoms warning of hypoxia after several hours; 50 ppm causes disturbances within an hour; 100 ppm becomes life-threatening after 30–60 min; and 300 ppm is rapidly fatal. Exposure causes histotoxic hypoxia, usually without cyanosis (Hb-O_2 saturation is normal), and with a burning sensation in throat if ingested. Low doses (cyanide <1 mg l^{-1} = 38 μmol l^{-1}, lactate <10 mmol l^{-1} blood) cause headache, nausea, confusion, drowsiness, tachypnea, and tachycardia. Moderate doses (cyanide 1–3 mg l^{-1} = 38–114 μmol l^{-1}, lactate 10–15 mmol l^{-1} blood) cause hyperglycemia, lactic acidosis, convulsions, bradypnea then bradycardia, paralysis, coma, and death. With high doses (cyanide >3 mg l^{-1} = 114 μmol l^{-1}, lactate >15 mmol l^{-1} blood), collapse may be instantaneous with death within 30 s of inhalation, or within 30 min of ingestion.

Chronic Toxicity, Immunotoxicity, Reproductive Toxicity, and Carcinogenicity

Animal

Dependence on cyanogenic plants such as cassava and sorghum as a source of carbohydrate has been associated with the development of goiter. Chronic cyanide exposure reduces levels of dopamine and 5-hydroxytryptamine, demyelinates white matter, and causes memory loss and Parkinsonian-like features in the rat.

Human

Dietary dependence on cassava can gradually lead to tropical ataxic neuropathy. This is characterized by optic atrophy, sensorineural deafness, and ataxia due to sensory spinal nerve involvement, sometimes in combination with scrotal dermatitis, stomatitis, and glossitis. Chronic cyanide exposure can also lead to myxedema, thyroid goiter, and cretinism (which can be transmitted to the fetus after maternal exposure) due to enhanced formation of thiocyanate, which blocks the uptake of iodide by the thyroid gland. Chronic effects from cyanide found in cigarette smoke include tobacco amblyopia, whereby optic atrophy occurs associated with central scotoma, loss of red-green distinction, and pupillary defect.

Clinical Management

HCN can mimic carbon monoxide poisoning (cf. convulsions and comatose), but this can be discounted by measuring Hb-CO. There is an effective nitrite–thiosulfate antidote regimen provided the patient survives the initial exposure: If unconscious but breathing then administer amyl nitrite (one ampule every 3 min for up to 20 min or until consciousness is regained). If not breathing then also inject 0.3 g sodium nitrite (10 ml of a 3% solution, intravenously at 2.5 ml min^{-1}), or 4–10 mg kg^{-1} for children (0.12–0.33 ml kg^{-1} of 3% solution) to convert Fe^{2+} Hb to Fe^{3+} methemoglobin and increase the sink for binding cyanide away from circulating cyanocytochrome *c* oxidase and into cyanomethemoglobin. The nitrite should be followed by 12.5 g thiosulfate (50 ml of a 25% solution, also injected at 2.5 ml min^{-1}), or 400 mg kg^{-1} for children (1.6 ml kg^{-1} of 25% solution), supplemented with 100% O_2. Cyanide from cyanomethemoglobin preferentially reacts with thiosulfate to produce thiocyanate, which is then excreted in urine (methemoglobin can then be converted back to Hb by a 1% methylene blue infusion). If exposure is severe, 300 mg dicobalt edetate (20 ml of 1.5%, intravenously over 1 min, can be administered twice without risking cobalt toxicity; followed by 50 ml of 50% dextrose) to chelate cyanide. Alternatively, 5 g hydroxocobalamin (intravenously over 15 min) may be used when exposure is associated with fire and smoke inhalation (as Hb will already be compromised). Dermal exposure requires disposal of clothing and decontamination of skin with soap and water for at least 10 min, in a well-ventilated area, combined with personal protective equipment for caregivers. Mouth-to-mouth pulmonary resuscitation should not be performed because of the risk of rescuer contamination. In cases of ingestion, gastric lavage and 1 g kg^{-1} activated charcoal slurry may be useful within the first hour, but emetics are generally avoided to restrict contamination. Useful symptomatic adjunct therapy includes intravenous $NaHCO_3$ for metabolic acidosis, and intravenous benzodiazepines for frequent or prolonged convulsions.

Ecotoxicology

Fish are sensitive to HCN below 0.05 mg l^{-1}.

Exposure Standards and Guidelines

HCN exposure limit is 10 ppm (11 mg m^{-3}) over 15 min; CH_3CN exposure limit is 60 ppm (102 mg m^{-3}) over 15 min, or 40 ppm (68 mg m^{-3}) over 8 h; KCN and NaCN exposure limit is 5 mg m^{-3} over 8 h.

See also: Cyanamide; Cyanogen Chloride.

Further Reading

Anderson, P.D., 2012. Emergency management of chemical weapons injuries. J. Pharm. Pract. 25 (1), 61–68.

Anseeuw, K., Delvau, N., Burillo-Putze, G., et al., 2013. Cyanide poisoning by fire smoke inhalation: a European expert consensus. Eur. J. Emerg. Med. 20 (1), 2–9.

Barillo, D.J., 2009. Diagnosis and treatment of cyanide toxicity. J. Burn Care Res. 30 (1), 148–152.

De La Calzada-Jeanlouie, M., Coombs, J., Shaukat, N., Olsen, D., 2013. Utility of sodium thiosulfate in acute cyanide toxicity. Ann. Emerg. Med. 61 (1), 124–125.

Grabowska, T., Skowronek, R., Nowicka, J., Sybirska, H., 2012. Prevalence of hydrogen cyanide and carboxyhaemoglobin in victims of smoke inhalation during enclosed-space fires: a combined toxicological risk. Clin. Toxicol. (Phila) 50 (8), 759–763.

Hamel, J., 2011. A review of acute cyanide poisoning with a treatment update. Crit. Care Nurse 31 (1), 72–82.

Ma, J., Dasgupta, P.K., 2010. Recent developments in cyanide detection: a review. Anal. Chim. Acta 673 (2), 117–125.

Redman, A., Santore, R., 2012. Bioavailability of cyanide and metal-cyanide mixtures to aquatic life. Environ. Toxicol. Chem. 31 (8), 1774–1780.

Schwertner, H.A., Valtier, S., Bebarta, V.S., 2012. Liquid chromatographic mass spectrometric (LC/MS/MS) determination of plasma hydroxocobalamin and cyanocobalamin concentrations after hydroxocobalamin antidote treatment for cyanide poisoning. J. Chromatogr. B Analyt. Technol. Biomed. Life Sci. 905, 10–16.

Thomas, C., Svehla, L., Moffett, B.S., 2009. Sodium-nitroprusside-induced cyanide toxicity in pediatric patients. Expert Opin. Drug Saf. 8 (5), 599–602.

Way, J.L., Leung, P., Cannon, E., et al., 2007. The mechanism of cyanide intoxication and its antagonism. In: Evered, D., Harnett, S. (Eds.), Cyanide Compounds In Biology: Ciba Foundation Symposium, vol. 140. John Wiley & Sons, Ltd, Chichester, UK.

Relevant Website

http://toxnet.nlm.nih.gov – TOXNET, Toxicology Data Network, National Library of Medicine, Search for cyanide.

Cyanogen Chloride

M Abdollahi and A Hosseini, Faculty of Pharmacy and Pharmaceutical Sciences Research Center, Tehran University of Medical Sciences, Tehran, Iran; and Razi Drug Research Center, Faculty of Medicine, Tehran University of Medical Sciences, Tehran, Iran

This article is a revision of the previous edition article by Leonard I. Sweet, volume 1, pp 701–703, © 2005, Elsevier Inc.

- Name: Cyanogen chloride
- Chemical Abstracts Service Registry Number: 506-77-4
- Synonyms: 4-03-00-00090 (Beilstein Handbook Reference), BRN 0969190, Caswell No. 267, Chlorcyan, Chlorine cyanide, Chlorine cyanide (ClCN), Chlorocyan, Chlorocyanide, Chlorocyanogen, Chlorure de cyanogene, Cyanogen chloride, EINECS 208-052-8, EPA Pesticide Chemical Code 025801, HSDB 917, RCRA waste number P033, UNII-697I61NSA0.
- Molecular Formula: CClN
- Chemical Structure:

Background (Significance/History)

Cyanide poisoning was first reported with the effects of extract of bitter almonds; then cyanide was identified and isolated from cherry laurel. Cyanogen chloride was first prepared in 1787 by the action of chlorine upon hydrocyanic acid (aka prussic acid) and was called 'oxidized prussic acid.' The correct formula for cyanogen chloride was first established in 1815. Cyanogen chloride was used in World War I in 1916.

Uses

Cyanogen chloride is used in chemical synthesis (military poison gas), as a warning agent in fumigant gases, and as a tear gas, metal cleaner (in ore refining or production of synthetic rubber), as well as for electroplating and photography. Because of cyanogen chloride's warning characteristics, it was much used as a pesticide formerly. It is now used in the preparation of tetracyanomethane and methane tetracarbonitrile by heating silver tricyanomethanide in liquid cyanogen chloride. It is also used in the Lonza process in the preparation of extremely pure malononitrile. Cyanogen chloride was widely used in industry in fumigating ships and warehouses and in ore-extracting processes. Cyanogen chloride generated by an auto analyzer from chloramine T and potassium cyanide was used instead of cyanogen bromide as a reagent for nicotine alkaloid determinations of tobacco extracts.

Environmental Fate and Behavior

Routes and Pathways

At room temperature, cyanogen chloride is a colorless gas with a pungent, biting odor that has been described as 'pepper-like.' Cyanogen chloride is soluble in both water ($6.00E+04$ mg l^{-1}) and most organic solvents (e.g., chloroform, ethanol, or benzene); however, such mixtures often are unstable. An estimated vapor pressure of 1230 mmHg at 25 °C indicates cyanogen chloride exists solely as a gas in the atmosphere. Based on the estimated Henry's law constant of 0.025 atm-m^3 mol^{-1} for cyanogen chloride, volatilization from moist soil surfaces and rapidly from water surfaces is expected to occur. Other physical properties of cyanogen chloride include an octanol/water partition coefficient as log P_{ow}: −0.380 and also a low boiling point (13 °C) and a melting point of −6.55 °C.

Partition Behavior in Water, Sediment, and Soil

Based on the high volatility and rapid hydrolysis of cyanogen chloride, its adsorption to soil and sediment is not an important environmental fate process. Estimated vapor pressure of 1230 mmHg suggests that cyanogen chloride will volatilize rapidly from water surfaces and it is expected to volatilize from dry soil surfaces.

Environmental Persistency (Degradation/Speciation)

Alkaline chlorination of water-containing cyanide produces cyanogen chloride and cyanogen chloride hydrolyzes to CNO(−) and also hydrolyzes rapidly to hydrochloric acid and cyanic acid under alkaline conditions. Cyanogen chloride is unstable in raw surface waters, with estimated half-lives ranging from 1 min 45 s to 10 h at 5 °C in ambient waters and 5.25 h at pH 8 at 20 °C. Cyanogen chloride is not expected to be susceptible to direct photolysis by sunlight because it does not contain chromophores that absorb at wavelengths >290 nm. The environmental fate of cyanogen chloride resulting from the inherent diversity that exists in nature is largely site specific in that the biotic and abiotic characteristics of soil and water greatly influence the ability of this compound to persist, absorb, degrade, dissociate, and bind. However, because of its high volatility and rapid hydrolysis, cyanogen chloride is considered a nonpersistent agent.

Long-Range Transport

Cyanogen chloride is highly volatile and hydrolyzes rapidly in the environment.

Bioaccumulation and Biomagnifications

Based on the high volatility and rapid hydrolysis of cyanogen chloride, its bioconcentration is not an important environmental fate process.

Exposure and Exposure Monitoring

Routes and Pathways (Including Environmental Release)

The manufacture of cyanogen chloride and its use in organic synthesis may cause its release into the environment through

 http://dx.doi.org/10.1016/B978-0-12-386454-3.00484-X

waste streams. Its use as a byproduct of the raw water chlorination, a warning agent in fumigant gases, and a chemical warfare agent will result in its direct release into the environment. The use of active chlorine for the treatment of cyanide-containing wastewater can produce cyanogen chloride that may be released into the environment.

Human Exposure

Human exposure to cyanogen chloride can occur by inhalation, ingestion, skin contact, or eye contact. The general population may be exposed to cyanogen chloride via ingestion of drinking water. Exposure to cyanogen chloride may occur to individuals coming in contact with it in regions in which it was once used as a chemical warfare agent. Cyanogen chloride has the potential to contaminate agricultural products when it is released into the air as a liquid spray (aerosol), but if it is released as a gas, it is highly unlikely to contaminate agricultural products. Occupational exposure may occur through inhalation and dermal contact with cyanogen chloride at workplaces where this compound is produced or used.

Environmental Exposure (Monitoring Data)

Humans are exposed to very low levels of cyanides from air. Generally, levels of cyanide in water sources are low but depend on the discharges and upstream sources. Data from the United States indicate that the mean cyanide concentration in most surface waters is $<3.5\ \mu g\ l^{-1}$. Low absorption of cyanogen chloride to soil and sediment because of its high volatility and rapid hydrolysis suggest that this compound does not have important environmental exposure through soil and sediment.

Toxicokinetics

Cyanide is readily absorbed through inhalation as well as skin and mucous membranes. Inhalation of the gas causes the most rapid onset of toxicity, whereas the effects of ingestion are often delayed because of gastrointestinal absorption. After cyanide is absorbed, it is rapidly distributed through the body through blood. The small quantity of cyanide always present in human tissues is metabolized primarily by the hepatic enzyme rhodanese, which catalyzes the irreversible reaction of cyanide and a sulfane to produce a relatively nontoxic compound (thiocyanate) excreted in the urine. Because of the ability of the body to detoxify small amounts of cyanide via the rhodanese-catalyzed reaction with sulfane, the lethal dose of cyanide is time dependent. An amount of cyanide administered over a very short period of time may be lethal whereas the same amount absorbed slowly may cause no biological effects. Cyanogen chloride reacts rapidly with both serum and red cells, but seemingly cyanogen chloride is converted to cyanide ion via reaction with hemoglobin and glutathione, which eventually liberates the CN ion. It seems that higher-percentage conversions of cyanogen chloride to cyanide are obtained with washed red cells than with whole blood. Cyanogen chloride reacts directly with glutathione, and the rate of reaction is of the same order as with hemoglobin. Because the rate of reaction of cyanogen chloride with glutathione and hemoglobin is of the same order, both reactions seem to contribute to the conversion of cyanogen chloride to cyanide.

Mechanism of Toxicity

The primary effect of cyanide poisoning results from the inhibition of the metal-containing enzymes, specifically, cytochrome oxidase a3 (containing iron) within the mitochondria. Cyanide poisons the mitochondrial electron transport chain within cells and renders the body unable to derive energy (ATP) from oxygen, therefore causing rapid death. Other mechanisms include pulmonary arteriolar and/or coronary vasoconstriction that results in cardiogenic shock and pulmonary edema. Cyanide can also directly stimulate chemoreceptors in the aorta and carotid artery, causing hyperpnea.

Acute and Short-Term Toxicity

Animal

Acute exposure to cyanogen chloride has caused marked irritation of the respiratory tract with hemorrhagic exudate from the trachea and bronchi, and pulmonary edema. The oral LD_{50} for cyanogen chloride in cat is 6 mg kg^{-1}. The acute LD_{50} of cyanogen chloride in dog, rabbit, and domestic animals (goat/sheep) has been estimated 3.3, 3.15, and 2.97 mg kg^{-1}, respectively.

Human

Acute exposure to cyanogen chloride can be rapidly fatal. It severely irritates the eyes, nose, and airways, as well as causes marked lacrimation, rhinorrhea, and bronchosecretions.

Acute exposure to cyanogen chloride can also produce systemic effects by interfering with oxygen use at the cellular level, with profound effects on the central nervous system (CNS), respiratory, and cardiovascular systems. Inhalation exposure to cyanogen chloride at 140 ppm for 60 min or 1500 ppm for 3 min has an estimated 50% mortality. Acute inhalation exposure to cyanogen chloride causes CNS effects: seizures, coma, and mydriasis; cardiovascular effects: shock, dysrhythmias, critically low blood pressure, and cardiac arrest; respiratory effects: abnormally rapid, followed by abnormally slow respirations, pulmonary edema, and respiratory arrest; and eye effects: inflammation of the surface of the eye, dilated pupils, and temporary blindness. Acute ingestion of cyanogen chloride causes a possible bitter, acrid burning taste, followed by constriction or numbness of the throat, salivation, nausea, and vomiting.

Chronic Toxicity

Animal

Chronic cyanide exposure studies showed decreased weight gain and thyroxin levels and myelin degeneration in rats at

30 mg kg^{-1} day^{-1}. Other chronic studies either used the sc route or gave higher-effect levels.

Human

Effects of repeated or chronic exposure to cyanogen chloride are similar to cyanide and other cyanide compounds. The effects of long-term exposure to cyanide are nebulous and include confusion, intellectual deterioration, and Parkinson-like syndromes. Chronically exposed workers may complain of headache, easy fatigue, chest discomfort, eye irritation, palpitations, anorexia, and epistaxis. Exposure to small amounts of cyanide compounds for a long time causes loss of appetite, weakness, headache, dizziness, nausea, and symptoms of irritation of the upper respiratory tract and eyes.

Reproductive Toxicity

Information is unavailable about reproductive or developmental toxicity from chronic or repeated exposure to cyanogen chloride in humans, but teratogenic effects have been observed in experimental animals exposed to cyanide and related compounds.

Genotoxicity

There is no evidence on genotoxicity of cyanogen chloride in animals or humans.

Carcinogenicity

Cyanogen chloride has not undergone a complete determination and evaluation under the US EPA's IRIS program for evidence of human carcinogenic potential.

Clinical Management

There is no role for home management of cyanide exposure, and any exposure to cyanide salts or cyanide gas should be referred to a health care facility. Management of oral exposure is symptomatic and supportive, and should not induce vomiting but should immediately administer 100% oxygen. In large ingestions, prehospital, activated charcoal can be considered wherever there will be a delay in definitive health care. In eye and dermal exposure, remove the patient from the source of exposure and then wash the eye with large amounts of tepid water for at least 15 min. In skin exposure, remove the clothes and wash the skin with water. In inhalation exposure, immediately remove the patient from the source of exposure and administer 100% oxygen. Airway management is needed in patients who are comatose or have altered mental status. In each of the types of exposure, a cyanide antidote, either hydroxocobalamin or the sodium nitrite/sodium thiosulfate kit, should be administered. The cyanide antidote kit (nitrites and thiosulfate) in clinical use consists of amyl nitrite, sodium nitrite, and sodium thiosulfate. Enhanced elimination can be performed with antidotes; however, the role of hemodialysis is uncertain.

Ecotoxicology

Freshwater/Sediment Organisms Toxicity

Marine Organisms Toxicity

No LOLI (List Of LIsts™) ecotoxicity data are available for this compound. Several sources of data were reported on cyanogen chloride, which were for freshwater fish and invertebrates and they found no information on the breakdown product of cyanic acid. In other studies, no additional toxicity data were identified for cyanogen chloride. Cyanogen chloride is very toxic to aquatic invertebrates and fish. Median lethal concentration (LC_{50}) values were estimated at 120–150 g l^{-1}. Cyanogen chloride causes mortality in zooplankton and is very highly toxic for *Daphnia magna* with an estimated LC_{50} of cyanogen chloride of 29 μg l^{-1} at 48-h exposure.

Terrestrial Organism Toxicity (Soil Microorganisms, Plants, Terrestrial Invertebrates, Terrestrial Vertebrates)

There are no acute or chronic toxicity data available for terrestrial organisms exposed to cyanogen chloride. Only a few studies addressing terrestrial plant uptake of cyanide (only in the form of NaCN) could be found. It seems that further studies need to be conducted to adequately evaluate the effect of cyanogen chloride on terrestrial organisms and its associated toxicity to higher plants and animals.

Other Hazards

It seems that cyanogen chloride has the additional hazard of being able to polymerize, usually explosively.

Exposure Standards and Guidelines

Based on ACGIH, threshold limit values: 0.3 ppm. According to NIOSH recommendations, recommended exposure limit: 15 min ceiling value: 0.3 ppm (0.6 mg m^{-3}). AIHA emergency response planning guidelines (ERPG): ERPG (1) not appropriate; ERPG (2) 0.4 ppm (without serious, adverse effects); and ERPG (3) 4 ppm (not life threatening) for up to 1-h exposure.

See also: Emergency Response and Preparedness; Pesticides; Cyanide; Volatile Organic Compounds; Sarin (GB); Soman; Tabun; Corrosives; Mitochondrial Toxicity.

Further Reading

Cyanogen Chloride – Compound Summary. PubChem Compound. USA: National Center for Biotechnology Information, 27 March 2005. Identification. http://pubchem.ncbi.nlm.nih.gov/summary/summary.cgi?cid=10477&loc=ec_rcs. Retrieved 5 June 2012.

NIOSH Pocket Guide to Chemical Hazards, September 2007. Department of Health and Human Services, Centers for Disease Control, National Institute for Occupational Safety & Health, p. 82.

Lide, David R (Ed.), 2006. CRC Handbook of Chemistry and Physics, eighty-seventh ed. CRC Press, Boca Raton, FL ISBN 0-8493-0487-3.

WHO, 2007. Cyanogen Chloride in Drinking-Water. Background Document for Development of WHO Guidelines for Drinking-Water Quality. World Health Organization, Geneva (WHO/SDE/WSH/XX.XX/XX).

Relevant Websites

http://toxnet.nlm.nih.gov – Toxicology Data Network, US National Library of Medicine

http://www.inchem.org – IPCS International Program on Chemical Safety

Cyclodienes

SE Koshlukova and NR Reed, California Environmental Protection Agency, Sacramento, CA, USA

This article is a revision of the previous edition article by Benny L. Blaylock, volume 1, pp 703–704, © 2005, Elsevier Inc.

Chemical Profile and Bioaccumulation

Cyclodienes are chlorinated hydrocarbon compounds with polycyclic structures manufactured as insecticides. They are a subclass of the organochlorine insecticides, generally grouped based on commonalities in several aspects, including common precursor, common mode of action, and similarity in pesticidal activity. The recognized cyclodienes are isodrin, endrin (isodrin epoxide), aldrin, dieldrin (aldrin epoxide), heptachlor, chlordane, telodrin (isobenzan), endosulfan, and toxaphene (**Figure 1**). With the exception of toxaphene, the precursor for the cyclodienes is hexachlorocyclopentadiene. Toxaphene, a mixture of about 200 related compounds, is formed by chlorination of camphene. Isodrin and endrin are stereoisomers of aldrin and dieldrin, respectively. Endrin and dieldrin are epoxides of isodrin and aldrin, respectively.

The principal chemical and physical properties of cyclodiene insecticides are low volatility, chemical stability, lipid solubility, slow rate of degradation in the environment, and ability to bioaccumulate and biomagnify throughout the terrestrial and aquatic food chain. The cyclodienes adsorb strongly to soil and sediment, resist leaching to groundwater, and persist for a very long time (>20 years). Due to their stability, cyclodienes released to the environment have traveled vast distances and contaminated areas remote from their use (e.g., Arctic regions). Bioconcentration factors in fish as high as 3.5 million are reported for persistent toxaphene congeners, 38 000 for chlordane, and 11 000–13 000 for endosulfan, heptachlor, and dieldrin. The cyclodienes and their metabolites persist in animal and human fat, serum, and breast milk.

Background and Uses

The cyclodienes were developed as insecticides in the 1940s and 1950s and were at one time widely used in large quantities to control termites in buildings by underground applications; as wood preservatives to control borers, termites, and dry rot; and for protective treatment of underground cables and as fumigating agents. They were extensively applied as insecticides on agricultural crops (e.g., corn, potatoes, citrus, bananas, cabbage, cotton, sugar cane, and tobacco) and lawns and gardens. Other major uses included control of fleas, flies, mites, lice, ants, locusts, and disease vectors (malaria, yellow fever). In addition to high insecticidal activity, some cyclodienes also possess other pesticidal properties. For example, endrin was used to control rodents (rodenticide) and birds (avicide). Toxaphene was used to eradicate undesirable fish species.

Prior to the 1980s, the estimated annual global production was 70 000 tons of chlordane, 24 000 tons of toxaphene, 20 000 tons of aldrin and dieldrin, 9000 tons of endosulfan, and 3000 tons of heptachlor. After the ban of dichlorodiphenyltrichloroethane (DDT) in the United States in 1972, several cyclodienes, in particular toxaphene, became the most important substitutes. However, around the same time, concerns regarding carcinogenicity potential, toxicity to the immune and developing nervous systems, environmental persistence, and bioaccumulation in the food chain led to the cancellation of most cyclodiene uses. Starting in the late 1970s, all cyclodienes except endosulfan were banned and their production ceased in the United States, the European Union, and most other countries worldwide. The production and all uses of endosulfan are scheduled to end in 2016 globally. Heptachlor is still registered in the United States for the control of fire ants in underground power transformers, however, the extent of this use is unclear.

The cyclodienes are on the UN Environment Programme list of persistent organic pollutants, for which international action is required to reduce risks to humans and the environment. Despite major international actions to eliminate or restrict their use, many cyclodienes are still produced and used as insecticides in China, India, and possibly elsewhere.

Exposure

Before their ban, human exposure to cyclodienes happened directly from their insecticidal use. Today, exposure continues due to persistence of their residues in certain foods, water, air, and soils. The main exposure route is through ingestion of contaminated water and foods (particularly fish and meat). Enforceable levels in water and foods are established for residues of aldrin, dieldrin, heptachlor, chlordane, and toxaphene, and some of their metabolites and components (heptachlor epoxide, oxychlordane, nonachlor, and chlordene). Action levels were established in 1990 for the unavoidable residues due to environmental contamination.

Inhalation of vapors from contaminated soil and water or direct dermal contact with residual cyclodienes from past pesticide applications is also possible. Indoor air exposure to chlordane, heptachlor, aldrin, and dieldrin over long periods may persist in homes previously treated for termite control.

Occupational exposure remains in countries where chlordane is produced and used as an insecticide. The exposure is likely higher for the general public living near hazardous waste sites where cyclodienes have been detected. Aldrin, chlordane, dieldrin, endosulfan, endrin, heptachlor, and toxaphene are found in many of the of the 1684 National Priorities List (NPL) sites, the most hazardous waste sites in the United States These chemicals are on the 2011 Comprehensive Environmental Response, Compensation, and Liability Act priority list for substances with the highest frequency, toxicity, and potential for human exposure at NPL sites.

Toxicokinetics

All cyclodienes are well absorbed orally and by inhalation in humans and animals. Dermal absorption is also significant,

 http://dx.doi.org/10.1016/B978-0-12-386454-3.00118-4

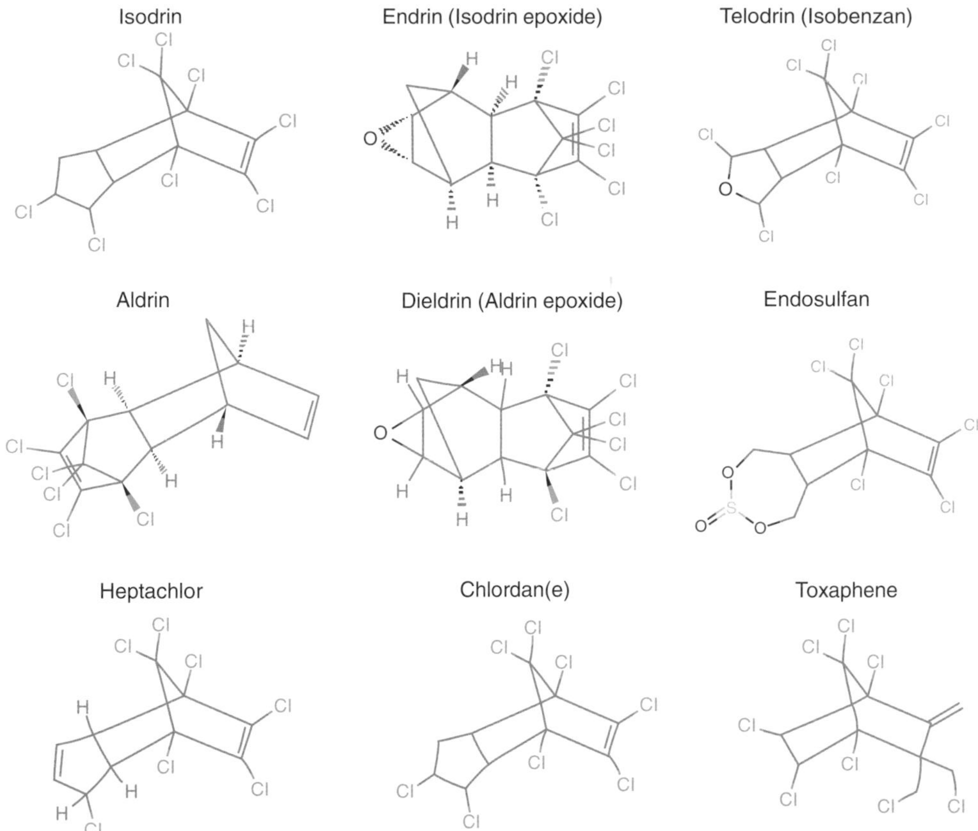

Figure 1 Cyclodiene pesticides. Reproduced from: http://pubchem.ncbi.nlm.nih.gov.

except for toxaphene, which is poorly absorbed through the skin. Absorption is evident by their detection in blood and tissues, and in the observed systemic toxicity, while the level of absorption is estimated in studies using radiolabeled cyclodienes. Typically, peak blood level of the parent compounds and their metabolites occurs between 2 and 8 h after dosing in animals.

The cyclodienes are extensively metabolized by the liver cytochrome P450 enzymes (CYP) to oxidized and dechlorinated metabolites, most with subsequent conjugation and distribution in the body. Many of the metabolites are equally or more toxic and persistent than the parent compounds. Examples of significant metabolites are oxychlordane and heptachlor epoxide (main metabolites of chlordane and heptachlor), dieldrin (epoxide of aldrin), and endosulfan sulfate (endosulfan metabolite). Isobenzan gamma-lactone is less toxic than the parent chemical telodrin.

Cyclodiene residues are highest in the fat (still present years after the last exposure) and lower in liver, kidneys, brain, and muscles. They are found in cow and human milk. Transplacental transport is evident in detecting the cyclodienes and their metabolites in maternal placenta, umbilical cord, and blood of newborns.

Mechanism of Toxicity

The cyclodienes represent the oldest generation of chloride channel-blocker insecticides that exhibit marked mammalian toxicity. To insects and mammals, they are highly toxic convulsants that cause hyperexcitation through blocking the gamma-aminobutyric acid (GABA)-gated chloride channels in the central nervous system.

The primary target for cyclodiene toxicity is the central nervous system. As noncompetitive antagonists of the chloride ion channel of the $GABA_A$-receptor, the cyclodienes interfere with the passage of chloride ions and thereby block the actions of the inhibitory neurotransmitter GABA. Seizures, vomiting, and convulsions are typical symptoms of excessive nerve stimulation associated with antagonism with GABA. The action of cyclodienes in the brain is very complex due to their biotransformation to more toxic metabolites and the presence of toxic components. In addition, all cyclodienes induce hepatic cytochrome CYP enzymes. Other potential targets include adenosine triphosphatase (ATPase) functions, Ca^{2+}, Na^+, and K^+ ion transporters, protein kinase C and mitogen-activated protein kinases, nervous system development, inflammatory cytokines, macromolecule synthesis, DNA methylation, steroid metabolism, testosterone and neurotransmitter receptors, and lipid peroxidation.

Toxicity

The cyclodienes are moderate (e.g., aldrin, dieldrin, heptachlor, chlordane, and toxaphene) to high acutely toxic (e.g., endrin, telodrin, and endosulfan) oral toxicants based on their reported LD_{50} values in animals.

Liver is the most common nonlethal target reported in chronic animal studies with cyclodienes except for endosulfan. The characteristic liver changes (increased liver weights, alterations in serum liver enzyme activities and triglycerides, necrosis, fat in the hepatocytes, and depletion of glycogen) are often referred to as of the chlorinated hydrocarbon insecticide rodent liver type.

Human deaths from accidental dermal exposure or intentional ingestion of cyclodienes are reported. Nonlethal acute poisoning signs in humans are headaches, tremors, seizures, numbness, nausea, fatigue, gastrointestinal symptoms, skin and eye irritation, unconsciousness, incoordination, excitability, hyporeflexia, and convulsions. Currently, there is no specific antagonist to the effects of cyclodiene insecticides. However, benzodiazepines and barbiturates are used to control the seizures.

Although generally negative in mutagenicity tests, the cyclodiene insecticides are associated with liver tumors in rodents. Taking into consideration their carcinogenicity profiles in animals, the International Agency for Research on Cancer classified several cyclodienes (e.g., chlordane, heptachlor, aldrin, dieldrin, and toxaphene) as possibly carcinogenic to humans.

Many cyclodiene insecticides, including chlordane and heptachlor, administered at environmentally relevant doses during the developmental period can alter the immune system in animals, or have lasting impact on immune functions in humans exposed at home or at work. Endocrine-disrupting properties, reproductive effects, and developmental neurotoxicity in animals and possibly in humans have recently become a significant concern. Exposure to more than one chlorinated cyclodiene with similar mechanisms of toxicity may result in cumulative effects. The cyclodiene insecticides are highly toxic to aquatic life, bees, earthworms, and birds.

See also: A-esterase; Carboxylesterases; Dichloropropene; Dithiocarbamates; Diuron; Furfural; Nithiazine; Permethrin; Thiram; The International Society for the Study of Xenobiotics; Methane.

Further Reading

Agency for Toxic Substances and Disease Registry (ATSDR), 2002. Toxicological Profile for Aldrin/Dieldrin. Public Health Service, U.S. Department of Health and Human Services. http://www.atsdr.cdc.gov/toxprofiles/tp1.pdf.

Agency for Toxic Substances and Disease Registry (ATSDR), 1994. Toxicological Profile for Chlordane. Public Health Service, U.S. Department of Health and Human Services. http://www.atsdr.cdc.gov/ToxProfiles/tp31.pdf.

Agency for Toxic Substances and Disease Registry (ATSDR), 1996. Toxicological Profile for Endrin. Public Health Service, U.S. Department of Health and Human Services. http://www.atsdr.cdc.gov/toxprofiles/tp89.pdf.

Agency for Toxic Substances and Disease Registry (ATSDR), 2007. Toxicological Profile for Heptachlor and Heptachlor Epoxide. Public Health Service, U.S. Department of Health and Human Services. http://www.atsdr.cdc.gov/ToxProfiles/tp12.pdf.

Agency for Toxic Substances and Disease Registry (ATSDR), 2010. Toxicological Profile for Toxaphene. Public Health Service, U.S. Department of Health and Human Services. http://www.atsdr.cdc.gov/toxprofiles/tp94.pdf.

Brooks, G., 2010. Interactions with the gamma-aminobutyric acid A-receptor: polychlorocycloalkanes and recent congeners and other ligands. In: Kreiger, R. (Ed.), Hayes' Handbook of Pesticide Toxicology, third ed. Elsevier, pp. 2065–2092.

USEPA, 2010. Endosulfan. The Health Effect Division's Human Health Risk Assessment. United States Environmental Protection Agency. EPA-HQ-OPP-2002-0262. http://www.regulations.gov/contentStreamer?objectId=0900006480afefa3&disposition=attachment&contentType=pdf.

World Health Organization (WHO), 1991. Isobenzan. Environmental Health Criteria 129. International Programme on Chemical Safety (IPCS), WHO. http://www.inchem.org/documents/ehc/ehc/ehc129.htm.

Relevant Websites

http://www.atsdr.cdc.gov/toxprofiles/index.asp – Agency for Toxic Substances and Disease Registry.

http://toxnet.nlm.nih.gov – Hazardous Substance Data Bank.

http://npic.orst.edu/ – National Pesticide Information Center.

http://www.epa.gov – United States Environmental Protection Agency.

Cycloheximide

V Lawana, Iowa State University, Ames, IA, USA
MC Korrapati, Medical University of South Carolina, Charleston, SC, USA
HM Mehendale, University of Louisiana at Monroe, Monroe, LA, USA

This article is a revision of the previous edition article by Midhun C. Korrapati, Harihara M. Mehendale, volume 1, pp 705–707, © 2005, Elsevier Inc.

- Name: Cycloheximide
- Chemical Abstracts Service Registry Number: 66-81-9
- Synonyms: 1S-(1a(S),3a,5b)-4-(2-(3,5-Dimethyl-2-oxo-cyclohexyl))-2-hydroxyethyl-2,6-piperidinedione; Actidione; Naramycin A; Actidone; Hizarocin; Neocycloheximide; CHX
- Molecular Formula: $C_{15}H_{23}NO_4$
- Chemical Structure:

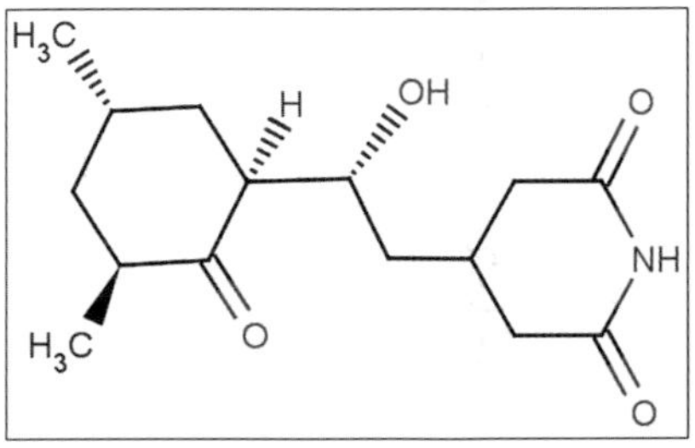

Background

Cycloheximide (CHX; mol. wt. 281.35) is a beige colored, crystal powdered, water-soluble, semisynthetic compound, isolated as a by-product from beers of streptomycin-producing strain of a *Streptomyces* species. CHX, a popular inhibitor of protein synthesis, also stimulates glycogenolysis, gluconeogenesis, and ureogenesis; therefore, it is extensively used in biomedical research. CHX exerts its effect by interfering with the translocation step in protein synthesis (movement of two tRNA molecules and mRNA in relation to the ribosome) thus blocking translational elongation. The effects of CHX were compared to those of norepinephrine in many systems. Both CHX and norepinephrine produce slight increases in the levels of cyclic adenosine monophosphate (AMP). The adrenergic activity of CHX should be considered when this drug is used as an inhibitor of protein synthesis.

Most prominent toxic effects of CHX include DNA damage, teratogenesis, and other reproductive effects (including birth defects and toxicity to male germ cells). CHX is mostly used only in *in vitro* experiments, and is not suitable for human use as a therapeutic compound. The best-known use of CHX is as an experimental tool in molecular biology to determine the half-life of a protein. Although its precise mechanism of action remains incompletely understood, CHX been shown to inhibit translation elongation through binding to the E-site of the 60S ribosomal unit and interfering with deacetylated tRNA. CHX's use as a fungicide in agricultural applications is increasingly becoming unpopular as the health risks of CHX have become better understood.

Uses

CHX is used as a fungicide, plant growth regulator, and as a protein synthesis inhibitor. This is also used in laboratory media as a selective agent to permit isolation of pathogenic and nonpathogenic fungi. In research, it has been frequently used in many protein biosynthetic and degradation studies. In the field of plant growth regulator, it is used to stimulate ethylene production. It is also used as a rodenticide and in beer manufacturing processes. In molecular biological field, it is also used for ribosome and translational profiling.

Environmental Fate and Behavior

CHX is formed as a by-product during the production of streptomycin and may be released to the environment through streptomycin production waste streams. CHX is also produced in nature by bacterial strains of *Streptomyces griseus*. If released to air, an estimated vapor pressure of 4.5×10^{-13} mm Hg at 25 °C indicates CHX will exist solely in the particulate phase in the ambient atmosphere. Particulate phase CHX will be removed from the atmosphere by wet and dry deposition. If released to soil, CHX is expected to have very high mobility based upon an estimated K_{oc} of 47. Volatilization from moist soil surfaces is not expected to be an important fate process based upon an estimated Henry's law constant of 3.5×10^{-15} atm-m^3 mole^{-1}. CHX is not expected to volatilize from dry soil surfaces based upon its estimated vapor pressure. If released into water, CHX is not expected to adsorb to suspended solids and sediment based upon the estimated K_{oc}. Volatilization from water surfaces is not expected to be an important fate process based upon this compound's estimated Henry's law constant. At a concentration of 50 μg l^{-1}, CHX had a bioconcentration factor (BCF) of <0.3 while at 5 μg l^{-1} it had a BCF of <2.8 in orange-red killi fish. According to a classification scheme, these BCF values suggest bioconcentration in aquatic organisms is very low. Occupational exposure to CHX may occur through dermal contact with this compound in the waste stream at workplaces where streptomycin is produced.

Exposure Routes and Pathways

CHX being produced as a by-product, waste releases to the environment from streptomycin production may contain CHX. Occupational exposure to CHX may occur through dermal contact with this compound found in the waste stream at workplaces where streptomycin is produced.

Toxicokinetics

CHX shows almost 90–100% absorption via gut, when orally ingested. Due to its lipophilic nature, CHX gets distributed preferentially to fat and to some extent other lipid-rich tissues. The studies have produced a rough estimate of its distribution as fat > lymph nodes, adrenal and thyroid glands > skin > bone marrow, nasal mucosa, gastrointestinal (GI) tract > liver, lung > kidney, brain, blood, heart, muscle, spleen, ovary, pancreas. CHX is slowly metabolized by hepatic cytochrome P450 system and gets converted to 4-(formylmethyl)-glutarimide and 2,4-dimethylcyclohexanone. Studies have been done to investigate the formation of epoxide and superoxide free radical formation during its metabolism. Following its metabolism to more polar metabolites, these metabolites tend to get excreted in urine.

Mechanism of Toxicity

CHX is a potent inhibitor of protein synthesis in animals. It binds to E-site of 70S ribosome-mRNA complex, blocking the translational step of protein biosynthesis. It causes an increase in adrenal RNA and increased production of glucocorticoids.

Acute/Short-Term and Chronic Toxicity

Animal

Animals given toxic doses exhibit salivation, bloody diarrhea, tremors, and excitement, leading to coma and death due to cardiovascular collapse. A single dose of CHX (2 mg kg^{-1}, ip) produced progressive decrease in bile flow in rats. The oral LD_{50} in monkeys and dogs is ~500 mg kg^{-1} and that for rats is only 2 mg kg^{-1}. In all the three species, toxic symptoms include excessive salivation and diarrhea. Bloodstained feces may arise from vascular lesions of colon (monkey) or stomach and small intestines (dogs). Rats and dogs show transient central nervous system (CNS) excitement with tremors and in the dog perhaps meningeal irritation. Death is due to cardiovascular collapse and is preceded by coma in all species. Autopsies on rat revealed enlarged adrenals, stomach hemorrhage, liver congestion, and kidney damage. LD_{50} values of CHX for some experimental animals are listed below.

Dog oral 65 mg kg^{-1}	
Monkey oral 60 mg kg^{-1}	
Rat oral 2 mg kg^{-1}	Mouse oral 133 mg kg^{-1}
Rat ip 3700 μg kg	Mouse ip 100 mg kg^{-1}
Rat sc 2500 μg kg	Mouse sc 160 mg kg^{-1}
Rat iv 2 mg kg^{-1}	Mouse iv 150 mg kg^{-1}

Source: NLM-HSDB.

Human

CHX is a potent irritant. When ingested, gastrointestinal symptoms of nausea, vomiting, diarrhea, and excessive salivation have been reported. Other signs of poisoning are transient CNS excitement and tremors.

Chronic Toxicity (or Exposure)

CHX has been shown to be mutagenic in both animals and humans.

Clinical Management

Intragastric administration of charcoal as a slurry (240 ml water for 30 g charcoal) should be undertaken to minimize absorption of life-threatening levels of CHX by ingestion.

Reproductive and Developmental Toxicity

CHX is a potent reproductive toxicant. It is a well-known spermicidal agent. Several miscarriage and stillbirths were reported among people with previous oral exposure to CHX, but no clear mechanistic evidence has been reported till date in humans. Animal studies using oral exposure have identified dose-dependent toxicity to reproductive system, such as ovarian lesions and hormonal and menstrual changes (in female rats and monkeys), reduced fertility (in rats), reduced mating index (in male rats), and testicular effects (in male rats and pigs). It is an established teratogen in animal models.

Genotoxicity

There are not many cases of genotoxicity reported, and human genotoxicity data for CHX are limited. CHX is shown to be a weak inducer of DNA fragmentation and micronuclei formation in human hepatocytes cell culture. However, it was not able to cause gene mutations or unscheduled DNA repair. Genomic adducts of its metabolites are too reported, but no data are still significant. Additional studies employing other *in vivo* and *in vitro* assays would be useful to determine the genotoxic potential of hexachlorobenzene.

Carcinogenicity

Cycloheximide is not a well-known carcinogen and not many cases of its tumorigenic potential have been reported. However, some researchers claim that it may interfere with p53-dependent cell cycle, by interrupting with p53 biosynthesis. More work in this field is needed in support of this claim.

Clinical Management

For inhalation exposure, management commonly includes moving the exposed individuals to fresh air and monitoring respiratory distress. Emesis is recommended in acute ingestion. Gastric lavage with subsequent administration of activated charcoal is highly recommended in acute management to reduce GI absorption. Charcoal should be administered as a slurry (240 ml water for 30 g charcoal); usual dose: 25–100 g in adults/adolescents, 25–50 g in children (1–12 years), and 1 g kg^{-1} in infants less than 1-year-old. Hydrocortisone (1 mg kg^{-1}) should be considered in symptomatic patients. Atropine may be useful for cholinergic effects. To reduce body burden, continuous administration of mineral oil can lead to increased depletion of CHX from both blood and adipose tissue. Acute high dose management can be done based on symptoms, such as ingestion of diuretic in case of kidney elimination. Patients exposed via inhalation must be moved rapidly to fresh air. Respiratory distress should be monitored, and eyes must be irrigated with copious amounts of room temperature water for at least 15 min in ocular exposure. If irritation, pain, swelling, lacrimation, or photophobia persists, the patient should be seen in a health care facility.

Ecotoxicology

CHX is expected to have very high mobility in soil. Volatilization from moist soil surfaces is not expected to be an important disbursement process. It is not expected to adsorb to suspended solids and sediment. Volatilization from water surfaces is not expected. It is expected to exist solely in the particulate phase in the ambient atmosphere. CHX is a highly biodegradable agent, hence, long-term effect in environmental toxicity is not seen. It causes aquatic toxicity and toxicity to birds, upon high-dose exposure to these areas. However, due to its restricted use, not many cases of CHX-induced ecotoxic cases are reported. LD_{50} values for orally administered CHX in male mallard duck and female pheasant are 82.5 and 9.38 mg kg^{-1}, respectively.

Exposure Standards and Guidelines

Extremely hazardous substances that are solids are subject to either of the two threshold planning quantities. The lower quantity applies only if the solid exists in powdered form and has a particle size less than 100 mm, or is handled in solution or in molten form. If the solid does not meet any of these criteria, it is subject to the upper threshold planning quantity. CHX is an extremely hazardous substance that is subject to reporting when stored in amounts in excess of its threshold planning quantity of 100 or 10 000 lb.

See also: Charcoal; LD_{50}/LC_{50} (Lethal Dosage 50/Lethal Concentration 50); Occupational Exposure Limits.

Further Reading

Chang, H.H., Tsai, P.H., Liu, C.W., et al., 2013. Cycloheximide stimulates suppressor of cytokine signaling-3 gene expression in 3T3-L1 adipocytes via the extracellular signal-regulated kinase pathway. Toxicol. Lett. 217 (1), 42–49.

Emmanouil-Nikoloussi, E.N., Nikoloussis, E., Manthou, M.E., et al., 2010. Breast tumor developed in a pregnant rat after treatment with the teratogen cycloheximide. Hippokratia 14 (2), 136–138.

Gold, P.E., Wrenn, S.M., 2012. Cycloheximide impairs and enhances memory depending on dose and footshock intensity. Behav. Brain Res. 233 (2), 293–297.

Mattson, M.P., Furukawa, K., 1997. Anti-apoptotic actions of cycloheximide: blockade of programmed cell death or induction of programmed cell life? Apoptosis 3, 257–264.

Nishide, S.Y., Ono, D., Yamada, Y., Honma, S., Honma, K., 2012. De novo synthesis of PERIOD initiates circadian oscillation in cultured mouse suprachiasmatic nucleus after prolonged inhibition of protein synthesis by cycloheximide. Eur. J. Neurosci. 35 (2), 291–299.

Pan, S.Y., Zhang, Y., Guo, B.F., Han, Y.F., Ko, K.M., 2011. Tacrine and bis(7)-tacrine attenuate cycloheximide-induced amnesia in mice, with attention to acute toxicity. Basic Clin. Pharmacol. Toxicol. 109 (4), 261–265.

Parry, E.W., 1981. Cycloheximide treatment modifies the pattern of 'metastasis' following intravenous injection of Ehrlich ascites tumour cells. Gann 72, 464–467.

Satav, J.G., Katyare, S.S., Fatterparker, P., Sreenivasan, A., 1997. Study of protein synthesis in rat liver mitochondria use of cycloheximide. Eur. J. Biochem. 73, 287–296.

Schneider-Poetsch, T., Ju, J., Eyler, D.E., et al., 2010. Inhibition of eukaryotic translation elongation by cycloheximide and lactimidomycin. Nat. Chem. Biol. 6 (3), 209–217.

Zhao, X., Cao, M., Liu, J.J., et al., February 10, 2011. Reactive oxygen species is essential for cycloheximide to sensitize lexatumumab-induced apoptosis in hepatocellular carcinoma cells. PLoS One 6 (2), e16966. http://dx.doi.org/10.1371/journal.pone.0016966.

Relevant Websites

http://www.cdph.ca.gov/programs/hesis/Documents/cyclohex.pdf – California.Gov.

http://toxnet.nlm.nih.gov/cgi-bin/sis/search/r?dbs+hsdb:@term+@rn+@rel+66-81-9 – National Library of Medicine.

http://toxnet.nlm.nih.gov/cgi-bin/sis/search/r?dbs+genetox:@term+@rn+@rel+%2266-81-9%22 – National Library of Medicine.

http://www.pesticideinfo.org/Detail_Chemical.jsp?Rec_Id=PC35038 – PAN Pesticide Database.

http://pubchem.ncbi.nlm.nih.gov/summary/summary.cgi?cid=6197#x351 – Pubchem.

http://datasheets.scbt.com/sc-3508.pdf – Santa Cruz Biotechnology.

Cyclohexane

SE Gad, Gad Consulting Services, Cary, NC, USA

- Name: Cyclohexane
- Chemical Abstracts Service Registry Number: 110-82-7
- Synonyms: Benzenehexahydride, Hexahydro-benzene, Hexamethylene, Hexanaphthene
- Molecular Formula: C_6H_{12}
- Chemical Structure:

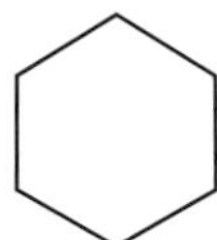

Background Information

Cyclohexane is obtained by the distillation of petroleum or by hydrogenation of benzene. It constitutes 0.5–1.0% of petroleum.

Uses

Cyclohexane is used as a nonpolar solvent for lacquers, resins, fats, oils, and waxes, in paint and varnish remover, in the manufacture of nylon, in the extraction of essential oils, and in analytical chemistry for molecular weight determination. In addition, it is used in the manufacture of adipic acid, benzene, cyclohexanone, cyclohexanol, cyclohexyl chloride, nitrocyclohexane, and solid fuel for camp stoves. Further, it is used in industrial recrystallization of steroids and in fungicidal formulations (it has a slight fungicidal action).

Environmental Fate and Behavior

If released to air, cyclohexane will exist solely as a vapor in the ambient atmosphere, and will be degraded in the atmosphere by reaction with photochemically produced hydroxyl radicals, though direct photolysis is not expected due to the lack of absorption in the environmental spectrum. Volatilization from water surfaces is expected to be an important fate for this compound, and half-lives in a model river and lake are expected to be 3 h and ~3.5 days respectively. Adsorption to suspended solids and sediments is also expected, though hydrolysis in the environment is unlikely due to the lack of hydrolyzable functional groups.

The potential for bioconcentration and bioaccumulation of cyclohexane in aquatic organisms is moderate. It is highly resistant to biodegradation and is catabolized chiefly by cooxidation.

Exposure and Exposure Monitoring

Cyclohexane was a predominant pollutant in shoe and leather factories in Italy, associated with the use of glue. Occupational exposure to cyclohexane may occur through inhalation and dermal contact with this compound where cyclohexane is produced or used. The general population may be exposed to cyclohexane via inhalation of ambient air, ingestion of drinking water, and dermal contact with products containing cyclohexane and due to its presence in gasoline. It has been found in mother's milk and has been detected in studies of the air in various cities.

Environmental Water Concentrations

Contamination has been found in several drinking water sources including bottled water and most commonly in wells, the highest concentration found was 540 ppb. Only trace quantities of cyclohexane have been detected in bedrock and groundwater. Surface waters are generally found to contain 0.5–4.0 ppb.

Toxicokinetics

Cyclohexane is readily absorbed via inhalation and the oral routes of exposure; it is rapidly absorbed into the blood through the lungs. Animal studies indicate dermal absorption to be high, probably due to the defatting action of the compound. Cyclohexane absorption into the lungs is rapid, with the concentration in the lungs reaching 42–62% of the air concentration. Cyclohexane administered to rats either by oral gavage or by intravenous injection was rapidly absorbed and distributed to the tissues. Cyclohexane partitions preferentially to lipid-rich tissues such as fat, liver, and brain. Cyclohexane is metabolized by cytochrome P450 enzymes in the liver and other tissues. Several metabolites have been identified including cyclohexanol and transcyclohexane-1,2-diol. These compounds have been identified in the urine of human subjects and experimental animals within 48 h of exposure. Inhaled cyclohexane is excreted primarily via expiration from the lungs. A small portion partitions to and is excreted in the urine. Metabolites of cyclohexane are conjugated, primarily to glucuronides and possibly to sulfates, and excreted in the urine.

Mechanism of Toxicity

The precise mechanism of toxicity of cyclohexane has not been identified, but is likely similar to other central nervous system (CNS) depressants and general anesthetics. These compounds are believed to exert their effects through a general interaction with the CNS, and interference with neuronal membrane functions has been postulated as a mechanism of action. Disruption of membrane enzymes and the corresponding alterations in cell functions may account for the behavioral and anesthetic effects observed following exposure to various solvents.

 http://dx.doi.org/10.1016/B978-0-12-386454-3.00835-6

Acute and Short-Term Toxicity

Animal

The reported oral LD_{50} in rabbits is 5.5–6.0 mg kg^{-1} indicating the relatively low oral acute toxicity of cyclohexane. Vapor concentrations of 92 000 mg m^{-1} produced rapid narcosis and death in rabbits. In mice, concentrations of 51 000 mg m^{-3} caused narcosis and death occurred at 61 200–71 400 mg m^{-3}. The oral LD_{50} was reported as 12 705 mg kg^{-1} for rats and 813 mg kg^{-1} for mice. Observations indicating CNS effects have been noted in many studies.

Human

Cyclohexane is a CNS depressant and may produce mild anesthetic effects. Inhalation exposure can cause headache, nausea, dizziness, drowsiness, and confusion. Very high concentrations may cause unconsciousness, convulsions, and death. Vapors may be irritating to the nose and throat. Severe lung irritation, damage to lung tissues, or death may result from aspiration into the lungs. Direct dermal contact with liquid may cause mild irritation, which may become more severe if exposure is prolonged. Eyes may become irritated upon exposure to vapors or liquid; however, the effect is generally mild and temporary unless exposure is prolonged. Ingestion of cyclohexane may cause sore throat, nausea, diarrhea, or vomiting.

Chronic Toxicity

Animal

Lower doses (1.0–5.5 mg kg^{-1}) produced mild to extensive hepatocellular degeneration and glomerulonephritis. Microscopic changes in the liver and kidneys were observed in rabbits exposed to 2700 mg m^{-3} for 50 exposures. No changes were noted at 1490 mg m^{-3}. In subchronic inhalation studies in rats and mice, the no observed effect level (NOEL) in rats for acute, transient effects was 500 ppm based on a diminished/absent response to an auditory alerting stimulus at 2000 ppm and above. The NOEL for subchronic toxicity in rats was 7000 ppm based on the lack of adverse effects on body weight, clinical chemistry, tissue morphology, and neurobehavioral parameters. In mice, the NOEL for acute, transient effects was 500 ppm based on behavioral changes during exposure at 2000 ppm and above. The NOEL for subchronic toxicity in mice was 2000 ppm based on hematological changes at 7000 ppm.

Human

Prolonged exposure may produce liver and kidney damage. Cyclohexane is not a carcinogen or a developmental toxicant.

Immunotoxicity

Cyclohexane is not known to be immunotoxic; however, there have been few studies performed.

Reproductive Toxicity

In a prospective study in Toronto, major congenital malformations were noted in 13 of 125 fetuses of mothers exposed to organic solvents (not just cyclohexane) during pregnancy. Studies in rats have shown reduced weights in pups and diminished response to audible stimuli at high dose levels. No observed adverse effect level (NOAEL) for maternal and fetal effects has been reported as over 20 000 mg m^{-3} in rodents.

Inhalation exposure to concentrations of 6886 and 24 101 mg m^{-3}cyclohexane resulted in maternal toxicity in Cesaraen-derived (CD) rats, as demonstrated by a significant reduction in body weight gain. There was no evidence of developmental toxicity in rat pups at the highest concentration tested, 24 101 mg m^{-3}. The NOAEL for developmental toxicity in rat pups was 24 101 mg m^{-3}. Inhalation exposure to the highest concentration of 24 101 mg m^{-3}cyclohexane resulted in no evidence of maternal or developmental toxicity in rabbits.

Genotoxicity

Negative results were obtained in Ames and sister chromatid exchange, mouse lymphoma, and unscheduled DNA synthesis assays.

Carcinogenicity

Cyclohexane is not a carcinogen.

Clinical Management

If inhalation exposure occurs, the source of contamination should be removed or the victim should be moved to fresh air. Artificial respiration should be administered or, if the heart has stopped, cardiopulmonary resuscitation should be provided. If dermal contact has occurred, contaminated clothing should be removed and the affected area should be washed with water and soap for at least 5 min or until the chemical is removed. Contaminated eyes should be flushed with lukewarm, gently flowing water for 5 min or until the chemical is removed. If ingestion occurs, vomiting should not be induced. Water should be given to dilute the compound. If vomiting occurs naturally, the victim should lean forward to reduce risk of aspiration. Aspiration of the compound into the lungs may produce chemical pneumonitis requiring antibiotic treatment and administration of oxygen and expiratory pressure.

Ecotoxicology

LC_{50} for fathead minnow is 95 mg l^{-1} (static).

TLm for Fathead minnow is 43–32 mg l^{-1} (24–96 h); conditions of bioassay not specified.

TLm for Bluegill is 43–34 mg l^{-1} (24–96 h); conditions of bioassay not specified.

TLm for Goldfish is 42.3 mg l^{-1} (24–96 h); conditions of bioassay not specified.

TLm for Guppy is 57.7 mg l^{-1} (24–96 h); conditions of bioassay not specified.

Coho salmon; no significant mortalities were observed up to 100 ppm after 96 h in artificial seawater at 8 °C.

Exposure Standards and Guidelines

The American Conference of Governmental Industrial Hygienists threshold limit value (TLV), 8 h time-weighted average (TWA), is 100 ppm.

Permissible exposure limit: Table Z-1 8 h TWA: 300 ppm (1050 mg m^{-3}).

8 h TWA: 100 ppm.

Excursion limit recommendation: Excursions in worker exposure levels may exceed three times the TLV–TWA for no more than a total of 30 min during a workday, and under no circumstances should they exceed five times the TLV–TWA, provided that the TLV–TWA is not exceeded.

Recommended exposure limit: 10 h TWA: 300 ppm (1050 mg m^{-3}).

Miscellaneous

Cyclohexane is an indirect food additive for use only as a component of adhesives.

See also: Cyclohexene; Hexane.

Further Reading

Baxter, C.S., 2001. Alicyclic hydrocarbons. In: Bingham, E., Cohrssen, B., Powell, C.H. (Eds.), Patty's Toxicology, fifth ed., vol. 4. Wiley, New York, pp. 161–165.

Bingham, E., Cohrssen, B., 2012. Patty's Toxicology, sixth ed. John Wiley and Sons, Hoboken, NJ.

Hissink, A.M., et al., 2009. Physiologically based pharmacokinetic modeling of cyclohexane as a tool for integrating animal and human test data. Int. J. Toxicol. 28 (6), 498–509.

Kreckmann, K.H., Baldwin, J.K., Roberts, L.G., et al., 2000. Inhalation developmental toxicity and reproduction studies with cyclohexane. Drug Chem. Toxicol. 23, 555–573.

Lammers, J.H., Emmen, H.H., Muijser, H., Hoogendijk, E.M., McKee, R.H., Owen, D.E., Kulig, B.M., 2009. Neurobehavioral effects of cyclohexane in rat and human. Int. J. Toxicol. 28 (6), 488–497.

Lewis Sr, R.J. (Ed.), 2000. Cyclohexane. Sax's Dangerous Properties of Industrial Materials, vol. 2. Wiley, New York, pp. 1037–1038.

Malley, L.A., Bamberger, J.R., Stadler, J.C., et al., 2000. Subchronic toxicity of cyclohexane in rats and mice by inhalation exposure. Drug Chem. Toxicol. 23, 513–537.

Rouvière, P.E., Chen, M.W., 2003. Isolation of *Brachymonas petroleovorans* CHX, a novel cyclohexane degrading proteobacterium. FEMS Microbiol. Lett. 227, 101–106.

Relevant Websites

http://www.echemportal.org/echemportal – OECD - The Global Portal to Information on Chemical Substances: Search for Cyclohexane.

http://echa.europa.eu/documents/10162/d99cee39-82e6-4754-aac1-497106c9bd7c – European Commission (2004) Cyclohexane. European Risk Assessment Report vol. 41.

http://www.epa.gov/iris/toxreviews/1005tr.pdf – Environmental Protection Agency Integrated Risk Information System.

http://www.toxnet.nlm.nih.gov – Toxnet homepage

Cyclohexene

S Mostafalou and H Bahadar, Tehran University of Medical Sciences, Tehran, Iran

This article is a revision of the previous edition article by Patricia J. Beattie, volume 1, pp 707–708, © 2005, Elsevier Inc.

- Name: Cyclohexene
- Chemical Abstracts Service Registry Number: CAS110-83-8
- Synonyms: 1,2,3,4-Tetrahydrobenzene; Tetrahydrobenzene; Cyclohex-1-ene
- Molecular Formula: C_6H_{10}
- Chemical Class: Cycloalkene
- Chemical Structure:

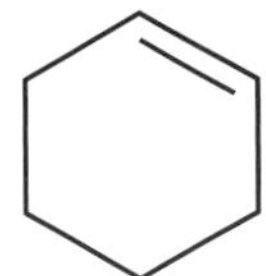

Background and Significant History

Cyclohexene is a hydrocarbon, mostly obtained from the hydrogenation of benzene.

Uses of Cyclohexene

Cyclohexene is as an intermediate used in the manufacture of tetrahydrobenzoic acid, adipic acid, maleic acid, and aldehydes. Cyclohexene is also used as a stabilizer in high-octane gasoline and as a catalyst in oil extraction.

Environmental Fate and Behavior

The release of cyclohexene into the air occurs in the form of waste streams from manufacturing units. Cyclohexene has a vapor pressure of 89 mm Hg at 25 °C, indicating that it exists as a vapor form in the environment and is degraded by reactions with photochemically induced hydroxyl radicals, ozone, and nitrate radicals. The half-life for these reactions in the air is 6, 2, and 4 h, respectively.

Estimated K_{oc} of 850 indicates that cyclohexene has low mobility in the soil. Cyclohexene has Henry's law constant of 4.55×10^{-2}atm-m^3 mol^{-1}. Based on this Henry's law constant, volatilization is expected to be the major process of removal of cyclohexene from moist soil and water, if released into it.

Exposure and Exposure Monitoring

Exposure to cyclohexene is expected through inhalation and dermal contact in workplaces where it is either produced or employed as an intermediate chemical. Cyclohexene is a volatile liquid, so inhalation, if handled in an unprotected manner, and dermal contact are the major human exposure routes. Cyclohexene is monitored in exposed individuals, as the hydroxylated and conjugated metabolites can be measured by high-pressure liquid chromatography.

Toxicokinetics

The absorption of cyclohexene is rapid through skin and from the respiratory tract after inhaling the vapors. Cyclohexene-like hydrocarbons are poorly absorbed into the gastrointestinal tract, and do not cause much toxicity after ingestion.

Mechanism of Toxicity

Cyclohexene is suspected to have an irritating effect on the skin. After exposure through inhalation, it can cause depression of the central nervous system. The mechanism for these toxicities is not fully understood.

Acute and Short-Term Toxicity

Animal

Sprague–Dawley rats were administered cyclohexene at doses of 500, 1000, and 2000 mg kg^{-1} by gavage. Three animals out of five in the last group demonstrated some clinical signs of abnormal gait, salivation, piloerection, and tremors, and death within 3 days. The cause of the death was revealed as pulmonary congestion by necropsy. The LD_{50} value for both male and female sexes has been established in the range of 1000–2000 mg kg^{-1}.

Chronic Toxicity

Animals

In a study conducted on rats, guinea pigs, and rabbits, cyclohexene was administered at 150, 300, or 600 ppm, 6 h per day for 6 months. A significant rise in alkaline phosphatase level was detected, but the other parameters of blood such as glucose, cellular components, hemoglobin, and biochemical profile (blood urea nitrogen, cholesterol, serum glutamic pyruvic transaminases, serum glutamic oxaloacetic transaminases, lactate dehydrogenase, electrolytes) remained the same.

Human

Chronic exposure of human to cyclohexene would likely cause pulmonary damage, CNS depression, hypoxia, pneumatocele formation, and chronic lung dysfunction.

Reproductive Toxicity

Rats were administered cyclohexene by gavage at doses of 50, 150, and 500 mg kg^{-1} day^{-1}. The males received it for 48 days and the females for 42–53 days. The treatment continued from 14 days before mating to day 4 of lactation. No harmful effect of cyclohexene on the reproductive system was observed.

Genotoxicity

Cyclohexene has been found not to be mutagenic by reverse mutation assay using *Salmonella typhimurium* TA100, TA1535, and TA1537 and *Escherichia coli* wp2 uvrA.

Clinical Management

Inhalation

The patient should be removed from the exposure site and given oxygen and artificial respiration if not breathing.

Ingestion

Swallowing of cyclohexene is rare; if swallowed, the patient should be given a large quantity of water. If the patient is unconscious, vomiting is contraindicated.

Skin Contact

After skin contact with cyclohexene, the contaminated area should be thoroughly washed with soap for at least 15 min.

Eye Contact

In the case of eyes affected by cyclohexene, they should be washed with water for at least 15 min.

Ecotoxicology

Aquatic Ecotoxicity

Regarding acute toxicity to aquatic organisms, an EC_{50} of 2.1–5.3 mg l^{-1} for *daphnids*, an LC_{50} of 5.8 mg l^{-1} for fish, *Oryzias latipes*, and an LC_{50} of 12.4 mg l^{-1} for fish, *Poecilia reticulata*, have been reported. The 48 h EC_{50} of 2.1 mg l^{-1} has been reported for *Daphnia magnia*.

Other Hazards

Cyclohexene is a flammable liquid and slightly toxic by ingestion.

Exposure Standards and Guidelines

Based on Occupational Safety and Health Administration standard, permissible exposure limit for cyclohexene is 300 ppm over an 8-h work shift.

Miscellaneous

Vapor pressure: 89 mm Hg.
Melting point: −1.04 °C.
Boiling point: 82.9 °C.
Henry's law constant: 0.0455 atm-m^3 mol^{-1}.
Log *p* (octanol–water): 2.86.

See also: Benzene; Occupational Safety and Health Administration; Gasoline.

Further Reading

Canton, J.H., Wegman, R.C.C., 1983. Studies on the toxicity of tribromoethene, cyclohexene and bromocyclohexane to different freshwater organisms. Water Res. 17, 743–747.

Material Safety Data Sheet; MSDS NO: 243. 2011. Cyclohexene. Scholar Chemistry 866, 5100 W. Henrietta Rd, Rochester, NY 14586, 260–0501. http://www.westliberty.edu/health-and-safety/files/2012/08/Cyclohexene.pdf.

Occupational Health Guidelines for Cyclohexene. US Department of Health and Human services, Centers for Disease Control. www.cdc.gov/niosh/docs/81-123/pdfs/0167.pdf.

UNEP Publication, SIDS Initial Assessment Report. 2002. Cyclohexene, CAS No. 110-83-8, National SIDS Contact Point in Sponsor Country: Ms. Mizuho Hayakawa. Ministry of Foreign Affairs, Japan. www.inchem.org/documents/sids/sids/110838.pdf.

Relevant Websites

http://www.inchem.org. – International Programme on Chemical Safety: INCHEM: Cyclohexene.

http://toxnet.nlm.nih.gov – Toxnet (Toxicology Data Network): search under Toxline for Cyclohexene.

Cyclopeptide *see* Mushrooms, Cyclopeptide

Cyclophosphamide

CM Stork and SM Schreffler, Upstate Medical University, Syracuse, NY, USA

This article is a revision of the previous edition article by Greene Shepherd, volume 1, pp 709–711, © 2005, Elsevier Inc.

- Name: Cyclophosphamide
- Chemical Abstracts Service Registry Numbers: 50-18-0; 6055-19-2 (monohydrate)
- Synonyms: 2H-1,3,2-oxazaphosphorin-2-amine, *N*,*N*-bis(2-chloroethyl)tetrahydro-2-oxide; 2H-1,3,2-oxazaphosphorine, 2-[bis(2-chloroethyl)amino]tetrahydro-, 2-oxide; Asta B 518; B 518; Bis(2-chloroethyl)phosphoramide cyclic propanolamide ester; Clafen; Claphene; Cyclophosphamid; Cyclophosphamide hydrate; Cyclophosphamide monohydrate; Cyclophosphamidum; Cyclophosphan; Cyclophosphane; Cyclophosphanum; Cyclostin; Cytophosphan; Cytophosphane; Cytoxan; Endoxan; Endoxan monohydrate; Genoxal; Hexadrin; Mitoxan; *N*,*N*-Bis(β-chloroethyl)-*N*′,O-trimethylenephosphoric acid ester diamide; *N*,*N*-bis (β-chloroethyl)-*N*′,O-propylenephosphoric acid ester diamide; Neosar; NSC 26271; Phosphorodiamidic acid, *N*,*N*-bis(2-chloroethyl)-*N*′-(3-hydroxypropyl)-, intramol ester; Procytox; Revimmune; Sendoxan
- Chemical/Pharmaceutical/Other Class: Nitrogen mustard alkylating agent
- Molecular Formula: $C_7H_{15}C_{12}N_2O_2P$
- Chemical Structures:

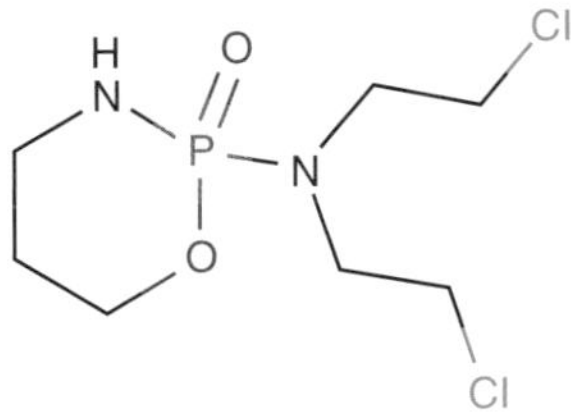

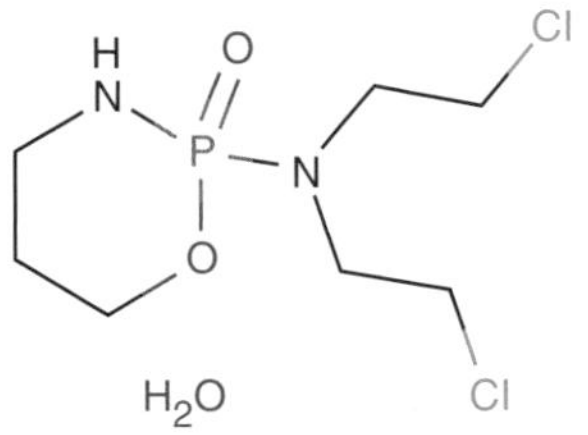

Background Information

Cyclophosphamide, a nitrogen mustard alkylating agent from the oxazophorines group, was first synthesized by Arnold Bourseaux and Norbert Brock in 1958. The first clinical trials involving cyclophosphamide were published at the end of the 1950s. It was reported that cyclophosphamide is converted to its active metabolites by mixed-function oxidase enzymes in the liver. These metabolites were demonstrated to slow cancerous cell growth by forming cross-linkages in the DNA of susceptible proliferating malignant cells and inhibiting replication. Unfortunately, normal cells were also affected, resulting in serious side effects. By mechanisms not fully understood, cyclophosphamide also induces effects on immune effector and suppressor cells, decreasing the immune system's response to various diseases. The US Food and Drug Administration approved its use in November 1959.

Uses

Cyclophosphamide is an effective single antineoplastic (anticancer) agent, but is more frequently used concurrently or sequentially with other antineoplastic drugs. Cyclophosphamide is also a potent immunosuppressive agent used to prevent transplant rejection and in the treatment of nonneoplastic autoimmune disorders, such as Wegener's granulomatosis, rheumatoid arthritis, 'minimal change' nephrotic syndrome, and multiple sclerosis. Cyclophosphamide is used rarely in veterinary practice for defleecing sheep and has been tested as an insect chemosterilant.

Environmental Fate

Cyclophosphamide may be released into the atmosphere secondary to production or through waste streams. If released into the air, it is expected to be present in both vapor and particulate phases at ambient temperature and pressure. Vapor-phase degradation by hydroxyl radicals in general produces a half-life of 5.5 h. Particulate cyclophosphamide will be broken down by both wet and dry decompositions as well as through photodegradation.

Physicochemical Properties

Cyclophosphamide is a solid compound at standard temperature and pressure. It has a melting point of 41–45 °C and is soluble in water at 1–5 g per 100 ml (23 °C; log *P* is 0.8 and log *S* is −1.2.)

Exposure Routes and Pathways

Exposure to this odorless, white, crystalline powder may occur during its manufacture, formulation, or distribution as an antineoplastic/immunosuppressive drug. During manufacture and experimental use, exposure may be by inhalation or skin absorption. Therapeutically, it is administered orally, intramuscularly, intraperitoneally, intravenously, and intrapleurally.

Toxicokinetics

Cyclophosphamide is rapidly absorbed, metabolized, and excreted. Peak plasma concentrations after an oral dose is approximately 1 h. It is distributed rapidly to all tissues and exhibits an elimination half-life of 3–12 h. It is eliminated primarily in the form of metabolites, but 5–25% of the dose is excreted unchanged in the urine. Plasma protein binding of unchanged drug is low, but some metabolites are bound to an extent greater than 60%. In humans, cyclophosphamide is metabolized by hepatic cytochrome P450 to the active metabolites acrolein, 4-aldophosphamide, 4-hydrocyclophosphamide, and nor-nitrogen mustard. The primary active metabolite is 4-hydroxycyclophosphamide, which exists in equilibrium with aldophosphamide, its ring-opened tautomer. Most of the aldophosphamide is oxidized by the enzyme aldehyde dehydrogenase (ALDH) to make carboxyphosphamide. A small proportion of aldophosphamide is converted into phosphoramide mustard and acrolein. Phosphamide mustard, acrolein, and nor-nitrogen mustard have all been proven to have toxic effects.

Mechanism of Toxicity

Cyclophosphamide works by interrupting the cell cycle in a nonphase-specific manner. The main effects of cyclophosphamide are due to the antitumor activity of its metabolite phosphoramide mustard. Phosphoramide mustard prevents cell division by forming cross-linkages in DNA both between and within DNA strands at guanine *N*-7 positions. This is irreversible and leads to cell death. Phosphoramide mustard is formed only in cells that have low levels of ALDH. ALDHs are abundant in rapidly proliferating tissues (bone marrow stem cells, liver, and intestinal epithelium) and are protective against the toxic effects of phosphoramide mustard and acrolein by driving the conversion of aldophosphamide to carboxyphosphamide. The toxic side effects are due to the phosphoramide mustard and acrolein. Nor-nitrogen mustard is responsible for the renal damage that occurs in some cases.

Acute and Short-Term Toxicity (or Exposure)

Animal

The LD in mice ranges from 370 mg kg^{-1} (subcutaneous) to 310 mg kg^{-1} (intravenous). The LD in rats was 160 mg kg^{-1} (intravenous), 180 mg kg^{-1} (oral), and 400 mg kg^{-1} (intraperitoneal in rats bearing tumors). The intravenous LD was 400 mg kg^{-1} in guinea pigs and 40 mg kg^{-1} in dogs. In mice, rats, and dogs, the predominant hematological effect of cyclophosphamide is leukopenia and thrombocytopenia. Prolonged treatment of rodents with cyclophosphamide has produced pathological structural changes in a variety of organs, including lung, gut, pancreas, and liver. In rats, cyclophosphamide given orally decreases mitosis in crypts, decreases the height of villi, and causes degeneration of the intestinal mucosa. A single intraperitoneal dose of cyclophosphamide caused marked necrosis of the bladder, renal tubular, and renal pelvic epithelium in mice, rats, and dogs. Cyclophosphamide is teratogenic in the rhesus monkey when given intramuscularly for various periods between 25 and 43 days of pregnancy at doses ranging from 2.5 to 20 mg kg^{-1} body weight. Placental transfer of cyclophosphamide has been demonstrated in mice, and a positive correlation between alkylation of embryonic DNA and the production of congenital abnormalities has been reported in mice.

Human

Patients treated with cyclophosphamide have been reported to exhibit various side effects such as flushing of the face, swollen lips, cardiotoxicity, pneumonitis or interstitial fibrosis, agitation, dizziness, tiredness, weakness, headache, nausea, vomiting, diarrhea, stomatitis, hemorrhagic colitis, hepatitis, hemorrhagic cystitis, fever, chills, sore throat, sweating, pancytopenia, leukopenia, alopecia, changes in the nucleoli of lymphocytes, water and sodium retention, pulmonary fibrosis, and visual blurring. Birth defects, such as limb reductions or pigmentation of the fingernails and skin, were also noted. Although the entire urinary tract is at risk of toxicity from the metabolite acrolein, the bladder is most susceptible because of its prolonged exposure. Cystitis, hemorrhagic cystitis, and fibrosis of the bladder wall have been reported in patients treated for cystitis, rheumatoid arthritis, lupus erythematosus, and neoplasia, respectively. Fatal cardiomyopathy may result when very large doses of cyclophosphamide are given as conditioning for bone marrow transplantation. Cyclophosphamide has teratogenic and mutagenic potential and can cause sterility of either sex. It can damage germ cells in prepubertal, pubertal, and adult males and cause premature ovarian failure in females. It is most toxic to the human fetus during the first 3 months, and congenital abnormalities have been detected after intravenous injections of large doses to pregnant women during this period of pregnancy. Mothers taking cyclophosphamide should avoid breastfeeding.

Chronic Toxicity (or Exposure)

Animal

Mice dosed at 7% of the LD_{50} cyclophosphamide per week subcutaneously for 1 year had higher rates of leukemias, mammary carcinomas, ovarian carcinomas, and lung tumors compared to controls.

Human

Chronic exposure to cyclophosphamide is associated with neoplasms, bone marrow suppression, and gonadal toxicity.

Depending on the total dose of cyclophosphamide, patients have a 1.6- to 2.4-fold overall increase in malignancies with a 5- to 30-fold increase in bladder carcinoma, up to 10.4-fold increase in skin cancer, up to 11-fold increase in lymphomas, and up to 5.7-fold increase for leukemia. Bone marrow suppression results in leukopenia, anemia, and thrombocytopenia. Myelodysplastic syndrome occurs in 2–8% of patients. Immune system suppression may result in serious and sometimes fatal infections. The spectrum of infections is wide and includes bacterial, viral, and fungal. The most commonly seen infections are pneumonia, endocarditis, spondylodiscitis, and catheter-associated *Staphylococcus aureus* sepsis. Alopecia and other toxic effects may develop in patients.

Immunotoxicity

Cyclophosphamide is an alkylating agent with significant immunosuppressive effects.

Genotoxicity

Cyclophosphamide is an alkylating agent and has been shown to cause DNA damage and genotoxicity. It can increase the rate of micronuclei abnormalities, seen in tests of genotoxicity. Cyclophosphamide stops tumor growth by the same mechanism; it can damage other DNA by cross-linking guanine bases in DNA double-helix strands and adds an alkyl group to electronegative bonds.

Reproductive Toxicity

Cyclophosphamide can cause reproductive toxicity in both males and females. It interferes with spermatogenesis and oogenesis. Sterility, sometimes reversible, can occur in both men and women with cyclophosphamide. Dose and duration of therapy are factors in the risk for sterility related to cyclophosphamide. Amenorrhea and decreases in estrogen and other hormone production can occur in women treated with cyclophosphamide. Cyclophosphamide has been shown to cause fetal abnormalities when administered during pregnancy in animals and in humans. In males, altered interest and sexual behavior, diminished fertility, and changes to sperm count and shape can occur.

Carcinogenicity

Cyclophosphamide is carcinogenic in humans and animals. Bladder cancer is seen at increased rates following therapy with cyclophosphamide for nonmalignant diseases and increases in acute nonlymphocytic leukemia are seen in patients treated with cyclophosphamide for non-Hodgkin's lymphoma. Cyclophosphamide has been found to cause tumor in animal models when given via various routes. Increases in several different types of tumor types were seen both at administration sites and at distant sites for different routes of administration.

Clinical Management

Treatment is largely supportive. Cyclophosphamide is adsorbed by activated charcoal, and charcoal should be used for substantial, recent ingestions. Patients may require aggressive fluid support. Standard supportive therapies, such as vasopressors, should be utilized as clinically indicated. Patients may require prolonged observation due to the delay in the development of adverse effects. Antibiotics may be needed to treat or minimize opportunistic infection due to the development of immunosuppression. Management of cyclophosphamide-induced hemorrhagic cystitis includes electrocauterization, systemic vasopressin, intravesical administration of silver nitrate, formalin, prostaglandin F2, and hydrostatic pressure. Preventative therapies that have been shown to reduce occurrence include aggressive hydration for dilutional effects, frequent bladder emptying, intravenous administration of 2-mercatoethane sulfonate sodium, and intravesical administration of *N*-acetylcysteine. Baseline electrocardiogram and echocardiograms should be obtained for all patients with large exposures. One case of cyclophosphamide-induced cardiomyopathy has been successfully treated with fluid restriction, digoxin and furosemide.

See also: Acrolein.

Further Reading

Aguiar Bjanda, D., Cabrera Suarez, M.A., Bohn Sarmiento, U., Aguiar Morales, J., 2006. Successful recovery after accidental overdose of cyclophosphamide. Ann. Oncol. 17 (8), 1334.

Braverman, A.C., Antin, J.H., Plappert, M.T., 1991. Cyclophosphamide cardiotoxicity in bone marrow transplantation. J. Clin. Oncol. 9, 1215–1223.

Colvin, O.M., August 1999. An overview of cyclophosphamide development and clinical applications. Curr. Pharm. Des. 5 (8), 555–560.

Nitharwal, R.K., Patel, H., Karchuli, M.S., Ugale, R.R., 2013. Chemoprotective potential of *Coccinia indica* against cyclophosphamide-induced toxicity. Indian J. Pharmacol. 45 (5), 502–507.

Pailoi, A., Luksch, R., Fagioli, F., Tamburini, A., Cesari, M., Palmerini, E., Abate, M.E., Marchesi, E., Balladelli, A., Pratelli, L., Ferrari, S., June 19, 2013. Chemotherapy-related toxicity in patients with non-metastatic Ewing sarcoma: influence of sex and age. J. Chemother. (Epub ahead of print).

Subramaniam, S.R., Cader, R.A., Mohd, R., Yen, K.W., Ghafor, H.A., 2013. Low-dose cyclophosphamide-induced acute hepatotoxicity. Am. J. Case Rep. 14, 345–349.

Thomas, L.L., Mertens, M.J., von dem Borne, A.E., van Boxtel, C.J., Veenhof, C.H., Veies, E.P., 1988. Clinical management of cytotoxic drug overdose. Med. Toxicol. Adverse Drug Exp. 3 (4), 253–263.

Wang, C.C., Weng, T.I., Lu, M.Y., Yang, R.S., Lin, K.H., Wu, M.H., Liu, S.H., July 20, 2013. Hemorrhagic cystitis in children treated with alkylating agent cyclophosphamide: the experience of a medical center in Taiwan. J. Formos. Med. Assoc. pii: S0929-6646(13)00206-4. (Epub ahead of print).

Relevant Websites

http://www.cancer.org/treatment/treatmentsandsideeffects/guidetocancerdrugs/cyclophosphamide – American Cancer Society online resource on cyclophosphamide.

http://www.cancer.gov/cancertopics/druginfo/cyclophosphamide – National Cancer Institute – Cancer Drug Information page – cyclophosphamide.

http://www.inchem.org/documents/iarc/suppl7/cyclophosphamide.html – Online resource for carcinogenicity related to cyclophosphamide.

http://www.hopkinsvasculitis.org/vasculitis-treatments/cyclophosphamide-cytoxan/ – Vasculitis Center – Johns Hopkins – online resource on cyclophosphamide.

Cyclosporine

T Dodd-Butera, California State University San Bernardino, San Bernardino, CA, USA
M Broderick, California Poison Control System, San Diego Division, San Diego, CA, USA

- Name: Cyclosporine
- Chemical Abstracts Service Registry Number*: 59865-13-3
- Synonyms: (*R*-(*R**,*R**-(*E*)))-Cyclic(L-alanyl-D-alanyl-*N*-methyl-L-leucyl-*N*-methyl-L-leucyl-*N*-methyl-L-valyl-3-hydroxy-*N*,4-dimethyl-L-2-amino-6-octenoyl-L-alpha-aminobutyryl-*N*-methylglycyl-*N*-methyl-L-leucyl-L-valyl-*N*-methyl-L-leucyl); Cyclosporin A; [Gengraf (modified); Neoral (modified); Sandimmune (nonmodified); Restasis (ocular)]
- Molecular Formula*: $C_{62}H_{111}N_{11}O_{12}$
- Chemical Structure†:

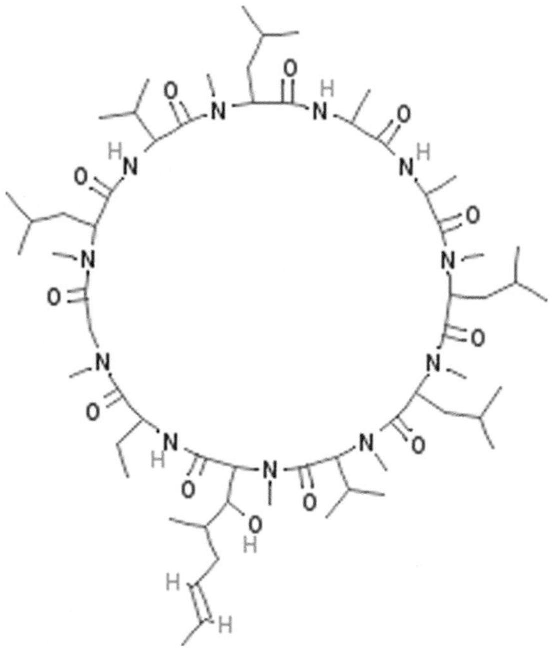

* All from ChemIDplus.

† PubChem http://pubchem.ncbi.nlm.nih.gov/summary/summary.cgi?cid=5280754#itabs-2d

Background

Cyclosporine (CAS 59865-13-3) is a neutral, lipophilic, cyclic polypeptide containing 11 amino acids. The drug has immunosuppressive properties, based on the ability to block transcription of cytokine genes in activated T cells. Since the introduction to clinical use in 1983 as an immunosuppressant, survival rates for patients receiving transplants and grafts have steadily improved. Ophthalmic formulations increase tears and have been used for chronic dry eye conditions.

Cyclosporine can be derived as a metabolite from the soil fungus, *Tolypocladium inflatum*. It was the first metabolite from any microorganism utilized clinically, to regulate growth and function of a normal mammalian cell. It can also be manufactured synthetically. Hazardous combustion and decomposition products include carbon monoxide, carbon dioxide, nitrogen oxide, hydrogen chloride gas, and phosgene.

Uses

Cyclosporine was approved for transplant immunosuppression in 1983. It is administered to prevent organ rejection after transplant of kidney, liver, lung, heart, or bone marrow and for suppression of graft-versus-host disease. In addition, it has been utilized for treatment of Crohn's disease, rheumatoid arthritis, and psoriasis. More recently, ophthalmic forms have been used to treat chronic dry eye conditions. Cyclosporine is available in modified and original forms; but prescriptions are not interchangeable, due to the difference in bioavailability.

Exposure and Exposure Monitoring

Exposure to cyclosporine in therapeutic settings is via oral or parenteral routes. Oral medications may be found in liquid or capsule form. Ocular exposure may also occur, generally via single-dose drop packs from therapeutic ophthalmic formulations.

There is a lack of correlation in some exposures between dose and therapeutic blood levels due to various factors, including absorption, metabolism, and product formulation. Thus, monitoring of exposure to therapeutic drug levels is ideally by investigation of the blood cyclosporine concentration versus time (or area under the curve – AUC, see example in **Figure 1**). Blood concentration at hour 2 (C_2) of dosing is

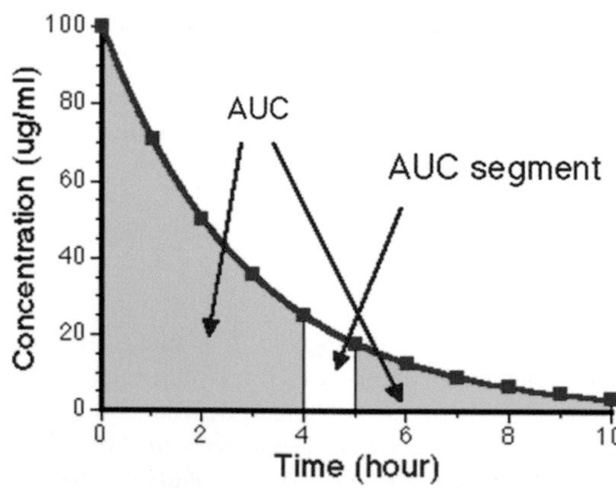

Figure 1 Example of linear plot of C_p versus time showing AUC and AUC segment permission granted Bourne, D.W.A., 2013. Calculation of AUC using the Trapezoidal Rule retrieved from http://www.boomer.org/c/p4/c02/c0208.html.

 http://dx.doi.org/10.1016/B978-0-12-386454-3.00013-0

sometimes utilized in clinical settings, as opposed to predose or initial monitoring, known as the trough level. Optimal clinical monitoring techniques for safety and efficacy are continuing to be investigated. Monitoring blood levels is important in order to insure cyclosporine levels are high enough in transplant patients to prevent rejection. Further, distinguishing between kidney rejection and kidney damage from elevated cyclosporine levels is critical in monitoring safe exposures and outcomes such as survival and symptom relief, as in the latter for usage in rheumatoid arthritis and psoriasis.

Occupational exposures require an exhaust system and protection to avoid worker inhalation of dust particles. Skin and eye protection is also required, with access to rinsing capabilities, if exposures occur. Transfer to a closed chemical waste container for disposal is recommended, in the event of a spill. Avoidance of spilled materials into a drain is advised, although exact ecological fate is undetermined.

Toxicokinetics

Cyclosporine is biotransformed primarily in the liver by CYP3A4; however, alternate metabolic pathways may yield toxic metabolites. Metabolites have both decreased toxicity and pharmacologic activity, when compared to the parent compound. Most of the cyclosporine dose is excreted in bile as an active metabolite. Less than 1% is excreted as unchanged drug. Cyclosporine has a biphasic elimination pattern from the blood, with a half-life range of 5–18 h. Inducers of CYP3A4 increase cyclosporine metabolism, whereas competitors may increase cyclosporine to potentially toxic levels. Interindividual and intraindividual variabilities in toxicokinetics exist for cyclosporine levels. Enhanced microemulsion techniques in some forms of cyclosporine improve consistency in absorption.

Variability in CYP3A4 expression due to environmental factors has been evaluated, along with genetic polymorphisms for impact on cyclosporine blood levels, clinical endpoints, and toxicity. Factors influencing levels include: age, body mass index, food intake, serum albumin, lipoproteins, and intestinal P-glycoprotein activity. Drugs and other substances that affect microsomal enzymes, especially the CYP3A system, may affect cyclosporine metabolism and blood concentrations. Cyclosporine influences the toxicokinetics of digoxin by increasing the volume of distribution, half-life, and eliminated renal fraction. It is essential that patients taking cyclosporine discuss exposure to over-the-counter, prescription, and herbal preparations (such as St. John's wort) with their health care provider to avoid toxicity from drug interaction and altered metabolism.

Mechanisms of Action

The exact mechanism of action is not fully elucidated, but the overall effect is a decrease in the activity of the immune system. The proposed mechanism appears to be due to inhibition of the action of calcineurin, which suppresses interleukin-2 levels and inhibits T-lymphocyte proliferation. The result is blocking of the translocation of the cytosolic component of the nuclear factor of activated T cells, ultimately suppressing the antigenic response. The high lipophilicity of cyclosporine allows access for binding to intracellular sites of action. Cyclosporine does not significantly impact myelosuppression or nonspecific biological defense systems.

Acute and Short-Term Toxicity

Animal

Animal studies show immunosuppression, renal glomerular and tubular damage, vascular smooth muscle targets, endothelial effects, and neurological toxicity.

Human

Acute cyclosporine intoxication after organ transplantation may occur during adjustment to therapeutic dosing regimen, miscalculation of dosage, or intentional overdose. As a calcineurin inhibitor, cyclosporine acts as a vasoconstrictor from a decrease in vasodilators, with interference in mitochondrial permeability transition pores causing direct toxicity to renal tubules. Headache and hypertension may result, along with diminished renal function. Other symptoms associated with exposure to cyclosporine may include decreased hepatic function. Some of these may occur as side effects of therapeutic doses or as a result of toxic levels. These may occur as acute or chronic toxicity. Allergic reactions may also occur in persons with sensitivity to the drug or vehicle of suspension or delivery. There is a potential for severe hepatotoxicity, nephrotoxicity, and neurotoxicity, with recorded cases of acute tubular necrosis, atrial fibrillation, and death with acute overdose.

Chronic Toxicity

Animal

Lymphoma was noted in grafted macaques and male mice receiving cyclosporine. Rats exposed to cyclosporine A developed renal and hepatocellular tumors. Nephrotoxicity may be experienced with acute or long-term exposure, as in humans. Endothelial cell toxicity was noted in studies with vascular endothelial growth factor as a cellular stress response.

Human

Patients who receive cyclosporine have underlying medical and surgical considerations, and additional drug exposures, that may contribute to patient symptoms and negative outcomes. Toxicity from the drug itself has been noted, though, due to underlying mechanisms of action. Adverse reactions include gingivitis which may become gum hyperplasia, gastrointestinal disturbances, hirsutism, hyperkalemia, hyperlipidemia, hypertension, renal dysfunction, and tremor. Due to the immunosuppressive actions of the drug, there is an increased risk of infections when on cyclosporine therapy, particular with use of adjunct medications. Nephrotoxicity, hepatoxicity, accelerated atherosclerosis, hypertension, and graft vascular disease are common complications of long-term cyclosporine administration. The primary indication for cessation or alteration of therapy is renal toxicity, in many patients taking cyclosporine. Related hypertension may occur in both renal and cardiac transplant recipients. Increased interstitial areas and accumulation of extracellular matrix have also been noted. Additionally, cyclosporine is considered a human carcinogen, due to increased risk of lymphoma and skin cancer in patients taking the drug for psoriasis. In some cases, tumor regression occurred after discontinuing cyclosporine.

The primary indication for cessation or alteration of therapy is renal toxicity, in many patients taking cyclosporine. Related hypertension may occur in both renal and cardiac transplant recipients.

Immunotoxicity

As previously discussed, cyclosporine is a potent immunosuppressive agent, so prolonged use can increase susceptibility to infections and result in other related effects.

Reproductive and Developmental Toxicity

Animal

Studies in rats and rabbits have shown that large doses may cause death to the fetus or birth defects, depending on timing of exposure in gestation. In rodent studies, embryonic exposure resulted in functional immunity impairment during postnatal maturation. Cyclosporine has been shown to cross the placenta.

Human

Women who take cyclosporine during pregnancy may be at increased risk for delivering prematurely, though controlled scientific studies in human developmental toxicity and teratogenicity are needed. The maternal disease process itself for which cyclosporine is required, may introduce risk to the pregnancy, so well-designed studies considering all factors would address the gap in information. Regarding lactation, cyclosporine has been detected in breast milk. Limited information indicates that variable levels found in breast milk, may expose infants to maternal cyclosporine. The potential risk, extrapolating from previous toxicity studies, is immunosuppression, renal effects, and carcinogenicity; however, controlled studies to assess the extent of risk have not been conducted to evaluate the impact, if any, on infant growth, development, and well-being. Short- and long-term adverse effects from exposure have not been well studied, and individual patients need to base decisions on advice of health care providers for use of cyclosporine during pregnancy and lactation.

Genotoxicity

Most *in vitro* tests were negative for genetic damage; however, there was a slight increase in sister chromatid exchange in human lymphocytes exposed *in vitro*. *In vitro* studies demonstrate apoptosis and antiproliferative effects on endothelial and epithelial cells. Tumor progression promotion was noted in calcineurin inhibitors.

Carcinogenicity

Cyclosporine is a known human carcinogen; malignancy after transplant surgery has contributed to patient morbidity and mortality. Lymphoma and skin cancer are two malignancies related to cyclosporine in the scientific literature. The risk of developing skin cancer has been linked to cyclosporine treatment and previous psoralen and UVA/UVB, in patients with psoriasis. Cyclosporine, along with other immunosuppressants that are calcineurin inhibitors, has been linked to posttransplant malignancies. However, immunosuppression may contribute to the mortality rates, as it disrupts both antitumor and antiviral activities. Studies in transplant patients have linked cyclosporine to both increased risk of malignancy and no increase in risk after treatment. Future studies elucidating mechanisms and patient outcomes are needed with regard to malignancy and cyclosporine use, as compared with newer immunosuppressants.

Clinical Management

In the event of an acute overdose, a health care provider, local emergency responders, and a poison control center should be contacted so that life-support measures may be instituted, if required. Clinical responses to cyclosporine overdose vary widely. Symptoms may include headache, nausea, central nervous system depression or excitation, respiratory depression, and cardiovascular events, such as hypertension or atrial fibrillation. Monitoring by a health care provider of cyclosporine blood levels, serum electrolytes, renal, and hepatic function with therapeutic use is indicated. Activated charcoal may be administered for drug adsorption, as determined by a health care provider. Observation of allergic reaction should also be noted in any exposure, in the event of patient sensitivity.

Ecotoxicology

Avoidance of spilled materials into a drain is advised, although exact ecological fate is undetermined. Bioaccumulation potential is considered low, although further studies on ecological fate would add to the scientific knowledge regarding cyclosporine in the environment.

See also: Carcinogen; Immune System; Kidney; St. John's Wort.

Further Reading

Chapman, J.R., 2011. Chronic calcineurin inhibitor nephrotoxicity – lest we forget. Am. J. Transplant. 11 (4), 693–697. http://dx.doi.org/10.1111/j.1600-6143.2011.03504.x.

Goodman and Gilman's, 1996. The Pharmacological Basis of Therapeutics, ninth ed. McGraw-Hill, New York, NY.

Ho, S., Clipstone, N., Timmermann, L., Northrop, J., Graef, I., Fiorentino, D., Nourse, J., Crabtree, G.R., September 1996. The mechanism of action of cyclosporin A and FK506. Clin. Immunol. Immunopathol. 80 (3 Pt 2), S40–S45.

Sweetman, S.C. (Ed.), 2011. Martindale: The Complete Drug Reference, thirty-seventh ed. Pharmaceutical Press, London.

Relevant Websites

http://www.ncbi.nlm.nih.gov/sites/entrez?cmd=search&db=pccompound&term=5284373 – National Library of Medicine.

http://ntp-apps.niehs.nih.gov/ntp_tox/index.cfm?fuseaction=ntpsearch.searchresults&searchterm=59865-13-3 – National Toxicology Program.

Cyfluthrin

S Karanth, Charles River Laboratories, Reno, NV, USA

- Name: Cyfluthrin
- Chemical Structure:

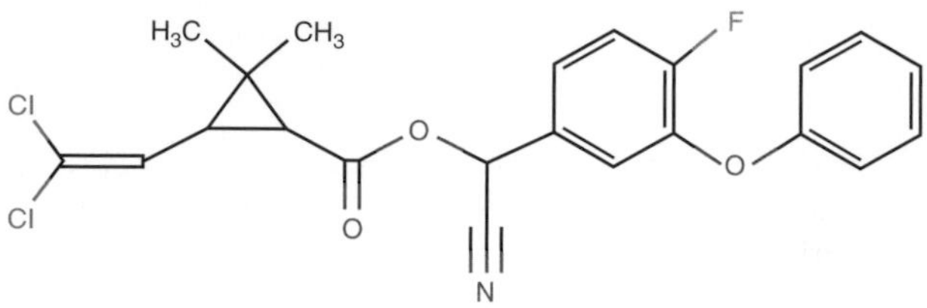

Background

Cyfluthrin was first registered for use by the US Environmental Protection Agency (EPA) in 1987. It is found in both restricted use and general use pesticides. Cyfluthrin is the active ingredient in many insecticide products, including Baythroid®, Attatox®, Contur®, Solfac®, and Tempo®. Commercial synthetic pyrethroids, including cyfluthrin, are a mixture of isomers and all of the isomers have the same mode of action.

Uses

Cyfluthrin is a broad-spectrum nonsystemic insecticide used in the control of cockroaches, ants, termites, mosquitoes, flies, tobacco budworms, and common chewing and sucking insects of cotton, cereals, potatoes, and peanuts. It is also used in the control of public health pests.

Environmental Fate

Cyfluthrin readily breaks down following exposure to sunlight. It is highly immobile in soil, unstable in water, and is not a groundwater contaminant. On soil surfaces its half-life is 2–3 days. Under anaerobic conditions, its half-life in soils is approximately 2 months. It rapidly breaks down in surface waters as it floats on the surface where it is subject to photodegradation.

Exposure and Exposure Monitoring

Common routes of cyfluthrin exposure include dermal, ingestion, and inhalation. Cyfluthrin degrades rapidly in soil and has shown little leaching potential.

Toxicokinetics

Toxicokinetic studies with ^{14}C-cyfluthrin in rats have shown that the initial step of biotransformation includes ester hydrolysis resulting in 3-phenoxy-4-fluorobenzyl alcohol intermediate and permethric acid. 3-Phenoxy-4-fluorobenzyl alcohol is further oxidized to 3-phenoxy-4-fluorobenzoic acid, which is either hydroxylated to 4′-hydroxy-3-phenoxy-4fluorobenzoic or conjugated with glycine to 4′-hydroxy-3-phenoxy-4-fluorobenzoic acid. Cyfluthrin is excreted mainly as urinary metabolites, but a portion of it is also excreted unchanged in feces.

Mechanism of Toxicity

Historically, pyrethroids were grouped into two subclasses, Types I and II, based on chemical structure and the production of either the T (tremor) or the CS (choreoathetosis with salivation) intoxication syndrome following intravenous or intracerebral administration to rodents. Cyfluthrin belongs to Type II (CS) subclass and elicits toxicity by modifying the voltage-sensitive sodium channels in neuronal membranes. It binds to a receptor site on the α-subunit of the sodium channel, which results in prolonged opening of sodium channels. This delay in the closure of sodium channels leads to a protracted sodium influx causing repetitive firing of sensory nerve endings and hyperexcitation. Higher doses of cyfluthrin may result in complete depolarization of the nerve membrane and blockade of nerve conduction.

Acute and Short-Term Toxicity

Animal

Cyfluthrin is moderately toxic to mammals with an oral LD_{50} of 850–1200 mg kg^{-1} in rats. Large doses of cyfluthrin cause excess salivation, irritability, tremors, incoordination, convulsions, and a fall in blood pressure. The acute toxicity of cyfluthrin increases at lower temperatures, and it is also acutely toxic when inhaled.

Human

Cyfluthrin is slightly irritating to skin and eyes in humans. One of the common symptoms of cyfluthrin poisoning is paresthesia (stinging, burning, and itching skin, particularly on the face), progressing to numbness. Dermal irritation may worsen if exposed to sun or heat. Large doses of cyfluthrin may cause excessive salivation, irritability, tremors, convulsions, and death. Inhalation exposure may result in labored breathing and nasal discharge.

Chronic Toxicity

Animal

Chronic exposure to cyfluthrin is reported to cause diarrhea, reduced body temperature, and weight loss in laboratory rats.

 http://dx.doi.org/10.1016/B978-0-12-386454-3.00119-6

A 24-month dietary exposure study showed no organ-specific toxicities in laboratory animals. Long-term inhalation of cyfluthrin is reported to cause adverse effects, including lower body temperature and weight loss.

Human

As cyfluthrin is commonly used on food crops, risks of dietary exposure and through water and air are relatively high. Exposure may also occur through inhalation and contact from indoor and outdoor uses.

Immunotoxicity

In oral dosing studies in rodents, several pyrethroids suppressed the cellular immune response or produced thymus atrophy; however, the significance of these immunological studies to humans is unclear.

Reproductive Toxicity

Cyfluthrin is reported to cause abortions and resorption of fetuses in rabbits, and in rats, it is reported to cause decreased pup viability and body weight.

Genotoxicity

There are no adequate data on genotoxic effects of cyfluthrin. The mutagenic potential of beta-cyfluthrin was studied in various *in vitro* and *in vivo* test systems and none of the test systems used revealed any evidence of mutagenic and/or genotoxic potential of beta-cyfluthrin.

Carcinogenicity

Mutagenicity and carcinogenicity studies have shown no evidence of potential effects in rats and mice.

Clinical Management

General decontamination procedures should be initiated in case of cyfluthrin exposure. In case of dermal exposure, the contaminated area must be washed with plenty of water and soap. Topical application of vitamin E preparations may help reduce the severity of skin reactions. The affected eye must be irrigated with lukewarm water for at least 10 min. The contaminated clothing should be removed and the airway cleared. In case of ingestion, gastric lavage is avoided as solvents present in cyfluthrin formulations may increase the risk of aspiration pneumonia. Atropine (adults and children >12 years: 2–4 mg kg^{-1}; children <12 years: 0.05–0.1 mg kg^{-1}, IV) may be useful to control excessive salivation but care should be taken to avoid excess administration. If prolonged and frequent seizures appear, diazepam should be used for treatment (5–10 mg kg^{-1}, IV).

Ecotoxicology

Cyfluthrin is highly toxic to bees with an $LD_{50} < 0.04$ μg bee^{-1}. It is also highly toxic to marine and freshwater organisms and is least toxic to birds.

Exposure Standards and Guidelines

Acceptable daily intake = 0.004 mg kg^{-1} bw^{-1}.

Chronic oral reference dose (US EPA) = 0.002 4 mg kg^{-1} day^{-1}.

See also: Atropine; Ecotoxicology; Neurotoxicity; Pesticides; Pyrethrins/Pyrethroids.

Further Reading

Laskowski, D.A., 2002. Physical and chemical properties of pyrethroids. Rev. Environ. Contam. Toxicol. 174, 49–170.

Soderlund, D.M., Clark, J.M., Sheets, L.P., Mullin, L.S., Piccirillo, V.J., Sargent, D., Stevens, J.T., Weiner, M.L., 2002. Mechanisms of pyrethroid neurotoxicity: implications for cumulative risk assessment. Toxicology 171, 3–59.

Spencer, J., O'Malley, M., 2006. Pyrethroid illnesses in California, 1996–2002. Rev. Environ. Contam. Toxicol. 186, 57–72.

Wolansky, M.J., Harrill, J.A., 2008. Neurobehavioral toxicology of pyrethroid insecticides in adult animals: a critical review. Neurotoxicol. Teratol. 30, 55–78.

Relevant Websites

http://www.epa.gov/oppsrrd1/reevaluation/pyrethroids-pyrethrins.html – Environmental protection Agency.

http://extoxnet.orst.edu/pips/cyfluthr.htm – Extension Toxicology Network.

http://www.pesticide.org/get-the-facts/pesticide-factsheets/factsheets/cyfluthrin – Journal of Pesticide Reform: Insecticide Fact Sheet - Cyfluthrin.

http://www.who.int/foodsafety/chem/jmpr/publications/pesticide_inventory_report_2010.pdf – Inventory of IPCS and other WHO pesticide evaluations and summary of toxicological evaluations performed by the Joint Meeting on Pesticide Residues (JMPR) through 2010.

http://www.who.int/whopes/quality/en/Cyfluthrin_spec_eval_WHO_Nov_2004.pdf – World Health Organization.

Cypermethrin

SA Burr, Plymouth University Peninsula Schools of Medicine and Dentistry, Plymouth, UK

This article is a revision of the previous edition article by Paul R. Harp, volume 1, pp 714–716, © 2005, Elsevier Inc.

- Chemical Abstracts Service Registry Number: CAS 52315-07-8
- Synonyms: [Cyano-(3-phenoxyphenyl)methyl] 3-(2,2-dichloroethenyl)-2,2-dimethylcyclopropane-1-carboxylate; Ammo; Asymmethrin; Barricade; Cymperator; Cypercopal; Cypermethrine; Hilcyperin; Neramethrin; Ripcord; CID 2912
- Classification: Type II pyrethroid insecticide
- Molecular Formula: $C_{22}H_{19}Cl_2NO_3$, molecular weight 416.29716
- Chemical Structure:

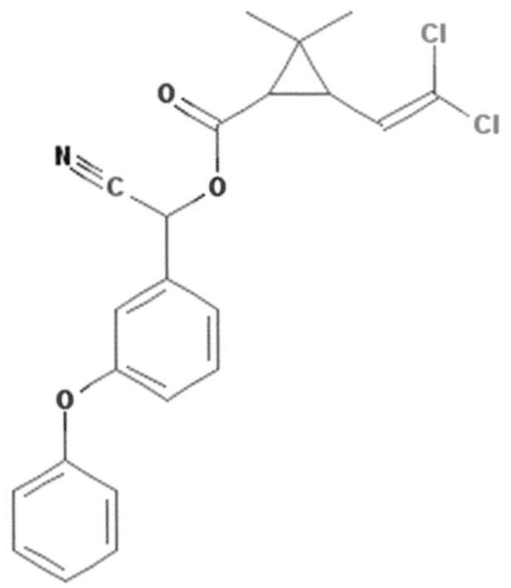

Uses

Cypermethrin is a potent broad-spectrum insecticide used in a range of agricultural, public health, and domestic applications. For arable farming, cypermethrin is one of the most widely used pesticides in terms of total land area treated. Cypermethrin is available as a powder, emulsion, or a concentrate for ultra-low-volume application. Technical cypermethrin is a mixture of eight isomers that includes two active isomers (1R *cis* S and 1S *cis* R isomers).

Environmental Fate

Cypermethrin is sixfold more persistent in soil than in aquatic environments. Depending on conditions, the environmental half-life ranges from 2 days (for hydrolysis at pH 9) to 165 days (for photolysis in soil).

Exposure

Dermal exposure is the most common route, although ingestion and inhalation can occur.

Toxicokinetics

Absorption of pyrethroids is poor through the skin and not much more effective through the gastrointestinal tract. Pyrethroids are rapidly metabolized through ester cleavage and hydroxylation. Pyrethroids accumulate in adipose tissue, which has a varying affinity for the different isomeric forms of cypermethrin. In rat, elimination half-lives of 3.4 and 18 days have been measured for *trans* and *cis* isomers, respectively. Urinary excretion is the primary route of elimination. Fecal excretion can also be significant depending on the animal species and isomeric form.

Mechanism of Toxicity

Cypermethrin is a type II pyrethroid: a functional neurotoxin slowing the inactivation of voltage-gated sodium channels leading to a state of hyperexcitability, which in turn causes fine tremor, salivation, and choreoathetosis. Other proposed contributory actions include antagonism of γ-aminobutyric acid A ($GABA_A$) inhibition, and voltage-gated chloride and calcium channels.

Acute and Short-Term Toxicity

Cypermethrin produces a syndrome in both insects and mammals known as chorea salivation. The effects are hyperexcitability, fine tremor, hypersalivation, choreoathetosis, ataxia, seizures, and death. Humans experience the same effects as other animals, but are also able to report paresthesia after dermal exposure and nausea after ingestion.

Chronic Toxicity, Genotoxicity, and Carcinogenicity

Studies of mice have demonstrated possible genotoxicity in spleen and bone marrow. The US Environmental Protection Agency has classified cypermethrin as a possible human carcinogen based on benign lung adenomas found in mice. Chronic effects following cypermethrin exposure have not been reported in humans.

Clinical Management

Dermal exposure can be treated by washing the contaminated skin with oils. Application of vitamin E cream preparations can be used for both prophylaxis and treatment of paresthesia. With cases of ingestion, gastric decontamination with activated charcoal may be of benefit within the first hour. Gastric lavage should be avoided when formulations contain solvents. If systemic toxicity does occur, the central signs of poisoning can be difficult to control and may be confused with intoxication by other pesticides such as anticholinesterases, which also cause hyperexcitability, although pyrethroids do not inhibit acetylcholinesterase. Respiratory support may be needed and control of metabolic acidosis may require sodium bicarbonate. Atropine may be useful to control

 http://dx.doi.org/10.1016/B978-0-12-386454-3.00120-2

hypersalivation. Single short-lived seizures may not require treatment. Since pyrethroids do not produce morphological damage, only symptomatic treatment is needed. Frequent or prolonged convulsions may be controlled with intravenous diazepam or lorazepam. If unresponsive, consider phenobarbital or phenytoin (before thiopental or general anesthesia). Pentobarbitone has been shown to be more effective than phenobarbitone in animal studies. Complete recovery usually occurs following symptomatic treatment in cases of mild–moderate intoxication.

Ecotoxicology

Birds have a comparatively low susceptibility to cypermethrin, whereas bees, crustaceans, and fish are all highly susceptible under experimental conditions. However, environmental factors such as sediment binding may reduce the actual susceptibility of nontarget aquatic species.

Exposure Standards and Guidelines

The acceptable daily intake set by the Food and Agriculture Organization (FAO)/World Health Organization (WHO) Joint Meeting on Pesticide Residues (JMPR) for cypermethrin is 0–0.02 mg kg^{-1} body weight.

See also: Cyfluthrin; Deltamethrin; Neurotoxicity; Permethrin; Pesticides; Pyrethrins/Pyrethroids.

Further Reading

WHO/IPCS, 1989. Environmental Health Criteria 82: Cypermethrin. World Health Organization, Geneva.

Relevant Websites

http://toxnet.nlm.nih.gov – TOXNET, Toxicology Data Network, National Library of Medicine, Search for Cypermethrin.
http://www.who.int – World Health Organization, Search for Cypermethrin.

Cysteine, *N*-Acetyl-L

SR Clough, Bedford, NH, USA

This article is a revision of the original print edition article by David M Krentz and Linda A Malley, volume 1, pp 392–393, © 1998, Elsevier Inc.

- Chemical Abstracts Service Registry Number: 616-91-1
- Synonyms: L-α-Acetamido-β-mercaptopropionic acid, Acetylcysteine, Airbron, Broncholysin, Brunac, Fabrol, Fluatox, Fluimucetin, Fluimucil, Fluprowit, Inspir, L-α-Acetamido-β-mercaptopropionic acid, Mercapturic acid, Mucocedyl; Mucolator, Mucolyticum, Mucomyst, Muco Sanigen, Mucosil, Mucosol, Mucosolvin, Mucret, *N*-Acetyl-L-cysteine (NAC), *N*-Acetyl-L-(β)-cysteine, *N*-Acetyl-3-mercaptoalanine (IUPAC), Neo-Fluimucil, Parvolex, Respaire, Tixair
- Chemical/Pharmaceutical/Other Class: Mucolytic, Antidote
- Chemical Formula: $C_5H_9NO_3S$
- Chemical Structure:

SH O OH H_3C NH O

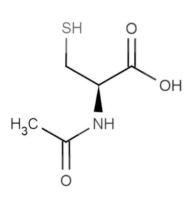

Uses

N-Acetyl-L-cysteine (NAC) is a white crystalline powder that melts in the range of 104–110 °C and has a very slight odor. It is a natural sulfur-containing compound that is produced in living organisms from the amino acid cysteine. It is involved in the intracellular synthesis of a chemical called glutathione (GSH). Cells (particularly liver cells) use GSH to detoxify chemicals by making them more water soluble and thus easier to excrete from the body. NAC is also a powerful antioxidant. NAC is primarily marketed and used as a mucolytic agent to break up mucus (by reducing disulfide bonds in mucoproteins) in persons having bronchopulmonary diseases including chronic bronchitis, cystic fibrosis, asthma, sinusitis, and pneumonia. It is also used extensively as an antidote for acetaminophen (paracetamol) overdose or toxicity. Because it is a precursor of GSH, it has been proven useful in replenishing depleted GSH levels in the liver. Other studies have shown it can be used as a chelating agent for the treatment of heavy metal (mercury, lead, cadmium) poisoning. Other reports (primarily animal studies) have suggested that NAC can find use as a detoxifying agent for a number of toxicants, such as paraquat, urethane, aflatoxin, *Escherichia coli*, carbon tetrachloride, chloroform, and carbon monoxide. NAC is also used for preventing alcoholic liver damage, for reducing toxicity of ifosfamide and doxorubicin (drugs that are used for cancer treatment), as a hangover remedy, for preventing kidney damage due to certain X-ray dyes, and for human immunodeficiency virus.

Exposure Routes and Pathways

The most common route of exposure to NAC is (voluntary) inhalation via the respiratory tract. Inhalation of 1–2 mL of a 10% solution may be given as often as every hour. Although not approved by the US Food and Drug Administration, it may be given intravenously in emergency situations. According to a National Institute for Occupational Safety and Health survey conducted between 1981 and 1983, over 30,000 workers in the United States are exposed to NAC on a daily basis. Over two-thirds of those people are inhalation therapists and clinical laboratory technicians, with the remaining majority in some type of medical profession.

Toxicokinetics

Oral administration of NAC has poor bioavailability, ranging from 4 to 10%. Following oral administration, peak plasma levels occur within 2 or 3 h. With intravenous administration, peak plasma levels occur immediately. Orally administered NAC appears to distribute primarily to the kidneys, liver, and lungs. It is detectable in pulmonary secretions for at least 5 h after the dose. Following respiratory exposure, NAC is rapidly absorbed and exists as the free species in plasma with a concomitant increase both in plasma L-acetylcysteine levels and in protein and nonprotein sulfhydryl concentrations. Protein binding is approximately 83%. The volume of distribution in humans is 0.337–0.47 $l\,kg^{-1}$. Thirty percent of intravenously administered NAC is renally cleared. NAC elimination is not impaired in patients with severe liver damage. The terminal half-life of NAC is 2–6 h and is increased to 11 h in newborns. This may be increased to 13 h after an intravenous injection.

Mechanism of Toxicity

Fatalities from normal doses and overdoses of intravenous NAC have not been reported. This is most probably due to the fact that the body produces this compound naturally and can rapidly metabolize it in the liver. Toxicity is usually limited to anaphylactoid reactions and nausea/vomiting. The average time for the onset of adverse effects following commencement

 http://dx.doi.org/10.1016/B978-0-12-386454-3.00485-1

of the infusion of NAC was 30 min (range, 5–70 min). *In vivo* and *in vitro* tests indicate that NAC is an inhibitor of allergen tolerance by inhibition of prostaglandin E synthesis. Adverse reactions are anaphylactoid in type and have been attributed to cause histamine release.

Acute and Short-Term Toxicity (or Exposure)

N-Acetylcysteine is used primarily in the treatment of acetaminophen (paracetamol) overdose and/or toxicity. It is also nebulized for mucolytic effects and less often used to treat corneal ulcers. It has a very low potential to cause acute toxicity in either animals or humans.

Animal

Oral formulations of *N*-acetylcysteine are used intravenously in the clinical treatment of animals, although it has not been approved for this use. The Registry of Toxic Effects of Chemical Substances (RTECS) lists an acute oral, intravenous, and intraperitoneal LD_{50} in dogs of 1.0, 0.7, and 0.7 g kg^{-1} body weight, respectively. For mice, RTECS lists an oral, intravenous, and intraperitoneal LD_{50} of 4.4, 3.8, and 0.4 g kg^{-1} body weight, respectively. For rats, RTECS lists an oral and intravenous LD_{50} of 5.05 and 1.14 g kg^{-1} body weight, respectively. Acute effects cited for mice include central nervous system depression and somnolence; rats showed gastrointestinal changes.

Human

The primary toxicity of NAC consists of nausea/vomiting, particularly after oral therapy, and an anaphylactoid reaction, particularly after IV administration, that may be life threatening. Many cases of anaphylactic reactions have been reported with symptoms primarily consisting of rash, nausea, hypotension, bronchospasm, angioedema, tachycardia, and respiratory distress. NAC may also have some neurological toxicity that includes dizziness, intracranial hypertension, hypoactivity, ataxia, and seizures. There have been reports of mucosal damage with full strength (20%) NAC, which causes hyperemia and hemorrhages of bowel mucosa. During inhalation therapy, irritation or soreness of the mouth may occur. The RTECS cites a 'lowest published toxic dose' reported for a child of 8.48 g kg^{-1} over a 3-day period. This is a relatively large dose and places this substance in the acute category of 'practically nontoxic.'

Chronic Toxicity (or Exposure)

Animal

NAC has not been shown to cause birth defects in rats or rabbits. When administered to rabbits during the critical phase of embryogenesis, no malformation resulted.

Human

Experience in 59 pregnant patients suggested that use of NAC in pregnancy did not result in toxic effects on the fetus. In practice, the risk to the mother and baby of paracetamol-induced liver damage probably far outweighs any potential risk of *N*-acetylcysteine, and pregnancy should not be considered a contraindication to the use of this agent.

In Vitro Toxicity Data

N-Acetylcysteine is negative in the Ames mutagenicity test and also reduces the mutagenic effect of chemical carcinogens in the same assay.

Clinical Management

Since 1974, it has been known, and generally accepted, that NAC is hepatoprotective, especially for treating overdoses of acetaminophen. Basic and advanced life-support measures should be utilized as necessary. For acetaminophen overdose, a 140 mg kg^{-1} dose followed by 70 mg kg^{-1} every 4 h for an additional 17 doses should be administered. Since NAC has not been approved for intravenous administration, assistance is available through the Rocky Mountain Poison Center. NAC should not be mixed with erythromycin lactobionate or tetracycline.

Environmental Fate

Because NAC is a natural compound that contains no halogen atoms or substitutions, it would be expected to be easily metabolized by microorganisms in the environment and thus not present a risk from the standpoint of persistence or bioaccumulation.

Ecotoxicology

NAC is produced naturally in the body and is therefore not anticipated to be a hazard to ecological receptors.

Exposure Standards and Guidelines

There are no regulatory exposure standards or guidelines for NAC. Acute doses of 140 mg kg^{-1} are recommended for the initial 'loading' dose in humans (i.e., for paracetamol poisoning) and 1330 mg kg^{-1} can be tolerated by humans over a 72-h period.

See also: Acetaminophen; Aflatoxin; Alcoholic Beverages and Health Effects; Carbon Tetrachloride; Chloroform; Carbon Monoxide; *Escherichia coli* (Escherichia Coli); Ethanol; Glutathione; Paraquat; Nitrite Inhalants.

Further Reading

Meredith, T.J., Jacobsen, T., Haines, J.A., Berger, J.C., (Eds.), 1995. IPCS/CES Evaluation of Antidotes Series. Antidotes for Poisoning by Paracetamol, vol. 3 Cambridge University Press on behalf of the World Health Organization and of the Commission of the European Communities.

Relevant Websites

http://www.drugs.com/ppa/acetylcysteine-n-acetylcysteine.html – Drugs.com (Drug Information Online)

http://www.intox.org – IPCS INTOX Data Bank.

http://www.rxlist.com – The Internet Drug Index.

http://chem.sis.nlm.nih.gov/chemidplus/ – US National Library of Medicine

http://www.fda.gov – US Food and Drug Administration.

http://www.webmd.com – WebMD.

Cytochrome P450

K Shankar, University of Arkansas for Medical Sciences, Little Rock, AR, USA
HM Mehendale, University of Louisiana at Monroe, Monroe, LA, USA

Introduction

Evolution of P450s: Cytochrome P450 proteins are one of the largest superfamily of enzyme proteins. Genes encoding cytochrome P450 (called CYP) are found in virtually all genomes. Sequence comparisons indicate that the diverse superfamily originated from a common ancestral gene some 3 billion years ago. The origin of the P450 superfamily lies in prokaryotes, before the advent of eukaryotes and before the accumulation of molecular oxygen in the atmosphere. As a comparison, *Mycobacterium tuberculosis* has 20 P450 genes, Baker's yeast has three and the fruit fly *Drosophila melanogaster* has 83 genes. Humans have 57 different active P450 genes and a similar number (58) of pseudogenes. There are particularly large number of P450 genes in the plants with 323 genes in the rice and 249 genes in the thale cress genomes. In the human genome, the P450 genes are arranged into 18 families and 42 subfamilies. The upregulation of specific forms of CYPs is mediated by numerous xenobiotics, steroid hormones, and their metabolites in addition to environmental carcinogens, such as polyaromatic hydrocarbons. Upon upregulation, cytochrome P450s biotransform the parent compounds as well as the exogenous substrates into toxic metabolites that increase the genotoxic and oxidative load on the cell ultimately influencing cell signaling. This explains the role of CYPs as to how they metabolize procarcinogens to carcinogens, or nontoxic drugs to toxic compounds, occasionally leading to neoplastic progression.

Biochemistry of P450 Enzymes

In vertebrates the liver is the richest source of P450 and is also the most active organ in the oxidation of xenobiotics. P450 enzymes are expressed in the microsomal fraction (smooth endoplasmic reticulum) of the cell where they are anchored in the lipid bilayer. Some P450 isozymes are also localized in the mitochondria. In addition to the liver, P450s are also ubiquitously expressed in the lung, kidney, skin, nasal mucosa, gastrointestinal tract, placenta, bladder, nervous system, blood platelets, among other tissues. Although they are expressed in a variety of tissues, the function of P450s seems to differ in each case. The liver, lung, and small intestine carry out mainly xenobiotic biotransformation. Placental P450s are devoid of ability to metabolize any appreciable xenobiotics but function mainly as a steroid hormone-metabolizing system. Kidney P450s are involved in some metabolism of xenobiotics, but are involved in cholecalciferol and salt balance regulation. Cytochrome P450s are heme–thiolate proteins (iron-containing) of the cytochrome *b* type and derive the name P450 from the wavelength (450 nm) at which the carbon monoxide derivative of the reduced cytochrome has an absorption maximum. Cytochrome P450s, like other monooxygenases, carry out oxidation reactions in which one atom of molecular oxygen is reduced to water while another is incorporated into the substrate. Reducing equivalents are transferred from NADPH to P450 by a flavoprotein enzyme called the NADPH–cytochrome P450 reductase (P450 reductase).

Reactions catalyzed by P450s: P450s catalyze a large number of substrates which may be exogenous or endogenous compounds. P450s carry out aliphatic and aromatic hydroxylations, aromatic epoxidations (leading to stable epoxides like dieldrin from aldrin, or arene oxides), *O*-, *N*-, and *S*-dealkylations and oxidations, oxidative deaminations and desulfurations, among other reactions. Although the primary evolutionary role of the P450 enzymes is to convert hydrophobic xenobiotics into more hydrophilic compounds and enhance their removal from the body, P450s also catalyze reactions, which lead to more reactive (and hence toxic) compounds. Several xenobiotics are converted into potential carcinogens via the cytochrome P450 system.

Major CYP Families

P450 enzymes may be broadly classified into three classes, tentatively designated by functional class (FC)-E, FC-S, and FC-X, based on the characteristics of their substrates and products. FC-E enzymes are essential for the synthesis and degradation of endogenous compounds such as hormones, prostaglandins, and vitamins. FC-X enzymes are directly involved in the detoxication of xenobiotics, whereas FC-S enzymes participate in the biosynthesis and catabolism of secondary metabolites. This categorization is not strict, and the boundaries between the functional classes are often ambiguous. For example, mammalian CYP1–CYP4 are usually considered to be detoxification enzymes; however, they are also involved in the metabolism of steroids and eicosanoids crucial for mammalian life processes. Human cytochrome P450s that metabolize xenobiotic compounds are almost exclusively in the CYP1–CYP4 and to a some degree CYP (5, 8, 19, 21, 26) families. **Table 1** shows all possible forms of CYP450s reported in humans compiled by Karolinska Institute (updated 2011).

The CYP1 family consists of three genes and two subfamilies. Genes in this family are controlled by the aryl hydrocarbon (Ah receptor), which is activated most notably by components of incineration products and cigarette smoke. CYP1A1 and CYP1B1 are expressed in varying amounts in different tissues and are most efficient in metabolizing polycyclic aromatic hydrocarbons, while CYP1A2 preferentially metabolizes arylamines and *N*-heterocyclics. In addition, CYP1A2 metabolizes about 10–20 drugs, whereas CYP1B1 and CYP1A1 do not seem to act mainly as drugs. The CYP2 family is the largest P450 family in humans containing 16 individual isozymes. Human CYP2C8, CYP2C9, CYP2C18, and CYP2C19 together metabolize to varying amounts greater than half of all frequently prescribed drugs. Results from *in vitro* assays show that CYP2D6 metabolizes more than 75 drugs. CYP2E1, a prominent bioactivator in toxicology, metabolizes several compounds

 http://dx.doi.org/10.1016/B978-0-12-386454-3.00299-2

Table 1 Human cytochrome P450s (CYP) allele nomenclature (Karolinska Institute)

Family name	*Name of the isozyme*	*References*
POR	Cytochrome P450 oxidoreductase	http://www.cypalleles.ki.se/por.htm
CYP1	CYP1A1; CYP1A2; CYP1B1	http://www.cypalleles.ki.se/cyp1a1.htm http://www.cypalleles.ki.se/cyp1a2.htm http://www.cypalleles.ki.se/cyp1b1.htm
CYP2	CYP2A6; CYP2A13; CYP2B6; CYP2C8; CYP2C9; CYP2C19; CYP2D6; CYP2E1; CYP2F1; CYP2J2; CYP2R1; CYP2S1; CYP2W1	http://www.cypalleles.ki.se/cyp2a6.htm http://www.cypalleles.ki.se/cyp2a13.htm http://www.cypalleles.ki.se/cyp2b6.htm http://www.cypalleles.ki.se/cyp2c8.htm http://www.cypalleles.ki.se/cyp2c9.htm http://www.cypalleles.ki.se/cyp2c19.htm http://www.cypalleles.ki.se/cyp2d6.htm http://www.cypalleles.ki.se/cyp2e1.htm http://www.cypalleles.ki.se/cyp2f1.htm http://www.cypalleles.ki.se/cyp2j2.htm http://www.cypalleles.ki.se/cyp2r1.htm http://www.cypalleles.ki.se/cyp2S1.htm http://www.cypalleles.ki.se/cyp2w1.htm
CYP3	CYP3A4; CYP3A5; CYP3A7; CYP3A43	http://www.cypalleles.ki.se/cyp3a4.htm http://www.cypalleles.ki.se/cyp3a5.htm http://www.cypalleles.ki.se/cyp3a7.htm http://www.cypalleles.ki.se/cyp3a43.htm
CYP4	CYP4A11; CYP4A22; CYP4B1; CYP4F2	http://www.cypalleles.ki.se/cyp4a11.htm http://www.cypalleles.ki.se/cyp4a22.htm http://www.cypalleles.ki.se/cyp4b1.htm http://www.cypalleles.ki.se/cyp4f2.htm
CYP>4	CYP5A1; CYP8A1; CYP19A1; CYP21A2; CYP26A1	http://www.cypalleles.ki.se/cyp5a1.htm http://www.cypalleles.ki.se/cyp8a1.htm http://www.cypalleles.ki.se/cyp19a1.htm http://www.cypalleles.ki.se/cyp21.htm http://www.cypalleles.ki.se/cyp26a1.htm

including acetaminophen, benzene, chloroform, carbon tetrachloride, butadiene, vinyl chloride, etc. The CYP3 family has four members and has the most abundantly expressed P450s in the liver. CYP3A4 and CYP3A5 are known to metabolize more than 120 frequently prescribed drugs. The CYP3A family is regulated via the pregnane-X-receptor, a nuclear receptor which can be induced by pregnenolone-related compounds.

Endogenous Functions of P450s

Following the sequencing of the human genome all the human P450s have been identified. However, while the endogenous physiological role of the majority of P450s remains unknown, as a group P450s are essential for mammalian development. Studies in mice lacking the microsomal NADPH–cytochrome P450 oxidoreductase and hence devoid of P450 activity, reveal a requirement for P450s around embryonic day 10.5, resulting in embryonic lethality by day 13.5. Deletion of P450 activity in the liver, on the other hand, does not lead to embryonic lethality, suggesting that hepatic microsomal P450-mediated steroid hormone metabolism is not essential for fertility. However, endogenous lipid metabolism and the ability to metabolize xenobiotics such as acetaminophen and phenobarbital are profoundly affected, highlighting the central role of hepatic P450s. The biological roles of several individual P450 isozymes are now becoming clear with the use of gene knockout and transgenic animals. Three important biological systems that are highly dependent on P450 enzymes require special mention.

Cholesterol Metabolism and Bile Acid Biosynthesis

At least seven cytochrome P450 enzymes play critical roles in conversion of acetate into sterols and bile acids. Key among these are the CYP51A1, CYP7A1, CYP7B1, and CYP39A1. The roles of each of these enzymes are beyond the scope of this article, but some excellent reviews and texts are available on the topic.

Steroid Synthesis and Metabolism

Six P450s participate in steroid synthesis. CYP11A1 catalyzes the synthesis of pregnenolone. CYP17A1 is required for the biosynthesis of cortisol, testosterone, and estrogen. CYP19A1 converts androgenic steroids to estrogens. CYP11B2, CYP21A1, and CYP21A2 are also involved in the intermediary steps in the formation of corticosterone and aldosterone.

Vitamin D_3 Biosynthesis and Metabolism

The vitamin D_3 system which acutely controls calcium status, in addition to a host of other physiological functions, is a classic example of P450 in multiple tissues, and it is also involved in the biosynthesis of a biologically active metabolite. Cholecalciferol is hydroxylated at the 25th position by either CYP27A1 or CYP2D25, both of which are expressed in the liver. The 25-hydroxycholecalciferol undergoes another P450-mediated hydroxylation at the 1-α position by the renal CYP27B1 to the active 1,25-dihydroxycholecalciferol (vitamin D_3). Most of the biological function is attributed to this metabolite, although recent studies suggest that even the 25-hydroxy metabolite may be exerting certain biological effects. The degradation of the active 1,25-vitamin D_3 is catalyzed by the renal CYP24A1 enzyme, which catalyzes a third 24-hydroxylation leading to 1,24,25-vitamin D_3 metabolite.

See also: Biotransformation; Mechanisms of Toxicity; Vitamin A; Vitamin C (Ascorbic Acid); Vitamin D; Vitamin E.

Further Reading

Cavallari, L.H., Jeong, H., Bress, A., 2011. Role of cytochrome P450 genotype in the steps toward personalized drug therapy. Pharmacogenomics Pers. Med. 4, 123–136.

Gotoh, O., 2012. Evolution of cytochrome P450 genes from the viewpoint of genome informatics. Biol. Pharm. Bull. 35 (6), 812–817.

McGraw, J., Waller, D., 2012. Cytochrome P450 variations in different ethnic populations. Exp. Opin. Drug Metabol. Toxicol. 8 (3), 371–382.

Nelson, D.R., 2009. The cytochrome P450 homepage. Hum. Genomics 4 (1), 59–65.

Nelson, D.R., 2011. Progress in tracing the evolutionary paths of cytochrome P450. Biochim. Biophys. Acta Protein Proteonomics 1814 (1), 14–18.

Sridhar, J., Liu, J., Foroozesh, M., Stevens, C.L., 2012. Insights on cytochrome P450 enzymes and inhibitors obtained through QSAR studies. Molecules 17 (8), 9283–9305.

Zanger, U.M., 2012. Cytochrome P450 Polymorphisms. Encyclopedia of Drug Metabolism and Interactions, Published Online: 31 Jan 2012, http://dx.doi.org/10.1002/9780470921920.edm009

Relevant Websites

http://drnelson.uthsc.edu/CytochromeP450.html – Cytochrome P450 Homepage.

http://www.humgenomics.com/content/pdf/1479-7364-4-1-59.pdf – GENOME DATABASES - The Cytochrome P450 Homepage.

http://www.genenames.org/genefamily/cyp.php – HUGO Gene Nomenclature Committee - Cytochrome P450s.

http://www.cypalleles.ki.se/ – The Human Cytochrome P450 (CYP) Allele Nomenclature Database.

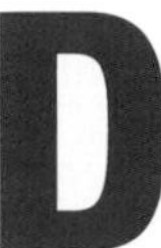

2,4-D (2,4-Dichlorophenoxy Acetic Acid)

KD Chadwick and RS Mangipudy, Bristol-Myers Squibb, Drug Safety Evaluation, New Brunswick, NJ, USA

This article is a revision of the previous edition article by Raja S. Mangipudy and Harihara M. Mehendale, volume 1, pp. 721–723, © 2005, Elsevier Inc.

- Name: 2,4-Dichlorophenoxy acetic acid
- Chemical Abstracts Service Registry Number: 94-75-7
- Synonyms: 2,4-Dichlorophenoxyacetic acid; 2,4-Di-chlorophenoxyacetic acid
- Molecular Formula: $C_8H_6Cl_2O_3$
- Chemical Structure:

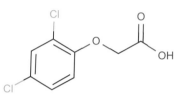

Background and Uses

2,4-D free acids, esters, amines, and salts are formulated in water suspensions or solutions, or in various organic solvents, for application as systemic herbicides that are used post-emergence for selective control of broadleaf weeds. 2,4-D is registered with the US Environmental Protection Agency (EPA) for use on a variety of food/feed sites, turf, lawn, aquatic sites, and forestry applications, and as a growth regulator in citrus crops. Residents and professional applicators may use 2,4-D on home lawns.

Environmental Fate and Behavior

2,4-D has a relatively short half-life and is rather immobile in soil. Soil half-lives have been estimated at 10 days for the acid, diethylamine, and ester forms. The half-life of 2,4-D in aerobic aquatic environments was estimated at 15 days and >41 days in anaerobic aquatic laboratory studies.

The acid, amine, and ester forms of 2,4-D are metabolized to compounds of nontoxicological significance and ultimately to forms of carbon. Therefore, 2,4-D is considered to be a biodegradable compound. Under normal conditions, 2,4-D residues are not persistent in soil, water, or vegetation.

Exposure

2,4-D may be encountered as a vapor, as a liquid, or in mixtures. It may cause damage at the point of contact (skin, eyes, lungs, or gastrointestinal tract (GI tract)). Occupational exposure may occur through inhalation and dermal contact when 2,4-D is produced or used.

Laboratory testing for 2,4-D is not widely available to physicians. The literature has reported the use of high performance liquid chromatography with tandem mass spectrometry to detect 2,4-D.

Toxicokinetics

Rapid and complete absorption of chlorophenoxy compounds from the GI tract has been reported. Nearly complete absorption of 2,4-D occurs within 24 h in humans. 2,4-D is primarily metabolized by acid hydrolysis, and a minor amount is conjugated. It is highly protein bound and widely distributed. The primary organs of deposition are kidneys, liver, and the central and peripheral nervous systems.

2,4-D is primarily excreted unchanged (90%) in the kidneys via the renal organic anion secretory system. It may be conjugated to glycine or taurine. A minor fraction of 2,4-D is filtered by the glomerulus. The estimated half-life of 2,4-D is ~18 h.

Mechanism of Toxicity

2,4-D is a plant-growth regulator that appears to function by causing uncontrolled cell division in vascular tissue. It stimulates nucleic acid and protein synthesis and affects enzyme activity and respiration. It is absorbed by plant leaves, stems, and roots, and moves throughout the plant. It accumulates in growing tips.

Acute and Short-Term Toxicity

Animal

2,4-D generally has low oral toxicity orally or dermally, or by inhalation. The oral LD_{50} values range from 639 to 1646 $mg\,kg^{-1}$ in rats depending on the chemical form of 2,4-D. Mice are more sensitive to 2,4-D, with an LD_{50} of 138 $mg\,kg^{-1}$. Acute dermal LD_{50} values are $\geq$1829 $mg\,kg^{-1}$ in rabbits, depending on the chemical form tested.

Acid and salt forms of 2,4-D are severe eye irritants. The ester and salt forms are considered slight skin irritants.

Dogs are more sensitive to chlorophenoxy acid herbicides than other animals. Signs of toxicity in dogs include

 http://dx.doi.org/10.1016/B978-0-12-386454-3.00300-6

myotonia, vomiting, and weakness. Rats demonstrated lack of coordination, central nervous system depression, and muscle weakness.

Subchronic oral exposure in rats causes damage to the eye, thyroid, kidney, adrenals, ovaries, and testes.

Human

Case reports and observational studies provide the majority of the information regarding exposure (poisoning) in humans. A 2004 report compiled medical cases of 69 people who ingested 2,4-D and other chlorophenoxy herbicides; 23 died. Symptoms of acute oral 2,4-D exposure include vomiting, abdominal pain, diarrhea, headache, confusion, aggressive or bizarre behavior, and hypotension. A peculiar breath odor is sometimes noted. Neuromuscular effects including twitching, weakness, and loss of tendon reflexes have lasted from several weeks to permanently.

Chronic Toxicity

Animal

Chronic toxicity in the eye, kidney, thyroid, and liver of the rat was comparable to the subchronic studies.

Human

No human data have been reported on chronic effects of 2,4-D except epidemiological studies of cancer occurrence; see Carcinogenicity section for further information.

Immunotoxicity

Based on the effects observed on the thyroid and gonads, there is concern about endocrine disruption potential. The US EPA has requested additional studies and assessments including immunotoxicity.

Reproductive Toxicity

Teratogenic effects of 2,4-D have been observed in the rat but only when maximal renal clearance has been met or exceeded. Developmental effects included increased incidence of skeletal abnormalities.

In rats dosed orally with $100\,\mathrm{mg\,kg^{-1}\,day^{-1}}$ 2,4-D from birth to 25 days of age had lower levels of acetylcholinesterase in the olfactory bulb and the hippocampus region of the brain. Monoamine neurotransmitters were also reduced. These results may account for slower learning in rats that were exposed to 2,4-D during postnatal development of the brain.

Genotoxicity

2,4-D has been active in many different short-term genetic assays, including DNA damage and repair, mutations in yeast and humans cells, sex-linked recessive mutations in fruit flies, and chromosome aberrations *in vitro*.

Carcinogenicity

No oncogenic effects were observed in mice or rats following 2 years of dietary exposure with 2,4-D.

The link between 2,4-D and non-Hodgkin's lymphoma in humans has been suggested based on epidemiologic data, but despite reviews of the epidemiologic data by US EPA, 2,4-D has been classified as 'not classifiable as to human carcinogenicity.' The most recent review in 2004 indicated that none of the recent epidemiological studies definitively linked human cancer cases to 2,4-D. The International Agency for Research on Cancer (IARC) had not assigned 2,4-D a cancer rating as of October 2011. However, in 1987, IARC placed the family of chlorophenoxy herbicides in the group of compounds that are 'possibly carcinogenic to humans.'

A confounding factor in determining the carcinogenicity of 2,4-D is the frequent use of 2,4-D in mixtures with other agents, especially 2,4,5-T and its contaminant TCDD (dioxin). The possibility that 2,4-D may be a human carcinogen will require further assessment.

Clinical Management

No specific antidote is available. The patient must be monitored for seizures, gastrointestinal irritation, possible liver, kidney, or muscle damage, arrhythmias, acidosis, dyspnea, headache, coma, hyperthermia, and hypotension. Gastric lavage and activated charcoal/cathartic are probably more useful decontamination methods.

Ecotoxicology

2,4-D is toxic to terrestrial and aquatic plants. 2,4-D is considered to be moderately to practically nontoxic to birds and slightly toxic to small mammals. 2,4-D acid and amine salts are slightly to practically nontoxic to freshwater or marine fish and aquatic invertebrates. 2,4-D esters are highly toxic to fish and freshwater and marine invertebrates.

Other Hazards

To keep residues of 2,4-D out of meat or milk, dairy cattle should not be grazed on treated areas for 7 days after application. Also, hay should not be cut for 30 days and meat animals should not be slaughtered for 3 days. Contact with dried residues on vegetation is not expected to be hazardous. Inert ingredients found in 2,4-D products may include ethylene glycol, methanol, sequestering agents, petroleum hydrocarbons, and surfactants. Ethylene glycol is moderately toxic to humans; it may cause tearing, anesthesia, headache, cough, respiratory stimulation, nausea or vomiting, and pulmonary, kidney, and liver changes. Methanol is moderately toxic to humans; it may cause damage to the optic nerve, tearing, headache, cough, difficult breathing, other respiratory effects, nausea, or vomiting. Some commercially formulated 2,4-D products have LD_{50} values that are much higher than the 2,4-D acid. This indicates that these formulations may have considerably less acute toxicity than the acid form. However, exposure to these formulated products may have other health effects similar to those reported for 2,4-D alone or for inert ingredients in commercial formulations. Some 2,4-D formulations may be contaminated with halogenated dibenzo-*p*-dioxins (but not TCDD), dibenzofurans, or *N*-nitrosamines. Dibenzodioxins and dibenzofurans may cause disorders of the skin, blood, and gastrointestinal tract; they may also cause headaches, numbness, birth defects, or fetal toxicity. Nitrosamines are carcinogenic.

The Material Safety Data Sheet should always be referred to for detailed information on handling and disposal.

Exposure Standards and Guidelines

- Acceptable daily intake is 0.3 $mg\,kg^{-1}\,day^{-1}$
- Maximum contaminant level is 0.07 $mg\,l^{-1}$
- Reference dose is 0.01 $mg\,kg^{-1}\,day^{-1}$
- Permissible exposure limit is 10 $mg\,m^{-3}$ (8 h)

See also: Chlorophenoxy Herbicides.

Further Reading

Burns, C.J., Swaen, G.M., 2012. Review of 2,4-dichlorophenoxyacetic acid (2,4-D) biomonitoring and epidemiology. Crit. Rev. Toxicol. 42 (9), 768–786.

Burns, C., Bodner, K., Swaen, G., Collins, J., Beard, K., Lee, M., 2011. Cancer incidence of 2,4-D production workers. Int. J. Environ. Res. Public Health 8 (9), 3579–3590.

Baharuddin, M.R., Sahid, I.B., Noor, M.A., Sulaiman, N., Othman, F., 2011. Pesticide risk assessment: a study on inhalation and dermal exposure to 2,4-D and Paraquat among Malaysian paddy farmers. J. Environ. Sci. Health Sec. B 46 (7), 600–607.

Gervais, J.A., Luukinen, B., Buhl, K., Stone, D., 2008. 2,4-D Technical Fact Sheet. National Pesticide Information Center, Oregon State University Extension Services. http://npic.orst.edu/factsheets/2,4-DTech.pdf.

Mazhar, F.M., Moawad, K.M., El-Dakdoky, M.H., Amer, A.S., 4 September 2012. Fetotoxicity of 2,4-dichlorophenoxyacetic acid in rats and the protective role of vitamin E. Toxicol. Ind. Health [Epub ahead of print].

Relevant Websites

http://www.aphis.usda.gov/publications/biotechnology/2012/faq_dow_tolerant_soybean.pdf – Animal and Plant Health Inspection Service.

http://www.cdpr.ca.gov/docs/risk/toxsums/toxsumlist.htm – California EPA Department of Pesticides Regulation. Search for 2,4-D under Toxicology Data Review Summaries.

http://www.npic.orst.edu/ – National Pesticide Information Center, maintained by Oregon State University. Search for 2,4-D Technical Fact Sheet.

http://toxnet.nlm.nih.gov – TOXNET, Specialized Information Services, National Library of Medicine. Search for 2,4-D.

http://www.epa.gov/pesticides – US Environmental Protection Agency website. Search for 2,4-D.

Dacarbazine

A Murray, Manchester University College of Pharmacy, Fort Wayne, IN, USA

- Name: Dacarbazine
- Representative Chemical: Triazene Alkylating Agent
- Chemical Abstracts Service Registry Number: 4342-03-4
- Synonyms: (Dimethyltriazeno)imidazolecarboxamide; 1*H*-imidazole-4-carboxamide, 5-(3,3-dimethyl-1-triazenyl); 4(5)-(3,3-Dimethyl-1-triazeno)imidazole-4-carboxamide; 4-(3,3-Dimethyl-1-triazeno)imidazole-5-carboxamide; 4-(5)-(3,3-Dimethyl-1-triazeno)imidazole-5(4)-carboxamide; 4-(Dimethyltriazeno)imidazole-5-carboxamide; 4-(or 5)-(3,3-Dimethyl-1-triazeno)imidazole-5(or 4)-carboxamide; 5-(3,3-Dimethyl-1-triazeno)imidazole-4-carboxamide; 5-(3,3-Dimethyltriazeno)imidazole-4-carboxamide; 5-Dimethyltriazeno)imidazole-4-carboxamide; AI3-52825; Biocarbazine; Biocarbazine R; CCRIS 190; Carboxamide, 5-(3,3-dimethyl-1-triazeno)imidazole-4; DIC; DTIC; DTIC-Dome; Dacarbazine; Dacarbazino; Dacarbazino [INN-Spanish]; Dacarbazinum; Dacarbazinum [INN-Latin]; Decarbazine; Deticene; Di-me-triazenoimidazolecarboxamide; EINECS 224-396-1; HSDB 3219; ICDMT; Imidazole-4-carboxamide, 5-(3,3-dimethyl-1-triazenyl); NCI-C04717; NSC 45388; NSC-45388; UNII-7GR28W0FJI
- Molecular Formula: $C_6H_{10}N_6O$
- Chemical Structure:

H3C, H3C, N, N, N, H, N, N, H2N, O

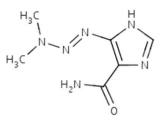

Background

Dacarbazine is a colorless to an ivory-colored solid belonging to the alkylating class of antineoplastic medications. Alkylating agents were the first anticancer molecules developed. Within this group of compounds, there are six major classes of agents; with dacarbazine categorized as part of the triazenes. The nitrogen mustards, the first of the alkylating agents, were approved for clinical use in the 1940s; while the triazene compound, dacarbazine, was not approved for use in humans until 1975. DTIC, or 5-(3,3-dimethyltriazeno) imidazole-4-carboxamide is an imidazole-carboxamide derivative synthesized for the first time in 1959. In order to synthesize the drug, nitrous acid was added to the 5-diazoimidazole derivative and this molecule was then treated in a solution of dimethylamine in methanol. Dacarbazine is used therapeutically primarily in melanoma and Hodgkin's disease.

Uses

Dacarbazine is used therapeutically to treat various oncologic malignancies, typically in combination regimens. The primary FDA-approved indication for this compound is in treatment of metastatic malignant melanoma. In addition, it is approved as a second line therapy in Hodgkin's disease when used in combination with other effective agents. Dacarbazine is also commonly used off-label in soft tissue sarcoma. Dacarbazine, like other chemotherapeutic treatment options, is being researched for its antineoplastic effects in other malignancies. In the future, dacarbazine may be useful as treatment for various oncology-related diseases.

Environmental Fate and Behavior

Dacarbazine is a colorless to an ivory-colored crystalline solid that must be reconstituted and administered as a parenteral agent for intravenous injection. It is available as a dry powder in 100, 200, and 500 mg vials that when reconstituted have a standard concentration of 10 mg dacarbazine per 1 ml solution and a pH of 3–4. Vials of dacarbazine should be refrigerated (2–8 °C) and protected from light. When exposed to light, dacarbazine is rapidly decomposed to 4-diazoimidazole-5-carboxamide. When exposed to high temperatures (250–255 °C) dacarbazine decomposes explosively. Dacarbazine is slightly soluble in water. Dacarbazine may be diluted in either normal saline or dextrose 5% water. Reconstituted solution is stable for 24 h at room temperature (20 °C) and 96 h under refrigeration (4 °C); however, it is recommended by the manufacturer to use the product within 8 and 72 h, respectively. Dacarbazine should not be used if it turns pink, as this is a sign of decomposition.

Exposure and Exposure Monitoring

Exposure Routes and Pathways

Exposure to dacarbazine may occur through dermal contact, inhalation, or accidental ingestion during its production, preparation, administration, or cleanup of medical waste. In addition, excretions of recipients who are administered dacarbazine also pose a risk of exposure to those who may clean up this type of waste. Appropriate work practices play an important role in avoiding occupational exposure.

Toxicokinetics

Oral absorption of dacarbazine is unpredictable and slow; and therefore this compound is only given intravenously. The volume of distribution following intravenous administration

 http://dx.doi.org/10.1016/B978-0-12-386454-3.01213-6

of dacarbazine is $0.63\,l\,kg^{-1}$, which exceeds total human body water content. This implies localization of the medication to body tissue, most notably the liver. Dacarbazine is extensively metabolized via the cytochrome P450 system and is a major substrate of both CYP1A2 and CYP2E1. Dacarbazine is primarily excreted renally via renal tubular secretion. The major inactive metabolite, AIC, and unchanged drug are both excreted renally. Dacarbazine exhibits a biphasic half-life with an initial half-life of 19 min and a terminal half-life of 5 h. In the presence of renal and hepatic dysfunction, the half-life may be extended up to 55 min and 7.2 h, respectively.

Mechanism of Toxicity

The exact mechanism of action of dacarbazine is unknown; however, several proposed mechanisms have been made including inhibition of DNA synthesis by acting as a purine analog, alkylating agent, and interference with sulfhydryl groups. It is most commonly classified as an alkylating agent in the triazene group. While the active compound of dacarbazine, DTIC, is structurally similar to purines, its primary mechanism of action precludes the agent from being classified as an antimetabolite. Dacarbazine is a synthetic compound that is metabolically activated to the active alkylating metabolite methyl-triazeno-imidazole-carboxamide (MTIC) via the cytochrome P450 system, primarily CYP1A1, CYP1A2, and CYP 2E1. MTIC is rapidly tautomerized into an inactive derivative, 5-aminoimidazole-4-carboxamide (AIC), which is renally excreted. The entire process of activating DTIC occurs within 15 min of intravenous infusion. DTIC exerts its actions throughout all phases of the cellular cycle. The antitumor effects of this compound are related to the induction of methyl adducts to DNA. The 70% of alkylation occurs at the N_7 position of guanine. The cytotoxic and mutagenic effects of MTIC are manifested through alkylation of DNA at the O_6 guanine position, accounting for 6–8% of methylated bases formed. This is primarily a result of generation of incorrect base pairing, leading to DNA double strand breaks and apoptosis.

Short- and Long-Term Toxicities

Animal

The following LD_{50} values were determined in rats and mice for oral, intravenous, and intraperitoneal administration, respectively: $2147\,mg\,kg^{-1}$, $411\,mg\,kg^{-1}$, and $350\,mg\,kg^{-1}$; $2032\,mg\,kg^{-1}$, $466\,mg\,kg^{-1}$, $567\,mg\,kg^{-1}$. Similar toxicity effects were observed in both rats and mice including changes in motor activity and antipsychotic behavioral effects.

Human

The primary toxicity to humans associated with dacarbazine is gastrointestinal effects including nausea and vomiting. More than 90% of patients will experience this effect within 1–3 h after treatment. During treatment, a flulike syndrome may occur including chills, fever, malaise, and myalgias. Upon administration, irritation to skin may occur. Extravasation is an additional risk of this medication which may lead to tissue necrosis. Like other cytotoxic agents, myelosuppression with both leukopenia and thrombocytopenia is an effect typically occurring on days 5–7 after treatment, with recovery occurring days 21–28. Severe, but rare toxicities with dacarbazine have been reported relating to liver failure and death. Cases presented in the literature confirmed by autopsy patients developing hepatic vein thrombosis leading to hepatic necrosis and ultimately death. Hepatic injury with dacarbazine is poorly understood and warrants further research.

Immunizations (vaccines), either during or after treatment with this drug can be harmful. Dacarbazine can influence the immune system, making vaccinations ineffective. It can lead to serious infections if a live virus vaccine is used during or soon after treatment. Close contact with people who have recently received a live virus vaccine must be avoided (oral polio vaccine or smallpox vaccine). Doctors approval is required is advised. Dacarbazine can make humans sensitive to sunlight or bright ultraviolet light, with redness, rash, hives, itching, or other symptoms. Because of the way this drug is administered, humans have a higher long-term risk of getting a second type of cancer, such as leukemia.

Reproductive Toxicity

Dacarbazine has been studied in animals for its reproductive effects in both male and female rats as well as rabbits. When male rats were given dosages up to $50\,mg\,kg^{-1}$ twice per week for 9 weeks of dacarbazine, no effect was noted on fertility. Similarly, no adverse effects were noted on fertility in female rats given dacarbazine dosages up to $30\,mg\,kg^{-1}\,day^{-1}$ for 2 weeks prior to mating. However, when evaluating effects on offspring of female rats administered dacarbazine, many abnormalities were observed. Various timing during pregnancy and dosing of dacarbazine was evaluated for effects on offspring. Administration of a single dose of dacarbazine (800 or $1000\,mg\,kg^{-1}$) to pregnant rats on day 11 or 12 of gestation produced skeletal reduction defects, craniofacial anomalies, and encephaloceles. Intraperitoneal administration at doses of $30\,mg\,kg^{-1}\,day^{-1}$ and higher throughout organogenesis was also related to skeletal defects. In addition, decreases in litter size were also observed. When higher dacarbazine doses of 50 and $70\,mg\,kg^{-1}\,day^{-1}$ were administered, major malformations occurred in rat offspring. When intraperitoneally administered at the end of pregnancy, tremors occurred. Rabbits were also evaluated for fetal abnormalities. Dacarbazine produced abortion and increased malformations when given at a dose of $10\,mg\,kg^{-1}\,day^{-1}$ in pregnant rabbits. Skeletal abnormalities were also noted in the offspring of rabbits when given a dose seven times the human dose on days 6–15 of gestation. No adverse effects were noted when the dacarbazine dose was $5\,mg\,kg^{-1}\,day^{-1}$. Dacarbazine was studied in a group of pregnant women in 1997. Healthy babies were born to these women; however, due to the effects noted in animal studies and limited human data, this compound should only be used in pregnancy if the potential benefit outweighs the potential risk to the fetus. In addition, it is not recommended to breast-feed while using dacarbazine due to the potential for serious adverse reactions to the nursing infant.

Genotoxicity

Genotoxicity is a concern with antineoplastic agents, which may go on to cause other malignancies in the host. Dacarbazine has been shown *in vitro* in rodent cell assays to interact with the genetic material of normal cells. The mechanism by which dacarbazine exerts genotoxic effects is not well understood, though it may be due in part by the methylation of DNA. The dacarbazine intermediary causes methylation at the N_7 and O_6 positions, as previously discussed. Genotoxicity occurring from the O_6 methylation has been shown in one study to account for approximately 12% of miscoding of DNA, suggesting this may only be a secondary cause of genotoxicity by dacarbazine. In addition, dacarbazine was shown in an *in vitro* study in human lymphocytes to be an inducer of genotoxic damage. Cytogenic assays were used to assess for chromosomal aberrations, breakage, and loss. At higher dacarbazine concentrations, higher levels of chromosomal aberrations were observed.

Carcinogenicity

Dacarbazine has demonstrated carcinogenicity in experimental cancer studies in both rats and mice. When given orally to either male or female rats, or intraperitoneally in female rats only, dacarbazine caused cancers of the mammary glands, spleen, and thymus. In addition, brain tumors occurred following oral administration in female rats. When administered intraperitoneally to both male and female mice, lung tumors occurred. Lymphoma and blood-vessel tumors occurred solely in male mice; while uterine tumors developed in female mice. Further study is needed to evaluate the carcinogenicity risk in humans administered dacarbazine. To date, two studies have evaluated this risk with no reported incidences. However, the first was a retrospective cohort study with a small number of patients evaluated. Dacarbazine is reasonably anticipated to be a human carcinogen based on studies in experimental animals; however, the human relationship between cancer and exposure to dacarbazine is inadequate at this time.

Clinical Management

The major limiting effect of dacarbazine is the nausea and vomiting induced within 1–3 h after infusion. Premedication with antinausea medication is typically administered to patients who receive dacarbazine in order to alleviate this side effect. Dacarbazine should be used in caution in patients with renal or hepatic impairment and monitored closely for toxicity. A complete blood count with differential and liver function tests should be monitored prior to each treatment of dacarbazine and throughout therapy.

Exposure Standards and Guidelines

As with other chemotherapeutic agents, handling of dacarbazine must take place in a separated, clearly marked working area. Personal protective precautions should take place when handling dacarbazine including respiratory, hand, eye, and skin precautions. In cases of accidental spills, clean-up measures should be in place including typical personal protective procedures as well as methods for effective cleanup and removal of the contamination. Dacarbazine should not enter drains or waterways to avoid environmental exposure. Waste materials should be disposed separately in containers and disposed off as hazardous waste.

See also: Chromosome Aberrations; Toxicity, Acute; Toxicity, Subchronic and Chronic; Cancer Chemotherapeutic Agents; Cytochrome P450; Genetic Toxicology; Carcinogen–DNA Adduct Formation and DNA Repair; Triazines.

Further Reading

Khan, F., Sherwani, A.F., Afzal, M., 2010. Analysis of genotoxic damage induced by dacarbazine: an in vitro study. Toxin Rev. 29, 130–136.

Marchesi, F., Turriziani, M., Tortorelli, G., et al., 2007. Triazene compounds: mechanism of action and related DNA repair systems. Pharmacol. Res. 56, 275–287.

Psaroudi, M.C., Kyrtopoulos, S.A., 2000. Toxicity, mutation frequency and mutation spectrum induced dacarbazine in CHO cells expressing different levels of O6-methylguanine-DNA methyltransferase. Mutat. Res. 447, 257–265.

US Department of Health and Human Services/National Toxicology Program, June 10, 2011. Report on Carcinogens, twelfth ed. Dacarbazine (4342-03-4).

Warr, D., 2012. Management of highly emetogenic chemotherapy. Curr. Opin. Oncol. 24 (4), 371–375.

Dalapon

DR Wallace, Oklahoma State University Center for Health Sciences, Tulsa, OK, USA

This article is a revision of the previous edition article by Priya Raman, volume 1, pp 723–724, © 2005, Elsevier Inc.

- Name: Dalapon
- Chemical Abstracts Service Registry Number: 75-99-0
- Synonyms: Alatex, Basinex P, Dalacide, Devipon, Ded-Weed, Dowpon, Dalapon 85, Dowpon-M, Radapon liquid, Revenge
- Chemical/Pharmaceutical/Other Class: Herbicide (halogenated aliphatic)
- Molecular Formula: $C_3H_4Cl_2O_2$
- Chemical Structure:

Background

Dalapon is a commonly used herbicide for the control of annual and perennial grasses in croplands. The US Environmental Protection Agency (EPA) has listed dalapon as a general use pesticide and categorized dalapon as a Class II toxic agent (moderately toxic). As such, any product that contains dalapon would be labeled with 'warning.' The moderate toxicity associated with dalapon is confined primarily to workers around dalapon and those individuals who are applying dalapon. Contact with the herbicide can be caustic to human skin, damaging to the conjunctiva of the human eye, and irritating/damaging to the upper respiratory system of humans. When used to control grasses in cropland as well as noncropland, dalapon is distributed via either aerial or ground equipment for foliage application. Some of the common croplands that have benefitted from dalapon application include corn, potatoes, legume crops, citrus, fruit, and nut trees. It is used extensively in the western United States to control a variety of grasses such as Bermuda, Johnson, Crab, and Quack grasses. Dalapon is translocated to the roots where it acts as a growth regulator. Although highly soluble with the ability to readily move through the environment, dalapon is relative safe and instances of dalapon intoxication are rare. The primary sources of toxicity are contact with the sodium or magnesium salt of dalapon, which is an irritant to the eyes, skin, and respiratory system. Cases of elevated levels of dalapon in drinking water or groundwater have also been rare, and little toxicity has been reported following dalapon exposure in water. Individuals who were exposed to high levels for extended periods of time can experience kidney dysfunction. Collectively, dalapon is a relatively safe herbicide for the control of many annual and perennial grasses.

Uses

Dalapon is used as an herbicide primarily to control annual and perennial grasses, including Bermuda grass and Johnson grass. Use of dalapon on food crops is primarily with sugarcane and sugar beets. Dalapon is also used on fruits, potatoes, carrots, asparagus, alfalfa, and flax, and in forestry, home gardening, and to control reed and sedge growth in aquatic environments.

Environmental Fate and Behavior

Dalapon is somewhat persistent in soil but does not readily adsorb to soil particles. It can remain active in soil for several months when applied at high rates. In general, dalapon is considered to have low to moderate persistence with detection in soil for 2–8 weeks. Due to its inability to bind to soil particles, dalapon has a relatively high mobility in soil, with leaching possible. Microorganisms in the soil are very efficient at degrading dalapon. The herbicide is usually not found below the first 6 inches of soil layer. Breakdown is relatively rapid and complete, leading to the production of compounds that are not naturally occurring. Soil microorganisms are efficient at degrading dalapon, however, such that dalapon is not typically found in groundwater. High temperatures and increased moisture accelerate dalapon degradation in soil. Dalapon can also be degraded by ultraviolet light. In aquatic environments, dalapon is degraded by microorganisms (most important), hydrolysis, and photolysis. In the absence of microbial degradation, the half-life of dalapon is several months or longer if the water temperature is below 25 °C, with the primary hydrolysis product being pyruvate. Dalapon is absorbed by both plant roots and leaves followed by translocation. With high applications, dalapon precipitates and leads to local corrosive effects on plants. Due to the ability of dalapon to be rapidly metabolized and degraded by microorganisms, hydrolyzed to pyruvate, rapidly translocated to plants, and quickly moved through the environment, it is not expected that dalapon will constitute any bioaccumulation hazard.

Exposure and Exposure Monitoring

Dermal inhalation and ocular exposures of liquid or vapor are the most common routes of exposure. If the chemical leaches into groundwater, there is the possibility of ingestion, although drinking water with levels in excess of the maximum contaminant level goal (MCLG) ($0.2\ mg\ l^{-1}$) has been reported to cause some kidney damages in a few people. Gas chromatography is the best method for the determination of dalapon exposure and for monitoring dalapon levels in humans (as well as plants and groundwater). Two methods of detection have been described, both with high levels of detection. Gas chromatography with electron capture detection can detect dalapon at 1 $\mu g\,l^{-1}$ in water, whereas methods describing mass spectrometry have reported nearly a tenfold greater (0.13 $\mu g\,l^{-1}$) sensitivity in detecting dalapon in water.

Toxicokinetics

As an herbicide, dalapon is considered to have a very high 'movement rating' suggesting its ability to rapidly move been environments such as soil and water. It has a relatively long half-life in soil of approximately 30 days and a very high solubility in water of 500–900 $g\,l^{-1}$. Although dalapon appears to readily move through the environment, it is a polar compound that is not readily absorbed by tissues. It causes irritation to the tissue with which it comes into contact. If absorbed in the gastrointestinal tract, it is principally eliminated as the parent compound in the urine.

Mechanism of Toxicity

The mechanism of action of dalapon is the same as for most acids. The acid denatures tissue proteins upon contact. At lower concentrations, the dalapon causes nonlethal yellowing of sensitive plants, which clearly distinguished them from resistant plants. The mode of action of chlorinated aliphatic acids is not known but they probably affect many enzyme pathways. Dalapon is readily absorbed into roots and leaves of plants and then translocated. Lower concentrations will inhibit plant growth and cause leaf chlorosis, followed by necrosis and death. Higher concentrations of dalapon will result in significant necrosis of areas of the plant in contact with dalapon. Although the direct mechanism of these effects has remained elusive, it is thought that dalapon may affect lipid, carbohydrate, and nitrogen metabolism as secondary effects. One prevailing hypothesis for the primary dalapon affect is that dalapon exerts direct effects on plant structural proteins leading to these secondary metabolic outcomes.

Acute and Short-Term Toxicity

In animals, the oral LD_{50} values were 7.5–9.3 $g\,kg^{-1}$ in male and female rats. Relatively similar high oral LD_{50} values were noted in rabbits and guinea pigs (3.9–4.6 $g\,kg^{-1}$). Dalapon is a moderate skin and eye irritant. The sodium salt of dalapon caused irritation, severe conjunctivitis, and corneal injury in rabbits, with recovery over several days. In humans, dalapon can cause corrosive injury to tissues. Burning and irritation are the predominant acute toxicities seen with acute exposure to dalapon. Skin lesions are more likely with moistened skin. Eye exposure can cause corneal destruction and conjunctiva edema accompanied by pain and tearing. Permanent eye damage can result from ocular exposure. Ingestion can lead to oral, throat, and gastrointestinal irritation. Inhalation of vapors causes irritation of the eyes, nose, and throat with destruction of mucus membranes. Severe inhalation exposure can cause respiratory distress accompanied by pulmonary edema. Some other symptoms of high acute exposure to dalapon include loss of appetite; slowed heartbeat; gastrointestinal disturbances such as vomiting, diarrhea, tiredness, and pain; and irritation of respiratory tract. When significant exposure to dalapon is not a consideration, there have been little to no effects of dalapon reported in humans. When proper personal protective equipment is worn to prevent ocular or respiratory exposure, dalapon is relatively safe in short-term or acute exposure.

Chronic Toxicity

In animals, the long-term feeding studies in dogs and rats indicated increased kidney weights at high dosages. The no observed adverse effect level (NOAEL) in a 2-year feeding study in rats was 15 $mg\,kg^{-1}\,day^{-1}$. The NOAEL in a 1-year feeding study in dogs was 50 $mg\,kg^{-1}\,day^{-1}$. In humans, long-term exposure may cause increased kidney and liver weights. Repeated or prolonged exposure to dalapon can cause irritation to the mucous membrane linings of the mouth, nose, throat, and lungs, and to the eyes. Chronic skin contact can lead to moderate irritation or even mild burns. Dalapon was negative in a variety of mutagenic test assays.

Immunotoxicity

There have been no reports of immunotoxicity following dalapon exposure in any species.

Reproductive Toxicity

Effects of dalapon on reproduction are negligible except at extremely high concentrations. The doses/concentrations utilized in studies to elicit changes in reproduction are nearly 10 000-fold higher than what is acceptable. Female rats receiving doses up to 2000 $mg\,kg^{-1}$ did not affect animal fertility or the ability to reproduce. Offspring receiving up to 1500 $mg\,kg^{-1}$ resulted in reduced rates of weight gain and lower weights. No other adverse effects have been reported.

Genotoxicity

There have been no reports of dalapon mutagenicity or teratogenicity. Rats receiving doses up to 2000 $mg\,kg^{-1}\,day^{-1}$ did not demonstrate observable teratogenic effects. Mutagenicity tests in variety of microorganisms suggest that dalapon does not exhibit any effects on gene mutation.

Carcinogenicity

Chronic administration of dalapon to rats at 5, 15, or 50 $mg\,kg^{-1}\,day^{-1}$ for 2 years did not elicit any carcinogenic effects. Microbial studies have also confirmed this finding with dalapon concentrations up to 1000-fold higher than what is considered acceptable.

Clinical Management

In the event of dermal exposure to dalapon, contaminated clothing should be removed quickly and the exposed area should be flushed with copious amounts of water for 15 min. With eye exposure, the affected eye should be flushed with water for 30 min, occasionally lifting the upper and lower lids. With inhalation exposure, the victim should be moved to fresh air. If the victim is not breathing, artificial respiration should be administered. If swallowed, vomiting should not be induced. If the victim is conscious, he or she should drink plenty of water or milk. If it is suspected that an individual has been exposed to extremely high concentrations for extended periods of time, kidney function tests should be performed at regular intervals to determine that renal function is maintained within normal values.

Ecotoxicity

The LC_{50} of dietary (5-day exposure) dalapon was more than 5000 ppm in mallards, ring-necked pheasants, and Japanese quail. The acute oral LD_{50} of dalapon in chickens is 45–56 g kg^{-1}. Reproduction may be affected in birds at nonlethal exposures. Mallard ducks exhibited a reduced reproduction rate at doses that were 25% of what is considered lethal. Gold fish exposed to 100 ppm had a 0% mortality rate after 24 h. This rate increased to 100% in the presence of 500 ppm dalapon. LC_{50} values for dalapon in a variety of fish species were 100 mg l^{-1}. This would suggest that dalapon has a low order of toxicity in most fish. Dalapon is only slightly toxic to mollusks. Crustaceans and insects are most sensitive of aquatic invertebrates. Dalapon is relatively nontoxic to honeybees and terrestrial insects.

Exposure Standards and Guidelines

The American Conference of Governmental Industrial Hygienists TLV is 1 ppm; the MCLG is 0.2 mg l^{-1}, or 200 ppb; and the RfD is 0.03 mg kg^{-1} day^{-1}. Both the Occupational Health and Safety Administration and the National Institute on Occupational Safety and Health (NIOSH) have established TLV–TWA levels of 1 ppm (5.8 mg m^{-3} as the inhalable fraction over an 8-h work shift). The US EPA has set both the MCL and the MCLG at 0.2 mg l^{-1} or 200 ppb. These levels were established in 1974 when the US Congress passed the Safe Drinking Water Act and later in 1994 following the passage of the Phase V Rule. If levels of dalapon exceed these recommended levels, the concentration in water can be reduced by the addition of activated granular carbon.

See also: Common Mechanism of Toxicity in Pesticides; Methyl Bromide; Environmental Risk Assessment, Pesticides and Biocides.

Further Reading

Ashton, F.M., DeVilliers, O.T., Glenn, R.K., Duke, W.B., 1977. Localization of metabolic sties of action of herbicides. Pest Biochem. Physiol. 7, 122–141.

Boutin, C., Aya, K.L., Carpenter, D., Thomas, P.J., Rowland, O., 2012. Phytotoxicity testing for herbicide regulation: shortcomings in relations to biodiversity and ecosystem series in agrarian systems. Sci. Total Environ. 415, 79–92.

Buchanan-Wollaston, V., Snape, A., Cannon, F., 1992. A plant selectable marker gene based on the detoxification of the herbicide dalapon. Plant Cell Rep. 11, 627–631.

Burge, W.D., 1969. Populations of dalapon-decomposing bacteria in soil as influenced by additions of dalapon or others carbon sources. Appl. Microbiol. 17, 545–550.

Busto, M.D., Smith, P.P., Perez-Mateos, M., Burns, R.G., 1992. Degradation of aliphatic halogen-substituted pesticides by dehalogenase isolated from *Pseudomonas alcaligenes*. Identification and properties of the enzyme. Sci. Total Environ. 123/124, 267–277.

Cantor, K.P., Villanueva, C.M., Silverman, D.T., Figueroa, J.D., Real, F.X., et al., 2010. Polymorphisms in GSTT1, GSTZ1, and CYP2E1, disinfection by-products and the risk of bladder cancer in Spain. Environ. Health Perspect. 118, 1545–1550.

Cardador, M.J., Gallego, M., 2010. Determination of haloacetic acids in human urine by headspace gas chromatography-mass spectrometry. J. Chromatogr. B Analyt. Technol. Biomed. Life Sci. 878, 1824–1830.

Carere, A., Ortali, V.A., Cardamone, G., Torracca, A.M., Raschetti, R., 1978. Microbiological mutagenicity studies of pesticides *in vitro*. Mutat. Res. 57, 277–286.

George, J.P., Hingorani, H.G., 1982. Herbicide toxicity to fish-food organisms. Environ. Pollut. Ser. A Ecol. Biol. 28, 183–188.

Greaves, M.P., Davies, H.A., Marsh, J.A., Wingfield, G.I., 1981. Effects of pesticides on soil microflora using dalapon as an example. Arch. Environ. Contam. Toxicol. 10, 437–449.

Hawker, D.W., Cumming, J.L., Neale, P.A., Bartkow, M.E., Escher, B.I., 2011. A screening level fate model of organic contaminants from advanced water treatment in a potable water supply reservoir. Water Res. 45, 768–780.

Lewis, T.E., Wolfinger, T.F., Barta, M.L., 2004. The ecological effects of trichloroacetic acid in the environment. Environ. Int. 30, 1119–1150.

Marsh, J.A.P., Greaves, M.P., 1979. The influence of temperature and moisture on the effects of the herbicide dalapon on nitrogen transformations in soil. Soil Biol. Biochem. 11, 279–285.

Newbold, C., 1975. Herbicides in aquatic systems. Biol. Conserv. 7, 97–118.

Ozawa, H., Tsukioka, T., 1992. Trifluoroanilide derivatization method for the gas chromatographic determination of propionic acid herbicides in water. Anal. Chim. Acta 267, 25–30.

Reigart, J.R., Roberts, J.R., 1999. Recognition and Management of Pesticide Poisonings, fifth ed. Office of Prevention, Pesticides and Toxic Substances, EPA 735-R-98-003, pp. 118–125.

Swarcewicz, M.K., Gregorczyk, A., 2012. The effects of pesticide mixtures on degradation of pendimethalin in soils. Environ. Monit. Assess. 184, 3077–3084.

Van Der Poll, J.M., De Vos, R.H., 1980. Improved determination of dalapon residues in plant tissues and natural water by derivatization and electron capture gas chromatography. J. Chromat. 187, 244–248.

Xie, Y., 2001. Analyzing haloacetic acids using gas chromatography/mass spectrometry. Water Res. 35, 1599–1602.

Relevant Websites

http://www.cdc.gov/niosh/npg/npgd0200.html.

http://www.epa.gov/safewater/pdfs/factsheets/soc/dalapon.pdf.

http://extoxnet.orst.edu/pips/dalapon.htm.

http://npic.orst.edu/RMPP/rmpp_main2a.pdf.

http://www.oehha.ca.gov/water/phg/dalapon061909.html.

http://pmep.cce.cornell.edu/profiles/extoxnet/carbaryl-dicrotophos/dalapon-ext.html.

http://pmep.cce.cornell.edu/profiles/herb-growthreg/dalapon-ethephon/dalapon/herb-prof-dalapon.html.

http://toxnet.nlm.nih.gov/cgi-bin/sis/search/r?dbs+toxline:@term+@DOCNO+RISKLINE/2002060067.

http://water.epa.gov/drink/contaminants/basicinformation/dalapon.cfm.

Danthron

N Yang, Manchester University, Fort Wayne, IN, USA

- Name: Danthron
- Chemical Abstracts Service Registry Number: 117-10-2
- Synonyms: Altan, Antrapurol, Chrysazin, Dantrona, Dantron
- Molecular Formula: $C_{14}H_8O_4$
- Chemical Structure:

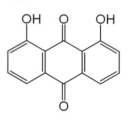

Background

Danthron, a natural product, was originally extracted from the roots and rhizome of Polygonaceae plant (**Figure 1**), also called Da Huang in traditional Chinese herbal medicine. Now it is synthesized in many countries, such as Germany, India, Japan, Poland, the United Kingdom, and the United States. Danthron is reasonably anticipated to be a human carcinogen.

Danthron is an anthraquinone that exists at room temperature as a red or orange crystalline powder. Some of the physical and chemical properties of danthron are in **Table 1**. It is practically insoluble in water, but soluble in a variety of solvents (acetone, chloroform, diethyl ether, ethanol) and alkaline hydroxide solutions. The stability of danthron is generally good. It is stable under room temperatures and normal pressures. Structural analogs and metabolites of danthron include 1,3,8-trihydroxy-6-methyl-9, 10-anthracenedione (emodin), and 1,8-dihydroxy-3-hydroxy-9,10-anthracenedione (aloe-emodin) (**Figure 2**). They share similar solubility properties as danthron.

Oral exposure to danthron caused tumors in two rodent species and at several different tissue sites. Dietary administration of danthron caused liver cancer (hepatocellular carcinoma) in male mice and benign and malignant intestinal tract tumors (adenoma and adenocarcinoma of the colon and adenoma of the cecum) in male rats.

Uses

Danthron has been widely administrated as a laxative since the 1900s. In the United States, danthron has been forbidden to continual use as laxative because it is considered to be a carcinogen. Food and Drug Administration (FDA) withdrew danthron from the market for this purpose in 1987. However, in the United Kingdom, it is only considered as a possible carcinogen. Therefore, danthron is only restricted to patients who have already been diagnosed as terminal cancer. Currently, danthron is being used to a lesser extent as an intermediate in the manufacture of alizarine and indanthrene dyes.

Environment Fate and Behavior

Danthron is discovered in several species of plants and insects. It has been isolated from dried leaves and stems of *Xyris semifuscata* harvested in Madagascar, and roots of Da Huang, a Chinese traditional herbal medicine. Danthron also appears to be biosynthesized by some insects. The presence of danthron in insects may be a way of protection from predators. Danthron can be manually synthesized by many countries. In the United States, danthron was available from 12 suppliers.

If released to the atmosphere, danthron will exist in both the vapor phase and the particulate phase. Vapor phase danthron has an estimated half-life of 11 days. Particulate phase danthron can be physically removed from air by wet and dry

Table 1 Physical and chemical properties of danthron

Property	*Information*
Molecular weight	240.2[a]
Specific gravity	1.54 g cm^{-3}[b]
Melting point	193 °C[a]
Boiling point	Sublimes[b]
Log K_{ow}	3.94[a]
Water solubility	9 mg l^{-1}[a]
Vapor pressure	7.6×10^{-11} mm Hg[a]
Vapor density relative to air	8.3[b]

Source: http://pubchem.ncbi.nlm.nih.gov/summary/summary.cgi?cid=2950.

(a)

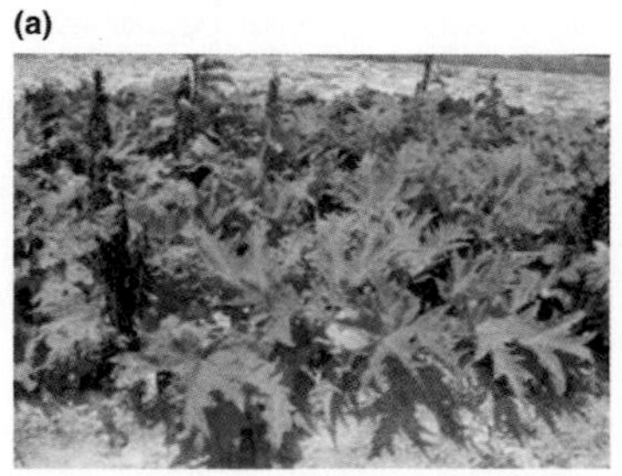

(b)

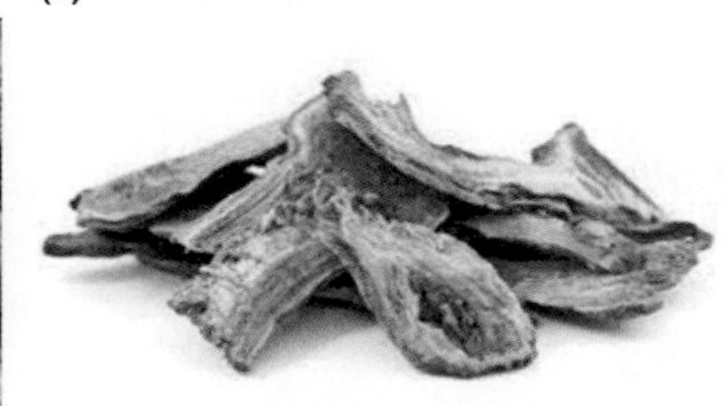

Figure 1 (a) Da Huang and (b) dried root of Da Huang.

 http://dx.doi.org/10.1016/B978-0-12-386454-3.01214-8

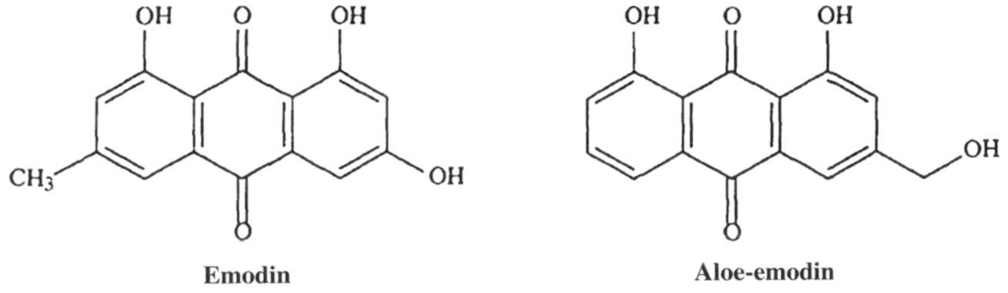

Figure 2 Structures of emodin and aloe-emodin.

deposition. It is expected to biodegrade with 68% degradation within 3 months.

If released to water, danthron is expected to adsorb to the surface of solid particle and sediment. Biodegradation is also a major pathway processed in water. It was reported that 82% of the added danthron was degraded by fresh water within 3 days. If added to seawater, 91% of danthron was reported as degraded. Danthron may bioconcentrate in aquatic organisms, such as fish and shrimps.

Exposure and Exposure Monitoring

Before danthron was withdrawn from the laxative market in 1987, this medicine was available from nine companies as 14 over-the-counter (OTC) products with the following trade names: (Danivac, Doctate-P, Dorbane, Dorbantyl, Dorbantyl Forte, Doxan, Doxidan, Magcyl, Modane, Tonelax, West-Ward Dioctyl with danthron, and Valax)®. In these medicines, tablet formulations contained 37.5, 50, or 75 mg danthron; capsule formulations, 25, 40, or 50 mg; and a liquid formulation, 37.5 mg per 5 ml. Occupational exposure to danthron can also occur during its application as a dye intermediate or as a catalytic agent in the paper pulping process.

Generally, the primary route for the population ingesting danthron is through drinking water and other related oral administration. The primary route of potential human exposure to danthron is oral administration. Potential occupational exposure may also occur for workers in dye and paper pulping companies, who use danthron as a dye intermediate or a catalytic agent. The National Occupational Exposure Survey (1981–83) indicated that 357 workers, including 187 women, were potentially exposed to danthron. Thirty years later, these numbers can only increase.

Toxicokinetics

After direct administration of danthron into the rat duodenum via a nonrecirculating perfusion system was significantly absorbed from rat duodenum, glucuronide and sulfate conjugates were formed. It is also considered that bacterial reduction of danthron in the colon did not play a major role in danthron metabolism. P450 is directly involved in the metabolism of this compound.

Administrating danthron to pregnant women the evening before the induction of labor, danthron was found in the babies' urine immediately after delivery. It was also found in a much lower concentration detectable in the amniotic fluid. The findings suggested that danthron was absorbed transplacentally and excreted via the fetal kidney into the amniotic fluid. Danthron is also specifically considered as a chemical with strong evidence of milk transfer in humans.

Mechanism of Toxicity

Danthron can cause DNA damage particularly at guanines in the 5′-GG-3′, 5′-GGGG-3′, 5′-GGGGG-3′ sequences in the presence of Cu(II), cytochrome P450 reductase and the nicotinamide adenine dinucleotide phosphate (NADPH)-generating system. H_2O_2 and Cu(I) may also be involved because this DNA damage can be inhibited by catalase and bathocuproine. The further mechanism is danthron is reduced by P450 reductase and generate reactive oxygen species through the redox cycle, leading to extensive Cu(II)-mediated DNA damage. The DNA damage also comes from similar topoisomerase II inhibitor behavior of danthron.

Genotoxicity

Danthron is genotoxic to several prokaryotic, lower eukaryotic, and mammalian *in vitro* species. Danthron induced gene mutations in several strains of *Salmonella typhimurium*. The Ames test revealed that danthron was mutagenic only toward *S. typhimurium* strain TA102 in the presence of an exogenous metabolic activation system (S9 mix). Various concentrations of danthron (25, 50, and 100 $\mu g\ ml^{-1}$) increased the frequencies of micronuclear cells with or without S9 mix, and the comet length, tail length, and Olive tail moment in comet assays without S9 mix in a dose-dependent manner. Danthron could also induce respiration-deficient mutations in the yeast *Saccharomyces cerevisiae* and inhibit gap-junction intercellular communication in Chinese hamster V79 cells. However, the inhibition on gap-junction intercellular communication was not proved in another V79 cell study as well as in human fibroblasts.

Carcinogenicity

Danthron is defined to be a reasonably anticipated human carcinogen based on evidence of carcinogenicity from studies majorly in experimental animals.

Oral administration of danthron caused tumors in two rodent species, several different organs, and tissues, such as liver cancer (hepatocellular carcinoma) in male mice and malignant intestinal tract tumors (adenoma and adenocarcinoma of the colon and adenoma of the cecum) in male rats. However, the data available in human studies are not adequate to determine how much the exposure to danthron affects the occurrence of human cancer. There is only one case reported, the clinical cancer case of the small intestine (leiomyosarcoma) in a female teenager with a long history of exposure to danthron.

Danthron was also evaluated for its ability to promote the induction of tumors by other chemicals. The incidence and multiplicity of colon tumors (adenoma or adenocarcinoma) and liver tumors (adenoma) were significant in male mice, treated by danthron following 1,2-dimethylhydrazine as a tumor initiator. However, no skin tumors were detected in female 7 weeks ICR/Ha Swiss mice, administrated by 7,12-dimethylbenz(*a*)anthracene and danthron, for up to 476 days.

Exposure Standards and Guidelines

FDA regulated that laxative containing danthron may no longer be marketed in the United States, on or after 28 March 1987. Another final rule amends part 310 (21 code of Federal Regulations (CFR) part 310) to include danthron by adding new Sec. 310.545(a)(12)(iv)(B). This final rule, effective from 29 January 1999, shows "no over-the-counter drug products that are subject to this final rule may be initially introduced or initially delivered for introduction into interstate commerce unless they are the subject of an approved application."

See also: Toxicity Testing, Inhalation.

Further Reading

Bennett, M., Cresswell, H., 2003. Factors influencing constipation in advanced cancer patients: a prospective study of opioid dose, dantron dose and physical functioning. Palliat. Med. 17 (5), 418–422.

Chiang, J.H., Yang, J.S., Ma, C.Y., et al., 2011. Danthron, an anthraquinone derivative, induces DNA damage and caspase cascades-mediated apoptosis in SNU-1 human gastric cancer cells through mitochondrial permeability transition pores and Bax-triggered pathways. Chem. Res. Toxicol. 24 (1), 20–29.

Chiou, S.M., Chiu, C.H., Yang, S.T., et al., 2012. Danthron triggers ROS and mitochondria-mediated apoptotic death in C6 rat glioma cells through caspase cascades, apoptosis-inducing factor and endonuclease G multiple signaling. Neurochem. Res. 37 (8), 1790–1800.

Jackson, T.C., Verrier, J.D., Kochanek, P.M., January 2013. Anthraquinone-2-sulfonic acid (AQ2S) is a novel neurotherapeutic agent. Cell Death Dis. 10 (4), e451. http://dx.doi.org/10.1038/cddis.2012.187.

Müller, S.O., Eckert, I., Lutz, W.K., Stopper, H., 1996. Genotoxicity of the laxative drug components emodin, aloe-emodin and danthron in mammalian cells: topoisomerase II mediated? Mutat. Res. 371 (3–4), 165–173.

National Toxicology Program, April 2012. Toxicology study of senna (CAS No. 8013-11-4) in C57BL/6NTAC mice and toxicology and carcinogenesis study of senna in genetically modified C3B6.129F1/Tac-Trp53tm1Brd haploinsufficient mice (feed studies). Natl. Toxicol. Program Genet. Modif. Model Rep. (15), 1–114.

National Toxicology Program, 2011. Danthron. Rep. Carcinog. 12, 128–129.

Nesslany, F., Simar-Meintières, S., Ficheux, H., Marzin, D., 2009. Aloe-emodin-induced DNA fragmentation in the mouse in vivo comet assay. Mutat. Res. 678 (1), 13–19.

Rossi, S., Tabolacci, C., Lentini, A., et al., 2010. Anthraquinones danthron and quinizarin exert antiproliferative and antimetastatic activity on murine B16-F10 melanoma cells. Anticancer Res. 30 (2), 445–449.

Sugie, S., Mori, Y., Okumura, A., Yoshimi, N., Okamoto, K., Sato, S., Tanaka, T., Mori, H., 1994. Promoting and synergistic effects of chrysazin on 1,2-dimethylhydrazine-induced carcinogenesis in male ICR/CD-1 mice. Carcinogenesis 15 (6), 1175–1179.

USFDA, January 29, 1999. Laxative drug products for over-the-counter human use. Food and drug administration, HHS. Final rule. Fed. Regist. 64 (19), 4535–4540.

Zhang, Z., Fu, J., Yao, B., Zhang, X., Zhao, P., Zhou, Z., 2011a. In vitro genotoxicity of danthron and its potential mechanism. Mutat. Res. 722 (1), 39–43.

Zhang, H., Zhou, R., Li, L., et al., 2011b. Danthron functions as a retinoic X receptor antagonist by stabilizing tetramers of the receptor. J. Biol. Chem. 286 (3), 1868–1875.

Relevant Websites

http://ntp.niehs.nih.gov/ntp/roc/twelfth/profiles/Danthron.pdf – National Institute of Environmental Health Sciences.

http://www.ncbi.nlm.nih.gov/pubmed/21850139 – National Toxicology Program.

DDT (Dichlorodiphenyltrichloroethane)

SA Burr, Plymouth University Peninsula Schools of Medicine and Dentistry, Plymouth, UK

This article is a revision of the previous edition article by Benny L. Blaylock, volume 1, pp 725–727, © 2005, Elsevier Inc.

- Chemical Abstracts Service Registry Number: 50-29-3
- Synonyms: 1-Chloro-4-[2,2,2-trichloro-1-(4-chlorophenyl) ethyl]benzene; *p,p*′-DDT; Arkotine; Bovidermol; Chlorophenothane; Clofenotane; Dicophane; Estonate; Parachlorocidum, Pentachlorin; CID 3036
- Classification: Synthetic organochlorine insecticide
- Molecular Formula: $C_{14}H_9Cl_5$, molecular weight 354.48626
- Chemical Structure:

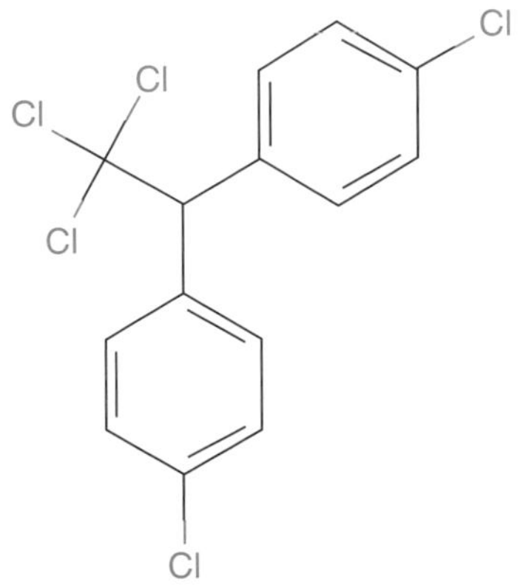

Cl Cl Cl Cl Cl

Background

Dichlorodiphenyltrichloroethane (DDT) was used worldwide as a potent insecticide and insect repellent, initially for the control of insects that spread disease (e.g., mosquitoes for malaria and lice for typhus) and later for agricultural and domestic purposes. DDT typically remains effective for 6–12 months, not only causing insect death, but at lower exposures having an irritant and spatial repellency effect that obliges insects to avoid contact, limiting human exposure to disease transmission. Due to low water solubility, DDT is retained in soil fractions with a high organic content and may accumulate with repeated applications extending the environmental half-life. Although cheap to produce, stable, and with low mammalian toxicity, concerns over environmental persistence and bioaccumulation led to the widespread banning of its use starting with Hungary in 1968 (reinforced in 2001 by the Stockholm Convention on Persistent Organic Pollutants, which has been ratified by most countries including the United States).

Uses

DDT continues to be used in a permitted restricted capacity for public health measures in some (mostly tropical and developing) parts of the world and in a few nonsignatory countries for agricultural purposes. Therefore, DDT continues to be used in some countries for indoor residual spraying of surfaces at 1–2 g m^{-2} (having a similar cost to implement as pyrethroids, which, due to their higher potency, are sprayed at 0.02–0.3 g m^{-2}). However, many insect populations have begun to develop resistance by preventing DDT binding via modifications to the sodium channel target site. There are also continuing concerns over genotoxic, reproductive, and developmental effects on human health. Synthetically produced, total DDT is a mixture of *p,p*′-DDT, *o,p*′-DDT, 1,1-dichloro-2,2-bis(*p*-chlorophenyl)ethylene (DDE), and 1,1-dichloro-2,2-bis(*p*-chlorophenyl)ethane (DDD). DDD is used clinically as an adjunctive treatment in patients with adrenocortical carcinoma after complete surgical resection.

Environmental Fate

DDT is persistent in the environment with a half-life of 2–30 years depending on conditions. Low solubility in water leads to absorption and retention in soil with losses through runoff, volatilization, photolysis, and biodegradation. DDT may eventually leach from soil into groundwater, especially in soil with little organic matter. DDT may reach surface water by runoff, atmospheric transport, drift, or direct application (e.g., to control mosquitoes). The reported half-life for DDT in watercourses is 28 days in rivers and 56 days in lakes, with losses through volatilization, photolysis, adsorption to water-borne particles, and sedimentation. Aquatic organisms also readily accumulate DDT and its metabolites.

Exposure

DDT exposure is most commonly through ingestion of contaminated food. DDT is ubiquitous in the atmosphere but present at such low levels that exposure via inhalation is negligible unless in an area of intensive use. There is minimal absorption of DDT through intact skin, even with high exposure levels.

Toxicokinetics

DDT is hydrophobic and lipophilic requiring an organic solvent (e.g., oil or fat) as a vehicle. Gastrointestinal absorption is slow with symptoms taking several hours to develop. DDT is metabolized slowly by liver microsomal enzymes initially dehydrochlorinating DDT to DDE and reducing to DDD.

In some rodents (rats and hamsters, but not mice) DDT induces microsomal liver enzymes to promote metabolism. DDD is converted to 2,2-bis(*p*-chlorophenyl)acetic acid (DDA) via hydroxylation to an acyl chloride intermediate followed by hydrolysis. DDA is the main route for DDT elimination, mostly being excreted in bile and some in urine. Lactating mothers may excrete up to 10% of DDT doses via breast milk. DDT accumulates in all tissues but the highest levels are in adipose tissue. Coexposure to DDT and dieldrin results in more DDT storage and less dieldrin storage than individual exposures. DDE is more strongly bound in tissue than DDT. The half-life of DDT in humans is 3–6 years and twice as long for DDE. Starvation mobilizes fat reserves, increasing nervous system deposition and neurotoxic effects.

Mechanism of Toxicity

DDT is primarily a functional neurotoxin: DDT keeps sodium ion channels open for longer peroid (acting at the same binding site as pyrethroids) and prolongs the recovery phase of action potentials, increasing excitability and inducing repetitive neuronal discharges to stimuli that would otherwise elicit a single response. The observed effects are muscle twitch and tremors (so-called DDT jitters), leading slowly to excitatory paralysis and death over hours–days. Insect knockdown rate and lethality are improved by application at lower ambient temperatures. Both DDT and pyrethroids also increase protein kinase C-induced phosphorylation of the sodium channel alpha subunit. The DDT metabolite *o,p*′-DDD decreases adrenocorticotrophic hormone-stimulated glucocorticoid secretion. DDE is an anti-androgen and *o,p*′-DDT is weakly estrogenic. Endocrine disruption has been linked to reduced reproductive success, increased prematurity and neurobehavioral problems. DDT is also both directly genotoxic and induces enzymes producing genotoxic intermediates and DNA adducts.

Acute and Short-Term Toxicity

Animal

Acute effects are incoordination, ataxia, fine tremor, myoclonic jerks, seizures, and death. The order of species susceptibility to DDT from least to most susceptible is: bird, goat, sheep, pig, monkey, dog, cat, rat, and mouse. Rat oral lethal dose 50% (LD_{50}) values are 113–800 mg kg^{-1} and mouse oral LD_{50} values are 150–300 mg kg^{-1}. Dermal LD_{50} values are 3–20 times higher than oral LD_{50} values (e.g., the rat dermal LD_{50} value is 2500 mg kg^{-1}).

Human

Single oral doses of 250 mg have no clinically measurable effect. Above 250 mg, effects on sensory and motor nerves develop: oral hyperesthesia, ataxia, fatigue, contact hypersensitivity, oral paresthesia, dizziness, nausea, vomiting, confusion, tremors, and seizures. Effects start after 0.5–6 h, with peak effects after 6–10 h, and recovery over 1 day to 5 weeks. The lowest exposures resulting in death are 50 mg kg^{-1} for DDT and 500 mg kg^{-1} for DDD.

Chronic Toxicity, Immunotoxicity, Reproductive Toxicity, and Carcinogenicity

Animal

Typical effects are weight loss, anemia, weakness, and tremors, before paralysis and death ensue. Additional developmental effects include impaired learning performance following gestational and lactational exposures in mice. Reproductive effects include sterility in rats and decreased fetal weight in rabbits. Immune effects include decreased antibody production in both chickens and mice. Cancer studies are equivocal. Liver effects include hepatocyte hypertrophy, centrilobular necrosis, and hepatoma in some rodent studies but not others. There is clearer evidence for DDT disrupting endogenous hormone action on ovary, oviduct, and uterine function, particularly for birds in which *o,p*-DDT disrupts reproductive tract development impairing eggshell quality. Furthermore, the DDT metabolite *p,p*′-DDE inhibits calcium ATPase in egg shell gland membranes and reduces the uptake of calcium carbonate from the blood, resulting in a dose-dependent reduction in eggshell thickness.

Human

DDT is routinely found in food and in blood samples. Normal background levels are unlikely to cause any adverse effects. Daily exposure to aerosolized DDT, sufficient to leave a white deposit on nasal hair causes moderate irritation of the nose, throat, and eyes. House spraying for several months has caused anemia and thrombocytopenia. Continued exposure to high doses can lead to nausea, vomiting, parasthesia, hypertonia, exaggerated reflexes, muscular fasciculations, ataxia, seizures, hyperpyrexia, and metabolic acidosis. There may be a link with premature parturition and low birth weight in mothers with high DDE blood levels. Infants may be exposed through breast milk. *p,p*′-DDT has a five-fold higher breast cancer incidence in the highest compared with the lowest exposure groups in women exposed before puberty. Increased risks for many forms of cancer have been reported, although causal effects have been difficult to establish. The International Agency for Research on Cancer has classified DDT as possibly carcinogenic to humans.

Clinical Management

With cases of ingestion, gastric decontamination with lavage and activated charcoal may be of benefit within the first hour. If systemic toxicity does occur, the central signs of poisoning can be difficult to control and may be confused with intoxication by other pesticides such as anticholinesterases, which also cause hyperexcitability; although DDT does not inhibit acetylcholinesterase. Single short-lived seizures may not require treatment. Since DDT does not produce morphological damage, only symptomatic treatment is needed. Frequent or prolonged convulsions may be controlled with intravenous diazepam or lorazepam. If unresponsive, phenobarbital or phenytoin (before thiopental or general anesthesia) may be considered. Respiratory support may be needed and control of metabolic acidosis may require sodium bicarbonate.

Ecotoxicology

DDT accumulates through the food chain to apex predators. DDT is toxic to aquatic invertebrates as well as insects. Early developmental stages of invertebrates have been shown to be particularly susceptible. The invertebrates are eaten by smaller populations of fish, many species of which have been shown to store the DDT from large numbers of invertebrates or other fish. In turn, the fish are eaten by an even smaller population of birds. The intensified DDT storage disrupts endocrine function. Birds produce thinner eggshells in proportion to their dose of DDT and have been reported to have altered mating behavior.

Exposure Standards and Guidelines

For humans, the World Health Organization's acceptable daily intake is 0.01 mg kg^{-1}, with a permissible exposure limit of 1.0 mg m^{-3} (over 8 h).

See also: Neurotoxicity; Organochlorine Insecticides; Pesticides.

Further Reading

Davies, T.G.E., Field, L.M., Usherwood, P.N.R., Williamson, M.S., 2007. DDT, pyrethrins, pyrethroids and insect sodium channels. IUBMB Life 59 (3), 151–162.

Jaga, K., Dharmani, C., 2003. Global surveillance of DDT and DDE levels in human tissues. Int. J. Occup. Med. Environ. Health 16 (1), 7–20.

Turusov, V., Rakitsky, V., Tomatis, L., 2002. Dichlorodiphenyltrichloroethane (DDT): ubiquity, persistence, and risk. Environ. Health Perspect. 110 (2), 125–128.

Relevant Websites

http://www.atsdr.cdc.gov/ToxProfiles/tp.asp?id=81&tid=20 – ATSDR Toxicological Profile for DDT, DDE, and DDD, updated 2008.

http://toxnet.nlm.nih.gov – TOXNET, Toxicology Data Network, National Library of Medicine, Search for DDT.

http://www.who.int – World Health Organization, Search for DDT.

Decane

SR Clough, Haley & Aldrich, Inc., Bedford, NH, USA

- Chemical Abstracts Service Registry Number: 124-18-5
- Synonyms: Decane, UN2247 (DOT), Alkane C(10), Decyl hydride, *n*-Decane
- Chemical/Pharmaceutical/Other Class: Aliphatic hydrocarbon (C10)
- Molecular Formula: $C_{10}H_{22}$
- Chemical Structure:

H_3C—(CH₂)₈—CH_3

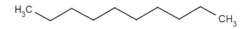

Uses

Decane is a constituent in the paraffin fraction of petroleum and is also present in low concentrations as a component of gasoline. It is used as a solvent in organic synthesis reactions as a hydrocarbon standard in the manufacture of petroleum products, in the rubber industry, and in the paper processing industry, and as a constituent in polyolefin manufacturing wastes. Decane is a flammable liquid (at room temperature) that is lighter than water.

Environmental Fate and Behavior

Decane has a molecular weight of 142.28 g mol^{-1}. At 20 °C, *n*-decane has solubility in water of 0.009 mg l^{-1}, a vapor pressure of 2.7 mm Hg, and a Henry's law constant of 5.15 atm-m^3 mol^{-1}. The odor threshold is around 11 mg m^{-3}. The log octanol/water partition coefficient is 5.01. Conversion factors for *n*-decane in air are as follows: 1 mg m^{-3} = 0.17 ppm and 1 ppm = 5.82 mg m^{-3}.

If released to air, *n*-decane will exist solely as a vapor in the ambient atmosphere. Vapor-phase *n*-decane will be degraded in the atmosphere by reaction with photochemically produced hydroxyl radicals, the half-life for this reaction in air is approximately 11.5 h.

Based on *n*-decane's vapor pressure, it may volatilize from dry soil surfaces. In biodegradation studies in soil, hydrocarbons with molecular weights equivalent to or lower than decane disappeared from the soil in both active and sterile treatments by the first sampling time (5 days), indicating that evaporation was a major removal process. Decane is expected to have low to no mobility in soil based on estimated organic carbon partition coefficient (Koc) values in the range of 1700–43 000. Volatilization from moist soil surfaces is expected to be an important fate process based on a Henry's law constant of 5.2 atm m^3 mol^{-1}, which is calculated from *n*-decane's vapor pressure and water solubility. Adsorption to soil, however, would be expected to attenuate due to volatilization.

According to output using US Environmental Protection Agency's (US EPA) EPI Suite computer program, *n*-decane would have a relatively short half-life in a river or open water body. Estimated volatilization half-lives for a model river and model lake are 1.2 h and 113 days, respectively; however, volatilization from water surfaces might be attenuated by adsorption to suspended solids in the water column. Seawater from Narragansett Bay, Rhode Island, was spiked with *n*-(1-14C)decane. Mass balance was calculated after a 2.5-week experiment and showed that 71–82% of the radiolabeled *n*-decane had been mineralized to $^{14}CO_2$. Hydrolysis is not expected to occur since *n*-decane lacks functional groups that hydrolyze under environmental conditions.

Although the predicted bioaccumulation and biomagnifications factors are moderate (~900), it would not be expected to be found in the tissues of fish or wildlife as: (1) *n*-decane contains no persistent functional groups (e.g., chlorine, bromine); (2) exposure would be expected to be low based on a low half-life in the environment; and (3) subsequent to exposure, *n*-decane would be rapidly metabolized by the liver (similar to what is seen with other organic compounds, such as polycyclic aromatic hydrocarbons). This is apparently the case as *n*-decane was not observed above the detection limit in most fish samples taken from the wild. The average *n*-decane concentration for oysters and clams, sampled from the Mississippi River near New Orleans, was 21 and 2.5 μg kg^{-1} of wet weight, respectively.

As *n*-decane is a volatile petroleum compound, it would have a propensity to migrate to the atmosphere following an environmental release. Oil-oxidizing microorganisms will degrade *n*-decane along with other alkanes, cycloalkanes, and aromatics. In wastewater, rotating disk contact aerators will remove >99% of the compound from the influent (Verschueren, 1996).

Exposure and Exposure Monitoring

National Institute for Occupational Safety and Health (NIOSH) has statistically estimated that >1600 workers are potentially exposed to *n*-decane in the USA. Occupational exposure to *n*-decane may occur through inhalation and dermal contact with this compound at workplaces where *n*-decane is used. Monitoring data indicate that the general population may be exposed to very low levels of *n*-decane *via* inhalation of ambient air, ingestion of food and drinking water, and dermal contact with consumer products containing *n*-decane.

Because *n*-decane can exist as a liquid and a vapor at normal temperature and pressure, exposure could occur either by dermal contact or by inhalation, and oral exposure would most likely be either incidental or accidental. *n*-Decane can be measured in air down to levels as low as 0.1 ppb. It has been measured and detected in both indoor air (2–800 μg m^{-3}) and outdoor air (0.6–10 μg m^{-3}) with the latter typically a result of automobile emissions. A review of indoor air concentrations of volatile organic compounds in North America found 0.44 ppb

 http://dx.doi.org/10.1016/B978-0-12-386454-3.00486-3

(2.56 μg m^{-3}) in 'existing' residences and 3 ppb (17.5 μg m^{-3}) in 'new' homes.

Toxicokinetics

Inhaled *n*-decane is rapidly distributed from the blood to different organs and tissues, particularly those with high fat content. The concentration of *n*-decane in the brains of rats exposed to 100 ppm, 12 h day^{-1} for 3 days, was 60.2 μmol kg^{-1}. Corresponding values for other tissues were 6.8 μmol kg^{-1} in blood, 45.9 μmol kg^{-1} in liver, 77.7 μmol kg^{-1} in kidneys, and 1230 μmol kg^{-1} in fat.

Aliphatic hydrocarbons, such as *n*-decane, undergo conversion to alcohols in liver cells, catalyzed by cytochrome P-450 monooxygenases. For *n*-alkanes with a carbon chain length of eight or more, only oxidation of the terminal carbon has been observed. After this conversion, conjugation of the hydroxy group to a glucuronic acid or sulfate ester may occur. Further oxidation to an aldehyde, ketone, or carboxylic acid by other enzyme systems may take place. The fatty acids formed from the *n*-alkanes can be degraded by β-oxidation.

Decane is oxidized by microsomes from the livers of mouse, rat, rabbit, and other species. The metabolites of this biochemical process, identified as excretion products in the urine, were decanol, decanoic acid, and decamethylene glycol. Decane hydroxylation took place in the liver, other organs, and microsomes isolated from the kidneys and lungs. Phenobarbital pretreatment in rats markedly increased *n*-decane hydroxylase activity in liver microsomes.

Decane has been shown to directly affect *in vitro* cytochrome P-450 enzyme activity toward other substrates. Decane caused reduced recovery of products of liver and lung 7-ethoxycoumarin deethylase and of lung benzo[a]pyrene hydroxylase activities in microsome preparations from Sprague Dawley rats. However, it did not reduce nicotinamide adenine dinucleotide phosphate (NADPH) formation and did not affect cytochrome P-450 reductase activity when the enzyme was assayed with the substrate, cytochrome *c*.

Mechanism of Toxicity

The mechanism of toxicity is suspected to be similar to other solvents that rapidly induce anesthesia-like effects, that is a 'nonspecific narcosis' due to disruption (solvation) of the integrity of the cellular membranes of the central nervous system.

Decane is generally considered to be relatively nontoxic compared to effects seen following exposure to other aliphatic hydrocarbons. This is probably due to the fact that it is less volatile than the shorter chain aliphatic hydrocarbons (e.g., pentane or heptane) and may not be as readily transferred across either the pulmonary alveoli or the blood–brain barrier. If it is aspirated into the lungs, however, *n*-decane will cause adverse effects similar to those seen with petroleum distillates.

Using *in vitro* and/or microbial systems, *n*-decane has been shown to be metabolized to decanol and is thus thought to be readily biodegradable in the natural environment.

Acute and Short-Term Toxicity (Animal/Human)

At very high concentrations involving acute exposure, *n*-decane is an asphyxiant and narcotic. Decane has been shown to have narcotic effects in both mice and rats, primarily in experiments documenting acute exposure at high concentrations. One study estimated a 2-h LC_{50} of 72 300 mg m^{-3} in rats. In mice, an intravenous dose of 912 mg kg^{-1} is expected to cause death in 50% of the experimental animals.

Acute adverse effects to humans would be expected to be similar to those seen in laboratory animals that are acutely exposed to petroleum solvents. Humans who are acutely exposed to hydrocarbon solvents show, in general, order of increasing exposure, disorientation, euphoria, giddiness, confusion, unconsciousness, paralysis, convulsion, and death. There is currently no regulatory/industrial air standard for occupational exposure to *n*-decane.

Human subjects exposed to *n*-decane (10, 35, or 100 μl l^{-1}) in a chamber for 6 h day^{-1}, 1 day week^{-1} for 4 weeks developed decreased tear film stability, increased number of conjunctival polymorphonuclear leukocytes, and irritation of mucous membranes of the eyes. Decane, in solutions as strong as 30%, produced no skin irritation in human subjects when applied for 24 h (NTP, 2002).

Chronic Toxicity (Animal/Human)

Dermal application of *n*-decane as an undiluted liquid to mice (0.1–0.15 g mouse^{-1}, three times per week for 50 weeks) caused fibrosis of the dermis, pigmentation, and some ulceration. Kidney effects and lung hemorrhaging were also observed in some of the animals.

A rat study showed that a concentration of 540 ppm in air (18 h day^{-1}, 7 days week^{-1}, 8 weeks) had a significant positive effect on weight gain. This exposure also caused some slight adverse effects (e.g., decreased white blood cell count) but no significant toxic effects overall.

Immunotoxicity

A comprehensive search on the adverse effects of decane on the immune system could not find any studies in the public domain. Pregnant women should, however, avoid inhalation of any type of petroleum solvent vapors.

Reproductive Toxicity

A comprehensive search on the adverse reproductive effects of decane could not find any studies in the public domain. Pregnant women should, however, avoid inhalation of any type of petroleum solvent vapors.

Genotoxicity

Decane was not mutagenic when tested (either with or without known mutagens) in five strains of *Salmonella typhimurium* at concentrations of up to 10 mg plate^{-1}. Mutagenicity was not enhanced by rodent liver S-9. An NTP study reported results for *n*-decane in *Salmonella* as 'nonmutagenic' and 'inconclusive' with no further details.

Carcinogenicity

No 2-year carcinogenicity studies of *n*-decane were identified in the available literature. Decane has been shown to have cocarcinogenic and tumor-promoting activities (skin painting) in several studies.

Clinical Management

Persons who are exposed to high concentrations of *n*-decane in air should vacate or be removed from the source and seek fresh air. Upon oral ingestion, vomiting should not be induced as pulmonary aspiration may occur, resulting in severe narcosis and/or death. In areas of expected increased concentration, extreme care must be taken to use explosion proof apparatus and keep the areas free from ignition sources, such as sparks from static electricity.

Ecotoxicology

The US EPA ECOTOX database has very few records for *n*-decane. An acute (48–96 h) no observed effect concentration of 500 mg l^{-1} was recorded for the sheepshead minnow (saltwater fish). An acute 96-h LC_{50} of 530 mg l^{-1} was reported for the bluegill fish (*Lepomis macrochirus*). The no observed effect concentration for the water flea (*Daphnia magna*) was 1.3 mg l^{-1}. The 24 and 48 h LC_{50} were 24 and 18 mg l^{-1}, respectively.

Other Hazards

Extreme care must be taken to keep areas of expected high concentration free from ignition sources, for example, sparks from static electricity. Only explosion proof equipment should be used in these areas. The lower and upper explosive limits for *n*-octane are 0.8 and 5.4% by volume, respectively.

See also: Petroleum Distillates; Propane; Pentane; Hexane; Heptane; Octane.

Further Reading

Hodgson, A.T., Levin, H., 2003. Volatile organic compounds in indoor air: a review of concentrations measured in North America since 1990. LBNL-51715. Revised October 2003.

HSDB, 2011. Decane. Hazardous Substances Databank, National Library of Medicine Toxnet system, [Record No. 63]. http://www.toxnet.nlm.nih.gov. Searched October 20, 2011.

National Toxicology Program, 2002. Summary of Data for Chemical Selection, Decane (124-18-5). Prepared for NCI by Technical Resources International, Inc. to support chemical nomination under contract no. N02-CB-07007 (11/02; 3/03).

Schultz, T.W., 1989. Nonpolar narcosis: a review of the mechanisms of action for baseline aquatic toxicity. ASTM STP 1027. In: Cowgill, U.M., Williams, L.R. (Eds.), Aquatic Toxicology and Hazard Assessment, vol. 12. American Society for Testing and Materials, Philadelphia, PA, pp. 104–109.

USEPA, 2011. United States Environmental Protection Agency, Office of Pollution Prevention Toxics and Syracuse Research Corporation. EPI Suite Quantitative Structure Activity Relationship Computer Program: http://www.epa.gov/oppt/exposure/pubs/episuite.htm – US EPA: Estimation Program Interface (EPI) Suite.

Verschueren, K., 1996. Handbook of Environmental Data on Organic Chemicals, third ed. Van Nostrand Reinhold, New York. ISBN 0-442-01916-5.

DEET (Diethyltoluamide)

ME Hilburn, Oklahoma State University, Stillwater, OK, USA

This article is a revision of the previous edition article by Mark L. Winter, volume 1, pp 728–729, © 2005, Elsevier Inc.

- Chemical Abstracts Service Registry Number: CAS 134-62-3
- Synonyms: Detamide; Autan; I-Delphene; Meta-delphene; Black Flag; Tabarad; Delphene; Dieltamide; Flypel; Muskol; Naugatuck Det; Off; 612 Plus; Jungle plus; Pellit; DETA; DET; *N,N*-Diethyl-3-methylbenzamide; *N,N*-Diethyl-*m*-toluamide
- Chemical/Pharmaceutical/Other Class: Methyl benzamide repellent
- Chemical Structure:

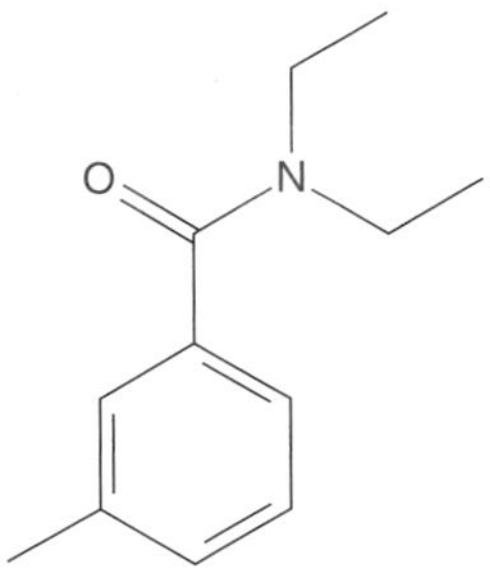

History/Background

DEET was first developed and patented by the US Army in 1946. It was approved for general public use by the US Environmental Protection Agency (EPA) in 1957 and was reregistered in 1998. It has been estimated that more than 1.8 million kg (~4 million pounds) of DEET are used in the United States every year in more than 225 registered products. DEET is often sold and used in lotions or sprays with concentrations up to 100%. However, the Center for Disease Control recommends only 30–50% DEET to reduce the incidence of vector-borne disease transmission. Registered products must contain at least 95% of the meta-isomer, but small amounts of the more toxic ortho-isomer and the less toxic para-isomer are permitted.

Uses

DEET is used as an insect repellent.

Environmental Fate

Little information is available on the environmental fate of DEET. DEET is stable to hydrolysis at environmental pH levels. The initial belief was that DEET was not likely to enter aquatic ecosystems because it was first registered for indoor use. It has been shown in several studies, however, that DEET is found in many waterways in the United States and around the world, such as groundwater, open water, sewage (influent and effluent), surface water, and septic waste in concentrations ranging from $30\,\mathrm{ng\,l^{-1}}$ to $13\,\mathrm{\mu g\,l^{-1}}$. A major source of introduction to aquatic environments is via sewage following washing and excretion by humans. The potential for DEET to be transported through soil is unknown. Although, some studies have shown that purification of water containing low concentrations of DEET using a combination of sand filtration, activated sludge treatment, and ozonation has a removal efficiency less than 69% (ozonation being the most efficient step). Sand filtration alone was inefficient, notably due to DEET's hydrophilic nature ($K_{ow} < 3$). This evidence suggests that DEET may not be retained in soil and other organic matter, but travels with groundwater into larger bodies of water, and more extreme measures than this must be taken to remove DEET from natural and domestic waters. On the other hand, one study noted that DEET 'has an estimated K_{oc} value of 536, indicating potential for sorption to suspended solids and sediment.'

Exposure and Monitoring

DEET is available in solutions, lotions, gels, aerosol sprays, sticks, impregnated towelettes, and wristbands. Dermal and ocular exposures are the most common exposure pathways. Inhalation is possible when using sprays and also ingestion if eating outdoors without proper hand washing.

Toxicokinetics

Approximately 50% of each topically applied dose of DEET is absorbed within 6 h. Peak plasma levels are attained within 1 h. DEET should not be applied to damaged skin or open wounds; this will increase the rate of absorption. Ingestion of DEET can result in symptoms within 30 min, implying very rapid absorption. Oxidative enzymes in the liver metabolize DEET. Two major metabolic pathways in humans have been determined: oxidation of the methyl group giving a carboxylic acid or methyl hydroxyl group on the benzene ring and dealkylation of the amide side chain. The two main metabolites in humans are *N*-ethyl-*m*-toluamide (ET) and *N,N*-diethyl-*m*-hydroxymethylbenzamide (BALC). The metabolites are produced by separate Cytochrome P450 isoforms. People will metabolize DEET differently based on the level of activity of these isoforms in each individual.

Following movement through the skin, DEET is absorbed and distributed rather rapidly. Some studies indicate, however, that DEET and metabolites can remain in the skin and fatty tissues for 1 or 2 months after topical application. About 3.8–8.33% of an applied dose is excreted in urine. Ingestion of 50 ml of 100% DEET by adolescents or adults has resulted in severe toxicity and death. Ingestion of 25 ml of 50% DEET by a 1-year-old child resulted in severe toxicity.

Mechanism of Toxicity

Historically, it was thought that DEET worked via blocking of insect olfactory receptors and that DEET masked the target to the insect senses so the insect would not detect a food source. Instead, however, recent evidence indicates that the odor of DEET is what acts as the true repellent. A specific type of an olfactory receptor neuron in the antennal sensilla of mosquitoes was identified, and this neuron is activated by DEET. This activity is responsible for the properties that give DEET its repellent ability.

DEET is also toxic to the central nervous system (CNS). DEET acts as an inhibitor to the enzyme acetylcholinesterase which is required for the proper functioning of the human nervous system, other vertebrates, and insects. The enzyme acetylcholinesterase hydrolyzes acetylcholine, which is important to muscle control. When this process is inhibited, acetylcholine builds up in the synaptic cleft and causes neuromuscular paralysis and death by asphyxiation.

Acute and Short-Term Toxicity (or Exposure)

Animal

The acute oral LD_{50} values were reported as 1800–2700 mg kg^{-1} in male rats and 1750–1800 mg kg^{-1} in females. Rats given an LD_{50} dose showed signs of toxicity that included lacrimation, chromodacryorrhea, depression, prostration, tremors, asphyxia convulsions, and respiratory failure. Ocular administration of DEET led to mild to moderate edema of the nictitating membrane, lacrimation, conjunctivitis, and corneal injury. These signs dissipated within 5 days. DEET is not a sensitizer in guinea pigs.

Human

A toxic syndrome consisting of ataxia, hypertonicity, tremor, and clonic jerking, and progressing to coma and seizures, can occur after dermal or oral exposure. Ingestion can cause gastrointestinal irritation with nausea, vomiting, and diarrhea. Symptoms can occur within 30 min after an acute ingestion. Dermal exposure can cause irritation, sensitization, and erythema. A study with volunteers using 75% DEET showed that 48% had severe dermal reactions at the crease of the elbow but not at other dermal application sites. Ocular exposure can cause eye irritation. Inhalation can cause respiratory tract irritation or irritation of the mucous membranes.

Chronic Toxicity (or Exposure)

Animal

Dietary exposure to DEET for 200 days at 10 000 ppm led to growth retardation. Relative increases in testes and liver weights were noted in male rats, liver and spleen in female rats, and kidneys of both sexes. No significant changes were noted at 500 ppm. Dermal application of DEET (1 g kg^{-1} day^{-1}) led to reproductive toxicity in rats. No teratogenic response was noted in rabbits treated with dermal dosages as high as 5 g kg^{-1} day^{-1}. DEET can cause testicular and renal hypertrophy with repeated dosing.

Human

Chronic application of 70% DEET solution caused paranoid psychosis, pressurized speech, flight of ideas, and delusions after 2 weeks of daily application for the inappropriate treatment of a skin rash. Repeated application causes erythema. Extensive daily dermal application of 10–15% DEET for 2 days to 3 months has resulted in encephalopathy in children. Toxic encephalopathy has been associated with DEET in children. Signs of toxicity included agitation, weakness, disorientation, ataxia, seizures, coma, and in three cases, death. As part of the Reregistration Eligibility Decision on DEET released in 1998, however, the US EPA reviewed all available data on the toxicity of DEET and concluded that "normal use of DEET does not present a health concern to the general US population."

Immunotoxicity

Little is known about the immunotoxicity of DEET. The results of one study suggested that DEET affects immune function at exposure levels reported in the occupational and military settings. In this study, the T-dependent IgM response was dose responsively suppressed by DEET in B6C3F1 mice. It was determined that when comparing the DEET doses used in this rodent study, the half-life is similar to that reported in humans. It is unclear if DEET is a potential health hazard for the general population.

Reproductive Toxicity

Some claims have been made that the application of DEET by pregnant mothers has cause some birth defects. At least two controlled studies, however, have shown that DEET was detected at concentrations up to 3.55 ng ml^{-1} in amniotic fluid and cord serum in pregnant women exposed, yet no clinical abnormalities or aberrant birth outcomes were observed in the newborns or up to 1 year after birth.

Genotoxicity

Little is known about the genotoxic effects of DEET. Although DEET is considered to be noncarcinogenic, there is some concern that it can cause some genotoxic effects. One study showed a concentration-dependent increase in genotoxic effects for DEET to middle turbinate human nasal mucosal cells. Exposure of 1.0 mM DEET (the highest dose given) showed a mean percentage of undamaged cells of 20.4 ± 5.2%. This result was compared to a positive control (MMNG) showing 0% undamaged cells at a concentration of 0.75 mM.

Carcinogenicity

DEET is not listed as a carcinogen by the American Conference of Governmental Industrial Hygienists (ACGIH), the International Agency for Research on Cancer (IARC), the National Toxicology Program (NTP), or the California Proposition 65 (CA Prop 65). More recent research has found that DEET shows a significant concentration-dependent genotoxic response with human nasal mucosal cells, suggesting potential carcinogenic properties.

Clinical Management

Basic life-support measures for respiratory and cardiovascular function should be used. Dermal decontamination should be accomplished by repeated washing with soap. Exposed eyes should be irrigated with copious amounts of room-temperature water for at least 15 min. If eye irritation persists after irrigation, medical assistance should be sought. Ipecac-induced emesis is not recommended in cases of accidental oral exposure because coma and seizures can occur rapidly within 30 min to 1 h of ingestion. Gastric lavage should be performed cautiously with a small-bore soft nasogastric tube with small aliquots of water or saline. Activated charcoal can also be used. Initial control of seizure activity may be attempted with a benzodiazepine. Respiratory depression, hypotension, dysrhythmias, and the need for endotracheal intubation should be monitored.

Ecotoxicology

A limited but increasing amount of data is available on the ecotoxicology of DEET. A few studies show that it is slightly toxic to birds, coldwater fish, and invertebrates, with typical toxicity values about 100–200 mg l^{-1}, but little or no evidence shows toxicity to small mammals. The acute LD_{50} in quail was 1375 mg kg^{-1}. The LC_{50} values for *Oncorhynchus mykiss* (rainbow trout), *Gammarus fasciatus* (scud), *Pimephales promelas* (fathead minnow), and *Gambusia affinis* (western mosquitofish) are 71.3 mg l^{-1} 96 h^{-1}, 100 mg l^{-1} 96 h^{-1}, 110 mg l^{-1} 96 h^{-1}, and 235 mg l^{-1} 48 h^{-1}, respectively. The DEET LC_{50} for *Daphnia magna* (water flea) is 160 mg l^{-1} 48 h^{-1}. The LC_{50} values for *N*,*N*-diethyl-*m*-toluamide-*N*-oxide (DEET metabolite) and *N*-ethyl-*m*-toluamide (DEET metabolite) for *D. magna* are >190 mg l^{-1} 96 h^{-1} and 109 mg l^{-1} 96 h^{-1}, respectively. Additionally, phytoplankton (*Chlorella protothecoides* or green microalgae) showed 20% inhibition in photosynthetic yield at 100 mg l^{-1} DEET with an EC_{50} of 388 mg l^{-1} 24 h^{-1}.

Miscellaneous

When combined with other agents such as carbamates and other insecticides, DEET can interact with them to give enhanced toxic effects. The dermal application of DEET and the pyrethroid fenvalerate can cause hypersalivation, ataxia, lethargy, seizures, and death in cats within 4–6 h. In rats, it has been shown that dermal exposure to DEET and permethrin increases permeability of the blood–brain and the blood–testis barrier compared to exposure to DEET alone.

DEET can also act as a solvent and should be not be used near some plastics, synthetic fabrics such as rayon or spandex, leather, or painted or varnished surfaces.

Further Reading

Aronson, D., Weeks, J., Meylan, B., Guiney, P.D., Howard, P.H., Jan 2012. Environmental release, environmental concentrations, and ecological risk of *N*, *N*-diethyl-*m*-toluamide (DEET). Integr. Environ. Assess. Manag. 8 (1), 135–166.

Committee on Gulf War and Health: Literature Review of Pesticides and Solvents, 2003. Gulf war and health: Insecticides and Solvents, vol. 2. National Academies Press, Washington, D.C.

Corbel, V., Stankiewicz, M., Pennetier, C., et al., 2009. Evidence for inhibition of cholinesterases in insect and mammalian nervous systems by the insect repellent DEET. BMC Biol. 7, article number 47.

Costanzo, S.D., Watkinson, A.J., Murby, E.J., Kolpin, D.W., Sandstrom, M.W., 2007. Is there a risk associated with the insect repellent DEET (*N*, *N*-diethyl-*m*-toluamide) commonly found in aquatic environments? Sci. Total Environ. 384, 214–220.

Keil, D.E., McGuinn, W.D., Dudley, A.C., et al., 2009. *N*, *N*-Diethyl-*m*-toluamide (DEET) suppresses humoral immunological function in B6C3F1 mice. Toxicol. Sci. 108 (1), 110–123.

Nakada, N., Shinohara, H., Murata, A., et al., 2007. Removal of selected pharmaceuticals and personal care products (PPCPs) and endocrine-disrupting chemicals (EDCs) during sand filtration and ozonation at a municipal sewage treatment plant. Water Res. 41, 4373–4382.

Plumlee, K.H., 2006. DEET. In: Peterson, M.E., Talcott, P.A. (Eds.), Small Animal Toxicology, second ed. Elsevier Inc, pp. 690–692.

Sudakin, D.L., Trevathan, W.R., 2003. DEET: a review and update of safety and risk in the general population. J. Toxicol. Clin. Toxicol. 41, 831–839.

Tisch, M., Schmezer, P., Faulde, M., Groh, A., Maier, H., 2002. Genotoxicity studies on permethrin, DEET and diazinon in primary human nasal mucosal cells. Eur. Arch. Otorhinolaryngol. 259, 150–153.

Weeks, J.A., Guiney, P.D., Nikiforov, A.I., Jan 2012. Assessment of the environmental fate and ecotoxicity of *N*, *N*-diethyl-*m*-toluamide (DEET). Integr. Environ. Assess. Manag. 8 (1), 120–134.

Yan, X., Lashley, S., Smulian, J.C., et al., 2009. Pesticide concentrations in matrices collected in the perinatal period in a population of pregnant women and newborns in New Jersey, USA. Hum. Ecol. Risk Assess. 15, 948–967.

Relevant Websites

http://www.atsdr.cdc.gov – Center for Disease Control.
http://pmep.cce.cornell.edu – Cornell University.
http://www.nap.edu/catalog.php?record_id=10628 – The National Academies Press.
http://www.epa.gov – US Environmental Protection Agency.
http://www.inchem.org/documents/pds/pds/pest80_e.htm – World Health Organization.

DEF (Butyl Phosphorotrithioate)

P Raman, Northeast Ohio Medical University, Rootstown, OH, USA

- Name: DEF (butyl phosphorotrithioate)
- Chemical Abstracts Service Registry Number: 78-48-8
- Synonyms: Tributyl *S,S,S*-phosphorothioate; Butiphos; De-Green; Tribuphos
- Molecular Formula: $C_{12}H_{27}OPS_3$
- Chemical Structure:

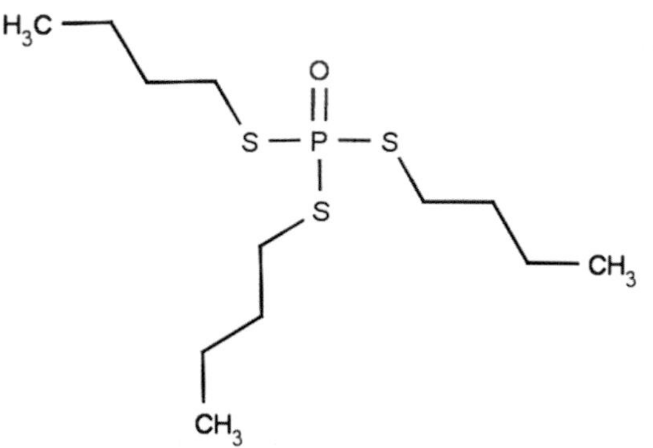

Background

DEF is a cholinesterase-inhibiting organophosphorus pesticide compound used as a cotton defoliant that was registered in 1960. DEF is a colorless to pale-yellow transparent liquid with a skunk-like odor. It has a molecular weight of 314.5, water solubility of 2.3 ppm at 20 °C, melting point of <−25 °C, and boiling point of 150 °C at 0.3 mm Hg, with a relative density of 1.057. It is completely miscible with *n*-hexane, dichloromethane, toluene, and 2-propanol and has an octanol–water partition coefficient of 3.31×10^5 at 25 °C. DEF toxicity is primarily attributed to inhibition of various esterases, including acetylcholinesterase (AChE), butyrylcholinesterase (BuChE), neuropathic target esterase (NTE), and carboxylesterase, resulting in increased accumulation of endogenous acetylcholine (ACh) in cholinergic nerve terminals and related effector organs. Acute DEF toxicity leads to muscarinic receptor stimulation characterized by increased intestinal motility, bronchial constriction and bronchial secretions, miosis, bladder contraction, and bradycardia. Nicotinic receptor activation causes muscle weakness, twitching, cramps, and general fasciculations. Severe cases of DEF poisoning may lead to slurred speech, tremors, ataxia, convulsion, and depression of respiratory and circulatory centers, eventually resulting in coma. DEF is also a potent liver arylamidase inhibitor *in vitro*. Based on an exposure assessment for DEF issued by the US Environmental Protection Agency (EPA) in an Interim Reregistration Eligibility Document in 2000, a reentry interval of 7 days was established to be adequate for protection of cotton field workers exposed to DEF. Some common names of DEF are tribufos, butifos, merphos oxide, and Folex.

Uses

DEF is an organophosphate chemical used as a cotton defoliant to facilitate mechanical harvesting. Recommended application rate is ~1–2.5 pints per acre per year applied as a diluted spray. Two products containing DEF as their active ingredient include DEF 6, manufactured by Bayer Corporation, and Folex 6 DC, manufactured by Amvac Chemical Co. Used for pest control in industrial agriculture (tends to be more toxic agents), organophosphates of low to intermediate toxicity are used to control ectoparasites on farm and companion animals and humans (head lice), and for home and garden pest control.

Environmental Fate and Behavior

DEF is relatively stable in aqueous solutions (pH 5 and 7) up to 32 days but slightly degraded at pH 9 with a half-life of 124 days. The hydrolytic breakdown product of DEF is known as desbutylthio tribufos. DEF is stable up to 30 days in sandy loam soil exposed to natural sunlight, but degrades in aqueous solution upon exposure to natural sunlight for 30 days, with an estimated half-life of 44 days. The estimated soil adsorption coefficient (K_d) for DEF ranges from 60.6 for sandy loam soil to 106 for clay loam. The estimated soil adsorption constant (K_{oc}) for DEF ranges from 4870 for silt loam to 12 684 for sand. DEF is highly persistent in soil with biodegradation half-lives of 745 and 389 days in sandy loam soil under aerobic and anaerobic conditions. Based on water solubility, high soil adsorption, hydrolysis, and aerobic soil metabolism data, DEF is not identified as a potential groundwater contaminant. However, DEF is likely to become airborne following aerial application or ground spraying. Also, while DEF itself is not significantly volatile, its degradation product, *n*-butyl mercaptan (nBM), is volatile and accounts for a skunk-like odor near areas where DEF has been applied. DEF is also formed via release of the defoliant merphos, which undergoes rapid oxidation under environmental conditions to tribufos. DEF has a vapor pressure of 5.3×10^{-6} mm Hg at 25 °C, suggesting its occurrence in both vapor and particulate phases in ambient atmosphere. Vapor-phase DEF degrades by interacting with photochemically produced hydroxyl radicals; half-life for this reaction in air is estimated to be 5 h. Particulate-phase DEF gets removed from atmosphere by wet and dry deposition. Volatilization of DEF from water surfaces is not an important fate process based on its Henry's Law constant of 2.9×10^{-7} atm m^3 mol^{-1} at 20 °C.

Exposure Routes and Pathways

The major route of exposure to DEF is skin contact. It is readily absorbed by oral exposure and rapidly metabolized.

 http://dx.doi.org/10.1016/B978-0-12-386454-3.00301-8

Toxicokinetics

DEF is readily absorbed through the skin and orally. It is metabolized to nBM in the gastrointestinal tract by hydrolysis. The metabolite is excreted in the urine. A urinary metabolic profiling following oral administration of DEF to a lactating goat revealed that DEF is efficiently metabolized to many metabolites. The amount of DEF in liver, kidney, and muscle represented 0.1% of the total residue. A major metabolite, 3-hydroxybutylmethyl sulfone, was found in the tissue, milk, and urine. The hydrolytic products of DEF, *S,S*-dibutyl phosphorodithioate and *S*-butyl phosphorothioate were identified as minor components in urine, comprising 5 and 4% of the total residue, respectively. Metabolism of DEF involves hydrolysis to *S,S*-dibutyl phosphorodithioate and nBM, the latter being converted to the fatty acid, butyric acid. *S,S*-dibutyl is susceptible to further metabolism to nBM and phosphate.

Mechanism of Toxicity

DEF is a relatively weak inhibitor of AChE. The compound is hydrolyzed to a large extent in the intestine to nBM, which is responsible for the late acute effects of DEF. The putative molecular target in neural tissue for initiation of delayed neuropathy is neurotoxic esterase or NTE. Metabolism proceeds by hydrolysis followed by methylation and successive oxidation of butylmercaptan, yielding the main metabolite (3-hydroxy)-butylmethylsulfone.

Several studies indicate that rodents metabolize and excrete delayed neurotoxic organophosphorus esters with great efficiency, whereas the adult chicken seems to have difficulty carrying out these processes. The feline (cat model) is intermediate between rodents and chickens. No human case of *O*-ethyl-*O*-nitrophenyl phenylphosphonothioate-induced delayed neurotoxicity has been reported despite the fact that it has been in use for over a quarter of a century. Some investigators propose that the cat may be a better model to extrapolate neurotoxicity results to humans. Analysis of the metabolism and residue levels of the defoliant *S,S,S*-tributylphosphorotrithioate in a goat model revealed that majority of the metabolites were excreted in the urine, although quantifiable amounts were recorded in the other tissues (e.g., liver, kidney, muscle), milk, and feces. Major metabolite was found to be 3-hydroxybutylmethyl sulfone, and the two minor components in the urine were *S,S*-dibutyl phosphorodithioate and *S*-butyl phosphorothioate.

Acute and Short-Term Toxicity (or Exposure)

Animal

DEF produces profound hypothermia in rats, mice, and guinea pigs by inhibition of thermogenesis. Its actions on heat conservation and motor control are, however, minimal. It is effective against both shivering and nonshivering thermogenesis and completely blocks the increase in body temperature evoked by anterior hypothalamic stimulation. The toxicological effect of DEF, the extent and permanence of injury, and the progression or improvement of clinical signs of toxicity depended on the dose, duration, and route of exposure. The acute effects of DEF in experimental animals are primarily attributed to inhibition of AChE, BuChE, NTE, and carboxylesterase. Neurological effects are most predominant following daily exposures ranging from 3 weeks to 3 months. Other adverse effects in animals include anemia, impaired renal function and reproductive toxicity such as reduced fertility, increased number of stillbirths, reduced birth weights, and increased postnatal deaths. LD_{50} values of DEF in different experimental models are listed below:

Animal model	*Gender*	*Route of administration*	*Dose*
Guinea pig	Male	Oral	260 mg kg^{-1}
Rabbit	N/A	Dermal	97 mg kg^{-1}
Mouse	N/A	i.p.	290 mg kg^{-1}
Mouse	N/A	Oral	77 mg kg^{-1}
Rat	N/A	i.p.	210 mg kg^{-1}
Rat	N/A	Dermal	168 mg kg^{-1}
Rat	Male	Oral	435 mg kg^{-1}
Rat	Female	Oral	234 mg kg^{-1}
Rat	Male	Inhalation	4.65 mg l^{-1} per 4 h
Rat	Female	Inhalation	2.46 mg l^{-1} per 4 h

Source: National Library of Medicine TOXNET.

Human

Late acute poisoning from DEF is related to the release of its breakdown product, nBM. Signs of toxicity appear within 1 h after exposure and include general weakness, malaise, sweating, nausea, vomiting, anxiety, and drowsiness. DEF affects the lymphocyte NTE in exposed workers. The most common clinical manifestations include cholinergic toxicity (such as lacrimation, salivation, diarrhea, pupillary constriction, tremors, convulsions, hypothermia), as well as delayed neuropathy such as loss of coordination and paralysis.

Chronic Toxicity (or Exposure)

Animal

A subchronic administration of DEF caused three toxicologic effects in hens, depending on the route of exposure: (1) an acute cholinergic effect resulting from inhibition of AChE, relieved by atropine, not associated with neuropathological lesions; (2) a late acute effect in chickens resulting from nBM toxicity 4 days after oral administration of daily large doses of DEF resulting in darkening and drooping of the comb, loss of appetite and weight, weakness, emaciation, paralysis, and death, not relieved by atropine nor associated with histopathological changes in nerve tissues; and (3) delayed neurotoxicity after a delay period following topical application causing axonal and myelin degeneration resulting in ataxia, paralysis, and death. Other adverse effects observed in animals following long-term (1–2 years) exposure to DEF include reduced body weight, hypothermia, brain AChE inhibition, and anemia. In addition, numerous noncarcinogenic as well as potentially precancerous microscopic changes have also been reported, primarily affecting gastrointestinal tract, liver, lungs, adrenals, and spleen.

Human

Both intensity and length of exposure play important roles in determining the extent of inhibition of NTE in lymphocytes; 50% of preexposed values of NTE activity were obtained when measured 3 or 4 weeks after the beginning of DEF exposure. However, there is no direct evidence of a correlation between a high level of lymphocyte NTE inhibition and development of neuropathy in humans. Blood AChE and plasma BuChE levels remained unchanged during the study period. There is no available weight-of-the-evidence summary assessment for DEF as a developmental or reproductive toxin.

In Vitro Toxicity Data

DEF has been reported to cause extensive alterations in morphological features of erythrocyte and nuclear membranes and affected the permeability properties of rat liver mitochondrial membrane. A reduction in the activity of cytochrome-c-oxidase and NADPH-oxidase has also been observed. Content of both DNA and RNA decreased in tissues studied within 1 month of DEF intoxication and was usually restored within 3 months. Histological study showed development of necrodystrophy in liver tissue and of fibroplastic glomerulonephritis in kidney. The deteriorating effect of DEF on cellular genome functions relates not only to its cytotoxicity but also to the cancerogenic and mutagenic properties of the pesticide.

Clinical Management

Supportive and symptomatic treatment should be provided to the patient following accidental or intentional exposure to DEF. Airway protection along with administration of either atropine sulfate (intravenous or intramuscular), pralidoxine, or glycopyrolate is probably the best antidote to deal with DEF poisoning.

Mutagenicity

All studies were negative.

Genotoxicity

Tribufos (98.5%) did not produce an increase in the mutation frequency in a mutagenicity assay using *Salmonella typhimurium* strains TA98, TA100, TA1535, TA1537, and TA1538 at concentrations ranging from 667 to 10 000 μg per plate with and without metabolic activation. No increase in chromosomal aberrations was seen in Chinese hamster ovary cells exposed to tribufos (98.5%) at concentrations of 0.007–0.1 μl ml^{-1} with metabolic activation and at 0.004–0.05 μl ml^{-1} without activation. Other investigators did not find any increase in sister chromatid exchanges in Chinese hamster V79 cells exposed to tribufos (95.7%) at concentrations from 2.5 to 20 μg ml^{-1} with and without metabolic activation. In an unscheduled DNA synthesis assay, no increase in the average grains per nucleus was observed in rat primary hepatocytes exposed to tribufos (98.5%) at concentrations between 0.000 1 and 0.03 μl ml^{-1}.

Carcinogenicity

US EPA classified tribufos as a likely high dose/not likely low dose carcinogen under its new carcinogenicity classification system. Their justification for this classification was that tumors were only increased at the highest dose level where severe toxicity occurred. Although not explicitly stated, this classification treats tribufos as a threshold carcinogen because they use a margin of exposure (MOE) approach to protect for oncogenicity rather than calculate an oncogenic potency factor. The no observed effect level (NOEL) they selected to calculate the MOEs for oncogenicity was 0.1 mg kg^{-1} day^{-1} based on plasma ChE inhibition in dogs, the most sensitive endpoint for chronic exposure (i.e., the same NOEL used for evaluating the chronic dietary exposure). US EPA had no concerns regarding the acute or chronic exposure to tribufos through drinking water.

Ecotoxicology (All Values Are at 95% Confidence Limit/Interval)

LC_{50} Values

Oncorhynchus mykiss (rainbow trout) 660 μg l^{-1} per 96 h at 13 °C (560–750 μg l^{-1} per 96 h). Static conditions without aeration.

Oncorhynchus mykiss (rainbow trout, weight 0.91 g) 1700 ppb per 96 h (1300–2300 ppb); flow-through, 96.2%.

Lepomis macrochirus (bluegill) 620 μg l^{-1} per 96 h at 18 °C (390–975 μg l^{-1} per 96 h). Static conditions without aeration.

Menidia beryllina (inland silverside) 455 μg l^{-1} per 96 h. Conditions of bioassay not specified in source examined.

Anas platyrhynchos (mallard duck, 7 days old) dietary >5000 ppm per 8 days.

Colinus virginianus (northern bobwhite, 14 days old) dietary 1519 ppm per 8 days.

Americamysis bahia (opossum shrimp, <24 h old) 11.5 ppb per 96 h (9.3–15.1 ppb); flow-through, 96.4% active ingredient (AI) formulated product.

Bufo woodhousei fowleri (Fowler's toad, tadpoles) 1200 μg l^{-1} per 24 h (900–2600 μg l^{-1}); static formulated product.

Bufo woodhousei fowleri (Fowler's toad, tadpoles) 760 μg l^{-1} per 48 h (460–820 μg l^{-1}); static formulated product.

Bufo woodhousei fowleri (Fowler's toad, tadpoles) 420 μg l^{-1} per 96 h (160–1100 μg l^{-1}); static formulated product.

Cyprinodon variegatus (sheepshead minnow, weight 0.10 g) 767 ppb per 96 h (56–1370 ppb); flow-through, 98.6% AI formulated product.

Lepomis macrochirus (bluegill, weight 1.9 g) 630 ppb per 96 h (500–780 ppb); flow-through, 96.2% AI formulated product.

Lepomis macrochirus (bluegill, weight 2.3 g) 610 ppb per 96 h; flow-through, 72.3% AI formulated product.

Exposure Standards and Guidelines

Children (1–6 years) have been reported to have the highest potential for both acute and chronic dietary exposure to DEF. DEF has an MOE that ranges from 40 to 11 000 for acute systemic effects, and from 1500 to 37 000 for acute dermal irritation. Allowable tolerances for residues of defoliant DEF in or on food commodities are established at 0.002–0.02 ppm.

See also: Delayed Neurotoxicity; Pesticides.

Further Reading

Abou-Donia, M.B., Graham, D.G., Abdo, K.M., Komeil, A.A., 1979. Delayed neurotoxic, late acute and cholinergic effects of *S,S,S*-tributyl phosphorotrithioate (DEF): subchronic (90 days) administration in hens. Toxicology 14 (3), 229–243.

Anderson, T.A., Salice, C.J., Erickson, R.A., et al., 2013. Effects of landuse and precipitation on pesticides and water quality in playa lakes of the southern high plains. Chemosphere 92 (1), 84–90.

Brausch, J.M., Smith, P.N., 2009. Mechanisms of resistance and cross-resistance to agrochemicals in the fairy shrimp *Thamnocephalus platyurus* (Crustacea: Anostraca). Aquat. Toxicol. 92 (3), 140–145.

Casida, J.E., Quistad, G.B., 2005. Serine hydrolase targets of organophosphorus toxicants. Chem. Biol. Interact. 157–158, 277–283.

Fujioka, K., Casida, J.E., 2007. Glutathione *S*-transferase conjugation of organophosphorus pesticides yields *S*-phospho-, *S*-aryl-, and *S*-alkylglutathione derivatives. Chem. Res. Toxicol. 20 (8), 1211–1217.

Kreft, W.D., Hoffert, J.R., Fromm, P.O., 1985. Action of organophosphates on the electroretinogram of rainbow trout. Exp. Biol. 44 (1), 19–27.

Mosallanejad, H., Smagghe, G., 2009. Biochemical mechanisms of methoxyfenozide resistance in the cotton leafworm *Spodoptera littoralis*. Pest Manage. Sci. 65 (7), 732–736.

Quistad, G.B., Fisher, K.J., Owen, S.C., Klintenberg, R., Casida, J.E., 2005. Platelet-activating factor acetylhydrolase: selective inhibition by potent *n*-alkyl methylphosphonofluoridates. Toxicol. Appl. Pharmacol. 205 (2), 149–156.

Quistad, G.B., Klintenberg, R., Casida, J.E., 2005. Blood acylpeptide hydrolase activity is a sensitive marker for exposure to some organophosphate toxicants. Toxicol. Sci. 86 (2), 291–299.

Shi, J., Zhang, L., Gao, X., January 11, 2011. Characterisation of spinosad resistance in the housefly *Musca domestica* (Diptera: Muscidae). Pest Manag. Sci. (Epub ahead of print).

Van Leeuwen, T., Van Pottelberge, S., Nauen, R., Tirry, L., 2007. Organophosphate insecticides and acaricides antagonise bifenazate toxicity through esterase inhibition in *Tetranychus urticae*. Pest Manag. Sci. 63 (12), 1172–1177.

Relevant Websites

http://www.cdpr.ca.gov/ – California Department of Pesticide Regulation: search for DEF.

http://www.epa.gov/oppsrrd1/REDs/factsheets/2145iredfact.pdf – US Environmental Protection Agency.

http://www.regulations.gov – regulations.gov – Your Voice in Federal Decision-Making: search for Propoxur.

Deferoxamine

SJ Miller, Grady Health System, Atlanta, GA, USA
BW Morgan, Georgia Poison Center, Atlanta, GA, USA

This article is a revision of the previous edition article by Greene Shepherd, volume 1, pp 731–733, © 2005, Elsevier Inc.

- Name: Deferoxamine
- Chemical Abstracts Service Registry Number: 70-51-9
- Synonyms: Desferrioxamine, DFO, Desferral, Deferrioxamine B, Propionohydroxamic acid
- Molecular Formula: $C_{25}H_{48}N_6O_8$
- Chemical Structure:

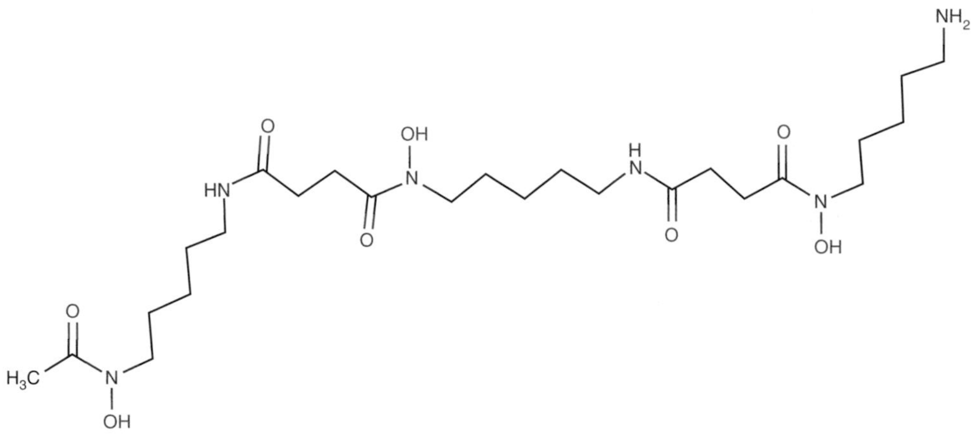

Background

Deferoxamine was introduced in the 1960s for chelation of iron. It is synthesized by removing a central iron molecule from ferrioxamine B, a compound obtained from the microorganism *Streptomyces pilosus*. Deferoxamine binds to iron from ferritin and forms ferrioxamine, a very stable and water-soluble chelate with a characteristic reddish color.

Uses

Deferoxamine is used for the treatment of both acute iron intoxication and chronic iron overload due to transfusion-dependent anemias. It has also been used in trials for malaria treatment and for aluminum chelation in hemodialysis patients. Studies of a rat model of intracerebral hemorrhage have noted that deferoxamine treatment reduced oxidative stress from iron release, indicating a possible role in preventing damage associated with hemorrhagic strokes.

Exposure and Exposure Monitoring

Routes and Pathways of Human Exposure

In cases of acute iron toxicity, intravenous injection and intramuscular injection are the approved routes of administration. Although it is no longer recommended, oral administration of a deferoxamine lavage solution was utilized at one time. Nightly subcutaneous infusions combined with monthly intravenous infusions are used in chronic iron overload.

Toxicokinetics

Deferoxamine alone is poorly absorbed from the gastrointestinal tract. When given orally in the setting of an iron overdose, ferrioxamine is formed in the gastrointestinal tract and seems to be well absorbed. The absorbed ferrioxamine is then cleaved during first-pass metabolism resulting in free iron capable of damaging the hepatic tissue. Deferoxamine metabolism takes place in primarily the plasma, where it is rapidly converted to multiple metabolites. Other organs may also have some metabolizing capacity. Deferoxamine has a very high affinity and specificity for the ferric iron and chelates it in a 1:1 molar ratio; that is, 100 mg of deferoxamine will bind to and eliminate 8.5 mg of elemental iron. Its elimination half-life in human plasma is between 10 and 30 min. With a volume of distribution of 0.6–1.2 $l\ kg^{-1}$, deferoxamine mainly distributes in blood. Renal clearance is the major elimination route of deferoxamine in humans, accounting for about one-third of the total body clearance; 0.296 and 0.234 $l\ h^{-1}$ in healthy and hemochromatotic adults, respectively. Once formed, ferrioxamine is rapidly excreted unchanged in the urine, which may acquire ferrioxamine's brown or reddish 'vin-rose' color. Its elimination half-life is 5.9 and 4.6 h in normal and hemochromatotic adults, respectively. Bile excretion also contributes to elimination.

 http://dx.doi.org/10.1016/B978-0-12-386454-3.00721-1

Mechanism of Toxicity

Localized infusion or injection site reactions may occur with deferoxamine administration, such as pain, urticaria and flushing of the skin. Hypersensitivity reactions have been documented with both acute and chronic administration of deferoxamine. Some of the more serious side effects include infusion rate-related hypotension, renal insufficiency, neurotoxicity, growth retardation, pulmonary toxicity, and infections. Deferoxamine may induce venous dilation when given at doses greater than 15 mg kg^{-1} h^{-1} leading to poor venous return, depressed cardiac output, and eventually hypotension. Increased levels of histamine have been noted during hypotensive episodes, although pretreatment with antihistamines has not been shown to stop the reaction. An acute decrease in glomerular filtration rate and renal plasma flow secondary to hypotension is the possible mechanism underlying the nephrotoxicity induced by deferoxamine. Depletion of iron, translocation of copper, and chelation of other trace elements including zinc may interfere with critical iron-dependent enzymes, causing oxidative damage within various tissues. These are possible mechanisms thought to be responsible for deferoxamine-induced neurotoxicity, growth retardation, and pulmonary toxicity. *In vitro* studies have shown that deferoxamine inhibits the synthesis of prostaglandin, hemoglobin, ferritin, collagen, and DNA. The iron–deferoxamine complex, ferrioxamine, is a growth factor for many bacteria and fungi. Deferoxamine has been associated with *Yersinia enterocolitica* overgrowth and fatal cases of mucormycosis with prolonged therapy.

Acute and Short-Term Toxicity

Animal

The LD_{50} of deferoxamine in mice and rats is greater than 280 mg kg^{-1} with intravenous administration and greater than 1000 mg kg^{-1} with oral administration. Deferoxamine-induced hypotension, tachycardia, and renal insufficiency have also been reported in rats and dogs.

Human

Rapid infusion of deferoxamine over 15 min results in hypotension and tachycardia. An infusion rate of 15 mg kg^{-1} h^{-1} or longer is recommended by the manufacturer. Intravenous deferoxamine administration has been reported to cause renal insufficiency indicated by a progressive increase in serum creatinine and decrease in creatinine clearance. Patients treated with deferoxamine chronically may develop neurotoxicity manifested as visual and hearing losses, growth retardation, and bacterial infections.

Chronic Toxicity

Animal

Dogs given subcutaneous injections of high-dose deferoxamine developed lens opacities.

Human

Patients with inherited or acquired anemias that require regular blood transfusions frequently have symptoms or laboratory evidence of iron overload. Deferoxamine given subcutaneously over 8–12 h has been the standard of therapy for these patients. Patients receiving higher doses (e.g., 125 mg kg^{-1}) demonstrated ocular toxicity of blurriness, loss of night vision, and optic neuropathy. Ototoxicity has been noted as well, with up to 25% of patients on chronic deferoxamine demonstrating some impairment of high-frequency hearing. Impaired cardiac function has been shown in patients receiving deferoxamine and high doses of vitamin C (more than 500 mg daily), although smaller doses (200 mg daily) seem to optimize efficacy of deferoxamine.

Immunotoxicity

There are cases reported in which patients experienced anaphylactic and/or anaphylactoid reactions.

Reproductive Toxicity

Deferoxamine is Food and Drug Administration Pregnancy Category C. Studies with mice and rabbits showed delayed ossification and skeletal abnormalities when doses more than four times the maximum daily human dose were used. *In vitro*, there seems to be little transfer of deferoxamine across the placenta, so effects may be due to chelation of trace metals on the maternal side. However, deferoxamine has been used safely and without adverse effects in pregnant women with thalassemia as treatment of iron overload.

Carcinogenicity

Although long-term carcinogenicity studies have not been performed with deferoxamine, it is possible that cytotoxicity may occur due to DNA synthesis inhibition.

Clinical Management

For patients who develop hypotension secondary to deferoxamine, the infusion should be discontinued and restarted at a slower rate after recovery of the blood pressure. Fluid resuscitation and vasopressors should be used as necessary to support the patient. Treatment of pulmonary toxicity should include ventilatory support and symptomatic care. Patients experiencing anaphylactic reactions should discontinue deferoxamine and start treatment with antihistamines and steroids. Patients who develop infections secondary to deferoxamine use should be started on antibiotics or antifungals (e.g., sulfamethoxazole-trimethoprim or amphotericin B) while cultures and sensitivities are pending. For patients receiving chronic treatment with deferoxamine, periodic evaluation of visual and auditory function is recommended; in patients currently experiencing these neurologic complications,

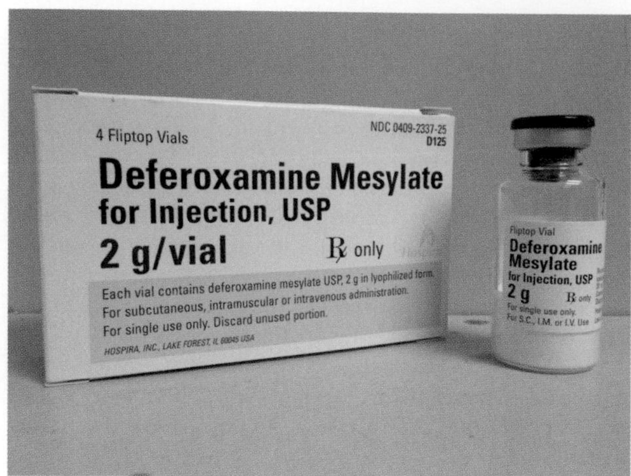

Figure 1 Commercially available deferoxamine mesylate

deferoxamine therapy should be discontinued and a neurologist should be consulted.

Exposure Standards and Guidelines

Deferoxamine is approved for intramuscular and intravenous administration in the setting of acute iron intoxication. Although the manufacturer states that intramuscular is the preferred route for all patients not in shock, most clinicians utilize intravenous infusions of deferoxamine as this is a more reliable delivery method and chelates more iron than intramuscular bolus dosing. The manufacturer recommends a maximum of 6 g of deferoxamine per day and a maximum infusion rate of 15 mg kg^{-1} h^{-1}. Indications for administering deferoxamine in these patients include clinical evidence of iron toxicity, such as shock, altered mental status, metabolic acidosis, or coma; laboratory indications of toxicity – serum iron level greater than 500 μg dl^{-1} or elevated anion gap; or radiologic evidence of a large number of pills in the gastrointestinal tract.

Miscellaneous

Deferoxamine is commercially available as deferoxamine mesylate (**Figure 1**).

See also: Iron.

Further Reading

Fine, J.S., 2000. Iron poisoning. Curr. Probl. Pediatr. Adolesc. Health Care 30, 71–90.
Freedman, M.H., Grisaru, D., Olivieri, N., et al., 1990. Pulmonary syndrome in patients with thalassemia major receiving intravenous deferoxamine infusions. Am. J. Dis. Child. 144, 565–569.
Howland, M.A., 1996. Risks of parenteral deferoxamine for acute iron poisoning. J. Toxicol. Clin. Toxicol. 34, 491–497.
Olivieri, N.F., Buncic, J.R., Chew, E., et al., 1986. Visual and auditory neurotoxicity in patients receiving subcutaneous deferoxamine infusions. N. Engl. J. Med. 314, 869–873.
Tenenbein, M., 1996. Benefits of parenteral deferoxamine for acute iron poisoning. J. Toxicol. Clin. Toxicol. 34, 485–489.

Relevant Website

http://www.pharma.us.novartis.com/product/pi/pdf/desferal.pdf – Novartis Pharmaceuticals Corporation.

Delaney Clause

RC Guy, Robin Guy Consulting, LLC, Lake Forest, IL, USA

Background Information

In 1958, the Food, Drug, and Cosmetic Act (FD&C Act) was amended to include a clause which essentially banned the use of food additives and pesticides which were shown to cause cancer in humans or animals. The Delaney Clause was contained in Section 409 [348(c)(3)(A)] of the FD&C Act. Section 409 lays out requirements for the use of food additives, including pesticide residues. The Delaney Clause states "no additive shall be deemed to be safe if it is found to induce cancer when ingested by man or animal, or if it is found, after tests which are appropriate for the evaluation of the safety of food additives, to induce cancer in man or animal."

This clause regulates pesticide residues in processed foods to mean that carcinogenicity potential is the only factor, and that any benefits of the pesticide or food additive may not be considered. In addition, it set up a 'zero-cancer-risk' standard for food additives. If residues of carcinogenic pesticides are found to concentrate in processed foods, the Environmental Protection Agency (EPA) cannot set a tolerance or maximum legal limit for that pesticide/food combination. Later, Congress added the same zero-cancer-risk clause for amendments governing new animal drugs, and color additives (1960 Color Additives Amendment).

The birth of the Delaney Clause can be traced back to a 1950 resolution in the US House of Representatives that charged a House select subcommittee to investigate the use of chemicals in foods. Among the subcommittee's responsibilities was an examination of the 'nature, extent, and effect' of 'chemicals, compounds, and synthetics' on all facets of food production. The subcommittee was chaired by James J. Delaney, a New York Democrat.

While the Delaney Clause prevented the use of possibly dangerous chemicals such as DES, some prospectively useful substances were banned because improved analytical testing procedures were able to detect very small quantities of possible carcinogens. When the Delaney Clause was introduced, analytical testing procedures detected substances in concentrations of parts per million. It later became possible to detect substances in concentrations of one part per billion or trillion, making it far more probable that traces of a carcinogen be detected. Worsening this problem was the fact that tested substances are administered to animals at the maximum tolerated dose (MTD), far more than would be normally ingested. The Delaney Clause was criticized by many scientists who believed that its zero-tolerance standard was impossibly high.

The Delaney Clause was eventually replaced with a new law, the Food Quality Protection Act (FQPA) of 1996, which advanced a new standard of 'reasonable certainty of no harm.' Prior to the passage of the FQPA, the FDA had been employing Delaney in the case of food additives and animal drugs in a similar manner, i.e., 'reasonable certainty of no harm.' FDA incorporated the idea of safety into its color additive regulations. Currently, under 21 CFR 70.3(i), a color additive is 'safe' if 'there is convincing evidence that establishes with reasonable certainty that no harm will result from the intended use of the color additive.' The EPA was following the zero-tolerance standard. The FQPA ended the application of the Delaney Clause to pesticide tolerance levels. FQPA would allow EPA to determine what level of risk will be adequate to protect the public health as long as the dietary risk posed to food consumers is negligible.

See also: The International Conference on Harmonisation; Micronucleus Assay; Mouse Lymphoma Assay; Toxicity Testing, Mutagenicity.

Relevant Websites

http://www.epa.gov – US Environmental Protection Agency.
http://www.fda.gov – US Food and Drug Administration.
http://nepis.epa.gov – US Environmental Protection Agency - National Center for Environmental Publications: Search for Delaney Clause.

 http://dx.doi.org/10.1016/B978-0-12-386454-3.00836-8

Deltamethrin

SA Burr, Plymouth University Peninsula Schools of Medicine and Dentistry, Plymouth, UK

This article is a revision of the previous edition article by Paul R. Harp, volume1, pp 736–737, © 2005, Elsevier Inc.

- Chemical Abstracts Service Registry Number: 52918-63-5
- Synonyms: [(*S*)-cyano-(3-phenoxyphenyl)methyl] (1*R*,3*R*)-3-(2,2-dibromoethenyl)-2,2-dimethylcyclopropane-1-carboxylate, Crackdown, Decamethrin, Decamethrine, Deltacide, Deltagran, Deltamethrine, Esbecythrin, Stricker, Suspend, CID 40585
- Classification: Type II pyrethroid insecticide
- Molecular Formula: $C_{22}H_{19}NO_3$
- Chemical structure:

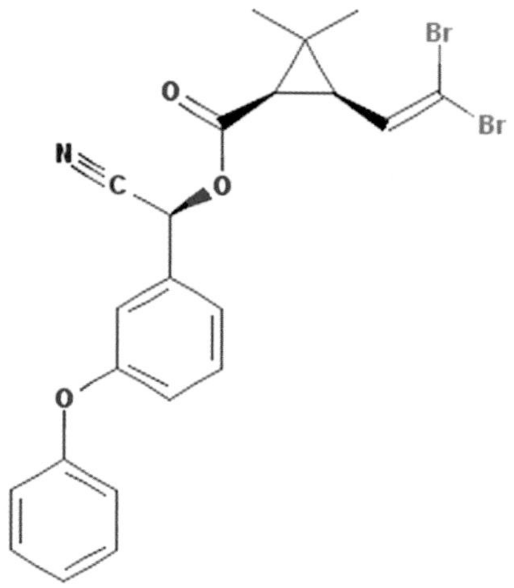

Uses

Deltamethrin is a potent broad-spectrum insecticide used in a range of agricultural, public health, and domestic applications. Deltamethrin is available as a powder, emulsion, thermal fogging concentrate, or concentrate for ultralow volume application. Deltamethrin is widely used particularly in domestic settings to control mosquitoes. However, many insect populations have begun to develop resistance. Technical deltamethrin is the single most active isomer (1*R*, *cis*, alpha-*S*).

Environmental Fate

Deltamethrin is twofold more persistent in aquatic environments than in soil. Depending on conditions the environmental half-life ranges from 2 days (for hydrolysis at pH 9) to 80 days (for degradation in an aquatic environment).

Exposure

Dermal, oral, and inhalational exposures can occur. Trace quantities have been measured in human breast milk.

Toxicokinetics

Absorption of pyrethroids is poor through the skin and not much more effective through the gastrointestinal tract. Pyrethroids are rapidly metabolized through ester cleavage and hydroxylation. Pyrethroids accumulate in adipose tissue. Urinary excretion is the primary route of elimination.

Mechanism of Toxicity

Deltamethrin is a type II pyrethroid, a functional neurotoxin slowing the inactivation of voltage-gated sodium channels leading to a state of hyperexcitability which in turn causes fine tremor, salivation, and choreoathetosis. Other proposed contributory actions include antagonism of gamma-aminobutyric acid A receptor inhibition and voltage-gated chloride and calcium channels.

Acute and Short-Term Toxicity

Deltamethrin produces a syndrome in both insects and mammals known as chorea salivation. The effects are hyperexcitability, fine tremor, hypersalivation, choreoathetosis, ataxia, seizures, and death. Humans experience the same effects as other animals but are also able to report paresthesia after dermal exposure and nausea after ingestion.

Chronic Toxicity

Chronic effects following deltamethrin exposure have been reported in neither animals nor humans.

Clinical Management

Dermal exposure can be treated by washing the contaminated skin with oils. Application of vitamin E cream preparations can be used for both prophylaxis and treatment of paresthesia. With cases of ingestion, gastric decontamination with activated charcoal may be of benefit within the first hour. Gastric lavage should be avoided where formulations contain solvents. If systemic toxicity does occur, the central signs of poisoning can be difficult to control and may be confused with

 http://dx.doi.org/10.1016/B978-0-12-386454-3.00124-X

intoxication by other pesticides such as anticholinesterases that also cause hyperexcitability – although pyrethroids do not inhibit acetylcholinesterase. Respiratory support may be needed and control of metabolic acidosis may require sodium bicarbonate. Atropine may be useful to control hypersalivation. Single short-lived seizures may not require treatment. Since pyrethroids do not produce morphological damage, only symptomatic treatment is needed. Frequent or prolonged convulsions may be controlled with intravenous diazepam or lorazepam. If unresponsive, consider phenobarbital or phenytoin (before thiopental or general anesthesia). Pentobarbitone has been shown to be more effective than phenobarbitone in animal studies. Complete recovery usually occurs following symptomatic treatment in cases of mild-to-moderate intoxication.

Ecotoxicology

Bees, crustaceans, and fish are all highly susceptible to deltamethrin under experimental conditions. However, environmental factors such as sediment binding may reduce the actual susceptibility of nontarget aquatic species.

Exposure Standards and Guidelines

The acceptable daily intake set by the Food and Agriculture Organization/World Health Organization Joint Meeting on Pesticide Residues (JMPR) for deltamethrin is 0–0.01 mg kg^{-1} body weight, with an acute oral reference dose of 0.05 mg kg^{-1} body weight.

See also: Cyfluthrin; Cypermethrin; Neurotoxicity; Permethrin; Pesticides; Pyrethrins/Pyrethroids.

Further Reading

Barlow, S.M., Sullivan, F.M., Lines, J., 2001. Risk assessment of the use of deltamethrin on bednets for the prevention of malaria. Food Chem. Toxicol. 39, 407–422.

He, F.S., Deng, H., Ji, X., Zhang, Z.W., Sun, J.X., Yao, P.P., 1991. Changes of nerve excitability and urinary deltamethrin in sprayers. Int. Arch. of Occup. Environ. Health 62, 587–590.

WHO/IPCS, 1990. Environmental Health Criteria 97: Tetramethrin, Cyhalothrin and Deltamethrin. World Health Organization, Geneva.

Relevant Websites

http://toxnet.nlm.nih.gov – TOXNET, Toxicology Data Network, National Library of Medicine, Search for Deltamethrin.

http://www.who.int – World Health Organization, Search for Deltamethrin.